Mechanism-of-Action Illustrations (cont.)

Drugs with illustrated mechanisms of action	Drugs with similar mechanisms of action
isosorbide dinitrate, isosorbide mononitrate	nitroglycerin
lanthanum carbonate	sevelamer hydrochloride
linezolid	none
memantine hydrochloride	none
milrinone lactate	none
nateglinide	repaglinide
olmesartan medoxomil	irbesartan, losartan potassium, valsartan
omeprazole	esomeprazole magnesium, lansoprazole, pantoprazole sodium, rabeprazole sodium
palonosetron hydrochloride	alosetron, dolasetron, granisetron, ondansetron
spironolactone	none

Discover the NDH App!

START YOUR FREE TRIAL TODAY!

Experience the convenience of having the trusted drug reference app with you everywhere you go. Designed for today's nurses, you'll love having this app for your classes, clinicals, and throughout your nursing career!

Download the **NDH app** to check out these features:

- Easy navigation and improved search
- Personalized note-taking & bookmarking
- Relevant news feed tailored to you
- Top trending drug searches in real-time
- Calculators for hard-to-remember formulas

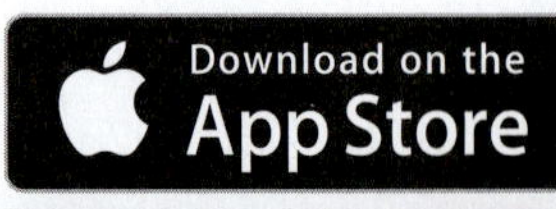

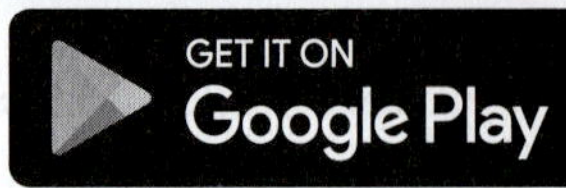

ATTENTION NURSING STUDENTS!

Scan to learn how you can **SAVE 25%** on your annual subscription.

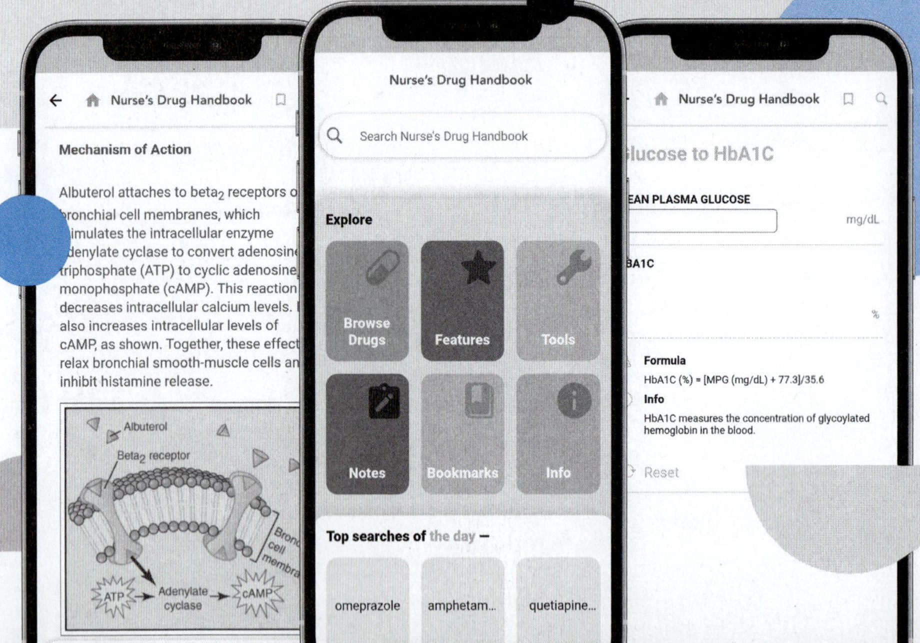

2026

NDH

NURSE'S DRUG HANDBOOK

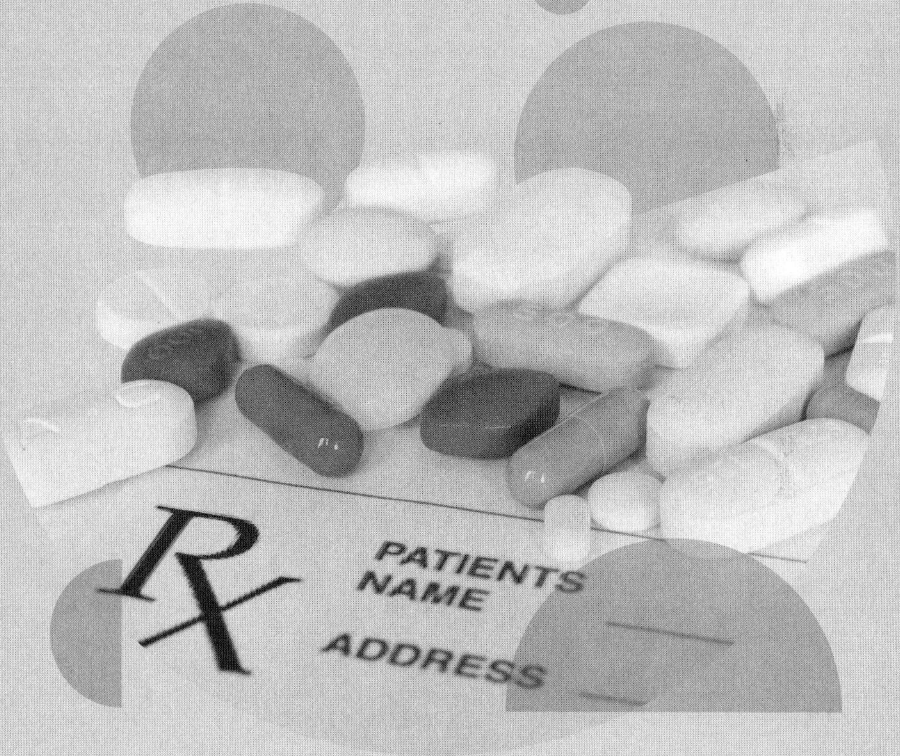

PATIENTS NAME

ADDRESS

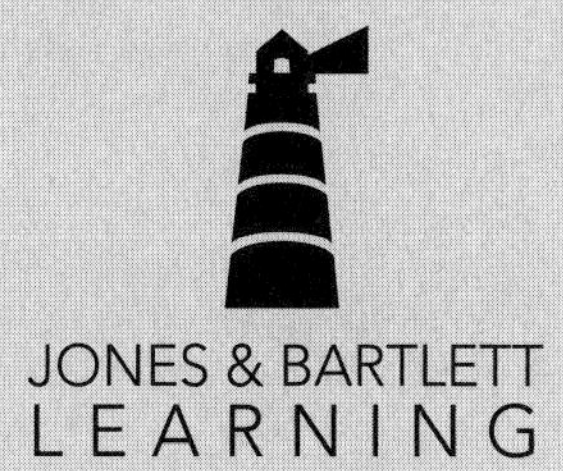

JONES & BARTLETT LEARNING

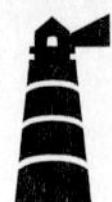

World Headquarters
Jones & Bartlett Learning
25 Mall Road
Burlington, MA 01803
978-443-5000
info@jblearning.com
www.jblearning.com

Jones & Bartlett Learning books and products are available through most bookstores and online booksellers. To contact Jones & Bartlett Learning directly, call 800-832-0034, fax 978-443-8000, or visit our website, www.jblearning.com.

Substantial discounts on bulk quantities of Jones & Bartlett Learning publications are available to corporations, professional associations, and other qualified organizations. For details and specific discount information, contact the special sales department at Jones & Bartlett Learning via the above contact information or send an email to specialsales@jblearning.com.

The manufacturer's authorised representative in the EU for product safety is Mare Nostrum Group B.V., Mauritskade 21D, 1091 GC Amsterdam, The Netherlands. Email: gpsr@mare-nostrum.co.uk

31488-5

Production Credits
Vice President, Innovative Learning and Assessment Solutions: Ada Woo
Senior Director, Content Production and Delivery: Christine Emerton
Director, Product: Melissa Kleeman Moy
Product Manager: Bill Lawrensen
Manager, Content Development: Carol Guerrero
Content Manager: Christina Freitas
Content Management: S4Carlisle Publishing Services
Manager, Intellectual Properties and Content Production: Kristen Rogers
Content Production Manager: Belinda Thresher
Senior Intellectual Property Specialist: Angela Dooley
Senior Product Marketing Manager: Lindsay White
Director, Product Fulfillment: Aaron McKinzie
Purchasing Manager: Wendy Kilborn
Composition: S4Carlisle Publishing Services
Project Management: S4Carlisle Publishing Services
Cover Design: MPS Limited
Intellectual Property Specialist: Faith Brosnan
Intellectual Property Specialist: Maria Leon Maimone
Cover Image (Title Page): © Soru_Epotok/Shutterstock
Printing and Binding: Lakeside Book Company

Library of Congress Cataloging-in-Publication Data
Library of Congress Control Number: 2025938584

6048

Printed in the United States of America
29 28 27 26 25 10 9 8 7 6 5 4 3 2 1

Contents

Online Resources

The following resources are available online.

How to Use This Text

The *Nurse's Drug Handbook* gives you what today's nurses and nursing students need: accurate, concise, and reliable drug facts. This text emphasizes the vital information you need to know before, during, and after drug administration. The information is presented in an easy-to-understand language and organized alphabetically, so you can quickly find what you need.

What's Special

In addition to the drug information you will find in each entry (see "Drug Entries" for details), the *Nurse's Drug Handbook* boasts these special features:

- The design makes it easy to find the most need-to-know drug information, such as indications, dosages, dosage adjustments, drug administration, contraindications, and warnings.
- Introductory material reviews essential general information you need to know to administer drugs safely and effectively, including an overview of pharmacology and the principles of drug administration. In addition, the five steps of the nursing process are explained and related specifically to drug therapy.
- Highly useful illustrations throughout the text help you visualize selected mechanisms of action by showing how drugs work at the cellular, tissue, and organ levels. In addition, the inside front cover features a table listing all the drugs whose mechanisms of action are illustrated, as well as other drugs with the same mechanisms of action.
- No-nonsense writing style speaks in everyday language and uses the terms and abbreviations you typically encounter in your practice and your studies.
- Up-to-date drug information includes the latest FDA-approved drugs marked with a special "NEW" icon to alert the reader of its recent approval, new and revised indications and dosages, latest drug administration instructions, updated contraindications, new drug interactions, newly reported adverse reactions, latest childbearing considerations, and changes in the nursing considerations and patient teachings to reflect new information.
- Dosage adjustment, headlined in color, alerts you to expected dosage changes for a patient with a specific condition or disorder, such as advanced age or renal impairment or concurrent drug therapy that may require an increase or decrease in dosage because of a potential interaction.
- Adverse drug reactions that are life-threatening are bolded and in color for quick identification.
- Warning, displayed in color, calls attention to important facts that you need to know before, during, and after drug administration. For example, in the beclomethasone entry, this feature states not to abruptly stop beclomethasone therapy because life-threatening adrenal insufficiency may occur causing fatigue, hypotension, lassitude, nausea, vomiting, and weakness. It also states to be watchful for adrenal insufficiency when the patient experiences severe asthma attacks or stress such as exposure to infection, surgery, trauma, or other stressors.
- Easy-to-use tables showing route, onset, peak, duration, and half-life of the drug (see page viii for more details), and other tables in the appendices provide a time-saving way to track and check information. Many of the appendices will give you an overview of the most important facts for important drug groups, including insulin preparations, interferons, pediatric immunizations and vitamins, as well as selected allergen oral extracts, antihistamines, antihypertensive combinations, combination antivirals, drugs to treat hemophilia, obstetrical drugs, ophthalmics, and topical drugs. You'll also find that several appendices provide handy instructions for calculating drug dosages and I.V. flow rates, common weights and measures used in drug administration, and syringe–drug compatibility. In addition, two of the appendices will help you gain an understanding of the FDA's emergency

authorization uses during times of a major health crisis as well as important guidelines to follow for safe opioid use.

Drug Entries

The *Nurse's Drug Handbook* clearly and concisely presents all the vital facts on the drugs that you'll typically administer. To help you find the information you need quickly, drug entries are organized alphabetically by generic drug name—from abacavir sulfate to zonisamide. For ease of use, every drug entry follows a consistent format.

GENERIC AND TRADE NAMES

First, each entry identifies the drug's main generic name, in color, as well as alternate generic names. (For drugs prescribed by trade name, you can quickly check the comprehensive index, which refers you to the appropriate generic name and page.)

Next, the entry lists the most common U.S. trade names for each drug. It also includes common trade names available only in Canada, marked "(CAN)."

CLASS AND SCHEDULE

Each entry lists the drug's pharmacologic and therapeutic classes. With this information, you can compare drugs in the same pharmacologic class but in different therapeutic classes, and vice versa.

Where appropriate, the entry also includes the drug's controlled substance schedule. (For details, see *Controlled substance schedules.*)

INDICATIONS AND DOSAGES

This section lists FDA-approved therapeutic indications. For each indication, you'll find the applicable drug form or route, age group (adults, adolescents, or children), and dosage, including amount per dose, timing, and duration when known and appropriate.

Drug Administration

This section provides you with what you need to know on how to safely administer the drug. The section clearly lists instructions for each route of administration that is possible and includes P.O., I.V., I.M., subcutaneous, inhaled, intranasal, topical, transdermal, or vaginal. The section under I.V. ends with a list of incompatibilities as indicated by the manufacturer.

ROUTE, ONSET, PEAK, DURATION, AND HALF-LIFE

Quick-reference tables show the drug's onset, peak, and duration (when known) for each administration route. The onset of action is the time a drug takes to be absorbed, reach a therapeutic blood level, and elicit an initial therapeutic response. The peak therapeutic effect occurs when a drug reaches its highest blood concentration, and the greatest amount of drug reaches the site of action to produce the maximum therapeutic response. The duration of action is the amount of time the drug remains at a blood level that produces a therapeutic response. The drug's half-life (when known) determines the time it takes for half of the drug to be eliminated from the body.

Controlled substance schedules

The Controlled Substances Act of 1970 mandated that certain prescription drugs be categorized in schedules based on their potential for abuse. The greater their potential for abuse, the greater the restrictions on their prescription. The controlled substance schedules range from I to V, signifying highest to lowest abuse potential.

I High potential for abuse

No accepted medical use exists for schedule I drugs, which include heroin and lysergic acid diethylamide (LSD).

II High potential for abuse

Use may lead to severe physical or psychological dependence. Examples include amphetamine, dextroamphetamine, fentanyl, hydrocodone, hydromorphone, meperidine, methadone, morphine, oxycodone, and oxymorphone. No renewals are permitted.

III Some potential for abuse

Use may lead to low-to-moderate physical dependence or high

psychological dependence. Examples include buprenorphine and opioid analgesics that contain no more than 90 mg of codeine per dosage unit. Up to five renewals are permitted within 6 months.

IV Low potential for abuse

Use may lead to limited physical or psychological dependence. Examples include alprazolam, clonazepam, clorazepate, diazepam, lorazepam, midazolam, temazepam, tramadol, and trizolam. Up to five renewals are allowed within 6 months.

V Subject to state and local regulation

Abuse potential is low. Examples include antidiarrheal drugs that contain atropine diphenosylate, ezogabine and pregabalin or cough medicines with less than 200 mg codeine/100 ml. Partial refills cannot occur more than 6 months after the issue date. When a partial fill occurs, it's treated in the same manner and with the same rules as a refill of the drug.

Every prescription for a controlled substance must include issue date; name and address of the patient; name, address, and DEA registration number of practitioner; drug name; strength of drug; dosage form; quantity prescribed; directions for use; refills (if authorized); and manual signature of the prescriber.

Most, but not all states, mandate the prescription for a controlled substance (schedules II-V) must be issued electronically to the pharmacy. In addition, medical providers who prescribe for patients having Medicare Part D and Medicare Advantage prescription insurance plans need to use e-prescribe for their controlled medications.

MECHANISM OF ACTION

This section concisely describes how a drug achieves its therapeutic effects at cellular, tissue, and organ levels, when known. Illustrations of selected mechanisms of action lend exceptional clarity to sometimes complex processes.

CONTRAINDICATIONS

An alphabetical list details the conditions and disorders that preclude administration of the drug.

INTERACTIONS

This section includes drugs, foods, and activities (such as alcohol use and smoking) that can cause important, problematic, or life-threatening interactions with the topic drug. For each interacting drug, food, or activity, you'll learn the effects of the interaction.

ADVERSE REACTIONS

Organized by body system, this section lists common, serious, and life-threatening adverse reactions. Life-threatening adverse reactions are bolded and in color for easy identification.

CHILDBEARING CONSIDERATIONS

All FDA-approved prescription drugs can no longer use the lettering system to categorize drugs based on their potential to cause fetal harm such as A, B, C, D, or X. Instead, a more comprehensive text is now required in the packaging label to explain the risks. Labeling of over-the-counter drugs will remain unchanged and is not affected by the FDA-mandated change.

The Childbearing Consideration section provides information using the new guidelines. This section is subdivided into four categories, with the first three categories consisting of pregnancy risks, labor and delivery risks, and lactation risks, if present, to the fetus or newborn and the fourth category indicating any reproductive risks the drug may pose.

NURSING CONSIDERATIONS

Warnings, general precautions, and key information that you must know before, during, and after drug administration are detailed in this section. Examples include cautions certain populations require and types of monitoring needed.

Patient-teaching information is also included here. You'll find important guidelines for patients, such as how and when to take each prescribed drug, how to spot and manage adverse reactions, which cautions to observe, when to call the prescriber, and more. To save your time, however, this section doesn't repeat basic patient-teaching points. (For a summary of those, see *Federal guidelines for drug disposal*, page xi, and *Teaching your patient about drug therapy*, page x.)

In short, the *Nurse's Drug Handbook* is designed expressly to give you more of what you need. It puts vital drug information at your fingertips and helps you always stay current in this critical part of your practice or studies.

Teaching your patient about drug therapy

Your teaching about drug therapy will vary with your patient's needs and your practice setting. To guide your teaching, each drug entry provides key information that you must teach your patient about that drug. For all patients, however, you also should:

- Teach the generic and trade name for each prescribed drug that they'll take after discharge—even if they took the drug before admission.
- Clearly explain why each drug was prescribed, how it works, and what it's supposed to do. To help your patient understand the drug's therapeutic effects, relate its action to their disorder or condition.
- Review the drug form, dosage, and route with the patient. Tell them whether the drug is an aerosol, tablet, spray, suppository, or other form, and explain how to take it correctly. Also, tell them how often to take the drug and for what length of time, if known. Emphasize that they should take the drug exactly as prescribed.
- Describe the drug's appearance and explain that scored tablets can be broken in half for safe, accurate dosing. Warn the patient not to break unscored tablets because doing so may alter the drug dosage. If your patient has trouble swallowing capsules, tell them to inquire if the capsule can be opened and sprinkled on food or mixed in a beverage; some can and some cannot. If the capsule should not be opened, have patient ask about being switched to a liquid form, if available. Also, warn them not to crush or chew enteric-coated, delayed-release (D.R.), extended-release (E.R.), sustained-release (S.R.), or similar drug forms.
- Teach the patient about common adverse reactions that may occur. Advise them to notify the prescriber at once if a dangerous adverse reaction, such as rash or syncope, occurs.
- Warn them not to suddenly stop taking a drug if they're bothered by unpleasant adverse reactions, such as diarrhea or nausea. Instead, encourage them to discuss the reactions with their prescriber, who may adjust the dosage or substitute a drug that causes fewer adverse reactions.
- Tell patient that if a drug is known to cause adverse reactions (such as dizziness and drowsiness) that can impair the patient's ability to perform activities that require alertness, warn them not to engage in such activities until the adverse effects are known and resolved. In some cases, helping them develop a dosing schedule that minimizes these adverse reactions can be helpful.
- Inform the patient as to which adverse reactions resolve with time.
- Teach the patient how to store the drug properly. Let them know if the drug is sensitive to light or temperature and how to protect it from these elements.
- Instruct the patient to store the drug in its original container, if possible, with the drug's name and dosage clearly printed on the label.
- Inform the patient which devices to use—and which to avoid—for drug storage or administration. For example, warn them not to take liquid cyclosporine with a plastic cup or utensils.
- Teach the patient what to do if they miss a dose. Generally, they should take a once-daily drug as soon as they

remember—provided it's not close to the end of the 24 hours when the next dose is due. Warn them never to double the dose to make up for a missed dose. If they have questions or concerns about missed doses, tell them to contact their prescriber.

- Provide information specific to the prescribed drug. For example, if a patient takes a diuretic to manage heart failure, instruct them to weigh themselves daily at the same time of day, using the same scale, and wearing the same amount of clothing. Or, if the patient takes digoxin or an antihypertensive drug, teach them how to measure their pulse and blood pressure and how to record the measurements. Then, instruct them to bring the diary to their regular appointments so the prescriber can monitor their response to the drug.
- Advise the patient to refill prescriptions promptly unless they no longer are prescribed the drug. Also, instruct them to discard expired drugs because they may become ineffective or even dangerous over time. For example, outdated tetracycline may cause life-threatening Fanconi's syndrome.
- Warn the patient to always keep all drugs out of the reach of children.

Federal guidelines for drug disposal

Give patients these important instructions for properly disposing of their unwanted prescription drugs:

- Consider mixing discarded prescription drugs with a substance like coffee grounds or used cat litter and putting them in impermeable, nondescript containers, such as empty cans or sealable bags.
- Flush prescription drugs down the toilet only if the label or accompanying patient information specifically says to do so.
- See if the community has a pharmaceutical take-back program that allows citizens to bring unused drugs to a central location for proper disposal.

Overview of Pharmacology

Understanding the basics of pharmacology is an essential nursing responsibility. Pharmacology is the science that deals with the physical and chemical properties as well as the biochemical and physiologic effects of drugs. It includes the areas of pharmacokinetics, pharmacodynamics, pharmacotherapeutics, pharmacognosy, and toxicodynamics.

The *Nurse's Drug Handbook* deals primarily with pharmacokinetics, pharmacodynamics, and pharmacotherapeutics—the information you need to administer safe and effective drug therapy (discussed as follows). Pharmacognosy is the branch of pharmacology that deals with the biological, biochemical, and economic features of naturally occurring drugs. Toxicodynamics is the study of the harmful effects that excessive amounts of a drug produce in the body; in a drug overdose or drug poisoning, large drug doses may saturate or overwhelm normal mechanisms that control absorption, distribution, metabolism, and excretion.

Drug Nomenclature

Most drugs are known by several names—chemical, generic, trade, and official—each of which serves a specific function. (See *How drugs are named.*) However, multiple drug names can also contribute to medication errors. You may find a familiar drug packaged with an unfamiliar name if your institution changes suppliers or if a familiar drug is newly approved in a different dose or for a new indication.

How drugs are named

A drug's chemical, generic, trade, and official names are determined at different phases of the drug development process and serve different functions. For example, the various names of the commonly prescribed anticonvulsant divalproex sodium are:

- Chemical name: pentanoic acid, 2-propyl-, sodium salt (2:1), or ($C_{16}H_{31}O_4Na$)
- Generic name: divalproex sodium
- Trade name: Depakote
- Official name: divalproex sodium delayed-release tablets, USP

A drug's chemical name describes its atomic and molecular structure. The chemical name of divalproex sodium—pentanoic acid, 2-propyl-, sodium salt (2:1), or $C_{16}H_{31}O_4Na$ (pronounced valproate semisodium)—indicates that the drug is a combination of two valproic acid compounds with a sodium molecule attached to only one side.

Once a drug successfully completes several clinical trials, it receives a generic name, also known as the nonproprietary name. The generic name is usually derived from, but shorter than, the chemical name. The United States Adopted Names Council is responsible for selecting generic names, which are intended for unrestricted public use.

Before submitting the drug for FDA approval, the manufacturer creates and registers a trade name (or brand name) when the drug appears ready to be marketed. Trade names are copyrighted and followed by the symbol® to indicate that they're registered and that their use is restricted to the drug manufacturer. Once the original patent on a drug has expired, any manufacturer may produce the drug under their own trade name.

A drug's official name is the name under which it is listed in the United States Pharmacopoeia (USP) and the National Formulary (NF).

Drug Classification

Drugs can be classified in various ways. Most pharmacology textbooks group drugs by their functional classification, such as psychotherapeutics, which is based on common characteristics. Drugs can also be classified according to their therapeutic use, such as antipanic or antiobsessional drugs. Drugs within a certain therapeutic class may be further divided into subgroups based on their mechanisms of action. For example, the therapeutic class antineoplastics according to the National Library of Medicine can be further classified as alkylating agents, antimetabolites, hormones and antagonists, natural products, and miscellaneous. However, in recent years, the miscellaneous group has come to include some of the most important drugs such as antibiotic antineoplastics, biologic response modifers, histone deacetylase inhibitors, monoclonal antibodies, protein kinase inhibitors, taxanes, topoisomerase inhibitors, and vica alkaloids.

Pharmacokinetics

Pharmacokinetics is the study of a drug's actions—or fate—as it passes through the body during absorption, distribution, metabolism, and excretion.

ABSORPTION

Before a drug can begin working, it must be transformed from its pharmaceutical dosage form to a biologically available (bioavailable) substance that can pass through various biological cell membranes to reach its site of action. This process is known as absorption. A drug's absorption rate depends on its route of administration, its circulation through the tissue into which it is administered, and its solubility—that is, whether it is more water soluble (*hydrophilic*) or fat soluble (*lipophilic*).

Although drugs may penetrate cellular membranes either actively or passively, most drugs do so by *passive diffusion*, moving inertly from an area of higher concentration to an area of lower concentration. Passive diffusion may occur through water or fat. Passive diffusion through water—*aqueous diffusion*—occurs within large water-filled compartments, such as interstitial spaces, and across epithelial membrane tight junctions and pores in the epithelial lining of blood vessels. Aqueous diffusion is driven by concentration gradients. Drug molecules that are bound to large plasma proteins, such as albumin, are too large to pass through aqueous pores in this way. Passive diffusion through fat—*lipid diffusion*—plays an important role in drug metabolism because of the large number of lipid barriers that separate the aqueous compartments of the body. The tendency of a drug to move through lipid layers between aqueous compartments often depends on the pH of the medium—that is, the ability of the water-soluble or fat-soluble drug to form weak acid or weak base.

Drugs with molecules that are too large to readily diffuse may rely on active *diffusion*, in which special carriers on molecules, including amino acids, glucose, and peptides, transport the drug through the membranes. However, some molecules with selective membrane carriers can expel foreign drug molecules; this is why many drugs can't cross the blood–brain barrier.

Drug absorption begins at the administration route. The three main administration route categories are enteral, parenteral, and transcutaneous. Depending on its nature or chemical makeup, a drug may be better absorbed from one site than from another.

Enteral Administration

Enteral administration consists of the oral, gastric or nasogastric, and rectal routes.

Oral: Drugs administered orally are absorbed in the GI tract and then proceed by the hepatic portal vein to the liver and into the systemic circulation. Although generally considered the preferred route, oral drug administration has several disadvantages:

- The oral route doesn't always yield sufficiently high blood concentrations to be effective.
- Bioavailability may be less than optimal because of incomplete absorption and first-pass elimination (the part of metabolism that occurs during transit through the liver before the drug reaches the general circulation).
- Drug absorption may be incomplete if the drug is degraded by digestive enzymes or the acidic pH in the stomach or if it is excreted from the liver into the bile.

- Food in the GI tract, gastric emptying time, and intestinal motility may also impede drug absorption.

Gastric or nasogastric: Drugs administered through a gastric or nasogastric tube enter the stomach directly and are absorbed in the GI tract.

Rectal: Rectal drugs and suppositories also enter the GI tract directly after being inserted in the rectum and absorbed through the rectal mucosa. After being absorbed into the lower GI tract, rectal drugs enter the circulation through the inferior vena cava, bypassing the liver and thus avoiding first-pass metabolism. Suppositories, however, tend to travel upward into the rectum, where veins, such as the superior hemorrhoidal vein, lead to the liver. As a result, drug absorption by this route is often unreliable and difficult to predict.

Parenteral Administration

Parenteral routes may be used whenever enteral routes are contraindicated, inadequate, or unavailable. These routes include intramuscular (I.M.), intravenous (I.V.), subcutaneous (SubQ), and intradermal (I.D.) administration. Drug absorption is much faster and more predictable after parenteral administration than after enteral administration.

I.M.: Drugs administered by the I.M. route are injected deep into the muscle, where they're absorbed relatively quickly. The rate of drug absorption depends on the vascularity of the injection site, the physiochemical properties of the drug, and the solution in which the drug is contained.

I.V.: I.V. drug administration involves injecting or infusing the drug directly into the blood circulation, allowing for rapid distribution throughout the body. This route usually provides the greatest bioavailability.

Subcutaneous: Drugs administered by the subcutaneous route are injected into the connective tissue just below the skin and are absorbed by simple diffusion from the injection site. The factors that affect I.M. absorption also affect subcutaneous absorption. Absorption by the subcutaneous route may be slower than by the I.M. route.

Intradermal: Drugs administered intradermally, such as purified protein derivative (PPD), are injected into the dermis, from which they diffuse slowly into the local microcapillary system.

Transcutaneous Administration

Transcutaneous drug administration allows drug absorption through the skin or soft-tissue surface. Drugs may be inhaled, inserted sublingually, applied topically, or administered to the eyes, ears, nose, or vagina.

Inhalation: Inhaled drugs may be given as a powder and aerosolized or mixed in solution and nebulized directly into the respiratory tract, where they're absorbed through the alveoli. Inhaled drugs are usually absorbed quickly because of the abundant blood flow in the lungs, though some inhaled drugs have low systemic absorption.

Sublingual: Sublingual drug administration involves placing a tablet, troche, or lozenge under the tongue. The drug is absorbed across the epithelial lining of the mouth, usually quickly. This route avoids first-pass metabolism.

Topical: Topical drugs—creams, lotions, ointments, and patches—are placed on the skin and then cross the epidermis into the capillary circulation. They may also be absorbed through hair follicles, sweat glands, and other skin structures. Absorption by the skin is enhanced if the drug is in a solution.

Ophthalmic: Ophthalmic drugs include solutions and ointments that are instilled or applied directly to the cornea or conjunctiva as well as small, elliptical disks that are placed directly on the eyeball behind the lower eyelid. The movements of the eyeball promote distribution of these drugs over the surface of the eye. Although ophthalmic drugs produce a local effect on the conjunctiva or anterior chamber, some preparations may be absorbed systemically and therefore produce systemic effects.

Otic: Drops administered into the external auditory canal, otic drugs are used to treat infection or inflammation and to soften and remove ear wax. Otic solutions exert a local effect and may result in minimal systemic absorption with no adverse effects.

Nasal: Nasal solutions and suspensions are applied directly to the nasal mucosa by instillation or inhalation to produce local effects, such as vasoconstriction to reduce nasal congestion. Some nasal solutions, such as mometasone furoate, are administered by this route specifically to produce systemic effects.

Vaginal: Vaginal drugs include creams, suppositories, and troches that are inserted into the vagina, sometimes using a special applicator. These drugs are administered locally to treat such conditions as bacterial and fungal infections.

DISTRIBUTION

Distribution is the process by which a drug is transported by the circulating fluids to various sites, including its sites of action. To ensure maximum therapeutic effectiveness, the drug must permeate all membranes that separate it from its intended site of action. Drug distribution is influenced by blood flow, protein binding, and tissue availability. Drugs that cannot distribute to the tissues in which they are needed are not effective.

METABOLISM

Drug metabolism is the enzymatic conversion of a drug's structure into substrate molecules or polar compounds that are either less active or inactive and are readily excreted. Drugs can also be synthesized to larger molecules. Metabolism may also convert a drug to a more toxic compound. Because the primary site of drug metabolism is the liver, children, older people, and patients with impaired hepatic function are at risk for altered therapeutic effects.

Biotransformation is the process of changing a drug into its active metabolite. Compounds that require metabolic biotransformation for activation are known as *prodrugs*. During phase I of biotransformation, the parent drug is converted into an inactive or partially active metabolite. Much of the original drug may be eliminated during this phase. During phase II, the inactive or partially active metabolite binds with available substrates, such as acetic acid, glucuronic acid, sulfuric acid, or water, to form its active metabolite. When biotransformation leads to synthesis, larger molecules are produced to create a pharmacologic effect.

EXCRETION

The body eliminates drugs by both excretion and metabolism. Drug metabolites—and, in some cases, the active drug itself—are eventually excreted from the body, usually through bile, feces, and urine. The primary organ for drug elimination is the kidney. Impaired renal function may alter drug elimination, thereby altering the drug's therapeutic effect. Other excretion routes include evaporation through the skin, exhalation from the lungs, and secretion into breast milk or salvia.

A drug's elimination half-life is the amount of time required for half of the drug to be eliminated from the body. The half-life roughly correlates with the drug's duration of action and is based on normal hepatic and renal function. Typically, the longer the half-life, the less often the drug has to be given and the longer it remains in the body.

Pharmacodynamics

Pharmacodynamics is the study of the biochemical and physiologic effects of drugs and their mechanisms of action. A drug's actions may be structurally specific or nonspecific. Structurally specific drugs combine with cell receptors, such as glycoproteins or proteins, to enhance or inhibit cellular enzyme actions. Drug receptors are the cellular components affected at the site of action. Many drugs form chemical bonds with drug receptors, but a drug can bond with a receptor only if it has a similar shape—much the same way that a key fits into a lock. When a drug combines with a receptor, channels are either opened or closed and cellular biochemical messengers, such as calcium or cyclic adenosine monophosphate ions, are activated. Once activated, cellular functions can be turned either on or off by these messengers.

Structurally nonspecific drugs, such as biological response modifiers, don't combine with cell receptors; rather, they produce changes within the cell membrane or interior.

The mechanisms by which drugs interact with the body are not always known. Drugs may work by physical action (such as the protective effects of a topical ointment), by chemical reaction (such as an antacid's effect on the gastric mucosa), by modifying the metabolic activity of invading pathogens (such as an antibiotic), or by replacing a missing biochemical substance (such as insulin).

AGONISTS

Agonists are drugs that interact with a receptor to stimulate a response. They alter cell physiology by binding to plasma membranes or intracellular structures. *Partial agonists* can't achieve maximal effects even though they may occupy all available receptor sites on a cell. *Strong agonists* can cause maximal effects while occupying only a small number of receptor sites on a cell. *Weak agonists* must occupy many more receptor sites than strong agonists to produce the same effect.

ANTAGONISTS

Antagonists are drugs that attach to a receptor but don't stimulate a response; instead, they inhibit or block responses that would normally be caused by agonists.

- Competitive antagonists bind to receptor sites that are also compatible with an agonist, thus preventing the agonist from binding to the site.
- Noncompetitive antagonists bind to receptor sites that aren't occupied by an agonist; this changes the receptor site so that it is no longer recognized by the agonist.
- Irreversible antagonists work in much the same way that noncompetitive ones do, except that they permanently bind with the receptor.

Antagonism plays an important role in drug interactions. When two agonists that cause opposite therapeutic effects are combined, such as a vasodilator and a vasoconstrictor, the effects cancel each other out. When two antagonists are combined, such as morphine and naloxone, both drugs may become inactive.

Pharmacotherapeutics

Pharmacotherapeutics is the study of how drugs are used to prevent or treat disease. Understanding why a drug is prescribed for a certain disease can assist in prioritizing drug administration with other patient care activities. Knowing a drug's desired and unwanted effects may help uncover problems not readily apparent from the admitting diagnosis. This information may also help prevent such problems as adverse reactions and drug interactions.

A drug's *desired effect* is the expected or intended clinical response to the drug. This is the response that should be evaluated as soon as a drug is given. Dosage adjustments and the continuation of therapy often depend on accurate evaluation and documentation of the patient's response.

An *adverse reaction* is any noxious and unintended response to a drug that occurs at therapeutic doses used for prophylaxis, diagnosis, or therapy. Adverse reactions associated with excessive amounts of a drug are considered drug overdoses. Be prepared to follow the institution's policy for reporting adverse drug reactions.

An *idiosyncratic response* is a genetically determined abnormal or excessive response to a drug that occurs in a particular patient. The unusual response may indicate that the drug has saturated or overwhelmed mechanisms that normally control absorption, distribution, metabolism, or excretion, thus altering the expected response. It is not always clear whether a reaction is adverse or idiosyncratic. Once the reaction is reported, the prescriber usually determines the appropriate course of action.

An *allergic reaction* is an adverse response that results from previous exposure to the same drug or to one that's chemically similar to it. The patient's immune system reacts to the drug as if it were a foreign invader and may produce a mild hypersensitivity reaction, characterized by localized dermatitis or photosensitivity. Allergic reactions should be reported to the prescriber immediately as some reactions may become serious or even life-threatening, requiring the drug to be discontinued. Follow-up care may include giving drugs, including antihistamines and corticosteroids, to counteract the allergic response.

An *anaphylactic reaction* involves an immediate hypersensitivity response characterized by angioedema, pruritus, and urticaria. Left untreated, an anaphylactic reaction can lead to systemic involvement, resulting in shock. It is often associated with life-threatening hypotension and respiratory distress. Be prepared to assist with emergency life-support measures, especially if the reaction occurs in response to I.V. drugs, which have the fastest rate of absorption.

A *drug interaction* occurs when one drug alters the pharmacokinetics of another drug—for example, when two or more drugs are given concurrently. Such concurrent administration can decrease or increase the therapeutic or adverse effects of either drug. Some drug interactions are beneficial. For example, when taken with penicillin, probenecid decreases the excretion rate of penicillin, resulting in higher blood levels of penicillin. Drug interactions also may occur when a drug's metabolism is altered, often owing to the induction of or competition for metabolizing enzymes. For example, H_2-receptor agonists, which reduce secretion of the enzyme gastrin, may alter the breakdown of enteric coatings on other drugs. Drug interactions due to carrier protein competition typically occur when a drug inhibits the kidneys' ability to reduce excretion of other drugs. For example, probenecid is completely reabsorbed by the renal tubules and is metabolized very slowly. It competes with the same carrier protein as sulfonamides for active tubular secretion and decreases the renal excretion of sulfonamides. This particular competition can lead to an increased risk of sulfonamide toxicity.

Special Considerations

Although every drug has a usual dosage range, certain factors such as a patient's age, weight, culture and ethnicity, gender, pregnancy status, and hepatic and renal function may contribute to the need for dosage adjustments. When special considerations such as these are encountered, be prepared to reassess the prescribed dosage to make sure that it is safe and effective for your patient.

CULTURE AND ETHNICITY

Certain drugs are more effective or more likely to produce adverse effects in particular ethnic groups or races. For example, Asian patients being treated for hyperlipidemia with rosuvastatin require a smaller dose to decrease the risk of adverse reactions, while African Americans have an increased risk of developing angioedema with ACE inhibitors. A patient's cultural or religious background also may call for special consideration. For example, a drug made from porcine products may be unacceptable to a Jewish or Muslim patient.

ELDERLY PATIENTS

Because aging produces certain changes in body composition and organ function, older patients present unique therapeutic and dosing problems that require special attention. For example, the weight of the liver, the number of functioning hepatic cells, and hepatic blood flow all decrease as a person ages, resulting in slower drug metabolism. Renal function may also decrease with aging. These processes can lead to the accumulation of active drugs and metabolites as well as increased sensitivity to the effects of some drugs in older patients. Because they're also more likely to have multiple chronic illnesses, many older patients take multiple prescription drugs each day, thus increasing the risk of drug interactions.

CHILDREN

Because their bodily functions aren't fully developed, children—particularly those under age 12—may metabolize drugs differently than do adults. In infants, immature hepatic and renal functions delay metabolism and excretion of drugs. As a result, pediatric drug dosages are very different from adult dosages.

The FDA has provided drug manufacturers with guidelines that define pediatric age categories. Unless the manufacturer provides a specific age range, use these categories as a guide when administering drugs:

- neonates—birth up to age 1 month
- infants—ages 1 month to 2 years
- children—ages 2 to 12
- adolescents—ages 12 to 16

CHILDBEARING CONSIDERATIONS

The many physiologic changes that take place in the body during the childbearing process may affect a drug's pharmacokinetics and alter its effectiveness. In addition, exposure to drugs may pose risks for the developing fetus. Before administering a drug to a pregnant patient, be sure to check the new more comprehensive text for drugs and intervene appropriately.

Principles of Drug Administration

Because there are thousands of drugs and hundreds of facts about each one, taking responsibility for drug administration can seem overwhelming. One way to enhance understanding of the principles of drug administration is to *associate, ask*, and *predict* during the critical thinking process. For example, associate each drug with general information already known about the drug or drug class. *Ask* why a drug is administered by a certain route and why it is given multiple times throughout the day rather than only once. Learn to *predict* a drug's actions, uses, adverse effects, and possible drug interactions based on knowledge of the drug's mechanism of action. As these principles are applied to drug administration, which facts are needed to make rational clinical decisions will become clear.

Prescriptions for patients in hospitals and other institutions are typically written by a physician, physician assistant, or nurse practitioner on a form called the *physician's order sheet* or they're directly input into a computerized system with an electronic signature. Drugs are prescribed based not only on their specific mechanisms of action but also on the patient's profile, which commonly includes age, ethnicity, gender, pregnancy status, smoking and drinking habits, and use of other drugs.

"Rights" of Drug Administration

Always keep in mind the following "rights" of drug administration: the right drug, right time, right dose, right patient, right route, right preparation and administration, and right documentation.

RIGHT DRUG

Many drugs have different concentrations, similar spellings, and several generic forms. Before administering any drug, compare the exact spelling and concentration of the prescribed drug that appears on the label with the information contained in the medication administration record or drug profile. Regardless of which drug distribution system your facility uses, read the drug label and compare it with the medication administration record at least three times:

- before removing the drug from the dispensing unit or unit dose cart.
- before preparing or measuring the prescribed dose.
- before opening a unit dose package (just before administering the drug to the patient).

RIGHT TIME

Various factors can affect the time that a drug is administered, such as the timing of meals and other drugs, scheduled diagnostic tests, standardized times used by the institution, and factors that may alter the consistency of blood levels and drug absorption. Before administering any p.r.n. drug, check the patient's chart to ensure that no one else has already administered it and that the specified time interval has passed. Also, document administration of a p.r.n. drug immediately.

RIGHT DOSE

Whenever you're dispensing an unfamiliar drug or are in doubt about a dosage, check the prescribed dose against the range specified in a reliable reference. Be sure to consider any reasons for a dosage adjustment that may apply to the particular patient. Also, make sure standard abbreviations the institution uses for writing prescriptions are familiar and understood.

RIGHT PATIENT

Always compare the name of the patient on the medication record with the name on the patient's identification bracelet. When using a unit dose system, compare the name on the drug profile with that on the identification bracelet.

RIGHT ROUTE

Each drug prescription should specify the administration route. If the administration route is missing from the prescription, consult the prescriber before giving the drug. Never substitute one route for another unless a prescription has been obtained for the change.

RIGHT PREPARATION AND ADMINISTRATION

For drugs that must be mixed, poured, or measured, be sure to maintain aseptic technique. Follow any specific directions included by the manufacturer regarding diluent amount and type and the use of filters, if needed. Clearly label any drug that has been reconstituted with the patient's name, the strength or dose, the date and time that the drug was prepared, the amount and type of diluent that was used, the expiration date, and your initials.

RIGHT DOCUMENTATION

It's crucial that documentation of drug administration appears on the right patient's medical record. Sometimes two patients on the same nursing unit may have the same last name, and even the same first initial. Documentation done in haste may cause the wrong medical record to be pulled. This could result in an apparent medication error as it would appear from the documentation—the patient who was supposed to get a drug did not and the patient who was not supposed to get the drug did. Always double-check the patient's full name and one other identifying factor such as the patient's age or prescriber name before documenting drug administration on the patient's medical record.

Administration Routes

Drugs may be administered by a variety of routes and dosage forms. A particular route may be chosen for convenience or to maximize drug concentration at the site of action, to minimize drug absorption elsewhere, to prolong drug absorption, or to avoid first-pass metabolism.

Different dosage forms of the same drug may have different drug absorption rates, times of onset, and durations of action. For example, nitroglycerin is a coronary vasodilator that may be administered by the I.V., sublingual, or translingual route, or as a topical ointment or patch. The I.V., sublingual, and translingual forms of nitroglycerin provide a rapid onset of action, whereas the ointment and patch forms have a slower onset and a prolonged duration of action.

Drug administration routes include the enteral, parenteral, and transcutaneous routes.

ENTERAL

The enteral route consists of oral, gastric or nasogastric, and rectal administration. Drugs administered enterally enter the blood circulation by way of the GI tract. This route is considered the most natural and convenient route as well as the safest. As a result, most drugs are taken enterally, usually to provide systemic effects.

Oral

- *Tablets:* Tablets, the most commonly used dosage form, come in a variety of colors, sizes, and shapes. Some tablets are specially coated for various purposes. Enteric coatings permit safe passage of a tablet through the stomach, where some drugs may be degraded or may produce unwanted effects, to the environment of the intestine. Some coatings protect the drug from the destructive influences of air, light, or moisture during storage; some coatings may contain the drug, while others conceal a bad taste. Coatings are also used to ensure appropriate drug release and absorption. Tablets with coatings shouldn't be crushed or broken because doing so may alter drug release.
- *Capsules:* Capsules are solid dosage forms in which the drug and other ingredients are enclosed in a hard or soft shell of varying size and shape. Drugs typically are released faster from capsules than from tablets.
- *Solutions:* Drugs administered in solution are absorbed more rapidly than many of those administered in solid form; however, they don't always produce predictable drug levels in the blood. Some drugs in solution should be administered with meals or snacks to minimize their irritating effect on the gastric mucosa.
- *Suspensions:* Suspensions are preparations consisting of finely divided drugs in a suitable vehicle, usually water. Suspensions should be shaken before administration to ensure the uniformity of the preparation and administration of the proper dosage.

Gastric or Nasogastric

Drugs administered through a gastrostomy or nasogastric tube enter the stomach directly, bypassing the mouth and esophagus. They're usually administered in liquid form because an intact tablet or capsule could cause an obstruction in a gastric or nasogastric tube. Sometimes, a tablet may be crushed, or a capsule opened for gastric or nasogastric administration; however, doing so will affect the drug's release. You may need to consult a pharmacist to determine which tablets can be crushed or capsules opened.

Rectal

Some enteral drugs are administered rectally—as ointments, solutions, or suppositories—to provide either local or systemic effects. When inserted into the rectum, suppositories soften, melt, or dissolve, releasing the drug contained inside them. The rectal route may be preferred for drugs that are destroyed or inactivated by the gastric or intestinal environment or that irritate the stomach. It also may be indicated when the oral route is contraindicated because of difficulty swallowing or vomiting. The drawbacks of rectal administration include inconvenience, noncompliance, and incomplete or irregular drug absorption.

PARENTERAL

In parenteral drug administration, a drug enters the circulatory system through an injection rather than through GI absorption. This administration route is chosen when rapid drug action is desired; when the patient is uncooperative, unconscious, or unable to accept medication by the oral route; or when a drug is ineffective by other routes. Drugs may be injected into joints, muscles, spinal column, and veins. However, the most common parenteral routes are the intradermal (I.D.), intramuscular (I.M.), intravenous (I.V.), and subcutaneous (SubQ) routes. Drugs administered parenterally may be mixed in either a solution or a suspension; those mixed in a solution typically act more rapidly than those mixed in a suspension. Parenteral administration has several disadvantages: The drug can't be removed, or the dosage reduced once it has been injected, and injections typically are more expensive to administer than other dosage forms because they require strict sterility.

Intradermal

Common sites for intradermal injection are the arm and the back. Because only about 0.1 ml may be administered intradermally, this route is rarely used except in diagnostic and test procedures, such as screening for allergic reactions.

Intramuscular

I.M. injections are administered deep into the anterolateral aspect of the thigh (vastus lateralis), the dorsogluteal muscle (gluteus maximus), the upper arm (deltoid), or the ventrogluteal muscle (gluteus medius). I.M. injections typically provide sustained drug action. This route is commonly chosen for drugs that irritate the subcutaneous tissue. The drug should be injected as far as possible from major nerves and blood vessels.

Intravenous

In I.V. drug administration, an aqueous solution is injected directly into the vein—typically of the forearm. Drugs may be administered as a single, small-volume injection or as a slow, large-volume infusion. Because drugs injected I.V. don't encounter absorption barriers, this route produces the most rapid drug action, making it vital in emergency situations. Except for I.V. fat emulsions used as nutritional supplements, oleaginous preparations aren't usually administered by this route because of the risk of fat embolism.

Subcutaneous

The subcutaneous route may be used to inject small volumes of medication, usually 1 ml or less. Subcutaneous injections typically are given below the skin in the abdominal area, lateral area of the anterior thigh, lateral lumbar area, or posterior surface of the upper arm. Injection sites should be rotated to minimize tissue irritation if the patient receives frequent subcutaneous injections—as, for example, in a patient who takes insulin.

TRANSCUTANEOUS

In transcutaneous administration, a drug crosses the skin layers from either the outside (dermal) or the inside (mucocutaneous).

This route includes inhalation, nasal, ophthalmic, otic, sublingual, topical, and vaginal administration.

Inhalation

Some drugs may be inhaled nasally or orally to produce a local effect on the respiratory tract or a systemic effect. Although drugs given by inhalation avoid first-pass hepatic metabolism, the lungs can also serve as an area of first-pass metabolism by providing respiratory conversion to more water-soluble compounds.

Nasal

Nasal solutions and suspensions are applied directly to the nasal mucosa for decreased systemic absorption and enhanced local penetration. These drugs are usually used to reduce the inflammation typically associated with perennial or seasonal rhinitis but may also be used for other purposes such as to elicit a systemic response.

Ophthalmic

Ophthalmic ointments and solutions are applied directly to the conjunctiva or cornea for enhanced local penetration and decreased systemic absorption. Ophthalmic solutions pose a greater risk of drug loss through the nasolacrimal duct into the nasopharynx than ophthalmic ointments do.

Otic

Otic solutions are instilled directly into the external auditory canal for decreased systemic absorption and local penetration. These drugs, which include anesthetics, antibiotics, and anti-inflammatory drugs, usually require occlusion of the ear canal with cotton after instillation.

Sublingual

In sublingual administration, tablets are placed under the tongue and allowed to dissolve. Nitroglycerin is commonly administered by this route, which allows rapid drug absorption and action. The sublingual route also avoids first-pass metabolism.

Topical

Topical drugs—including creams, lotions, pastes, and ointments—are applied directly to the skin. Transdermal delivery systems, usually in the form of a disk or an adhesive patch, are among the latest developments in topical drug administration. Because they provide slow drug release, these systems are typically used to avoid first-pass metabolism and ensure prolonged duration of action.

Vaginal

Vaginal creams, suppositories, and troches are inserted into the vagina for slow, localized absorption. Body pH that differs from blood pH causes drug trapping or reabsorption, which delays drug excretion through the renal tubules. Vaginal secretions are alkaline, with a pH of 3.4 to 4.2, whereas blood has a pH of 7.35 to 7.45.

Drug Therapy and the Nursing Process

A systematic approach to nursing care, the nursing process helps guide the development, implementation, and evaluation of care and ensures delivery of consistent, effective, and safe drug therapy to the patient. The nursing process consists of five steps, including assessment, nursing diagnosis, planning, implementation, and evaluation. Even though documentation is not a step in the nursing process, documenting all aspects of care before, during, and after drug administration is a legal and professional responsibility.

Assessment

The first step in the nursing process, assessment involves gathering information that's essential to guide the patient's drug therapy. This information includes the patient's allergies, drug and medical history, present drug use, and physical examination findings. Assessment is an ongoing process that serves as a baseline against which to compare any changes in the patient's condition; it's also the basis for developing and individualizing the patient's plan of care.

ALLERGIES

Find out if the patient is allergic to any drugs or foods. If they have an allergy, explore it further by determining the type of drug or food that triggers a reaction, the first time they experienced a reaction, the characteristics of the reaction, and other related information. Keep in mind that some patients consider annoying symptoms, such as indigestion, an allergic reaction. However, be sure to document a true allergy according to the facility's policy to ensure that the patient doesn't receive that drug or any related drug that may cause a similar reaction. Also, document allergies to foods because they may lead to adverse drug reactions or drug interactions. For example, sulfite is a food additive as well as a drug additive, so a patient with a known allergy to sulfite-containing foods is likely to react to sulfite-containing drugs.

DRUG HISTORY

The patient's drug history is critical in the planning of drug-related care. Ask about their previous use of over-the-counter and prescription drugs, as well as herbal remedies. For each drug, determine:

- the reason the patient took it.
- the prescribed dosage.
- the administration route.
- the frequency of administration.
- the duration of the drug therapy.
- any adverse reactions the patient may have experienced and how they handled them.

Also determine if the patient has a history of drug abuse or addiction. Depending on their emotional and physical state, a drug history may need to be obtained from other sources, such as family members, friends, other caregivers, and the medical record.

MEDICAL HISTORY

While reviewing the patient's medical history, determine if they have any acute or chronic conditions that may interfere with their drug therapy. Certain disorders involving major body systems, such as the cardiovascular, GI, hepatic, and renal systems, may affect a drug's absorption, transport, metabolism, or excretion and interfere with its action; they also may increase the incidence of adverse reactions and lead to toxicity. For each disorder identified, try to determine when the condition was diagnosed, what drugs were prescribed, and who prescribed them. This information can help determine whether the patient is receiving incompatible drugs and whether more than one prescriber is managing their drug therapy.

Ask females of childbearing age if they are or may be pregnant. Also, inquire if females of childbearing age are using a contraceptive and, if so, what type is being used. Some drugs such as isotretinoin require females of childbearing age to use an effective contraceptive, or the drug cannot be given. In other instances, the type of contraceptive used may need to be changed or a second type of contraceptive added such as with rifampin therapy. Ask mothers if they are breastfeeding. Many drugs are safe to use during pregnancy, but others may harm the fetus. Also, some drugs are distributed into breast milk. If the patient is or might be pregnant, check the FDA's recommendation for the prescribed drug and notify the prescriber if the drug may pose a risk to the fetus. If the patient is breastfeeding, find out if the drug is distributed in breast milk and intervene appropriately.

PRESENT DRUG USE

Ask about the patient's current use of over-the-counter and prescription drugs, as well as herbal remedies. As with the drug history, find out the specific details for each drug (dosage, route, frequency, and reason for taking). Also, ask the patient if they think the drug has been effective and when they took the last dose.

If the patient uses herbal remedies, explore the use of these products because herbs may interact with certain drugs. Also, ask about the patient's use of illegal drugs, such as heroin, as well as recreational drugs, such as alcohol and tobacco. If the patient acknowledges use of these drugs, be alert for possible drug interactions. This information also may provide insight about the patient's response—or lack of response—to their current drug treatment plan.

Try to find out if the patient has any other problems that might affect their compliance with the drug treatment plan and intervene appropriately. For instance, a patient who is unemployed and has no health insurance may fail to fill a needed prescription. In such a case, contact an appropriate individual such as a social worker who may be able to help the patient obtain financial assistance.

Be sure to ask the patient if their drug treatment plan requires special monitoring or follow-up laboratory tests. For example, patients who take antihypertensives need to have their blood pressure checked routinely, and those who take warfarin must have their prothrombin time tested regularly. Other patients must undergo periodic blood tests to assess their hepatic and renal function. Determine whether the patient has complied with this part of their treatment plan and ask them if they know the results of the latest monitoring or laboratory tests.

PHYSICAL EXAMINATION FINDINGS

As part of the physical examination, note the patient's age and weight. Be aware that age determines the dosage of certain drugs, such as sedatives and hypnotics, whereas weight determines the dosage of others, including some I.V. antibiotics and antivirals. As the physical examination is performed, note any abnormal findings that may point to body organ or system dysfunction. For example, if ascites and liver enlargement are detected, the patient may have impaired hepatic function, which can affect the metabolism of a drug they're taking and lead to harmful adverse or toxic effects. Also, note whether a body organ or system appears to be responding to drug treatment. For example, if a patient has been taking an antibiotic to treat chronic bronchitis, thoroughly evaluate their respiratory status to measure their progress. Be sure to assess the patient for possible adverse reactions to the drugs they're taking.

Assess the patient's neurologic function to make sure that they can understand their drug regimen and carry out required tasks, such as performing a fingerstick to obtain blood for glucose measurement. If the patient can't understand essential drug information, a family member or another person will need to be identified who is willing to become involved in the teaching process.

Nursing Diagnosis

Based on information derived from the assessment and physical examination findings, the nursing diagnoses are statements of actual or potential problems that a nurse is licensed to treat or manage alone or in collaboration with other members of the healthcare team. They're worded according to guidelines established by the North American Nursing Diagnosis Association (NANDA) International.

One of the most common nursing diagnoses related to drug therapy is *knowledge deficit*, which indicates that the patient doesn't have sufficient understanding of their drug regimen. However, adverse reactions are the basis for most nursing diagnoses related to drug administration. For example, a patient receiving an opioid analgesic might have a nursing diagnosis of *constipation* related to decreased intestinal motility or *ineffective breathing* pattern related to respiratory depression. A patient receiving long-term, high-dose corticosteroids may have a risk for *impaired skin integrity* related to cortisone acetate or *self-concept disturbance* related to physical changes from prednisone therapy. Many antiarrhythmics cause orthostatic hypotension and thus may place an older patient at *high risk for injury* related to possible syncope. Broad-spectrum antibiotics, especially penicillin, may lead to the overgrowth of *Clostridioides difficile*, a bacterium that is normally present in the intestine. This overgrowth in turn may lead to pseudomembranous colitis, characterized by abdominal pain and severe diarrhea. The nursing diagnoses in such a case might include *alteration in comfort* related to abdominal pain, *fluid balance deficit* related to diarrhea, and *potential for infection* related to bacterial overgrowth.

Planning

During the planning phase, establish expected outcomes—or goals—for the patient and then develop specific nursing interventions to achieve them. Expected outcomes are observable or measurable goals that should occur as a result of nursing interventions and sometimes in conjunction with medical interventions. Developed in collaboration with the patient, the outcomes should be objective and realistic and should clearly communicate the direction of the plan of care to other nurses. They should be written as behaviors or responses for the patient, not the nurse, to achieve and should include a time frame for measuring the patient's progress. An example of a typical expected outcome is, *the patient will accurately demonstrate self-administration of insulin before discharge*. Based on each outcome statement established, develop appropriate nursing interventions, which might include calculation of drug dosages based on weight, drug administration techniques, monitoring of vital signs, patient teaching, and recording of intake and output.

Implementation

As the nursing interventions are implemented, be sure to stringently follow the classic rule of drug administration: Administer the right dose of the right drug by the right route to the right patient at the right time and on the right patient record. Also, keep in mind the legal and professional need to follow institutional policy regarding standing orders, prescription renewal, and the use of nursing judgment. During the implementation phase, also begin to evaluate the nursing interventions and patient's expected outcomes and make necessary changes to the plan of care.

Evaluation

Evaluation is an ongoing process rather than a single step in the nursing process. During this phase, evaluate each expected outcome to determine whether it has been achieved, whether the original plan of care is working, or if it should be modified. In evaluating a patient's drug treatment plan, determine whether the drug is controlling the signs and symptoms for which it was prescribed. Also evaluate the patient for physiologic or psychological responses to the drug, especially adverse reactions. This constant monitoring allows appropriate and timely suggestions to be made for changes to the plan of care, such as dosage adjustments or changes in delivery routes, until each expected outcome has been achieved.

Documentation

You're responsible for documenting all your actions related to the patient's drug therapy, from the assessment phase to evaluation. And, remember it must appear on the correct medical record for the right patient. Each time you administer a drug, document the drug name, dose, time given, and your evaluation of its effect. When you administer drugs that require additional nursing judgment, such as those prescribed on an as-needed basis, document the rationale for administering the drug and follow-up assessment or interventions for each dose administered.

If a prescribed drug is withheld based on nursing judgment, document the action and the rationale for it, and notify the prescriber of the action in a timely manner. Whenever a prescriber is notified about a significant finding related to drug therapy, such as an adverse reaction, document the date and time, the person contacted, what was discussed, and the intervention(s) taken.

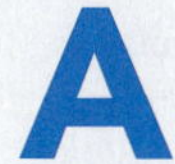

abacavir sulfate

Ziagen

Class and Category

Pharmacologic class: Nucleoside reverse transcriptase inhibitor (NRTI)
Therapeutic class: Antiretroviral

Indications and Dosages

✱ *As adjunct to treat human immunodeficiency virus (HIV-1) infection*

ORAL SOLUTION

Adults. 600 mg once daily or 300 mg twice daily.
Children, infants ages 3 mo and older. 16 mg/kg once daily or 8 mg/kg twice daily. *Maximum*: 600 mg daily.

TABLETS

Children weighing 25 kg (55 lb) or more. 300 mg in a.m. and 300 mg in p.m.
Children weighing 20 kg (44 lb) to less than 25 kg (55 lb). 150 mg in a.m. and 300 mg in p.m.
Children weighing 14 kg (30.8 lb) to less than 20 kg (44 lb). 150 mg in a.m. and 150 mg in p.m.

± **DOSAGE ADJUSTMENT** For patients with mild hepatic impairment, dosage reduced to 200 mg twice daily and only oral solution used to ensure accurate dosage.

Drug Administration

P.O.

- Be aware that a scored tablet is available for pediatric patients weighing 14 kg or more, provided the child can swallow tablets.
- Oral solution is a clear to opalescent, yellowish solution, which may turn brown over time.
- May be stored in refrigerator or at room temperature.
- Use a calibrated device to measure oral solution to ensure accurate dosing.
- Abacavir is given in combination with other antiretroviral agents.

Route	Onset	Peak	Duration
P.O.	Unknown	07–1.7 hr	Unknown

Half-life: 1.5 hr

Mechanism of Action

Blocks an HIV enzyme called reverse transcriptase, which is responsible for starting or increasing the speed of a chemical reaction. By blocking this enzyme, HIV is prevented from multiplying.

Contraindications

Hypersensitivity to abacavir or its components, moderate or severe hepatic impairment, presence of HLA-B*5701 allele

Interactions

DRUGS

methadone: Possibly increased methadone clearance
riociguat: Increased riociguat exposure, increasing risk of riociguat adverse reactions

Adverse Reactions

CNS: Anxiety, chills, depression, dizziness, fatigue, fever, headache, lethargy, malaise, migraines, paresthesia, sleep disorders
CV: Edema, elevated triglyceride levels, **hypotension**, **MI**
EENT: Conjunctivitis, ENT infections, mouth ulcerations, pharyngitis
ENDO: Cushingoid appearance, fat redistribution, hyperglycemia
GI: Abdominal pain, diarrhea, elevated liver enzymes, gastritis, hyperamylasemia, **liver failure**, nausea, **pancreatitis**, **severe hepatomegaly with steatosis**, vomiting
GU: Renal dysfunction, **renal failure**
HEME: Anemia, **leukopenia**, **neutropenia**, **thrombocytopenia**
MS: Achiness, arthralgia, elevated CPK levels, musculoskeletal pain, myalgia, myolysis
RESP: **Adult respiratory distress syndrome**, bronchitis, cough, dyspnea, pneumonia, **respiratory failure**, viral respiratory infections
SKIN: **Erythema multiforme**, rash, **Stevens-Johnson syndrome**, **toxic epidermal necrolysis**
Other: **Anaphylaxis**, **immune reconstitution syndrome**, **lactic acidosis**,

lymphadenopathy, **multiorgan failure**, nonspecific pain

Childbearing Considerations

PREGNANCY

- Pregnancy exposure registry: 1-800-258-4263.
- It is not known if drug can cause fetal harm although it does cross the placental barrier.
- Use with caution only if benefit to mother outweighs potential risk to fetus.

LACTATION

- Drug is present in breast milk.
- The Centers for Disease Control and Prevention recommends that HIV-1-infected mothers not breastfeed to avoid risking postnatal transmission of HIV-1 infection in HIV-negative infants or developing viral resistance in HIV-positive infants. They also do not recommend breastfeeding because of potential drug-induced adverse reactions in the infant.

Nursing Considerations

! **WARNING** Ensure all patients have been screened for HLA-B*5701 allele before therapy begins because carriers of the HLA-B*5701 allele are at greater risk of developing serious and sometimes fatal hypersensitivity reactions to abacavir.

- Know that a past medical history of an allergic reaction to any abacavir-containing product is a contraindication for the use of abacavir therapy.
- Use caution when administering abacavir to patients with known risk factors for liver disease.
- Use cautiously in patients with coronary artery disease because an increase in myocardial infarctions have occurred within 6 months of initiating abacavir therapy.

! **WARNING** Monitor patient closely for any hypersensitivity reaction. If present, notify prescriber immediately and expect drug to be discontinued, especially if a hypersensitivity reaction cannot be ruled out. Being a woman, obesity, and prolonged nucleoside exposure have been identified as risk factors. Know that a hypersensitivity reaction to abacavir usually presents with at least 2 of the following signs or symptoms: constitutional symptoms (achiness, fatigue, generalized malaise), fever, GI symptoms (abdominal pain, diarrhea, nausea, vomiting), rash, or respiratory symptoms (cough, dyspnea, pharyngitis). Other signs and symptoms that may be present include arthralgia, edema, headache, lethargy, myalgia, myolysis, and paresthesia. Know that adult respiratory distress syndrome, anaphylaxis, hypotension, renal failure, and respiratory failure have also occurred in association with an abacavir-induced hypersensitivity reaction and death has occurred.

- Monitor patient's liver enzymes periodically, as ordered, and monitor patient for any signs and symptoms of lactic acidosis or liver dysfunction such as severe hepatomegaly with steatosis, which may become life-threatening. Be aware that incidence is higher in women and in the presence of obesity. If present, notify prescriber, and expect abacavir therapy to be discontinued even in the absence of marked transaminase elevations.

! **WARNING** Be aware that immune reconstitution syndrome has occurred in patients treated with combination antiretroviral therapy, including abacavir. The inflammatory response predisposes susceptible patients to opportunistic infections such as cytomegalovirus infection, *Mycobacterium avium* infection, *Pneumocystis jiroveci* pneumonia, or tuberculosis. Autoimmune disorders such as Graves' disease, Guillain-Barré syndrome, or polymyositis have also occurred. Report sudden or unusual adverse reactions to prescriber.

- Observe patient for redistribution of body fat, including breast enlargement, central obesity, development of buffalo hump, facial wasting, and peripheral wasting, which may produce a cushingoid-type appearance.

PATIENT TEACHING

- Instruct patient and family or caregiver to administer drug exactly as prescribed. If a dose is missed, patient should take it as soon as it is remembered. Stress importance of not doubling the next dose or taking more than the prescribed dose.

! **WARNING** Review the warning card and medication guide with patient and family member or caregiver on how to recognize a hypersensitivity reaction. Stress importance of stopping abacavir at the first sign of a hypersensitivity reaction and notifying prescriber. If reaction is serious, urge patient to seek immediate medical care.

- Instruct patient and family or caregiver on the signs and symptoms of lactic acidosis and liver dysfunction. Advise patient to stop taking abacavir, if present, and notify prescriber.
- Advise patient and family or caregiver to inform prescriber of any signs or symptoms of an infection, as well as any persistent, severe, or unusual adverse reactions.
- Instruct mothers not to breastfeed while they are receiving abacavir therapy.
- Warn patient that fat distribution may occur with abacavir therapy.
- Tell females of childbearing age to report pregnancy. Encourage patient to enroll in the pregnancy exposure registry if pregnancy occurs.

abaloparatide

Tymlos

Class and Category

Pharmacologic class: Parathyroid hormone analogue
Therapeutic class: Antiosteoporotic

Indications and Dosages

* *To treat postmenopausal women with osteoporosis who are at high risk for fracture, such as a history of multiple risk factors for fracture, have already sustained an osteoporotic fracture, or who have failed or are intolerant to other available osteoporosis therapy; to increase bone density in men with osteoporosis at high risk for fracture, such as a history of multiple risk factors for fracture, have already sustained an osteoporotic fracture, or who have failed or are intolerant to other available osteoporosis therapy*

SUBCUTANEOUS INJECTION

Adult men and postmenopausal women. 80 mcg once daily.

Drug Administration

SUBCUTANEOUS

- Remove prefilled pen from refrigerator before first use (pen delivers 30 doses of drug). Solution should be clear and colorless. If not, discard the solution.
- Administer into the periumbilical region of abdomen, rotating site every day. Never give intramuscularly or intravenously.
- Give first several doses with patient lying down or sitting, in case orthostatic hypotension occurs. Monitor patient for at least 4 hr after each dose.
- Give at about the same time every day.
- After first use of pen, store at room temperature. Do not freeze or subject pen to heat.
- Discard pen after 30 days, regardless of any drug remaining in pen.

Route	Onset	Peak	Duration
SubQ	Unknown	0.51 hr	Unknown

Half-life: 1.7 hr

Mechanism of Action

Acts as an agonist at the PTH1 receptor, which activates the cAMP signaling pathway in target cells to increase bone mineral density and content. This, in turn, increases bone strength at vertebral and/or nonvertebral sites.

Contraindications

Hypersensitivity to abaloparatide or its components

Interactions

DRUGS

None reported by manufacturer.

Adverse Reactions

CNS: Asthenia, dizziness, fatigue, headache, insomnia, lethargy, malaise, vertigo
CV: Orthostatic hypotension, palpitations, tachycardia
GI: Abdominal distention or pain (upper), constipation, diarrhea, nausea, vomiting
GU: Hypercalciuria, urolithiasis
MS: Arthralgia, bone, back, extremity, and joint pain; muscle spasms of back and leg
RESP: Dyspnea (context of allergic reaction)
SKIN: Pruritus, rash, urticaria
Other: **Anaphylaxis or other hypersensitivity reactions**,

anti-abaloparatide antibodies, elevated serum uric acid levels, **hypercalcemia**, injection-site reactions (bruising, hemorrhage, pain, pruritus, rash, redness, severe edema, swelling)

Childbearing Considerations

PREGNANCY

- No human data with drug use in pregnant women is available.
- Drug is not indicated for use in females of childbearing age.

LACTATION

- There is no information on drug being present in breast milk, effects on the breastfed infant, or the effects on milk production.
- Drug is not indicated for use in breastfeeding mothers.

Nursing Considerations

- Know that abaloparatide and/or parathyroid hormone analogues should not be given for more than 2 years cumulatively during patient's lifetime because of the potential risk of osteosarcoma.
- Be aware that abaloparatide should not be given to patients at increased risk for osteosarcoma. These risks include bone metastases or skeletal malignancies, hereditary disorders predisposing to osteosarcoma, metabolic bone diseases other than osteoporosis (including Paget's disease of the bone), open epiphyses, or prior external beam or implant radiation therapy involving the skeleton.

! **WARNING** Assess patient for signs of a hypersensitivity reaction that could become life-threatening such as anaphylaxis. Notify prescriber immediately, if present, and be prepared to provide suportive emergency care, as needed and ordered.

! **WARNING** Know that abaloparatide should not be given to patients with preexisting hypercalcemia or who have an underlying hypercalcemic disorder, such as primary hyperparathyroidism, because of the risk of exacerbating hypercalcemia.

- Monitor patient's serum calcium levels, as ordered, because drug may increase calcium levels, causing hypercalcemia, hypercalciuria, and urolithiasis. If preexisting hypercalciuria or urolithiasis is suspected, expect to measure the patient's urinary calcium excretion, as ordered.
- Ensure that patient is receiving supplemental calcium and vitamin D if dietary intake is inadequate.

PATIENT TEACHING

! **WARNING** Inform patient that abaloparatide should not be given more than 2 years cumulatively in patient's lifetime because of a potential risk for osteosarcoma. Tell patient to immediately report persistent localized pain or occurrence of a new soft-tissue mass that is tender to touch.

- Instruct patient, family, or caregiver how to administer a subcutaneous injection using the abaloparatide pen and how to properly dispose of the needle and pen.
- Emphasize the importance of not sharing the drug or needles with others. Also, tell patient not to transfer the contents of the pen to a syringe.
- Tell patient the pen must be discarded after 30 days of use, even if it still contains unused solution.
- Advise patient to change positions slowly for at least 4 hours after abaloparatide has been given and to watch for a drop in her blood pressure with position changes. Symptoms to be alert for include dizziness, nausea, or a rapid heart rate. If present, tell patient to lie down or sit down until symptoms pass.

! **WARNING** Review allergic reactions with patient and stress importance of seeking immediate medical attention if signs of anaphylaxis, dyspnea, hives, itching, or rash occurs.

! **WARNING** Instruct patient to report signs and symptoms of high calcium levels such as constipation, lethargy, muscle weakness, nausea, or vomiting. Inform patient that she will need to have her calcium level checked routinely.

- Review dietary sources of calcium and vitamin D. Inform patient that calcium and vitamin D supplementation will be needed if dietary intake is insufficient.

abatacept

Orencia

Class and Category

Pharmacologic class: Selective co-stimulation modulator

Therapeutic class: Antiarthritic (psoriatic, rheumatic)

Indications and Dosages

* *To treat moderate to severe active rheumatoid arthritis as monotherapy or concomitantly with disease-modifying antirheumatic drugs (DMARDs) other than Janus kinase (JAK) inhibitors or biologic disease-modifying antirheumatic drugs (bDMARDs), such as tumor necrosis factor (TNF) antagonists*

I.V. INFUSION

Adults weighing more than 100 kg (220 lb). *Initial:* 1,000 mg, repeated at 2 and 4 wk after the first infusion and every 4 wk thereafter.

Adults weighing 60 to 100 kg (132 to 220 lb). *Initial:* 750 mg, repeated at 2 and 4 wk after the first infusion and every 4 wk thereafter.

Adults weighing less than 60 kg (132 lb). *Initial:* 500 mg, repeated at 2 and 4 wk after the first infusion and every 4 wk thereafter.

I.V. INFUSION FOLLOWED BY SUBCUTANEOUS INJECTION

Adults receiving a loading dose and weighing more than 100 kg (220 lb). *Loading dose:* 1,000 mg I.V. followed by 125 mg given as a subcutaneous injection within a day after the loading dose. *Maintenance:* 125 mg once/wk.

Adults receiving a loading dose and weighing 60 to 100 kg (132 to 220 lb). *Loading dose:* 750 mg I.V. followed by 125 mg given as a subcutaneous injection within a day after the loading dose. *Maintenance:* 125 mg once/wk.

Adults receiving a loading dose and weighing less than 60 kg (132 lb). *Loading dose:* 500 mg I.V. followed by 125 mg given as a subcutaneous injection within a day after the loading dose. *Maintenance:* 125 mg once/wk.

SUBCUTANEOUS INJECTION

Adults. 125 mg once/wk.

* *To treat active psoriatic arthritis (PsA) with or without nonbiologic disease-modifying antirheumatic drugs (DMARDs)*

I.V. INFUSION

Adults weighing more than 100 kg (220 lb). *Initial:* 1,000 mg, repeated at 2 and 4 wk after the first infusion and every 4 wk thereafter.

Adults weighing 60 to 100 kg (132 to 220 lb). *Initial:* 750 mg, repeated at 2 and 4 wk after the first infusion and every 4 wk thereafter.

Adults weighing less than 60 kg (132 lb). *Initial:* 500 mg, repeated at 2 and 4 wk after the first infusion and every 4 wk thereafter.

SUBCUTANEOUS INJECTION

Adults. 125 mg once weekly.

* *To treat psoriatic arthritis (PsA) as monotherapy or concomitantly with methotrexate*

SUBCUTANEOUS INJECTION

Children ages 2 and older weighing 50 kg (110 lb) or more. 125 mg once weekly.

Children ages 2 and older weighing 25 kg to less than 50 kg (55 lb to 110 lb). 87.5 mg once weekly.

Children ages 2 and older weighing 10 kg to less than 25 kg (22 lb to 55 lb). 50 mg once weekly.

* *To treat moderate to severe active polyarticular juvenile idiopathic arthritis as monotherapy or concomitantly with methotrexate*

I.V. INFUSION

Children ages 6 to 17 weighing more than 100 kg (220 lb). *Initial:* 1,000 mg, repeated at 2 and 4 wk after the first infusion and every 4 wk thereafter.

Children ages 6 to 17 weighing 75 to 100 kg (165 to 220 lb). *Initial:* 750 mg, repeated at 2 and 4 wk after the first infusion and every 4 wk thereafter.

Children ages 6 to 17 weighing less than 75 kg (165 lb). *Initial:* 10 mg/kg, repeated at 2 and 4 wk after the first infusion and every 4 wk thereafter.

SUBCUTANEOUS INJECTION

Children ages 2 and older weighing 50 kg (110 lb) or more. 125 mg once/wk.

Children ages 2 and older weighing 25 kg (55 lb) to less than 50 kg (110 lb). 87.5 mg once/wk.

Children ages 2 and older weighing 10 kg (22 lb) to less than 25 kg (55 lb). 50 mg once/wk.

∗ *To prevent acute graft versus host disease (aGVHD), in combination with a calcineurin inhibitor and methotrexate in patients undergoing hematopoietic stem cell transplantation (HSCT) from a matched or one allele-mismatched unrelated donor*

I.V. INFUSION

Adults and children ages 6 and older. 10 mg/kg on the day before transplantation (day 1), followed by 10 mg/kg on days 5, 14, and 28 after transplantation.

Children ages 2 to less than 6 yr. 15 mg/kg on the day before transplantation (day 1), followed by 12 mg/kg on days 5, 14, and 28 after transplantation.

±**DOSAGE ADJUSTMENT** For patients transitioning from I.V. therapy to subcutaneous injection, first subcutaneous dose should be administered instead of the next scheduled I.V. dose.

Drug Administration

I.V.

- Prepare I.V. injection by reconstituting each vial with 10 ml of Sterile Water for Injection, directing the stream of Sterile Water for Injection to the inside glass wall of vial to minimize foaming. Use only the silicone-free disposable syringe with an 18G to 21G needle provided with each vial because a siliconized syringe may cause translucent particles to form in solution. If the drug is accidently reconstituted with a siliconized syringe, the solution should be discarded. If the provided silicone-free disposable syringe is contaminated or dropped, a new silicone-free disposable syringe should be used. If needed, call 1-800-ORENCIA to obtain silicone-free syringes.
- After injecting Sterile Water for Injection into vial, gently swirl vial until contents are completely dissolved. The solution should appear clear and colorless to pale yellow. To minimize foaming, don't shake and don't prolong or use vigorous agitation. Vent the vial with a needle to dissipate any foam that may be present.
- Dilute the reconstituted solution with 0.9% Sodium Chloride Injection to achieve a final solution volume of 100 ml. To do so, first withdraw a volume equal to the volume of the reconstituted drug solution required for patient dose from a 100-ml infusion bag or bottle. Then, slowly add the reconstituted solution into the infusion bag or bottle using the same silicone-free disposable syringe provided with each vial. Mix gently. Do not shake the bag or bottle.
- Give I.V. dose after dilution over 30 min (60 min for prevention of aGVHD) using an infusion set and a sterile, nonpyrogenic, low protein-binding filter with a pore size of 0.2 to 1.2 µm. Drug infusion must be completed within 24 hr of reconstitution.
- Be aware that once fully diluted, I.V. solution must be administered within 24 hr. Diluted solution may be kept for up to 24 hr at room temperature or refrigerated. If reconstituted solution isn't used within 24 hr, discard.
- *Incompatibilities:* Other drugs in the same intravenous line concurrently

SUBCUTANEOUS

- Administer subcutaneous injection using only the supplied single-dose prefilled glass syringe or the prefilled 125-mg/ml ClickJect autoinjector. Solution should appear clear to slightly opalescent and colorless to pale yellow.
- Know that the autoinjector or prefilled syringe is never to be used for intravenous infusion.
- Rotate sites and never give in areas where the skin is bruised, hard, red, or tender.

Route	Onset	Peak	Duration
I.V./SubQ	Unknown	Unknown	Unknown

Half-life: 13.1 days

Mechanism of Action

Inhibits T-cell activation by binding to CD80 and CD86 to block interaction with CD28. CD28 is part of the costimulatory signal needed for full activation of T cells. Activated T cells have been implicated in the pathogenesis of rheumatoid arthritis. With decreased proliferation of T cells, inflammation and other evidence of rheumatoid arthritis decrease.

Contraindications

Hypersensitivity to abatacept or its components

Interactions

DRUGS

live-virus vaccines: Possibly decreased response to vaccine, and risk of infection with live virus
tumor necrosis factor antagonists: Increased risk of serious infection

Adverse Reactions

CNS: Dizziness, fever, headache
CV: Hypertension, **hypotension**
EENT: Epistaxis, nasopharyngitis, rhinitis, sinusitis
GI: Abdominal pain, diarrhea, diverticulitis, dyspepsia, nausea
GU: **Acute pyelonephritis**, UTI
HEME: Anemia, **decreased CD4 lymphocyte count**
MS: Back or limb pain
RESP: Bronchitis, COPD worsening, cough, dyspnea, **hypoxia**, pneumonia, upper respiratory tract infection, wheezing
SKIN: Cellulitis, flushing, pruritus, rash, urticaria
Other: **Anaphylaxis**, **angioedema**, antibody formation against abatacept, cytomegalovirus (CMV) infection or reactivation, Epstein-Barr virus (EBV) reactivation, herpes simplex, herpes-zoster infection, flu-like symptoms, hypermagnesemia, **immunosuppression**, **malignancies**, serious infections such as **sepsis**, varicella infection

Childbearing Considerations

PREGNANCY

- Pregnancy exposure registry: 1-877-311-8972.
- It is not known if drug can cause fetal harm, including reaction to a live vaccine administered to the infant after exposure in utero.
- Use with caution only if benefit to mother outweighs potential risk to fetus.

LACTATION

- It is not known if drug is present in breast milk.
- Mothers should check with prescriber before breastfeeding.

Nursing Considerations

- Screen patient for latent tuberculosis (TB) with a tuberculin skin test before starting abatacept. If test is positive, expect to provide treatment, as ordered, before starting abatacept. Also, screen patient for hepatitis B. If present, expect abatacept to be withdrawn because antirheumatic therapies such as abatacept may reactivate hepatitis B. For patient receiving drug to prevent aGVHD, expect patient to be prescribed antiviral prophylactic treatment for Epstein-Barr virus reactivation and to continue it for 6 months following HSCT. Be aware that patient may also receive prophylactic antivirals for cytomegalovirus (CMV) infection/reactivation during treatment and for 6 months following HSCT.
- Review patient's immunization record, and make sure all immunizations are current before therapy starts. Know that while non-live vaccines may be administered during abatacept therapy, live vaccines should not be given during therapy and for 3 months after drug is discontinued.
- Use cautiously in patients with a history of recurrent infections; underlying conditions that may predispose them to infection; or existing chronic, latent, or localized infection. They have an increased risk of infection with abatacept therapy.
- Use cautiously in patients with COPD and monitor respiratory status closely because abatacept may worsen COPD and increase the risk of adverse respiratory reactions.
- Know that TNF antagonists shouldn't be given with abatacept because of an increased risk of serious infection.
- Watch patient closely for infusion-related reactions that may occur within 1 hour of the start of the infusion. Adverse reactions to be alert for include dizziness, headache, and hypertension. Less commonly a patient may experience cough, dyspnea, flushing, hypersensitivity, hypotension, nausea, pruritus, rash, and wheezing. Notify prescriber if present but know that most patients need not discontinue abatacept because of these events unless severe.

! WARNING Monitor adult patient closely for anaphylaxis and angioedema after the first infusion of the drug, which may become life-threatening or even fatal and may occur within 1 hour of the start of the infusion. Angioedema has also occurred with subsequent intravenous doses as early as after the dose or delayed for days before being exhibited. If a serious hypersensitivity reaction occurs, notify prescriber, expect drug to be discontinued, and provide emergency supportive care, as needed and ordered.

! **WARNING** Monitor patient closely for evidence of infection or malignancy throughout therapy because abatacept inhibits T-cell activation, increasing the risk of both.

PATIENT TEACHING

- Instruct patient, family, or caregiver how to administer abatacept subcutaneously.
- Instruct patient not to receive immunizations with live vaccines during abatacept therapy and for 3 months afterward.
- Advise patient to tell prescriber of all medications being taken, including over-the-counter drugs and other biologic drugs before therapy begins.

! **WARNING** Emphasize need to report any evidence of hypersensitivity to prescriber.

! **WARNING** Alert patient that abatacept may increase the risk of malignancy. Instruct patient to notify prescriber of any persistent, serious, or unusual adverse effects.

- Review signs and symptoms of infection and notify prescriber if present. Warn patient to avoid crowds and people with infections.
- Inform females of childbearing age to report pregnancy. Encourage patient to register with the pregnancy exposure registry if pregnancy occurs.

abrocitinib

Cibinqo

Class and Category

Pharmacologic class: Janus kinase (JAK) inhibitor

Therapeutic class: Anti-inflammatory

Indications and Dosages

* *To treat refractory, moderate-to-severe atopic dermatitis in patients whose disease is not adequately controlled with other systemic drug products, including biologics, or when use of those therapies is inadvisable*

TABLETS

Adults and children ages 12 and older. 100 mg once daily, increased to 200 mg once daily, as needed.

± **DOSAGE ADJUSTMENT** For patients with moderate renal impairment (eGFR of 30 to 59 ml/min), poor CYP2C19 metabolizers, or patients who are receiving strong CYP2C19 inhibitors, initial dosage reduced to 50 mg once daily with dosage doubled, as needed.

Drug Administration

P.O.

- Tablets should not be chewed, crushed, or split and should be swallowed whole.
- Missed dose may be administered immediately unless it is less than 12 hr before the next dose.

Route	Onset	Peak	Duration
P.O.	Unknown	1 hr	Unknown

Half-life: 5 hr

Mechanism of Action

Reduces inflammation by inhibiting Janus kinase1 through the blockage of the adenosine triphosphate binding site.

Contraindications

Concurrent treatment with antiplatelet therapies, except for low-dose aspirin (less than or equal to 81 mg daily), during the first 3 months of treatment; hypersensitivity to abrocitinib or its components

Interactions

DRUGS

antiplatelets: Possibly increased risk of bleeding with thrombocytopenia

combination of CYP2C19 and CYP2C9 inhibitors (moderate to strong), CYP2C19 inhibitors (strong): Possibly increased risk of adverse reactions to abrocitinib

CYP2C9 or CYP2C19 inducers (strong): Possibly loss or reduced effectiveness of abrocitinib

live vaccines: Increased risk of adverse effects

P-gp substrates such as digoxin: Increased plasma concentrations of P-gp substrates, possibly resulting in increased risk of adverse reactions of the P-gp substrate where small concentration changes may lead to serious or life-threatening toxicity

Adverse Reactions

CNS: Dizziness, fatigue, headache
CV: **Deep vein thrombosis**, elevated lipids, hypertension, **major adverse cardiovascular events (MACE)**
EENT: Nasopharyngitis, oropharyngeal pain
GI: Abdominal discomfort or upper quadrant pain, gastroenteritis, nausea, vomiting
GU: UTI
HEME: Lymphopenia, **thrombocytopenia**
MS: Elevated creatine phosphokinase (CPK)
RESP: Pneumonia, **pulmonary embolism**
SKIN: Acne, contact dermatitis, impetigo
Other: Flu-like symptoms, herpes simplex infections, herpes zoster infection, **malignancy**, serious infections

Childbearing Considerations

PREGNANCY

- Pregnancy exposure registry: 1-877-311-3770.
- It is not known if drug can cause fetal harm.
- Use with caution only if benefit to mother outweighs potential risk to fetus.

LACTATION

- Drug may be present in breast milk.
- Mothers should not breastfeed during therapy and for one day after the last dose.

REPRODUCTION

- Females of childbearing age may have possible impaired fertility based on animal studies that may be reversible.

Nursing Considerations

- Be aware abrocitinib should not be used in patients with severe or end-stage renal disease or severe hepatic impairment.
- Know that abrocitinib should not be used in patients with an active, serious infection including localized infections or in patients receiving concurrent therapy with other biologic immunomodulators or other immunosuppressants or JAK inhibitors.
- Determine that screening for tuberculosis (TB) and viral hepatitis have been done before abrocitinib therapy is begun because drug is not recommended in patients with active hepatitis B or C or active TB. Patients with latent TB or those with a negative latent TB test who are at high risk for TB will need preventative therapy for latent TB prior to starting abrocitinib. Know that hepatitis B virus reactivation may occur during drug therapy; monitor patient closely.
- Ensure a CBC is done prior to starting abrocitinib therapy, again 4 weeks after therapy started, and 4 weeks after a dosage increase. Drug is not recommended to be started or, if therapy has begun, drug should be discontinued, for patients with an absolute lymphocyte count less than 500/mm3, an absolute neutrophil count less than 1,000 mm3, or a hemoglobin value less than 8 g/dL. Also, drug should not be started in patients with a platelet count less than 150,000/mm3 or drug discontinued, if therapy already started if patient experiences a platelet count below 500,000/mm3.
- Expect to complete any necessary immunizations such as herpes zoster vaccinations, as needed, prior to starting abrocitinib therapy. Avoid use of live vaccines immediately prior to, during, and immediately after drug therapy.
- Know that drug can be used with topical corticosteroids, as needed.
- Know that blood lipids should be checked 4 weeks after abrocitinib therapy is begun because increases may occur. If hyperlipidemia occurs, notify prescriber and expect treatment to begin.

! **WARNING** Monitor patient for major adverse cardiovascular events such as a CVA, MI, or thrombosis and expect drug to be discontinued, if present. Also, be aware that abrocitinib should be avoided in patients at risk for thrombosis. Patients may be at higher risk for sudden cardiovascular death if 50 years of age and older and have at least one cardiovascular risk factor.

! **WARNING** Monitor patient closely for signs and symptoms of infection during therapy. Other drugs known as JAK inhibitors used to treat inflammatory conditions have caused active TB (extrapulmonary or pulmonary disease); invasive fungal infections such as cryptococcosis and pneumocystosis; and opportunistic infections such a bacterial, viral, and other infections. If a serious or opportunistic infection develops, alert prescriber, and expect abrocitinib to be discontinued. Be aware that patients who have tested negative for latent TB may still develop TB during drug therapy.

! **WARNING** Monitor patient, especially current or past smokers, for signs and symptoms of a malignancy because malignancies have been reported in patients treated with abrocitinib. Perform a skin assessment regularly because skin malignancies, including nonmelanoma skin cancer, also have occurred.

- Assess patient regularly for viral reactivation, including herpes simplex or herpes zoster. If herpes zoster occurs, notify prescriber as drug therapy may need to be halted until infection has resolved.

PATIENT TEACHING

- Instruct patients how to take tablets.
- Stress importance of complying with ordered blood tests before abrocitinib therapy begins and periodically throughout drug therapy.

! **WARNING** Tell patient about the increased risk of major adverse cardiovascular events and that the risk is increased in patients who are or who have smoked or have other cardiovascular risk factors. Review the signs and symptoms of major cardiovascular events and stress importance of seeking immediate emergency care, if suspected.

! **WARNING** Alert patient that drug may increase risk of developing certain cancers, including skin cancer. Advise patient to limit sunlight and UV light exposure, use broad-spectrum sunscreen, and wear protective clothing when outdoors. Also, tell patient to report any persistent, severe, or unusual signs and symptoms to prescriber.

! **WARNING** Review signs and symptoms of a deep vein thrombosis and pulmonary embolism with patient and urge patient to seek immediate emergency care, if suspected.

! **WARNING** Advise patient to seek immediate medical attention if patient notices any change in vision while taking abrocitinib therapy.

- Review signs and symptoms of infection with the patient stressing importance of notifying prescriber, if an infection occurs. Inform patient that there is a greater risk of developing herpes zoster that could become serious while taking abrocitinib.
- Tell patient to inform all prescribers of abrocitinib therapy prior to receiving any vaccination because live vaccines should not be given immediately before, during, or after abrocitinib therapy.
- Inform females of childbearing age that drug may affect fertility.
- Tell mothers not to breastfeed while taking drug and for one day after drug is discontinued.

acamprosate calcium

Class and Category

Pharmacologic class: Amino acid neurotransmitter analogue
Therapeutic class: Alcohol deterrent

Indications and Dosages

* *To maintain abstinence from alcohol for alcohol-dependent patients who are abstinent at the start of treatment*

D.R. TABLETS

Adults. 666 mg 3 times daily. Alternatively, 3 daily doses divided as 666 mg in morning, 333 mg in afternoon, and 333 mg in evening.

± **DOSAGE ADJUSTMENT** For patients with moderate renal impairment (creatinine clearance of 30 to 50 ml/min), initial dosage reduced to 333 mg 3 times daily.

Drug Administration

P.O.

- Have patient swallow tablets whole and do not break, crush, or split the tablets.

Route	Onset	Peak	Duration
P.O.	Unknown	3–8 hr	Unknown

Half-life: 20–33 hr

Contraindications

Hypersensitivity to acamprosate or its components, severe renal impairment (creatinine clearance 30 ml/min or less)

Interactions

DRUGS

None reported by manufacturer.

Adverse Reactions

CNS: Abnormal thinking, amnesia, anxiety, asthenia, chills, depression, dizziness, headache, insomnia, paresthesia, somnolence, **suicidal ideation**, syncope, tremor
CV: Chest pain, hypertension, palpitations, peripheral edema, vasodilation
EENT: Abnormal vision, dry mouth, pharyngitis, rhinitis, taste perversion
GI: Abdominal pain, anorexia, constipation, diarrhea, flatulence, increased appetite, indigestion, nausea, vomiting
GU: **Acute renal failure**, decreased libido, impotence
HEME: **Leukopenia**, lymphocytosis, **thrombocytopenia**
MS: Arthralgia, back pain, myalgia
RESP: Bronchitis, cough, dyspnea
SKIN: Diaphoresis, pruritus, rash
Other: Flu-like symptoms, infection, weight gain

Childbearing Considerations

PREGNANCY

- It is not known if drug causes fetal harm but animal studies suggest it may.

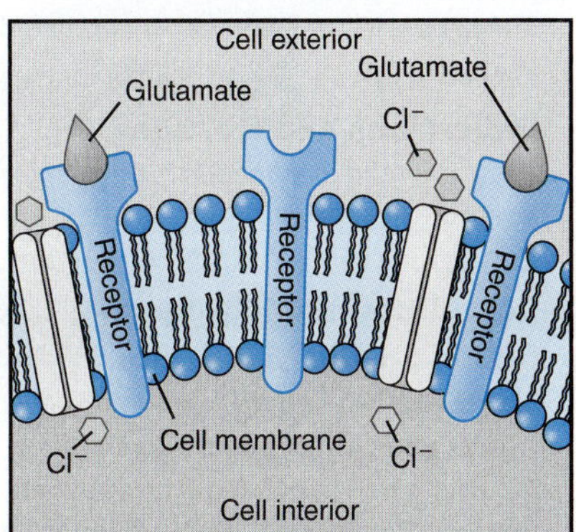

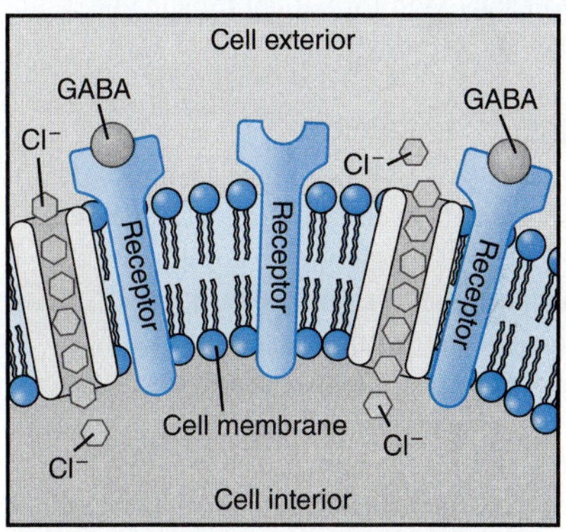

Mechanism of Action

May restore the altered balance between excitation and inhibition in neurons in the brain that may occur because of chronic alcoholism.

Binding of the neurotransmitter gamma-aminobutyric acid (GABA) to its receptors in the CNS opens the chloride ion channel and releases chloride (Cl^-) into the cell (below left), thereby reducing neuronal excitability by inhibiting depolarization.

By interacting with GABA receptor sites, acamprosate prevents GABA from binding (below right).

Binding of glutamate to its receptors closes the chloride ion channel, increasing neuronal excitability by promoting depolarization (below left). This imbalance fosters a craving for alcohol. By interacting with glutamate receptor sites, acamprosate prevents glutamate from binding (below right).

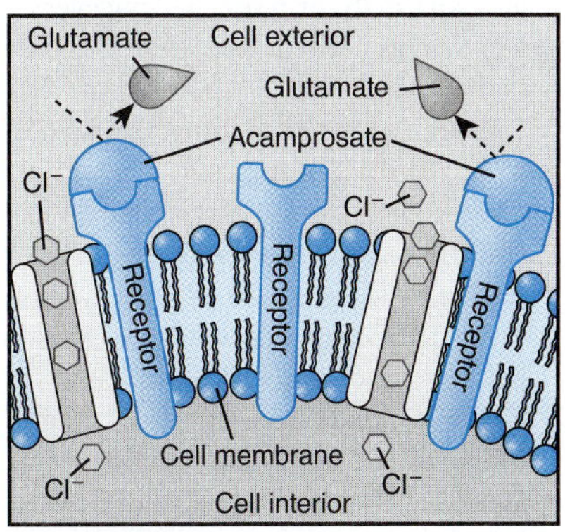

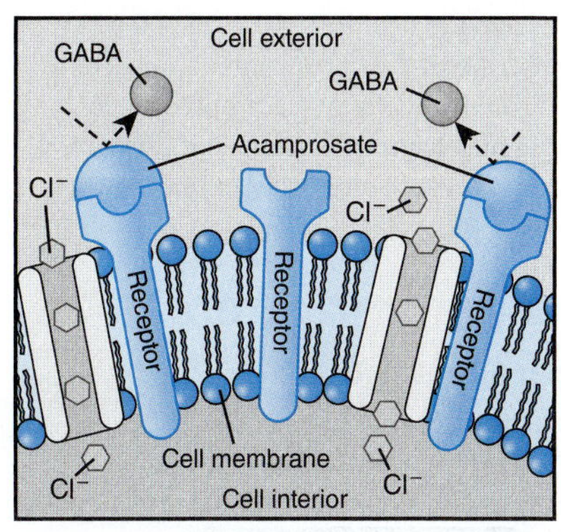

- Use with caution only if benefit to mother outweighs potential risk to fetus.

LACTATION

- It is not known if drug is present in breast milk.
- Mothers should check with prescriber before breastfeeding.

Nursing Considerations

- Know that acamprosate should start as soon as possible after patient has undergone alcohol withdrawal and achieved abstinence.
- Continue to give acamprosate even during periods of alcohol relapse, as ordered.

! **WARNING** Monitor patient for suicidal behavior or thoughts.

PATIENT TEACHING

- Inform patient how to take acamprosate. Advise patient to take drug with meals if patient is struggling with compliance and regularly eats 3 meals a day; otherwise drug can be taken without regards to eating.
- Instruct patient to take acamprosate exactly as prescribed, even if a relapse occurs, and to seek help for a relapse.
- Warn patient that acamprosate won't reduce symptoms of alcohol withdrawal if relapse occurs followed by cessation.

! **WARNING** Urge family or caregiver to monitor patient for evidence of depression (difficulty concentrating, excessive sleeping, fatigue, lack of appetite or interest in life), or suicidal tendencies because a small number of patients taking acamprosate have attempted suicide.

- Advise patient to use caution when performing hazardous activities until adverse CNS effects of drug are known.
- Tell females of childbearing age to notify prescriber if they are or intend to become pregnant while taking acamprosate; the drug may have to be stopped if pregnancy occurs because fetal risks are unknown.

acetaminophen (paracetamol)

Oral or rectal: Abenol (CAN), Acephen, Actamin Maximum Strength, Actimol Children's (CAN), Actimol infant (CAN), Altenol, Aminofen, Apra, Atasol (CAN), Cetafen, Children's Mapap, Children's Nortemp, Children's Tylenol Meltaways, Dolono, Febrol, Feverall, Genapap, Genebs, Junior Tylenol Meltaways, Mapap, Pediaphen (CAN), Pyrecot, Pyrigesic, Redutemp, Silapap, Tylenol, Tylenol 8-hr Arthritis Pain Caplets, Tylenol Extra Strength Caplets; ***Parenteral:*** Acetaminophen

Class and Category

Pharmacologic class: Nonsalicylate, para-aminophenol derivative
Therapeutic class: Antipyretic, nonopioid analgesic

Indications and Dosages

* *To relieve mild to moderate pain; to relieve fever*

REGULAR STRENGTH (325 MG): CAPLETS, CAPSULES, CHEWABLE TABLETS, ELIXIR, GELCAPS, LIQUID SOLUTION, SPRINKLES, SUSPENSION, TABLETS

Adults and children ages 12 and older. 325 mg to 640 or 650 mg every 4 to 6 hr, as needed. *Maximum:* 3,250 mg (5 doses) in 24 hr.

EXTRA STRENGTH (500 MG) CAPLETS OR TABLETS

Adults. 1,000 mg every 6 hr, as needed. *Maximum:* 3,000 mg in 24 hr.

8-HR (650 MG) CAPLETS

Adults. 1,300 mg every 8 hr, as needed. *Maximum:* 3,900 mg in 24 hr.

CHEWABLE TABLETS, DISINTEGRATING TABLETS, ORAL SUSPENSION, SYRUP

Children ages 12 and older weighing 43.5 kg (96 lb) or more. 640 mg every 4 to 6 hr, as needed. *Maximum:* 3,200 mg (5 doses) in 24 hr.
Children ages 11 weighing 32.6 kg (72 lb) to 43 kg (95 lb). 480 mg every 4 hr, as needed. *Maximum:* 2,400 mg (5 doses) in 24 hr.
Children ages 9 to 10 weighing 27 kg (60 lb) to 32 kg (71 lb). 400 mg every 4 hr, as needed. *Maximum:* 2,000 mg (5 doses) in 24 hr.
Children ages 6 to 8 weighing 21.5 kg (48 lb) to 26.5 kg (59 lb). 320 mg every 4 hr, as needed. *Maximum:* 1,600 mg (5 doses) in 24 hr.

Children ages 4 to 5 weighing 16.4 kg (36 lb) to 21 kg (47 lb). 240 mg every 4 hr, as needed. *Maximum:* 1,200 mg (5 doses) in 24 hr.
Children ages 2 to 3 weighing 10.9 kg (24 lb) to 16 kg (35 lb). 160 mg every 4 hr, as needed. *Maximum:* 800 mg (5 doses) in 24 hr.

ORAL SUSPENSION, SYRUP

Children ages 12 to 23 mo weighing 8 to 10.9 kg (17.6 to 24 lb). 120 mg every 4 hr, as needed.
Infants ages 4 to 11 mo weighing 5 to 8 kg (11 to 17.6 lb). 80 mg every 4 hr, as needed.
Infants ages 3 mo or less weighing 2.7 to 5 kg (6 to 11 lb). 40 mg every 4 hr, as needed.

SUPPOSITORIES

Adults and adolescents. 325 mg to 650 mg every 4 to 6 hr, as needed. *Maximum:* 3,900 mg in 24 hr.
Children ages 6 to 12. 325 mg every 4 to 6 hr, as needed. *Maximum:* 1,625 mg in 24 hr.
Children ages 3 to 6. 120 mg every 4 to 6 hr, as needed. *Maximum:* 600 mg in 24 hr.
Children ages 1 to 3. 80 mg every 4 to 6 hr, as needed. *Maximum:* 400 mg in 24 hr.
Children ages 6 to 11 mo. 80 mg every 6 hr, as needed. *Maximum:* 320 mg in 24 hr.

* *To relieve mild to moderate pain; to manage moderate to severe pain with adjunctive opioid analgesics*

I.V. INFUSION

Adults and adolescents ages 13 and older weighing 50 kg (110 lb) or more. 650 mg every 4 hr, as needed, or 1,000 mg every 6 hr, as needed. *Maximum:* 1,000 mg as a single dose, a minimum dosing interval of 4 hr, and a maximum dosage of 4,000 mg in 24 hr.
Adults and children ages 2 and older weighing less than 50 kg (110 lb). 12.5 mg/kg every 4 hr, as needed, or 15 mg/kg every 6 hr, as needed. *Maximum:* 15 mg/kg (up to 750 mg) in a single dose, a minimum dosing interval of 4 hr, and a maximum dose of 75 mg/kg (up to 3,750 mg) in 24 hr.

* *To reduce fever*

I.V. INFUSION

Adults and adolescents ages 13 and older weighing 50 kg (110 lb) or more. 650 mg every 4 hr, as needed, or 1,000 mg every 6 hr, as needed. *Maximum:* 1,000 mg as a single dose, a minimum dosing interval of 4 hr, and a maximum dosage of 4,000 mg in 24 hr.
Adults and children ages 2 and older weighing less than 50 kg (110 lb). 12.5 mg/kg every 4 hr, as needed, or 15 mg/kg every 6 hr, as needed. *Maximum:* 15 mg/kg (up to 750 mg) in a single dose, a minimum dosing interval of 4 hr, and a maximum dose of 75 mg/kg (up to 3,750 mg) in 24 hr.
Infants 29 days to 2 yr. 15 mg/kg every 6 hr, as needed. *Maximum:* 60 mg/kg/day with minimum dosing interval of 6 hr.
Premature neonates at least 32 wk gestational age and up to chronological age of 28 days. 12.5 mg/kg every 6 hr, as needed. *Maximum:* 50 mg/kg/day with minimum dosing interval of 6 hr.

± **DOSAGE ADJUSTMENT** For patients with severe renal impairment (creatinine clearance 30 ml/min or less), dosing interval increased, and total daily dosage reduced. For patients with mild to moderate hepatic impairment, total daily dosage reduced.

Drug Administration

P.O.

- Extended-release forms should be swallowed whole. Do not crush or split extended-release forms and make sure patient does not chew these forms.
- Shake liquid forms well before measuring dose. Use liquid form for children and adults who have difficulty swallowing. Use a calibrated device to measure dosage.
- Place disintegrating tablets on patient's tongue and allow to dissolve in mouth or tablets can be chewed before swallowing. Tablets may be given with or without water after swallowing.

I.V.

- Do not confuse a dose in milligrams with a dose in milliliters when preparing and administering I.V. acetaminophen. Also, make sure the dose is based on the patient's weight and infusion pumps are properly programmed.
- Solution should be clear and container and seals intact before using. Do not use plastic container in series connection.
- Be aware that patients weighing 50 kg (110 lb) or more and requiring 1,000-mg doses of parenteral acetaminophen can have the dose administered by inserting a vented intravenous set through the septum of the 100-ml vial. Further dilution is not required.

- For doses less than 1,000 mg, the dose must be withdrawn from the vial and placed into a separate container prior to administration to prevent inadvertent overdose.
- Administer over 15 min.
- Place small-volume pediatric doses up to 60 ml in a syringe and administer over 15 min using a syringe pump.
- Use parenteral drug within 6 hr once vacuum seal of glass vial has been penetrated or contents transferred to another container.
- *Incompatibilities:* Other drugs, including chlorpromazine and diazepam

P.R.

- If suppository is too soft to administer, either run it under cold water while still in wrapper or refrigerate it for at least 15 min.
- Do not take wrapper off until ready to administer.
- Store suppositories under 26.6°C (80°F).

Route	Onset	Peak	Duration
P.O.	30–45 min	30–60 min	4–6 hr
I.V.	15–30 min	15–20 min	4–6 hr
P.R.	1 hr	1.5–3 hr	6+ hr

Half-life: 2–5 hr (neonates: 4–10 hr)

Mechanism of Action

Inhibits the enzyme cyclooxygenase, blocking prostaglandin production and interfering with pain impulse generation in the peripheral nervous system. Acetaminophen also acts directly on temperature-regulating center in the hypothalamus by inhibiting synthesis of prostaglandin E_2.

Contraindications

Hypersensitivity to acetaminophen or its components, severe active liver disease or impairment

Interactions

DRUGS

anticholinergics: Decreased onset of acetaminophen action
barbiturates, carbamazepine, hydantoins, isoniazid, rifampin, sulfinpyrazone: Decreased therapeutic effects and increased hepatotoxic effects of acetaminophen
dasatinib, imatinib: Possibly increased risk of hepatotoxicity
lamotrigine: Possibly decreased therapeutic effects of these drugs
oral contraceptives: Decreased effectiveness of acetaminophen
probenecid: Possibly increased therapeutic effects of acetaminophen
propranolol: Possibly increased action of acetaminophen
warfarin: Possibly increased international normalized ratio
zidovudine: Possibly decreased zidovudine effects

ACTIVITIES

alcohol use: Increased risk of hepatotoxicity

Adverse Reactions

CNS: Agitation, anxiety, fatigue, fever, headache, insomnia
CV: **Hypotension**, hypertension, peripheral edema
EENT: **Stridor (parenteral form)**
ENDO: **Hypoglycemic coma**
GI: Abdominal pain, constipation, diarrhea, **hepatotoxicity**, jaundice, nausea, vomiting
GU: Oliguria (parenteral form)
HEME: **Hemolytic anemia (with long-term use)**, **leukopenia**, **neutropenia**, **pancytopenia**, **thrombocytopenia**
MS: Muscle spasm (parenteral form)
RESP: Parenteral form: **atelectasis**, dyspnea, plural effusion, **pulmonary edema**, wheezing
SKIN: **Acute generalized exanthematous pustulosis**, blisters, pruritus, rash, reddening, **Stevens-Johnson syndrome**, **toxic epidermal necrolysis**, urticaria
Other: **Anaphylaxis**, **angioedema**, hypersensitivity reactions; for parenteral form: hypoalbuminemia, **hypokalemia**, **hypomagnesemia**, **hypophosphatemia**, injection-site pain

Childbearing Considerations

PREGNANCY

- It is not known if drug can cause fetal harm.
- Use with caution only if benefit to mother outweighs potential risk to fetus.

LACTATION

- Drug may be present in breast milk.
- Mothers should check with prescriber before breastfeeding.

REPRODUCTION
- Drug may reduce fertility in females and males.

Nursing Considerations
- Use acetaminophen cautiously in patients with active hepatic disease or hepatic impairment, alcoholism, chronic malnutrition, severe hypovolemia, or severe renal impairment.
- Know that before and during long-term therapy, including parenteral therapy, liver function test results such as ALT, AST, and bilirubin levels, as ordered, must be monitored because acetaminophen may cause hepatotoxicity.
- Monitor the end of a parenteral infusion to prevent possibility of air embolism.
- Calculate total daily intake of acetaminophen, including other products that may contain acetaminophen so maximum daily dosage is not exceeded.

! **WARNING** Monitor patient for hypersensitivity reactions that may become life-threatening such as anaphylaxis or angioedema. If present, notify prescriber immediately, withhold drug as ordered, and provide supportive care, as needed and ordered.

- Monitor renal function in patient on long-term therapy. Keep in mind that albumin or blood in urine may indicate nephritis; dark brown urine may indicate presence of the metabolite phenacetin; and decreased urine output may indicate renal failure.

PATIENT TEACHING
- Teach patient and family or caregiver how to administer oral form of acetaminophen prescribed.
- Instruct patient and family or caregiver to read manufacturer's label and follow dosage guidelines precisely. Explain that infants' and children's acetaminophen liquid aren't equal in drug concentration and aren't interchangeable. Tell them to use only the measuring device that comes with the bottle to help ensure accurate dosage.
- Caution patient and family or caregiver not to exceed recommended dosage or take other drugs containing acetaminophen at the same time because of risk of liver damage. Teach them signs and symptoms of liver damage, such as bleeding, easy bruising, and malaise, which commonly occurs with chronic overdose. Stress importance of reporting to prescriber if signs and symptoms appear.

! **WARNING** Alert patient and family or caregiver that an allergic reaction may occur with drug use. Stress importance of notifying prescriber if an allergic reaction occurs and to seek immediate medical care, if severe.

! **WARNING** Caution patient that serious skin reactions, although rare, may occur even with first-time use and any time acetaminophen is used, even if no skin reactions occurred with a previous use of drug. Tell patient that if blisters, redness, or a skin rash occur, they should stop using drug and seek emergency treatment immediately.

acetylcysteine

Acetadote, Acetylcysteine 10% or 20%

Class and Category
Pharmacologic class: L-cysteine derivative
Therapeutic class: Antidote (for acetaminophen overdose), mucolytic

Indications and Dosages
* *To liquefy abnormal, thickened, or viscid mucus secretions in chronic pulmonary disorders (including bronchiectasis, bronchitis, cystic fibrosis, and emphysema) and in pneumonia, pulmonary complications of cardiovascular or thoracic surgery, and tracheostomy care*

SOLUTION BY DIRECT INSTILLATION INTO TRACHEOSTOMY (ACETYLCYSTEINE)

Adults and children. 1 to 2 ml of 10% or 20% solution instilled every 1 to 4 hr, as needed.

SOLUTION BY INHALATION (ACETYLCYSTEINE)

Adults and children. 1 to 10 ml of 20% solution or 2 to 20 ml of 10% solution nebulized through face mask, mouthpiece, or tracheostomy every 2 to 6 hr. *Usual:* 3 to 5 ml of 20% solution or 6 to 10 ml of 10% solution 3 or 4 times daily.

* *To treat acetaminophen overdose*

DILUTED INHALATION SOLUTION GIVEN ORALLY (ACETYLCYSTEINE)

Adults and children. *Loading dose:* 140 mg/kg. *Maintenance:* 70 mg/kg 4 hr after loading dose and then every 4 hr for a total of 17 doses.

I.V. INFUSION (ACETADOTE)

Adults weighing 100 kg (220 lb) or more. 15,000 mg in 200 ml diluent infused over 1 hr followed by 5,000 mg in 500 ml of diluent infused over 4 hr, followed by 10,000 mg in 1,000 ml of diluent infused over 16 hr. Alternatively, 20,000 mg in 1,000 ml diluent infused over 4 hr followed by 10,000 mg in 500 ml of diluent infused over 16 hr.
Adults and children weighing 41 kg (90.2 lb) to 100 kg (220 lb). 150 mg/kg in 200 ml of diluent infused over 60 min, followed by 50 mg/kg in 500 ml of diluent infused over 4 hr, followed by 100 mg/kg in 1,000 ml of diluent infused over 16 hr. Alternatively, 200 mg/kg in 1,000 ml diluent infused over 4 hr followed by 100 mg/kg in 500 ml diluent infused over 16 hr.
Adults and children weighing 21 kg (46.2 lb) to 41 kg (90.2 lb). 150 mg/kg in 100 ml of diluent infused over 60 min, followed by 50 mg/kg in 250 ml of diluent infused over 4 hr, followed by 100 mg/kg in 500 ml of diluent infused over 16 hr.
Children weighing 5 kg (11 lb) to 20 kg (44 lb). 150 mg/kg in 3 ml/kg of diluent infused over 60 min, followed by 50 mg/kg in 7 ml/kg of diluent infused over 4 hr, followed by 100 mg/kg in 14 ml/kg of diluent infused over 16 hr.

Drug Administration

P.O. (INHALATION SOLUTION)

- Dilute 20% solution to 5% solution with soda such as diet coke or water by adding 3 ml of soda or water for every 1 ml of drug.
- Be aware that drug smells strongly of sulfur.
- Repeat dose, as prescribed, if patient vomits loading dose or any maintenance dose within 1 hour of administration.
- Solution (drug mixed with water) may be administered by nasogastric tube or Miller-Abbott tube, as needed.

I.V.

- Dilute parenteral solution (Acetadote) with 0.45% Sodium Chloride Injection, 5% Dextrose in Water, or Sterile Water for Injection following manufacturer's guidelines because dilution is based on dosage. Acetadote may turn from colorless to slight pink or purple once the stopper is punctured, but color change has no effect on product quality.
- Treating acetaminophen overdose with intravenous therapy may require adjusting total administered volume, as ordered, for patients weighing less than 40 kg (88 lb) and for those who need fluid restriction, to avoid fluid overload and possibly fatal hyponatremia or seizures.
- Infuse drug according to weight following manufacturer's guidelines.
- Diluted solution can be stored for 24 hr at room temperature.
- Discard unused drug.
- *Incompatibilities:* None reported by manufacturer

INHALATION

- It may be necessary to dilute 20% inhalation or instillation solution with normal saline solution or Sterile Water when acetylcysteine is used to liquefy secretions. The 10% solution may be used undiluted.
- Use nebulizers made of aluminum, glass, plastic, or stainless steel. Don't give acetylcysteine with nebulization equipment if drug could come into contact with copper, iron, or rubber.
- Be aware hand bulbs are not recommended to administer drug because output is too small and, in some cases, the particle size is too large.
- Have patient wash his face and rinse his mouth at the end of each nebulization treatment because nebulization causes sticky residue on face and in mouth.
- *Incompatibilities for direct instillation or nebulization:* All antibiotics, chymotrypsin, hydrogen peroxide, iodized oil, trypsin

Route	Onset	Peak	Duration
P.O.	Unknown	1–3.5 hr	Unknown
I.V.	Unknown	30–60 min	Unknown
Inhalation	5–10 min	1–2 hr	Unknown

Half-life: 5.6 hr

Mechanism of Action

Decreases viscosity of pulmonary secretions by breaking disulfide links that bind glycoproteins in mucus. Reduces liver damage from acetaminophen overdose. Usually, acetaminophen's toxic metabolites bind with glutathione in the liver, which detoxifies them. When acetaminophen overdose depletes glutathione stores, toxic metabolites bind with protein in liver cells, killing them. Acetylcysteine maintains or restores levels of glutathione or acts as its substitute, which reduces liver damage from acetaminophen overdose.

Contraindications

Hypersensitivity to acetylcysteine or its components (no contraindications when used as an antidote)

Interactions

DRUGS

activated charcoal: Possibly adsorption and decreased effectiveness of oral acetylcysteine
nitroglycerin: Increased effects of nitroglycerin and possibly significant headache and hypotension

Adverse Reactions

CNS: Chills, dizziness, drowsiness, fever, headache
CV: Edema, hypertension, **hypotension**, tachycardia
EENT: Rhinorrhea, stomatitis, **stridor**, tooth damage
GI: Anorexia, constipation, **hepatotoxicity**, nausea, vomiting
RESP: **Bronchospasm**, chest tightness, cough, **hemoptysis**, **respiratory distress**, shortness of breath, wheezing
SKIN: Clammy skin, erythema, facial flushing, pruritus, rash, urticaria
Other: **Anaphylaxis**, **angioedema**

Childbearing Considerations

PREGNANCY

- It is not known if drug can cause fetal harm.
- Use with caution only if benefit to mother outweighs potential risk to fetus.

LACTATION

- It is not known if drug is present in breast milk.
- Mothers should check with prescriber before breastfeeding. Breastfeeding mothers may consider pumping and discarding their milk for 30 hr after drug administration.

Nursing Considerations

- Know that acetylcysteine should be used cautiously in patients with asthma or a history of bronchospasm because drug may adversely affect respiratory function.
- Keep in mind that acetylcysteine is most effective if given within 24 hours of acetaminophen ingestion. For specific instructions, contact a regional poison center at 1-800-222-1222 or a special health professional assistance hotline at 1-800-525-6115.
- Know that alternative dosing using only 2 doses instead of 3 for patients with higher weights are used to prevent or lessen potential liver damage from acetamininphen overdose.
- Be aware that suicidal patient may not provide reliable information about vomiting. Watch such a patient to ensure that he ingests all prescribed dosage.

! WARNING Know that when drug is given intravenously, acute flushing and erythema of the skin may occur within 30 to 60 minutes of administration and often resolves spontaneously even with continued infusion of drug. However, monitor patient closely for acute hypersensitivity reactions regardless of form of drug administered, such as hypotension, rash, shortness of breath, and wheezing. If present, immediately stop administration of drug, notify prescriber, and provide supportive care, as needed and ordered. Be aware that for less severe hypersensitivity reactions when drug is administered intravenously, a temporary interruption of the infusion and/or administration of an antihistamine with resolution of symptoms may allow the infusion to be carefully restarted. However if symptoms return or increase in severity, drug should be discontinued and an alternative treatment given.

- Watch for signs of hepatotoxicity (altered coagulation, easy bruising, and prolonged bleeding time) during treatment for acetaminophen overdose.
- Be aware that acetylcysteine may have a disagreeable odor, which disappears as treatment progresses.
- Assess characteristics, frequency, and type of patient's cough when drug is used to liquefy secretions. Particularly note sputum. If cough does not clear secretions, prepare to perform mechanical suctioning.

- Monitor patient for adverse drug reactions, especially a significant change in blood pressure or appearance of tachycardia.

PATIENT TEACHING

! **WARNING** Alert patient and family or caregiver that drug may cause an allergic reaction that could be quite serious. If an allergic reaction occurs, have patient notify prescriber, and if servere, to seek immediate medical attention.

- Tell patient receiving acetylcysteine intravenously that facial redness or flushing may occur but usually resolves on its own.
- Instruct patient to notify prescriber immediately about nausea, rash, or vomiting, as well as feeling dizzy or light-headed, shortness of breath, or wheezing.
- Warn patient about acetylcysteine's unpleasant smell; reassure him that it subsides as treatment progresses.
- Urge patient prescribed drug to loosen mucus, to consume 2 to 3 liters of fluid daily unless contraindicated by another condition, to decrease mucus viscosity.
- Instruct mothers who are breastfeeding to consider pumping and discarding their milk for 30 hours after acetylcysteine administration.

acyclovir

Sitavig

acyclovir sodium

Class and Category

Pharmacologic class: Nucleoside analogue
Therapeutic class: Antiretroviral

Indications and Dosages

* *To treat initial episodes of herpes genitalis*

CAPSULES, ORAL SUSPENSION, TABLETS

Adults. 200 mg every 4 hr, 5 times daily for 10 days.

OINTMENT 5%

Adults. Applied to completely cover all lesions every 3 hr, 6 times daily for 7 days.

* *To treat severe initial episodes of herpes genitalis*

I.V. INFUSION

Adults and adolescents. 5 mg/kg every 8 hr for 5 days.

* *To suppress unusually frequent recurrent episodes of herpes genitalis (6 or more episodes per year)*

CAPSULES, ORAL SUSPENSION, TABLETS

Adults. 200 mg 3 times daily, increased if breakthrough occurs up to 200 mg, 5 times daily for up to 12 mo. Alternatively, 400 mg twice daily for up to 12 mo.

* *To treat recurrent episodes of herpes genitalis intermittently*

CAPSULES, ORAL SUSPENSION, TABLETS

Adults. 200 mg every 4 hr, 5 times daily for 5 days.

* *To treat recurrent herpes labialis in immunocompetent patients*

BUCCAL TABLETS (SITAVIG)

Adults. 50 mg as a single dose.

CREAM 5%

Adults and adolescents. Applied 5 times daily for 4 days and initiated as soon as possible following onset of signs and symptoms.

* *To treat non-life-threatening mucocutaneous herpes simplex virus infections in immunocompromised patients*

OINTMENT 5%

Adults. Applied to completely cover all lesions every 3 hr, 6 times daily for 7 days.

* *To treat cutaneous and mucosal herpes simplex (HSV-1 and HSV-2) infections in immunocompromised patients*

I.V. INFUSION

Adults and adolescents. 5 mg/kg every 8 hr for 7 days.
Infants and children ages 3 mo to 12 yr. 10 mg/kg every 8 hr for 7 days.

* *To treat herpes simplex encephalitis*

I.V. INFUSION

Adults and adolescents. 10 mg/kg every 8 hr for 10 days.
Infants and children ages 3 mo to 12 yr. 20 mg/kg every 8 hr for 10 days.

* *To treat neonatal herpes simplex virus infections*

I.V. INFUSION

Neonates postmenstrual age of at least 34 weeks. 20 mg/kg every 8 hr for 21 days.
Neonates postmenstrual age of less than 34 weeks. 20 mg/kg every 12 hr for 21 days.

∗ *To treat herpes zoster in immunocompetent patients*

CAPSULES, ORAL SUSPENSION, TABLETS

Adults. 800 mg every 4 hr, 5 times daily for 7 to 10 days with treatment initiated within 72 hr of onset of lesions.

∗ *To treat varicella-zoster infection in immunocompetent patients*

CAPSULES, ORAL SUSPENSION, TABLETS

Adults and children weighing over 40 kg (88 lb). 800 mg 4 times daily for 5 days.
Children ages 2 and older weighing less than 40 kg (88 kg). 20 mg/kg 4 times daily for 5 days.

∗ *To treat varicella-zoster infection in immunocompromised patients*

I.V. INFUSION

Adults and adolescents. 10 mg/kg every 8 hr for 7 days.
Obese adults. Ideal body weight used to calculate dose. *Maximum:* 20 mg/kg every 8 hr.
Children. 20 mg/kg every 8 hr for 7 days.

±**DOSAGE ADJUSTMENT** For patients with renal impairment who have genital herpes or herpes-zoster infection, oral dosage reduced, or dosage interval increased as follows: If dosage is normally 200 mg every 4 hours 5 times daily and creatinine clearance is less than 10 ml/min, dosage interval increased to every 12 hours; if dosage is normally 400 mg every 12 hours and creatinine clearance is less than 10 ml/min, dosage reduced to 200 mg every 12 hours; if dosage is normally 800 mg every 4 hours and creatinine clearance is 10 to 25 ml/min, dosage interval increased to every 8 hours, and if creatinine clearance is less than 10 ml/min, dosage interval increased to every 12 hours. For patients receiving intravenous dosing, dosage reduced, or dosage interval increased as follows: if creatinine clearance is 25 to 50 ml/min, dosage interval increased to every 12 hours; if creatinine clearance is 10 to 25 ml/min, dosage interval increased to every 24 hours; if creatinine clearance is 0 to 10 ml/min, dosage is reduced by 50% and dosage interval increased to every 24 hours. For patients receiving hemodialysis, an additional dose given after each dialysis.

Drug Administration

P.O.

- Drug can be given with food if GI upset occurs.
- Shake oral suspension well before using. Use a calibrated measuring device when measuring dose of oral suspension. Store at room temperature and protect from light.

Buccal

- Apply within 1 hr after onset of symptoms and before the appearance of herpes labialis.
- Apply tablet, on same side as the herpes labialis symptoms, to upper gum region just above the incisor tooth using a dry finger covered in a finger cot immediately after taking tablet out of the blister.
- Hold in place with slight pressure over the upper lip for 30 sec to ensure adhesion of tablet so tablet will remain in position as it gradually dissolves during the day.
- While either side of the tablet can be applied, the rounded side may be more comfortable for the patient.
- Tablet should not be chewed, crushed, sucked on, or swallowed. Food and drink can be taken normally, but brushing teeth, chewing gum, pressing or touching the tablet after placement, and wearing upper dentures should be avoided.
- Replace tablet if it does not adhere or falls off within the first 6 hr.
- If tablet is swallowed within first 6 hr, have patient drink a glass of water and apply a new tablet.
- Know that if tablet falls out or is swallowed after the first 6 hr, it does not need to be reapplied.

I.V.

- Prepare intravenous infusion if product being used comes in powder form by first dissolving the contents of a 10-ml vial containing 500 mg of acyclovir in 10 ml of Sterile Water for Injection or a 20-ml vial containing 1,000 mg of acyclovir in 20 ml of Sterile Water for Injection (do not use Bacteriostatic Water for Injection containing benzyl alcohol or parabens). The result is a concentration of 50 mg acyclovir per ml. Shake vial well to ensure that drug has been dissolved.
- Use reconstituted solution within 12 hr. Know that if refrigerated, a precipitate may form but will redissolve at room temperature.
- Remove reconstituted solution from vial and add to any appropriate intravenous solution to deliver concentration needed. Use diluted solution within 24 hr.

- If drug vial comes as a sterile aqueous solution, it does not need to be reconstituted as the vial is ready for further dilution prior to infusion. Add vial contents for dose required to any appropriate intravenous solution to deliver concentration needed. Use diluted solution within 24 hrs.
- Infuse over 1 hr at a constant rate to reduce risk of renal tubular damage.
- Never administer drug intramuscularly, subcutaneously, as an I.V. bolus or rapid injection.
- Know that infusion concentrations of about 7 mg/ml or lower are recommended, as higher concentrations may cause inflammation or phlebitis at the injection site if inadvertent extravasation occurs.
- *Incompatibilities*: None listed by manufacturer

TOPICAL

- Apply with a rubber glove or finger cot, covering all lesions thoroughly.
- Apply about 0.5-inch ribbon of ointment per 4 square inches of surface area.
- Keep topical product away from eyes.

Route	Onset	Peak	Duration
P.O.	Unknown	1.5–2 hr	Unknown
P.O. (buccal)	Unknown	7 hr	Unknown
I.V.	Immediate	1 hr	Unknown
Topical	Unknown	Unknown	Unknown

Half-life: 2–3 hr

Mechanism of Action

Inhibits herpes virus replication through several combined actions (inhibition of DNA polymerase, premature termination of DNA synthesis, and thymidine kinase specificity).

Contraindications

Hypersensitivity to acyclovir or valacyclovir or any of their components

Interactions

DRUGS

cimetidine, probenecid: Possibly increased acyclovir plasma concentrations
mycophenolate mofetil: Increased plasma concentration of both drugs

Adverse Reactions

CNS: Agitation, asthenia, ataxia, **coma**, confusion, dizziness, **encephalopathy**, fever, hallucinations, headache, malaise, paresthesia, psychotic symptoms, **seizures**, somnolence, tremor
CV: Peripheral edema
EENT: Visual abnormalities
GI: Diarrhea, elevated liver enzymes, gastrointestinal distress, **hepatitis**, hyperbilirubinemia, jaundice, nausea, vomiting
GU: **Acute renal failure**, elevated blood creatinine and blood urea nitrogen, hematuria, **hemolytic uremic syndrome**, renal pain
HEME: Anemia, leukocytosis, **leukopenia**, lymphadenopathy, **neutropenia**, **thrombocytopenia**, **thrombotic thrombocytopenic purpura**
MS: Myalgia
RESP: Dyspnea
SKIN: Alopecia, contact dermatitis (topical), eczema (topical), **erythema multiforme**, photosensitivity, pruritus, rash, **Stevens-Johnson syndrome**, **toxic epidermal necrolysis**, urticaria
Other: **Anaphylaxis**, **angioedema**, generalized pain, injection-site reactions (inflammation, phlebitis)

Childbearing Considerations

PREGNANCY

- It is not known if drug can cause fetal harm.
- Use with caution only if benefit to mother outweighs potential risk to fetus.

LACTATION

- Drug is present in breast milk (not known for buccal form).
- Mothers should check with prescriber before breastfeeding.

Nursing Considerations

- Know that acyclovir therapy should be initiated as soon as possible after signs and symptoms appear.
- Use caution when administering acyclovir to patients with dehydration or preexisting renal disease or who are receiving other nephrotoxic drugs because of increased risk of renal impairment. Also, use cautiously in patients with underlying neurologic disorders as well as electrolytc abnormalities, hepatic dysfunction, or significant hypoxia because, although uncommon, encephalopathic changes have occurred with acyclovir administration.
- Ensure that patient receiving acyclovir is adequately hydrated before drug is given, to decrease risk of renal impairment.

! **WARNING** Monitor patient closely for hypersensitivity reactions that can become life-threatening such as anaphylaxis and angioedema. Notify prescriber at first sign of hypersensitivity and provide supportive care, as needed and ordered.

! **WARNING** Know that hemolytic uremic syndrome and thrombotic thrombocytopenic purpura have occurred in immunocompromised patients receiving acyclovir therapy and have resulted in death. Report any hematologic or renal dysfunction signs and symptoms to prescriber immediately.

PATIENT TEACHING

- Inform patient that acyclovir does not cure herpes infections but helps to manage the signs and symptoms.
- Instruct patient on how to take prescribed form of drug.
- Advise patient who requires acyclovir therapy to manage recurrent genital herpes to initiate therapy at the first sign or symptom of an episode.
- Stress importance of maintaining adequate hydration throughout acyclovir therapy to reduce risk of kidney damage.

! **WARNING** Stress importance of stopping drug therapy and seeking immediate medical attention if any signs and symptoms of an allergic reaction occur.

- Instruct patient to seek medical attention if he experiences persistent, severe, or unusual adverse reactions.
- Tell females of childbearing age to notify prescriber if pregnancy occurs.
- Advise patient with genital herpes to avoid contact, including intercourse, when lesions and/or symptoms are present, to avoid infecting partner.

adalimumab
Humira

adalimumab-aacf
Idacio

adalimumab-aaty
Yflyma

adalimumab-adaz
Hyrimoz

adalimumab-adbm
Cyltezo

adalimumab-afzb
Abrilada

adalimumab-aqvh
Yusimry

adalimumab-atto
Amjevita

adalimumab-bwwd
Hadlima

adalimumab-fkjp
Hulio

adalimumab-ryvk
Simlandi

Class and Category

Pharmacologic class: Monoclonal antibody
Therapeutic class: Tumor necrosis factor (TNF) blocker

Indications and Dosages

✱ *To reduce signs and symptoms, induce major clinical response, inhibit progression of structural damage, and improve physical function in patients with moderate to severe active rheumatoid arthritis; to reduce signs and symptoms, inhibit progression of structural damage, and improve physical function in patients with psoriatic arthritis; to reduce signs and symptoms in patients with active ankylosing spondylitis*

SUBCUTANEOUS INJECTION (ABRILADA, AMJEVITA, CYLTEZO, HADLIMA, HULIO, HUMIRA, HYRIMOZ, IDACIO, SIMLANDI, YUFLYMA, YUSIMRY)

Adults. 40 mg every other wk.

±**DOSAGE ADJUSTMENT** For patients with rheumatoid arthritis not taking concomitantly methotrexate, dosage may be increased to 40 mg every week or 80 mg every other week, as needed.

* *To reduce signs and symptoms of moderately to severely active polyarticular juvenile idiopathic arthritis*

SUBCUTANEOUS INJECTION (ABRILADA, AMJEVITA, CYLTEZO, HADLIMA, HULIO, HUMIRA, HYRIMOZ, IDACIO, SIMLANDI, YUFLYMA, YUSIMRY)

Children ages 2 and older weighing 30 kg (66 lb) or more. 40 mg every other wk.

SUBCUTANEOUS INJECTION (ABRILADA, AMJEVITA, CYLTEZO, HADLIMA, HULIO, HUMIRA, SIMLANDI)

Children ages 2 and older weighing less than 30 kg (66 lb) but at least 15 kg (33 lb). 20 mg every other wk.

SUBCUTANEOUS INJECTION (ABRILADA, HADLIMA, HUMIRA, HYRIMOZ)

Children ages 2 and older weighing 10 kg (22 lb) to less than 15 kg (33 lb). 10 mg every other wk.

* *To treat adult patients with moderately to severely active Crohn's disease*

SUBCUTANEOUS INJECTION (ABRILADA, AMJEVITA, CYLTEZO, HADLIMA, HULIO, HUMIRA, HYRIMOZ, IDACIO, SIMLANDI, YUFLYMA, YUSIMRY)

Adults. *Initial:* 160 mg given as four 40-mg injections for 1 day or 80 mg given as two 40-mg injections for 2 consecutive days, followed by 80 mg given as two 40-mg injections on day 15. *Maintenance:* 40 mg every other wk starting on day 29.

* *To treat pediatric patients with moderately to severely active Crohn's disease*

SUBCUTANEOUS INJECTION (ABRILADA, AMJEVITA, CYLTEZO, HADIMA, HULIO, HUMIRA, HYRIMOZ, IDACIO, SIMLANDI, YUFLYMA, YUSIMRY)

Children ages 6 and older weighing 40 kg (88 lb) or more. *Initial*: 160 mg given as four 40-mg injections on day 1 or 80 mg given as two 40-mg injections for 2 consecutive days, followed by 80 mg given as two 40-mg injections on day 15. *Maintenance*: 40 mg every other wk starting on day 29.

SUBCUTANEOUS INJECTION (ABRILADA, AMJEVITA, CYLTEZO, HADIMA, HULIO, HUMIRA, SIMLANDI)

Children ages 6 and older weighing less than 40 kg (88 lb) but at least 17 kg (37 lb). *Initial*: 80 mg given as two 40-mg injections on day 1 followed by 40 mg on day 15. *Maintenance*: 20 mg every other wk starting on day 29.

* *To treat adult patients with moderately to severely active ulcerative colitis*

SUBCUTANEOUS INJECTION (ABRILADA, AMJEVITA, CYLTEZO, HADLIMA, HULIO, HUMIRA, HYRIMOZ, IDACIO, SIMLANDI, YUFLYMA, YUSIMRY)

Adults. *Initial:* 160 mg given as four 40-mg injections on day 1 or 80 mg given as two 40-mg injections on day 1 and repeated on day 2, followed by 80 mg given as two 40-mg injections on day 15. *Maintenance*: 40 mg every other wk starting on day 29.

±**DOSAGE ADJUSTMENT** For patients showing no evidence of clinical remission by 8 weeks, drug discontinued.

* *To treat pediatric patients with moderately to severely active ulcerative colitis*

SUBCUTANEOUS INJECTION (HUMIRA)

Children ages 5 and older weighing 40 kg (88 lb) or more. *Initial:* 160 mg given as four 40-mg injections on day 1 or given as two 40-mg injections on day 1 and repeated on day 2, followed by 80 mg given as two 40-mg injections on days 8 and 15. *Maintenance:* 40 mg every wk starting on day 22 or 80 mg every other wk starting on day 29.

Children ages 5 and older weighing less than 40 kg (88 lb) but at least 20 kg (44 lb). *Initial:* 80 mg given as two 40-mg injections on day 1 followed by 40 mg on days 8 and 15. *Maintenance*: 20 mg every wk starting on day 22 or 40 mg every other wk starting on day 29.

A

* *To treat moderate to severe chronic plaque psoriasis in patients who are candidates for phototherapy or systemic therapy, and when other systemic therapies are less appropriate*

SUBCUTANEOUS INJECTION (ABRILADA, AMJEVITA, CYLTEZO, HADLIMA, HULIO, HUMIRA, HYRIMOZ, IDACIO, SIMLANDI, YUFLYMA, YUSIMRY)

Adults. *Initial:* 80 mg given as two 40-mg injections on day 1. *Maintenance:* 40 mg every other wk starting on day 8.

* *To treat moderate to severe hidradenitis suppurativa*

SUBCUTANEOUS INJECTION (HUMIRA)

Adults and adolescents ages 12 and older weighing 60 kg (132 lb) or more. *Initial:* 160 mg given as four 40-mg injections on day 1 or two 40-mg injections on day 1 and repeated on day 2, followed by 80 mg given as two 40-mg injections on day 15. *Maintenance:* 40 mg weekly or 80 mg every other wk starting on day 29.
Adolescents ages 12 and older weighing 30 kg (66 lb) to 60 kg (132 lb). *Initial:* 80 mg given as two 40-mg injections on day 1 followed by 40 mg on day 8. *Maintenance:* 40 mg every other wk starting on day 22.

SUBCUTANEOUS INJECTION (ABRILADA, CYLTEZO, HULIO, SIMLANDI, YUFLYMA)

Adults. *Initial:* 160 mg given as four 40-mg injections on day 1 or two 40-mg injections on day 1 and repeated on day 2, followed by 80 mg given as two 40-mg injections on day 15. *Maintenance:* 40 mg weekly or 80 mg every other wk starting on day 29.

* *To treat noninfectious intermediate, posterior, and panuveitis*

SUBCUTANEOUS INJECTION (ABRILADA, AMJEVITA, CYLTEZO, HADLIMA, HULIO, HUMIRA, SIMLANDI, YUSIMRY)

Adults. *Initial:* 80 mg given as two 40-mg injections on day 1. *Maintenance:* 40 mg every other wk starting on day 8.

SUBCUTANEOUS INJECTION (HUMIRA)

Children ages 2 and older weighing 30 kg (66 lb) or more. 40 mg every other wk.
Children ages 2 and older weighing less than 30 kg (66 lb) but at least 15 kg (33 lb). 20 mg every other wk.
Children ages 2 and older weighing less than 15 kg (33 lb) but at least 10 kg (22 lb). 10 mg every other wk.

Drug Administration

SUBCUTANEOUS

- Follow the manufacturer's instructions on how to prepare and administer the adalimumab product prescribed for the patient.
- Know that adalimumab products must be refrigerated but may be left at room temperature with cap or cover on for about 15 to 30 min before injecting.
- Inject doses in separate sites in the abdomen or thigh.
- Rotate injection sites and do not give injections into an area where the skin is bruised, hard, red, or tender.
- Activate the protection device on needles of prefilled syringes delivered to institutions by holding the syringe in one hand and, with the other hand, sliding outer protective shield over exposed needle until it locks into place.
- Know that adalimumab may come in a single-use glass vial containing 40 mg (0.8 ml) of adalimumab referred to as an "institutional use vial" because the drug should only be given in a medical institution. Withdraw only 1 dose when using the "institutional use vial" and administer promptly. Because the vial does not contain preservatives, discard any unused drug. Be aware that the only dosage form for HADLIMA allowing for weight-based dosing in pediatric patients weighing below 30 kg is the "institutional use" vial.
- Protect drug from light.
- Check product being used to determine if latex may be contained in the pen or prefilled syringe. Do not handle if allergic to latex.

Route	Onset	Peak	Duration
SubQ	Unknown	131–187 hr	Unknown

Half-life: 10–20 days

Mechanism of Action

Binds to tumor necrosis factor (TNF) to block interaction with p55 and p75 cell surface TNF receptors, and lyses surface TNF-expressing cells in the presence of complement. TNF may be a major component of rheumatoid arthritis inflammation and joint destruction. Reduced TNF level in synovial fluid improves signs and symptoms and prevents further structural damage in rheumatoid arthritis. It also causes a decrease in levels of acute phase reactants of inflammation such as C-reactive protein, which may explain why it is useful in alleviating signs and symptoms in other inflammatory disease processes.

Contraindications

Active infection, hypersensitivity to adalimumab or its components

Interactions

DRUGS

abatacept, anakinra, rituximab: Possibly increased risk of serious infection and neutropenia in patients with rheumatoid arthritis

CYP450 substrates with narrow therapeutic index such as cyclosporine, theophylline, warfarin: Possibly altered effectiveness of these drugs

live vaccines: Increased risk of adverse vaccine effects

Adverse Reactions

CNS: Confusion, **CVA**, demyelinating disorders such as **Guillain-Barré syndrome** or multiple sclerosis, fever, headache, **hypertensive encephalopathy**, paresthesia, **subdural hematoma**, syncope, tremor

CV: **Arrhythmias, atrial fibrillation, cardiac arrest**, chest pain, **congestive heart failure**, coronary artery disease, **deep vein thrombosis**, hypercholesterolemia, hyperlipidemia, hypertension, **MI**, palpitations, **pericardial effusion, pericarditis**, peripheral edema, **systemic vasculitis**, tachycardia

EENT: Cataract, optic neuritis, otitis media, pharyngitis, sinusitis

ENDO: **Ketosis**, parathyroid disorder

GI: Abdominal pain, cholecystitis, cholelithiasis, diverticulitis, elevated alkaline phosphatase level, elevated liver enzymes, esophagitis, gastroenteritis, **gastrointestinal hemorrhage, hepatic failure or necrosis, hepatitis or reactivation of hepatitis B, large bowel perforation**, nausea, **pancreatitis**, vomiting

GU: Cystitis, hematuria, kidney calculus, menstrual disorder, paraproteinemia, **pyelonephritis**, UTI

HEME: **Agranulocytosis, aplastic anemia, granulocytopenia, leukopenia**, lymphocytosis, **neutropenia, pancytopenia**, polycythemia, **thrombocytopenia**

MS: Arthritis (including pyogenic or septic arthritis); back, extremity, pelvic, or thorax pain; bone disorder, fracture, or necrosis; muscle spasms; myasthenia; myositis, prosthetic infections; septic arthritis, synovitis

RESP: **Asthma**, bronchitis, **bronchospasm**, decreased pulmonary function, dyspnea, interstitial lung disease, pleural effusion, pneumonia, **pulmonary embolism**, tuberculosis (new or reactivation), upper respiratory tract infection

SKIN: Alopecia, cellulitis, cutaneous vasculitis, erysipelas (red skin), **erythema multiforme**, herpes zoster, **lichenoid reaction, melanoma, Merkel cell carcinoma**, new or worsening psoriasis, **nonmelanoma skin cancer**, rash, **Stevens-Johnson syndrome**, urticaria

Other: **Anaphylaxis**; **angioedema**; antibody formation against adalimumab; bacterial, mycobacterial, fungal, parasitic, viral, and other opportunistic infections; benign or unspecified cysts or polyps; dehydration; flare-up of disease process; flu-like symptoms; healing abnormalities; injection-site erythema, hemorrhage, itching, pain, or swelling; **leukemias, lymphomas and other malignancies, such as breast, colon, lung, and prostate**; lupus-like symptoms; postsurgical infection; sarcoidosis; **sepsis**

Childbearing Considerations

PREGNANCY

- It is not known if drug can cause fetal harm. However, monoclonal antibodies increasingly cross the placental barrier as pregnancy progresses.
- Infants exposed to drug in utero should have risks and benefits considered before being given live or live-attenuated vaccines.
- Use with caution only if benefit to mother outweighs potential risk to fetus.

LACTATION

- Drug is present in breast milk.
- Mothers should check with prescriber before breastfeeding.

Nursing Considerations

! **WARNING** Use adalimumab products cautiously in patients with recurrent infection or increased risk of infection and in patients who live in regions where tuberculosis and certain mycoses, such as *Histoplasma*, are endemic. Be aware that *Legionella* and *Listeria*, 2 bacterial infections, also have occurred with tumor necrosis factor–alpha-blockers such as adalimumab. Assess patient for signs and symptoms of an active infection before beginning adalimumab therapy. If patient has evidence of an active infection, drug therapy shouldn't start until the infection has been treated. Monitor patient closely throughout adalimumab therapy because infections associated with tumor necrosis factor–alpha-blocker therapy may involve multiple organ systems and become life-threatening. Be aware that patients over age 65 years, patients with other diagnoses, and patients taking concomitant immunosuppressants may be at greater risk of infection. If a serious infection develops during drug therapy, expect drug to be discontinued.

- Note if patient's past medical history includes hepatitis B virus infection (HBV). Chronic carriers of this virus may be at increased risk of reactivation of HBV when exposed to adalimumab products. Risk becomes even higher if patient is also receiving other drugs that suppress the immune system. Monitor patient closely throughout adalimumab therapy and for several months after therapy is discontinued. Notify prescriber if patient develops signs and symptoms of HBV reactivation during or after adalimumab therapy. If confirmed, expect drug to be discontinued if HBV reactivation occurs during adalimumab therapy. Provide supportive care, as needed.
- Ensure that children with juvenile idiopathic arthritis are up to date with current immunization guidelines prior to adalimumab therapy being started. However, know that they may receive vaccinations, except for live vaccines, while taking adalimumab, as needed. Be aware that the safety of administering live or live-attenuated vaccines in infants exposed to drug in utero is unknown.
- Use cautiously in a patient with a preexisting or recent onset of a central or peripheral nervous system demyelinating disorders such as Guillain-Barré, multiple sclerosis, or optic neuritis because, although rare, new onset or exacerbation of demyelinating disorders have occurred with adalimumab therapy. If this occurs, know that drug should be discontinued.
- Make sure patient has a tuberculin skin test before therapy starts. If skin test is positive, treatment of latent tuberculosis (TB) will start before adalimumab, as prescribed. Also, ensure that patient previously treated for TB, including prophylactic treatment, has a tuberculin skin test periodically throughout therapy, as adalimumab products may induce new onset or reactivate TB. Also, monitor patient for signs and symptoms of TB, as tests for latent TB infection may be falsely negative while taking adalimumab.

! **WARNING** Stop adalimumab immediately and tell prescriber if patient has an allergic reaction such as an anaphylactoid reaction, angioneurotic edema, rash, urticaria, or other allergic signs and symptoms. Expect drug to be discontinued for life-threatening or serious allergic reactions and provide supportive care, as needed and ordered.

- Watch closely for evidence of congestive heart failure (anxiety; crackles; dyspnea; sudden, unexplained weight gain) and notify prescriber if present.
- Monitor patient's CBC, as ordered, because adalimumab products may have adverse hematologic effects. Notify prescriber about persistent bleeding, bruising, fever, or pallor.

! **WARNING** Be aware that, although rare, malignancies such as breast, colon, lung, and prostate but especially leukemias and lymphomas, have occurred in patients receiving TNF blockers such as adalimumab products. These malignancies have also occurred in children. Patients with rheumatoid arthritis and other chronic inflammatory disease, especially those with very active disease or chronic exposure to immunosuppressant therapies may be at greatest risk for the development of lymphomas. Monitor patients closely.

- Be aware that adalimumab may cause formation of autoantibodies, and rarely, a lupus-like syndrome. Monitor drug's effectiveness and notify prescriber if patient's signs and symptoms of condition being treated with adalimumab worsens. Also, expect drug to be discontinued if patient develops a lupus-like syndrome.

PATIENT TEACHING

- Inform patient, family, or caregiver that the first injection of adalimumab must take place with a healthcare professional present.
- Teach patient, family, or caregiver how to give adalimumab as a subcutaneous injection at home, if applicable, using the adalimumab product prescribed. Emphasize importance of injecting the full amount to obtain the correct dose, rotating sites, and storing the drug properly at home and when traveling. Also, instruct how to properly dispose of needles, pens, and syringes.
- Advise patient, family, or caregiver that the needle cover may contain rubber and can cause a latex-induced allergic reaction if touched with bare hands. Have patient allergic to latex check if product prescribed contains a rubber needle cover before using.

! **WARNING** Review signs and symptoms of an allergic reaction (difficulty breathing, rash, swollen face), and tell patient to seek emergency care immediately if these occur.

- Tell patient, family, or caregiver that injection-site reactions (such as bruising, itching, rash, redness, and swelling) may occur but are usually mild and transient. If present, advise the application of a towel soaked with cold water on the injection site if it hurts or remains swollen. If reaction does not disappear or seems to worsen, prescriber should be notified immediately.
- Review signs and symptoms of infection and infection control measures for patient to take during adalimumab therapy.
- Inform patient, family, or caregiver that TB may occur during adalimumab therapy. Prescriber should be notified if a low-grade fever, persistent cough, and wasting or weight loss occurs.
- Teach patient, family, or caregiver how to recognize evidence of bleeding disorders and to tell prescriber if present; drug may have to be stopped. Advise patient to comply with all prescribed laboratory tests.

! **WARNING** Inform patient, family, or caregiver that the risk of certain kinds of cancer, especially leukemias and lymphomas, is higher in patients taking adalimumab but still rare. Emphasize the importance of follow-up visits and reporting a sudden onset or unusual signs or symptoms.

- Caution patient against receiving live-virus vaccines while taking adalimumab because doing so may adversely affect the immune system.
- Inform patient, family, or caregiver that blood samples may be needed periodically, but especially around week 24 of therapy, to check for autoantibody development. Explain that adalimumab therapy will have to be stopped if it is detected.
- Instruct patient, family, or caregiver to report lupus-like signs and symptoms that, although rare, may occur during therapy, such as chest pain that does not go away, joint pain, a rash on arms or cheeks that is sensitive to the sun, or shortness of breath. Explain that drug may be stopped if these occur.
- Advise patient, family, or caregiver to inform all healthcare providers about adalimumab use and to inform prescriber about any over-the-counter medications being taken, including herbal remedies and mineral and vitamin supplements. Also, patient should report to prescriber any new or worsening medical conditions.
- Instruct females of childbearing age to notify prescriber immediately if pregnancy occurs, as adalimumab products may affect the immune response of utero-exposed newborn or infant.
- Encourage mothers wishing to breastfeed infant to discuss with prescriber before doing so. Also, emphasize the importance of telling pediatrician if an adalimumab product was taken any time during pregnancy, prior to having infant receive any vaccines.

adefovir dipivoxil

Hepsera

Class and Category

Pharmacologic class: Nucleotide analogue
Therapeutic class: Antiviral

Indications and Dosages

✷ *To treat chronic hepatitis B in patients with evidence of active viral replication and either evidence of persistent elevations in serum aminotransferases (ALT or AST) or histologically active disease*

TABLETS

Adults and children ages 12 and older. 10 mg once daily.

± **DOSAGE ADJUSTMENT** For patients with a creatinine clearance between 30 and 49 ml/min, dosage interval changed to every 48 hours. For patients with a creatinine clearance between 10 and 29 ml/min, dosage interval changed to 72 hours. For patients receiving hemodialysis, dosage interval changed to every 7 days following dialysis.

Drug Administration

P.O.

- Administer drug at the same time every day.
- Drug may be administered with or without food.

Mechanism of Action

Inhibits hepatitis B virus (HBV) by competing with the natural substrate deoxyadenosine triphosphate and by causing DNA chain termination after its incorporation into viral DNA, which prevents replication.

Contraindications

Hypersensitivity to adefovir dipivoxil or its components

Interactions

DRUGS

drugs that are excreted renally or known to affect renal function, such as aminoglycosides, cyclosporine, NSAIDs, tacrolimus, and vancomycin: Possibly increased serum concentrations of adefovir or these drugs or both, increasing risk of adverse reactions

Adverse Reactions

CNS: Asthenia, headache
GI: Abdominal pain, diarrhea, dyspepsia, flatulence, nausea, **pancreatitis**, **severe acute exacerbations of hepatitis**, **severe hepatomegaly with steatosis**, vomiting
GU: Abnormal renal function, elevated creatinine level, **Fanconi syndrome**, **nephrotoxicity**, **proximal renal tubulopathy**, **renal failure**
MS: Bone pain, myopathy, osteomalacia
SKIN: Pruritus, rash
Other: **HIV resistance**, **hypophosphatemia**, **immune reconstitution syndrome**, **lactic acidosis**

Childbearing Considerations

PREGNANCY

- Pregnancy exposure registry: 1-800-258-4263.
- It is not known if drug can cause fetal harm.
- Use with caution only if benefit to mother outweighs potential risk to fetus.

LACTATION

- It is not known if drug is present in breast milk.
- Mothers should check with prescriber before breastfeeding.

Nursing Considerations

- Check to be sure HIV antibody testing has been done prior to starting adefovir therapy because treatment with anti-hepatitis B therapies, such as adefovir, may cause an emergence of HIV resistance.
- Use with extreme caution in patients with renal dysfunction. Check to ensure that patient's creatinine clearance is known before adefovir therapy begins and then rechecked periodically throughout therapy because adefovir may cause a delayed nephrotoxicity that may require dosage interval to be lengthened or drug discontinued. Know that patients at higher risk include those having underlying renal dysfunction and patients taking concomitant nephrotoxic agents such as aminoglycosides, cyclosporine, NSAIDs, tacrolimus, and vancomycin.
- Use caution when administering adefovir to patient with liver dysfunction or known risk factors for liver disease.

! **WARNING** Know that lactic acidosis and severe hepatomegaly with steatosis have occurred with adefovir therapy and death has occurred in some patients. Risk factors include being a woman, presence of obesity, and prolonged nucleoside exposure. However, know that lactic acidosis and severe hepatomegaly with steatosis have also occurred in patients with no known risk factors. Expect drug to be discontinued in any patient who develops clinical or laboratory findings suggestive of lactic acidosis or pronounced hepatotoxicity, even in the absence of marked transaminase elevations.

! **WARNING** Monitor patient for signs and symptoms of hepatitis such as abdominal pain, dark urine, fatigue, fever, jaundice, nausea, and vomiting. Notify prescriber if hepatitis is suspected. Also, expect patient to be closely monitored for at least several months after adefovir has been discontinued because exacerbation of hepatitis may occur with some cases being severe.

- Monitor patient throughout treatment for evidence of loss of therapeutic response. Indicators include increasing levels of HBV DNA over time after an initial decline below assay limit, progression of clinical signs or symptoms of hepatic disease and/or worsening of hepatic necro inflammatory findings or return of persistently elevated ALT levels. These findings may require drug to be discontinued.

! **WARNING** Be aware that immune reconstitution syndrome has occurred in patients treated with combination antiretroviral therapy, including adefovir. The inflammatory response predisposes susceptible patients to opportunistic infections such as cytomegalovirus infection, *Mycobacterium avium* infection, *Pneumocystis jiroveci* pneumonia, or tuberculosis. Autoimmune disorders such as Graves' disease, Guillain-Barré syndrome, or polymyositis have also occurred. Report sudden or unusual adverse reactions to prescriber.

PATIENT TEACHING

- Instruct patient with hepatitis B on the importance of testing for HIV before therapy begins and then periodically throughout therapy to avoid development of resistance to HIV treatment.
- Instruct patient how to take adefovir and what to do if he misses a dose.
- Advise patient that treatment with adefovir does not reduce the risk of transmission of HBV to others.

! **WARNING** Alert patient that severe adverse reactions may develop while taking adefovir. Encourage him to stop taking drug and seek medical attention immediately if he experiences any persistent, severe, or unusual symptoms.

! **WARNING** Tell patient to report any new or worsening symptoms suggestive of liver dysfunction to prescriber immediately because emergence of resistant hepatitis B virus may occur, or disease may worsen during treatment. Also, warn patient with hepatitis B that acute severe exacerbations of hepatitis B may occur following discontinuation of adefovir. He should not discontinue drug without prescriber knowledge.

adenosine

Class and Category

Pharmacologic class: Nucleoside
Therapeutic class: Class V antiarrhythmic, diagnostic aid

Indications and Dosages

* *To convert paroxysmal supraventricular tachycardia (PSVT) to normal sinus rhythm*

I.V. INJECTION

Adults and children weighing 50 kg (110 lb) or more. *Initial:* 6 mg injected over 1 to 2 sec. If PSVT continues after 1 to 2 min, 12 mg given and repeated in 1 to 2 min, as needed. *Maximum:* 12 mg as a single dose.
Children weighing less than 50 kg. *Initial:* 0.05 to 0.1 mg/kg injected over 1 to 2 sec. If PSVT continues after 1 to 2 min, additional bolus injections are given, incrementally increasing dose by 0.05 to 0.1 mg/kg. Administration continued until PSVT converts to normal sinus rhythm or until patient reaches maximum single dose. *Maximum:* 0.3 mg/kg (12 mg) as a single dose.

✱ As adjunct to thallium-201 myocardial perfusion scintigraphy in patients unable to exercise adequately during testing

I.V. INJECTION

Adults. 140 mcg/kg/min (total infused dose of 0.84 mg/kg).

Drug Administration

I.V.

✱ For use to convert paroxysmal supraventricular tachycardia (PSVT) to normal sinus rhythm

- Do not refrigerate drug as crystals may occur. If crystals are present, dissolve crystals by warming drug to room temperature. The solution must be clear at the time of use.
- Give by rapid I.V. bolus over 1 to 2 sec. Slower delivery can cause reflex tachycardia and systemic vasodilation.
- Administer either directly into a central or peripheral vein or, if given into an I.V. line, give as close to patient as possible and follow with a rapid saline flush.
- Don't give more than 12 mg as a single dose.
- *Incompatibilities:* None listed by manufacturer

✱ For use as adjunct to thallium-201 myocardial perfusion scintigraphy

- Give drug used as an adjunct to thallium-201 myocardial perfusion scintigraphy as a continuous peripheral intravenous infusion over 6 min. Know that the required dose of thallium-201 should be injected at the midpoint of the drug infusion. It is compatible with the drug and may be injected directly into the drug infusion set.
- Store drug at room temperature.
- Discard any unused drug.
- *Incompatibilities:* None listed by manufacturer

Route	Onset	Peak	Duration
I.V.	Immediate	Immediate	Unknown

Half-life: >10 sec

Mechanism of Action

Slows conduction time through the AV node and can interrupt AV node reentry pathways to restore normal sinus rhythm.

Contraindications

Hypersensitivity to adenosine or its components; second- or third-degree heart block or sick sinus syndrome, except in patients with a functioning artificial pacemaker

Interactions

DRUGS

carbamazepine: Increased degree of heart block
digoxin, verapamil: Possibly increased depressant effect on SA or AV node and increased risk of ventricular fibrillation
dipyridamole: Increased adenosine effects
methylxanthines, such as theophylline: Antagonized adenosine effects

FOODS

caffeine: Antagonized adenosine effects

Adverse Reactions

CNS: Apprehension, **CVA**, dizziness, headache, heaviness in arms, light-headedness, nervousness, paresthesia, **seizures**
CV: **Atrial fibrillation**, **bradycardia**, **cardiac arrest**, chest pain or pressure, **heart block**, hypertension, **hypotension**, **MI**, palpitations, **prolonged asystole**, **sinus exit block or pause**, **sustained ventricular tachycardia**, tachycardia, **torsades de pointes**, transient hypertension, **ventricular fibrillation**
EENT: Blurred vision, metallic taste, **throat tightness**
GI: Nausea, vomiting
MS: Jaw, neck, and back pain
RESP: **Bronchoconstriction**, **bronchospasm**, dyspnea, hyperventilation, **respiratory arrest**
SKIN: Diaphoresis, erythema, facial flushing, rash
Other: Injection-site reactions, including pain, sensitivity reactions

Childbearing Considerations

PREGNANCY

- It is not known if drug can cause fetal harm.
- Use with caution only if benefit to mother outweighs potential risk to fetus.

LACTATION

- It is not known if drug is present in breast milk.
- A decision should be made to discontinue breastfeeding or the drug to avoid potential serious adverse reactions in the breastfed infant.

Nursing Considerations

! WARNING Know that drug should not be given to patients with signs and symptoms of acute myocardial ischemia, as these patients may be at greater risk for serious cardiovascular reactions, including a myocardial infarction during a medical stress test.

- Monitor blood pressure, heart rate and rhythm, and respiratory status often during adenosine therapy.
- Be aware that at the time of conversion to normal sinus rhythm, arrhythmias such as AV block, premature atrial or ventricular contractions, sinus bradycardia, or sinus tachycardia may occur for a few seconds, but they don't usually require intervention.

! **WARNING** Stop drug and notify prescriber immediately if severe respiratory difficulties develop or patient develops signs of hypersensitivity such as chest discomfort, erythema, flushing, or rash.

PATIENT TEACHING

- Inform patient how drug will be administered.
- Inform patient of increased risk for serious adverse effects. Instruct patient to report chest pain, difficulty breathing, palpitations, or severe headache during adenosine therapy.
- Warn patient that mild, temporary reactions may occur, such as dizziness, flushing, and nausea.

albuterol sulfate

(salbutamol sulfate)

ProAir Digihaler, ProAir RespiClick, Ventolin HFA

Class and Category

Pharmacologic class: Adrenergic
Therapeutic class: Bronchodilator

Indications and Dosages

✱ *To prevent exercise-induced bronchospasm*

INHALATION POWDER (PROAIR DIGIHALER, PROAIR RESPICLICK)

Adults and children ages 4 and older. 2 inhalations 15 to 30 min before exercise.

INHALATION AEROSOL (VENTOLIN HFA)

Adults and children ages 4 and older. 2 inhalations 15 to 30 min before exercise.

✱ *To prevent or treat bronchospasm in patients with reversible obstructive airway disease*

E.R. TABLETS

Adults and children over age 12. *Initial:* 4 or 8 mg every 12 hr. *Maximum:* 32 mg daily in divided doses every 12 hr.
Children ages 6 to 12. *Initial:* 4 mg every 12 hr. *Maximum:* 24 mg daily in divided doses every 12 hr.

SYRUP

Adults and adolescents over age 14. *Initial:* 2 or 4 mg (1 to 2 tsp) 3 or 4 times daily. Dosage increased stepwise up to 8 mg 4 times daily, as needed. *Maximum:* 32 mg daily in divided doses.
Children ages 6 to 14. *Initial:* 2 mg (1 tsp) 3 or 4 times daily. Dosage increased stepwise up to maximum dose, as needed. *Maximum:* 24 mg daily in divided doses.
Children ages 2 to 6. *Initial:* 0.1 mg/kg 3 times daily (not to exceed 2 mg 3 times daily), increased to 0.2 mg/kg 3 times daily (not to exceed 4 mg 3 times daily), as needed. *Maximum:* 12 mg daily in divided doses.

TABLETS

Adults and adolescents over age 12. *Initial:* 2 or 4 mg 3 or 4 times daily. Dosage increased stepwise up to 8 mg 4 times daily, as needed. *Maximum:* 32 mg daily in divided doses.
Children ages 6 to 12. *Initial:* 2 mg 3 or 4 times daily. Dosage increased stepwise up to maximum dose, as needed. *Maximum:* 24 mg daily in divided doses.

± **DOSAGE ADJUSTMENT** For elderly patients and patients sensitive to beta-adrenergic stimulation, initial dosage reduced to 2 mg (1 tsp) of syrup 3 or 4 times daily or 2 mg of tablets 3 or 4 times daily and then slowly increased, as needed, to as much as 8 mg 3 or 4 times daily, not exceeding total daily dose of 32 mg in adults and children ages 12 years and older and not exceeding total daily dose of 24 mg in children ages 6 to 12.

INHALATION SOLUTION

Adults, children ages 12 and older and children ages 2 to 12 weighing 15 kg (33 lb) or more. 2.5 mg 3 or 4 times daily, as needed, by nebulization.
Children ages 2 to 12 weighing 10 kg (22 lb) to less than 15 kg (33 lb). *Initial:* 0.63 mg or 1.25 mg 3 or 4 times daily, as needed, by nebulization.

A

INHALATION POWDER (PROAIR DIGIHALER, PROAIR RESPICLICK)

Adults and children ages 4 and older.
1 inhalation every 4 hr or 2 inhalations every 4 to 6 hr.

INHALATION AEROSOL (VENTOLIN HFA)

Adults and children ages 4 and older.
1 inhalation every 4 hr or 2 inhalations every 4 to 6 hr.

Drug Administration

P.O.

- Do not break, crush, or split extended-release tablets or mix with food for administration. E.R. tablets should be swallowed whole.
- Use an accurate measuring device when measuring syrup dosage.

INHALATION

- Use entire contents of a 1-unit-dose vial when administering by nebulization. Adjust flow rate to deliver drug solution over 5 to 15 min. Do not administer any other drugs in nebulizer. Care for nebulizer following manufacturer's instructions.
- Administer pressurized inhalations of albuterol during inspiration, when airways are open wider and aerosol distribution is more effective.
- Advise patient to wait at least 1 min between inhalations if dosage requires more than 1 inhalation.
- There is no need to prime ProAir Digihaler or ProAir RespiClick device. Do not use these devices with a spacer or volume holding chamber. Do not wash or put these devices in water. Instead, they should be cleaned by gently wiping the mouthpiece with a dry cloth or tissue, as needed.
- Prime Ventolin HFA before first use, when not used for more than 2 wk, or when inhaler has been dropped by releasing 4 sprays. Shake the Ventolin HFA inhaler well before each spray. Wash actuator with warm water and let air dry completely at least once a week and store mouthpiece in downward position.
- Discard the ProAir Digihaler device 13 mo from opening the foil pouch or after the expiration date, whichever comes first. The ProAir RespiClick device should also be discarded 13 mo from opening the foil pouch when the dose counter displays 0 or after the expiration date, whichever comes first. Discard Ventolin HFA inhaler when counter reaches 000.

Route	Onset	Peak	Duration
P.O.	15–30 min	2–3 hr	4–8 hr
P.O. (E.R.)	30 min	2–3 hr	< 12 hr
P.O. (Syrup)	5–15 min	2 hr	< 6 hr
Inhalation (powder)	5–15 min	30 min	4–6 hr
Inhalation (solution)	5–15 min	0.5–2 hr	4–6 hr

Half-life: 3.8–9.3 hr

Contraindications

Hypersensitivity to albuterol or its components

Interactions

DRUGS

beta-blockers: Inhibited effects of albuterol

Mechanism of Action

Attaches to $beta_2$ receptors on bronchial cell membranes, which stimulates the intracellular enzyme adenylate cyclase to convert adenosine triphosphate (ATP) to cyclic adenosine monophosphate (cAMP). This reaction decreases intracellular calcium levels. It also increases intracellular levels of cAMP, as shown. Together, these effects relax bronchial smooth muscle cells and inhibit histamine release.

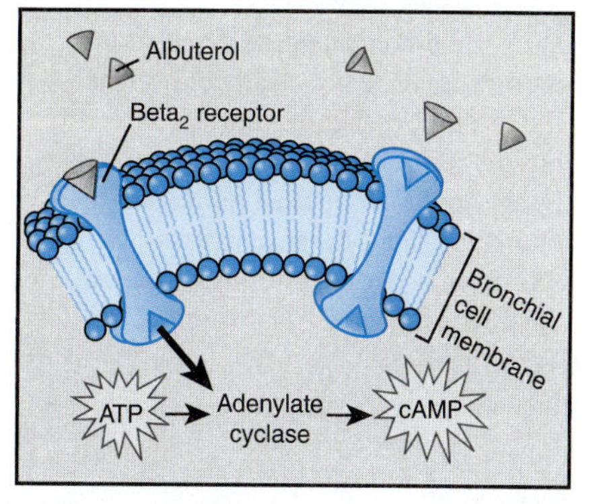

bronchodilators (sympathomimetics), such as theophylline: Possibly adverse CV effects
digoxin: Decreased serum digoxin level
MAO inhibitors, tricyclic antidepressants: Increased vascular effects of albuterol
potassium-lowering drugs: Possibly hypokalemia
potassium-wasting diuretics: Possibly increased hypokalemia

Adverse Reactions

CNS: Anxiety, dizziness, drowsiness, headache, hyperkinesia, insomnia, irritability, nervousness, tremor, vertigo, weakness
CV: **Angina**, **arrhythmias**, chest pain, hypertension, **hypotension**, palpitations
EENT: Altered taste, dry mouth and throat, ear pain, glossitis, hoarseness, **oropharyngeal edema**, pharyngitis, rhinitis, taste perversion
ENDO: Hyperglycemia
GI: Anorexia, diarrhea, dysphagia, heartburn, nausea, vomiting
GU: UTI
MS: Muscle cramps
RESP: **Bronchospasm**, cough, dyspnea, **paradoxical bronchospasm**, **pulmonary edema**
SKIN: Diaphoresis, flushing, pallor, pruritus, rash, urticaria
Other: **Anaphylaxis**, **angioedema**, **hypokalemia**, infection, **metabolic acidosis**

Childbearing Considerations

PREGNANCY

- Pregnancy exposure registry: 1-877-311-8972 or http://mothertobaby.org/pregnancy studies/.
- It is not known if drug can cause fetal harm.
- Use with caution only if benefit to mother outweighs potential risk to fetus.

LABOR AND DELIVERY

- Drug should only be used if benefit to mother during labor clearly outweighs the risk for beta agonist interference with uterine contractility.
- Drug should not be used for management of preterm labor because serious adverse reactions, including pulmonary edema, have been reported in the mother.

LACTATION

- It is not known if drug is present in breast milk.
- A decision should be made to discontinue breastfeeding or the drug to avoid potential serious adverse reactions in the breastfed infant.

Nursing Considerations

! **WARNING** Use cautiously in patients with cardiac disorders, diabetes mellitus, digitalis intoxication, hypertension, hyperthyroidism, or history of seizures. Albuterol can worsen these conditions.

! **WARNING** Monitor patient for signs and symptoms of a hypersensitivity reaction that could become life-threatening such as anaphylaxis and angioedema. Also, monitor patient for other adverse reactions, which also may be quite serious such as angina, arrhythmias, bronchospasm, and metabolic acidosis. Notify prescriber immediately if serious adverse reactions occur, expect drug to be withheld and a different drug prescribed, and provide supportive care, as needed and ordered.

- Monitor serum potassium level because albuterol may cause transient hypokalemia.
- Monitor effectiveness of drug to prevent or relieve patient's respiratory symptoms. Be aware that drug tolerance can develop with prolonged use.

PATIENT TEACHING

- Teach patient how to use type of inhaler or oral form prescribed.
- Advise patient prescribed an inhaler to wait at least 1 minute between inhalations if dosage requires more than one inhalation, and to check with prescriber before using other inhaled drugs.
- Warn patient not to exceed prescribed dose or frequency. If doses become less effective, tell patient to contact his prescriber.

! **WARNING** Tell patient to immediately report signs and symptoms of allergic reaction, such as difficulty swallowing, itching, and rash. Stress importance of seeking immediate medical care if allergic reaction is severe.

- Advise patient to notify prescriber of any persistent, serious, or unusual adverse reactions.

- Alert mothers that breastfeeding should not be undertaken during albuterol therapy to prevent serious adverse reactions in the breastfed infant.

alemtuzumab

Lemtrada

Class and Category

Pharmacologic class: Monoclonal antibody
Therapeutic class: Immunomodulator

Indications and Dosages

∗ *To treat relapsing forms of multiple sclerosis, to include active relapsing progressive disease and active secondary progressive disease*

I.V. INFUSION

Adults. *First treatment course:* 12 mg/day on 5 consecutive days for 60 mg total dose. *Second treatment course:* 12 mg/day on 3 consecutive days for 36 mg total dose administered 12 mo after first treatment course. *Subsequent treatment courses:* 12 mg/day on 3 consecutive days, as needed, for 36 mg total dose administered 12 mo after last dose of any prior treatment course.

Drug Administration

I.V.

- Premedicate patient with high-dose corticosteroids such as 1,000 mg of methylprednisolone or equivalent, as prescribed, immediately prior to alemtuzumab infusion and for first 3 days of each treatment course to decrease risk of infusion reactions. Antihistamines and/or antipyretics may be prescribed and given prior to infusion.
- Administer antiviral prophylaxis for herpetic viral infections, as prescribed, starting on the first day of each treatment course and continuing for a minimum of 2 mo following treatment or until CD4+ lymphocyte count is at least 200 cells per microliter, whichever occurs later.
- Do not freeze or shake vials prior to use. Solution should not be discolored or contain particulate matter.
- Withdraw 1.2 ml from drug vial into a syringe and inject into a 100-ml bag of sterile 0.9% Sodium Chloride, USP or 5% Dextrose in Water, USP. Gently invert bag to mix solution.
- Ensure the sterility of the prepared solution because it contains no antimicrobial preservatives. Also, protect it from light. Diluted solution may be stored for up to 8 hr refrigerated or at room temperature.
- Infuse alemtuzumab over 4 hr starting within 8 hr after dilution. Know that duration of infusion may be extended if clinically indicated.
- Do not give drug as a bolus or I.V. push.
- Check vital signs before infusion and frequently during infusion.
- *Incompatibilities:* Other drugs through the same intravenous line

Route	Onset	Peak	Duration
I.V.	Unknown	Unknown	Unknown

Half-life: 2 wk

Mechanism of Action

Binds possibly to CD52, a cell surface antigen present on T and B lymphocytes and on natural killer cells, macrophages, and monocytes. This results in antibody-dependent cellular cytolysis and complement-mediated lysis.

Contraindications

Hypersensitivity to alemtuzumab or its components, presence of active infections or HIV infection

Interactions

DRUGS

antineoplastics, immunosuppressants: Increased risk of immunosuppression
live viral vaccines: Increased risk of infection
myelosuppressive agents: Enhanced myelosuppressive effects

Adverse Reactions

CNS: Anxiety, asthenia, **autoimmune encephalitis**, chills, **CVA**, dizziness, fatigue, fever, **Guillain-Barré syndrome**, headache, insomnia, Lambert-Eaton myasthenia gravis, myasthenic syndrome, paresthesia, **progressive multifocal leukoencephalopathy**, **suicidal ideation**
CV: **Cervicocephalic arterial dissection**, **MI**, **myocardial ischemia**, peripheral edema, tachycardia, vasculitis

EENT: Epistaxis, nasopharyngitis, oropharyngeal pain, retinal pigment epitheliopathy, sinusitis, taste distortion
ENDO: New onset of type 1 diabetes mellitus, thyroid dysfunction
GI: Abdominal pain, **autoimmune hepatitis**, cholecystitis, diarrhea, dyspepsia, nausea, vomiting
GU: Abnormal uterine bleeding, **glomerular nephropathies including anti-glomerular basement membrane disease**, hematuria, membranous glomerulonephritis, UTI
HEME: **Acquired hemophilia A**, **autoimmune hemolytic anemia and pancytopenia**, **decreased CD4 and CD8 lymphocytes and T-lymphocyte count**, **hemophagocytic lymph histiocytosis**, **immune thrombocytopenia**, **lymphopenia**, **neutropenia**, **thrombotic thrombocytopenic purpura**
MS: Arthralgia; back, extremity, or neck pain; muscle weakness; myalgia; rheumatoid arthritis
RESP: Cough, dyspnea, **hypersensitivity pneumonitis**, **pneumonitis with fibrosis**, **pulmonary alveolar hemorrhage**, upper respiratory infection
SKIN: Alopecia, dermatitis, erythema, flushing, pruritus, rash, urticaria, vitiligo
Other: **Adult-onset Still's disease (AOSD)**; alemtuzumab antibody formation; **anaphylaxis**; autoimmune conditions; **bacterial**, **fungal**, **herpes**, **opportunistic, or other viral infections** (serious to **life-threatening**); flu-like symptoms; **infusion reactions** (serious to **life-threatening**); **malignancies (lymphoma**, **lymphoproliferative disorders**, **melanoma**, **thyroid cancer)**; **sarcoidosis**; undifferentiated connective tissue disorders

Childbearing Considerations

PREGNANCY

- Pregnancy exposure registry: 1-800-745-4447, option 2.
- Drug may cause fetal harm, as placental transfer of antithyroid antibodies to fetus may result in neonatal Graves' disease.
- Use with caution only if benefit to mother outweighs potential risk to fetus.

LACTATION

- It is not known if drug is present in breast milk.
- Mothers should check with prescriber before breastfeeding.

REPRODUCTION

- Females of childbearing age should use effective contraceptive measures during drug therapy and for 4 mo following that course of treatment.
- Animal studies have shown adverse effects on sperm parameters in males and reduced number of corpora lutea and implantations in females.

Nursing Considerations

- Know that alemtuzumab is only available through a restricted distribution under a Risk Evaluation Mitigation Strategy Program because of the risk of autoimmunity, infusion reactions, and malignancies.
- Know that Lemtrada and Campath contain the same generic drug, alemtuzumab, but are used to treat different disorders as Campath has an orphan designation to only treat B-cell chronic lymphocytic leukemia and Lemtrada only treats multiple sclerosis. Do not confuse the two drugs because they are not interchangeable. If patient has been previously treated with Campath, monitor patient for additive and long-lasting effects on the immune system.
- Complete any necessary immunizations at least 6 weeks prior to treatment, as prescribed. Ensure tuberculosis screening has been done prior to drug therapy.

! WARNING Assess patient for signs and symptoms of an infection prior to beginning therapy, and then before each infusion. Know that infections frequently occur with alemtuzumab treatment and can become life-threatening. Examples of infections that may occur include serious infections such as appendicitis, gastroenteritis, pneumonia, and tooth infections; Epstein-Barr viral infection; fungal infections; herpes viral infections; human papilloma virus infections; *Listeria monocytogenes* infections; opportunistic infections; and tuberculosis. Know that treatment may be delayed until active infection is under control.

- Screen patients at high risk for hepatitis B or C virus prior to initiating therapy. Be aware patients at high risk for hepatitis B or C virus may be at risk of irreversible liver damage caused by a potential virus reactivation.

- Expect baseline laboratory tests to be performed prior to alemtuzumab therapy and periodically thereafter as follows: Complete blood count (CBC) with differential prior to and then monthly; serum creatinine levels prior to and then monthly; thyroid function test, such as a thyroid-stimulating hormone level, prior to and then every 3 months; and urinalysis with urine cell counts, including urine protein-to-creatinine ratio, prior to and then monthly. Also expect to check total bilirubin and serum transaminase levels prior to and then periodically and to perform a baseline skin examination followed by yearly exams for melanoma. Expect to continue monitoring these test results for up to 48 months after last dose is infused.

! **WARNING** Be aware that despite premedicating patient with high-dose corticosteroids as well as antihistamines and/or antipyretics prior to therapy, a serious infusion reaction may still occur that could become life-threatening. Infusion reactions may include anaphylaxis, angioedema, bradycardia, bronchospasm, chest pain, fever, headache, hypertension or hypotension, rash, tachycardia (including atrial fibrillation), or transient neurologic symptoms. Additional infusion adverse reactions may include chills, dizziness, dyspepsia, dyspnea, fatigue, insomnia, nausea, pain, pruritus, pulmonary infiltrates, and urticaria. Observe patient during and for at least 2 hours after each infusion. Question patient frequently regarding symptoms they may be experiencing. Be prepared to manage anaphylaxis or serious infusion reactions immediately, if present. Be aware that immediate discontinuation of drug should be considered if a serious infusion reaction occurs.

! **WARNING** Monitor patient for signs and symptoms of a CVA because drug may cause hemorrhagic and ischemic stroke from cervicocephalic arterial dissection involving multiple arteries and can occur within 3 days of infusion, with most occurring within 1 day.

! **WARNING** Monitor patient for signs and symptoms of neurologic disorders such as Guillain-Barré or progressive multifocal leukoencephalopathy (PML). If any occur, notify prescriber immediately and withhold drug while diagnostic evaluation is ongoing. If confirmed, provide appropriate and supportive care, as prescribed.

! **WARNING** Know that alemtuzumab causes serious, sometimes fatal, autoimmune conditions such as anti-glomerular basement membrane disease and immune thrombocytopenia. Expect to monitor CBC with differential, serum creatinine levels, and urinalysis with urine cell counts at periodic intervals for 48 months after last dose. Also, be aware that AOSD, a rare inflammatory disease, may occur with alemtuzumab therapy. Monitor patient for arthritis (pain, stiffness, and possible swelling of multiple joints), fever (> 39°C or 102.2°F lasting more than a week), leukocytosis, and rash with patient having no history or signs and symptoms of infections, malignancies, or other rheumatic conditions. If suspected, notify prescriber and expect drug to be discontinued, if confirmed. In addition, monitor patient for thrombotic thrombocytopenic purpura (fever, microangiopathic hemolytic anemia, neurologic signs and symptoms, renal impairment, and thrombocytopenia). If suspected, notify prescriber immediately and expect drug to be discontinued, if the disorder is confirmed.

! **WARNING** Monitor patient for suicidal behavior or thoughts. Notify prescriber if any concerns arise.

! **WARNING** Be aware that alemtuzumab may cause an increased risk of malignancies, including lymphoproliferative disorders, melanoma, and thyroid cancer. Expect baseline exam and yearly follow-ups to be done.

- Monitor patient's renal function, as ordered. Notify prescriber immediately of any abnormalities, because urgent evaluation and treatment can improve the preservation of renal function. Know that glomerular nephropathies can occur up to 40 months after the last dose of alemtuzumab. Expect patient's urine protein-to-creatinine ratio to be measured if urine dipstick shows 1+ protein or greater.

- Monitor patient for liver dysfunction because drug can cause significant liver injury, including autoimmune hepatitis. Patients should also be monitored for Graves' disease.
- Be aware that acquired hemophilia A has occurred in patients taking alemtuzumab. Assess patient frequently for spontaneous subcutaneous hematomas and extensive bruising in addition to epistaxis, gastrointestinal or other types of bleeding, and hematuria. Report findings immediately to prescriber.

PATIENT TEACHING

! **WARNING** Inform patient that alemtuzumab may cause serious to life-threatening infusion reactions requiring patient to stay at infusion center for 2 hours after each infusion. Patient should seek immediate medical attention if a reaction occurs after leaving infusion center because reactions can occur for up to 72 hours after infusion.

! **WARNING** Review signs of an MI or stroke with patient. Instruct patient to seek immediate medical attention if symptom occur. Also, instruct patient to report any signs and symptoms of infection, as well as other persistent, severe, or unusual signs and symptoms that are not common to patient, such as cough, hemoptysis, shortness of breath, or wheezing. In addition, review signs and symptoms of AOSD and thrombotic thrombocytopenic purpura and stress importance to immediately notify prescriber if suspected.

! **WARNING** Tell family or caregiver to monitor patient for suicidal behavior or thoughts. If present, prescriber should be notified immediately.

- Instruct patients to avoid potential sources of *Listeria monocytogenes*, such as dairy products made with unpasteurized milk, deli meat, poultry, seafood, soft cheeses, or undercooked meat. Review signs and symptoms for *Listeria* infection because risk of when patient can become infected is unknown. Some cases have been reported up to 8 months after last dose.
- Stress importance of having a yearly skin exam.
- Advise patient to notify prescriber if bleeding, blood in urine, bruising, dark or bloody stools, or nosebleeds occur, or painful or swollen joints develop.
- Encourage female patients to have an annual human papilloma virus screening done.
- Advise females of childbearing age of risk to fetus and to notify prescriber when pregnancy is suspected or known.

alendronate sodium

Binosto, Fosamax

Class and Category

Pharmacologic class: Bisphosphonate
Therapeutic class: Bone resorption inhibitor

Indications and Dosages

∗ *To prevent postmenopausal osteoporosis*

TABLETS (FOSAMAX)

Adult women. 5 mg daily or 35 mg once/wk.

∗ *To treat postmenopausal osteoporosis*

ORAL SOLUTION, TABLETS (FOSAMAX)

Adult women. 10 mg (tablet) daily or 70 mg (oral solution or tablet) once/wk.

EFFERVESCENT TABLETS (BINOSTO)

Adult women. 70 mg once/wk.

∗ *To treat patients with Paget's disease of the bone who have an alkaline phosphatase level at least 2 times the upper limit of normal, patients who are symptomatic, or patients at risk for further complications*

TABLETS (FOSAMAX)

Adults. 40 mg daily for 6 mo. Treatment repeated following a 6-mo posttreatment evaluation period, as needed, in patients who have failed to normalize their serum alkaline phosphatase levels or have relapsed based on increases in alkaline phosphatase.

∗ *To increase bone mass in men with osteoporosis*

ORAL SOLUTION, TABLETS (FOSAMAX)

Adult men. 10 mg (tablet) daily or 70 mg (oral solution or tablet) once/wk.

EFFERVESCENT TABLETS (BINOSTO)

Adult men. 70 mg once/wk.

✱ *To treat glucocorticoid-induced osteoporosis in men and women who receive a daily glucocorticoid dosage of 7.5 mg or greater of prednisone and who have low bone mineral density*

TABLETS (FOSAMAX)

Adults. 5 mg daily.

± **DOSAGE ADJUSTMENT** For postmenopausal women not receiving estrogen, dosage for glucocorticoid-induced osteoporosis increased to 10 mg daily.

Drug Administration

P.O.

- Use only plain water, not flavored or mineral water, that is at room temperature when administering drug.
- Administer after patient awakens and at least 30 min before patient drinks, eats, or is given other drugs.
- Administer effervescent form of alendronate by dissolving 1 tablet in 4 ounces of plain water. Wait at least 5 min after effervescence stops and then stir the solution for about 10 sec before handing to patient to ingest.
- Give tablet form with 6 to 8 ounces of plain water in the morning.
- Give patient at least 2 ounces of plain water following ingestion of oral solution.
- Keep patient in an upright position for 30 min after administering drug.

Route	Onset	Peak	Duration
P.O.	Unknown	Unknown	Unknown

Half-life: >10 yr

Mechanism of Action

Reduces activity of cells that cause bone loss, slows rate of bone loss after menopause, and increases amount of bone mass. May act by inhibiting osteoclast activity on newly formed bone resorption surfaces, which reduces the number of sites where bone is remodeled. Bone formation then exceeds bone resorption at these remodeling sites, which gradually increases bone mass. May also inhibit bone dissolution by binding to hydroxyapatite crystals, which are composed of calcium, phosphate, and hydroxide and give bone its rigid structure.

Contraindications

Esophageal abnormalities that delay esophageal emptying, such as achalasia or stricture; hypersensitivity to alendronate or its components; hypocalcemia; inability to sit upright or stand for at least 30 min

Interactions

DRUGS

antacids, calcium, iron, multivalent cations: Decreased absorption of alendronate

aspirin: Increased risk of GI distress

levothyroxine: Possibly slight decrease in bioavailability of alendronate

FOODS

any food: Delayed absorption and decreased serum level of alendronate

Adverse Reactions

CNS: Asthenia, dizziness, headache, vertigo

CV: Peripheral edema

EENT: Cholesteatoma of external auditory canal

GI: Abdominal distention and pain, constipation, diarrhea, dysphagia, **esophageal perforation** or ulceration, esophagitis, flatulence, gastritis, gastroesophageal reflux disease, heartburn, indigestion, **melena**, nausea, vomiting

MS: Arthralgia; femoral shaft or subtrochanteric fractures; focal osteomalacia; jaw osteonecrosis; joint swelling; muscle spasms; myalgia; severe bone, joint, and/or muscle pain

RESP: **Asthma exacerbation**

SKIN: Photosensitivity, pruritus, rash, **Stevens-Johnson syndrome**, **toxic epidermal necrolysis**

Other: **Anaphylaxis**, **hypocalcemia**

Childbearing Considerations

PREGNANCY

- It is not known if drug can cause fetal harm.
- Drug should be discontinued as soon as pregnancy is known.
- Know that there is a theoretical risk of fetal harm, especially skeletal, if a woman becomes pregnant after completing a course of bisphosphonate therapy. Time between cessation of drug therapy to conception, the particular bisphosphonate used, and route of administration causing fetal harm is unknown.

LACTATION

- It is not known if drug is present in breast milk.
- Mothers should check with prescriber before breastfeeding.

Nursing Considerations

- Know that alendronate should not be administered to patients who have esophageal disorders, hypocalcemia, or are unable to sit upright or stand for at least 30 minutes.
- Monitor patient's serum calcium level before, during, and after treatment. Expect hypocalcemia to be treated before alendronate therapy begins. If hypocalcemia occurs during therapy, expect prescriber to order a calcium supplement.
- Ensure adequate dietary intake of calcium and vitamin D before, during, and after treatment.

! **WARNING** Monitor patient for a hypersensitivity reaction, which could become life-threatening such as anaphylaxis. If present, notify prescriber, expect drug to be discontinued, and provide supportive care, as needed and ordered.

! **WARNING** Monitor patient closely, as alendronate may irritate upper GI mucosa causing esophageal ulceration, which could lead to hemorrhage.

- Be aware that oral osteoporosis drugs such as alendronate may have the potential to increase the risk of esophageal cancer. While studies are underway to determine this potential, assess patient regularly for chest pain, difficulty or painful swallowing, or new or worsening heartburn; notify prescriber if present.
- Monitor patient for jaw pain because alendronate may cause osteonecrosis of the jaw, with risk increasing as therapy duration becomes longer. Patients at increased risk include those who have poor oral hygiene, preexisting dental or periodontal disease, require an invasive dental procedure, or wear ill-fitting dentures. Patients are also at increased risk if they have a cancer diagnosis, concomitant therapy such as chemotherapy or corticosteroid therapy, or other illnesses, such as anemia, coagulopathy, infection or preexisting dental or periodontal disease.

PATIENT TEACHING

- Advise patient how to take the form of alendronate prescribed.
- Teach patient to remain upright for 30 minutes after taking alendronate and until she has eaten the first food of the day.
- Inform patient receiving the effervescent tablet form to be aware that each tablet contains 650 mg sodium, which is equivalent to approximately 1,650 mg of salt (sodium chloride) per tablet.
- Encourage patient to consume adequate daily amounts of calcium and vitamin D.

! **WARNING** Alert patient that drug may cause an allergic reaction that could become quite serious. Tell patient to notify prescriber, if present, and to seek immediate medical care, if serious.

! **WARNING** Instruct patient to report any chest pain, difficulty swallowing or pain when swallowing, or new or worsening heartburn to prescriber.

- Instruct patient to report to prescriber any new or unusual pain in hip or thigh.
- Tell patient to inform dentist of alendronate therapy prior to dental work and to notify dentist of delayed healing or any signs of infection after an extraction.
- Warn females of childbearing age to notify prescriber if pregnancy occurs.

aliskiren hemifumarate

Rasilez (CAN), Tekturna

Class and Category

Pharmacologic class: Direct renin inhibitor
Therapeutic class: Antihypertensive

Indications and Dosages

* *To treat hypertension*

TABLETS

Adults and children ages 6 to 17 weighing 50 kg (110 lb) or more. 150 mg once daily, increased to 300 mg once daily, as needed.

Drug Administration

P.O.

- Avoid giving drug with a high-fat meal, as effectiveness may be reduced.
- Drug should be given at same time every day.

Route	Onset	Peak	Duration
P.O.	Unknown	1–3 hr	Unknown

Half-life: 24 hr

Mechanism of Action

Inhibits renin secreted by the kidneys in response to decreased blood volume and renal perfusion. Renin cleaves angiotensinogen to form angiotensin I, which is converted to angiotensin II by ACE and non-ACE pathways. Angiotensin II is a powerful vasoconstrictor that induces release of catecholamines from the adrenal medulla and prejunctional nerve endings. It also promotes aldosterone secretion and sodium reabsorption. Together, these actions increase blood pressure. By inhibiting renin release, aliskiren impairs the renin–angiotensin–aldosterone system. Without the vasoconstrictive effect of angiotensin II, blood pressure decreases.

Contraindications

Children under the age of 2, hypersensitivity to aliskiren or its components, presence of diabetes and concurrent ACE inhibitor or angiotensin receptor blocker (ARB) therapy, pregnancy

Interactions

DRUGS

ACE inhibitors, ARBs: Increased risk of hyperkalemia, hypotension, or renal dysfunction, especially in the elderly and patients who are volume-depleted or already have renal impairment
atorvastatin, cyclosporine, itraconazole, ketoconazole, verapamil: Increased aliskiren blood level
furosemide: Decreased blood furosemide levels
irbesartan: Decreased blood aliskiren level
NSAIDs: Increased risk of decreased renal function and hypotension
P-glycoprotein: Possible alteration in absorption and disposition of aliskiren at P-gp site
potassium-sparing diuretics, potassium supplements: Increased risk of hyperkalemia

FOODS

high-fat food: Decreased aliskiren absorption substantially

Adverse Reactions

CNS: Dizziness, fatigue, headache, **seizures**
CV: **Hypotension**, peripheral edema
EENT: Nasopharyngitis
GI: Abdominal pain, diarrhea, dyspepsia, elevated liver enzymes, gastroesophageal reflux, **hepatic dysfunction**, nausea, vomiting
GU: Elevated blood creatinine, renal calculi
HEME: Decreased hemoglobin and hematocrit
MS: Back pain
RESP: Increased cough, upper respiratory tract infection
SKIN: Erythema, pruritus, rash, **Stevens-Johnson syndrome**, **toxic epidermal necrolysis**, urticaria
Other: **Anaphylaxis**, **angioedema**, elevated creatine kinase or uric acid level, gout, **hyperkalemia**, **hyponatremia**

Childbearing Considerations

PREGNANCY

- Drug can cause fetal harm, especially if exposure occurs during the second or third trimester.
- Drug reduces fetal renal function, leading to anuria and renal failure, and increases fetal and neonatal morbidity and death. It can also cause fetal lung hypoplasia, hypotension, and skeletal deformations such as skull hypoplasia.
- Drug is contraindicated in pregnant women and should be discontinued as soon as possible when pregnancy occurs.

LACTATION

- It is not known if drug is present in breast milk.
- Drug is not recommended for use in breastfeeding mothers, to avoid potential serious adverse reactions, including hyperkalemia, hypotension, and renal impairment in the breastfed infant.

Nursing Considerations

- Be aware that aliskiren should not be used in patients with diabetes who are concurrently taking ACE inhibitors or ARBs because of the increased risk of serious adverse effects such as renal dysfunction, hyperkalemia, hypotension, and renal dysfunction. Also, know that aliskiren should not be given to patients with moderate renal impairment (glomerular filtration rate of less than 60 ml/min) who are also receiving ACE inhibitor or ARB therapy because renal impairment may worsen.

- Monitor patient's renal function closely, especially in patients receiving drugs such as ACE inhibitors, ARBs, NSAIDs, potassium-sparing diuretics, or potassium supplements that affect the renin–angiotensin system. Use aliskiren cautiously in patients whose renal function may depend in part on the activity of this system such as those with post MI, renal artery stenosis, or severe heart failure or who are elderly or experiencing volume depletion because aliskiren therapy increases the risk of renal dysfunction in these patients that could lead to acute renal failure.
- Take measures to correct volume or salt depletion from high-dose diuretic therapy before starting aliskiren, as ordered, to prevent hypotension. If hypotension occurs during aliskiren therapy, place patient in a supine position and give 0.9% Sodium Chloride solution intravenously, as needed and prescribed.

! WARNING Monitor patient for a hypersensitivity reaction, which could become life-threatening such as anaphylaxis or angioedema. If present, notify prescriber, expect drug to be discontinued, and provide supportive care, as needed and ordered. Be aware that patient shouldn't receive aliskiren again.

- Monitor serum electrolytes, especially potassium levels, as ordered in patients who already are experiencing renal insufficiency or who have diabetes because of increased risk for hyperkalemia in the presence of aliskiren therapy. Also, monitor patients who are taking ACE inhibitors, ARBs, or NSAIDs along with aliskiren because of increased risk of hyperkalemia.
- Monitor blood pressure regularly to determine effectiveness of the drug.

PATIENT TEACHING

- Advise patient to avoid high-fat meals while taking aliskiren because fat decreases drug absorption significantly.

! WARNING Alert patient that drug may cause an allergic reaction that could become serious. Tell patient to notify prescriber, if present, and to seek immediate medical care if serious.

- Explain that decreased blood pressure could lead to light-headedness, especially in the first few days of therapy. Advise patient to change positions slowly and, if light-headedness persists or fainting occurs, to notify prescriber. Explain that light-headedness and fainting could also result from dehydration caused by excessive perspiration, diarrhea, inadequate fluid intake, or vomiting. Instruct patient on how to prevent dehydration.
- Instruct patient to avoid using potassium supplements or potassium salt substitutes while taking aliskiren.
- Advise patient to inform all prescribers about aliskiren therapy as well as any ACE inhibitor or angiotensin receptor blockers therapy patient may be taking.
- Instruct females of childbearing age to notify prescriber immediately if she is pregnant because drug will have to be discontinued and another antihypertensive chosen.
- Inform mothers that breastfeeding is not recommended while taking aliskiren, as drug can cause high potassium level, kidney impairment, and low blood pressure in a nursing infant.

allopurinol

Purinol (CAN), Zyloprim

allopurinol sodium

Aloprim

Class and Category

Pharmacological class: Xanthine oxidase inhibitor
Therapeutic class: Antigout

Indications and Dosages

∗ *To treat primary gout and hyperuricemia*

TABLETS

Adults. *For mild gout:* 200 to 300 mg daily. *For moderately severe tophaceous gout:* 400 to 600 mg daily. Dosages above 300 mg daily given in divided doses. *Minimum:* 100 to 200 mg daily. *Maximum:* 800 mg daily.

✱ *To reduce flare-up of acute gouty attacks*

TABLETS

Adults. 100 mg daily, increased by 100 mg/wk until serum uric acid level is 6 mg/dl or less.

✱ *To prevent uric acid nephropathy in patients with leukemia, lymphoma, and other malignancies such as solid tumors who are receiving chemotherapy that causes elevations of serum and urinary uric acid levels*

TABLETS

Adults. 300 to 800 mg daily for 2 to 3 days, then adjusted to keep serum uric acid level within normal limits.

Children ages 6 to 10. 300 mg daily, adjusted after 48 hr, depending on response to treatment.

Children under age 6. 150 mg daily, adjusted after 48 hr, depending on response to treatment.

I.V. INFUSION

Adults. 200 to 400 mg/m^2 daily as a single infusion or in equally divided doses every 6, 8, or 12 hr beginning 24 to 48 hr before initiation of chemotherapy. *Maximum:* 600 mg daily.

Children. *Initial:* 200 mg/m^2 daily as a single infusion or in equally divided doses every 6, 8, or 12 hr beginning 24 to 48 hr before initiation of chemotherapy. Dosage then titrated according to uric acid levels. *Maximum:* 400 mg daily.

✱ *To treat recurrent calcium oxalate calculi*

TABLETS

Adults. 200 to 300 mg daily as a single dose or in divided doses, adjusted based on 24-hr urine urate level.

± **DOSAGE ADJUSTMENT** For adult patients with impaired renal function with gout, dosage adjusted according to eGFR as follows: between 30 and 60 ml/min, dosage reduced to 50 mg daily; between 15 to 30 ml/min, dosage reduced to 50 mg and given every other day; between 5 to15 ml/min, dosage reduced to 50 mg and given twice weekly; and if less than 5 ml/min, dosage reduced to 50 mg and given once weekly. For adult patients with impaired renal function associated with cancer therapy, dosage adjusted to 200 mg daily if eGFR is 10 to 20 ml/min, 100 mg daily if eGFR is less than 10 ml/min, or 50 mg every 12 hours or 100 mg every 24 hours if patient is on dialysis.

Drug Administration

P.O.

- Drug better tolerated if given after meals.

I.V.

- Administer 24 to 48 hr before chemotherapy, if possible.
- Reconstitute each 30-ml vial with 25 ml of Sterile Water for Injection. Solution should appear clear, almost colorless with no more than a slight opalescence. Further dilute to desired concentration, but no greater than 6 mg/ml, with 0.9% Sodium Chloride Injection or 5% Dextrose in Water for Injection.
- Infuse at a rate based on the volume of the infusion solution.
- If not used immediately, diluted solution may be stored for up to 10 hr but storage time must include time that will be used to give infusion. Store only at room temperature that does not exceed 25°C (77°F).
- *Incompatibilities:* Amikacin sulfate, amphotericin B, carmustine, cefotaxime sodium, chlorpromazine hydrochloride, cimetidine hydrochloride, clindamycin phosphate, cytarabine, dacarbazine, daunorubicin hydrochloride, diphenhydramine hydrochloride, doxorubicin hydrochloride, doxycycline hyclate, droperidol, floxuridine, gentamicin sulfate, haloperidol lactate, hydroxyzine hydrochloride, idarubicin hydrochloride, imipenem-cilastatin sodium, mechlorethamine hydrochloride, meperidine hydrochloride, metoclopramide hydrochloride, methylprednisolone sodium succinate, minocycline hydrochloride, nalbuphine hydrochloride, netilmicin sulfate, ondansetron hydrochloride, prochlorperazine edisylate, promethazine hydrochloride, sodium bicarbonate, streptozocin, tobramycin sulfate, vinorelbine tartrate

Route	Onset	Peak	Duration
P.O.	Unknown	1.5 hr	1–2 wk
I.V.	Unknown	30 min	Unknown

Half-life: 1–2 hr

Mechanism of Action

Inhibits uric acid production by inhibiting xanthine oxidase, the enzyme that converts hypoxanthine and xanthine to uric acid. Allopurinol is metabolized to oxipurinol, which also inhibits xanthine oxidase.

Contraindications

Hypersensitivity to allopurinol or its components

Interactions

DRUGS

ACE inhibitors: Increased risk of hypersensitivity reactions
amoxicillin, ampicillin: Increased risk of rash
azathioprine, mercaptopurine: Increased plasma levels of these drugs with increased risk of toxicity
chlorpropamide: Increased risk of hypoglycemia in patients with renal insufficiency
cyclophosphamide, other cytotoxic drugs: Enhanced bone marrow suppression
dicumarol: Increased half-life and anticoagulant action of dicumarol
thiazide diuretics: Possibly increased risk of allopurinol toxicity
uricosuric agents: Increased urinary excretion of uric acid

Adverse Reactions

CNS: Chills, drowsiness, fever, headache, neuritis, paresthesia, peripheral neuropathy, somnolence
CV: Vasculitis
EENT: Epistaxis, loss of taste
GI: Abdominal pain, diarrhea, dysphagia, elevated liver enzymes, gastritis, **granulomatous hepatitis**, hepatic necrosis, hepatomegaly, **hepatotoxicity**, jaundice, nausea, vomiting
GU: Exacerbated renal calculi, **renal failure or impairment**
HEME: **Agranulocytosis**, anemia, **aplastic anemia, bone marrow depression**, eosinophilia, leukocytosis, **leukopenia**, **thrombocytopenia**
MS: Arthralgia, exacerbation of gout, myopathy
SKIN: Alopecia; ecchymosis; **exfoliative rash**; maculopapular, purpuric or scaly **rash**; pruritus; **Stevens-Johnson syndrome (SJS)**; **toxic epidermal necrolysis (TEN)**; urticaria
Other: **Drug hypersensitivity syndrome (DHA), drug reaction with eosinophilia and systemic symptoms (DRESS)**

Childbearing Considerations

PREGNANCY

- Drug may cause fetal harm.
- Use with caution only if benefit to mother outweighs potential risk to fetus.

LACTATION

- Drug is present in breast milk.
- Mothers should not breastfeed during drug therapy and for 1 wk after last dose.

Nursing Considerations

- Be aware allopurinol is not recommended for patients with HLA-B*58:01 allele, which is a genetic marker for severe skin hypersensitivity reactions to allopurinol. The frequency is higher in patients of African, Asian (e.g., Han Chinese, Korean, Thai), and Native Hawaiian/Pacific Islander ancestry.
- Obtain baseline CBC and uric acid level, as ordered, before and during allopurinol therapy. Cytopenias have occurred as early as 6 weeks and as late as 6 years after the start of allopurinol therapy. Concurrent therapy with drugs associated with myelosuppression increases risk. In these patients, expect CBC evaluation to be done more frequently. Expect allopurinol to be discontinued if cytopenias occur during therapy.
- Monitor BUN and serum creatinine at least daily during early allopurinol administration. Monitor patient for signs and symptoms of renal impairment, especially in patients with a history of kidney stones or renal dysfunction. This is because formation of xanthine calculi or precipitation or urates in patients receiving concomitant uricosuric agents may cause or worsen renal impairment. Maintain a fluid intake to produce a daily urinary output of 2 liters daily. Also, vitamin C should not be given to patient because the pH of urine should be kept neutral to slightly alkaline. Expect dosage to be adjusted if renal impairment occurs.

! **WARNING** Monitor patient for a rash, which may be the first sign of a hypersensitivity reaction that may precede a life-threatening reaction such as DRESS, SJS, or TEN. A skin rash may occur 1 week or more after allopurinol therapy is initiated.

Patients at increased risk include those who are receiving amoxicillin, ampicillin, bendamustine, or thiazide diuretics concurrently. In addition, patients with decreased renal function receiving diuretics concurrently are at greater risk. If present, notify prescriber immediately. Expect drug to be discontinued.

- Monitor patients for hepatotoxicity (anorexia, pruritus, weight loss). If symptoms are present, obtain an order for liver enzymes. If patient has preexisting liver disease, expect to monitor liver enzymes periodically during the early treatment with allopurinol. If liver enzymes become elevated, notify prescriber and expect drug to be discontinued.

PATIENT TEACHING

- Advise patient how to take oral form of drug.
- Stress importance of drinking enough water (8 to 10 full glasses) to produce a daily urinary output of at least 2 liters.
- Inform patient that acute gout attacks may occur more often early in allopurinol treatment and that effectiveness of the drug may not be noticeable for 2 weeks or longer.

! **WARNING** Tell patient to notify prescriber immediately if a rash develops and to stop taking drug until the rash is evaluated.

- Instruct patient to report persistent, severe, or unusual signs and symptoms.
- Instruct patient not to drive or perform hazardous tasks because drug may cause drowsiness.
- Urge patient not to take allopurinol with alcohol or other CNS depressants.
- Warn females of childbearing age that drug may cause harm to fetus. Encourage reporting known or suspected pregnancy to prescriber.
- Alert mothers that breastfeeding should not be done during allopurinol therapy and for 1 week after last dose.

almotriptan malate

Class and Category

Pharmacologic class: Selective serotonin receptor agonist (5-HT_1)

Therapeutic class: Antimigraine drug

Indications and Dosages

∗ *To treat acute migraine in adults with history of migraine and in adolescents with history of migraine usually lasting more than 4 hr when untreated*

TABLETS

Adults and adolescents ages 12 to 17. *Initial:* 6.25 or 12.5 mg as a single dose, repeated in 2 hr, as needed. *Maximum:* 25 mg/24 hr or 4 migraine treatments/mo.

± **DOSAGE ADJUSTMENT** For patients with impaired hepatic or renal function or patients receiving potent CYP3A4 inhibitors such as ketoconazole, initial dose reduced to 6.25 mg with maximum daily dose of 12.5 mg.

Drug Administration

P.O.

- Expect to give first dose of almotriptan in a medical facility for patients with risk factors for coronary artery disease (CAD) but no known cardiovascular abnormalities.
- Obtain an ECG immediately after first dose of almotriptan, as ordered, in patients with risk factors for CAD because cardiac ischemia can occur without causing clinical symptoms.
- Repeat dose after 2 hr if patient's migraine continues. Do not administer more than 4 doses in a 30-day period.

Route	Onset	Peak	Duration
P.O.	Rapid	1–3 hr	Unknown

Half-life: 3–4 hr

Mechanism of Action

May stimulate 5-HT_1 receptors on intracranial blood vessels and sensory nerves in trigeminal vascular system. By activating these receptors, almotriptan selectively constricts dilated and inflamed cranial blood vessels and inhibits production of proinflammatory neuropeptides. It also interrupts transmission of pain signals to the brain.

Contraindications

Basilar or hemiplegic migraine, cerebrovascular or peripheral vascular disease, hypersensitivity to almotriptan or its components, hypertension (uncontrolled), ischemic or vasospastic coronary artery disease (CAD), use within 24 hr of ergotamine-containing or ergot-type drugs or other serotonin receptor agonists

Interactions

DRUGS

ergotamine-containing drugs: Prolonged vasospastic reactions
erythromycin, itraconazole, ketoconazole, MAO inhibitors, ritonavir, verapamil: Possibly increased blood almotriptan level
selective serotonin reuptake inhibitors (such as citalopram, escitalopram, fluoxetine, fluvoxamine, paroxetine, sertraline), serotonin norepinephrine reuptake inhibitors (such as duloxetine, venlafaxine): Increased risk of serotonin syndrome

Adverse Reactions

CNS: Confusion, dizziness, headache, hemiplegia, hypoesthesia, malaise, paresthesia, restlessness, **seizures**, **serotonin syndrome**, somnolence, syncope, vertigo
CV: Angina pectoris, **coronary artery vasospasm**, hypertension, **ischemia**, **MI**, palpitations, tachycardia, vasodilation, **ventricular fibrillation or tachycardia**
EENT: Blepharospasm, dry mouth, oral hypoesthesia, swollen tongue, visual impairment
GI: Abdominal pain or discomfort, colitis, nausea
MS: Arthralgia, extremity coldness or pain, myalgia
SKIN: Cold sweat, diaphoresis, erythema
Other: **Anaphylaxis**, **angioedema**

Childbearing Considerations

PREGNANCY

- It is not known if drug can cause fetal harm.
- Use with caution only if benefit to mother outweighs potential risk to fetus.

LACTATION

- It is not known if drug is present in breast milk.
- Mothers should check with prescriber before breastfeeding.

Nursing Considerations

! **WARNING** Monitor patient with CAD for angina because almotriptan can cause coronary artery vasospasm. Also, monitor patient for abdominal pain and bloody diarrhea because drug may cause peripheral vasospastic reactions, such as ischemic bowel disease.

! **WARNING** Monitor patient for hypersensitivity reactions, especially in patients hypersensitive to sulfonamides because cross-sensitivity may occur. If patient develops signs and symptoms of anaphylaxis or angioedema, stop drug, notify prescriber, and expect to provide supportive care, as needed and ordered.

! **WARNING** Monitor patient for evidence of serotonin syndrome, such as agitation, chills, confusion, diaphoresis, diarrhea, fever, hyperactive reflexes, poor coordination, restlessness, shaking, talking or acting with uncontrolled excitement, tremor, and twitching. In its most severe form, serotonin syndrome can resemble neuroleptic malignant syndrome, which includes autonomic instability with possible fluctuations in vital signs, as well as high fever, mental status changes, and muscle rigidity.

- Monitor blood pressure regularly during therapy in patients with hypertension because almotriptan may produce a transient increase in blood pressure.
- Evaluate effectiveness of drug to relieve migraines on a regular basis.

PATIENT TEACHING

- Inform patient that almotriptan is used to treat acute migraine and that he shouldn't take it to treat nonmigraine headaches.
- Advise patient not to take more than maximum prescribed dosage, as medication overuse can cause migraine-like daily headaches or a marked increase in frequency of migraine attacks requiring detoxification to treat, which could lead to withdrawal symptoms.

! **WARNING** Instruct patient to seek emergency care immediately for signs of hypersensitivity such as breathing difficulties, itching, or a rash; cardiac symptoms (such as heaviness, pain, pressure or tightness in chest, jaw, neck, or throat); or if multiple new symptoms develop (such as diarrhea, high fever, incoordination, mental changes, nausea, vomiting) after taking the drug.

- Caution patient that drug may cause adverse CNS reactions and advise him to avoid hazardous activities until he knows how drug affects him.
- Advise patient to consult prescriber before taking any over-the-counter or prescription drugs.

alogliptin benzoate

Nesina

Class and Category

Pharmacologic class: Dipeptidyl peptidase-4 (DPP-4) inhibitor
Therapeutic class: Oral antidiabetic

Indications and Dosages

✱ *As adjunct to diet and exercise to achieve control of glucose levels in type 2 diabetes mellitus as monotherapy or in conjunction with combination therapy*

TABLETS

Adults. 25 mg once daily.

±**DOSAGE ADJUSTMENT** For patients with moderate renal impairment (creatinine clearance less than 60 ml/min but equal to or greater than 30 ml/min), dosage decreased to 12.5 mg once daily. For patients with severe renal impairment (creatinine clearance less than 30 ml/min but equal to or greater than 15 ml/min) or patients with end-stage renal disease or who are on hemodialysis, dosage decreased to 6.25 mg once daily.

Drug Administration

P.O.

- Administer drug at about the same time every day.

Route	Onset	Peak	Duration
P.O.	Unknown	1–2 hr	Unknown

Half-life: 21 hr

Mechanism of Action

Inhibits the dipeptidyl peptidase-4 enzyme to slow inactivation of incretin hormones. These hormones are released by the intestine in response to a meal. When blood glucose level is increased, incretin hormones increase insulin synthesis and release from pancreatic beta cells. One type of incretin hormone, glucagon-like peptide (GLP-1), also lowers glucagon secretion from pancreatic alpha cells, which reduces hepatic glucose production. These combined actions decrease blood glucose level in type 2 diabetes.

Contraindications

Diabetic ketoacidosis; hypersensitivity to alogliptin or its components, including anaphylaxis, angioedema, or severe cutaneous adverse reactions; type 1 diabetes

Interactions

DRUGS

insulin, sulfonylureas: Possibly increased risk of hypoglycemia

Adverse Reactions

CNS: Headache
CV: **Heart failure**
EENT: Nasopharyngitis
ENDO: **Hypoglycemia**
GI: **Acute pancreatitis**, constipation, diarrhea, elevated liver enzymes, **fulminant hepatic failure**, ileus, nausea
GU: Tubulointerstitial nephritis
MS: Arthralgia (disabling and severe), joint pain (severe), **rhabdomyolysis**
RESP: Upper respiratory tract infection
SKIN: Bullous pemphigoid, rash, **Stevens-Johnson syndrome**, urticaria
Other: **Anaphylaxis and other hypersensitivity reactions**, **angioedema**, serum sickness

Childbearing Considerations

PREGNANCY

- It is not known if drug can cause fetal harm.
- Use with caution only if benefit to mother outweighs potential risk to fetus.

LACTATION

- It is not known if drug is present in breast milk.
- Mothers should check with prescriber before breastfeeding.

Nursing Considerations

- Use alogliptin cautiously in patients with a history of angioedema to another drug in the same class because it is not known if patient will be predisposed to angioedema with alogliptin therapy.
- Determine patient's history for heart failure because drug may increase risk for heart

failure. Monitor patient closely throughout drug therapy.

- Assess patient's history for renal dysfunction and check renal function before starting alogliptin therapy, as ordered, because dosage may need to be adjusted. Monitor renal function, as ordered, throughout drug therapy for evidence of dysfunction.
- Assess patient's liver function before starting alogliptin therapy. If abnormalities are present, monitor patient closely for signs and symptoms of liver dysfunction. If patient develops anorexia, dark urine, fatigue, jaundice, or right upper abdominal discomfort during therapy, notify prescriber and expect liver enzymes to be assessed. If elevated, expect drug to be discontinued.

! **WARNING** Monitor patient for serious hypersensitivity reactions, including severe cutaneous adverse reactions. If present, notify prescriber, expect alogliptin to be discontinued, and provide supportive care, as needed and ordered.

! **WARNING** Monitor patient for signs and symptoms of acute pancreatitis, such as acute upper abdominal pain, fever, nausea, and vomiting. If suspected, notify prescriber and expect alogliptin to be discontinued, if confirmed.

- Monitor patient also receiving insulin or insulin secretagogues, such as sulfonylureas, for hypoglycemia. Follow protocol for treating hypoglycemia if it occurs. Notify prescriber if hypoglycemia occurs and expect dosage of insulin or insulin secretagogue to be reduced.
- Check patient's blood glucose level and hemoglobin A1C, as ordered, to determine effectiveness of alogliptin therapy.

PATIENT TEACHING

- Emphasize the need to follow an exercise program and a diet control program during alogliptin therapy. Tell patient to take drug at about the same time every day.
- Teach patient how to monitor blood glucose level and when to report changes.

! **WARNING** Advise patient to notify prescriber immediately if skin reactions such as blisters, erosions, hives, rash or other cutaneous abnormalities occur. Also, instruct patient to seek immediate medical care if difficulty breathing or swallowing occurs or swelling of face, throat, or tongue is present.

! **WARNING** Instruct patient to stop taking alogliptin and to report persistent severe abdominal pain, possibly radiating to the back, that may or may not be accompanied by vomiting. Also, instruct patient to notify prescriber if anorexia, fatigue, nausea, vomiting, or yellowing of skin or whites of the eye occurs.

! **WARNING** Review signs and symptoms of heart failure with patient and instruct her to notify prescriber immediately if present.

- Caution patient that taking other drugs used to decrease blood glucose level may lead to hypoglycemia. Review signs and symptoms and appropriate treatment.
- Alert patient that if severe joint pain occurs, he should notify prescriber as alogliptin may have to be discontinued.
- Instruct patient to contact prescriber if he develops other illnesses, such as infection, or experiences surgery or trauma because his diabetes medication may need adjustment.
- Inform patient that periodic blood tests will be done to determine effectiveness of drug.

alprazolam

Alprazolam Intensol, Apo-Alpraz (CAN), Xanax, Xanax TS (CAN), Xanax XR

Class, Category, and Schedule

Pharmacologic class: Benzodiazepine
Therapeutic class: Anxiolytic, antipanic
Controlled substance schedule: IV

Indications and Dosages

✱ *To treat generalized anxiety disorder*

ORAL SOLUTION, ORALLY DISINTEGRATING TABLETS, TABLETS

Adults. *Initial:* 0.25 to 0.5 mg 3 times daily and increased, as needed, every 3 to 4 days. *Maximum:* 4 mg daily in divided doses.

✱ *To treat panic disorder*

ORAL SOLUTION, ORALLY DISINTEGRATING TABLETS, TABLETS

Adults. *Initial:* 0.5 mg 3 times daily, increased every 3 to 4 days by no more than 1 mg daily, based on patient response. *Maximum:* 10 mg in equally divided doses 3 or 4 times daily.

E.R. TABLETS

Adults. *Initial:* 0.5 to 1 mg daily, increased every 3 to 4 days by no more than 1 mg daily, based on patient response. *Usual:* 3 to 6 mg once daily. *Maximum:* 10 mg daily as single dose.

±**DOSAGE ADJUSTMENT** For debilitated or elderly patients or patients with advanced hepatic disease taking immediate-release form, initial dosage decreased to 0.25 mg twice daily or 3 times daily and increased gradually, as needed and tolerated; initial dose of extended-release form kept at 0.5 mg daily, then gradually increased, as needed. For patients starting ritonavir therapy, dosage decreased by 50%, then dosage increased to target dose after 10 to 14 days (immediate-release form) or gradually (extended-release form), as needed.

Drug Administration

P.O.

- Use dry, gloved hands to remove orally disintegrating tablet from bottle just prior to administration. Have patient immediately place tablet on top of the tongue to dissolve. There is no need for patient to drink a liquid beverage after taking this form of drug.
- Use calibrated dropper provided with drug to measure dosage of oral solution. Administer oral solution with either a beverage or semisolid food such as applesauce or pudding. Give drug immediately after mixing.
- Do not break, crush, or split extended-release tablet.
- Administer extended-release tablets in morning.
- Dosage should be reduced slowly when drug is discontinued because of potential dependency.

Route	Onset	Peak	Duration
P.O.	15–30 min	1.5 hr	6 hr
P.O. (E.R.)	Unknown	1.6 hr	11.3 hr

Half-life: 6.3–26.9 hr

Mechanism of Action

May increase effects of gamma-aminobutyric acid (GABA) and other inhibitory neurotransmitters by binding to specific benzodiazepine receptors in cortical and limbic areas of the CNS. GABA inhibits excitatory stimulation, which helps control emotional behavior. The limbic system contains many benzodiazepine receptors, which may help explain drug's antianxiety effects.

Contraindications

Acute angle-closure glaucoma; hypersensitivity to alprazolam, other benzodiazepines, or their components; strong CYP3A inhibitors (except for ritonavir) such as itraconazole or ketoconazole

Interactions

DRUGS

anticonvulsants; antidepressants; antihistamines; other benzodiazepines, CNS depressants, psychotropics: Possibly increased CNS depressant effects

CYP3A inducers such as carbamazepine, phenytoin: Decreased plasma level of alprazolam and potential decreased effectiveness

CYP3A inhibitors (except for ritonavir) such as itraconazole, ketoconazole: Possibly profound effect on clearance of alprazolam, causing elevated concentrations of alprazolam and increased risk of adverse reactions

digoxin: Possibly increased serum digoxin level, causing digitalis toxicity

opioids: Increased risk of significant respiratory depression

ritonavir: Administration for less than 14 days possibly increases alprazolam exposure

ACTIVITIES

alcohol use: Enhanced adverse CNS effects of alprazolam; increased risk of significant sedation and somnolence, especially if combined with an opioid

Adverse Reactions

CNS: Abnormal involuntary movements, agitation, akathisia, anxiety, confusion, cognitive disorder, depersonalization, depression, derealization, disinhibition, dizziness, drowsiness, fatigue, hallucinations, headache, hypomania, insomnia, irritability, lack of coordination, light-headedness, mania, memory loss, muscle twitching, nervousness, paresthesia, rigidity, sedation, **seizures**, speech problems, **suicidal ideation**, syncope, talkativeness, tremor, weakness

CV: Chest pain, edema, **hypotension**, nonspecific ECG changes, palpitations, peripheral edema, tachycardia
EENT: Altered salivation or taste, blurred vision, diplopia, dry mouth, nasal congestion, tinnitus
ENDO: Galactorrhea, gynecomastia, hyperprolactinemia
GI: Abdominal discomfort, anorexia, constipation, diarrhea, elevated bilirubin or liver enzymes, **hepatic failure**, **hepatitis**, jaundice, nausea, vomiting
GU: Altered libido, incontinence, menstrual disorders, urinary hesitancy
MS: Dysarthria, muscle rigidity and spasms
RESP: **Apnea**, **hypoventilation**, **respiratory depression**, upper respiratory tract infection
SKIN: Dermatitis, diaphoresis, photosensitivity, pruritus, rash, **Stevens-Johnson syndrome**
Other: **Angioedema**, physical and psychological dependence, protracted withdrawal syndrome, weight gain or loss

Childbearing Considerations

PREGNANCY

- Pregnancy exposure registry: 1-866-961-2388 or https://womensmentalhealth.org/clinical-and-research-programs/pregnancyregistry/othermedications/.
- Drug can potentially cause fetal harm, During late in pregnancy, neonatal sedation (respiratory depression, hypotonia, lethargy) and/or withdrawal symptoms (feeding difficulties, hyperreflexia, inconsolable crying, irritability, restlessness, tremors) may occur at birth.
- Use with caution only if benefit to mother outweighs potential risk to fetus.

LABOR AND DELIVERY

- Drug has no established use during labor and delivery.

LACTATION

- Drug is present in breast milk.
- A decision should be made to discontinue breastfeeding or the drug to avoid potential adverse reactions in the breastfed infant.

Nursing Considerations

! **WARNING** Use cautiously in patients with underlying hepatic dysfunction because alprazolam may cause severe liver dysfunction. Monitor liver enzymes, as ordered and notify prescriber if patient exhibits any signs and symptoms of liver dysfunction.

! **WARNING** Be aware that opioid therapy should only be used concomitantly with alprazolam in patients for whom other treatment options are inadequate. If prescribed together, expect dosing and duration of the opioid to be limited. Monitor patient closely for signs and symptoms of decrease in consciousness, including coma; profound sedation; and significant respiratory depression. If present, notify prescriber immediately and provide emergency supportive care, as death may occur.

! **WARNING** Monitor patient for signs and symptoms of hypersensitivity reactions such as angioedema. If present, notify prescriber, withhold drug, and provide supportive care, as needed and ordered.

! **WARNING** Monitor patient with impaired respiratory function closely because severe pulmonary dysfunction may occur. Notify prescriber immediately if apnea, hypoventilation, or respiratory depression occurs and provide supportive care.

! **WARNING** Monitor patient closely if depression occurs because of the potential for episodes of hypomania, mania, and suicidal ideation.

- Be aware that alprazolam therapy can result in significant dependence even with short-term use and dosages less than 4 mg daily. Monitor patient closely. A sudden cessation of therapy can result in acute withdrawal reactions. In certain individuals, withdrawal symptoms may last for weeks to up to more than 12 months. Notify prescriber if physical and psychological dependence is suspected.

PATIENT TEACHING

- Instruct patient how to take form of drug prescribed.
- Instruct patient never to increase prescribed dose or increase frequency because of risk of dependency.
- Warn against stopping drug abruptly because withdrawal symptoms may occur.

! **WARNING** Warn patient not to consume alcohol or take an opioid during alprazolam treatment without prescriber knowledge, as severe respiratory depression can occur and may lead to death. Instruct patient to inform all prescribers of alprazolam use, especially if pain medication may be prescribed.

! **WARNING** Alert patient that drug may cause an allergic reaction. If an allergic reaction occurs, tell patient to notify prescriber. If reaction is severe, stress importance of seeking immediate medical care.

! **WARNING** Tell family or caregiver to watch patient for changes in behavior or thoughts and to notify prescriber if any occurs, especially suicidal behavior or thoughts.

- Advise patient to avoid activities that require alertness such as driving until alprazolam's effects are known.
- Instruct females of childbearing age to notify prescriber immediately if she is or becomes pregnant as drug may cause sedation or withdrawal in neonate at birth.
- Inform mothers that breastfeeding should not be undertaken during alprazolam therapy because of risk of adverse reactions in the breastfed infant.

alteplase

(tissue plasminogen activator, recombinant)

Activase, Activase rt-PA (CAN), Cathflo Activase

Class and Category

Pharmacologic class: Tissue plasminogen activator (tPA)
Therapeutic class: Thrombolytic

Indications and Dosages

∗ *To treat acute MI for reduction of incidence of heart failure and mortality*

ACCELERATED I.V. INFUSION COMBINED WITH I.V. INJECTION

Adults weighing more than 67 kg (148 lb). 15-mg bolus given over 1 to 2 min, followed by 50 mg infused over 30 min, and then 35 mg infused over next 60 min. *Maximum:* 100 mg.
Adults weighing 67 kg (148 lb) or less. 15-mg bolus given over 1 to 2 min, followed by 0.75 mg/kg (up to 50 mg) infused over 30 min, and then, 0.5 mg/kg (up to 35 mg) infused over next 60 min. *Maximum:* 100 mg.

I.V. INJECTION COMBINED WITH 3-HOUR I.V. INFUSION

Adults weighing 65 kg (143 lb) or more. 6 to 10 mg by bolus over first 1 to 2 min, then as an infusion, 50 to 54 mg over remainder of first hr, 20 mg over second hr, and 20 mg over third hr. *Maximum:* 100 mg.
Adults weighing less than 65 kg (143 lb). 0.075 mg/kg by bolus over first 1 to 2 min, then as an infusion, 0.675 mg/kg over remainder of first hr, 0.25 mg/kg over second hr, and 0.25 mg/kg over third hr. *Maximum:* 100 mg.

∗ *To treat acute ischemic stroke within 3 hours after onset of stroke symptoms and only after computed tomography or other diagnostic imaging method excludes intracranial hemorrhage*

I.V. INFUSION COMBINED WITH I.V. INJECTION

Adults. 0.9 mg/kg infused over 60 min, with 10% of total dose given as bolus over first min. *Maximum:* 90 mg.

∗ *To treat acute massive pulmonary embolism*

I.V. INFUSION

Adults. 100 mg infused over 2 hr.

∗ *To restore function of occluded central venous access devices*

I.V. INJECTION (CATHFLO ACTIVASE)

Adults and children weighing 30 kg (66 lb) or more. 2 mg/2 ml instilled into occluded catheter; if unsuccessful, may repeat once after 2 hr.
Adults and children weighing less than 30 kg (66 lb). 110% of the lumen volume (not to exceed 2 mg/2 ml) instilled into occluded catheter; if unsuccessful, may repeat once after 2 hr.

Drug Administration

I.V.

Activase

- Know that drug may be given to treat acute ischemic stroke prior to availability of coagulation results in patients without recent use of heparin or oral anticoagulants.
- Do not use drug vial if vacuum is not present.

- Reconstitute 50-mg vial using an 18 G needle and a syringe by adding the contents of the accompanying 50-ml vial of Sterile Water for Injection. Direct the stream into the lyophilized cake in the drug vial. If slight foaming occurs, let stand undisturbed for several minutes to allow large bubbles to dissipate. Administer as reconstituted at 1 mg/ml or it can be further diluted immediately before administration in an equal volume of 0.9% Sodium Chloride Injection or 5% Dextrose Injection to yield a concentration of 0.5 mg/ml, using either polyvinyl chloride bags or glass vials. Avoid excessive agitation during dilution. Instead mix by gently swirling and/ or slow inversion.
- Reconstitute 100-mg vial using only preservative-free Sterile Water for Injection (100-ml vial) and the transfer device that comes with the drug. Remove one of the protective caps from the transfer device and insert the piercing pin vertically into the center of the stopper of the Sterile Water for Injection vial, keeping the vial upright. Remove the protective cap from the other end of the transfer device. Do not invert the vial of Sterile Water for Injection. Holding the drug vial upside down, position it so that the center of the stopper is directly over the exposed pin of the transfer device. Push drug vial down onto the transfer device, ensuring that the piercing pin is inserted through the center of the stopper. Invert the 2 vials so that the drug vial is on the bottom (upright) and the vial of Sterile Water for Injection is upside down. Allow the entire contents of the vial of Sterile Water for Injection to flow down through the transfer device into the drug vial. Remove the transfer device and the empty Sterile Water for Injection vial from the drug vial. Discard both. Mix solution with a gentle swirl. Do not shake. Know that slight foaming may occur; this is normal. Leave solution undisturbed for several min to allow any large bubbles to dissipate. Resultant solution should be colorless to pale yellow transparent looking.
- The bolus dose should be prepared by removing the appropriate volume from the vial of the reconstituted (1 mg/ml) drug using a syringe and needle. If a 50-mg vial is used, the syringe should not be primed with air and the needle should be inserted into the drug vial stopper. If the 100-mg drug vial is used, the needle should be inserted away from the puncture mark made by the transfer device. Remove the appropriate volume from a port on the infusion line after the infusion set is primed. Program an infusion pump to deliver the bolus over 1 to 2 min.
- After the bolus has been given, follow with the infusion. If using 50-mg vials, administer the infusion using either a polyvinyl chloride bag or glass vial and infusion set. If using 100-mg vials for the infusion, remove any amount of drug in excess of the dose to be given from the drug vial. Insert the spike end of an infusion set through the same puncture site created by the transfer device in the stopper of the vial of the reconstituted drug. Peel the clear plastic hanger from the vial label. Hang the drug vial from the resulting loop. Program the infusion to deliver the infusion at the rate prescribed for the condition being treated.
- Reconstituted solution should be discarded if not used within 8 hr; if further diluted, solution must be used immediately.
- Monitor I.V. infusion site. If extravasation occurs causing ecchymosis or inflammation, stop the infusion and apply local therapy. Move I.V. drug site to another location.

Cathflo Activase

- Reconstitute Cathflo Activase to a final concentration of 1 mg/ml immediately before administration.
- Withdraw 2.2 ml of Sterile Water for Injection. Do not use Bacteriostatic Water for Injection. Inject the 2.2 ml of Sterile Water for Injection into the drug vial, directing the diluent stream into the powder. Slight foaming may occur but is not unusual. Leave drug undisturbed for several minutes to allow large bubbles to dissipate.
- Mix by gently swirling contents until completely dissolved, usually within 3 min. Do not shake. Solution should be colorless to pale yellow transparent.
- Solution may be stored for up to 8 hr following reconstitution when stored at 2–30°C (36–86°F).

- Withdraw 2 mg/2 ml solution from vial and instill the dose prescribed into the occluded catheter. Do not use excessive pressure while instilling drug into catheter, to avoid rupturing the catheter or expelling a clot into the circulation. Wait 30 min and check catheter function by attempting to aspirate blood. If still occluded, expect to wait an additional 90 min before assessing again. If still occluded, expect to repeat dose.
- Once catheter function is restored, aspirate 4 to 5 ml of blood in patients weighing 10 kg (22 lb) or more or 3 ml in patients weighing less than 10 kg (22 lb) to remove the drug and residual clot, then gently irrigate the catheter with 0.9% Sodium Chloride Injection.
- *Incompatibilities:* Other drugs

Route	Onset	Peak	Duration
I.V.	Unknown	Unknown	Unknown

Half-life: <5 min

Mechanism of Action

Binds to fibrin in a thrombus and converts trapped plasminogen to plasmin. Plasmin breaks down fibrin, fibrinogen, and other clotting factors, which dissolves the thrombus.

Contraindications

For all indications: Active internal bleeding, arteriovenous malformation or aneurysm, bleeding diathesis, hypersensitivity to alteplase or its components, intracranial neoplasm, severe uncontrolled hypertension

For acute MI and pulmonary embolism only: History of stroke, intracranial or intraspinal surgery or trauma in past 3 mo

For acute ischemic stroke only: Recent head trauma, recent intracranial or intraspinal surgery or trauma in past 3 mo, recent stroke, seizure activity at onset of stroke, subarachnoid hemorrhage, suspicion or history of intracranial hemorrhage

Interactions

DRUGS

ACE inhibitors: Possible increased risk of angioedema

anticoagulants, antiplatelets, vitamin K antagonists: Increased risk of bleeding

Adverse Reactions

CNS: **Cerebral edema or herniation**, **CVA**, fever, **seizures**

CV: **Arrhythmias (including bradycardia and electromechanical dissociation)**, **cardiac arrest**, **cardiac tamponade**, **cardiogenic shock**, **cholesterol embolism**, **coronary thrombolysis**, **heart failure**, **hypotension**, mitral insufficiency, **myocardial reinfarction or rupture**, **pericardial effusion**, **pericarditis**, **venous embolism or thrombosis**

EENT: Epistaxis, gingival bleeding, **laryngeal edema**

GI: **GI bleeding**, nausea, **retroperitoneal bleeding**, vomiting

GU: **GU bleeding**

HEME: **Bleeding that may be severe**

RESP: Pleural effusion, **pulmonary edema**, **pulmonary reembolization**

SKIN: Bleeding at puncture sites, ecchymosis, rash, urticaria

Other: **Anaphylaxis**, **angioedema**

Childbearing Considerations

PREGNANCY

- It is not known if drug may cause fetal harm, but some evidence suggests the possibility exists.
- Drug should only be used in pregnant women in life-threatening situations if no other safer alternative is available, as pregnancy increases risk of bleeding.

LACTATION

- It is not known if drug is present in breast milk.
- Mothers should check with prescriber before breastfeeding, once condition has stabilized, as its effect on the breastfed infant is unknown.

Nursing Considerations

- Apply pressure at puncture site for at least 30 minutes, followed by a pressure dressing after administering alteplase.

! WARNING Know that treatment for acute ischemic stroke must begin within 3 hours after onset of stroke symptoms and only after computed tomography or other diagnostic imaging method excludes intracranial hemorrhage to avoid complications.

! WARNING Monitor continuous ECG for arrhythmias during drug therapy because alteplase therapy may cause arrhythmias from sudden reperfusion of the myocardium.

! **WARNING** Monitor patient closely for hypersensitivity reactions which may be life-threatening (angioedema, laryngeal edema, rash, shock) during alteplase administration and for several hours after infusion is completed. If hypersensitivity occurs, discontinue the alteplase infusion immediately and institute appropriate emergency interventions such as administering antihistamines, epinephrine, or intravenous corticosteroids, as prescribed.

! **WARNING** Know that the most common complication of alteplase is bleeding, including internal bleeding that could be severe and sometimes fatal, as well as external bleeding, especially at arterial and venous puncture sites. Avoid intramuscular injections and trauma to patient receiving drug. Discontinue alteplase immediately if serious bleeding occurs. Be aware that the following conditions increase risk: acute pericarditis; advanced age, especially if patient is currently receiving anticoagulant therapy; cerebrovascular disease; diabetic hemorrhagic retinopathy or other hemorrhagic ophthalmic conditions; hemostatic defects, including those secondary to severe hepatic or renal disease; hypertension (diastolic above 110 mm Hg or systolic above 175 mm Hg); pregnancy; recent GI or GU bleeding, intracranial hemorrhage, or trauma; septic thrombophlebitis or occluded AV cannula at seriously infected site; significant hepatic dysfunction; or subacute bacterial endocarditis.

- Be aware that the use of thrombolytics such as alteplase can increase the risk of thromboembolic events in patients with high risk of left heart thrombus, such as patients with atrial fibrillation or mitral stenosis. Also, know that the drug does not adequately treat underlying deep vein thrombosis in patients with a pulmonary embolism. Watch this type of patient closely for reembolization.
- Assess blood pressure and heart rate and rhythm frequently during and after therapy.
- Know that pregnancy may increase risk of bleeding. Monitor pregnant patient closely.

PATIENT TEACHING

- Tell patient how drug will be administered.
- Inform patient that pressure will be applied to the puncture site of drug administration for at least 30 minutes followed by a pressure dressing being applied.
- Reassure patient that he will be monitored closely during and after drug administration.

! **WARNING** Instruct patient to notify staff immediately if difficulty breathing occurs or a feeling of swelling in tongue and throat as well as any other hypersensitivity reactions such as itchiness.

! **WARNING** Tell patient to immediately report bleeding, including from the gums or nose. Also, stress importance of alerting staff of any persistent, severe, or unusual adverse reactions.

- Advise patient to limit physical activity during alteplase administration to reduce risk of bleeding and injury.

aluminum carbonate

Basalgel

aluminum hydroxide

Alternagel, Amphojel

Class and Category

Pharmacologic class: Aluminum salt
Therapeutic class: Antacid, phosphate binder

Indications and Dosages

* *To treat hyperacidity*

CAPSULES, ORAL SUSPENSION, TABLETS (ALUMINUM CARBONATE)

Adults. 2 capsules or tablets or 10-ml suspension every 2 hr up to 12 times daily, as needed.

ORAL SUSPENSION (ALUMINUM HYDROXIDE)

Adults. 640 mg (10 ml) up to 5 or 6 times daily after meals and at bedtime. *Maximum:* 3,840 mg (60 ml) daily.

Drug Administration

P.O.

- Have patient chew tablets thoroughly before swallowing and then have patient drink a full glass of water. Also, have patient drink a full glass of water with capsule form.
- Shake suspension well before administering and use a calibrated measuring device to measure dose.
- Administer aluminum hydroxide after meals and at bedtime.
- Don't give aluminum hydroxide within 1 to 2 hr of other oral drugs.

Route	Onset	Peak	Duration
P.O.	20 min	Unknown	20–180 min

Half-life: Unknown

Mechanism of Action

Neutralizes or reduces gastric acidity, increasing stomach and duodenal alkalinity. Protects stomach and duodenum lining by inhibiting pepsin's proteolytic activity. Binds with phosphate ions in intestine to form insoluble aluminum–phosphate compounds, which lower blood phosphate level.

Contraindications

Hypersensitivity to aluminum or its components

Interactions

DRUGS

allopurinol, chloroquine, corticosteroids, diflunisal, digoxin, ethambutol, H_2-receptor blockers, iron, isoniazid, phenothiazines, tetracyclines, thyroid hormones, ticlopidine: Decreased effects of these drugs

benzodiazepines: Increased benzodiazepine effects

Adverse Reactions

CNS: **Encephalopathy**

GI: Constipation, **intestinal obstruction**, white-speckled stool

MS: Osteomalacia, osteoporosis

Other: **Aluminum intoxication**, **electrolyte imbalances**

Childbearing Considerations

PREGNANCY

- It is not known if drug can cause fetal harm.
- Use with caution only if benefit to mother outweighs potential risk to fetus.

LACTATION

- It is not known if drug is present in breast milk.
- Mothers should check with prescriber before breastfeeding.

Nursing Considerations

- Know that two 0.6-g aluminum hydroxide tablets can neutralize 16 mEq of acid.
- Monitor patient's serum levels of phosphate, sodium, and other electrolytes, as appropriate and ordered.

! **WARNING** Monitor patient for uncommon but life-threatening adverse reactions such as aluminum intoxication, electrolyte imbalances, encephalopathy, and intestinal obstruction. If present, notify prescriber at once and provide supportive care, as needed and ordered.

PATIENT TEACHING

- Instruct patient how to take form of drug prescribed.
- Warn patient not to take maximum dosage for more than 2 weeks unless prescribed because doing so may cause stomach to secrete excess hydrochloric acid.

! **WARNING** Instruct patient to notify prescriber if persistent, severe, or unusual adverse reactions occur that could require immediate medical attention.

- Teach patient to prevent constipation with a high-fiber diet and increased fluid intake (2 to 3 liters daily), if appropriate.
- Advise patient to notify prescriber about taking other medications and supplements before taking aluminum because of risk of interactions.
- Advise patient to notify prescriber if symptoms worsen or don't subside.

amantadine hydrochloride

Gocovri, Osmolex ER

Class and Category

Pharmacologic class: Dopamine agonist

Therapeutic class: Antidyskinetic, antiviral

Indications and Dosages

∗ *To manage symptoms of Parkinson's disease, including arteriosclerotic parkinsonism, idiopathic Parkinson's disease, and postencephalitic parkinsonism types; to relieve signs and symptoms of parkinsonism caused by carbon monoxide poisoning*

CAPSULES, ORAL SOLUTION, TABLETS

Adults who do not have serious medical illnesses or who are not receiving other antiparkinson drugs. 100 mg twice daily and increased, as needed. *Maximum:* 300 mg daily in divided doses.

Adults with serious associated medical illnesses or who are receiving other antiparkinson drugs. 100 mg once daily, increased after 1 to several wk to 100 mg twice daily, as needed. *Maximum:* 400 mg daily in divided doses.

∗ *To treat drug-induced extrapyramidal reactions*

CAPSULES, ORAL SOLUTION, TABLETS

Adults. *Initial:* 100 mg twice daily and then increased, as needed. *Maximum:* 300 mg daily in divided doses.

±**DOSAGE ADJUSTMENT** *For all indications above:* For adult patients receiving immediate-release form with a creatinine clearance of 30 to 50 ml/min, 200 mg on day 1 and then 100 mg daily. For patients with a creatinine clearance of 15 to 29 ml/min, 200 mg on day 1 and then 100 mg every other day. For patients with creatinine clearance less than 15 ml/min or patients on hemodialysis, 200 mg weekly. For patients with congestive heart failure, orthostatic hypotension, or peripheral edema, dosage may have to be reduced. For patients developing central nervous system adverse effects or other effects while taking 200-mg daily dose, dosage decreased to 100 mg once daily.

∗ *To treat dyskinesia in patients with Parkinson's disease receiving levodopa-based therapy; as adjunct to patients receiving levodopa/carbidopa for Parkinson's disease and experiencing "off" episodes*

E.R. CAPSULES (GOCOVRI)

Adults. *Initial:* 137 mg once daily. After 1 wk, increased to 274 mg once daily.

±**DOSAGE ADJUSTMENT** (Gocovri) For patients with a creatinine clearance of 30 to 59 ml/min, initial dosage reduced to 68.5 mg once daily at bedtime, with maximum dosage not to exceed 137 mg once daily at bedtime. For patients with a creatinine clearance of 15 to 29 ml/min, dosage reduced to 68.5 mg once daily at bedtime with no increased dosage adjustment.

∗ *To treat Parkinson's disease; to treat drug-induced extrapyramidal reactions*

E.R. TABLETS (OSMOLEX ER)

Adults. *Initial:* 129 mg once daily with dosage increased weekly to 322 mg, as needed. *Maximum:* 322 mg given as a 129-mg and 193-mg tablet in morning.

±**DOSAGE ADJUSTMENT** (Osmolex ER) For patients with a creatinine clearance of 30 to 59 ml/min, dosage titration done every 3 weeks instead of weekly and dosing frequency increased to 1 dose every 48 hours. For patients with a creatinine clearance of 15 to 29 ml/min, dosage titration interval increased to every 4 weeks instead of weekly, and dosing frequency increased to 1 dose every 96 hours.

Drug Administration

P.O.

- Use a calibrated device to measure dosage of oral solution.
- Administer immediate-release capsules and tablets whole. Do not break, crush, or split tablets or open capsules.
- E.R. capsules and tablets should not be chewed, crushed, or split but swallowed whole.
- E.R. capsules may be opened, and contents sprinkled on a teaspoon of soft food, such as applesauce, and then administered immediately. Mixture should be swallowed immediately without chewing and not stored for future use.
- Administer E.R. capsules at bedtime and E.R. tablets in the morning.

Route	Onset	Peak	Duration
P.O.	Unknown	1–4 hr	Unknown
P.O. (E.R.)	Unknown	12 hr	Unknown

Half-life: 10–31 hr

Mechanism of Action

Affects dopamine, a neurotransmitter that is synthesized and released by neurons leading from substantia nigra to basal ganglia and is essential for normal motor function. In Parkinson's disease, progressive degeneration of these neurons reduces intrasynaptic dopamine. Amantadine may cause dopamine to accumulate in the basal ganglia by increasing dopamine release or by blocking dopamine reuptake into the presynaptic neurons of the CNS. Amantadine also may stimulate dopamine receptors or make postsynaptic receptors more sensitive to dopamine. These actions help control alterations in involuntary muscle movements, such as tremors and rigidity, that are associated with Parkinson's disease.

Contraindications

End-stage renal disease, hypersensitivity to amantadine or its components

Interactions

DRUGS

anticholinergics or other drugs with anticholinergic activity: Possibly increased anticholinergic effects and risk of paralytic ileus
CNS stimulants: Excessive CNS stimulation, possibly causing arrhythmias, insomnia, irritability, nervousness, or seizures
live-virus vaccines: Possibly interference with vaccine effectiveness
quinidine, quinine, trimethoprim-sulfamethoxazole: Increased blood amantadine level
urine acidifying drugs: Increased elimination of amantadine with possible decrease in effectiveness
urine alkaline drugs: Decreased elimination of amantadine with possible increase in adverse reactions

ACTIVITIES

alcohol use: Possibly increased risk of CNS effects such as confusion, dizziness, light-headedness, and orthostatic hypotension

Adverse Reactions

CNS: Agitation, amnesia, anxiety, ataxia, confusion, depression, dizziness, dream abnormalities, drowsiness, euphoria, fatigue, fever, hallucinations, headache, hypokinesia, insomnia, irritability, light-headedness, mental impairment, nervousness, **neuroleptic malignant syndrome**, nightmares, psychiatric behavior, **seizures**, slurred speech, somnolence, **suicidal ideation**, syncope, weakness
CV: **Arrhythmias**, **cardiac arrest**, **congestive heart failure**, hypertension, orthostatic hypotension, peripheral edema, tachycardia
EENT: Blurred vision; corneal edema or opacity; dry mouth, nose, or throat; keratitis; light sensitivity; mydriasis; optic nerve palsy
GI: Anorexia, constipation, diarrhea, dysphagia, nausea, vomiting
GU: Decreased libido, dysuria, urinary retention
HEME: **Agranulocytosis**, **leukopenia**, **neutropenia**
RESP: **Acute respiratory failure**, **pulmonary edema**, tachypnea
SKIN: Diaphoresis, eczematoid dermatitis, livedo reticularis (purplish, netlike rash), pruritus, rash
Other: **Anaphylaxis**; intense urges to perform certain activities, such as gambling or sexual acts

Childbearing Considerations

PREGNANCY

- It is not known if drug can cause fetal harm, although some evidence exists that drug may have the potential to cause developmental issues, including cardiovascular, skeletal, and visceral malformations when administered in the first trimester.
- Use with caution only if benefit to mother outweighs potential risk to fetus.

LACTATION

- Drug is present in breast milk.
- Drug may alter breast milk excretion or production.
- Breastfeeding should not be undertaken with immediate-release drug therapy; mothers should check with prescriber if taking extended-release form before breastfeeding.

Nursing Considerations

- Be aware that patients receiving more than 200 mg daily are more likely to experience adverse or toxic reactions.

! **WARNING** Monitor patient for hypersensitivity reactions such as anaphylaxis. If present, notify prescriber immediately, withhold drug, and provide supportive care, as needed and ordered.

! **WARNING** Monitor patients who have a history of psychiatric illness or substance abuse because amantadine may worsen these conditions. Some patients taking amantadine have attempted suicide or had suicidal ideation.

- Be aware that amantadine may increase seizure activity in patients with a history of seizures.

! **WARNING** Monitor patient for evidence of neuroleptic malignant syndrome during dosage reduction or discontinuation of therapy. These include fever, hypertension or hypotension, involuntary motor activity, mental changes, muscle rigidity, tachycardia, and tachypnea. Be prepared to provide supportive treatment and additional drug therapy, as prescribed.

- Monitor patient for edema and weight gain because drug may cause redistribution of body fluid.
- Assess patient regularly for skin changes because melanoma risk is higher in those with Parkinson's disease. It isn't clear whether the risk is increased by the disease or by its treatment.
- Monitor patient for decreased drug effectiveness over time. If therapeutic response declines, expect to increase dosage or discontinue drug temporarily, as ordered.

PATIENT TEACHING

- Instruct patient to take amantadine exactly as prescribed and not to stop drug abruptly.
- Instruct patient how to take drug form prescribed.

! **WARNING** Alert patient that amantadine may cause an allergic reaction. Tell patient to notify prescriber immediately, if present and to seek immediate medical care if severe.

! **WARNING** Advise patient, family, or caregiver to notify prescriber immediately if patient reveals thoughts of suicide.

- Encourage patient to avoid consuming alcohol during amantadine therapy because alcohol may increase the risk of confusion, dizziness, light-headedness, or orthostatic hypotension.
- Advise patient to avoid driving and other activities that require a high level of alertness until he knows how the drug affects him because it may cause blurred vision and mental impairment.
- Advise patient to change positions slowly to minimize effects of orthostatic hypotension.
- Tell patient to use ice chips or sugarless candy or gum to relieve dry mouth.
- Caution patient to resume physical activities gradually as signs and symptoms improve.
- Urge patient to have regular skin examinations by a dermatologist or other qualified healthcare professional.
- Instruct patient to notify prescriber about intense urges, such as for gambling or sex, because dosage may have to be reduced or drug discontinued.

amikacin sulfate

Arikayce

Class and Category

Pharmacologic class: Aminoglycoside
Therapeutic class: Antibiotic

Indications and Dosages

* *To treat serious gram-negative bacterial infections (including bone, burns, CNS, joint, intra-abdominal, postoperative infections, respiratory tract, skin and soft tissue; neonatal sepsis; septicemia; and serious, complicated, and recurrent UTI) caused by* Acinetobacter, Enterobacter, Escherichia coli, Klebsiella, Proteus, Providencia, Pseudomonas, or Serratia; *and susceptible strains of staphylococci in patients allergic to other antibiotics, and in mixed staphylococcal/gram-negative infections*

I.M. INJECTION, I.V. INFUSION

Adults, children and older infants. 15 mg/kg daily in equal doses at equally spaced intervals (7.5 mg/kg every 12 hr or 5 mg/kg every 8 hr) for 7 to 10 days. *Maximum: For normal weight patients:* 15 mg/kg daily. *For obese patients*: 1.5 g/day.
Neonates. *Loading dose:* 10 mg/kg. *Maintenance:* 7.5 mg/kg every 12 hr for 7 to 10 days.

± **DOSAGE ADJUSTMENT** For patients with impaired renal function, dosage reduced but given at the normal interval or dosage unchanged but dosing interval prolonged.

∗ *To treat uncomplicated UTI when causative organisms are not susceptible to antibiotics having less potential toxicity*

I.M. INJECTION, I.V. INFUSION

Adults. 250 mg twice daily for 7 to 10 days.

±**DOSAGE ADJUSTMENT** For patients with impaired renal function, dosage reduced but given at the normal interval or dosage unchanged but dosing interval prolonged.

∗ *To treat refractory* Mycobacterium avium *complex (MAC) lung disease for patients who did not achieve negative sputum cultures after a minimum of 6 consecutive months of a multidrug background regimen therapy*

ORAL INHALATION (ARIKAYCE)

Adults. 590 mg once daily using the Lamira Nebulizer System.

Drug Administration

I.M.

- Give I.M. injection in large muscle mass.

I.V.

- Prepare amikacin I.V. solution by adding contents of 500-mg vial to 100 or 200 ml of sterile diluent such as 0.9% Sodium Chloride Injection, 5% Dextrose Injection, or other compatible solutions listed in manufacturer's guidelines. Store at room temperature if not used immediately for up to 24 hr. When stored in refrigerator allow solution to warm to room temperature before administration.
- Infuse drug over 30 to 60 min for adults and children and 1 to 2 hr for neonates.
- *Incompatibilities:* Other drugs

ORAL INHALATION

- Know that oral inhalation of drug is limited to adults who have limited or no alternative treatment options.
- Know that Arikayce is for oral inhalation use only and should be at room temperature before administration.
- Administer by nebulization only using the Lamira Nebulizer System. The handset and aerosol head must be cleaned and disinfected before using them for the first time, as well as after every use.
- Administer bronchodilator, if prescribed, before administering amikacin oral inhalation.
- Prior to opening glass vial, shake vial well for at least 10 to 15 sec until the contents appear uniform and well mixed. Open the vial by flipping up the plastic top of the vial then pulling downward to loosen the metal ring. The metal ring and rubber stopper should be removed carefully. Then, pour contents of vial into the medication reservoir of the nebulizer handset.
- Expect the inhalation treatment to take about 14 min, although it may take as long as 20 min.
- After 7 uses, the aerosol head will have to be replaced.

Route	Onset	Peak	Duration
I.V.	Immediate	30 min	8–12 hr
I.M.	Rapid	1 hr	8–12 hr
Oral inhalation	Unknown	Unknown	Unknown

Half-life: 2 hr (oral inhalation: 5.9–19.5 hr)

Mechanism of Action

Binds to negatively charged sites on bacteria's outer cell membrane, disrupting cell integrity. Also, binds to bacterial ribosomal subunits and inhibits protein synthesis. Both actions lead to cell death.

Contraindications

Hypersensitivity to amikacin, other aminoglycosides, or their components

Interactions

DRUGS

general anesthetics: Increased risk of neuromuscular blockade
loop diuretics: Increased risk of ototoxicity
neuromuscular blockers: Possibly increased neuromuscular blockade and prolonged respiratory depression
penicillins: Possibly inactivation of or synergistic effects with amikacin
other nephrotoxic drugs: Increased risk of nephrotoxicity

Adverse Reactions

CNS: Drowsiness, headache, loss of balance, **neuromuscular blockade**, tremor, vertigo
EENT: Hearing loss, ototoxicity, tinnitus
GI: Nausea, vomiting
GU: **Azotemia**, dysuria, **nephrotoxicity**, oliguria or polyuria, proteinuria
MS: **Acute muscle paralysis**; arthralgia; muscle fatigue, spasms, and weakness
RESP: **Apnea**; *Inhalation form:* **bronchospasm**, exacerbation of underlying

pulmonary disease, **hemoptysis**, **hypersensitivity pneumonitis**
Other: **Anaphylaxis**, **angioedema**, **hyperkalemia**, **hypersensitivity reactions**

Childbearing Considerations

PREGNANCY

- Drug may cause fetal harm such as total, irreversible, bilateral deafness in pediatric patients exposed in utero.
- Drug should not be given to pregnant women unless no other alternative is available.

LACTATION

- It is not known if drug is present in breast milk.
- A decision should be made to discontinue breastfeeding or the drug to avoid potential adverse reactions in the breastfed infant.

Nursing Considerations

- Expect to obtain results of culture and sensitivity testing before therapy begins.

! **WARNING** Assess renal function before drug therapy is begun and then daily during therapy, as ordered because amikacin may produce nephrotoxic effects. To minimize renal tubule irritation, maintain hydration during therapy.

- Obtain patient's weight prior to treatment given as an I.M. injection or I.V. infusion (except for uncomplicated UTI) for calculation of correct dosage.

! **WARNING** Monitor patient for hypersensitivity reactions, which can be life-threatening. Notify prescriber if an allergic reaction occurs and, if serious, expect drug to be discontinued and supportive care provided, as needed and ordered.

- Measure serum amikacin concentrations as ordered, usually 30 to 90 minutes after injection (for peak concentration) and just before administering next parenteral dose (for trough concentration).
- Watch for signs of ototoxicity, such as tinnitus and vertigo, especially during high-dosage or prolonged amikacin therapy. However, know that ototoxicity has occurred in some patients even when serum aminoglycoside levels were normal. Patients with a maternal history of ototoxicity due to aminoglycoside use or have a known mitochondrial DNA variant are at a higher risk for ototoxicity.
- Be aware that amikacin may exacerbate muscle weakness in such conditions as myasthenia gravis and Parkinson's disease.

PATIENT TEACHING

- Instruct patient how to administer oral inhalation form of amikacin, if prescribed.

! **WARNING** Tell patient to report any signs and symptoms of an allergic reaction such as difficulty breathing immediately and, if using oral inhalation form, to seek immediate medical care.

- Tell patient that daily laboratory tests are necessary during treatment. Stress importance of compliance.
- Instruct patient to report changes in urination, headache, hearing changes, nausea, ringing in ears, and vomiting.
- Caution females of childbearing age to alert prescriber if pregnancy occurs.
- Advise mothers that breastfeeding should not be undertaken while receiving amikacin therapy.

amiloride hydrochloride

Midamor (CAN)

Class and Category

Pharmacologic class: Potassium-sparing diuretic
Therapeutic class: Diuretic

Indications and Dosages

* *As adjunct to loop or thiazide diuretic therapy in patient with heart failure or hypertension to correct diuretic-induced hypokalemia or to prevent diuretic-induced hypokalemia that increases the risk of arrhythmias or other complications*

TABLETS

Adults. 5 mg daily as single dose; if hypokalemia persists, increased to 10 mg. If hypokalemia continues to persist, increased to 15 mg daily and then 20 mg daily, as needed.

Drug Administration

P.O.

- Administer with food to reduce GI upset.

Route	Onset	Peak	Duration
P.O.	2 hr	3–4 hr	24 hr

Half-life: 6–9 hr

Mechanism of Action

Inhibits sodium reabsorption in distal convoluted tubules and cortical collecting ducts, causing sodium and water loss and enhancing potassium retention.

Contraindications

Hypersensitivity to amiloride or its components; impaired renal function; serum potassium level above 5.5 mEq/L; therapy with another potassium-sparing diuretic, such as spironolactone or triamterene, or a potassium supplement

Interactions

DRUGS

ACE inhibitors, angiotensin II receptor antagonists, cyclosporine, enalapril, lisinopril, potassium products, spironolactone: Increased risk of hyperkalemia
digoxin: Decreased effectiveness of digoxin
lithium: Reduced renal clearance of lithium and increased risk of lithium toxicity
NSAIDs: Reduced diuretic effect of amiloride

FOODS

high-potassium food: Increased risk of hyperkalemia

Adverse Reactions

CNS: Confusion, depression, dizziness, drowsiness, **encephalopathy**, fatigue, headache, insomnia, nervousness, paresthesia, somnolence, tremor, vertigo
CV: Angina, **arrhythmias**, orthostatic hypotension, palpitations
EENT: Dry mouth, increased intraocular pressure, nasal congestion, tinnitus, vision disturbances
GI: Abdominal pain or fullness, anorexia, appetite changes, constipation, diarrhea, **GI bleeding**, heartburn, indigestion, jaundice, nausea, thirst, vomiting
GU: Bladder spasms, dysuria, impotence, loss of libido, polyuria
HEME: **Aplastic anemia**, **neutropenia**
MS: Arthralgia, muscle spasms, or weakness
RESP: Cough, dyspnea
SKIN: Alopecia, pruritus, rash
Other: Dehydration, hyperchloremia, **hyperkalemia**, **hypernatremia**, **metabolic acidosis**

Childbearing Considerations

PREGNANCY

- It is not known if drug can cause fetal harm.
- Use with caution only if benefit to mother outweighs potential risk to fetus.

LACTATION

- It is not known if drug is present in breast milk.
- A decision should be made to discontinue breastfeeding or the drug to avoid potential adverse reactions in the breastfed infant.

Nursing Considerations

- Monitor fluid intake and output, renal function test results, and weight. Also, monitor serum potassium level to detect hyperkalemia and sodium levels to detect hypernatremia.

! WARNING Don't administer amiloride with other potassium-sparing diuretics.

! WARNING Monitor patient for changes in neurologic status because drug can cause multiple neurologic adverse reactions. Also monitor patient for GI disturbances, especially bleeding, and electrolyte imbalances. If present, notify prescriber immediately.

! WARNING Expect periodic complete blood counts to be performed to monitor patient for possible aplastic anemia and neutropenia.

PATIENT TEACHING

- Instruct patient to take drug with food.
- Warn patient to avoid high-potassium food and salt substitutes that contain potassium.

! WARNING Tell patient to notify prescriber of any persistent, severe, or unusual adverse reactions because drug can cause serious adverse reactions.

- Advise patient to consult prescriber before taking other drugs, including over-the-counter remedies, especially sympathomimetics.

- Advise patient to increase fiber and fluid intake to prevent constipation.
- Warn patient to expect reversible hair loss and impotence.
- Tell mothers that breastfeeding should not be undertaken while receiving amiloride.

amiodarone hydrochloride

Nexterone, Pacerone

Class and Category

Pharmacologic class: Benzofuran derivative
Therapeutic class: Class III antiarrhythmic

Indications and Dosages

∗ *To treat life-threatening, recurrent ventricular fibrillation and hemodynamically unstable ventricular tachycardia when these arrhythmias don't respond to other drugs or when patient can't tolerate other drugs*

TABLETS (PACERONE)

Adults. *Loading:* 800 to 1,600 mg daily in divided doses for 1 to 3 wk. Once arrhythmia is controlled or side effects become prominent, dosage reduced to 600 to 800 mg daily in divided doses for 1 mo and then reduced to 400 mg daily if cardiac rhythm is stable. *Maintenance:* 400 mg daily.

∗ *To treat or prevent life-threatening, recurrent ventricular fibrillation and hemodynamically unstable ventricular tachycardia when these arrhythmias don't respond to other drugs, when patient can't tolerate other drugs, or when oral amiodarone is indicated but patient is unable to take oral medication*

I.V. INFUSION (NEXTERONE)

Adults. *Loading:* 150 mg (15 mg/min) of 150-mg/100-ml solution infused over 10 min followed by 360 mg (1 mg/min) of 360-mg/200-ml solution infused over 6 hr followed by 540 mg (0.5 mg/min) of 360-mg/200-ml infused over remaining 18 hr. *Maintenance:* 720 mg (0.5 mg/min) of 360-mg/200-ml solution infused over 24 hr and repeated every 24 hr for up to 2 to 3 wk, as needed. Changed to oral form as soon as possible.

∗ *To treat breakthrough episodes of ventricular fibrillation or hemodynamically unstable ventricular tachycardia*

I.V. INFUSION (NEXTERONE)

Adults. 150 mg (15 mg/min) of 150-mg/100-ml solution infused over 10 min.

Drug Administration

P.O.

- Administer consistently with regard to meals because food affects absorption.
- Doses should be divided for total daily doses of 1,000 mg or higher, or when GI intolerance develops.
- Expect dosage to be reduced if excessive GI intolerance occurs.

I.V.

- Know that Nexterone is already premixed and does not require further dilution. Solution should appear clear. Check for minute leaks prior to use by squeezing the bag firmly.
- Use an in-line filter during administration. Also, use a central venous catheter whenever possible. A central venous catheter is required when infusion rate exceeds 2 mg/ml because drug may cause peripheral vein phlebitis at higher rates.
- Use only a volumetric infusion pump to administer drug.
- Don't use plastic containers in series connections because this could result in an air embolism.
- Infusions exceeding 2 hr must be administered in glass or polyolefin bottles containing 5% Dextrose in Water. Avoid using evacuated glass containers for admixing, as incompatibility with a buffer in the container may cause precipitation.
- Know that after the initial rate, subsequent infusions are given at different rates depending on the dose and sequence given.
- Monitor patient's blood pressure and pulse rate frequently throughout infusion as bradycardia and hypotension may occur and may require infusion rate to be decreased and possibly additional supportive care given, as prescribed. Expect to have a temporary pacemaker available if patient is at risk for AV block or bradycardia.
- Protect from light until ready to use; does not have to be protected from light during administration.
- Drug should be changed to oral form as soon as possible.

- *Incompatibilities:* Aminophylline, amoxicillin sodium-clavulanic acid, ampicillin sodium/sulbactam sodium, argatroban, bivalirudin, cefamandole nafate, cefazolin sodium, ceftazidime, digoxin, furosemide, heparin sodium, imipenem-cilastatin sodium, magnesium sulfate, mezlocillin sodium, micafungin, piperacillin tazobactam sodium, potassium phosphates, sodium bicarbonate, sodium nitroprusside, and sodium phosphates

Route	Onset	Peak	Duration
P.O.	2 days–3 wk	3–7 hr	Weeks–months
I.V.	Hours–3 days	Unknown	Weeks–month

Half-life: 26–107 days (I.V.: 9–36 days)

Mechanism of Action

Acts on cardiac cell membranes, prolonging repolarization and the refractory period and raising ventricular fibrillation threshold. Drug relaxes vascular smooth muscles, mainly in coronary circulation, and improves myocardial blood flow. It relaxes peripheral vascular smooth muscles, decreasing peripheral vascular resistance and myocardial oxygen consumption.

Contraindications

Bradycardia that causes syncope (unless pacemaker present), cardiogenic shock, hypersensitivity to amiodarone or its components, SA node dysfunction, second- and third-degree AV block (unless pacemaker present)

Interactions

DRUGS

anticoagulants: Increased anticoagulant response and possibly serious bleeding
anesthetic agents, azole antifungals, class I and III antiarrhythmics, fluoroquinolones (selected ones), halogenated inhalation, lithium, loratadine, macrolide antibiotics (selected ones), phenothiazines (selected ones), trazodone, tricyclic antidepressants: Increased risk of prolonged QT interval and life-threatening arrhythmias, such as torsades de pointes
beta-blockers, clonidine, digoxin, diltiazem, ivabradine: Potentiate amiodarone effects with increased risk of AV block, bradycardia, and hypotension
calcium channel blockers: Increased serum levels of these drugs and increased risk of AV block, bradycardia, and hypotension
cholestyramine, phenytoin, rifampin: Decreased amiodarone level
cimetidine, protease inhibitors (selected ones): Increased amiodarone level
cyclosporine: Increased cyclosporine level
CYP450 inducers such as St. John's wort: Reduced exposure of amiodarone
CYP450 inhibitors such as azole antifungals, cimetidine, and selected fluoroquinolone and macrolide antibiotics: Increased exposure of amiodarone
dabigatran, dextromethorphan, phenytoin: Possible increased serum levels of these drugs
dextromethorphan, methotrexate, phenytoin: Increased serum levels of these drugs and increased risk of toxicity
digoxin: Increased serum digoxin level and risk of digitalis toxicity
fentanyl: Increased serum fentanyl level with increased risk of bradycardia, decreased cardiac output, and hypotension
flecainide procainamide, quinidine: Increased serum levels of these drugs
HMG-CoA reductase inhibitors such as atorvastatin, lovastatin, and simvastatin: Increased risk of myopathy and rhabdomyolysis
ledipasvir/sofosbuvir, sofosbuvir/simeprevir: May cause serious symptomatic bradycardia
protease inhibitors: Possibly increased risk of elevated amiodarone levels and toxicity
sofosbuvir: Increased risk of symptomatic bradycardia requiring possible pacemaker insertion
theophylline: Increased serum theophylline level; increased risk of theophylline toxicity
warfarin: Potentiated anticoagulant response with possible serious or fatal bleeding

FOODS

grapefruit juice: Increased amiodarone level

Adverse Reactions

CNS: Abnormal gait, ataxia, confusion, delirium, demyelinating polyneuropathy, disorientation, dizziness, fatigue, fever, hallucinations, headache, insomnia, involuntary motor activity, lack of coordination, malaise, paresthesia, parkinsonian symptoms, peripheral neuropathy, **pseudotumor cerebri**, sleep disturbances, tremor
CV: **Arrhythmias (including AV block**, **bradycardia**, **electromechanical**

dissociation, torsades de pointes, and ventricular tachycardia or fibrillation), cardiac arrest, cardiogenic shock, edema, **heart failure, hypotension, QT prolongation,** vasculitis
EENT: Abnormal salivation, abnormal taste and smell, blurred vision, corneal microdeposits, dry eyes or mouth, halo vision, lens opacities, macular degeneration, optic neuritis, optic neuropathy, papilledema, permanent blindness, photophobia, scotoma
ENDO: Hyperthyroidism, hypothyroidism, syndrome of inappropriate ADH secretion, thyroid nodules, **thyroid cancer**
GI: Abdominal pain, anorexia, **cirrhosis,** constipation, diarrhea, elevated bilirubin or liver enzymes, **hepatic failure, hepatitis,** nausea, **pancreatitis,** vomiting
GU: **Acute renal failure,** decreased libido, epididymitis, impotence, **renal insufficiency**
HEME: **Agranulocytosis, aplastic or hemolytic anemia, coagulation abnormalities, neutropenia, pancytopenia,** spontaneous bruising, **thrombocytopenia**
MS: Muscle weakness, myopathy, **rhabdomyolysis**
RESP: **Acute respiratory distress syndrome in postoperative setting;** bronchiolitis obliterans organizing pneumonia; bronchospasm; crackles and wheezing; **eosinophilic pneumonia; infiltrates that lead to** dyspnea, cough, **hemoptysis, hypoxia, pulmonary fibrosis, pulmonary alveolar hemorrhage, pulmonary interstitial pneumonitis;** pleural effusion; pleuritis; pneumonia; pulmonary inflammation, **pulmonary fibrosis; respiratory arrest or failure**
SKIN: Alopecia, bluish gray pigmentation, bullous dermatitis, eczema, **erythema multiforme, exfoliative dermatitis,** flushing, photosensitivity, pruritus, rash, **skin cancer,** solar dermatitis, **Stevens-Johnson syndrome, toxic epidermal necrolysis,** urticaria
Other: **Anaphylaxis including shock, angioedema, drug reaction with eosinophilia and systemic symptoms (DRESS),** lupus-like syndrome

Childbearing Considerations

PREGNANCY

- Drug crosses the placental barrier and has the possibility to cause fetal harm.
- Fetal adverse effects may include arrhythmias such as bradycardia, periodic ventricular extrasystoles, and QT prolongation; growth restriction; neurodevelopmental abnormalities, such as ataxia, delayed motor development, jerk nystagmus, and speech delay with difficulties with written language and math later in childhood; premature birth; and thyroid dysfunction.
- Drug should not be given to pregnant women unless benefit to the mother outweighs potential risk to fetus.

LABOR AND DELIVERY

- Newborn should be monitored for signs and symptoms of cardiac arrhythmias and thyroid dysfunction.

LACTATION

- Drug is present in breast milk.
- Breastfeeding is not recommended during drug therapy.

REPRODUCTION

- Drug may reduce female and male fertility, but it is not known if this effect is reversible.
- Females of childbearing age should use effective contraception to avoid pregnancy.

Nursing Considerations

- Check patient's implantable cardiac device (if present), as ordered, at the start of and during amiodarone therapy because drug may affect defibrillating or pacing thresholds.
- Monitor all patients but especially elderly patients closely when conversion to oral amiodarone is made for continued effectiveness.

! **WARNING** Monitor patient for hypersensitivity reactions that may become life-threatening. If present, notify prescriber immediately and provide supportive care, as needed and ordered. Also, monitor patient for serious adverse reactions as amiodarone can adversely affect many systems. Report any persistent, severe, or unusual signs and symptoms promptly to prescriber.

! **WARNING** Be aware that amiodarone may cause or worsen pulmonary disorders that may develop days to weeks after therapy and progress to respiratory failure or even death. Expect to obtain chest x-ray and pulmonary function tests before therapy starts and then chest x-ray and follow-up exams every 3 to 6 months during therapy.

! **WARNING** Monitor continuous ECG for arrhythmias, heart rate below 60 beats/min, and increased PR and QRS intervals because amiodarone may cause sinus arrest or symptomatic bradycardia and new ventricular arrhythmias or worsen existing arrhythmias as well as increasing resistance to cardioversion. Electrolyte imbalance or use of concomitant antiarrhythmics or other interacting drugs may increase the development of these arrhythmias. Expect to correct electrolyte imbalance, as ordered, prior to initiating treatment with amiodarone.

- Monitor oxygen level and vital signs often during and after giving amiodarone. Keep emergency equipment and drugs nearby.
- Monitor serum amiodarone level periodically, as ordered, which normally ranges from 1.0 to 2.5 mcg/ml.
- Assess thyroid hormone levels, as ordered; drug inhibits conversion of T_4 to T_3 and may cause drug-induced hyperthyroidism, thyrotoxicosis, and new or worsened arrhythmias. If new signs of arrhythmias or thyroid dysfunction occur, notify prescriber at once.
- Monitor liver enzymes, as ordered. If elevations become persistent and significant, notify prescriber and expect maintenance dosage to be reduced or drug discontinued.
- Be aware that patient should undergo regular ophthalmic examinations including fundoscopy and slit-lamp examination during amiodarone therapy because drug can cause serious visual impairment including permanent blindness.

PATIENT TEACHING

- Inform patient how drug will be administered.
- Instruct patient to take oral drug consistently with regard to meals.
- Advise patient to avoid drinking grapefruit juice or taking St. John's wort while receiving amiodarone.

! **WARNING** Alert patient that drug may cause an allergic reaction. If present, tell patient to alert prescriber immediately. If allergic reaction is severe, stress importance of seeking immediate medical care.

- Explain that patient will need frequent monitoring and laboratory tests during treatment. Encourage compliance.
- Advise patient to report cough, dark urine, dyspnea, fainting, fatigue, lightheadedness, nausea, sudden change in quality or rapidity of pulse, swollen feet and hands, vomiting, wheezing, or yellow sclerae or skin.
- Instruct patient to report abnormal bleeding or bruising. Also, tell patient to report any sign of visual impairment or decreased or increased levels of energy.
- Stress importance of alerting prescriber if persistent, severe, or unusual adverse reactions occur during drug therapy. Inform patient that adverse interactions or reactions may persist following the discontinuation of amiodarone. If serious, prescriber also should be notified.
- Stress importance of informing all prescribers of amiodarone use, as serious drug interactions may occur.
- Advise patient to avoid corneal refractive laser surgery while taking drug.
- Warn females of childbearing age that amiodarone can cause fetal harm. Instruct them to use effective contraceptive measures and report suspected or known pregnancy immediately.
- Advise mothers who have been breastfeeding to discontinue nursing because drug is excreted in human milk and may cause potential harm.

amisulpride

Barhemsys

Class and Category

Pharmacologic class: Dopamine-2 receptor antagonist
Therapeutic class: Antiemetic

Indications and Dosages

✱ *To prevent postoperative nausea and vomiting, either alone or in combination with an antiemetic of a different class*

I.V. INJECTION

Adults. 5 mg injected over 1 to 2 min at the time of induction of anesthesia.

* *To treat postoperative nausea and vomiting in patients who have received antiemetic prophylaxis with an antiemetic of a different class or who have not received prophylaxis*

I.V. INJECTION

Adults. 10 mg injected over 1 to 2 min as a single dose.

Drug Administration

I.V.

- Dilution not required.
- Compatible with 0.9% Sodium Chloride Injection, 5% Dextrose Injection, Lactated Ringer's Solution or Water for Injection, which may be used to flush I.V. line before and after administration.
- Protect from light.
- Administer within 12 hr of removal of vial from the protective carton.
- Inject over 1 to 2 min as a single I.V. injection.
- *Incompatibilities:* None reported by manufacturer

Route	Onset	Peak	Duration
I.V.	Immediate	1–2 min	Unknown

Half-life: 12 hr

Mechanism of Action

Blocks the dopamine-2 receptor sites located in the chemoreceptor trigger zone. Inhibition of these sites prevents stimulation of the vomiting center, which prevents or stops nausea and vomiting.

Contraindications

Hypersensitivity to amisulpride or its components

Interactions

DRUGS

dopamine agonists: Reciprocal antagonism of effects between amisulpride and dopamine agonists, especially with levodopa, which should not be given with amisulpride

drugs prolonging QT interval: Potential additive effects; droperidol should not be administered with amisulpride and other drugs that prolong QT interval and require ECG monitoring

Adverse Reactions

CNS: Chills

CV: **Hypotension**

ENDO: Elevated prolactin levels

GI: Abdominal distention

Other: **Hypokalemia**, infusion-site pain

Childbearing Considerations

PREGNANCY

- It is not known if drug can cause fetal harm.
- Use with caution only if benefit to mother outweighs potential risk to fetus.

LACTATION

- Drug is present in breast milk.
- Pumping breast milk and discarding for 48 hr after drug is given will help minimize drug exposure of breastfed infant. However, mothers should check with prescriber before breastfeeding.

Nursing Considerations

- Be aware that amisulpride should not be given to patients with severe renal impairment (eGFR less than 30 ml/min) because it is substantially excreted by the kidneys and may increase risk of adverse reactions. It may be used in patients with mild to moderate renal impairment.

! **WARNING** Know that amisulpride should not be given to patients receiving concurrent therapy with droperidol or to patients with congenital long QT syndrome because of risk of QT prolongation.

! **WARNING** Expect to monitor patient's ECG in patients with concurrent therapy of drugs known to prolong QT interval or for patients with conditions known to prolong QT interval. ECG monitoring is also recommended in patients with congestive heart failure, electrolyte abnormalities such as hypokalemia or hypomagnesemia, or in the presence of preexisting arrhythmias/ cardiac conduction disorders.

PATIENT TEACHING

- Advise patient to inform anesthesiologist about drugs being taken prior to surgery.

! **WARNING** Instruct patient to immediately report a change in heart rate or if he feels faint or light-headed.

- Instruct mothers to check with prescriber before continuing breastfeeding during amisulpride therapy as pumping of breast milk and discarding for 48 hours after drug is given may be required.

amitriptyline hydrochloride

Elavil (CAN)

Class and Category

Pharmacologic class: Tricyclic antidepressant
Therapeutic class: Antidepressant

Indications and Dosages

* *To relieve depression, especially when accompanied by anxiety and insomnia*

TABLETS

Adults. *Outpatient:* 75 mg daily in divided doses, increased to 150 mg daily, as needed. Alternatively, 50 to 100 mg at bedtime, increased by 25 to 50 mg, as needed, to 150 mg daily. *Inpatient:* 100 mg daily, gradually increased to 200 mg daily and then 300 mg daily, as needed. *Maintenance:* 40 to 100 mg daily at bedtime.

± **DOSAGE ADJUSTMENT** For adolescent and elderly patients at bedtime, dosage reduced to 10 mg 3 times daily plus 20 mg at bedtime.

Drug Administration

P.O.

- Increase in dosage made preferably in late afternoon and/or bedtime doses to decrease daytime sedation.

Route	Onset	Peak	Duration
P.O.	7–14 days	2–5 hr	Unknown

Half-life: 13–36 hr

Contraindications

Acute recovery phase after MI, concurrent therapy with cisapride, hypersensitivity to amitriptyline or its components, MAO inhibitor therapy within 14 days

Interactions

DRUGS

anticholinergics, epinephrine, norepinephrine: Increased effects of these drugs
barbiturates: Decreased amitriptyline level
carbamazepine: Decreased serum amitriptyline level and increased serum carbamazepine level, which increases therapeutic and toxic effects of carbamazepine
cimetidine, disulfiram, fluoxetine, fluvoxamine, haloperidol, H_2-receptor antagonists, methylphenidate, oral contraceptives, paroxetine, phenothiazines, sertraline: Increased serum amitriptyline level

Mechanism of Action

Releases serotonin and norepinephrine from their storage sites normally when an impulse reaches adreneric nerves. Most of this is taken back into the nerves and stored by the reuptake mechanism, as shown below on the left.

Blocks serotonin and norepinephrine reuptake by adrenergic nerves. By doing so, amitriptyline raises serotonin and norepinephrine levels at nerve synapses. This action may elevate mood and reduce depression.

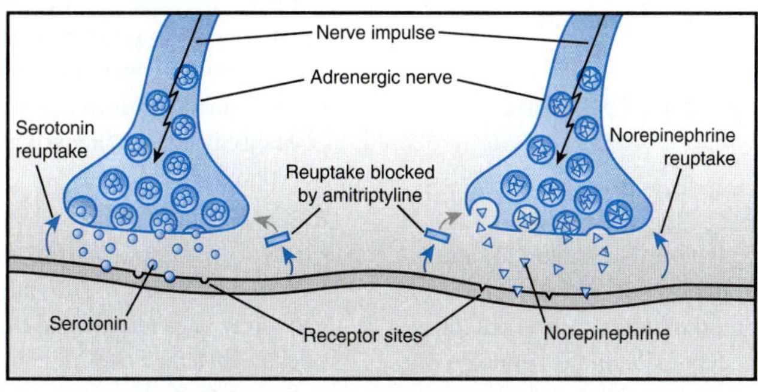

cisapride: Possibly prolonged QT interval and increased risk of arrhythmias
clonidine, guanethidine, and other antihypertensives: Decreased antihypertensive effects
dicumarol: Increased anticoagulant effect
levodopa: Decreased levodopa absorption; sympathetic hyperactivity, sinus tachycardia, hypertension, agitation
MAO inhibitors: Possibly seizures and death
thyroid replacement drugs: Arrhythmias and increased antidepressant effects

ACTIVITIES

alcohol use: Enhanced CNS depression
smoking: Decreased amitriptyline effects

Adverse Reactions

CNS: Anxiety, ataxia, **coma**, chills, delusions, disorientation, drowsiness, extrapyramidal reactions, fatigue, fever, headache, insomnia, nightmares, peripheral neuropathy, **suicidal ideation**, tremor
CV: **Arrhythmias (including prolonged AV conduction**, **heart block**, and tachycardia), **cardiomyopathy**, hypertension, **MI**, nonspecific ECG changes, orthostatic hypotension, palpitations
EENT: Abnormal taste, black tongue, blurred vision, dry mouth, increased salivation, nasal congestion, tinnitus
ENDO: Gynecomastia, hyperglycemia, **hypoglycemia**, increased prolactin level, syndrome of inappropriate ADH secretion
GI: Abdominal cramps, constipation, diarrhea, flatulence, ileus, increased appetite, nausea, vomiting
GU: Impotence, libido changes, menstrual irregularities, testicular swelling, urinary hesitancy, urine retention
HEME: **Agranulocytosis**, **bone marrow depression**, eosinophilia, **leukopenia**, **thrombocytopenia**
SKIN: Alopecia, flushing, purpura
Other: Weight gain

Childbearing Considerations

PREGNANCY

- It is not known if drug can cause fetal harm, but limited studies suggest it may.
- Know that drug is a tricyclic antidepressant. This type of antidepressant has been known to cause withdrawal symptoms such as agitation and respiratory depression in the neonate when given to the mother during the last trimester of pregnancy. Also, urinary retention in the neonate has been reported when mother has taken drug during pregnancy.
- Use with caution only if benefit to mother outweighs potential risk to fetus.

LACTATION

- Drug is present in breast milk.
- A decision should be made to discontinue breastfeeding or the drug to avoid potential adverse reactions in the breastfed infant.

Nursing Considerations

! WARNING Don't give an MAO inhibitor within 14 days of amitriptyline because of the risk of seizures and death.

- Use caution if patient has a history of angle-closure glaucoma, seizures, or urine retention because of amitriptyline's atropine-like effects.

! WARNING Watch patients closely (especially adolescents and young adults), for suicidal tendencies, particularly when therapy starts and dosage changes. Depression may worsen temporarily during these times.

! WARNING Monitor patient for arrhythmias, including heart block and tachycardia, especially in patients with cardiovascular disorders.

- Monitor blood pressure for hypertension or hypotension.
- Expect to monitor patient's complete blood count regularly, as ordered, because drug may cause serious hematological reactions. Also monitor patient for persistent, severe, or unusual adverse reactions because drug can cause many different types of adverse reactions.
- Stay alert for behavior changes, such as decreased interest in personal appearance or hallucinations. Be aware that psychosis may develop in schizophrenic patients, and symptoms may increase in paranoid patients.
- Avoid abrupt withdrawal after long use because headache, nausea, nightmares, and vertigo may occur.

PATIENT TEACHING

- Instruct patient how to take amitriptyline. Warn patient not to stop taking drug abruptly because adverse effects can occur. Instead, encourage patient to notify prescriber of any concerns.

- Instruct patient to avoid using alcohol or over-the-counter drugs that contain alcohol during amitriptyline therapy because alcohol enhances CNS depressant effects.

! **WARNING** Urge family or caregiver to watch patient closely for suicidal tendencies, especially when therapy starts or dosage changes and particularly if patient is an adolescent or young adult.

- Advise patient and family or caregiver to report to prescriber any persistent, severe, or unusual adverse reactions.
- Tell females of childbearing age to alert prescriber if pregnancy occurs.
- Advise mothers breastfeeding should not be undertaken during amitriptyline therapy.

amlodipine benzoate

Katerzia

amlodipine besylate

Norliqva, Norvasc

Class and Category

Pharmacologic class: Calcium channel blocker
Therapeutic class: Antianginal, antihypertensive

Indications and Dosages

✶ *To control hypertension*

ORAL SOLUTION (NORLIQVA), ORAL SUSPENSION (KATERZIA), TABLETS (NORVASC)

Adults. *Initial:* 5 mg once daily, increased gradually over 7 to 14 days, as needed. *Maximum:* 10 mg once daily.
Children ages 6 to 17. 2.5 to 5 mg once daily. *Maximum*: 5 mg once daily.

±**DOSAGE ADJUSTMENT** For elderly, fragile, or small adult patients with impaired hepatic function, initial dosage decreased to 2.5 mg once daily. Then increased gradually over 7 to 14 days based on response.

✶ *To treat chronic stable angina and vasospastic angina (Prinzmetal's or Variant angina); to reduce risk of hospitalization for angina and the risk of coronary revascularization procedure in patients with recently documented coronary artery disease without heart failure or an ejection fraction less than 40%*

ORAL SOLUTION (NORLIQVA), ORAL SUSPENSION (KATERZIA), TABLETS (NORVASC)

Adults. 5 to 10 mg once daily.

±**DOSAGE ADJUSTMENT** For elderly patients and those with impaired hepatic function, dosage maintained at 5 mg once daily.

Drug Administration

P.O.

- Shake oral suspension container before measuring dose. Store oral suspension in refrigerator and protect from light. Store oral solution at room temperature. Use a calibrated device to measure dosage of solution or suspension.
- Administer with food if GI upset occurs.

Route	Onset	Peak	Duration
P.O.	Unknown	6–12 hr	24 hr

Half-life: 30–50 hr

Mechanism of Action

Binds to dihydropyridine and nondihydropyridine cell membrane receptor sites on myocardial and vascular smooth muscle cells and inhibits influx of extracellular calcium ions across slow calcium channels. This decreases intracellular calcium level, inhibiting smooth muscle cell contractions and relaxing coronary and vascular smooth muscles, decreasing peripheral vascular resistance, and reducing systolic and diastolic blood pressure. Decreased peripheral vascular resistance also decreases myocardial workload, oxygen demand, and possibly angina. Also, by inhibiting coronary artery muscle cell contractions and restoring blood flow, drug may relieve Prinzmetal's angina.

Contraindications

Hypersensitivity to amlodipine or its components

Interactions

DRUGS

ACE inhibitors, aliskiren (in patients with diabetes or renal impairment): Increased risk of hyperkalemia, hypotension, and renal dysfunction

cyclosporine, simvastatin, tacrolimus: Possibly increased blood levels of these drugs
CYP3A4 inhibitors such as diltiazem, ketoconazole, itraconazole, and ritonavir: Possibly increased blood amlodipine level
sildenafil: Possibly excessive hypotension

Adverse Reactions

CNS: Anxiety, dizziness, extrapyramidal disorder, fatigue, headache, lethargy, lightheadedness, paresthesia, somnolence, syncope, tremor
CV: **Arrhythmias**, chest pain, **hypotension**, palpitations, peripheral edema
EENT: Dry mouth, gingival hyperplasia, pharyngitis
ENDO: Hot flashes
GI: Abdominal cramps or pain, anorexia, constipation, diarrhea, dysphagia, elevated liver enzymes, esophagitis, flatulence, indigestion, jaundice, nausea, **pancreatitis**, vomiting
GU: Decreased libido, impotence, urinary frequency
MS: Myalgia
RESP: Dyspnea
SKIN: Dermatitis, flushing, rash
Other: Weight loss

Childbearing Considerations

PREGNANCY

- It is not known if drug can cause fetal harm.
- Use with caution only if benefit to mother outweighs potential risk to fetus.

LACTATION

- Drug is present in breast milk.
- Mothers should check with prescriber before breastfeeding.

Nursing Considerations

- Use amlodipine cautiously in patients with heart block, heart failure, hepatic disorder, impaired renal function, or severe aortic stenosis because of increased risk of adverse reactions.

! **WARNING** Assess patient frequently for chest pain when starting or increasing the dose of amlodipine because an acute MI or worsening of angina can occur, especially in patients with severe obstructive coronary artery disease.

- Monitor patient with impaired hepatic function closely because amlodipine is extensively metabolized by the liver and expect to titrate dosage slowly when administering drug to patients with severe hepatic impairment.
- Monitor blood pressure while adjusting dosage, especially in patients with heart failure or severe aortic stenosis because symptomatic hypotension may occur.

PATIENT TEACHING

- Instruct patient how to take form of amlodipine prescribed.

! **WARNING** Tell patient to immediately notify prescriber of arm or leg swelling, difficulty breathing, dizziness, hives, rash, or any other persistent, severe, or unusual adverse reactions. Stress importance of reporting chest pain immediately to prescriber and to seek immediate medical care.

- Advise patient to have blood pressure checked routinely for possible hypotension.

amoxicillin trihydrate

(amoxycillin)

Amoxil, Apo-Amoxi (CAN), Novamoxin (CAN)

Class and Category

Pharmacologic class: Aminopenicillin
Therapeutic class: Antibiotic

Indications and Dosages

∗ *To treat ear, nose, and throat infections caused by* Haemophilus influenzae, Staphylococcus *spp,* Streptococcus pneumoniae, *or* Streptococcus *species; to treat GU tract infections caused by* Enterococcus faecalis, Escherichia coli, *or* Proteus mirabilis; *to treat skin and soft-tissue infections caused by* E. coli, Staphylococcus *spp, or* Streptococcus *spp; and to treat pharyngitis, tonsillitis, or both secondary to* Streptococcus pyogenes *infection*

CAPSULES, CHEWABLE TABLETS, ORAL SUSPENSION, TABLETS

Adults and children weighing 40 kg (88 lb) or more. 250 mg every 8 hr or 500 mg every 12 hr. *For severe infection;* 500 mg every 8 hr or 875 mg every 12 hr. Given at least 10 days for pharyngitis and tonsillitis.

Children ages 12 wk and older weighing less than 40 kg (88 lb). 20 mg/kg daily in divided doses every 8 hr or 25 mg/kg daily in divided doses every 12 hr. *For severe infections*: 40 mg/kg daily in divided doses every 8 hr or 45 mg/kg daily in divided doses every 12 hr. Given at least 10 days for pharyngitis and tonsillitis.
Children under age 12 wk. Up to 30 mg/kg/day in divided doses every 12 hr. Given at least 10 days for pharyngitis and tonsillitis.

✱ *To treat lower respiratory tract infections caused by* H. influenzae, Staphylococcus *spp or* Streptococcus *spp.*

CAPSULES, CHEWABLE TABLETS, ORAL SUSPENSION, TABLETS

Adults and children weighing 40 kg (88 lb) or more. 875 mg every 12 hr. Alternatively, 500 mg every 8 hr.
Children ages 12 wk and older weighing less than 40 kg (88 lb). 40 mg/kg in divided doses every 8 hr. Alternatively, 45 mg/kg in divided doses every 12 hr.
Children under age 12 wk. Up to 30 mg/kg daily in divided doses every 12 hr.

✱ *As adjunct to eradicate* Helicobacter pylori *to reduce risk of duodenal ulcer recurrence*

CAPSULES, CHEWABLE TABLETS, ORAL SUSPENSION, TABLETS

Adults. 1 g every 12 hr with 500 mg of clarithromycin every 12 hr and 30 mg of lansoprazole every 12 hr for 14 days. Alternatively, 1 g every 8 hr with 30 mg of lansoprazole every 8 hr for 14 days.

±**DOSAGE ADJUSTMENT** For patients with impaired renal function with an eGFR less than 30 ml/min, dosage reduced to less than 875 mg; for an eGFR of 10 to 30 ml/min, dosage reduced to 500 mg or 250 mg every 12 hours; and for an eGFR less than 10 ml/min, dosage reduced to 500 mg or 250 mg and frequency reduced to every 24 hours.

Drug Administration

P.O.

- Shake oral suspension well before each use. Use a calibrated device to measure dosage.
- Administer oral suspension form to children by dropping directly on child's tongue to swallow. If this does not work, mix dose of suspension with a cold drink (fruit juice, ginger ale, milk, water) or formula and have child drink it immediately.
- Reconstituted suspension may be refrigerated but not required. Discard after 14 days.
- Chewable tablets should not be swallowed whole.
- Each 200-mg chewable tablet contains 1.82 mg phenylalanine; each 400-mg chewable tablet contains 3.64 mg phenylalanine. Suspension does not contain phenylalanine.

Route	Onset	Peak	Duration
P.O.	Unknown	1–2 hr	6–8 hr

Half-life: 9–11 hr

Mechanism of Action

Kills bacteria by binding to and inactivating penicillin-binding proteins on the inner bacterial cell wall, weakening the bacterial cell wall and causing lysis.

Contraindications

Hypersensitivity to amoxicillin, other beta-lactam antibiotics, or their components

Interactions

DRUGS

allopurinol: Increased risk of rash
chloramphenicol, erythromycins, sulfonamides, tetracyclines: Reduced bactericidal effect of amoxicillin
methotrexate: Increased risk of methotrexate toxicity
oral anticoagulants: Possible prolonged prothrombin time (increased international normalized ratio)
oral contraceptives with estrogen: Possibly reduced effectiveness of contraceptive
probenecid: Increased amoxicillin effects

Adverse Reactions

CNS: Agitation, anxiety, **aseptic meningitis**, behavioral changes, confusion, dizziness, insomnia, reversible hyperactivity, **seizures**
CV: Hypersensitivity vasculitis
EENT: Black, hairy tongue; mucocutaneous candidiasis; tooth discoloration
GI: ***Clostridium difficile*-associated diarrhea**, diarrhea, **drug-induced enterocolitis syndrome (DIES)**, elevated liver enzymes, **hemorrhagic or pseudomembranous colitis**, **hepatic dysfunction**, jaundice, nausea, vomiting

GU: Crystalluria, vaginal mycosis
HEME: **Agranulocytosis**, anemia (including **hemolytic anemia**), eosinophilia, granulocytosis, **leukopenia**, **thrombocytopenia**, **thrombocytopenic purpura**
SKIN: **Acute generalized exanthematous pustulosis (AGEP)**, **erythema multiforme**, erythematous maculopapular rash, **exfoliative dermatitis**, generalized rash, linear IgA bullous dermatosis, mucocutaneous candidiasis, pruritus, **Stevens-Johnson syndrome**, **toxic epidermal necrolysis**, urticaria
Other: **Anaphylaxis and other hypersensitivity reactions**, **angioedema**, **drug reaction with eosinophilia and systemic symptoms (DRESS)**, serum sickness-like reaction (such as arthralgia, arthritis, fever, myalgia, rash, and urticaria)

Childbearing Considerations

PREGNANCY

- It is not known if drug can cause fetal harm.
- Use with caution only if benefit to mother outweighs potential risk to fetus.

LABOR AND DELIVERY

- It is not known if drug given to mother during labor has immediate or delayed adverse effects on the fetus.

LACTATION

- Drug is present in breast milk and may lead to sensitization in infant.
- Mothers should check with prescriber before breastfeeding.

Nursing Considerations

- Know that patients with mononucleosis shouldn't receive amoxicillin because this class of drugs may cause an erythematous rash.
- Use drug cautiously in patients with hepatic impairment. Monitor CBC and hepatic and renal function, as ordered, in patients on prolonged therapy. Also, use cautiously in breastfeeding and elderly patients.
- Expect to start therapy before culture and sensitivity test results are known.

! **WARNING** Stop amoxicillin immediately and provide emergency care as indicated and ordered if a hypersensitivity reaction occurs. Also, monitor patient for a rash, which could be the first sign of a severe cutaneous adverse reaction. However, DRESS may initially present with only fever or swollen lymph nodes. Monitor patient closely and alert prescriber as drug will need to be discontinued. Expect to provide supportive care, as needed and ordered.

! **WARNING** Monitor patient closely for diarrhea, which may indicate pseudomembranous colitis caused by *Clostridium difficile*. It can range from mild to life-threatening. If diarrhea occurs, notify prescriber and expect testing to be done to confirm presence of *C. difficile*. If confirmed, expect to withhold amoxicillin, and treat with an antibiotic effective against *C. difficile* along with electrolytes, fluids, and protein, as needed and ordered.

! **WARNING** Monitor patient, especially children, for DIES, a non-IgE mediated hypersensitivity reaction that presents as protracted vomiting occurring 1 to 4 hours after amoxicillin is given. It may be accompanied by diarrhea (within 24 hours of amoxicillin being given), hypotension, lethargy, pallor, and shock. If suspected, immediately notify prescriber, discontinue drug, and provide supportive care, as needed and ordered.

- Monitor patient for superinfection. If it occurs, expect to discontinue drug and provide treatment, as needed and ordered.

PATIENT TEACHING

- Instruct patient, family, or caregiver how to administer the amoxicillin product prescribed. If patient is a child, instruct on how to administer drug if placing drug directly on child's tongue for child to swallow doesn't work.
- Alert patient, family, or caregiver that chewable tablets of amoxicillin contain phenylalanine and should not be given to a patient with phenylketonuria.
- Urge patient to take amoxicillin for full length of time prescribed, even if he feels better.

! **WARNING** Instruct patient, family, or caregiver to notify prescriber immediately if an allergic reaction or a rash occurs. Stress importance of seeking immediate medical care if allergic reaction is severe or rash is present.

- Teach patient to notify prescriber if infection worsens or does not improve after 72 hours.

! **WARNING** Urge patient to tell prescriber about diarrhea that is severe or lasts longer than 3 days. Remind patient that bloody or watery stools can occur 2 or more months after antibiotic therapy is discontinued and may be serious, requiring prompt treatment.

- Inform patient with diabetes who is using glucose tests based on the Benedict's copper reduction reaction that false-positive reactions may occur when testing for glucose in urine. Advise patient to use glucose tests based on enzymatic glucose oxidase reaction instead.

amphetamine

Adzenys XR-ODT, Dyanavel XR

amphetamine sulfate

Evekeo, Evekeo ODT

dextroamphetamine

Xelstrym

dextroamphetamine sulfate

Dexedrine ER, ProCentra, Zenzedi

methamphetamine hydrochloride

Desoxyn

Class, Category, and Schedule

Pharmacologic class: Phenethylamine
Therapeutic class: CNS stimulant
Controlled substance schedule: II

Indications and Dosages

✶ *To treat attention deficit hyperactivity disorder (ADHD)*

ORAL SOLUTION (PROCENTRA), TABLETS (ZENZEDI)

Children ages 6 and older. *Initial:* 5 mg daily or twice daily. Increased by 5 mg daily at 1-wk intervals until desired response occurs. Rarely, dosage above 40 mg daily is needed.
Children ages 3 to 6. *Initial:* 2.5 mg daily. Increased by 2.5 mg daily at 1-wk intervals until desired response occurs.

TABLETS (EVEKEO)

Children ages 6 and older. *Initial:* 5 mg daily upon awakening. Alternatively, twice daily once upon awakening and once 4 to 6 hr later. Increased by 5 mg daily at 1-wk intervals until desired response occurs. Rarely, dosage above 40 mg daily is needed.
Children ages 3 to 5. *Initial:* 2.5 mg daily upon awakening. Increased by 2.5 mg daily at 1-wk intervals until desired response occurs.

TABLETS (DESOXYN)

Children ages 6 and older. *Initial:* 5 mg once or twice daily, increased in increments of 5 mg at weekly intervals, as needed. *Usual:* 20 to 25 mg daily in 1 or 2 divided doses.

ORAL DISINTEGRATING TABLETS (EVEKEO ODT)

Children ages 6 and older. *Initial:* 5 mg once daily or twice daily. An additional dose given 4 to 6 hr later, as needed. Increased by 2.5 mg or 5 mg at 1-wk intervals until desired response occurs. Rarely, dosage above 40 mg daily is needed.
Children ages 3 to 6. *Initial:* 2.5 mg once daily or twice daily. An additional dose given 4 to 6 hr later, as needed. Increased by 2.5 mg at 1-wk intervals until desired response occurs.

ORAL DISINTEGRATING E.R. TABLETS (ADZENYS XR-ODT)

Adults. 12.5 mg once daily.
Children ages 6 to 17. *Initial:* 6.3 mg once daily in the morning and then increased in increments of 3.1 mg or 6.3 mg weekly, as needed. *Maximum:* 18.8 mg once daily for children ages 6 to 12; 12.5 mg once daily for children ages 12 to 17.

E.R. CAPSULES (DEXEDRINE ER)

Children ages 6 and older. *Initial:* 5 mg daily or twice daily. Increased by 5 mg daily at 1-wk intervals until desired response occurs.

E.R. ORAL SUSPENSION (DYANAVEL XR), E.R. TABLETS (DYANAVEL XR)

Children ages 6 and older. *Initial:* 2.5 or 5 mg once daily. Increased by 2.5 to 10 mg every 4 to 7 days. *Maximum:* 20 mg daily.

±**DOSAGE ADJUSTMENT** For patients receiving acidifying agents such as ascorbic acid or alkalinizing agents such as sodium bicarbonate, a dosage adjustment may be needed.

TRANSDERMAL SYSTEM (XELSTRYM)

Adults. 9 mg/9 hr applied 2 hr before an effect is needed and removed within 9 hr. Increased to 18 mg/9 hr, as needed. *Maximum:*18 mg/9 hr and only 1 transdermal system applied per 24 hr.
Children ages 6 to 17. *Initial:* 4.5 mg/9 hr applied 2 hr before an effect is needed and removed within 9 hr. Dosage titrated in weekly increments of 4.5 mg, as needed. *Maximum:* 18 mg/9 hr and only 1 transdermal system applied per 24 hr.

±**DOSAGE ADJUSTMENT** For patients using transdermal system and have severe renal impairment (eGFR 15 to less than 30 ml/min), maximum dose is 13.5 mg/9 hours. For patients using transdermal system and have end stage renal disease (eGFR less than 15 ml/min), maximum dose is 9 mg/9 hours.

✱ *To treat narcolepsy*

E.R. CAPSULES (DEXEDRINE ER), ORAL SOLUTION (PROCENTRA), TABLETS (EVEKEO, ZENZEDI)

Adults. 5 to 60 mg daily in divided doses, depending on response.
Children ages 12 and older. *Initial:* 10 mg daily. Increased by 10 mg daily at 1-wk intervals until desired response occurs.
Children ages 6 to 12. *Initial:* 5 mg daily. Increased by 5 mg daily at 1-wk intervals until desired response occurs.

±**DOSAGE ADJUSTMENT** For patients with narcolepsy developing adverse reactions such as anorexia or insomnia, dosage reduced.

✱ *As adjunct to weight reduction program to treat exogenous obesity short term*

TABLETS (EVEKEO)

Adults and adolescents. *Usual:* Up to 30 mg daily in divided doses of 5 to 10 mg, 30 to 60 min before meals.

TABLETS (DESOXYN)

Adults and adolescents. 5 mg one-half hr before each meal. *Maximum:* Few weeks duration.

Drug Administration

P.O.

- Do not substitute 1 amphetamine product for another on a milligram-per-milligram basis because of different amphetamine salt compositions and differing pharmacokinetic profiles. The exception is Dyanavel XR tablets and Dyanavel XR suspension, which may be used interchangeably.
- Administer first dose in the morning. Give additional doses 4 to 6 hr apart. Do not administer the last dose, if more than 1 daily dose is prescribed, late in evening because insomnia may occur.
- Each 5 ml of oral solution contains 5 mg of dexamphetamine.
- Use a calibrated measuring device for accurate dosing of oral solution or suspension. Shake oral suspension bottle before measuring dose. Wash oral dosing syringe or measuring device after each use.
- Dyanavel XR tablets may be chewed or swallowed whole.
- Administer disintegrating tablets by first carefully removing tablets from package (avoid pushing tablets through the foil) with gloved hand. Tablet should be immediately placed on patient's tongue and allowed to dissolve without chewing or crushing.
- E.R. capsules should be swallowed whole.

TRANSDERMAL

- Apply 1 transdermal system 2 hr before an effect is needed and remove system within 9 hr after application. Apply to a clean, dry, intact skin area void of gels, lotions, or oils on the patient's chest, flank, hip, or upper arm or back. Do not apply with dressings, tape, or other common adhesives. Change application site when applying a new transdermal system.
- Avoid touching the adhesive side of the drug to avoid absorption of the drug. If touched, immediately wash hands with soap and water.
- Reattach lifted edges of the system by pressing firmly and smoothing down the edges of the system. Do not use dressings, tape, or other common adhesives to reattach

edges. If the system comes off completely, apply a new system.

- Do not substitute for other amphetamine products on a mg/mg basis because different amphetamine products have different base compositions and pharmacokinetic profiles.

Route	Onset	Peak	Duration
P.O.	20–90 min	1–2 hr	3–6 hr
P.O. (E.R.)	Unknown	4–5 hr	Unknown
Transdermal	Unknown	6-9 hr	Unknown

Half-life: 9–12 hr (transdermal: 6.4–11.5 hr)

Mechanism of Action

May produce its CNS stimulant effects by facilitating release and blocking reuptake of norepinephrine at adrenergic nerve terminals and by direct stimulation of alpha and beta receptors in the peripheral nervous system. It also releases and blocks reuptake of dopamine in limbic regions of the brain. The drug's main action appears to be in the cerebral cortex and, possibly, the reticular activating system. These actions cause decreased motor restlessness, increased alertness, and diminished drowsiness and fatigue. Its peripheral actions include increased blood pressure and mild bronchodilation and respiratory stimulation.

Contraindications

Advanced arteriosclerosis; agitation (for narcolepsy treatment); glaucoma; history of drug abuse; hypersensitivity to amphetamines or their components; hypersensitivity or idiosyncratic reaction to sympathomimetic amines; hyperthyroidism; MAO inhibitor therapy, including I.V. methylene blue or linezolid within 14 days; moderate to severe hypertension; symptomatic cardiovascular disease

Interactions

DRUGS

acetazolamide, alkalinizers (such as sodium bicarbonate), some thiazides: Increased blood level and effects of amphetamine
adrenergic blockers: Inhibited adrenergic blockade
antihistamines: Possibly reduced sedation from antihistamine
antihypertensives: Possibly decreased antihypertensive effect
buspirone, CYP206 inhibitors, fentanyl, lithium, MAO inhibitors, selective serotonin reuptake inhibitors, serotonin norepinephrine reuptake inhibitors, St. John's wort, tramadol, tricyclic antidepressants, triptans: Increased risk of serotonin syndrome
chlorpromazine: Inhibited CNS stimulant effects of amphetamine
ethosuximide: Possibly delayed ethosuximide absorption
GI acidifiers (such as ascorbic acid), reserpine: Decreased amphetamine absorption
guanethidine: Decreased antihypertensive effect and decreased amphetamine absorption
haloperidol: Decreased CNS stimulation
lithium carbonate: Possibly decreased anorectic and stimulant effects of amphetamine
MAO inhibitors: Potentiated effects of amphetamine; possibly hypertensive crisis
meperidine: Increased analgesia
methenamine: Increased urine excretion and decreased effects of amphetamine
norepinephrine: Possibly increased adrenergic effect of norepinephrine
phenobarbital, phenytoin: Synergistic anticonvulsant action
propoxyphene: Increased CNS stimulation, potentially fatal seizures
proton pump inhibitors: Possibly decreased effectiveness of amphetamines
tricyclic antidepressants: Possibly enhanced antidepressant effects and decreased effects of amphetamine
urinary acidifiers (such as ammonium chloride, ascorbic acid, sodium acid phosphate): Increased amphetamine excretion and decreased amphetamine blood level and effects
veratrum alkaloids: Decreased hypotensive effect

ACTIVITIES

alcohol: Possibly increased release of dose into bloodstream

FOODS

acidic fruit juices: Decreased amphetamine absorption

Adverse Reactions

CNS: Aggression, anger, anxiety, depression, dizziness, dyskinesia, dysphoria, euphoria, exacerbation of motor and phonic tics and

Tourette's syndrome, excessive talkativeness, hallucinations, headache, insomnia, irritability, overstimulation, paranoia, paresthesia, psychotic episodes, restlessness, **serotonin syndrome**, tremor
CV: **Cardiomyopathy**, hypertension, **MI**, palpitations, Raynaud's phenomenon, **sudden death**, tachycardia
EENT: Blurred vision, dry mouth, mydriasis, teeth grinding, unpleasant taste
ENDO: Growth suppression in children and teens (long-term use)
GI: Anorexia, constipation, diarrhea, GI disturbances, intestinal ischemia
GU: Frequent or prolonged erections, impotence, libido changes
MS: **Rhabdomyolysis**
SKIN: Alopecia, application site reactions with transdermal system (burning, discomfort, edema, erythema, pain, pruritus, swelling), excessive skin picking, rash, **Stevens-Johnson syndrome**, **toxic epidermal necrolysis**, urticaria
Other: **Anaphylaxis**, **angioedema**, physical and psychological dependence, weight loss

Childbearing Considerations

PREGNANCY

- Pregnancy exposure registry: 1-866-961-2388 or https://womensmentalhealth.org/research/pregnancyregistry/adhd-medications/.
- Drug may cause fetal harm because amphetamines cause vasoconstriction, which results in decreased placental perfusion.
- Use with caution only if benefit to mother outweighs potential risk to fetus.

LABOR AND DELIVERY

- Know that infants born to mothers dependent on amphetamines have an increased risk of premature delivery and low birth weight because amphetamines can cause contractions.
- Monitor infants born to mothers dependent on amphetamines for withdrawal symptoms such as agitation and significant lassitude as well as feeding difficulties and irritability in the postnatal period.

LACTATION

- Drug is present in breast milk. Large doses of amphetamines may interfere with milk production, especially in mothers whose lactation is not well established.
- A decision should be made to discontinue breastfeeding or the drug to avoid potential adverse reactions in the breastfed infant.

Nursing Considerations

- Keep in mind that when symptoms of ADHD occur with acute stress reactions, treatment with amphetamines usually isn't indicated.

! **WARNING** Don't give amphetamine during or for up to 14 days after MAO therapy to prevent hypertensive crisis. Also, know that amphetamine therapy should be avoided in patients with structural cardiac abnormalities or other serious cardiac disease such as cardiomyopathy, coronary artery disease, or serious cardiac arrhythmias as sudden death may occur.

! **WARNING** Assess all patients for risk for abuse, addiction, and misuse before starting amphetamine therapy as drug has a high potential for addiction leading to abuse and misuse of drug. During drug therapy be alert for evidence of abuse and misuse as overdose or even death may occur. Report signs and symptoms of abuse such as hyperactivity, irritability, marked insomnia, personality changes, and severe dermatoses.

- Assess patient for personal and family history for tics or Tourette's syndrome before amphetamine therapy is initiated. Also, monitor patient during drug therapy for new or exacerbation of motor or verbal tics or worsening of Tourette's syndrome.
- Screen patient with bipolar disorder for risk factors for developing a manic episode such as a history of depression or family history of bipolar disorder, depression, or suicide. Also monitor all patients for manic or psychotic symptoms throughout amphetamine therapy because even patients without a prior history of psychotic illness or mania may exhibit manic or psychotic symptoms. If symptoms occur, notify prescriber, and expect drug to be discontinued.

! **WARNING** Monitor patient for hypersensitivity reactions that could become life-threatening such as anaphylaxis and angioedema. If present, notify prescriber immediately, withhold drug as ordered, and provide supportive care, as needed and ordered.

! **WARNING** Monitor patient closely for evidence of serotonin syndrome, such as agitation, coma, diarrhea, hallucinations, hyperreflexia, hyperthermia, incoordination, labile blood pressure, nausea, tachycardia, and vomiting. Notify prescriber immediately because serotonin syndrome reactions may be life-threatening. Expect to discontinue amphetamine therapy and any other serotonergic agents a patient may be taking. Be prepared to provide supportive care.

- Monitor patient for hypertension and tachycardia as amphetamine therapy may increase blood pressure and heart rate.
- Assess patients' fingers and toes for digital changes because amphetamine can cause peripheral vasculopathy, including Raynaud's phenomenon. While signs and symptoms are usually intermittent and mild, digital ulceration and/or soft tissue breakdown can occur. If suspected or evident, notify prescriber and expect dosage to be reduced or drug discontinued.
- Expect to decrease dosage if patient has bothersome adverse reactions, such as anorexia and insomnia. To minimize insomnia, administer drug earlier in day.
- Monitor children and teens receiving drug long term for growth suppression or not gaining weight.

PATIENT TEACHING

- Instruct patient, family, or caregiver how to administer form of amphetamine prescribed.

! **WARNING** Explain drug's abuse and addiction potential, and caution against altering dosage or frequency unless prescribed. Remind patient that misuse can lead to an overdose or even death. Encourage patient to keep amphetamine in a safe place, preferably locked, and not to share the drug with anyone. Review proper disposal of drug when no longer used.

- Stress importance of avoiding alcohol while taking amphetamine therapy.

! **WARNING** Alert patient, family, or caregiver drug may cause an allergic reaction. Stress importance of notifying prescriber, if present, and to seek immediate medical care if serious.

- Tell patient to report any new or worsening behavior and thought problems; new or worsening bipolar illness; new manic symptoms; or new psychotic symptoms such as believing things that are not true, feeling suspicious, or hearing voices. Also advise patient to report any persistent, severe, or unusual adverse effects to prescriber, such as motor and verbal tics or worsening of Tourette's syndrome.
- Advise patient to notify prescriber if fingers or toes begin to feel cool, numb, or painful and/or change color from pale to blue to red. Tell patient to notify prescriber immediately if ulcers appear on fingers or toes.
- Inform family or caregiver, long-term use of amphetamines may cause suppression of growth and weight loss.
- Urge patient to avoid hazardous activities until drug's effects are known and resolved.
- Instruct patient to notify prescriber before taking any new drugs, including over-the-counter preparations.
- Advise females of childbearing age to notify prescriber if pregnancy occurs.
- Instruct breastfeeding mothers to avoid breastfeeding during amphetamine therapy because drug is excreted in breast milk.

amphotericin B

amphotericin B lipid complex

Abelcet

amphotericin B liposomal complex

AmBisome

Class and Category

Pharmacologic class: Amphoteric polyene
Therapeutic class: Antifungal

Indications and Dosages

∗ To treat severe life-threatening fungal infections

I.V. INFUSION (AMPHOTERICIN B)

Adults and adolescents. *Initial:* 1-mg test dose in 20 ml of D_5W infused over 20 to 30 min; if test dose is tolerated, then 0.25 to 0.3 mg/kg daily, given over 2 to 6 hr. Increased in 5- to 10-mg increments, based on patient tolerance and infection severity, to a final daily dose of 0.5 to 0.7 mg/kg but not to exceed a total daily dose of 1.5 mg/kg. *Usual range:* Up to 1 mg/kg daily or 1.5 mg/kg every other day.

∗ To provide empirical therapy for presumed fungal infection in febrile, neutropenic patients

I.V. INFUSION (AMBISOME)

Adults and children. 3 mg/kg daily.

∗ To treat invasive fungal infections in patients who are refractory to or intolerant of conventional amphotericin B therapy

I.V. INFUSION (ABELCET)

Adults and children. 5 mg/kg daily.

∗ To treat severe Aspergilus *species,* Candida *species or* Cryptococcus *species refractory to amphotericin B deoxycholate or in patients whose renal impairment or unacceptable toxicity precludes the use of amphotericin B deoxycholate*

I.V. INFUSION (AMBISOME)

Adults and children. 3 to 5 mg/kg daily.

∗ To treat visceral leishmaniasis

I.V. INFUSION (AMBISOME)

Immunocompetent adults and children. 3 mg/kg daily on days 1 through 5 and on days 14 and 21. A repeat course of therapy given, as needed.

Immunocompromised adults and children. 4 mg/kg daily on days 1 through 5 and days 10, 17, 24, 31, and 38.

∗ To treat Cyptococcal *meningitis in patients with HIV*

I.V. INFUSION (AMBISOME)

Adults and children. 6 mg/kg daily.

Drug Administration

I.V.

- Expect to give an antihistamine, antipyretic, or corticosteroid, if prescribed, just before infusing amphotericin B to help minimize fever and shaking chills.
- Each product of amphotericin B is not interchangeable on a milligram-per-milligram basis with other amphotericin B products.
- Avoid rapid infusion because arrhythmias, hypokalemia, hypotension, and shock may occur.
- *Incompatibilities for all products:* Other I.V. drugs, electrolytes, saline products

Amphotericin B

- Under no circumstances should the total daily dose of 1.5 mg/kg be exceeded.
- Under no circumstances should the total daily dose of 1.5 mg/kg be exceeded.
- Reconstitute drug by rapidly directing 10 ml Sterile Water for Injection without a bacteriostatic agent into the lyophilized cake, using a 20G needle. Shake vial immediately until the colloidal solution is clear.
- Further dilute with 5% Dextrose Injection with a pH above 4.2 to yield a concentration of 0.1 mg/ml of amphotericin B. The pH of each container of Dextrose Injection should be ascertained before use. If the pH is below 4.2, then a buffer should be added before it is used to dilute the concentrated solution of amphotericin B following the manufacturer's guidelines.
- An in-line membrane filter may be used as long as it is not less than 1.0 micron to ensure passage of the antibiotic dispersion.
- Administer by slow infusion over 2 to 6 hr (depending on the dose).

Amphotericin B Liposomal Complex (AmBisome)

- An in-line membrane filter may be used if the mean pore diameter is more than 1 micron to prevent significant drug removal because reconstituted amphotericin B liposomal complex is a colloidal suspension.
- To reconstitute, add 12 ml of Sterile Water for Injection to each drug vial to obtain a concentration of 4 mg/ml. Do not reconstitute with saline or add saline to reconstituted concentration. The use of any solution other than Sterile Water for Injection, including Bacteriostatic Water, may cause precipitation of drug. Shake drug vial vigorously for 30 sec to completely disperse the drug. It will form a yellow, translucent suspension.
- The reconstituted drug concentrate may be stored for up to 24 hr at 2–8°C (36–46°F). Do not freeze.
- Withdraw amount needed from drug vial. Attach the 5-micron filter provided to the syringe. Inject the syringe contents through

the filter into the appropriate amount of 5% Dextrose Injection (use only one filter per drug vial) to obtain a final concentration of 1 to 2 mg/ml prior to administration. Lower concentrations (0.2 to 0.5 mg/ml) may be used for infants and small children to provide sufficient volume for infusion.

- Administer the diluted solution within 6 hr.
- Flush existing intravenous line with 5% Dextrose in Water before administering drug. If this is not possible, a separate intravenous line must be used.
- Infuse over 2 hr using a controlled infusion device. Time may be reduced to 1 hr in patients in whom drug is well tolerated, or the infusion time may be increased if patient experiences discomfort during infusion.

Amphotericin B Lipid Complex (Abelcet)

- Prepare amphotericin B lipid complex by shaking vial gently until no yellow sediment is seen. Using an 18G needle, withdraw prescribed dose from required number of vials into 1 or more 20-ml syringes. Replace needle with 5-micron filter needle supplied with each vial.
- Empty syringe contents into a bag of 5% Dextrose in Water so that final concentration is 1 mg/ml. Expect to use a concentration of 2 mg/ml for children and patients with cardiovascular disease. Before infusing, shake bag until contents are mixed thoroughly.
- Do not use an in-line filter.
- Flush an existing I.V. line with 5% Dextrose Injection before infusion or use a separate infusion line for drug administration.
- Infuse at 2.5 mg/kg/hr.
- If infusion exceeds 2 hr, shake infusion bag every 2 hr.
- The admixed drug in 5% Dextrose Injection may be stored for up to 48 hr at 2–8°C (36–46°F) and an additional 6 hr at room temperature. Do not freeze.

Route	Onset	Peak	Duration
I.V.	Immediate	Unknown	Unknown

Half-life: 24 hr–15 days

Mechanism of Action

Binds to sterols in fungal cell plasma membranes, which changes membrane permeability and allows loss of potassium and small molecules from cells. This action results in fungal cell impairment or death.

Contraindications

Hypersensitivity to amphotericin B or its components

Interactions

DRUGS

antineoplastics: Increased risk of bronchospasm, hypotension, and nephrotoxicity
corticosteroids, corticotropin: Increased risk of hypokalemia and cardiac dysfunction
cyclosporine, nephrotoxic drugs: Increased risk of nephrotoxicity
digitalis glycosides: Possibly hypokalemia and more severe digitalis toxicity
flucytosine: Possibly increased flucytosine toxicity
imidazoles, such as clotrimazole, fluconazole, ketoconazole, miconazole: Possibly induced resistance to amphotericin
leukocyte transfusion: Possibly acute pulmonary toxicity
skeletal muscle relaxants: Possibly hypokalemia and increased muscle relaxation

Adverse Reactions

CNS: Fever, headache, shaking chills, tiredness, weakness
CV: Chest pain, **hypotension**, irregular heartbeat
EENT: Difficulty swallowing, pharyngitis
GI: Abdominal pain, anorexia, diarrhea, **hepatic failure**, indigestion, jaundice, nausea, vomiting
GU: Decreased or increased urine output, hemorrhagic cystitis, impaired renal function
HEME: **Agranulocytosis**, anemia, **leukopenia**, **thrombocytopenia**, **unusual bleeding** or bruising
MS: Arthralgia, muscle spasms, myalgia, **rhabdomyolysis**
RESP: **Apnea**, **bronchospasm**, **cyanosis**, dyspnea, **hypoventilation**, **hypoxia**, **pulmonary edema**, tachypnea
SKIN: Erythema, flushing, maculopapular rash, pruritus and redness especially around ears, urticaria
Other: **Anaphylaxis**, **angioedema**, **hypocalcemia**, **hypokalemia**, **hypomagnesemia**, infusion-site pain, thrombophlebitis

Childbearing Considerations

PREGNANCY

- It is not known if drug can cause fetal harm.

- Use with caution only if benefit to mother outweighs potential risk to fetus.

LACTATION

- It is not known if drug is present in breast milk.
- Breastfeeding should be discontinued during drug therapy.

Nursing Considerations

- Assess I.V. insertion site regularly to detect extravasation of amphotericin B, which may cause severe local irritation. To minimize local thrombophlebitis, obtain an order to add heparin to infusion or expect to administer amphotericin on alternate days, which also may help prevent anorexia, as prescribed. Alternate-day dose shouldn't exceed 1.5 mg/kg.

! **WARNING** Monitor patient for hypersensitivity reactions. If present, notify prescriber immediately, withhold drug as ordered, and provide supportive care, as needed and ordered.

- Monitor renal function, as ordered, because of the risk of renal impairment. Plan to obtain serum creatinine level every other day while amphotericin B dosage is increasing and then at least twice weekly during therapy. If BUN or serum creatinine levels increase significantly, expect amphotericin B to be withheld until renal function improves. Know that a cumulative dose of more than 4 g may cause irreversible renal dysfunction.
- Expect to monitor CBC and platelet count weekly during therapy to detect adverse hematologic effects. Also, monitor serum calcium, magnesium, and potassium levels twice weekly to detect abnormalities.
- Be aware that false elevations of serum phosphate may occur when samples are analyzed using the PHOSm assay.

PATIENT TEACHING

- Inform patient that amphotericin B will be given intravenously. Stress importance of alerting staff immediately if any discomfort or swelling is felt at the insertion site.

! **WARNING** Tell patient to immediately alert staff if difficulty breathing, a feeling of throat constriction or tongue swelling occurs or any other signs and symptoms of an allergic reaction. Also, tell patient to report any other adverse effects that are persistent, severe, or unusual while receiving the drug.

- Alert patient that frequent blood tests will be needed during amphotericin B therapy.
- Inform mothers who are breastfeeding that breastfeeding should be discontinued during amphotericin B therapy.

ampicillin

ampicillin sodium

ampicillin trihydrate

Class and Category

Pharmacologic class: Aminopenicillin
Therapeutic class: Antibiotic

Indications and Dosages

✶ *To treat GI infections and GU infections (other than gonorrhea) caused by susceptible strains of enterococci,* Escherichia coli, Salmonella typhi *and other species,* Shigella, *or* Proteus mirabilis

CAPSULES, ORAL SUSPENSION

Adults and children weighing more than 20 kg (44 lb). 500 mg every 6 hr.
Children weighing 20 kg (44 lb) or less. 100 mg/kg daily in divided doses every 6 hr.

I.M. INJECTION, I.V. INFUSION, I.V. INJECTION

Adults and children weighing 40 kg (88 lb) or more. 500 mg every 6 hr.
Children weighing less than 40 kg (88 lb). 50 mg/kg daily in divided doses every 6 to 8 hr.

✶ *To treat uncomplicated gonorrhea caused by susceptible strains of non–penicillinase-producing* Neisseria gonorrhoeae

CAPSULES, ORAL SUSPENSION

Adults and children weighing more than 20 kg (44 lb). 3.5 g as a single dose with 1 g of probenecid.

✶ *To treat respiratory tract infections caused by susceptible strains of non–penicillinase-producing* Haemophilus influenzae, *staphylococci, or streptococci, including* Streptococcus pneumoniae

CAPSULES, ORAL SUSPENSION

Adults and children weighing more than 20 kg (44 lb). 250 mg every 6 hr.
Children weighing 20 kg (44 lb) or less. 50 mg/kg daily in divided doses every 6 to 8 hr.

I.M. INJECTION, I.V. INFUSION, I.V. INJECTION

Adults and children weighing 40 kg (88 lb) or more. 250 to 500 mg every 6 hr.
Children weighing less than 40 kg (88 lb). 25 to 50 mg/kg daily in divided doses every 6 to 8 hr.

∗ *To treat soft-tissue infections caused by susceptible strains of staphylococci or streptococci organisms*

I.M. INJECTION, I.V. INFUSION, I.V. INJECTION

Adults and children weighing 40 kg (88 lb) or more. 250 to 500 mg every 6 hr.
Children weighing less than 40 kg (88 lb). 25 to 50 mg/kg daily in divided doses every 6 to 8 hr.

∗ *To treat septicemia; to treat bacterial meningitis caused by susceptible strains of* Neisseria meningitidis

I.M. INJECTION, I.V. INFUSION, I.V. INJECTION

Adults and children. 150 to 200 mg/kg daily in divided doses every 3 to 4 hr. Dosage may initially be administered I.V. for at least 3 days and then continued I.M.
Neonates greater than 34 wk gestation and less than or equal to 28 days postnatal. 150 mg/kg daily in divided doses every 8 hr.
Neonates less than or equal to 34 wk gestation but greater than or equal to 8 days but less than 28 days postnatal. 150 mg/kg daily in divided doses every 12 hr.
Neonates less than or equal to 34 wk gestation but less than or equal to 7 days postnatal. 100 mg/kg daily in divided doses every 12 hr.

∗ *To treat urethritis in males due to* N. gonorrhoeae

I.M. INJECTION, I.V. INFUSION, I.V. INJECTION

Adult men. 2 doses of 500 mg at 8- or 12-hr intervals. May repeat or extend treatment, as needed.

Drug Administration

P.O.

- Give with 8 ounces of water 30 min before or 2 hr after meals.
- Shake suspension well before each use and keep bottle tightly closed between uses. Use a calibrated device to measure dosage. Store in refrigerator and discard unused portion after 14 days.

I.V.

- For direct I.V. administration, reconstitute by adding 5 ml of Bacteriostatic Water for Injection or Sterile Water for Injection to 250- or 500-mg vial and administer slowly over 3 to 5 min or dilute with 7.4-ml to 1-g vial or 14.8 ml to 2-g vial and administer over 10 to 15 min. Do not exceed 100 mg/min. More rapid administration may cause seizures.
- Do not reconstitute using Bacteriostatic Water for Injection if giving drug to newborns.
- For intermittent infusion, reconstitute solution as outlined above and then dilute with 50 to 100 ml of intravenous solution such as 0.9% Sodium Chloride Injection or Lactated Ringer's Injection (see manufacturer's list for other suitable solutions). Infuse over 15 to 30 min. Check manufacturer's guidelines and adjust infusion rate, as needed, so that the total dose of ampicillin is administered before the drug loses its stability in the solution used for dilution.
- *Incompatibilities:* None reported by manufacturer

I.M.

- Reconstitute by adding 1 ml of Bacteriostatic Water for Injection or Sterile Water for Injection to each 250-mg vial, 1.8 ml of diluent to each 500-mg vial, 3.5 ml of diluent to each 1-g vial, or 6.8 ml of diluent to each 2-g vial.
- Do not use Bacteriostatic Water for Injection when drug will be given to newborns.
- Use within 1 hr after preparation because potency may decrease significantly after this period.

Route	Onset	Peak	Duration
P.O.	Unknown	1–2 hr	6–8 hr
I.V.	Immediate	Unknown	Unknown
I.M.	Unknown	1 hr	Unknown

Half-life: 1–1.8 hr

Mechanism of Action

Inhibits bacterial cell wall synthesis. The rigid, cross-linked cell wall is assembled in several steps. Ampicillin exerts its effects on susceptible bacteria in the final stage of the cross-linking process by binding with and inactivating penicillin-binding proteins (enzymes responsible for linking the cell wall strands). This action causes bacterial cell lysis and death.

Contraindications

Hypersensitivity to ampicillin, other penicillins, or their components; infection caused by penicillinase-producing organism

Interactions

DRUGS

allopurinol: Increased risk of rash, particularly in hyperuricemic patient
aminoglycosides: Possibly inactivated action
bacteriostatic antibiotics such as chloramphenicol, erythromycins, sulfonamides, tetracyclines: Possibly impaired action of ampicillin
live-virus vaccines such as BCG (intravesical) and typhoid: May decrease effectiveness of vaccine
oral anticoagulants: Increased risk of bleeding
oral contraceptives: Possibly reduced contraceptive effectiveness and breakthrough bleeding

Adverse Reactions

CNS: Chills, fatigue, fever, headache, malaise
CV: Chest pain, edema, thrombophlebitis
EENT: Epistaxis, glossitis, **laryngeal stridor**, mucocutaneous candidiasis, stomatitis, **throat tightness**
GI: Abdominal distention, ***Clostridium difficile*-associated diarrhea**, diarrhea, enterocolitis, flatulence, gastritis, nausea, **pseudomembranous colitis**, vomiting
GU: Dysuria, urine retention, vaginal candidiasis
HEME: **Agranulocytosis**, anemia, eosinophilia, **leukopenia**, **thrombocytopenia**, **thrombocytopenic purpura**
SKIN: **Erythema multiforme**; erythematous, mildly pruritic maculopapular rash or other types of rashes; **exfoliative dermatitis**; pruritus; urticaria
Other: **Anaphylaxis**, **angioedema**, injection-site pain

Childbearing Considerations

PREGNANCY

- It is not known if drug can cause fetal harm.
- Use with caution only if benefit to mother outweighs potential risk to fetus.

LABOR AND DELIVERY

- Oral drug is poorly absorbed during labor.
- It is not known if drug has any immediate or delayed adverse effects on the fetus, prolongs the duration of labor, or increases the likelihood that forceps delivery or other obstetrical intervention or resuscitation of the newborn will be needed.

LACTATION

- Drug is present in breast milk.
- Mothers should check with prescriber before breastfeeding.

Nursing Considerations

- Know that ampicillin should be avoided in patients with mononucleosis because of increased risk of rash.
- Expect to give ampicillin for 48 to 72 hours after patient becomes asymptomatic. For streptococcal infection, expect to give ampicillin for at least 10 days after cultures show streptococcal eradication to reduce risk of glomerulonephritis or rheumatic fever.

! WARNING Monitor patient closely for hypersensitivity reactions such as anaphylaxis, which may be life-threatening. Patients at greatest risk are those with a history of asthma, hay fever, or urticaria; history of multiple allergies; or hypersensitivity to cephalosporins. Stop drug if a hypersensitivity reaction occurs, notify prescriber immediately, expect drug to be discontinued and provide supportive care, as needed and ordered.

- Closely monitor results of CBC and liver and renal function tests if high-dose or long-term ampicillin therapy is required.

! WARNING Monitor patient closely for diarrhea, which may be pseudomembranous colitis caused by *Clostridium difficile.* It can range from being mild to life-threatening. If diarrhea occurs, notify prescriber and expect testing to be done. If *C. difficile* is confirmed, expect to withhold ampicillin and administer an antibiotic effective against *C. difficile* and electrolytes, fluids, and protein, as needed and ordered.

- Notify prescriber if patient has evidence of superinfection; expect to stop drug and provide appropriate treatment.

PATIENT TEACHING

- Instruct patient how to take the prescribed oral form of ampicillin. Emphasize the importance of taking the full course of ampicillin exactly as prescribed.

! **WARNING** Review signs and symptoms of an allergic reaction. Tell patient to stop taking ampicillin and notify prescriber immediately, if any occurs. If reaction is severe, stress importance of seeking immediate medical care.

! **WARNING** Urge patient to tell prescriber about diarrhea that's severe or lasts longer than 3 days. Remind patient that bloody or watery stools may occur 2 or more months after antibiotic therapy and may be serious, requiring prompt treatment.

- Tell patient to notify prescriber if other persistent, severe, or unusual adverse reactions occur.

angiotensin II

Giapreza

Class and Category

Pharmacologic class: Peptide hormone of the renin–angiotensin–aldosterone system
Therapeutic class: Antihypertensive

Indications and Dosages

∗ *To increase blood pressure in patients with septic or other distributive shock*

I.V. INFUSION

Adults. *Initial:* 20 ng/kg/min continuously then increased in increments of up to 15 ng/kg/min every 5 min, as needed, to achieve or maintain target blood pressure. When no longer needed, dosage decreased in increments of up to 15 ng/kg/min every 5 to 15 min, with adjustments made based upon blood pressure. *Maximum:* For first 3 hr, dosage should not exceed 80 ng/kg/min; maintenance dosage should not exceed 40 ng/kg/min.

± **DOSAGE ADJUSTMENT** For patients sensitive to angiotensin II effects, dosage may be decreased to as low as 1.25 ng/kg/min.

Drug Administration

I.V.

- Dilute drug in 0.9% Sodium Chloride solution prior to use to achieve a final concentration of 5,000 ng/ml or 10,000 ng/ml.
- Administer as a continuous infusion and preferably through a central venous line. Adjust dosage every 5 min, as needed.
- Know that diluted solution may be stored at room temperature or in refrigerator. Discard unused prepared solution after 24 hr regardless of how it was stored.
- *Incompatibilities:* None reported by manufacturer

Route	Onset	Peak	Duration
I.V.	Within 1 min	5 min	Unknown

Half-life: > 1 min.

Mechanism of Action

Binds to the G-protein-coupled angiotensin II receptor type I on vascular smooth muscle cells, which stimulates myosin and causes smooth muscle contraction. These actions raise blood pressure by increasing aldosterone release and causing vasoconstriction.

Contraindications

Hypersensitivity to angiotensin II components

Interactions

DRUGS

ACE inhibitors: Possibly increased response to angiotensin II
angiotensin II receptor blockers (ARBs): Possibly decreased response to angiotensin II

Adverse Reactions

CNS: Delirium
CV: **Arterial and venous thrombotic events, deep vein thrombosis**, peripheral ischemia, tachycardia
ENDO: Hyperglycemia
HEME: **Thrombocytopenia**
Other: **Acidosis**, fungal infection

Childbearing Considerations

PREGNANCY

- It is not known if drug can cause fetal harm.

- Use with caution only if benefit to mother outweighs potential risk to fetus.

LACTATION

- It is not known if drug is present in breast milk.
- Mothers should check with prescriber before breastfeeding, once condition has stabilized.

Nursing Considerations

- Take blood pressure every 5 minutes for the first 3 hours and monitor blood pressure every 5 to 15 minutes thereafter, as needed.

! **WARNING** Monitor patient closely for thrombotic events. Take precautions to prevent these events, especially deep venous thromboses. If suspected, notify prescriber, and provide supportive care, as needed and ordered.

- Monitor patient's blood glucose level for hyperglycemia and, if present, provide treatment as needed and ordered.

PATIENT TEACHING

- Instruct patient on angiotensin II use if patient's condition allows for understanding.
- Tell patient to report any abnormal symptoms unless patient is not coherent because of the presence of shock.

apixaban

Eliquis

Class and Category

Pharmacologic class: Factor Xa inhibitor
Therapeutic class: Anticoagulant

Indications and Dosages

✱ *To reduce the risk of stroke and systemic embolism in patients with nonvalvular atrial fibrillation*

TABLETS

Adults. 5 mg twice daily.

± **DOSAGE ADJUSTMENT** For patients with at least 2 of the following characteristics: age 80 or older, having a serum creatinine of 1.5 mg/dl or greater, or weighing 60 kg (132 lb) or less; dosage decreased to 2.5 mg twice daily.

✱ *To prevent deep vein thrombosis following hip or knee replacement surgery*

TABLETS

Adults. 2.5 mg twice daily beginning 12 to 24 hr after surgery and lasting 12 days for knee replacement and 35 days for hip replacement.

✱ *To treat deep vein thrombosis and pulmonary embolism*

TABLETS

Adults. 10 mg twice daily for 7 days followed by 5 mg twice daily.

✱ *To reduce risk of recurrence of deep vein thrombosis and pulmonary embolism*

TABLETS

Adults. 2.5 mg twice daily following 6 mo of treatment for deep vein thrombosis or pulmonary embolism.

± **DOSAGE ADJUSTMENT** For patients receiving 5-mg or 10-mg dosage twice daily, dosage reduced by 50% if patient also receiving combined strong dual inhibitors of cytochrome P450 3A4 (CYP3A4) and P-glycoprotein (P-gp) such as itraconazole, ketoconazole, or ritonavir. For patients receiving 2.5-mg dosage twice daily, coadministration with combined strong CYP3A4 and P-gp inhibitors are avoided.

Drug Administration

P.O.

- Crush tablet and mix with apple juice or water or put in applesauce and administer immediately for patient unable to swallow whole tablets.
- For patient with a nasogastric tube, crush tablet and suspend in 60 ml of 5% Dextrose in Water or plain water and immediately administer through the nasogastric tube.
- Be aware that crushed tablets are stable in apple juice, 5% Dextrose in Water, plain water, or applesauce for up to 4 hr.

Route	Onset	Peak	Duration
P.O.	Rapid	3–4 hr	Unknown

Half-life: 12 hr

Mechanism of Action

Inhibits free and clot-bound factor Xa and prothrombinase activity. Although apixaban has no direct effect on platelet aggregation, it does indirectly inhibit platelet aggregation induced by thrombin. By inhibiting factor Xa, apixaban decreases thrombin generation and thrombus development.

Contraindications

Active pathological bleeding, severe hypersensitivity to apixaban or its components

Interactions

DRUGS

antiplatelets, aspirin, fibrinolytics, heparin NSAIDs (chronic use): Increased risk of bleeding
strong dual inducers of CYP3A4 and P-gp, such as carbamazepine, phenytoin, rifampin, St. John's wort: Decreased effectiveness of apixaban
strong dual inhibitors of CYP3A4 and P-gp, such as itraconazole, ketoconazole, ritonavir: Increased effects of apixaban

Adverse Reactions

CNS: **Hemorrhagic stroke**, syncope
CV: **Hypotension**
EENT: Epistaxis, gingival bleeding, ocular hemorrhage
GI: Elevated bilirubin and liver enzymes, **fresh bleeding from rectum**, **GI bleeding or hemorrhage**, **hematemesis**, **melena**, **rectal hemorrhage**
GU: Hematuria, **vaginal hemorrhage**
HEME: **Excessive bleeding**, **including hemorrhage**, **hemorrhagic anemia**, **thrombocytopenia**
SKIN: Ecchymosis, petechiae, rash
MS: Muscle hemorrhage
RESP: **Hemoptysis**
Other: **Anaphylaxis**, **angioedema**, elevated alkaline phosphatase, hematomas at injection sites

Childbearing Considerations

PREGNANCY

- It is not known if drug can cause fetal harm but there is the potential for hemorrhage.
- Drug use is not recommended during pregnancy unless no other alternative is available.

LABOR AND DELIVERY

- Use with caution only if absolutely necessary and no other alternative is available because there is a potential for hemorrhage. A shorter acting anticoagulant should be considered as delivery approaches.

LACTATION

- It is not known if drug is present in breast milk.
- A decision should be made to discontinue breastfeeding or the drug to avoid potential adverse reactions in the breastfed infant.

REPRODUCTION

- Drug may cause significant abnormal uterine bleeding, possibly requiring surgical intervention. If females are of childbearing age, plans for a pregnancy should be made known to the prescriber.

Nursing Considerations

- Know that apixaban should not be given to patients with severe hepatic dysfunction. Drug should also not be given to patient with triple positive antiphospholipid syndrome because drug therapy has been associated with increased rates of recurrent thrombotic events.

! WARNING Monitor patient for a hypersensitivity reaction that could become life-threatening. At first sign of an allergic reaction, notify prescriber, withhold drug as ordered, and provide supportive care, as needed, and ordered.

! WARNING Monitor patient closely for bleeding, as apixaban may cause life-threatening bleeding. Expect drug to be discontinued with active pathological hemorrhage and expect to give the antidote, coagulation factor Xa (recombinant), inactivated-zhzo (Andexxa) to reverse effects of anticoagulation. Know that effects of apixaban may persist for at least 24 hours after the last dose, but that activated oral charcoal can reduce the absorption of apixaban, thereby lowering apixaban plasma concentration if given close to last dose of apixaban.

- Expect apixaban to be discontinued 48 hours before an invasive procedure or surgery if patient has a moderate or high risk of hemorrhage and 24 hours before an invasive procedure or surgery if patient has a mild risk of hemorrhage.
- Be aware that if apixaban is discontinued prematurely and adequate alternative anticoagulation is not present, the risk of thrombosis increases.
- Be aware that manufacturer's guidelines should be followed when patient is switching from or to other anticoagulants. For example, when patient is switching from warfarin to apixaban therapy, expect warfarin to be discontinued and apixaban started when the international normalized ratio (INR) is

below 2. When switching from apixaban to warfarin, expect apixaban to be discontinued and both a parenteral anticoagulant and warfarin given at the time the next dose of apixaban would have been given. Then, the parenteral anticoagulant is discontinued when INR reaches an acceptable range. When switching between apixaban and anticoagulants other than warfarin, expect to discontinue the one being taken and begin the other at the next scheduled dose.

PATIENT TEACHING

- Instruct patient how to take apixaban tablets and what to do if a dose is missed.
- Emphasize the importance of taking apixaban exactly as prescribed.
- Tell patient not to stop taking apixaban without first consulting prescriber.

! WARNING Instruct patient to alert prescriber if an allergic reaction occurs. If severe, stress importance of seeking immediate medical attention.

! WARNING Advise patient to report any unusual bleeding or bruising to the prescriber. Inform patient that it may take longer for her to stop bleeding and to take bleeding precautions, such as avoiding the use of a razor and using a soft-bristle toothbrush. Instruct patient that if bleeding is excessive, to apply pressure to site if possible, and seek immediate medical care.

- Tell patient to alert all prescribers to use of apixaban therapy before any invasive procedure, including dental work, is scheduled.
- Tell females of childbearing age to discuss plans for a possible pregnancy with prescriber. Advise female patient to notify prescriber immediately if pregnancy occurs.
- Inform mothers breastfeeding should not be undertaken during apixaban therapy.

apremilast

Otezla

Class and Category

Pharmacologic class: Phosphodiesterase 4 inhibitor
Therapeutic class: Antirheumatic

Indications and Dosages

✱ *To treat active psoriatic arthritis; to treat moderate to severe plaque psoriasis in patients who are candidates for phototherapy or systemic therapy; to treat oral ulcers associated with Behçet's disease.*

TABLETS

Adults. *Initial:* 10 mg in a.m. on day 1; 10 mg in a.m. and p.m. on day 2; 10 mg in a.m. and 20 mg in p.m. on day 3; 20 mg in a.m. and p.m. on day 4; 20 mg in a.m. and 30 mg in p.m. on day 5; and 30 mg in a.m. and p.m. on day 6 and thereafter. *Maintenance:* 30 mg in a.m. and p.m.

✱ *To treat pediatric moderate to severe plaque psoriasis who are candidates for phototherapy or systemic therapy*

TABLETS

Children ages 6 and older weighing 50 kg (110 lb) or more. *Initial:* 10 mg in a.m. on day 1; 10 mg in a.m. and 10 mg in p.m. on day 2; 10 mg in a.m. and 20 mg in p.m. on day 3; 20 mg in a.m. and 20 mg in p.m. on day 4; 20 mg in a.m. and 30 mg in p.m. on day 5; and 30 mg in a.m. and 30 mg in p.m. on day 6 and thereafter. *Maintenance:* 30 mg in a.m. and 30 mg in p.m.
Children ages 6 and older weighing 20 kg (44 lb) to less than 50 kg (110 lb). *Initial:* 10 mg in a.m. on day 1; 10 mg in a.m. and 10 mg in p.m. on day 2; 10 mg in a.m. and 20 mg in p.m. on day 3; 20 mg in a.m. and 20 mg in p.m. on day 4; 20 mg in a.m. and 20 mg in p.m. on day 5; and 20 mg in a.m. and 20 mg in p.m. on day 6 and thereafter. *Maintenance:* 20 mg in a.m. and 20 mg in p.m.

±**DOSAGE ADJUSTMENT** For adult patients with severe renal impairment (creatinine clearance less than 30 ml/min), dosage titration decreased to once daily using only the morning titration schedule and maintenance dosage kept at 30 mg once daily in the morning. For pediatric patients with severe renal impairment (creatinine clearance less than 30 ml/min), dosage titration decreased to once daily using only the morning titration and maintenance dosage kept at 30 mg once daily for children weighing 50 kg (110 lb) or more and to 20 mg once daily for children weighing 20 kg (44 lb) to less than 50 kg (110 lb).

Drug Administration

P.O.

- Do not have patient chew tablets and do not crush or split tablets. Tablets should be swallowed whole.

Route	Onset	Peak	Duration
P.O.	Unknown	2.5 hr	Unknown

Half-life: 6–9 hr

Mechanism of Action

Inhibits phosphodiesterase 4, which is specific for cyclic adenosine monophosphate (cAMP). This action results in increased intracellular cAMP levels, which are thought to help relieve symptoms of psoriatic arthritis.

Contraindications

Hypersensitivity to apremilast or its components

Interactions

DRUGS

strong CYP450 inducers such as rifampin: Decreased apremilast exposure with loss of effectiveness

Adverse Reactions

CNS: Depression, fatigue, headache, insomnia, migraine, **suicidal ideation**
EENT: Nasopharyngitis
GI: Abdominal pain, anorexia, diarrhea, dyspepsia, gastroesophageal reflux disease, nausea, upper abdominal pain, vomiting
MS: Arthralgia, back pain
RESP: Bronchitis, cough, upper respiratory infection
SKIN: Infected hair follicles, rash
Other: **Anaphylaxis**, **angioedema**, weight loss

Childbearing Considerations

PREGNANCY

- Pregnancy exposure registry: 1-877-311-8972 or https://mothertobaby.org/ongoing-study/otezla/.
- It is not known if drug can cause fetal harm although some studies suggest an increased risk for fetal loss.
- Use with caution only if benefit to mother outweighs potential risk to fetus.

LACTATION

- It is not known if drug is present in breast milk.
- Mothers should check with prescriber before breastfeeding.

Nursing Considerations

! WARNING Monitor patient for hypersensitivity reactions that could include anaphylaxis and angioedema. If a hypersensitivity reaction occurs, notify prescriber immediately, expect drug to be discontinued, and provide supportive care, as needed and prescribed.

! WARNING Watch patient closely for evidence of depression, especially when apremilast therapy begins because apremilast therapy may increase risk of depression and possibly lead to suicidal thinking or behavior.

- Monitor patient for persistent, severe or unusual adverse reactions and notify prescriber, if present. Monitor patients ages 65 or older for signs and symptoms of dehydration or hypotension that may occur as a result of severe diarrhea, nausea, or vomiting.
- Monitor patient's weight regularly because apremilast may cause weight loss. Notify prescriber if weight loss occurs that is unexplained or is significant.

PATIENT TEACHING

- Instruct patient how to take tablets. Tell patient to follow titration schedule exactly, as this will help reduce the incidence and severity of GI symptoms associated with initial therapy.

! WARNING Review allergic reactions with patient and stress importance of notifying prescriber, if present, and seeking emergency medical care, if severe.

! WARNING Instruct family or caregiver to watch patient closely for evidence of suicidal tendencies, especially when therapy starts, and to report concerns to prescriber immediately.

- Advise patient to notify prescriber if severe diarrhea, nausea, or vomiting occurs as well as any other persistent, severe, or unusual adverse reactions.
- Instruct patient to weigh themselves regularly and report any significant weight loss.

aprepitant

Aponvie, Cinvanti, Emend

fosaprepitant dimeglumine

Emend for Injection

Class and Category

Pharmacologic class: Substance P/neurokinin 1 (NK1) receptor antagonist
Therapeutic class: Antiemetic

Indications and Dosages

* *As adjunct to prevent acute and delayed nausea and vomiting associated with moderately to highly emetogenic chemotherapy, including high-dose cisplatin*

CAPSULES (EMEND)

Adults and children ages 12 and older. 125 mg 1 hr before chemotherapy treatment, followed by 80 mg daily 1 hr before chemotherapy on day 2 and 3, or if no chemotherapy, 80 mg in a.m. on day 2 and 3.

ORAL SUSPENSION (EMEND)

Adults and children ages 12 and older who cannot swallow oral capsules and children ages 6 mo to less than 12 yr weighing at least 6 kg (13.2 lb). 3 mg/kg (maximum 125 mg) on day 1, followed by 2 mg/kg (maximum 80 mg) 1 hr before chemotherapy on days 2 and 3, or if no chemotherapy, 2 mg/kg (maximum 80 mg) in a.m. on days 2 and 3.

I.V. INFUSION (EMEND FOR INJECTION)

Adults receiving a single-dose regimen. 150 mg as a single dose infused over 20 to 30 min before chemotherapy.

I.V. INFUSION (CINVANTI)

Adults receiving a single-dose regimen. 130 mg as a single dose infused over 30 min and completed about 30 min prior to chemotherapy on day 1 only.

I.V. INJECTION (CINVANTI)

Adults receiving a single-dose regimen. 130 mg as a single dose administered over 2 min and given 30 min prior to chemotherapy.

* *As adjunct to prevent acute and delayed nausea and vomiting associated with moderately emetogenic chemotherapy*

I.V. INFUSION (EMEND)

Adults receiving a single-dose regimen. 150 mg as a single dose infused over 20 to 30 min before chemotherapy.

I.V. INFUSION (CINVANTI)

Adults receiving a single-dose regimen. 130 mg as a single dose infused over 30 min and completed about 30 min prior to chemotherapy on day 1 only.

I.V. INJECTION (CINVANTI)

Adults receiving a single-dose regimen. 130 mg as a single dose administered over 2 min and given 30 min prior to chemotherapy.

I.V. INFUSION (CINVANTI) FOLLOWED BY CAPSULES (EMEND)

Adults receiving moderately emetogenic cancer chemotherapy as a 3-day regimen. 100 mg as a single dose infused over 30 min about 30 min prior to chemotherapy on day 1, followed by 80 mg of oral aprepitant on days 2 and 3.

I.V. INJECTION (CINVANTI) FOLLOWED BY CAPSULES (EMEND)

Adults receiving moderately emetogenic cancer chemotherapy as a 3-day regimen. 100 mg as a single dose administered over 2 min and given 30 min before chemotherapy on day 1, followed by 80 mg of oral aprepitant on days 2 and 3.

* *To prevent nausea and vomiting associated with moderately to highly emetogenic chemotherapy with single-day pediatric chemotherapy regimens*

I.V. INFUSION (EMEND FOR INJECTION)

Adolescents ages 12 to 17. 150 mg as a single dose infused over 30 min and completed about 30 min prior to chemotherapy on day 1 only.
Children ages 2 to less than 12. 4 mg/kg (maximum 150 mg) as a single dose infused over 60 min and completed about 30 min prior to chemotherapy on day 1 only.
Children ages 6 mo to less than 2 yr weighing at least 6 kg (13.2 lb). 5 mg/kg (maximum 150 mg) as a single dose infused over 60 min and completed about 30 min prior to chemotherapy on day 1 only.

* *To prevent nausea and vomiting associated with moderately to highly emetogenic chemotherapy with multi-day pediatric chemotherapy regimens*

CAPSULES (EMEND), I.V. INFUSION (EMEND FOR INJECTION), ORAL SUSPENSION (EMEND)

Adolescents ages 12 to 17. 115 mg as a single dose infused over 30 min and completed about 30 min prior to chemotherapy on day 1 followed by 80 mg daily of oral aprepitant on days 2 and 3.

Children ages 6 mo to less than 12 yr weighing at least 6 kg (13.2 lb). 3 mg/kg (maximum 115 mg) as a single dose infused over 60 min and completed about 30 min prior to chemotherapy on day 1, followed by 2 mg/kg (maximum 80 mg) daily of oral aprepitant in suspension form on days 2 and 3.

* *To prevent postoperative nausea and vomiting*

CAPSULES (EMEND)

Adults. 40 mg within 3 hr prior to induction of anesthesia.

I.V. INJECTION (APONVIE)

Adults. 32 mg administered over 30 sec prior to induction of anesthesia.

Drug Administration

- Expect to administer aprepitant with dexamethasone and a 5-HT_3 antagonist, such as dolasetron, granisetron, or ondansetron, for maximum antiemetic effects.

P.O.

- Administer 1 hr before chemotherapy.
- Administer capsule form only to children ages 12 and older. Suspension form should be administered to children under age 12 or to an older patient who cannot swallow capsules.
- Capsules must be swallowed whole.
- Oral suspension will be prepared by a healthcare provider following manufacturer's instructions and put in an oral dispenser after mixing.
- Administer by first taking cap off the dispenser and then placing the dispenser in the patient's mouth along the inner cheek on either the left or right side. Slowly dispense the drug.
- Refrigerate prepared oral suspension until administered. May be stored at room temperature for up to 3 hr before use. Discard any doses remaining after 72 hr.

I.V.

Aponvie

- Inspect vial for particulate matter and discoloration prior to administering drug; if present discard. Solution should appear opaque and off-white to amber in color.
- Withdraw 4.4 ml from the drug vial and administer as an I.V. injection over 30 seconds prior to the induction of anesthesia.
- Remember to flush I.V. line with 0.9% Sodium Chloride Injection before and after administration of drug.
- *Incompatibilities for Aponvie only:* Solutions other than 0.9% Sodium Chloride Injection; 5% Dextrose Injection; and solutions containing divalent cations (calcium, magnesium), including Lactated Ringer's Solution.

Cinvanti

- *For 30-min I.V. infusion:* Reconstitute by withdrawing 18 ml for 130-mg dose or 14 ml for 100-mg dose from drug vial and transfer it into an infusion bag containing 100 ml of 0.9% Sodium Chloride Injection or 5% Dextrose for Injection. Use only non- Di (2-ethyhexyl) phthalate (DEHP) tubing, non-polyvinylchloride (PVC) infusion bags.
- Gently invert the bag 4 or 5 times. Avoid shaking. Before administration, inspect bag for particulate matter and discoloration.
- Diluted solution is stable at ambient room temperature for up to 6 hr if mixed in 0.9% Sodium Chloride Injection or 12 hr if mixed in 5% Dextrose Injection or up to 72 hr if stored under refrigeration with either solution.
- *For 2-min I.V. push:* Prepare by withdrawing 18 ml for the 130-mg dose or 14 ml for the 100-mg dose from the vial. Do not dilute. Flush infusion line with 0.9% Sodium Chloride for Injection solution before and after administration.

Emend

- Reconstitute by injecting 5 ml 0.9% Sodium Chloride for Injection along vial wall to prevent foaming. Avoid jetting the 0.9% Sodium Chloride solution into the vial. Swirl vial gently. Avoid shaking. Withdraw contents from vial and add to an infusion bag containing 145 ml 0.9% Sodium Chloride Injection. Gently invert the bag 2 or 3 times.
- Determine volume to be administered based on dosage prescribed. For adults, the entire prepared infusion bag of 150 ml should be administered. For patients 12 and older, the volume to be administered is calculated as follows: Volume to administer

(ml) = the recommended dose (mg). In patients 6 mo of age to less than 12 yr, the volume to be administered is calculated as follows: Volume to administer (ml) = recommended dose (mg/kg) × weight (kg). For pediatric patients the entire volume in the infusion bag may not be required. The dose to be administered should never exceed the maximum dose. If necessary, for volumes less than 150 ml, the calculated volume can be transferred to an appropriate size bag or syringe prior to administration.

- Administer by infusion at the rate given under Indications and Dosages section for the indication and age of patient being treated.
- Reconstituted solution may be stored at room temperature for 24 hr.
- *Incompatibilities for Cinvanti and Emend products:* Any solution containing divalent cations such as calcium and magnesium, including Hartmann's Solution and Lactated Ringer's Solution.

Route	Onset	Peak	Duration
P.O.	1 hr	4 hr	24 hr
I.V.	Unknown	>1 hr	Unknown

Half-life: 9–13 hr

Mechanism of Action

Crosses the blood–brain barrier to occupy brain NK1 receptors, which prevents nerve transmission of signals that cause nausea and vomiting.

Contraindications

Concurrent use of pimozide, hypersensitivity to aprepitant or its components

Interactions

DRUGS

carbamazepine, other CYP3A4 inducers, phenytoin, rifampin: Possibly decreased blood aprepitant level
CYP3A4 inhibitors (such as clarithromycin, diltiazem, itraconazole, ketoconazole, nefazodone, nelfinavir, ritonavir, and troleandomycin): Increased blood aprepitant level
CYP3A4 substrates (such as astemizole, benzodiazepines, cisapride, docetaxel, etoposide, imatinib, irinotecan, paclitaxel, pimozide, terfenadine, vinblastine, vincristine, and vinorelbine): Increased level of CYP3A4 substrates, resulting in possibly serious or life-threatening adverse reactions
dexamethasone, methylprednisolone: Increased effects of these drugs and risk of adverse reactions
ifosfamide: Increased risk of neurotoxicity and possibly other serious or life-threatening adverse reactions
oral contraceptives: Possibly decreased effectiveness of hormonal contraceptives
paroxetine: Possibly decreased blood level of both drugs
warfarin: Decreased effectiveness of warfarin and decreased prothrombin time

Adverse Reactions

CNS: Anxiety, asthenia, confusion, depression, dizziness, fatigue, fever, headache, hypoesthesia, hypothermia, insomnia, malaise, peripheral or sensory neuropathy, rigors, somnolence, syncope, tremor
CV: **Bradycardia, deep vein thrombosis,** edema, hypertension, **hypotension, MI,** palpitations, peripheral edema, tachycardia, thrombophlebitis at injection site
EENT: Conjunctivitis, dry mouth, increased salivation, mucous membrane alteration, nasal discharge, oral candidiasis, oropharyngeal pain, pharyngitis, stomatitis, taste perversion, tinnitus, vocal disturbance
ENDO: Hot flashes, hyperglycemia
GI: Abdominal pain, anorexia, constipation, diarrhea, dysphagia, elevated liver enzymes, epigastric discomfort, flatulence, gastritis, gastroesophageal reflux, heartburn, hiccups, nausea, obstipation (intractable constipation), vomiting
GU: Dysuria, elevated BUN and serum creatinine levels, hematuria, leukocyturia, proteinuria, **renal insufficiency**, UTI
HEME: Anemia, **febrile neutropenia**, hematoma, leukocytosis, **leukopenia, neutropenia, thrombocytopenia**
MS: Arthralgia, back pain, muscle weakness, musculoskeletal pain, myalgia, pelvic pain
RESP: Cough, dyspnea, **hypoxia, non–small-cell lung carcinoma, pneumonitis, pulmonary embolism, respiratory depression or insufficiency**, respiratory tract infection
SKIN: Acne, alopecia, diaphoresis, flushing, pruritus, rash, **Stevens-Johnson syndrome, toxic epidermal necrolysis**, urticaria

Other: **Anaphylaxis**, **anaphylactic shock**, **angioedema**, candidiasis, dehydration, elevated alkaline phosphatase, herpes simplex, **hypokalemia**, **hyponatremia**, infusion-site pain or induration, **malignant neoplasm**, **septic shock**, weight loss

Childbearing Considerations

PREGNANCY

- It is not known if drug can cause fetal harm.
- Aponvie should be avoided in pregnant females due to the alcohol content, which can cause fetal harm. Use Cinvanti and Emend with caution only if benefit to mother outweighs potential risk to fetus.

LACTATION

- It is not known if drug is present in breast milk.
- Mothers should check with prescriber before breastfeeding.

REPRODUCTION

- Drug may reduce hormonal contraceptive effectiveness.
- Females of childbearing age should be instructed to use an effective alternative or backup nonhormonal contraceptive, such as spermicides or male partners' use of condoms, during therapy and for 1 mo following last dose.

Nursing Considerations

- Use caution when giving aprepitant to patients with severe hepatic insufficiency because drug's effects on such patients aren't known.

! **WARNING** Monitor patient closely for hypersensitivity reactions, which could include anaphylaxis and anaphylactic shock during or soon after administration of drug. Symptoms to be alert for include dyspnea, erythema, flushing, hypotension, and syncope. If a hypersensitivity reaction occurs, stop infusion or injection if still being given, notify prescriber, expect drug to be discontinued, and be prepared to provide supportive care, as needed and ordered.

- Be aware that ifosfamide-induced neurotoxicity may occur after aprepitant and ifosfamide have been coadministered. Monitor patient closely.
- Monitor patient for persistent, severe, or unusual adverse reactions because drug can adversely affect multiple systems.

PATIENT TEACHING

- Instruct cancer patient how to administer the form of aprepitant prescribed.
- Inform family or caregiver drug may be given different ways for children with cancer ages 6 months and older. Review the type of dosage regimen prescribed.
- Reassure patients receiving drug to prevent nausea and vomiting after surgery that drug will be given prior to anesthesia.

! **WARNING** Instruct patient to report an allergic reaction such as difficulty breathing or swallowing, dizziness, fainting, flushing, hives, itching, or rash and seek immediate medical attention if not in a healthcare setting.

- Tell patient to notify prescriber if persistent, severe, or unusual adverse reactions occur as drug can adversely affect multiple systems.
- Tell patient taking chronic warfarin therapy to have clotting status monitored closely especially at 7 to 10 days during each chemotherapy cycle in which the drug is used.
- Caution patient to inform prescriber of any drugs he is taking, including over-the-counter drugs and herbal preparations because they may interact with aprepitant.
- Tell females of childbearing age taking hormonal contraceptives to use an alternative or backup method of contraception during aprepitant therapy and for 1 month after last dose because drug reduces effectiveness of hormonal contraceptives. Also, alert females of childbearing age that Aponvie should not be used to prevent nausea and vomiting after surgery if pregnancy is known.

NEW!

aprocitentan

Tryvio

Class and Category

Pharmacologic class: Endothelin receptor antagonist
Therapeutic class: Antihypertensive

Indications and Dosages

✷ As adjunct to treat hypertension in combination with other antihypertensive drugs for patients who are not adequately controlled on other drugs

TABLETS

Adults. 12.5 mg once daily.

Drug Administration

P.O.

- For all females of childbearing age, ensure a negative pregnancy test has been obtained before administering drug; monthly while administering drug, and 1 mo after drug is discontinued.
- Tablets should be swallowed whole.
- If dose is missed, skip missed dose and give the next dose at the regular time the next day. Never administer 2 doses on the same day.
- Protect tablets from light and moisture.

Route	Onset	Peak	Duration
P.O.	Unknown	4-5 hr	Unknown

Half-life: 41 hr

Mechanism of Action

Inhibits binding of endothelin (ET)-1 to ET_A and ET_B receptors to prevent cell proliferation, fibrosis, inflammation, and vasoconstriction, which results in decreased blood pressure.

Contraindications

Hypersensitivity to aprocitentan or its components, pregnancy

Interactions

DRUGS

None listed by manufacturer.

Adverse Reactions

CV: Fluid retention, peripheral edema
GI: Elevated liver enzymes, **hepatotoxicity**
GU: Decreased sperm counts
HEME: Anemia
SKIN: Allergic dermatitis or edema, erythema, rash
Other: **Angioedema**

Childbearing Considerations

PREGNANCY

- Pregnancy exposure registry: 1-866-429-8964.
- Drug can cause fetal harm such as major birth defects and fetal death.
- Drug is contraindicated in pregnancy.

LACTATION

- It is not known if drug is present in breast milk.
- Breastfeeding should not be undertaken during drug therapy.

REPRODUCTION

- Females of childbearing age should use effective contraception prior to beginning drug therapy, during drug therapy and for one month after drug is discontinued.
- Males may experience impaired fertility, and it is not known if this effect is reversible.

Nursing Considerations

! WARNING Be aware the use of aprocitentan requires a Risk Evaluation and Mitigation Strategy (REMS) before drug can be dispensed, to ensure that the benefits outweigh the risk of embryo-fetal toxicity. Know that drug must be discontinued immediately if pregnancy occurs.

! WARNING Know that aprocitentan is not recommended for patients with heart failure (New York Heart Association stage III-IV), unstable cardiac function or patients with NTproBNP 500 pg/ml or greater because drug was not studied in these patients.

! WARNING Be aware that drug is not recommended for patients with an eGFR less than 15 ml/min or who are on dialysis. Know that patients with renal impairment (eGFR of 15 ml/min or greater) are at greater risk for edema and fluid retention as well as older patients. Monitor patient for fluid retention and peripheral edema and, if present, notify prescriber as drug may need to be discontinued.

! WARNING Be aware that aprocitentan is not recommended for patients with moderate to severe hepatic impairment or who have elevated aminotransferases greater than 3 times the upper limit of normal (ULN) because of increased risk for hepatotoxicity. Expect to obtain serum aminotransferase levels and a total bilirubin before therapy is begun and periodically during therapy, as ordered. Notify prescriber if patient develops signs and symptoms of hepatotoxicity (anorexia, dark urine, fatigue, fever, itching, jaundice, nausea, right upper abdominal pain, vomiting), or if aminotransferase elevations occur with an increase of bilirubin greater than 2 times ULN. Expect drug to be discontinued.

- Know that aprocitentan is not recommended for patients with severe anemia. Expect to obtain a hemoglobin level prior to therapy beginning and then periodically during therapy, as ordered.

! **WARNING** Monitor patient closely for any hypersensitivity reaction such as angioedema, which could become life-threatening. If present, notify prescriber immediately and expect drug to be discontinued. Provide supportive care, as needed and ordered.

PATIENT TEACHING

! **WARNING** Inform females of childbearing age a negative pregnancy test must be obtained before aprocitentan therapy is begun, then monthly while on therapy, and for one month after drug is discontinued. Advise patient to use effective contraception (one hormone method with a barrier method or two barrier methods) throughout drug therapy and for one month after drug is discontinued. Inform patient that if her partner has had a vasectomy, a hormone or barrier method must still be used. Stress importance of notifying prescriber immediately if menses is delayed or pregnancy occurs.

- Instruct patient how to administer aprocitentan, what to do if a dose is missed, and how to store drug.

! **WARNING** Alert patient that aprocitentan may cause an allergic reaction. If present, tell patient to notify prescriber promptly and, if severe, to seek immediate medical care.

! **WARNING** Review signs and symptoms of hepatotoxicity. Tell patient to notify prescriber, if present.

- Instruct patient to notify prescriber if patient develops unusual weight gain or ankle or feet swelling.
- Alert male patients about the possibility of impaired fertility because of aprocitentan therapy. Encourage patient to discuss any concerns with prescriber.
- Stress importance of complying with periodically ordered laboratory tests to check for adverse effects that may occur with aprocitentan therapy.

argatroban

Class and Category

Pharmacologic class: Direct thrombin inhibitor
Therapeutic class: Anticoagulant

Indications and Dosages

* *To prevent or treat thrombosis in patients with heparin-induced thrombocytopenia (HIT)*

I.V. INFUSION

Adults without hepatic impairment. 2 mcg/kg/min. *Maximum:* 10 mcg/kg/min.

± **DOSAGE ADJUSTMENT** For patients with moderate or severe hepatic impairment, dosage adjusted to maintain patient's APTT at 1.5 to 3 times the initial baseline value, not to exceed 100 seconds. Initial dosage reduced to 0.5 mcg/kg/min.

* *To prevent or treat thrombosis in patients with or at risk for HIT when undergoing percutaneous coronary intervention (PCI)*

I.V. INFUSION, I.V. INJECTION

Adults without hepatic impairment. *Initial:* 350 mcg/kg bolus injected over 3 to 5 min followed by 25 mcg/kg/min infusion.

± **DOSAGE ADJUSTMENT** For all patients, dosage adjusted to keep activated clotting time (ACT) at 300 to 450 seconds. If ACT is less than 300 seconds, additional I.V. bolus dose of 150 mcg/kg given and infusion increased to 30 mcg/kg/min; if ACT exceeds 450 seconds, dosage reduced to 15 mcg/kg/min. For patients with dissection, impending abrupt closure, thrombus formation during PCI, or inability to reach or keep ACT above 300 seconds, additional bolus doses of 150 mcg/kg may be given, and infusion increased to 40 mcg/kg/min.

Drug Administration

I.V.

- Ensure all parenteral anticoagulants are discontinued before drug is administered.

- The 250-mg/2.5-ml single-dose vial must be diluted 100-fold prior to infusion. Dilute each 2.5-ml vial with 250 ml of room-temperature diluent using 0.9% Sodium Chloride Injection, 5% Dextrose Injection, or Lactated Ringer's Injection to a final concentration of 1 mg/ml. Drug solution should appear clear, colorless to pale yellow.
- Invert diluent bag repeatedly for 1 min to mix completely before administering. Initially the solution may appear to have a slight haziness, but this rapidly disappears upon mixing. Final solution should be clear.
- Give bolus dose over 3 to 5 min.
- Solution is stable at room temperature of 20–25°C (68–77°F) in ambient indoor light for 24 hr. Prepared solution does not require light-resistant measures such as foil protection for I.V. tubing when administering drug. However, drug should not be exposed to direct sunlight.
- *Incompatibilities:* Other I.V. drugs

Route	Onset	Peak	Duration
I.V.	Immediate	1–3 hr	2–4 hr

Half-life: 39–51 min

Mechanism of Action

Exerts its anticoagulant effects by inhibiting thrombin-catalyzed or induced reactions, including fibrin formation, activation of coagulation factors V, VIII, and XIII; protein C; and platelet aggregation.

Contraindications

Active major bleeding, hypersensitivity to argatroban or its components

Interactions

DRUGS

heparin, oral anticoagulants: Increased risk of bleeding

Adverse Reactions

CNS: **Cerebrovascular bleeding**, fever, headache
CV: **Atrial fibrillation**, **cardiac arrest**, **hypotension**, **unstable angina**, **ventricular tachycardia**
GI: Abdominal pain, anorexia, diarrhea, elevated liver enzymes, **GI bleeding**, **melena**, nausea, vomiting
GU: Elevated BUN and serum creatinine levels, hematuria (microscopic), UTI
HEME: **Hemorrhage**, **hypoprothrombinemia**, **unusual bleeding** or bruising
RESP: Cough, dyspnea, **hemoptysis**, pneumonia
SKIN: Bleeding at puncture site, rash
Other: **Sepsis**

Childbearing Considerations

PREGNANCY

- Drug may cause fetal harm due to increased risk of bleeding.
- Use with caution only if benefit to mother outweighs potential risk to fetus.

LABOR AND DELIVERY

- Use with caution during labor and delivery.
- Use of drug increases risk of bleeding for both the mother and fetus/neonate.

LACTATION

- It is not known if drug is present in breast milk.
- Mothers should check with prescriber before breastfeeding.

Nursing Considerations

- Know that argatroban isn't recommended for PCI patients with significant hepatic disease or AST/ALT levels 3 times or more the upper limits of normal.
- Expect to perform blood coagulation tests before and 2 hours after start of therapy because of the major risk of bleeding associated with argatroban. Be aware that coagulopathy must be ruled out before therapy starts. When giving drug to a patient undergoing PCI, expect to check ACT 5 to 10 minutes after each bolus and each infusion rate change and every 20 to 30 minutes during the PCI procedure. Be aware that thrombin times may not be helpful for monitoring argatroban activity because the drug affects all thrombin-dependent coagulation tests.

! WARNING Monitor patients with thrombocytopenia or those receiving daily doses of salicylates greater than 6 g for signs and symptoms of bleeding; these patients are at increased risk of bleeding from hypoprothrombinemia.

! **WARNING** Monitor the following patients for signs and symptoms of bleeding, which may become severe and occur at any site in the body because they are at increased risk during argatroban therapy: patients who have recently had a large vessel puncture or organ biopsy, lumbar puncture, major bleeding (including GI, intracranial, intraocular, retroperitoneal, or pulmonary bleeding), major surgery (including brain, eye, or spinal cord surgery), spinal anesthesia, or stroke; patients with organ or vascular abnormalities, such as advanced renal disease, dissecting aortic aneurysm, diverticulitis, hemophilia, hepatic disease (especially if associated with a deficiency of vitamin K–dependent clotting factors), infective endocarditis inflammatory bowel disease, peptic ulcer disease or severe uncontrolled hypertension; and women with active menstruation. Risk of bleeding, especially hemorrhage, is also increased with concomitant use with other anticoagulants, antiplatelets, and thrombolytics.

- Avoid I.M. injections, whenever possible, in patients receiving argatroban, to decrease the risk of bleeding.
- Monitor pregnant women during labor and delivery for excessive bleeding or unexpected changes in coagulation parameters. Know that exposure to argatroban may increase the risk of bleeding in the fetus and neonate. Monitor closely.
- Expect dosage to be tapered before stopping to prevent the risk of rebound hypercoagulopathy; drug's effects last only a short time once drug is discontinued.

! **WARNING** Monitor patient for evidence of cardiac dysfunction that could become life-threatening. Notify prescriber immediately of any concerns and be prepared to provide supportive care, as needed and ordered.

PATIENT TEACHING

- Inform patient that argatroban is a blood thinner that's given in the hospital into a vein. If he needs long-term anticoagulation, he'll be switched to another drug before discharge.

! **WARNING** Advise patient to report immediately any unexplained or unusual bleeding, such as blood in urine, easy bruising, nosebleeds, tarry stools, and vaginal bleeding.

- Instruct patient to avoid injury while receiving argatroban. For example, suggest that he brush his teeth gently, using a soft-bristled toothbrush, and take special care when flossing.

! **WARNING** Instruct patient to notify prescriber immediately if his pulse becomes irregular or he develops chest pain or feeling faint. If relief is not obtained quickly, stress importance of seeking immediate medical care.

aripiprazole

Abilify, Abilify Asimtufii, Abilify Maintena, Abilify Mycite

aripiprazole lauroxil

Aristada, Aristada Initio

Class and Category

Pharmacologic class: Atypical antipsychotic
Therapeutic class: Antipsychotic

Indications and Dosages

∗ *To treat schizophrenia; to maintain monotherapy treatment of bipolar I disorder*

I.M. INJECTION (ABILIFY ASIMTUFII)

Adults receiving oral aripiprazole or another oral antipsychotic but known to tolerate aripiprazole. *Initial:* 960 mg given once concomitantly with oral aripiprazole 10 to 20 mg given for 14 consecutive days. *Maintenance:* 960 mg every 2 mo (56 days after previous injection).
Adults receiving Abilify Maintena once a month. *Initial:* 960 mg in place of next scheduled injection of Abilify Maintena. *Maintenance:* 960 mg every 2 mo (56 days after previous injection).

± **DOSAGE ADJUSTMENT** For patients who develop adverse reactions, dosage may be reduced to 720 mg once every 2 months. For patients missing a dose and it is less than 14 weeks, next dose administered as soon as possible and then once every

2-month schedule resumed. For patients missing a dose and it is more than 14 weeks, concomitant oral aripiprazole restarted and given for 14 consecutive days with the next administered injection of Abilify Asimtufii. For patients who are CYP2D6 poor metabolizers, dosage reduced to 720 mg once every 2 months. For patients who are CYP2D6 poor metabolizers taking concomitant CYP3A4 inhibitors, administration of Abilify Asimtufii should be avoided. For patients who are taking concomitant CYP2D6 or CYP3A4 inhibitors, dosage reduced to 720 mg every 2 months. For patients taking strong CYP2D6 and strong CYP3A4 inhibitors or CYP3A4 inducers, administration of Abilify Asimtufii should be avoided.

∗ *To treat schizophrenia*

TABLETS (ABILIFY)

Adults. *Initial:* 10 or 15 mg once daily. Increased, as needed, with dosage adjustments at 2-wk intervals. *Maximum:* 30 mg daily.
Adolescents. *Initial:* 2 mg once daily for 2 days, then increased to 5 mg once daily for 2 days, then increased to 10 mg once daily. Further increased in 5-mg increments, as needed. *Maximum:* 30 mg once daily.

I.M. INJECTION (ABILIFY MAINTENA), TABLETS (ABILIFY)

Adults stabilized on a daily dose of oral aripiprazole. *Initial:* 400 mg monthly (no sooner than 26 days after the previous injection) into the deltoid or gluteal muscle followed by 10 to 20 mg P.O. of drug or another oral antipsychotic for 14 consecutive days. *Maintenance:* 400 mg monthly (no sooner than 26 days after the previous injection) into the deltoid or gluteal muscle.

±**DOSAGE ADJUSTMENT** For patients experiencing adverse reactions with the 400-mg dose of Abilify Maintena, dosage reduced to 300 mg once monthly.

I.M. INJECTION (ARISTADA), TABLETS (ABILIFY)

Adults stabilized on a daily dose of oral aripiprazole. *Initial dose for patient stabilized on 10 mg daily of oral aripiprazole:* 441 mg every month I.M. into the deltoid or gluteal muscle. *Initial dose for patient stabilized on 15 mg daily of oral aripiprazole:* 662 mg every month, 882 mg every 6 wk, or 1,064 mg every 2 mo I.M. into the gluteal muscle. *Initial dose for patient stabilized on 20 mg or higher daily dose of oral aripiprazole:* 882 mg each month I.M. into the gluteal muscle. Aristada dosage regimen initiated in one of two ways. *Option 1:* First I.M. injection administered along with one 30-mg oral dose of drug plus one 675-mg I.M. injection of Aristada Initio. *Option 2:* Oral aripiprazole administered for 21 consecutive days in conjunction with the first I.M. injection of Aristada. After initial dose of Aristada given, future doses adjusted, as needed.

TABLET (ABILIFY MYCITE)

Adults. *Initial:* 10 or 15 mg once daily, with dosage increased no sooner than every 2 wk. *Maximum:* 30 mg once daily.

∗ *As adjunct with oral aripiprazole to initiate Aristada treatment for patients with schizophrenia*

I.M. INJECTION (ARISTADA, ARISTADA INITIO), TABLETS (ABILIFY)

Adults with established tolerability with oral aripiprazole. 675 mg (Aristada Initio) as a single dose into the deltoid or gluteal muscle and given at the same time as a 30-mg oral dose of aripiprazole. First dose of Aristada (441 mg, 662 mg, 882 mg, or 1,064 mg) is then administered on the same day or up to 10 days thereafter. Alternatively, initial dose of Aristada is based on current oral daily dose. If patient is taking 10 mg P.O. daily, 441 mg of Aristada is given every month; if patient is taking 15 mg P.O.daily, 662 mg is given every month, 882 mg is given every 6 wk, or 1064 mg is given every 2 mo; and if patient is taking 20 mg P.O. or higher daily, 882 mg of Aristada is given every mo.

∗ *To treat acute manic and mixed episodes in bipolar I disorder; as adjunct with lithium or valproate in patients with bipolar I disorder*

TABLETS (ABILIFY)

Adults. *Initial:* 15 mg once daily (10 to 15 mg if lithium or valproate coadministered), increased to 30 mg once daily, as needed. *Maximum:* 30 mg once daily.
Children ages 10 to 17. *Initial:* 2 mg once daily, increased after 2 days to 5 mg once daily and then after 2 days to 10 mg once daily. Increased in 5-mg increments, as needed. *Maximum:* 30 mg once daily.

TABLETS (ABILIFY MYCITE)

Adults with acute and mixed episodes of bipolar I disorder. *Initial:* 15 mg once daily and then increased, as needed. *Maximum:* 30 mg once daily.

Adults with bipolar I disorder receiving adjunct treatment with lithium or valproate. *Initial:* 10 to 15 mg once daily and then increased, as needed. *Maximum:* 30 mg once daily.

∗ *To maintain stability with monotherapy treatment of bipolar I disorder*

I.M. INJECTION (ABILIFY MAINTENA), TABLETS (ABILIFY)

Adults stabilized on a daily dose of oral aripiprazole. *Initial:* 400 mg monthly (no sooner than 26 days after the previous injection) into the deltoid or gluteal muscle followed by 10 to 20 mg P.O. of drug or another oral antipsychotic for 14 consecutive days. *Maintenance:* 400 mg monthly (no sooner than 26 days after the previous injection) into the deltoid or gluteal muscle.

±**DOSAGE ADJUSTMENT** For patients experiencing adverse reactions with the 400-mg dose of Ability Maintena, dosage reduced to 300 mg monthly. Dosage reduced to 300 mg monthly if adverse reactions occur.

∗ *As adjunct to treat depression in patients already taking an antidepressant*

TABLETS (ABILIFY)

Adults. *Initial:* 2 to 5 mg once daily, with dosage increased by 5 mg daily at 1-wk intervals, as needed. *Maximum:* 15 mg once daily.

TABLETS (ABILIFY MYCITE)

Adults. *Initial:* 2 to 5 mg once daily, increased, as needed, in increments of up to 5 mg daily no less than once a wk. *Maximum:* 15 mg once daily.

∗ *To treat irritability associated with autistic disorder*

TABLETS (ABILIFY)

Children ages 6 to 17. *Initial:* 2 mg once daily, with dosage increased after 1 wk to 5 mg once daily and then after 1 wk to 10 mg once daily and then after 1 wk to 15 mg once daily, as needed.

∗ *To treat Tourette's disorder*

TABLETS (ABILIFY)

Children ages 6 to 18 weighing 50 kg (110 lb) or more. *Initial:* 2 mg once daily for 2 days, then 5 mg once daily for 5 days, followed by dosage increased to 10 mg once daily on day 8. Dosage increased 5 mg once daily at weekly intervals, as needed, to control tics. *Maximum:* 20 mg once daily.

Children ages 6 to 18 weighing less than 50 kg (110 lb). *Initial:* 2 mg once daily for 2 days, with dosage increased to 5 mg once daily on day 3. Dosage increased to 10 mg/kg once daily after at least 1 wk, as needed, to control tics. *Maximum:* 10 mg once daily.

∗ *To treat agitation associated with bipolar mania or schizophrenia*

I.M. INJECTION (ABILIFY)

Adults. 5.25 to 9.75 mg, repeated, as needed, after 2 or more hr. *Maximum:* Cumulative daily doses up to 30 mg with dosing intervals of 2 hr or more.

±**DOSAGE ADJUSTMENT** For patients who are known CYP2D6 poor metabolizers or patients taking strong CYP2D6 or CYP3A4 inhibitors or strong CYP3A4 inducers, Aristada Initio administration avoided because dosage adjustment cannot be made, as product is only available in a single strength. For patients who are known CYP2D6 poor metabolizers and patients taking concomitant CYP2D6 inhibitors, CYP3A4 inhibitors, and/or CYP3A4 inducers for more than 14 days, dosage reductions made for other aripiprazole products. For patients taking strong CYP3A4 inducers, such as carbamazepine or rifampin, dosage reduction individualized with current dosage prescribed and type of aripiprazole formulation being used taken into account. For patients taking strong CYP3A4 inducers such as carbamazepine or rifampin, dosage of Abilify formulation doubled over 1 to 2 weeks except for Abilify Asimtufii which requires concomitant therapy to be avoided.

Drug Administration

P.O.

Abilify

- Have patient swallow tablets whole.

P.O./PATCH

Abilify Mycite

- Be aware that Abilify Mycite is a tablet-patch combination. The tablets have an embedded ingestible event marker (IEM) to track drug ingestion and a patch that is worn containing a sensor that detects the signal from the IEM after the patient ingests the tablet and transmits data to a smartphone, which the smartphone application (app) then displays patient information and uses a Web-based portal for healthcare professionals, families, and caregivers.
- There are two types of Mycite patches. For the 1-component patch, apply only when instructed by the app to the left side of the body just above the lower edge of the rib cage. For the 2-component patch, apply only when instructed by the app to the left or right side of the body just above the lower edge of the rib cage.
- Do not place the patch in areas where the skin is cracked, inflamed, irritated, or scraped or in a location that overlaps the area of the most recently removed patch.
- If patient develops skin irritation, the patch should be removed. The patch is kept on when patient is exercising, showering, or swimming. However, the patch should be removed when patient undergoes an MRI and replaced with a new patch as soon as possible.
- Be aware the app will prompt the patient to change the patch at least weekly or sooner and it will tell the patient how to correctly apply and remove the patch.
- Abilify Mycite tablets should be swallowed whole. These tablets should not be chewed, crushed, or split because tablet contains a sensor to track patient compliance.

I.M.

- Tolerability must be established with oral form for patients who have never taken aripiprazole prior to initiating parenteral therapy.
- Do not confuse the various types of I.M. preparations. They are not interchangeable.

Abilify

- Draw up the required volume of solution into a syringe as follows: 0.7 ml for a 5.25-mg single dose; 1.3 ml for a 9.75-mg dose; and 2 ml for a 15-mg dose.
- Inject slowly and deeply into the muscle mass.
- Do not administer intravenously or subcutaneously.

Abilify Maintena

- After first dose of Abilify Maintena, expect to continue to administer oral aripiprazole (10 to 20 mg) for 14 consecutive days to achieve a therapeutic level during the initiation of the I.M. injection.
- Abilify Maintena comes in two types of kits: prefilled chamber syringe or single-use vial.
- Reconstitute Abilify Maintena lyophilized powder in prefilled dual-chamber syringe by pushing plunger rod slightly to engage threads. Then, rotate plunger rod until the rod stops rotating to release diluent. After plunger rod is at a complete stop, middle stopper will be at the indicator line. Vertically shake the syringe vigorously for 20 sec until drug is uniformly milky white.
- Reconstitute Abilify Maintena using a single-use vial by using the syringe with the pre-attached needle to withdraw 1.9 ml of Sterile Water for Injection for a 400-mg vial and 1.5 ml of Sterile Water for Injection for a 300-mg vial. Slowly inject the solution into the drug vial. Withdraw air to equalize the pressure, then remove the needle from the vial. Engage the needle safety device by using the one-handed technique. Gently press the sheath against a flat surface until the needle is firmly engaged in the needle protection sheath and discard appropriately. Shake the drug vial vigorously for 30 sec until the reconstituted suspension appears uniform. It should be opaque and milky white in color. If the injection is not given immediately after reconstitution, keep the vial at room temperature and shake the vial vigorously for at least 60 sec to resuspend prior to administration. Do not store the reconstituted suspension in a syringe.
- Prepare Abilify Maintena prior to injection after reconstituting from a single-use vial by removing cover from the vial adapter package, but do not remove the vial adapter from the package. Using the vial adapter package to handle the vial adapter, attach the prepackaged BD Luer-Lok syringe to the vial adapter. Use the syringe to remove the vial adapter from the package and discard the vial adapter package. Do not touch the spike tip of the adapter at any time. Determine the recommended volume

for injection using the manufacturer's chart for size vial being used and dosage prescribed. After wiping top of vial with a sterile alcohol swab, place and hold vial of the reconstituted suspension on a hard surface. Attach the adapter syringe assembly to the vial by holding the outside of the adapter and pushing the adapter's spike firmly through the rubber stopper until the adapter snaps in place. Slowly withdraw the recommended volume from the vial into the syringe. Prior to injection, detach the Luer-Lok syringe containing the recommended volume of reconstituted Abilify Maintena suspension from the vial.

- Once the drug is reconstituted, select the appropriate hypodermic safety needle provided by the manufacturer to use for the injection. When selecting the deltoid site for a nonobese patient, use a 23G, 1-inch needle; for an obese patient use a 22G, 1.5-inch needle. When selecting the gluteal site, for a nonobese patient, use a 22G, 1.5-inch needle; for an obese patient use a 21G, 2-inch needle.
- Inject Abilify Maintena dosage slowly, deep into the deltoid or gluteal muscle, and never I.V. or subcutaneously. Do not massage the injection site.
- Use the following guide for determining when to administer missed doses of the long-acting formulation, Abilify Maintena:
  - If a second or third dose is missed and it's been more than 4 wk but less than 5 wk since the last injection, administer the injection as soon as possible. If more than 5 wk have elapsed since the last injection, restart concomitant oral aripiprazole, as ordered, for 14 days with the next administered injection.
  - If a fourth or subsequent doses are missed and it's been more than 4 wk but less than 6 wk since the last injection, administer the injection as soon as possible. If more than 6 wk have elapsed since the last injection, restart concomitant oral aripiprazole, as ordered, for 14 days with the next administered injection.

Aristada

- Prepare Aristada for injection by first tapping the syringe at least 10 times and then shaking syringe vigorously for 30 sec to ensure a uniform suspension. If pen is not used within 15 min, shake again for 30 sec. Select needle length based on injection site and attach to syringe using a clockwise twisting motion. For administration in the deltoid muscle, use a 21G, 1-inch or 20G, 1½-inch needle; for administration in the gluteal muscle, use a 20G, 1½-inch or 20G, 2-inch needle. Prime the syringe to remove air.
- Administer Aristada formulation into the gluteal muscle by I.M. injection only for all dosages except the 441-mg dose, which may also be administered into the deltoid muscle. Inject in a rapid and continuous manner in less than 10 sec.
- Follow manufacturer's guidelines when a dose of Aristada is missed; these are based upon the dosage missed and length of time that has elapsed. However, be aware that Aristada Initio may have to be used to reinitiate treatment with Aristada.

Aristada Initio

- Prepare Aristada Initio for injection in the same manner as Aristada. The kit contains 3 safety needles (a 20G, 2-inch needle with a yellow needle hub, a 20G, 1½-inch needle with a yellow needle hub, and a 21G, 1-inch needle with a green needle hub). Select the injection needle to use (deltoid administration requires a 20G to 21G needle and gluteal administration requires a 20G needle). Avoid overtightening the needle when attaching to syringe because needle hub may crack.
- Inject in a rapid and continuous manner intramuscularly into the deltoid or gluteal muscle. Do not inject by any other route.

Aristada Asimtufii

- Remove pre-filled syringe from package.
- Inspect suspension in pre-filled syringe, which should be opaque and milky-white in color. Discard if suspension appears discolored or particulate matter is present.
- Prepare syringe by first tapping the syringe at least 10 times and then shake syringe vigorously for at least 10 sec until the suspension is uniform.
- Select the appropriate needle size. For non-obese patients, select the 22G, 1.5 inch (38 mm) from black package. For obese patients select the 21G, 2-inch (51 mm) needle from green package.
- Twist and pull off the pre-filled syringe tip cap. While holding the base of the needle, ensure the needle is firmly seated on the

safety device by pushing it. Gently twist clockwise until securely fitted.

- Once ready to inject, hold the pre-filled syringe upright and remove the needle-cap straight up. Do not twist the needle-cap, as this may cause the needle to loosen from the syringe. Slowly advance the plunger rod upward to expel the air and until the suspension fills needle base.
- Slowly inject entire contents of syringe into the gluteal muscle as an I.M. injection. Do not administer by any other route.
- Do not massage the injection site.
- After injection, press the safety shield on a hard surface to cover and lock shield over the needle. Discard used syringe and needle along with the unused needle.

Route	Onset	Peak	Duration
P.O.	Unknown	3–5 hr	Unknown
I.M.	Unknown	4–7 days	Unknown

Half-life: 75–94 hr

Mechanism of Action

May produce antipsychotic effects through partial agonist and antagonist actions. Aripiprazole acts as a partial agonist at dopamine (especially D_2) receptors and serotonin (especially 5-HT_{1A}) receptors. The drug acts as an antagonist at 5-HT_{2A} serotonin receptor sites.

Contraindications

Hypersensitivity to aripiprazole or its components

Interactions

DRUGS

antihypertensives: Possibly enhanced antihypertensive effects

benzodiazepines such as lorazepam: Increased risk of orthostatic hypotension and sedation

strong CYP3A4 inducers such as carbamazepine, rifampin: Possibly increased clearance and decreased blood level of aripiprazole

strong CYP34A inhibitors such as clarithromycin, itraconazole; strong CYP2D6 inhibitors such as fluoxetine, quinidine, paroxetine: Increased exposure of aripiprazole and increased risk of adverse reactions

ACTIVITIES

alcohol use: Increased CNS depression

Adverse Reactions

CNS: Abnormal gait, aggression, agitation, akathisia, anxiety, asthenia, catatonia, cognitive and motor impairment, confusion, **CVA (elderly)**, delusions, depression, dizziness, dream disturbances, dystonia, extrapyramidal reactions, fatigue, fever, hallucinations, headache, **homicidal ideation**, hostility, insomnia, **intracranial hemorrhage**, lethargy, light-headedness, mania, nervousness, **neuroleptic malignant syndrome**, paranoia, parkinsonism, restlessness, schizophrenic reaction, **seizures**, sleep walking, somnolence, **suicidal ideation**, tardive dyskinesia, transient ischemic attack (elderly), tremor

CV: Angina pectoris, **arrhythmias**, **bradycardia**, **cardiopulmonary arrest**, chest pain, **circulatory collapse**, **deep vein thrombosis**, dyslipidemia, elevated serum CK levels, **heart failure**, hyperlipidemia, hypertension, **MI**, orthostatic hypotension, palpitations, peripheral edema, **prolonged QT interval**, tachycardia

EENT: Blurred vision, conjunctivitis, diplopia, dry mouth, hiccups, increased salivation, **laryngospasm**, nasal congestion, nasopharyngitis, oculogyric crisis, **oropharyngeal spasm**, pharyngitis, photophobia, rhinitis, sinusitis

ENDO: Blood glucose fluctuation, breast pain, decreased prolactin levels, gynecomastia, hyperglycemia, diabetes mellitus

GI: Abdominal discomfort, constipation, decreased appetite, diarrhea, difficulty swallowing, **GI bleeding**, gastroesophageal reflux disease, **hepatitis**, hiccups, indigestion, jaundice, nausea, vomiting

GU: Decreased or increased libido, erectile dysfunction, menstrual disorders, nocturia, priapism, **renal failure**, urinary incontinence or retention

HEME: **Agranulocytosis**, anemia, **leukopenia**, **neutropenia**, **thrombocytopenia**

MS: Arthralgia, joint stiffness, muscle spasms or weakness, musculoskeletal pain, myalgia, neck and limb rigidity, **rhabdomyolysis**, trismus

RESP: **Apnea**, **aspiration**, **asthma**, cough, dyspnea, pneumonia, **pulmonary edema or embolism**, **respiratory failure**

SKIN: Alopecia, diaphoresis, dry skin, ecchymosis, photosensitivity, pruritus, rash, ulceration, urticaria
Other: **Anaphylaxis**; **angioedema**; dehydration; **drug reaction with eosinophilia and systemic symptoms (DRESS)**; elevated blood creatine phosphokinase (Aristada); flu-like symptoms; **heat stroke**; injection-site induration, pain, redness, swelling (Aristada); **hypokalemia**; **hyponatremia**; intense uncontrollable urges to perform certain activities, such as gambling and sexual acts; weight gain

Childbearing Considerations

PREGNANCY

- Pregnancy exposure registry: 1-866-961-2388 or http://womensmentalhealth.org/clinical-and-research-programs/pregnancyregistry/.
- Drug may cause fetal harm. Neonates exposed to drug during the third trimester of pregnancy are at risk for extrapyramidal and withdrawal symptoms.
- Use with caution only if benefit to mother outweighs potential risk to fetus and no other alternative is available.

LACTATION

- Drug is present in human milk.
- Mothers should check with prescriber before breastfeeding.

Nursing Considerations

- Know that aripiprazole shouldn't be used to treat dementia-related psychosis in the elderly because of an increased risk of death.
- Use cautiously in patients with cardiovascular disease, cerebrovascular disease, or conditions that would predispose them to hypotension. Also, use cautiously in those with a history of seizures or with conditions that lower the seizure threshold, such as Alzheimer's disease.
- Use cautiously in elderly patients because of increased risk of serious adverse cerebrovascular effects, such as stroke and transient ischemic attack.
- Know that most ingestions can be tracked with Abilify Mycite within 30 minutes, but it may take up to 2 hours for the smartphone app and web portal to detect that the tablet has been taken.
- Monitor patient for difficulty swallowing or excessive somnolence, which could predispose to accidental injury or aspiration. For patients with medical conditions or who are taking medications that could exacerbate CNS effects, complete a fall risk assessment and institute safety measures.

! **WARNING** Monitor patient for hypersensitivity reactions which could become life-threatening such as anaphylaxis or angioedema. Also, be on the alert for severe skin reactions such as DRESS, which may present first as a rash although sometimes it initially presents with only a fever or swollen lymph nodes. If present, notify prescriber immediately, expect drug to be withheld as ordered, and provide supportive care, as needed and ordered.

! **WARNING** Watch patients closely (especially children, adolescents, and young adults) for suicidal tendencies, particularly when therapy starts and dosage changes because depression may worsen temporarily during these times.

! **WARNING** Monitor patient's CBC, as ordered, because serious adverse hematologic reactions may occur, such as agranulocytosis, leukopenia, and neutropenia. Assess more often during first few months of therapy if patient has a history of drug-induced leukopenia or neutropenia or a significantly low WBC count. If abnormalities occur during therapy, watch for fever or other signs of infection, notify prescriber and, if severe, expect drug to be stopped.

! **WARNING** Be aware that aripiprazole rarely may cause neuroleptic malignant syndrome, seizures, and tardive dyskinesia. Monitor patient closely throughout therapy and take safety precautions as needed. Be aware that tardive dyskinesia may resolve, partially or completely, if aripiprazole is discontinued.

- Monitor patient's blood glucose level, lipid levels, and weight, as ordered, because atypical antipsychotic drugs such as aripiprazole may cause metabolic changes. If patient is already a diabetic, monitor blood glucose levels more closely.
- Assess effectiveness of aripiprazole regularly and notify prescriber if drug is ineffective or patient has become noncompliant.

PATIENT TEACHING

- Instruct patient how to take the oral formulation of aripiprazole prescribed. Stress importance of patient receiving drug intramuscularly to comply with appointments for administration.
- Instruct patient how to use the Abilify Mycite system, which will have to be downloaded and compatibility with patient's smartphone checked. Once downloaded, patient should follow manufacturer's instructions. Inform patient that a functioning pod will be needed before using the Maintenance Kit. Tell patient that most ingestions will be detected within 30 minutes on the app; however, it can take more than 2 hours for the smartphone app and web portal to detect ingestion. In some cases, the ingestion of the tablet may not be detected. If it is not, stress that dose should not be repeated.
- Alert patient that the patch which is part of the Abilify Mycite system must be removed if undergoing an MRI and a new one applied after the test.
- Urge patient to avoid alcohol during aripiprazole therapy.

! **WARNING** Alert patient that drug can cause an allergic reaction or a severe skin reaction. Tell patient to notify prescriber if an allergic reaction occurs or a rash, fever, or swollen lymph nodes occur. If reaction is severe, stress importance of seeking immediate medical care.

! **WARNING** Urge family or caregiver to watch patient closely for suicidal tendencies, especially when therapy starts or dosage changes, and particularly if patient is a child, adolescent or young adult.

- Instruct patient to notify prescriber promptly if persistent, serious, or unusual adverse reactions occur because drug can adversely affect many body systems.
- Urge patient to avoid activities that raise body temperature suddenly, such as exposure to extreme heat or strenuous exercise, and to compensate for situations that cause dehydration, such as diarrhea or vomiting.
- Instruct patient, family or caregiver to notify prescriber about intense urges, such as for gambling or sex, because dosage may have to be reduced or drug discontinued.
- Advise patient to get up slowly from a lying or sitting position during aripiprazole therapy to minimize orthostatic hypotension.
- Instruct patient to avoid hazardous activities until drug's effects are known and resolved. Also, alert patient and family of increased risk for falls, especially if patient has other medical conditions or takes medication that may affect the nervous system.
- Instruct diabetic patient to monitor blood glucose levels closely, especially if taking the oral solution form because each milliliter of solution contains 400 mg of sucrose and 200 mg of fructose.
- Instruct patient to inform all prescribers of any drugs he is taking, including over-the-counter drugs, because of risk of interactions.
- Advise females of childbearing age to notify prescriber if they intend to become or are pregnant.

asenapine

Secuado

asenapine maleate

Saphris

Class and Category

Pharmacologic class: Dopamine-serotonin antagonist
Therapeutic class: Atypical antipsychotic

Indications and Dosages

* *To treat schizophrenia*

SUBLINGUAL TABLETS (SAPHRIS)

Adults. *Initial:* 5 mg twice daily, increased to 10 mg twice daily after 1 wk, as needed and tolerated. *Maximum:* 10 mg twice daily.

TRANSDERMAL (SECUADO)

Adults. *Initial:* 3.8 mg/24 hr, increased to 5.7 mg/24 or 7.6/24 hr after 1 wk, as needed and tolerated.

* *To treat manic or mixed episodes associated with bipolar I disorder as monotherapy*

SUBLINGUAL TABLETS (SAPHRIS)

Adults. 5 or 10 mg twice daily and then if 5-mg dose is used it may be increased to

10 mg twice daily, as needed and tolerated. *Maximum:* 10 mg twice daily.
Children ages 10 and older. *Initial:* 2.5 mg twice daily increased after 3 days to 5 mg twice daily and after an additional 3 days to 10 mg twice daily, as needed and tolerated. *Maximum:* 10 mg twice daily.

✶ *To provide maintenance monotherapy in adults in the treatment of bipolar I disorder*

SUBLINGUAL TABLETS (SAPHRIS)

Adults. 5 or 10 mg twice daily, depending on dosage patient was stabilized on. A dose of 10 mg twice daily decreased to 5 mg twice daily, as needed. *Maximum:* 10 mg twice daily.

✶ *As adjunct therapy with lithium or valproate to treat bipolar I disorder*

SUBLINGUAL TABLETS (SAPHRIS)

Adults. *Initial:* 5 mg twice daily, increased to 10 mg twice daily, as needed. *Maximum:* 10 mg twice daily.

±**DOSAGE ADJUSTMENT** For patients experiencing adverse reactions, dosage may be decreased to 5 mg twice daily.

Drug Administration

P.O.

- Sublingual tablet should be removed from package only when ready for administration, using dry, gloved hands. Firmly press and hold thumb button, and then pull out the tablet pack from case. Then, peel back the colored tab, being careful not to push tablet through the tab because doing so could damage tablet. Also, do not cut or tear the tablet pack. Gently remove the tablet. Have patient place whole tablet under the tongue and let it dissolve completely. Slide tablet pack back into case until it clicks.
- Sublingual tablets should not be chewed, crushed, or swallowed. Do not cut or split the sublingual tablet.
- Patient should not eat or drink for at least 10 min after taking oral asenapine.

TRANSDERMAL

- Each transdermal system is to be worn for 24 hr only and only 1 transdermal system should be worn at a time.
- Apply to a clean, dry, and intact skin area on the abdomen, hip, or upper arm or back. The transdermal system should be applied to a different application site each time a new transdermal system is applied.
- Do not cut open the pouch until ready to apply. Do not cut the transdermal system.
- If the transdermal system lifts at the edges, reattach by pressing firmly and smoothing down the edges. However, if it comes off, a new transdermal system should be applied.
- Be aware patient can shower but not swim or take a tub bath while wearing the transdermal system.
- Discard each used transdermal system by folding it so the adhesive side sticks to itself and then discard.

Route	Onset	Peak	Duration
P.O.	Unknown	30–90 min	Unknown
Transdermal	Unknown	12–24 hr	Unknown

Half-life: 24 hr (Transdermal: 30 hr)

Mechanism of Action

May produce antipsychotic effects through antagonist actions at dopamine receptors, especially D_2, and serotonin receptors, especially 5-HT_{2A}.

Contraindications

Hypersensitivity to asenapine or its components, severe hepatic impairment

Interactions

DRUGS

antihypertensives, CNS depressants: Possibly enhanced effects
class I A and III antiarrhythmics, gatifloxacin, moxifloxacin, other antipsychotic drugs: Increased risk of prolonged QT interval
paroxetine: Possibly increased paroxetine effect

ACTIVITIES

alcohol use: Possibly enhanced effect

Adverse Reactions

CNS: Agitation, akathisia, anger, anxiety, depression, dizziness, dyskinesia, dystonia, extrapyramidal symptoms, fatigue, fever, gait disturbance, headache, hyperkinesia, insomnia, irritability, mania, masked facies, **neuroleptic malignant syndrome**, parkinsonism, **seizures**, somnolence, **suicidal ideation**, syncope, tardive dyskinesia, torticollis, tremor
CV: Hyperlipidemia, hypertension, orthostatic hypotension, peripheral edema, **prolonged QT interval**, tachycardia, temporary bundle branch block

EENT: Accommodation disorder; blepharospasm; blurred vision; **choking**; diplopia; dry mouth; nasal congestion; nasopharyngitis; oral hypoesthesia or paresthesia; oropharyngeal pain; salivary hypersecretion; sublingual application-site reactions such as blisters, inflammation, oral ulcers, peeling, or sloughing; swollen tongue; taste perversion; toothache
ENDO: Diabetes mellitus, hyperglycemia, hyperprolactinemia
GI: Abdominal pain, constipation, dyspepsia, dysphagia, elevated liver enzymes, gastroesophageal reflux disease, increased appetite, stomach discomfort, vomiting
GU: Dysmenorrhea, enuresis (children)
HEME: Anemia, **leukopenia**, **neutropenia**, **thrombocytopenia**
MS: Arthralgia, dysarthria, extremity pain, muscle rigidity, myalgia
RESP: Dyspnea
SKIN: Photosensitivity reaction
Other: **Anaphylaxis**, **angioedema**, dehydration, elevated creatine kinase, **hyponatremia**, weight gain

Childbearing Considerations

PREGNANCY

- Pregnancy exposure registry: 1-866-961-2388 or http://womensmentalhealth.org/clinical-and-research-programs/pregnancyregistry/.
- Drug may cause fetal harm. Neonates exposed to drug during the third trimester of pregnancy are at risk for extrapyramidal and withdrawal symptoms.
- Use with caution only if benefit to mother outweighs potential risk to fetus.

LACTATION

- It is not known if drug is present in breast milk.
- Mothers should check with prescriber before breastfeeding.

Nursing Considerations

- Avoid asenapine in patients with a history of cardiac arrhythmias; conditions that might prolong the QT interval, such as bradycardia, hypokalemia, or hypomagnesemia; or congenital QT interval prolongation because of increased risk of torsades de pointes or sudden death.
- Know that asenapine is not approved to treat dementia-related psychosis in elderly patients because of an increased risk of death.
- Use cautiously in patients with mild to moderate hepatic impairment.
- Use cautiously in patients with a history of seizures or who have conditions that may lower the seizure threshold, such as Alzheimer's dementia, because drug increases risk of seizures in these patients.

! WARNING Monitor patient closely even with the first dose for life-threatening hypersensitivity reactions that may include anaphylaxis and angioedema. If present, withhold drug, notify prescriber, and provide supportive care, as needed and tolerated.

! WARNING Monitor patient for suicidal behavior or thinking as drug can cause suicidal ideation. If present, notify prescriber immediately and expect drug to be discontinued. Take measures to keep patient safe.

! WARNING Monitor patient for excessive somnolence or trouble swallowing, which could predispose him to aspiration, choking, or injury.

! WARNING Know that asenapine rarely may cause neuroleptic malignant syndrome. Monitor patient closely throughout therapy and take safety precautions as needed. Expect to stop drug, if present.

- Know that the smallest dose of asenapine and the shortest duration of treatment should be used to minimize the risk of the patient developing tardive dyskinesia, which may become irreversible. If signs and symptoms appear, notify the prescriber, and know that the drug may have to be discontinued.
- Monitor patient's blood glucose level, lipid levels and weight, as ordered, because atypical antipsychotic drugs such as asenapine may cause metabolic changes. If patient is already diabetic, monitor blood glucose levels more closely.
- Monitor patient's CBC regularly, as ordered. Notify prescriber of any change because drug may have to be stopped if serious hematologic adverse reactions occur.

PATIENT TEACHING

- Instruct patient how to administer either the oral form or transdermal system of asenapine prescribed.
- Inform patient taking sublingual form that application-site reactions may occur in the sublingual area, which may include blisters, inflammation, oral ulcers, peeling, or sloughing of tissue. Also, inform patient that numbness or tingling of his mouth or throat may occur after administration of asenapine, but that it usually resolves within 1 hour.
- Tell patient using the transdermal system that if burning or irritation occurs, the transdermal system should be removed and a new one applied in a different site. Caution patient not to apply external heat sources over the transdermal system.

! **WARNING** Teach patient the signs and symptoms of a serious allergic reaction and to seek immediate emergency treatment if present. Also, inform patient of other serious adverse reactions and tell patient to report any persistent, severe, or unusual effects to prescriber immediately, including abnormal movements.

- Urge patient to avoid alcohol while taking asenapine.
- Urge patient to avoid activities that raise body temperature suddenly, such as exposure to extreme heat or strenuous exercise, and to compensate for situations that cause dehydration, such as diarrhea or vomiting.
- Tell patient that if he has a preexisting low WBC or a history of drug-induced low WBC, he should have his CBC monitored throughout asenapine therapy.
- Instruct diabetic patient taking asenapine to monitor blood glucose levels closely because hyperglycemia may occur.
- Advise patient to get up slowly from lying or sitting position during asenapine therapy to minimize orthostatic hypotension.
- Caution patient to avoid hazardous activities until drug's effects are known and resolved. Also, alert patient and family or caregiver of increased risk for falls, especially if patient has other medical conditions or takes medication that may affect the nervous system.
- Inform prescriber of any new medication being prescribed or use of any over-the-counter drugs.
- Advise females of childbearing age to notify prescriber if she intends to become or is pregnant during therapy because drug may affect the fetus. Inform her that if she does become pregnant, she should contact the prescriber and notify the pregnancy registry.

aspirin
(acetylsalicylic acid, ASA)

Aspir-81, Aspirin, Aspir-Low, Bayer, Durlaza, Ecotrin, Empirin, Miniprin, Novasen (CAN), St. Joseph Children's, Supasa (CAN), Vazalore, Zorprin

Class and Category

Pharmacologic class: Salicylate
Therapeutic class: NSAID (anti-inflammatory, antiplatelet, antipyretic, nonopioid analgesic)

Indications and Dosages

* *To relieve mild pain or fever*

CHEWABLE TABLETS, CONTROLLED-RELEASE TABLETS, ENTERIC-COATED TABLETS, SOLUTION, TABLETS, TIMED-RELEASE TABLETS

Adults and adolescents weighing 50 kg (110 lb) or more. 325 to 650 mg every 4 to 6 hr, as needed; or 500 mg every 3 hr, as needed; or 1,000 mg every 6 hr, as needed. *Maximum:* 4,000 mg daily.

Children ages 2 to 12 weighing less than 50 kg (110 lb). 10 to 15 mg/kg/dose every 4 to 6 hr, increased up to 90 mg/kg/day or 4,000 mg/day, whichever is less.

SUPPOSITORIES

Adults and adolescents. 300 or 600 mg every 4 hr for no more than 10 days.

* *To relieve mild to moderate pain from inflammation, as in osteoarthritis and rheumatoid arthritis*

CAPSULES (VAZALORE), CHEWABLE TABLETS, CONTROLLED-RELEASE TABLETS, ENTERIC-COATED TABLETS, SOLUTION, TABLETS, TIMED-RELEASE TABLETS, SUPPOSITORIES

Adults and adolescents. 3 g daily in divided doses.

∗ *To treat juvenile rheumatoid arthritis*

CAPSULES (VAZALORE), CHEWABLE TABLETS, CONTROLLED-RELEASE TABLETS, ENTERIC-COATED TABLETS, SOLUTION, TABLETS, TIMED-RELEASE TABLETS, SUPPOSITORIES

Children. 90 to 130 mg/kg daily in divided doses every 6 to 8 hr.

∗ *To reduce the risk of ischemic stroke or recurrent transient ischemic attacks*

CAPSULES (VAZALORE), TABLETS

Adults. 50 to 325 mg once daily.

∗ *To reduce the severity of or prevent acute MI*

TABLETS (NON-ENTERIC-COATED)

Adults. *Initial:* 160 to 325 mg as soon as MI is suspected. *Maintenance:* 160 to 325 mg daily for 30 days.

∗ *To treat suspected acute MI*

CAPSULES (VAZALORE), TABLETS

Adults. 160 mg to 162.5 mg given as soon as infarction is suspected, then once daily for 30 days postinfarction.

∗ *To reduce risk of MI in patients with previous MI, stable angina, or unstable angina*

CAPSULES (VAZALORE), TABLETS

Adults. 75 to 325 mg daily.

∗ *To reduce the risk of death and MI in patients with chronic coronary artery disease; to reduce risk of death and recurrent stroke in patients who have had an ischemic stroke or transient ischemic attack*

E.R. CAPSULES (DURLAZA)

Adults. 162.5 mg once daily.

∗ *To prepare patient for carotid endarterectomy*

CAPSULES (VAZALORE), TABLETS

Adults. 80 mg once daily to 650 mg twice daily, started presurgery.

∗ *As adjunct therapy with coronary artery bypass graft*

CAPSULES (VAZALORE), TABLETS

Adults. 81 mg to 325 mg daily starting 6 hr after procedure and continued for 1 yr.

∗ *As adjunct treatment for percutaneous transluminal coronary angioplasty*

CAPSULES (VAZALORE), TABLETS

Adults. 325 mg 2 hr before procedure, then 160 to 325 mg daily.

∗ *To treat spondyloarthropathies*

CAPSULES (VAZALORE), TABLETS

Adults. Up to 4 g daily in divided doses.

∗ *To treat arthritis and pleurisy of systemic lupus erythematosus (SLE)*

CAPSULES (VAZALORE), TABLETS

Adults. *Initial:* 3 g daily, then dosage adjusted, as needed.

Drug Administration

P.O.

- Administer with food and a full glass of water to reduce adverse GI effects.
- Have patient swallow E.R. or enteric-coated forms. These forms should not be chewed, crushed, or split.
- E.R. capsules should be taken with a full glass of water at the same time every day. Capsules should be swallowed whole.
- For suspected MI, patient should chew immediate-release, non-enteric-coated aspirin to speed its anti-blood-clotting properties.
- Use calibrated device to measure dosage when administering solution form.

RECTAL

- Suppositories should be refrigerated until time of administration.

Route	Onset	Peak	Duration
P.O. (chewable)	20 min	20 min	1–4 hr
P.O. (tabs)	5–30 min	25–40 min	1–4 hr
P.O. (buffered)	5–30 min	1–2 hr	1–4 hr
P.O. (E.R.)	5–30 min	1–4 hr	4–6 hr
P.O. (Enteric)	5–30 min	Unknown	1–4 hr
P.O. (Solution)	5–30 min	15–40 min	1–4 hr
P.R.	Unknown	3–4 hr	Unknown

Half-life: 15 min–6 hr

Mechanism of Action

Blocks the activity of cyclooxygenase, the enzyme needed for prostaglandin synthesis. Prostaglandins, important mediators in the inflammatory response, cause local vasodilation with swelling and pain. With blocking of cyclooxygenase and inhibition of prostaglandins, inflammatory symptoms subside. Pain is also relieved because prostaglandins play a role in pain transmission from the periphery to the spinal cord. Aspirin inhibits platelet aggregation by interfering with production of thromboxane A2, a substance that stimulates platelet aggregation. Aspirin acts on the heat-regulating center in the hypothalamus and causes peripheral vasodilation, diaphoresis, and heat loss.

Contraindications

Active bleeding or coagulation disorders; breastfeeding (continuous high dose); fever, chickenpox, or flu-like symptoms in children and teens; current or recent GI bleed or ulcers; hypersensitivity to aspirin, aspirin products, other NSAIDs, tartrazine dye, or their components; third trimester of pregnancy

Interactions

DRUGS

ACE inhibitors, beta-blockers: Decreased antihypertensive effect
acetazolamide: Possibly acetazolamide toxicity
ammonium chloride and other urine acidifiers: May increase level of aspirin with possibility of aspirin toxicity
antacids, urine alkalinizers: Decreased aspirin effectiveness
anticoagulants, antiplatelets: Increased risk of bleeding; prolonged bleeding time
corticosteroids: Increased excretion and decreased blood level of aspirin
digoxin: Increased risk of digitalis toxicity
diuretics: Possibly decreased diuretic effectiveness, especially in patients with renal impairment
heparin: Increased risk of bleeding
ibuprofen, naproxen: Possibly reduced cardioprotective and stroke preventive effects of aspirin
methotrexate: Increased blood level and decreased excretion of methotrexate, causing toxicity
oral antidiabetic agents: Possibly enhanced hypoglycemic effects
other NSAIDs: Possibly decreased blood NSAID level and increased risk of adverse GI effects
selective serotonin reuptake inhibitors (SSRIs): Increased risk of upper gastrointestinal bleeding
uricosuric agents: Decreased uricosuric effect
valproic acid: Possibly increased valproic acid level and incidence of adverse reactions

ACTIVITIES

alcohol use: Increased risk of ulcers

Adverse Reactions

CNS: Confusion, **CNS depression**
EENT: Hearing loss, tinnitus
GI: Diarrhea, **GI bleeding**, heartburn, **hepatotoxicity**, nausea, stomach pain, vomiting
HEME: Decreased blood iron level, **leukopenia**, **prolonged bleeding time**, shortened life span of RBCs, **thrombocytopenia**
RESP: **Bronchospasm**
SKIN: Ecchymosis, rash, urticaria
Other: **Angioedema**, **Reye's syndrome**, salicylism (CNS depression, confusion, diaphoresis, diarrhea, difficulty hearing, dizziness, headache, hyperventilation, lassitude, tinnitus, and vomiting) with regular use of large doses

Childbearing Considerations

PREGNANCY

- Drug can cause fetal harm especially in the third trimester, as drug may cause premature closure of the ductus arteriosus in the fetus.
- Salicylates have also been associated with altered maternal and neonatal hemostasis mechanisms, decreased birth weight, and perinatal mortality.
- Drug is generally not recommended for use during pregnancy and drug should not be used at 20 wk gestation or later. Low-dose aspirin (60 to 100 mg daily) may be used sometimes with clotting disorders, preeclampsia, or recurrent pregnancy loss.

LABOR AND DELIVERY

- Drug should not be used 1 wk before and during labor and delivery because of the potential for bleeding at delivery.

LACTATION

- Drug is present in breast milk.
- A decision should be made to discontinue breastfeeding or the drug to avoid potential adverse reactions in the breastfed infant unless low-dose aspirin is prescribed as an antiplatelet.
- If low-dose aspirin is used, infant should be monitored for bleeding and bruising.

Nursing Considerations

! **WARNING** Never administer aspirin to a child or adolescent with chickenpox or flu-like symptoms because of the risk of a rare but life-threatening reaction called Reye's syndrome.

! **WARNING** Monitor patient closely for hypersensitivity reactions such as angioedema. If present, withhold aspirin, notify prescriber, and provide supportive care, as needed and tolerated.

- Monitor patient for serious adverse reactions such as bronchospasms, bleeding, or liver dysfunction. Notify prescriber immediately if present and expect to provide emergency care as ordered and indicated by the type of adverse reaction present.
- Monitor patient for signs of salicylate toxicity. Be aware that dehydrated febrile children and elderly patients are at higher risk for toxicity. Monitor salicylate level in patients receiving high doses or long-term therapy. Ask about tinnitus. This reaction usually occurs when blood aspirin level reaches or exceeds maximum dosage for therapeutic effect.
- Expect aspirin therapy to be temporarily halted 5 to 7 days before elective surgery to reduce risk of bleeding.

PATIENT TEACHING

! **WARNING** Caution caregivers not to give aspirin to a child or adolescent with chickenpox or flu symptoms because of risk of Reye's syndrome (rare life-threatening reaction). Tell them to consult prescriber for alternative drugs.

- Instruct patient, family, or caregiver how to administer form of aspirin prescribed.
- Tell patient not to use aspirin if it has a strong vinegar-like odor.
- Instruct patient to take aspirin with food or after meals because it may cause GI upset if taken on an empty stomach.
- Advise adult patient taking low-dose aspirin not to also take ibuprofen or naproxen because these drugs may reduce the cardioprotective and stroke preventive effects of aspirin.
- Caution patient not to increase dose or take aspirin more often than prescribed as toxicity can occur. Tell patient to notify prescriber if tinnitus occurs.

! **WARNING** Review signs and symptoms of an allergic reaction with patient, family, or caregiver. Stress importance of stopping aspirin therapy if an allergic reaction occurs and to seek immediate medical attention. Advise patient with tartrazine allergy not to take aspirin.

- Advise patient to avoid alcohol while taking aspirin to decrease risk of ulcers.

! **WARNING** Instruct patient to stop taking aspirin and notify prescriber if any symptoms of stomach or intestinal bleeding occur, such as passage of bloody or tarry stools or if patient is coughing up blood or vomit that looks like coffee grounds.

- Tell patient to consult prescriber before taking aspirin with any prescription drug for arthritis, blood disorder, diabetes, or gout.
- Advise pregnant women to check with prescriber before taking aspirin at 20 weeks or later.
- Tell mothers breastfeeding is usually not recommended with aspirin use. If low-dose aspirin is prescribed, caution mother to monitor breastfed infant for bleeding and bruising.

atazanavir sulfate

Reyataz

Class and Category

Pharmacologic class: Protease inhibitor
Therapeutic class: Antiretroviral

Indications and Dosages

* *As adjunct to treat HIV-1 infection*

CAPSULES, ORAL POWDER

Adults, including pregnant women, who are treatment-experienced or treatment-naïve. 300 mg once daily in combination with ritonavir 100 mg once daily.
Adults who are HIV treatment-naïve and cannot tolerate ritonavir. 400 mg once daily.
Adults who are HIV treatment-naïve and taking efavirenz, adults who are treatment-experienced and taking both H2RA and tenofovir DF. 400 mg once daily

in combination with ritonavir 100 mg once daily.

Children ages 13 to 18 weighing at least 40 kg (88 lb) and are HIV treatment-naïve and cannot tolerate ritonavir. 400 mg once daily.

Children ages 6 to 18 weighing at least 35 kg (77 lb) who are treatment-experienced or treatment-naïve. 300 mg once daily in combination with ritonavir 100 mg once daily.

Children ages 6 to 18 weighing less than 35 kg (77 lb) but at least 15 kg (33 lb) who are treatment-experienced or treatment-naïve. 200 mg once daily in combination with ritonavir 100 mg once daily.

ORAL POWDER

Children up to age 6 weighing less than 25 kg (55 lb) but at least 15 kg (33 lb) who are treatment-experienced or treatment-naïve. 250 mg once daily in combination with ritonavir 80 mg once daily.

Infants ages 3 mo and older weighing less than 15 kg (33 lb) but at least 5 kg (11 lb) who are treatment-experienced or treatment-naïve. 200 mg once daily in combination with ritonavir 80 mg once daily.

± **DOSAGE ADJUSTMENT** For HIV treatment-experienced pregnant patients who are in the second or third trimester and also being treated with either H2RA or tenofovir DF, atazanavir dosage increased to 400 mg once daily and given with ritonavir 100 mg once daily. For HIV treatment-naïve adult patients with mild hepatic impairment, atazanavir dosage increased to 400 mg once daily and given without ritonavir. For HIV treatment-naïve adult patients with moderate hepatic impairment, atazanavir dosage kept at 300 mg once daily but given without ritonavir. For HIV treatment-naïve patients with end-stage renal disease managed with hemodialysis, dosage kept at 300 mg with ritonavir 100 mg. For pediatric patients weighing 5 kg (11 lb) to less than 10 kg (22 lb) and do not tolerate the 200-mg (4 packets) dose of oral powder and have not previously taken an HIV protease inhibitor, dosage may be decreased to 150 mg (3 packets) with close HIV viral load monitoring.

Drug Administration

P.O.

- Do not administer atazanavir at the same time as H_2-receptor antagonists or proton pump inhibitors.
- Administer atazanavir capsule form and ritonavir simultaneously with food. Know that capsule form without ritonavir is not recommended for treatment-experienced patients with prior virologic failure.
- If patient changes from capsule form to oral powder or vice versa, dosage adjustment may be needed.
- Capsules should be swallowed whole by the patient. Do not open.
- Mix oral powder as follows: Determine number of packets needed and tap each packet to settle powder. Using a clean pair of scissors, cut each packet along the dotted line. Mix with food such as applesauce or yogurt using a minimum of 1 tablespoon of food mixed in a container and then administered to patient. Follow with mixing second tablespoon in container with food and administering the residual mixture.
- For infants, oral powder may be mixed with 30 ml of infant formula, milk, or water if infant can drink from a cup. After administering drug in this way, add 15 ml of liquid to the cup and have child drink the residual mixture. If water was used to mix the drug, the child should immediately be given something to eat.
- For infants less than 6 mo old who cannot drink from a cup or eat solid food, mix with 10 ml of infant formula in a medicine cup and give using an oral dosing syringe and administer into either inner cheek of infant. Add an additional 10 ml of formula to cup used to mix drug and formula, draw up residual mixture, and administer to infant.
- Do not use an infant bottle to administer drug because full dose may not be delivered.
- When drug is mixed with food or liquid, it must be administered within 1 hr of preparation. Mixture may remain at room temperature during this time.
- Administer ritonavir immediately after atazanavir powder administration.
- Oral powder contains 35 mg of phenylalanine, which can be harmful if patient has phenylketonuria. Capsules contain no phenylalanine.

Route	Onset	Peak	Duration
P.O.	Unknown	2–3 hr	Unknown

Half-life: 7–8 hr

Mechanism of Action

Inhibits the virus-specific processing of specific polyproteins selectively in HIV-1-infected cells to prevent formation of mature virions.

Contraindications

Concurrent therapy with drugs that are highly dependent on CYP3A or UGT1A for clearance, and when elevated plasma concentrations of the interacting drugs are associated with serious and/or life-threatening events (alfuzosin, amiodarone [with ritonavir], apalutamide, carbamazepine, cisapride, dihydroergotamine, elbasvir/grazoprevir, encorafenib, ergonovine, ergotamine, glecaprevir/pibrentasvir, indinavir, irinotecan, ivosidenib, lomitapide, lovastatin, lurasidone [with ritonavir], methylergonovine, midazolam (oral), nevirapine, phenobarbital, phenytoin, pimozide, quinidine [with ritonavir], rifampin, sildenafil (when used for treatment of pulmonary arterial hypertension), simvastatin, St. John's wort, triazolam); concurrent therapy with CYP3A strong inducers; hypersensitivity to atazanavir or any of its components

Interactions

DRUGS

amiodarone, atorvastatin, bepridil, buprenorphine, colchicine, diltiazem, ethinyl and norethindrone, felodipine, fluticasone, ketoconazole, itraconazole, immunosuppressants, lidocaine (systemic) lurasidone, midazolam, nicardipine, nifedipine, norbuprenorphine, PDE5 inhibitors (sildenafil, tadalafil, vardenafil), quetiapine, rifabutin, quinidine, rosuvastatin, salmeterol, trazodone, tricyclic antidepressants, verapamil, voxilaprevir: Increased plasma concentrations of these drugs with possible increased risk of adverse effects that could be serious or life-threatening

antacids, buffered medications, CYP3A4 strong inducers, efavirenz, H_2-receptor antagonists, proton pump inhibitors: Decreased plasma concentration of atazanavir, decreasing effectiveness

boceprevir: Decreased plasma concentrations of both atazanavir and ritonavir when administered together, decreasing effectiveness of both drugs

bosentan: Decreased plasma concentration of atazanavir and increased plasma concentration of bosentan

carbamazepine: Decreased plasma concentration of atazanavir and increased plasma concentration of carbamazepine, increasing risk of serious carbamazepine-induced adverse reactions

clarithromycin: Increased plasma concentration of both atazanavir and clarithromycin, increasing risk of QT prolongation

didanosine: Decreased plasma concentration of both atazanavir and didanosine, with decreased effectiveness

ethinyl estradiol and norgestimate: Decreased plasma concentration of ethinyl estradiol and increased plasma concentration of norgestimate, possibly affecting contraceptive effectiveness

lamotrigine: Possibly decreased plasma concentration of lamotrigine, with increased risk of seizure activity

other protease inhibitors such as saquinavir: Possibly increased plasma concentration of protease inhibitor

phenobarbital, phenytoin: Decreased plasma concentration of atazanavir, phenobarbital, and phenytoin, decreasing effectiveness and increasing risk of seizures

ritonavir: Increased plasma concentration of atazanavir and risk of serious adverse reactions

tenofovir disoproxil fumarate: Decreased plasma concentration of atazanavir; increased plasma concentration of tenofovir

voriconazole: Decreased plasma concentrations of both atazanavir and voriconazole in patients with a functional CYP2C19 allele; decreased plasma concentration of atazanavir and increased plasma concentration of voriconazole in patients without a functional CYP2C19 allele

warfarin: Increased plasma concentration of warfarin, increasing risk of serious or life-threatening bleeding

Adverse Reactions

CNS: Depression, dizziness, fever, headache, insomnia, peripheral nervous system abnormalities

CV: **Cardiac conduction abnormalities (second- or third-degree AV block, left bundle branch block)**, edema, elevated cholesterol and triglyceride levels, peripheral edema, **QT prolongation**

EENT: Nasal congestion (children), oropharyngeal pain (children), rhinorrhea (children), scleral icterus
ENDO: Diabetes mellitus, fat redistribution, hyperglycemia, **hypoglycemia (children)**
GI: Abdominal pain, cholecystitis, cholelithiasis, cholestasis, diarrhea, elevated liver and pancreatic enzymes, **hepatic dysfunction**, hyperbilirubinemia, jaundice, nausea, **pancreatitis**, vomiting
GU: **Chronic kidney disease**, **granulomatous interstitial nephritis**, **interstitial nephritis**, nephrolithiasis
HEME: Decreased hemoglobin or platelet count, **neutropenia**
MS: Arthralgia, elevated creatine kinase, extremity pain (children), myalgia
RESP: Cough (children), wheezing (children)
SKIN: Alopecia, **erythema multiforme**, pruritus, rash, **Stevens-Johnson syndrome**, **toxic skin eruptions**
Other: **Angioedema**, **drug reaction with eosinophilia and systemic symptoms (DRESS)**, **immune reconstitution syndrome**

Childbearing Considerations

PREGNANCY

- Pregnancy exposure registry: 1-800-258-4263.
- It is not known if drug can cause fetal harm.
- Use with caution only if benefit to mother outweighs potential risk to fetus.
- Drug has potential to increase risk for hyperbilirubinemia and lactic acidosis syndrome in mother during pregnancy.

LABOR AND DELIVERY

- Drug can cause increased risk of adverse reactions in mother during the first 2 mo after delivery because drug exposure could be higher during this time.
- Neonate may develop severe hyperbilirubinemia during the first few days following birth if exposed to drug in utero.

LACTATION

- Drug is present in breast milk.
- The Centers for Disease Control and Prevention recommends that HIV-1 infected mothers not breastfeed to avoid risking postnatal transmission of HIV-1 infection as well as the possibility of potential drug-induced adverse reactions in the infant.

Nursing Considerations

- Be aware that atazanavir is not recommended for HIV treatment-experienced patients with end-stage renal disease managed with hemodialysis. Expect all patients to have renal laboratory testing prior to atazanavir being initiated and periodically throughout drug therapy. Testing should include estimated creatinine clearance, serum creatinine, and urinalysis with microscopic examination. If kidney disease occurs and becomes progressive, expect that atazanavir may be discontinued.
- Expect patients with marked elevations in transaminases or underlying hepatitis B or C viral infections that have occurred before atazanavir treatment to have hepatic function evaluated prior to start of therapy and periodically during treatment because these patients may experience further hepatic decompensation or transaminase elevations while taking atazanavir.
- Be aware that patients with preexisting conduction system disease should be monitored by ECG.

! **WARNING** Be aware that severe, life-threatening, or fatal events as well as serious adverse reactions may occur with greater exposure to drugs that are CYP3A inhibitors. Monitor patient closely for serious drug interactions if CYP3A inhibitors are administered concomitantly.

! **WARNING** Monitor patient closely for signs of a hypersensitivity reaction such as angioedema. Notify prescriber immediately if present, expect drug to be discontinued, and provide supportive care, as needed and ordered.

! **WARNING** Monitor patient for the appearance of a rash. Although common and usually not affecting the use of atazanavir, some rashes may become severe and life-threatening. Although rash is usually the first symptom of DRESS, the condition may initially present with only fever or swollen lymph noses. At the first sign of any of these symptoms, notify prescriber, expect drug to be discontinued and provide supportive care, as needed and ordered.

- Monitor patients with hemophilia for increased bleeding because spontaneous skin hemarthrosis and hematomas have occurred in these patients while taking atazanavir. Provide supportive care, as needed.
- Report signs or symptoms suggestive of cholelithiasis or nephrolithiasis to prescriber, as drug may have to be temporarily interrupted or discontinued if confirmed.
- Monitor patient's blood glucose level throughout atazanavir therapy because drug has been associated with the development of newly onset diabetes mellitus or exacerbation of preexisting diabetes mellitus. Notify prescriber if hyperglycemia occurs and provide care, as prescribed.

! **WARNING** Be aware that immune reconstitution syndrome has occurred in patients treated with combination antiretroviral therapy, including atazanavir. The inflammatory response predisposes susceptible patients to opportunistic infections such as cytomegalovirus infection, *Mycobacterium avium* infection, *Pneumocystis jiroveci* pneumonia, or tuberculosis. Autoimmune disorders such as Graves' disease, Guillain-Barré syndrome, or polymyositis have also occurred. Report sudden or unusual adverse reactions to prescriber.

PATIENT TEACHING

- Instruct patient, family, or caregiver how to administer form of atazanavir prescribed.
- Alert patient, family, or caregiver using the oral powder form of atazanavir that it contains 35 mg of phenylalanine, which can be harmful if patient has phenylketonuria. The capsule form of drug contains no phenylalanine.
- Stress importance of maintaining adequate hydration while taking drug because of risk of chronic kidney disease.

! **WARNING** Instruct patient to notify prescriber immediately if an allergic reaction occurs and to seek emergency medical care, if severe.

! **WARNING** Advise patient to report the appearance of a fever, rash, or swollen lymph nodes to prescriber immediately and stop taking drug.

! **WARNING** Stress importance of informing all prescribers of atazanavir therapy because drug interacts with many other drugs and may cause life-threatening interactions. Tell patient not to take any over-the-counter medication, including herbals, without consulting prescriber first.

- Advise patient to report dizziness or lightheadedness to prescriber because drug may cause changes in how the heart functions. Also, tell patient to report any yellowing of the skin or whites of the eyes.
- Review signs and symptoms of the presence of gallbladder or kidney stones with patient and advise patient to notify prescriber if any such signs and symptoms develop, as drug may have to be temporarily withheld or discontinued.
- Tell patient with diabetes mellitus to monitor glucose levels during atazanavir therapy, as adjustments in her diabetes treatment regimen may be needed. Also, review signs and symptoms of diabetes mellitus with all patients because newly onset diabetes mellitus has occurred during atazanavir therapy.
- Instruct patient to report any signs and symptoms of infection or persistent or unusual adverse effects to prescriber.
- Alert patient that atazanavir may redistribute or cause accumulation of body fat, which may include breast enlargement, a buffalo hump on the back of the neck, central obesity, and wasting appearance of extremities and face.
- Encourage females of childbearing age who become pregnant to register on the pregnancy exposure registry through their prescriber.
- Instruct mothers not to breastfeed while taking atazanavir.

atenolol

Tenormin

Class and Category

Pharmacologic class: Beta-adrenergic blocker (beta$_1$ and at high doses beta$_2$)
Therapeutic class: Antianginal, antihypertensive

Indications and Dosages

✱ To treat angina pectoris; to treat hypertension

TABLETS

Adults. 50 mg once daily increased after 7 days for angina and 7 to 14 days for hypertension to 100 mg once daily, as needed. *Maximum:* 100 mg for treatment of hypertension; 200 mg for treatment of angina pectoris.

✱ To treat acute MI in hemodynamically stable patients to reduce cardiovascular mortality

TABLETS

Adults. 100 mg once daily or 50 mg twice daily for at least 7 days.

±**DOSAGE ADJUSTMENT** For elderly patients and for patients with a creatinine clearance of 15 to 35 ml/min, dosage usually not increased above 50 mg daily P.O. For patients with creatinine clearance less than 15 ml/min, dosage reduced to 25 mg daily.

Drug Administration

P.O.

- Take patient's apical pulse and blood pressure before each dose.
- Administer at about the same time each day.
- Do not discontinue abruptly.

Route	Onset	Peak	Duration
P.O.	1 hr	2–4 hr	24 hr

Half-life: 6–7 hr

Mechanism of Action

Inhibits stimulation of $beta_1$-receptor sites, located mainly in the heart, decreasing cardiac excitability, cardiac output, and myocardial oxygen demand. Atenolol also acts to decrease release of renin from the kidneys, aiding in reducing blood pressure. At high doses, it inhibits stimulation of $beta_2$ receptors in the lungs, which may cause bronchoconstriction.

Contraindications

Anesthesia with agents that produce myocardial depression; cardiogenic shock; heart block greater than first degree; hypersensitivity to atenolol, other beta-blockers or their components; hypotension; metabolic acidosis; overt heart or uncontrolled failure; pheochromocytoma in the absence of alpha-blockade; right ventricular failure secondary to pulmonary hypertension; severe peripheral arterial disorders; sick sinus syndrome; sinus bradycardia

Interactions

DRUGS

amiodarone and class I antiarrhythmics such as disopyramide: Additive atenolol effects with increased risk of asystole, heart failure, and severe bradycardia
anesthetic agents: Possibly induced hypotensive state with associated reflex tachycardia
calcium channel blockers such as verapamil and diltiazem: Possibly symptomatic bradycardia and conduction abnormalities
catecholamine-depleting drugs such as guanethidine, reserpine: Additive antihypertensive effect
clonidine: Possible rebound hypertension following discontinuation of clonidine
digoxin, fingolimod: Possible potentiate bradycardia
dihydropyridines such as nifedipine: Increased risk of cardiac failure and hypotension in patients with latent cardiac insufficiency
NSAIDs: Possible blunting of the antihypertensive effect of atenolol

Adverse Reactions

CNS: Depression, disorientation, dizziness, drowsiness, emotional lability, fatigue, fever, lethargy, light-headedness, short-term memory loss, vertigo
CV: **Arrhythmias, including bradycardia and heart block**; **cardiogenic shock**; cold arms and legs; **mitral insufficiency**; **myocardial reinfarction**; orthostatic hypotension; Raynaud's phenomenon
EENT: Dry eyes, **laryngospasm**, pharyngitis
ENDO: **Hypoglycemia**
GI: Diarrhea, **ischemic colitis**, **mesenteric artery thrombosis**, nausea
GU: **Renal failure**
HEME: **Agranulocytosis**
MS: Leg pain
RESP: **Bronchospasm**, dyspnea, **pulmonary emboli**, **respiratory distress**, wheezing
SKIN: Erythematous rash
Other: **Hypersensitivity reactions**

Childbearing Considerations

PREGNANCY

- Drug crosses placental barrier and can cause fetal harm.
- Use of drug starting in the second trimester has caused a lower birth rate for gestational

age of fetus; in the third trimester bradycardia may occur in the fetus.
- Use with caution only if benefit to mother outweighs potential risk to fetus.

LABOR AND DELIVERY
- Newborns are at risk for bradycardia and hypoglycemia if exposed to drug in utero.

LACTATION
- Drug is present in breast milk.
- Mothers should check with prescriber before breastfeeding because breastfed infant may be at risk for bradycardia and hypoglycemia.

Nursing Considerations

- Use atenolol cautiously in patients with arterial circulatory disorders, patients with conduction abnormalities or left ventricular dysfunction who take diltiazem or verapamil, patients with heart failure controlled by digitalis glycosides or diuretics, and patients with impaired renal function.

! **WARNING** Monitor patient for hypersensitivity reactions. If present, notify prescriber, expect atenolol to be discontinued and another drug substituted, and provide supportive care, as needed and ordered. Also, notify prescriber if patient develops serious adverse reactions such as bradycardia, hypotension, or other serious adverse reaction.

! **WARNING** Monitor patients for hypoglycemia that may become prolonged or severe, especially in patients who are diabetic or patients who are fasting because of not eating regularly, having surgery, or are vomiting. Be aware that beta-blockers such as atenolol may mask early warning signs of hypoglycemia, such as tachycardia. Monitor patient's blood glucose level closely. If hypoglycemia occurs, notify prescriber and expect to administer glucose or glucagon, as ordered and needed.

! **WARNING** Monitor patient for heart failure. At first sign of heart failure, expect patient to receive a digitalis glycoside, a diuretic, or both and to be monitored closely. If failure continues, expect to stop atenolol.

! **WARNING** Closely monitor patient with hyperthyroidism because atenolol may mask some signs of thyrotoxicosis. Abrupt withdrawal of atenolol may precipitate thyrotoxicosis.

- Know that if patient also receives clonidine, expect to stop atenolol several days before gradually withdrawing clonidine. Then, expect to restart atenolol therapy several days after clonidine has been discontinued.
- Be aware that chronic beta-blocker therapy such as atenolol is not routinely withheld prior to major surgery because the benefits outweigh the risks associated with its use with general anesthesia and surgical procedures.

PATIENT TEACHING
- Instruct patient how to take atenolol and what to do if a dose is missed.

! **WARNING** Caution patient not to stop taking atenolol abruptly. Otherwise, angina may worsen, and an arrhythmia or MI may occur. Also tell patient with hyperthyroidism not to stop taking drug abruptly as serious adverse effects can occur that could become life-threatening.

! **WARNING** Advise patient to notify prescriber if an allergic reaction occurs. Stress importance of seeking immediate medical attention if reaction is severe.

! **WARNING** Alert patient that atenolol may cause hypoglycemia that could become severe even if patient is not diabetic. Risk is increased if patient is fasting or vomiting or has diabetes. Stress that hypoglycemia may become severe quickly and to seek immediate medical care if present.

! **WARNING** Review signs and symptoms of heart failure with patient and instruct to notify prescriber if shortness of breath or sudden weight gain over a period of a few days occurs.

- Inform the patient that he may experience fatigue and reduced tolerance to exercise and that he should notify his prescriber if this interferes with his normal lifestyle. Tell him to perform minimal physical activity to prevent chest pain when he is being weaned from atenolol therapy.
- Advise females of childbearing age to notify prescriber if pregnancy occurs.

atogepant

Qulipta

Class and Category

Pharmacologic class: Calcitonin gene-related peptide (CGRP) receptor antagonist
Therapeutic class: Antimigraine drug

Indications and Dosages

✱ *To prevent episodic migraine*

TABLETS

Adults. 10 mg, 30 mg, or 60 mg once daily.

✱ *To prevent chronic migraine*

TABLETS

Adults. 60 mg once daily.

±**DOSAGE ADJUSTMENT** For patients with episodic migraine who have severe renal impairment and end-stage renal disease (creatinine clearance less than 30 ml/min), dosage limited to 10 mg once daily. For patients with chronic migraine who have severe renal impairment and end-stage renal disease (creatinine clearance less than 30 ml/min), the drug should be avoided. For patients with episodic migraine taking strong CYP3A4 inhibitors, dosage limited to 10 mg once daily or if taking CYP3A4 inducers, dosage limited to 30 mg or 60 mg once daily. For patients with chronic migraine taking CYP3A4 inducers or strong CYP3A4 inhibitors, drug should be avoided. For patients with episodic migraine who are taking OATP inhibitors, dosage limited to 10 mg or 30 mg once daily. For patients with chronic migraines who are taking OATP inhibitors, dosage limited to 30 mg once daily. For patients ages 65 and older with episodic migraine, dosage usually initiated at the low end of the dosing range.

Drug Administration

P.O.

- Do not administer drug with grapefruit juice.
- Administer drug after dialysis for patients with episodic migraine and end-stage renal disease undergoing intermittent dialysis.

Route	Onset	Peak	Duration
P.O.	Unknown	1–2 hr	Unknown

Half-life: 11 hr

Mechanism of Action

Blocks the CGRP protein from attaching to receptors to prevent migraine headaches.

Contraindications

Hypersensitivity to atogepant or its components

Interactions

DRUGS

CYP3A4 strong or moderate inducers, such as carbamazepine, efavirenz, etravirine, phenytoin, rifampin, St. John's wort: Decreased exposure to atogepant with decreased effectiveness

FOODS

grapefruit, grapefruit juice: Increased exposure of atogepant with increased risk of adverse reactions

Adverse Reactions

CNS: Dizziness, fatigue, somnolence
GI: Anorexia, constipation, elevated liver enzymes, nausea
RESP: Dyspnea
SKIN: Pruritus, rash, urticaria
Other: **Anaphylaxis**, **facial angioedema**, weight loss

Childbearing Considerations

PREGNANCY

- It is not known if drug can cause fetal harm.
- Use with caution only if benefit to mother outweighs potential risk to fetus.
- Be aware that females of childbearing age with migraine may be at increased risk of gestational hypertension and preeclampsia during pregnancy.

LACTATION

- It is not known if drug is present in breast milk.
- Mothers should check with prescriber before breastfeeding.

Nursing Considerations

- Know that atogepant should not be administered to patients with severe hepatic impairment.

! **WARNING** Monitor patient for hypersensitivity reactions such as pruritus, rash, and urticaria that may become life-threatening causing anaphylaxis and angioedema of the face. Be aware that the reaction may occur days after the drug was administered. If present, stop drug, notify prescriber, and provide supportive care, as needed and ordered.

PATIENT TEACHING

- Instruct patient how to take atogepant.
- Instruct patient to avoid eating grapefruit or drinking grapefruit juice while taking atogepant.

! **WARNING** Inform patient atogepant may cause an allergic reaction that could become severe and may occur days after the drug has been administered. Stress importance of stopping atogepant therapy and notifying prescriber immediately if an allergic reaction occurs. If reaction is severe, instruct patient to seek immediate medical care.

- Advise patient to report all drug use to prescriber, including over-the-counter medication and herbal products.

atomoxetine hydrochloride

Strattera

Class and Category

Pharmacologic class: Selective norepinephrine reuptake inhibitor
Therapeutic class: Anti-ADHD agent

Indications and Dosages

✶ *To treat attention deficit hyperactivity disorder (ADHD)*

CAPSULES

Adults and children weighing more than 70 kg (154 lb). *Initial:* 40 mg daily, increased after at least 3 days to 80 mg daily given either as a single daily dose in the morning or as evenly divided doses in the morning and late afternoon or early evening. After 2 to 4 additional wk, dosage may be increased to 100 mg daily if optimal response has not been achieved. *Maximum:* 100 mg daily.
Adults and children weighing 70 kg (154 lb) or less. *Initial:* 0.5 mg/kg daily, increased after at least 3 days to 1.2 mg/kg daily given either as a single daily dose in the morning or as evenly divided doses in the morning and late afternoon or early evening, as needed. *Maximum:* 1.4 mg/kg or 100 mg daily, whichever is less.

± **DOSAGE ADJUSTMENT** For patients with moderate (Child-Pugh class B) hepatic impairment, dosage reduced by 50%. For patients with severe (Child-Pugh class C) hepatic impairment, dosage reduced by 75%. For patients weighing more than 70 kg and taking strong CYP2D6 inhibitors (fluoxetine, paroxetine, or quinidine), initial dosage of 40 mg daily increased to 80 mg daily only if symptoms fail to improve after 4 weeks. For patients weighing 70 kg or less and taking strong CYP2D6 inhibitors or are CYP2D6 poor metabolizers, initial dosage of 0.5 mg/kg daily increased to 1.2 mg/kg daily only if symptoms fail to improve after 4 weeks.

Drug Administration

P.O.

- Administer capsules whole. Do not open capsules for administration.
- If capsule inadvertently opens, immediately wash hands and any surface drug touched.

Route	Onset	Peak	Duration
P.O.	Unknown	1–2 hr	> 24 hr

Half-life: 5.2 hr

Mechanism of Action

Inhibits presynaptic norepinephrine transport selectively in the nervous system to increase attention span and produce a calming effect.

Contraindications

Angle-closure glaucoma, hypersensitivity to atomoxetine or its components, pheochromocytoma, severe cardiovascular disorders, use within 14 days of MAO inhibitor therapy

Interactions

DRUGS

albuterol and other beta$_2$ agonists: May potentiate action of albuterol and other beta$_2$ agonists on cardiovascular system
antihypertensives, pressor agents: Possibly increased blood pressure
CYP2D6 inhibitors (such as fluoxetine, paroxetine, and quinidine): Increased blood atomoxetine level

MAO inhibitors: Possibly induced hypertensive crisis

Adverse Reactions

CNS: Aggressiveness, anxiety, chills, crying, **CVA**, delusional thinking, depression, dizziness, early morning awakening, fatigue, hallucinations, headache, hostility, hypoesthesia, insomnia, irritability, jittery feeling, lethargy, mania, mood changes, paresthesia (children and adolescents), peripheral coldness, pyrexia, rigors, sedation, **seizures**, sensory disturbances, sleep disturbance, somnolence, **suicidal ideation**, syncope, tics, tremor, unusual dreams
CV: Chest pain, hypertension, orthostatic hypotension, **MI**, palpitations, **QT interval prolongation**, Raynaud's phenomenon, tachycardia
EENT: Blurred vision, conjunctivitis, dry mouth, ear infection, mydriasis, nasal congestion, nasopharyngitis, pharyngitis, rhinorrhea, sinus congestion
ENDO: Hot flashes
GI: Abdominal pain (upper), anorexia, constipation, diarrhea, dyspepsia, elevated liver enzymes, flatulence, gastroenteritis (viral), indigestion, nausea, **severe hepatic dysfunction**, vomiting
GU: Decreased libido, dysmenorrhea, dysuria, ejaculation disorders, erectile dysfunction, impotence, male pelvic pain, menstrual irregularities, orgasm abnormality, priapism, prostatitis, urinary hesitancy (children and adolescents), urine retention (children and adolescents)
MS: Arthralgia, back pain, myalgia, **rhabdomyolysis**
RESP: Cough, upper respiratory tract infection
SKIN: Alopecia, dermatitis, diaphoresis, hyperhidrosis, pruritus, rash, urticaria
Other: **Anaphylaxis**, **angioedema**, flu-like symptoms, weight loss

Childbearing Considerations

PREGNANCY

- Pregnancy exposure registry: 1-866-961-2388 or https://womensmentalhealth.org/adhd-medications/.
- It is not known if drug can cause fetal harm although some animal studies suggest adverse developmental risks may occur.
- Drug is not recommended during pregnancy unless benefit to mother outweighs potential risk to fetus.

LACTATION

- It is not known if drug is present in breast milk.
- Mothers should check with prescriber before breastfeeding.

REPRODUCTION

- Females of childbearing age should avoid pregnancy during drug therapy by using an effective contraceptive.

Nursing Considerations

- Know that patient should be screened for a family or personal history of bipolar disorder, hypomania, or mania before atomoxetine therapy is begun. This is because drug can increase risk for exacerbation of these disorders. In addition, drug may cause manic or psychotic symptoms even in patients without a prior history at normal doses. Monitor patient carefully throughout therapy, and if symptoms such as delusional thinking, hallucinations, mania, or onset or worsening of aggressive behavior or hostility occur, notify prescriber and expect drug to be discontinued.
- Use atomoxetine cautiously in patients with cardiovascular or cerebrovascular disease (especially hypertension or tachycardia) because drug may increase blood pressure and heart rate. Also, use cautiously in those prone to orthostatic hypotension and those with cardiomyopathy, serious heart rhythm abnormalities, serious structural cardiac abnormalities or other serious cardiac problems because drug may increase risk of sudden death from these conditions.
- Obtain baseline blood pressure and heart rate before starting therapy. Monitor patient's vital signs after dosage increases and periodically during therapy.

! **WARNING** Monitor patient closely for hypersensitivity reactions that could become life-threatening such as anaphylaxis or angioedema. If these occur, notify prescriber immediately, withhold drug, and provide supportive care, as needed and ordered.

! **WARNING** Monitor patient closely for evidence of suicidal thinking and behavior because atomoxetine increases the risk of suicidal ideation.

- Monitor patient's liver function studies, as ordered. Notify prescriber immediately if enzyme levels are elevated or patient has evidence of hepatic dysfunction. Expect to stop drug permanently.
- Monitor child's or adolescent's growth and weight. Expect to interrupt therapy, as prescribed, if patient isn't growing or gaining weight appropriately.

PATIENT TEACHING

- Instruct patient how to take atomoxetine. If drug gets in his eyes, tell him to flush immediately with water and seek medical care.
- Reassure patient or caregiver that drug does not cause physical or psychological dependence.

! **WARNING** Instruct patient, family, or caregiver to immediately report to prescriber if an allergic reaction occurs such as difficulty breathing or swallowing or if facial swelling occurs and seek immediate medical care.

! **WARNING** Urge family or caregiver to watch the child or adolescent closely for evidence of abnormal behavior or thinking or increased aggression or hostility. Emphasize need to notify prescriber about unusual changes.

- Urge patient to tell prescriber immediately about dark urine, flu-like symptoms, itchiness, right upper abdominal pain, or yellowing of his skin or eyes. Also, tell patient to notify prescriber immediately if he experiences exertional chest pain, unexplained syncope, or other symptoms suggestive of heart disease.
- Urge male patient to seek immediate medical attention for a penile erection that becomes painful or prolonged.
- Advise patient to report urinary hesitancy or urine retention to prescriber.
- Caution patient to assume sitting or standing position slowly because of drug's potential effect on blood pressure.
- Remind patient of the importance of alerting all prescribers to any over-the-counter drugs, including dietary supplements, or herbal remedies he is taking.
- Caution patient to avoid hazardous activities until drug's CNS effects are known and resolved.
- Instruct patient or caregiver to monitor weight during therapy.
- Inform females of childbearing age to use an effective contraception during drug therapy and to report pregnancy immediately to prescriber.

atorvastatin calcium

Atorvaliq, Lipitor

Class and Category

Pharmacologic class: HMG-CoA reductase inhibitor

Therapeutic class: Antihyperlipidemic

Indications and Dosages

✱ *To control lipid levels as adjunct to diet in mixed dyslipidemia and primary (heterozygous familial and nonfamilial) hypercholesterolemia*

ORAL SUSPENSION, TABLETS

Adults. *Initial:* 10 or 20 mg once daily; then increased according to lipid level. *Maintenance:* 10 to 80 mg once daily.

± **DOSAGE ADJUSTMENT** For patients who need cholesterol level reduced more than 45%, initial dose may be increased to 40 mg once daily.

✱ *As adjunct to control lipid levels in homozygous familial hypercholesterolemia*

ORAL SUSPENSION, TABLETS

Adults. *Initial:* 10 mg to 20 mg once daily, increased, as needed. *Maintenance:* 10 to 80 mg once daily.

ORAL SUSPENSION

Adolescents and children ages 10 and older. *Initial:* 10 mg to 20 mg once daily, increased, as needed. *Maintenance:* 10 mg to 80 mg once daily.

✱ *As adjunct to control lipid levels in pediatric heterozygous familial hypercholesterolemia*

ORAL SUSPENSION, TABLETS

Adolescents and children ages 10 and older. *Initial:* 10 mg once daily, adjusted at intervals of 4 wk or more, as needed. *Maximum:* 20 mg once daily.

✱ *To reduce risk of acute cardiovascular events such as angina, CVA, or MI and to reduce risk for revascularization procedures or hospitalization for congestive heart failure in patients with coronary heart disease (CAD); to reduce risk of angina, CVA, or MI in patients without clinical evidence of CAD but with multiple risk factors for CAD such as age, family history of early CAD, hypertension, low HDL-C, or smoking; to reduce risk of CVA or MI in patients with type 2 diabetes without clinical evidence of CAD but with multiple risk factors for CAD such as albuminuria, hypertension, retinopathy, or smoking*

ORAL SUSPENSION, TABLETS

Adults. *Initial:* 10 mg to 20 mg once daily, increased, as needed. *Maintenance:* 10 to 80 mg once daily.

± **DOSAGE ADJUSTMENT** *For all indications:* For patients taking clarithromycin, darunavir plus ritonavir, elbasvir plus grazoprevir, fosamprenavir, fosamprenavir plus ritonavir, itraconazole, letermovir, or saquinavir plus ritonavir, dosage not to exceed 20 mg once daily. For patients taking nelfinavir, dosage should not exceed 40 mg once daily.

Drug Administration

P.O.

- Give drug at the same time of day to maintain effects.
- Oral suspension is available in the concentration of 20 mg/5 ml. Use a calibrated device to measure dosage.
- Administer oral suspesnion on an empty stomach either 1 hr before or 2 hr after a meal.
- Store oral suspension at room temperature. Use within 60 days of first opening bottle, then discard regardless if any suspension remains.
- Do not administer a missed dose but resume dosing with next scheduled dose.

Route	Onset	Peak	Duration
P.O.	Unknown	1–2 hr	Unknown

Half-life: 14 hr

Mechanism of Action

Reduces plasma cholesterol and lipoprotein levels by inhibiting HMG-CoA reductase and cholesterol synthesis in the liver and by increasing the number of LDL receptors on liver cells to enhance LDL uptake and breakdown.

Contraindications

Acute liver failure or decompensated cirrhosis, hypersensitivity to atorvastatin or its components

Interactions

DRUGS

azole antifungals, colchicine, erythromycin, gemfibrozil, lipid-modifying doses of niacin, other fibrates: Increased risk of myopathy and rhabdomyolysis

cyclosporine, CYP3A4 and/or OATP1B1 strong inhibitors such as clarithromycin, HIV and HCV protease inhibitors, including combination drugs, itraconazole, letermovir: Possibly increased plasma concentrations of atorvastatin and adverse reactions such as myopathy and rhabdomyolysis

digoxin: Increased digoxin level and increased risk of toxicity

efavirenz, rifampin, other CYP450 3A4 inducers: Possible decreased plasma atorvastatin level and effectiveness

oral contraceptives such as ethinyl estradiol and norethindrone: Increased hormone levels

FOODS

grapefruit juice: Increased blood atorvastatin level

Adverse Reactions

CNS: Abnormal dreams, amnesia, asthenia, cognitive impairment, confusion, depression, dizziness, emotional lability, facial paralysis, fatigue, fever, forgetfulness, headache, hyperkinesia, insomnia, lack of coordination, malaise, memory impairment or loss, nightmare, paresthesia, peripheral neuropathy, somnolence, syncope, weakness

CV: **Arrhythmias**, orthostatic hypotension, palpitations, phlebitis, vasodilation

EENT: Amblyopia, altered refraction, blurred vision, dry eyes or mouth, epistaxis, eye hemorrhage, gingival hemorrhage, glaucoma, glossitis, hearing loss, lip swelling, loss of taste, nasopharyngitis, ocular myasthenia, pharyngitis, pharyngolaryngeal pain, sinusitis, stomatitis, taste perversion, tinnitus

ENDO: Hyperglycemia, **hypoglycemia**

GI: Abdominal or biliary discomfort or pain, anorexia, cholestasis, colitis, constipation, diarrhea, duodenal or stomach ulcers, dyspepsia, dysphagia, elevated liver

enzymes, eructation, esophagitis, flatulence, gastroenteritis, **hepatic dysfunction or failure** (fatal and nonfatal), **hepatitis,** increased appetite, indigestion, jaundice, melena, nausea, **pancreatitis, rectal hemorrhage,** vomiting
GU: Abnormal ejaculation; cystitis; decreased libido; dysuria; epididymitis; hematuria; impotence; nephritis; nocturia; renal calculi; urinary frequency, incontinence, or urgency; urine retention; UTI; vaginal hemorrhage; WBCs in urine
HEME: Anemia, **thrombocytopenia**
MS: Arthralgia; back, extremity, neck, or other musculoskeletal pain; bursitis; elevated creatine kinase; gout; **immune-mediated necrotizing myopathy**; joint swelling; leg cramps; muscle spasm; myalgia; myasthenia gravis; myopathy; myositis; neck rigidity; **rhabdomyolysis**; tendon contracture or rupture; tenosynovitis; torticollis
RESP: Dyspnea, interstitial lung disease, pneumonia
SKIN: Acne, alopecia, contact dermatitis, diaphoresis, dry skin, ecchymosis, eczema, **erythema multiforme**, petechiae, photosensitivity, pruritus, rash, seborrhea, **Stevens-Johnson syndrome, toxic epidermal necrolysis**, ulceration, urticaria
Other: Anaphylaxis, angioedema, elevated alkaline phosphatase level, flu-like symptoms, infection, lymphadenopathy, weight gain

Childbearing Considerations

PREGNANCY

- Drug may cause fetal harm.
- Drug is not recommended for use during pregnancy.

LACTATION

- It is not known if drug is present in breast milk.
- Drug is not recommended for use during breastfeeding because of potential for serious adverse reactions in breastfed infant.

REPRODUCTION

- Females of childbearing age should use effective contraception during drug therapy.

Nursing Considerations

- Know that atorvastatin should not be used in patients taking cyclosporine, gemfibrozil, telaprevir, or tipranavir plus ritonavir because of high risk for rhabdomyolysis with acute renal failure.

! **WARNING** Be aware that patients who do not have coronary artery disease but had a stroke or TIA within 6 months preceding atorvastatin therapy in which the 80 mg dosage was prescribed have an increased risk for hemorrhagic stroke.

- Use atorvastatin with extreme caution in patients who consume substantial quantities of alcohol or have a history of liver disease because atorvastatin use increases risk of liver dysfunction.
- Expect liver function tests to be performed before atorvastatin therapy starts and then thereafter as clinically necessary. If clinical symptoms such as hyperbilirubinemia and jaundice occur, notify prescriber and expect atorvastatin therapy to be discontinued until cause of liver dysfunction has been identified. If no cause can be found, expect drug to be discontinued permanently.

! **WARNING** Monitor patient for hypersensitivity reactions that could become life-threatening such as anaphylaxis and angioedema. If present, withhold drug, notify prescriber, and provide supportive care, as needed and ordered.

! **WARNING** Notify prescriber immediately and expect to withhold atorvastatin therapy if patient develops an acute condition suggestive of a myopathy (unexplained muscle pain, tenderness or weakness, especially if accompanied by elevated CPK level, fever, or malaise) or has a risk factor predisposing to the development of renal failure secondary to rhabdomyolysis, such as an acute severe infection; hypotension; major surgery; severe electrolyte, endocrine, or metabolic disorder; or uncontrolled seizures.

- Monitor patients who are 65 or older or patients with renal impairment because these are risk factors for atorvastatin-induced myopathy and rhabdomyolysis.
- Expect to measure lipid levels as early as 4 weeks after therapy starts, to adjust dosage as directed, and to repeat periodically until lipid levels are within desired range.
- Monitor diabetic patient's blood glucose levels because atorvastatin therapy can affect blood glucose control.

PATIENT TEACHING

- Emphasize that atorvastatin is an adjunct to—not a substitute for—a low-cholesterol diet.
- Instruct patient how to take type of atorvastatin prescribed and what to do if a dose is missed.
- Reinforce the benefits of therapy and urge patient to comply.

! **WARNING** Alert patient drug may cause an allergic reaction. Instruct patient to notify prescriber if an allergic reaction occurs and to seek immediate medical care if the reaction is severe.

! **WARNING** Advise patient to notify prescriber immediately if he develops unexplained muscle pain, tenderness, or weakness, especially if accompanied by fatigue or fever. Also instruct patient to notify prescriber of any persistent, severe, or unusual signs and symptoms because atorvastatin may cause serious adverse reactions.

- Instruct patient to consult prescriber before taking over-the-counter niacin because of increased risk of rhabdomyolysis
- Warn patient to limit alcohol intake during atorvastatin therapy.
- Advise patient with diabetes to monitor blood glucose levels closely.
- Inform females of childbearing age to use effective contraception while taking atorvastatin because atorvastatin is contraindicated in pregnancy. Tell her to notify prescriber immediately if pregnancy occurs, as drug will have to be discontinued.
- Advise mothers that breastfeeding is not recommended during atorvastatin therapy.

atovaquone

Mepron

Class and Category

Pharmacologic class: Ubiquinone analogue
Therapeutic class: Antiprotozoal

Indications and Dosages

∗ *To prevent* Pneumocystis jiroveci *pneumonia in patients who can't tolerate trimethoprim-sulfamethoxazole*

ORAL SUSPENSION

Adults and adolescents. 1,500 mg (10 ml) once daily.

∗ *To treat mild to moderate* P. jiroveci *pneumonia in patients who can't tolerate trimethoprim-sulfamethoxazole*

ORAL SUSPENSION

Adults and adolescents. 750 mg (5 ml) twice daily for 21 days. *Maximum:* 1,500 mg/day.

Drug Administration

P.O.

- Administer with meals to enhance absorption.
- Shake bottle gently before opening to measure dose. Use a calibrated device to measure dosage.
- If administering drug from a foil pouch, open pouch by removing tab at perforation and tear at notch. Administer entire contents from pouch directly into the patient's mouth, or it can be poured into a dosing spoon or cup prior to administration. Expect to use the entire contents of 2 pouches for a 10-ml dose.

Route	Onset	Peak	Duration
P.O.	Unknown	Unknown	Unknown

Half-life: 2–4 days

Mechanism of Action

May destroy *P. jiroveci* organisms by inhibiting the enzymes needed to synthesize nucleic acid and adenosine triphosphate.

Contraindications

Hypersensitivity to atovaquone or its components

Interactions

DRUGS

indinavir: Possible loss of efficacy of indinavir
metoclopramide, rifabutin, rifampin, tetracycline: Possibly decreased blood atovaquone level

Adverse Reactions

CNS: Fever, headache, insomnia
EENT: Rhinitis, **throat tightness**, vortex keratopathy
GI: Abdominal pain, diarrhea, elevated liver enzymes, **hepatic failure**, **hepatitis**, nausea, **pancreatitis**, vomiting
GU: **Acute renal dysfunction**
HEME: Anemia, **thrombocytopenia**
RESP: **Bronchospasm**, cough, dyspnea

SKIN: Desquamation, **erythema multiforme**, rash, **Stevens-Johnson syndrome**, urticaria
Other: **Angioedema**, **hypersensitivity reactions**, **methemoglobinemia**

Childbearing Considerations

PREGNANCY

- It is not known if drug can cause fetal harm.
- Use with caution only if benefit to mother outweighs potential risk to fetus.

LACTATION

- It is not known if drug is present in breast milk.
- Centers for Disease Control and Prevention recommend mothers infected with HIV-1 not breastfeed their infant to avoid risking postnatal transmission of HIV-1.

Nursing Considerations

- Use atovaquone cautiously in patient with severe hepatic impairment because, although rare, serious adverse reactions affecting liver function may occur.

> ! **WARNING** Monitor patient for hypersensitivity reactions that could become life-threatening such as angioedema. If present, notify prescriber, withhold drug, and provide supportive care, as needed and ordered.

- Monitor patient for serious adverse reactions because drug can adversely affect many body systems. Notify prescriber if patient experiences persistent, severe, or unusual adverse effects.
- Monitor blood test results because atovaquone may decrease hemoglobin levels, neutrophil count, and serum sodium; and may increase ALT, AST, alkaline phosphatase, and serum amylase levels.

PATIENT TEACHING

- Instruct patient how to take oral suspension form of the drug and what to do if a dose is missed.
- Tell patient to notify prescriber if his condition does not improve in a few days.

> ! **WARNING** Alert patient the drug may cause an allergic reaction. Tell him to notify prescriber if he develops signs of an allergic reaction, such as fever or rash and to seek immediate medical care if reaction become severe.

- Advise patient to notify prescriber if persistent, severe, or unusual adverse reactions occur while taking atovaquone.
- Inform mothers with HIV that breastfeeding is not recommended during drug therapy.

atropine

AtroPen

atropine sulfate

Class and Category

Pharmacologic class: Anticholinergic
Therapeutic class: Antiarrhythmic, antimuscarinic

Indications and Dosages

✶ *To treat bradyasystolic cardiac arrest*

I.V. INJECTION (ATROPINE SULFATE)

Adults. 1 mg, repeated every 3 to 5 min, as needed. *Maximum*: 3 mg total dose.

✶ *To provide temporary blockade of severe or life-threatening muscarinic anticholinesterase effects from muscarinic mushroom or organophosphorus poisoning*

I.V. INJECTION (ATROPINE SULFATE)

Adults. 2 to 3 mg, repeated every 20 to 30 min, as needed, until signs of poisoning are significantly lessened, or signs of atropine toxicity occur.

✶ *To treat exposure to chemical nerve agent or insecticide*

I.M. INJECTION (ATROPINE)

Adults and children weighing over 41 kg (90 lb) with 2 or more mild symptoms. 2 mg. If severe symptoms develop at any time after injection, 2 more 2-mg injections given in rapid succession.
Adults and children weighing over 41 kg (90 lb) who are unconscious or have other severe symptoms. 2 mg given immediately 3 times in rapid succession.
Children weighing 18 to 41 kg (40 to 90 lb) with 2 or more mild symptoms. 1 mg. If severe symptoms develop at any time after injection, 2 more 1-mg injections given in rapid succession.
Children weighing 18 to 41 kg (40 to 90 lb) who are unconscious or exhibit any other

severe symptoms. 1 mg given immediately 3 times in rapid succession.
Children weighing 7 to 18 kg (15 to 40 lb) with 2 or more mild symptoms. 0.5 mg. If severe symptoms develop at any time after injection, 2 more 0.5-mg injections given in rapid succession.
Children weighing 7 to 18 kg (15 to 40 lb) who are unconscious or exhibit any other severe symptoms. 0.5 mg given immediately 3 times in rapid succession.
Children weighing less than 7 kg (15 lb) with 2 or more mild symptoms. 0.25 mg. If severe symptoms develop at any time after injection, 2 or more 0.25-mg injections given in rapid succession.
Children weighing less than 7 kg (15 lb) who are unconscious or exhibit any other severe symptoms. 0.25 mg given immediately 3 times in rapid succession.

± **DOSAGE ADJUSTMENT** For patients experiencing mild symptoms to either a chemical nerve agent or insecticide, no additional doses are recommended if no severe symptoms develop after 10 to 15 min.

Drug Administration

I.V.

- Be aware atropine sulfate is available as a 1 mg/10ml single-dose syringe.
- Administer into a large vein or I.V. tubing over 1 to 2 min.
- *Incompatibilities:* None listed by manufacturer

I.M.

- AtroPen has no absolute contraindications when used to treat life-threatening insecticide exposure or nerve gas. However, the 2-mg atropine autoinjector should not be used in children weighing 41 kg (90 lb) or less for any indication, as its effectiveness and safety have not been established.
- Can be given through clothing.
- Administer by firmly jabbing tip into midlateral thigh at a 90-degree angle. If patient is thin, pinch the skin before injecting into the site.
- Hold the AtroPen firmly in place for at least 10 sec to allow the injection to finish. After removing, massage the injection site for several seconds.
- After injection, make sure needle is visible on autoinjector. If not, repeat administration, jabbing more firmly than first time.

Route	Onset	Peak	Duration
I.V.	Immediate	2–4 min	Brief
I.M.	Rapid	3 min	Brief

Half-life: 2–10 hr, and age-dependent

Mechanism of Action

Inhibits acetylcholine's muscarinic action at the neuroeffector junctions of smooth muscles, cardiac muscles, exocrine glands, SA and AV nodes, and the urinary bladder. In small doses, atropine inhibits salivary and bronchial secretions and diaphoresis. In moderate doses, it increases impulse conduction through the AV node and increases heart rate. In large doses, it decreases GI and urinary tract motility and gastric acid secretion.

Contraindications

Hypersensitivity to atropine or other belladonna alkaloids or their components

Interactions

DRUGS

amantadine, anticholinergics, antidyskinetics, glutethimide, meperidine, muscle relaxants, phenothiazines, tricyclic antidepressants and other drugs with anticholinergic properties, including antiarrhythmics (disopyramide, procainamide, quinidine), antihistamines, buclizine: Increased atropine effects
barbiturates: Potentiated effects of barbiturates
ketoconazole: Decreased ketoconazole absorption
levodopa: Decreased plasma levodopa concentration and effectiveness
opioid analgesics: Increased risk of ileus, severe constipation, and urine retention
potassium chloride, especially wax-matrix forms: Possibly GI ulcers
pralidoxime: May potentiate the effect of atropine causing atropinization (dryness of mouth and nose, flushing, mydriasis, and tachycardia)
urinary alkalizers (calcium or magnesium antacids, carbonic anhydrase inhibitors, citrates, sodium bicarbonate): Delayed excretion, increased risk of adverse atropine effects

Adverse Reactions

CNS: Agitation, amnesia, anxiety, ataxia, Babinski's or Chaddock's reflex, behavioral

changes, CNS stimulation (at high doses), **coma**, confusion, decreased concentration, decreased tendon reflexes, delirium, dizziness, drowsiness, EEG abnormalities, excessive thirst, fatigue, fever, hallucinations, headache, **hyperpyrexia**, hyperreflexia, insomnia, lethargy, mania, mental disorders, nervousness, paranoia, restlessness, **seizures**, sensation of intoxication, somnolence, stupor, syncope, vertigo, weakness
CV: **Arrhythmias**, **bradycardia (at low doses)**, **cardiac dilation**, chest pain, hypertension, **hypotension**, **left ventricular failure**, **MI**, palpitations, tachycardia (at high doses), **weak or impalpable peripheral pulses**
EENT: Acute angle-closure glaucoma, altered taste, blepharitis, blindness, blurred vision, conjunctivitis, cyclophoria, cycloplegia, decreased visual acuity or accommodation, dry eyes or conjunctiva, dry mucous membranes, dry mouth, eye irritation, eyelid crusting, heterophoria, increased intraocular pressure, keratoconjunctivitis, lacrimation, laryngitis, **laryngospasm**, mydriasis, nasal congestion, oral lesions, photophobia, pupils poorly reactive to light, strabismus, tongue chewing
ENDO: Hyperglycemia, **hypoglycemia**
GI: Abdominal distention and pain, bloating, constipation, decreased bowel sounds or food absorption, delayed gastric emptying, dysphagia, heartburn, ileus, nausea, vomiting
GU: Bladder distention, difficulty urinating, elevated BUN, enuresis, impotence, loss of libido, polydipsia, urinary hesitancy, urinary urgency, urine retention
HEME: Anemia, elevated erythrocytes and hemoglobin, leukocytosis
MS: Dysarthria, hypertonia, muscle twitching
RESP: **Bradypnea**, **exacerbation of chronic lung disease**, dyspnea, **inspiratory stridor**, **pulmonary edema**, **respiratory failure**, **shallow breathing**, **subcostal recession**, tachypnea
SKIN: Cold skin, decreased or excessive sweating, dermatitis, **exfoliative dermatitis**, flushing, rash, urticaria
Other: **Anaphylaxis**, dehydration, **hypokalemia**, **hyponatremia**, injection-site pain, sensations of warmth

Childbearing Considerations

PREGNANCY

- It is not known if drug can cause fetal harm, although it does cross the placental barrier.
- Use with caution only if benefit to mother outweighs potential risk to fetus.

LACTATION

- Drug is present in breast milk.
- Mothers should check with prescriber before breastfeeding.

Nursing Considerations

- Be aware that high-dose atropine sulfate should not be used in patients with ulcerative colitis because of risk of toxic megacolon or in patients with hiatal hernia and reflux esophagitis because of risk of esophagitis.
- Use caution when atropine is given to patients with known cardiac conduction problems or cardiovascular disease because of its effect on the heart. Caution should also be used when atropine is given to patients with acute glaucoma, partial pyloric stenosis, or significant bladder outflow obstruction.
- Know that for patient prescribed atropine for insecticide exposure or suspected nerve gas, dosage is determined by severity of symptoms. Mild symptoms include acute onset of blurred vision, bradycardia, chest tightness, difficulty breathing, excessive unexplained teary eyes or runny nose, increased salivation, miosis, muscle twitching, nausea, stomach cramps, tachycardia, unexplained coughing or wheezing, and vomiting. Severe symptoms include confusion or other strange behavior, extreme secretions from airway or lungs, involuntary defecation and urination, seizures, severe difficulty breathing, severe muscle twitching and general weakness, tremors, and unconsciousness.

! **WARNING** Monitor patient closely for hypersensitivity reactions, including anaphylaxis, after drug is given. If present, notify prescriber and provide supportive care, as needed and ordered.

! **WARNING** Assess for symptoms of toxic doses of atropine, such as agitation, confusion, drowsiness, and excitement, which are likely to affect elderly patients even with low doses. If symptoms occur, take safety precautions to prevent injury.

- Monitor patients with chronic lung disease because atropine may cause thickening of bronchial secretions and formation of dangerous viscid plugs.
- Monitor elderly patients receiving atropine closely because they are more susceptible to the effects of the drug.
- Assess bladder and bowel elimination. Notify prescriber of constipation, diarrhea, urinary hesitancy, or urine retention.

PATIENT TEACHING

- Teach patient prescribed an AtroPen when and how to self-administer the drug. Remind patient that if the AtroPen is used, this is only an initial emergency treatment, and they still need to seek additional emergency care.

! **WARNING** Alert patient that atropine may cause an allergic reaction or other serious adverse reactions. If an allergic reaction is present or patient experiences persistent, severe, or unusual adverse reactions, patient should notify prescriber promptly and seek immediate medical care if adverse reactions are severe.

- Advise patient to notify prescriber if he has constipation, difficulty urinating, or persistent or severe diarrhea.
- Encourage patient with lung disease to maintain adequate hydration in order to keep secretions from becoming thick.
- Inform patient that atropine may inhibit sweating. Advise patient to avoid excessive exercise or heat exposure, which can lead to heat injury.

azathioprine

Azasan, Imuran

azathioprine sodium

Imuran I.V.

Class and Category

Pharmacologic class: Purine antagonist
Therapeutic class: Immunosuppressant, antirheumatic

Indications and Dosages

✱ *As adjunct to prevent kidney rejection after homotransplantation*

TABLETS (AZASAN, IMURAN)

Adults and children. *Initial:* 3 to 5 mg/kg daily as a single dose on, or 1 to 3 days before, day of transplantation then decreased according to patient's response and tolerance to 1 to 3 mg/kg daily following surgery. *Maintenance:* 1 to 3 mg/kg daily.

I.V. INFUSION (IMURAN I.V.)

Adults unable to tolerate oral dosage. *Initial:* 3 to 5 mg/kg as a single dose on, or 1 to 3 days daily before, day of transplantation, then decreased according to patient's response and tolerance to 1 to 3 mg/kg daily following surgery until P.O. dose is tolerated (usually 1 to 4 days).

± **DOSAGE ADJUSTMENT** For patients with oliguria (as from tubular necrosis) after transplantation and in patients with heterozygous deficiency of either nucleotide diphosphatase (NUDT15) or thiopurine *S*-methyl transferase (TPMT), dosage reduced with reduction being greater if both heterozygous deficiency of NUDT15 and TPMT are present.

✱ *To reduce signs and symptoms of acute rheumatoid arthritis*

TABLETS (AZASAN, IMURAN)

Adults. *Initial:* 1 mg/kg (50 to 100 mg) daily as a single dose or on a twice-daily schedule for 6 to 8 wk. *Maintenance:* If initial therapy does not produce therapeutic effects or no serious adverse effects occur after 6 to 8 wk, dosage increased every 4 wk in 0.5-mg/kg increments up to 2.5 mg/kg/daily.

± **DOSAGE ADJUSTMENT** For patients with heterozygous deficiency of either nucleotide diphosphatase (NUDT15) or thiopurine *S*-methyl transferase (TPMT), dosage reduced with reduction being greater if both heterozygous deficiency of NUDT15 and TPMT are present. For patients who are relatively oliguric, especially patients with tubular necrosis in the immediate postcadaveric transplant period, lower doses are usually given.

Drug Administration

- Expect to use lowest possible maintenance dosage for rheumatoid arthritis, reducing it gradually in 0.5-mg/kg (about 25-mg) increments at 4-wk intervals, as ordered.
- Follow procedure for proper handling and disposal of this immunosuppressive antimetabolite drug.

P.O.

- Give with meals if GI upset occurs.
- Know that drug can be stopped abruptly, but its effects may persist for several days.

I.V.

- Use restricted to patients who can't tolerate oral form of drug.
- Reconstitute by adding 10 ml of Sterile Water for Injection and swirl until solution is clear.
- Further dilute in 0.9% Sodium Chloride or 5% Dextrose in Water, with final volume dependent on infusion time. Use within 24 hr after reconstitution.
- Infuse over 30 to 60 min (most common) but know that it may be infused as short as 5 min and as long as 8 hr for the daily dose.
- Drug switched to oral form as soon as patient can tolerate it, which is usually in 1 to 4 days.
- *Incompatibilities:* None reported by manufacturer

Route	Onset	Peak	Duration
P.O./I.V.	Unknown	1–2 hr	Unknown

Half-life: 5 hr

Mechanism of Action

May prevent proliferation and differentiation of activated B and T cells by interfering with purine (protein) and nucleic acid (DNA and RNA) synthesis.

Contraindications

Hypersensitivity to azathioprine or its components, pregnancy (treatment of rheumatoid arthritis)

Interactions

DRUGS

ACE inhibitors and drugs that affect bone marrow and cell development in bone marrow such as trimethoprim-sulfamethoxazole: Possibly severe leukopenia
cyclosporine: Possibly decreased plasma cyclosporine level
ribavirin: Possibly induced severe pancytopenia and possibly increased risk of azathioprine-related myelotoxicity
xanthine oxidase inhibitors such as allopurinol, febuxostat: Increased plasma azathioprine levels possibly leading to azathioprine toxicity
warfarin: Possibly inhibited anticoagulant effect of warfarin

Adverse Reactions

CNS: Fever, malaise, **progressive multifocal leukoencephalopathy**
GI: Abdominal pain, diarrhea, **hepatotoxicity**, nausea, **pancreatitis**, steatorrhea, vomiting
HEME: Immunosuppression (severe), **leukopenia**, macrocytic anemia, **pancytopenia**, **thrombocytopenia**
MS: Arthralgia, myalgia
SKIN: Acute febrile neutrophilic dermatosis (Sweet's syndrome), alopecia, **cancer**, rash
RESP: **Interstitial pneumonitis**
Other: Infection, **lymphomas and other neoplasms**, negative nitrogen balance

Childbearing Considerations

PREGNANCY

- Drug can cause fetal harm.
- Drug is contraindicated for use during pregnancy for treatment of rheumatoid arthritis.
- Use should be avoided to treat renal homotransplantation during pregnancy, if possible.

LACTATION

- Drug is present in breast milk.
- A decision should be made to discontinue breastfeeding or the drug because of the potential risk for tumor formation in the infant.

REPRODUCTION

- Females of childbearing age should be advised to avoid becoming pregnant during drug therapy.

Nursing Considerations

- Obtain results of baseline laboratory tests, including platelet, RBC, and WBC counts. Expect to monitor results once a week during first month of therapy, twice a month during second and third months, and once a month or more thereafter.

! **WARNING** Expect to reduce dosage or discontinue azathioprine if WBC count decreases rapidly or remains significantly and consistently low.

! **WARNING** Be aware that patients with low or absent NUDT15 or TPMT levels are at risk for developing severe and life-threatening myelosuppression. Expect patient to be tested for these disorders if significant myelosuppression occurs. If confirmed, expect dosage to be decreased in the presence of heterozygous deficiency and drug discontinued in the presence of homozygous deficiency.

! **WARNING** Monitor patient closely for abnormal signs and symptoms suggestive of lymphomas, especially in adolescent and young adult males who have a history of inflammatory bowel disease, in patients who have received a renal transplant, or in patients with rheumatoid arthritis because the majority of patients who develop a lymphoma fall into one of these categories.

! **WARNING** Be aware that azathioprine therapy increases risk of bacterial, fungal, protozoal, and viral infections. Watch for evidence of infection such as fever, chills, mouth sores, or sore throat. Expect to administer aggressive antibiotic, antiviral, or other drug therapy, and reduce azathioprine dosage. Minimize the risk of infection. If patient has severe leukopenia, take precautions, such as limiting visitors and placing him in a private room.

- Know that hematologic reactions typically are dose-related and may occur late in therapy, especially in patients with transplant rejection. Act quickly if patient develops thrombocytopenia, by taking bleeding precautions, such as avoiding I.M. injections and venipunctures, applying ice to areas of trauma, and checking I.V. infusion sites every 2 hours for bleeding.
- Monitor patient's prothrombin time if he also receives an oral anticoagulant.
- Monitor liver enzymes, as ordered, for early signs of hepatotoxicity.
- Know that rheumatoid arthritis requires at least 12 weeks of azathioprine therapy. During this time, continue other pain-relief measures, such as physical therapy, rest, and other drugs, such as corticosteroids and salicylates, as ordered.

PATIENT TEACHING

- Instruct patient how to take oral azathioprine.
- Encourage patient to comply with frequent laboratory appointments.

! **WARNING** Teach patient to recognize and report signs of infection such as fever and sore throat. Review infection control measures to take to minimize infection risk. If infection occurs, tell patient to notify prescriber at once and seek immediate medical care if infection is severe.

! **WARNING** Inform patient that drug may cause cancer. Tell patient to seek medical attention for any abnormal signs and symptoms that might be suggestive of a malignancy. Also stress importance of alerting prescriber of any persistent, severe, or unusual adverse reactions.

- Encourage patient who develops significant myelosuppression to be tested for possible causes.
- Teach patient how to reduce the risk of bleeding and falling.
- Inform females of childbearing age to use effective contraception during drug therapy.
- Advise mothers not to breastfeed.

azelastine hydrochloride

Astelin, Astepro

Class and Category

Pharmacologic class: H_1-receptor antagonist
Therapeutic class: Antihistamine

Indications and Dosages

✶ *To treat symptoms of seasonal allergic rhinitis*

NASAL SPRAY (ASTELIN)

Adults and children ages 12 and older. 1 or 2 sprays in each nostril twice daily.
Children ages 5 to 11. 1 spray in each nostril twice daily.

NASAL SPRAY (ASTEPRO)

Adults and children ages 12 and older. 1 or 2 sprays (0.1% or 0.15%) in each nostril twice daily. Alternatively, 0.15% solution may be administered as 2 sprays in each nostril once daily.

Children ages 6 to 11. 1 spray (0.1% or 0.15%) in each nostril twice daily.

Children ages 2 to 5. 1 spray (0.1%) in each nostril twice daily.

∗ *To treat symptoms of perennial allergic rhinitis*

NASAL SPRAY (ASTEPRO)

Adults and children ages 12 and older. 2 sprays (0.15%) in each nostril twice daily.

Children ages 6 to 11. 1 spray (0.1% or 0.15%) in each nostril twice daily.

Children ages 6 mo to 5 yr. 1 spray (0.1%) in each nostril twice daily.

∗ *To treat symptoms of vasomotor rhinitis*

NASAL SPRAY (ASTELIN)

Adults and adolescents ages 12 and older. 2 sprays in each nostril twice daily.

Drug Administration

INTRANASAL

- Prime pump before administering for first time by placing thumb on base and the index and middle fingers on shoulder area of bottle and then pressing thumb firmly and quickly against bottle 4 times (Astelin) or 6 times (Astepro), or until fine mist appears.
- If spray hasn't been used in more than 3 days, the container will have to be reprimed by pumping 2 sprays or until fine mist appears.
- Have patient clear nostrils gently, if needed, before using spray. Then have patient tilt head downward. Have patient place spray tip about ¼ to ½ inch into 1 nostril. Then have patient aim spray tip toward back of nose, closing other nostril. Patient should then press pump 1 time and sniff gently at the same time. Procedure repeated in other nostril if a second spray is prescribed.
- Wipe tip of spray container with a clean tissue after each use.
- Store bottle upright and keep it tightly closed.

Route	Onset	Peak	Duration
Intranasal	30 min	2–3 hr	12 hr

Half-life: 22–25 hr

Mechanism of Action

Binds nonselectively to central and peripheral H_1 receptors, preventing histamine from reaching its site of action, which reduces or prevents most of histamine's physiologic effects. By blocking histamine at its site of action, azelastine inhibits GI, respiratory, and vascular smooth muscle contraction; decreases capillary permeability, which reduces flares, itching, and wheals; and decreases lacrimal and salivary gland secretions.

Contraindications

Hypersensitivity to azelastine or its components

Interactions

DRUGS

cimetidine: Possibly increased blood azelastine level

CNS depressants: Possibly increased sedative effects and reduced mental alertness

ACTIVITIES

alcohol use: Possibly increased sedative effects and reduced mental alertness

Adverse Reactions

CNS: Dizziness, fatigue, headache, somnolence

CV: **Atrial fibrillation**, palpitations

EENT: Bitter taste, dry mouth, epistaxis, nasal burning, paroxysmal sneezing, pharyngitis, rhinitis

GI: Nausea

Other: Weight gain

Childbearing Considerations

PREGNANCY

- It is not known if drug can cause fetal harm.
- Use with caution only if benefit to mother outweighs potential risk to fetus.

LACTATION

- It is not known if drug is present in breast milk.
- Mothers should check with prescriber before breastfeeding.
- Breastfed infants should be monitored for signs of milk rejection.

Nursing Considerations

- Monitor patient for an irregular, fast heartbeat because drug can cause palpitations and atrial fibrillation.
- Assess for changes in alertness, and take safety precautions, as needed.

PATIENT TEACHING

- Teach patient how to use the product of azelastine nasal spray prescribed.
- Caution patient not to use alcohol while taking azelastine.

! **WARNING** Emphasize that patient must consult prescriber before taking any over-the-counter drugs, such as a cold remedy or cough syrup because of the risk of extreme CNS depression.

- Tell patient to alert prescriber if palpations occur or pulse becomes irregular.
- Inform patient that decreased alertness may occur. Advise him to avoid hazardous activities or those that require alertness, such as driving or operating machinery, until drug's effects are known.
- Inform breastfeeding mothers to monitor infant for milk rejection because drug may cause a bitter taste in breast milk.

azithromycin

Zithromax

azithromycin dihydrate

Zmax

Class and Category

Pharmacologic class: Macrolide
Therapeutic class: Antibiotic

Indications and Dosages

* *To treat mild community-acquired pneumonia caused by* Chlamydophila pneumoniae, Haemophilus influenzae, Mycoplasma pneumoniae, *or* Streptococcus pneumoniae; *pharyngitis and tonsillitis caused by* Streptococcus pyogenes; *and uncomplicated skin and soft-tissue infections caused by* Staphylococcus aureus, S. pyogenes, *or* Streptococcus agalactiae

ORAL SUSPENSION, TABLETS (ZITHROMAX)

Adults. 500 mg as a single dose on day 1, followed by 250 mg once daily on days 2 through 5.

* *To treat pediatric community-acquired pneumonia caused by* C. pneumoniae, H. influenzae, M. pneumoniae, *or* S. pneumoniae

ORAL SUSPENSION (ZITHROMAX)

Children ages 6 and older. 10 mg/kg as a single dose (not to exceed 500 mg daily) on day 1, followed by 5 mg/kg (not to exceed 250 mg daily) once daily on days 2 through 5.

* *To treat pediatric otitis media caused by* H. influenzae, Moraxella catarrhalis, *or* S. pneumoniae

ORAL SUSPENSION (ZITHROMAX)

Children ages 6 mo and older. 30 mg/kg as a single dose. Alternatively, 10 mg/kg once daily for 3 days, or 10 mg/kg as a single dose on day 1 followed by 5 mg/kg once daily on days 2 through 5.

* *To treat pediatric pharyngitis or tonsillitis caused by* S. pyogenes

ORAL SUSPENSION (ZITHROMAX)

Children ages 2 and older. 12 mg/kg once daily for 5 days.

* *To treat community-acquired pneumonia caused by* C. pneumoniae, H. influenzae, Legionella pneumophila, M. catarrhalis, M. pneumoniae, S. aureus, *or* S. pneumoniae *and requiring initial I.V. therapy*

I.V. INFUSION, ORAL SUSPENSION, TABLETS (ZITHROMAX)

Adults. 500 mg I.V. as a single dose daily for at least 2 days, followed by 500 mg P.O. as a single dose daily until patient completes 7 to 10 days of therapy.

* *To treat community-acquired pneumonia caused by* C. pneumoniae, H. influenzae, M. pneumoniae, *or* S. pneumoniae

E.R. ORAL SUSPENSION (ZMAX)

Adults and children weighing 34 kg (75 lb) or more. 2 g as a single dose.
Children ages 6 mo and older weighing less than 34 kg (75 lb). 60 mg/kg as a single dose.

* *To treat acute bacterial sinusitis caused by* H. influenzae, M. catarrhalis, *or* S. pneumoniae

ORAL SUSPENSION, TABLETS (ZITHROMAX)

Adults. 500 mg once daily for 3 days.
Children ages 6 mo and older. 10 mg/kg once daily for 3 days.

E.R. ORAL SUSPENSION (ZMAX)

Adults and children weighing 34 kg (75 lb) or more. 2 g as a single dose.
Children ages 6 mo and older weighing less than 34 kg (75 lb). 60 mg/kg as a single dose.

∗ *To treat acute bacterial exacerbations of COPD, including chronic bronchitis caused by* H. influenzae, M. catarrhalis, *or* S.pneumoniae

ORAL SUSPENSION, TABLETS (ZITHROMAX)

Adults. 500 mg once daily for 3 days, or 500 mg as a single dose on day 1, followed by 250 mg once daily on days 2 through 5.

∗ *To treat nongonococcal cervicitis and urethritis caused by* Chlamydia trachomatis

ORAL SUSPENSION, TABLETS (ZITHROMAX)

Adults. 1 g as a one-time dose.

∗ *To treat cervicitis or urethritis caused by* Neisseria gonorrhoeae

ORAL SUSPENSION, TABLETS (ZITHROMAX)

Adults. 2 g as a one-time dose.

∗ *To prevent* Mycobacterium avium *complex (MAC) in patients with advanced HIV infection*

ORAL SUSPENSION, TABLETS (ZITHROMAX)

Adults. 1.2 g once weekly, as needed.

∗ *As adjunct to treat MAC in patients with advanced HIV infection*

ORAL SUSPENSION, TABLETS (ZITHROMAX)

Adults. 600 mg daily in combination with ethambutol 15 mg/kg daily.

∗ *To treat pelvic inflammatory disease caused by* C. trachomatis, N. gonorrhoeae, *or* Mycoplasma hominis *and requiring initial I.V. therapy*

I.V. INFUSION, ORAL SUSPENSION, TABLETS (ZITHROMAX)

Adults. 500 mg I.V. as a single dose daily for 1 to 2 days, followed by 250 mg P.O. as a single dose daily until patient completes 7 days of therapy.

Drug Administration

P.O.

- Administer Zmax on an empty stomach at least 1 hr before or 2 hr following a meal. Zithromax can be administered with or without food.
- Reconstitute Zmax oral suspension by adding 60 ml of water to the container. Shake well before administering. Do not refrigerate. Constituted suspension should be consumed within 12 hr. Any suspension remaining after dosing must be discarded.
- Reconstitute Zithromycin oral suspension as follows: add 9 ml of water to either 300-mg or 600-mg bottles, 12-ml to 900-mg bottle, and 15-ml to 1,200-mg bottle. Shake well after constituting and before each dose. Store at room temperature and use within 10 days. Discard any drug left in bottle after drug has been discontinued.
- For children weighing less than 34 kg (75 lb) and prescribed either type of oral suspension, use a calibrated dosing device to measure dose.

I.V.

- Reconstitute by adding 4.8 ml of Sterile Water for Injection to the 500-mg drug vial and shaking until all the drug is dissolved. Each ml of reconstituted solution contains 100 mg of azithromycin. Solution is stable for 24 hr when stored below 30°C (86°F).
- Use a standard (non-automated) 5-ml syringe to ensure that an accurate amount of 4.8 ml is withdrawn for reconstitution.
- Dilute further to provide a concentration range of 1–2 mg/ml by transferring 5 ml of the reconstituted solution into 0.9% Sodium Chloride Injection, 5% Dextrose in Water, or any of the other solutions recommended by the manufacturer. To achieve a final infusion solution concentration of 1 mg/ml, use 500 ml of diluting solution; to achieve 2 mg/ml, use 250 ml of diluting solution.
- Infuse a 2 mg/ml infusion over 1 hr and a 1 mg/ml infusion over 3 hr. Do not give as a bolus or as an intramuscular injection.
- Diluted drug may be stored at or below room temperature of 30°C (86°F) for 24 hr or for 7 days if refrigerated.
- *Incompatibilities:* Other intravenous additives or drugs

Route	Onset	Peak	Duration
P.O.	Unknown	2.5–4.5 hr	Unknown
I.V.	Unknown	1–2 hr	Unknown

Half-life: 2–3 days

Mechanism of Action

Binds to a ribosomal subunit of susceptible bacteria, blocking peptide translocation and inhibiting RNA-dependent protein synthesis. Drug concentrates in phagocytes, macrophages, and fibroblasts, which release it slowly and may help move it to infection sites.

Contraindications

History of cholestatic jaundice or hepatic dysfunction associated with prior use of azithromycin; hypersensitivity to azithromycin, erythromycin, ketolide antibiotics, other macrolide antibiotics, or their components

Interactions

DRUGS

antacids that contain aluminum or magnesium: Possibly decreased peak blood azithromycin level
nelfinavir: Possibly increased blood levels of these drugs
oral anticoagulants such as warfarin: Possibly potentiated effects of oral anticoagulants
other macrolides: Possible adverse effects

FOODS

any food: Altered absorption rate of azithromycin

Adverse Reactions

CNS: Aggressiveness, agitation, anxiety, asthenia, dizziness, fatigue, headache, hyperactivity, malaise, nervousness, paresthesia, **seizures**, somnolence, syncope, vertigo
CV: **Arrhythmias**, chest pain, edema, **hypotension**, palpitations, **prolonged QT interval**, **torsades de pointes**, **ventricular tachycardia**
EENT: Hearing loss, oral candidiasis, perversion or loss of taste or smell, tinnitus, tongue discoloration
ENDO: Hyperglycemia
GI: Abdominal pain, anorexia, cholestatic jaundice, ***Clostridioides difficile*–associated diarrhea**, constipation, diarrhea, dyspepsia, elevated liver enzymes, flatulence, **hepatic necrosis or failure**, **hepatitis**, nausea, **pancreatitis**, pyloric stenosis, **pseudomembranous colitis**, vomiting
GU: **Acute renal failure**, elevated BUN and serum creatinine levels, nephritis, vaginal candidiasis
HEME: **Leukopenia**, **neutropenia**, **thrombocytopenia**
MS: Arthralgia, elevated creatine kinase levels
SKIN: Acute generalized exanthematous pustulosis, **erythema multiforme**, photosensitivity, pruritus, rash, **Stevens-Johnson syndrome**, **toxic epidermal necrolysis**, urticaria
Other: **Anaphylaxis**, **angioedema**, **drug reaction with eosinophilia and systemic symptoms (DRESS)**, elevated serum phosphorus level, **hyperkalemia**, infusion-site reaction (such as pain and redness), new or worsening myasthenia syndrome, superinfection

Childbearing Considerations

PREGNANCY

- It is not known if drug can cause fetal harm.
- Use with caution only if benefit to mother outweighs potential risk to fetus.

LACTATION

- Drug is present in breast milk.
- Mothers should check with prescriber before breastfeeding.
- If breastfeeding occurs, mother should monitor breastfed infant for diarrhea, rash, or vomiting.

Nursing Considerations

! WARNING Be aware that azithromycin should not be used in patients with bradyarrhythmias, congenital long QT syndrome, history of torsades de pointes, known QT prolongation, or uncompensated heart failure; patients with ongoing proarrhythmic conditions such as significant bradycardia or uncorrected hypokalemia or hypomagnesemia; or patients receiving drugs known to prolong the QT interval such as class IA (procainamide, quinidine) or class III (amiodarone, dofetilide, sotalol) antiarrhythmic agents because of increased risk of life-threatening arrhythmias such as torsades de pointes.

! WARNING Know that azithromycin should not be used in patients who have undergone donor stem cell transplant for cancer of the blood or lymph nodes because of an increased risk for cancer relapse and possibly death.

- Obtain culture and sensitivity test results, if possible, before starting therapy.
- Use azithromycin cautiously in patients with hepatic dysfunction not associated with prior use of azithromycin (drug is metabolized in the liver) or renal dysfunction (effects are unknown in this group). Monitor patient's liver enzymes and renal function closely during azithromycin

therapy and expect drug to be discontinued if signficiant hepatic or renal dysfunction occurs.

! **WARNING** Be aware that azithromycin therapy has been linked to an increased risk for acute cardiovascular death, with the risk being greatest during the first 5 days of therapy. The risk can occur in patients with or without a history of preexisting cardiovascular disease.

! **WARNING** Monitor patient for hypersensitivity reactions that could become life-threatening such as anaphylaxis and angioedema. Notify prescriber if an allergic reaction occurs, withhold drug, and provide supportive care, as needed and ordered.

! **WARNING** Monitor elderly patients closely for arrhythmias because they are more susceptible to drug effects on the QT interval.

! **WARNING** Monitor bowel elimination for diarrhea; if needed, obtain stool culture to rule out pseudomembranous colitis caused by *Clostridium difficile*. It may be mild or become life-threatening. If it occurs, expect to stop azithromycin and give antibiotics effective with *C. difficile* as well as electrolytes, fluid, and protein, as needed and ordered.

- Assess patient for bacterial or fungal superinfection, which may occur with prolonged or repeated therapy. If it occurs, expect to give another antibiotic or antifungal.
- Be aware that laboratory abnormalities may occur during azithromycin therapy. If present, alert prescriber, as changes can be reversible.

PATIENT TEACHING

- Instruct patient how to take form of azithromycin therapy prescribed.
- Urge patient to consult prescriber before taking over-the-counter drugs, including antacids. If they're prescribed, tell patient to take azithromycin 1 hour before or 2 to 3 hours after taking antacids. Also, advise patient to inform all prescribers of azithromycin therapy.

! **WARNING** Tell patient to report signs and symptoms of allergic reaction (such as chest tightness, hives, itching, rash, and trouble breathing) immediately and, if severe, to seek immediate medical care.

! **WARNING** Inform patient that drug may cause serious heart rhythm changes. Stress importance of seeking immediate emergency help if chest discomfort, dizziness, or feeling faint occurs or heart feels like it's pounding, racing, or the heartbeat is irregular.

! **WARNING** Warn patient that abdominal pain and loose, watery stools may occur. If diarrhea persists or becomes severe, urge him to contact prescriber and replace fluids.

- Teach patient to watch for and immediately report signs of superinfection, such as white patches in the mouth.
- Tell breastfeeding mothers to monitor their babies for diarrhea, rash, or vomiting.

aztreonam

Azactam, Cayston

Class and Category

Pharmacologic class: Monobactam
Therapeutic class: Antibiotic

Indications and Dosages

✻ *To improve respiratory symptoms in cystic fibrosis patients with* Pseudomonas aeruginosa

INHALATION (CAYSTON)

Adults and children ages 7 and older. 75 mg (1 vial) 3 times daily with doses at least 4 hr apart for 28 days (followed by 28 days off therapy).

✻ *To treat infections of the female reproductive tract, including endometritis and pelvic cellulitis caused by* Enterobacter *species including* E. cloacae, Escherichia coli, Klebsiella pneumoniae, *or* Proteus miraabilis; *intra-abdominal infections caused by* Citrobacter *species including* C. freundii, Enterobacter *species including* E. cloacae, K. pneumoniae, Pseudomonas aeruginosa, *or* Serratia *species including* S. marcescens; *lower respiratory tract including bronchitis and penumonia caused by* Enterobacter *species* E. coli, Haemophilus influenzae, K. pneumoniae, P. aeruginosa, P. mirabilis, *or* S. marcescens; *skin or soft tissue, caused by* Citrobacter *species* Enterobacter *species,* E. coli, K. pneumoniae, P. aeruginosa, P. mirabilis, *or* S. marcescens *or urinary tract including complicated and uncomplicated caused by* Citrobacter *species,* E. cloacae, E. coli, K. oxytoca, K. pneumoniae, P. mirabilis, P. aeruginosa, *or* S. marcescens; *septicemia caused by* Enterobacter *species,* E. coli, K. pneumoniae, P. mirabilis, P. aeruginosa, *or* S. marcescens; *and surgical abscesses caused by susceptible strains of gram-negative bacteria*

I.V. INFUSION, I.V. INJECTION, I.M. INJECTION (AZACTAM)

Adults with a urinary tract infection. 500 mg or 1 g every 8 or 12 hr.

Adults with moderately severe systemic infections. 1 or 2 g given every 8 to 12 hr.

Adults with severe systemic or life-threatening infections or an infection due to *Pseudomonas aeruginosa*. 2 g every 6 or 8 hr. *Maximum:* 8 g daily.

I.V. INFUSION, I.V. INJECTION (AZACTAM)

Children ages 9 mo and older with mild to moderate infections. 30 mg/kg every 8 hr. *Maximum:* 120 mg/kg daily.

Children ages 9 mo and older with moderate to severe infections. 30 mg/kg every 6 to 8 hr up to 120 mg/kg daily. *Maximum:* 120 mg/kg/daily.

±**DOSAGE ADJUSTMENT** For adult patients with a creatinine clearance of 10 to 30 ml/min, initial dose is 1 to 2 g; then 50% of usual dose at usual interval. For adult patients with a creatinine clearance of less than 10 ml/min, initial dose is 500 mg, 1 g, or 2 g; then 25% of the usual dose every 6, 8, or 12 hours. For hemodialysis adult patients with serious or life-threatening infections, in addition to the maintenance doses, one-eighth of the initial dose given after each hemodialysis session.

Drug Administration

I.M.

- Reconstitute with at least 3 ml of 0.9% Sodium Chloride Injection, Bacteriostatic Sodium Chloride Injection, Sterile Water for Injection, or Sterile Bacteriostatic Water for Injection for each gram of aztreonam to be administered.
- Do not admix with any local anesthetic agent.
- Administer as a deep injection into a large muscle mass (such as the lateral part of the thigh or upper outer quadrant of the gluteus maximus).

I.V.

- For bolus injection, reconstitute by injecting 6 to 10 ml of Sterile Water for Injection into drug vial. Immediately shake vial vigorously to mix. After withdrawing prescribed dose, discard unused solution. Reconstituted solution will be colorless to light straw yellow but may turn light pink on standing at room temperature. This does not affect drug potency.
- Give I.V. bolus injection directly into I.V. tubing slowly over 3 to 5 min after flushing line with a compatible solution, if needed. Once administered, flush I.V. line again, if necessary.
- If drug is to be administered as an I.V. infusion, the 15-ml drug vial should first be reconstituted with at least 3 ml of Sterile Water for Injection for each gram of aztreonam to be administered. Immediately shake vial vigorously to mix. After withdrawing prescribed dose, discard unused solution. Reconstituted solution will be colorless to light straw yellow but may turn light pink on standing at room temperature. This does not affect drug potency. Further dilute drug with an I.V. solution such as 0.9% Sodium Chloride, 5% Dextrose in Water, Lactated Ringer's Injection, or any other solution recommended by manufacturer.
- Administer I.V. infusion over 20 to 60 min.
- Flush I.V. tubing with a solution such as 0.9% Sodium Chloride for Injection before and after administering I.V. infusion, if necessary.
- If drug solution is frozen, thaw it, but do not immerse drug in water baths or microwave irradiation to thaw it. After thawing is complete, invert the container to ensure a well-mixed solution. Administer only as an I.V. infusion.
- *Incompatibilities:* Cephradine, metronidazole, or nafcillin sodium; other admixtures except for ampicillin sodium, cefazolin sodium, clindamycin phosphate, cloxacillin sodium, gentamicin sulfate, tobramycin sulfate, and vancomycin hydrochloride

INHALATION

- Dilute each vial of inhalation solution with 1 ampule of the diluent that comes with drug. To do so, open the glass drug vial carefully, remove metal ring by pulling the tab, and remove the gray rubber stopper. Twist the tip off the diluent ampule and squeeze the liquid into the glass drug vial. Replace the rubber stopper, then gently swirl the vial until contents have been completely dissolved.
- Administer immediately, using only an Altera Nebulizer System. After placing the diluted drug into the handset of the nebulizer, turn the unit on. Then, place the mouthpiece of the handset into the patient's mouth. Have patient breathe normally through his mouth. Expect to administer drug over 2 to 3 min.
- Bronchodilators should be given prior to aztreonam inhalation therapy. A short-acting bronchodilator should be used at least 15 min before but no sooner than 4 hr prior to aztreonam inhalation therapy, or a long-acting bronchodilator at least 30 min before but no longer than 12 hr prior to aztreonam inhalation therapy. If patient is receiving multiple inhaled therapies, administer the bronchodilator first, followed by mucolytics, and last aztreonam.

Route	Onset	Peak	Duration
I.V.	Unknown	Immediate	Unknown
I.M.	Unknown	60 min	Unknown
Inhalation	Unknown	60 min	Unknown

Half-life: 1.5–2 hr

Mechanism of Action

Inhibits bacterial cell wall synthesis in susceptible aerobic gram-negative bacteria. These bacteria assemble rigid, cross-linked cell walls in several steps. Aztreonam affects the final cross-linking step by inactivating penicillin-binding protein 3 (the enzyme that links cell wall strands), which causes cell lysis and death.

Contraindications

Hypersensitivity to aztreonam or its components

Interactions

DRUGS

None reported by manufacturer.

Adverse Reactions

CNS: Confusion, dizziness, **encephalopathy**, fever, headache, insomnia, malaise, paresthesia, **seizures**, vertigo
CV: Chest pain, **hypotension**, transient ECG changes
EENT: Altered taste, diplopia, halitosis, mouth ulcers, mucocutaneous candidiasis, nasal congestion, sneezing, tinnitus, tongue numbness
GI: Abdominal cramps, diarrhea, elevated enzymes, **GI bleeding**, **hepatitis**, jaundice, nausea, **pseudomembranous colitis**, vomiting
GU: Breast tenderness, elevated serum creatinine level, vaginal candidiasis
HEME: Anemia, eosinophilia, leukocytosis, **neutropenia**, **pancytopenia**, positive Coombs' test, **prolonged PT and APTT**, **thrombocytopenia**, thrombocytosis
MS: Arthralgia, joint swelling, myalgia
RESP: **Bronchospasm**, dyspnea, wheezing
SKIN: Diaphoresis, **erythema multiforme**, **exfoliative dermatitis**, flushing, petechiae, pruritus, purpura, rash, **toxic epidermal necrolysis**, urticaria
Other: **Anaphylaxis**, **angioedema**, injection-site reaction (pain, phlebitis, swelling, or thrombophlebitis)

Childbearing Considerations

PREGNANCY

- It is not known if drug can cause fetal harm although it does cross the placental barrier.
- Cystic fibrosis may increase the risk for preterm delivery.
- Use with caution only if benefit to mother outweighs potential risk to fetus.

LACTATION

- Drug is present in breast milk.
- Breastfeeding should be withheld during drug therapy when Azactam is used. Mothers should check with prescriber before breastfeeding when Cayston is used.

Nursing Considerations

- Obtain culture and sensitivity test results, if possible, before starting aztreonam therapy.

If patient is acutely ill, expect to begin therapy before results are available.

- Keep in mind that other antimicrobials may be used with aztreonam in seriously ill patients at risk for gram-positive infection.
- Expect to use I.V. route for patients who need single doses over 1 g and those with life-threatening systemic infections, such as peritonitis or septicemia.
- Evaluate patient's liver and renal function test results, as ordered, before therapy begins if patient has hepatic or renal impairment. Continue to monitor throughout drug therapy, and especially if patient is receiving an aminoglycoside because of the increased risk for nephrotoxicity.

! **WARNING** Monitor patient for a hypersensitivity reaction, which could become life-threatening such as anaphylaxis or angioedema. If present, notify prescriber immediately, withhold drug, and provide supportive care, as needed and ordered.

- Assess for signs of bacterial or fungal superinfection, which may occur with prolonged or repeated therapy. If superinfection occurs, treat it as prescribed.

! **WARNING** Monitor bowel elimination for diarrhea; if needed, obtain stool culture to rule out pseudomembranous colitis caused by *Clostridium difficile*. It could be mild or become life-threatening. If it occurs, expect to discontinue aztreonam and administer antibiotics effective against *C. difficile* as well as electrolytes, fluids, and protein, as needed and ordered.

PATIENT TEACHING

- Emphasize the need to take full course of aztreonam exactly as prescribed, even if patient feels better before finishing it.
- Instruct patient how to dilute and administer inhalation form of drug, if ordered.

! **WARNING** Teach patient to recognize and immediately report signs and symptoms of allergic reactions, such as chest tightness, difficulty breathing, hives, itching, and rash. Tell patient to seek immediate medical care if allergic reaction is severe.

- Warn patient that abdominal pain and loose, watery stools may occur 2 months or more after aztreonam therapy stops. If diarrhea persists or becomes severe, urge him to contact prescriber and replace fluids.
- Teach patient to watch for and immediately report signs of superinfection, such as white patches in mouth.
- Instruct patient to notify prescriber if persistent, severe, or unusual adverse reactions occur as drug may adversely affect many body systems.

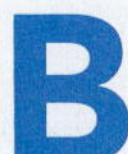

baloxavir marboxil

Xofluza

Class and Category

Pharmacologic class: Polymerase acidic endonuclease inhibitor
Therapeutic class: Influenza antiviral

Indications and Dosages

✶ *To treat acute uncomplicated influenza in patients who have been symptomatic for no more than 48 hours and who are otherwise healthy or at high risk of developing influenza-related complications; to prevent influenza following contact with an individual who has influenza*

TABLETS

Adults and children ages 5 and older weighing at least 80 kg (176 lb). 80 mg as a single dose.
Adults and children ages 5 and older weighing 20 kg (44 lb) to less than 80 kg (176 lb). 40 mg as a single dose.

ORAL SUSPENSION

Adults and children ages 5 and older weighing at least 80 kg (176 lb). 40 ml (80 mg) as a single dose.
Adults and children ages 5 and older weighing 20 kg (44 lb) to less than 80 kg (176 lb). 20 ml (40 mg) as a single dose.
Children weighing less than 20 kg (44 lb). 2 mg/kg as a single dose.

Drug Administration

P.O.

- Do not give drug with antacids, calcium-fortified beverages, dairy products, oral supplements (calcium, iron, magnesium, selenium, or zinc), or polyvalent cation-containing laxatives.
- Tablets should be swallowed whole.
- Store oral granules (used to make oral suspension) at room temperature. Gently tap the bottom of the bottle to loosen the granules. Constitute granules with 20 ml of plain or Sterile Water to a volume of suspension of 40 mg/20 ml (2 mg/ml). Gently swirl the suspension. Do not shake. More than one bottle may be needed for adults and adolescents weighing at least 80 kg (176 lb) and less than one bottle may be needed for children weighing less than 20 kg (44 lb).
- Use a calibrated measuring device to ensure correct dosage.
- For enteral administration, flush tube with 1 ml of water, administer the suspension with an enteral syringe, and reflush tube with 1 ml of water after administration.
- Drug does not contain preservatives and must be administered within 10 hr after constitution. During that time, it may be stored at room temperature. Discard if not used within 10 hr or if suspension has been stored above 25°C (77°F).

Route	Onset	Peak	Duration
P.O.	Unknown	4 hr	Unknown

Half-life: 79.1 hr

Mechanism of Action

Inhibits the endonuclease activity of the polymerase acidic protein, an influenza virus-specific enzyme required for viral gene transcription. This action prevents the influenza virus from being replicated.

Contraindications

Hypersensitivity to baloxavir marboxil or its components

Interactions

DRUGS

antacids, laxatives, oral supplements, and other polyvalent cation-containing products (e.g., calcium, iron, magnesium, selenium, or zinc): Possibly decreased plasma concentrations of baloxavir, which may reduce its effectiveness
live attenuated intranasal influenza vaccine: Possibly decreased effectiveness of vaccination

FOODS

calcium-fortified beverages, dairy products: Possibly decreased effectiveness of baloxavir

Adverse Reactions

CNS: Abnormal behavior, delirium, hallucinations, headache
EENT: Nasopharyngitis, sinusitis

GI: Colitis, diarrhea, melena, nausea, **rectal bleeding**, vomiting
RESP: Bronchitis
SKIN: **Erythema multiforme**, rash, urticaria
Other: **Anaphylactic shock, anaphylaxis, angioedema, other hypersensitivity reactions**

Childbearing Considerations

PREGNANCY

- It is not known if drug can cause fetal harm.
- Use with caution only if benefit to mother outweighs potential risk to fetus.

LACTATION

- It is not known if drug is present in breast milk.
- Mothers should check with prescriber before breastfeeding.

Nursing Considerations

- Be aware that baloxavir is not effective in treating infections other than influenza. Also, drug should not be given to children under the age of 5 because treatment-emergent resistance is increased in this age group.

! **WARNING** Monitor patient closely for hypersensitivity reactions that could be life-threatening. If present, notify prescriber, expect drug to be withheld, as ordered, and provide supportive care, as needed and ordered.

PATIENT TEACHING

- Inform patient that baloxavir will be administered only once.
- Instruct patient, family, or caregiver how to administer oral form of drug prescribed.
- Caution patient that drug must not be taken with a calcium-fortified beverage or a meal containing dairy products. Also, tell patient to alert prescriber if he is taking any drugs that contain calcium, iron, magnesium, selenium, or zinc because baloxavir may not be as effective when taken with such drugs.

! **WARNING** Warn patient that drug can cause severe allergic reactions. If an allergic reaction occurs, tell patient, family, or caregiver to notify prescriber and, if severe, to seek immediate medical attention.

- Advise patient to check with prescriber before receiving live attenuated influenza vaccines after taking drug.

baricitinib

Olumiant

Class and Category

Pharmacologic class: Janus kinase (JAK) inhibitor
Therapeutic class: Antirheumatic

Indications and Dosages

* *To treat moderate to severe active rheumatoid arthritis as monotherapy or in combination with methotrexate or other non-biologic disease-modifying antirheumatic drugs (DMARDs) in patients who have had an inadequate response to one or more tumor necrosis factor (TNF) antagonist therapies*

TABLETS

Adults. 2 mg once daily.

* *To treat severe alopecia areata*

TABLETS

Adults. *Initial:* 2 mg once daily, increased to 4 mg once daily, as needed, and then decreased back to 2 mg once daily once an adequate response has occurred with the 4-mg dosage. *Initial dosage for patients with nearly complete or complete scalp hair loss:* 4 mg once daily and then decreased to 2 mg once daily once an adequate response has occurred.

± **DOSAGE ADJUSTMENT** For patients with rheumatoid arthritis or alopecia areata who have moderate renal impairment (estimated glomerular filtration rate between 30 and 60 ml/min) or are taking strong organic anion transporter 3 (OAT3) inhibitors, such as probenecid, dosage reduced to 1 mg (2 mg if initial dosage for alopecia areata was 4 mg) once daily. For patients developing an absolute lymphocyte count (ALC) less than 500 cells/mm^3, drug withheld until ALC is 500 cells/mm^3 or greater. For patients developing an absolute neutrophil count (ANC) less than 1,000 cells/mm^3, drug withheld until ANC is 1,000 cells/mm^3 or greater. For patients developing a hemoglobin value less than 8 g/dl, drug withheld until hemoglobin is 8 g/dl or greater.

* *To treat COVID-19 in hospitalized patients requiring supplemental oxygen, non-invasive or invasive mechanical ventilation, or extracorporeal membrane oxygenation (ECMO)*

TABLETS

Adults. 4 mg once daily for 14 days or until hospital discharge, whichever occurs first.

±**DOSAGE ADJUSTMENT** For patients with COVID-19 who have moderate renal impairment (estimated glomerular filtration rate between 30 and 60 ml/min) or are taking strong organic anion transporter 3 (OAT3) inhibitors, such as probenecid, dosage reduced to 2 mg once daily. For patients developing an absolute lymphocyte count (ALC) less than 200 cells/mm^3, drug withheld until ALC is 200 cells/mm^3 or greater. For patients developing an absolute neutrophil count (ANC) less than 500 cells/mm^3, drug withheld until ANC is 500 cells/mm^3 or greater.

Drug Administration

P.O.

- Administer drug with or without food.
- For patients who cannot swallow tablet form, mix tablets with 5 to 10 ml of room temperature water in a ventilated enclosure or while wearing a N95 respirator. Swirl the tablet(s) gently and then administer immediately. Rinse container with an additional 5 to 10 ml of room temperature water and give to patient to drink so that the entire contents is swallowed. Drug is stable in water for up to 4 hr.
- To administer through a gastrostomy (G) tube, prepare solution the same as for oral administration except mix with 10 to 15 ml of room temperature water. Draw entire solution into a syringe and administer through the G tube immediately. Rinse container with an additional 10 to 15 ml of room temperature water and administer through the G tube again.
- To administer drug though a nasogastric (NG) tube or an orogastric (OG) tube, prepare solution the same as for oral administration except mix with 30 ml of room temperature water. Draw entire solution into a syringe and administer through the NG or OG tube immediately. Rinse container with an additional 15 ml of room temperature water and administer through the tube again. To avoid clogging smaller diameter tubes (smaller than 12 Fr), the syringe can be held horizontally and shaken during administration.

Route	Onset	Peak	Duration
P.O.	Unknown	1 hr	Unknown

Half-life: 12 hr

Mechanism of Action

Interferes with cellular processes of hematopoiesis and immune cell function, thereby reducing the signs and symptoms of rheumatoid arthritis, which is thought to be an autoimmune disorder.

Contraindications

Hypersensitivity to baricitinib or its components

Interactions

DRUGS

strong OAT3 inhibitors, such as probenecid: Increased baricitinib exposure, increasing risk of adverse reactions

live vaccines: Decreased effectiveness of vaccine

Adverse Reactions

CNS: Fatigue, headache

CV: Elevated lipid levels, **thrombosis (including arterial and deep vein thrombosis)**

GI: Abdominal pain, elevated liver enzymes, **gastrointestinal perforation**, nausea

GU: Genital candida infections, UTI

HEME: Anemia, **elevated platelet count**, **lymphopenia**, **neutropenia**

MS: Elevated creatine phosphokinase (CPK) levels

RESP: Bronchitis, pneumonia, **pulmonary embolus**, respiratory infections

SKIN: Acne, **nonmelanoma skin cancers**, rash, urticaria

Other: **Angioedema**; infections, such as bacterial, fungal (invasive), mycobacterial, viral, or other opportunistic infections; **lymphomas and other malignancies**, **weight gain**

Childbearing Considerations

PREGNANCY

- Pregnancy exposure registry: 1-800-545-5979.
- Drug can cause fetal harm based on animal studies.
- Use with caution only if benefit to mother outweighs potential risk to fetus.

LACTATION

- It is not known if drug is present in breast milk.
- Breastfeeding should be avoided during drug therapy and for 4 days after last dose.

REPRODUCTION

- Females of childbearing age should use effective contraception throughout drug therapy.

Nursing Considerations

- Know that baricitinib is not recommended to be used concurrently with biologic immunomodulators, cyclosporine or other potent immunosuppressants, or other JAK inhibitors. Know that baricitinib therapy should also be avoided in patients with an active, serious infection, including localized infections. In addition, drug is not recommended in patients with a glomerular filtration rate less than 30 ml/min or patients who have severe hepatic impairment.
- Be aware that patients hospitalized with COVID-19 may not be able to have preliminary testing or test results available as outlined below before drug is initiated because of the emergent situation caused by the virus.

! **WARNING** Expect patient to have a baseline CBC done prior to starting baricitinib therapy. Be aware that the drug should not be initiated in patients with an ALC less than 500 cells/mm^3 (200 cells/mm^3 for COVID-19 infection), ANC less than 1,000 cells/mm^3 (500 cells/mm^3 for COVID-19 infection), or hemoglobin level less than 8 g/dl (no restriction for COVID-19 infection). Monitor patient's CBC results closely throughout drug therapy, as drug may cause anemia, lymphopenia, or neutropenia.

! **WARNING** Use baricitinib cautiously in patients who may be at increased risk for GI perforation or thrombosis, as drug use may increase the risk for these life-threatening disorders.

- Know that patients should be screened for viral hepatitis before initiating therapy with baricitinib. Expect liver enzymes to be determined prior to baricitinib therapy and periodically throughout therapy because drug can affect liver function. Know that if increases in liver enzymes occur and liver injury is suspected, drug therapy should be stopped until drug-induced liver dysfunction is ruled out.
- Test patients for latent tuberculosis (TB), as ordered, prior to initiating baricitinib therapy. If positive, expect patient to receive treatment. Monitor all patients for signs and symptoms of TB throughout therapy, including patients who were negative for latent TB infection prior to initiating therapy. Know that TB therapy also may be prescribed for patients with a history of active or latent TB in whom an adequate course of treatment cannot be confirmed and for patients with a negative test for latent tuberculosis but who have risk factors for tuberculosis (TB).
- Ensure patient is up to date on immunizations before starting baricitinib therapy.

! **WARNING** Monitor patient closely for hypersensitivity reactions, such as angioedema, rash, and urticaria. Reactions may become serious. If present, notify prescriber and expect baricitinib to be discontinued. Provide supportive care, as needed and ordered.

! **WARNING** Be aware that patients who are 50 years or older with at least one cardiovascular risk factor, including being a current or past smoker, may have a higher risk for sudden cardiovascular death, MI, stroke , or thrombosis (including arterial deep venous thrombosis and pulmonary embolism) because higher rates have occurred with use of another JAK inhibitor. Monitor patient closely for cardiovascular abnormalities and expect drug to be discontinued if any occurs.

! **WARNING** Assess patient regularly for signs and symptoms of infection during and after therapy because serious and sometimes fatal infections due to bacterial, invasive fungal, mycobacterial, viral, or other opportunistic pathogens may occur. Patients at higher risk are those who are taking immunosuppressants, such as corticosteroids or methotrexate. Notify prescriber if infection is suspected and expect antibiotic therapy to be prescribed, if confirmed. Know that baricitinib may be temporarily stopped if patient is not responding to antibiotic therapy and not restarted until the infection is under control.

! **WARNING** Be aware that baricitinib increases the risk of cancer. Assess patient regularly, especially for nonmelanoma skin cancers. Also, know that higher rates of lung cancers and lymphomas have occurred with use of another JAK inhibitor.

- Assess patient for viral reactivation, including herpes zoster, during drug therapy. If patient develops herpes zoster during therapy with baricitinib, expect drug therapy to be interrupted until the episode has been resolved.
- Monitor patient for new-onset abdominal symptoms, especially patients with a history of diverticulitis because baricitinib increases the risk for GI perforation.
- Monitor patient's lipid profile periodically, as ordered, during baricitinib therapy. Know that a lipid profile should be performed about 12 weeks into baricitinib therapy to determine if management of hyperlipidemia is needed.
- Avoid giving patient live vaccines during baricitinib therapy because drug may reduce effectiveness of the vaccination.

PATIENT TEACHING

- Instruct patient how to administer baricitinib and to take drug exactly as prescribed.

! **WARNING** Stress importance of seeking immediate medical attention if an allergic reaction, such as hives; rash; or swelling of lips, throat, or tongue occurs, and to stop taking baricitinib.

! **WARNING** Inform patient of risk for infections. Review signs and symptoms of infection and stress importance of notifying prescriber if an infection is suspected or develops. Also, tell patient that herpes zoster may also occur. Because it could become quite serious, it should be reported.

! **WARNING** Review signs and symptoms of a blood clot, MI, or stroke with patient and stress importance of seeking immediate medical attention if suspected.

! **WARNING** Stress importance of seeking immediate emergency care if a new onset of abdominal pain, chills, fever, nausea, or vomiting occurs.

! **WARNING** Tell patient that baricitinib therapy increases the risk of certain cancers. Encourage her to report any persistent, severe, or unusual signs or symptoms to prescriber. Also, instruct patient to periodically examine her skin for signs of skin cancer.

- Alert patient that laboratory abnormalities such as an elevated lipid profile or liver enzymes may occur during baricitinib therapy and may require treatment. Stress importance of complying with ordered laboratory tests.
- Instruct patient not to receive vaccinations containing live virus during baricitinib therapy.
- Encourage females of childbearing age to use effective contraception during baricitinib therapy. If pregnancy occurs, prescriber should be notified.
- Advise mothers not to breastfeed during treatment with baricitinib and for 4 days after last dose.

beclomethasone dipropionate

QNASL, QVAR Redihaler

beclomethasone dipropionate monohydrate

Beconase AQ

Class and Category

Pharmacologic class: Corticosteroid
Therapeutic class: Antiasthmatic, anti-inflammatory

Indications and Dosages

* *To maintain treatment of asthma as prophylactic therapy*

ORAL INHALATION AEROSOL (QVAR REDIHALER)

Adults and adolescents who are not on an inhaled corticosteroid. *Initial:* 1 to 2 inhalations (40 to 80 mcg) twice daily, depending on strength used. *Maximum:* 4 to 8 inhalations (up to 320 mcg) twice daily, depending on strength used.
Adults and adolescents switching from another inhaled corticosteroid. *Dependent on strength of previous inhaled corticosteroid and disease severity:* 1 inhalation (40 mcg), 1 or 2 inhalations (80 mcg) depending on dosage strength, 2 to 4 inhalations (160 mcg) depending on dosage strength, or 4 inhalations (320 mcg) using 80-mcg strength twice daily. *Maximum:* 320 mcg twice daily.
Children ages 4 to 11. 1 inhalation (40 mcg) twice daily, increased after 2 wk to 2 inhalations (80 mcg) twice daily, as needed. *Maximum:* 2 inhalations (80 mcg) twice daily.

* *To relieve symptoms of perennial or seasonal allergic and nonallergic (vasomotor) rhinitis; to prevent recurrence of nasal polyps after surgical removal*

NASAL SPRAY (BECONASE AQ)

Adults and children ages 12 and older. 1 or 2 inhalations (42 or 84 mcg) in each nostril twice daily for total dose of 168 or 336 mcg daily.
Children ages 6 to 12. *Initial:* 1 spray (42 mcg) in each nostril twice daily, increased to 2 sprays (84 mcg) in each nostril twice daily, as needed. Once control is achieved, dosage decreased to 1 spray (42 mcg) in each nostril twice daily. *Maximum:* 336 mcg (2 sprays in each nostril) daily given in 2 divided doses 12 hr apart.

* *To treat nasal symptoms associated with perennial or seasonal allergic rhinitis*

NASAL SPRAY (QNASL)

Adults and children ages 12 and older. 2 inhalations (using 80-mcg strength) in each nostril once daily for a total dose of 320 mcg daily. *Maximum:* 4 inhalations (320 mcg) per day.
Children ages 4 to and including 11. 1 inhalation (using 40-mcg strength) in each nostril once daily for a total dose of 80 mcg daily. *Maximum:* 2 inhalations (80 mcg) per day.

Drug Administration

NASAL SPRAY

- Daily dosages given twice daily should be spaced about 12 hr apart.
- Have patient blow nose and then hand device to patient to hold upright and insert actuator tip into one nostril. Have patient point device slightly away from the nasal septum while holding other nostril closed.
- Have patient hold breath while pressing down completely on the canister to release 1 spray. The patient should hold breath for 5 sec and then breathe out through the mouth. Then, device should be removed from nostril. Steps are repeated for the dose in the other nostril.
- Do not allow patient to blow nose for the next 15 min.

Beconase AQ

- Pump nasal spray 6 times or until a fine mist is seen before using for the first time. If drug has not been used for a week, repeat priming.
- Shake well before using.
- Clean nasal applicator by washing in cold water, dry, and replace cap and safety clip back in position.

QNASL

- Does not have to be primed. Before using a new container, spray counter should read 120.
- Use a clean, dry tissue to clean tip. Do not wash in water.

ORAL INHALATION

QVAR Redihaler

- Do not use with a spacer or volume holding chamber.
- Does not require priming or shaking before administration.
- Before using a new container, spray counter should read 120.
- Inhaler should be held in an upright position with the mouthpiece positioned down. There is no button to push. The white cap on the inhaler must be closed before each inhalation. Have patient insert mouthpiece into mouth and close lips around it. Have patient inhale deeply to release drug. Then, have patient remove

inhaler and hold breath for 5 to 10 sec, then breathe out slowly. If more than 1 inhalation is required, repeat the same steps.
- Have patient rinse mouth with water without swallowing after each dose.
- Clean mouthpiece weekly by gently wiping with a dry cloth or tissue. Never place inhaler in water.

Route	Onset	Peak	Duration
Inhalation	1–2 wk	30 min	Unknown
Intranasal	2 wk	Unknown	Unknown

Half-life: 2.9–4 hr

Mechanism of Action

May decrease number and activity of cells involved in the inflammatory response of allergies, asthma, and rhinitis, such as basophils, eosinophils, lymphocytes, macrophages, mast cells, and neutrophils. May also inhibit production or secretion of chemical mediators, such as cytokines, eicosanoids, histamine, and leukotrienes. May produce direct smooth-muscle cell relaxation and decrease airway hyperresponsiveness.

Contraindications

Hypersensitivity to beclomethasone or its components, relief of acute asthma or acute bronchospasm, status asthmaticus (QVAR)

Interactions

DRUGS

None reported by manufacturer.

Adverse Reactions

CNS: Aggression, depression, fatigue, fever, headache, insomnia, light-headedness, mania, psychomotor hyperactivity, sleep disorders, **suicidal ideation**
CV: Chest pain, tachycardia
EENT: Blurred vision, burning sensation in nasal passages, cataracts, central serous chorioretinopathy, dry mouth, dysphonia, earache, elevated intraocular pressure, epistaxis, glaucoma, hoarseness, lacrimation, loss of smell and taste, nasal congestion or ulceration, nasal septal perforation, nose and throat dryness and irritation, nose and oral candidiasis (inhaler), pharyngitis, rhinorrhea, sinusitis, sneezing, unpleasant smell and taste
ENDO: **Adrenal insufficiency**, cushingoid symptoms
GI: Diarrhea, indigestion, nausea, **rectal hemorrhage**
GU: Dysmenorrhea, UTI
MS: Arthralgia, growth suppression in children, reduction in bone mineral density (long-term therapy)
RESP: Bronchitis, **bronchospasm**, chest congestion, cough, **pulmonary infiltrates**, upper respiratory tract infection, wheezing
SKIN: Acne, eczema, pruritus, rash, skin discoloration, urticaria
Other: **Anaphylaxis**, **angioedema**, flu-like symptoms, impaired wound healing, lymphadenopathy, weight gain

Childbearing Considerations

PREGNANCY

- It is not known if drug can cause fetal harm.
- Use with caution only if benefit to mother outweighs potential risk to fetus.

LACTATION

- Drug may be present in breast milk.
- Mothers should check with prescriber before breastfeeding.

Nursing Considerations

- Be aware that beclomethasone should not be used with patients who have experienced recent nasal septal ulcers, nasal surgery, or nasal trauma because of corticosteroids' adverse effects on wound healing.
- Know that drug should be used with extreme caution but preferably not at all in patients with active or quiescent respiratory tuberculosis, untreated bacterial, parasitic, fungal, or viral infections, or in the presence of ocular herpes simplex. Monitor patient closely throughout therapy for signs and symptoms of infection because immunosuppression occurs with corticosteroid therapy.
- Know that if patient also takes an oral corticosteroid, expect to taper dosage slowly (by decreasing daily dosage or taking drug every other day, as ordered) about 1 week after beclomethasone therapy begins. However, expect to resume oral corticosteroid during a severe asthma attack or stressful period.

! **WARNING** Be aware that when gradually switching patient from oral corticosteroid to inhaled beclomethasone, watch for signs of life-threatening adrenal insufficiency, such as fatigue, hypotension, lassitude, nausea, vomiting, and weakness during transition period and when exposed to infection, surgery, trauma, or other stressors. If signs occur, notify prescriber immediately. Also, watch for signs of adrenal insufficiency during periods of stress because beclomethasone inhalation or nasal spray may not be able to meet the increased corticosteroid need.

! **WARNING** Be prepared to give a fast-acting bronchodilator, as prescribed, if patient has an acute asthma attack or increased wheezing after receiving beclomethasone, Expect beclomethasone to be discontinued if this occurs.

! **WARNING** Monitor patient for hypersensitivity reactions that could become life-threatening such as anaphylaxis or angioedema. If present, notify prescriber immediately, withhold drug if ordered, and provide supportive care, as needed and ordered.

! **WARNING** Monitor patient closely for altered thinking, such as suicidal thoughts. If present, notify prescriber because drug will have to be discontinued.

- Monitor patient for infection because drug can cause immunosuppression. Assess for signs of candidiasis, such as plaques or thick white coating on tongue and sides of mouth. Have patient rinse mouth with water without swallowing after inhalation; this may help to prevent oral candidiasis. If present, notify prescriber and expect to reduce dose or frequency or to stop beclomethasone. Also, anticipate treatment with antifungal drug.
- Assess nasal discharge regularly when patient is prescribed nasal spray. Look for color or consistency changes, which may indicate infection when patient is using beclomethasone nasal spray.
- Monitor patients with a change in vision or a history of blurred vision, cataracts, glaucoma, or intraocular pressure because use of inhaled and intranasal corticosteroids may cause eye abnormalities. If adverse eye symptoms develop, notify prescriber and expect patient to be referred to an ophthalmologist.
- Monitor the growth of children receiving beclomethasone nasally.

PATIENT TEACHING

- Instruct patient how to administer form of beclomethasone prescribed.
- Advise patient prescribed 2 inhalations to wait a minute between them.
- Tell patient prescribed an inhaled bronchodilator with beclomethasone oral inhalation to use bronchodilator first, wait for 5 minutes, and then use beclomethasone.

! **WARNING** Warn patient that beclomethasone isn't intended to relieve acute bronchospasm. Instead, instruct patient to administer a fast-acting bronchodilator, as prescribed, if bronchospasms or increased wheezing occurs after administering beclomethasone. Tell patient to notify prescriber of the occurrence because beclomethasone will need to be discontinued.

- Urge patient to notify prescriber if asthma symptoms don't respond to beclomethasone therapy.

! **WARNING** Alert patient that drug can cause an allergic reaction. If an allergic reaction occurs, tell patient to notify prescriber and, if severe, to seek immediate medical care.

! **WARNING** Advise patient not to abruptly stop taking beclomethasone because adrenal sufficiency may occur. Urge her to notify prescriber if she develops signs of adrenal insufficiency, such as anorexia, dizziness, dyspnea, fainting, fatigue, fever, hypotension, malaise, or nausea. Advise patient to wear medical identification that states need for supplemental oral corticosteroids during severe asthma attack or stress.

! **WARNING** Warn patient and family or caretaker to report any abnormal thinking, such as suicidal thoughts, immediately to prescriber. Tell family or caregiver to take suicidal precautions.

- Caution patient to avoid exposure to chickenpox and measles because drug may cause immunosuppression. If she's exposed to these disorders, urge her to notify prescriber immediately. Also, review signs and symptoms of infection to report to prescriber and infection control precautions to take.

- Tell patient to report any changes in vision to prescriber.

belimumab

Benlysta

Class and Category

Pharmacologic class: Monoclonal antibody
Therapeutic class: Immunosuppressant

Indications and Dosages

∗ *To treat active lupus nephritis in patients who are receiving standard therapy; to treat active systemic lupus erythematosus (SLE) in patients who are receiving standard therapy*

I.V. INFUSION

Adults and children ages 5 and older. 10 mg/kg at 2-wk intervals for the first 3 doses and at 4-wk intervals thereafter.

∗ *To treat active lupus nephritis in patients who are receiving standard therapy*

SUBCUTANEOUS INJECTION

Adults. *Initial:* 400 mg (given as two 200-mg injections) once/wk for 4 doses, then 200 mg thereafter.
Adults transitioning from intravenous therapy. 200 mg once/wk with first two doses given I.V. then first subcutaneous dose, given 1 to 2 wk after the last I.V. dose.

∗ *To treat active systemic lupus erythematosus (SLE) in patients receiving standard therapy*

SUBCUTANEOUS INJECTION

Adults. 200 mg once/wk.
Adults transitioning from intravenous therapy. 200 mg once/wk, with first dose given 1 to 4 wk after the last I.V. dose.
Children ages 5 and older weighing 40 kg (88 lb) or more. 200 mg once/wk.
Children ages 5 and older weighing 15 kg (33 lb) to less than 40 kg (88 lb). 200 mg once every 2 wk.

Drug Administration

- Be aware that vials containing belimumab are intended for intravenous use only and autoinjectors and prefilled syringes are intended for subcutaneous use only. The single-dose autoinjector is for use in adults and children ages 5 and older. The single-dose prefilled syringe is for use in adults.

I.V.

- Patient should be premedicated prior to receiving each dose of belimumab to prevent hypersensitivity and infusion reactions, as prescribed.
- Remove vial from refrigerator and allow to stand 10 to 15 min prior to reconstitution.
- Reconstitute with 1.5 ml of Sterile Water for Injection, USP for a 120-mg vial and 4.8 ml of Sterile Water for Injection, USP when reconstituting a 400-mg vial. When injecting diluent solution into the vial, direct stream of Sterile Water for Injection toward the side of the vial to minimize foaming. Gently swirl vial for 60 sec every 5 min until the powder is dissolved. Do not shake or refrigerate during this process. It typically takes 10 to 15 min for powder to dissolve but may take as long as 30 min. Protect reconstituted solution from sunlight.
- When using a mechanical reconstitution device (swirler), do not exceed 500 rpm, and swirl no longer than 30 min.
- Solution should appear opalescent and colorless to pale yellow without particles. Small air bubbles may be present and are acceptable.
- Use only 0.45% Sodium Chloride Injection, 0.9% Sodium Chloride Injection, or Lactated Ringer's Injection to further dilute the drug to a volume of 250 ml (100 ml for patients weighing less than or equal to 40 kg (88 lb). Withdraw amount of solution from the infusion bag (compatible with polyolefin or polyvinylchloride bags) or bottle equivalent to the vial contents of reconstituted drug required for patient's dose. Then, add the required volume of the reconstituted solution of the drug into the infusion bag or bottle. Gently invert bag or bottle to mix the solution. Discard any unused solution left in the vial(s).
- The reconstituted solution should be stored in the refrigerator, protected from direct sunlight, if not used immediately. The diluted solution may be stored in the refrigerator or at room temperature.
- Infuse over 1 hr. The total time from reconstitution to completion of infusion,

including any storage time, should not exceed 8 hr.

- If an infusion reaction occurs, slow the rate of infusion, or stop it temporarily, as ordered.
- *Incompatibilities:* Dextrose intravenous solutions; other drugs infused concomitantly in the same I.V. line

SUBCUTANEOUS

- First subcutaneous injection should be given under the supervision of a healthcare professional.
- Remove the autoinjector or prefilled syringe from the refrigerator and allow it to sit at room temperature for 30 min prior to administering. Do not warm the drug any other way. Solution should appear clear to opalescent and colorless to pale yellow. Discard if product exhibits discoloration or particulate matter or if the autoinjector or prefilled syringe is accidentally dropped on a hard surface.
- Inject into the abdomen or thigh. When administering a 400-mg dose in the same area, administer the 2 injections at least 5 cm (2 inches) apart. Use a different injection site for each injection; do not give the injection into areas where the skin is bruised, hard, red, or tender.

Route	Onset	Peak	Duration
I.V.	Unknown	Unknown	Unknown
SubQ	Unknown	2–6 days	Unknown

Half-life: 18–19 days

Mechanism of Action

Blocks the binding of soluble B-cell lymphocyte stimulator protein, a B-cell survival factor, to its receptors on B cells. This action causes cell death, which helps to relieve the signs and symptoms of active, autoantibody-positive, systemic lupus erythematosus.

Contraindications

Hypersensitivity to belimumab or its components

Interactions

DRUGS

live virus vaccines: Possibly suppressed immune response and increased adverse effects of vaccine

other biologics such as rituximab (in patients with SLE): Increased risk of serious infections and post-injection systemic reactions

Adverse Reactions

CNS: Anxiety, depression, fatigue, fever, headache, insomnia, migraines, myalgia, **progressive multifocal leukoencephalopathy, suicidal ideation**
CV: **Bradycardia, hypotension**
EENT: Nasopharyngitis, pharyngitis, sinusitis
GI: Diarrhea, nausea
GU: Cystitis, lupus nephritis, UTI
HEME: **Leukopenia**
MS: Extremity pain, myalgia
RESP: Bronchitis, dyspnea, pneumonia, upper respiratory tract infection
SKIN: Cellulitis, nonmelanoma skin cancers, pruritus, rash, urticaria
Other: Anti-belimumab antibody formation, flu-like symptoms, **hypersensitivity reactions** (**anaphylaxis**, **angioedema**, dyspnea, **hypotension**, pruritus, rash, urticaria), infusion reactions (**bradycardia**, headache, **hypotension**, myalgia, nausea, rash, urticaria), injection-site reactions (erythema, hematoma, induration, pain, pruritus), **malignancies**, serious infections

Childbearing Considerations

PREGNANCY

- Pregnancy exposure registry: 1-877-311-8972 or https://mothertobaby.org/ongoing-study/benlysta-belimumab/.
- Drug may cause fetal harm. Drug actively crosses placental barrier with largest amount transferred in the third trimester, which may affect fetal immune response in utero.
- Use with caution only if the benefit to the mother outweighs the potential risk to the fetus.
- Monitor neonate and infant if drug exposure occurred in utero for B-cell reduction and other immune dysfunction.

LACTATION

- It is not clear if drug is present in breast milk.
- Mothers should check with prescriber before breastfeeding.

REPRODUCTION

- Females of childbearing age should avoid pregnancy by using effective contraception during drug therapy and for at least 4 mo after final dose of the drug.

Nursing Considerations

- Be aware that other biologic therapies, such as B-cell targeted therapies or intravenous cyclophosphamide therapy, are not recommended during belimumab therapy because potential drug interactions are unknown.
- Know that belimumab should not be used to treat patients who are receiving drug therapy to treat a chronic infection.
- Do not administer live vaccines to patient during 30 days before or concurrently with belimumab because safety has not been established.
- Monitor African American patients closely during belimumab therapy for decreased effectiveness because clinical trials have shown the response rate may be lower in these patients.

! **WARNING** Monitor patient for hypersensitivity and infusion reactions. Be aware that patients with a history of multiple drug allergies or significant hypersensitivity may be at increased risk for a hypersensitivity or infusion reaction. Know that it may be difficult to tell the difference between a hypersensitivity reaction and an infusion reaction. Monitor patient closely. If a serious reaction occurs such as anaphylaxis or angioedema, slow or temporarily stop the infusion or withhold further subcutaneous injections of the drug, as ordered, because death has occurred with some patients experiencing hypersensitivity reactions. Expect to provide emergency medical treatment as ordered and indicated by the severity of the reaction. Non-acute reactions include fatigue, headache, myalgia, nausea, and skin reactions and may occur up to 1 week after the drug has been administered. Be aware that reactions may occur in patients who have previously tolerated belimumab administration.

! **WARNING** Monitor patient for abnormal behavior or thinking because belimumab may cause depression and suicidal ideation.

! **WARNING** Watch for evidence of infection (such as cough, fever, malaise, pain) because patients receiving immunosuppressants, such as belimumab, are at increased risk for serious infections, such as bronchitis, cellulitis, pneumonia, and urinary tract infection. Although rare, belimumab may cause the serious infection, progressive multifocal leukoencephalopathy (PML), exhibited by new-onset or deteriorating neurological signs and symptoms. If patient develops an infection, notify prescriber, monitor patient closely, and know that drug therapy may be interrupted until infection is gone unless PML is diagnosed in which case, expect belimumab to be discontinued.

! **WARNING** Monitor patient with SLE receiving rituximab concomitantly for increased risk of adverse reactions such as post-injection systemic reactions and adverse reactions, including serious infections.

! **WARNING** Be aware that belimumab increases the risk of cancer because it causes immunosuppression. Assess patient regularly, especially for nonmelanoma skin cancers.

PATIENT TEACHING

- Instruct patient who will be self-injecting belimumab, as a subcutaneous injection, how to administer the injection and dispose of needle and syringe after injection. Tell patient what to do if a dose is missed.
- Instruct patient to notify prescriber if effectiveness of drug decreases, especially if patient is African American.

! **WARNING** Instruct patient to report any signs of a hypersensitivity reaction such as hives, itching, or rash. If patient develops difficulty breathing or swallowing or swelling of face, throat, or tongue, medical attention should be sought immediately.

! **WARNING** Caution patient, family, or caregiver to report new or worsening depression, suicidal thoughts, or other mood changes.

! **WARNING** Encourage patient to report any persistent, severe, or unusual signs and symptoms to prescriber because drug may increase risk for cancer and infections. Also, review infection control measures to take while receiving belimumab.

- Advise patient not to receive any immunization with live vaccines for 30 days before or concurrently with belimumab and to avoid contact with anyone who has an infection.
- Tell females of childbearing age to use effective contraception during treatment and for at least 4 months after the final treatment because of potential adverse effects to infants exposed to drug in utero. Advise her to notify prescriber if pregnancy occurs and encourage her to enroll in the belimumab pregnancy registry.

benazepril hydrochloride

Lotensin

Class and Category

Pharmacologic class: ACE inhibitor
Therapeutic class: Antihypertensive

Indications and Dosages

* *To control hypertension alone or with a thiazide diuretic*

SUSPENSION, TABLETS

Adults who aren't receiving a diuretic. *Initial:* 10 mg daily. *Maintenance:* 20 to 40 mg daily as a single dose or in 2 equally divided doses.

Adults who are receiving a diuretic. 5 mg daily.

± **DOSAGE ADJUSTMENT** For adult patients with impaired renal function and creatinine clearance less than 30 ml/min, the initial dosage should be 5 mg/day and then increased gradually until blood pressure is controlled or dosage reaches maximum of 40 mg daily.

SUSPENSION, TABLETS

Children ages 6 and older with eGFR of 30 ml/min or higher. *Initial:* 0.2 mg/kg daily and increased, as needed. *Maximum:* 0.6 mg/kg daily or 40 mg daily.

Drug Administration

P.O.

- Shake suspension before each use. Use calibrated device when measuring dosage.
- Suspension should be refrigerated and can be stored for up to 30 days.

Route	Onset	Peak	Duration
P.O.	1 hr	1–2 hr	24 hr

Half-life: 10–11 hr

Mechanism of Action

May reduce blood pressure by affecting renin–angiotensin–aldosterone system. By inhibiting angiotensin-converting enzyme, benazepril:

- prevents conversion of angiotensin I to angiotensin II, a potent vasoconstrictor that also stimulates aldosterone release.
- may inhibit renal and vascular production of angiotensin II.
- decreases serum angiotensin II level and increases serum renin activity. This decreases aldosterone secretion, slightly increasing serum potassium level and fluid loss.
- decreases vascular tone and blood pressure.
- inhibits aldosterone release, which reduces sodium and water resorption, increases their excretion, and reduces blood pressure.

Contraindications

Aliskiren therapy in patients with diabetes; concurrent therapy with a neprilysin inhibitor (e.g., sacubitril) or within 36 hr of switching to or from sacubitril/valsartan combination; history of angioedema; hypersensitivity to benazepril, other ACE inhibitors, or their components

Interactions

DRUGS

aliskiren (in patients with diabetes or renal impairment), angiotensin receptor blockers, other ACE inhibitors: Increased risk of hyperkalemia, hypotension, and renal dysfunction
antidiabetics (oral), insulin: Possibly increased risk of hypoglycemia
diuretics: Possibly excessive hypotension
gold salts: Possibly nitritoid reaction, including facial flushing, hypotension, nausea, and vomiting
lithium: Increased serum lithium level and risk of lithium toxicity
mTOR inhibitors (everolimus, sirolimus, temsirolimus), neprilysin inhibitors: Increased risk for angioedema
NSAIDs: Possible decreased renal function in patients who are elderly, volume depleted,

or have a compromised renal function; may increase antihypertensive effect of benazepril
potassium preparations, potassium-sparing diuretics: Possibly increased serum potassium level

Adverse Reactions

CNS: Anxiety, asthenia, dizziness, drowsiness, fatigue, headache, hypertonia, insomnia, nervousness, paresthesia, sleep disturbance, somnolence, syncope, weakness
CV: Angina, **ECG changes**, **hypotension**, orthostatic hypotension, palpitations, peripheral edema
EENT: Sinusitis
ENDO: Hyperglycemia
GI: Abdominal pain, **acute liver failure**, **cholestatic hepatitis**, constipation, elevated liver enzymes, gastritis, **hepatic necrosis**, **melena**, nausea, **pancreatitis**, small bowel angioedema, vomiting
GU: **Acute renal failure**, decreased libido, elevated BUN and serum creatinine levels, frequent urination, impotence, **nephrotic syndrome**, oliguria, **progressive azotemia**, proteinuria, **renal insufficiency**, UTI
HEME: **Agranulocytosis**, decreased hemoglobin level, **hemolytic anemia**, **leukopenia**, **neutropenia**, **thrombocytopenia**
MS: Arthralgia, arthritis, myalgia
RESP: ACE cough, **asthma**, bronchitis, **bronchospasm**, dyspnea
SKIN: Alopecia, dermatitis, diaphoresis, flushing, pemphigus, photosensitivity, pruritus, rash, **Stevens-Johnson syndrome**
Other: **Anaphylaxis**, **angioedema**, **hyperkalemia**, **hyponatremia**

Childbearing Considerations

PREGNANCY

- Drug can cause fetal harm, especially during the second and third trimesters of pregnancy.
- Oligohydramnios that occurs in pregnant females as a result of the drug can cause reduced fetal renal function leading to anuria and renal failure, fetal lung hypoplasia, and skeletal deformations, including skull hypoplasia. In addition, hypotension and death may occur.
- Drug should not be given during pregnancy and drug should be discontinued as soon as possible if pregnancy occurs.

LACTATION

- Drug is present in breast milk.
- Mothers should check with prescriber before breastfeeding.

REPRODUCTION

- Females of childbearing age should be advised to avoid pregnancy by using effective contraception during drug therapy.

Nursing Considerations

- Evaluate blood pressure with patient lying down, sitting, and standing before starting benazepril and then regularly, as appropriate, to monitor effectiveness.
- Evaluate BUN and serum creatinine levels and urine output, as ordered, before therapy and then during therapy, especially in patients post-MI or who have renal artery stenosis, severe heart failure, or are volume depleted. Monitor patients closely who are also receiving angiotensin receptor blocker or NSAID therapy because these patients may be at increased risk for developing acute renal failure.

! WARNING Monitor patient for hypersensitivity reactions, that may become life-threatening such as anaphylaxis and angioedema. Angioedema can occur even after the first dose. Especially monitor African American patients closely because of a higher incidence of angioedema in these patients. Also, monitor patients receiving dialysis closely because sudden and potentially life-threatening anaphylactoid reactions have occurred in some patients dialyzed with high-flux membranes while receiving an ACE inhibitor like benazepril. If anaphylaxis occurs, notify prescriber immediately, stop dialysis, withhold drug, and provide supportive care, as needed and ordered.

! WARNING Monitor patient's WBC count periodically, as ordered, to detect serious hematological adverse reactions such as agranulocytosis and neutropenia. Also, monitor patient's electrolytes, as ordered to detect electrolyte imbalances.

- Monitor liver enzymes regularly, as ordered. Assess patient routinely for signs and symptoms of liver dysfunction, such as fatigue and jaundice. Notify prescriber if patient develops jaundice or exhibits elevated liver enzyme levels, as drug will have to be discontinued.

- Take safety precautions, such as having patient change positions slowly and sit on edge of bed before arising, to prevent injury caused by orthostatic hypotension.

PATIENT TEACHING

- Instruct patient how to administer benazepril.
- Teach patient how to monitor blood pressure, if appropriate, and how to recognize signs of hypertension and hypotension.

! **WARNING** Instruct patient to contact prescriber immediately if she has an allergic reaction. Stress importance of seeking immediate medical care if reaction is severe such as swelling of the face, eyes, lips, or tongue.

! **WARNING** Review signs and symptoms of blood disorders to be watchful for during drug therapy and to notify prescriber if any occur. Stress importance of complying with laboratory appointments.

! **WARNING** Urge patient to contact prescriber before using any over-the-counter salt substitutes, which may contain potassium, or potassium supplements. These substances increase the risk of hyperkalemia.

! **WARNING** Advise patient to stop benazepril and notify prescriber as soon as possible if she experiences syncope.

- Explain that a dry, persistent cough may develop and may not subside unless benazepril is stopped. If cough becomes bothersome or interferes with activities or sleep, patient should notify prescriber.
- Caution patient to avoid sudden position changes and to rise slowly from lying or sitting position to minimize orthostatic hypotension.
- Caution females of childbearing age to use reliable contraception during drug therapy and to notify prescriber immediately if pregnancy occurs because drug will need to be discontinued.

benralizumab

Fasenra

Class and Category

Pharmacologic class: Monoclonal antibody
Therapeutic class: Antiasthmatic

Indications and Dosages

* *As adjunct to treat severe asthma as an add-on maintenance treatment in patients with eosinophilic phenotype*

SUBCUTANEOUS INJECTION

Adults, children ages 12 and older, children ages 6 to 11 weighing 35 kg (77 lb) or more. 30 mg once every 4 wk for the first 3 doses, then once every 8 wk.
Children ages 6 to 11 weighing less than 35 kg (77 lb). 10 mg every 4 wk for the first 3 doses, then once every 8 wk.

* *To treat eosinophilic granulomatosis with polyangiitis*

SUBCUTANEOUS INJECTION

Adults. 30 mg once every 4 wk.

Drug Administration

SUBCUTANEOUS

- Administer drug using the prefilled syringe or the autoinjector pen. Know that the autoinjector pen should not be used to self-administer drug by children ages 6 to 11.
- Prior to administration, warm drug by leaving carton at room temperature for about 30 min. Drug should appear clear to opalescent, colorless to slightly yellow, and may contain a few translucent or white to off-white particles. Do not use if solution is cloudy, discolored, or large particles or foreign particulate matter is visible.
- Do not expel any small air bubbles prior to administration.
- Gently pinch the skin and insert the needle into the abdomen, thigh, or upper arm.
- When using the prefilled syringe, inject by pushing plunger all the way until the plunger head is completely between the needle guard activation clips, which is needed to activate the needle guard. After injection, maintain pressure on the plunger head and remove the needle. Release pressure on the plunger head to allow the needle guard to cover the needle.

- When using the autoinjector pen, be careful not to shake it. Remove the cap and inject into the injection site pressing firmly. A click will be heard that indicates injection has begun and the green plunger will start to fill the viewing window. Hold for 15 sec. A second click will be heard indicating the injection is complete. The green plunger will also have filled the viewing window. Remove the needle.
- While prefilled syringe and autoinjector pen are usually stored in the refrigerator in the original carton, the devices may be stored at room temperature in the original carton, if needed, for a maximum of 14 days.
- Be aware that the single-dose autoinjector pen device is intended for use by the patient, family, or caregiver.

Route	Onset	Peak	Duration
SubQ	Rapid	Unknown	Unknown

Half-life: 15.5 days

Mechanism of Action

Binds to the alpha subunit of the human interleukin-5 receptor, which is expressed on the surface of basophils and eosinophils. Eosinophils play a part in the inflammatory process, which is present in the pathogenesis of asthma. When binding to the interleukin-5 receptor occurs, eosinophils are reduced through an antibody-dependent cell-mediated cytotoxicity to help relieve inflammation found in asthma.

Contraindications

Hypersensitivity to benralizumab or its components

Interactions

DRUGS

None reported by manufacturer.

Adverse Reactions

CNS: Fever, headache
EENT: Pharyngitis
SKIN: Rash, urticaria
Other: **Anaphylaxis**, **angioedema**, benralizumab antibody formation, injection-site reactions (erythema, pain, papule, pruritus)

Childbearing Considerations

PREGNANCY

- Pregnancy exposure registry: 1-877-311-8972 or mothertobaby.org/Fasenra.
- It is not known if drug can cause fetal harm. Drug actively crosses placental barrier with largest amount transferred in the third trimester.
- Use cautiously only if the benefit to the mother outweighs the potential risk to the fetus.

LACTATION

- It is not clear if drug is present in breast milk.
- Mothers should check with prescriber before breastfeeding.

Nursing Considerations

- Expect to treat patients with preexisting parasitic (helminth) infections before starting benralizumab therapy because it is not known if the drug will influence a patient's response to treatment for such an infection. If patient develops a parasitic infection while taking benralizumab and does not respond to treatment, expect benralizumab to be discontinued until the infection is resolved.

! WARNING Know that benralizumab should never be used to treat acute asthma symptoms, acute bronchospasms, acute exacerbations of asthma, or status asthmaticus.

! WARNING Monitor patient closely for hypersensitivity reactions that may occur within hours after benralizumab has been administered and may become life-threatening such as anaphylaxis or angioedema. If present, notify prescriber, expect drug to be discontinued, and provide supportive care, as needed and ordered.

- Expect inhaled or systemic corticosteroids used to treat asthma to be gradually withdrawn, if no longer needed. Corticosteroid therapy should never be withdrawn abruptly.

PATIENT TEACHING

- Teach patient, family, or caregiver how to administer benralizumab device prescribed.

! WARNING Instruct patient that benralizumab is not effective in treating acute asthma symptoms or acute exacerbations. If asthma remains uncontrolled or worsens after benralizumab therapy is begun, tell patient to notify prescriber or seek emergency medical care.

! **WARNING** Tell patient to report any signs of an allergic reaction, such as difficulty breathing, hives, or rash immediately. Remind patient that although an allergic reaction usually occurs within hours after benralizumab is administered, a delayed reaction could occur even days later. Stress importance of seeking immediate medical care if reaction is severe.

- Emphasize importance of not decreasing any prescribed inhaled or systemic corticosteroid dosage without prescriber knowledge.

NEW!

benzgalantamine

Zunveyl

Class and Category

Pharmacologic class: Cholinesterase inhibitor
Therapeutic class: Anti-dementia

Indications and Dosages

✱ *To treat mild to moderate dementia of the Alzheimer's type*

D.R. TABLETS

Adults. *Initial:* 5 mg twice daily for a minimum of 4 wk then increased to maintenance dose of 10 mg twice daily. Increased to 15 mg twice daily, if needed, after an additional 4 wk on maintenance dose.

± **DOSAGE ADJUSTMENT** For patients with moderate hepatic impairment, or patients with renal impairment (creatine clearance of 9 to 59 ml/min), dosage should not exceed 10 mg twice daily. Drug not recommended for patients with severe hepatic impairment or in patients with renal impairment who have a creatine clearance of less than 9 ml/min.

Drug Administration

P.O.

- Can be administered with or without food
- Tablets should be swallowed whole and not chewed, crushed, or split.
- Ensure adequate fluid intake.
- Do not administer with any products containing alcohol.
- If therapy is interrupted for more than 3 days, expect patient to be restarted at the lowest dosage and then increased according to dosing guidelines to reach current dose.

Route	Onset	Peak	Duration
P.O.	Unknown	2.5 to 3 hr	Unknown

Half-life: 7 hr

Mechanism of Action

Enhances cholinergic function as a prodrug of galantamine by increasing the concentration of acetylcholine through reversible inhibition of its hydrolysis by cholinesterase. This action compensates for the acetylcholine-producing neurons that degenerate in the brains of patients with Alzheimer's disease thereby improving cognitive function.

Contraindications

Hypersensitivity to benzgalantamine or its components

Interactions

DRUGS

anticholinergics: Altered effects of anticholinergic drugs
cholinergic agonists such as bethanechol, other cholinesterase inhibitors, similar neuromuscular blocking agents, succinylcholine: Synergistic effect may occur

Adverse Reactions

CNS: Asthenia, depression, dizziness, dysgeusia, extrapyramidal disorder, fatigue, hallucinations, headache, hypersomnia, lethargy, malaise, paresthesia, **seizures**, somnolence, syncope, tremor
CV: **Bradycardia**, **complete atrioventricular block**, first degree atrioventricular block, hypertension, **hypotension**, palpitations, supraventricular extrasystoles
EENT: Altered sense of taste, blurred vision, tinnitus
GI: Abdominal discomfort or pain, decreased appetite, diarrhea, dyspepsia, elevated hepatic enzymes, **hepatitis**, nausea, vomiting
MS: Muscle spasms or weakness
SKIN: Acute generalized exanthematous pustulosis, **erythema multiforme**, flushing, hyperhidrosis, **Stevens-Johnson syndrome**
Other: Decreased weight, dehydration, **hypersensitivity reactions**

Childbearing Considerations

PREGNANCY

- It is not known if drug can cause fetal harm.
- Use with caution only if benefit to mother outweighs potential risk to fetus.

LACTATION

- It is not known if drug is present in breast milk.
- Mothers should check with prescriber before breastfeeding.

Nursing Considerations

- Use caution when administering benzgalantamine to patients with a history of chronic obstructive pulmonary disease or severe asthma because of the drug's cholinomimetic action. Monitor patient's respiratory function throughout drug therapy for changes.

! **WARNING** Monitor patient for a hypersensitivity reaction. If present, notify prescriber, expect drug to be discontinued, and provide supportive care, as needed and ordered.

! **WARNING** Monitor patient for a serious skin reaction, which may become life-threatening, such as Stevens-Johnson syndrome. Notify prescriber immediately at the first sign of a rash and expect drug to be discontinued unless rash is clearly not drug related.

! **WARNING** Monitor patient for seizure activities and institute seizure precautions, as needed, because drug may cause seizures.

! **WARNING** Monitor patient for increased active or occult GI bleeding because drug can increase gastric acid secretion, and it has been known to cause active or occult GI bleeding in patients taking other cholinomimetics. Patients who may be at increased risk include patients with a history of ulcer disease and those who are currently using NSAIDs.

! **WARNING** Monitor patient's heart rate and rhythm closely because drug may have vagotonic effects on the sinoatrial and atrioventricular nodes. This could lead to atrioventricular block and bradycardia.

- Monitor patient's weight because drug can cause weight loss.

PATIENT TEACHING

- Instruct patient, family, or caregiver how to administer benzgalantamine.
- Stress importance of patient consuming an adequate fluid intake and avoiding alcohol during benzgalantamine therapy.

! **WARNING** Alert patient, family, or caregiver that drug may cause an allergic reaction or a serious skin reaction. If an allergy, rash, or other skin abnormalities occur, tell patient to stop taking drug and notify prescriber immediately. If serious, advise to seek immediate medical attention.

! **WARNING** Inform patient, family, or caregiver that drug can cause serious adverse reactions such as a change in heart rhythm, possible GI bleeding, and seizures. If present, alert patient, family, or caregiver to notify prescriber promptly and to seek immediate medical care.

- Tell patient, family, or caregiver to alert prescriber if significant weight loss occurs.

benztropine mesylate

Class and Category

Pharmacologic class: Anticholinergic
Therapeutic class: Antiparkinsonian, central-acting anticholinergic

Indications and Dosages

* *As adjunct, to treat all forms of Parkinson's disease*

I.M. OR I.V. INJECTION, TABLETS

Adults with idiopathic Parkinson's disease. *Initial:* 0.5 to 1 mg once daily at bedtime and increased in increments of 0.5 mg at 5- to 6-day intervals, as needed. *Maximum:* 6 mg daily.

Adults with postencephalitic Parkinson's disease. *Initial:* 2 mg daily in 1 or more divided doses and increased in increments of 0.5 mg at 5- to 6-day intervals, as needed. *For sensitive patients:* 0.5 mg at bedtime and increased, as needed. *Maximum:* 6 mg daily.

✱ *To control extrapyramidal symptoms (except tardive dyskinesia) caused by phenothiazines and other neuroleptics*

I.M. OR I.V. INJECTION, TABLETS

Adults. 1 to 4 mg once or twice daily.

±**DOSAGE ADJUSTMENT** For patients who develop drug-induced extrapyramidal reactions shortly after antipsychotic therapy is begun, dosage changed to 1 to 2 mg 2 to 3 times daily.

✱ *To treat acute dystonic reactions*

I.M. OR I.V. INJECTION

Adults. *Initial:* 1 to 2 mg as a single dose.

✱ *To prevent recurrence of acute dystonic reactions*

TABLETS

Adults. 1 to 2 mg twice daily.

Drug Administration

P.O.

- May be administered before or after meals but is most often administered at bedtime.

I.M.

- Use a filtered needle when drawing drug up from vial.
- Administer into large muscle mass.

I.V.

- Rarely used because I.M. administration is just as effective.
- Manufacturer does not provide specific instructions for administration because there usually is no need to use this route.

Route	Onset	Peak	Duration
P.O.	1 hr	7 hr	24 hr
I.M., I.V.	15 min	Unknown	24 hr

Half-life: Unknown

Mechanism of Action

Blocks acetylcholine's action at cholinergic receptor sites. This restores the brain's normal dopamine and acetylcholine balance, which relaxes muscle movement and decreases drooling, rigidity, and tremor. Benztropine also may inhibit dopamine reuptake and storage, which prolongs dopamine's action.

Contraindications

Children younger than age 3, hypersensitivity to benztropine mesylate or its components

Interactions

DRUGS

amantadine, phenothiazines, tricyclic antidepressants: Possibly increased adverse anticholinergic effects
haloperidol: Possibly decreased haloperidol effects and development of tardive dyskinesia

Adverse Reactions

CNS: Agitation, confusion, delirium, delusions, depression, disorientation, dizziness, drowsiness, euphoria, excitement, fever, hallucinations, headache, light-headedness, listlessness, memory loss, nervousness, paranoia, psychosis, weakness
CV: **Hypotension**, mild bradycardia, orthostatic hypotension, palpitations, tachycardia
EENT: Blurred vision, diplopia, dry mouth, increased intraocular pressure, mydriasis, narrow-angle glaucoma, suppurative parotitis
GI: Constipation, duodenal ulcer, epigastric distress, ileus, nausea, vomiting
GU: Dysuria, urinary hesitancy, urine retention
MS: Muscle spasms, muscle weakness
SKIN: Decreased sweating, dermatoses, flushing, rash, urticaria

Childbearing Considerations

PREGNANCY

- It is not known if drug can cause fetal harm.
- Use with caution only if benefit to mother outweighs potential risk to fetus.

LACTATION

- It is not known if drug is present in breast milk.
- Mothers should check with prescriber before breastfeeding as drug may suppress lactation.

Nursing Considerations

- Assess muscle rigidity and tremor at baseline. Then, monitor patient often during drug therapy for improvement, which indicates drug's effectiveness.

! **WARNING** Monitor patient's cumulative drug effect, which increases risk of adverse reactions and overdose.

! **WARNING** Know that when giving drug to patient with drug-induced extrapyramidal reactions, watch for worsening psychiatric symptoms.

- Monitor patient's movements closely. High-dose benztropine therapy may cause inability to move specific muscle groups as well as weakness. If this occurs, expect to reduce benztropine dosage.
- Know that benztropine therapy should not be abruptly discontinued.

PATIENT TEACHING

- Instruct patient, family, or caregiver how to administer benztropine.

! **WARNING** Warn patient that drug has a cumulative effect, increasing risk of adverse reactions and overdose. Stress importance of notifying prescriber if persistent, serious, or unusual adverse reactions occur.

! **WARNING** Alert patient, family, or caregiver if patient has a psychiatric history that drug may worsen psychiatric symptoms. Prescriber should be notified if this occurs.

! **WARNING** Know that because benztropine decreases sweating, urge patient to avoid extremely hot or humid conditions to reduce risk of heatstroke and severe hyperthermia. This is especially important for elderly patients and those who abuse alcohol or have chronic illness or CNS disease.

- Caution against driving and similar activities until benztropine's effects are known and resolved because it may cause blurred vision, dizziness, or drowsiness.
- Stress need for periodic eye examinations and intraocular pressure measurements because drug may cause increase intraocular pressure causing narrow-angle glaucoma.

bethanechol chloride

Duvoid, Urecholine

Class and Category

Pharmacologic class: Cholinergic agonist
Therapeutic class: Urinary tract stimulant

Indications and Dosages

∗ *To treat acute postoperative and postpartum nonobstructive (functional) urine retention; to treat neurogenic atony of bladder with retention*

TABLETS

Adults. 10 to 50 mg 3 or 4 times daily. *To determine minimum effective dose:* 5 to 10 mg repeated every hr until response is obtained or maximum of 50 mg is reached.

Drug Administration

P.O.

- Give drug 1 hr before or 2 hr after meals. If taken soon after eating, nausea and vomiting may occur.

Route	Onset	Peak	Duration
P.O.	30 min	60–90 min	1 hr

Half-life: Unknown

Mechanism of Action

Acts directly on muscarinic receptors of the parasympathetic nervous system, increasing detrusor muscle tone in the bladder and allowing contraction strong enough to start voiding. Like natural neurotransmitter acetylcholine, bethanechol stimulates gastric motility, increases gastric tone, and enhances peristalsis.

Contraindications

Acute inflammatory lesions of GI tract, bronchial asthma, coronary artery disease, epilepsy, hypersensitivity to bethanechol or its components, hyperthyroidism, marked vagotonia, mechanical obstruction of GI or GU tract, Parkinson's disease, peptic ulcer disease, peritonitis, pronounced bradycardia or hypotension, questionable integrity of GI or GU mucosa, spastic GI disorders, vasomotor instability

Interactions

DRUGS

cholinergic drugs: Possibly increased effects of bethanechol
ganglionic blockers: Possibly severe hypotension, usually first manifested by severe adverse GI reactions
procainamide, quinidine: Possibly decreased effects of bethanechol

Adverse Reactions

CNS: Headache, malaise
CV: **Hypotension** with reflex tachycardia, vasomotor response
EENT: Excessive salivation, lacrimation, miosis

GI: Abdominal cramps, colicky pain, diarrhea, eructation, nausea, vomiting
GU: Urinary urgency
RESP: **Asthma attack, bronchoconstriction**

Childbearing Considerations

PREGNANCY

- It is not known if drug can cause fetal harm.
- Use with caution only if benefit to mother outweighs potential risk to fetus.

LACTATION

- It is not known if drug is present in breast milk.
- A decision should be made to discontinue breastfeeding or the drug to avoid potential serious adverse reactions in the breastfed infant.

Nursing Considerations

! **WARNING** Be aware that patient must have a functioning urinary sphincter because a sphincter that doesn't relax when bladder contracts can push urine upward into renal pelvis and cause reflux infection.

- Assess urine elimination before starting bethanechol therapy to attain a baseline. Then monitor patient's voiding pattern and check for urinary retention after voiding to determine effectiveness of drug.

! **WARNING** Monitor patient's respiratory status for bronchoconstriction that could lead to an asthma attack. If patient develops difficulty breathing and wheezing, notify prescriber at once and provide supportive care, as needed and ordered to relieve bronchoconstriction.

PATIENT TEACHING

- Instruct patient how to administer bethanechol.
- Tell patient to notify prescriber or seek urgent care if unable to void.

! **WARNING** Alert patient that drug may cause difficulty breathing and wheezing. If present, stress importance of stopping drug and seeking immediate medical care.

- Inform mothers breastfeeding should not be done during drug therapy.

bexagliflozin

Brenzavvy

Class and Category

Pharmacologic class: Sodium-glucose co-transporter 2 (SGLT2) inhibitor
Therapeutic class: Antidiabetic

Indications and Dosages

∗ *As adjunct to diet and exercise to improve glycemic control in patients with type 2 diabetes mellitus*

TABLETS

Adults. 20 mg once daily in morning.

Drug Administration

P.O.

- Administer in morning with or without food, ideally taken at the same time each day.
- Tablet should not be crushed or chewed.

Route	Onset	Peak	Duration
P.O.	Unknown.	2–4 hr.	Unknown

Half-life: 12 hrs

Mechanism of Action

Inhibits sodium-glucose co-transporter 2 in the kidneys (where the majority of glucose absorption from the renal glomerular filtrate occurs in the proximal tubule), thereby preventing glucose reabsorption. This decreases blood glucose levels.

Contraindications

Dialysis therapy, hypersensitivity to bexagliflozin or its components

Interactions

DRUGS

insulin, insulin secretagogues: Increased risk of hypoglycemia
lithium: Possibly decreased serum lithium concentrations
UGT enzyme inducers: Possibly significant reduction in exposure to bexagliflozin, reducing its effectiveness.

Adverse Reactions

CNS: Polydipsia
CV: Elevated low-density lipoprotein cholesterol
ENDO: **Hypoglycemia, ketoacidosis**
GU: Decreased estimated glomerular filtration rate, elevated serum creatinine

levels, genital mycotic infections, **necrotizing fasciitis of perineum (Fournier's gangrene)**, nocturia, polyuria, **pyelonephritis**, urinary urgency, **urosepsis**, UTI
MS: Lower limb amputation
SKIN: Dermatitis, rash
Other: Volume depletion

Childbearing Considerations

PREGNANCY

- Drug may cause adverse renal effects in developing fetuses according to animal studies.
- Drug is not recommended for use during the second and third trimester of pregnancy.

LACTATION

- It is not known if drug is present in breast milk.
- Mothers should not breastfeed while taking this drug because kidney maturation continues through the first 2 years of life.

Nursing Considerations

! WARNING Use is not recommended for patients who have type 1 diabetes mellitus due to increased risk of diabetic ketoacidosis.

- Assess patient's volume status and correct, if needed and ordered, prior to starting bexagliflozin therapy because drug can cause intravascular volume contraction leading to symptomatic hypotension and acute kidney injury. Continue to monitor patient throughout therapy for dehydration and renal dysfunction. Patients at highest risk include the elderly and patients with chronic renal insufficiency, congestive heart failure, and hypovolemia or patients who take loop diuretics. Notify prescriber immediately if patient has fluid losses or reduced oral intake increasing risk of acute kidney injury. Expect drug to be temporarily withheld until fluid balance is restored.
- Obtain serum creatinine level, as ordered, prior to starting bexagliflozin therapy to obtain a baseline of renal function. Know that drug is not recommended for patients with an eGFR <30 ml/min. Be aware that the elderly and patients with existing impaired renal function are at higher risk for adverse renal effects. Continue to monitor renal function throughout therapy, as ordered.

! WARNING Monitor patient for hypersensitivity reactions because anaphylaxis and angioedema have occurred with other SGLT2 inhibitors. If present, withhold drug, notify prescriber immediately, and be prepared to provide emergency supportive care, as needed and ordered.

! WARNING Monitor patient closely for ketoacidosis that have occurred in patients with diabetes taking bexagliflozin. Be aware that ketoacidosis can become life-threatening quickly even when blood glucose levels are less than 250 mg/dl. Notify prescriber immediately if ketoacidosis is suspected and expect drug to be discontinued. Be prepared to treat patient's ketoacidosis, as ordered. Be aware that patients at higher risk include patients with a history of alcohol abuse or who have a pancreatic insulin deficiency from any cause or have reduced caloric intake. Expect drug to be temporarily discontinued if patient must undergo prolonged fasting due to acute illness or for at least 3 days prior to surgery.

! WARNING Know that bexagliflozin increases risk of fractures, lower-limb amputation, and sepsis or septic shock events. Monitor patient closely.

! WARNING Monitor patient for a rare but life-threatening necrotizing infection of the perineum called Fournier's gangrene. Notify prescriber immediately if patient develops erythema, pain, swelling or tenderness in the genital or perineal area, along with fever or malaise. Expect treatment with broad-spectrum antibiotics and, if needed, surgical debridement of the area. Expect bexagliflozin to be discontinued if this occurs. Monitor patient's blood glucose levels closely and expect an alternative treatment for glycemic control.

- Monitor patient's cholesterol level throughout bexagliflozin therapy because drug may increase low-density lipoprotein cholesterol.
- Be aware that patients receiving insulin or insulin secretagogues may require a lower dose of these agents because bexagliflozin used in combination increases the risk of hypoglycemia. Monitor patient closely for hypoglycemia. If present, treat according to standard of care and notify prescriber.

- Monitor patients for genital mycotic infections or urinary tract infections, especially those with a history of such. If present, notify prescriber and treat, as prescribed.
- Be aware bexagliflozin increases urinary glucose excretion and will lead to positive urine glucose tests. Use only blood tests to monitor glucose control. Also, know that measurements using 1,5-AG assay is not recommended because it is unreliable in the presence of SGLT2 inhibitors such as bexagliflozin. Other methods should be used to monitor the patient's glycemic control.

PATIENT TEACHING

- Inform patient that bexagliflozin is not a replacement for diet and exercise therapy.
- Instruct patient how to administer bexagliflozin.
- Advise patient to maintain adequate fluid intake throughout bexagliflozin therapy. However, tell patient to notify prescriber if he is unable to take a normal amount of daily fluids due to fasting or illness or experiences an excessive loss of fluids from perspiration or gastrointestinal illnesses as drug may need to be temporarily withheld. Stress importance of paying attention to signs of dehydration and seeking medical attention quickly.

! **WARNING** Alert patient that drug may cause a serious allergic reaction. If patient experiences swelling of eyes, face, throat, or tongue or other serious allergic reactions such as hives, immediate emergency treatment should be sought.

! **WARNING** Review signs and symptoms of ketoacidosis with patient and urge him to seek immediate medical attention, if present, even if blood glucose level is less than 250 mg/dl.

- Educate patient also taking insulin or insulin secretagogues on the signs and symptoms of hypoglycemia and emergency treatment. Advise patient to notify prescriber if hypoglycemia occurs frequently or is severe.
- Advise patient of the importance of maintaining adequate fluid intake to prevent dehydration that can lead to dizziness, light-headednesss, and even fainting upon rising from a supine position. If symptoms of dehydration occur, tell patient to rise slowly from a lying or sitting position and to alert the prescriber.
- Instruct patient to notify prescriber of persistent, severe, or unusual adverse reactions.
- Tell patient to take fall precautions and other safety measures because bexagliflozin increases risk for fractures.
- Tell patient to monitor blood glucose level using blood tests instead of urine tests because drug increases urinary glucose excretion and will lead to positive urine glucose tests.
- Advise female patients of childbearing age to notify prescriber if pregnancy occurs as the drug is not recommended during the second and third trimester of pregnancy.
- Inform mothers that breastfeeding should not be undertaken during bexagliflozin therapy.
- Instruct patient on the importance of routine foot care. Tell patient to watch for any new pain or tenderness, sores or ulcers, or infections involving the leg or foot and to see immediate medical attention if present.

bezlotoxumab

Zinplava

Class and Category

Pharmacologic class: Monoclonal antibody
Therapeutic class: Clostridium difficile recurrence inhibitor

Indications and Dosages

* *To reduce recurrence of* Clostridium difficile *infection (CDI) in patients who are receiving antibacterial drug treatment for CDI and are at a high risk for CDI recurrence*

I.V. INFUSION

Adults and children ages 1 and older. 10 mg/kg infused over 60 min as a single dose.

Drug Administration

I.V.

- Prepare diluted solution immediately after removal of the vial(s) from refrigerator. Alternatively, drug can be left at room temperature (no longer than 24 hr) prior to dilution but it must be protected from light.

- Vial contents should appear clear to moderately opalescent, colorless to pale yellow. Do not use if solution is discolored or contains visible particles.
- Dilute by withdrawing the required volume from drug vial based on patient's weight in kg and transfer into an intravenous bag containing either 0.9% Sodium Chloride Injection or 5% Dextrose Injection with a final concentration ranging from 1 to 10 mg/ml.
- Mix diluted solution by gentle inversion. Do not shake.
- Store diluted solution at room temperature up to 16 hr or under refrigeration for up to 24 hr prior to administration. If refrigerated, allow the intravenous bag to come to room temperature before administering. Do not allow total time following mixture, including duration of infusion, to exceed 16 hr if kept at room temperature or 24 hr if refrigerated.
- Use a low-protein binding, nonpyrogenic, sterile 0.2-micron to 5-micron in-line or add-on filter and infuse over 60 min.
- May be infused through a central line or peripheral catheter. Do not administer as an intravenous bolus or push.
- *Incompatibilities:* Other drugs infused simultaneously through same infusion line

Route	Onset	Peak	Duration
I.V.	Unknown	Unknown	Unknown

Half-life: 19 days

Mechanism of Action

Binds to *C. difficile* toxin B and neutralizes its effects.

Contraindications

Hypersensitivity to bezlotoxumab or its components

Interactions

DRUGS

None reported by manufacturer.

Adverse Reactions

CNS: Fever, headache
CV: **Heart failure**, **ventricular tachyarrhythmia**
GI: Nausea
Other: Anti-bezlotoxumab antibodies, infusion-related reactions (dizziness, dyspnea, fatigue, fever, headache, hypertension, nausea)

Childbearing Considerations

PREGNANCY

- It is not known if drug can cause fetal harm.
- Use with caution only if benefit to mother outweighs potential risk to fetus.

LACTATION

- It is not known if drug is present in breast milk.
- Mothers should check with prescriber before breastfeeding.

Nursing Considerations

- Be aware that bezlotoxumab alone is not to be used to treat *C. difficile* infection (CDI), as it is not an antibacterial drug. It should only be used in conjunction with antibacterial drug treatment of CDI.

! **WARNING** Use with extreme caution in patients with a history of congestive heart failure, as drug may exacerbate congestive heart failure and may become severe enough to cause death. Notify prescriber immediately if signs and symptoms of congestive heart failure occur and expect to provide supportive care, as needed and ordered.

- Monitor patient for adverse reactions, especially infusion reactions that may include dizziness, dyspnea, fatigue, fever, hypertension, and nausea. Know that these reactions usually resolve within 24 hours.

PATIENT TEACHING

- Remind patient that bezlotoxumab does not take the place of the prescribed antibacterial therapy. Reinforce need to continue taking the antibacterial agent as prescribed.
- Tell patient drug will be administered as an I.V. infusion as a single dose.
- Reassure patient that although infusion reactions may occur, they usually resolve within 24 hours and are not usually serious.

! **WARNING** Urge patient to seek immediate medical attention if signs and symptoms of congestive heart failure occur.

bimekizumab-bkzx

Bimzelx

Class and Category

Pharmacologic class: Humanized interleukin-17A and F antagonist
Therapeutic class: Anti-psoriatic agent

Indications and Dosages

✱ *To treat moderate to severe plaque psoriasis in patients who are candidates for phototherapy or systemic therapy*

SUBCUTANEOUS INJECTION

Adults. *Initial:* 320 mg at wk 0, 4, 8, 12, and 16 followed by 320 mg (two 160-mg injections) every 8 wk.

±**DOSAGE ADJUSTMENT** For patients weighing 120 kg (264 lb) or greater, dosage frequency may be decreased to every 4 wk after wk 16.

✱ *To treat active psoriatic arthritis, to treat non-radiographic axial spondyloarthritis, to treat ankylosing spondylitis*

SUBCUTANEOUS INJECTION

Adults. 160 mg every 4 wk.

±**DOSAGE ADJUSTMENT** For patients with coexisting moderate to severe plaque psoriasis, dosage for plaque psoriasis is used.

✱ *To treat hidradenitis suppurativa*

SUBCUTANEOUS INJECTION

Adults. 320 mg at wk 0, 2, 4, 6, 8, 10, 12, 14, and 16, followed by 320 mg every 4 wk.

Drug Administration

SUBCUTANEOUS

- Remove drug carton from refrigerator and wait for 30 to 45 minutes to allow drug to reach room temperature before removing the prefilled syringe or autoinjector from carton to protect drug from light. Do not shake drug.
- Solution should be clear to slightly opalescent and colorless to pale brownish-yellow. Discard if solution contains visible particles, is discolored, or appears cloudy.
- If administering a 320 mg dose using the single-dose prefilled syringe or single-dose prefilled autoinjector containing only 160 mg/ml of the drug, 2 injections will be necessary. The drug is available as a 320 mg/2ml in a single-dose prefilled syringe or single-dose prefilled autoinjector requiring only 1 injection.
- Inject subcutaneously in locations such as the abdomen, thighs, or upper arm (back). If using abdomen, do not inject within 5 cm (2 in) of the navel or into areas where skin is affected by psoriasis or is bruised, hard, red, scaly, tender, or thick. If two injections are being given to achieve the dose, administer in two different anatomic locations.
- If a dose is missed, administer the dose as soon as possible and then resume dosing at the regularly scheduled interval.
- Store cartons of drug in refrigerator 2°C to 8°C (36°F to 46°F), or the prefilled syringes or autoinjectors may be stored at room temperature up to 30 days and then must be discarded, if not used. However, once the drug has reached room temperature, it should not be put back into the refrigerator.

Route	Onset	Peak	Duration
SubQ	Unknown	3–4 days	Unknown

Half-life: 23 days

Mechanism of Action

Inhibits the release of proinflammatory cytokines (IL-17A and IL-17F) and chemokines (IL-AF) selectively to improve psoriatic signs and symptoms.

Contraindications

Hypersensitivity to bimekizumab-bkzx or its components

Interactions

DRUGS

CYP450 substrates: Possibly modulation of the serum levels of some cytokines affecting effectiveness or drug concentration of the CYP450 substrates
live vaccines: Increased risk of serious infection

Adverse Reactions

CNS: Fatigue, fever, headache, **suicidal ideation**
EENT: Esophageal or oral candidiasis, nasopharnygitis, oropharyngeal pain, otitis externa or media, stomatitis
GI: Diarrhea, elevated alkaline phosphatase, bilirubin, and liver enzymes; gastroenteritis; inflammatory bowel disease
GU: Genital candidiasis, UTI, vulvovaginal candidiasis, vulvovaginal mycotic infection
HEME: **Neutropenia**

RESP: Bronchitis, upper respiratory infection
SKIN: Acne, eczema, folliculitis, skin candida, tinea infections
Other: Herpes simplex infections and other infections, injection site reactions (bruising, edema, erythema, pain, swelling)

Childbearing Considerations

PREGNANCY

Pregnancy exposure registry: 1-877-311-8972 or http://mothertobaby.org/pregnancy-studies/.

- It is not known if drug may cause fetal harm although the human IgG antibody does cross to the placenta increasingly as pregnancy progresses and peaks during the third trimester.
- Use with caution only if benefit to mother outweighs potential risk to fetus.

LACTATION

- It is not known if drug is present in breast milk.
- Mother should check with prescriber before breastfeeding.

Nursing Considerations

- Ensure that patient has been checked for tuberculosis (TB) infection before bimekizumab-bkzx therapy is begun. Be aware that bimekizumab-bkzx should not be administered to a patient with an active TB infection. Expect treatment for latent TB to be initiated before drug therapy is begun. Closely monitor patient throughout therapy for signs and symptoms of active TB before and after drug therapy.

! **WARNING** Be aware that patients with active liver disease or cirrhosis should not receive bimekizumab-bkzx therapy because drug may cause severe hepatic injury in these patients. Expect liver function to be evaluated before bimekizumab-bkzx is begun in all other patients with values of alkaline phosphatase, bilirubin, and liver enzymes obtained. Continue to monitor liver function periodically throughout drug therapy, as ordered and report any elevations in laboratory results. Monitor patient for signs and symptoms of liver dysfunction and notify prescriber if suspected. Expect drug to be to be withheld until it is determined liver injury has not occurred because of the drug.

! **WARNING** Know that patients with active inflammatory bowel disease should not receive bimekizumab-bkzx. Monitor other patients for signs and symptoms of inflammatory bowel disease. If new onset or worsening of signs and symptoms occurs, notify prescriber and expect drug to be discontinued.

! **WARNING** Know that bimekizumab-bkzx therapy increases the risk of infection and should not be initiated in a patient with a serious active infection until the infection resolves or is adequately treated. Institute infection control measures. Monitor patient for signs and symptoms of infection throughout therapy and notify prescriber if infection is suspected. Expect drug to be withheld during treatment for the infection.

- Check that patient is up to date on immunization before bimekizumab-bkzx therapy is begun. Do not administer any live vaccines to patient while receiving drug.

! **WARNING** Use with extreme caution in patients with severe depression or a history of suicidal ideation because higher rates of suicidal ideation have occurred in patients treated with bimekizumab-bkzx. Monitor patient closely for suicidal ideation or behavior. If present, notify prescriber and know that the drug may be discontinued.

PATIENT TEACHING

- Instruct patient or family or caregiver how to administer a bimekizumab-bkzx subcutaneous injection if drug will be administered at home. Tell patient what to do if a dose is missed.

! **WARNING** Advise patient and family or caregiver to be alert for signs of depression, worsening depression, suicidal ideation, or other mood changes. If present, stress importance of seeking medical attention promptly.

- Review infection control measures to follow during bimekizumab-bkzx therapy. Also, instruct patient to notify prescriber if signs and symptoms of infection occur as drug may need to be withheld during treatment of the infection.

- Inform patient and family or caregiver of the possibility of drug adversely affecting liver function. Review signs and symptoms of liver dysfunction and stress importance of notifying prescriber if present. Encourage patient to be compliant with laboratory appointments.
- Instruct patient on the signs and symptoms of inflammatory bowel disease and to alert prescriber if a new onset or worsening of signs and symptoms occurs.
- Advise patient not to receive any live vaccines while taking bimekizumab-bkzx. Instruct mothers who received drug during pregnancy to alert pediatrician to withhold live virus immunizations for a minimum of 4 months after baby's birth.

bisoprolol fumarate

Class and Category

Pharmacologic class: Beta$_1$-adrenergic blocker
Therapeutic class: Antihypertensive

Indications and Dosages

✱ *To treat hypertension, alone or with other antihypertensives*

TABLETS

Adults. 2.5 to 5 mg daily, increased to 10 to 20 mg daily if blood pressure doesn't respond to lower dosage.

± **DOSAGE ADJUSTMENT** For patients who have bronchospastic disease; for patients with impaired renal function and creatinine clearance less than 40 ml/min; or for patients who have impaired hepatic function, as from cirrhosis or hepatitis, dosage reduced to 2.5 mg daily initially and then increased gradually.

Drug Administration

P.O.

- Store at room temperature.
- Keep in tight container to protect from moisture.

Route	Onset	Peak	Duration
P.O.	1–2 hr	2–4 hr	Unknown

Half-life: 9–12 hr

Mechanism of Action

Inhibits stimulation of beta$_1$-receptors primarily in the heart, which decreases cardiac excitability, cardiac output, and myocardial oxygen demand. Bisoprolol also decreases renin release from kidneys, which helps reduce blood pressure.

Contraindications

Cardiogenic shock, hypersensitivity to bisoprolol or its components, overt heart failure, second- or third-degree heart block, sinus bradycardia

Interactions

DRUGS

antiarrhythmics, such as disopyramide; calcium channel blockers, such as diltiazem, verapamil: Increased risk of conduction delay and decreased heart rate
beta-blockers, digoxin: Increased risk of bradycardia
catecholamine-depleting drugs, such as guanethidine, reserpine: Increased risk of bradycardia or hypotension
clonidine: Possibly severe hypertension from withdrawal of clonidine or both drugs
rifampin: Possibly increased bisoprolol metabolism with decreased bisoprolol effects

Adverse Reactions

CNS: Anxiety, confusion, depression, dizziness, emotional lability, fatigue, fever, hallucinations, headache, insomnia, malaise, nightmares, paresthesia, sleep disturbances, syncope, tremor, unsteadiness, vertigo
CV: **Bradycardia, heart block, and other arrhythmias**; chest pain; claudication; edema; **heart failure**; hypercholesterolemia; hyperlipidemia; **hypotension**; **MI**; orthostatic hypotension; palpitations; peripheral vascular insufficiency
EENT: Altered taste, blurred vision, dry mouth, eye pain or pressure, hearing loss, increased salivation, **laryngospasm**, pharyngitis, rhinitis, sinusitis, tinnitus
GI: Constipation, diarrhea, epigastric pain, gastritis, indigestion, **ischemic colitis**, **mesenteric artery thrombosis**, nausea, vomiting
GU: Cystitis, decreased libido, impotence, Peyronie's disease, **renal artery thrombosis**, renal colic
HEME: **Agranulocytosis**, eosinophilia, **leukopenia**, **thrombocytopenia**, **thrombocytopenic purpura**
MS: Arthralgia, cold extremities, gout, muscle twitching, neck pain

RESP: **Asthma**, bronchitis, **bronchospasm**, cough, dyspnea, **respiratory distress**, upper respiratory tract infection
SKIN: Alopecia, dermatitis, diaphoresis, eczema, **exfoliative dermatitis**, flushing, pruritus, psoriasis, rash
Other: **Angioedema**, **hyperkalemia**, hyperuricemia, weight gain

Childbearing Considerations

PREGNANCY

- It is not known if drug can cause fetal harm.
- Use with caution only if benefit to mother outweighs potential risk to fetus.

LACTATION

- It is not known if drug is present in breast milk.
- Mothers should check with prescriber before breastfeeding.

Nursing Considerations

- Administer bisoprolol cautiously in patients with peripheral vascular disease because reduced cardiac output can cause or worsen arterial insufficiency. Assess patient's arms and legs for changes in color and temperature; check pulses; and ask about numbness, pain, and tingling.
- Measure blood pressure with patient lying, sitting, and standing before starting bisoprolol and then every 4 to 8 hours, as appropriate, to evaluate effectiveness. If systolic blood pressure falls to less than 90 mm Hg during drug therapy, notify prescriber as dosage may need to be reduced or drug discontinued.

! **WARNING** Monitor patient for hypersensitivity reactions such as angioedema or other serious reactions because drug can adversely affect many body systems which could cause life-threatening adverse effects such as angioedema and laryngospasm, arrythmias including heart block, hematologic disturbances, hyperkalemia, hypotension, mesenteric or renal artery thrombosis, MI, respiratory distress, or severe skin disorder. Notify prescriber immediately if a serious adverse reaction occurs including hypersensitivity and provide supportive care, as needed and ordered. Expect drug to be discontinued and replaced with a different type of drug.

! **WARNING** Avoid abrupt discontinuation of bisoprolol in patients with coronary artery disease because serious cardiovascular adverse reactions may be precipitated such as angina pectoris, MI, or ventricular arrhythmia. Also, avoid abrupt withdrawal of bisoprolol in patients with hyperthyroidism because doing so may cause or worsen thyroid storm. When drug is to be discontinued, expect it to be slowly discontinued over 1 to 2 weeks.

- Monitor patient with diabetes because bisoprolol may mask signs of hypoglycemia. Also monitor patient with hyperthyroidism closely because bisoprolol may mask signs of hypertension and tachycardia if condition worsens.
- Be aware that chronic beta-blocker therapy, such as bisoprolol, is not routinely withheld prior to major surgery because the benefits outweigh the risks associated with its use with general anesthesia and surgical procedures.

PATIENT TEACHING

- Instruct patient how to administer bisoprolol.
- Teach patient how to monitor blood pressure, if appropriate, and to recognize signs of hypertension and hypotension.

! **WARNING** Caution patient not to abruptly stop taking bisoprolol because serious or even life-threatening adverse reactions may occur. Encourage patient to discuss any concerns or questions with prescriber and not to alter dosage or frequency of administration without prescriber knowledge.

! **WARNING** Alert patient that bisoprolol may cause an allergic reaction as well as possibly adversely affect various body systems. Stress importance of notifying prescriber of persistent, severe, or unusual adverse reactions, including allergic reactions. If allergic or other adverse reactions become severe, tell patient to seek immediate medical care.

- Instruct patient to avoid sudden position changes and to rise slowly from a lying or sitting position to minimize the effects of orthostatic hypotension.

- Advise patient to avoid driving and other activities that require mental alertness until bisoprolol's CNS effects are known and resolved.
- Instruct patient to contact prescriber before using any over-the-counter product, such as a cold remedy or nasal decongestant.

bivalirudin

Angiomax, Angiomax RTU

Class and Category

Pharmacologic class: Direct thrombin inhibitor
Therapeutic class: Anticoagulant

Indications and Dosages

* *To provide anticoagulation in patients undergoing percutaneous coronary intervention (PCI), including patients with heparin-induced thrombocytopenia and patients with heparin-induced thrombocytopenia and thrombosis syndrome*

I.V. INFUSION, I.V. INJECTION

Adults. *Initial:* Immediately before procedure, 0.75-mg/kg bolus; then 1.75-mg/kg/hr infusion for duration of procedure. Five min after bolus dose and with continuous infusion running, another 0.3-mg/kg bolus may be given, as needed. After procedure, 1.75 mg/kg/hr may be continued for up to 4 hr for patients with ST segment elevation MI (STEMI).

±**DOSAGE ADJUSTMENT** For patients with severe renal impairment (eGFR less than 30 ml/min), infusion dosage reduced to 1 mg/kg/hr; for patients on hemodialysis, dosage reduced to 0.25 mg/kg/hr.

Drug Administration

I.V.

- Expect to give 300 to 325 mg of aspirin P.O. daily with bivalirudin therapy.

Angiomax

- Thaw frozen premixed solution at room temperature or under refrigeration. Do not thaw by bath immersion or in microwave.
- For bolus dose and continuous infusion, reconstitute by adding 5 ml Sterile Water for Injection to 250-mg vial and swirl gently until dissolved. Solution should appear slightly opalescent, colorless to slightly yellow.
- Withdraw and discard 5 ml from a 50-ml infusion bag of either 0.9% Sodium Chloride Injection or 5% Dextrose in Water. Then, add reconstituted contents of vial to infusion bag to yield 5 mg/ml.
- Use diluted solution to administer bolus dose first and then immediately follow with a continuous infusion at a rate of 1.75 mg/kg/hr. After 5 min, administer another reduced bolus, as needed, with continuous infusion running.
- If a low-rate infusion is ordered following initial infusion, dilute reconstituted drug in 500 ml of 0.9% Sodium Chloride Injection or 5% Dextrose in Water to yield a final concentration of 0.5 mg/ml.

Angiomax RTU

- Store in refrigerator. Remove only when ready to administer.
- This form need not be reconstituted or diluted.
- Administer initial bolus followed by the continuous infusion at a rate of 1.75 mg/kg/hr. After 5 min another reduced bolus may be given, as needed, with continuous infusion running.
- *Incompatibilities for both products:* Alteplase, amiodarone, amphotericin B, chlorpromazine HCl, diazepam, dobutamine, prochlorperazine edisylate, reteplase, streptokinase, vancomycin HCl

Route	Onset	Peak	Duration
I.V.	Rapid	Immediate	1 hr after end of infusion

Half-life: 25 min

Mechanism of Action

Binds selectively to thrombin, including thrombin trapped in established clots. Without thrombin, fibrinogen can not convert to fibrin, producing an anticoagulation effect.

Contraindications

Active major bleeding, hypersensitivity to bivalirudin or its components

Interactions

DRUGS

glycoprotein IIb/IIIa inhibitors, heparin, thrombolytics, warfarin: Risk of bleeding

Adverse Reactions

CNS: Headache, **intracranial hemorrhage**

CV: **Acute stent thrombosis (patients with ST segment elevation myocardial infarction), cardiac tamponade, hypotension, thrombosis during PCI**
EENT: Epistaxis, gingival bleeding
GI: Abdominal cramps, diarrhea, **GI or retroperitoneal bleeding**, nausea, vomiting
GU: Hematuria, vaginal bleeding
HEME: **Absence of anticoagulant effect, bleeding events**, decreased hemoglobin, **increased INR, severe bleeding**
MS: Back pain
RESP: Hemoptysis, **hemothorax, pulmonary hemorrhage**
SKIN: Ecchymosis
Other: **Anaphylaxis**, antibody formation to bivalirudin, injection-site bleeding, hematoma, or pain

Childbearing Considerations

PREGNANCY

- It is not known if drug can cause fetal harm.
- Use with caution only if benefit to mother outweighs potential risk to fetus.

LABOR AND DELIVERY

- Drug should not be used during labor and delivery because of the potential for drug-induced hemorrhage during delivery.

LACTATION

- It is not known if drug is present in breast milk.
- Mothers should check with prescriber before breastfeeding.

Nursing Considerations

- Be aware drug should be given with aspirin.

! **WARNING** Monitor blood coagulation tests before and regularly during therapy; bleeding is a major bivalirudin risk. Be aware that drug affects international normalized ratio (INR), so INR may not be useful for determining an appropriate warfarin dose.

! **WARNING** Monitor patient often for bleeding because there's no antidote for bivalirudin. All patients with unexplained drop in blood pressure or hematocrit should be evaluated for bleeding. If life-threatening bleeding occurs, notify prescriber immediately, stop drug, and monitor APTT and other coagulation tests as ordered. Blood transfusions may be needed. Patients with increased bleeding risk include menstruating females; patients with large vessel or lumbar puncture; major bleeding (including GI, intracranial, intraocular, pulmonary bleeding, or retroperitoneal); major surgery (including brain, eye, or spinal cord); organ biopsy; recent stroke; or spinal anesthesia; and patients with organ or vascular abnormalities, such as advanced renal disease, dissecting aortic aneurysm, diverticulitis, hemophilia, hepatic disease (especially from deficient vitamin K–dependent clotting factors), infective endocarditis, inflammatory bowel disease, peptic ulcer disease, or severe uncontrolled hypertension. These patients should be monitored more frequently for bleeding. Patients with unstable angina also may experience major bleeding events, such as intracranial bleeding, retroperitoneal bleeding, or a drop in hemoglobin of 3 g/dl or more.

! **WARNING** Know that if patient is receiving gamma brachytherapy, watch closely for evidence of thrombosis (absent or weak pulse, pain, pallor); use of bivalirudin may increase the risk in these patients.

! **WARNING** Monitor patient for hypersensitivity reactions that could become life-threatening such as anaphylaxis. If present, notify prescriber immediately and provide supportive care, as needed and ordered.

- Institute bleeding precautions such as avoiding I.M. or subcutaneous injections of any kind, if possible, to decrease the risk of bleeding.

PATIENT TEACHING

- Inform patient that bivalirudin is a blood thinner administered only in the hospital through an I.V.

! **WARNING** Alert patient that bivalirudin may cause an allergic reaction and to inform staff immediately if adverse reactions occur.

! **WARNING** Inform patient that bivalirudin increases risk of bleeding. Urge patient to check her skin for bruising or red spots and to immediately report dizziness, fainting, stomach pain, trouble breathing, and unusual bleeding (black, tarry stool; blood in urine; coughing blood; heavy menses; nosebleeds). Drug may have to be stopped.

B

- Encourage patient to reduce the risk of injury while receiving bivalirudin, such as by brushing her teeth gently with a soft-bristled toothbrush.
- Caution patient not to take anti-inflammatories, such as aspirin or aspirin-like products, ibuprofen, ketoprofen, and naproxen, or other blood thinners, such as warfarin, while receiving bivalirudin, unless directed.

brexpiprazole

Rexulti

Class and Category

Pharmacologic class: Atypical antipsychotic
Therapeutic class: Antipsychotic

Indications and Dosages

✱ As adjunct treatment of major depressive disorder

TABLETS

Adults. *Initial:* 0.5 or 1 mg once daily, then increased to 1 or 2 mg once daily after 1 wk. Further increased in 1-mg increments weekly, as needed. *Maximum:* 3 mg once daily.

✱ To treat schizophrenia

TABLETS

Adults. *Initial:* 1 mg once daily for 4 days, followed by 2 mg once daily for 3 days, then increased to 4 mg once daily. *Maximum:* 4 mg once daily.

Adolescents ages 13 and older. *Initial:* 0.5 mg once daily on days 1 to 4, followed by 1 mg once daily on days 5 to 7, then 2 mg once daily beginning on day 8 and onward. Increased in 1-mg increments weekly, as needed. *Maximum:* 4 mg once daily.

✱ To treat agitation associated with dementia due to Alzheimer's disease

TABLETS

Adults. *Initial:* 0.5 mg once daily on days 1 to 7 followed by 1 mg on days 8 through 14, then 2 mg once daily on day 15 and thereafter. Increased to 3 mg once daily after at least 14 days, as needed. *Maximum:* 3 mg once daily.

±**DOSAGE ADJUSTMENT** For patients with moderate to severe hepatic impairment or renal impairment (creatinine clearance less than 60 ml/min), maximum dosage should not exceed 2 mg once daily for patients with major depressive disorder or for agitation associated with dementia due to Alzheimer's disease and 3 mg for patients with schizophrenia. For patients who are poor CYP2D6 metabolizers or for patients taking strong CYP2D6 or CYP3A4 inhibitors, dosage reduced by 50%. For patients who are poor CYP2D6 metabolizers also taking moderate to strong CYP3A4 inhibitors or for patients taking both a moderate to strong CYP2D6 inhibitor and a moderate to strong CYP3A4 inhibitor, dosage reduced by 75%. For patients taking strong CYP3A4 inducers, dosage doubled over 1 to 2 weeks.

Drug Administration

P.O.

- Store at room temperature.

Route	Onset	Peak	Duration
P.O.	Unknown	4 hr	Unknown

Half-life: 91 hr

Mechanism of Action

May produce antipsychotic effects through partial agonist and antagonist actions. Brexpiprazole acts as a partial agonist at dopamine (especially D_2) receptors and serotonin (especially 5-HT1A) receptors. The drug acts as an antagonist at 5-HT2A serotonin receptor sites.

Contraindications

Hypersensitivity to brexpiprazole or its components

Interactions

DRUGS

clarithromycin, itraconazole, ketoconazole, and other strong CYP3A4 inhibitors; combination of a strong CYP3A4 inhibitor/strong CYP2D6 inhibitor (itraconazole/quinidine), moderate CYP3A4 inhibitor/strong CYP2D6 inhibitor (fluconazole/paroxetine), strong CYP3A4 inhibitor/moderate CYP2D6 inhibitor (itraconazole/duloxetine), moderate CYP3A4 inhibitor/moderate CYP2D6 inhibitor (fluconazole/duloxetine) fluoxetine, paroxetine, quinidine, and other strong CYP2D6 inhibitors: Increased brexpiprazole

exposure and possibly increased adverse brexpiprazole-related reactions
rifampin, St. John's wort, and other strong CYP3A4 inducers: Decreased brexpiprazole exposure and effectiveness

Adverse Reactions

CNS: Abnormal dreams, akathisia, anxiety, body temperature dysregulation, **CVA**, dizziness, dyskinesia, dystonia, extrapyramidal symptoms, fatigue, headache, impaired cognitive and motor skills, insomnia, **neuroleptic malignant syndrome**, restlessness, **seizures**, somnolence, **suicidal ideation**, syncope, tardive dyskinesia, tremor
CV: Dyslipidemia, orthostatic hypotension
EENT: Blurred vision, dry mouth, excessive salivation, nasopharyngitis
ENDO: Decreased blood cortisol levels, diabetes mellitus, elevated prolactin levels, hyperglycemia
GI: Abdominal pain, constipation, diarrhea, dyspepsia, flatulence, increased appetite, nausea
GU: UTI
HEME: **Agranulocytosis**, **leukopenia**, **neutropenia**
MS: Myalgia
SKIN: Hyperhidrosis
Other: Increased blood creatine phosphokinase level, pathological gambling and other compulsive behaviors, weight gain

Childbearing Considerations

PREGNANCY

- Pregnancy exposure registry: 1-866-961-2388 or http://womensmentalhealth.org/clinical-and-research-programs/pregnancyregistry/.
- It is not known if drug can cause fetal harm. However, extrapyramidal and/or withdrawal symptoms have been reported in neonates whose mothers were exposed to antipsychotic drugs during the third trimester of pregnancy.
- Use with caution only if benefit to mother outweighs potential risk to fetus.

LACTATION

- It is not known if drug is present in breast milk.
- Mothers should check with prescriber before breastfeeding.

Nursing Considerations

! **WARNING** Be aware that brexpiprazole should not be used to treat dementia-related psychosis in the elderly because of an increased risk of death.

- Use brexpiprazole cautiously in patients with a history of seizures or with conditions that lower the seizure threshold. Also, use cautiously in patients at risk for aspiration pneumonia because esophageal dysphagia has been associated with antipsychotic drug use.

! **WARNING** Watch patients closely for suicidal tendencies, especially in adolescents and young adults and particularly when therapy starts and dosage changes because depression may worsen temporarily during these times.

- Monitor patient for the development of dystonia (dyspnea, difficulty swallowing, protrusion of the tongue, and/or spasm of the neck muscles sometimes leading to tightness of the throat), especially during the first few days of treatment. Males and younger age groups are at higher risk for acute dystonia.

! **WARNING** Monitor patient's CBC, as ordered, because serious adverse hematologic reactions, such as agranulocytosis, leukopenia, and neutropenia, may occur with atypical antipsychotic therapy. Assess more often during first few months of therapy if patient has a history of drug-induced leukopenia or neutropenia or a significantly low WBC count. If abnormalities occur during therapy, watch for fever or other signs of infection, notify prescriber and, if severe, expect drug to be stopped.

! **WARNING** Monitor patient's blood glucose level, lipid levels, and weight, as ordered, because atypical antipsychotic drugs, such as brexpiprazole may cause metabolic changes. Monitor blood glucose levels closely because hyperglycemia has become extreme with other atypical antipsychotics, in some cases, causing hyperosmolar coma, ketoacidosis, or even death. Know that even in patients with no history of diabetes mellitus, hyperglycemia may develop.

! **WARNING** Know that antipsychotic drugs may cause neuroleptic malignant syndrome exhibited by altered mental state, autonomic instability, hyperpyrexia, and muscle rigidity. Monitor patient closely throughout brexpiprazole therapy. If suspected, notify prescriber immediately, be prepared to provide emergency supportive care, and expect drug to be discontinued.

- Be aware that atypical antipsychotic drugs such as brexpiprazole can cause orthostatic hypotension and syncope with the risk being the greatest when drug therapy is initiated, and dosage increase occurs. Patients at higher risk include the elderly, patients with a history of cardiovascular or cerebrovascular disease, and patients who also take antihypertensive drugs.
- Monitor patient for tardive dyskinesia, especially in elderly women. Know that it has the potential to be irreversible. The risk for developing tardive dyskinesia increases the longer brexpiprazole is used and the higher the total cumulative dose becomes. However, it may occur even after a somewhat brief time of brexpiprazole therapy and at low doses. It may also occur after the drug has been discontinued. If tardive dyskinesia develops, notify prescriber and expect drug to be discontinued, if possible.

PATIENT TEACHING

- Instruct patient on how to administer brexipiprazole and to follow dosage increases exactly as ordered.

! **WARNING** Tell family or caregiver to watch patient closely for suicidal tendencies, especially when therapy starts or dosage changes.

! **WARNING** Instruct patient on the signs and symptoms of an elevated blood glucose level that could become dangerously high. Tell diabetic patient to monitor blood glucose levels closely. If abnormalities occur, prescriber should be notified.

! **WARNING** Review signs and symptoms of adverse blood reactions and to promptly report to prescriber as some may be come quite serious. Stress importance of complying with laboratory appointments.

- Urge patient to avoid activities that raise body temperature suddenly, such as exposure to extreme heat or strenuous exercise, and to compensate for situations that cause dehydration, such as diarrhea or vomiting.
- Advise patient to get up slowly from a lying or sitting position during brexpiprazole therapy to minimize a drop in blood pressure.
- Instruct patient to avoid hazardous activities until drug's effects are known and resolved. Also, alert patient and family or caregiver of increased risk for falls, especially if patient has other medical conditions or takes medication that may affect the nervous system.
- Advise patient to report any persistent, severe, or unusual signs and symptoms to prescriber, especially abnormal movements.
- Inform patient and family or caregiver that drug may cause intense urges, particularly for gambling, but may also cause binge eating, sexual urges, or uncontrollable shopping as well as other compulsive or impulsive behaviors. These behaviors may not be recognized as abnormal by patient. Urge the reporting of such behaviors, as a dosage reduction or discontinuation of the drug may be required to protect patient from these harmful effects.
- Instruct patient to inform all prescribers of any drugs he's taking, including over-the-counter drugs because of risk of interactions.
- Advise females of childbearing age to notify prescriber if she intends to become or becomes pregnant during therapy.

brodalumab

Siliq

Class and Category

Pharmacologic class: Monoclonal IgG2 antibody
Therapeutic class: Antipsoriatic

Indications and Dosages

✱ *To treat moderate to severe plaque psoriasis in patients who are candidates for phototherapy or systemic therapy and have failed to respond or have lost response to other systemic therapies*

SUBCUTANEOUS INJECTION

Adults. *Initial:* 210 mg followed by 210 mg repeated at wk 1 and 2, and then 210 mg every 2 wk.

Drug Administration

SUBCUTANEOUS

- Allow prefilled syringe to reach room temperature before administering, which is about 30 min. Do not warm any other way and do not remove the gray needle cap on the prefilled syringe while allowing it to reach room temperature.
- Do not shake the prefilled syringe.
- Solution in the pen should appear clear to slightly opalescent, colorless to slightly yellow, and may have a few translucent to white particles. Do not use if cloudy or discolored or if foreign matter is present.
- Do not use the prefilled syringe if it has been dropped on a hard surface.
- Administer only as a subcutaneous injection into the patient's abdomen, thigh, or outer area of upper arm, injecting the full amount in the syringe to provide the correct dosage. Do not rub injection site after administering drug.
- Do not inject into an area that is affected by psoriasis or is bruised, hard, red, scaly, tender, or thick.
- Store in original carton to protect from light in refrigerator or at room temperature. However, do not place back into refrigerator if stored at room temperature; carton must be discarded after 14 days if stored at room temperature.

Route	Onset	Peak	Duration
SubQ	Unknown	3 days	Unknown

Half-life: Unknown

Mechanism of Action

Binds to human IL-17RA and inhibits its interactions with selective cytokines. This inhibits the release of proinflammatory chemokines and cytokines, which are thought to be part of the pathogenesis of plaque psoriasis.

Contraindications

Crohn's disease, hypersensitivity to brodalumab or its components

Interactions

DRUGS

CYP450 substrates, such as cyclosporine or warfarin: Possibly altered effectiveness of these drugs

live vaccines: Failure to produce an adequate immune response

Adverse Reactions

CNS: Headache, fatigue, **suicidal ideation**

EENT: Nasopharyngitis, oropharyngeal pain, pharyngitis

GI: Crohn's disease, diarrhea, nausea

GU: UTI

HEME: **Neutropenia**

MS: Arthralgia, myalgia

RESP: Bronchitis, upper respiratory infections

SKIN: Eczematous eruptions, tinea infections, urticaria

Other: **Anaphylaxis and other hypersenstivity reactions**, anti-brodalumab antibody formation, flu-like symptoms, fungal and other infections, injection-site reactions (bruising, erythema, hemorrhage, pain, pruritus)

Childbearing Considerations

PREGNANCY

- It is not known if drug can cause fetal harm. However, human IgG antibodies are known to cross the placental barrier; therefore, drug may be transmitted from the mother to the fetus.
- Use with caution only if benefit to mother outweighs potential risk to fetus.

LACTATION

- It is not known if drug is present in breast milk.
- Mothers should check with prescriber before breastfeeding.

Nursing Considerations

- Expect patient to be evaluated for tuberculosis (TB) before brodalumab therapy is begun. If present, know that brodalumab should not be initiated until treatment for latent TB has been given. Monitor all patients for signs and symptoms of TB during and after brodalumab therapy.
- Use cautiously in patients with a chronic infection or who have a history of recurrent infections because brodalumab increases the risk of infections, especially fungal infections. If an infection occurs and does

not respond to standard therapy for the infection, expect brodalumab to be withheld until the infection is resolved.

! **WARNING** Know that brodalumab is only available through a restricted program because of its potential to cause suicidal behavior and thoughts. Monitor patient closely and expect drug to be discontinued if suicidal ideation is present.

! **WARNING** Monitor patient closely for hypersensitivity reactions which could become life-threatening such as anaphylaxis. If present, notify prescriber, expect drug to be discontinued, and provide supportive care, as needed and ordered.

- Monitor patient for Crohn's disease and know that brodalumab must be discontinued if patient develops this disease while taking the drug.
- Monitor patient for eczematous eruptions that could become severe and in some cases require hospitalization. If present, notify prescriber as drug may need to be discontinued to resolve the skin condition.
- Avoid administering live vaccines while patient is receiving brodalumab because vaccines may not be effective.

PATIENT TEACHING

- Instruct patient self-administering brodalumab how to administer the drug as a subcutaneous injection.

! **WARNING** Alert patient and family or caregiver that drug may produce suicidal behavior or thoughts. If present, suicide precautions should be undertaken, prescriber notified, and drug discontinued.

! **WARNING** Alert patient that drug may cause an allergic or serious skin reaction. Tell patient to notify prescriber if present and if serious to seek immediate medical care.

- Advise patient to seek medical attention if signs or symptoms of infection occur.
- Tell patient to notify prescriber if persistent or severe bowel problems develop. If Crohn's disease is diagnosed, inform patient that brodalumab therapy must be discontinued.
- Advise patient not to receive live vaccines while taking brodalumab.

budesonide

Entocort EC, Eohilia, Pulmicort Flexhaler, Pulmicort Respules, Rhinocort Allergy, Tarpeyo, Uceris

Class and Category

Pharmacologic class: Corticosteroid
Therapeutic class: Antiasthmatic, anti-inflammatory

Indications and Dosages

∗ *To manage symptoms of perennial or seasonal allergic rhinitis*

NASAL SPRAY (BUDESONIDE)

Adults and children ages 6 and older. *Initial:* 32 mcg (1 spray) in each nostril once daily. *Maintenance:* Lowest dosage that controls symptoms. *Maximum for adults and children ages 12 and over:* 256 mcg once daily administered as 4 sprays (32 mcg/spray) per nostril. *Maximum for children ages 6 to less than 12:* 128 mcg once daily administered as 2 sprays (32 mcg/spray) per nostril.

NASAL SPRAY (RHINOCORT ALLERGY)

Adults and children ages 12 and older. *Initial:* 64 mcg (2 sprays) in each nostril once daily, reduced to 32 mcg (1 spray) in each nostril once daily when symptoms improve. **Children ages 6 to under 12.** *Initial:* 32 mcg (1 spray) in each nostril once daily, increased to 64 mcg (2 sprays) in each nostril once daily, as needed. Once symptoms are under control, dosage reduced back to 32 mcg (1 spray) in each nostril once daily.

∗ *To provide maintenance therapy as prophylactic therapy in asthma*

ORAL INHALATION (PULMICORT FLEXHALER)

Adults and adolescents ages 18 and older. *Initial:* 180 or 360 mcg twice daily, increased as needed. *Maximum:* 720 mcg twice daily. **Children ages 6 to 17.** *Initial:* 180 or 360 mcg twice daily. *Maximum:* 360 mcg twice daily.

NEBULIZED INHALATION (PULMICORT RESPULES)

Children ages 1 to 8 previously on bronchodilators alone. 0.25 mg twice daily by jet nebulizer. Alternatively, 0.5 mg once daily by jet nebulizer. *Maximum:* 0.5 mg/day. **Children ages 1 to 8 previously on inhaled steroids.** 0.25 mg twice daily by jet nebulizer.

Alternatively, 0.5 mg daily inhaled by jet nebulizer. *Maximum:* 1 mg/day.
Children ages 1 to 8 previously on oral corticosteroids. 0.5 mg twice daily by jet nebulizer. Alternatively, 1 mg daily inhaled by jet nebulizer. *Maximum:* 1 mg/day.

✱ *To treat mild to moderate active Crohn's disease involving the ileum, the ascending colon, or both*

D.R. CAPSULES (ENTOCORT EC)

Adults. 9 mg once daily for up to 8 wk. Course may be repeated for recurring episodes of active disease.
Children ages 8 to 17 weighing more than 25 kg (55 lb). 9 mg once daily for 8 wk, followed by 6 mg once daily for 2 wk.

±**DOSAGE ADJUSTMENT** For adult patients with moderate hepatic impairment, dosage reduced to 3 mg once daily for duration of treatment.

✱ *To maintain clinical remission of mild to moderate Crohn's disease involving the ileum, the ascending colon, or both*

D.R. CAPSULES (ENTOCORT EC)

Adults. 6 mg daily for up to 3 mo.

±**DOSAGE ADJUSTMENT:** For patients with moderate hepatic impairment, dosage reduced to 3 mg once daily for duration of treatment.

✱ *To induce remission in patients with active, mild to moderate ulcerative colitis*

E.R. TABLETS (UCERIS)

Adults. 9 mg daily for up to 8 wk.

✱ *To induce remission in patients with active, mild to moderate distal ulcerative colitis extending up to 40 cm from the anal verge*

RECTAL FOAM (UCERIS)

Adults. 1 metered dose (2 mg) twice daily for 2 wk followed by 1 metered dose (2 mg) once daily for 4 wk.

✱ *To reduce loss of kidney function in patients with primary immunoglobulin A nephropathy who are at risk for disease progression*

D.R. CAPSULES (TARPEYO)

Adults. 16 mg once daily in the morning at least 1 hr before a meal for 9 mo. After 9 mo, dosage decreased to 8 mg once daily for 2 wk and then discontinued.

✱ *To treat eosinophilic esophagitis*

ORAL SUSPENSION (EOHILIA)

Adults and children ages 11 and older. 2 mg twice daily for 12 wk.

Drug Administration

P.O.

EXTENDED-RELEASE TABLETS (UCERIS)

- Administer in morning.
- Tablets should be swallowed whole with water and not broken, chewed, or crushed.
- Do not administer with grapefruit juice.

D.R. CAPSULES (ENTOCORT EC)

- Administer in morning.
- Do not administer with grapefruit juice.
- Capsules should be swallowed whole and not chewed or split.
- Capsules may be opened and granules sprinkled onto 1 tablespoon of applesauce (not hot). Mix the granules with the applesauce and administer entire contents within 30 min of mixing. Stress importance of not chewing or crushing the granules.
- After administration either way, have patient drink 8 ounces of water.
- Mixture should not be saved for future use.

D.R. CAPSULES (TARPEYO)

- Administer in morning at least 1 hr before a meal.
- Capsules should be swallowed whole and not chewed, crushed, or opened.

ORAL SUSPENSION (EOHILIA)

- Administer on an empty stomach. Do not mix oral suspension with food or liquid.
- Shake drug stick pack for at least 10 sec before opening. Squeeze the stick pack from the bottom to the top directly into the patient's mouth. Repeat 2 to 3 times until the stick pack is empty. Have patient swallow the susupension.
- Ensure patient doses not drink or eat anything for 30 min after administration. After 30 min have the patient rinse mouth with water and spit out the contents without swallowing.

NASAL SPRAY (BUDESONIDE, RHINOCORT ALLERGY)

- Prime bottle before first use by pumping the bottle 8 times or until a fine spray comes out. If bottle is not used for 2 days, it will have to be primed again. If bottle is not used for more than 14 days, clean the spray tip, and prime it again by releasing 2 sprays.
- Shake bottle before each use. Have patient blow her nose, tilt her head slightly forward,

and insert tip into a nostril, pointing toward inner corner of eye, away from nasal septum. The other nostril should be held closed while patient inhales gently. Then, repeat in the other nostril.

ORAL INHALER (PULMICORT FLEXHALER)

- Prime oral inhaler before using it for first time by holding canister upright with mouthpiece on top and twisting base of device fully to right and then fully to left until it clicks.
- Load each dose just before use in the same way. Once loaded, do not shake device.
- Do not use with a spacer device.
- Have patient turn head away from device and exhale. Then, have her hold device upright, place her lips around mouthpiece, and inhale deeply. Device will discharge a dose. Have her remove her lips from mouthpiece to exhale.
- Have patient rinse mouth with water without swallowing after each dose.
- Keep canister away from heat sources, as its contents are flammable.

NEBULIZED INHALATION (PULMICORT RESPULES)

- Use with a compressed-air–driven jet nebulizer only. It must have an adequate air flow and a suitable face mask or nose piece.
- Do not mix other drugs in the nebulizer.
- Have patient rinse mouth with water after each treatment without swallowing the water.
- Discard ampules if not used within 2 wk of opening the protective aluminum foil envelope.
- Do not refrigerate or freeze drug.

RECTAL (UCERIS)

- Have patient empty bowels before administering rectal foam. Although product is lubricated, use additional petroleum jelly, as needed.
- Warm the canister in hands while shaking it vigorously for 10 to 15 sec prior to use.
- Administer in the morning and evening for the first 2 wk, then once daily in the evening.
- When administering in the evening, do so immediately before bedtime. Patient should not try to empty bowels again until morning.

Route	Onset	Peak	Duration
P.O./D.R.	Unknown	0.5–10 hr	Unknown
P.O./E.R.	Unknown	7.4–19.2 hr	Unknown
Intranasal	10 hr	30 min	Unknown
Nebulization	2–8 days	2 min	Unknown
Oral inhalation	24 hr	10–30 min	Unknown
P.R.	Unknown	Unknown	Unknown

Half-life: 2–3.6 hr

Mechanism of Action

Inhibits inflammatory cells and mediators, possibly by decreasing influx into nasal passages, bronchial walls, or the intestines. As a result, nasal or airway inflammation decreases. Oral inhalation form also inhibits mucus secretion in airways, decreasing the amount and viscosity of sputum.

Contraindications

Hypersensitivity to budesonide or its components, recent nasal surgery, septal ulcers, or trauma (nasal spray); status asthmaticus or other acute asthma episodes (oral inhalation)

Interactions

DRUGS

antacids, H2 blockers, proton pump inhibitors (oral Uceris): Dissolution of the coating of oral Uceris may be altered

clarithromycin, erythromycin, itraconazole, ketoconazole, and other strong CYP3A4 inhibitors, such as atazanavir, clarithromycin, indinavir, itraconazole, nefazodone, nelfinavir, ritonavir, saquinavir, telithromycin: Possibly increased blood budesonide level

FOODS

grapefruit juice: Possibly increased blood budesonide level

Adverse Reactions

CNS: Amnesia, asthenia, **benign intracranial hypertension**, changes in mood, dizziness, fatigue, fever, headache

CV: Hypertension, peripheral edema

EENT: Bad taste, cataracts, dry mouth, epistaxis, glaucoma, nasal irritation, oral or pharyngeal candidiasis, pharyngitis, rhinitis, sinusitis

ENDO: **Adrenal insufficiency**, growth suppression in children, hypercorticism

GI: Abdominal pain, diarrhea, dyspepsia, flatulence, indigestion, nausea, **pancreatitis**, **rectal bleeding**, vomiting
GU: UTI
HEMA: Increased WBC count
MS: Arthralgia, back pain, muscle cramps and spasms
RESP: **Bronchospasm**, increased cough, respiratory tract infection
SKIN: Acne, allergic or contact dermatitis, maculopapular rash, pruritus, purpura, rash, urticaria
Other: **Anaphylaxis**, **angioedema**, **immunosuppression**, increased risk of infection, (bacterial, fungal, helminthic, protozoan, or viral), **Kaposi's sarcoma**, weight gain

Childbearing Considerations

PREGNANCY

- Drug may cause fetal harm, as it crosses the placental barrier.
- Hypoadrenalism in infants may occur when mothers have received substantial doses of corticosteroids during pregnancy, especially oral forms. Inhaled corticosteroids pose less risk.
- Use with caution only if benefit to mother outweighs potential risk to fetus.

LACTATION

- Drug is present in breast milk following inhalation of the drug. It is unknown if drug is present in breast milk following oral administration.
- Mothers should check with prescriber before breastfeeding.

Nursing Considerations

- Use budesonide cautiously if patient has ocular herpes simplex; tubercular infection; or untreated bacterial, fungal, or systemic viral infection.

! **WARNING** Determine if patient has a milk allergy. Pulmicort Flexhaler contains small amounts of lactose, which may trigger bronchospasm, coughing, or wheezing in a patient with a severe milk-protein allergy.

! **WARNING** Monitor patient for evidence of hypersensitivity. If present, notify prescriber immediately. Expect to stop budesonide and provide supportive care, as needed and ordered.

! **WARNING** Assess patient who switches from a systemic corticosteroid to inhaled budesonide for adrenal insufficiency (fatigue, hypotension, lassitude, nausea, vomiting, weakness), which may be life-threatening. Hypothalamic–pituitary–adrenal axis function may take several months to recover after stopping systemic corticosteroids. Stopping budesonide abruptly may cause adrenal insufficiency. Also, be aware that drug can reduce the response of the hyypothalamus-pituitary-adrenal axis to stress such as surgery or infection. Monitor patient closely during stressful situations and notify prescriber of any concerns as supplementation with a systemic corticosteroid may be needed.

! **WARNING** Monitor patient for signs and symptoms of infection because budesonide suppresses the immune system and reduces resistance to new infections or exacerbates existing infections. Budesonide therapy can also increase the risk of disseminated infections, reactivation or exacerbation of latent infections, or mask some signs of infection. While some infections may be mild others can become severe or even fatal. Know that the infectious complications increases with increasing budesonide dosages. Notify prescriber immediately if patient develops an infection as drug may need to be discontinued and another drug substituted.

- Monitor patient exposed to chickenpox and expect to administer pooled I.V. immunoglobulin or varicella zoster immune globulin, if ordered. If chickenpox develops, give antiviral as ordered. A patient exposed to measles may need pooled I.M. immunoglobulin.
- Assess patient for effectiveness of budesonide therapy, especially if being weaned from a systemic corticosteroid. If patient has increased asthma or an immunologic condition previously suppressed by systemic corticosteroid—such as arthritis, conjunctivitis, an eosinophilic condition, eczema, or rhinitis—notify prescriber.
- Monitor patients with conditions, such as cataracts, diabetes mellitus, glaucoma,

hypertension, osteoporosis, or peptic ulcer, as glucocorticoid therapy may increase adverse effects. Also, monitor patients with a family history of diabetes or glaucoma.

- Monitor closely a child's growth pattern; budesonide may stunt growth.

PATIENT TEACHING

- Instruct patient, family, or caregiver how to administer form of budesonide prescribed. Tell patient to avoid grapefruit juice during drug therapy.

! **WARNING** Instruct patient not to use budesonide as a rescue inhaler.

- Caution patient not to use an oral inhaler with a spacer device.
- Tell patient to contact prescriber if symptoms persist or have worsened after 3 weeks. Caution against increasing the dose without consulting prescriber first.
- Inform family or caregiver of small children using nebulized Respules that improvement may begin within 2 to 8 days, but that full effect may not be evident for 4 to 6 weeks.

! **WARNING** Alert patient, family, or caregiver that drug may cause an allergic reaction. Instruct to notify prescriber if an allergic reaction occurs. Stress importance of seeking immediate medical care if reaction is severe.

! **WARNING** Review signs and symptoms of adrenal insufficiency with patient, family, or caregiver. Caution not to abruptly stop form of budesonide therapy prescribed as adrenal insufficiency may occur, which can be life-threatening. Inform patient who is switching from a systemic corticosteroid to the inhaled form of budesonide that risk also exists for adrenal insufficiency. Tell patient to notify prescriber immediately if adrenal insufficiency is suspected.

- Caution patient to avoid exposure to chickenpox and measles and, if exposed, to contact prescriber immediately.
- Instruct patient on long-term therapy to have regular eye examinations.

bumetanide

Bumex

Class and Category

Pharmacologic class: Loop diuretic as sulfonamide derivative
Therapeutic class: Diuretic

Indications and Dosages

∗ *To treat edema caused by heart failure, hepatic disease, and renal disease, including nephrotic syndrome*

TABLETS

Adults. 0.5 to 2 mg daily, increased, as needed, with a second or third dose every 4 to 5 hr. Alternatively, 0.5 to 2 mg every other day or daily for 3 or 4 days each week. *Maximum:* 10 mg daily.

I.M. OR I.V. INJECTION, I.V. INFUSION

Adults. 0.5 to 1 mg daily, increased, as needed, with a second or third dose every 2 to 3 hr. *Maximum:* 10 mg daily.

Drug Administration

P.O.

- Administer a single daily dose in the morning although administering in the evening may provide a greater diuretic effect.
- Administer on an empty stomach as food may delay absorption.

I.V.

- Given only if impaired absorption is suspected or oral administration is not practical.
- Administer I.V. injection undiluted as an injection over 1 to 2 min.
- Prepare I.V. infusion for intermittant administration by diluting drug in 0.9% Sodium Chloride, 5% Dextrose, or Lactated Ringer's Injection following manufacturer guidelines.
- Discard unused solution 24 hr after preparation.
- *Incompatibilities:* None reported by manufacturer

I.M.

- Given only if impaired absorption is suspected or oral administration is not practical.

Route	Onset	Peak	Duration
P.O.	30–60 min	1–2 hr	4–6 hr
I.V.	> 5 min	15–30 min	3.5–4 hr
I.M.	30–60 min	30 min	4–5 hr

Half-life: 1–1.5 hr

Mechanism of Action

Inhibits reabsorption of sodium, chloride, and water in the ascending limb of the loop of Henle, which promotes their excretion and reduces fluid volume.

Contraindications

Anuria, hepatic coma, hypersensitivity to bumetanide or its components, marked increase in BUN or creatinine levels or development of oliguria if progressive renal disease is present, severe electrolyte depletion

Interactions

DRUGS

aminoglycosides: Increased risk of ototoxicity
antihypertensives: Increased hypotensive effect
indomethacin: Slowed increase in urine and sodium excretion, inhibited plasma renin activity
lithium: Reduced lithium renal clearance, increased risk of lithium toxicity
nephrotoxic drugs: Potential for adverse renal effects
probenecid: Reduced sodium excretion

Adverse Reactions

CNS: Dizziness, **encephalopathy**, headache
CV: **Hypotension**
EENT: Ototoxicity
ENDO: Hyperglycemia
GI: Nausea
GU: **Azotemia**, elevated serum creatinine level
MS: Muscle spasms
SKIN: **Stevens-Johnson syndrome**, **toxic epidermal necrolysis**
Other: Hypersensitivity reactions, hyperuricemia, **hypocalcemia**, hypochloremia, **hypokalemia**, **hyponatremia**, hypovolemia

Childbearing Considerations

PREGNANCY

- It is not known if drug can cause fetal harm.
- Use with caution only if benefit to mother outweighs potential risk to fetus.

LACTATION

- It is not known if drug is present in breast milk.
- Breastfeeding is not recommended during drug therapy.

Nursing Considerations

! WARNING Know that a patient hypersensitive to sulfonamides may be hypersensitive to bumetanide. Monitor such a patient closely when starting therapy. If a hypersensitivity reaction occurs, notify prescriber, expect drug to be discontinued, as ordered, and provide supportive care, as needed and ordered.

! WARNING Monitor patient for skin abnormalities because drug can cause reactions that could become life-threatening. Notify prescriber immediately if skin alterations occur, expect drug to be discontinued as ordered, and provide supportive care, as needed and ordered.

! WARNING Assess fluid and electrolyte balance closely because bumetanide is a potent diuretic (40 to 60 times more potent than furosemide). Monitor fluid intake and output once every 8 hours, evaluate serum electrolyte levels when ordered, and assess for imbalances. Be aware that high-dose or too-frequent administration can cause profound diuresis and electrolyte and water depletion, especially in elderly patients.

! WARNING Know that patients at higher risk for hypokalemia are patients who take digitalis glycoside for heart failure or has aldosteronism, ascites, diarrhea, hepatic cirrhosis, potassium-losing nephropathy, or a history of ventricular arrhythmias.

- Assess for evidence of ototoxicity, such as tinnitus. Although rare, tinnitus may occur with I.V. use, high doses, or increased frequency of dosing in a patient with renal impairment.
- Monitor results of renal function tests during therapy to detect renal dysfunction.
- Monitor blood glucose levels in patients who are diabetic because drug can cause hyperglycemia.

PATIENT TEACHING

- Instruct patient how to administer oral bumetanide. Stress importance of not increasing the dose or frequency of taking it because drug is very potent.
- Review potassium-rich foods and urge patient to include them in her daily diet.

! **WARNING** Alert patient that bumetanide may cause an allergic reaction, especially if patient is already allergic to sulfonamides. Tell patient to notify prescriber immediately if an allergic reaction occurs and to seek immediate medical care if severe.

! **WARNING** Tell patient to notify prescriber immediately if skin changes occur because drug will need to be discontinued and additional medical care may be required.

! **WARNING** Stress importance of monitoring fluid intake and output and watching for evidence of electrolyte imbalance, such as hypokalemia (dizziness, headache, and muscle spasms).

- Review other potential adverse reactions and tell patient to report persistent, severe, or unusual reactions to prescriber.
- Advise patient to avoid hazardous activities until drug's CNS effects are known and resolved.
- Tell diabetic patient to monitor blood glucose level regularly and to notify prescriber about persistent hyperglycemia.
- Urge patient to return for appropriate follow-up care, especially if she's receiving bumetanide for a chronic condition.

buprenorphine

Brixadi, Butrans, Sublocade

buprenorphine hydrochloride

Belbuca, Buprenex

Class, Category, and Schedule

Pharmacologic class: Opioid
Therapeutic class: Opioid analgesic
Controlled substance schedule: III

Indications and Dosages

✶ *To control pain severe enough to require opioid treatment and for which alternative treatment options (i.e., nonopioid analgesics or opioid combination products) are inadequate or not tolerated*

I.M. OR I.V. INJECTION (BUPRENEX)

Adults and adolescents. 0.3 mg as a single dose. A second 0.3-mg dose may be given 30 to 60 min after first dose, as needed. Subsequent doses of 0.3 mg given up to 6-hr intervals, as needed. I.V. injection given slowly over at least 2 min. *Maximum:* 0.6 mg as a single dose.

Children ages 2 to 12. 2 to 6 mcg/kg every 4 to 6 hr, as needed although remedicating may not be needed for 6 to 8 hr. I.V. injection given slowly over at least 2 min. *Maximum:* 6 mcg/kg.

± **DOSAGE ADJUSTMENT** For adult patients not at high risk for opioid toxicity, I.M. dose increased to 0.6 mg and given as a single dose, as needed, depending on pain severity and patient response. For debilitated or elderly patients and patients who have respiratory disease or also use another CNS depressant, I.M. or I.V. dose kept to minimum.

✶ *To control severe chronic pain in patients requiring a continuous, around-the-clock opioid analgesic for an extended period of time for which alternative treatment options are inadequate*

TRANSDERMAL PATCH (BUTRANS)

Opioid-naïve adults. *Initial:* 5 mcg/hr with dosage titrated every 72 hr, as needed, to achieve pain relief with patch changed every 7 days. *Maximum*: 20 mcg/hr.

Adults whose daily dose of oral morphine or equivalent was less than 30 mg. *Initial:* 5 mcg/hr, increased after 72 hr, as needed, to 10 mcg/hr with patch changed every 7 days. *Maximum:* 20 mcg/hr.

Adults whose daily dose of oral morphine or equivalent was between 30 and 80 mg. *Initial:* Current around-the-clock opioid use tapered for up to 7 days to no more than 30 mg of morphine or equivalent per day. Then, a 10 mcg/hr patch applied, increased after 72 hr, as needed, to 20 mcg/hr with patch changed every 7 days. *Maximum:* 20 mcg/hr.

BUCCAL FILM (BELBUCA)

Opioid-naïve and opioid-nontolerant adults. *Initial:* 75 mcg once daily or, if tolerated, every 12 hr for at least 4 days, then increased to 150 mcg every 12 hr. Dosage further titrated, as needed, in increments of 150 mcg every 12 hr every 4 or more days. *Maximum:* 450 mcg every 12 hr.

Adults already on opioids. *Initial:* 75 mcg once daily or every 12 hr for patients whose daily dose of oral morphine sulfate equivalent (MSE) is less than 30 mg; 150 mcg every 12 hr for patients whose daily dose of oral MSE is between 30 and 89 mg; and 300 mcg every 12 hr for patients whose daily dose of oral MSE is between 90 and 160 mg. Then, dosage titrated, as needed, no more than every 4 days in increments of 150 mcg every 12 hr. *Maximum:* 900 mcg every 12 hr.

± **DOSAGE ADJUSTMENT** For patients with oral mucositis or severe hepatic impairment, initial dose and subsequent titrations, dosage decreased by half.

✶ *To treat opioid dependence*

SUBLINGUAL TABLETS (BUPRENORPHINE HYDROCHLORIDE)

Adults. *Induction:* 8 mg daily on day 1 followed by 16 mg daily on day 2 and thereafter. *Maintenance:* 4 to 24 mg daily, increased or decreased in 2- to 4-mg increments, as needed. *Maximum:* 24 mg daily.

± **DOSAGE ADJUSTMENT** For patients with severe hepatic impairment, initial dose and subsequent titrations, dosage decreased by half.

✶ *To treat moderate to severe opioid use disorder in patients who have initiated treatment with a buprenorphine-containing product, followed by dose adjustment for a minimum of 7 days*

E.R. SUBCUTANEOUS INJECTION (SUBLOCADE)

Adults. 300 mg monthly for first 2 mo followed by maintenance dose. *Maintenance:* 100 mg monthly. Maintenance dose may be increased to 300 mg monthly, as needed.

✶ *To treat moderate to severe opioid use disorder in patients who have initiated treatment with a single dose of a transmucosal buprenorphine product or who are already being treated with buprenorphine*

E.R. SUBCUTANEOUS INJECTION (BRIXADI)

Adults who are not currently receiving buprenorphine and after test dose of 4 mg of transmucosal buprenorphine that was tolerated without precipitating withdrawal. 16 mg followed by 8 mg within 3 days of first dose to achieve a total first wk dose of 24 mg. An additional 8 mg given at least 24 hr after previous injection within first wk, if needed for a total first wk dose of 32 mg. *Maintenance:* 24 mg or 32 mg every 7 days thereafter, whichever dose was established during wk 1. *Maximum:* 32 mg every 7 days.

Adults switching from transmcosal form to weekly subcutaneous injection. *For patients taking 6 mg or less of sublingual form daily:* 8 mg weekly. *For patient taking 8 to 10 mg of sublingual form daily:* 16 mg weekly. *For patient taking 12 to 16 mg of sublingual form daily:* 24 mg weekly. *For patient taking 18 to 24 mg of sublingual form daily*: 32 mg weekly.

Adults who are switching from transmucosal form to monthly subcutaneous injection. *For patient taking 8 to 10 mg of sublingual form daily:* 64 mg monthly. *For patient taking 12 to 16 mg of sublingual form daily*: 96 mg monthly. *For patient taking 18 to 24 mg daily:* 128 mg monthly.

Adults transitioning from weekly to monthly dosing schedule. *For patient taking 16 mg weekly:* 64 mg given monthly. *For patient taking 24 mg weekly:* 96 mg given monthly. *For patient taking 32 mg weekly:* 128 mg given monthly.

Adults transitioning from monthly to weekly dosing schedule. *For patient taking 64 mg monthly:* 16 mg given weekly. *For patient taking 96 mg monthly*, 24 mg given weekly. *For patient taking 128 mg monthly:* 32 mg given weekly.

Drug Administration

P.O.

Buccal film (Belbuca)

- Have patient wet the inside of cheek. Have patient place the yellow side of the film against the inside of cheek immediately after removing film from the package. Using clean, dry fingers, it should be held in place for 5 sec. The film will dissolve, usually within 30 min. Patient should not eat or drink until film is dissolved, nor should patient try to manipulate film with fingers or tongue while it is dissolving.

- After film is dissolved, have patient take a sip of water, swish gently around gums and teeth, and swallow. Patient should not brush teeth for at least 1 hr afterwards.
- Dispose of unused film by removing from the foil packages. Dispose of foil packages in the trash.

Sublingual tablets (Buprenorphine)

- Have patient place sublingual tablets under the tongue until dissolved. If more than 2 tablets per dose are prescribed, all tablets are placed under the tongue at the same time. If they won't fit, 2 tablets at a time can be placed under the tongue until full dose has been given.
- Sublingual tablets should not be swallowed. nor should the tablets be chewed or cut.
- After tablet has been completely dissolved, have patient take a sip of water, swish gently around the teeth and gums and then swallow the water. Ensure patient waits for at least 1 hr after receiving the sublingual tablets before brushing teeth.

I.V. (BUPRENEX)

- Give I.V. injection slowly over at least 2 min.
- Store avoiding excessive heat and prolonged exposure to light.
- *Incompatibilities:* None reported by manufacturer

I.M. (BUPRENEX)

- Administer as a deep intramuscular injection.

SUBCUTANEOUS (SUBLOCADE)

- Administer monthly with a minimum of 26 days between doses.
- Remove subcutaneous form from refrigerator at least 15 min prior to administration to allow drug to reach room temperature. Then, remove the foil pouch and safety needle from the carton. Open pouch and remove the syringe only immediately before administering drug. Check the solution, which should be colorless to yellow to amber. Attach the safety needle twisting it clockwise until it is tight and firmly attached. Do not remove the plastic cover from the needle at this time.
- Choose an injection site on patient's abdomen between the transpyloric and transtubercular planes that has adequate subcutaneous tissue that is free of excessive pigment, lesions, or nodules. Also, do not inject into an area where the skin is bruised, infected, irritated, reddened, or scarred in any way.
- Have patient assume a supine position.
- Clean injection site with an alcohol swab.
- Remove excess air from syringe and administer drug. Pinch the skin around the injection area pinching enough to accommodate the size of the needle. Use a slow, steady push to inject drug until all of the drug is given. Withdraw the needle, lock the needle guard, and discard the syringe.
- Do not massage or rub injection site.
- Never inject intradermally, I.M., or I.V.
- Monitor site for appearance of a lump that may take several wk to decrease in size. Ensure patient does not place any belts or clothing waistbands over injection site.

SUBCUTANEOUS (BRIXADI)

- BRIXADI is available in two formulations, a weekly formulation and a monthly formulation. Do not confuse the two and do not combine to yield a monthly dose.
- Drug is contained in a prefilled, single-dose syringe with a 23G 1/2-inch needle attached.
- If patient is not currently receiving buprenorphine, expect a test dose of 4 mg transmucosal to be given first. If test dose tolerated, and withdrawal not precipitated, patient transitioned to weekly dose. Weekly dosing must be done for this patient before monthly dosing is used.
- For patients currently receiving other buprenorphine-containing formulations, treatment can be initiated with either weekly or monthly dosing.
- Have naloxone on hand for emergency treatment of opioid overdose.
- Inspect solution in prefilled syringe. It should appear yellowish to yellow-clear. Discard if solution contains visible particles or is cloudy. Do not use after expiration date.
- Assemble safety syringe after washing hands by removing the safety syringe components from the carton. Insert the plunger into the

body of the syringe and rotate clockwise until it is attached to the stopper inside the syringe. A small air bubble may be visible.
- Put on gloves and select subcutaneous tissue site using abdomen, buttock, thigh, or upper arm. However, for patients who are not currently receiving buprenorphine treatment, the upper arm site should only be used after 4 consecutive doses have been given in other sites because the arm site has been associated with lower plasma levels compared to the other sites.
- Clean injection site with an alcohol wipe using a circular motion.
- Grasp the syringe and carefully pull the needle cap straight off. Immediately dispose of needle cap. A small drop of liquid may be seen at the tip of the needle, which is normal.
- Administer as a single injection. Do not divide dose. Administer weekly dose every 7 days; monthly dose every 28 days.
- To administer, first pinch skin at injection site and insert the needle on the syringe into the site at a 90-degree angle making sure to fully insert the needle. Then release skin that was pinched. Slowly press down on the plunger until it latches in the safety device wings. This will make certain all the drug has been injected. Keep plunger pressed fully down for an additional 2 sec.
- Keep plunger fully depressed while carefully lifting needle straight out from the injection site. Once needle has been removed from the injection site, slowly take your thumb off the plunger. This will allow the syringe guard to automatically cover the exposed needle. If there is a small amount of blood at the injection site, wipe away with a cotton ball or gauze. Do not rub injection site. Apply adhesive bandage to site, if needed.
- Monitor injection site for excessive swelling, redness, heat, or drainage. If present, notify prescriber.
- Rotate sites for weekly doses making sure same site is not used for at least 8 wk; monthly doses do not require sites to be rotated.
- For a missed dose, administer as soon as possible. The weekly dose may be administered up to 2 days before or after the weekly time frame; monthly dose may be administered up to 1 wk before or after the monthly time frame.
- Never inject drug in any manner other than as a subcutaneous injection.

TRANSDERMAL (BUTRANS)

- Place patch only on intact skin that is clean (washed with water only), dry, and hairless. If a hairless site is not available, clip, not shave, area prior to application. Do not apply patch to irritated skin.
- Apply patch immediately after its removal from pouch to side of chest, upper back, upper chest, or upper outer arm. Rotate sites and wait at least a minimum of 21 days before reapplying to the same site.
- If problems with adhesion occur, tape the edges of the patch with first-aid tape. If the patch should fall off during the 7-day interval, dispose of the patch and apply a new one at a different skin site.
- When removing the patch, fold it over on itself and discard.

Route	Onset	Peak	Duration
P.O.: Buccal	Unknown	2.5–3 hr	Unknown
P.O.: Sublingual	Unknown	3–4 hr	Unknown
I.V.	Immediate	2 min	6 hr
I.M.	15 min	1–2 hr	6 hr
SubQ	Unknown	24 hr	Unknown
Transdermal	17 hr	Unknown	7 days

Half-life: Depends on route; up to 60 days

Mechanism of Action

May bind with CNS receptors to alter the perception of and emotional response to pain. Buprenorphine may act by displacing narcotic agonists from their binding sites and competitively inhibiting their actions.

Contraindications

Acute or severe bronchial asthma in an unmonitored setting or in the absence of resuscitative equipment; hypersensitivity to buprenorphine or its components; known or suspected GI obstruction, including paralytic ileus; significant respiratory depression

Interactions

DRUGS

anticholinergic drugs: Increased risk of urinary retention and/or severe constipation that could lead to paralytic ileus *antimigraine agents; cyclobenzaprine; dextromethorphan; dolasetron; granisetron; linezolid; MAO inhibitors; methylene blue; ondansetron; palonosetron; selected psychiatric drugs, such as amoxapine, buspirone, lithium, mirtazapine, nefazodone, trazodone, vilazodone; selective serotonin reuptake inhibitors; serotonin-norepinephrine reuptake inhibitors; St. John's wort; tricyclic antidepressants; tryptophan:* Increased risk of serotonin syndrome

benzodiazepines, CNS depressants, other opioids, sedating antihistamines, tricyclic antidepressants: Increased risk of profound sedation, significant respiratory depression, and other life-threatening adverse effects

CNS depressants, MAO inhibitors: Additive hypotensive and respiratory and CNS depressant effects of these drugs that may be life-threatening

CYP3A4 inducers, such as carbamazepine, phenytoin, rifampin: Possibly decreased plasma concentration of buprenorphine

CYP3A4 inhibitors, such as azole-antifungals (ketoconazole), macrolide antibiotics (erythromycin), protease inhibitors (ritonavir): Increased plasma concentration of buprenorphine, causing increased or prolonged opioid effects

diuretics: Possibly reduced effectiveness of diuretics

mixed agonist/antagonist and partial agonist opioid analgesics, such as butorphanol, nalbuphine, pentazocine: Possibly reduced analgesic effect of buprenorphine and/or precipitate withdrawal symptoms

muscle relaxants: Possibly enhanced neuromuscular blocking action of skeletal muscle relaxants; increased degree of respiratory depression

non-nucleoside reverse transcriptase inhibitors (NNRTIs), such as delavirdine, efavirenz: Significant pharmacokinetic interactions that have potential to affect action of buprenorphine

protease inhibitors, such as atazanavir, ritonavir: Increased levels of buprenorphine causing symptoms of opioid excess, including increased sedation

ACTIVITIES

alcohol use: Increased serum buprenorphine levels possibly resulting in fatal overdose owing to CNS and respiratory depression

Adverse Reactions

CNS: **CNS depression**, dizziness, headache, sedation, **seizures**, syncope, vertigo
CV: **Bradycardia**, hypertension, **hypotension**, **QT prolongation**
EENT: Miosis; *Buccal form:* Dental abscesses, caries, or infection with tooth erosion or fracture, fillings falling out, and total tooth loss. *Sublingual form:* Burning mouth syndrome, glossitis, mucosal erythema, oral hypoesthesia, stomatitis
ENDO: **Adrenal insufficiency (rare)**, **hypoglycemia**
GI: Elevated liver enzymes or serum amylase level, **hepatitis**, **hepatotoxicity**, jaundice, nausea, spasm of the sphincter of Oddi, vomiting
GU: Androgen deficiency with chronic use, decreased libido, erectile dysfunction, impotency, infertility, lack of menstruation
RESP: **Bronchospasm**, **hypoventilation**, **respiratory depression**
SKIN: Diaphoresis, pruritus, rash, urticaria
Other: **Anaphylaxis**; **angioedema**; application-site inflammation, burns, discharge, and vesicle occurrence; injection site pain, pruritus, redness, and swelling; opioid-induced allodynia (pain from ordinarily non-painful stimuli) and hyperalgesia (paradoxical increase in pain); physical and psychological dependence

Childbearing Considerations

PREGNANCY

- It is not known if drug can cause fetal harm, but neonatal opioid withdrawal syndrome may occur in newborn infants of mothers receiving the drug for an extended period of time.
- Use with caution only if benefit to mother outweighs potential risk to fetus.

LABOR AND DELIVERY

- Mothers who are opioid-dependent on buprenorphine maintenance therapy may require additional analgesia during labor.
- Be aware that, as with all opioids, use of the drug prior to delivery may result in respiratory depression in the newborn.

LACTATION

- Drug is present in breast milk.
- Breastfeeding is usually not recommended.
- If breastfeeding occurs, mothers should be instructed to monitor infant for breathing difficulties and drowsiness.

REPRODUCTION

- Chronic use of opioids may cause reduced fertility in females of childbearing age and in males when used for an extended period of time.
- It is not known whether these effects on fertility are reversible.

Nursing Considerations

! **WARNING** Evaluate patient's risk for abuse and addiction prior to the start of buprenorphine therapy, as excessive use of drug may lead to abuse, addiction, misuse, overdose, and possibly death. Be prepared to monitor patient's intake throughout therapy. Because of the potential risks associated with buprenorphine therapy, be aware that the FDA now requires a Risk Evaluation and Mitigation Strategy (REMS) for buprenorphine use.

! **WARNING** Be aware that opioids like buprenorphine used for an extended period of time should not be given to females during pregnancy because the newborn may experience neonatal opioid withdrawal syndrome (NOWS), which may be life-threatening if not recognized and treated. This syndrome may exhibit as excessive or high-pitched crying, poor feeding, rapid breathing, or trembling. Also, buprenorphine should not be administered during labor because it may cause respiratory depression in the newborn.

! **WARNING** Be aware that opioid therapy like buprenorphine should be used with extreme caution only concomitantly with benzodiazepine therapy in patients for whom other treatment options are inadequate. If prescribed together, expect dosing and duration of the opioid to be limited. Monitor patient closely for signs and symptoms of decrease in consciousness, including coma; profound sedation; and significant respiratory depression. Notify prescriber immediately and provide emergency supportive care, as death may occur.

- Use buprenorphine cautiously in patients with acute alcoholism, adrenal insufficiency, alcohol withdrawal syndrome, biliary tract dysfunction, CNS depression, coma, hypothyroidism, kyphoscoliosis, myxedema, prostatic hypertrophy, psychosis, severe hepatic or renal impairment, toxic psychosis, or urethral stricture. Also, use cautiously in patients who take a drug that decreases hepatic clearance, are known drug abusers, or have a history of opioid addiction.
- Use drug cautiously in patients with head injury, intracranial lesions, or other conditions that could increase CSF pressure. Be particularly cautious when administering drug to patients with COPD or cor pulmonale and in patients who have decreased respiratory reserve, hypoxia, hypercapnia, or preexisting respiratory depression.
- Know that to avoid causing withdrawal, drug should not be given for opioid dependence until early signs of withdrawal occur.
- Be aware that the transdermal patch should not be used in patients whose prior total daily dose of opioid use is greater than 80 mg of oral morphine equivalents per day because the maximum 20 mcg/hr dosage may not provide adequate analgesia. An alternate analgesic should be considered.
- Know that if Brixadi or Sublocade is discontinued, monitor patient for several months for signs and symptoms of withdrawal and treat, as prescribed.
- Expect to obtain liver function tests prior to initiation of buprenorphine therapy and periodically throughout therapy because drug may cause hepatic dysfunction ranging from transient asymptomatic elevations in liver enzymes to hepatic failure and death. Acute hepatitis may also occur and, in some cases, require the drug to be discontinued, although in other cases even a dosage reduction of buprenorphine may not be needed. Monitor patient closely and report any signs and symptoms of hepatic dysfunction to prescriber.
- Monitor response to drug and vital signs often, especially after giving first dose and if patient develops a fever. Be aware that drug may cause severe hypotension, including orthostatic hypotension and syncope in ambulatory patients.

! **WARNING** Monitor patient for hypersensitivity reactions that could become life-threatening such as anaphylaxis or angioedema. If present, notify prescriber immediately, expect drug to be withheld or changed to a different drug, and provide supportive care, as needed and ordered.

! **WARNING** Monitor patient closely for respiratory depression, especially in cachectic, debilitated, or elderly patients; patients with chronic pulmonary disease, when initiating and titrating dosages; or when other drugs that depress respiration are given together. Immediately report respiratory depression because respiratory arrest may occur. Be prepared to provide emergency supportive care.

! **WARNING** Assess elderly patients for signs and symptoms of toxicity or overdose, as these patients may be at increased risk because of decreased cardiac, hepatic, or renal function and the presence of concomitant disease and other drug therapy. Have naloxone readily available to treat overdose.

! **WARNING** Know that many drugs may interact with opioids like buprenorphine to cause serotonin syndrome. Monitor patient closely for signs and symptoms, such as agitation, diaphoresis, diarrhea, fever, hallucinations, labile blood pressure, muscle twitching or stiffness, nausea, shakiness, shivering, tachycardia, trouble with coordination, or vomiting. Notify prescriber at once because serotonin syndrome may be life-threatening. Be prepared to discontinue drug, if possible and ordered, and provide supportive care.

! **WARNING** Monitor patient for adrenal insufficiency. Although rare, this can be life-threatening. Monitor patient for anorexia, dizziness, fatigue, hypotension, nausea, vomiting, or weakness. Notify prescriber if adrenal insufficiency is suspected and expect diagnostic testing to be done to determine if present. If diagnosis is confirmed, expect to administer corticosteroids and wean patient off buprenorphine, if possible.

- Monitor patient with a seizure disorder, as buprenorphine may worsen seizure control.
- Monitor the injection site when administering E.R. suspension form subcutaneously for injection-site reactions, such as pain, pruritis, and redness. However, know that injection-site reactions may also include abscess formation, necrosis, and ulceration that may require antibiotic therapy and debridement or surgical removal. Know that the drug (Sublocade) may be removed from a subcutaneous site surgically under local anesthesia within 14 days of the injection, but removal is not recommended with Brixadi. If Sublocade is removed, monitor patient for signs and symptoms of withdrawal and treat appropriately, as prescribed. Be aware that serious injection-site reactions may be increased with inadvertent intradermal or intramuscular administration. This form of drug should only be injected subcutaneously.
- Monitor patient for opioid-induced allodynia (pain from ordinarily non-painful stimuli) and hyperalgesia (paradoxical increase in pain), which is different from tolerance. Assess patient for increase in pain when buprenorphine dosage is increased or decrease in pain when buprenorphine dosage is decreased, Notify prescriber if opioid-induced allodynia and hyperalgesia occurs as dosage may need to be decreased or opioid rotation used.

! **WARNING** Monitor patient for hypoglycemia, especially patients with at least one predisposing risk factor such as diabetes mellitus. If present, treat according to institutional protocol. If recurring or severe investigate underlying cause with presciber and institute preventative measures.

- Do not discontinue therapy abruptly when buprenorphine therapy is no longer needed. Instead, expect a gradual downward titration of the dose to prevent signs and symptoms of withdrawal.

PATIENT TEACHING

- Instruct patient or family or caregiver how to administer form of buprenorphine prescribed and what to do if a dose is missed. Warn patient not to take more drug than prescribed and not to take it longer than absolutely needed because excessive or prolonged use can lead to abuse, addiction, misuse, overdose, and possibly death.
- Instruct family or caregiver on the use of naloxone and stress importance of having

drug in the home for emergency use in the event an overdose occurs.

- Warn patient not to stop taking drug abruptly. Instead, encourage patient to talk to prescriber about questions or concerns with the drug therapy.

! **WARNING** Instruct patient not to crush or dissolve tablet form of drug and then inject it, as life-threatening infections, precipitated withdrawal, and other serious health problems could occur.

- Inform patient wearing a buprenorphine patch not to expose it to any external heat source, such as electric blankets, heat lamps, heated water beds, heating pads, hot tubs, or saunas as absorption may be affected.

! **WARNING** Alert patient that drug can cause an allergic reaction. Tell patient to notify prescriber if an allergic reaction occurs and to seek immediate medical care if reaction is severe.

! **WARNING** Warn patient not to consume alcohol or take benzodiazepines or other CNS depressants, including other opioids, during buprenorphine therapy without prescriber knowledge, as severe respiratory depression can occur that may lead to death.

- Advise patient to report any persistent, severe, or unusual signs and symptoms to prescriber, including hypoglycemia.
- Alert patient that buprenorphine may cause feelings of pain from stimuli that doesn't usually cause pain or paradoxically pain may be increased, especially if dosage increased. Tell patient to notify prescriber if these types of reactions are experienced.
- Advise patient to get up slowly from a lying or sitting position to avoid a sudden drop in blood pressure.
- Caution patient to avoid hazardous activities while receiving buprenorphine until adverse effects are resolved.
- Inform patient that long-term use of opioids like buprenorphine may decrease sex hormone levels causing decreased libido, erectile dysfunction, impotence, infertility, or lack of menstruation. Encourage patient to report any such symptoms.
- Stress importance of good dental care and regular dental checkups. If dental problems occur, advise patient to notify prescriber and see a dentist. Tell patient to inform dentist that an oral form of buprenorphine therapy is being taken.
- Tell patient receiving the drug as an E.R. subcutaneous injection that a lump may appear at injection site and last for several weeks. Tell patient not to massage or rub the injection site and to be careful of the placement of any belts or clothing waistbands so as not to irritate the site. If other symptoms develop, instruct patient to have prescriber evaluate injection site.

! **WARNING** Caution patient to keep drug out of the reach of others, especially children, including patch form, as exposure to even one dose or patch could be fatal. Instruct patient to keep buprenorphine in a safe place and to protect it from theft because of it being an opioid.

- Advise females of childbearing age to notify prescriber if pregnancy occurs.
- Inform mothers wishing to breastfeed that breastfeeding is usually not recommended during buprenorphine therapy. However, if mother does breastfeed, caution her to monitor the infant for breathing difficulties and increased drowsiness. If present, tell mothers to stop breastfeeding and notify prescriber.
- Caution patient to dispose of expired, unused, or unwanted drug properly. Tell patients to visit the website: www.fda.gov/drugdisposal for instructions. The drug can also be flushed down the toilet after removing foil, if present, if a drug take-back option is not available.

bupropion hydrobromide

Aplenzin

bupropion hydrochloride

Forfivo XL, Wellbutrin SR, Wellbutrin XL

Class and Category

Pharmacologic class: Aminoketone
Therapeutic class: Antidepressant, smoking cessation adjunct

Indications and Dosages

* *To treat depression*

E.R. TABLETS (WELLBUTRIN SR)

Adults. *Initial:* 150 mg daily for 3 days; then 150 mg twice daily with at least 8 hr between successive doses and, after several wk, increased to 200 mg twice daily, as needed and tolerated. *Maximum:* 400 mg daily, given as 200 mg twice daily. Single doses should not exceed 200 mg/dose.

E.R. TABLETS (WELLBUTRIN XL)

Adults. *Initial:* 150 mg daily in the morning for 4 days; then 300 mg daily in the morning.

E.R. TABLETS (APLENZIN)

Adults. *Initial:* 174 mg daily in the morning for 4 days. Then, if tolerated well, dosage increased to 348 mg daily in the morning.

E.R. TABLETS (FORFIVO XL)

Adults. *Initial:* 300 mg daily of another bupropion product for at least 2 wk before maintenance with Forfivo XL is begun. *Maintenance:* 450 mg once daily.

TABLETS (BUPROPION)

Adults. *Initial:* 100 mg twice daily, increased after 3 or more days to 100 mg 3 times daily with at least 6 hr between successive doses, as needed. *Maximum:* 450 mg daily given as 150 mg 3 times daily.

* *To aid in smoking cessation*

E.R. TABLETS (BUPROPION)

Adults. *Initial:* 150 mg daily for 3 days and then 150 mg twice daily with at least 8 hr between each dose for 7 to 12 wk. *Maximum:* 300 mg daily given as 150 mg 2 times daily.

* *To prevent seasonal major depressive episodes in patient with seasonal affective disorder*

E.R. TABLETS (WELLBUTRIN XL)

Adults. *Initial:* 150 mg once daily starting in autumn, increased after 1 wk to 300 mg once daily in morning, as tolerated and needed. Decreased to 150 mg once daily 2 wk before stopping in early spring if dosage was 300 mg once daily.

E.R. TABLETS (APLENZIN)

Adults. *Initial:* 174 mg once daily starting in autumn, increased after 1 wk to 348 mg once daily, as tolerated and needed. Decreased to 174 mg once daily 2 wk before stopping in early spring if dosage was 348 mg once daily.

±**DOSAGE ADJUSTMENT** For patients with severe hepatic cirrhosis, no more than 75 mg daily of bupropion, 100 mg daily or 150 mg every other day of Wellbutrin SR, or 150 mg every other day of Wellbutrin XL, and 174 mg every other day of Aplenzin. For patients with renal impairment, dosage or frequency decreased on an individual basis.

Drug Administration

P.O.

- Use of drug for smoking cessation should be started a week or two before patient quits smoking.
- Administer daily doses or first dose of the day in the morning.
- E.R. tablets should be swallowed whole and not chewed, crushed, or cut.
- Adhere to manufacturer instructions on length of time to wait between doses, if applicable.
- Store tablets at room temperature while keeping tablets dry and out of the light.

Route	Onset	Peak	Duration
P.O.	Unknown	2 hr	1–2 days
P.O./E.R.	Unknown	5 hr	1–2 days
P.O./SR	Unknown	3 hr	1–2 days

Half-life: 21 hr

Mechanism of Action

May inhibit dopamine, norepinephrine, and serotonin uptake by neurons, which significantly relieves evidence of depression.

Contraindications

Hypersensitivity to bupropion or its components; seizure disorder or conditions that increase risk of seizures (i.e., abrupt discontinuation of alcohol, antiepileptic drugs, barbiturates, or benzodiazepines); anorexia nervosa or bulimia; use within 14 days of an MAO inhibitor (MAOI), including reversible MAOIs, such as linezolid or intravenous methylene blue; use of another form of bupropion concurrently

Interactions

DRUGS

amantadine, levodopa: Increased CNS adverse reactions to bupropion

antidepressants, antipsychotics, concurrent use of other bupropion products, systemic corticosteroids, theophylline: Increased risk of seizures

carbamazepine, phenobarbital, phenytoin: Increased bupropion metabolism resulting in decreased bupropion exposure
CYP2B6 inducers, such as efavirenz, lopinavir, ritonavir: Possibly decreased bupropion exposure and subsequent effectiveness
CYP2B6 inhibitors, such as clopidogrel, ticlopidine: Possibly increased bupropion exposure and risk of adverse reactions
digoxin: Possibly decreased digoxin levels
drugs metabolized by CYP2D6, such as certain antidepressants (i.e., desipramine, fluoxetine, imipramine, nortriptyline, paroxetine, sertraline, venlafaxine), antipsychotics (i.e., haloperidol, risperidone, thioridazine), beta-blockers (i.e., metoprolol), type IC antiarrhythmics (i.e., flecainide, propafenone): Increased blood exposure of these drugs and risk of adverse reactions
MAO inhibitors, including reversible MAOIs, such as linezolid and intravenous methylene blue: Increased risk of acute bupropion toxicity and serious hypertensive reactions
tamoxifen: Possibly reduced effectiveness of tamoxifen

ACTIVITIES

alcohol use, recreational drug abuse: Possible rare adverse neuropsychiatric events; reduced alcohol tolerance

Adverse Reactions

CNS: Abnormal coordination, abnormal EEG, aggression, agitation, akathisia, akinesia, anxiety, aphasia, asthenia, CNS stimulation, **coma**, confusion, **CVA**, decreased concentration or memory, delirium, delusions, depersonalization, depression, dizziness, dream abnormalities, emotional lability, euphoria, extrapyramidal syndrome, fever, general or migraine headache, hallucinations, **homicidal ideation**, hostility, hyperesthesia, hyperkinesia, hypertonia, insomnia, irritability, mania, nervousness, neuralgia, neuropathy, paranoia, panic, paresthesia, parkinsonism, psychosis and other neuropsychiatric reactions, restlessness, **seizures**, sleep disorder, somnolence, **suicidal ideation**, syncope, tremor, unmasking tardive dyskinesia, vertigo
CV: **Arrhythmias**, **Brugada pattern/syndrome**, chest pain, **complete AV block**, **extrasystoles**, hypertension, **MI**, orthostatic hypotension, palpitations, phlebitis, tachycardia, vasodilation
EENT: Acute-angle glaucoma, altered taste, amblyopia, blurred vision, dry mouth, gum hemorrhage, hearing loss, increased ocular pressure, increased salivation, mydriasis, pharyngitis, sinusitis, taste perversion, tinnitus
ENDO: Hyperglycemia, **hypoglycemia**, syndrome of inappropriate ADH secretion
GI: Abdominal pain, anorexia, colitis, constipation, diarrhea, dysphagia, esophagitis, flatulence, **GI hemorrhage**, GI ulceration, **hepatic dysfunction**, **hepatitis**, increased appetite, **intestinal perforation**, nausea, **pancreatitis**, vomiting
GU: Abnormal ejaculation, cystitis, decreased or increased libido, dyspareunia, dysuria, incontinence, painful erection, prostate disorder, salpingitis, urinary frequency and urgency, UTI, vaginal hemorrhage, vaginitis
HEME: Anemia, leukocytosis, **leukopenia**, lymphadenopathy, **pancytopenia**, **thrombocytopenia**
MS: Arthralgia; arthritis; muscle rigidity, twitching, and weakness; myalgia; **rhabdomyolysis**
RESP: **Bronchospasm**, cough, dyspnea, pneumonia, **pulmonary embolism**
SKIN: Acute generalized exanthematous pustulosis, alopecia, diaphoresis, **erythema multiforme**, **exfoliative dermatitis**, flushing, hirsutism, maculopapular rash, pruritus, rash, **Stevens-Johnson syndrome**, urticaria
Other: **Anaphylaxis**, **angioedema**, **drug reaction with eosinophilia and systemic symptoms (DRESS)**, generalized pain, hot flashes, **hyponatremia**, infection, serum sickness–like reaction, weight loss

Childbearing Considerations

PREGNANCY

- Pregnancy exposure registry: 1-844-405-6185 or visit https://womensmentalhealth.org/clinical-and-research-programs/pregnancyregistry/antidepressants/.
- It is not known if drug can cause fetal harm.
- Use with caution only if benefit to mother outweighs potential risk to fetus.

LACTATION

- Drug is present in breast milk.
- Mothers should check with prescriber before breastfeeding.

Nursing Considerations

- Know that certain forms of bupropion are not approved for smoking cessation treatment, such as Aplenzin, Forfivo XL, Wellbutrin SR, and Wellbutrin XL.
- Know that Forfivo XL should never be used to initiate treatment of depression because the dose is too high. Only after the patient has received other bupropion products first and then requires a 450-mg dose should Forfivo XL be used.
- Be aware that Forfivo XL should not be used in patients with hepatic or renal impairment because the only dosage available for Forfivo XL is 450 mg once daily, which may be too high a dose for the kidneys or liver to handle.
- Use cautiously in patients with renal impairment (all other brands); drug is excreted by kidneys.
- Assess patient's blood pressure before bupropion therapy begins and monitor periodically during therapy because bupropion may cause hypertension.

! **WARNING** Monitor patient for hypersensitivity reactions that could become life-threatening such as anaphylaxis or angioedema. If present, notify prescriber, expect drug to be discontinued, and provide supportive care, as needed and ordered.

! **WARNING** Monitor patient for serious skin reactions that could become life-threatening such as DRESS. Know that although first sign of DRESS is usually a rash, DRESS may only present with fever or swollen lymph nodes. If present, notify prescriber, expect drug to be discontinued, and provide supportive care, as needed and ordered.

! **WARNING** Monitor depressed patients closely for worsened depression and increased suicide risk, especially when therapy starts or dosage changes. Also monitor patient taking drug to stop smoking for neuropsychiatric symptoms, including suicidal ideation. If present, notify prescriber immediately, begin safety measures, and expect to discontinue drug.

! **WARNING** Monitor patient for seizures. To reduce seizure risk, allow at least 4 hours (tablets) or 8 hours (E.R. tablets) between doses. Know that maximum dosage should not be exceeded, and dosage reduction should be gradual because risk of seizures is dose-related. Use seizure precautions, especially in patients who are addicted to cocaine, opioids, or stimulants; have a history of CNS tumors, head trauma, or seizures; have hyponatremia, hypoxia, or severe hepatic cirrhosis; take drugs that lower the seizure threshold; take insulin or an oral antidiabetic; take over-the-counter anorectics or stimulants; or use excessive alcohol, benzodiazepines, hypnotics, or sedatives.

- Know that using transdermal nicotine with bupropion may cause hypertension. Monitor patient's blood pressure closely.

PATIENT TEACHING

- Instruct patient how to administer the form of bupropion prescribed. If used for smoking cessation, advise patient to take bupropion for 7 or more days before stopping smoking.

! **WARNING** Alert patient that drug may cause an allergic reaction or serious skin reactions. Advise patient to seek medical help immediately and stop taking drug if signs of chest pain, fever, hives, itching, rash, shortness of breath, swelling, (especially of face), or swollen lymph nodes occurs.

! **WARNING** Urge patient to avoid or minimize consuming alcohol and sedatives during therapy and not to stop drug abruptly or exceed dosage prescribed because seizures may occur. Also, warn patient not to abruptly stop taking antiseizure drugs or prescribed benzodiazepines or sedatives.

! **WARNING** Urge family or caregiver to monitor depressed patient closely for worsened depression, especially when therapy starts or dosage changes. Also, inform family or caregiver that drug may cause a variety of neuropsychiatric adverse events that could be serious, including suicidal behavior and thoughts even when used just for smoking cessation. If changes in behavior or thought patterns emerge with bupropion use, instruct family or caregiver to notify prescriber immediately.

- Alert patient that drug may cause mild pupillary dilation, which can lead to an episode of acute-closure glaucoma. Encourage him to have an eye exam to determine if he is susceptible to angle closure.
- Alert patient that bupropion therapy may produce a false-positive urine screening test for amphetamines even after drug has been discontinued. Other tests may be required to distinguish bupropion from amphetamines.

buspirone hydrochloride

Class and Category

Pharmacologic class: Azapirone
Therapeutic class: Anxiolytic

Indications and Dosages

✻ To manage anxiety

TABLETS

Adults. *Initial:* 7.5 mg twice daily increased by 5 mg daily at 2- to 3-day intervals until desired response occurs. *Maintenance:* 20 to 30 mg daily (usual therapeutic range) in divided doses. *Maximum:* 60 mg daily.

±**DOSAGE ADJUSTMENT** For patients using CYP3A4 inhibitors, dosage reduced. For patients receiving concomitant therapy with nefazodone, dosage decreased to 2.5 mg daily. For patients receiving concomitant therapy with CYP3A4 inducers, dosage may need to be increased.

Drug Administration

P.O.

- Administer consistently, either always with or always without food.
- Do not administer with grapefruit juice.

Route	Onset	Peak	Duration
P.O.	Slow	40–90 min	Unknown

Half-life: 18 hr

Mechanism of Action

May act as a partial agonist at serotonin 5-hydroxytryptamine$_{1A}$ receptors in the brain, producing antianxiety effects.

Contraindications

Hypersensitivity to buspirone or its components, severe hepatic or renal impairment

Interactions

DRUGS

CYP3A4 inducers, such as certain anticonvulsants (carbamazepine, phenobarbital, phenytoin) and dexamethasone: Possibly increased rate of buspirone metabolism and decreased effectiveness of buspirone
CYP3A4 inhibitors, such as ketoconazole and ritonavir: Possibly inhibited buspirone metabolism and increased blood level of buspirone
diltiazem, erythromycin, itraconazole, nefazodone, nordiazepam, verapamil: Increased blood level and adverse effects of buspirone
haloperidol: Increased haloperidol level
MAO inhibitors: Increased risk of hypertension
rifampin: Decreased blood buspirone level and pharmacodynamic effects

FOODS

any food: Possibly decreased buspirone clearance
grapefruit juice: Increased blood buspirone level

Adverse Reactions

CNS: Akathisia, anger, ataxia, cogwheel rigidity, confusion, decreased concentration, depression, dizziness, dream disturbances, drowsiness, dyskinesias, dystonia, excitement, extrapyramidal symptoms, fatigue, headache, hostility, insomnia, lack of coordination, light-headedness, mood swings, nervousness, paresthesia, parkinsonism, restless leg syndrome, restlessness, **serotonin syndrome**, transient recall impairment, tremor, weakness
CV: Chest pain, palpitations, tachycardia
EENT: Blurred vision, dry mouth, nasal congestion, pharyngitis, tinnitus, tunnel vision
GI: Abdominal or gastric distress, constipation, diarrhea, nausea, vomiting
GU: Urine retention
MS: Myalgia
SKIN: Diaphoresis, ecchymosis, rash, urticaria
Other: **Angioedema**

Childbearing Considerations

PREGNANCY

- It is not known if drug can cause fetal harm.
- Use with caution only if benefit to mother outweighs potential risk to fetus.

LACTATION

- It is not known if drug is present in breast milk.
- Drug use during breastfeeding is not recommended.

Nursing Considerations

- Use buspirone cautiously in patients with mild to moderate hepatic or renal impairment. Know that drug is not recommended in patients with severe hepatic or renal impairment.

! **WARNING** Monitor patient for hypersensitivity reaction that could become life-threatening such as angioedema. If present, notify prescriber, expect drug to be discontinued, and provide supportive care, as needed and ordered.

- Institute safety precautions because of possible adverse CNS reactions.
- Follow closely if patient is being withdrawn from long-term therapy with benzodiazepines or other sedative-hypnotic drugs while starting buspirone because buspirone won't prevent withdrawal symptoms.

PATIENT TEACHING

- Instruct patient how to administer buspirone. Emphasize the importance of not taking more of the drug than prescribed.
- Caution patient to avoid drinking large amounts of grapefruit juice.
- Inform patient that 1 to 2 weeks of therapy may be needed before drug's antianxiety effect is known.

! **WARNING** Alert patient that drug may cause an allergic reaction. Tell patient to notify prescriber if an allergic reaction occurs. If swelling of face, throat, or tongue occurs or other severe adverse reactions, stress importance of seeking immediate medical care.

- Advise patient to avoid hazardous activities until drug's CNS effects are known and resolved.
- Inform mothers breastfeeding is not recommended during buspirone therapy.

butorphanol tartrate

Class, Category, and Schedule

Pharmacologic class: Opioid agonist–antagonist
Therapeutic class: Anesthesia adjunct, opioid analgesic
Controlled substance schedule: IV

Indications and Dosages

✶ *To manage pain severe enough to require an opioid analgesic and for which alternative treatments are inadequate*

I.V. INJECTION

Adults. 0.5 to 2 mg (usually 1 mg) every 3 to 4 hr, as needed.

I.M. INJECTION

Adults. 1 to 4 mg (usually 2 mg) every 3 to 4 hr, as needed. *Maximum:* 4 mg/single dose.

NASAL SPRAY

Adults. 1 mg (1 spray) in one nostril. Dose repeated after 60 to 90 min, as needed; 2-dose sequence repeated every 3 to 4 hr after the second dose of the sequence, as needed. *For severe pain:* 2 mg (1 spray in each nostril) every 3 to 4 hr, as needed.

± **DOSAGE ADJUSTMENT** For elderly patients and those with impaired hepatic or renal function, dose maintained at 1 spray in one nostril. Dose repeated after 90 to 120 minutes, as needed; 2-dose sequence repeated every 6 hours or more, as needed.

✶ *As adjunct to provide preoperative anesthesia*

I.M. INJECTION

Adults. Individualized. *Usual:* 2 mg 60 to 90 min before surgery.

✶ *As adjunct to balanced anesthesia*

I.V. INJECTION

Adults. 2 mg shortly before induction and/or 0.5 to 1 mg in increments during anesthesia, as needed. Increments may be increased up to 0.06 mg/kg, as needed. *Usual range:* 4 mg to 12.5 mg.

✶ *To relieve pain during labor*

I.M. INJECTION, I.V. INJECTION

Pregnant females at full term in early labor. 1 to 2 mg repeated in 4 hr.

± **DOSAGE ADJUSTMENT** For elderly patients and patients with impaired hepatic or renal function, initial parenteral dose kept at 1 mg followed, as needed, by 1 mg in 90 to 120 minutes and dosage interval for subsequent doses increased to at least 6 hours or more.

Drug Administration

I.V.

- Administer by direct injection. following manufacturer guidelines.
- Protect from light.
- If skin contact occurs, rinse skin with cool water.
- *Incompatibilities:* None reported by manufacturer

I.M.

- Protect vial from light.
- If skin contact occurs, rinse skin with cool water.

NASAL INHALATION

- Have patient blow nose.
- Pull clear cover from the pump unit and remove protective clip from its neck.
- Prime pump unit by placing the nozzle between first and second fingers with thumb on the bottom of the bottle. Then, pump sprayer unit firmly and quickly until a fine spray appears (7 or 8 strokes). Re-prime the pump unit if it has not been used for 48 hr or longer.
- Insert spray tip about 1 cm (one-third inch) into one nostril, pointing tip toward the back of the nose. Close other nostril with one finger and tilt head slightly forward. Then, pump sprayer firmly and quickly by pushing down on the pump unit's finger grips and against the thumb at the bottom of the bottle.
- Have patient sniff gently with mouth closed.
- After spraying, remove pump from nose, have patient tilt head back, and sniff gently for a few more seconds.
- Replace protective clip and clear cover.

Route	Onset	Peak	Duration
I.V.	1–3 min	30–60 min	3–4 hr
I.M.	5–10 min	30–60 min	3–4 hr
Inhalation	15 min	1–2 hr	4–5 hr

Half-life: 4–10 hr

Mechanism of Action

Binds with specific CNS receptors to alter the perception of and emotional response to pain.

Contraindications

Acute or severe bronchial asthma in an unmonitored setting or in the absence of resuscitative equipment; GI obstruction, including paralytic ileus; hypersensitivity to butorphanol or its components (including the preservative benzethonium chloride); significant respiratory depression

Interactions

DRUGS

benzodiazepines, other CNS depressants: Additive CNS depression that can be significant, causing coma, prolonged sedation, or significant respiratory depression
Nasal vasoconstrictors, such as oxymetazoline: Decreased absorption rate and delayed onset of butorphanol
serotonergic drugs: Increased risk of serotonin syndrome

ACTIVITIES

alcohol use: Additive CNS depression that could be significant

Adverse Reactions

CNS: Anxiety, confusion, difficulty making purposeful movements, difficulty speaking, dizziness, euphoria, floating feeling, headache, insomnia (with nasal form), lethargy, nervousness, paresthesia, sensation of heat, somnolence, syncope, tremor, vertigo
CV: Chest pain, **hypotension**, palpitations, tachycardia, vasodilation
EENT: Blurred vision, dry mouth, ear pain, epistaxis, nasal congestion or irritation (with nasal form), pharyngitis, rhinitis, sinus congestion, sinusitis, tinnitus, unpleasant taste
ENDO: **Adrenal insufficiency (rare)**
GI: Anorexia, constipation, epigastric pain, nausea, vomiting
RESP: **Apnea**, bronchitis, cough, dyspnea, **respiratory depression**, **shallow breathing**, upper respiratory tract infection
SKIN: Clammy skin, pruritus
Other: **Anaphylaxis**, opioid-induced allodynia (pain from ordinarily non-painful stimuli) or hyperalgesia (paradoxical increase in pain), physical and psychological dependence

Childbearing Considerations

PREGNANCY

- Drug can cause fetal harm resulting in neonatal opioid withdrawal syndrome

(NOWS) shortly after birth if drug used for extended period of time during pregnancy.
- Use with caution only if benefit to mother outweighs potential risk to fetus.

LABOR AND DELIVERY
- Drug may prolong labor.
- If mother took butorphanol for an extended period of time during pregnancy, monitor neonate for excessive sedation or respiratory depression shortly after birth.

LACTATION
- Drug may be present in breast milk.
- Mothers should check with prescriber before breastfeeding.
- If breastfeeding occurs, mother should be instructed to monitor infant for breathing difficulties and drowsiness.
- Withdrawal symptoms can occur in breastfed infants when mother stops taking drug or breastfeeding stops.

REPRODUCTION
- Females of childbearing age should avoid pregnancy during drug use.
- Chronic use of opioids may reduce fertility if taken for an extended period of time and it is not known if effects on fertility are reversible.

Nursing Considerations

- Know that butorphanol should be used cautiously, if at all, in patients with depression, history of drug abuse, hepatic or renal dysfunction, or suicidal tendency.
- Use drug cautiously, if at all, in patients with head injury because drug can raise CSF pressure. Because it can increase cardiac workload, use with extreme caution in patients with acute MI, coronary insufficiency, or ventricular dysfunction.
- Monitor patient after first dose of nasal form; hypotension and syncope may occur.

! **WARNING** Assess patient for addiction tendency that could result in abuse and misuse of butorphanol because it is an opioid. Know that drug requires an Opioid Analgesic Risk Evaluation and Mitigation Strategy (REMS) before drug can be administered. Monitor patient throughout drug therapy for evidence of physical and/or psychological dependency. Notify prescriber of any concerns.

! **WARNING** Monitor patient for hypersensitivity reactions that could become life-threatening such as anaphylaxis. If present, notify prescriber immediately, expect drug to be withheld or changed to a different drug, and provide supportive care, as needed and ordered.

! **WARNING** Monitor patient closely for respiratory depression, especially during initiation of drug therapy or following a dosage increase. Know that patients at risk for respiratory depression include cachectic, debilitated, or elderly patients; patients with chronic pulmonary disease; or in patients using concomitantly other drugs such as benzothiazines or other CNS drugs including alcohol that depress respiration and are given together. Immediately report respiratory depression because respiratory arrest may occur. Be prepared to provide emergency supportive care.

! **WARNING** Monitor blood pressure often after giving drug. If severe hypertension develops (rare), stop drug at once and notify prescriber. If patient isn't narcotic-dependent, expect to administer naloxone to reverse butorphanol's effects.

! **WARNING** Assess elderly patients for signs and symptoms of toxicity or overdose, as these patients may be at increased risk because of decreased cardiac, hepatic, or renal function and the presence of concomitant disease and other drug therapy. Have naloxone readily available to treat overdose.

! **WARNING** Know that many drugs may interact with opioids like butorphanol to cause serotonin syndrome. Monitor patient closely for signs and symptoms, such as agitation, diaphoresis, diarrhea, fever, hallucinations, labile blood pressure, muscle twitching or stiffness, nausea, shakiness, shivering, tachycardia, trouble with coordination, or vomiting. Notify prescriber at once because serotonin syndrome may be life-threatening. Be prepared to discontinue drug, if possible and ordered, and provide supportive care.

! **WARNING** Monitor patient for adrenal insufficiency. Although rare, this can be life-threatening. Monitor patient for anorexia, dizziness, fatigue, hypotension, nausea, vomiting, or weakness. Notify prescriber if adrenal insufficiency is suspected and expect diagnostic testing to be done to determine if present. If diagnosis is confirmed, expect to administer corticosteroids and wean patient off butorphanol if possible.

- Monitor patient for opioid-induced allodynia (pain from ordinarily non-painful stimuli) and hyperalgesia (paradoxical increase in pain), which is different from tolerance. Assess patient for increase in pain when butorphanol dosage is increased or decrease level of pain when butorphanol dosage is decreased, Notify prescriber if opioid-induced allodynia and hyperalgesia occurs as dosage may need to be decreased or opioid rotation used.
- Take safety precautions because butorphanol causes CNS depression.

PATIENT TEACHING

- Instruct patient how to administer butorphanol nasal spray. Emphasize the importance of taking butorphanol exactly as prescribed because it can be addictive. Warn patient not to increase the dose or decrease the dosage interval without consulting prescriber.

! WARNING Tell family or caregiver how to administer naloxone in the event of an overdose and the importance of always having naloxone readily available at home.

! WARNING Alert patient that butorphanol may cause an allergic reaction. If an allergic occurs, instruct patient to notify prescriber and to immediately seek medical care, if severe.

! WARNING Tell patient to avoid alcohol and other CNS depressants, including over-the-counter drugs, while taking butorphanol because of additive adverse CNS reactions and risk of respiratory depression.

! WARNING Stress importance of patient keeping butorphanol out of reach of children as even one dose can cause a fatal overdose.

- Alert patient that butorphanol may cause feelings of pain from stimuli that doesn't usually cause pain or paradoxically pain may be increased, especially if dosage increased. Tell patient to notify prescriber if these types of reactions are experienced.
- Advise patient to avoid hazardous activities until drug's CNS effects are known and resolved.
- Tell females of childbearing age to notify prescriber if pregnancy occurs. Encourage to use effective contraception throughout butorphanol therapy.
- Inform mothers wishing to breastfeed of the risks to their infant such as difficulty breathing and drowsiness. Also alert mothers that if breastfeeding takes place while taking butorphanol, infant may experience withdrawal when breastfeeding stops or mother discontinues taking the drug.

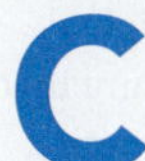

cabotegravir

Apretude, Vocabria

Class and Category

Pharmacologic class: HIV-1 integrase strand transfer inhibitor (INSTI)
Therapeutic class: Antiviral

Indications and Dosages

∗ *As adjunct with rilpivirine therapy for short-term treatment of HIV-1 infection for patients who are virologically suppressed (HIV-1 RNA less than 50 copies/ml) and on a stable antiretroviral regimen with no history of treatment failure and with no known or suspected resistance to either cabotegravir or rilpivirine in order to assess tolerability of cabotegravir prior to administration of cabotegravir and rilpivirine, as E.R. injectable suspensions*

TABLETS (VOCABRIA)

Adults and children ages 12 and older weighing at least 35 kg (77 lb). 30 mg in combination with 25 mg of rilpivirine once daily for at least 28 days with last oral dose given on the same day injections of cabotegravir and rilpivirine are started.

∗ *As adjunct with rilpivirne therapy for short-term treatment of HIV-1 infection for patients who are virologically suppressed (HIV-1 RNA less than 50 copies/ml) and on a stable antiretroviral regimen with no history of treatment failure and with no known or suspected resistance to either cabotegravir or rilpivirine when planned injection dosing with cabotegravir and rilpivirine will be missed for more than 7 days*

TABLETS (VOCABRIA)

Adults and children ages 12 and older weighing at least 35 kg (77 lb). *Initial:* 30 mg in combination with 25 mg of rilpivirine once daily initiated about 1 mo (+/– 7 days) after the last injection doses of cabotegravir and rilpivirine if on a monthly dosing schedule or 2 mo (+/– 7 days) if on a 2-mo dosing schedule and continued until the day the injections of cabotegravir and rilpivirine are restarted. *Maximum:* Replacement for missed injection therapy given no longer than 2 mo.

±**DOSAGE ADJUSTMENT** For patients planning to miss injection dosing with cabotegravir and rilpivirine for more than 2 mo, an alternative oral regimen is required.

∗ *To reduce the risk of sexually acquired HIV-1 infection short-term as pre-exposure prophylaxis for at-risk patients*

E.R. I. M. INJECTION (APRETUDE) AND TABLETS (VOCABRIA)

Adults and adolescents weighing at least 35 kg (77 lb) using an oral lead-in. *Initial:* 30 mg P.O. for at least 28 days followed by 600 mg I.M. administered on the last day or within 3 days of P.O. dosing followed by 600 mg I.M. given 1 mo later (+/– 7 days before or after the scheduled injection date). *Maintenance:* 600 mg I.M. given every 2 mo starting on the 5th mo (+/– 7 days before or after the scheduled injection date).

E.R. I. M. INJECTION (APRETUDE)

Adults and adolescents weighing at least 35 kg (77 lb) without an oral lead-in. *Initial:* 600 mg followed 1 mo later with 600 mg (+/– 7 days before or after the scheduled injection date). *Maintenance:* 600 mg every 2 mo starting on mo 4 (+/– 7 days before or after the scheduled injection date).

±**DOSAGE ADJUSTMENT** For patients planning to miss an I.M. dose by more than 7 days from when it is normally given, oral cabotegravir therapy begun at a dose of 30 mg daily for a duration of up to 2 months to replace 1 missed scheduled 2-month injection. The first dose of oral drug given approximately 2 months after the last injection dose. Injection dose restarted on the day or within 3 days of oral dosing being completed; if oral dosing is required for more than 2 months, an alternative oral regimen is required. For patients with an unplanned missed injection dose that is missed or delayed by more than 7 days and oral dosing has not been taken in the interim, patient reassessed to determine if resumption of injection dosing remains appropriate. If injection dosing is to be continued, manufacturer's guidelines followed to re-initiation Apretude therapy.

Drug Administration

P.O.

- Administer drug at about the same time each day.
- Administer with a meal.

I.M. INJECTION

- Ensure patient has been tested for HIV-1 infection prior to initiating drug and with each subsequent injection. The test used must be approved or cleared by the FDA for the diagnosis of acute or primary HIV-1 infection. If an antigen/antibody-specific test is used and provides negative results, the negative results should be confirmed using an RNA-specific assay, even if the results of the RNA assay are not available until after drug therapy is begun.
- Patient must agree to the required injection dosing and testing schedule prior to initiating drug therapy to help reduce the risk of acquiring HIV-1 infection or development of resistance.
- Initiate first injection on the last day of oral lead-in or within 3 days thereafter, if an oral lead-in dosing schedule is being used. Second injection given one mo later. The second injection may be given up to 7 days before or after the date the individual is scheduled to receive the injection.
- Store drug in refrigerator, allowing it to warm up to room temperature before administration. Do not dilute or reconstitute drug prior to administration. Shake the vial vigorously so that the suspension looks uniform before withdrawing drug from the vial. Small air bubbles are expected and acceptable. Once the suspension has been drawn into the syringe, administer injection as soon as possible. However, drug may remain in the syringe for up to 2 hr, if needed. Do not place the filled syringe in the refrigerator during this time. If more than 2 hr passes, the filled syringe and needle must be discarded.
- Administer in the ventrogluteal site (preferred) or the dorsogluteal site (less preferred). Do not administer in any other anatomical site or by any other route. Determine the patient's body mass index (BMI) to ensure that the needle length is sufficient to reach the gluteus muscle. Longer needle lengths (not included in the dosing kit) may be required for patients with higher BMI (e.g., >30 kg/m^2) to ensure that the injection is administered intramuscularly as opposed to subcutaneously.
- Store drug in refrigerator in the original carton until ready to use but exposure up to 30°C (86°F) is permitted. Do not freeze.

Route	Onset	Peak	Duration
P.O./I.M.	Unknown	Unknown	Unknown

Half-life: 40 hr

Mechanism of Action

Binds to the integrase active site and blocks the strand transfer step of retroviral deoxyribonucleic acid (DNA) integration, which is essential for HIV replication.

Contraindications

Concurrent use of anticonvulsants (carbamazepine, oxcarbazepine, phenobarbital, phenytoin), antimycobacterials (rifampin, rifapentine), and the drugs, cabotegravir and rilpivirine E.R. injectable suspensions with rifabutin; hypersensitivity to cabotegravir or its components; unknown or positive HIV-status (Apretude)

Interactions

DRUGS

antacids containing polyvalent cations, such as aluminum, calcium carbonate, or magnesium hydroxide: Decreased absorption of cabotegravir decreasing effectiveness
anticonvulsants, such as carbamazepine, oxcarbazepine, phenobarbital, phenytoin: Decreased cabotegravir plasma concentrations leading to potential for loss of effectiveness and increased risk of development of resistance
antimycobacterials, such as rifampin, rifapentine: Decreased cabotegravir plasma concentration decreasing effectiveness
methadone: Possibly decreased methadone levels possibly requiring dosage adjustment of methadone
UGT1A1 or 1A9 inducers: Possibly decreased cabotegravir plasma concentrations decreasing effectiveness

Adverse Reactions

CNS: Abnormal dreams, anxiety, asthenia, depression, fever, headache, insomnia, mood swings, **suicidal ideation**
CV: Elevated lipids
GI: Elevated liver enzymes, **hepatotoxicity**, nausea
MS: Myalgia
SKIN: Rash, urticaria

Other: **Angioedema and other hypersensitivity reactions**, flu-like symptoms, injection site reactions (abscess, bruising, discoloration, erythema, induration, nodules, numbness, pain, pruritis, redness, swelling, warmth), weight increase

Childbearing Considerations

PREGNANCY

- Pregnancy exposure registry: 1-800-258-4263.
- Potential increased risk for fetal neural tube defects when administered at the time of conception or in early pregnancy.
- Be aware that Apretude brand of drug is detected in maternal systemic circulation for up to 12 months or longer after drug therapy has ended increasing risk for fetal exposure if pregnancy occurs during this time frame.
- Use with caution only if benefit to mother outweighs potential risk to fetus.

LACTATION

- It is not known if drug is present in breast milk.
- The Centers for Disease Control and Prevention recommends that HIV-1-infected mothers not breastfeed, to avoid risking postnatal transmission of HIV-1 infection to infants. They also do not recommend breastfeeding because of potential drug-induced adverse reactions in the infant.
- Mothers receiving Apretude therapy should check with prescriber before breastfeeding because drug may still be present in the body for up to 12 months or longer after last dose.

Nursing Considerations

- Determine seronegative patients recent (in past month) potential HIV-1 infection exposure events (e.g., condomless sex or condom breaking during sex with a partner of unknown HIV-1 status or unknown viremic status, or a recent sexually transmitted infection [STI]). Evaluate for current or recent signs or symptoms consistent with acute HIV-1 infection (e.g., fever, fatigue, myalgia, skin rash) prior to initiating cabotegravir therapy.
- Use a test approved or cleared by the FDA if recent (less than 1 month) exposures to HIV-1 are suspected or clinical symptoms consistent with acute HIV-1 infection are present. When administering Apretude, HIV-1 testing should be repeated prior to each injection and upon diagnosis of any other STIs.
- Know that if an HIV-1 test indicates possible HIV-1 infection, or if symptoms consistent with acute HIV-1 infection develop following an exposure event while patient is receiving cabotegravir therapy, additional HIV testing to determine HIV status is needed. If an individual has confirmed HIV-1 infection, then the individual must be transitioned to a complete HIV-1 treatment regimen.

! WARNING Monitor patient closely for hypersensitivity reaction because other integrase inhibitors have caused hypersensitivity reactions. At the first sign of a hypersensitivity reaction (angioedema, blisters, conjunctivitis, difficulty breathing, eosinophilia, facial edema, fatigue, general malaise, hepatitis, joint or muscle aches, oral blisters or lesions), stop administering drug and notify prescriber. Provide supportive care, as needed and ordered.

! WARNING Monitor patient for depressive disorders, such as depression and mood swings that could lead to suicidal ideation. Institute suicide precautions, if needed. Report changes to prescriber, as cabotegravir may have to be discontinued.

! WARNING Know that patients with underlying liver disease or who have marked elevations in liver enzymes before cabotegravir therapy is initiated may develop worsening of liver function or further increased liver enzymes during cabotegravir therapy. Monitor closely for decreased liver function even in patients without known hepatic disease and expect liver enzymes to be monitored throughout drug therapy.

PATIENT TEACHING

- Explain need for testing and dosing schedule when cabotegravir therapy is used prior to initiating the drug and obtain patient's consent to comply with the schedule in order to reduce the risk of HIV-1 acquisition and the potential development of resistance.

C

! **WARNING** Alert patient that cabotegravir should not be taken if patient already has a HIV-1 infection or does not know HIV-1 status.

- Instruct patient how to administer cabotegravir and what to do if dose is missed.
- Counsel patient on the use of other HIV-1 infection prevention measures (e.g., consistent and correct condom use; knowledge of partner(s)' HIV-1 status, including viral suppression status; and regular testing for sexually transmitted infections (STIs) that can facilitate HIV-1 transmission). Encourage patients to reduce sexual risk behavior.

! **WARNING** Instruct patient to notify prescriber immediately if an allergic reaction occurs or a rash develops. Tell patient to stop drug and seek immediate medical attention if rash is accompanied by any other symptoms or allergic reaction is severe.

! **WARNING** Inform patient, family, or caregiver that cabotegravir may affect patient's mood enough to cause depression or even suicidal ideology. If present, review suicide precautions with family or caregiver and to notify prescriber immediately. Explain patient should be reevaluated to determine if drug should be discontinued.

! **WARNING** Stress importance of complying with ordered blood tests used to monitor liver function. Tell patient to watch for signs of liver dysfunction, such as dark or tea-colored urine, loss of appetite, nausea, pale-colored stools, pain or sensitivity on the right side below the ribs, or yellowing of the skin or whites of the eyes. If present, stress importance of notifying prescriber, as liver function will have to be assessed through laboratory tests and additional treatment may be needed.

- Tell patient to keep prescriber informed of all drug use, including prescribed drugs, over-the-counter drugs, and herbal products being taken.
- Advise mother receiving cabotegravir not to breastfeed her infant if HIV-1 infection is present and to check with prescriber regarding breastfeeding before taking Apretude form of drug.

calcitonin, salmon

Miacalcin, Miacalcin Nasal Spray

Class and Category

Pharmacologic class: Hormone
Therapeutic class: Antihypercalcemic, anti-osteoporotic

Indications and Dosages

✶ *To treat an early hypercalcemic emergency*

I.M. OR SUBCUTANEOUS INJECTION (MIACALCIN)

Adults. *Initial:* 4 USP Units/kg every 12 hr. Increased after 1 or 2 days, as needed, to 8 USP Units/kg every 12 hr and then 8 USP Units/kg every 6 hr after 2 more days, as needed. *Maximum:* 8 USP Units/kg every 6 hr.

✶ *To treat postmenopausal osteoporosis in women who are at least 5 years postmenopausal*

I.M. OR SUBCUTANEOUS INJECTION (MIACALCIN)

Adult women. *Initial:* 100 USP Units (0.5 ml) daily.

NASAL SPRAY (MIACALCIN NASAL SPRAY)

Adult women. 200 international units (1 spray) daily, alternating nostrils.

✶ *To treat symptomatic Paget's disease of the bone*

I.M. OR SUBCUTANEOUS INJECTION (MIACALCIN)

Adults. *Initial:* 100 USP Units (0.5 ml) daily.

Drug Administration

- Expect to perform a skin test following manufacturer's guidelines before giving drug if sensitivity to drug is suspected. Observe the site for 15 min after test injection. If evidence of sensitivity is detected, such as more than mild erythema or a wheal, notify prescriber.

I.M.

- Route preferred if dose volume exceeds 2 ml with total dose distributed across multiple injection sites. Solution should appear clear and colorless. Store drug in refrigerator.

NASAL SPRAY

- If using unopened bottle for the first time, remove from refrigerator and allow to reach room temperature. Solution should appear clear and colorless without particles.

- Lift up the blue plastic tab and carefully pull the metal safety seal off the bottle. Keep the bottle upright and remove the rubber stopper from the bottle. Hold the nose spray pump and gently remove the plastic protective cap from the bottom of the nose spray pump. Do not push down on the pump when it is not attached to the bottle. Hold the bottle upright and insert the nose spray pump into the bottle. Turn the pump clockwise to tighten it until it is securely attached to the bottle. Gently pull the clear protective cap to remove it from the top of the nose spray pump.
- Before first use, activate nasal pump by holding bottle upright and depressing the 2 white side arms of the pump toward the bottle. When bottle emits a full spray, pump is activated.
- Have patient gently blow nose first.
- Insert tip of bottle into 1 nostril while patient holds head upright.
- Depress pump firmly. Patient should not sniff, inhale deeply, or blow nose for a few min afterwards.
- Alternate nostrils daily.
- Wipe the nose spray pump with a clean, damp cloth 1 to 2 times a week. Dry the nose spray pump with a clean cloth.
- Gently put the protective cap back on the nasal spray pump. Hold the bottle with 2 fingers under the 2 side arms of the pump. Be careful not to push down on the pump while putting cap on. Do not refrigerate once bottle has been opened. Store upright and do not shake bottle. Bottle should be discarded after 30 doses regardless of any drug still left in bottle.

SUBCUTANEOUS

- Route can be used if dose volume is less than 2 ml. Store drug in refrigerator.

Route	Onset	Peak	Duration
I.M., SubQ	15 min	4 hr	8–24 hr
Nasal spray	> 10 min	31–39 min	Unknown

Half-life: 43–60 min

Mechanism of Action

Inhibits bone resorption directly. Besides reducing the serum calcium level, this action slows bone metabolism (a major factor in the development of Paget's disease) and calcium loss from the bone (a major factor in the development of osteoporosis).

Contraindications

Hypersensitivity to calcitonin salmon or its components

Interactions

DRUGS

lithium: Possibly decreased lithium level

Adverse Reactions

CNS: Agitation, anxiety, **CVA**, dizziness, fatigue, headache, insomnia, neuralgia, paresthesia, tremor, vertigo
CV: **Bundle branch block**, hypertension, **MI**, palpitations, peripheral edema, tachycardia, thrombophlebitis
EENT: Blurred vision; dry mouth; earache; epistaxis; eye pain; hearing loss; nasal irritation or ulceration (nasal spray), lesions, or redness; pharyngitis; rhinitis; salty taste; sinusitis; taste perversion; tinnitus; vitreous floaters
ENDO: Goiter, hyperthyroidism
GI: Abdominal pain, anorexia, cholelithiasis, diarrhea, epigastric discomfort, flatulence, gastritis, **hepatitis**, increased appetite, nausea, thirst, vomiting
GU: Hematuria, nocturia, polyuria, **pyelonephritis**, renal calculi
HEME: Anemia
MS: Arthralgia, arthrosis, back or musculoskeletal pain, joint stiffness, polymyalgia rheumatica
RESP: Bronchitis, **bronchospasm**, cough, dyspnea, pneumonia, upper respiratory tract infection
SKIN: Alopecia, diaphoresis, eczema, flushing of face or hands, pruritus of earlobes, rash, ulceration, urticaria
Other: **Anaphylaxis**, **anaphylactic shock**, **angioedema**, antibody formation, feverish sensation, **hypocalcemia**, influenza-like symptoms, injection-site inflammation, lymphadenopathy, **malignancies**, mild tetanic symptoms

Childbearing Considerations

PREGNANCY

- It is not known if drug can cause fetal harm.
- Use with caution only if benefit to mother outweighs potential risk to fetus.

LACTATION

- It is not known if drug is present in breast milk.

- Breastfeeding is not recommended because drug may interfere with lactation.

Nursing Considerations

- Know that mineral metabolism disorders, such as vitamin D deficiency, must be corrected before calcitonin therapy begins. These patients should also be monitored during therapy for signs and symptoms of hypocalcemia, such as muscle cramps, seizures, and twitching. Also, expect to give 1.5 g of supplemental calcium carbonate and at least 400 units of vitamin D daily. Plan to provide a balanced diet that includes foods high in calcium and vitamin D.
- Assess for nausea, especially with the first dose. Nausea tends to decrease or disappear with continued use.

! **WARNING** Monitor serum calcium level, as ordered, if patient receives calcitonin for hypercalcemia. During first several doses, keep parenteral calcium available in case the calcium level is inadvertently overcorrected.

! **WARNING** Monitor patient for hypersensitivity reactions, which could become life-threatening such as anaphylaxis or angioedema. Notify prescriber, expect drug to be discontinued, and provide supportive care, as needed and ordered.

- Periodically examine patient using nasal spray for nasal ulcers. If severe ulceration of the nasal mucosa occurs (ulcers causing heavy bleeding, ulcers greater than 1.5 mm, or ulcers penetrating below the mucosa), notify prescriber and expect nasal spray form to be discontinued. Also, know that nasal spray should not be used if smaller or less severe ulcers are present until healing occurs.
- Be aware if patient with Paget's disease relapses after treatment, check for antibody formation, as ordered.

PATIENT TEACHING

- Instruct patient how to administer form of calcitonin prescribed, including how to administer subcutaneous injections, if required.
- Stress importance of eating a diet high in calcium and vitamin D if patient is receiving drug for postmenopausal osteoporosis.
- Reassure patient experiencing nausea that it usually disappears with continued use.

! **WARNING** Review signs and symptoms of hypercalcemia and hypocalcemia. Urge patient to notify prescriber immediately, if present, or seek immediate medical care, if severe. Stress importance of complying with routine blood tests to monitor calcium level.

! **WARNING** Alert patient that drug may cause an allergic reaction, which could become severe. If present, instruct patient to notify prescriber promptly and to seek immediate medical care, if severe.

- Instruct patient prescribed nasal spray to report adverse nasal symptoms to prescriber.
- Inform mothers that breastfeeding is not recommended during calcitonin therapy because it may adversely affect being able to breastfeed.

calcitriol

(1,25-dihydroxy-cholecalciferol)

Rocaltrol

Class and Category

Pharmacologic class: Vitamin D analogue
Therapeutic class: Antihypocalcemic

Indications and Dosages

∗ *To treat hypocalcemia in predialysis patients*

CAPSULES, ORAL SOLUTION (ROCALTROL)

Adults and children ages 3 and older. *Initial:* 0.25 mcg daily. Increased, as needed, to 0.5 mcg daily.

ORAL SOLUTION

Children up to age 3. *Initial:* 10 to 15 mg/kg daily.

∗ *To treat hypocalcemia in dialysis patients*

CAPSULES, ORAL SOLUTION (ROCALTROL)

Adults. *Initial:* 0.25 mcg daily. Increased by 0.25 mcg daily every 4 to 8 wk, as needed. *Usual:* 0.5 to 1 mcg daily.

I.V. INJECTION (CALCITRIOL)

Adults. *Initial:* 1–2 mcg 3 times wk, approximately every other day, increased in increments of 0.5 to 1 mcg at 2- to 4-wk intervals, as needed.

±**DOSAGE ADJUSTMENT** For patients receiving drug I.V., initial doses depend on the severity of the hypocalcemia and may begin as little as 0.5 mcg or as much as 4 mcg 3 times a week, as needed. For patients with normal or only slightly reduced serum calcium levels and receiving oral therapy, dosage kept at 0.25 mcg, but dosage frequency increased to every other day.

✱ *To treat hypoparathyroidism, and pseudohypoparathyroidism*

CAPSULES, ORAL SOLUTION (ROCALTROL)

Adults and children ages 6 and older. *Initial:* 0.25 mcg daily in the morning. Increased every 2 to 4 wk, as needed. *Usual:* 0.5 to 2 mcg daily.

✱ *To treat hyypoparathyroidism*

ORAL SOLUTION

Children ages 1 to 5. *Usual:* 0.25 to 0.75 mcg daily in the morning.

Drug Administration

P.O.

- Measure dosage of oral solution using a calibrated device.
- Capsules should be swallowed whole and not chewed, crushed, or opened.

I.V.

- No dilution is needed.
- Administer rapidly as a bolus at the end of hemodialysis.
- *Incompatibilities:* None reported by manufacturer.

Route	Onset	Peak	Duration
P.O.	2.6 hr	3–6 hr	3–5 days
I.V.	Immediate	Unknown	3–5 days

Half-life: 5–8 hr

Mechanism of Action

Binds to specific receptors on intestinal mucosa to increase calcium absorption from intestine. Drug may also regulate calcium ion transfer from bone to blood and stimulate calcium reabsorption in the distal renal tubules, making more calcium available in the body.

Contraindications

Hypercalcemia, hypersensitivity to calcitriol or its components, vitamin D toxicity

Interactions

DRUGS

calcium supplements: Increased risk of hypercalcemia
cholestyramine: Decreased calcitriol absorption
corticosteroids: Possibly inhibits calcium absorption
digitalis glycosides: Possibly arrhythmias
ketoconazole: Decreased calcitriol level
magnesium-containing antacids Hypermagnesemia
mineral oil: Decreased blood calcitriol level (with prolonged use of mineral oil)
phenobarbital, phenytoin: Decreased synthesis and blood level of calcitriol
phosphate-binding agents: Possibly altered phosphate transport in bone, intestine, and kidneys
thiazide diuretics: Hypercalcemia
vitamin D: Additive effects, including possible hypercalcemia

Adverse Reactions

SKIN: **Erythema multiforme**, lip swelling, pruritus, rash, urticaria
Other: **Anaphylaxis**

Childbearing Considerations

PREGNANCY

- It is not known if drug can cause fetal harm. However, upon birth, the neonate may exhibit mild signs and symptoms of hypercalcemia for several days.
- Use with caution only if benefit to mother outweighs potential risk to fetus.

LACTATION

- Drug may be present in breast milk.
- Breastfeeding should not be done during drug therapy.

Nursing Considerations

- Check to be sure patient receives enough calcium.

! **WARNING** Monitor patient for a hypersensitivity reaction or skin changes that could become severe such as the development of anaphylaxis or erythema multiforme. If present, notify prescriber immediately, expect drug to be withheld as ordered, and provide supportive care, as needed and ordered.

! **WARNING** Monitor patient closely. In high-dose or long-term calcitriol therapy, be alert for vitamin D toxicity. Early evidence includes abdominal or bone pain, constipation, dry mouth, headache, metallic taste, myalgia, nausea, somnolence, vomiting, and weakness. Late evidence includes albuminuria, anorexia, arrhythmias, azotemia, conjunctivitis, decreased libido, elevated ALT and AST levels, elevated BUN level, hypercholesterolemia, hypertension, hyperthermia, irritability, mild acidosis, nephrocalcinosis, nocturia, pancreatitis, photophobia, polydipsia, polyuria, pruritus, rhinorrhea, vascular calcification, and weight loss.

PATIENT TEACHING

- Caution patient not to take other forms of vitamin D while taking calcitriol.
- Instruct patient how to take calcitriol and what to do if a dose is missed.

! **WARNING** Alert patient that calcitriol may cause an allergic reaction or a serious skin condition. If either occurs, stress importance of notifying prescriber promptly and seeking immediate medical care, if severe.

! **WARNING** Advise patient to notify prescriber immediately about possible vitamin D toxicity, such as headache, irritability, nausea, photophobia, vomiting, weakness, and weight loss.

- Inform mothers breastfeeding should not be done during drug therapy.

calcium acetate

Calphron, Phoslyra

calcium carbonate

Apo-Cal (CAN), Calci-Mix, Calsan (CAN), Liqui-Cal, Liquid Cal-600, Titralac

calcium chloride

Calciject (CAN)

calcium citrate

Cal-C Cap, Cal-Cee, Citracal

calcium gluconate

calcium lactate

Cal-Lac

Class and Category

Pharmacologic class: Calcium salts
Therapeutic class: Antacid, antihypermagnesemic, antihyperphosphatemic, antihypocalcemic, calcium replacement, cardiotonic

Indications and Dosages

✱ *To treat hyperphosphatemia*

CAPSULES, TABLETS (CALCIUM ACETATE)

Adults. *Initial:* 1,334 mg (2 capsules or tablets) 3 times daily with meals. Dosage increased every 2 to 3 wk to reduce serum phosphorus level below 6 mg/dl as long as hypercalcemia doesn't develop. *Usual:* 2,001 to 2,668 mg (3 or 4 capsules or tablets) 3 times daily with meals.

ORAL SOLUTION (CALCIUM ACETATE)

Adults. *Initial:* 1,334 mg (10 ml) 3 times daily with meals. Dosage increased every 2 to 3 wk to reduce serum phosphorus levels to the target range, as long as hypercalcemia doesn't develop. *Usual:* 2,001 to 2,668 mg (15 to 20 ml) 3 times daily with meals.

✱ *To prevent hypocalcemia with oral supplementation*

CAPSULES, ORAL SUSPENSION, TABLETS (CALCIUM CARBONATE); EFFERVESCENT TABLETS, TABLETS (CALCIUM CITRATE); TABLETS (CALCIUM GLUCONATE OR LACTATE)

Adults. 1,000 to 1,200 mg daily RDA elemental calcium.
Pregnant females and breastfeeding mothers. 1,000 to 1,300 mg daily RDA elemental calcium.
Children ages 9 to 18. 1,300 mg daily RDA elemental calcium.
Children ages 4 to 8. 1,000 mg daily RDA elemental calcium.

Children ages 1 to 3. 700 mg daily RDA elemental calcium.
Children ages 7 mo to 12 mo. 260 mg daily RDA elemental calcium.
Infants up to 6 mo. 200 mg daily RDA elemental calcium.

∗ *To provide antacid effects*

CHEWABLE TABLETS, ORAL SUSPENSION, TABLETS (CALCIUM CARBONATE)

Adults. 1,000 to 3,531 mg up to 4 times daily, as needed. *Maximum:* 6,750 to 7,500 mg daily for up to 2 wk.
Children ages 12 and older. 1,000 to 2,000 mg up to 3 times daily, as needed. *Maximum:* 7,500 mg daily up to 2 wk.
Children ages 6 to 11 or children weighing 22 to 43 kg (48 to 95 lb). 800 mg up to 3 times daily, as needed. *Maximum:* 2,400 mg daily up to 2 wk.

CHEWABLE TABLETS, ORAL SUSPENSION

Children ages 2 to 5 or children weighing 10.5 to 21 kg (24 to 47 lb). 400 mg up to 3 times daily, as needed. *Maximum:* 1200 mg daily up to 2 wk.

∗ *To provide emergency treatment for acute symptomatic hypocalcemia*

I.V. INFUSION (10% CALCIUM CHLORIDE)

Adults. 200 to 1,000 mg infused at 1 ml/min (100 mg/min), repeated, as needed, in intervals of 1 to 3 days.
Children. 2.7 mg/kg to 5 mg/kg, repeated, as needed.

±**DOSAGE ADJUSTMENT** For adult patients with renal impairment, initial dosage kept at 200 mg. For pediatric patients with renal impairment, initial dosage kept at 2.7 mg/kg.

I.V. INFUSION, I.V. INJECTION (CALCIUM GLUCONATE)

Adults. *Initial:* 500 to 2,000 mg (5 to 20 ml) not to exceed a rate of 0.5 to 2 ml/min. Dosage increased, as needed, in intervals of 1 to 3 days. *Usual daily dose, as needed:* 1,000 to 1,500 mg in divided doses as a bolus or continuous infusion initiated at a rate not to exceed 0.5 to 2 ml/min, with adjustments made, as needed.
Children ages more than 1 mo to 17 yr. *Initial:* 29–60 mg/kg. *Subsequent doses, as needed:* 29–60 mg/kg every 6 hr as a bolus or continuous infusion initiated at 8 to 13 mg/kg/hr, with adjustments made, as needed.
Neonates 1 mo or less. *Initial:* 100–200 mg/kg. *Subsequent doses, as needed:* 100 to 200 mg/kg every 6 hr as a bolus or continuous infusion initiated at 17–33 mg/kg/hr, with adjustments made, as needed.

∗ *As adjunct to treat magnesium intoxication*

I.V. INFUSION (CALCIUM GLUCONATE)

Adults. 1,000 to 2,000 mg as a one-time dose not to exceed a rate of 0.5 to 2 ml/min. Dosage repeated in severe cases.

∗ *To treat hyperkalemia*

I.V. INFUSION (CALCIUM GLUCONATE)

Adults. 500 to 3,000 mg as a one-time dose not to exceed a rate of 0.5 to 2 ml/min. Dosage repeated in extreme hyperkalemia cardiotoxicity.

∗ *To provide calcium during exchange transfusion*

I.V. INFUSION (CALCIUM GLUCONATE)

Adults. 300 mg with each 100 ml of citrated blood not to exceed a rate of 0.5 to 2 ml/min.

Drug Administration

P.O.

- Administer calcium acetate and calcium carbonate with meals.
- Chewable tablets must be chewed thoroughly before swallowing and followed with a glass of water.
- Shake suspension bottle well before each use.
- Use a calibrated device to measure oral solution or suspension dosage.
- Dissolve calcium citrate effervescent tablets in water and have patient drink immediately.
- Avoid administering calcium within 2 hr of other drugs.
- Store oral calcium at room temperature away from heat, light, and moisture. Do not freeze oral solution or suspension.

I.V.

- Administer calcium chloride and calcium gluconate only intravenously. Do not administer as an I.M. or subcutaneous injection.
- Warm solution to body temperature, if time permits.
- Administer through a small needle into a central or large vein or through a free-flowing compatible I.V. solution. Do not administer in a small foot or hand vein or into a scalp vein in neonates.

C

- Administer 10% calcium chloride slowly as an infusion in a central or deep vein, not exceeding 1 ml/min because rapid administration may cause arrthymias, bradycardia, hypotension, and syncope. Do not administer as a bolus.
- For calcium gluconate bolus administration, dilute in a compatible I.V. solution, such as 0.9% Sodium Chloride Injection or 5% Dextrose Injection to a concentration of 10–50 mg/ml. Solution should appear clear and colorless to slightly yellow. Use immediately. Administer slowly and do not exceed a rate of 200 mg/min in adults and 100 mg/min in pediatric patients, including neonates.
- For calcium gluconate continuous infusion, dilute drug in 0.9% Sodium Chloride Injection or 5% Dextrose Injection to a concentration of 5.8 to 10 mg/ml. For adults, initiate rate at 5.4 to 21.5 mg/kg/hr; for children older than 1 mo to 17 yr, initiate at 8–13 mg/kg/hr; and for neonates 1 mo or less, initiate at 17–33 mg/kg/hr. Rate then adjusted according to serum calcium levels.
- Check infusion site often. Stop infusion if patient experiences discomfort or pain at infusion site and notify prescriber. Should perivascular infiltration occur, immediately discontinue infusion at that site, notify prescriber and provide localized supportive care, as needed and ordered.
- Keep patient in a recumbent position for at least 15 min after I.V. administration.
- *Incompatibilities:* Calcium chloride: ceftriaxone, other drugs; calcium gluconate: ceftriaxone, I.V. fluids containing bicarbonate or phosphate, minocycline

Route	Onset	Peak	Duration
P.O.	Unknown	Unknown	Unknown
I.V.	Immediate	Immediate	30–120 min

Half-life: Unknown

Mechanism of Action

Increases levels of intracellular and extracellular calcium, which is needed to maintain homeostasis, especially in the nervous and musculoskeletal systems. Also, plays a role in normal cardiac and renal function, respiration, coagulation, and cell membrane and capillary permeability. Helps regulate the release and storage of neurotransmitters and hormones. Oral forms also neutralize or buffer stomach acid to relieve discomfort caused by hyperacidity.

Contraindications

Cardiac resuscitation with risk of existing digitalis toxicity, concurrent use of calcium supplements, hypercalcemia, hypersensitivity to calcium salts or their components, hypophosphatemia, newborns (up to 28 days) requiring or expected to require ceftriaxone I.V. therapy (I.V.), presence of asystole and electromechanical dissociation or ventricular fibrillation (I.V.), renal calculi

Interactions

DRUGS

bisphosphonates (alendronate, etidronate, ibandronate, risedronate): Possibly decreased absorption of bisphosphonates
calcium supplements, magnesium-containing preparations: Increased serum calcium or magnesium level, especially in patients with impaired renal function
digitalis glycosides: Increased risk of arrhythmias
fluoroquinolones: Reduced fluoroquinolone absorption by calcium carbonate
iron salts: Decreased gastric iron absorption
levothyroxine: Decreased absorption of levothyroxine
tetracyclines: Decreased tetracycline absorption and blood level, leading to decreased anti-infective response
thiazide diuretics: Possibly hypercalcemia
verapamil: Reversed verapamil effects
vitamin D (high doses): Excessively increased calcium absorption

ACTIVITIES

alcohol use (excessive), smoking: Possibly decreased calcium absorption

FOODS

caffeine, high-fiber food: Possibly decreased calcium absorption

Adverse Reactions

CNS: Paresthesia (parenteral form)
CV: **Hypotension**, irregular heartbeat (parenteral form), peripheral vasodilatation
EENT: Calcium taste
GI: Nausea or vomiting (parenteral form)
SKIN: Diaphoresis, flushing, or sensation of warmth (parenteral form)

Other: **Aluminum toxicity**; **hypercalcemia**; injection-site burning, pain, rash, or redness (parenteral form)

Childbearing Considerations

PREGNANCY

- It is not known if drug can cause fetal harm.
- Be aware that pregnancy may alter dosage needs for mother.
- Use with caution only if benefit to mother outweighs potential risk to fetus.

LACTATION

- Drug is present in breast milk.
- Mothers should check with prescriber before breastfeeding. Dosage needs for mother may change if breastfeeding.

Nursing Considerations

! **WARNING** Do not administer calcium chloride intravensously to newborns (up to 28 days) who require or are expected to require ceftriaxone intravenous therapy because of the risk of precipitation of ceftriaxone-calcium that may occur even if both drugs are given at different times or through separate intravenous lines. For infants older than 28 days, know that calcium chloride injection and ceftriaxone intravenous solutions may be administered sequentially one after another if infusion lines are at different sites, infusion lines are replaced, or infusion lines are thoroughly flushed between infusions with 0.9% Sodium Chloride solution.

! **WARNING** Monitor patient for signs and symptoms of hypercalcemia. Be aware that calcium chloride injection contains 3 times as much calcium per milliliter as calcium gluconate injection. Monitor serum calcium level in all patients, as ordered, and evaluate therapeutic response by assessing for Chvostek's and Trousseau's signs, which shouldn't appear. If present, notify prescriber immediately and, if severe, be prepared to provide emergency supportive care, as needed and ordered.

! **WARNING** Be aware that patients with kidney failure on dialysis may develop hypercalcemia when treated with calcium. Monitor patient closely. Know that these patients should not take calcium supplements, including antacids containing calcium.

! **WARNING** Monitor patient for aluminum toxicity, especially patients receiving prolonged parenteral administration in the presence of impaired renal function. CNS and bone toxicity may occur. Expect patients receiving parenteral nutrition solutions to have aluminum exposure limited to no more than 5 mcg/kg/day.

- Monitor patient closely receiving calcium chloride intravenously who has local trauma. Assess patient for abnormal dermal deposits of calcium salts and appearance of papules, plaques, or nodules that may occur with erythema, induration, and swelling. If present, notify prescriber immediately to minimize occurrence of tissue necrosis, secondary infection, and ulceration.

PATIENT TEACHING

- Instruct patient how to take oral form of calcium prescribed.
- Remind patient to take calcium separate from other prescribed drugs. For example, tell the patient to take fluoroquinolone at least 2 hours before or 6 hours after calcium; to take levothyroxine at least 4 hours before or after calcium; and to take a tetracycline at least 1 hour before calcium. Advise patient to avoid taking calcium within 2 hours of other oral drugs.
- Tell patient to avoid excessive consumption of alcoholic beverages, caffeine-containing products, and high-fiber foods and excessive use of tobacco because these substances may decrease calcium absorption.

! **WARNING** Review signs and symptoms of aluminum toxicity and hypercalcemia with patient. Stress importance of complying with routine blood tests to monitor calcium level. Tell patient to notify prescriber promptly if patient experiences signs and symptoms of aluminum toxicity or hypercalcemia and, if severe, to seek immediate medical care.

- Urge patient to ask prescriber before taking over-the-counter drugs because of risk of interactions.
- Inform mothers who are breastfeeding to alert prescriber as calcium needs for mothers may change during breastfeeding.

C

canagliflozin

Invokana

Class and Category

Pharmacologic class: Sodium-glucose co-transporter 2 (SGLT2) inhibitor
Therapeutic class: Antidiabetic

Indications and Dosages

✶ *As adjunct to control blood glucose level in type 2 diabetes mellitus*

TABLETS

Adults and children ages 10 and older with an eGFR of 60 ml/min or more. 100 mg once daily before the first meal of the day, followed by dosage increased up to 300 mg once daily, as needed. *Maximum:* 300 mg once daily.

✶ *To reduce the risk of major adverse cardiovascular events, such as nonfatal CVA or MI in patients with type 2 diabetes mellitus and established cardiovascular disease; to reduce the risk of end-stage kidney disease (ESKD), doubling of serum creatinine, cardiovascular death, and hospitalization for heart failure in patients with type 2 diabetes mellitus and diabetic nephropathy with albuminuria greater than 300 mg/day.*

TABLETS

Adults with an eGFR of 60 ml/min or more. 100 mg once daily.

± **DOSAGE ADJUSTMENT** For patients with eGFR less than 60 ml/min but at least 30 ml/min, dosage limited to 100 mg once daily. For patients with eGFR less than 30 ml/min, initiation is not recommended but patients with albuminuria greater than 300 mg/day may continue 100 mg once daily to reduce the risk of CV death, doubling of serum creatinine, end-stage kidney disease, and hospitalization for heart failure. For patients receiving an UGT enzyme inducer, such as phenobarbital, phenytoin, rifampin, or ritonavir and have eGFR of 60 ml/min or greater, dosage may be increased to 200 mg once daily if patients are tolerating 100 mg daily or increased to maximum of 300 mg once daily if patients are tolerating 200 mg daily. For patients receiving an UGT enzyme inducer and the eGFR is less than 60 ml/min, dosage increased to maximum of 200 mg once daily in patients tolerating 100 mg once daily.

Drug Administration

P.O.

- Administer before first meal of the day.

Route	Onset	Peak	Duration
P.O.	> 24 hr	1–2 hr	Unknown

Half-life: 10.6–13.1 hr

Mechanism of Action

Inhibits sodium-glucose co-transporter 2 (SGLT2) responsible for the majority of the reabsorption of filtered glucose from the tubular lumen in the kidneys. By inhibiting SGLT2, reabsorption of filtered glucose is reduced along with a lowering of the renal threshold for glucose, which increases urinary glucose excretion.

Contraindications

Hypersensitivity to canagliflozin or its components, use of dialysis

Interactions

DRUGS

digoxin: Possibly increased serum digoxin levels and digitalis toxicity
insulin, insulin secretagogues: Possibly increased risk of hypoglycemia
lithium: Decreased lithium concentration with reduced effectiveness of lithium
phenobarbital, phenytoin, rifampin, ritonavir: Decreased effectiveness of canagliflozin
UGT enzyme inducers: Decreased canagliflozin exposure, which may decrease effectiveness of canagliflozin

Adverse Reactions

CNS: Asthenia, fatigue, polydipsia, postural dizziness, syncope
CV: Elevation of low-density lipoprotein cholesterol (LDL-C) and non-high-density lipoprotein cholesterol (non-HDL-C), **hypotension**, orthostatic hypotension
ENDO: **Diabetic ketoacidosis and other ketoacidosis, hypoglycemia**
EENT: Dry mouth
GI: Abdominal pain, constipation, nausea, **pancreatitis**
GU: **Acute renal failure**, decreased eGFR, elevated serum creatinine levels, genital mycotic infections, **necrotizing fasciitis of the perineum (Fournier's gangrene)**, **pyelonephritis**, polyuria, renal impairment, UTIs, vulvovaginal pruritus, **urosepsis**

HEME: Elevated hemoglobin
MS: Bone fracture, decreased bone density, lower-limb amputation
SKIN: Erythema, photosensitivity, pruritus, rash, urticaria
Other: **Anaphylaxis**, **angioedema**, dehydration, **hyperkalemia**, **hyperphosphatemia**, **hypermagnesemia**

Childbearing Considerations

PREGNANCY

- Drug may cause fetal harm by adversely affecting kidney function of the fetus.
- Drug is not recommended during the second and third trimester of pregnancy.

LACTATION

- It is not known if drug is present in breast milk.
- Drug should not be given to mothers who are breastfeeding since kidney maturation in infant continues for 2 yr following birth.

Nursing Considerations

! **WARNING** Know that patients with volume depletion should have the condition corrected before canagliflozin therapy is begun because drug causes intravascular volume contraction. Patients especially at risk for symptomatic hypotension caused by volume depletion include the elderly, patients taking either diuretics or drugs that interfere with the renin–angiotensin–aldosterone system, patients with impaired renal function, or patients with low systolic blood pressure.

- Use drug cautiously in patients with chronic kidney insufficiency, congestive heart failure, decreased blood volume, and in patients taking medications such as ACE inhibitors and angiotensin receptor blockers, diuretics, and NSAIDs because these conditions and treatments may predispose patient to acute kidney injury while receiving canagliflozin. Patients with renal impairment taking drug for glycemic control may be at increased risk for hypotension and acute kidney injury. Ensure that kidney function has been assessed prior to start of canagliflozin therapy and then periodically thereafter. Expect drug to be discontinued if acute kidney injury occurs.

! **WARNING** Assess patient for hypersensitivity reactions such as angioedema and generalized urticaria, especially within hours to days after canagliflozin therapy is begun. The hypersensitivity reaction can become severe, causing anaphylaxis. If hypersensitivity to canagliflozin occurs, expect drug to be discontinued and provide supportive care as ordered.

! **WARNING** Expect drug to be temporarily discontinued to reduce the risk of acute kidney injury in patients who develop a reduced oral intake, such as in an acute illness or fasting, or who experience excessive fluid losses because of GI illness or significant heat exposure. Also, expect to withhold drug, as ordered and if possible, at least 3 days prior to surgery for procedures associated with prolonged fasting. Drug therapy may be resumed once patient has resumed oral intake.

! **WARNING** Monitor patient closely for ketoacidosis that may occur despite the patient having type 2 diabetes and may be present even if a blood glucose level is less than 250 mg/dl. If signs and symptoms occur such as dehydration, fruity odor to breath, malaise, nausea, shortness of breath, and vomiting, notify prescriber and expect drug to be discontinued. Provide supportive care, as needed and ordered.

! **WARNING** Report immediately signs and symptoms of necrotizing fasciitis of the perineum (Fournier's gangrene), a rare but serious and life-threatening necrotizing infection that has been linked to canagliflozin therapy. Report patient's complaints of erythema, pain or tenderness, or swelling in the genital or perineal area, along with fever or malaise, as treatment requires urgent surgical intervention along with immediate broad-spectrum antibiotic therapy. If confirmed, expect canagliflozin to be discontinued and an alternative treatment for glycemic control prescribed.

! **WARNING** Be aware that canagliflozin has been linked to an increase in foot and leg amputations in patients receiving the drug. Assess patient's feet and legs regularly for any abnormalities and notify prescriber immediately, if present. Be aware that patients may be at higher risk of lower-limb amputation if they have had blocked or narrowed blood vessels (usually in leg), have had damage to the nerves (neuropathy) in the leg; have had diabetic foot sores or ulcers; or have a history of amputation, heart disease, or are at risk for heart disease. Know that canagliflozin may be discontinued if abnormalities develop.

! **WARNING** Monitor patient for a UTI because canagliflozin increases risk of UTIs. Report promptly and expect to treat because the UTI can quickly become serious, developing into pyelonephritis and urosepsis.

- Monitor patient's blood glucose levels to determine effectiveness of canagliflozin therapy. Be aware that canagliflozin dosage should only be increased in patients who have at least an estimated glomerular filtration rate of 60 ml/min and need greater glucose control (unless patient is receiving an UGT enzyme inducer).
- Know that canagliflozin can increase urinary glucose excretion, leading to positive urine glucose tests, and should not be used to monitor glucose levels in patients with diabetes mellitus. Assess patient also receiving insulin or insulin secretagogues for hypoglycemia.
- Monitor serum potassium levels regularly, as ordered, during canagliflozin therapy in patients with impaired renal function and in patients predisposed to hyperkalemia due to medications or other medical conditions.
- Be aware that patients with a history of genital mycotic infections, as well as uncircumcised males, are at greater risk for developing genital mycotic infections.
- Monitor patient's lipid levels and expect to treat if an elevation occurs.
- Institute safety precautions to prevent falls because falls may cause a bone fracture. The risk of bone fracture may occur as early as 12 weeks after therapy is begun.

PATIENT TEACHING

- Inform patient that canagliflozin is not a substitute for diet and exercise management.
- Instruct patient how to administer canagliflozin and what to do if a dose is missed.

! **WARNING** Urge patient not to skip doses or increase dosage without consulting prescriber. However, tell patient to notify prescriber if he is unable to take a normal amount of daily fluids due to fasting or illness or experiences an excessive loss of fluids from excessive perspiration or GI illnesses, as drug may have to be temporarily withheld.

! **WARNING** Alert patient that drug may cause an allergic reaction. Tell patient if an allergic reaction occurs to notify prescriber promptly and, if severe, to seek immediate medical care.

- Teach patient how to monitor his blood glucose level. Advise patient with diabetes mellitus not to use urine glucose tests to monitor his glycemic control, as drug will cause a false-positive result.

! **WARNING** Review signs and symptoms of ketoacidosis with patient and urge him to seek immediate medical attention, if present, even if blood glucose level is less than 250 mg/dl. Emphasize importance of reporting signs of hypoglycemia, such as anxiety, confusion, dizziness, excessive sweating, headache, and nausea.

! **WARNING** Advise patient to seek medical care promptly if pain or tenderness, redness, or swelling of the genitals or the area from the genitals back to the rectum occurs, along with a fever above 38°C (100.4°F) or malaise develops.

! **WARNING** Instruct patient to notify prescriber right away if he notices any new pain or tenderness, sores or ulcers, or symptoms of infections in his feet or legs. Tell patient this is very important because canagliflozin therapy increases the risk of lower-limb amputations.

! **WARNING** Review signs and symptoms of a UTI with patient. Stress importance of notifying prescriber promptly, if present, so treatment can begin to prevent the infection from becoming severe.

- Inform patient that drug may increase his risk for bone fractures and to take safety precautions to prevent falls.
- Advise patient to avoid direct sunlight and to wear sunscreen when outdoors.
- Instruct females of childbearing age to notify prescriber if pregnancy occurs as drug will need to be discontinued by the second trimester.
- Inform mothers not to breastfeed their infant while taking canagliflozin.

candesartan cilexetil

Atacand

Class and Category

Pharmacologic class: Angiotensin receptor blocker

Therapeutic class: Antihypertensive

Indications and Dosages

∗ *To manage, or as adjunct in managing, hypertension*

ORAL SUSPENSION, TABLETS

Adults. *Initial:* 16 mg once daily. *Maintenance:* 8 to 32 mg once daily or 4 to 16 mg twice daily. *Maximum:* 32 mg daily.

Children ages 6 to 17 weighing more than 50 kg (110 lb). *Initial:* 8 to 16 mg daily. *Maintenance:* 4 to 32 mg once daily or 2 to 16 mg twice daily. *Maximum:* 32 mg daily.

Children ages 6 to 17 weighing 50 kg (110 lb) or less. *Initial:* 4 to 8 mg daily. *Maintenance:* 2 to 16 mg once daily or 1 to 8 mg twice daily. *Maximum:* 16 mg daily.

ORAL SUSPENSION

Children ages 1 to 6. *Initial:* 0.20 mg/kg daily. *Maintenance:* 0.05 to 0.4 mg/kg daily or 0.025 to 0.2 mg/kg twice daily. *Maximum:* 0.4 mg/kg daily.

± **DOSAGE ADJUSTMENT** For adult patients with moderate hepatic impairment, initial dosage reduced to 8 mg daily.

∗ *To treat heart failure in patients with an ejection fraction of 40% or less and NYHA class II–IV to reduce the risk of death from cardiovascular causes and reduce hospitalizations for heart failure*

ORAL SUSPENSION, TABLETS

Adults. *Initial:* 4 mg once daily for 2 wk; then doubled every 2 wk, as tolerated, until reaching target dose of 32 mg once daily.

Drug Administration

P.O.

- Tablets should be swallowed whole.
- Administer oral suspension to patients who cannot swallow tablets.
- Shake suspension well before each dose and use a calibrated device to measure dose.
- Store suspension at room temperature. Use within 30 days of opening bottle or discard. Also, discard after 100 days if not opened.

Route	Onset	Peak	Duration
P.O.	2–3 hr	6–8 hr	> 24 hr

Half-life: 5–9 hr, dose-dependent

Mechanism of Action

Blocks binding of angiotensin (AT) II to AT_1 receptor sites selectively in many tissues, including adrenal glands and vascular smooth muscle. This inhibits vasoconstrictive and aldosterone-secreting effects of AT II, which reduces blood pressure.

Contraindications

Concurrent aliskiren therapy in presence of diabetes, hypersensitivity to candesartan or its components

Interactions

DRUGS

aliskiren (in presence of diabetes or renal impairment), ACE inhibitors, angiotensin receptor blockers: Increased risk of hypotension, hyperkalemia, and renal dysfunction

lithium: Increased blood lithium level

NSAIDs: Possible decreased renal function in patients who are elderly, volume-depleted, or have a compromised renal function

potassium-sparing diuretics, potassium supplements, potassium-containing salt substitutes: Possibly increased risk of hyperkalemia

Adverse Reactions

CNS: Dizziness, headache

CV: **Hypotension**

EENT: Pharyngitis, rhinitis

GI: Elevated liver enzymes, **hepatitis**, impaired liver function

GU: Elevated BUN and serum creatinine levels

HEME: **Agranulocytosis**, **leukopenia**, **neutropenia**

MS: Back pain, **rhabdomyolysis**

RESP: Cough, upper respiratory tract infection
SKIN: Pruritus, rash, urticaria
Other: **Angioedema**, **hyperkalemia**, **hyponatremia**

Childbearing Considerations

PREGNANCY

- Drug can cause fetal harm.
- Drug given during the second or third trimester reduces fetal renal function and increases fetal and neonatal morbidity and death. Resulting oligohydramnios can cause fetal lung hypoplasia and skeletal malformations.
- Drug is contraindicated during pregnancy.

LACTATION

- It is not known if drug is present in breast milk.
- Breastfeeding is not recommended during drug therapy.

Nursing Considerations

! **WARNING** Determine if patient has fluid or salt depletion prior to starting candesartan. If patient has known or suspected hypovolemia and/or salt depletion such as may occur with prolonged diuretic therapy, dietary salt restriction, dialysis, diarrhea, or vomiting, expect to provide treatment such as 0.9% Sodium Chloride Injection I.V., as ordered, to correct it before starting candesartan. Continue to monitor blood pressure throughout candesartan therapy, especially after a dosage increase.

! **WARNING** Monitor patient for hypotension. If patient develops hypotension, expect to stop drug temporarily. Immediately place patient in supine position and prepare to give 0.9% Sodium Chloride Injection I.V., as prescribed. Expect to resume therapy after blood pressure stabilizes. Know that if patient is elderly, receiving concurrent antihypertensive or diuretic therapy with candesartan, or has heart failure, assess blood pressure often because of added risk of hypotension. Also, monitor patient closely during anesthesia and major surgery because candesartan increases risk of hypotension by blocking renin–angiotensin system.

! **WARNING** Monitor patient for hypersensitivity reactions that could become life-threatening, such as angioedema. If present, notify prescriber immediately, withhold drug as ordered, and provide supportive care, as needed and ordered.

! **WARNING** Watch for elevated BUN and serum creatinine levels, especially if patient has heart failure or impaired renal function; drug may cause acute renal failure. Also monitor patient's CBC, as ordered because drug can cause serious hematologic adverse reactions. Report persistent or significant increases immediately.

- Monitor patient for fluid deficit throughout drug therapy. If patient is receiving a diuretic, provide hydration, as ordered, to help prevent hypovolemia. Watch for evidence, such as hypotension with dizziness and fainting. If patient has heart failure and develops hypotension, dosage of diuretic, candesartan, or both may need to be reduced until blood pressure stabilizes and therapy resumes.

PATIENT TEACHING

- Instruct patient how to administer form of candesartan prescribed.
- Advise patient that full effects of candesartan may not occur for 4 to 5 weeks.

! **WARNING** Teach patient how to monitor blood pressure, if appropriate. Tell patient to notify prescriber if low blood pressure occurs.

! **WARNING** Alert patient that drug may cause an allergic reaction. If present, stress importance of notifying prescriber promptly and, if severe, to seek immediate medical care.

- Tell patient to report any persistent, serious, or unusual adverse reactions to prescriber promptly. Caution patient to comply with laboratory appointments to detect serious adverse reactions.
- Advise females of childbearing age to immediately report pregnancy. Explain that if she becomes pregnant, candesartan will have to be discontinued as soon as possible and treatment started with another antihypertensive that is safe to use during pregnancy.
- Inform mothers breastfeeding is not recommended during candesartan therapy.

cangrelor

Kengreal

Class and Category

Pharmacologic class: $P2Y_{12}$ platelet inhibitor
Therapeutic class: Antiplatelet

Indications and Dosages

✱ *As adjunct to percutaneous coronary intervention (PCI) to reduce risk of periprocedural MI, repeat coronary revascularization, and stent thrombosis in patients who have not been treated with a $P2Y_{12}$ platelet inhibitor and are not being given a glycoprotein IIb/IIIa inhibitor*

I.V. INFUSION, I.V. INJECTION

Adults. 30 mcg/kg I.V. bolus prior to PCI followed immediately by a 4 mcg/kg/min infusion for at least 2 hr or for the duration of PCI, whichever is longer.

Drug Administration

I.V.

- Reconstitute each 50-mg vial by adding 5 ml of Sterile Water for Injection. Swirl gently until all material is dissolved. Avoid vigorous mixing. Allow any foam to settle. Ensure that contents are fully dissolved, and the reconstituted material is clear and colorless to pale yellow.
- Dilute reconstituted solution immediately with 0.9% Sodium Chloride Injection or 5% Dextrose Injection. Withdraw the contents from 1 reconstituted vial and add to one 250-ml bag of I.V. solution. Mix the bag thoroughly. This will result in a concentration of 200 mcg/ml and last for about a 2-hr infusion. Know that patients weighing 100 kg or more will require a minimum of 2 bags.
- Diluted cangrelor is stable for 12 hr if diluted in 5% Dextrose Injection and 24 hr if diluted in 0.9% Sodium Chloride Injection and kept at room temperature.
- Administer via a dedicated I.V. line.
- Administer the bolus rapidly in less than 1 min from the diluted bag via manual I.V. push or pump. Make sure the bolus is completely administered before the start of PCI and then start infusion immediately after administration of the bolus at a rate of 4 mcg/kg/min.
- *Incompatibilities:* None reported by manufacturer.

Route	Onset	Peak	Duration
I.V.	2 min	2 min	1 hr after infusion stopped

Half-life: 3–6 min

Mechanism of Action

Blocks ADP-induced platelet activation and aggregation by binding selectively and reversibly to the $P2Y_{12}$ receptor to prevent further signaling and platelet activation.

Contraindications

Hypersensitivity to cangrelor or its components, significant active bleeding

Interactions

DRUGS

thienopyridines, such as clopidogrel, prasugrel: Elimination effect of these drugs if given during cangrelor infusion; these drugs should be administered after cangrelor infusion is discontinued

Adverse Reactions

CNS: Intracranial bleeding or hemorrhage
CV: Coronary artery dissection or perforation
EENT: Stridor
GU: Decreased renal function
HEME: Bleeding events
RESP: Bronchospasm, dyspnea
Other: Anaphylaxis, **including shock**, **angioedema**

Childbearing Considerations

PREGNANCY

- It is not known if drug can cause fetal harm.
- Use with caution only if benefit to mother outweighs potential risk to fetus.

LABOR AND DELIVERY

- Drug may increase risk of maternal bleeding and hemorrhage.
- Drug should be discontinued 1 hr prior to labor, delivery, or neuraxial blockade, if possible.

LACTATION

- It is not known if drug is present in breast milk.
- Mothers should check with prescriber before breastfeeding.

C

Nursing Considerations

! **WARNING** Monitor patient closely for bleeding that can range from minor to severe. Be prepared to treat bleeding events immediately and notify prescriber. Know that once cangrelor is discontinued, there is no antiplatelet effect after an hour.

! **WARNING** Monitor patient closely for hypersensitivity reactions following administration which could become life-threatening such as anaphylaxis or angioedema. Alert prescriber immediately, if present, and be prepared to discontinue drug and provide supportive emergency care, as needed and ordered.

! **WARNING** Montior patient for difficulty breathing because drug may cause bronchospasms or dyspnea.

- Be aware that after cangrelor is discontinued, an oral $P2Y_{12}$ platelet inhibitor should be administered such as clopidogrel 600 mg after discontinuation of cangrelor, prasugrel 60 mg immediately after discontinuation of cangrelor, or ticagrelor 180 mg at any time during cangrelor infusion or immediately after discontinuation.

PATIENT TEACHING

- Explain to patient how drug will be administered.

! **WARNING** Tell patient to alert medical staff immediately if an allergic reaction, difficulty breathing or bleeding occurs.

- Inform patient that the effects of cangrelor are gone after 1 hour of the drug being discontinued.

captopril

Class and Category

Pharmacologic class: ACE inhibitor
Therapeutic class: Antihypertensive, vasodilator

Indications and Dosages

∗ *To control hypertension*

TABLETS

Adults. *Initial:* 25 mg twice daily or 3 times daily. Increased to 50 mg twice daily or 3 times daily after 1 to 2 wk, as needed. If blood pressure is not well controlled at this dosage after an additional 1–2 wk, diuretic added. If blood pressure is still not controlled, dosage increased to 100 mg twice daily or 3 times daily and then, as needed, to 150 mg twice daily or 3 times daily while continuing diuretic. *Maximum:* 450 mg daily.

∗ *To control accelerated or malignant hypertension when prompt titration of blood pressure is needed*

TABLETS

Adults. *Initial:* 25 mg 2 or 3 times daily while continuing diuretic but discontinuing other current antihypertensive drug. Increased every 24 hr or less, as needed, until satisfactory response is obtained, or maximum dosage is reached. *Maximum:* 450 mg daily.

∗ *To treat congestive heart failure*

TABLETS

Adults. *Initial:* 25 mg 3 times daily. Increased to 50 mg 3 times daily, as needed. After 14 days, increased to 100 mg 3 times daily and then to 150 mg 3 times daily, as needed. *Maximum:* 450 mg daily.

± **DOSAGE ADJUSTMENT** For patients with normal or low blood pressure, who have been vigorously treated with diuretics, initial dosage reduced to 6.25 mg or 12.5 mg 3 times daily, then increased gradually over several days to 50 mg 3 times daily. Further increases done in 2-wk intervals, as needed. Maximum dosage not to exceed 450 mg daily.

∗ *To treat left ventricular dysfunction after MI*

TABLETS

Adults. *Initial:* 6.25 mg as a single dose starting 3 days after MI and then 12.5 mg 3 times daily. Increased to 25 mg 3 times daily over several days and then again to maintenance dosage over next several wk. *Maintenance:* 50 mg 3 times daily.

∗ *To treat diabetic nephropathy*

TABLETS

Adults. 25 mg 3 times daily.

± **DOSAGE ADJUSTMENT** For patients with renal impairment, initial dosage reduced, and smaller increments utilized for titration.

Drug Administration

P.O.

- Administer on an empty stomach 1 hr before meals.

Route	Onset	Peak	Duration
P.O.	> 15 min	60–90 min	Unknown

Half-life: 1.7 hr

Mechanism of Action

Inhibiting angiotensin-converting enzyme, captopril:

- prevents conversion of angiotensin I to angiotensin II, a potent vasoconstrictor that also stimulates the adrenal cortex to secrete aldosterone. Inhibiting aldosterone increases sodium and water excretion, reducing blood pressure and water retention.
- may inhibit renal and vascular production of angiotensin II.
- decreases serum angiotensin II level and increases renin activity. This decreases aldosterone secretion, slightly increasing serum potassium level and fluid loss.
- decreases vascular tone and blood pressure.

Contraindications

Combination therapy with a neprilysin inhibitor (e.g., sacubitril) or within 36 hr of switching to or from sacubitril/valsartan; concurrent aliskiren use in patients with diabetes or patients with renal impairment (GFR less than 60 ml/min); hypersensitivity to captopril, other ACE inhibitors, or their components

Interactions

DRUGS

adrenergic neuron-blocking drugs, beta adrenergic drugs, ganglionic blocking drugs: Possibly increased risk of hypotension

aliskiren in patients with diabetes, other ACE inhibitors, angiotensin receptor blockers: Increased risk of hypotension, hyperkalemia, and renal impairment

antacids: Possibly impaired captopril absorption

capsaicin: Possibly cause or worsening of cough from ACE inhibitor

diuretics; hypotension-producing drugs, such as hydralazine: Additive hypotensive effects

gold: Increased risk of nitritoid reaction, including facial flushing, hypotension, nausea, and vomiting

lithium: Increased risk of lithium toxicity

mTOR (everolimus, sirolimus, temsirolimus), neprilysin inhibitor, such as sacubitril: Increased risk for angioedema

nitrates, other vasodilators: Possibly potentiated effects

NSAIDs: Decreased antihypertensive response to captopril; possible decreased renal function in elderly patients or those who are volume-depleted or already have existing impaired renal function

potassium-containing drugs, potassium-sparing diuretics, potassium supplements: Increased risk of hyperkalemia

ACTIVITIES

alcohol use: Additive hypotensive effects

FOOD

moderate to high-potassium-containing foods: Possibly increased risk of hyperkalemia

Adverse Reactions

CNS: Fever

CV: Chest pain, **hypotension**, orthostatic hypotension, palpitations, tachycardia

EENT: Loss of taste

GU: Dysuria, impotence, **nephrotic syndrome**, nocturia, oliguria, polyuria, proteinuria, urinary frequency

HEME: Eosinophilia

MS: Arthralgia

RESP: Cough

SKIN: Photosensitivity, pruritus, rash

Other: **Angioedema**, **hyperkalemia**, **hyponatremia**, positive ANA titer

Childbearing Considerations

PREGNANCY

- Drug can cause fetal harm.
- Drug given during the second or third trimester reduces fetal renal function and increases fetal and neonatal morbidity and death. Resulting oligohydramnios can cause fetal lung hypoplasia and skeletal malformations.
- Drug is contraindicated in pregnancy and should not be given to a pregnant female unless no alternative is available.

LACTATION

- Drug is present in breast milk.
- A decision should be made to discontinue breastfeeding or the drug to avoid potential serious adverse reactions in the breastfed infant.

Nursing Considerations

! WARNING Monitor patient's blood pressure closely, especially when therapy starts and dosage increases. Also, know that excessive hypotension, although rare, may occur in hypertensive patients when captopril is used in patients with heart failure or those who are undergoing renal dialysis or in patients with salt/volume depletion (such as occurs with vigorous treatment with diuretics). Notify prescriber and keep patient supine if hypotension occurs.

! **WARNING** Monitor patient for hypersensitivity reactions that could become life-threatening, such as angioedema. If present, notify prescriber immediately, withhold drug, as ordered, and provide supportive care, as needed and ordered.

! **WARNING** Monitor patient's electrolytes routinely if patient is receiving other drugs that also affect the renin–angiotensin system because hyperkalemia may occur.

- Monitor renal function tests for signs of nephrotic syndrome, such as increased BUN and serum creatinine levels and proteinuria. Also, watch for such renal evidence as oliguria, polyuria, and urinary frequency or other signs of impaired renal function, especially in patients receiving other drugs that also affect the renin–angiotensin system.
- Monitor WBC regularly, as ordered, especially if patient has collagen vascular disease or renal disease.

PATIENT TEACHING

- Instruct patient how to administer captopril.
- Urge patient not to use salt substitutes that contain potassium and to consult prescriber before increasing potassium intake, to avoid increasing risk of hyperkalemia.

! **WARNING** Warn patient not to stop taking drug abruptly.

! **WARNING** Alert patient that captopril can cause an allergic reaction. Tell patient to notify prescriber immediately if an allergic reaction occurs. Stress importance of seeking immediate medical care if reaction is severe.

- Tell patient to rise slowly from a lying or sitting position to minimize orthostatic hypotension.
- Tell patient to avoid sunlight or wear sunscreen in direct sunlight because photosensitivity may occur.
- Urge patient to tell prescriber about signs and symptoms of infection, such as fever or sore throat.
- Advise females of childbearing age to notify prescriber immediately if pregnancy occurs.
- Inform mothers that breastfeeding should not be undertaken while receiving captopril therapy.

carbamazepine

Carbatrol, Epitol, Equetro, Tegretol, Tegretol-XR

Class and Category

Pharmacologic class: Iminostilbene derivative
Therapeutic class: Analgesic, anticonvulsant

Indications and Dosages

* *To treat epilepsy with generalized tonic–clonic seizures, mixed seizure patterns, and partial seizures with complex symptomatology*

E.R. TABLETS (TEGRETOL-XR)

Adults and children ages 12 and older. *Initial:* 200 mg twice daily. Increased weekly by up to 200 mg daily, as needed, and given in divided doses twice daily. *Maximum:* 1,600 mg daily in adults, 1,200 mg daily in children ages 16 to 18, and 1,000 mg daily in children ages 12 to 15.
Children ages 6 to 12. *Initial:* 100 mg twice daily. Increased weekly by 100 mg daily, as needed, and given in divided doses twice daily. *Maximum:* 1,000 mg daily.

E.R. CAPSULES (CARBATROL, EQUETRO)

Adults and children ages 12 and older. *Initial:* 200 mg twice daily. Increased weekly by up to 200 mg daily, as needed, and given in divided doses twice daily. *Maximum:* 1,600 mg daily in adults, 1,200 mg daily in children ages 16 to 18, and 1,000 mg daily in children ages 12 to 15.
Children under the age of 12. Individualized and based on body weight. *Maximum:* 35 mg/kg/24 hr.

ORAL SUSPENSION (TEGRETOL)

Adults and children ages 12 and older. *Initial:* 100 mg 4 times daily. Increased weekly by up to 200 mg daily, as needed, given in divided doses 3 times daily or 4 times daily.

Maximum: 1,600 mg daily in adults, 1,200 mg daily in children ages 16 and older, and 1,000 mg daily in children ages 12 to 15.
Children ages 6 to 12. *Initial:* 50 mg 4 times daily. Increased weekly by 100 mg daily, as needed, given in divided doses 3 times daily or 4 times daily. *Maximum:* 1,000 mg daily.
Children up to age 6. *Initial:* 10 to 20 mg/kg/day in divided doses 4 times daily. *Maximum:* 35 mg/kg daily.

CHEWABLE TABLETS, TABLETS (TEGRETOL)

Adults and children ages 12 and older. *Initial:* 200 mg twice daily. Increased weekly by up to 200 mg/day, as needed, given in divided doses 3 times daily or 4 times daily. *Maximum:* 1,600 mg daily in adults, 1,200 mg daily in children ages 16 and older, and 1,000 mg daily in children ages 12 to 15.
Children ages 6 to 12. *Initial:* 100 mg twice daily. Increased weekly by up to 100 mg daily, as needed, given in divided doses 3 times daily or 4 times daily. *Maximum:* 1,000 mg daily.
Children up to age 6. *Initial:* 10 to 20 mg/kg daily in divided doses twice daily or 3 times daily. Increased weekly, as needed, divided and given 3 or 4 times daily. *Maximum:* 35 mg/kg/day.

✶ *To relieve pain in trigeminal neuralgia*

CHEWABLE TABLETS (TEGRETOL), E.R. TABLETS (TEGRETOL-XR), TABLETS (TEGRETOL)

Adults. *Initial:* 100 mg twice daily. Increased by up to 200 mg daily, as needed, in increments of 100 mg every 12 hr. *Maintenance:* Ranging from 200 to 1,200 mg daily although usual maintenance dosage is 400 to 800 mg/day. *Maximum:* 1,200 mg daily.

E.R. CAPSULES (CARBATROL, EQUETRO)

Adults. *Day 1:* 200 mg given as one 200-mg capsule. Increased by up to 200 mg/day, as needed, in increments of 100 mg every 12 hr. *Maintenance*: Ranging from 200 mg to 1,200 mg daily with usual dosage between 400 to 800 mg daily. *Maximum:* 1,200 mg daily.

ORAL SUSPENSION (TEGRETOL)

Adults. 50 mg 4 times daily. Increased by up to 200 mg daily, as needed, in increments of 50 mg 4 times daily. *Maintenance:* 400 to 800 mg daily. *Maximum:* 1,200 mg daily.

✶ *To treat acute manic and mixed episodes in bipolar disorder*

E.R. CAPSULES (EQUETRO)

Adults. *Initial:* 200 mg twice daily, increased, as needed, in 200-mg increments. *Maximum:* 1,600 mg daily.

Drug Administration

P.O.

- Shake oral suspension well before administering and use a calibrated device to measure dosage. Do not administer with any other drugs that are in liquid form. Administer before, during, or after meals.
- Examine tablets before administration for chips or cracks. If present, discard and obtain a new tablet. Administer with food.
- E.R. capsules or tablets should not be chewed or crushed. In addition, tablets should not be split. Examine E.R. tablets before administration for chips or cracks. If present, discard and obtain a new tablet. Administer E.R. tablets with food. E.R. capsules may be taken with or without food.
- Oral suspension may be given or E.R. capsules may be opened and sprinkled over a teaspoon of soft food, such as applesauce, for administration if patient has difficulty swallowing.
- Incompatibility with oral suspension: Other diluents or liquid medications, especially liquid chlorpromazine or thioridazine (a precipitate may form).

Route	Onset	Peak	Duration
P.O.	Unknown	4.5 hr	Unknown
P.O./E.R.	Unknown	3–12 hr	Unknown
P.O./susp.	Unknown	1.5 hr	Unknown

Half-life: 10–40 hr

Contraindications

Concurrent therapy with boceprevir, delavirdine, or other non-nucleoside reverse transcriptase inhibitors, or nefazodone; history of bone marrow depression; hypersensitivity to carbamazepine, tricyclic compounds, or their components; MAO inhibitor therapy within 14 days

Mechanism of Action

May prevent or halt seizures by closing or blocking sodium channels, as shown here, thus preventing sodium from entering the cell. Keeping sodium out of the cell may slow nerve impulse transmission, thus slowing the rate at which neurons fire.

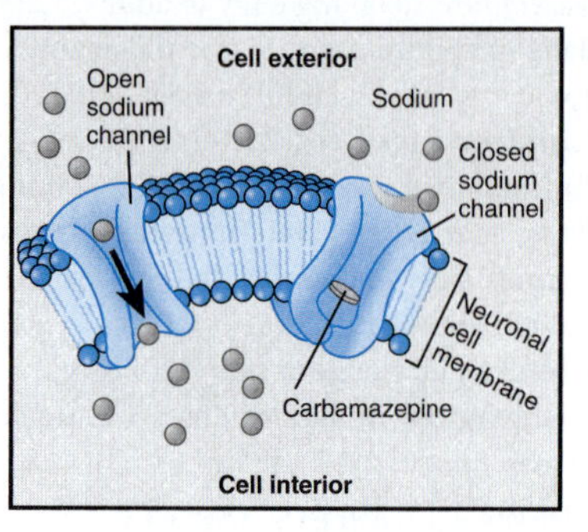

Interactions

DRUGS

acetaminophen (long-term use): Increased metabolism, leading to acetaminophen-induced hepatotoxicity or decreased acetaminophen effectiveness
albendazole, alprazolam, amitriptyline, apixaban, aripiprazole, buprenorphine, bupropion, buspirone, citalopram, clobazam, clonazepam, clozapine, corticosteroids, cyclosporine, dabigatran, desipramine, diazepam, dicumarol, doxycycline, edoxaban, eslicarbazepine, ethosuximide, everolimus, felbamate, felodipine, haloperidol, imatinib, itraconazole, lamotrigine, levothyroxine, lorazepam, methadone, methsuximide, midazolam, mirtazapine, nefazodone, nortriptyline, olanzapine, oxcarbazepine, paliperidone, praziquantel, protease inhibitors, quetiapine, risperidone, rivaroxaban, sertraline, sirolimus, tadalafil, theophylline, topiramate, tramadol, trazodone, triazolam, valproate, ziprasidone, zonisamide: Decreased blood levels of these drugs
chloroquine, mefloquine: Possibly antagonized activity of carbamazepine
clomipramine: Increased concentration of clomipramine
cyclophosphamide: Possibly increased cyclophosphamide toxicity
CYP3A4 inducers such as aminophylline, cisplatin, doxorubicin, felbamate, fosphenytoin, methsuximide, phenobarbital, rifampin, theophylline: Decreased blood carbamazepine level
CYP3A4 inhibitors such as acetazolamide, aprepitant, cimetidine, ciprofloxacin, clarithromycin, dalfopristin, danazol, dantrolene, delavirdine or other non-nucleoside reverse transcriptase inhibitors, diltiazem, erythromycin, fluconazole, fluoxetine, fluvoxamine, ibuprofen, isoniazid, itraconazole, ketoconazole, loratadine, loxapine, macrolides, nefazodone, niacinamide, nicotinamide, olanzapine, omeprazole, oxybutynin, propoxyphene, protease inhibitors, quetiapine, quinine, quinupristin, terfenadine, ticlopidine, trazodone, troleandomycin, valproate, valproic acid, verapamil, voriconazole, zileutone: Increased blood carbamazepine level
delavirdine: Possibly loss of virologic reaponse; development of resistance to delavirdine or to the class of non-nucleoside reverse treanscriptase inhibitors
drugs metabolized by CYP1A2, CYP2B6, CYP2C8/9/19, CYP3A4: Decreased concentrations of these drugs
furosemide, hydrochlorothiazide: Possibly increased risk of symptomatic hyponatremia
isoniazid: Increased risk of carbamazepine toxicity and isoniazid hepatotoxicity
hormonal contraceptives: Possibly less effectiveness of hormonal contraceptives
lithium: Increased risk of CNS toxicity
MAO inhibitors: Increased risk of serotonin syndrome
nondepolarizing neuromuscular blockers: Possibly reduced duration or decreased effectiveness of neuromuscular blocker
oral anticoagulants (direct acting, such as apixaban, dabigatran, edoxaban, rivaroxaban; warfarin): Increased metabolism and decreased effectiveness of anticoagulant
other anticonvulsant drugs: Possible alterations of thyroid function

other CNS depressants: Increased risk of CNS depression causing hypotension, profound sedation, respiratory depression, syncope
phenytoin: Decreased carbamazepine level; decreased or increased phenytoin level
primidone: Decreased carbamazepine level; increased primidone level

ACTIVITIES

alcohol use: Increased sedative effect

FOODS

grapefruit juice: Increased blood carbamazepine level

Adverse Reactions

CNS: Chills, confusion, dizziness, drowsiness, fatigue, fever, headache, **suicidal ideation**, syncope, talkativeness, unsteadiness, visual hallucinations
CV: **Arrhythmias, including AV block**; edema; **heart failure**; hypertension; **hypotension**; **thromboembolism**; thrombophlebitis; worsened coronary artery disease
EENT: Blurred vision, conjunctivitis, dry mouth, glossitis, **laryngeal edema**, nystagmus, oculomotor disturbances, stomatitis, tinnitus, transient diplopia
ENDO: Syndrome of inappropriate ADH secretion, water intoxication
GI: Abdominal pain, anorexia, constipation, diarrhea, dyspepsia, elevated liver enzymes, **hepatic failure**, **hepatitis**, jaundice, nausea, **pancreatitis**, vanishing bile duct syndrome, vomiting
GU: Abnormal spermatogenesis, acute urine retention, albuminuria, **azotemia**, elevated blood urea nitrogen, glycosuria, impaired male fertility, impotence, oliguria, **renal failure**, urinary frequency
HEME: Acute intermittent porphyria, **agranulocytosis**, **aplastic anemia**, **bone marrow depression**, eosinophilia, leukocytosis, **leukopenia**, **pancytopenia**, **thrombocytopenia**
MS: Arthralgia, leg cramps, myalgia, osteoporosis
RESP: Pulmonary hypersensitivity (dyspnea, fever, pneumonia, or pneumonitis)
SKIN: Acute generalized exanthematous pustulosis (AGEP), aggravation of disseminated lupus erythematosus, alopecia, altered skin pigmentation, diaphoresis, **erythema multiforme**, erythema nodosum, **exfoliative dermatitis**, hirsutism, nail shedding or separation of nail plate from nail matrix (onychomadesis), photosensitivity reactions, pruritic and erythematous rash, purpura, **Stevens-Johnson syndrome**, **toxic epidermal necrolysis**, urticaria
Other: Adenopathy, **anaphylaxis**, **angioedema**, **drug reaction with eosinophilia and systemic symptoms (DRESS)**, **hyperammonemia**, **multiorgan hypersensitivity or other hypersensitivity**, **hypocalcemia**, **hypogammaglobulinemia**, **hyponatremia**, lymphadenopathy

C

Childbearing Considerations

PREGNANCY

- Pregnancy exposure registry: 1-888-233-2334 or http://www.aedpregnancyregistry.org/.
- Drug can cause fetal harm, including anomalies of various body systems, such as cardiovascular malformations, congenital malformations (spina bifida), and developmental disorders.
- Drug should not be used in pregnancy unless the benefit to the mother outweighs the potential risk to the fetus.
- Be aware that drug should not be discontinued abruptly if used to prevent major seizures in mother because of potential for status epilepticus.
- There is a higher incidence of teratogenic effects associated with the use of anticonvulsants in combination therapy so if therapy must be continued in pregnancy, monotherapy is recommended.

LACTATION

- Drug is present in breast milk.
- Mothers should check with prescriber before breastfeeding.

REPRODUCTION

- Females of childbearing age taking hormonal contraceptives should use other forms of contraception to prevent pregnancy.
- Decreased sperm count may occur in males.

Nursing Considerations

- Avoid using carbamazepine in patients with a history of hepatic porphyria because it may prompt an acute attack. Also, be aware that the Tegretol brand suspension contains sorbitol and should not be given to a patient with fructose intolerance.

! **WARNING** Note patient's ancestry. If patient has Asian ancestry, make sure he has been evaluated for the genetic allelic variant HLA-B 1502 before starting carbamazepine therapy. If patient has African American; Chinese; European; Indian, including Native American; Japanese; Korean; Latin American; Taiwanese; or Thai ancestry, make sure he has been evaluated for the genetic allelic variant HLA-A 3101 before starting carbamazepine therapy. Patients positive for HLA-A 3101 or HLA-B 1502 shouldn't take carbamazepine because of the risk of serious, sometimes fatal, dermatologic reactions. The risk is between 5% and 15% in patients with these variants.

- Know that carbamazepine should be used with extreme caution, if at all, for a patient who has a history of cardiac conduction disturbance, including second- and third-degree atrioventricular (AV) block; cardiac, hepatic, or renal damage; adverse hematologic or hypersensitivity to other drugs including reactions to other anticonvulsants; or interrupted courses of therapy with carbamazepine.

! **WARNING** Obtain a CBC prior to initating carbamazepine therapy to obtain a baseline because hematologic adverse reactions may occur during therapy with many of them serious and some becoming life-threatening, such as agranulocytosis and apastic anemia. Monitor WBC and platelet counts monthly for first 2 months and then periodically thereafter, as ordered. Decreased counts may indicate bone marrow depression.

! **WARNING** Monitor patient for hypersensitivity and skin reactions that could become life-threatening, such as anaphylaxis and DRESS. Be aware that anaphylaxis and angioedema may occur in patients after taking the first dose or may occur after taking multiple doses. Notify prescriber at the first sign of a hypersensitivity reaction or fever, rash, or swollen lymph nodes. Expect drug to be discontinued and provide supportive care, as needed and ordered.

! **WARNING** Monitor liver function tests, as ordered. Assess patient for signs and symptoms of liver dysfunction such as fatigue and jaundice. Notify prescriber even if only slight elevations in liver enzymes occur or signs and symptoms of liver dysfunction are noted because, although rare, adverse hepatic effects may progress even if drug is discontinued and may become severe causing hepatic failure.

! **WARNING** Monitor patient closely for evidence of suicidal thinking or behavior, especially when therapy starts or dosage changes. Notify prescriber, if present, and expect drug to be discontinued.

- Monitor blood carbamazepine level periodically, as ordered, to assess for therapeutic and toxic levels; a blood level of 6 to 12 mcg/ml is optimal for anticonvulsant effects.
- Monitor patient's electrolytes, especially sodium level, as ordered. Hyponatremia may occur, especially in the elderly and patients treated with diuretics. Assess patient regularly for signs and symptoms of hyponatremia, such as confusion, difficulty concentrating, headache, memory impairment, unsteadiness, and weakness. If present, notify prescriber and expect drug to be discontinued.
- Withdraw carbamazepine gradually to minimize risk of seizures.

PATIENT TEACHING

! **WARNING** Stress importance of patient with Asian ancestry to be evaluated for the genetic allelic variant HLA-B 1502 before starting carbamazepine therapy.

- Instruct patient how to take form of carbamazepine prescribed.

! **WARNING** Alert patient that carbamazepine may cause an allergic reaction or serious skin reactions. Instruct patient to notify prescriber promptly, if present, and stress importance of seeking immediate medical care and to stop taking carbamazepine if difficulty in breathing or swallowing occurs or swelling of eyes, face, lips, or tongue develops. Also, instruct patient to stop carbamazepine and seek immediate care if a fever, rash, swollen lymph nodes or other abnormal skin manifestations occur.

! **WARNING** Instruct family or caregiver to watch patient closely for evidence of suicidal tendencies, especially when therapy starts or dosage changes, and to report such tendencies to prescriber immediately. Review suicide precautions with family or caregiver.

! **WARNING** Inform patient that carbamazepine therapy may cause serious adverse reactions. Review signs and symptoms of blood, liver, and renal disorders and electrolyte imbalance to report as well as any adverse reaction that is persistent, severe, or unusual.

- Encourage patient to comply with laboratory appointments.
- Urge patient to wear sunscreen and protective clothing to reduce photosensitivity.
- Tell females of childbearing age that drug decreases oral contraceptive effectiveness and urge her to use a different contraception. Because drug may cause fetal harm, tell her to notify prescriber if pregnancy occurs.
- Warn patient taking drug to treat seizures not to abruptly stop carbamazepine therapy. Encourage patient to discuss concerns or ask questions about the drug with prescriber.

cariprazine hydrochloride

Vraylar

Class and Category

Pharmacologic class: Atypical antipsychotic
Therapeutic class: Antipsychotic

Indications and Dosages

∗ *To treat schizophrenia*

CAPSULES

Adults. *Initial:* 1.5 mg once daily, then increased to 3 mg once daily on day 2, as needed, with further increases in 1.5-mg to 3-mg increments, as needed. *Usual:* 1.5 mg to 6 mg once daily. *Maximum:* 6 mg once daily.

∗ *To treat acute manic or mixed episodes associated with bipolar I disorder*

CAPSULES

Adults. *Initial:* 1.5 mg once daily, then increased to 3 mg once daily on day 2, with further increases in 1.5- to 3-mg increments, as needed. *Usual:* 3 mg to 6 mg once daily. *Maximum:* 6 mg once daily.

∗ *To treat depressive episodes associated with bipolar I disorder; as adjunctive therapy to antidepressants for the treatment of major depressive disorder (MDD)*

CAPSULES

Adults. *Initial:* 1.5 mg once daily, increased to 3 mg once daily on day 15, as needed and tolerated. *Maximum:* 3 mg once daily.

±**DOSAGE ADJUSTMENT** For patients with bipolar mania or schizophrenia initiating cariprazine therapy while already taking a strong CYP3A4 inhibitor, a cariprazine dose of 1.5 mg given every 3 days and increased to 1.5 mg every other day, as needed; if initiating therapy with a moderate CYP3A4 inhibitor, cariprazine dosage initiated at 1.5 mg every other day and increased to 1.5 mg daily, as needed. For patients with bipolar depression or receiving adjunctive therapy for treatment of major depressive disorder initiating cariprazine therapy while already taking a strong CYP3A4 inhibitor, a cariprazine dose of 1.5 mg given every 3 days; if initiating therapy with a moderate CYP3A4 inhibitor, a cariprazine dose of 1.5 mg given every other day. For patients currently taking 1.5 or 3 mg once daily of cariprazine and initiating treatment with a strong CYP3A4 inhibitor, cariprazine dosage changed to 1.5 mg every 3 days; if initiating therapy with a moderate CYP3A4 inhibitor cariprazine dosage changed to 1.5 mg every other day. For patient currrently taking 4.5 or 6 mg once daily of cariprazine and initiating treatment with a strong CYP3A4 inhibitor, cariprazine dosage changed to 1.5 mg every other day; if initiating therapy with a moderate CYP3A4 inhibitor cariprazine dosage changed to 1.5 mg once daily.

Drug Administration

P.O.

- Administer with or without food.
- Capsules should be swallowed whole and not chewed, crushed, or opened.
- Protect 3-mg and 4.5-mg capsules from light to prevent potential color fading.

Route	Onset	Peak	Duration
P.O.	Unknown	3–6 hr	Unknown

Half-life: 2–4 days

Mechanism of Action

May produce antipsychotic effects through partial agonist and antagonist actions. Cariprazine acts as a partial agonist at dopamine (especially D2) receptors and serotonin (especially 5-HT_{1A}) receptors. The drug acts as an antagonist at 5-HT_{2A} serotonin receptor sites.

Contraindications

Hypersensitivity to cariprazine or its components

Interactions

DRUGS

CYP3A4 inducers, such as carbamazepine, rifampin: Possibly decreased effectiveness of cariprazine
CYP3A4 moderate or strong inhibitors, such as itraconazole, ketoconazole: Increased exposure of cariprazine and risks of adverse reactions

Adverse Reactions

CNS: Agitation, akathisia, anxiety, body temperature dysregulation, cognitive and motor impairment, **CVA**, dystonia, dizziness, extrapyramidal symptoms, fatigue, fever, headache, insomnia, **neuroleptic malignant syndrome**, parkinsonism, restlessness, **seizures**, somnolence, **suicidal ideation**, syncope, tardive dyskinesia
CV: Edema, hyperlipidemia, hypertension, orthostatic hypotension, palpitations, tachycardia
EENT: Blurred vision, dry mouth, nasopharyngitis, oropharyngeal pain
ENDO: **Diabetic ketoacidosis**, hyperglycemia **(may be extreme)**, **hyperosmolar coma**
GI: Abdominal pain, anorexia, constipation, diarrhea, dyspepsia, dysphagia, elevated liver enzymes, gastritis, **hepatitis**, nausea, vomiting
GU: Pollakiuria, UTI
HEME: **Agranulocytosis**, **leukopenia**, **neutropenia**
MS: Arthralgia, back or extremity pain, elevated creatine phosphokinase, musculoskeletal stiffness, myalgia, **rhabdomyolysis**
RESP: Cough
SKIN: Excessive diaphoresis, rash, **Stevens-Johnson syndrome**
Other: **Hyponatremia**, weight gain

Childbearing Considerations

PREGNANCY

- Pregnancy exposure registry: 1-866-961-2388 or http://womensmentalhealth.org/clinical-and-research-programs/pregnancyregistry/.
- It is not known if drug can cause fetal harm. However, neonates exposed to antipsychotic drugs such as cariprazine during the third trimester are at risk for extrapyramidal and/or withdrawal symptoms following delivery.
- Use with caution only if the benefit to the mother outweighs the potential risk to the fetus.

LACTATION

- It is not known if drug is present in breast milk.
- Mothers should check with prescriber before breastfeeding.

Nursing Considerations

! **WARNING** Know that cariprazine should not be given to patients with severe hepatic or renal impairment nor to patients receiving a CYP3A4 inducer. Also, drug should not be used to treat dementia-related psychosis in the elderly because of an increased risk of death.

! **WARNING** Use cautiously in patients with cardiovascular disease, cerebrovascular disease, seizure disorders, or conditions that would predispose them to hypotension. Also, use cautiously in elderly patients because of increased risk of serious adverse effects, such as MI or stroke.

! **WARNING** Watch patient closely for suicidal tendencies, particularly when therapy starts and with dosage changes.

! **WARNING** Know that atypical antipsychotics such as cariprazine rarely may cause neuroleptic malignant syndrome, seizures, or tardive dyskinesia. Monitor patient closely throughout therapy and take safety precautions as needed.

! **WARNING** Monitor patient's CBC, as ordered, because serious adverse hematologic reactions that could become life-threatening may occur, such as agranulocytosis, leukopenia, and neutropenia. Expect to assess more often during first few months of therapy if patient has a history of drug-induced leukopenia or neutropenia or a significantly low WBC count. If abnormalities occur during therapy, watch for fever or other signs of infection, notify prescriber, and, if severe, expect drug to be discontinued.

! **WARNING** Monitor blood glucose levels closely and watch for signs and symptoms of abnormally high blood glucose levels or presence of ketones in urine because drug may cause serious complications such as diabetic ketoacidosis or hyperosmolar coma. Notify prescriber promptly, if present, and expect to provide supportive care to decrease blood glucose level safely, as needed and ordered.

! **WARNING** Monitor patient for difficulty swallowing or excessive somnolence, which could predispose to accidental injury or aspiration.

- Monitor all patient's lipid levels and weight, as ordered, because atypical antipsychotic drugs such as cariprazine may cause metabolic changes.
- Assess patient for late-occurring adverse reactions, especially akathisia or extrapyramidal symptoms that may first appear several weeks after cariprazine therapy begins. Also, be on the alert for an increase in adverse reactions after each dosage increase. If late-effect adverse reactions occur, notify prescriber, and expect dosage to be reduced or drug discontinued.

PATIENT TEACHING

- Instruct patient how to administer cariprazine.

! **WARNING** Urge family or caregiver to watch patient closely for suicidal tendencies, especially when therapy is started, and dosage changes are made. Tell them to take suicide precautions, if needed, and notify prescriber.

! **WARNING** Tell patient to notify prescriber promptly if persistent, severe, or unusual adverse reactions occurs because drug can cause significant adverse reactions that if left untreated could become life-threatening.

! **WARNING** Alert patient with diabetes to monitor blood glucose level closely. Review signs and symptoms of diabetic ketoacidosis and hyperosmolor coma with patient, family, or caregiver and to notify prescriber immediately if suspected. If patient feels acutely ill, tell family or caregiver to get patient immediate medical care.

- Advise patient to get up slowly from a lying or sitting position during cariprazine therapy to minimize orthostatic hypotension and syncope.
- Instruct patient to avoid hazardous activities until drug's effects are known and resolved. Also, alert patient and family or caregiver of increased risk for falls, especially if patient has other medical conditions or takes medication that may affect the nervous system.
- Urge patient to avoid activities that raise body temperature suddenly such as with strenuous exercise or exposure to situations that cause dehydration.
- Instruct patient to inform all prescribers of any drugs she's taking, including over-the-counter drugs because of risk of interactions.
- Advise females of childbearing age to notify prescriber if pregnancy occurs.

carvedilol

Coreg

carvedilol phosphate

Coreg CR

Class and Category

Pharmacologic class: Nonselective beta-blocker and alpha-1 blocker
Therapeutic class: Antihypertensive, heart failure treatment adjunct

Indications and Dosages

* *To control hypertension*

TABLETS (COREG)

Adults. 6.25 mg twice daily for 7 to 14 days, as tolerated. Then, dosage increased to 12.5 mg twice daily for 7 to 14 days, and then up to 25 mg twice daily, as needed and tolerated. *Maximum:* 50 mg daily.

E.R. CAPSULES (COREG CR)

Adults. *Initial:* 20 mg once daily. After 7 to 14 days, increased to 40 mg once daily. After another 7 to 14 days, increased to 80 mg once daily. *Maximum:* 80 mg once daily.

* *As adjunct to treat mild to severe chronic heart failure of cardiomyopathic or ischemic origin*

TABLETS (COREG)

Adults. 3.125 mg twice daily for 2 wk; then increased to 6.25, then 12.5, and then 25 mg twice daily at successive 2-wk intervals, as tolerated. *Maximum for patients weighing 85 kg (187 lb) or less:* 25 mg twice daily. *Maximum for patients weighing more than 85 kg (187 lb):* 50 mg twice daily.

E.R. CAPSULES (COREG CR)

Adults. *Initial:* 10 mg once daily for 2 wk. Then, increased to 20 mg once daily, as needed. Subsequent dosage increased by 20 mg every 2 wk, as needed. *Maximum:* 80 mg once daily.

±**DOSAGE ADJUSTMENT** For patients experiencing a heart rate less than 55 beats/min, dosage reduced.

* *To reduce cardiovascular mortality after acute phase of MI in patients with left ventricular ejection fraction of 40% or less*

TABLETS (COREG)

Adults. 6.25 mg twice daily for 3 to 10 days, as tolerated. Then, dosage increased to 12.5 mg twice daily for 3 to 10 days and then up to 25 mg twice daily, as needed and tolerated.

E.R. CAPSULES (COREG CR)

Adults. *Initial:* 20 mg once daily. After 3 to 10 days, increased to 40 mg once daily. Increased again, as needed, every 3 to 10 days until reaching tolerance or target dose of 80 mg once daily. *Maximum:* 80 mg once daily.

±**DOSAGE ADJUSTMENT** For patients with fluid retention or low blood pressure or heart rate, starting dosage may be decreased to 3.125 mg twice daily for tablet form and 10 mg for capsule form, titration may be slowed, or both. For patients controlled on tablet form, a switch to E.R. capsule form may occur as follows: patient taking 3.125 mg twice daily switched to 10 mg once daily; patient taking 6.25 mg twice daily switched to 20 mg once daily; patient taking 12.5 mg twice daily switched to 40 mg once daily; and patient taking 25 mg twice daily switched to 80 mg once daily. For elderly patients and patients at increased risk for dizziness, hypotension, or syncope switching from 12.5 twice daily dose, dosage of E.R. form decreased to 20 mg once daily and if taking 25 mg twice daily, dosage of E.R. form decreased to 40 mg once daily.

Drug Administration

P.O.

- Administer tablets with food.
- Administer E.R. capsules with food in the morning.
- E.R. capsules should be swallowed whole and not chewed or crushed. Capsule may be opened, and contents sprinkled on a spoonful of cold applesauce if swallowing a capsule is difficult. Administer immediately. Mixture should not be chewed.

Route	Onset	Peak	Duration
P.O.	30 min	1–2 hr	7–10 hr
P.O./E.R.	30 min	5 hr	24 hr

Half-life: 7–10 hr

Mechanism of Action

Reduces cardiac output and tachycardia, causes vasodilation, and decreases peripheral vascular resistance, which reduces blood pressure and cardiac workload. When given for at least 4 wk, carvedilol reduces plasma renin activity.

Contraindications

Bronchial asthma or related bronchospastic conditions; cardiogenic shock; decompensated heart failure that requires I.V. inotropic agents; history of serious hypersensitivity reactions, such as anaphylaxis, angioedema, or Stevens-Johnson syndrome; hypersensitivity to carvedilol or its components; second- or third-degree AV block, severe bradycardia, or sick sinus syndrome unless pacemaker is in place; severe hepatic impairment

Interactions

DRUGS

amiodarone; other CYP2C9 inhibitors, such as fluconazole: Increased risk of bradycardia or heart block
anesthetic agents that depress myocardial function (such as cyclopropane, trichloroethylene): Increased risk of depressed myocardial function
beta blockers, digoxin: Increased risk of bradycardia and hypotension
calcium channel blockers (especially diltiazem and verapamil): Abnormal cardiac conduction
catecholamine-depleting drugs (such as MAO inhibitors, reserpine): Additive effects, increased risk of severe bradycardia and hypotension
cyclosporine, digoxin: Increased blood levels of these drugs
insulin, oral antidiabetics: Increased risk of hypoglycemia
potent CYP2D6 inhibitors, such as fluoxetine, paroxetine, propafenone, quinidine: Possibly increased blood carvedilol levels
rifampin: Decreased significantly blood carvedilol level

Adverse Reactions

CNS: Asthenia, **CVA**, depression, dizziness, fatigue, fever, headache, hypesthesia, hypotonia, insomnia, light-headedness, malaise, paresthesia, somnolence, syncope, vertigo
CV: Angina, **AV block**, **bradycardia**, edema, **heart failure**, hyperglycemia, hypertension, hypertriglyceridemia, orthostatic hypotension, palpitations, peripheral vascular disorder
EENT: Blurred vision, dry eyes, periodontitis, pharyngitis, rhinitis
ENDO: Hyperglycemia, **hypoglycemia**
GI: Abdominal pain, diarrhea, elevated liver enzymes, jaundice, **melena**, nausea, vomiting
GU: Albuminuria, hematuria, elevated BUN and creatinine levels, impotence, incontinence, **renal insufficiency**, UTI
HEME: Anemia, **aplastic anemia**, **decreased PT**, **thrombocytopenia**, **unusual bleeding** or bruising
MS: Arthralgia, arthritis, back pain, muscle cramps
RESP: Dyspnea, increased cough, **interstitial pneumonitis**, **pulmonary edema**
SKIN: **Erythema multiforme**, pruritus, purpura, **Stevens-Johnson syndrome**, **toxic epidermal necrolysis**, urticaria
Other: **Anaphylaxis**, **angioedema**, flu-like syndrome, gout, **hyperkalemia**, hyperuricemia, **hyponatremia**, hypovolemia, viral infection, weight gain or loss

Childbearing Considerations

PREGNANCY

- It is not known if drug can cause fetal harm. However, use of beta blockers during the third trimester of pregnancy may increase the risk of neonatal bradycardia, hypoglycemia, hypotension, and respiratory depression.
- Use with caution only if benefit to mother outweighs potential risk to fetus.

LACTATION

- It is not known if drug is present in breast milk.
- Mothers should check with prescriber before breastfeeding.

Nursing Considerations

- Use with extreme caution in patients with bronchospastic disease such as chronic bronchitis or emphysema because although beta blockers are not usually used in these patients, carvedilol may be needed if there is a poor response or patient can't tolerate other antihypertensive drugs. Expect the smallest dose that is effective to be prescribed to minimize adverse effects.

! **WARNING** Monitor patient for hypersensitivity reactions, which could become life-threatening, such as anaphylaxis and angioedema. Notify prescriber promptly, if present, withhold drug as ordered, and provide supportive care, as needed and ordered.

! **WARNING** Be aware that beta blockers such as carvedilol may mask early warning signs of hypoglycemia, such as tachycardia and increase the risk for severe or prolonged hypoglycemia at any time during drug therapy, especially in patients with diabetes mellitus or patients who are fasting because of not eating regularly, surgery, or are vomiting. Monitor patient closely and if hypoglycemia occurs, treat promptly according to institutional protocal. If severe, expect to provide additional supportive care, as needed and ordered.

! **WARNING** Avoid stopping drug abruptly in patients with hyperthyroidism because thyroid storm may occur, and in patients with angina because it may worsen, or MI may occur.

- Monitor patient with heart failure and diabetes for hyperglycemia, especially when drug is initiated, dosage is adjusted, or drug discontinued.
- Monitor patient with a history of heart failure for worsening heart failure or fluid retention, especially during dosage increases.
- Monitor patients with peripheral vascular disease closely because drug may aggravate symptoms of arterial insufficiency.
- Be aware that chronic beta blocker therapy such as carvedilol is not routinely withheld prior to major surgery because the benefits outweigh the risks associated with its use with general anesthesia and surgical procedures.

PATIENT TEACHING

- Instruct patient how to administer form of carvedilol prescribed.

! **WARNING** Stress importance of not stopping drug therapy abruptly, especially if patient has angina or hyperthyroidism, as serious or even life-threatening adverse reactions may occur.

! **WARNING** Alert patient that drug may cause an allergic reaction. If present, tell patient to notify prescriber and to seek immediate medical care, if severe.

! **WARNING** Alert patient and family or caregiver that drug may cause a low blood glucose level at any time during drug therapy, especially if patient has diabetes or is fasting because of not eating regularly, undergoing surgery, or vomiting. Review signs and symptoms of hypoglycemia with patient and family or caregiver but warn that drug may prevent early warning signs. Instruct them how to treat a low blood glucose level. Stress importance of notifying prescriber promptly and seeking immediate medical care, if severe or happens frequently. Alert patient with heart failure and diabetes that drug may also increase blood glucose level, especially when drug is started, dosage changed, or drug discontinued.

- Tell patient with heart failure to notify prescriber if he gains 5 lb or more in 2 to 3 days or if shortness of breath increases, which may signal worsening heart failure.
- Warn patient that drug may cause dizziness, light-headedness, and orthostatic hypotension; advise him to take safety precautions and avoid performing hazardous activities, including driving until adverse effects are resolved. Tell patient to notify prescriber if present because dosage may need to be adjusted.
- Advise patient to notify ophthalmologist of carvedilol therapy because if cataract surgery is required, modifications of the surgical technique may be necessary. Inform patient wearing contact lens that tear flow may be decreased.
- Tell patient to notify prescriber of all medications taken, including over-the-counter preparations, before using them.

caspofungin acetate

Cancidas

Class and Category

Pharmacologic class: Echinocandins
Therapeutic class: Antifungal

Indications and Dosages

∗ *To treat invasive aspergillosis in patient's refractory to or intolerant of other therapies*

I.V. INFUSION

Adults. *Initial:* 70 mg on day 1, followed by 50 mg once daily with duration of therapy based upon clinical response, recovery from immunosuppression, and severity of underlying disease.
Children ages 3 mo to 17 yr. *Initial:* 70 mg/m^2 on day 1, followed by 50 mg/m^2 once daily and increased to 70 mg/m^2 once daily, as needed and tolerated. Duration of therapy based upon clinical response, recovery from immunosuppression, and severity of underlying disease.
Maximum: 70 mg once daily for both initial and maintenance doses.

∗ *To treat candidemia and other* Candida *infections such as intra-abdominal abscesses, peritonitis, and pleural space infections*

I.V. INFUSION

Adults. *Initial:* 70 mg on day 1, followed by 50 mg once daily and continued for at least 14 days after the last positive culture. Patients with neutropenia who remain persistently neutropenic may require a longer course of therapy pending resolution of the neutropenia.

Children ages 3 mo to 17 yr. *Initial:* 70 mg/m^2 on day 1, followed by 50 mg/m^2 once daily and increased to 70 mg/m^2 once daily, as needed and tolerated, and continued for at least 14 days after the last positive culture. Patients with neutropenia who remain persistently neutropenic may require a longer course of therapy pending resolution of the neutropenia. *Maximum:* 70 mg once daily for both initial and maintenance doses.

∗ *To treat presumed fungal infections in febrile, neutropenic patients*

I.V. INFUSION

Adults. *Initial:* 70 mg on day 1, followed by 50 mg once daily. Increased to 70 mg once daily, as needed. Duration of treatment based upon the patient's clinical response and resolution of neutropenia. Usually, treatment given for at least 14 days and continued for at least 7 days after neutropenia and symptoms have resolved. *Maximum:* 70 mg once daily.

Children ages 3 mo to 17 yr. *Initial:* 70 mg/m^2 on day 1, followed by 50 mg/m^2 once daily for at least 14 days, and continued for at least 7 days after neutropenia and symptoms have resolved. *Maximum:* 70 mg once daily for both initial and maintenance doses.

∗ *To treat esophageal candidiasis*

I.V. INFUSION

Adults. 50 mg once daily for 7 to 14 days after symptoms have resolved.

Children ages 3 mo to 17 yr. *Initial:* 70 mg/m^2 on day 1, followed by 50 mg/m^2 once daily and increased to 70 mg/m^2, as needed. Continued for 7 to 14 days after symptoms have resolved. *Maximum:* 70 mg once daily for both initial and maintenance doses.

±**DOSAGE ADJUSTMENT** For adult patients with moderate hepatic insufficiency, dosage reduced to 35 mg daily after initial 70-mg dose, if an initial dose is required. For patients receiving hepatic CYP enzyme inducers such as carbamazepine, dexamethasone, efavirenz, nevirapine, phenytoin, or rifampin, dosage may be increased to 70 mg once daily for adults and 70 mg/m^2 once daily for children (not to exceed 70 mg daily).

Drug Administration

I.V.

- Reconstitute vial by adding 10.8 ml of 0.9% Sodium Chloride Injection, Bacteriostatic Water for Injection with 0.9% benzyl alcohol, Bacteriostatic Water for Injection with methylparaben and propylparaben, or Sterile Water for Injection to the vial. Mix gently until a clear solution is obtained. Concentration will be 5 mg/ml for a 50-mg vial; 7 mg/ml for a 70-mg vial. A 50-mg vial should be used for children requiring a dose of 50 mg or less (with a concentration of 5 mg/ml) and the 70-mg vial used for a dose greater than 50 mg.

Mechanism of Action

- Interferes with fungal cell membrane synthesis by inhibiting the synthesis of β (1, 3)-D-glucan. A polypeptide, β (1, 3)-D-glucan is the essential component of the fungal cell membrane that makes it rigid and protective. Without it, fungal cells rupture and die. This mechanism of action is most effective against susceptible filamentous fungi, such as *Aspergillus*.

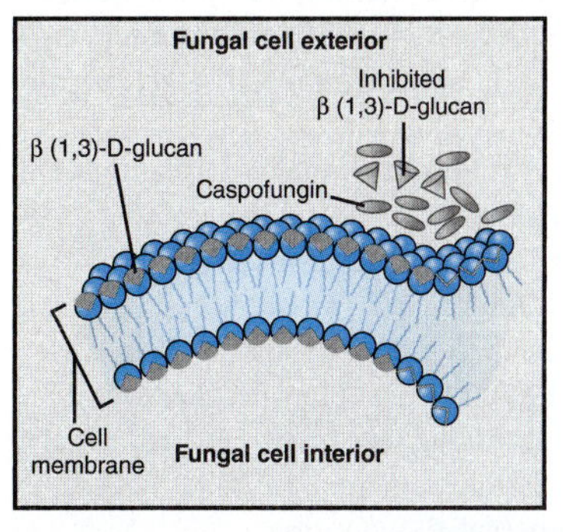

C

- Reconstituted solution may be stored for up to 1 hr at room temperature after reconstitution and prior to dilution.
- Dilute reconstituted solution by withdrawing prescribed dose from drug vial and adding to 250 ml of 0.225%, 0.45%, or 0.9% Sodium Chloride Injection or Lactated Ringer's Injection. Alternatively, drug can be added to a reduced volume of I.V. solution, not to exceed a final concentration of 0.5 mg/ml. Use within 24 hr if stored at room temperature or within 48 hr if refrigerated.
- Infuse slowly over 1 hr. Never administer as an I.V. bolus.
- *Incompatibilities:* Diluents containing dextrose, other drugs infused at the same time

Route	Onset	Peak	Duration
I.V.	Unknown	Unknown	Unknown

Half-life: 9–11 hr

Contraindications

Hypersensitivity to caspofungin acetate or its components

Interactions

DRUGS

carbamazepine, dexamethasone, efavirenz, nelfinavir, nevirapine, phenytoin, rifampin: Possibly decreased blood caspofungin level
cyclosporine: Transient increases in ALT and AST levels
tacrolimus: Possibly decreased blood tacrolimus level

Adverse Reactions

CNS: Asthenia, anxiety, chills, confusion, depression, dizziness, fatigue, fever, headache, insomnia, paresthesia, **seizures**, somnolence, tremor, warmth sensation
CV: Hypertension, **hypotension**, peripheral edema, phlebitis, tachycardia, thrombophlebitis
EENT: Epistaxis, mucosal inflammation, **stridor**
ENDO: Hyperglycemia
GI: Abdominal distention or pain, anorexia, constipation, diarrhea, dyspepsia, elevated bilirubin or liver enzymes, **hepatic dysfunction or necrosis**, hepatomegaly, hyperbilirubinemia, jaundice, nausea, **pancreatitis**, vomiting
GU: Elevated BUN or serum creatinine level, hematuria, proteinuria, **renal failure or insufficiency**, UTI
HEME: Decreased hemoglobin, hematocrit, and WBC count
MS: Arthralgia, back or extremity pain, myalgia
RESP: **Adult respiratory distress syndrome**, **bronchospasm**, cough, crackles, dyspnea, **hypoxia**, pleural effusion, pneumonia, **pulmonary edema**, **respiratory failure**, tachypnea
SKIN: Diaphoresis, erythema, **erythema multiforme**, flushing, petechiae, pruritus, rash, sensation of warmth, skin exfoliation, **Stevens-Johnson syndrome**, **toxic epidermal necrolysis**, urticaria
Other: **Anaphylaxis**, **angioedema**, **bacteremia**, **decreased serum bicarbonate level**, elevated alkaline phosphatase, elevated gamma-glutamyl transferase level, **hypercalcemia**, **hyperkalemia**, **hyperphosphatemia**, **hypokalemia**, **hypomagnesemia**, infusion-site reaction, **sepsis**, **septic shock**

Childbearing Considerations

PREGNANCY

- Drug may cause fetal harm based on animal studies.
- Use with caution only if benefit to mother outweighs potential risk to fetus.

LACTATION

- It is not known if drug is present in breast milk.
- Mothers should check with prescriber before breastfeeding.

Nursing Considerations

! **WARNING** Use cautiously in patients with a history of allergic skin reactions because caspofungin may cause serious skin reactions such as Stevens-Johnson syndrome and toxic epidermal necrolysis, which can be life-threatening.

! **WARNING** Monitor patient for possible histamine-mediated hypersensitivity adverse reactions, such as angioedema, bronchospasm, facial swelling, pruritus, rash, or warmth sensation. Report these symptoms immediately and expect caspofungin therapy to be discontinued. Provide supportive care, as needed and ordered.

! **WARNING** Montior patient for evidence of respiratory distress that could become life-threatening. Also monitor patient for other serious adverse reactions because drug can adversely affect many systems.

- Watch for flushed skin and assess patient often for unexplained temperature elevation.
- Monitor patient's liver function test results, as ordered, and report abnormalities.

PATIENT TEACHING

- Inform patient how drug will be administered.

! **WARNING** Review signs and symptoms of an allergic reaction and skin abnormalities. If present, tell patient to notify staff immediately.

! **WARNING** Instruct patient to notify staff immediately if difficult breathing occurs or any persistent, severe, or unusual adverse reaction is experienced.

cefazolin sodium

Class and Category

Pharmacologic class: First-generation cephalosporin
Therapeutic class: Antibiotic

Indications and Dosages

✱ *To treat biliary tract infections caused by* Escherichia coli, Proteus mirabilis, Staphylococcus aureus, *or various strains of* streptococci; *bone and joint infections caused by* S. aureus; *endocarditis caused by* S. aureus *or group A beta-hemolytic streptococci; genital infections, such as epididymitis and prostatitis, caused by* E. coli, Klebsiella *species,* P. mirabilis, *or some strains of* enterococci; *respiratory tract infections caused by* Haemophilus influenzae, Klebsiella *species,* S. aureus, Streptococcus pneumoniae, *or group A beta-hemolytic* streptococci; *septicemia caused by* E. coli, Klebsiella *species,* P. mirabilis S. aureus, *or* S. pneumoniae; *skin and soft-tissue infections caused by* S. aureus, *group A beta-hemolytic* streptococci, *or other strains of* streptococci; *or urinary tract infections caused by* E. coli, P. mirabilis, *or* Klebsiella *species*

I.V. INFUSION, I.M. OR I.V. INJECTION

Adults with a creatinine clearance equal to or greater than 55 ml/min. *For mild infections caused by susceptible gram-positive cocci*: 250 to 500 mg every 8 hr. *For moderate to severe infections*: 500 to 1,000 mg every 6 to 8 hr. *For severe, life-threatening infections*: 1,000 to 1,500 mg every 6 hr. *Maximum for severe, life-threatening infections:* 12 g daily in divided doses.

Infants 1 mo of age and older, children with a creatinine clearance equal to or greater than 70 ml/min. *For mild to moderate infections*: 25 to 50 mg/kg daily divided equally and given 3 times daily or 4 times daily. *For severe infections*: 100 mg/kg daily divided equally and given 3 times daily or 4 times daily.

✱ *To treat pneumococcal pneumonia*

I.V. INFUSION, I.M. OR I.V. INJECTION

Adults. 500 mg every 12 hr.

✱ *To treat acute uncomplicated UTI caused by* E. coli, Klebsiella *species,* P. mirabilis, *or some strains of* Enterobacter *or* Enterococcus

I.V. INFUSION, I.M. OR I.V. INJECTION

Adults. 1 g every 12 hr.

✱ *To provide surgical prophylaxis*

I.V. INFUSION, I.M. OR I.V. INJECTION

Adults with a creatinine clearance equal to or greater than 55 ml/min. 1 g 30 to 60 min before surgery; 0.5 to 1 g every 6 to 8 hr for 24 hr after surgery. *For surgeries expected to last 2 hr or longer:* 2 g 30 to 60 min before surgery; 0.5 to 1 g during surgery; and 0.5 to 1 g every 6 to 8 hr for 24 hr after surgery although drug therapy may continue for 3 to 5 days after surgery if the occurrence of an infection may be devastating, such as open-heart surgery or prosthetic arthroplasty.

I.V. INFUSION (CEFAZOLIN AND DEXTROSE)

Adults with a creatinine clearance equal to or greater than 55 ml/min and weighs less than 120 kg (264 lb). 1 to 2 g 30 to 60 min before surgery; 0.5 to 1 g every 6 to 8 hr for 24 hr after surgery. *For a surgical procedure expected to last 2 hr or longer:* 1 to 2 g 30 to 60 min before surgery, 0.5 to 1 g during surgery, and 0.5 to 1 g every 6 to 8 hr for 24 hr after surgery, although drug therapy may continue for 3 to 5 days after surgery if the occurrence

C

of an infection may be devastating, such as open-heart surgery or prosthetic arthroplasty. **Adults with a creatinine clearance equal to or greater than 55 ml/min and weighs 120 kg (264 lb) or greater.** 3 g 30 to 60 min before surgery and 0.5 to 1 g every 6 to 8 hr for 24 hr after surgery. *For a surgical procedure expected to last 2 hr or longer:* 3 g 30 to 60 min before surgery, 0.5 to 1 g during surgery, and 0.5 to 1 g every 6 to 8 hr after surgery, although drug therapy may continue for 3 to 5 days after surgery if the occurrence of an infection may be devastating, such as open-heart surgery or prosthetic arthroplasty. **Children ages 10 to 17 with a creatinine clearance equal to or greater than 70 ml/min weighing 50 kg (110 lb) but less than 120 kg (264 lb).** 2 g 30 to 60 min before surgery and 0.5 to 1 g every 6 to 8 hr for 24 hr after surgery. *For a surgical procedure expected to last 2 hr or longer:* 2 g 30 to 60 min before surgery, 0.5 to 1 g during surgery, and 0.5 to 1 g every 6 to 8 hr for 24 hr after surgery, although drug therapy may continue for 3 to 5 days after surgery if the occurrence of an infection may be devastating. **Children ages 10 to 17 with a creatinine clearance equal to or greater than 70 ml/min and weighing less than 50 kg (110 lb).** 1 g 30 to 60 min before surgery and 0.5 to 1 g every 6 to 8 hr for 24 hr after surgery. *For a surgical procedure expected to last 2 hr or longer:* 1 g 30 to 60 min before surgery, 0.5 to 1 g during surgery, and 0.5 to 1 g every 6 to 8 hr for 24 hr after surgery, although drug therapy may continue for 3 to 5 days after surgery if the occurrence of an infection may be devastating.

±**DOSAGE ADJUSTMENT** For adult patients with creatinine clearance of 35 to 54 ml/min, after initial dose appropriate to infection's severity, dosage interval restricted to at least 8 hours or longer; for adult patients with a creatine clearance of 11 to 34 ml/min, dosage reduced by 50% and given every 12 hours; and for adult patients with a creatinine clearance of 10 ml/min or less, dosage reduced by 50% and given every 18 to 24 hours. For infants one month of age and older and children with a creatinine clearance of 40 to 70 ml/min, dosage reduced to 60% and given in divided doses every 12 hr; for infants 1 month of age and older and children with a creatinine clearance of 20 to 40 ml/min, dosage reduced to 25% and given in divided doses every 12 hours; and for infants 1 month of age and older and children with a creatinine clearance of 5 to 20 ml/min, dosage reduced to 10% and given every 24 hours.

Drug Administration

I.V.

- Be aware that cefazolin for injection, 2 g/vial is only to be used for I.V. administration. It is not to be used for I.M. administration. Cefazolin for injection, 3 g/vial is for use only for I.V. infusion; it is not to be used for I.V. bolus injection or I.M. administration.

Single-use regular vials

- To prepare I.V. bolus administration, use the 2 g/vial only. First reconstitute the drug with Sterile Water for Injection following manufacturer guidelines. Shake well until dissolved.
- Further dilute vials with an additional 11 ml Sterile Water for Injection and shake well.
- Inject the solution as an I.V. bolus slowly, directly, or through tubing for patients receiving parenteral fluids as follows: for 1 g dose, inject slowly over 3 to 5 min and for 2 g dose, inject slowly over 7 to 11 min.
- To prepare drug for intermittent or continuous I.V. infusion, first reconstitute using 15 ml of Sterile Water for Injection. Then dilute reconstituted solution with 0.9% Sodium Chloride Injection or 5% Dextrose Injection using 50 or 100 ml of diluent for a 2 g dose and 100 ml of diluent for a 3 g dose.
- Reconstituted or diluted solution is stable for 24 hr at room temperature or for 7 days if refrigerated.
- Administer intermittent I.V. infusion over 30 to 60 min.

Duplex container

- Keep container in folded position until activation is intended. Remove from refrigerator and allow to come to room temperature.
- Unlatch side tab and unfold container. Visually inspect diluent chamber. Use only if container and seals are intact.
- Inspect drug powder by peeling foil strip from drug chamber. Protect from light after removal of foil strip. If foil strip is removed

but administration is delayed, refold container and latch side tab. Product then must be used within 7 days.

- To reconstitute, unfold container and point the set port in a downward direction. Starting at the hanger tab end, fold the container just below the diluent meniscus, trapping all air above the fold. To activate, squeeze the folded diluent chamber until the seal between the diluent and powder opens, releasing diluent into the drug powder chamber. Agitate the liquid-powder mixture until completely dissolved. Once dissolved, drug must be used within 24 hr if stored at room temperature or 7 days if refrigerated.
- To administer, point the set port in a downward direction. Starting at the hanger tab end, fold the container just below the solution meniscus, trapping all air above the fold. Squeeze the folded container until the seal between the reconstituted drug and set port opens, releasing the solution to set port. Squeeze container firmly to check for minute leaks. Then, peel foil cover from the set port and attach administration set.
- Do not use in series connections.
- Do not introduce additives to the container.
- Administer as an infusion over 30 min.

Plastic Container

- Thaw frozen container at room temperature or under refrigeration. Do not thaw by using a microwave or water baths and do not force thawing process. Be aware that precipitates may be present in frozen solution but will dissolve when solution reaches room temperature with little or no agitation. Potency of drug is not affected. Agitate after solution has reached room temperature. If solution remains cloudy, an insoluble precipitate is noted, or if any seals are not intact, discard container.
- Do not dilute. Check for minute leaks by squeezing container firmly. If leaks are detected, discard solution as sterility may be impaired. Do not add any other medication to container.
- Thawed solution is stable for 30 days if refrigerated or 48 hr if stored at room temperature. Do not refreeze once solution has thawed.
- Administer as an IV infusion over 30 min.
- Monitor I.V. site for extravasation, irritation, and phlebitis.
- *Incompatibilities:* None reported by manufacturer.

I.M.

- Reconstitute with 2 ml of Sterile Water for Injection for 500-mg vial and 2.5 ml of Sterile Water for Injection for 1-g single-dose vial. Shake well until dissolved. Solution will appear pale yellow to yellow.
- Administer I.M. injection deep into large muscle mass, such as the gluteus maximus.

Route	Onset	Peak	Duration
I.V.	Immediate	Immediate	Unknown
I.M.	Unknown	1–2 hr	Unknown

Half-life: 1.8 hr

Mechanism of Action

Interferes with bacterial cell wall synthesis by inhibiting the final step in the cross-linking of peptidoglycan strands. Peptidoglycan makes cell membranes rigid and protective. Without it, bacterial cells rupture and die.

Contraindications

Hypersensitivity to cefazolin, other cephalosporins, other beta-lactams, pencillins, or their components

Interactions

DRUGS

aminoglycosides, loop diuretics: Additive nephrotoxicity

probenecid: Increased and prolonged blood cefazolin level due to renal excretion of cefazolin being inhibited

Adverse Reactions

CNS: Chills, confusion, dizziness, fainting, fever, headache, light-headedness, **seizures**, somnolence, tiredness, weakness

CV: Edema, **hypotension**

EENT: Hearing loss, mouth ulcers, oral candidiasis

GI: Abdominal cramps, anal pruritus, anorexia, cholestasis, ***Clostridioides difficile*-associated diarrhea**, diarrhea, dyspepsia, elevated liver enzymes, epigastric pain, flatus, **hepatic failure**, **hepatitis**, hepatomegaly, nausea, **pseudomembranous colitis**, vomiting

GU: Acute tubulointerstitial nephritis, elevated BUN and serum creatinine levels, genital or vulvar pruritus, **nephrotoxicity**, **renal failure**, vaginal candidiasis
HEME: **Aplastic anemia**, eosinophilia, **hemolytic anemia**, **hemorrhage**, **hypoprothrombinemia**, **neutropenia**, **pancytopenia**, **thrombocytopenia**, **unusual bleeding**
MS: Arthralgia
RESP: Dyspnea
SKIN: Acute generalized exanthematous pustulosis (AGEP), ecchymosis, erythema, **erythema multiforme**, pruritus, rash, **Stevens-Johnson syndrome**, **toxic epidermal necrolysis**, urticaria
Other: **Anaphylaxis**; drug fever; injection-site induration, pain, phlebitis, redness, and swelling; serum sickness–like reaction; superinfection

Childbearing Considerations

PREGNANCY

- It is not known if drug can cause fetal harm but drug does cross the placenta.
- Use with caution only if benefit to mother outweighs potential risk to fetus.

LACTATION

- Drug is present in breast milk.
- Mothers should check with prescriber before breastfeeding.

Nursing Considerations

- Use cefazolin cautiously in patients with a history of GI disease, particularly colitis or in patients with impaired renal function. Also, use cautiously in patients hypersensitive to penicillin because cross-sensitivity has occurred in about 10% of such patients. In addition, cefazolin mixed in dextrose-containing solutions should be used cautiously in patients with diabetes mellitus or carbohydrate intolerance.
- Obtain culture and sensitivity test results, if possible and as ordered, before giving drug.

! WARNING Monitor patient for hypersensitivity reactions that could become life-threatening, such as anaphylaxis. Notify prescriber, if present, withhold drug, and provide supportive care, as needed and ordered.

! WARNING Monitor patient closely for diarrhea, which may indicate pseudomembranous colitis caused by *Clostridioides difficile*–associated diarrhea. It may be mild or become life-threatening. If diarrhea occurs, notify prescriber and expect testing to be done to confirm presence of *C. difficile*. If confirmed, expect to withhold drug, and treat with an antibiotic effective against *C. difficile* along with electrolytes, fluids, and protein, as needed and ordered.

! WARNING Institute seizure precautions and monitor patient closely for seizures, especially patients with renal impairment. If seizures occur, manage according to institutional protocol and notify prescriber. Drug may have to be discontinued or dosage adjusted.

- Monitor patient's CBC, as ordered. Assess for arthralgia, bleeding, or ecchymosis; they may indicate a blood dyscrasia. Know that patients at risk for hypoprothrombinemia include patients with hepatic or renal impairment, or poor nutritional state, patients receiving a protracted course of antibiotic therapy, or patients previously stabilized on anticoagulant therapy. Expect to administer vitamin K, as ordered and needed.
- Monitor BUN and serum creatinine for early signs of nephrotoxicity. Also, monitor fluid intake and output; decreasing urine output may indicate nephrotoxicity.
- Watch for evidence of superinfection: cough, drainage, fever, malaise, or perineal itching.

PATIENT TEACHING

- Inform patient drug will be administered either as an I.M. injection or intravenously. Instruct patient to complete the prescribed course of therapy.
- Reassure patient receiving drug as an I.M. injection that it doesn't typically cause pain.

! WARNING Alert patient to potential for serious allergic reactions. If present, have patient notify prescriber and if severe to seek immediate medical attention.

! WARNING Tell patient to report bloody, watery stools to prescriber immediately, even up to 2 months after drug therapy has ended.

! **WARNING** Warn patient of the possibility of seizures. Review seizure precautions and advise patient to notify prescriber if any occur, as dosage may need to be adjusted or drug discontinued.

- Instruct patient to notify prescriber if arthralgia bleeding, or ecchymosis occurs.
- Advise diabetic patient who is testing urine for glucose to use an enzymatic glucose oxidase test while taking drug, to avoid false-positive reactions.
- Inform patient that superinfection may occur and to notify prescriber if cough, diarrhea, discharge, fever, malaise, or perineal itching occurs.

cefdinir

Class and Category

Pharmacologic class: Third-generation cephalosporin
Therapeutic class: Antibiotic

Indications and Dosages

✱ *To treat acute exacerbations of chronic bronchitis caused by* H. influenzae *(including beta-lactamase–producing strains),* H. parainfluenzae *(including beta-lactamase–producing strains),* S. pneumoniae *(penicillin-susceptible strains only), or* M. catarrhalis *(including beta-lactamase–producing strains); to treat community-acquired pneumonia caused by* Haemophilus influenzae *(including beta-lactamase–producing strains),* H. parainfluenzae *(including beta-lactamase–producing strains),* Moraxella catarrhalis *(including beta-lactamase–producing strains), or* Streptococcus pneumoniae *(penicillin-susceptible strains only)*

CAPSULES

Adults and adolescents. *For acute exacerbations of chronic bronchitis:* 300 mg every 12 hr for 5–10 days or 300 mg every 24 hr for 10 days. *For community-acquired pneumonia:* 300 mg every 12 hr for 10 days. *Maximum:* 600 mg daily.

✱ *To treat pharyngitis or tonsillitis caused by* Streptococcus pyogenes

CAPSULES

Adults and adolescents. 300 mg every 12 hr for 5 to 10 days or 600 mg every 24 hr for 10 days. *Maximum:* 600 mg daily.

ORAL SUSPENSION

Children ages 6 mo to 12 yr. 7 mg/kg every 12 hr for 5 to 10 days or 14 mg/kg every 24 hr for 10 days.

✱ *To treat acute maxillary sinusitis caused by* H. influenzae *(including beta-lactamase–producing strains),* S. pneumoniae *(penicillin-susceptible strains only), or* M. catarrhalis *(including beta-lactamase–producing strains)*

CAPSULES

Adults and adolescents. 300 mg every 12 hr or 600 mg every 24 hr for 10 days. *Maximum:* 600 mg daily.

ORAL SUSPENSION

Children ages 6 mo to 12 yr. 7 mg/kg every 12 hr or 14 mg/kg every 24 hr for 10 days.

✱ *To treat uncomplicated skin and soft-tissue infections caused by* Staphylococcus aureus *(including beta-lactamase–producing strains) or* S. pyogenes

CAPSULES

Adults and adolescents. 300 mg every 12 hr for 10 days. *Maximum:* 600 mg daily.

ORAL SUSPENSION

Children ages 6 mo to 12 yr. 7 mg/kg every 12 hr for 10 days.

✱ *To treat acute bacterial otitis media caused by* H. influenzae *(including beta-lactamase–producing strains),* S. pneumoniae *(penicillin-susceptible strains only), or* M. catarrhalis *(including beta-lactamase–producing strains)*

ORAL SUSPENSION

Children ages 6 mo to 12 yr. 7 mg/kg every 12 hr for 5 to 10 days or 14 mg/kg every 24 hr for 10 days.

± **DOSAGE ADJUSTMENT** For adult patients with creatinine clearance less than 30 ml/min, dosage not to exceed 300 mg daily; for children with creatinine clearance less than 30 ml/min, dosage not to exceed 7 mg/kg (up to 300 mg) daily. For patients undergoing intermittent hemodialysis, dosage is 300 mg (adults) or 7 mg/kg (children) every other day in addition to 300 mg (adults) or 7 mg/kg (children) given at the conclusion of each hemodialysis session.

Drug Administration

P.O.

- Reconstitute cefdinir powder for oral suspension by tapping bottle to loosen powder,

C

and then dilute with water in 2 portions (38 ml for a final volume of 60 ml or 63 ml for a final volume of 100 ml) to make a concentration of 125 mg/5 ml or 250 mg/5 ml. Shake well after each portion of dilution.

- Shake well before each use and use a calibrated device to measure dose.
- Keep suspension bottle tightly closed and store it at room temperature. Discard any unused portion after 10 days.
- Capsules should be swallowed whole and not chewed, crushed, or opened.
- Give antacids that contain aluminum or magnesium and iron salts at least 2 hr before or after cefdinir.

Route	Onset	Peak	Duration
P.O.	Unknown	2–4 hr	Unknown

Half-life: 1.75 hr

Mechanism of Action

Interferes with bacterial cell wall synthesis by inhibiting the final step in the cross-linking of peptidoglycan strands. Peptidoglycan makes cell membranes rigid and protective. Without it, bacterial cells rupture and die.

Contraindications

Hypersensitivity to cefdinir, other cephalosporins, or their components

Interactions

DRUGS

antacids that contain aluminum or magnesium: Decreased cefdinir absorption if given within 2 hr of antacid
iron salts: Reduced cefdinir absorption if given within 2 hr of iron
probenecid: Increased blood level and prolonged half-life of cefdinir

Adverse Reactions

CNS: Asthenia, dizziness, drowsiness, headache, insomnia, somnolence
EENT: Dry mouth, pharyngitis, rhinitis
GI: Abdominal pain, anorexia, constipation, ***Clostridioides difficile*–associated diarrhea**, diarrhea, flatulence, indigestion, nausea, **pseudomembranous colitis**, stool discoloration, vomiting
GU: Leukorrhea, vaginal candidiasis, vaginitis
HEME: **Leukopenia**
SKIN: Pruritus, rash
Other: **Anaphylaxis**, serum sickness–like reaction

Childbearing Considerations

PREGNANCY

- It is not known if drug can cause fetal harm.
- Use with caution only if benefit to mother outweighs potential risk to fetus.

LACTATION

- It is not known if drug is present in breast milk.
- Mothers should check with prescriber before breastfeeding.

Nursing Considerations

! **WARNING** Monitor patient for hypersensitivity reaction that could become life-threatening, such as anaphylaxis, especially patients allergic to penicillin because cross-sensitivity can occur. If present, notify prescriber, withhold drug, and provide supportive care, as needed and ordered.

! **WARNING** Monitor patient closely for diarrhea, which may indicate pseudomembranous colitis caused by *Clostridioides difficile*–associated diarrhea. It can be mild or become life-threatening. If diarrhea occurs, notify prescriber and expect testing to be done to confirm presence of *C. difficile*. If confirmed, expect to withhold drug, and treat with an antibiotic effective against *C. difficile* along with electrolytes, fluids, and protein, as needed and ordered.

- Monitor patient with a chronic GI condition, such as colitis, for signs and symptoms of a drug-related exacerbation.
- Assess for evidence of superinfection, including cough, diarrhea, fever, malaise, or perineal itching; and vaginal drainage.

PATIENT TEACHING

- Instruct patient how to administer oral form of cedinir prescribed.
- Instruct patient to complete entire course of therapy, even if feeling better.
- Advise patient to take aluminum- or magnesium-containing antacids and iron salts at least 2 hours before or after taking cefdinir.

! WARNING Alert patient to potential for serious allergic reactions. If present, have patient notify prescriber and, if severe, to seek immediate medical attention.

! WARNING Tell patient to report bloody, watery stools to prescriber immediately, even up to 2 months after drug therapy has ended.

- Inform patient with history of colitis that cefdinir may worsen it; urge him to notify prescriber promptly if symptoms develop.
- Inform patient with diabetes mellitus that oral suspension contains 2.86 g of sucrose per teaspoon; advise him to monitor his blood glucose levels more frequently.
- Teach patient to recognize and report evidence of superinfection, such as cough, diarrhea, fever, malaise, perineal itching, and vaginal drainage. Inform patient that buttermilk and yogurt can help prevent superinfection.

cefepime hydrochloride

Class and Category

Pharmacologic class: Fourth-generation cephalosporin
Therapeutic class: Antibiotic

Indications and Dosages

∗ *To treat mild to moderate UTI caused by* Escherichia coli, *Klebsiella pneumoniae, or* Proteus mirabilis

I.M. INJECTION (ONLY FOR UTI CAUSED BY *E. COLI*), I.V. INFUSION

Adults and adolescents ages 16 and older with a creatinine clearance greater than 60 ml/min. 500 to 1,000 mg every 12 hr for 7 to 10 days.
Children ages 2 mo to 16 yr weighing up to 40 kg (88 lb) with a creatinine clearance greater than 60 ml/min. 50 mg/kg/dose every 12 hr for 7 to 10 days. *Maximum:* Not to exceed adult dose.

∗ *To treat severe UTI caused by* E. coli *or* K. pneumoniae; *to treat uncomplicated skin and soft-tissue infections caused by* Staphylococcus aureus *or* Streptococcus pyogenes

I.V. INFUSION

Adults and adolescents ages 16 and older with a creatinine clearance greater than 60 ml/min. 2 g every 12 hr for 10 days.
Children ages 2 mo to 16 yr weighing up to 40 kg (88 lb) with a creatinine clearance greater than 60 ml/min. 50 mg/kg/dose every 12 hr for 10 days. *Maximum:* Not to exceed adult dose.

∗ *To treat moderate to severe pneumonia caused by* Enterobacter *species,* K. pneumoniae, *or* Streptococcus pneumoniae

I.V. INFUSION

Adults and adolescents ages 16 and older with a creatinine clearance greater than 60 ml/min. 1 to 2 g every 8 to 12 hr for 10 days.
Children ages 2 mo to 16 yr weighing up to 40 kg (88 lb) with a creatinine clearance greater than 60 ml/min. 50 mg/kg/dose every 12 hr for 10 days. *Maximum:* Not to exceed adult dose.

∗ *To treat moderate to severe pneumonia caused by* P. aeruginosa

I.V. INFUSION

Adults and adolescents ages 16 and older with a creatinine clearance greater than 60 ml/min. 2 g every 8 hr for 10 days.
Children ages 2 mo to 16 yr weighing up to 40 kg (88 lb) with a creatinine clearance greater than 60 ml/min. 50 mg/kg/dose every 8 hr for 10 days. *Maximum:* Not to exceed adult dose.

∗ *To treat febrile neutropenia*

I.V. INFUSION

Adults and adolescents ages 16 and older with a creatinine clearance greater than 60 ml/min. 2 g every 8 hr for 7 days or until neutropenia resolves.
Children ages 2 mo to 16 yr weighing up to 40 kg (88 lb) with a creatinine clearance greater than 60 ml/min. 50 mg/kg/dose every 8 hr for 7 days or until neutropenia resolves. *Maximum:* Not to exceed adult dose.

∗ *To treat complicated intra-abdominal infections (together with metronidazole) caused by* Bacteroides fragilis, E. coli, Enterobacter *species,* K. pneumoniae, P. aeruginosa, *or viridans group* streptococci

I.V. INFUSION

Adults and adolescents ages 16 and older with a creatinine clearance greater than 60 ml/min. 2 g every 8 to 12 hr for 7 to 10 days.

±**DOSAGE ADJUSTMENT** For adult patients with creatinine clearance between 30 and 60 m/min, dosing interval increased to every 24 hours if dosing interval had been every 12 hours, and dosing interval increased to every 12 hours if dosing interval had been every 8 hours. For adult patients with creatinine clearance between 11 and 29 ml/min, dosage interval increased to 24 hr if dosage had been 500 mg every 12 hr; dosage decreased to 500 mg and dosage interval increased to every 24 hr if dosage had been 1 g every 12 hr; dosage decreased to 1 g and dosage interval increased to every 24 hr if dosage had been 2 g every 12 hr; and dosage interval increased to every 24 hr if dosage had been 2 g every 8 hr. For adult patients with creatinine clearance less than 11 ml/min, dosage decreased to 250 mg every 24 hours if dosage had been 500 mg or 1 g every 12 hours; dosage decreased to 500 mg every 24 hours if dosage had been 2 g every 12 hours; and dosage decreased to 1 g every 24 hours if dosage had been 2 g every 8 hours. For adult patients on continuous abdominal peritoneal dialysis or hemodialysis, dosage interval and dosage further altered. For pediatric patients, dosage decreased, and dosage interval increased in similar proportion as adults.

Drug Administration

I.V.

- For I.V. infusion, reconstitute using manufacturer's guidelines. Reconstitution varies with product used.
- Use only solutions recommended by manufacturer, as type of diluent varies with the product used.
- Use a Y-type administration set but discontinue primary I.V. solution during cefepime infusion.
- Infuse over 30 min.
- Reconstituted solution is stable for 24 hr at room temperature or 7 days in refrigerator with selected diluents (see manufacturer's guidelines).
- Color of solution may darken while stored but product potency is not affected.
- *Incompatibilities:* Solutions that contain ampicillin in a concentration of more than 40 mg/ml; solutions that contain aminophylline, gentamycin, metronidazole, netilmicin sulfate, tobramycin, or vancomycin

I.M.

- Reconstitute vials by following manufacturer's guidelines.
- Reconstituted solution is stable for 24 hr at room temperature or 7 days in refrigerator with selected diluents (see manufacturer's guidelines).
- Color of solution may darken while stored but product potency is not affected.

Route	Onset	Peak	Duration
I.V.	Unknown	30 min	Unknown
I.M.	Unknown	1–2 hr	Unknown

Half-life: 2–2.3 hr

Mechanism of Action

Interferes with bacterial cell wall synthesis by inhibiting the final step in the cross-linking of peptidoglycan strands. Peptidoglycan makes cell membranes rigid and protective. Without it, bacterial cells rupture and die.

Contraindications

Hypersensitivity to cefepime, other beta-lactam or cephalosporin antibacterials, penicillins, or their components

Interactions

DRUGS

aminoglycosides: Increased risk of nephrotoxicity and ototoxicity
potent diuretics, such as furosemide: Increased risk of nephrotoxicity

Adverse Reactions

CNS: Aphasia, chills, **coma**, confusion, **encephalopathy**, fever, hallucinations, headache, myoclonus, **neurotoxicity**, **nonconvulsive status epilepticus**, **seizures**, stupor
CV: Edema
EENT: Hearing loss, oral candidiasis
GI: Abdominal cramps, ***Clostridioides difficile*-associated diarrhea**, diarrhea, elevated liver enzymes and total bilirubin, **hepatic failure**, hepatomegaly, nausea, **pseudomembranous colitis**, vomiting
GU: Elevated BUN and creatinine levels, **nephrotoxicity**, **renal failure**, vaginal candidiasis
HEME: **Agranulocytosis**; anemia; **decreased** hematocrit, platelets, and **prothrombin activity**; eosinophilia; **hemolytic anemia**; **hypoprothrombinemia**; **leukopenia**; **neutropenia**; positive direct Coombs tests;

thrombocytopenia; **unusual bleeding or hemorrhage**
MS: Arthralgia
RESP: Dyspnea
SKIN: Ecchymosis, erythema, **erythema multiforme**, pruritus, rash, **Stevens-Johnson syndrome**, urticaria
Other: **Anaphylaxis**; elevated alkaline phosphatase, **hyperkalemia**, **hypocalcemia**, injection-site pain, redness, and swelling; superinfection

Childbearing Considerations

PREGNANCY

- It is not known if drug can cause fetal harm.
- Use with caution only if benefit to mother outweighs potential risk to fetus.

LACTATION

- Drug is present in breast milk.
- Mothers should check with prescriber before breastfeeding.

Nursing Considerations

- Use cefepime cautiously in patients with a history of GI disease, particularly colitis, or in patients with impaired renal function. Also, use cautiously in patients hypersensitive to other beta-lactam or cephalosporin antibacterials or penicillins because cross-sensitivity has occurred.
- Obtain culture and sensitivity test results, if possible and as ordered, before giving drug.

! **WARNING** Monitor patient closely for hypersensitivity reactions which could become life-threatening such as anaphylaxis. Be aware that an allergic reaction may occur even up to a few days after therapy starts. Notify prescriber immediately and expect cefepime to be discontinued. Provide supportive care, as needed and ordered.

! **WARNING** Monitor patient closely for diarrhea, which may indicate pseudomembranous colitis caused by *Clostridioides difficile*–associated diarrhea. It may be mild or become life-threatening. If diarrhea occurs, notify prescriber and expect testing to be done to confirm presence of *C. difficile*. If confirmed, expect to withhold drug, and treat with an antibiotic effective against *C. difficile* along with electrolytes, fluids, and protein, as needed and ordered.

! **WARNING** Monitor patient for evidence of neurotoxicity, such as aphasia, encephalopathy, myoclonus, nonconvulsive status epilepticus, or seizures. Be aware that although most cases occurred in patients with renal impairment who did not receive appropriate dosage adjustment, some did not. If neurotoxicity occurs, expect drug to be discontinued and provide supportive care, as prescribed.

! **WARNING** Monitor patient's bleeding time and complete CBC, as ordered, and assess patient for adverse blood reactions that could become life-threatening. Be aware that positive direct Coombs tests may occur with cefepime use. Expect drug to be discontinued and appropriate therapy instituted if patient develops a serious adverse hematologic reaction.

- Be aware that prothrombin time activity may decrease, especially in patients with hepatic or renal impairment, or poor nutritional state. A protracted course of antimicrobial therapy may also decrease prothrombin activity. Expect to monitor prothrombin time in patients at risk and have exogenous vitamin K ready for administration, as needed.
- Monitor BUN and serum creatinine levels for early signs of nephrotoxicity. Also, monitor fluid intake and output; decreasing urine output may indicate nephrotoxicity.
- Assess for signs of superinfection, such as cough or sputum changes, diarrhea, drainage, fever, malaise, or perineal itching.

PATIENT TEACHING

- Inform patient how drug will be administered.

! **WARNING** Instruct patient on the signs and symptoms of an allergic reaction and to notify prescriber, if present. If severe, urge patient to seek immediate emergency care.

! **WARNING** Tell patient to immediately report severe diarrhea to prescriber, even if it occurs as late as 2 or more months after the last dose was taken.

! **WARNING** Instruct family or caregiver to immediately seek emergency care for any change in mental status, development of seizure activity, difficulty speaking or understanding spoken or written words, or sudden jerking movements. Cefepime should be stopped until patient is evaluated.

- Alert patients with diabetes that cefepime therapy may result in a false-positive reaction for glucose in the urine when using methods based on Benedict's copper reduction reaction. Tell patients to use glucose tests based on enzymatic glucose oxidase if they are opposed to doing blood glucose tests.

cefixime

Class and Category

Pharmacologic class: Third-generation cephalosporin
Therapeutic class: Antibiotic

Indications and Dosages

∗ *To treat acute bronchitis and acute exacerbations of chronic bronchitis caused by* H. influenzae *or* Streptococcus pneumoniae; *pharyngitis and tonsillitis caused by* S. pyogenes; *and uncomplicated UTI caused by* Escherichia coli *or* Proteus mirabilis

CAPSULES, CHEWABLE TABLETS, ORAL SUSPENSION, TABLETS

Adults and children weighing 45 kg (99 lb) or more. 400 mg once daily or 200 mg every 12 hr.

CHEWABLE TABLETS, ORAL SUSPENSION

Children ages 6 mo to 12 yr weighing less than 45 kg (99 lb). 8 mg/kg once daily or 4 mg/kg every 12 hr.

∗ *To treat otitis media caused by* Haemophilus influenzae, Moraxella catarrhalis, *or* Streptococcus pyogenes

CHEWABLE TABLETS, ORAL SUSPENSION

Adults and children weighing 45 kg (99 lb) and more. 400 mg once daily or 200 mg every 12 hr.
Children ages 6 mo to 12 yr weighing less than 45 kg (99 lb). 8 mg/kg once daily or 4 mg/kg every 12 hr.

∗ *To treat uncomplicated gonorrhea caused by* Neisseria gonorrhoeae

CAPSULES, TABLETS

Adults. 400 mg as a single dose.

±DOSAGE ADJUSTMENT For patients with renal impairment with a creatinine clearance less than 60 ml/min, and patients on hemodialysis or continuous ambulatory peritoneal dialysis, dosage reduced.

Drug Administration

P.O.

- Shake oral suspension well before pouring dose and use a calibrated device to obtain an accurate dose.
- Store oral suspension at room temperature or in refrigerator and discard unused portion after 14 days.
- Chewable tablets should be chewed completely and swallowed.
- Chewable tablets contain aspartame, a source of phenylalanine, which can be harmful to patients with phenylketonuria (PKU).
- Capsules and tablets shouldn't be substituted for chewable tablets or oral suspension because these forms produce a higher peak blood level than do tablets when administered at the same dose.
- Tablets are scored and may be cut in half to obtain correct dosage, as needed.

Route	Onset	Peak	Duration
P.O.	Unknown	4 hr	Unknown

Half-life: 3–4 hr

Mechanism of Action

Interferes with bacterial cell wall synthesis by inhibiting the final step in the cross-linking of peptidoglycan strands. Peptidoglycan makes cell membranes rigid and protective. Without it, bacterial cells rupture and die.

Contraindications

Hypersensitivity to cefixime, other cephalosporins, or their components

Interactions

DRUGS

anticoagulants, such as warfarin: Increased prothrombin time; increased risk of bleeding
carbamazepine: Increased blood carbamazepine level

Adverse Reactions

CNS: Chills, dizziness, fever, headache, **seizures**
CV: Edema, elevated LDH level
EENT: Hearing loss, oral candidiasis

GI: Abdominal cramps, ***Clostridioides difficile*-associated diarrhea**, diarrhea, elevated liver enzymes, **hepatic failure**, **hepatitis**, hepatomegaly, hyperbilirubinemia, jaundice, nausea, **pseudomembranous colitis**, vomiting
GU: Elevated BUN or creatinine levels, genital pruritus, **nephrotoxicity**, **renal failure**, vaginal candidiasis
HEME: **Agranulocytosis**, eosinophilia, **hemolytic anemia**, **hypoprothrombinemia**, **leukopenia**, **neutropenia**, **pancytopenia**, **prolonged prothrombin time**, **thrombocytopenia**, **unusual bleeding**
MS: Arthralgia
RESP: Dyspnea
SKIN: Ecchymosis, erythema, **erythema multiforme**, pruritus, rash, **Stevens-Johnson syndrome**, **toxic epidermal necrolysis**, urticaria
Other: **Anaphylaxis**, **angioedema**, drug fever, serum sickness–like reactions, superinfection

Childbearing Considerations

PREGNANCY

- It is not known if drug can cause fetal harm.
- Use with caution only if benefit to mother outweighs potential risk to fetus.

LACTATION

- It is not known if drug is present in breast milk.
- Mothers should check with prescriber before breastfeeding.

Nursing Considerations

- Use cefixime cautiously in patients with a history of GI disease, especially colitis, or in patients with impaired renal function.
- Obtain culture and sensitivity test results, if possible and as ordered, before giving drug.

! WARNING Monitor patient for hypersensitivity reaction that could become life-threatening, such as anaphylaxis, especially patients allergic to penicillin because cross-sensitivity can occur. If present, notify prescriber, withhold drug, and provide supportive care, as needed and ordered.

! WARNING Monitor patient closely for diarrhea, which may indicate pseudomembranous colitis caused by *Clostridioides difficile*–associated diarrhea. It may be mild or become life-threatening. If diarrhea occurs, notify prescriber and expect testing to be done to confirm presence of *C. difficile*. If confirmed, expect to withhold drug, and treat with an antibiotic effective against *C. difficile* along with electrolytes, fluids, and protein, as needed and ordered.

! WARNING Monitor patient's bleeding time, complete CBC, and prothrombin time, as ordered and assess patient for adverse blood reactions that could become life-threatening. Expect drug to be discontinued and appropriate therapy instituted if patient develops a serious adverse hematologic reaction.

- Monitor BUN and serum creatinine for early signs of nephrotoxicity. Also, monitor fluid intake and output; decreasing urine output may indicate nephrotoxicity.
- Assess for signs of superinfection, such as cough or sputum changes, diarrhea, drainage, fever, malaise, or perineal itching.

PATIENT TEACHING

- Instruct patient how to administer oral form of cefixime prescribed.
- Stress importance to complete the prescribed course of therapy.
- Alert patient that chewable tablets contain aspartame, a source of phenylalanine, which can be harmful to patients with phenylketonuria (PKU).

! WARNING Inform patient that drug may cause an allergic reaction and to notify prescriber, if present. If serious urge patient to seek immediate emergency care.

! WARNING Tell patient to report severe diarrhea to prescriber immediately; this may occur even up to 2 months after cefixime therapy has been discontinued.

- Teach patient to recognize and report signs of superinfection, such as diarrhea, furry tongue, and perineal itching. If present, advise patient to notify prescriber.
- Inform patient that buttermilk and yogurt can help maintain intestinal flora and decrease diarrhea.

cefotaxime sodium

Class and Category

Pharmacologic class: Third-generation cephalosporin
Therapeutic class: Antibiotic

Indications and Dosages

∗ *To provide perioperative prophylaxis in contaminated or potentially contaminated surgery*

I.V. INFUSION, I.M. OR I.V. INJECTION

Adults and children weighing 50 kg (110 lb) or more. 1 g 30 to 90 min before surgery.

∗ *To provide perioperative prophylaxis related to cesarean section*

I.V. INFUSION, I.M. OR I.V. INJECTION

Adult females. 1 g as soon as cord is clamped I.V., then 1 g I.M. or I.V. at 6 and 12 hr after first dose.

∗ *To treat gonococcal urethritis and cervicitis in men and women*

I.M. INJECTION

Adults. 500 mg as a single dose.

∗ *To treat rectal gonorrhea in women*

I.M. INJECTION

Adult women. 500 mg as a single dose.

∗ *To treat rectal gonorrhea in men*

I.M. INJECTION

Adult men. 1 g as a single dose.

∗ *To treat uncomplicated infections caused by susceptible organisms*

I.V. INFUSION, I.M. OR I.V. INJECTION

Adults and children weighing 50 kg (110 lb) or more. 1 g every 12 hr.
Children ages 1 mo to 12 yr weighing less than 50 kg. 50 to 180 mg/kg daily in 4 to 6 divided doses.
Neonates ages 1 to 4 wk. 50 mg/kg I.V. every 8 hr.
Neonates ages under 1 wk. 50 mg/kg I.V. every 12 hr.

∗ *To treat moderate to severe infections caused by susceptible organisms*

I.V. INFUSION, I.M. OR I.V. INJECTION

Adults and children weighing 50 kg (110 lb) or more. 1 to 2 g every 8 hr.
Children ages 1 mo to 12 yr weighing less than 50 kg. 50 to 180 mg/kg daily in 4 to 6 divided doses. *For more serious infections, including meningitis,* higher dosages used.
Neonates ages 1 to 4 wk. 50 mg/kg I.V. every 8 hr.
Neonates ages under 1 wk. 50 mg/kg I.V. every 12 hr.

∗ *To treat septicemia and other infections that commonly require antibiotics in higher doses than those used to treat moderate to severe infections*

I.V. INFUSION OR INJECTION

Adults and children weighing 50 kg (110 lb) or more. 2 g every 6 to 8 hr. I.V. infusion given over longer than 5 min.

∗ *To treat life-threatening infections caused by susceptible organisms*

I.V. INFUSION OR INJECTION

Adults and children weighing 50 kg (110 lb) or more. 2 g every 4 hr. *Maximum:* 12 g daily.
Children ages 1 mo to 12 yr weighing less than 50 kg. 50 to 180 mg/kg daily in 4 to 6 divided doses.
Neonates ages 1 wk to 4 wk. 50 mg/kg every 8 hr.
Neonates ages under 1 wk. 50 mg/kg every 12 hr.

± **DOSAGE ADJUSTMENT** For patients with estimated creatinine clearance below 20 ml/min, dosage reduced by 50%.

Drug Administration

I.V.

- Reconstitute each 0.5-, 1-, or 2-g vial with 10 ml of Sterile Water for Injection. Shake to dissolve. Color should be a very pale yellow to light amber.
- Administer I.V. injection over 3 to 5 min through tubing of a free-flowing compatible I.V. solution. Temporarily stop other solutions being given through same I.V. site while drug is being administered.
- For intermittent I.V. infusion, further dilute in 50 to 100 ml of 0.9% Sodium Chloride Injection or 5% Dextrose Injection. Administer over 15 to 30 min while temporarily stopping other solutions being given through same I.V. site.
- For continuous I.V. infusion, further dilute reconstituted solution up to 1,000 ml with any of the solutions recommended by manufacturer. Also, see manufacturer guidelines for storage of diluted solution, which is based on type of fluid used for dilution.

- Monitor I.V. site for signs of extravasation or phlebitis.
- *Incompatibilities:* Aminoglycosides, diluents having a pH above 7.5, such as Sodium Bicarbonate Injection.

I.M.

- Reconstitute each 500-mg vial with 2 ml Bacteriostatic Water for Injection or Sterile Water for Injection; each 1-g vial with 3 ml diluent; and each 2-g vial with 5 ml diluent. Shake to dissolve. Do not use diluent that contains benzyl alcohol when preparing drug for a neonate.
- Inject deep into a large muscle, such as the gluteus maximus or lateral side of thigh. Use the anterolateral thigh for neonates and infants under 12 months of age. Aspirate to avoid inadvertent injection into a blood vessel. Doses of 2 g divided and injected into different sites.
- Protect powder and solution from heat and light.

Route	Onset	Peak	Duration
I.V.	Unknown	Unknown	Unknown
I.M.	Unknown	30 min	Unknown

Half-life: 1–1.5 hr

Mechanism of Action

Interferes with bacterial cell wall synthesis by inhibiting cross-linking of peptidoglycan strands. Peptidoglycan makes cell membranes rigid and protective. Without it, bacterial cells rupture and die.

Contraindications

Hypersensitivity to cefotaxime, other cephalosporins, or their components

Interactions

DRUGS

aminoglycosides, loop diuretics, NSAIDs: Increased risk of nephrotoxicity
probenecid: Increased and prolonged blood cefotaxime level

Adverse Reactions

CNS: Chills, fever, headache, **seizures**
CV: Edema
EENT: Hearing loss, oral candidiasis
GI: Abdominal cramps, cholestasis, ***Clostridioides difficile*-associated diarrhea**, diarrhea, elevated enzymes, **hepatic failure**, **hepatitis**, hepatomegaly, jaundice, nausea, **pseudomembranous colitis**, vomiting
GU: Elevated BUN level, **nephrotoxicity**, **renal failure**, vaginal candidiasis
HEME: Eosinophilia, **hemolytic anemia**, **hypoprothrombinemia**, **neutropenia**, **thrombocytopenia**, **unusual bleeding**
MS: Arthralgia
RESP: Dyspnea
SKIN: Ecchymosis, erythema, **erythema multiforme**, pruritus, rash, **Stevens-Johnson syndrome**, **toxic epidermal necrolysis**
Other: **Anaphylaxis**; injection-site pain, redness, and swelling; superinfection

Childbearing Considerations

PREGNANCY

- It is not known if drug can cause fetal harm.
- Use with caution only if benefit to mother outweighs potential risk to fetus.

LACTATION

- Drug is present in breast milk.
- Mothers should check with prescriber before breastfeeding.

Nursing Considerations

- Use cefotaxime cautiously in patients with a history of GI disease (especially colitis) or in patients with impaired renal function.
- Obtain culture and sensitivity test results, if possible and as ordered, before giving drug.

! **WARNING** Monitor patient for a hypersensitivity reaction that could become life-threatening, such as anaphylaxis, especially patients allergic to penicillin because cross-sensitivity can occur. If present, notify prescriber, withhold drug, and provide supportive care, as needed and ordered.

! **WARNING** Monitor patient closely for diarrhea, which may indicate pseudomembranous colitis caused by *Clostridioides difficile*–associated diarrhea. It may be mild or become life-threatening. If diarrhea occurs, notify prescriber and expect testing to be done to confirm presence of *C. difficile*. If confirmed, expect to withhold drug, and treat with an antibiotic effective against *C. difficile* along with electrolytes, fluids, and protein, as needed and ordered.

! **WARNING** Monitor patient's bleeding time, CBC, and prothrombin time, as ordered and assess patient for adverse blood reactions that could become life-threatening. Expect drug to be discontinued and appropriate therapy instituted if patient develops a serious adverse hematologic reaction.

- Be aware that cephalosporins, such as cefotaxime, may produce a positive direct Coombs test.
- Monitor BUN and serum creatinine levels and fluid intake and output for signs of nephrotoxicity.
- Monitor patient closely for superinfection. If evidence appears, notify prescriber and expect to stop drug and provide care.

PATIENT TEACHING

- Inform patient how drug will be adminsitered. Explain that I.M. injection may be painful.

! **WARNING** Inform patient that drug may cause an allergic reaction. Tell patient to notify prescriber if present. If serious, urge patient to seek immediate emergency care.

! **WARNING** Instruct patient to report watery, bloody stools to prescriber immediately, even up to 2 months after drug therapy has ended.

! **WARNING** Inform patient that drug may cause adverse blood reactions. Encourage compliance with laboratory tests and alert prescriber if bleeding or ecchymosis occurs.

- Teach patient to recognize and report signs of superinfection, such as diarrhea, furry tongue, and perineal itching. If present, advise patient to notify prescriber.

cefpodoxime proxetil

Class and Category

Pharmacologic class: Third-generation cephalosporin
Therapeutic class: Antibiotic

Indications and Dosages

✱ *To treat acute community-acquired pneumonia caused by* Haemophilus influenzae *or* Streptococcus pneumoniae

ORAL SUSPENSION, TABLETS

Adults and adolescents. 200 mg every 12 hr for 14 days.

✱ *To treat acute bacterial exacerbation of chronic bronchitis caused by* H. influenzae, Moraxella catarrhalis, *or* S. pneumoniae

ORAL SUSPENSION, TABLETS

Adults and adolescents. 200 mg every 12 hr for 10 days.

✱ *To treat rectal gonococcal infections in women and uncomplicated gonorrhea in men and women caused by* Neisseria gonorrhoeae

ORAL SUSPENSION, TABLETS

Adults. 200 mg as a single dose.

✱ *To treat uncomplicated UTI caused by* Escherichia coli, Klebsiella pneumoniae, Proteus mirabilis, *or* Staphylococcus saprophyticus

ORAL SUSPENSION, TABLETS

Adults and adolescents. 100 mg every 12 hr for 7 days.

✱ *To treat uncomplicated skin and soft-tissue infections caused by* S. aureus *or* S. pyogenes

ORAL SUSPENSION, TABLETS

Adults and adolescents. 400 mg every 12 hr for 7 to 14 days.

✱ *To treat acute otitis media caused by* H. influenzae, M. catarrhalis, S. pneumoniae, *or* S. pyogenes

ORAL SUSPENSION, TABLETS

Children ages 2 mo through 12 yr. 5 mg/kg every 12 hr for 5 days. *Maximum:* 200 mg/dose.

✱ *To treat pharyngitis and tonsillitis caused by* S. pyogenes

ORAL SUSPENSION, TABLETS

Adults and adolescents. 100 mg every 12 hr for 5 to 10 days.
Children ages 2 mo through 12 yr. 5 mg/kg every 12 hr for 5 to 10 days. *Maximum:* 100 mg/dose.

✱ *To treat acute maxillary sinusitis caused by* H. influenzae, M. catarrhalis, *or* S. pneumoniae

ORAL SUSPENSION, TABLETS

Adults and adolescents. 200 mg every 12 hr for 10 days.

Children ages 2 mo through 12 yr.
5 mg/kg every 12 hr for 10 days. *Maximum:* 200 mg/dose.

±**DOSAGE ADJUSTMENT** For patients with creatinine clearance less than 30 ml/min, dosing interval increased to 24 hours. For patients on hemodialysis, dosage frequency reduced to 3 times a week and given after hemodialysis.

Drug Administration

P.O.

- Administer tablets with food to enhance absorption.
- Oral suspension may contain aspartame, depending on the manufacturer. Check for absence of aspartame before administering to a patient with phenylketonuria.
- Shake oral suspension bottle well before pouring dose and use a calibrated device to ensure accurate doses. It need not be given with food.
- Refrigerate oral suspension and discard after 14 days.

Route	Onset	Peak	Duration
P.O.	Unknown	1 hr	Unknown

Half-life: 2–3 hr

Mechanism of Action

Interferes with bacterial cell wall synthesis by inhibiting the final step in the cross-linking of peptidoglycan strands. Peptidoglycan makes cell membranes rigid and protective. Without it, bacterial cells rupture and die.

Contraindications

Hypersensitivity to cefpodoxime, other cephalosporins, or their components

Interactions

DRUGS

aminoglycosides, loop diuretics: Increased risk of nephrotoxicity
antacids (high doses of aluminum hydroxide or sodium bicarbonate), H_2-receptor antagonists: Reduced bioavailability and blood level of cefpodoxime
probenecid: Possibly increased and prolonged blood cefpodoxime level

Adverse Reactions

CNS: Chills, fever, headache, **seizures**
CV: Edema
EENT: Hearing loss, oral candidiasis
GI: Abdominal cramps, ***Clostridioides difficile*–associated diarrhea**, diarrhea, elevated liver enzymes, **hepatic failure**, hepatomegaly, nausea, **pseudomembranous colitis**, vomiting
GU: Elevated BUN level, **nephrotoxicity**, **renal failure**, vaginal candidiasis
HEME: Eosinophilia, **hemolytic anemia**, **hypoprothrombinemia**, **neutropenia**, **thrombocytopenia**, **unusual bleeding**
MS: Arthralgia
RESP: Dyspnea
SKIN: Ecchymosis, erythema, **erythema multiforme**, pruritus, rash, **Stevens-Johnson syndrome**
Other: **Anaphylaxis**, superinfection

Childbearing Considerations

PREGNANCY

- It is not known if drug can cause fetal harm.
- Use with caution only if benefit to mother outweighs potential risk to fetus.

LACTATION

- Drug is present in breast milk.
- A decision should be made to discontinue breastfeeding temporarily during drug therapy or discontinue the drug to avoid potential serious adverse reactions in the breastfed infant.

Nursing Considerations

- Use cefpodoxime cautiously in patients who have impaired renal function or are receiving potent diuretics.
- Obtain culture and sensitivity test results, if possible and as ordered, before giving cefpodoxime.

! **WARNING** Monitor patient for hypersensitivity reaction that could become life-threatening, such as anaphylaxis, especially patients allergic to penicillin because cross-sensitivity can occur. Be aware that an allergic reaction may occur even a few days after therapy starts. If present, notify prescriber, withhold drug, and provide supportive care, as needed and ordered.

! **WARNING** Monitor patient closely for diarrhea, which may indicate pseudomembranous colitis caused by *Clostridioides difficile*–associated diarrhea. It may be mild or become life-threatening. If diarrhea occurs, notify prescriber and expect testing to be done to confirm presence of *C. difficile*. If confirmed, expect to withhold drug, and treat with an antibiotic effective against *C. difficile* along with electrolytes, fluids, and protein, as needed and ordered.

! **WARNING** Monitor patient's bleeding time, complete CBC, and prothrombin time, as ordered. Assess patient for adverse blood reactions that could become life-threatening. Expect drug to be discontinued and appropriate therapy instituted if patient develops a serious adverse hematologic reaction.

! **WARNING** Monitor patient for seizures and institute seizure precautions.

- Monitor BUN and serum creatinine for early signs of nephrotoxicity. Also, monitor fluid intake and output; decreasing urine output may indicate nephrotoxicity.

PATIENT TEACHING

- Instruct patient how to administer form of cefpodoxime prescribed.
- Urge patient to complete the prescribed course of therapy.
- Ensure patient with phenylketonuria checks if product contains aspartame before taking drug, as some oral suspension products do.
- Warn patient not to take an antacid within 2 hours before or after taking cefpodoxime.

! **WARNING** Inform patient drug may cause an allergic reaction. Tell patient to notify prescriber, if present and to seek immediate emergency care, if serious.

! **WARNING** Tell patient to report watery, bloody stools to prescriber immediately, even up to 2 months after drug therapy has ended.

! **WARNING** Inform patient that drug may cause adverse blood reactions. Encourage compliance with laboratory tests and alert prescriber if bleeding or ecchymosis occurs.

! **WARNING** Warn patient and family or caregiver drug may cause seizures. Review seizure precautions and stress importance of seeking immediate medical care, if a seizure occurs.

- Teach patient to recognize and report signs of superinfection, such as diarrhea, furry tongue, and perineal itching. If present, advise patient to notify prescriber.
- Inform patient that buttermilk and yogurt can help maintain intestinal flora and decrease diarrhea.
- Tell mothers breastfeeding should not be undertaken during drug therapy.

cefprozil

Class and Category

Pharmacologic class: Second-generation cephalosporin
Therapeutic class: Antibiotic

Indications and Dosages

✱ *To treat secondary bacterial infections in patients with acute bronchitis and acute bacterial exacerbations of chronic bronchitis caused by* Haemophilus influenzae, Moraxella catarrhalis, *or* Streptococcus pneumoniae

ORAL SUSPENSION, TABLETS

Adults and adolescents. 500 mg every 12 hr for 10 days.

✱ *To treat uncomplicated skin and soft-tissue infections caused by* Staphylococcus aureus *or* Streptococcus pyogenes

ORAL SUSPENSION, TABLETS

Adults and adolescents. 250 mg every 12 hr or 500 mg every 12 or 24 hr for 10 days.
Children ages 2 to 12. 20 mg/kg every 24 hr for 10 days. *Maximum:* Not to exceed adult dose.

✱ *To treat pharyngitis and tonsillitis caused by* S. pyogenes

ORAL SUSPENSION, TABLETS

Adults and adolescents. 500 mg every 24 hr for 10 days.
Children ages 2 to 12. 7.5 mg/kg every 12 hr for 10 days. *Maximum:* Not to exceed adult dose.

✱ *To treat otitis media caused by* H. influenzae, M. catarrhalis, *or* S. pneumoniae

ORAL SUSPENSION, TABLETS

Children ages 6 mo to 12 yr. 15 mg/kg every 12 hr for 10 days. *Maximum:* Not to exceed adult dose of 500 mg/dose or 1,000 mg/day.

✱ *To treat acute sinusitis caused by* H. influenzae, M. catarrhalis, *or* S. pneumoniae

ORAL SUSPENSION, TABLETS

Adults and adolescents. 250 mg every 12 hr for 10 days. *For moderate to severe infections:* 500 mg every 12 hr for 10 days.

Children ages 6 mo to 12 yr. 7.5 mg/kg every 12 hr for 10 days. *For moderate to severe infections:* 15 mg/kg every 12 hr for 10 days. *Maximum:* Not to exceed adult dose.

±**DOSAGE ADJUSTMENT** For patients with creatinine clearance less than 30 ml/min, dosage reduced by half and given at usual intervals.

Drug Administration

P.O.

- Administer without regard to meals.
- Check oral suspension for aspartame that is added by some manufacturers. Patients with phenylketonuria should only be given oral suspension without aspartame.
- Shake oral suspension well before pouring and use a calibrated measuring device to ensure accurate doses.
- Tell patient to refrigerate oral suspension and discard after 14 days.

Route	Onset	Peak	Duration
P.O.	Immediate	1.5 hr	Unknown

Half-life: 1.25 hr

Mechanism of Action

Interferes with bacterial cell wall synthesis by inhibiting the final step in the cross-linking of peptidoglycan strands. Peptidoglycan makes the cell membrane rigid and protective. Without it, bacterial cells rupture and die.

Contraindications

Hypersensitivity to cefprozil, other cephalosporins, or their components

Interactions

DRUGS

aminoglycosides, loop diuretics: Increased risk of nephrotoxicity
probenecid: Increased blood cefprozil level

Adverse Reactions

CNS: Chills, fever, headache, **seizures**
CV: Edema
EENT: Hearing loss, oral candidiasis
GI: Abdominal cramps, ***Clostridioides difficile*-associated diarrhea**, diarrhea, elevated liver enzymes, **hepatic failure**, hepatomegaly, nausea, **pseudomembranous colitis**, vomiting
GU: Elevated BUN level, **nephrotoxicity**, **renal failure**, vaginal candidiasis
HEME: Eosinophilia, **hemolytic anemia**, **hypoprothrombinemia**, **neutropenia**, **thrombocytopenia**, **unusual bleeding**
MS: Arthralgia
RESP: Dyspnea
SKIN: Ecchymosis, erythema, **erythema multiforme**, pruritus, rash, **Stevens-Johnson syndrome**
Other: **Anaphylaxis**, superinfection

Childbearing Considerations

PREGNANCY

- It is not known if drug can cause fetal harm.
- Use with caution only if benefit to mother outweighs potential risk to fetus.

LACTATION

- Drug is present in breast milk.
- Mothers should check with prescriber before breastfeeding.

Nursing Considerations

- Use cefprozil cautiously in patients who have a history of GI disease, especially colitis or in patients with impaired renal function.
- Obtain culture and sensitivity test results, if possible and as ordered, before giving drug.

! **WARNING** Monitor patient for hypersensitivity reaction that could become life-threatening, such as anaphylaxis, especially patients allergic to penicillin because cross-sensitivity can occur. Be aware that an allergic reaction may occur even a few days after therapy starts. If present, notify prescriber, withhold drug, and provide supportive care, as needed and ordered.

! **WARNING** Monitor patient closely for diarrhea, which may indicate pseudomembranous colitis caused by *Clostridioides difficile*–associated diarrhea. It may be mild or become life-threatening. If diarrhea occurs, notify prescriber and expect testing to be done to confirm presence of *C. difficile*. If confirmed, expect to withhold drug, and treat with an antibiotic effective against *C. difficile* along with electrolytes, fluids, and protein, as needed and ordered.

! **WARNING** Monitor patient's bleeding time, complete CBC, and prothrombin time, as ordered. Assess patient for adverse blood reactions that could become life-threatening. Expect drug to be discontinued and appropriate therapy instituted if patient develops a serious adverse hematologic reaction.

! **WARNING** Monitor patient for seizures and institute seizure precautions.

- Monitor BUN and serum creatinine for early signs of nephrotoxicity. Also, monitor fluid intake and output; decreasing urine output may indicate nephrotoxicity.

PATIENT TEACHING

- Instruct patient how to administer oral form of drug prescribed.
- Urge patient to complete the prescribed course of therapy.
- Alert patient with phenylketonuria that oral suspension may contain aspartame, depending on manufacturer.

! **WARNING** Inform patient that an allergic reaction may occur even a few days after therapy begins. Stress importance of notifying prescriber or seeking immediate emergency care, if severe.

! **WARNING** Tell patient to report watery, bloody stools to prescriber immediately, even up to 2 months after drug therapy has ended.

! **WARNING** Inform patient that drug may cause adverse blood reactions. Encourage compliance with laboratory tests and alert prescriber if bleeding or ecchymosis occurs.

! **WARNING** Warn patient and family or caregiver drug may cause seizures. Review seizure precautions and stress importance of seeking immediate medical care, if a seizure occurs.

- Teach patient to recognize and report signs of superinfection, such as diarrhea, furry tongue, and perineal itching. If present, advise patient to notify prescriber.
- Inform patient that buttermilk and yogurt can help maintain intestinal flora and decrease diarrhea.

ceftaroline fosamil

Teflaro

Class and Category

Pharmacologic class: Fifth-generation cephalosporin
Therapeutic class: Antibiotic

Indications and Dosages

∗ *To treat acute bacterial skin and skin structure infection caused by* Escherichia coli, Klebsiella oxytoca, K. pneumoniae, Staphylococcus aureus, Streptococcus agalactiae, *or* S. pyogenes

I.V. INFUSION

Adults. 600 mg every 12 hr for 5 to 14 days.
Children ages 2 to 18 weighing more than 33 kg (72.5 lb). 400 mg every 8 hr or 600 mg every 12 hr for 5 to 14 days.
Children ages 2 to 18 weighing 33 kg (72.5 lb) or less. 12 mg/kg every 8 hr for 5 to 14 days.
Children ages 2 mo to less than 2 yr. 8 mg/kg every 8 hr for 5 to 14 days.
Newborns (gestational ages 34 wk and older and postnatal ages 12 days and older) to less than 2 mo of age. 6 mg/kg every 8 hr for 5 to 14 days.

∗ *To treat community-acquired bacterial pneumonia caused by* E. coli, Haemophilus influenzae, K. oxytoca, K. pneumoniae, S. aureus, *or* S. pneumoniae

I.V. INFUSION

Adults. 600 mg every 12 hr for 5 to 7 days.
Children ages 2 to 18 weighing more than 33 kg (72.5 lb). 400 mg every 8 hr or 600 mg every 12 hr for 5 to 14 days.
Children ages 2 to 18 weighing 33 kg (72.5 lb) or less. 12 mg/kg every 8 hr for 5 to 14 days.
Children ages 2 mo to less than 2 yr. 8 mg/kg every 8 hr for 5 to 14 days.

± **DOSAGE ADJUSTMENT** For adult patients with a creatinine clearance above 30 ml/min but no higher than 50 ml/min, dosage reduced to 400 mg every 12 hours; for adult patients with a creatinine clearance above 15 ml/min but no higher than 30 ml/min, dosage reduced to 300 mg every 12 hours; for adult patients with a creatinine clearance of less than 15 ml/min, including those on hemodialysis, dosage reduced to 200 mg every 12 hours. For pediatric patients, dosage adjustment is unknown if creatinine clearance is below 50 ml/min.

Drug Administration

I.V.

- Reconstitute each drug vial with 20 ml of 0.9% Sodium Chloride Injection, 5% Dextrose in Water, Lactated Ringer's Injection, or Sterile Water for Injection. Mix gently to ensure drug is completely dissolved. Color may range from clear to light or dark yellow depending on the concentration and storage conditions.
- Drug must be diluted after reconstitution with 0.45% or 0.9% Sodium Chloride Injection, 2.5% or 5% Dextrose Injection, or Lactated Ringer's Injection. Do not use Sterile Water for Injection for dilution.
- If diluting 600 mg of reconstituted solution in a 50-ml infusion bag for adult administration, withdraw 20 ml of diluent from the infusion bag. Then, inject entire content of the drug vial into the bag to provide a total volume of 50 ml. Concentration will be 12 mg/ml.
- If diluting 400 mg of reconstituted solution in a 50-ml infusion bag for adults or pediatric patients weighing more than 33 kg (72.5 lb), withdraw 20 ml of diluent from the infusion bag. Inject entire content of drug vial into the bag to provide a total volume of 50 ml. Concentration will be 8 mg/ml.
- If diluting reconstituted solution for pediatric patients weighing 33 kg (72.5 lb) or less, amount of solution withdrawn from the reconstituted drug vial for dilution in infusion bag will vary according to the age and weight of the child (see manufacturer's guidelines). The concentration should not exceed 12 mg/ml.
- Reconstituted drug may also be diluted in 250 ml of recommended solution for adult administration.
- Color of infusion solution varies from clear to light or dark yellow depending on the concentration and storage.
- Infuse diluted solution within 6 hr of mixing if stored at room temperature or within 24 hr if refrigerated.
- For adults and children 2 mo of age and older, infuse over 5 to 60 min; for infants less than 2 mo of age, infuse over 30 to 60 min.
- *Incompatibilities:* Other drugs

Route	Onset	Peak	Duration
I.V.	Unknown	5 min after infusion	Unknown

Half-life: 2.6 hr

Mechanism of Action

Interferes with bacterial cell wall synthesis by inhibiting the final step in the cross-linking of peptidoglycan strands. Peptidoglycan makes the cell membrane rigid and protective. Without it, bacterial cells rupture and die.

Contraindications

Hypersensitivity to ceftaroline, other cephalosporins, or their components

Drug Reactions

None reported by manufacturer.

Adverse Reactions

CNS: Dizziness, **encephalopathy**, fever, headache, **seizures**
CV: **Bradycardia**, palpitations, phlebitis
ENDO: Hyperglycemia
GI: Abdominal pain, ***Clostridioides difficile*–associated diarrhea**, constipation, diarrhea, elevated liver enzymes, **hepatitis**, nausea, vomiting
GU: **Renal failure**
HEME: **Agranulocytosis**, anemia, eosinophilia, **hemolytic anemia**, **leukopenia**, **neutropenia**, **thrombocytopenia**
RESP: **Eosinophilic pneumonia**
SKIN: Pruritus, rash, urticaria
Other: **Anaphylaxis**, direct Coombs test seroconversion, **hyperkalemia**, **hypokalemia**, **hypersensitivity reactions**

Childbearing Considerations

PREGNANCY

- It is not known if drug can cause fetal harm.
- Use with caution only if benefit to mother outweighs potential risk to fetus.

LACTATION

- It is not known if drug is present in breast milk.
- Mothers should check with prescriber before breastfeeding.

Nursing Considerations

- Obtain culture and sensitivity results, if possible and as ordered, before giving drug.

! **WARNING** Monitor patient for hypersensitivity reaction that could become life-threatening, such as anaphylaxis, especially patients allergic to carbapenems or penicillin because cross-sensitivity can occur. Be aware that an allergic reaction may occur even a few days after therapy starts. If present, notify prescriber, withhold drug, and provide supportive care, as needed and ordered.

! **WARNING** Monitor patient closely for diarrhea, which may indicate pseudomembranous colitis caused by *Clostridioides difficile*–associated diarrhea. It may be mild or become life-threatening. If diarrhea occurs, notify prescriber and expect testing to be done to confirm presence of *C. difficile*. If confirmed, expect to withhold drug, and treat with an antibiotic effective against *C. difficile* along with electrolytes, fluids, and protein, as needed and ordered.

! **WARNING** Monitor patient's bleeding time, complete CBC, and prothrombin time, as ordered. Assess patient for adverse blood reactions that could become life-threatening. Expect drug to be discontinued and appropriate therapy instituted if patient develops a serious adverse hematologic reaction. Also be aware that seroconversion from a negative to a positive direct Coombs test result may occur. If anemia develops during or after ceftaroline therapy, expect a direct Coombs test to be ordered. If drug-induced hemolytic anemia is suspected, expect to discontinue drug and provide supportive care, as indicated.

! **WARNING** Monitor patient for adverse neurological reactions such as encephalopathy and seizures, especially in patients with renal impairment. Institute seizure precautions. If present, notify prescriber, as drug may have to be discontinued or dosage adjusted.

- Monitor BUN and serum creatinine for early signs of nephrotoxicity. Also, monitor fluid intake and output; decreasing urine output may indicate nephrotoxicity.

PATIENT TEACHING

- Inform patient that drug will be given intravenously.

! **WARNING** Inform patient that drug may cause an allergic reaction. Tell patient to report serious allergic reactions, such as a rash, immediately.

! **WARNING** Instruct patient to report watery, bloody stools to prescriber immediately, even up to 2 months after drug therapy has ended.

! **WARNING** Warn patient that adverse neurological adverse reactions may occur, such as seizures. Review seizure precautions. If any occur, tell patient to notify prescriber immediately, as dosage may have to be changed or drug discontinued.

! **WARNING** Inform patient that drug may cause adverse blood reactions. Encourage compliance with laboratory tests and alert prescriber if bleeding or ecchymosis occurs.

- Teach patient to recognize and report signs of superinfection, such as diarrhea, furry tongue, and perineal itching. If present, advise patient to notify prescriber.
- Inform patient that buttermilk and yogurt can help maintain intestinal flora and decrease diarrhea.

ceftazidime

Tazicef

Class and Category

Pharmacologic class: Third-generation cephalosporin
Therapeutic class: Antibiotic

Indications and Dosages

∗ *To treat UTI caused by* Enterobacter *species,* Escherichia coli, Klebsiella species, Proteus mirabilis *or other species, such as indole-positive* Proteus, *or* Pseudomonas aeruginosa

I.V. INFUSION, I.M OR I.V. INJECTION

Adults and children ages 12 and older. *For uncomplicated UTI:* 250 mg every 12 hr. *For complicated UTI:* 500 mg every 8 to 12 hr.

I.V. INFUSION, I.V. INJECTION

Children ages 1 mo to 12 yr. 30 to 50 mg/kg every 8 hr. *Maximum:* 6 g daily.

Neonates up to 4 wk. 30 mg/kg every 12 hr.

* *To treat mild skin and skin structure infections caused by* Enterobacter *species,* E. coli, Klebsiella species, P. mirabilis *and other* Proteus *species, including indole-positive* Proteus, P. aeruginosa, Serratia *species,* Staphylococcus aureus, *or* Streptococcus pyogenes *(group A beta-hemolytic* streptococci*); uncomplicated pneumonia, caused by* Citrobacter *species,* Enterobacter *species,* E. coli, Haemophilus influenzae, Klebsiella *species,* P. mirabilis, P. aeruginosa *and other* Pseudomonas *species,* Serratia *species,* Staphylococcus pneumoniae, *or* Streptococcus pneumoniae

I.V. INFUSION, I.M. OR I.V. INJECTION

Adults and children ages 12 and older. 0.5 to 1 g every 8 hr.

I.V. INFUSION, I.V. INJECTION

Children ages 1 mo to 12 yr. 30 to 50 mg/kg every 8 hr. *Maximum:* 6 g daily.

Neonates up to 4 wk. 30 mg/kg every 12 hr.

* *To treat bone and joint infections caused by* Enterobacter *species,* Klebsiella *species,* P. aeruginosa, *or* S. aureus

I.V. INFUSION, I.V. INJECTION

Adults and children ages 12 and older. 2 g every 12 hr.

Children ages 1 mo to 12 yr. 30 to 50 mg/kg every 8 hr. *Maximum:* 6 g daily.

Neonates up to 4 wk. 30 mg/kg every 12 hr.

* *To treat serious gynecologic infections caused by* E. coli*; to treat intra-abdominal infections caused by* E. coli, Klebsiella *species,* or S. aureus*; to treat meningitis caused by* H. influenzae *or* Neisseria meningitidis*; and life-threatening infections, such as bacterial septicemia caused by* E. coli, H. influenzae, Klebsiella *species,* P. aeruginosa, Serratia *species,* S. aureus, *or* S. pneumoniae *especially in immunocompromised patients*

I.V. INFUSION, I.V. INJECTION

Adults and children ages 12 and older. 2 g every 8 hr.

Children ages 1 mo to 12 yr. 30 to 50 mg/kg every 8 hr. *Maximum:* 6 g daily.

Neonates up to 4 wk. 30 mg/kg every 12 hr.

* *To treat pseudomonal lung infection in patients with cystic fibrosis and normal renal function*

I.V. INFUSION, I.V. INJECTION

Adults and children 1 mo and older. 30 to 50 mg/kg every 8 hr. *Maximum:* 6 g daily.

Neonates from birth to 4 wk. 30 mg/kg every 12 hr.

± **DOSAGE ADJUSTMENT** For adult patients with creatinine clearance of 31 to 50 ml/min, dosage reduced to 1 g every 12 hours; for adult patients with creatinine clearance of 16 to 30 ml/min, dosage reduced to 1 g every 24 hours; for adult patients with creatinine clearance of 6 to 15 ml/min, dosage reduced to 0.5 g every 24 hours; for adult patients with creatinine clearance of less than 5 ml/min, dosage reduced to 0.5 g every 48 hours. For hemodialysis adult patients, a loading dose of 1 g given followed by 1 g after each session. For adult patients undergoing continuous ambulatory peritoneal dialysis or intraperitoneal dialysis, a loading dose of 1 g may be given, followed by 500 mg every 24 hours or 250 mg may be added to the 2-liter dialysis fluid. For pediatric patients with renal impairment, dosage adjustment made based on body surface area or lean body mass and dosing frequency reduced.

Drug Administration

I.V.

- Administration of fractional doses is not recommended.

Vials

- Do not use pharmacy bulk package for I.V. injection.
- Protect ceftazidime powder and reconstituted drug from heat and light; both tend to darken during storage.
- Thaw frozen solution at room temperature, not in water bath or microwave. Do not refreeze.
- Don't use diluents containing benzyl alcohol when administering to neonates.
- All drug vials are under reduced pressure. Carbon dioxide will be released during dissolution, causing positive pressure to develop in the drug vial.
- Consult recommended manufacturer's instructions to reconstitute drug, as instructions vary among products.
- Administer I.V. injection slowly over 3 to 5 min through tubing of a flowing compatible I.V. fluid. Temporarily stop other solutions being given through the same I.V. site while drug is being administered.

C

- For intermittent infusion, administer over 30 min.
- Avoid using Sodium Bicarbonate Injection as a diluent because drug is least stable in it.
- Rotate I.V. sites every 72 hr.
- Store solution for up to 12 hr at room temperature or 7 days in refrigerator.

Duplex

- Keep container in folded position until activation is intended. Remove from refrigerator and allow to come to room temperature.
- Unlatch side tab and unfold container. Visually inspect diluent chamber. Use only if container and seals are intact.
- Inspect drug powder by peeling foil strip from drug chamber. Protect from light after removal of foil strip. If foil strip is removed but administration is delayed, refold container and latch side tab. Product then must be used within 7 days.
- To reconstitute, unfold container and point the set port in a downward direction. Starting at the hanger tab end, fold the container just below the diluent meniscus, trapping all air above the fold. To activate, squeeze the folded diluent chamber until the seal between the diluent and powder opens, releasing diluent into the drug powder chamber. Agitate the liquid-powder mixture until completely dissolved. Once dissolved, drug must be used within 24 hr if stored at room temperature or 7 days if refrigerated.
- To administer, point the set port in a downward direction. Starting at the hanger tab end, fold the container just below the solution meniscus, trapping all air above the fold. Squeeze the folded container until the seal between the reconstituted drug and set port opens, releasing the solution to set port. Squeeze container firmly to check for minute leaks. Then, peel foil cover from the set port and attach administration set.
- Temporarily stop other solutions being given through the same I.V. site while drug is being administered.
- Do not use in series connections.
- Do not introduce additives to the container.
- Administer as an infusion over 30 min.
- *Incompatibilities:* Aminoglycosides, vancomycin

I.M.

- Reconstitute each gram with 3 ml of 0.5% or 1% Lidocaine Hydrochloride Injection, Bacteriostatic Water for Injection, or Sterile Water for Injection.
- Give I.M. injection deep into large muscle mass, such as the gluteus maximus or lateral part of the thigh. Lateral part of the thigh is the preferred site for neonates and infants up to 12 mo.

Route	Onset	Peak	Duration
I.V.	Immediate	30 min	Unknown
I.M.	Unknown	1 hr	Unknown

Half-life: 2 hr

Mechanism of Action

Interferes with bacterial cell wall synthesis by inhibiting the cross-linking of peptidoglycan strands. Peptidoglycan makes the cell membrane rigid and protective. Without it, bacterial cells rupture and die.

Contraindications

Hypersensitivity to ceftazidime, other beta-lactam or cephalosporins, penicillins or their components

Interactions

DRUGS

aminoglycosides, loop diuretics: Increased risk of nephrotoxicity
chloramphenicol: Antagonistic effect on ceftazidime
oral combined estrogen–progesterone contraceptives: Decreased effectiveness of oral contraceptive

Adverse Reactions

CNS: Chills, **coma**, **encephalopathy**, fever, headache, irregular lapses of posture, **nonconvulsive status epilepticus**, myoclonus, neuromuscular excitability, **seizures**
CV: Edema
EENT: Hearing loss, oral candidiasis
GI: Abdominal cramps, ***Clostridioides difficile*–associated diarrhea**, diarrhea, elevated liver enzymes, **hepatic failure**, hepatomegaly, nausea, **pseudomembranous colitis**, vomiting
GU: Elevated BUN level, **nephrotoxicity**, **renal failure**, vaginal candidiasis
HEME: Eosinophilia, **hemolytic anemia**, **hypoprothrombinemia**, **neutropenia**, **thrombocytopenia**, **unusual bleeding**

MS: Arthralgia
RESP: Dyspnea
SKIN: Ecchymosis, erythema, **erythema multiforme**, pruritus, rash, **Stevens-Johnson syndrome**
Other: **Anaphylaxis**; injection-site pain, redness, and swelling; superinfection

Childbearing Considerations

PREGNANCY

- It is not known if drug can cause fetal harm.
- Use with caution only if benefit to mother outweighs potential risk to fetus.

LACTATION

- Drug is present in breast milk.
- Mothers should check with prescriber before breastfeeding.

Nursing Considerations

- Use cautiously in patients with a history of GI disease, particularly colitis because risk of pseudomembranous colitis is increased.

! **WARNING** Use cautiously in patients with renal insufficiency because high and prolonged serum ceftazidime concentrations can occur from usual dosages. This can lead to asterixis, coma, encephalopathy, myoclonia, neuromuscular excitability, nonconvulsive status epilepticus, and seizures. Ensure that patients with significant renal insufficiency are receiving reduced dosage based on their creatinine clearance. Also monitor BUN and serum creatinine for early signs of nephrotoxicity. Also, monitor fluid intake and output; decreasing urine output may indicate nephrotoxicity.

- Obtain culture and sensitivity test results, if possible and as ordered, before giving drug.

! **WARNING** Monitor patient for a hypersensitivity reaction that could become life-threatening, such as anaphylaxis, especially patients allergic to carbapenems or penicillin because cross-sensitivity can occur. Be aware that an allergic reaction may occur even a few days after therapy starts. If present, notify prescriber, withhold drug, and provide supportive care, as needed and ordered.

! **WARNING** Monitor patient closely for diarrhea, which may indicate pseudomembranous colitis caused by *Clostridioides difficile*–associated diarrhea. It may be mild or become life-threatening. If diarrhea occurs, notify prescriber and expect testing to be done to confirm presence of *C. difficile*. If confirmed, expect to withhold drug, and treat with an antibiotic effective against *C. difficile* along with electrolytes, fluids, and protein, as needed and ordered.

! **WARNING** Monitor patient's bleeding time, complete CBC, and prothrombin time, as ordered. Assess patient for adverse blood reactions that could become life-threatening. Expect drug to be discontinued and appropriate therapy instituted if patient develops a serious adverse hematologic reaction. If drug-induced hemolytic anemia is suspected, expect to discontinue drug and provide supportive care, as indicated.

- Monitor ALT, AST, bilirubin, CBC, hematocrit, LD, and serum alkaline phosphatase levels during long-term therapy.
- Assess for signs of superinfection, such as cough or sputum changes, diarrhea, drainage, fever, malaise, pain, perineal itching, rash, redness, and swelling.

PATIENT TEACHING

- Inform patient that drug will either be given by an I.M. injection or intravenously.
- Stress importance of completing course of therapy.

! **WARNING** Alert patient that allergic reactions can occur, especially after a few days of drug therapy. Instruct patient to notify prescriber if present and seek immediate medical attention if severe.

! **WARNING** Urge patient to report watery, bloody stools to prescriber immediately, even up to 2 months after drug therapy has ended.

! **WARNING** Instruct patient to monitor urine output. Review signs and symptoms of types of neurologic adverse reactions that may occur with ceftazidime therapy. Review seizure precautions. If present, or urine output decreases, urge patient to notify prescriber.

! **WARNING** Inform patient that drug may cause adverse blood reactions. Encourage compliance with laboratory tests and alert prescriber if bleeding or ecchymosis occurs.

- Teach patient to recognize and report signs of superinfection, such as diarrhea, furry tongue, and perineal itching. If present, advise patient to notify prescriber.
- Inform patient that buttermilk and yogurt can help maintain intestinal flora and decrease diarrhea.
- Urge diabetic patients testing urine for glucose to use an enzymatic glucose oxidase reactor during drug therapy.

NEW!

ceftobiprole medocaril sodium

Zevtera

Class and Category

Pharmacologic class: Fifth-generation cephalosporin
Therapeutic class: Antibiotic

Indications and Dosages

∗ *To treat* Staphylococcus aureus *bloodstream infections (SAB) (bacteremia), including those with right-sided infective endocarditis caused by methicillin-susceptible and methicillin-resistant isolates*

I.V. INFUSION

Adults. 667 mg infused over 2 hr at a concentration of 2.67 mg/ml every 6 hr on days 1 to 8 increased to every 8 hr beginning on day 9 up to day 42.

∗ *To treat acute bacterial skin and skin structure infections (ABSSSI) caused by* Klebsiella pneumoniae, S. aureus *(methicillin-susceptible and methicillin-resistant isolates) or* Streptococcus pyrogenes

I.V. INFUSION

Adults. 667 mg infused over 2 hr at a concentration of 2.67 mg/ml every 8 hr for 5 to 14 days.

∗ *To treat community-acquired bacterial pneumonia (CABP) caused by* Escherichia coli, Haemophilus influenzae, H.parainfluenzae, K. pneumoniae, S.aureus *(methicillin-susceptible isolates), or* Streptococcus pneumoniae

I.V. INFUSION

Adults. 667 mg infused over 2 hr at a concentration of 2.67 mg/ml every 8 hr for 5 to 14 days

Children ages 12 to less than 18. 13.3 mg/kg (up to 667 mg/dose) infused over 2 hr at a concentration of 2.67 mg/ml every 8 hr for 7 to 14 days.

Children ages 3 mo to less than 12 yr. 20 mg/kg (up to 667 mg dose) infused over 2 hr at a concentration of 5.33 mg/ml every 8 hr for 7 to 14 days.

±**DOSAGE ADJUSTMENT** For adult patients with a creatinine clearance greater than 150 ml/min, dosage interval increased to every 6 h for all indications. For adult patients with SAB and a creatine clearance of 30 ml/min to less than 50 ml/min, dosage interval increased to every 8 hr on days 1 to 8 and every 12 hr from day 9 up to 42 days. For adult patients with SAB and a creatinine clearance of 15 ml/min to less than 30 ml/min, dosage reduced to 333 mg given every 8 hr on days 1 to 8 and 333 mg given every 12 hr from day 9 up to day 42. For adult patients with SAB and a creatine clearance of less than 15 ml/min, including hemodialysis, dosage reduced to 333 mg given every 24 hr for duration of therapy. For adult patients with ABSSSI or CABP with a creatinine clearance of 30 ml/min to less than 50 ml/min dosage interval increased to every 12 hr. For adult patients with ABSSSI or CABP with a creatinine clearance of 15 ml/min to less than 30 ml/min, dosage reduced to 333 mg given every 12 hr. For adult patients with ABSSSI or CABP and a creatinine clearance less than 15 ml/min, including hemodialysis, dosage reduced to 333 mg given every 24 hr. For pediatric patients with CABP ages 12 yr to less than 18 yr and an eGFR of 30 ml/min to less than 50 ml/min, dosage reduced to 10 mg/kg (up to 667 mg) given every 12 hr. For pediatric patients with CABP ages 12 yr to less than 18 yr and an eGFR of 15 ml/min to less than 30 ml/min, dosage reduced to 10 mg/kg (up to 333 mg) given every 12 hr. For pediatric patients with CABP ages 6 yr to less than 12 yr and an eGFR of 30 ml/min to less than 50 ml/min, dosage reduced to 10 mg/kg (up to 667 mg) given every 12 hr. For pediatric patients with CABP ages 6 yr to less than 12 yr and an eGFR of 15 ml/min to less than 30 ml/min, dosage reduced to 10 mg/kg (up to 333 mg) given every 24 hr. For pediatric patients with CABP ages 2 yr to less than 6 yr and an eGFR of 30 ml/min to less than 50 ml/min, dosage reduced to 13.3 mg/kg (up to 667 mg) given every 12 hr. For pediatric patients with CABP ages 2 yr to less than 6 yr and an eGFR of 15 ml/min to less than 30 ml/min, dosage reduced to 13.3 mg/kg (up to 333 mg) given every 24 hr. Dosage adjustment is unknown for pediatric patients less than 2 yr of age with any degree of renal impairment.

Drug Administration

I.V.

- For adults and pediatric patients 12 yr and older, reconstitute drug powder with 10 ml of Sterile Water or 10 ml of 5% Dextrose Injection; for pediatric patients ages 3 mo to less than 12 yr, reconstitute drug powder in vial with ONLY 10 ml of 5% Dextrose Injection.
- Shake reconstituted vial vigorously until dissolution is complete, which may take up to 10 min. Solution should appear clear to slightly opalescent and yellowish in color after any foam has dissipated. The volume of the reconstituted solution is about 10.6 ml.
- Further dilute the reconstituted solution following manufacturer's instructions closely using 0.9% Sodium Chloride or 5% Dextrose Injection for adults and children 12 yr and older or ONLY 5% Dextrose Injection for children 3 mo to less than 12 yr. Once diluted, gently invert infusion bag 5 to 10 times to form a homogenous solution. Avoid vigorous agitation to prevent foaming.
- Be aware that the concentration and final volume of diluted drug for adults 18 yr and older without renal failure should be 2.67 mg/ml in a 250 ml infusion bag or with renal failure (creatinine clearance less than 30 ml/min) 2.67 mg/ml in a 125 ml infusion bag.
- Be aware that the concentration and final volume of diluted drug for children is calculated based on patient weight. For pediatric patients 12 yr to less than 18 yr with or without renal impairment, final concentration and volume to be administered should be 2.67 mg/ml in a maximum of 250 ml; for pediatric patients 3 mo to less than 12 yr without renal impairment or pediatric patients ages 2 yr to less than 12 yr with renal impairment, final concentration and volume to be administered should be 5.33 mg/ml in a maximum of 125 ml.
- Store reconstituted solution that cannot be used immediately in the refrigerator for up to 24 hr or at room temperature up to 1 hr.
- Store diluted solution in refrigerator or at room temperature following manufacturer's instructions for length of storage time. If diluted solution is stored in the refrigerator, allow it to warm to room temperature before administration. Do not expose infusion solution to direct sunlight but know that the infusion solution does not need to be protected from light during administration. Never freeze drug solution.
- *Incompatibilities:* Calcium-containing solutions, I.V. solutions other than 0.9% Sodium Chloride or 5% Dextrose Injection, other drug products

Route	Onset	Peak	Duration
I.V.	Unknown	2-4 hr	Unknown

Half-life: 3.3 hr

Mechanism of Action

Interferes with bacterial cell wall synthesis by inhibiting the cross-linking of peptidoglycan strands. Peptidoglycan makes the cell membrane rigid and protective. Without it, bacterial cells rupture and die.

Contraindications

Hypersensitivity to ceftobiprole, other cephalosporins, or their components

Interactions

DRUGS

organic anion transporting polypeptide 1B1/1B3 (OATP1B1/OATP1B3) substrates: Possibly increased plasma concentrations of these substrates

Adverse Reactions

CNS: Anxiety, chills, dizziness, fatigue, fever, headache, insomnia, irritability, myoclonus, **seizures**
CV: Elevated LDH and triglycerides, hypertension, phlebitis, **thrombosis**
EENT: Impaired taste
GI: Abdominal pain, cholestasis, **Clostridioides difficile–associated diarrhea** diarrhea, dyspepsia, dysphagia, elevated bilirubin and liver enzymes, hepatic dysfunction, nausea, vomiting

GU: Benign idiopathic urinary frequency (pollakiuria), elevated blood creatinine, renal dysfunction, **toxic nephropathy**
HEME: **Agranulocytosis**, anemia, **aplastic anemia, hemorrhage, leukopenia, prolonged prothrombin time, thrombocytopenia, thrombocytosis**
RESP: **Bronchospasms**, dyspnea, pleuritis, pneumonia (aggravated), **wheezing**
SKIN: Mucocutaneous fungal infections, pruritus, rash, urticaria
Other: **Anaphylaxis including shock**, angioedema, drug fever, **hypokalemia**, hyponatremia, injection site reaction (pain), serum sickness-like reaction,

Childbearing Considerations

PREGNANCY

- It is not known if drug can cause fetal harm.
- Use with caution only if benefit to mother outweighs potential risk to fetus.

LACTATION

- It is not known if drug is present in breast milk.
- Mothers should check with prescriber before breastfeeding.

Nursing Considerations

! **WARNING** Be aware that ceftobiprole should not be used to treat ventilator-associated bacterial pneumonia because of a possible increase in mortality.

- Question patient about previous hypersensitivity reactions to other beta-lactam antibacterial, other cephalosporins, and penicillins before ceftobiprole therapy begins because cross-sensitivity may occur.

! **WARNING** Monitor patient for hypersensitivity reactions that could become life-threatening, such as anaphylaxis and angioedema. If present, notify prescriber, withhold drug, and provide supportive care, as needed and ordered.

! **WARNING** Monitor patient closely for diarrhea, which may indicate *Clostridioides difficile–associated diarrhea* that may range from being mild to life-threatening. If diarrhea occurs, notify prescriber and expecting testing for *C. difficile*. If confirmed, expect to withhold drug, and treat with an antibiotic effective against *C. difficile* along with electrolytes, fluids, and protein, as needed and ordered.

! **WARNING** Institute seizure precautions as needed. If patient develops adverse CNS reactions, including seizures, expect patient to undergo a neurological evaluation to see if ceftobiprole therapy needs to be discontinued.

- Be aware that ceftobiprole may cause false-positive results in dipstick tests for glucose, ketones, occult blood or urine protein. While patient is receiving ceftobiprole therapy, plan to use alternate methods for testing to confirm positive results. Also be aware that the drug may interfere with serological testing, such as the Coombs test.

PATIENT TEACHING

- Inform patient that ceftobiprole is administered intravenously.

! **WARNING** Instruct patient to notify the staff (if in hospital) or prescriber (if at home) immediately of any allergic reactions such as the development of difficulty breathing, facial swelling, hives, itching, or a rash. If reaction is severe, and patient is at home, stress importance of stopping drug and seeking immediate medical attention.

! **WARNING** Alert patient that ceftobiprole may cause serious CNS reactions, including seizures. Review seizure precautions with patient. Stress importance of alerting staff or prescriber, if a seizure occurs or any other serious CNS reactions.

! **WARNING** Inform patient that diarrhea is a common occurrence with antibiotic therapy and may occur more than 2 months after drug was discontinued. However, urge patient to report watery, bloody stools to staff or prescriber immediately.

- Tell patient that dipstick tests used to detect glucose, ketones, or occult blood may cause a false-positive result while taking ceftobiprole. Advise patient to alert prescriber of ceftobiprole therapy if a positive result occurs.

ceftriaxone sodium

Class and Category

Pharmacologic class: Third-generation cephalosporin
Therapeutic class: Antibiotic

Indications and Dosages

* *To treat infections such as bacterial septicemia caused by* Escherichia coli, Haemophilus influenzae, Klebsiella pneumoniae, Staphylococcus aureus, *or* Streptococcus pneumoniae; *bone and joint infections caused by* Enterobacter *species,* E. coli, K. pneumoniae, Proteus mirabilis, S. aureus, *or* S. pneumoniae; *intra-abdominal infections caused by* Bacteroides fragilis, Clostridium *species,* E. coli, K. pneumoniae, *or* Peptostreptococcus *species; lower respiratory tract infections caused by* Enterobacter aerogenes, E. coli, H.influenzae, H. parainfluenzae, K. pneumoniae, P. mirabilis, Serratia marcescens, S. aureus, *or* S. pneumoniae; *pelvic inflammatory disease caused by* Neisseria gonorrhoeae; *skin and soft-tissue infections caused by* Acinetobacter calcoaceticus, B. fragilis, E. cloacae, E. coli, K. pneumoniae, K. oxytoca, Morganella morganii, Peptostreptococcus *species,* P. mirabilis, Pseudomonas aeruginosa, Serratia marcescens, S. aureus, S. epidermidis, S. pyogenes, *or viridans group* streptococci; *and urinary tract infections caused by* E. coli, K. pneumoniae, M. morganii, P. mirabilis, *or* P. vulgaris

I.V. INFUSION

Adults. *For moderate to severe infections:* 1 to 2 g daily or in equally divided doses twice daily for 4 to 14 days, although complicated infections may require higher doses or longer therapy. Infections caused by *Streptococcus pyogenes* should be continued for at least 10 days. *Maximum:* 4 g daily.
Children. *For serious infections:* 50 to 75 mg/kg in divided doses every 12 hr for 4 to 14 days. Infections caused by *Streptococcus pyogenes* should be continued for at least 10 days. *Maximum:* 2 g daily.

* *To treat meningitis caused by* H. influenzae, Neisseria meningitidis, *or* S. pneumoniae

I.V. INFUSION

Adults. 1 to 2 g daily or in equally divided doses twice daily for 4 to 14 days, although a complicated infection may require higher doses and longer therapy. *Maximum:* 4 g daily.
Children. *Initial:* 100 mg/kg (not to exceed 4 g) once daily followed by 100 mg/kg once daily or in equally divided doses every 12 hr for 7 to 14 days. *Maximum:* 4 g daily.

± **DOSAGE ADJUSTMENT** For patients with both severe hepatic and renal impairment, dosage limited to 2 g daily.

* *To treat acute bacterial otitis media caused by* M. catarrhalis *(including beta-lactamase producing strains),* H. influenzae *(including beta-lactamase producing strains), or* S. pneumoniae

I.M. INJECTION

Children. 50 mg/kg as a single dose. *Maximum:* 1 g.

* *To treat uncomplicated gonorrhea (cervical/urethral, pharyngeal, or rectal) caused by* Neisseria gonorrhoeae

I.M. INJECTION

Adults. 250 mg as a single dose.

* *To provide surgical prophylaxis before biliary tract surgery, coronary artery bypass surgery or hysterectomy*

I.V. INFUSION

Adults. 1 g 30 min to 2 hr before surgery.

Drug Administration

I.V.

ADD-Vantage vials

- Be aware that the ADD-Vantage vial container is used to deliver a 1 or 2 g dose. To avoid an accidental overdose, do not use this product for children who require less than the full adult dose.
- Open diluent container by peeling overwrap at corner and remove solution container. Some opacity of the plastic may be present, but this is normal. The opacity will diminish gradually.
- Assemble vial and flexible diluent container by removing the protective covers from the top of the vial and the vial port on the diluent container. To remove the breakaway vial cap swing the pull ring over the top of the vial and pull down far enough to start the opening; then pull straight up to remove the cap. To remove the vial port cover, grasp the tab on the pull ring, pulling

up to break the 3 tie strings, then pull back to remove the cover. Screw the vial into the vial port until it will go no further. The vial must be screwed in tightly to assure a seal, which occurs about a 1/2 turn (180 degrees) after the first audible click. Label appropriately.

- Squeeze the bottom of the diluent container gently to inflate the portion of the container surrounding the end of the drug vial. With the other hand, push the drug vial down into the container, telescoping the walls of the container. Grasp the inner cap of the vial through the walls of the container. Pull the inner cap from the drug vial, allowing the drug and diluent to mix. Mix thoroughly.
- Prepare to administer by checking for leaks by squeezing container firmly. If present, discard and obtain a new one. Attach administration set. Lift the free end of the hanger loop on the bottom of the vial, breaking the 2 tie strings. Bend loop outward to lock it in the upright position, then suspend from hanger. Attach to I.V.
- Do not use plastic containers in series connections.
- Administer over 30 min.

Single-use regular vials

- If using, drug vials, reconstitute with an appropriate diluent, such as Sterile Water for Injection, 0.9% Sodium Chloride for Injection, or 5% Dextrose Injection (see manufacturer's guidelines for other solutions that can be used) as follows: for 250-mg vial, add 2.4 ml; for 500-mg vial, add 4.8 ml; for 1-g vial, add 9.6 ml; and for 2-g vial, add 19.2 ml to yield 100 mg/ml.
- After reconstitution, further dilute to 50 to 100 ml with diluent indicated above and infuse over 30 min (60 min for neonates).
- Do not use plastic containers in series connections.
- If administering with a pump, take care to discontinue pumping action before the container runs dry, or an air embolism may result.
- Store drug powder at room temperature and protect from light. After reconstitution, protection from light is not necessary. Check manufacturer's guidelines for length of storage based upon concentration and diluent used.

Duplex

- Be aware the duplex container is used to deliver a 1- or 2-g dose. To avoid an accidental overdose, this product should not be used for children who require less than the full adult dose.
- Keep container in folded position until activation is intended. Remove from refrigerator and allow to come to room temperature.
- Unlatch side tab and unfold container. Visually inspect diluent chamber. Use only if container and seals are intact.
- Inspect drug powder by peeling foil strip from drug chamber. Protect from light after removal of foil strip. If foil strip is removed but administration is delayed, refold container and latch side tab. Product then must be used within 7 days.
- To reconstitute, unfold container and point the set port in a downward direction. Starting at the hanger tab end, fold the container just below the diluent meniscus, trapping all air above the fold. To activate, squeeze the folded diluent chamber until the seal between the diluent and powder opens, releasing diluent into the drug powder chamber. Agitate the liquid-powder mixture until completely dissolved. Once dissolved, drug must be used within 24 hr if stored at room temperature or 7 days if refrigerated.
- To administer, point the set port in a downward direction. Starting at the hanger tab end, fold the container just below the solution meniscus, trapping all air above the fold. Squeeze the folded container until the seal between the reconstituted drug and set port opens, releasing the solution to set port. Squeeze container firmly to check for minute leaks. Then, peel foil cover from the set port and attach administration set.
- Do not use in series connections.
- Do not introduce additives to the container.
- Administer as an infusion over about 30 min.
- *Incompatibilities for all I.V. forms:* Aminoglycosides; amsacrine; calcium solutions such as Ringer's solution or Hartmann's solution, including parenteral nutrition; fluconazole; vancomycin. For patients other than neonates, ceftriaxone and calcium-containing solutions may

be given sequentially if infusion lines are thoroughly flushed with a compatible fluid between infusions.

I.M.

- Reconstitute with an appropriate diluent, such as Sterile Water for Injection or 0.9% Sodium Chloride for Injection, by adding 1.8 ml to a 500-mg vial to make a concentration of 250 mg/ml and 1 ml to a 500-mg vial to make a 350-mg/ml concentration. Using a 1-g vial, add 3.6 ml to make a 250-mg/ml concentration and 2.1 ml to make a 350-mg/ml concentration.
- Shake well.
- Inject deep into large muscle mass, such as the gluteus maximus.
- Know that 1% Lidocaine Solution (without epinephrine) can be used instead of Sterile Water for Injection as a diluent to lessen the pain of an I.M. injection (follow manufacturer's instructions when doing so). However, it is not without risk.
- Store drug powder at room temperature and protect from light. After reconstitution, protection from light is not necessary. Check manufacturer's guidelines for length of storage based upon concentration and diluent used.

Route	Onset	Peak	Duration
I.V.	Immediate	30 min	Unknown
I.M.	Unknown	1.5–4 hr	Unknown

Half-life: 5–9 hr

Mechanism of Action

Interferes with bacterial cell wall synthesis by inhibiting cross-linking of peptidoglycan strands. Peptidoglycan makes the cell membrane rigid and protective. Without it, bacterial cells rupture and die.

Contraindications

Hyperbilirubinemic or premature neonates (up to a postmenstrual age of 41 wk); hypersensitivity to ceftriaxone, other beta-lactam antibacterials or cephalosporins, penicillins, or their components; intravenous administration of ceftriaxone solutions containing lidocaine; neonates who are 28 days old or less if they're expected to need calcium-containing solutions, including parenteral nutrition.

Interactions

DRUGS

aminoglycosides, loop diuretics: Increased risk of nephrotoxicity

Adverse Reactions

CNS: Chills, **encephalopathy**, fever, headache, hypertonia, myoclonus, neurotoxicity, **nonconvulsive status epilepticus**, reversible hyperactivity, **seizures**
CV: Edema
EENT: Glossitis, hearing loss, stomatitis
GI: Abdominal cramps, cholestasis, ***Clostridioides difficile*-associated diarrhea**, diarrhea, elevated liver enzymes, gallbladder dysfunction, **hepatic failure**, **hepatitis**, hepatomegaly, nausea, oral candidiasis, **pancreatitis**, pseudolithiasis, **pseudomembranous colitis**, vomiting
GU: **Acute renal failure**, elevated BUN level, **nephrotoxicity**, oliguria, vaginal candidiasis, ureteric obstruction, urolithiasis
HEME: **Agranulocytosis**, **aplastic anemia**, eosinophilia, **hemolytic anemia**, **hemorrhage**, **hypoprothrombinemia**, **leukopenia**, **neutropenia**, **thrombocytopenia**
MS: Arthralgia
RESP: **Allergic pneumonitis**, dyspnea
SKIN: Allergic dermatitis, ecchymosis, erythema, **erythema multiforme**, exanthema, pruritus, rash, **Stevens-Johnson syndrome**, **toxic epidermal necrolysis**, urticaria
Other: **Anaphylaxis**; drug fever; injection-site pain, redness, and swelling; serum sickness; superinfection

Childbearing Considerations

PREGNANCY

- It is not known if drug can cause fetal harm.
- Use with caution only if benefit to mother outweighs potential risk to fetus.

LACTATION

- Drug is present in breast milk.
- Mothers should check with prescriber before breastfeeding.

Nursing Considerations

! **WARNING** Be aware that calcium-containing products must not be given I.V. within 48 hours of ceftriaxone, including solutions given through a different I.V. line and

C

at a different site, in neonates because a ceftriaxone-calcium salt may precipitate in the lungs and kidneys and could be fatal.

- Obtain culture and sensitivity results, if possible and as ordered, before giving drug.

! WARNING Use cautiously in patients with renal insufficiency because high and prolonged serum ceftazidime concentrations can occur from usual dosages. This can lead to asterixis, coma, encephalopathy, myoclonia, neuromuscular excitability, nonconvulsive status epilepticus, and seizures. Ensure that patients with significant renal insufficiency are receiving reduced dosage based on their creatinine clearance. Also monitor BUN and serum creatinine for early signs of nephrotoxicity. Also, monitor fluid intake and output; decreasing urine output may indicate nephrotoxicity.

! WARNING Be aware that local anesthetics such as lidocaine used to lessen the pain of an I.M. injection may cause methemoglobinemia as late as several hours after the injection. Monitor patient closely.

! WARNING Monitor patient for hypersensitivity reaction that could become life-threatening, such as anaphylaxis, especially patients allergic to penicillin because cross-sensitivity can occur. Be aware that an allergic reaction may occur even a few days after therapy starts. If present, notify prescriber, withhold drug, and provide supportive care, as needed and ordered.

! WARNING Monitor patient closely for diarrhea, which may indicate pseudomembranous colitis caused by *Clostridioides difficile*–associated diarrhea. It may be mild or become life-threatening. If diarrhea occurs, notify prescriber and expect testing to be done to confirm presence of *C. difficile*. If confirmed, expect to withhold drug, and treat with an antibiotic effective against *C. difficile* along with electrolytes, fluids, and protein, as needed and ordered.

! WARNING Monitor patient's bleeding time, complete CBC, and prothrombin time, as ordered.Assess patient for adverse blood reactions that could become life-threatening. Expect drug to be discontinued and appropriate therapy instituted if patient develops a serious adverse hematologic reaction. If drug-induced hemolytic anemia is suspected, expect to discontinue drug and provide supportive care, as indicated.

- Assess ALT, AST, bilirubin, CBC, hematocrit, LD, and serum alkaline phosphatase levels during long-term therapy. If abnormalities occur, notify prescriber. Drug may have to be discontinued.
- Assess for signs of superinfection, such as cough or sputum changes, diarrhea, drainage, fever, malaise, or perineal itching.
- Monitor patient for evidence of gallbladder disease (abdominal pain, nausea, vomiting) because drug may cause ceftriaxone-calcium salt to deposit in the gallbladder, which may mimic gallstones. Expect drug to be discontinued if gallbladder disorders arise.

PATIENT TEACHING

- Inform patient drug may be given either as an I.M. injection or intravenously.
- Stress importance of completing course of therapy.
- Tell patient that if he received drug as an I.M. injection that used lidocaine as the diluent, he should watch for signs and symptoms such as fatigue; headache; light-headedness; skin color change of blue, gray, or pale; rapid heart rate; or shortness of breath. If present, patient should seek immediate medical attention.

! WARNING Alert patient that allergic reactions can occur, especially after a few days of drug therapy. Instruct patient to notify prescriber, if present, and seek immediate medical attention if severe.

! WARNING Urge patient to report watery, bloody stools to prescriber immediately, even up to 2 months after drug therapy has ended.

! WARNING Instruct patient to monitor urine output. Review signs and symptoms of types of neurologic adverse reactions that may occur with ceftazidime therapy. Review seizure precautions. If urine output drops or neurologic adverse reactions occur, urge patient to notify prescriber.

! **WARNING** Inform patient that drug may cause adverse blood reactions. Encourage compliance with laboratory tests and alert prescriber if bleeding or ecchymosis occurs.

- Teach patient to recognize and report signs of superinfection, such as diarrhea, furry tongue, and perineal itching. If present, advise patient to notify prescriber.
- Inform patient that buttermilk and yogurt can help maintain intestinal flora and decrease diarrhea.

cefuroxime axetil

cefuroxime sodium

Class and Category

Pharmacologic class: Second-generation cephalosporin
Therapeutic class: Antibiotic

Indications and Dosages

* *To treat pharyngitis and tonsillitis caused by* Streptococcus pyogenes

TABLETS

Adults and adolescents. 250 mg every 12 hr for 10 days.

ORAL SUSPENSION

Children ages 3 mo to 12 yr. 10 mg/kg twice daily for 10 days. *Maximum:* 500 mg daily.

* *To treat acute otitis media caused by* Haemophilus influenzae, Moraxella catarrhalis, Streptococcus pneumoniae, *or* S. pyogenes

TABLETS

Children under age 13 who can swallow tablets. 250 mg every 12 hr for 10 days.

ORAL SUSPENSION

Children ages 3 mo to 12 yr. 15 mg/kg twice daily for 10 days. *Maximum:* 1 g daily.

* *To treat acute bacterial maxillary sinusitis caused by* H. influenzae *or* S. pneumoniae

TABLETS

Adults, adolescents, and children under age 13 who can swallow tablets. 250 mg every 12 hr for 10 days.

ORAL SUSPENSION

Children ages 3 mo to 12 yr. 15 mg/kg twice daily for 10 days. *Maximum:* 1 g daily.

* *To treat acute bacterial exacerbations of chronic bronchitis (mild to moderate) caused by* H. influenzae, Haemophilus parainfluenzae, *or* S. pneumoniae

TABLETS

Adults and adolescents. 250 or 500 mg every 12 hr for 10 days.

* *To treat uncomplicated skin and skin structure infections caused by* Enterobacter *species,* E. coli, Klebsiella *species,* S. aureus, *or* S. pyogenes

TABLETS

Adults and adolescents. 250 or 500 mg every 12 hr for 10 days.

* *To treat impetigo caused by* S. aureus *(including beta-lactamase-producing strains) or* S. pyogenes

ORAL SUSPENSION

Children ages 3 mo to 12 yr. 15 mg/kg twice daily for 10 days. *Maximum:* 1 g daily.

* *To treat lower respiratory tract infections, including pneumonia, caused by* E. coli, H. influenzae, Klebsiella *species,* S. aureus, S. pneumoniae, *or* S. pyogenes

I.V. INFUSION, I.M. OR I.V. INJECTION

Adults. *Uncomplicated infection:* 750 mg every 8 hr for 5 to 10 days. *Complicated or severe infections:* 1.5 g every 8 hr.
Children over age 3 mo. 50 to 100 mg/kg/day in equally divided doses every 6 to 8 hr. *Maximum:* Not to exceed adult dosage.

* *To treat early Lyme disease caused by* Borrelia burgdorferi

TABLETS

Adults and adolescents. 500 mg every 12 hr for 20 days.

* *To treat uncomplicated UTI caused by* E. coli *or* Klebsiella pneumoniae

TABLETS

Adults and adolescents. 250 mg every 12 hr for 7 to 10 days.

I.V. INFUSION, I.M. OR I.V. INJECTION

Adults. 750 mg every 8 hr for 5 to 10 days.
Children over age 3 mo. 50 to 100 mg/kg/day in equally divided doses every 6 to 8 hr. *Maximum:* Not to exceed adult dosage.

* *To treat uncomplicated gonorrhea caused by* Neisseria gonorrhoeae

TABLETS

Adults. 1 g as a single dose.

I.M. INJECTION

Adults. 1.5 g as a single dose and given with oral probenecid 1 g.

∗ *To treat bone and joint infections caused by* S. aureus

I.V. INFUSION, I.M. OR I.V. INJECTION

Adults. 1.5 g every 8 hr.
Children over age 3 mo. 50 mg/kg every 8 hr. *Maximum:* Adult dose.

∗ *To treat bacterial meningitis caused by* H. influenzae, Neisseria meningitidis, S. aureus, *or* S. pneumoniae

I.V. INFUSION, I.V. INJECTION

Adults. 1.5 mg every 6 hr. every 8 hr. *Maximum:* 3 g every 8 hr.
Children over age 3 mo. 200 to 240 mg/kg/daily in divided doses every 6 to 8 hr.

∗ *To treat moderate infections other than those listed above*

I.V. INFUSION, I.M. OR I.V. INJECTION

Adults. 750 mg to 1.5 g every 8 hr for 5 to 10 days.

I.V. INFUSION, I.V. INJECTION

Children over age 3 mo. 50 mg/kg daily in equally divided doses every 6 to 8 hr.

∗ *To treat complicated or life-threatening infections other than those listed above*

I.V. INFUSION, I.V. INJECTION

Adults. 1.5 g every 6 hr.
Children over age 3 mo. 100 mg/kg daily in equally divided doses every 6 to 8 hr.

∗ *To provide perioperative prophylaxis*

I.M. OR I.V. INJECTION

Adults. 1.5 g I.V. 30 to 60 min before surgery (at induction of anesthesia for open-heart surgery), and then 0.75 g every 8 hr for prolonged procedures (1.5 g every 12 hr for total of 6 g with open-heart surgery).

I.V. INJECTION

Children over age 3 mo. 50 mg/kg as a single dose. An additional 50 mg/kg dose given if surgery lasts longer than 4 hr. *Maximum:* 1.5 g/dose.

± **DOSAGE ADJUSTMENT** For parenteral dosage for adults with a creatinine clearance of 10 to 20 ml/min, dosage reduced to 0.75 g and given every 12 hours. For parenteral dosage for adults with a creatinine clearance of less than 10/ml/min, dosage reduced to 0.75 g and given every 24 hours. For parenteral dosage for children with renal impairment, dosage adjustment similar to the recommendations for adults. For adults receiving oral drug with a creatinine clearance of 10 to 30 ml/min, dosage interval increased to every 24 hr. For adults receiving oral drug with a creatinine clearance of less than 10 ml/min (without hemodialysis), dosage interval increased to every 48 hr. For adults receiving oral drug on hemodialysis, standard dose given at the end of each dialysis. No recommendations given by manufacturer for children with renal impairment receiving oral therapy.

Drug Administration

P.O.

- Oral suspension and tablets are not interchangeable and cannot be substituted on a milligram-per-milligram basis for one another.
- Oral suspension contains phenylalanine as a component of aspartame and should not be given to patients with PKU.
- To prepare oral suspension, shake the bottle to loosen the powder. Add amount of water required for reconstitution according to manufacturer guidelines. After reconstitution wait 1 hr before administering oral suspension to patient.
- Shake oral suspension well before each use. Use a calibrated device to measure dosage. Administer with food. Replace cap securely after each opening. Store oral suspension in refrigerator. Discard reconstituted oral suspension after 10 days.
- Tablet should be swallowed whole and not chewed, crushed, or split.
- Administer tablets with or without food. Make sure lid on container is put on tightly after each opening.

I.V.

Vials

- Reconstitute each 750-mg vial with 8.3 ml of Sterile Water for Injection and each 1.5-g vial with 16 ml of Sterile Water for Injection.
- For I.V. injection, administer slowly into a vein over 3 to 5 min through the tubing system of a free-flowing intravenous solution.

- For intermittent I.V. infusion with a Y-type administration set, temporarily discontinue administration of any other solution at the same site. Dilute reconstituted drug with 100 ml of 0.9% Sodium Chloride Injection, 5% Dextrose Injection, or other compatible solutions (see manufacturer guidelines) and infuse over 15 to 60 min.
- Follow manufacturer's instructions for use of TwistVials when used to prepare an intermittent I.V. infusion.
- For continuous I.V. infusion, add reconstituted drug to 0.9% Sodium Chloride Injection or 5% Dextrose Injection (see manufacturer's guidelines for other solutions that may be used) to provide a concentration between 1 and 30 mg/ml.
- Store reconstituted solution for 24 hr at room temperature or 48 hr refrigerated; store reconstituted solutions that have been further diluted for 24 hr at room temperature or 7 days refrigerated.

Galaxy Plastic Containers

- Follow manufacturer's instructions on use of Galaxy plastic containers used for intermittent or continuous infusions.

Duplex

- Keep container in folded position until activation is intended. Remove from refrigerator and allow to come to room temperature.
- Unlatch side tab and unfold container. Visually inspect diluent chamber. Use only if container and seals are intact.
- Inspect drug powder by peeling foil strip from drug chamber. Protect from light after removal of foil strip. If foil strip is removed but administration is delayed, refold container and latch side tab. Product then must be used within 7 days.
- To reconstitute, unfold container and point the set port in a downward direction. Starting at the hanger tab end, fold the container just below the diluent meniscus, trapping all air above the fold. To activate, squeeze the folded diluent chamber until the seal between the diluent and powder opens, releasing diluent into the drug powder chamber. Agitate the liquid-powder mixture until completely dissolved. Once dissolved, drug must be used within 24 hr if stored at room temperature or 7 days if refrigerated.
- To administer, point the set port in a downward direction. Starting at the hanger tab end, fold the container just below the solution meniscus, trapping all air above the fold. Squeeze the folded container until the seal between the reconstituted drug and set port opens, releasing the solution to set port. Squeeze container firmly to check for minute leaks. Then, peel foil cover from the set port and attach administration set.
- Do not use in series connections.
- Do not introduce additives to the container.
- For intermittent infusion, administer over 15 to 60 min.
- *Incompatibilities:* Aminoglycosides, sodium bicarbonate

I.M.

- Reconstitute 750-mg vial with 3 ml of Sterile Water for Injection and shake gently.
- Inject deeply into a large muscle mass such as the gluteus maximus or the lateral side of the thigh.
- Store reconstituted solution for 24 hr at room temperature or 48 hr refrigerated.

Route	Onset	Peak	Duration
P.O.	Unknown	2–3 hr	Unknown
I.V.	Immediate	2–3 min	Unknown
I.M.	Unknown	15–30 min	Unknown

Half-life: 1–2 hr

Mechanism of Action

Interferes with bacterial cell wall synthesis by inhibiting the final step in the cross-linking of peptidoglycan strands. Peptidoglycan makes the cell membrane rigid and protective. Without it, bacterial cells rupture and die.

Contraindications

Hypersensitivity to cefuroxime, other cephalosporins or their components

Interactions

DRUGS

aminoglycosides, loop diuretics: Increased risk of nephrotoxicity
antacids, histamine-2 antagonists, proton pump inhibitors: Possibly lower bioavailability of oral cefuroxime
oral combined estrogen–progesterone contraceptives: Decreased effectiveness of oral contraceptive

C

Adverse Reactions

CNS: Chills, fever, headache, **seizures**
CV: **Acute myocardial ischemia with or without MI**, edema
EENT: Hearing loss, oral candidiasis
GI: Abdominal cramps, ***Clostridioides difficile*-associated diarrhea**, diarrhea, elevated liver enzymes, **hepatic failure**, hepatomegaly, nausea, **pseudomembranous colitis**, vomiting
GU: Elevated BUN level, **nephrotoxicity**, **renal failure**, vaginal candidiasis
HEME: Eosinophilia, **hemolytic anemia**, **hypoprothrombinemia**, **neutropenia**, **thrombocytopenia**, **unusual bleeding**
MS: Arthralgia
RESP: Dyspnea
SKIN: Cutaneous vasculitis, ecchymosis, erythema, **erythema multiforme**, pruritus, rash, **Stevens-Johnson syndrome**
Other: **Anaphylaxis**; **angioedema**; injection-site edema, pain, and redness; serum sickness–like reaction; superinfection

Childbearing Considerations

PREGNANCY

- It is not known if drug can cause fetal harm.
- Use with caution only if benefit to mother outweighs potential risk to fetus.

LACTATION

- Drug is present in breast milk.
- Mothers should check with prescriber before breastfeeding.

Nursing Considerations

- Obtain culture and sensitivity results, if possible and as ordered, before giving drug.
- Monitor I.V. site for extravasation and phlebitis.

! **WARNING** Monitor patient for a hypersensitivity reaction that could become life-threatening, such as anaphylaxis, especially patients allergic to penicillin because cross-sensitivity can occur. Be aware that an allergic reaction may occur even a few days after therapy starts. Know that acute myocardial ischemia with or without MI can be part of the allergic reaction. If hyersenstivity or chest pain is present, notify prescriber, withhold drug, and provide supportive care, as needed and ordered.

! **WARNING** Monitor patient closely for diarrhea, which may indicate pseudomembranous colitis caused by *Clostridioides difficile*-associated diarrhea. It may be mild or become life-threatening. If diarrhea occurs, notify prescriber and expect testing to be done to confirm presence of *C. difficile*. If confirmed, expect to withhold drug, and treat with an antibiotic effective against *C. difficile* along with electrolytes, fluids, and protein, as needed and ordered.

! **WARNING** Monitor patient's bleeding time, complete CBC, and prothrombin time, as ordered. Assess patient for adverse blood reactions that could become life-threatening. Expect drug to be discontinued and appropriate therapy instituted if patient develops a serious adverse hematologic reaction. If drug-induced hemolytic anemia is suspected, expect to discontinue drug and provide supportive care, as indicated.

! **WARNING** Monitor patient for seizures. Instittue seizure precautions. Be prepared to provide immediate treatment, as ordered, if a seizure occurs, expect drug to be discontinued and provide supportive care, as needed and ordered.

- Monitor BUN and serum creatinine levels to detect early signs of nephrotoxicity. Also, monitor fluid intake and output; decreasing urine output may indicate nephrotoxicity. Also, be alert for precipitates in the patient's urine, especially children. If any sign of renal dysfunction occurs, notify prescriber, expect drug to be discontinued, and provide supportive care, as prescribed.
- Assess for signs of superinfection, such as cough or sputum changes, diarrhea, drainage, fever, malaise, or perineal itching.

PATIENT TEACHING

- Inform patient that drug will either be administered as an I.M. injection or given intravensously.
- Stress importance of completing course of therapy.

! **WARNING** Alert patient that allergic reactions can occur, especially after a few days of drug therapy. If present, instruct patient to notify prescriber and seek immediate medical attention if severe.

! **WARNING** Urge patient to report watery, bloody stools to prescriber immediately, even up to 2 months after drug therapy has ended.

! **WARNING** Review signs and symptoms of types of neurologic adverse reactions that may occur with ceftazidime therapy. Review seizure precautions. If present, urge patient to notify prescriber.

! **WARNING** Inform patient that drug may cause adverse blood reactions. Encourage compliance with laboratory tests and alert prescriber if bleeding or ecchymosis occurs.

- Teach patient to recognize and report signs of superinfection, such as diarrhea, furry tongue, and perineal itching. If present, advise patient to notify prescriber.
- Inform patient that buttermilk and yogurt help maintain intestinal flora and can decrease diarrhea during therapy.

celecoxib

Celebrex, Elyxyb

Class and Category

Pharmacologic class: NSAID
Therapeutic class: Analgesic, anti-inflammatory, antirheumatic

Indications and Dosages

∗ *To relieve signs and symptoms of osteoarthritis*

CAPSULES

Adults. 200 mg daily or 100 mg twice daily.

∗ *To relieve signs and symptoms of rheumatoid arthritis*

CAPSULES

Adults. 100 to 200 mg twice daily.

∗ *To relieve signs and symptoms of juvenile rheumatoid arthritis*

CAPSULES

Children ages 2 and older weighing more than 25 kg (55 lb). 100 mg twice daily. **Children ages 2 and older weighing 10 to 25 kg (22 to 55 lb).** 50 mg twice daily.

∗ *To treat signs and symptoms of ankylosing spondylitis*

CAPSULES

Adults. 200 mg daily or 100 mg twice daily. Dosage increased to 400 mg daily or 200 mg twice daily after 6 wk, as needed.

∗ *To manage acute pain, to treat primary dysmenorrhea*

CAPSULES

Adults. 400 mg, followed by 200 mg, as needed, on day 1. On subsequent days, 200 mg twice daily, as needed.

∗ *To treat acute migraine*

ORAL SOLUTION (ELYXYB)

Adults. 120 mg as a single dose. *Maximum:* 120 mg in a 24-hr period.

± **DOSAGE ADJUSTMENT** For patients with moderate hepatic impairment, daily dosage reduced by 50%. For adult patients who are poor CYP2C9 metabolizers, starting dosage half the lowest recommended dose and the maximum dose for the treatment of migraine headaches should not exceed 60 mg in a 24-hour period. For children who are poor CYP2C9 metabolizers, alternative treatment recommended.

Drug Administration

P.O.

- Capsule may be opened and sprinkled onto a level teaspoon of cool or room-temperature applesauce and given with water, if capsule cannot be swallowed whole. Mixture should not be chewed.
- Drug-and-applesauce mixture may be stored up to 6 hr in refrigerator.
- Use a calibrated device to measure dose of oral solution. The concentration is 120 mg/4.8 ml. Store at room temperature.

Route	Onset	Peak	Duration
P.O.	Unknown	3 hr	Unknown

Half-life: 11 hr

Mechanism of Action

Inhibits the enzymatic activity of cyclooxygenase-2 (COX-2), the enzyme needed to convert arachidonic acid to prostaglandin. It does this selectively. Prostaglandins are responsible for mediating the inflammatory response and causing local vasodilation, swelling, and pain. Prostaglandins also play a role in peripheral pain transmission to the spinal cord. By inhibiting COX-2 activity and prostaglandin production, this reduces inflammatory symptoms and relieves pain.

Contraindications

Allergic reaction (such as anaphylaxis or angioedema) to aspirin, other NSAIDs, or sulfonamide derivatives or history of aspirin-induced nasal polyps with bronchospasm; hypersensitivity to celecoxib or its components; treatment of pain after coronary artery bypass graft surgery

Interactions

DRUGS

ACE inhibitors, angiotensin II receptor antagonists, beta-blockers: Decreased antihypertensive effect of these drugs, increased risk of renal failure in patients who are elderly, have existing renal dysfunction, or are volume-depleted
anticoagulants, such as warfarin, antiplatelet drugs such as aspirin and other salicylates, corticosteroids, selective serotonin reuptake inhibitors: Increased risk of GI ulceration and other GI complications, increased risk of bleeding
cyclosporine: Increased risk of cyclosporine-induced nephrotoxicity
CYP2C9 inducers, such as rifampin: Possibly decreased effectiveness of celecoxib
CYP2C9 inhibitors such as fluconazole: Possibly increased risk of celecoxib toxicity
CYP2D6 substrates: Possibly enhance the exposure and toxicity of these drugs
digoxin: Increased risk of digitalis toxicity
furosemide, thiazide diuretics: Reduced diuretic effects of these drugs, increased risk of renal failure
lithium: Possibly elevated blood lithium level
methotrexate: Increased risk of methotrexate toxicity (neutropenia, renal dysfunction, thrombocytopenia)
pemetrexed: Increased risk of myelosuppression, GI, and renal toxicity

ACTIVITIES

alcohol, smoking: Increased risk of adverse GI reactions

Adverse Reactions

CNS: **Aseptic meningitis**, **cerebral hemorrhage**, **CVA**, depression, dizziness, fever, headache, insomnia, **suicidal ideation**, syncope, transient ischemic attacks, vertigo
CV: **Aortic valve incompetence**, **bradycardia**, chest pain, **congestive heart failure**, **deep vein thrombosis**, fluid retention, hypertension, **MI**, palpitations, peripheral edema, tachycardia, **thrombosis**, **unstable angina**, vasculitis, **ventricular fibrillation**, **ventricular hypertrophy**
EENT: Conjunctival hemorrhage, deafness, labyrinthitis, nasopharyngitis, pharyngitis, rhinitis, sinusitis, vitreous floaters
ENDO: Hyperglycemia, **hypoglycemia**
GI: Abdominal pain, diarrhea, elevated liver enzymes, **esophageal perforation**, flatulence, **GI bleeding** or ulceration, **hepatic failure**, ileus, indigestion, jaundice, nausea, **pancreatitis**, **perforation of intestines or stomach**, vomiting
GU: **Acute renal failure**, interstitial nephritis, ovarian cyst, proteinuria, urinary incontinence, UTI
HEME: **Agranulocytosis**, **aplastic anemia**, decreased hematocrit and hemoglobin, **leukopenia**, **pancytopenia**, **prolonged APTT**, **thrombocytopenia**
MS: Arthralgia, back pain, elevated serum creatine kinase level, epicondylitis, tendon rupture
RESP: **Bronchospasm**, cough, dyspnea, pneumonia, **pulmonary embolism**, upper respiratory tract infection
SKIN: Acute generalized exanthematous pustulosis, **erythema multiforme**, **exfoliative dermatitis**, fixed drug eruptions, phototoxicity, rash, **Stevens-Johnson syndrome**, **toxic epidermal necrolysis**, urticaria
Other: **Anaphylaxis**, **angioedema**, **drug reaction with eosinophilia and systemic symptoms (DRESS)**, **hyperkalemia**, **hypernatremia**, **hyponatremia**, **sepsis**

Childbearing Considerations

PREGNANCY

- Drug increases risk of premature closure of the fetal ductus arteriosus if given during the third trimester of pregnancy and fetal renal dysfunction causing oligohydramnios and possibly neonatal renal impairment if given during the second or third trimester of pregnancy.
- Drug is not recommended in pregnant women starting at 20 wk of gestation.

LACTATION

- Drug may be present in breast milk in low concentrations.
- Mothers should check with prescriber before breastfeeding.

REPRODUCTION

- Drug may delay or prevent rupture of ovarian follicles, which may result in infertility that is reversible once drug therapy has been discontinued.
- Drug may have to be withheld in females of childbearing age who are having difficulty conceiving or who are being tested for infertility.

Nursing Considerations

- Know that NSAIDs like celecoxib should be avoided in patients with a recent MI because risk of reinfarction increases with NSAID therapy. If therapy is unavoidable, monitor patient closely for signs of cardiac ischemia.
- Be aware that NSAIDs such as celecoxib should not be given to patients with severe heart failure because risk of heart failure increases with NSAID use. If use is unavoidable, monitor patient for worsening of heart failure.
- Use celecoxib cautiously in patients with hypertension and monitor blood pressure closely throughout therapy because drug can increase blood pressure or worsen hypertension.
- Use celecoxib cautiously in adult patients known to be poor CYP2C9 metabolizers based on history or experience with other CYP2C9 substrates, such as phenytoin or warfarin.

! **WARNING** Use celecoxib cautiously in children with systemic onset juvenile rheumatoid arthritis because serious adverse reactions can occur, including disseminated intravascular coagulation.

! **WARNING** Monitor patient for hypersensitivity reactions that may become life-threatening such as anaphylaxis or angioedema. If present, notify prescriber immediately, withhold drug, and provide supportive care, as needed and ordered.

! **WARNING** Assess patient's skin regularly for signs of rash or other adverse skin manifestations because celecoxib is a sulfur drug and may cause serious skin reactions without warning even in patients with no history of sensitivity to sulfur. Drug may also cause DRESS, often with early symptoms of a fever, lymphadenopathy, and rash, which can proceed to severe signs and symptoms. At first sign of reaction, stop drug and notify prescriber immediately.

! **WARNING** Know that use of NSAIDs such as celecoxib increases risk of serious cardiovascular thrombotic events, including MI and stroke, which can be life-threatening. These events may occur early in treatment and risk increases with duration of use. Be aware that these events have occurred even in patients who do not have a history or known risk factors for cardiovascular disease. Monitor patient for warning signs such as chest pain, shortness of breath, slurring of speech, or weakness. If any signs and symptoms develop, withhold celecoxib, alert prescriber immediately, and provide supportive care, as prescribed.

! **WARNING** Be aware that serious GI tract ulceration and bleeding as well as perforation of intestine or stomach can occur without warning or symptoms. Debilitated or elderly patients are at greatest risk along with patients with a prior history of GI bleeding and/or peptic ulcer disease who used NSAIDs. Other patients who may be at risk include patients with advanced liver disease and/or coagulopathy, patients in poor health, smokers, use of certain drugs (anticoagulants, antiplatelets, oral corticosteroids, selective serotonin reuptake inhibitors), and use of alcohol. If patient develops GI distress, withhold celecoxib and notify prescriber immediately.

- Monitor patient—especially if elderly or receiving long-term celecoxib therapy—for less common but serious adverse GI reactions, including anorexia, constipation, diverticulitis, dysphagia, esophagitis, gastritis, gastroenteritis, gastroesophageal reflux disease, hemorrhoids, hiatal hernia, melena, stomatitis, and vomiting.

! **WARNING** Monitor liver enzymes because, in rare cases, elevation may progress to a severe hepatic reaction, including fatal hepatitis or hepatic failure or necrosis.

! **WARNING** Expect to monitor laboratory results (including WBC) and assess for infection in patient who has bone marrow suppression, such as occurs with antineoplastic therapy because celecoxib's anti-inflammatory and antipyretic actions may mask signs and symptoms of infection, including fever and pain.

- Monitor BUN and serum creatinine levels in elderly patients; patients taking ACE inhibitors, angiotensin II receptor antagonists, or diuretics; and patients with heart failure, impaired hepatic dysfunction or renal function because drug may cause hepatic or renal failure.
- Monitor CBC for decreased hemoglobin level and hematocrit because drug may worsen anemia.

PATIENT TEACHING

- Instruct patient how to administer form of celcoxib prescribed.
- Tell patient to take celecoxib exactly as prescribed and not to increase dosage or take drug longer than prescribed because serious adverse reactions can occur.
- Advise patient not to take other NSAIDs or salicylates while taking celecoxib. Also, advise patient to consult prescriber before taking low-dose aspirin.
- Advise patient to notify prescriber if pain continues or is poorly controlled.

! **WARNING** Alert patient that celcoxib may cause an allergic or skin reaction that could become severe. Tell patient to notify prescriber immediately if present including a rash and to seek emergency medical care, if severe.

! **WARNING** Explain that celecoxib may increase the risk of serious adverse cardiovascular events; urge patient to seek immediate medical attention if signs or symptoms arise, such as chest pain, shortness of breath, slurred speech, and weakness. Inform patient that the risk of congestive heart failure increases with NSAID use. Instruct patient to promptly report any evidence of edema, shortness of breath, or unexplained weight gain.

! **WARNING** Tell patient that celecoxib may increase the risk of serious adverse GI reactions. Stress the need to seek immediate medical attention if signs or symptoms develop, such as abdominal or epigastric, black or tarry stools, indigestion, and vomiting blood or material that resembles coffee grounds.

- Urge patient to avoid alcohol consumption and smoking during celecoxib therapy because they may increase the risk of adverse GI reactions.
- Inform pregnant women of fetal risks if taking drug. Stress importance of not taking celecoxib if pregnant, especially at 20 weeks or later.

cenobamate

Xcopri

Class, Category, and Schedule

Pharmacologic class: Sodium channel antagonist
Therapeutic class: Anticonvulsant
Controlled substance schedule: V

Indications and Dosages

✱ *To treat partial-onset seizures as adjunct or monotherapy*

TABLETS

Adults. *Initial:* 12.5 mg once daily for 2 wk, then titrated as follows: 25 mg once daily for wk 3 and wk 4, 50 mg once daily for wk 5 and wk 6, 100 mg once daily for wk 7 and wk 8, and 150 mg once daily for wk 9 and wk 10. *Maintenance:* 200 mg once daily beginning wk 11. Dosage further increased above 200 mg in increments of 50 mg once daily every 2 wk, based on response and tolerability. *Maximum:* 400 mg once daily.

± **DOSAGE ADJUSTMENT** For patients with mild to moderate hepatic impairment, maximum dosage 200 mg once daily with additional dosage reduction may be required.

Drug Administration

P.O.

- Tablets should be swallowed whole and taken with a liquid.
- Tablets can also be crushed for patients who cannot swallow the tablets. Mix crushed tablet with 25 ml of water. Swirl to suspend the crushed particles. After administering, add 25 ml to container and have patient drink to ensure no tablet residue is left in the container. Repeat if tablet residue is still visible in container.

- Crushed tablet mixed with water can also be administered through a nasogastric (NG) tube. Mix crushed tablets with 25 ml of water and swirl to suspend the crushed tablets. Instill the suspension with a cather-tip syringe into the NG tube. Refill the syringe again with 10 ml of water, swirl gently, and administer. If particles remain in syringe, repeat again.
- Maintain titration schedule, as rapid titration may cause adverse reactions that could be serious.
- Be aware drug should be discontinued slowly with dosage gradually reduced over a period of at least 2 wk unless drug must be discontinued abruptly because of a safety concern such as a serious allergic reaction.

Route	Onset	Peak	Duration
P.O.	Unknown	1–4 hr	Unknown

Half-life: 50–60 hr

Mechanism of Action

May reduce repetitive neuronal firing by inhibiting voltage-gated sodium currents. It also is a positive allosteric modulator of the γ-aminobutyric acid ($GABA_A$) ion channel.

Contraindications

Familial short QT interval, hypersensitivity to cenobamate or its components

Interactions

DRUGS

carbamazepine, CYP2B6 substrates, CYP3A substrates, lamotrigine, oral contraceptives: Decreased plasma concentrations of these drugs, decreasing effectiveness

clobazam, CYP2C19 substrates, phenobarbital, phenytoin: Increased plasma concentrations of these drugs, increasing risk of adverse reactions

CNS depressants: Increased risk of neurological adverse reactions, including sedation and somnolence

drugs that shorten QT interval: Potential greater shortening of QT interval

ACTIVITIES

alcohol use: Increased risk of neurological adverse reactions, including sedation and somnolence

Adverse Reactions

CNS: Aggression, aphasia, asthenia, ataxia, balance disorder, confusion, delusions, dizziness, euphoric mood, fatigue, gait disturbance, hallucinations, hostility, irritability, headache, memory impairment, migraine, paranoia, psychosis, sedation, somnolence, **suicidal ideation**, tremor, vertigo

CV: Palpitations, **QT shortening**

EENT: Blurred vision, diplopia, dry mouth, nasopharyngitis, nystagmus, pharyngitis, taste distortion

GI: Abdominal pain, anorexia, constipation, diarrhea, dyspepsia, elevated liver enzymes, **hepatic failure**, nausea, vomiting

GU: Dysmenorrhea, pollakiuria, UTI

MS: Back pain, dysarthria, musculoskeletal chest pain

RESP: Dyspnea, hiccups

SKIN: Pruritus, rash

Other: Appendicitis, **drug reaction with eosinophilia and systemic symptoms (DRESS)/multiorgan hypersensitivity**, **hyperkalemia**, physical and/or psychological dependence, weight loss

Childbearing Considerations

PREGNANCY

- Pregnancy exposure registry: 1-888-233-2334 or visit http://www.aedpregnancyregistry.org.
- It is not known if drug causes fetal harm.
- Use with caution only if benefit to mother outweighs potential risk to fetus.

LACTATION

- It is not known if drug is present in breast milk.
- Mothers should check with prescriber before breastfeeding.

REPRODUCTION

- Females of childbearing age taking an oral contraceptive will need to use an additional alternative nonhormonal method during drug therapy.

Nursing Considerations

! WARNING Know that cenobamate should not be given to patients with familial short QT syndrome because of risk of synergistic effect on the QT interval that would increase the risk of sudden death or ventricular arrhythmias.

- Use cenobamate cautiously in patients also receiving other medications known to shorten QT intervals, as a synergistic effect could occur.

! **WARNING** Monitor patient for signs and symptoms of a hypersensitivity reaction, including drug reaction with eosinophilia and systemic symptoms (DRESS), such as facial swelling, fever, lymphadenopathy, and rash in addition to other organ system involvement, such as hematological abnormalities, hepatitis, myocarditis, myositis, or nephritis. Eosinophilia is often present. Early manifestations such as fever or lymphadenopathy may be present without a rash. Notify prescriber immediately if suspected, as a hypersensitivity rection, including DRESS can be life-threatening. Expect cenobamate to be discontinued. Provide supportive care, as needed and ordered.

! **WARNING** Monitor patient for emergence of or worsening depression, suicidal thoughts or behavior, and/or any unusual changes in behavior or mood because cenobamate increases risk of suicidal behavior and thoughts. Suicidal ideation has occurred as early as 1 week after starting drug therapy and can persist for duration of therapy.

- Be aware that patient may develop a tolerance to drug and potentially abuse it. Discuss any concerns with prescriber.

PATIENT TEACHING

- Instruct patient how to administer cenobamate.

! **WARNING** Warn patient that drug can cause physical and psychological dependence. Stress importance of not altering dosage or frequency of administration. Also warn patient not to abruptly stop taking drug without consulting prescriber because seizures can occur.

- Tell patient alcohol should be avoided while taking cenobamate.

! **WARNING** Instruct patient to notify prescriber of persistent, severe, or unusual signs and symptoms, especially if a fever or rash, along with other signs or symptoms, is present.

! **WARNING** Urge family or caregiver to monitor patient closely for suicidal tendencies, especially when therapy starts or dosage changes, and report any concerns to prescriber.

! **WARNING** Tell family or caregiver to seek immediate emergency care if patient becomes unconscious or experiences prolonged palpitations.

- Instruct patient to inform prescriber of all drugs taken, including over-the-counter and herbal preparations.
- Urge patient to avoid hazardous activities until drug's CNS and visual effects are known and resolved.
- Advise females of childbearing age using oral contraceptives to use additional or an alternative nonhormonal contraceptive during cenobamate therapy. Cenobamate may reduce the efficacy of oral contraceptives.

cephalexin hydrochloride

cephalexin monohydrate

Class and Category

Pharmacologic class: First-generation cephalosporin
Therapeutic class: Antibiotic

Indications and Dosages

* *To treat bone infections caused by* Proteus mirabilis *or* Staphylococcus aureus; *genitourinary tract infections caused by* Escherichia coli, Klebsiella pneumoniae, *or* P. mirabilis; *respiratory infections caused by* Streptococcus pneumoniae *or* S. pyogenes; *and skin and skin structure infections caused by* S. aureus *or* S. pyogenes

CAPSULES, ORAL SUSPENSION, TABLETS

Adults and adolescents ages 15 and older. 250 mg every 6 hr or 500 mg every 12 hr for 7 to 14 days. *For severe infections:* Up to 4 g daily in 2 to 4 equally divided doses for 7 to 14 days.

Children older than 1 to age 15. 25 to 50 mg/kg daily given in equally divided doses for 7 to 14 days. For beta-hemolytic streptococcal infections, duration of at least 10 days is recommended. *For severe infections:* 50 to 100 mg/kg daily given in equally divided doses for 7 to 14 days.

∗ *To treat otitis media caused by* Haemophilus influenzae, Moraxella catarrhalis, S. aureus, S. pneumoniae, *or* S. pyogenes

ORAL SUSPENSION

Children. 75 to 100 mg/kg daily in equally divided doses every 6 hr.

±**DOSAGE ADJUSTMENT** For patients ages 15 and older with a creatinine clearance of 30 to 59 ml/min, maximum dosage not to exceed 1 g; for creatinine clearance of 15 to 29 ml/min, dosage reduced to 250 mg every 8 or 12 hours; for creatinine clearance of 5 to 14 ml/min and patient not yet on dialysis, dosage reduced to 250 mg every 24 hours; and for creatinine clearance of 1 to 4 ml/min and patient not yet on dialysis, dosage reduced to 250 mg every 48 or 60 hours.

Mechanism of Action

Interferes with bacterial cell wall synthesis, like all cephalosporins, by inhibiting the final step in the cross-linking of peptidoglycan strands. Peptidoglycan makes the cell membrane rigid and protective. Without it, bacterial cells rupture and die. This mechanism of action is most effective against bacteria that divide rapidly, including many gram-positive and gram-negative bacteria.

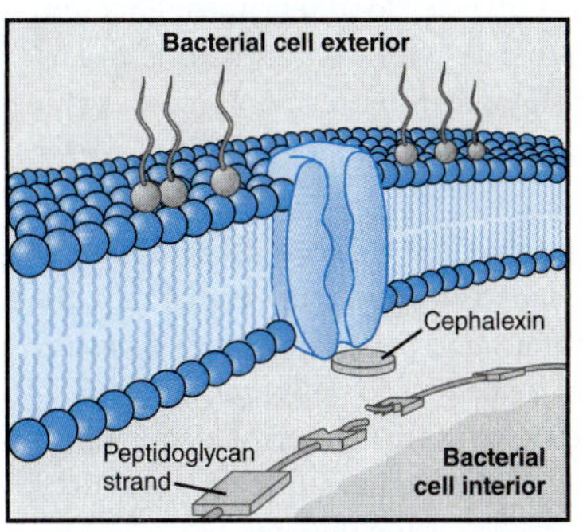

Drug Administration

P.O.

- Capsules and tablets should be swallowed whole without chewing or crushing.
- Prepare oral suspension as follows: Tap bottle to loosen powder. Then, add 70 ml of water to 125 mg/5 ml or 250 mg/5 ml bottle to make a 100-ml suspension or add 140 ml to 125 mg/5 ml or 250 mg/5 ml to make a 200-ml suspension. Add the water in 2 portions, shaking well after each addition.
- Shake oral suspension well before measuring each dose and use a calibrated device to ensure an accurate dose.
- Store oral suspension in refrigerator. Discard after 14 days.

Route	Onset	Peak	Duration
P.O.	Unknown	1 hr	Unknown

Half-life: 30–75 min

Contraindications

Hypersensitivity to cephalexin, other cephalosporins, or their components

Interactions

DRUGS

metformin: Increased plasma metformin levels and increased risk of adverse reactions

probenecid: Increased and prolonged blood cephalexin level

Adverse Reactions

CNS: Chills, fever, headache, **seizures**

CV: Edema

EENT: Hearing loss, oral candidiasis

GI: Abdominal cramps, ***Clostridioides difficile*–associated diarrhea**, diarrhea, elevated liver enzymes, **hepatic failure**, hepatomegaly, nausea, **pseudomembranous colitis**, vomiting

GU: Elevated BUN level, **nephrotoxicity**, **renal failure**, vaginal candidiasis

HEME: Eosinophilia, **hemolytic anemia**, **hypoprothrombinemia**, **neutropenia**, **thrombocytopenia**, **unusual bleeding**

MS: Arthralgia

RESP: Dyspnea

SKIN: Ecchymosis, erythema, **erythema multiforme**, pruritus, rash, **Stevens-Johnson syndrome**

Other: **Anaphylaxis**, superinfection

C

Childbearing Considerations

PREGNANCY

- It is not known if drug can cause fetal harm.
- Use with caution only if benefit to mother outweighs potential risk to fetus.

LACTATION

- Drug is present in breast milk.
- Mothers should check with prescriber before breastfeeding.

Nursing Considerations

- Obtain culture and sensitivity test results, if possible and as ordered, before giving drug.

! WARNING Monitor patient for a hypersensitivity reaction that could become life-threatening, such as anaphylaxis, especially patients allergic to penicillin because cross-sensitivity can occur. Be aware that an allergic reaction may occur even a few days after therapy starts. If hyersenstivity occurs, notify prescriber, withhold drug, and provide supportive care, as needed and ordered.

! WARNING Monitor patient closely for diarrhea, which may indicate pseudomembranous colitis caused by *Clostridioides difficile*–associated diarrhea. It may be mild or become life-threatening. If diarrhea occurs, notify prescriber and expect testing to be done to confirm presence of *C. difficile*. If confirmed, expect to withhold drug, and treat with an antibiotic effective against *C. difficile* along with electrolytes, fluids, and protein, as needed and ordered.

! WARNING Monitor patient's bleeding time, complete CBC, and prothrombin time, as ordered. Assess patient for adverse blood reactions that could become life-threatening. Expect drug to be discontinued and appropriate therapy instituted if patient develops a serious adverse hematologic reaction. If drug-induced hemolytic anemia is suspected, expect to discontinue drug and provide supportive care, as indicated.

! WARNING Monitor patient for seizures. Institute seizure precautions. Be prepared to provide immediate treatment, as ordered if a seizure occurs, expect drug to be discontinued and provide supportive care, as needed and ordered.

- Monitor patient's BUN and serum creatinine levels to detect early signs of nephrotoxicity. Also, monitor fluid intake and output; decreasing urine output may indicate nephrotoxicity. Expect to monitor a patient who already has renal impairment more frequently for nephrotoxicity because drug clearance is slowed.
- Assess ALT, AST, bilirubin, CBC, hematocrit, and serum alkaline phosphatase levels during long-term therapy.

PATIENT TEACHING

- Instruct patient on how to administer the oral form of drug prescribed.
- Advise patient to complete prescribed course of therapy.

! WARNING Inform patient that an allergic reaction may occur with drug use. Tell patient to notify prescriber, if present and to seek immediate medical care, if serious.

! WARNING Urge patient to report watery, bloody stools to prescriber immediately, even if they occur up to 2 months after cephalexin therapy has ended.

! WARNING Review signs and symptoms of types of neurologic adverse reactions that may occur with ceftazidime therapy. Review seizure precautions. If present, urge patient to notify prescriber.

! WARNING Inform patient that drug may cause adverse blood reactions. Encourage compliance with laboratory tests and tell patient to alert prescriber if bleeding or ecchymosis occurs.

- Teach patient to recognize and report signs of superinfection, such as diarrhea, furry tongue, and perineal itching. If present, advise patient to notify prescriber.
- Tell patient that buttermilk and yogurt can help maintain intestinal flora and decrease diarrhea during therapy.

certolizumab pegol

Cimzia

Class and Category

Pharmacologic class: Tumor necrosis factor (TNF) blocker

Therapeutic class: Immunomodulator, disease modifying antirheumatic drug (DMARD)

Indications and Dosages

✱ *To reduce signs and symptoms of Crohn's disease and maintain clinical response in patients with moderately to severely active disease who have had an inadequate response to conventional therapy*

SUBCUTANEOUS INJECTION

Adults. *Initial:* 400 mg (given as two 200-mg injections) and repeated at wk 2 and 4. *Maintenance:* 400 mg (given as two 200-mg injections) every 4 wk, if clinical response occurs.

✱ *To treat active ankylosing spondylitis, active psoriatic arthritis, moderate to severe active rheumatoid arthritis, and nonradiographic axial spondyloarthritis*

SUBCUTANEOUS INJECTION

Adults. *Initial:* 400 mg (given as two 200-mg injections) and repeated at wk 2 and 4 followed by 200 mg every other week. *Maintenance:* 200 mg every other wk, or 400 mg (given as two 200-mg injections) every 4 wk, if clinical response occurs.

✱ *To treat moderate to severe plaque psoriasis in patients who are candidates for phototherapy or systemic therapy*

SUBCUTANEOUS INJECTION

Adults. 400 mg (given as two 200-mg injections) every other wk.

± **DOSAGE ADJUSTMENT** For patients with plaque psoriasis who weigh 90 kg (198 lb) or less, dosage may be changed to 400 mg (given as two 200-mg injections) and repeated at weeks 2 and 4, followed by 200 mg every other week.

✱ *To treat active polyarticular juvenile idiopathic arthritis*

SUBCUTANEOUS INJECTION

Children ages 2 and older weighing 40 kg (88 lb) or more. *Initial:* 400 mg (given as two 200-mg injections) and repeated at wk 2 and 4. *Maintenance:* 200 mg every 2 wk.

Children ages 2 and older weighing 20 kg (44 lb) to less than 40 kg (88 lb). *Initial:* 200 mg and repeated at wk 2 and 4. *Maintenance:* 100 mg every 2 wk.

Children ages 2 and older weighing 10 kg (22 lb) to less than 20 kg (44 lb). *Initial:* 100 mg and repeated at wk 2 and 4. *Maintenance:* 50 mg every 2 wk.

Drug Administration

SUBCUTANEOUS

- Allow drug to be at room temperature for 30 min before reconstituting. Do not warm drug any other way. Reconstitute two 200-mg certolizumab vials for each 400-mg dose and one 200-mg vial for a 200-mg dose.
- Inject 1 ml Sterile Water for Injection into each vial needed, using the 20 G needle provided. Direct the stream at the vial wall rather than directly onto drug.
- Gently swirl vial(s) without shaking for about 1 min. Continue swirling every 5 min as long as undissolved particles are observed, which may take as long as 30 min. Solution should be clear to opalescent, colorless to pale yellow. The final reconstituted solution will be 200 mg/ml.
- Do not leave at room temperature, once reconstituted, for more than 2 hr before administration. If administration will be delayed, reconstituted drug can be refrigerated for up to 24 hr. Do not let drug freeze.
- Administer drug only when solution has reached room temperature.
- Using a 20 G needle, withdraw drug from vial using a separate syringe and needle for each vial.
- Switch to a 23 G needle, pinch the skin at the injection site, and administer subcutaneously into patient's abdomen (staying at least 2 inches away from navel) or thigh. Do not exceed 200 mg per site and do not inject into skin that is bruised, hard, red, or tender or where there are scars or stretch marks.
- If prefilled syringe is refrigerated, have it warm up to room temperature before administering drug. Know that the needle shield inside the removable cap of the prefilled syringe contains a derivative

of natural rubber latex, which may cause allergic reactions if touched by latex-sensitive persons.

Route	Onset	Peak	Duration
SubQ	Unknown	54–171 hr	Unknown

Half-life: 14 days

Mechanism of Action

Binds to human tumor necrosis factor (TNF) alpha, inhibiting it. TNF alpha stimulates production of inflammatory mediators, including interleukin-1, nitric oxide, platelet activating factor, and prostaglandins. TNF alpha level is increased in patients with Crohn's disease and rheumatoid arthritis. Inhibition of TNF alpha causes C-reactive protein level to decline in patients with Crohn's disease, and the disease improves.

Contraindications

Hypersensitivity to certolizumab or its components

Interactions

DRUGS

abatacept, anakinra, natalizumab, rituximab: Possibly increased risk of serious infection and neutropenia
immunosuppressants: Possibly increased risk of infection
live-virus vaccines: Increased risk of adverse vaccine effects

Adverse Reactions

CNS: Anxiety, bipolar disorder, **CVA**, dizziness, fatigue, fever, headache, malaise, **suicidal ideation**, syncope, transient ischemic attack (TIA)
CV: Angina, **arrhythmias**, **atrial fibrillation**, **cardiac failure**, **congestive heart failure**, hypertension, **hypotension**, **MI**, **pericardial effusion**, **pericarditis**, peripheral edema, thrombophlebitis, vasculitis
EENT: Laryngitis, nasopharyngitis, optic neuritis, pharyngitis, retinal hemorrhage, uveitis
ENDO: Hot flashes
GI: Abdominal pain, diarrhea, elevated liver enzymes, **hepatitis**, **hepatitis B virus (HBV) reactivation**, **intestinal obstruction**
GU: Menstrual dysfunction, **nephrotic syndrome**, **pyelonephritis**, **renal failure**, UTI
HEME: Anemia, **bleeding**, **leukemia**, **leukopenia**, lymphadenopathy, **pancytopenia**, thrombophilia
MS: Arthralgia, back and extremity pain
RESP: Acute bronchitis, cough, dyspnea, pneumonia, upper respiratory infection
SKIN: Allergic dermatitis, alopecia, change of plaque psoriasis into a different psoriasis subtype, **erythema multiforme**, erythema nodosum, lichenoid skin reaction, **melanoma**, **Merkel cell carcinoma**, new or worsening psoriasis, rash, **Stevens-Johnson syndrome**, **toxic epidermal necrolysis**, urticaria
Other: **Anaphylaxis**; **angioedema**; antibody formation to certolizumab; bacterial, invasive fungal, mycobacterial, parasitic, viral or other opportunistic infections including aspergillosis, blastomycosis, candidiasis, coccidioidomycosis, histoplasmosis, legionellosis, listeriosis, pneumocystosis, and tuberculosis; herpes infections; injection-site reactions (bruising, discoloration, pain, redness, swelling); **lymphomas and other malignancies**; lupus-like syndrome; sarcoidosis; serum sickness

Childbearing Considerations

PREGNANCY

- Pregnancy exposure registry: 1-877-311-8972 or http://mothertobaby.org/pregnancy-studies/.
- It is not known if drug can cause fetal harm, although it may affect fetal immune responses.
- Use with caution only if benefit to mother outweighs potential risk to fetus.
- Know that the safety of administering live or live-attenuated vaccines in neonates exposed to drug in utero is unknown.

LACTATION

- Drug is present in breast milk.
- Mothers should check with prescriber before breastfeeding.

Nursing Considerations

- Be aware that certolizumab should not be initiated in a patient with an active infection, including serious localized infections.
- Use certolizumab cautiously in patients with recurrent or increased risk of infection, patients who live in regions where histoplasmosis and tuberculosis (TB) are endemic, and patients with a history of CNS demyelinating disorders because any of these disorders can occur, rarely, during certolizumab therapy. Be aware that a falsely

negative antigen and antibody test for histoplasmosis may occur in some patients during certolizumab therapy, even when an active infection is present. Patient should be monitored closely throughout therapy.

- Use cautiously in patients who are chronic carriers of HBV because drug may reactivate the virus. Assess patient for evidence of HBV infection before starting and periodically throughout certolizumab therapy. If HBV reactivation occurs, notify prescriber, stop drug, and start appropriate therapy, as ordered.
- Make sure patient has a tuberculin skin test before therapy starts. If skin test is positive (induration 5 mm or greater), treatment of latent TB must start before certolizumab is given, as prescribed. In addition, expect antituberculosis therapy to be given to a patient with a history of latent or active TB in whom an adequate course of treatment cannot be confirmed and for patients with a negative test for latent TB but having risk factors for TB infection. Be aware that a falsely negative test for latent TB may occur during certolizumab therapy, so any signs and symptoms suggestive of TB should be carefully evaluated.
- Ensure patient is up to date with immunizations before beginning certolizumab therapy. Do not administer live vaccines immediately before therapy is begun or during therapy.

! **WARNING** Monitor patient for a hypersensitivity reaction that could become life-threatening, such as anaphylaxis and angioedema. If present, notify prescriber immediately, withhold drug as ordered, and provide supportive care, as needed and ordered.

! **WARNING** Assess patient's skin regularly, especially for patients who are at risk for skin cancer, as drug may cause melanomas and Merkel cell carcinoma as well as other life-threatening disorders such as Stevens-Johnson syndrome. At the first sign of a rash, notify prescriber.

! **WARNING** Monitor patient's CBC, as ordered, because certolizumab may have adverse hematologic effects. Notify prescriber about persistent bleeding, bruising, fever, or pallor.

- Monitor all patients for infection during therapy, especially those who are at higher risk for infection, such as patients receiving immunosuppressants, those who are over 65 years of age, or who have comorbid conditions. If serious infection develops, expect prescriber to stop drug.
- Monitor patient closely for evidence of congestive heart failure (anxiety; crackles; dyspnea; sudden, unexplained weight gain), and notify prescriber if they occur.

! **WARNING** Be aware that certolizumab is a TNF inhibitor. Although rare, malignancies (especially lymphomas and leukemias) have been reported in patients receiving these drugs. Patients with rheumatoid arthritis, especially those with very active disease, and patients with other disorders that certolizumab treats are at greatest risk. Monitor these patients closely.

PATIENT TEACHING

- Instruct patient on how to administer drug as a subcutaneous injection using the prefilled syringe, if appropriate.
- Inform patient that injection-site reactions such as pain or redness may occur and usually are mild and transient. Instruct him to apply a towel soaked in cold water to the site if it hurts. Tell patient to call prescriber if reaction persists or worsens.
- Tell patient not to receive immunizations using live vaccines during certolizumab therapy.

! **WARNING** Review signs and symptoms of allergic reaction (rash, swollen face, trouble breathing), and tell patient to stop taking drug, notify prescriber, and seek emergency care immediately if these occur.

! **WARNING** Tell patient to report evidence of bleeding disorders to prescriber; drug may have to be stopped. Advise patient to comply with all prescribed tests.

! **WARNING** Inform patient that certain kinds of cancer, especially leukemias and lymphomas, are more likely in patients taking certolizumab but are still rare. Emphasize need to keep follow-up visits and to report persistent, serious, or unusual signs or symptoms. Also, advise patient to have periodic skin examinations, especially if they are at risk for skin cancer.

- Instruct patient to notify prescriber if persistent, severe, or unusual adverse reactions occur.
- Inform patient that drug may lower the ability of the immune system to fight infections. Tell patient to report any signs and symptoms of infection, including TB or reactivation of HBV infections that may occur during therapy. Instruct him to avoid people with an infection and report fever, including a low-grade fever, persistent cough, or wasting or weight loss to prescriber.
- Instruct patient to report lupus-like signs and symptoms that, although rare, may occur during therapy, such as chest pain that doesn't go away, joint pain, rash on cheeks or arms that's sensitive to the sun, or shortness of breath. Explain that drug may have to be discontinued if these occur.
- Advise patient to inform all healthcare providers about certolizumab use and to inform prescriber about any herbal remedies, vitamin and mineral supplements, and over-the-counter medications being taken.

cetirizine hydrochloride

Quzyttir, Zyrtec

Class and Category

Pharmacologic class: Histamine-1 (H-1) receptor antagonist
Therapeutic class: Antihistamine

Indications and Dosages

✱ To treat acute urticaria

I.V. INJECTION (QUZYTTIR)

Adults and adolescents ages 12 and older. 10 mg every 24 hr, as needed.
Children ages 6 to 11. 5 or 10 mg, depending on severity, every 24 hr, as needed.
Children 6 mo to 5 yr with normal hepatic and renal function. 2.5 mg every 24 hr, as needed.

✱ To treat chronic urticaria, perennial allergic rhinitis, or seasonal allergic rhinitis

CHEWABLE TABLETS, DISSOLVE TABLETS, SYRUP, TABLETS (ZYRTEC)

Adults and children ages 6 and older. 5 or 10 mg once daily.
Children ages 2 to 5. 2.5 mg once daily, increased to 5 mg once daily or 2.5 mg every 12 hr, as needed.

SYRUP

Children ages 6 mo to 23 mo. 2.5 mg once daily. *For children that are between 12 and 23 mo*: Dosage increased to 2.5 mg every 12 hr, as needed.

±**DOSAGE ADJUSTMENT** For adult and adolescent patients 12 years of age and older with decreased renal function (creatinine clearance 11–31 ml/min), patients on hemodialysis (creatinine clearance less than 7 ml/min), patients with hepatic impairment, patients 77 years and older, and pediatric patients ages 6 to 11 with impaired hepatic or renal function, dosage limited to 5 mg once daily. Pediatric patients below the age of 6 with impaired hepatic or renal function should not receive certirizine.

Drug Administration

P.O.

- Chewable tablets should be chewed completely before swallowing.
- Dissolve tablets are meant to be dissolved in mouth, but the tablets can be chewed or swallowed. May be taken with or without water.
- Syrup should be measured with a calibrated device to ensure accurate dose.

I.V.

- Withdraw dosage from a single-use vial. Each ml contains 10 mg of cetirizine hydrochloride.
- Administer only as an I.V. injection over 1 to 2 min.
- Do not administer to children under the age of 6 yr with impaired hepatic or renal function.
- *Incompatibilities:* None listed by manufacturer.

Route	Onset	Peak	Duration
P.O.	Unknown	1 hr	Unknown
I.V.	Unknown	Unknown	Unknown

Half-life: 8.3 hr

Mechanism of Action

Mediated via selective inhibition of peripheral H_1-receptors to alleviate urticaria.

Contraindications

Hypersensitivity to cetirizine, hydroxyzine, levocetirizine, or their components

Interactions

DRUGS

CNS depressants: Increased CNS impairment
theophylline: Possibly decreased clearance of cetirizine, increasing plasma cetirizine levels

ACTIVITIES

alcohol use: Increased CNS impairment

Adverse Reactions

CNS: Dizziness, fatigue, feeling hot, headache, insomnia, irritability, paresthesia, presyncope, sedation, somnolence
EENT: Dry mouth, epistaxis, pharyngitis, taste alteration
GI: Abdominal pain, diarrhea, dyspepsia, nausea, vomiting
RESP: **Bronchospasm**, cough
SKIN: Diaphoresis

Childbearing Considerations

PREGNANCY

- It is not known if drug causes fetal harm.
- Use with caution only if benefit to mother outweighs potential risk to fetus.

LACTATION

- Drug may be present in breast milk.
- Mothers should check with prescriber before breastfeeding.

Nursing Considerations

! **WARNING** Monitor patient's respiratory status because drug can cause bronchospasms. If present, notify prescriber and exect drug to be discontinued.

- Institute safety precautions because drug can cause sedation and somnolence.
- Monitor patient for adverse reactions. If persistent, severe, or unusual adverse reactions occur, notify prescriber.

PATIENT TEACHING

- Instruct patient on how to take form of drug prescribed.
- Warn patient not to drink alcohol while receiving cetirizine because alcohol also increases sedation and somnolence.

! **WARNING** Tell patient to keep drug out of reach of small children.

- Instruct patient to avoid hazardous activities until drug's CNS effects are known and resolved. Warn her that taking other CNS depressants, including over-the-counter products, increases sedation and somnolence.
- Instruct patient to report any persistent, severe, or unusul adverse reactions to prescriber.

C

ciclesonide

Alvesco, Omnaris, Zetonna

Class and Category

Pharmacologic class: Corticosteroid
Therapeutic class: Antiasthmatic, anti-inflammatory

Indications and Dosages

* *To provide prophylactic maintenance therapy for patients with asthma*

INHALATION AEROSOL (ALVESCO)

Adults and children ages 12 and older who received bronchodilator therapy. *Initial:* 80 mcg twice daily, increased after 4 wk, as needed and then adjusted to lowest effective dose when stabilized. *Maximum:* 160 mcg twice daily.
Adults and children ages 12 and older who received inhaled corticosteroid. *Initial:* 80 mcg twice daily, increased after 4 wk, as needed and then adjusted to lowest effective dose when stabilized. *Maximum:* 320 mcg twice daily.
Adults and children ages 12 and older who received oral corticosteroid therapy. *Initial and maximum:* 320 mcg twice daily, adjusted to lowest effective dose when stabilized. *Maximum:* 320 mcg twice daily.

* *To treat nasal congestion in seasonal allergic rhinitis*

NASAL SPRAY (OMNARIS)

Adults and children ages 6 and older. 200 mcg once daily as 2 sprays in each nostril.

NASAL AEROSOL (ZETONNA)

Adults and children ages 12 and older. 74 mcg once daily as 1 spray (37 mcg) in each nostril.

∗ *To treat nasal congestion in perennial allergic rhinitis*

NASAL SPRAY (OMNARIS)

Adults and children ages 12 and older. 200 mcg once daily as 2 sprays in each nostril.

NASAL AEROSOL (ZETONNA)

Adults and children ages 12 and older. 74 mcg once daily as 1 spray (37 mcg) in each nostril.

Drug Administration

INHALATION

- Use inhalation form only with the actuator supplied with the product.
- Prime Alvesco before first use by actuating the inhaler 3 times while holding the actuator upright; repeat priming if inhaler is not used for more than 10 days.
- To administer drug, have patient hold the actuator upright, then have patient breathe out fully before closing lips around mouthpiece keeping tongue below it. Then while breathing in deeply and slowly, have patient press down on the center of the dose indicator and keep pressed until the canister stops moving in the actuator. When finished, have patient hold breath for about 10 sec, if possible. Tell patient a soft click may be heard from the indicator as it counts down during use.
- Have patient gargle and rinse mouth after each dose to help prevent dry mouth and throat, relieve throat irritation, and prevent oral yeast infection.
- Clean mouthpiece weekly with a clean, dry tissue, both inside and out. Wipe over the front of the small hole where the drug comes out with a dry, folded tissue. Do not wash or put any part of the unit in water or any other liquid.
- When the dose indicator shows a red zone in the window, this indicates a need for a refill. When the indicator shows 0, discard the inhaler.

INTRANASAL

- Avoid spraying drug directly onto the nasal septum.

Omnaris

- Gently shake nasal spray before each use. On first use, spray 8 times into the air, looking for a fine mist. If drug hasn't been used for more than 4 days, it should be primed again with 1 spray or until a fine mist appears.
- Have patient blow nose gently before inserting tip of bottle into 1 nostril while keeping head upright and other nostril closed by pressing finger on it. Have patient breathe in quickly and gently while spraying drug into the nostril. Repeat for second spray. Then have patient repeat procedure in other nostril. Remind patient not to blow nose for at least a few minutes after using the nasal spray.
- After daily use, wipe the nozzle tip with a clean tissue and replace cap. Follow manufacturer guidelines if the nozzle is clogged or requires more thorough cleaning.
- Discard after 120 actuations following initial priming or 4 mo after bottle is removed from the foil pouch, whichever occurs first.

Zetonna

- Nasal spray should be primed before first use, by actuating 3 times. If drug hasn't been used for 10 days or more, it should be primed again by actuating 3 times. If canister is dropped and actuator becomes separated, reassemble and test spray once into the air before using.
- Have patient blow nose gently followed by having patient insert the tip of the bottle into 1 nostril while keeping head upright and pressing other nostril closed with a finger. Have patient breathe in quickly and gently while spraying the drug 1 time into the nostril. Have patient repeat procedure in other nostril. Remind patient not to blow nose for at least 15 min after using the nasal spray.
- Clean outside of nose piece with a clean, dry tissue or cloth weekly; do not wash or put in water.
- When the Zetonna dose indicator shows a red zone in the window, this indicates a need for a refill. When the indicator shows 0, discard the canister.

Route	Onset	Peak	Duration
Inhalation	> 4 wk	1 hr	Unknown
Intranasal	1–2 days	1–5 wk	Unknown

Half-life: Inhalation, 0.7 hr; intranasal, unknown

Mechanism of Action

Inhibits cells involved in the asthma inflammatory response, such as basophils, eosinophils, lymphocytes, macrophages, mast cells, and neutrophils. Ciclesonide also inhibits production or secretion of chemical mediators, such as cytokines, eicosanoids, histamine, and leukotrienes.

Contraindications

Hypersensitivity to ciclesonide or its components, primary treatment of status asthmaticus or other acute asthma episodes that require intensive measures (Alvesco)

Interactions

DRUGS

ketoconazole: Increased exposure time of ciclesonide

Adverse Reactions

CNS: Dizziness, fatigue, headache
EENT: Cataracts, conjunctivitis, dry mouth or throat, dysphonia, epistaxis, glaucoma, hoarseness, nasal congestion or ulceration, nasal septal perforation, nasopharyngitis, oropharyngeal candidiasis, pharyngolaryngeal pain, sinusitis
ENDO: **Adrenal insufficiency**, cushingoid symptoms, decreased bone mineral density, hypercorticism, hyperglycemia, slower growth in children
GI: Nausea
MS: Arthralgia, back or limb pain, musculoskeletal chest discomfort or pain, reduction in bone mineral density
RESP: **Bronchospasm**, cough, pneumonia, upper respiratory tract infection
SKIN: Urticaria
Other: **Angioedema (immediate or delayed)**, flu-like symptoms, **immunosuppression**, infections

Childbearing Considerations

PREGNANCY

- It is not known if drug can cause fetal harm although hypoadrenalism may occur in neonates born of mothers receiving corticosteroids during pregnancy.
- Use with caution only if benefit to mother outweighs potential risk to fetus.

LACTATION

- It is not known if drug is present in breast milk.
- Mothers should check with prescriber before breastfeeding.

Nursing Considerations

- Know that ciclesonide should not be used in patients with recent nasal septal ulcers, nasal surgery, or nasal trauma until healing has occurred.
- Use cautiously in patients with tuberculosis; bacterial, fungal, parasitic, or viral infection; ocular herpes simplex; or chickenpox or measles because these conditions may worsen with ciclesonide therapy. If exposure occurs to chickenpox during drug treatment, expect patient to receive varicella zoster immune globulin (VZIG) and if chickenpox develops, expect patient to be treated with an antiviral agent. If exposure to measles occurs, patient may be given pooled I.M. immunoglobulin therapy. Monitor patient closely during therapy because drug causes immunosuppression and increases risk of infection.
- Use cautiously in patients with a history of cataracts, glaucoma, or increased intraocular pressure because ciclesonide may increase intraocular pressure or cause cataract formation. Also, use cautiously in patients with major risk factors for decreased bone mineral content, such as family history of osteoporosis, prolonged immobilization, or long-term use of drugs that can reduce bone mass, such as anticonvulsants and oral corticosteroids.

! WARNING Monitor patient for a hypersensitivity reaction that may become life-threatening such as angioedema that can occur immediately after exposure to ciclesonide or reaction may be delayed. If angioedema or any other hypersensitivity reactions occurs, notify prescriber; withhold drug, if ordered; expect another corticosteroid drug to replace ciclesonide; and provide supportive care, as needed and ordered.

- Inspect patient's oral cavity if using inhaler form, or nasal cavity if using nasal spray regularly for abnormalities. If nasal candidiasis occurs, expect to continue ciclesonide therapy, unless severe. If nasal erosion, perforation, or ulceration occurs, notify prescriber and expect nasal spray to be discontinued. To prevent oral candidiasis in patients taking oral inhalation form, have patient rinse mouth after the inhalation. If oral candidiasis occurs with oral inhalation form of drug despite rinsing mouth, expect drug to be discontinued.

- Be aware that if patient takes a systemic corticosteroid, expect to taper dosage by no more than 2.5 mg/day at weekly intervals, starting 1 week after ciclesonide therapy begins. Monitor these patients closely for symptoms of withdrawal such as depression, joint and/or muscular pain, and lassitude. Also monitor patient for appearance of conditions that may have been masked by systemic corticosteroids such as conjunctivitis, arthritis, eczema, eosinophilic conditions, or rhinitis and appears when patient is switched to ciclesonide.

! **WARNING** Know that if patient is switched from systemic corticosteroid to ciclesonide, assess for adrenal insufficiency (fatigue, hypotension, lassitude, nausea, vomiting, weakness) early in therapy and whenever patient has infection, stress, surgery, or trauma, or other steroid-depleting conditions or procedures. Notify prescriber immediately if signs or symptoms develop.

! **WARNING** Administer a fast-acting inhaled bronchodilator, as prescribed, if an acute asthma attack occurs. Ciclesonide inhalation is not a bronchodilator, and its action takes longer than needed to abort acute asthma symptoms. If bronchospasm occurs immediately after ciclesonide use, expect to stop drug and notify prescriber as another drug will need to replace ciclesonide therapy.

- Monitor growth in children because ciclesonide may suppress growth.

PATIENT TEACHING

- Instruct patient how to administer form of ciclesonide prescribed.
- Urge patient to use ciclesonide regularly, as prescribed, but not for acute bronchospasm. Also, tell her never to decrease or increase the dosage without consulting prescriber.
- Instruct patient to gargle and rinse her mouth after each dose of inhaler to help prevent dry mouth and throat, relieve throat irritation, and prevent oral yeast infection.
- Explain that the full effect of drug may not occur for 4 weeks or more.
- Stress importance of notifying prescriber if symptoms continue or worsen.

! **WARNING** Alert patient that ciclesonide may cause an allergic reaction. If present, tell patient to notify prescriber and if severe (such as swelling of the lips, pharynx, or tongue) to seek immediate medical care.

! **WARNING** Instruct patient to notify prescriber immediately if asthma attacks don't respond to bronchodilators during ciclesonide inhaler use.

! **WARNING** Review signs and symptoms of adrenal insufficiency with patient. Stress importance of alerting prescriber if present or seeking immediate medical care if severe. Make patient aware that if she is switching from an oral corticosteroid to inhaled ciclesonide, she should carry medical identification indicating the need for supplemental systemic corticosteroids during a severe asthma attack or stress.

! **WARNING** Caution patient to avoid contact with people who have infections because drug suppresses the immune system, increasing the risk of infection. Instruct patient to notify prescriber about exposure to chickenpox, measles, or other infections because additional treatment may be needed.

- Encourage patient to inspect nasal cavity if taking nasal form of ciclesonide and oral cavity if taking oral inhalation of drug for abnormalities. Tell patient to notify prescriber if any abnormalities are observed or nose bleeds occur.
- Warn patient that drug may affect bone mineral density in patients at risk for decreased bone mineral density and to take precautions against falling or injuries.
- Alert parents or caregivers that drug may decrease growth in children. Encourage contacting prescriber with questions or concerns.

cilostazol

Class and Category

Pharmacologic class: Phosphodiesterase 3 (PDE 3) inhibitor
Therapeutic class: Antiplatelet

Indications and Dosages

∗ *To reduce symptoms of intermittent claudication*

TABLETS

Adults. 100 mg twice daily.

±**DOSAGE ADJUSTMENT** For patients taking a moderate or strong CYP3A4 inhibitor (diltiazem, erythromycin, itraconazole, ketoconazole) or taking a CYP2C19 inhibitor (fluconazole, omeprazole, ticlopidine), dosage reduced to 50 mg twice daily.

Drug Administration

P.O.

- Administer at least 30 min before or 2 hr after breakfast and dinner.
- Don't administer with grapefruit juice.

Route	Onset	Peak	Duration
P.O.	Unknown	Unknown	Unknown

Half-life: 11–13 hr

Mechanism of Action

May inhibit phosphodiesterase, decreasing phosphodiesterase activity and suppressing cyclic adenosine monophosphate (cAMP) degradation. This action increases cAMP in platelets and blood vessels, which inhibits platelet aggregation and causes vasodilation. This in turn relieves symptoms of claudication.

Contraindications

Heart failure, hypersensitivity to cilostazol or its components

Interactions

DRUGS

CYP2C19 inhibitors (e.g., fluconazole, omeprazole, ticlopidine) or CYP3A4 inhibitors (e.g., diltiazem, erythromycin, omeprazole, ticlopidine): Increased plasma cilostazol level

ACTIVITIES

smoking: Decreased cilostazol effects by about 20%

FOODS

grapefruit: Increased risk of adverse reactions
high-fat foods: Faster cilostazol absorption and increased risk of adverse reactions

Adverse Reactions

CNS: **Cerebral hemorrhage**, dizziness, headache, paresthesia
CV: Angina, chest pain, hypertension, **hypotension**, **left ventricular outflow tract obstruction** (patients with sigmoid-shaped interventricular septum), palpitations, peripheral edema, **prolonged QT interval**, **supraventricular or ventricular tachycardia**, **thrombosis**, **torsades de pointes**
EENT: Pharyngitis, rhinitis
ENDO: Diabetes mellitus, hot flashes, hyperglycemia
GI: Abdominal pain, abnormal stool, diarrhea, elevated liver enzymes, flatulence, **GI hemorrhage**, **hepatic dysfunction**, indigestion, jaundice, vomiting
GU: Elevated BUN level, hematuria
HEME: **Agranulocytosis**, **aplastic anemia**, **bleeding tendency**, **decreased platelet count**, **granulocytopenia**, **leukopenia**, **pancytopenia**, **thrombocytopenia**
MS: Back pain, myalgia
RESP: Cough, **interstitial pneumonia**, **pulmonary hemorrhage**
SKIN: Eruptions, pruritus, rash, **Stevens-Johnson syndrome**
Other: Infection, increased blood uric acid level

Childbearing Considerations

PREGNANCY

- It is not known if drug can cause fetal harm.
- Use with caution only if benefit to mother outweighs potential risk to fetus.

LACTATION

- It is not known if drug is present in breast milk.
- A decision should be made to discontinue breastfeeding or the drug to avoid potential serious adverse reactions in the breastfed infant.

Nursing Considerations

! **WARNING** Monitor patient's cardiovascular status and vital signs closely because cilostazol may cause cardiovascular lesions, which could lead to problems, such as endocardial hemorrhage.

! WARNING Monitor patient for persistent, serious, or unusual adverse reactions because drug can adversely affect many systems. Expect to monitor patient's bleeding time, CBC, and prothrombin time, as ordered. At the first sign of a significant adverse reaction, notify prescriber and provide supportive care, as needed and ordered.

- Be aware that left ventricular outflow tract obstruction has been reported in patients with sigmoid-shaped interventricular septum. Monitor patients for development of new cardiac symptoms, including a systolic murmur, after starting cilostazol.
- Monitor blood glucose level in all patients to detect hyperglycemia. Also, assess for signs of type 2 diabetes mellitus, such as fatigue, polydipsia, polyphagia, and polyuria.

PATIENT TEACHING

- Instruct patient how to administer cilostazol.
- Warn patent to avoid grapefruit juice during therapy because it can increase the risk of adverse reactions.
- Urge patient not to smoke because it decreases drug's effects.
- Explain that assessment of drug effectiveness is based on ability to walk increased distances. Stress that drug effects won't appear until 2 to 4 weeks after therapy starts and that full effects may take up to 12 weeks.

! WARNING Inform patient that drug may cause serious adverse reactions. Stress importance of notifying prescriber if adverse reactions occur. Also, review signs and symptoms of hyperglycemia and, if present, to report to prescriber.

cimetidine

Tagamet HB

cimetidine hydrochloride

Class and Category

Pharmacologic class: Histamine H_2 antagonist
Therapeutic class: Antiulcer agent

Indications and Dosages

✶ To treat duodenal ulcer

ORAL SOLUTION, TABLETS

Adults and adolescents ages 16 and older. *Initial:* 800 mg (or 1,600 mg if ulcer is greater than 1.0 cm and patient is heavy smoker) once daily. Alternatively, 300 mg 4 times daily, or 400 mg twice daily for 4 to 6 wk. *Maintenance:* 400 mg once daily.

I.M. INJECTION

Adults. *Initial:* 300 mg every 6 to 8 hr.

I.V. INJECTION, I.V. INTERMITTENT INFUSION

Adults. *Initial:* 300 mg every 6 to 8 hr. Frequency of a 300-mg dose increased, as needed. *Maximum:* 2,400 mg daily.

I.V. CONTINUOUS INFUSION

Adults. 37.5 mg/hr. *Maximum:* 900 mg daily.

✶ To prevent recurrence of duodenal ulcer

ORAL SOLUTION, TABLETS

Adults and adolescents ages 16 and older. 400 mg once daily for as long as 5 yr after treatment for a duodenal ulcer.

✶ To treat active, benign gastric ulcer

ORAL SOLUTION, TABLETS

Adults and adolescents ages 16 and older. 800 mg once daily or 300 mg 4 times daily for up to 8 wk.

I.M. INJECTION

Adults and adolescents ages 16 and older. 300 mg every 6 to 8 hr.

I.V. INJECTION, I.V. INTERMITTENT INFUSION

Adults. *Initial:* 300 mg every 6 to 8 hr. Frequency of a 300-mg dose increased, as needed. *Maximum:* 2,400 mg daily.

I.V. CONTINUOUS INFUSION

Adults and adolescents ages 16 and older. *Initial:* 37.5 mg/hr. *Maximum:* 900 mg daily.

✶ To manage erosive gastroesophageal reflux disease

ORAL SOLUTION, TABLETS

Adults. 1,600 mg daily in divided doses (800 mg twice daily or 400 mg 4 times daily) for up to 12 wk.

✶ To treat pathological hypersecretory conditions, such as Zollinger-Ellison syndrome

ORAL SOLUTION, TABLETS

Adults and adolescents ages 16 and older. 300 mg 4 times daily increased in dosage and/or frequency, as needed. *Maximum:* 2,400 mg daily.

I.M. INJECTION

Adults and adolescents ages 16 and older. 300 mg every 6 to 8 hr.

I.V. INJECTION, I.V. INTERMITTENT INFUSION

Adults. *Initial:* 300 mg every 6 to 8 hr. Frequency of a 300-mg dose increased, as needed. *Maximum:* 2,400 mg daily.

I.V. CONTINUOUS INFUSION

Adults. *Initial:* 37.5 mg/hr. *Maximum:* 900 mg daily.

∗ *To treat heartburn and acid indigestion*

ORAL SOLUTION, TABLETS

Adults and children ages 12 and older. *Initial:* 200 mg, as needed, up to twice daily. *Maximum:* 400 mg every 24 hr for no more than 2 wk unless prescribed longer.

∗ *To prevent stress-related upper GI bleeding during hospitalization*

I.V. CONTINUOUS INFUSION

Adults. 37.5 mg/hr for 7 days.

±**DOSAGE ADJUSTMENT** For patients with severe renal impairment, dosage reduced to 300 mg and frequency lengthened to every 12 hours (but increased to every 8 hours with caution, as needed). For patients with both renal and liver impairment, dosage decreased even further. For patients with a creatinine clearance less than 30 ml/min and being treated to prevent stress-related upper GI bleeding during hospitalization, dosage reduced by 50%.

Drug Administration

- Oral forms are preferred method of administration. However, patients unable to take oral drug, may have drug given parenterally.

P.O.

- For treatment other than use as an antacid or for acid indigestion, once-daily doses given at bedtime; twice-daily doses given in morning and at bedtime; 4-times-a-day doses given with meals and at bedtime.
- For use as an antacid or for acid indigestion, administer with water at onset of symptoms or up to 30 min before eating.
- Use calibrated device when measuring oral solution dosage.
- Do not administer an antacid within 1 hr of administering cimetidine.

I.V.

- Solutions compatible for use to dilute drug include 0.9% Sodium Chloride Injection, 5% Dextrose Injection, 5% Sodium Bicarbonate Injection, and Lactated Ringer's.
- Diluted solutions may be stored for up to 48 hr at room temperature.
- For I.V. injection, dilute to a total volume of 20 ml. Inject over 5 min or more. Do not administer rapidly.
- For intermittent infusion, dilute in at least 50 ml I.V. solution. Infuse over 15 to 20 min.
- For continuous infusion, dilute 900 mg in 100- to 1,000-ml I.V. solution (volume used individualized). Use a volumetric pump to infuse drug if volume is less than 250 ml. Administer at a rate of 37.5 mg/hr.
- *Incompatibilities:* None listed by manufacturer.

I.M.

- Administer undiluted.
- Inform patient the injection may be painful.

Route	Onset	Peak	Duration
P.O.	1 hr	45–90 min	4–5 hr
I.V.	30 min	Immediate	4–5 hr
I.M.	Unknown	15 min	4–5 hr

Half-life: 2 hr

Mechanism of Action

Blocks histamine's action at H_2-receptor sites on stomach's parietal cells. This action reduces gastric fluid volume and acidity. Cimetidine also decreases the amount of gastric acid secreted in response to betazole, caffeine, food, insulin, or pentagastrin.

Contraindications

Hypersensitivity to cimetidine or its components

Interactions

DRUGS

antacids, metoclopramide: Decreased cimetidine absorption

chlordiazepoxide, diazepam, lidocaine, metronidazole, nifedipine, phenytoin, propranolol, quinidine, theophylline, tricyclic antidepressants (certain ones), warfarin: Reduced metabolism and increased blood

levels and effects of these drugs, possibly toxicity from these drugs
digoxin, ketoconazole: Altered absorption of these drugs
warfarin: Increased risk of bleeding

ACTIVITIES

alcohol use: Possibly increased blood alcohol level

FOODS

caffeine: Reduced metabolism and increased blood level and effects of caffeine

Adverse Reactions

CNS: Confusion, dizziness, hallucinations, headache, peripheral neuropathy, somnolence
ENDO: Mild gynecomastia if used longer than 1 mo
GI: Mild and transient diarrhea
GU: Impotence, transiently elevated serum creatinine level
SKIN: Rash
Other: Pain at I.M. injection site

Childbearing Considerations

PREGNANCY

- It is not known if drug can cause fetal harm.
- Use with caution only if benefit to mother outweighs potential risk to fetus.

LACTATION

- Drug is present in breast milk.
- Breastfeeding is not recommended during drug therapy.

Nursing Considerations

- Be alert for confusion in debilitated or elderly patients who receive cimetidine.
- Monitor patient for adverse reactions, which are usually mild. However, if patient develops a rash, notify prescriber.

PATIENT TEACHING

- Instruct patient how to take oral form of cimetidine prescribed. If patient unable to take drug orally, tell patient it will be administered as an I.M. injection, which could be painful or intravenously.
- Tell patient to avoid taking antacids within 1 hour of taking cimetidine.
- Caution patient not to take drug for more than 14 days, unless prescribed for a longer time.
- Advise patient to avoid alcohol while taking cimetidine, to prevent interactions.
- Warn patient who smokes that cigarette smoking increases gastric acid secretion and can worsen gastric disease.
- Inform mothers wishing to breastfeed that breastfeeding is not recommended during drug therapy.

cinacalcet hydrochloride

Sensipar

Class and Category

Pharmacologic class: Calcimimetic
Therapeutic class: Calcium reducer

Indications and Dosages

✱ *To treat secondary hyperparathyroidism in patients with chronic renal disease who are on dialysis*

TABLETS

Adults. *Initial:* 30 mg once daily and then increased to 60 mg once daily 2 to 4 wk later, as needed. Dosage increased after 2 to 4 wk to 90 mg once daily, as needed, followed by 120 mg once daily 2 to 4 wk later, as needed, and then to maximum dose of 180 mg once daily 2 to 4 wk later, as needed. *Maximum:* 180 mg daily.

✱ *To treat hypercalcemia in patients with parathyroid carcinoma; to treat primary hyperparathyroidism in patients who are unable to undergo parathyroidectomy*

TABLETS

Adults. *Initial:* 30 mg twice daily, increased in 2 to 4 wk to 60 mg twice daily, then in 2 to 4 wk to 90 mg twice daily, and then in 2 to 4 wk to 90 mg 3 times daily or 4 times daily, as needed to normalize serum calcium level.

± **DOSAGE ADJUSTMENT** For patients who start or stop therapy with a strong CYP3A4 inhibitor, such as itraconazole or ketoconazole, cinacalcet dosage may have to be adjusted.

Drug Administration

P.O.

- Administer drug with food or shortly after a meal.

- Tablet should be swallowed whole and not chewed, crushed, or split.

Route	Onset	Peak	Duration
P.O.	Unknown	2–6 hr	Unknown

Half-life: 30–40 hr

Mechanism of Action

Increases sensitivity of calcium-sensing receptors on the surface of parathyroid cells to extracellular calcium. This sensitivity directly reduces parathyroid hormone (PTH) level, which in turn decreases serum calcium level.

Contraindications

Hypersensitivity to cinacalcet or its components, hypocalcemia

Interactions

DRUGS

CYP2D6 substrates, such as carvedilol, desipramine, metoprolol; drugs that have a narrow therapeutic index, flecainide, tricyclic antidepressants (most): Possibly increased blood level of these drugs
other calcium-lowering drugs, including other calcium-sensing receptor agonists: Increased risk of severe hypocalcemia
strong CYP3A4 inhibitors, such as itraconazole, ketoconazole: Possibly increased blood cinacalcet level

Adverse Reactions

CNS: Asthenia, dizziness, **seizures**
CV: **Arrhythmias**, hypertension, **hypotension** (in the presence of impaired cardiac function), **worsening heart failure** (in the presence of impaired cardiac function)
GI: Anorexia, diarrhea, **gastrointestinal bleeding**, nausea, vomiting
MS: Adynamic bone disease, myalgia
SKIN: Rash, urticaria
Other: Acute pseudogout, **angioedema**, **hypersensitivity reaction**, **hypocalcemia**, noncardiac chest pain

Childbearing Considerations

PREGNANCY

- It is not known if drug can cause fetal harm.
- Use with caution only if benefit to mother outweighs potential risk to fetus.

LACTATION

- It is not known if drug is present in breast milk.
- Mothers should check with prescriber before breastfeeding.

Nursing Considerations

- Be aware that cinacalcet is not recommended for use in patients with chronic kidney disease who are not on dialysis because of an increased risk of hypocalcemia.
- Use cinacalcet cautiously in patients with a history of seizures because reduced blood calcium level may lower seizure threshold. Also, use cautiously in patients with hepatic insufficiency because cinacalcet metabolism may be reduced.

! WARNING Monitor patient for a hypersensitivity reaction that may become life-threatening such as angioedema. If present, notify prescriber promptly; expect to withhold drug, as ordered; and provide supportive care, as needed and ordered.

! WARNING Monitor patient for hypocalcemia exhibited by cramping, myalgia, paresthesia, prolonged QT interval that may cause ventricular arrhythmias, seizures, and tetany. Also, monitor patient's blood calcium and phosphorus levels within 1 week after starting therapy and when adjusting dosage. If hypocalcemia develops, notify prescriber immediately because treatment to raise calcium level will be needed. Treatment may include giving supplemental calcium, starting or increasing dosage of calcium-based phosphate binder or vitamin D sterols, or temporarily withholding cinacalcet.

- Monitor dialysis patient's intact PTH levels 1 to 4 weeks after therapy starts and when dose is adjusted and then every 1 to 3 months thereafter, as ordered. Keep in mind that adynamic bone disease may develop if iPTH levels drop below 100 mg/ml. Expect to reduce dosage or discontinue cinacalcet, as ordered, in a patient whose intact PTH level falls below the target range of 150 to 300 pg/ml.

! **WARNING** Monitor patient for worsening of common GI adverse reactions of nausea and vomiting and for signs and symptoms of GI bleeding and ulcerations. Risk factors include esophagitis, gastritis, severe vomiting, or ulcers. Notify prescriber if such symptoms are present and provide supportive care, as ordered.

PATIENT TEACHING

- Instruct patient how to administer cinacalcet.

! **WARNING** Alert patient that drug may cause an allergic reaction. If present, tell patient to notify prescriber and to seek immediate medical care, if severe.

! **WARNING** Review signs and symptoms of hypocalcemia with patient and urge him to notify prescriber, if signs/symptoms present.

! **WARNING** Advise patient to report any symptoms of GI bleeding, nausea, or vomiting to prescriber.

- Alert patient with heart failure that cinacalcet may worsen heart failure, requiring additional monitoring of their condition or treatment.
- Inform patient that regular blood tests will be ordered to monitor the safe use of cinacalcet. Stress importance of complying with testing schedule.

ciprofloxacin

Cipro, Cipro I.V.

Class and Category

Pharmacologic class: Fluoroquinolone derivative
Therapeutic class: Antibiotic

Indications and Dosages

✱ *To prevent inhalation anthrax after exposure*

I.V. INFUSION FOLLOWED BY ORAL SUSPENSION OR TABLETS

Adults. 400 mg I.V. every 12 hr and then switched to 500 mg P.O. every 12 hr, as soon as possible, for a total of 60 days.
Children. 10 mg/kg I.V. every 12 hr and then switched to 15 mg/kg P.O. every 12 hr, as soon as possible, for a total of 60 days. *Maximum:* 400 mg per dose I.V.; 500 mg per dose P.O.

✱ *To treat acute sinusitis caused by susceptible organisms*

ORAL SUSPENSION, TABLETS

Adults. 500 mg every 12 hr for 10 days.

I.V. INFUSION

Adults. 400 mg every 12 hr for 10 days.

✱ *To treat bone and joint infections caused by susceptible organisms*

ORAL SUSPENSION, TABLETS

Adults. *For mild to moderate infections:* 500 mg every 12 hr for 4 to 8 wk. *For severe or complicated infections:* 750 mg every 12 hr for 4 to 8 wk.

I.V. INFUSION

Adults. *For mild to moderate infections:* 400 mg every 12 hr for 4 to 8 wk. *For severe or complicated infections:* 400 mg every 8 hr for 4 to 8 wk.

✱ *To treat skin and soft-tissue infections caused by susceptible organisms*

ORAL SUSPENSION, TABLETS

Adults. *For mild to moderate infections:* 500 mg every 12 hr for 7 to 14 days. *For severe or complicated infections:* 750 mg every 12 hr for 7 to 14 days.

I.V. INFUSION

Adults. *For mild to moderate infections:* 400 mg every 12 hr for 7 to 14 days. *For severe or complicated infections:* 400 mg every 8 hr for 7 to 14 days.

✱ *To treat chronic bacterial prostatitis caused by susceptible organisms*

ORAL SUSPENSION, TABLETS

Adults. 500 mg every 12 hr for 28 days.

I.V. INFUSION

Adults. 400 mg every 12 hr for 28 days.

✱ *To treat infectious diarrhea caused by susceptible organisms*

ORAL SUSPENSION, TABLETS

Adults. 500 mg every 12 hr for 5 to 7 days.

✱ *To treat UTI caused by susceptible organisms*

ORAL SUSPENSION, TABLETS

Adults. *For mild to moderate infections:* 250 mg every 12 hr for 7 to 14 days. *For severe or complicated infections:* 500 mg every 12 hr for 7 to 14 days.

I.V. INFUSION

Adults. *For mild to moderate infections:* 200 mg every 12 hr for 7 to 14 days. *For* *severe or complicated infections:* 400 mg every 8 hr for 7 to 14 days.

∗ *To treat complicated UTI or pyelonephritis*

ORAL SUSPENSION, TABLETS

Children from ages 1 to 17. *For mild to moderate infections:* 10 mg/kg every 12 hr for 10 to 21 days. *For severe infections*: 20 mg/kg every 12 hr for 10 to 21 days. *Maximum:* 750 mg per dose.

I.V. INFUSION

Children ages 1 to 17. 6 to 10 mg/kg every 8 hr for 10 to 21 days.

∗ *To treat acute uncomplicated cystitis*

ORAL SUSPENSION, TABLETS

Adults. 250 mg every 12 hr for 3 days.

∗ *To treat or prevent plague, including pneumonic and septicemic plague, due to* Yersinia pestis

ORAL SUSPENSION, TABLETS

Adults. 500 to 750 mg every 12 hr for 14 days.
Children. 15 mg/kg every 8 to 12 hr for 14 days. *Maximum:* 500 mg/dose.

I.V. INFUSION

Adults. 400 mg every 8 to 12 hr for 14 days.
Children. 10 mg/kg every 8 to 12 hr for 14 days. *Maximum:* 400 mg/dose.

∗ *To treat lower respiratory tract infections caused by susceptible organisms*

ORAL SUSPENSION, TABLETS

Adults. *For mild to moderate infections:* 500 mg every 12 hr for 7 to 14 days. *For severe or complicated infections:* 750 mg every 12 hr for 7 to 14 days.

I.V. INFUSION

Adults. *For mild to moderate infections:* 400 mg every 12 hr for 7 to 14 days. *For severe or complicated infections:* 400 mg every 8 hr for 7 to 14 days.

∗ *To treat nosocomial pneumonia caused by susceptible organisms*

I.V. INFUSION

Adults. 400 mg every 8 hr for 10 to 14 days.

∗ *To treat complicated intra-abdominal infections caused by susceptible organisms*

ORAL SUSPENSION, TABLETS

Adults. 500 mg every 12 hr for 7 to 14 days.

I.V. INFUSION

Adults. 400 mg every 12 hr for 7 to 14 days.

∗ *To treat typhoid fever caused by susceptible organisms*

ORAL SUSPENSION, TABLETS

Adults. 500 mg every 12 hr for 10 days.

∗ *To treat uncomplicated urethral or cervical gonococcal infections caused by* N. gonorrhoeae

ORAL SUSPENSION, TABLETS

Adults. 250 mg as a single dose.

∗ *To provide empirical therapy in febrile neutropenic patients*

I.V. INFUSION

Adults. 400 mg every 8 hr for 7 to 14 days given concomitantly with piperacillin.

∗ *To treat acute otitis externa caused by* Pseudomonas aeruginosa *or* Staphylococcus aureus

OTIC SUSPENSION 0.2%

Children ages 1 yr and older. Contents of one single-dose container (0.25 ml) instilled into the affected ear twice daily about 12 hr apart for 7 days.

±**DOSAGE ADJUSTMENT** For adult patients with a creatinine clearance of 30 to 50 ml/min taking oral suspension or tablets, dosage reduced to 250 to 500 mg every 12 hours; if creatinine clearance is 5 to 29 ml/min, dosage reduced to 250 to 500 mg every 18 hours. For adult patients on dialysis, dosage reduced to 250 mg to 500 mg every 24 hours and given after dialysis. For adult patients receiving drug intravenously and who have a creatinine clearance between 5 to 29 ml/min, dosage reduced to 200 to 400 mg every 18 to 24 hours. No manufacturer's guidelines given for dosage adjustment in children with impaired renal function.

Drug Administration

- Ensure patient is adequately hydrated throughout therapy to prevent formation of highly concentrated urine that could lead to crystalluria.

P.O.

- E.R. and immediate-release tablets aren't interchangeable.
- Tablets are scored and may be split in half to provide correct dosage. Tablets should be swallowed without chewing or crushing.
- Administer with a main meal, preferably the evening meal.
- To mix oral suspension, know that the small bottle contains the microcapsules and the large bottle contains the diluent. Open both bottles and pour the microcapsules

completely into the larger bottle of diluent. Do not add water to the suspension. Remove the top layer of the diluent bottle label to reveal the Cipro Oral Suspension label. Close the large bottle according to the directions on the cap and shake vigorously for about 15 sec. Write expiration date on bottle label.

- Reconstituted drug may be stored at room temperature for 14 days. Avoid freezing suspension.
- To administer oral suspension, shake bottle vigorously for 15 sec prior to dose. Use the co-packaged graduated teaspoon provided. Tell patient not to chew the microcapsules in the suspension but to swallow them whole. Give patient water to drink after administration.
- Wash the graduated spoon afterwards with soap and water and dry thoroughly.
- Oral suspension should not be administered through a feeding or nasogastric tube.
- Administer at least 2 hr before or 6 hr after aluminum/magnesium antacids; polymeric phosphate binders (lanthanum carbonate, sevelamer) or sucralfate; didanosine chewable or buffered tablets or pediatric powder for oral solution; other highly buffered drugs; or products containing calcium, iron, or zinc.
- Do not administer drug with dairy products or calcium-fortified juices; however, drug may be given with a meal that contains these products.
- For missed dose, administer as soon as possible but no later than 6 hr prior to the next scheduled dose. If less than 6 hr remains before the next dose, missed dose should be skipped.

I.V.

- Intravenous drug comes in a premixed solution in flexible containers of 200 ml. The solution in the flexible containers need not be diluted.
- Administer infusion over 60 min.
- Slowing infusion and administering drug into a larger vein will minimize patient discomfort and reduce the risk of venous irritation.
- *Incompatibilities:* Aminophylline, amoxicillin, cefepime, clindamycin, dexamethasone, floxacillin, furosemide, heparin, phenytoin

OTIC DROPS

- Warm solution by holding container in hands for at least 1 min, to minimize dizziness that may occur from instilling a cold solution into the ear canal.
- Have patient lie with the affected ear upward. Instill solution. Have patient maintain position for at least 1 min. Repeat, if needed for the opposite ear.
- Discard unused portion.

Route	Onset	Peak	Duration
P.O.	Unknown	1–2 hr	Unknown
P.O./E.R.	Unknown	1–4 hr	Unknown
I.V.	Unknown	Unknown	Unknown
Otic	Unknown	Unknown	Unknown

Half-life: 3–5 hr

Mechanism of Action

Inhibits the enzyme DNA gyrase, which is responsible for the unwinding and supercoiling of bacterial DNA before it replicates. By inhibiting this enzyme, ciprofloxacin causes bacterial cells to die.

Contraindications

Concurrent therapy with tizanidine; hypersensitivity to ciprofloxacin, other quinolones, or their components

Interactions

DRUGS

antacids, didanosine, iron supplements, multivitamins that contain iron or zinc sucralfate: Decreased ciprofloxacin absorption
caffeine, clozapine, duloxetine, methotrexate, methylxanthines, olanzapine, ropinirole, sildenafil, zolpidem: Increased plasma levels of these drugs and increased risk of serious adverse reactions, including toxicity
cyclosporine: Elevated serum creatinine
drugs that prolong QT interval, such as class IA or III antiarrhythmics, antipsychotics, macrolides, tricyclic antidepressants: Increased risk of further QT prolongation
NSAIDs (except acetylsalicylic acid): Increased risk of seizures with high doses of ciprofloxacin
oral anticoagulants: Enhanced anticoagulant effects
oral hypoglycemics: Possibly increased risk of hypoglycemia that may be severe (especially with glyburide)

phenytoin: Increased or decreased blood phenytoin level
probenecid: Increased blood ciprofloxacin level and, possibly, toxicity
theophylline: Increased risk of CNS or other serious adverse reactions
tizanidine: Potentiation of hypotensive and sedative effects of tizanidine

FOODS

caffeine: Increased caffeine effects
dairy products: Delayed drug absorption

Adverse Reactions

CNS: Abnormal gait, agitation, anxiety, ataxia, **cerebral thrombosis**, confusion delirium, depersonalization, depression, disorientation, disturbance in attention, dizziness, drowsiness, fever, hallucinations, headache, **increased intracranial pressure (pseudotumor cerebri)**, insomnia, irritability, lethargy, light-headedness, malaise, manic reaction, memory impairment, migraine, nervousness, nightmares, paranoia, paresthesia, peripheral neuropathy, phobia, restlessness, **seizures**, **status epilepticus**, **suicidal ideation**, syncope, tremor, toxic psychosis, unresponsiveness, weakness
CV: Angina, **aortic aneurysm and dissection**, **atrial flutter**, **cardiopulmonary arrest**, **cardiovascular collapse**, hypertension, **MI**, orthostatic hypotension, palpitations, phlebitis, **QT prolongation**, tachycardia, **torsades de pointes**, vasculitis, **ventricular arrhythmia or ectopy**
EENT: Oral candidiasis
ENDO: Hyperglycemia, **hypoglycemia**
GI: Abdominal pain, anorexia, ***Clostridioides difficile*–associated diarrhea**, constipation, diarrhea, dysphagia, elevated liver enzymes, flatulence, **GI bleeding**, **hepatic failure or necrosis**, **hepatitis**, indigestion, **intestinal perforation**, jaundice, nausea, **pancreatitis**, **pseudomembranous colitis**, vomiting
GU: **Acute renal failure or insufficiency**, crystalluria, hematuria, increased serum creatinine level, interstitial nephritis, **nephrotoxicity**, renal calculi, urine retention, vaginal candidiasis
HEME: **Agranulocytosis**, **aplastic or hemolytic anemia**, **bone marrow depression**, **leukopenia**, lymphadenopathy, **pancytopenia**, **thrombocytopenia**
MS: Arthralgia, myalgia, tendinitis, tendon rupture
RESP: **Allergic pneumonitis**, **bronchospasm**, **pulmonary embolism**, **respiratory arrest**
SKIN: Acute generalized exanthematous pustulosis (AGEP), **erythema multiforme**, **exfoliative dermatitis**, photosensitivity, rash, **Stevens-Johnson syndrome**, **toxic epidermal necrolysis**, urticaria
Other: **Acidosis**, **anaphylaxis**, **angioedema**, serum sickness–like reaction

Childbearing Considerations

PREGNANCY

- It is not known if drug can cause fetal harm.
- Use with caution only if benefit to mother outweighs potential risk to fetus.

LACTATION

- Drug is present in breast milk.
- A decision should be made to discontinue breastfeeding temporarily during drug therapy or discontinue the drug to avoid potential serious adverse reactions in the breastfed infant except for postexposure with inhalation anthrax. If breastfeeding is temporarily stopped, mother could consider pumping and discarding breast milk during therapy and for an additional 2 days after the last dose.
- If breastfeeding does occur, mother should monitor her breastfed infant for bloody or loose stools and candidiasis (diaper rash, thrush).

Nursing Considerations

- Obtain culture and sensitivity test results, as ordered, before giving ciprofloxacin.
- Know that ciprofloxacin should not be used in a patient with myasthenia gravis as it may exacerbate muscle weakness.

! **WARNING** Know that ciprofloxacin should not be given to patients with a known aortic aneurysm or patients who are at greater risk for aortic aneurysms, unless no alternative antibacterial treatment is available. This is because studies suggest an increased risk of aortic aneurysm and dissection within 2 months following use of fluoroquinolones, especially in the elderly.

! **WARNING** Use drug with extreme caution in patients who may be more susceptible to drug's effect on QT interval, such as those taking class IA or III antiarrhythmics; those with uncorrected hypokalemia or hypomagnesemia; or in the presence of a history of cardiac disease, such as heart failure, QT-interval prolongation, or torsades de pointes.

! **WARNING** Use drug cautiously in patients with CNS disorders and disorders that may predispose patient to seizures, such as history of epilepsy or conditions that may lower the seizure threshold, such as history of altered brain structure, reduced cerebral blood flow, severe cerebral arteriosclerosis, or stroke. Take seizure precautions. If a seizure occurs, expect ciprofloxacin to be discontinued immediately.

- Be aware that patient should be well hydrated during therapy to help prevent alkaline urine, which may lead to crystalluria and nephrotoxicity.

! **WARNING** Monitor patient for hypersensitivity reactions, which may become life-threatening such as anaphylaxis or angioedema. A hypersensitivity reaction may occur as soon as after the first dose. Some reactions maybe accompanied by acute myocardial ischemia with or without MI, cardiovascular collapse, dyspnea, facial or pharyngeal edema, itching, loss of consciousness, tingling, or urticaria. If a hypersensitivity reaction occurs, notify prescriber immediately, stop drug administration, and be prepared to provide supportive care, as needed and ordered.

! **WARNING** Monitor patient closely for diarrhea, which may indicate pseudomembranous colitis caused by *Clostridioides difficile*–associated diarrhea. It may be mild or become life-threatening. If diarrhea occurs, notify prescriber and expect testing to be done to confirm presence of *C. difficile*. If confirmed, expect to withhold drug, and treat with an antibiotic effective against *C. difficile* along with electrolytes, fluids, and protein, as needed and ordered.

! **WARNING** Monitor patient closely for changes in behavior or mood that may be caused by ciprofloxacin-induced depression or worsening psychotic reactions potentially resulting in self-injurious behavior, such as suicide. Be aware these reactions may occur even after just 1 dose. If present, notify prescriber immediately and expect to discontinue ciprofloxacin therapy, and institute precautions to keep patient safe until adverse effects have disappeared.

! **WARNING** Monitor patient's bleeding time, complete CBC, and prothrombin time, as ordered. Assess patient for adverse blood reactions that could become life-threatening. Expect drug to be discontinued and appropriate therapy instituted if patient develops a serious adverse hematologic reaction. If drug-induced hemolytic anemia is suspected, expect to discontinue drug and provide supportive care, as indicated.

! **WARNING** Assess patient's hepatic and renal functions periodically, as ordered. Report any abnormalities, including signs and symptoms of dysfunction, to prescriber. For example, severe liver toxicity has occurred with ciprofloxacin use (within 1 to 39 days of therapy) and has been associated more frequently with hypersensitivity reactions. If dysfunction occurs, expect drug to be discontinued and provide supportive care, as ordered and needed.

! **WARNING** Monitor patient's blood glucose levels, especially diabetic patients, for signs and symptoms of changes in blood glucose levels. Both symptomatic hyperglycemia and hypoglycemia may occur as a result of ciprofloxacin therapy. Be aware that severe hypoglycemia has occurred when drug has been administered intravenously. If a hypoglycemic reaction occurs in a patient receiving drug intravenously, discontinue administration immediately, notify prescriber, and initiate appropriate emergency treatment for hypoglycemia.

- Assess patient for evidence of peripheral neuropathy. Notify prescriber and expect to stop drug if patient complains of burning, numbness, pain, tingling, or weakness in extremities or if physical examination reveals deficits in light touch, motor strength, pain, position sense, temperature, or vibratory sensation.

- Monitor patients (especially children, elderly patients, patients receiving corticosteroids, and patients who have renal failure or who have had a heart, kidney, or lung transplant) for evidence of tendon rupture, such as inflammation, pain, and swelling at the site. Be aware that tendon rupture may occur within the first 48 hours of therapy, throughout therapy, or months after ciprofloxacin therapy. Notify prescriber about suspected tendon rupture and have patient rest and refrain from exercise until tendon rupture has been ruled out. If present, expect to provide supportive care as ordered.

PATIENT TEACHING

- Instruct patient how to administer oral form of ciprofloxacin prescribed.
- Urge patient to complete the prescribed course of therapy, even if he feels better before it's finished.
- Tell patient not to take drug with calcium-fortified juices or dairy products.
- Advise patient to take ciprofloxacin 2 hours before or 6 hours after antacids, iron supplements, or multivitamins that contain iron or zinc.
- Encourage patient to drink plenty of fluids during therapy to help prevent crystalluria.
- Urge patient to avoid caffeinated products because caffeine may accumulate in the body during ciprofloxacin therapy and cause excessive stimulation.

! **WARNING** Inform patient that an allergic reaction may occur with drug use. Tell patient to notify prescriber, if present and to seek immediate medical care, if serious.

- Urge patient to report watery, bloody stools to prescriber immediately, even if they occur up to 2 months after cephalexin therapy has ended.

! **WARNING** Review signs and symptoms of types of neurologic adverse reactions that may occur with ciprofloxacin therapy. Review seizure precautions. If present, urge patient to notify prescriber. Also inform patient and family or caregiver, depression may occur and become severe causing suicidal ideation. Stress importance of keeping patient safe and seeking immediate medical care for patient if suicidal behavior or thoughts are present.

! **WARNING** Inform patient that drug may cause adverse blood reactions. Encourage compliance with laboratory tests and alert prescriber if bleeding or ecchymosis occurs.

! **WARNING** Instruct patient to seek emergency medical help immediately if sudden back, chest, or stomach pain occurs. Tell patient to stop taking drug and to notify prescriber at first sign of rash or other hypersensitivity reaction.

- Stress importance of notifying prescriber if other persistent, severe, or unusual adverse reactions occur.
- Caution patient to avoid excessive exposure to sunlight or artificial ultraviolet light because severe sunburn may result. Tell patient to notify prescriber if sunburn develops; drug will have to be stopped.
- Urge patient to avoid hazardous activities until CNS effects of drug are known.
- Advise patient to notify prescriber about changes in limb movement or sensation and about inflammation, pain, or swelling over a joint. Urge patient to rest the affected limb at the first sign of discomfort.
- Warn patient, especially diabetic patient, that ciprofloxacin may alter blood glucose levels. Review signs and symptoms of hyperglycemia and hypoglycemia. Tell patient to report symptomatic changes in blood glucose levels immediately to prescriber and review how to treat hypoglycemia.
- Inform mothers who are breastfeeding to consider pumping and discarding breast milk during treatment and an additional 2 days after the last dose. If breastfeeding does occur, mother should monitor her breastfed infant for bloody or loose stools and candidiasis (diaper rash, thrush).

citalopram hydrobromide

Celexa

Class and Category

Pharmacologic class: Selective serotonin reuptake inhibitor (SSRI)
Therapeutic class: Antidepressant

Indications and Dosages

∗ *To treat depression*

ORAL SOLUTION, TABLETS

Adults. *Initial:* 20 mg once daily. Increased to 40 mg daily, after 1 wk, as needed. *Maximum:* 40 mg daily.

CAPSULES

Adults. 30 mg once daily.

±**DOSAGE ADJUSTMENT** For patients taking concomitant CYP2C19 inhibitors, who are poor CYP2C19 metabolizers, who have hepatic impairment, or who are older than 60 years of age, dosage should not exceed 20 mg daily.

Drug Administration

P.O.

- Use calibrated measuring device to measure dose of oral solution.
- Be aware that drug therapy cannot be initiated with capsule form because it is only available in a 30 mg strength and drug therapy is initiated with 20 mg once daily. Also when drug therapy is discontinued, other forms of the drug will need to be used because gradual dosage reduction is required.

Route	Onset	Peak	Duration
P.O.	1–2 wk	4 hr	1–2 days

Half-life: 24–48 hr

Mechanism of Action

Blocks serotonin reuptake by adrenergic nerves, which normally release this neurotransmitter from their storage sites when activated by a nerve impulse. This blocked reuptake increases serotonin levels at nerve synapses, which may elevate mood and reduce depression.

Contraindications

Hypersensitivity to citalopram or its components, pimozide therapy, use within 14 days of MAO inhibitor therapy, including I.V. methylene blue or linezolid

Interactions

DRUGS

amphetamines, antidepressants, buspirone, fentanyl, isoniazid, linezolid, lithium, MAO inhibitors, methylene blue, other selective serotonin reuptake inhibitors (escitalopram, fluoxetine, fluvoxamine, paroxetine, sertraline), opioids, pentamidine, selegiline, serotonin norepinephrine reuptake inhibitors (desvenlafaxine, duloxetine, milnacipran, venlafaxine), St. John's wort, tramadol, triptans, tryptophan: Increased risk of life-threatening serotonin syndrome

anticoagulants, antiplatelets, NSAIDs: Increased risk of bleeding

antipsychotics, class IA and class III antiarrhythmics, CYP2C19 inhibitors, gatifloxacin, methadone, moxifloxacin, pimozide: Increased risk of QT prolongation and torsades de pointes

aspirin, NSAIDs, warfarin: Increased risk of bleeding ranging from ecchymoses to life-threatening hemorrhage

carbamazepine: Possibly increased clearance of citalopram

cimetidine: Possibly increased blood citalopram level and increased risk of QT prolongation

clozapine: Substantial increases in plasma clozapine levels

CNS depressants: Possible potentiated CNS effect

diuretics: Possibly increased risk of hyponatremia

ketoconazole: Decreased peak concentrations of ketoconazole

metoprolol; tricyclic antidepressants, such as desipramine or imipramine: Possibly increased blood levels of these drugs; possibly life-threatening serotonin syndrome

Adverse Reactions

CNS: Agitation, akathisia, amnesia, anxiety, apathy, asthenia, confusion, **CVA**, delirium, depression, dizziness, drowsiness, dyskinesia, fatigue, fever, hypomania, impaired concentration, insomnia, mania, migraine, myoclonus, **neuroleptic malignant syndrome**, paresthesia, **seizures**, **serotonin syndrome**, somnolence, **suicidal ideation**, tremor

CV: Angina, bundle branch block, chest pain, **heart failure**, **MI**, orthostatic hypotension, **prolonged QT interval**, tachycardia, **thrombosis**, **torsades de pointes**, **ventricular arrhythmias**

EENT: Abnormal accommodation, acute-angle glaucoma, blurred vision, decreased sense of smell, dry mouth, epistaxis, nystagmus, rhinitis, sinusitis, stuffy nose, taste perversion

ENDO: Hypoprolactinemia
GI: Abdominal pain, anorexia, diarrhea, flatulence, **GI bleeding or hemorrhage**, **hepatic necrosis**, indigestion, nausea, **pancreatitis**, vomiting
GU: **Acute renal failure**, amenorrhea, anorgasmia, decreased libido, dysmenorrhea, ejaculation disorders, erectile dysfunction, impotence, polyuria, priapism, UTI
HEME: **Abnormal bleeding**, **decreased PT**, **hemolytic anemia**, **thrombocytopenia**
MS: Arthralgia, myalgia, **rhabdomyolysis**
RESP: Cough, upper respiratory tract infection
SKIN: Diaphoresis, ecchymosis, **epidermal necrolysis**, **erythema multiforme**, hematoma, petechiae, pruritus, rash, **Stevens-Johnson syndrome**
Other: **Anaphylaxis and other hypersensitivity reactions**, **angioedema**, discontinuation syndrome, **hyponatremia**, **life-threatening hemorrhages**, weight gain or loss

Childbearing Considerations

PREGNANCY

- Pregnancy exposure registry: 1-844-405-6185 or https://womensmentalhealth.org/research/pregnancyregistry/antidepressants.
- Drug may cause fetal harm if given late in the third trimester. It can be evident as early as immediately after birth with neonate exhibiting constant crying and irritability, feeding difficulty, temperature instability, respiratory distress and/or seizures. Drug may also cause a spontaneous abortion.
- Use with caution only if benefit to mother outweighs potential risk to fetus.

LABOR AND DELIVERY

- Monitor mother exposed to a selective serotonin reuptake inhibitor like citaloram, especially in the month before delivery, for postpartum hemorrhage.

LACTATION

- Drug is present in breast milk.
- Mothers should check with prescriber before breastfeeding.
- If breastfeeding occurs, mother should monitor infant for decreased feeding, excessive somnolence, irritability, restlessness, and weight loss.

Nursing Considerations

! **WARNING** Be aware that citalopram should not be given to patients with congenital long QT syndrome, bradycardia, hypokalemia or hypomagnesemia, recent acute MI, or uncompensated heart failure because of increased risk of prolonged QT interval and torsades de pointes. It should also not be given to patients who are taking other drugs that prolong the QT interval. Expect hypokalemia and hypomagnesemia to be corrected before citalopram therapy is begun. Maximum dosage of 40 mg once a day should not be exceeded because of increased risk for patient to develop a prolonged QT. Also, use citalopram cautiously in patients with other cardiac conditions. ECG monitoring may be ordered to monitor the patient's QT interval and detect the development of serious arrhythmias.

- Know that citalopram therapy should not be prescribed for patients with untreated angle-closure glaucoma because drug may trigger an angle closure attack in a patient with anatomically narrow angles who does not have a patent iridectomy.
- Use citalopram cautiously in patients with hepatic impairment because citalopram clearance is affected and can lead to increased plasma citalopram levels.

! **WARNING** Use cautiously in patients with a history of seizures because drug may cause seizures. Monitor patient closely and institute seizure precautions.

! **WARNING** Monitor patient for a hypersensitivity reaction that could become life-threatening, such as anaphylaxis. or angioedema. If present, notify prescriber promptly, expect to withhold drug, as ordered, and provide supportive care, as needed and ordered.

! **WARNING** Monitor patient for suicidal tendencies, especially when therapy starts and dosage changes.

! **WARNING** Monitor patient for bleeding events because citalopram increases risk of bleeding. Bleeding can range from being mild to causing life-threatening hemorrhages. Concomitant use of aspirin, NSAIDs, other anticoagulants or antiplatelet drugs, and warfarin increases bleeding risk. Also, patients taking selective serotonin reuptake inhibitors are especially at increased risk for GI bleeding. Monitor patient closely throughout drug therapy and notify prescriber at first sign of bleeding.

! WARNING Monitor patient for adverse neurologic reactions that could be quite serious, including change in patient's mood leading to suicidal ideation, especially when drug therapy starts and when dosage changes occur. Also, monitor patient for possible serotonin syndrome, when dosage increases. Signs and symptoms may include agitation, chills, confusion, diaphoresis, diarrhea, fever, hyperactive reflexes, poor coordination, restlessness, shaking, talking, or acting with uncontrolled excitement, tremor, and twitching. In its most severe form, serotonin syndrome can resemble neuroleptic malignant syndrome, which includes autonomic instability, a high fever, or muscle rigidity with possible changes in mental status and vital signs.

! WARNING Assess patients for signs and symptoms suggesting hyponatremia and monitor patient's serum sodium level closely. Be aware that in many cases the syndrome of inappropriate secretion of antidiuretic hormone is the underlying cause. Know that elderly patients, those who are volume depleted, and those taking diuretics are at increased risk for developing hyponatremia. If hyponatremia develops, notify prescriber, expect drug to be discontinued, and expect to provide treatment prescribed to raise the serum sodium level.

- Be aware that effective antidepressant therapy may activate hypomania or mania in predisposed people. If patient develops symptoms of hypomania or mania, notify prescriber immediately and expect to discontinue citalopram.
- Expect to reduce dosage gradually when drug is no longer needed to avoid serious adverse reactions associated with discontinuation syndrome such as agitation, anxiety, confusion, dizziness, dysphoric mood, emotional lability, headache, hypomania, insomnia, irritability, lethargy, nausea, sweating, sensory disturbances, seizures, tinnitus, and tremor.

PATIENT TEACHING

- Instruct patient how to administer citalopram.
- Inform patient that citalopram's full effects may take up to 4 weeks.

! WARNING Caution patient to never abruptly discontinue taking citalopram because withdrawal syndrome may occur that could be quite serious.

! WARNING Alert patient that drug may cause an allergic reaction. Tell patient to notify prescriber if an allergic reaction occurs and to seek immediate medical care, if reaction is severe.

! WARNING Urge family or caregiver to monitor patient closely for suicidal tendencies, especially when therapy starts or dosage changes. Also, tell them drug may activate hypomania or mania. Instruct them to notify prescriber, if present.

! WARNING Urge patient, family, or caregiver to report persistent, severe, sudden, or unusual adverse reactions promptly to prescriber. Although uncommon, life-threatening adverse effects may occur such as GI hemorrhage. Advise patient to seek immediate emergency care if adverse effects are serious.

- Caution against taking over-the-counter aspirin, NSAIDs, or other remedies (including herbal products, such as St. John's wort) while taking citalopram because they may increase the risk of bleeding. Advise patient not to self-medicate for allergies, colds, or coughs without consulting prescriber because these preparations can increase the risk of adverse reactions.
- Advise patient that drug may cause mild pupillary dilation, which may lead to an episode of acute closure glaucoma. Encourage patient to have an eye exam before starting therapy to see if he is at risk.
- Alert patient that use of drug may cause symptoms of sexual dysfunction in both

females and males. Tell patient to discuss concerns with prescriber.

- Advise females of childbearing age to notify prescriber if pregnancy occurs.
- Instruct mothers who are breastfeeding to monitor their infant for excess sedation, irritability, poor feeding, poor weight gain, and restlessness. If present, the mother should notify pediatrician.

cladribine

Mavenclad

Class and Category

Pharmacologic class: Purine antimetabolite
Therapeutic class: Anti-multiple sclerosis

Indications and Dosages

✱ *To treat relapsing forms of multiple sclerosis (MS), to include active secondary progressive disease and relapsing-remitting disease, in patients who have had an inadequate response to, or are unable to tolerate, an alternate drug indicated for the treatment of MS*

TABLETS

Adults. 3.5 mg/kg divided into 2 yearly treatment courses (1.75 mg/kg/treatment course with each treatment course further divided into 2 treatment cycles). First course/first cycle is begun at any time, followed by first course/second cycle administered 23 to 27 days after last dose of first course/first cycle. Second course/first cycle administered at least 43 wk after last dose of first course/second cycle. Second course/second cycle administered 23 to 27 days after last dose of second course/first cycle. Each cycle dosage divided over 4 to 5 consecutive days with once-daily dose given as one or two 10-mg tablets. No more than 20 mg given once daily. Cycle dosage based on weight as follows:
For adults weighing 110 kg (242 lb) or above. 100 mg for cycle one and 100 mg for cycle two.
For adults weighing 100 kg (220 lb) to less than 110 kg (242 lb). 100 mg for cycle one and 90 mg for cycle two.
For adults weighing 90 kg (198 lb) to less than 100 kg (220 lb). 90 mg for cycle one and 80 mg for cycle two.
For adults weighing 80 kg (176 lb) to less than 90 kg (198 lb). 80 mg for cycle one and 70 mg for cycle two.
For adults weighing 70 kg (154 lb) to less than 80 kg (176 lb). 70 mg for cycle one and 70 mg for cycle two.
For adults weighing 60 kg (132 lb) to less than 70 kg (154 lb). 60 mg for cycle one and 60 mg for cycle two.
For adults weighing 50 kg (110 lb) to less than 60 kg (132 lb). 50 mg for cycle one and 50 mg for cycle two.
For adults weighing 40 kg (88 lb) to less than 50 kg (110 lb). 40 mg for cycle one and 40 mg for cycle two.

Drug Administration

P.O.

- Drug is a cytotoxic drug and requires special handling and disposal procedures. The patient should handle the tablets with dry hands. Ensure patient washes hands after touching tablets.
- If tablet is left on a surface, or if a broken or fragmented tablet is released from the blister pack, the area must be thoroughly washed with water.
- Upon removal from blister pack, tablets should immediately be swallowed whole and taken with water.
- Tablets should not be chewed or crushed.
- Have patient avoid prolonged skin contact with tablets.
- Separate doses of drug from other oral drugs by at least 3 hr during the 4- to 5-day treatment cycles.

Route	Onset	Peak	Duration
P.O.	Unknown	0.5–1.5 hr	Unknown

Half-life: 24 hr

Mechanism of Action

May involve cytotoxic effects on B and T lymphocytes through impairment of DNA synthesis, resulting in depletion of lymphocytes.

Contraindications

Active chronic infections such as hepatitis or tuberculosis (TB), breastfeeding (avoid for 10 days following last dose), females and males of childbearing age who do not plan to use effective contraception during cladribine therapy and for 6 mo after last dose in each treatment course, HIV infection, hypersensitivity to cladribine or its components, current malignancy, pregnancy

Interactions

DRUGS

antiviral and antiretroviral drugs, such as lamivudine, ribavirin, stavudine, zalcitabine, zidovudine: Possible interference with cladribine effectiveness

hepatotoxic drugs: Increased risk of serious adverse reactions because of additive hematological effects

immunomodulatory, immunosuppressive, myelosuppressive drugs: Increased risk of serious adverse reactions because of additive effects on immune system

interferon-beta: Possibly increased lymphopenia risk

potent BCRP CNT, ENT transporter inhibitors, such as cilostazol, curcumin, cyclosporine, dilazep, dipyridamole, eltrombopag, nifedipine, reserpine, ritonavir, sulindac: Possible alteration of bioavailability, intracellular distribution, and renal elimination of cladribine

potent BCRP and P-gp transporter inducers: Possible decreased exposure of cladribine, decreasing effectiveness

Adverse Reactions

CNS: Depression, fever, headache, insomnia, **seizures**, vertigo
CV: **Cardiac failure**, hypertension
EENT: Diplopia, mucous membrane ulceration, oral herpes, **throat swelling**
GI: **Activation of latent hepatitis infections**, anorexia, elevated bilirubin and liver enzymes, **fulminant hepatitis**, jaundice, **liver injury**, nausea
GU: Pyelonephritis
HEME: Anemia, **decreased platelet count**, **lymphopenia**, **neutropenia**, **pancytopenia**, **thrombocytopenia**
MS: Arthralgia, back pain
RESP: Bronchitis, upper respiratory infection
SKIN: Alopecia, dermatitis, pruritus, rash
Other: Bacterial, fungal, herpes viral, opportunistic, TB infections; **hypersensitivity reactions**; **malignancies**

Childbearing Considerations

PREGNANCY

- Pregnancy exposure registry: 1-800-283-8088, ext 5563 or FAX: 1-781-681-2961.
- A negative pregnancy test must be obtained before drug therapy begins.
- Drug causes fetal harm.
- Drug is contraindicated during pregnancy.
- If pregnancy occurs during treatment, drug must be discontinued.

LACTATION

- It is not known if drug is present in breast milk.
- Drug is contraindicated in breastfeeding mothers.

REPRODUCTION

- Females of childbearing age should use effective contraception during cladribine therapy and for at least 6 months after last dose of each yearly treatment course because drug interferes with DNA synthesis. A barrier method should be added during drug dosing and for 4 weeks after last dose in each treatment course if females of childbearing age are using systematically acting hormonal contraceptives because it is unknown if cladribine may reduce effectiveness of this type of contraception.
- Male patients should take precautions to prevent pregnancy in their female partner of childbearing age by using effective contraception during cladribine therapy and for 6 months after last dose in each yearly treatment course because drug interferes with DNA synthesis.
- Pregnancy should immediately be reported to prescriber.

Nursing Considerations

- Know that cladribine is not recommended for patients with clinically isolated syndrome because drug is deemed unsafe in the treatment of this syndrome.

! **WARNING** Be aware that cladribine may increase the risk of malignancy and is contraindicated in patients who currently have a malignancy. Expect patient to be screened for cancer before cladribine therapy begins and follow standard cancer screening guidelines during and after drug therapy. Know that as an antineoplastic drug, the intravenous form of drug is used to treat hairy cell leukemia.

! **WARNING** Know that drug is not recommended for patients with moderate to severe hepatic impairment as drug may cause significant and even life-threatening liver injury. Expect to obtain alkaline phosphatase, serum aminotransferase, and total bilirubin levels prior to each treatment cycle and course. Monitor patients, especially patients with mild hepatic impairment or patients taking other hepatotoxic drugs for liver dysfunction (abdominal pain, anorexia, dark urine, fatigue, jaundice, unexplained nausea, or vomiting). If present, notify prescriber and expect serum transaminases and total bilirubin to be measured. If elevated, expect drug therapy to be interrupted or discontinued.

! **WARNING** Ensure that all females of childbearing age as well as partners who are of childbearing age of male patients have had a negative pregnancy test prior to cladribine therapy because drug can cause fetal harm.

- Ensure that CBCs, with differential, including lymphocyte count, are performed as follows: before initiating first course, before initiating second course, 2 to 3 months after starting treatment in each treatment course (if lymphocyte count at month 2 is below 200 cells/microliter, expect monthly monitoring until month 6), and periodically thereafter and when clinically indicated. Lymphocytes must be within normal limits before initiating first treatment course and at least 800 cells/microliter before initiating second treatment course. Expect drug to be withheld if lymphocyte count is below 200 cells/microliter. Expect to administer antiherpes prophylaxis in patients with lymphocyte counts less than 200 cells/microliter, as ordered. Second treatment course may have to be delayed for up to 6 months to allow for recovery of lymphocytes to reach at least 800 cells/microliter. However, if recovery takes longer than 6 months, expect drug to be discontinued.

! **WARNING** Be aware that serious and sometimes life-threatening infection may occur with cladribine therapy. Assess patient for the presence of infection prior to starting cladribine therapy. This includes evaluating patient for acute infection (cladribine therapy may have to be delayed until infection is under control). HIV infection, active TB, and active hepatitis must be excluded before initiation of each treatment course. Then monitor patient closely throughout drug therapy for evidence of an infection. Notify prescriber if signs and symptoms of an infection are present.

- Expect to obtain a baseline (within 3 months) magnetic resonance imaging prior to first treatment course because of risk of progressive multifocal leukoencephalopathy (PML). Also, expect to assess alkaline phosphatase, total bilirubin, and serum aminotransferase levels prior to starting cladribine therapy.
- Administer all immunizations, as ordered, according to immunization guidelines prior to starting cladribine therapy. Vaccination of patients who are seronegative for varicella zoster virus is recommended prior to drug treatment. Vaccination with zoster vaccine recombinant adjuvanted is recommended for patients who are seropositive to varicella zoster virus. either prior to initiation or during drug treatment, including when patient's lymphocyte counts are less than or equal to 500 cells/microliter. Expect to administer live-attenuated or live vaccines at least 4 to 6 weeks prior to starting drug therapy.

! **WARNING** Monitor patient for hypersensitivity reactions, which may become severe such as swelling of the throat. If present, stop cladribine immediately and notify prescriber. Provide supportive emergency care, as needed and ordered.

- Monitor patient for heart failure such as edema, irregular or rapid heartbeat, or shortness of breath because cladribine may induce heart failure.

! **WARNING** Monitor patient for signs and symptoms of progressive multifocal leukoencephalopathy (PML), such as changes in memory, orientation, or thinking leading to confusion and personality changes, as well as clumsiness of limbs, progressive weakness on one side of the body, and visual disturbances. Although no reports of PML have occurred with cladribine for treating relapsing forms of

MS, it is a possibility. At first sign of PML, notify prescriber, expect cladribine to be withheld, and ensure that appropriate diagnostic evaluation is done. Know that MRI findings may reveal problems before clinical signs or symptoms appear.

! **WARNING** Be aware that if patient requires a blood transfusion, irradiation of cellular blood components is recommended, prior to administration, to decrease risk of transfusion-related graft-versus-host disease. Expect a hematologist to be consulted.

! **WARNING** Be aware that following the administration of 2 treatment courses, drug should not be administered during the next 2 years because of risk of malignancy.

- Monitor patient for signs and symptoms of infection throughout drug therapy, especially if lymphocyte count is below 500 cells/microliter. Know that infections occur in about half of patients, with the most serious being herpes zoster and pyelonephritis. At first sign of infection, notify prescriber because drug therapy may have to be delayed or interrupted. Institute infection control measures.

PATIENT TEACHING

- Instruct patient how to administer cladribine and what to do if a dose is missed.
- Tell patient to separate taking cladribine from all other oral drugs by at least 3 hours during the 4- or 5-day treatment cycles.

! **WARNING** Warn patient that drug is contraindicated in pregnancy because it can cause fetal harm. Tell females of childbearing age and men with female partners of childbearing age to use effective contraception during cladribine therapy and for 6 months after the last dose in each treatment course. If females of childbearing age are using systemically acting hormonal contraceptives, tell them to add a barrier method during cladribine therapy and for at least 4 weeks after the last dose in each treatment course. Stress importance of informing prescriber immediately if pregnancy is suspected or confirmed, as drug must be discontinued.

! **WARNING** Inform patient that once two courses of therapy is given, the drug cannot be administered again for 2 years.

! **WARNING** Alert patient that drug may cause an allergic reaction. If an allergic reaction occurs, tell patient to notify prescriber and if severe, to seek immediate medical care.

! **WARNING** Tell patient to notify prescriber immediately if edema, irregular or rapid heartbeat, or shortness of breath occurs.

! **WARNING** Inform patient that liver injury may occur with drug therapy. Review signs and symptoms of liver dysfunction with patient and stress importance of notifying prescriber, if present.

- Stress importance of complying with laboratory appointments and cancer screening.
- Review infection control measures to take while receiving cladribine. Tell patient to notify prescriber immediately if an infection occurs.
- Advise patient to notify prescriber if persistent, severe, or unusual adverse reactions occur as drug can cause many adverse reactions, some of which could be serious.
- Advise patient to avoid receiving live virus vaccinations during cladribine therapy and to check with prescriber before receiving any vaccinations immediately after drug therapy.
- Tell mothers breastfeeding is contraindicated during drug therapy.

clarithromycin

Class and Category

Pharmacologic class: Macrolide
Therapeutic class: Antibiotic

Indications and Dosages

✱ *To treat pharyngitis and tonsillitis caused by* Streptococcus pyogenes

ORAL SUSPENSION, TABLETS

Adults. 250 mg every 12 hr for 10 days.
Children ages 6 mo and older. 7.5 mg/kg every 12 hr for 10 days.

✱ *To treat acute maxillary sinusitis caused by* Haemophilus influenzae, Moraxella catarrhalis, *or* Streptococcus pneumoniae

ORAL SUSPENSION, TABLETS

Adults. 500 mg every 12 hr for 14 days.
Children ages 6 mo and older. 7.5 mg/kg every 12 hr for 10 days.

E.R. TABLETS

Adults. 1,000 mg every 24 hr for 14 days.

✱ *To treat acute exacerbations of chronic bronchitis caused by* H. influenzae, H. parainfluenzae, M. catarrhalis, *or* S. pneumoniae

ORAL SUSPENSION, TABLETS

Adults. 250 mg every 12 hr for 7 to 14 days if caused by *M. catarrhalis* or *S. pneumoniae*, 500 mg every 12 hr for 7 to 14 days if caused by *H. influenzae*, or 500 mg every 12 hr for 7 days if caused by *H. parainfluenzae*.

E.R. TABLETS

Adults. 1,000 mg every 24 hr for 7 days.

✱ *To treat uncomplicated skin and soft-tissue infections caused by* Staphylococcus aureus *or* S. pyogenes

ORAL SUSPENSION, TABLETS

Adults. 250 mg every 12 hr for 7 to 14 days.
Children ages 6 mo and older. 7.5 mg/kg every 12 hr for 10 days.

✱ *To treat community-acquired pneumonia caused by* Chlamydia pneumoniae, Mycoplasma pneumoniae, *or* S. pneumoniae

ORAL SUSPENSION, TABLETS

Adults. 250 mg every 12 hr for 7 to 14 days.
Children ages 6 mo and older. 7.5 mg/kg every 12 hr for 10 days.

E.R. TABLETS

Adults. 1,000 mg every 24 hr for 7 days.

✱ *To treat community-acquired pneumonia caused by* H. influenzae

ORAL SUSPENSION, TABLETS

Adults. 250 mg every 12 hr for 7 days.

E.R. TABLETS

Adults. 1,000 mg every 24 hr for 7 days.

✱ *To treat community-acquired pneumonia caused by* H. parainfluenzae *or* M. catarrhalis

E.R. TABLETS

Adults. 1,000 mg every 24 hr for 7 days.

✱ *To treat acute otitis media caused by* H. influenzae, M. catarrhalis, *or* S. pneumoniae

ORAL SUSPENSION, TABLETS

Children ages 6 mo and older. 7.5 mg/kg every 12 hr for 10 days.

✱ *To reduce the risk of active duodenal ulcer recurrence caused by* Helicobacter pylori

ORAL SUSPENSION, TABLETS

Adults. 500 mg every 8 hr for 14 days with omeprazole 40 mg daily in the morning for 14 days. Then, omeprazole continued at 20 mg daily in the morning from days 15 through 28. Alternatively, 500 mg every 12 hr for 14 days with lansoprazole 30 mg and amoxicillin 1 g every 12 hr for 10 to 14 days or 500 mg every 12 hr with omeprazole 20 mg and amoxicillin 1 g every 12 hr for 10 days.

✱ *To prevent or treat* Mycobacterium avium *complex in patients with advanced HIV infection*

ORAL SUSPENSION, TABLETS

Adults. 500 mg every 12 hr.
Children ages 20 mo and older. 7.5 mg/kg every 12 hr.

± **DOSAGE ADJUSTMENT** For patients with severe renal impairment (creatinine clearance less than 30 ml/min), dosage reduced by 50%. For patients with moderate renal impairment (creatinine clearance 30 to 60 ml/min) also taking atazanavir or ritonavir, dosage reduced by 50%. For patients with severe renal impairment (creatinine clearance less than 30 ml/min) also taking atazanavir or ritonavir, dosage reduced by 75%.

Drug Administration

P.O.

- To reconstitute oral granules to make an oral suspension, add 29.5 ml (50 ml volume) or 59 ml (100 ml volume) of water to make a concentration of 125 mg/5 ml or add 28.5 ml (50 ml volume) or 57 ml (100 ml volume) of water to make a concentration of 250 mg/5 ml. Add half amount of water first and shake vigorously followed by second half of water amount and shake again.
- Shake oral suspension well before each use and use a calibrated device to measure dose.
- Oral suspension does not have to be taken with food.
- Store oral suspension at room temperature; do not refrigerate.
- Discard after 14 days.
- Administer E.R. tablets with food. E.R. tablets should not be chewed or crushed but must be swallowed whole.
- Immediate-release tablets can be taken with or without food.

Route	Onset	Peak	Duration
P.O.	Unknown	2–3 hr	Unknown
P.O./E.R.	Unknown	5–8 hr	Unknown

Half-life: 3–7 hr

Mechanism of Action

Inhibits RNA-dependent protein synthesis in many types of aerobic, anaerobic, gram-negative, and gram-positive bacteria. By binding with the 50S ribosomal subunit of the bacterial 70S ribosome, clarithromycin causes bacterial cells to die.

Contraindications

Concurrent therapy with cisapride, colchicine (in patients with renal or hepatic impairment), dihydroergotamine, ergotamine, lomitapide, lovastatin, pimozide, or simvastatin; history of cholestatic jaundice or hepatic dysfunction; hypersensitivity to clarithromycin, erythromycin, or any macrolide antibiotic or their components

Interactions

DRUGS

alfentanil, bromocriptine, cilostazol, cyclosporine, methylprednisolone, phenobarbital, St. John's wort, tacrolimus, vinblastine: Possibly increased risk of adverse reactions
alprazolam, midazolam (oral), triazolam: Possibly increased effects of these triazolobenzodiazepines, including increased and/or prolonged sedation
antiarrhythmics, such as amiodarone, disopyramide, dofetilide, procainamide, quinidine, sotalol: Increased risk of prolonged QT interval, torsades de pointes, or other life-threatening arrhythmias
atazanavir, ritonavir: Increased clarithromycin levels
calcium channel blockers: Increased risk of acute kidney dysfunction and hypotension, especially in patients 65 yr or older
carbamazepine, other drugs metabolized by cytochrome P450 enzyme system, tolterodine: Increased blood levels of these drugs
cisapride, pimozide: Increased risk of cardiac arrhythmias
colchicine: Increased risk of colchicine toxicity
colchicine: Increased risk of life-threatening colchicine toxicity
digoxin: Increased serum digoxin level, increasing risk of toxicity
dihydroergotamine, ergotamine: Risk of acute ergot toxicity
disopyramide: Hypoglycemia, increased risk of torsades de pointes
efavirenz, nevirapine, rifampicin, rifabutin, rifapentine: Decreased concentration of clarithromycin with decreased effectiveness
hexobarbital, phenytoin, valproate: Increased risk of adverse reactions
insulin, oral hypoglycemics such as nateglinide, pioglitazone, repaglinide, rosiglitazone: Increased risk of severe hypoglycemia
itraconazole: Increased plasma concentration of clarithromycin and itraconazole with increased risk of adverse reactions that may become prolonged
lomitapide: Markedly increased transaminases levels
maraviroc: Possibly increased maraviroc exposure, resulting in increased risk of adverse reactions
nifedipine: Potential for hypotension and peripheral edema
omeprazole: Increased clarithromycin concentrations in gastric tissue and mucus
oral anticoagulants: Potentiated anticoagulant effects
quetiapine: Increased quetiapine exposure and related toxicity
rifabutin: Decreased clarithromycin serum levels, increased rifabutin serum levels, increased risk of uveitis
sildenafil, tadalafil, vardenafil: Possibly increased exposure of these phosphodiesterase inhibitors
statins, such as atorvastatin, lovastatin, pravastatin, simvastatin: Increased risk of rhabdomyolysis
theophylline: Increased blood theophylline level
tolterodine: Significant increase in tolterodine level in patients with a deficiency in CYP2D6 activity
verapamil: Increased risk of bradyarrhythmias, hypotension, and lactic acidosis
zidovudine: Decreased blood zidovudine level

Adverse Reactions

CNS: Anxiety, confusion, disorientation, dizziness, fatigue, hallucinations, headache, insomnia, mania, nightmares, **seizures**, somnolence, tremor, vertigo

CV: **Prolonged QT interval**, **ventricular arrhythmias**
EENT: Altered smell, altered taste, glossitis, hearing loss, oral moniliasis, stomatitis, tinnitus, tongue or tooth discoloration
ENDO: **Hypoglycemia**
GI: Abdominal pain, anorexia, **cholestatic hepatitis**, ***Clostridioides difficile*-associated diarrhea**, diarrhea, elevated liver enzymes, **hepatic dysfunction**, **hepatitis**, **hepatotoxicity**, indigestion, jaundice, nausea, **pancreatitis**, **pseudomembranous colitis**, vomiting
GU: Elevated BUN level
HEME: **Increased prothrombin time**, **leukopenia**, **neutropenia**, **thrombocytopenia**
MS: **Rhabdomyolysis**
SKIN: Acute generalized exanthematous pustulosis, Henoch–Schönlein purpura, pruritus, rash, **Stevens-Johnson syndrome**, **toxic epidermal necrolysis**, urticaria
Other: **Anaphylaxis**, **angioedema**, **drug reaction with eosinophilia and systemic symptoms (DRESS)**, new or worsening myasthenia gravis symptoms, superinfection

Childbearing Considerations

PREGNANCY

- It is not known if drug can cause fetal harm.
- Drug should be used with caution during pregnancy only if benefit to mother outweighs potential risk to fetus and if no alternative therapy is available.

LACTATION

- Drug is present in breast milk.
- Mothers should check with prescriber before breastfeeding.

Nursing Considerations

- Expect to obtain a specimen for culture and sensitivity tests before giving first dose.
- Know that clarithromycin therapy should be avoided in patients at risk for QT prolongation, such as uncorrected hypokalemia or hypomagnesemia or significant bradycardia, and in patients receiving class IA or class III antiarrhythmias. Elderly patients are more susceptible to clarithromycin's effect on the QT interval.

! WARNING Be aware that use of clarithromycin in patients with coronary artery disease is not recommended because of an increased risk of heart problems or death that may occur even years after exposure to drug.

! WARNING Monitor patient closely for acute hypersensitivity reactions such as anaphylaxis and serious skin disorders. If a hypersensitivity reaction or skin disorder is present, especially a fever, rash, or swollen lymph nodes, notify prescriber, expect clarithromycin therapy to be discontinued immediately, and provide supportive care, as needed and ordered.

! WARNING Monitor patient for neurological adverse reactions such as seizures that may occur as a result of clarithromycin therapy. Institute seizure precautions.

! WARNING Monitor patient for signs and symptoms of liver dysfunction, especially hepatitis (anorexia, dark urine, jaundice, pruritus, or tender abdomen). Notify prescriber immediately if signs and symptoms are present and expect clarithromycin to be discontinued.

! WARNING Monitor patients with diabetes who are also receiving insulin or oral hypoglycemics closely for hypoglycemia, which could be severe.

! WARNING Monitor patient's hematological status closely and expect bleeding time, CBC, and prothrombin time to be monitored because drug can cause serious adverse reactions such as bleeding that could become life-threatening.

! WARNING Assess patient's bowel pattern daily; severe diarrhea may indicate pseudomembranous colitis caused by *Clostridioides difficile*. It may be mild or become life-threatening. If diarrhea occurs, notify prescriber and expect testing to be done to confirm presence of *C. difficile*. If confirmed, expect to withhold clarithromycin and treat with an antibiotic effective against *C. difficile*, as ordered. Also expect to administer electrolytes, fluids, and protein, as ordered.

- Monitor patient's renal function closely, especially in patients with renal impairment. Be aware that patients with renal impairment may need decreased dosage.

- Assess for signs of superinfection, such as cough or sputum changes, diarrhea, drainage, fever, malaise, or perineal itching.

PATIENT TEACHING

- Instruct patient on how to administer form of clarithromycin prescribed.
- Emphasize importance of taking the full course of clarithromycin exactly as prescribed, even after feeling better because skipped doses or not completing the full course prescribed may hinder drug from eliminating the bacterial infection and increases risk of bacterial resistance.

! **WARNING** Tell patient to report an allergic reaction such as fever, itching, rash, severe nausea, or swollen lymph nodes, and any other persistent, severe, or unusual reaction to prescriber immediately and if severe to seek emergency medical care.

! **WARNING** Urge patient to report bloody, watery stools to prescriber immediately, even if they occur 2 months or more after therapy has ended.

! **WARNING** Advise patient who has coronary artery disease to continue lifestyle modifications and medications for the heart condition because clarithromycin may be associated with increased risk for worsening heart problems or mortality years after the end of clarithromycin therapy. Review signs and symptoms of heart disease with all patients because some patients may not know coronary artery disease is present. Emphasize importance of reporting such signs and symptoms to prescriber even if it is years after exposure to clarithromycin.

! **WARNING** Alert patient and family or caregiver that clarithromycin may cause seizures. Stress importance of notifying prescriber if a seizure occurs and to seek immediate medical attention.

! **WARNING** Advise patient to report signs and symptoms of liver dysfunction immediately to prescriber.

! **WARNING** Instruct patient with diabetes who is also taking insulin or an oral hypoglycemic agent to monitor his blood glucose level closely as changes may occur, especially hypoglycemia. Review how to treat hypoglycemia and instruct patient to notify prescriber if hypoglycemia is severe or occurs frequently.

- Instruct patient not to take over-the-counter or prescription drugs without consulting prescriber.
- Instruct patient not to perform hazardous activities, including driving, until effects on the nervous system, such as confusion and dizziness, are known and resolved.
- Tell patient drug may cause superinfection. Review signs and symptoms with patient and to alert prescriber if they occur.
- Inform patient that buttermilk and yogurt can help maintain intestinal flora and decrease diarrhea.

clindamycin hydrochloride

Cleocin, Dalacin C (CAN)

clindamycin palmitate hydrochloride

Cleocin Pediatric, Dalacin C Flavored Granules (CAN)

clindamycin phosphate

Cleocin, Dalacin C Phosphate (CAN)

Class and Category

Pharmacologic class: Lincosamide
Therapeutic class: Antibiotic

Indications and Dosages

* *To treat gynecological infections caused by anaerobes that occur with endometritis, nongonococcal tubo-ovarian abscess, pelvic cellulitis, and postsurgical vaginal cuff infection; intra-abdominal infections caused by anaerobes, such as occur with intra-abdominal abscess and peritonitis; serious respiratory*

tract infections caused by anaerobes, such as occur with anaerobic pneumonitis, empyema, and lung abscess and those caused by pneumococci, staphylococci, or streptococci; septicemia caused by anaerobes; and serious skin and soft-tissue infections caused by anaerobes, staphylococci, or streptococci

CAPSULES, ORAL SOLUTION

Adults and adolescents. *For serious infections:* 150 to 300 mg every 6 hr. *For severe infections:* 300 to 450 mg every 6 hr. **Children.** *For serious infections:* 8 to 16 mg/kg daily in equally divided doses 3 times daily or 4 times daily. *For severe infections:* 16 to 20 mg/kg/day in equally divided doses 3 times daily or 4 times daily.

I.V. INFUSION, I.M. INJECTION

Adults and adolescents ages 16 and older. *For serious infections:* 600 to 1,200 mg daily in equally divided doses twice daily to 4 times daily. *For severe infections:* 1,200 to 2,700 mg daily in equally divided doses twice daily to 4 times daily. *For life-threatening infections:* Up to 4,800 mg daily in equally divided doses twice daily to 4 times daily.
Children ages 1 mo to 16 yr. 20 to 40 mg/kg daily in equally divided doses 3 times daily or 4 times daily, depending on severity of infection.
Neonates less than age 1 mo. 15 to 20 mg/kg daily in equally divided doses 3 times daily or 4 times daily, depending on severity of infection.
Neonates with postmenstrual age (PMA) greater than or equal to 32 wk but less than or equal to 40 wk. 7 mg/kg every 8 hr.
Neonates with a PMA less than 32 wk. 5 mg/kg every 8 hr.

* *To treat bone and joint infections including acute hematogenous osteomyelitis caused by* Staphylococcus aureus; *as adjunct therapy in surgical treatment of chronic bone and joint infections due to susceptible organisms*

I.V. INFUSION, I.M. INJECTION

Adults and adolescents ages 16 and older. *For serious infections:* 600 to 1,200 mg daily in equally divided doses twice daily to 4 times daily. *For severe infections:* 1,200 to 2,700 mg daily in equally divided doses twice daily to 4 times daily. *For life-threatening infections:* 4,800 mg daily in equally divided doses twice daily to 4 times daily.

Drug Administration

P.O.

- Capsules should be swallowed whole and not chewed, crushed, or opened. Avoid administering capsule form with patient lying down and give drug with at least 8 ounces of water to avoid risk of esophagitis and esophageal ulcer.
- Prepare oral solution 100-ml bottles by adding a large portion but not all of 75 ml of water. Shake vigorously and then add remainder of water for a total of 75 mg/5 ml and shake until the solution is uniform.
- Store at room temperature. Do not refrigerate reconstituted solution, as it may thicken and be difficult to pour.
- Use a calibrated measuring device when measuring oral solution dosage and shake container before measuring dose.
- Discard oral solution after 2 wk.

I.V.

- Be aware drug solution contains benzyl alcohol, which can cause Gasping syndrome in neonates and premature infants. Premature and low birth weight infants may be more likely to develop toxicity.
- Solutions used for diluting drug include 0.9% Sodium Chloride Injection, 5% Dextrose Injection, or Lactated Ringer's Injection (see manufacturer's instructions for complete list).
- The concentration of clindamycin in diluent for infusion should not exceed 18 mg/ml. Infusion rate should not exceed 30 mg/min.
- For intermittent infusion, dilute 300-mg dose with 50 ml and infuse over 10 min; 600-mg dose diluted with 50 ml and infused over 20 min; 900-mg dose diluted with 50 to 100 ml and infused over 30 min; and 1,200-mg dose diluted in 100 ml and infused over 40 min.
- Administration of more than 1,200 mg in a single 1-hr infusion is not recommended.
- Alternatively, a rapid I.V. infusion given over 30 min for first dose followed by a continuous infusion rate that varies between 0.75 mg/min and 1.25 mg/min, depending on the clindamycin level to be maintained, can be administered, if prescribed.
- Prepare drug to be used in the ADD-Vantage system according to manufacturer's guidelines.

C

- Frozen solutions should be thawed at room temperature before use and not refrozen.
- Premixed drug solution for I.V. administration is available in the GALAXY plastic container. Check for minute leaks prior to use by squeezing bag firmly. Do not add add supplementary drugs to solution. Do not use unless solution is clear, and seal is intact.
- Do not use plastic containers in series connections, which could result in air embolism.
- Check I.V. site often for irritation and phlebitis.
- *Incompatibilities:* Aminophylline, ampicillin sodium, barbiturates, calcium gluconate, magnesium sulfate, phenytoin sodium

I.M.

- Single injections greater than 600 mg are not recommended.
- Administer undiluted.

Route	Onset	Peak	Duration
P.O.	Unknown	45–60 min	Unknown
I.V.	Immediate	Immediate	Unknown
I.M.	Unknown	1–3 hr	Unknown

Half-life: 2–3 hr

Mechanism of Action

Inhibits protein synthesis in susceptible bacteria by binding to the 50S subunits of bacterial ribosomes and preventing peptide bond formation, which causes bacterial cells to die.

Contraindications

Hypersensitivity to clindamycin or any of its components

Interactions

DRUGS

CYP3A4 and CYP3A5 inducers: Possibly decreased plasma concentrations of clindamycin decreasing its effectiveness
CYP3A4 and CYP3A5 inhibitors: Possibly increase plasma concentrations of clindamycin with potential for adverse reactions
erythromycin: Possibly blocked access of clindamycin to its site of action
kaolin-pectin antidiarrheals: Decreased absorption of oral clindamycin
neuromuscular blockers: Increased neuromuscular blockade

Adverse Reactions

CNS: Fatigue, headache
CV: **Hypotension**, thrombophlebitis (after I.V. injection)
EENT: Esophagitis, esophageal ulcer, eye pain (topical), glossitis, metallic or unpleasant taste (with high I.V. doses), stomatitis
GI: Abdominal pain, acute kidney injury, ***Clostridioides difficile*–associated diarrhea**, diarrhea, elevated liver enzymes, esophagitis, jaundice, nausea, **pseudomembranous colitis**, vomiting
GU: **Acute renal injury**, cervicitis, renal dysfunction, vaginitis, and vulvar irritation (with vaginal form)
HEME: **Agranulocytosis**, eosinophilia, **leukopenia**, **neutropenia**, **thrombocytopenic purpura**
MS: Polyarthritis
SKIN: Acute generalized exanthematous pustulosis, contact dermatitis (topical), **erythema multiforme**, **exfoliative dermatitis**, irritation, maculopapular rash, pruritus, rash, **Stevens-Johnson syndrome**, **toxic epidermal necrolysis**, urticaria
Other: **Anaphylaxis**; **angioedema**; **drug reaction with eosinophilia and systemic symptoms (DRESS)**; induration, pain, or sterile abscess after injection; superinfection

Childbearing Considerations

PREGNANCY

- It is not known if drug can cause fetal harm.
- Drug should be used with caution during pregnancy, especially during the first trimester, only if benefit to mother outweighs potential risk to fetus.

LACTATION

- Drug is present in breast milk.
- Mothers should check with prescriber before breastfeeding.
- An alternative drug should be substituted if breastfeeding occurs. If this is not possible, infant should be monitored for blood in the stool, diarrhea, and candidiasis (thrush, diaper rash).

Nursing Considerations

- Expect to obtain a specimen for culture and sensitivity testing before giving first dose.
- Use clindamycin cautiously in patients who have a history of asthma, GI disease, or significant allergies; in those with hepatic

or renal dysfunction; and in atopic or elderly patients. Infants and children should be monitored closely for organ system dysfunction.

! **WARNING** Monitor patient closely for acute hypersensitivity reactions such as anaphylaxis or angioedema and serious skin disorders such as DRESS. If a hypersensivity reaction or skin disorder is present, especially a fever, rash, or swollen lymph nodes, notify prescriber, expect drug therapy to be discontinued immediately, and provide supportive care, as needed and ordered.

! **WARNING** Monitor patient's hematological status closely and expect CBC to be monitored because drug can cause serious adverse reactions that could become life-threatening.

! **WARNING** Assess patient's bowel pattern daily; severe diarrhea may indicate pseudomembranous colitis caused by *Clostridioides difficile*. It may be mild or become life-threatening. If diarrhea occurs, notify prescriber and expect testing to be done to determine if diarrhea is caused by *C. difficile*. If confirmed, expect to withhold clindamycin and treat with an antibiotic effective against *C. difficile*, as ordered. Also expect to administer electrolytes, fluids, and protein, as ordered.

- Monitor renal function during drug therapy, particularly in patients with pre-existing renal dysfunction or those taking concomitant nephrotoxic drugs. In case of acute kidney injury, notify prescriber and expect drug to be discontinued when no other etiology is identified.
- Monitor results of CBC, liver enzymes, and platelet counts during prolonged therapy.
- Observe patient for signs and symptoms of superinfection, such as sore mouth and vaginal itching, which may occur 2 to 9 days after therapy begins.

PATIENT TEACHING

- Instruct patient how to take oral form of clindamycin prescribed. If oral form not prescribed, tell patient drug will be administered as an I.M. injection or intraveneously.
- Tell patient to complete the prescribed course of therapy, even if he feels better before it's finished.
- Inform patient that I.M. injection may be painful.

! **WARNING** Tell patient to immediately report an allergic reaction or skin abnormalities such as a fever, rash, or swollen lymph nodes. Instruct patient to notify prescriber if present and to seek immediate medical care, if severe.

! **WARNING** Urge patient to report bloody, watery stools to prescriber immediately, even up to 2 months after drug therapy has ended.

- Tell patient drug may cause superinfection. Review signs and symptoms with patient and to alert prescriber if they occur.
- Inform patient that buttermilk and yogurt can help maintain intestinal flora and decrease diarrhea.
- Advise mothers not to breastfeed because drug does appear in breast milk and cause adverse GI effects for infant. If breastfeeding does occur, tell mother to monitor infant for blood in the stool, diarrhea, and candidiasis (thrush, diaper rash). If present, mother should notify pediatrician.

clonazepam

Klonopin, Klonopin ODT

Class, Category, and Schedule

Pharmacologic class: Benzodiazepine
Therapeutic class: Anticonvulsant, antipanic
Controlled substance schedule: IV

Indications and Dosages

* *As adjunct or to treat Lennox-Gastaut syndrome (petit mal variant) and akinetic and myoclonic seizures; to treat absence seizures (petit mal) in patients who have failed to respond to succinimides*

ORAL DISINTEGRATING TABLETS, TABLETS

Adults and children ages 10 and older or weighing more than 30 kg (66 lb). *Initial:* 1.5 mg daily in divided doses 3 times daily. Increased by 0.5 to 1 mg every 3 days, as needed, until seizures are controlled, or adverse reactions make further increases undesirable. *Maximum:* 20 mg daily.

Children under age 10 weighing 30 kg (66 lb) or less. *Initial:* 0.01 to 0.03 mg/kg daily (not to exceed 0.05 mg/kg/day) in divided doses 2 or 3 times daily. Increased by 0.25 to 0.5 mg every third day up to maintenance dosage unless seizures are controlled, or adverse reactions make further increases undesirable. *Maintenance:* 0.1 to 0.2 mg/kg daily, preferably in 3 equal doses.

* *To treat panic disorder*

ORALLY DISINTEGRATING TABLETS, TABLETS

Adults. *Initial:* 0.25 mg twice daily. Increased, as needed, to 1 mg daily after 3 days. If more than 1 mg daily is required, dosage increased in increments of 0.125 to 0.25 mg twice daily every 3 days until panic disorder is controlled or adverse reactions make further increases undesirable. *Maximum:* 4 mg daily.

Drug Administration

P.O.

- To administer an orally disintegrating tablet, first peel back the foil on the blister. Do not push tablet through foil. Immediately, and using dry gloved hands, remove tablet and place in patient's mouth or have patient place in mouth. It can be swallowed with or without water.
- Regular tablet should be swallowed whole with water. Tablet should not be broken, chewed, or crushed.
- Drug should not be stopped abruptly. When used to treat panic disorder, expect to taper dosage gradually by 0.125 mg twice daily every 3 days, until the drug is completely discontinued.

Route	Onset	Peak	Duration
P.O.	20–40 min	1–4 hr	6–12 hr

Half-life: 17–60 hr

Mechanism of Action

Acts to prevent panic and seizures through unknown mechanisms. However, it is thought drug may potentiate the effects of gamma-aminobutyric acid (GABA), which is an inhibitory neurotransmitter. This action is also thought to suppress the spread of seizure activity caused by seizure-producing foci in the cortex, limbic, and thalamus structures.

Contraindications

Acute–narrow-angle glaucoma; hepatic disease; hypersensitivity to clonazepam, other benzodiazepines, or their components

Interactions

DRUGS

anesthetics, anticonvulsants, antidepressants, antipyschotics, anxiolytics, barbiturates, opioids, other benzodiazepines and CNS depressants, sedative antihistamines, sedative/hypnotics: Increased risk of CNS depression, including significant change in mental status possibly leading to coma, respiratory depression, sedation, and somnolence

carbamazepine, lamotrigine, phenobarbital, phenytoin: Possibly decreased plasma clonazepam levels with potential for interference with its effectiveness

fluconazole: Possibly impaired clonazepam metabolism with potential for exaggerated concentrations and effects

opioids: Increased risk of severe respiratory depression

phenytoin: Possibly altered plasma concentrations of phenytoin

ACTIVITIES

alcohol use: Increased CNS depression, including severe respiratory depression and significant sedation and somnolence

Adverse Reactions

CNS: Abnormal dreams, aggression, agitation, amnesia, anxiety, apathy, ataxia, attention disturbance, confusion, depersonalization, depression, dizziness, drowsiness, emotional lability, excessive dreaming, fatigue, hallucinations, headache, hostility, hysteria, insomnia, irritability, memory loss, nervousness, nightmares, organic disinhibition, psychosis, reduced intellectual ability, sedation, sleep disturbances, **suicidal ideation**

CV: Palpitations

EENT: Blurred vision, eyelid spasm, increased salivation, loss of taste, pharyngitis, rhinitis, sinusitis, yawning

GI: Abdominal pain, anorexia, constipation, increased appetite

GU: Altered libido, difficult ejaculation, dysmenorrhea, dysuria, enuresis, impotence, nocturia, urine retention, UTI

HEME: Anemia, eosinophilia, **leukopenia**, **thrombocytopenia**

MS: Dysarthria, myalgia

RESP: Bronchitis, cough, **respiratory depression**
Other: **Hypersensitivity reaction**, physical and psychological dependence

Childbearing Considerations

PREGNANCY

- Pregnancy exposure registry: 1-888-233-2334 or http://www.aedpregnancyregistry.org/.
- Administration immediately before or during childbirth can cause a syndrome of difficulty feeding, hypothermia, hypotonia, and respiratory depression in the infant after birth. Also, know that if mothers have taken clonazepam during the later stages of pregnancy, their infants can develop neonatal abstinence syndrome or withdrawal that can occur within hours to weeks after birth and persist for hours to months.
- Drug should be used with caution during pregnancy, especially in third trimester, only if benefit to mother outweighs potential risk to fetus.

LABOR AND DELIVERY

- Administration immediately prior to or during childbirth can cause floppy infant syndrome (difficulty feeding, hypothermia, hypotonia, respiratory depression), sedation, and withdrawal which can last up to 14 days.
- Drug is not recommended during labor and delivery.

LACTATION

- Drug is present in breast milk.
- Mothers should check with prescriber before breastfeeding.
- If breastfeeding takes place, monitor infant for drowsiness, poor sucking, poor weight gain, and sedation.

Nursing Considerations

- Assess patient before therapy is begun and throughout therapy for patient's risk for abuse, misuse, and addiction, such as physical and psychological dependence (strong desire or need to increase dose to maintain drug effects) especially in patients with a history of substance abuse. Alert prescriber, if present.
- Use clonazepam cautiously in patients with mixed seizure disorder (because drug can increase the risk of generalized tonic–clonic seizures), renal failure, or troublesome secretions (because clonazepam increases salivation) and in elderly patients (because they're more sensitive to drug's CNS effects). Also, use cautiously in patients with compromised respiratory function and porphyria.
- Monitor patient closely for signs of loss of effectiveness of anticonvulsant activity, especially within the first 3 months of administration. If noted, notify prescriber because a dosage adjustment may reestablish effectiveness.

! WARNING Monitor patient for a hypersensitivity reaction. If present, notify prescriber promptly, withhold drug, as ordered, and provide supportive care, as needed and ordered.

! WARNING Be aware that benzodiazepine therapy like clonazepam should only be used concomitantly with opioids in patients for whom other treatment options are inadequate. If prescribed together, expect dosing and duration of the opioid to be limited. Monitor patient closely for signs and symptoms of decrease in consciousness, including coma, profound sedation, and significant respiratory depression. Notify prescriber immediately and provide emergency supportive care, as death may occur.

! WARNING Monitor patient closely for evidence of suicidal thinking or behavior, especially when therapy starts or dosage changes.

! WARNING Know that chronic maternal use of drug over an extended period of time during pregnancy can result in neonatal opioid withdrawal syndrome (NOWS), which may be life-threatening, if not recognized and treated appropriately. NOWS occurs when a newborn was exposed to opioid drugs like codeine for a prolonged period while in utero.

- Monitor blood drug level, CBC, and liver enzymes during long-term or high-dose therapy, as ordered.
- Be aware that paradoxical and psychiatric reactions have occurred with benzodiazepines. Because clonazepam is a benzodiazepine, monitor patient for aggression, agitation, anger, anxiety,

C

hallucinations, irritability, nightmares, and psychoses. Children and elderly patients are at greater risk of developing paradoxical reactions. If noted, notify prescriber and expect drug to be discontinued gradually.

PATIENT TEACHING

- Instruct patient how to take form of drug prescribed.
- Tell patient to take drug exactly as prescribed. Explain that stopping drug abruptly can cause seizures and withdrawal symptoms. Inform patient that in some cases, protracted withdrawal syndromes have occurred lasting weeks to more than a year.

! **WARNING** Warn patient not to consume alcohol or take an opioid during clonazepam therapy without prescriber knowledge, as severe respiratory depression can occur and may lead to death. Instruct patient to inform all prescribers of clonazepam use, especially if pain medication may be prescribed.

! **WARNING** Alert patient that drug may cause an allergic reaction. If present, tell patient to notify prescriber promptly and if severe to seek immediate medical care.

! **WARNING** Urge family or caregiver to watch patient closely for evidence of suicidal tendencies, especially when therapy starts or dosage changes, and to report concerns to prescriber immediately.

- Instruct patient to report difficulty urinating, palpitations, persistent drowsiness, seizure activity, severe dizziness, and other disruptive adverse reactions.
- Suggest that family or caregiver monitor child's performance in school because clonazepam can cause drowsiness or inattentiveness.
- Warn females of childbearing age who become pregnant while taking clonazepam to notify prescriber of pregnancy.
- Advise mother undertaking breastfeeding to monitor infant for drowsiness, poor sucking, poor weight gain, and sedation. Tell her to notify pediatrician if present.
- Tell patient to let prescriber know about any new drug prescribed by another healthcare provider or before using any new over-the-counter preparations.
- Urge patient to carry medical identification of his seizure disorder and drug therapy.

clonidine

Catapres-TTS

clonidine hydrochloride

Catapres, Dixarit (CAN), Duraclon, Kapvay, Onyda XR

Class and Category

Pharmacologic class: Centrally acting alpha agonist
Therapeutic class: Analgesic, antihypertensive, behavior modifier

Indications and Dosages

✶ To manage hypertension

TABLETS

Adults. *Initial:* 0.1 mg twice daily, increased by 0.1 mg/wk to produce desired response. *Maintenance:* 0.2 to 0.6 mg daily in divided doses. *Maximum:* 2.4 mg daily.

TRANSDERMAL PATCH (CATAPRES-TTS)

Adults. *Initial:* 0.1-mg patch applied every 7 days. After 1 to 2 wk, if blood pressure isn't controlled, two 0.1-mg patches or one 0.2-mg patch applied. Dosage adjusted, as needed, every 7 days. *Maximum:* Two 0.3-mg patches worn at same time.

± **DOSAGE ADJUSTMENT** For elderly patients and patients with renal failure, dosage may be initially reduced. For patients switching from oral form to transdermal patch, on day 1 patch applied and 100% of oral dose given; on second day 50% of oral dose given; on third day 25% of oral dose given; and on fourth day, oral dose discontinued.

✶ To treat attention deficit hyperactivity disorder (ADHD) alone or as adjunct therapy with stimulant drugs

E.R. TABLETS (KAPVAY)

Children ages 6 to 17. *Initial:* 0.1 mg at bedtime, increased in increments of 0.1 mg daily at weekly intervals, as needed, with total daily dosage equally divided and given 2 times daily with equal or higher dose given at bedtime. *Maximum:* 0.4 mg/day.

E.R ORAL SUSPENSION (ONYDA XR)

Children ages 6 and older. *Initial:* 0.1 mg once daily at bedtime, increased in increments of 0.1 mg daily at weekly intervals, as needed. *Maximum:* 0.4 mg once daily.

✳ *As adjunct to relieve severe pain (in cancer patients) that isn't adequately relieved by opioid analgesics alone*

CONTINUOUS EPIDURAL INFUSION (DURACLON)

Adults. *Initial:* 30 mcg/hr. Titrated up or down, as needed, depending on comfort. *Maximum:* 40 mcg/hr.

Children old enough to tolerate epidural infusion. *Initial:* 0.5 mcg/kg/hr. Dosage then adjusted cautiously, as needed.

Drug Administration

P.O.

- E.R. tablets are not interchangeable with immediate-release tablets. E.R. oral suspension is not interchangeable with other clonidine products.
- E.R. tablets should be swallowed whole and never chewed, crushed, or cut.
- Administer once-a-day E.R. tablets at bedtime. If more than 1 daily dose is ordered, administer second dose of an equal or higher split at bedtime.
- Use the oral dosing dispenser and bottle adapter provided with E.R. oral suspension. Ensure that bottle adapter is firmly inserted into the bottle before first use and keep the adapter in place for the duration of the usage of the bottle.
- Gently shake E.R. oral suspension bottle with a smooth up and down motion (to avoid foaming) for at least 10 sec before each administration.
- Discard any unused E.R. oral suspension remaining in bottle after 60 days of first opening bottle.
- Dosage should be decreased by 0.1 mg every 3 to 7 days when it is being discontinued.

TRANSDERMAL

- Apply patch to a nonhairy site of intact skin on chest or upper outer arm.
- If a transdermal patch loosens during 7-day application period, place adhesive overlay directly over patch to ensure adhesion.
- Rotate transdermal sites.
- Remove patch and place a fresh one on another site if skin irritation, rash, or redness develops at patch site.
- Fold used transdermal patch in half with adhesive sides together and discard it out of the reach of children.

EPIDURAL INFUSION

- Dilute 500-mcg/ml strength to final concentration of 100 mcg/ml with 0.9% Sodium Chloride Injection prior to administration. Drug should not be used with a preservative.
- Administered as a continuous infusion by healthcare professional familiar with epidural techniques and patient management problems associated with this route.
- A controlled-infusion device should be used for administration.
- Monitor infusion pump function and inspect the catheter tubing for obstruction or dislodgement to reduce risk of inadvertent abrupt withdrawal of the epidural infusion.

Route	Onset	Peak	Duration
P.O.	30–60 min	1–3 hr	6–10 hr
P.O./E.R.	1–2 wk	7–8 hr	Unknown
Transdermal	2–3 days	2–3 days	7–8 days
Epidural	Unknown	30–60 min	Unknown

Half-life: 12–20 hr

Mechanism of Action

Stimulates peripheral alpha-adrenergic receptors in the CNS to produce transient vasoconstriction and then stimulates central alpha-adrenergic receptors in the brain stem to reduce heart rate, peripheral vascular resistance, and systolic and diastolic blood pressure. Although alpha$_2$ adrenergic receptors in the brain are stimulated, the precise action that calms children with ADHD is unknown. May produce analgesia by preventing transmission of pain signals to the brain at presynaptic and postjunctional alpha$_2$-adrenoreceptors in the spinal cord. With epidural administration, clonidine produces analgesia in body areas innervated by the spinal cord segments in which the drug concentrates.

C

Contraindications

Anticoagulant therapy (epidural infusion); bleeding diathesis (epidural infusion); hypersensitivity to clonidine or its components, including adhesive used in transdermal patch; injection-site infection (epidural infusion)

Interactions

DRUGS

barbiturates, other CNS depressants: Increased depressant effects of these drugs
beta-blockers, calcium channel blockers, digoxin: Additive effects, such as bradycardia and AV block; increased risk of worsened hypertensive response when clonidine is withdrawn (beta-blockers only)
diuretics, other antihypertensive drugs: Increased hypotensive effect
epidural local anesthetics: Prolonged effects of epidural local anesthetics when used with epidural clonidine
fluphenazine: Possible development of acute delirium
tricyclic antidepressants: Decreased antihypertensive effect of clonidine

ACTIVITIES

alcohol use: Enhanced CNS depressant effects of alcohol

Adverse Reactions

CNS: Agitation, delusional perception, depression, dizziness, drowsiness, fatigue, hallucinations, headache, malaise, nervousness, paresthesia, sedation, syncope, weakness, tremor
CV: **Arrhythmias**, **AV block**, **bradycardia (severe)**, chest pain, **congestive heart failure**, orthostatic hypotension, Raynaud's phenomenon
EENT: Accommodation disorder, blurred vision, burning eyes, decreased lacrimation, dry eyes and mouth, salivary gland pain
GI: Constipation, **hepatitis**, mildly elevated liver enzymes, nausea, vomiting
GU: Decreased libido, erectile dysfunction, nocturia
HEME: **Thrombocytopenia**
SKIN: Pruritus, rash, urticaria
Other: **Angioedema**, weight gain, withdrawal symptoms

Childbearing Considerations

PREGNANCY

- Pregnancy exposure registry: 1-866-961-2388 or https://womensmentalhealth.org/adhd-medications/.
- It is not known if drug can cause fetal harm.
- Drug (except for epidural clonidine) should be used with caution during pregnancy only if benefit to mother outweighs potential risk to fetus. Epidural clonidine is contraindicated for use in obstetric, postpartum, or perioperative pain management because it may cause hemodynamic instability.

LACTATION

- Drug is present in breast milk.
- Mothers should check with prescriber before breastfeeding for oral clonidine but breastfeeding or the drug should be discontinued when epidural clonidine is used.
- If breastfeeding occurs, infant should be monitored for symptoms of bradycardia or hypotension, such as lethargy, poor feeding, rapid breathing, or sedation.

REPRODUCTION

- Drug may impair fertility in females and males according to animal studies.

Nursing Considerations

! **WARNING** Be aware that clonidine should not be used in most patients with severe cardiovascular disease or in those who are not hemodynamically stable because of the potential for severe hypotension.

- Use clonidine cautiously in elderly patients, who may be more sensitive to its hypotensive effect.

! **WARNING** Monitor patient for a hypersensitivity reaction which could become life-threatening, such as angioedema. If present, notify prescriber promptly; expect drug to be withheld, as ordered; and provide supportive care, as needed and ordered.

! **WARNING** Be aware that stopping drug abruptly can elevate serum catecholamine levels and cause such withdrawal symptoms as agitation, confusion headache, nervousness, rebound hypertension (could be severe), and tremor.

! WARNING Monitor blood pressure and heart rate often during clonidine therapy because clonidine may worsen AV block and sinus node dysfunction, especially if patient is taking another sympatholytic drug. If severe bradycardia occurs, be prepared to administer I.V. atropine or isoproterenol and assist with insertion of temporary cardiac pacing.

- Expect transdermal clonidine to take 2 to 3 days to lower blood pressure.
- Remove patch before patient has an MRI to avoid possible burns at the patch site.
- Expect blood pressure to rise within 48 hours after drug is discontinued.

PATIENT TEACHING

- Instruct patient how to administer form of drug prescribed.

! WARNING Advise patient to take drug exactly as prescribed and not to stop abruptly because severe hypertension and withdrawal symptoms may occur.

! WARNING Alert patient that drug may cause an allergic reaction. Tell patient to notify prescriber promptly and, if severe, to seek immediate medical care.

- Advise patient to avoid hazardous activities until drug's CNS effects are known and resolved. Caution patient that these effects are increased by concomitant use of alcohol, barbiturates, or other sedating drugs.
- Advise men that libido may decrease, or erectile dysfunction may occur.
- Instruct patient to report chest pain, dizziness with position changes, excessive drowsiness, rash, urine retention, and vision changes. As needed, tell patient to rise slowly to avoid hypotensive effects.
- Inform patient who wears contact lenses that clonidine may cause dry eyes.
- Advise patient who has a history of syncope or has a condition that predisposes him to syncope such as bradycardia, dehydration, hypotension, or orthostatic hypotension to avoid becoming dehydrated or overheated during therapy.
- Instruct mothers who are breastfeeding to monitor infant for symptoms of bradycardia or hypotension, such as lethargy, poor feeding, rapid breathing, or sedation. If present, pediatrician should be notified and breastfeeding or the drug discontinued.

clopidogrel bisulfate

Plavix

Class and Category

Pharmacologic class: $P2Y_{12}$ platelet inhibitor
Therapeutic class: Platelet aggregation inhibitor

Indications and Dosages

* *To reduce the rate of CVA and MI in patients with established peripheral arterial disease or a history of recent CVA or MI*

TABLETS

Adults. 75 mg once daily.

* *To reduce rate of CVA and MI in patients with non-ST-segment elevation acute coronary syndrome (unstable angina/non-ST-elevation MI) [NSTEMI], including patients who are to be managed medically and those who are to be managed with coronary revascularization; to reduce rate of CVA and MI in patients with acute ST-elevation MI (STEMI) who are to be managed medically*

TABLETS

Adults. *Initial:* 300 mg as a single dose followed by 75 mg once daily with aspirin therapy.

Drug Administration

P.O.

- Drug should not be discontinued abruptly.
- Expect drug to be given with aspirin.
- Do not administer drug with grapefruit products.

Route	Onset	Peak	Duration
P.O.	2 hr	45 min	5 days

Half-life: 6 hr

Mechanism of Action

Binds to adenosine diphosphate (ADP) receptors on the surface of activated platelets. This action blocks ADP, which deactivates nearby glycoprotein IIb/IIIa receptors and prevents fibrinogen from attaching to receptors. Without fibrinogen, platelets can't aggregate and form thrombi.

Contraindications

Active pathological bleeding, including intracranial hemorrhage and peptic ulcer; hypersensitivity to clopidogrel or its components

Interactions

DRUGS

anticoagulants, chronic use of NSAIDs, other antiplatelets such as aspirin: Increased risk of bleeding
CYP1C19 inducers (strong), such as rifampin: Increased plasma clopidogrel level increasing risk of bleeding
CYP2C19 inhibitors, such as dexlansoprazole, esomeprazole, lansoprazole, omeprazole, pantoprazole: Decreased plasma clopidogrel level, decreased platelet inhibition
NSAIDs, serotonin norepinephrine reuptake inhibitors (SNRIs), selective serotonin reuptake inhibitors (SSRIs): Increased risk of GI bleeding
opioid agonists: Delayed and reduced absorption of clopidogrel
repaglinide and other CYP2C8 inhibitors: Increased repaglinide and other CYP2C8 inhibitors exposure possibly increasing risk of adverse reactions, especially hypoglycemia
warfarin: Prolonged bleeding time, increased risk of bleeding

FOODS

grapefruit products: Inhibits metabolic activation of clopidogrel possibly impairing its effectiveness

Adverse Reactions

CNS: Confusion, depression, dizziness, **fatal intracranial bleeding**, fatigue, fever, hallucinations, headache
CV: Chest pain, edema, hypercholesterolemia, hypertension, **hypotension**, vasculitis
EENT: Altered or loss of taste; conjunctival, ocular, or retinal bleeding; epistaxis; rhinitis; stomatitis; taste disorders
ENDO: **Insulin autoimmune syndrome, severe hypoglycemia**
GI: Abdominal pain; **acute liver failure**; colitis; diarrhea; duodenal, gastric, or peptic ulcer; elevated liver enzymes; gastritis; **gastrointestinal and retroperitoneal hemorrhage**; indigestion; nausea; **noninfectious hepatitis, pancreatitis**
GU: Elevated serum creatinine level, **glomerulopathy**, UTI
HEME: **Acquired hemophilia A, agranulocytosis, aplastic anemia, neutropenia, pancytopenia, prolonged bleeding time, thrombocytopenic purpura, thrombotic thrombocytopenic purpura, unusual bleeding** or bruising
MS: Arthralgia, back pain, musculoskeletal bleeding, myalgia
RESP: Bronchitis, **bronchospasm**, cough, dyspnea, **eosinophilic pneumonia, interstitial pneumonitis, respiratory tract bleeding**, upper respiratory tract infection
SKIN: Acute generalized exanthematous pustulosis, bullous dermatitis, eczema, **erythema multiforme, exfoliative dermatitis**, lichen planus, pruritus, skin bleeding, **Stevens-Johnson syndrome, toxic epidermal necrolysis**, urticaria
Other: **Anaphylaxis, angioedema, drug reaction with eosinophilia and systemic symptoms (DRESS)**, flu-like symptoms, serum sickness

Childbearing Considerations

PREGNANCY

- It is not known if drug can cause fetal harm.
- Drug should be used with caution during pregnancy and given only if benefit to mother outweighs potential risk to fetus.

LABOR AND DELIVERY

- Drug may cause maternal bleeding and hemorrhage if given during labor and delivery.
- Know that drug should be temporarily withheld for 5 to 7 days prior to labor, delivery, or use with neuraxial anesthesia, if possible.

LACTATION

- It is not known if drug is present in breast milk.
- Mothers should check with prescriber before breastfeeding.

Nursing Considerations

! WARNING Avoid clopidogrel in patients who have a genetic variation in CYP2C19 or are receiving CYP2C19 inhibitors. Platelet inhibition may decline, increasing the risk of adverse cardiovascular effects after MI.

- Use clopidogrel cautiously in patients with severe hepatic or renal disease, risk of bleeding from surgery or trauma, or conditions that predispose to bleeding (such as peptic ulcer disease or thrombotic thrombocytopenic purpura).

! **WARNING** Determine if patient has a history of hypersensitivity that may have included a hematologic reaction to any other thienopyridine drug, such as prasugrel or ticlopidine, because allergic cross-reactivity has been reported. Monitor patient for a hypersensitivity reaction, which could become severe such as anaphylaxis or angioedema. Also monitor patient for skin reactions such as a rash that could indicate the beginning of a severe reaction. Be aware that DRESS may only present with a fever or swollen lymph nodes although rash is the most common initial presentation. If a hypersensitivity or skin reaction is present, notify prescriber promptly, expect drug to be withheld as ordered, and provide supportive care, as needed and ordered.

! **WARNING** Monitor patient closely for increased bleeding that could become life-threatening, such as intracranial bleeding. Know that concurrent anticoagulant, chronic NSAIDs, and other antiplatelets such as aspirin therapy increases the risk.

! **WARNING** Monitor patient's blood glucose level closely, especially if diabetic, because drug can cause severe hypoglcemia.

- Obtain blood cell count, as ordered, whenever signs and symptoms suggest a hematologic problem.
- Be aware that clopidogrel prolongs bleeding time; expect to stop it 5 days before elective surgery.

PATIENT TEACHING

- Instruct patient how to administer clopidogrel.
- Instruct patient not to take drug with any grapefruit products.
- Instruct patient not to discontinue clopidogrel abruptly or without first consulting prescriber.
- Remind patient to adhere to aspirin therapy, as prescribed.

! **WARNING** Alert patient that drug may cause an allergic reaction. Tell patient to notify prescriber, if present, and to seek immediate medical care if severe. Also warn patient that drug may cause skin reactions that could become severe. Tell patient to notify prescriber if a fever, rash, swollen lymph nodes, or other skin reactions appear.

! **WARNING** Warn patient that drug may cause low blood sugar levels. Review signs and symptoms of hypoglycemia and how to treat. Tell patient to notify prescriber if hypoglycemia occurs because it can cause persistent hypoglycemia, which could become severe.

! **WARNING** Caution patient that bleeding may continue longer than usual. Instruct him to report unusual bleeding or bruising because it could become severe. Caution patient not to use over-the-counter preparations, such as NSAIDs or proton pump inhibitors, during clopidogrel therapy because of potential for bleeding.

- Instruct patient to notify prescriber of any persistent, severe, or unusual adverse reactions because drug can affect many body systems.
- Urge patient to inform all other healthcare providers, including dentists, that he takes clopidogrel. This is especially important before patient has surgery or other procedures or before taking a new drug because of an increased risk for bleeding.

clozapine

Clozaril, Versacloz

Class and Category

Pharmacologic class: Atypical antipsychotic
Therapeutic class: Atypical antipsychotic

Indications and Dosages

✱ *To treat severe schizophrenia unresponsive to standard drugs; to reduce risk of recurrent suicidal behavior in schizophrenia or schizoaffective disorders*

ORALLY DISINTEGRATING TABLETS, ORAL SUSPENSION, TABLETS

Adults. *Initial:* 12.5 mg once or twice daily. Increased by 25 to 50 mg daily to 300 to 450 mg daily in divided doses by the end of 2 wk.

Subsequently, dosage increased in increments of 100 mg or less, once or twice weekly. *Maximum:* 900 mg daily in divided doses.

±**DOSAGE ADJUSTMENT** For patient who has had even a brief interruption in drug therapy, dosage reduced as follows: if 1 day's dosing is missed, treatment resumed at 40% to 50% of the established dose; if 2 days dosing is missed, dose resumed at 25% of the established dosage; and for longer interruptions, dosage re-initiated at 12.5 mg once or twice daily with dosage increased to previous dosage more quickly than done for initial treatment. For patients receiving a strong CYP1A2 inhibitor, such as ciprofloxacin, enoxacin, or fluvoxamine concurrently, dosage decreased by two-thirds and then adjusted according to clinical response. For patients experiencing adverse reactions during concomitant therapy with a moderate or weak CYP1A2 inhibitor such as caffeine or oral contraceptives or a CYP2D6 or CYP3A4 inhibitor such as bupropion, cimetidine, duloxetine, erythromycin, escitalopram, fluoxetine, paroxetine, quinidine, sertraline, or terbinafine, clozapine dosage may need to be decreased. For patients receiving a CYP1A2 inducer (tobacco smoking) or CYP3A4 inducers, such as carbamazepine, phenytoin, rifampin, or St. John's wort concurrently, clozapine dosage may have to be increased if clinical response is ineffective. For patients with significant renal or hepatic impairment or patients are a CYP2D6 poor metabolizer, clozapine dosage may be decreased if patient develops significant adverse reactions. For patients experiencing neutropenia, drug therapy may need to be interrupted depending on degree of neutropenia.

Drug Administration

P.O.

- Administer single daily doses at bedtime. If more than 1 dose is given daily, the dose may be split unequally so a larger dose is given at bedtime.
- Administer orally disintegrating tablets by peeling foil back to remove tablet (rather than pushing tablet through foil) with a dry, gloved hand and then immediately place or have patient place tablet in mouth and let it dissolve. Patient also may chew the tablet before swallowing. No water is needed.
- Shake oral suspension container for 10 sec before every use. The oral dosing syringe provided with the product should be the only device used to measure dosage. Firmly insert adapter into the neck of the bottle before the first use and keep it there. Then, fill the syringe with air equivalent to the dose being withdrawn from the bottle. To withdraw the dose, insert the dosing syringe into the adapter and push air from syringe into the bottle. Then, invert bottle and slowly pull back the plunger to the prescribed dose. After removing the syringe from the bottle adapter, slowly squirt the suspension into patient's mouth. Replace the cap over the adapter until next dose is due and rinse syringe well with warm water and dry. Store at room temperature. Do not refrigerate or freeze. Protect from light. Discard in 100 days after initial opening of bottle.
- Expect to reduce dosage gradually over a period of 1 to 2 weeks if termination of drug therapy is planned.

Route	Onset	Peak	Duration
P.O.	15 min	1.5–2.5 hr	4–12 hr

Half-life: 12 hr

Mechanism of Action

May produce antipsychotic effects by interfering with dopamine binding to dopamine—especially D_4—receptors in the limbic region of the brain and by antagonizing adrenergic, cholinergic, histaminic, and serotoninergic receptors.

Contraindications

Absolute neutrophil count (ANC) below 1,500/mm^3 for general population and at least 1,000/mm^3 for patients with Benign Ethnic Neutropenia, hypersensitivity to clozapine or its components

Interactions

DRUGS

antidepressants (selected ones); carbamazepine; class IC antiarrhythmics, such as encainide, flecainide, propafenone; phenothiazines: Increased levels of these drugs with possible increased adverse reactions

bupropion, cimetidine, ciprofloxacin, duloxetine, enoxacin, erythromycin, escitalopram, fluoxetine, fluvoxamine, oral contraceptives,

paroxetine, quinidine, sertraline, terbinafine: Possibly increased blood clozapine level and increased risk of adverse reactions
carbamazepine, phenytoin, rifampin, St. John's wort: Decreased blood clozapine level with decreased effectiveness
chlorpromazine, class 1a antiarrhythmias, such as quinidine or procainamide, class III antiarrhythmias, such as amiodarone or sotalol, dolasetron, droperidol, erythromycin, gatifloxacin, halofantrine, iloperidone, levomethadyl, mesoridazine, mefloquine, methadone, moxifloxacin, pentamidine, pimozide, probucol, sparfloxacin, tacrolimus, thioridazine ziprasidone: Possible increased risk of prolonged QT interval
CNS depressants: Increased CNS depression
other anticholinergic drugs: Increased risk for anticholinergic toxicity or severe GI adverse reactions

ACTIVITIES

alcohol use: Increased CNS depression
caffeine: Increased blood clozapine level
smoking: Decreased blood clozapine level

Adverse Reactions

CNS: Agitation, akinesia, anxiety, ataxia, cholinergic rebound adverse reactions after discontinuation, confusion, delirium, depression, dizziness, drowsiness, dystonia, EEG abnormality, fatigue, fever, headache, hyperkinesia, hypokinesia, insomnia, lethargy, myoclonic jerks, **neuroleptic malignant syndrome**, nightmares, obsessive–compulsive symptoms, paresthesia, possible cataplexy, restlessness, restless leg syndrome, rigidity, sedation, **seizures**, sleep disturbance **(sleep apnea)**, slurred speech, **status epilepticus**, syncope, tardive dyskinesia, tremor, vertigo, weakness
CV: **Atrial or ventricular fibrillation**, **bradycardia**, **cardiac arrest**, **cardiomyopathy**, chest pain, **deep vein thrombosis**, dyslipidemia, **ECG changes**, hypercholesterolemia, hypertension, hypertriglyceridemia, **hypotension**, leukocytoclastic vasculitis, **MI**, **mitral valve incompetence**, **myocarditis**, orthostatic hypotension, palpitations, **pericarditis**, **QT-interval prolongation**, tachycardia, **torsades de pointes**, vasculitis, **ventricular tachycardia**
EENT: Blurred vision, dry mouth, increased nasal congestion, increased salivation, narrow-angle glaucoma, periorbital edema, pharyngitis, salivary gland swelling, tongue numbness or soreness
ENDO: **Ketoacidosis**, **pseudopheochromocytoma**, **severe hyperglycemia**
GI: Abdominal discomfort; **acute pancreatitis**; anorexia; **bowel perforation, necrosis, or ulceration**; cholestasis; colitis; constipation; diarrhea; dysphagia; elevated liver enzymes; heartburn; **hepatic cirrhosis or fibrosis**; **hepatitis**; **hepatotoxicity**; **hypomotility with severe complications**; **intestinal ischemia or infarction**; jaundice; **liver failure or injury**; **megacolon**; nausea; **pancreatitis**; vomiting
GU: Abnormal ejaculation, including retrograde; acute interstitial nephritis; nocturnal enuresis; priapism; **renal failure**; urinary frequency, urgency, and incontinence; urine retention
HEME: **Agranulocytosis**; elevated hemoglobin, hematocrit and erythrocyte sedimentation rate; eosinophilia; **granulocytopenia**; **leukopenia**; **neutropenia (may become severe)**; **thrombocytopenia**; thrombocytosis
MS: Back or leg pain, elevated creatine phosphokinase, muscle spasm or weakness, myalgia, myasthenic syndrome, **rhabdomyolysis**
RESP: **Aspiration**, dyspnea, lower respiratory tract infection, pleural effusion, pneumonia, **pulmonary embolism**, **respiratory arrest**
SKIN: **Erythema multiforme**, photosensitivity, pigmentation disorder, pruritus, rash, **Stevens-Johnson syndrome**, urticaria
Other: **Angioedema**, anticholinergic toxicity, **hypersensitivity reactions**, hyperuricemia, **hyponatremia**, inflammation of serous membranes, **sepsis**, systemic lupus erythematosus, weight gain or loss

Childbearing Considerations

PREGNANCY

- Pregnancy exposure registry: 1-866-961-2388 or http://womensmentalhealth.org/clinical-and-research-programs/pregnancyregistry/.
- It is not known if drug can cause fetal harm. However, neonates exposed to drug during the third trimester are at risk for extrapyramidal and/or withdrawal symptoms following delivery.

- Drug should be used with caution during pregnancy only if benefit to mother outweighs potential risk to fetus.

LACTATION

- Drug is present in breast milk.
- Mothers should check with prescriber before breastfeeding. If breastfeeding occurs, infant should be monitored for the development of neutropenia and excessive sedation.

Nursing Considerations

- Be aware that clozapine should not be given to elderly patients with dementia-related psychosis.

! **WARNING** Use clozapine cautiously in patients with cardiovascular, hepatic, or renal disease because they have an increased risk of serious or fatal adverse reactions. Also, use cautiously in patients with risk factors for a stroke because drug use may increase risk of cerebrovascular adverse events.

! **WARNING** Use cautiously in patients with a history of prolonged QT syndrome or who have existing conditions that might prolong the QT interval, such as a recent MI, serious cardiac arrhythmia, or uncompensated heart failure. Drug should also be used cautiously in patients with cardiovascular disease or a family history of prolonged QT syndrome because clozapine therapy may increase the QT interval enough to cause life-threatening arrhythmias such as torsades de pointes, especially in patients who are hypokalemic. Know that hypokalemia should be corrected, if present, before clozapine therapy begins and the serum potassium level monitored closely throughout therapy. If QT prolongation occurs, notify prescriber and expect drug to be discontinued if the QT interval exceeds 500 m/sec.

- Use clozapine cautiously in patients with a clinically significant prostatic hypertrophy, urinary retention, or other conditions in which anticholinergic effects can lead to significant adverse reactions.
- Be aware that because of the risk of severe neutropenia, clozapine is available only through a restricted program called the Clozapine REMS Program.

! **WARNING** Check patient's baseline CBC, including differential before therapy and weekly for first 6 months, as ordered. Know that the baseline absolute neutrophil count (ANC) must be at least 1,500/µl for the general population; and must be at least 1,000/µl for patients with documented Benign Ethnic Neutropenia (BEN) before therapy can begin. If ANC remains equal to or greater than 1,500/µl during the first 6 months, expect to check the patient's ANC every 2 weeks for next 6 months, as ordered. If counts remain stable, expect to continue checking patient's ANC every 4 weeks thereafter. Also, know that laboratory monitoring may be reduced for hospice patients with an estimated life expectancy of 6 months or less.

! **WARNING** Monitor patient for a hypersensitivity reaction that could become life-threatening, such as angioedema. If present, notify prescriber promptly; withhold drug, as ordered; and provide supportive care, as needed and ordered.

! **WARNING** Monitor patient for bradycardia, cardiac arrest, orthostatic hyotension, and syncope, especially when drug is initiated, and during rapid dosage increases. Be alert for these adverse reactions even with the first dose, with doses as low as 12.5 mg per day, and when restarting patient on clozapine who has had even a brief interruption in drug treatment. Know that risk increases in patients with cardiovascular or cerebrovascular disease or conditions predisposing patient to hypotension such as dehydration or use of antihypertensive drugs.

! **WARNING** Know that, rarely, clozapine causes severe or life-threatening adverse reactions, such as agranulocytosis, or cardiac or respiratory arrest, deep vein thrombosis, myocarditis (especially in first month), neuroleptic malignant syndrome, pericarditis, and severe hyperglycemia with ketoacidosis in nondiabetic patients. It also may cause seizures and tardive dyskinesia. Monitor patient closely. Know that these risks are often dose related. Expect therapy to begin with a dose as low as 12.5 mg with titration done slowly and divided daily dosing possibly used.

! **WARNING** Monitor patient for GI hypomotility caused by an anticholinergic effect that may exhibit a wide range of complications ranging from constipation to paralytic ileus. Notify prescriber immediately, if present, because a delay in diagnosis and treatment increases risk of severe complications such as fecal impaction, intestinal obstruction, ischemia, infarction, megacolon, necrosis, or ulceration that have resulted in hospitalization and surgery as well as death.

! **WARNING** Monitor patient for signs and symptoms of cardiomyopathy, mitral valve incompetence, or myocarditis such as chest pain, dyspnea, ECG changes, fever, flu-like symptoms, hypotension, palpitations, or tachycardia. If present, notify prescriber immediately and expect drug to be discontinued and a cardiac evaluation done promptly.

- Monitor patients, especially male patients and younger patients, for dystonia, particularly during the first few days of treatment. Be alert for complaints of neck spasms, which sometimes may progress to throat tightness, trouble breathing or swallowing, and tongue protrusion.
- Monitor patient's neutrophil count, as ordered. If patient develops mild neutropenia (1,000 to 1,499/μl), treatment should be expected to continue but ANC monitoring should be increased to 3 times weekly until level reaches 1,500/μl. If patient develops moderate neutropenia (500 to 999/μl), expect treatment to be interrupted and daily monitoring of the patient's ANC done until the level reaches 1,000/μl, then 3-times-a-week monitoring until level reaches 1,500/μl. Expect therapy to be resumed once ANC reaches 1,000/μl. If patient develops severe neutropenia (less than 500/μl), expect drug to be discontinued, and daily monitoring of ANC until it reaches 1,000/μl, then 3 times weekly until it is normal. Be aware that clozapine therapy should not be restarted unless the benefits outweigh future risks and if restarted, the patient should resume treatment as a new patient receiving drug for the first time.
- Monitor patient's temperature. Expect to withhold clozapine if patient develops a fever of 38.5°C (101.3°F) or higher and obtain an ANC level immediately, as fever is often the first sign of neutropenic infection.
- Monitor patient's liver enzymes, as ordered. Report any signs of liver dysfunction, such as anorexia, fatigue, jaundice, malaise, or nausea to prescriber. Expect clozapine to be discontinued if liver enzymes become elevated in combination with symptoms or patient develops hepatitis.
- Monitor patient for CNS and peripheral anticholinergic toxicity, especially at higher dosages or in overdose situation.

PATIENT TEACHING

- Instruct patient how to administer form of clozapine prescribed. Tell patient that he'll receive only a 1-week supply at a time.
- Tell patient to avoid alcohol while taking clozapine because alcohol can depress nervous system.
- Advise patient and family or caregiver that drug may increase risk of orthostatic hypotension and syncope, especially during initial dosage titration. Warn patient that if he stops drug for more than 2 days, he will need to contact prescriber for instructions; dosage will have to be changed.

! **WARNING** Alert patient that an allergic reaction can occur to clozapine. If present, tell patient to notify prescriber and, if severe, to seek immediate medical care.

! **WARNING** Tell patient drug may cause blood dyscrasias that could become quite serious. Inform patient that he'll need at least weekly blood tests. Encourage compliance with laboratory appointments. Review evidence of dyscrasias (fatigue, fever, sore throat, weakness); urge patient to report them to prescriber if they occur.

! **WARNING** Stress importance of notifying prescriber promptly if persistent, severe, or unusual adverse reactions occur because drug can affect many body systems and can cause serious adverse reactions that would warrant immediate medical attention.

! **WARNING** Tell patient that drug-induced constipation may occur. Advise appropriate hydration, increased fiber intake, and physical activity. Patient should alert prescriber if constipation develops or other adverse effects such as abdominal distention or pain, nausea, or vomiting develop because, if left unchecked, severe complications could occur.

- Instruct patient to avoid hazardous activities until drug's CNS effects are known and resolved.
- Alert patient and family or caregiver of increased risk for falls, especially if patient has other medical conditions or takes medication that may affect the nervous system.
- Advise patient to rise slowly from lying or sitting position to minimize orthostatic hypotension.
- Tell patient to consult prescriber before taking over-the-counter drugs.
- Tell females of childbearing age to notify prescriber if pregnancy occurs.
- Tell mothers who are breastfeeding to monitor their infant for excess sedation and to notify the pediatrician so that infant can be monitored for neutropenia.

coagulation factor Xa, inactivated-zhzo

Andexxa

Class and Category

Pharmacologic class: Human coagulation factor Xa, recombinant
Therapeutic class: Factor Xa inhibitor antidote

Indications and Dosages

∗ *To reverse life-threatening or uncontrolled bleeding induced by apixaban or rivaroxaban therapy*

I.V. INFUSION, I.V. INJECTION

Adults. *For low dose (used if last dose of apixaban was 5 mg or less, rivaroxaban was 10 mg or less, and last dose of either drug was taken less than 8 hr or unknown):* 400 mg as an I.V. bolus, followed by 4 mg/min for up to 120 min. *For high dose (used if last dose of apixaban was greater than 5 mg or unknown or rivaroxaban was greater than 10 mg or unknown and last dose of either drug was taken less than 8 hr or unknown):* 800 mg as an I.V. bolus, followed by 8 mg/min for up to 120 min. If either drug was taken 8 hr or more, regardless of dosage, low-dose regimen used.

Drug Administration

I.V.

- Store unopened vials in refrigerator. Do not freeze.
- Prepare I.V. bolus by reconstituting each 200-mg vial of drug by slowly injecting 20 ml of Sterile Water for Injection, using a 20 G needle or higher and directing the solution onto the inside wall of the vial to minimize foaming. Gently swirl each vial until powder is completely dissolved. Do not shake, to avoid foaming. This takes about 3 to 5 min. Use a 60-ml syringe or larger with a 20 G needle to withdraw the reconstituted solution from each of the vials until the required dosing volume is achieved. Transfer the solution from the syringe into an empty polyolefin or polyvinyl chloride I.V. bag with a volume of 250 ml or less. Use a 0.2- or 0.22-micron in-line polyethersulfone or equivalent low-protein-binding filter and administer the bolus at a rate of 30 mg/min.
- Prepare continuous I.V. infusion following the same procedure for I.V. bolus preparation. Use a 0.2- or 0.22-micron inline polyethersulfone or equivalent low-protein-binding filter. Within 2 min following the bolus dose, begin I.V. infusion and infuse for up to 120 min, as prescribed.
- Know that vials that have been reconstituted are stable at room temperature for up to 8 hr or may be stored for up to 24 hr if refrigerated. Reconstituted solution in I.V. bags is stable at room temperature for up to 8 hr.
- *Incompatibilities:* None listed by manufacturer.

Route	Onset	Peak	Duration
I.V.	2–5 min (bolus)	4 hr	2 hr (following infusion)

Half-life: 5–7 hr

Mechanism of Action

Binds and sequesters the factor Xa inhibitors apixaban and rivaroxaban, thereby exerting its procoagulant effect.

Contraindications

Hypersensitivity to coagulation factor Xa, inactivated-zhzo or its components

Interactions

DRUGS

None reported by manufacturer.

Adverse Reactions

CV: Thromboembolic events
EENT: Altered sense of taste
GU: UTI
RESP: Cough, dyspnea, pneumonia
SKIN: Flushing, urticaria
Other: Anticoagulation factor Xa, inactivated-zhzo antibodies; feeling hot

Childbearing Considerations

PREGNANCY

- It is not known if drug can cause fetal harm.
- Use with caution during pregnancy only if benefit to mother outweighs potential risk to fetus.

LACTATION

- It is not known if drug is present in breast milk.
- Mothers should check with prescriber before breastfeeding.

Nursing Considerations

- Be aware that the dosing of coagulation factor Xa, inactivated-zhzo is based on the specific drug that had been administered (apixaban or rivaroxaban), dose of the drug taken, and the time since the patient's last dose of the drug.

! **WARNING** Monitor patient closely for thrombosis because patients treated with coagulation factor Xa, inactivated-zhzo have underlying disease states that predispose them to thromboembolic events that can occur up to 30 days after drug has been administered. Expect patient to resume anticoagulant therapy as soon as possible following use of coagulation factor Xa, inactivated-zhzo to reduce the risk of thrombosis.

PATIENT TEACHING

- Inform patient that coagulation factor Xa, inactivated-zhzo is administered in 2 steps: first, as an intravenous bolus; then followed by a continuous intravenous infusion that may last up to 2 hours after the bolus has been given.

! **WARNING** Inform patient that reversing the effects of the prescribed apixaban or rivaroxaban increases the risk of thromboembolic events for up to 30 days following the administration of coagulation factor Xa, inactivated-zhzo. Review the signs and symptoms of a blood clot that may occur in various areas of the body. Urge patient to seek immediate medical attention if a blood clot is suspected.

C

codeine sulfate

Class, Category, and Schedule

Pharmacologic class: Opioid
Therapeutic class: Opioid analgesic
Controlled substance schedule: II

Indications and Dosages

∗ *To treat mild to moderate pain that requires opioid treatment and for which alternative treatment options (e.g., nonopioid analgesics or opioid combination products) are inadequate or not tolerated*

TABLETS

Adults. 15 to 60 mg (usual, 30 mg) every 4 hr, as needed. *Maximum:* 360 mg in 24 hr.

± **DOSAGE ADJUSTMENT** For elderly patients and patients with hepatic or renal failure, initial dosage started at lowest dose or dosing intervals increased and then titrated slowly depending on the appearance of adverse reactions.

Drug Administration

P.O.

- Administer drug with food.
- Expect to administer dosage at the lowest dose necessary to achieve pain relief.
- Drug should not be discontinued abruptly after chronic use.
- Protect drug from light and moisture.

Route	Onset	Peak	Duration
P.O.	30–45 min	1 hr	4–6 hr

Half-life: 3 hr

Mechanism of Action

May produce analgesia through partial metabolism to morphine. Drug binds with delta, kappa, and mu receptors in the spinal cord and with $kappa_3$ and mu_1 receptors higher in the CNS, decreasing intracellular cAMP, which inhibits adenylate cyclase activity and prevents release of pain neurotransmitters, such as dopamine and substance P, and altering perception of and emotional response to pain.

Contraindications

Acute or severe bronchial asthma in an unmonitored setting or absence of resuscitative equipment; children under the age of 12 for all uses and adolescents under the age of 18 for use with cold and cough medications as well as for pain management after adenoidectomy and/or tonsillectomy; GI obstruction, including paralytic ileus; hypersensitivity to codeine, other opioids, or their components; significant respiratory depression; use of MAO inhibitors or within past 14 days

Interactions

DRUGS

anticholinergics: Increased risk of severe constipation and urinary retention
antihypertensives, diuretics: Potentiated hypotensive effects
benzodiazepines, CNS depressants, muscle relaxants, other opioids, sedating antihistamines, tricyclic antidepressants: Increased risk of severe respiratory depression and significant sedation and somnolence
buprenorphine, butorphanol, nalbuphine, pentazocine: Possibly reduces analgesic effect of codeine and/or precipitate withdrawal symptoms
CYP2D6 inhibitors (such as bupropion, fluoxetine, paroxetine, quinidine): Possibly decreased effectiveness of codeine that may cause some patients to experience opioid withdrawal
CYP2D6 inhibitor that is being discontinued: Possibly increase or prolong adverse reactions and potentially fatal respiratory depression
CYP3A4 inducers (such as carbamazepine, phenytoin, rifampin) or discontinuation of a CYP3A4 inhibitor (such as azole antifungals, macrolide antibiotics, protease inhibitors): Decreased plasma codeine concentration with possible decreased effectiveness, causing some patients to experience opioid withdrawal
CYP3A4 inhibitors or discontinuation of a CYP3A4 inducer: Increased plasma codeine concentration leading to increased or prolonged adverse reactions and potentially fatal respiratory depression
diuretics: Reduced effectiveness of diuretics
MAO inhibitors, such as linezolid, tranylcypromine: Increased risk of unpredictable, severe, and sometimes fatal reactions
muscle relaxants: Possibly enhanced neuromuscular blocking action of skeletal muscle relaxants; increased severity of respiratory depression
naloxone: Antagonized codeine effect
naltrexone: Precipitated withdrawal symptoms in codeine-dependent patients
serotonergic drugs such as 5-HT_{3A} receptor antagonists, cyclobenzaprine, I.V. methylene blue, linezolid, MAO inhibitors, metaxalone, mirtazapine, selective serotonin reuptake inhibitors (SSRIs), serotonin and norepinephrine reuptake inhibitors (SNRIs), tramadol, trazodone, tricyclic antidepressants, triptans: Increased risk of serotonin syndrome

ACTIVITIES

alcohol use: Additive CNS effects, including severe respiratory depression and significant sedation and somnolence

Adverse Reactions

CNS: **Coma**, delirium, depression, disorientation, dizziness, drowsiness, euphoria, hallucinations, headache, lack of coordination, lethargy, light-headedness, mental and physical impairment, mood changes, restlessness, sedation, **seizures**, tremor
CV: **Bradycardia**, **heart block**, hypertension, **hypotension (may be severe)**, orthostatic hypotension, palpitations, tachycardia
EENT: Altered taste, blurred vision, diplopia, dry mouth, **laryngeal edema**, **laryngospasm**, miosis
ENDO: **Adrenal insufficiency (rare)**, androgen deficiency (over extended period of time), **hypoglycemia**
GI: Abdominal cramps and pain, anorexia, constipation, flatulence, gastroesophageal reflux, ileus, indigestion, nausea, vomiting
GU: Decreased libido, difficult ejaculation, dysuria, erectile dysfunction, impotence, infertility with prolonged use, lack of

menstruation, oliguria, ureteral spasm, urinary incontinence, urine retention
MS: Muscle rigidity
RESP: **Apnea**, **bronchoconstriction**, **bronchospasm**, **depressed cough reflex**, **respiratory depression**, **sleep-related breathing disorders (sleep apnea, sleep-related hypoxemia)**
SKIN: Diaphoresis, flushing, pallor, pruritus, rash, urticaria
Other: **Anaphylaxis**, **angioedema**, opioid-induced allodynia (pain from ordinarily non-painful stimuli) and hyeralgesia (increased pain), physical and psychological dependence, withdrawal

Childbearing Considerations

PREGNANCY

- It is not known if drug can cause fetal harm, but drug does cross the placental barrier. However, prolonged use of drug during pregnancy may cause physical dependence in the neonate resulting in neonatal opioid withdrawal syndrome shortly after birth.
- Drug should be used with caution during pregnancy only if benefit to mother outweighs potential risk to fetus.

LABOR AND DELIVERY

- Infants exposed to codeine during labor should be assessed for excess sedation and respiratory depression.
- An opioid antagonist, such as naloxone, must be readily available to reverse neonatal adverse effects, if present.

LACTATION

- Drug is present in breast milk.
- Breastfeeding is not recommended during drug therapy.
- If breastfeeding occurs, mother should monitor breastfed infant for breathing difficulties and drowsiness as well as withdrawal symptoms when breastfeeding ceases or drug is discontinued.

REPRODUCTION

- Chronic use of opioids over extended period of time such as codeine sulfate may reduce fertility in both men and women. It is not known if this effect is reversible.

Nursing Considerations

- Evaluate patient's risk for abuse and addiction prior to the start of codeine therapy as excessive use of the drug may lead to abuse, addiction, misuse, overdose, and possibly death. Be prepared to monitor patient's intake throughout therapy. Because of the potential risks associated with codeine therapy, be aware that the FDA now requires a Risk Evaluation and Mitigation Strategy (REMS) for codeine use to educate the patient.
- Evaluate patient for therapeutic response, including decreased facial grimacing and pain.

! **WARNING** Know that the safety and effectiveness of codeine therapy in pediatric patients have not been established. Codeine should not be given to children under the age of 12 for any reason and for adolescents under the age of 18 when used in cold or cough preparations, as well as following adenoidectomy and/or tonsillectomy. Also, know that codeine should not be given to children ages 12 to 18 if they have other risk factors that may increase their sensitivity to the respiratory depressant effects of codeine. Risk factors include conditions associated with hypoventilation, such as concomitant use of other medications that cause respiratory depression or the presence of neuromuscular disease, obesity, obstructive sleep apnea, or severe pulmonary disease. In addition, codeine should not be given to patients who are known ultrarapid metabolizers of codeine, including mothers who are breastfeeding, as breastfed infants have died when exposed to high levels of morphine (codeine converts to morphine) in breast milk.

! **WARNING** Monitor respiratory depth, effort, and rate because codeine can cause respiratory depression that could become life-threatening, especially in patients with chronic pulmonary disease or in patients who are cachectic, debilitated, or elderly. Notify prescriber immediately if respiratory rate drops below 10 breaths/min.

! **WARNING** Monitor patient's blood pressure closely because codeine may cause severe hypotension including orthostatic hypotension and syncope, especially if experiencing reduced blood volume or receiving concurrent therapy with other CNS depressants. Monitor blood pressure, particularly after initiating codeine therapy or when titrating dosage. Know that codeine therapy should be avoided in patients with circulatory shock.

! **WARNING** Monitor any patient receiving codeine closely, especially the patient who has never received a narcotic like codeine or morphine, for signs of overdose, such as confusion, extreme sleepiness, or shallow breathing because patient may not know he is an ultrarapid metabolizer. Some patients are ultrarapid metabolizers because of a CYP2D6 polymorphism. How prevalent this phenotype is varies widely. It is estimated that 0.5% to 1% Chinese, Hispanics, and Japanese; 1% to 10% Caucasians; 3% African Americans; and 16% to 28% of Arabs, Ethiopians, and North Africans may carry the CYP2D6 genotype. Keep naloxone readily available.

! **WARNING** Monitor patient for a hypersensitivity reaction, which could become life-threatening, such as anaphylaxis or angioedema. If present, notify prescriber, expect codeine to be discontinued, and provide supportive care, as needed and ordered.

! **WARNING** Be aware that opioid therapy like codeine should only be used concomitantly with benzodiazepine therapy in patients for whom other treatment options are inadequate. If prescribed together, expect dosing and duration of the opioid to be limited. Monitor patient closely for signs and symptoms of decrease in consciousness, including coma, profound sedation, and significant respiratory depression. If present, notify prescriber immediately and provide emergency supportive care, as death may occur.

! **WARNING** Know that chronic maternal use of codeine during pregnancy can result in neonatal opioid withdrawal syndrome (NOWS), which may be life-threatening, if not recognized and treated appropriately. NOWS occurs when a newborn was exposed to opioid drugs like codeine for a prolonged period while in utero.

! **WARNING** Know that many drugs may interact with opioids like codeine to cause serotonin syndrome. Monitor patient closely for signs and symptoms, such as agitation, diaphoresis, diarrhea, fever, hallucinations, labile blood pressure, muscle twitching or stiffness, nausea, shakiness, shivering, tachycardia, trouble with coordination, or vomiting. Notify prescriber at once because serotonin syndrome may be life-threatening. Be prepared to discontinue drug, if possible, and provide supportive care.

! **WARNING** Monitor patient for adrenal insufficiency. Although rare, it can be life-threatening. Monitor patient for anorexia, dizziness, fatigue, hypotension, nausea, vomiting, or weakness. Notify prescriber if adrenal insufficiency is suspected and expect diagnostic testing to be done to confirm. If diagnosis is confirmed, expect to administer corticosteroids and wean patient off codeine, if possible.

! **WARNING** Monitor patient's blood glucose level, especially if patient is a diabetic, because codeine has caused hypoglycemia in patients taking opioids like codeine.

- Take safety precautions, as needed.
- Assess urine output to detect retention.
- Monitor patient for opioid induced allodynia and hyeralgesia. Be aware these symptoms differ from tolerance and may occur with both short-term and long-term use of opioid analgesics. If present, notify prescriber as dosage may need to be decreased or opioid rotation tried.

PATIENT TEACHING

- Instruct patient, family, or caregiver how to administer form of codeine prescribed.
- Instruct patient to take codeine exactly as prescribed and not to adjust dose or frequency without consulting prescriber because misuse increases risk of addiction

! **WARNING** Tell patient, family, or caregiver to notify prescriber if respiratory rate drops below normal, patient's respirations become abnormal, or patient develops syncope. Stress importance of seeking immediate medical care, if severe.

! **WARNING** Warn patient not to consume alcohol or take a benzodiazepine during codeine therapy without prescriber knowledge, as severe respiratory depression can occur and may lead to death.

! **WARNING** Advise patient, family, or caregiver that naloxone should be readily available to use in the home in the event of an opioid overdose, especially if patient uses concomitant CNS depressants, has a history of opioid use disorder, prior opioid overdose, or there are household members or other close contacts at risk for accidental ingestion or overdose. Provide instruction on how to administer naloxone.

! **WARNING** Alert patient that codeine may cause an allergic reaction. Tell patient to notify prescriber, if present, and to seek immediate medical care, if severe.

! **WARNING** Alert patient, family, or caregiver that codeine may cause a low blood sugar, especially if patient is a diabetic. Review signs and symptoms of hypoglycemia and how to treat. Tell them to notify prescriber if a low blood sugar occurs and stress importance of seeking immediate medical care, if severe.

! **WARNING** Warn patient to keep codeine out of the reach of children to prevent accidental ingestion that could be life-threatening.

- Alert patient that codeine may cause pain to worsen or cause pain from stimuli that usually doesn't cause pain. If patient experiences increased pain, tell patient to notify prescriber.
- Caution pregnant patient not to increase dosage or take codeine for a prolonged period because infant may experience withdrawal when born.
- Urge breastfeeding mothers to notify prescriber before taking codeine because drug appears in breast milk and could cause breathing difficulties and drowsiness in the infant as well as withdrawal symptoms when breastfeeding ceases or drug is discontinued.
- Advise patient to avoid hazardous activities until drug's CNS effects are known.
- Caution patient to get up slowly from a lying or sitting position.
- Urge patient to consume plenty of fluids and high-fiber foods, if not contraindicated, to prevent constipation.
- Inform patient that long-term use of opioids like codeine may decrease sex hormone levels, causing decreased libido, erectile dysfunction, impotence, infertility, or lack of menstruation. Encourage patient to report any such symptoms.
- Instruct patient to tell all prescribers of codeine use and not to take any over-the-counter medication, including herbal medicines, without prescriber knowledge.
- Instruct patient how to safely dispose of unused codeine. Tell patient to mix drug with an unpalatable substance such as cat litter, dirt, or used coffee grounds and then place mixture in a sealed plastic bag, which can be thrown into the household trash. Tell patient to remove all personal information on the prescription bottle before throwing away bottle.

colchicine

Colcrys, Gloperba, Lodoco, Mitigare

Class and Category

Pharmacologic class: Colchicum alkaloid derivative

Therapeutic class: Antigout

Indications and Dosages

To prevent gouty arthritis attacks

CAPSULES, ORAL SOLUTION, TABLETS

Adults and adolescents ages 16 and older. 0.6 mg once or twice daily. *Maximum:* 1.2 mg daily.

To treat acute gouty arthritis flares

TABLETS (COLCRYS)

Adults. *Initial:* 1.2 mg at first sign of flare; then 0.6 mg 1 hr later. *Maximum:* 1.8 mg over a 1-hr period.

To treat familial Mediterranean fever (FMF)

TABLETS (COLCRYS)

Adults and adolescents ages 12 and older. 1.2 mg to 2.4 mg daily, given in 1 to 2 divided doses, with dosage increments made in 0.3 mg/day to maximum dose or dosage decrements made in 0.3 mg/day for intolerable adverse reactions. *Maximum:* 2.4 mg daily in 1 or 2 divided doses.

Children ages 6 to 12. 0.9 to 1.8 mg daily, given in 1 or 2 divided doses.

Children ages 4 to 6. 0.3 to 1.8 mg daily, given in 1 or 2 divided doses.

±**DOSAGE ADJUSTMENT** (Colcrys) For patients experiencing a gout flare during prophylactic treatment, dosage not to exceed 1.2 mg at the first sign of flare, followed by 0.6 mg 1 hour later, and then prophylactic dose resumed 12 hours later. For patients taking strong CYP3A4 inhibitors (atazanavir, clarithromycin, darunavir/ritonavir, indinavir, itraconazole, ketoconazole, lopinavir/ritonavir, nefazodone, nelfinavir, ritonavir, saquinavir, telithromycin, tipranavir/ritonavir) within 14 days, moderate CYP3A4 inhibitors (amprenavir, aprepitant, diltiazem, erythromycin, fluconazole, fosamprenavir, grapefruit juice, verapamil) within 14 days, P-gp inhibitors (cyclosporine, ranolazine) within 14 days, or protease inhibitors (atazanavir, darunavir, fosamprenavir, fosamprenavir/ritonavir, indinavir, lopinavir/ritonavir, nelfinavir, ritonavir, saquinavir, tipanavir), dosage may be reduced, dosage interval may be increased, and dose not repeated for 3 days. For patients with hepatic or renal impairment and receiving concomitant therapy with strong CYP3A4 or P-gp inhibitors, drug not given. For patients with severe renal impairment, including patients receiving dialysis, dosage adjustment may be required and interval between treatment courses may be increased. For patients with severe hepatic impairment receiving colchicine prophylactically, dosage decreased. For patients with severe hepatic impairment receiving colchicine treatment for acute gout flare, dosage not adjusted but treatment course not repeated more than once every 2 weeks. For patients with FMF who have moderate or severe renal impairment, undergoing dialysis, or have severe hepatic impairment, dosage reduced.

∗ *To reduce risk of CVA, cardiovascular death, coronary revascularization, and MI in patients with established atherosclerotic disease or with multile risk factors for cardiovascular disease*

TABLETS (LODOCO)

Adults. 0.5 mg once daily.

Drug Administration

P.O.

- Use a calibrated device to measure oral solution dosage.
- Store oral solution at room temperature.
- Capsules and tablets should be swallowed whole with water and not chewed or crushed.
- If a dose is missed for patient taking drug for treatment of a gout flare during prophylaxis, the missed dose should be given immediately, then wait 12 hr, and resume previous dosing schedule. For all other missed doses, drug should be given as soon as possible. Dose should never be doubled.
- Do not administer drug with grapefruit juice.

Route	Onset	Peak	Duration
P.O.	18–24 hr	42–72 hr	Unknown

Half-life: 27–31 hr

Contraindications

Concurrent use with strong CYP3A4 inhibitors or P-glycoprotein inhibitors in patients with hepatic or renal impairment;

Mechanism of Action

Helps stop the process of leukocytes phagocytose urate crystals being deposited in affected joints, a process that releases chemotactic factors, degradation enzymes, and other inflammatory substances. The process is probably halted by disrupting microtubules in leukocytes. Normally, microtubules contribute to cell structure and movement. When colchicine binds to tubulin (protein from which microtubules are made), the microtubule falls apart, as shown. This process disrupts cell function and prevents leukocytes from invading joints and causing inflammation.

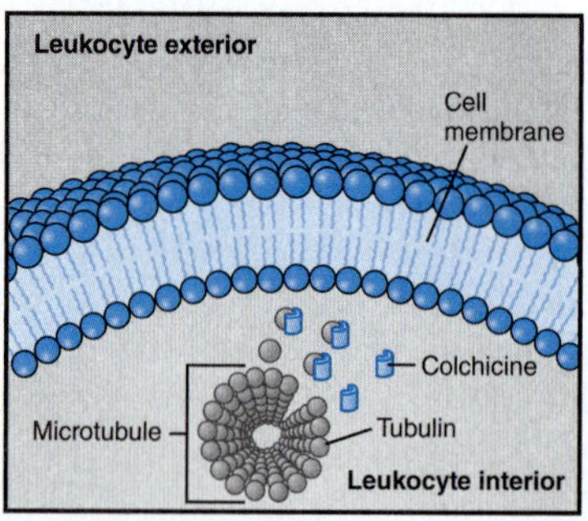

hepatic or renal impairment both being present; hypersensitivity to colchicine or its components; pre-existing blood dyscrasias

Interactions

DRUGS

clarithromycin, cyclosporin, ranolazine: Significant increase in colchicine plasma levels with possible fatal colchicine toxicity

digoxin; HMG-CoA reductase inhibitors, such as atorvastatin, fluvastatin, lovastatin, pravastatin, simvastatin; other lipid-lowering drugs, such as fibrates, gemfibrozil: Increased risk of myopathy and rhabdomyolysis

diltiazem, verapamil: Significant increase in colchicine plasma concentration with increased risk of colchicine toxicity; neuromuscular toxicity

moderate CYP3A4 inhibitors, such as amprenavir, aprepitant, erythromycin, fluconazole, fosamprenavir: Increased risk of colchicine toxicity

strong CYP3A4 inhibitors, such as atazanavir, darunavir/ritonavir, indinavir, itraconazole, ketoconazole, lopinavir/ritonavir, nefazodone, nelfinavir, ritonavir, saquinavir, telithromycin, tipranavir/ritonavir: Significant increase in colchicine plasma levels with high risk of toxicity

ACTIVITIES

alcohol use: Increased risk of adverse GI effects

FOOD

grapefruit juice: Increased risk of colchicine toxicity

Adverse Reactions

CNS: Peripheral neuropathy

GI: Abdominal pain, anorexia, diarrhea, nausea, vomiting

HEME: **Agranulocytosis**, **aplastic anemia**, **thrombocytopenia**

MS: Myopathy, **neuromuscular toxicity**, **rhabdomyolysis**

SKIN: Alopecia, rash

Childbearing Considerations

PREGNANCY

- It is not known if drug can cause fetal harm, but it does cross the placental barrier.
- Drug should be used with caution during pregnancy only if benefit to mother outweighs potential risk to fetus.

LACTATION

- Drug is present in breast milk.
- Mothers should check with prescriber before breastfeeding.

REPRODUCTION

- Drug may cause infertility in males, although rare and possibly reversible.

Nursing Considerations

- Know that debilitated or elderly patients and those with a history of cardiac disease or impaired hepatic or renal function are at increased risk for cumulative toxicity.
- Expect to monitor CBC and platelet and reticulocyte counts at baseline and every 3 months after therapy starts.

! WARNING Notify prescriber immediately and expect to stop colchicine if patient develops evidence of toxicity, such as abdominal pain, diarrhea, nausea, or vomiting.

! WARNING Be aware that drug can cause blood dyscrasias that could become life-threatening or even cause death. Monitor patient closely, especially patients with hepatic or renal dysfunction or in patients taking concomitant drugs that reduce the metabolism of colchicine.

! WARNING Know that neuromuscular toxicity and rhabdomyolysis may occur in patients receiving chronic treatment at therapeutic doses. Monitor patient closely for signs and symptoms of neuromuscular toxicity and rhabdomyolysis, especially in elderly patients (even those who have normal hepatic and renal function) and patients with renal dysfunction. In addition, concurrent drug therapy with bezafibrate, cyclosporine, fenofibrate, fenofibric acid, and statins may increase risk of myopathy. If neuromuscular signs and symptoms occur, notify prescriber and expect drug to be discontinued. After drug has been discontinued, symptoms usually resolve within one week to several months.

PATIENT TEACHING

- Instruct patient how to administer colchicine and what to do if a dose is missed.
- Caution patient not to take drug with grapefruit juice.

- Explain that gouty arthritis pain and swelling typically subside in 24 to 48 hours after therapy begins.

! **WARNING** Stress importance of having blood tests every 3 months, as ordered, during therapy to detect adverse blood reactions. Tell patient to notify prescriber if bleeding, bruising, or fatigue occurs.

! **WARNING** Advise patient to notify prescriber immediately if abdominal pain, diarrhea, nausea, or vomiting occurs.

! **WARNING** Review signs and symptoms of neuromuscular adverse effects. If present, stress importance of notifying prescriber.

- Tell patient to inform all prescribers of colchicine therapy, especially if patient has kidney or liver dysfunction because of potential drug interactions.

cortisone acetate

Class and Category

Pharmacologic class: Glucocorticoid
Therapeutic class: Anti-inflammatory, corticosteroid replacement, immunosuppressant

Indications and Dosages

* *To treat allergic and inflammatory disorders, collagen disorders, dermatologic disorders, edema (from nephrotic syndrome or systemic lupus erythematosus), endocrine disorders, GI disorders, hematologic disorders, multiple sclerosis (acute exacerbations), neoplastic diseases, ophthalmic disorders, respiratory disorders, rheumatic disorders, trichinosis with myocardial or neurologic involvement, and tuberculous meningitis*

TABLETS

Adults and adolescents. *Initial:* 25 to 300 mg daily. *Maintenance:* Dosage decreased or increased based on patient's response.

Drug Administration

P.O.

- Administer with food.

Route	Onset	Peak	Duration
P.O.	1–2 hr	2–4 hr	30–36 hr

Half-life: 30–60 min

Mechanism of Action

Binds to intracellular glucocorticoid receptors and suppresses inflammatory and immune responses by:

- inhibiting neutrophil and monocyte accumulation at the inflammation site and suppressing their phagocytic and bactericidal activity.
- stabilizing lysosomal membranes.
- suppressing the antigen response of macrophages and helper T cells.
- inhibiting synthesis of cellular mediators of inflammatory response, such as cytokines, interleukins, and prostaglandins.

Contraindications

Hypersensitivity to cortisone or its components, systemic fungal infection

Interactions

DRUGS

ephedrine, phenobarbital, phenytoin, rifampin: Deceased blood levels of cortisone
live-*virus vaccines:* Possibly serum antibody response not obtained in the presence of cortisone
oral anticoagulants: Possibly obstructed anticoagulant effects
potassium-wasting diuretics: Possibly hypokalemia

Adverse Reactions

CNS: Ataxia, behavior changes, depression, dizziness, euphoria, fatigue, headache, **increased intracranial pressure with papilledema**, insomnia, lassitude, malaise, mood swings, paresthesia, **seizures**, steroid psychosis, syncope, vertigo
CV: **Arrhythmias**, **fat embolism**, **heart failure**, hypertension, **hypotension**, thrombophlebitis
EENT: Exophthalmos, glaucoma, increased intraocular pressure, nystagmus, posterior subcapsular cataracts
ENDO: **Adrenal insufficiency**, Cushing's syndrome, diabetes mellitus, growth suppression in children, hyperglycemia, negative nitrogen balance from protein catabolism
GI: Abdominal distention, hiccups, increased appetite, nausea, **pancreatitis**, peptic ulcer, ulcerative esophagitis, vomiting
GU: Glycosuria, menstrual irregularities, perineal burning or tingling

HEME: Leukocytosis
MS: Arthralgia; aseptic necrosis of femoral and humeral heads; compression fractures; muscle atrophy, twitching, and weakness; myalgia; osteoporosis; spontaneous fractures; steroid myopathy; tendon rupture
SKIN: Acne; diaphoresis; ecchymosis; erythema; hirsutism; hyperpigmentation; hypopigmentation; necrotizing vasculitis; petechiae; purpura; rash; scarring; sterile abscesses; striae; subcutaneous fat atrophy; thin, fragile skin; urticaria
Other: **Anaphylaxis**, **hypocalcemia**, **hypokalemia**, **hypokalemic alkalosis**, impaired wound healing, masking of infection, **metabolic alkalosis**, suppressed skin test reaction, weight gain

Childbearing Considerations

PREGNANCY

- It is not known if drug can cause fetal harm.
- Drug should be used with caution during pregnancy only if benefit to mother outweighs potential risk to fetus.
- Monitor infant for hypoadrenalism if mother has received large doses of cortisone during pregnancy.

LACTATION

- Drug is present in breast milk.
- Breastfeeding should not be undertaken with drug therapy because of potential serious adverse reactions in breastfed infant.

Nursing Considerations

- Use cortisone cautiously in patients with ocular herpes simplex because corneal perforation may occur.
- Expect prescriber to order baseline ophthalmologic examination before therapy starts because prolonged use of cortisone may result in glaucoma, increased intraocular pressure, and damage to optic nerve.

! **WARNING** Assess patient for signs and symptoms of infection before giving cortisone because drug may mask them or make patients more susceptible to new infections because cortisone suppresses the immune system. If a new infection develops, expect to administer appropriate antibiotics. Also, know that chickenpox and measles can have more serious or even a fatal outcome in non-immune children or adults taking cortisone. If patient is exposed to chickenpox, expect to administer varicella zoster immune globulin prophylactically or if exposed to measles, expect to administer pooled I.M. immunoglobulin prophylactically. If chickenpox develops, expect an antiviral drug to be prescribed.

! **WARNING** Obtain serum electrolyte levels before therapy, as ordered, and monitor results often during therapy to detect electrolyte imbalances. Increased calcium excretion, potassium depletion, and sodium and water retention may occur with large doses of cortisone. Anticipate the need for calcium and potassium supplementation and sodium restriction, as needed.

- Keep in mind that prescriber will order lowest effective dose.
- Expect patient to receive concurrent antacid or antihistamine therapy to prevent the development of a peptic ulcer from cortisone administration.

! **WARNING** Monitor patient for a severe hypersensitivity reaction such as anaphylaxis. If present, notify prescriber immediately and prepare to provide supportive care, as needed and ordered.

! **WARNING** Assess for adrenal insufficiency (fatigue, hypotension, lassitude, nausea, vomiting, and weakness) or suppression in patient exposed to stress or receiving prolonged cortisone therapy. Notify prescriber immediately if patient has evidence of this life-threatening adverse reaction. Expect to taper oral cortisone dosage slowly to prevent adrenal insufficiency and withdrawal syndrome (abdominal or back pain, anorexia, dizziness, fever, headache, and syncope).

- Be aware that live-virus vaccines shouldn't be given during cortisone therapy because serum antibody response may not be obtained.
- Watch for signs and symptoms of steroid psychosis (confusion, delirium, euphoria, insomnia, mood swings, personality changes, severe depression), which may develop 15 to 30 days after starting drug. Be prepared to stop drug if such signs occur. If

stopping isn't possible, expect to administer a psychotropic drug.

- Watch for cushingoid signs, such as acne, buffalo hump, central obesity, ecchymosis, moon face, striae, and weight gain. Notify prescriber if they occur.

PATIENT TEACHING

- Instruct patient how to administer cortisone prescribed.
- Stress importance to take oral cortisone exactly as prescribed.

! **WARNING** Caution patient not to stop drug abruptly because doing so may lead to adrenal insufficiency, withdrawal symptoms, or both, which could become life-threatening. Inform patient about adrenal insufficiency and need for possible dosage increases during stress. Advise him to notify prescriber immediately if signs or symptoms develop or if he's exposed to stress.

! **WARNING** Tell patient to be alert for an allergic reaction to cortisone that could be severe. Stress importance of seeking immediate medical care, if present.

! **WARNING** Caution patient to avoid exposure to people with infections because cortisone can cause immunosuppression. Also, teach him to recognize and immediately report signs and symptoms of infection.

- Teach patient to recognize and report persistent, severe, or unsual adverse reactions.
- Urge patient receiving long-term cortisone therapy to carry medical identification.
- Recommend regular eye examinations.
- Tell mothers breastfeeding is not recommended during cortisone therapy.
- Urge patient to keep follow-up appointments with prescriber, which may include laboratory tests, to evaluate effects of therapy.

crizanlizumab-tmca

Adakveo

Class and Category

Pharmacologic class: Monoclonal antibody (P-selectin blocker)
Therapeutic class: Anti-vaso-occlusive

Indications and Dosages

* *To reduce the frequency of vaso-occlusive crises in patients with sickle cell disease*

I.V. INFUSION

Adults and adolescents ages 16 and older. 5 mg/kg at wk 0, wk 2, and every 4 wk thereafter.

Drug Administration

I.V.

- Calculate the number of vials needed for administration. 1 vial is needed for every 100 mg (10 ml) of crizanlizumab-tmca. Bring vials to room temperature for a maximum of 4 hr prior to the start of preparation (piercing the first vial).
- Visually inspect vials. Solution should be clear to opalescent, colorless, or may have a slightly brownish-yellow tint.
- Obtain a 100-ml 0.9% Sodium Chloride Injection or 5% Dextrose Injection infusion bag/container made of polyvinyl chloride (PVC), polyethylene (PE), or polypropylene (PP).
- Remove a volume of solution from the infusion bag/container that is equal to the required volume of the drug. Withdraw the necessary amount of drug solution and dilute by adding to the infusion bag/container. The volume added to the infusion bag/container should not exceed 96 ml.
- Gently invert infusion bag to mix diluted solution. Do not shake. Discard unused portion in drug vials.
- Administer diluted drug solution as soon as possible. If not administered immediately, store prepared solution at room temperature for no more than 4.5 hr from the start of preparation (piercing the first vial) to the completion of infusion, or refrigerate for no more than 24 hr from the start of preparation (piercing the first vial) to the completion of infusion. This includes storage of the diluted solution and time to warm up to room temperature. Protect diluted solution from light during storage under refrigeration.
- Infuse diluted solution over a period of 30 min through an intravenous line, which must contain a sterile, nonpyrogenic 0.2-micron inline filter.
- After administration of drug, flush the line with at least 25 ml of 0.9% Sodium Chloride Injection or 5% Dextrose Injection.

- Adjust dosage schedule for missed doses. If a dose is missed, it should be administered as soon as possible. If drug is administered within 2 wk after the missed dose, dosage schedule continues according to patient's original schedule. If dose is administered more than 2 wk after it was missed, dosing is continued every 4 wk thereafter.
- *Incompatibilities:* Other drugs through the same intravenous line

Route	Onset	Peak	Duration
I.V.	Unknown	Unknown	Unknown

Half-life: 10.6 days

Mechanism of Action

Binds to P-selectin to block interactions with its ligands, including P-selectin glycoprotein ligand 1. Binding P-selectin on the surface of the activated endothelium and platelets blocks interactions between endothelial cells, leukocytes, platelets, and red blood cells, which reduces vaso-occlusion.

Contraindications

Hypersensitivity to crizanlizumab-tmca or its components

Interactions

DRUGS

None reported by manufacturer.

Adverse Reactions

CNS: Fever
EENT: Oropharyngeal pain
GI: Abdominal discomfort, pain, or tenderness; diarrhea; nausea; vomiting
GU: Vulvovaginal pruritus
MS: Arthralgia, back pain, musculoskeletal chest pain, myalgia
SKIN: Pruritus
Other: Crizanlizumab-tmca–induced antibodies, infusion-related reactions (chills, dizziness, fatigue, fever, nausea, pruritus, shortness of breath, sweating, urticaria, vomiting, wheezing), infusion-site reactions (extravasation, pain, swelling)

Childbearing Considerations

PREGNANCY

- Drug has potential to cause fetal harm, based on animal studies.
- Use with caution only if benefit to mother outweighs potential risk to fetus.

LACTATION

- It is not known if drug is present in breast milk.
- Mothers should check with prescriber before breastfeeding.

Nursing Considerations

- Know that crizanlizumab-tmca may be given with or without hydroxyurea.

C

! **WARNING** Monitor patient for infusion-related reactions. If severe, notify prescriber, discontinue infusion, and institute treatment protocol, as needed and ordered.

- Be aware that crizanlizumab-tmca interferes with automated platelet counts (platelet clumping), particularly when blood samples are collected in tubes containing EDTA, which may lead to unevaluable or falsely decreased platelet counts. Blood samples should be run within 4 hours of blood collection, or blood samples should be collected in tubes containing citrate. If needed, estimate platelet count via peripheral blood smear.

PATIENT TEACHING

- Inform patient how drug will be administered and answer any questions or address any concerns patient may have.

! **WARNING** Inform patient that infusion-related reactions may occur. Review these reactions with patient. Advise patient to immediately report any signs or symptoms of an infusion-related reaction, including after leaving the healthcare facility.

- Instruct patient to inform healthcare provider that they are receiving crizanlizumab-tmca prior to any blood tests, due to the potential interference with laboratory tests used to measure platelet counts.

crofelemer

Mytesi

Class and Category

Pharmacologic class: Botanical
Therapeutic class: Antidiarrheal

Indications and Dosages

✶ *To provide symptomatic relief of noninfectious diarrhea in patients with HIV/AIDS on antiretroviral therapy*

D.R. TABLETS

Adults. 125 mg twice daily.

Drug Administration

P.O.

- D.R. tablets should be swallowed whole and not chewed, crushed, or split.

Route	Onset	Peak	Duration
P.O./D.R.	45–60 min	> 2 hr	3–4 hr

Half-life: Not significantly absorbed

Mechanism of Action

Inhibits both the cyclic adenosine monophosphate (cAMP)–stimulated cystic fibrosis transmembrane conductance regulator (CFTR) chloride ion channel, and the calcium-activated chloride channel (CaCC) at the luminal membrane of enterocytes. By blocking chloride secretion and accompanying high-volume water loss in diarrhea, the flow of chloride and water in the GI tract becomes normalized.

Contraindications

Hypersensitivity to crofelemer or its components

Interactions

DRUGS

None reported by manufacturer.

Adverse Reactions

CNS: Anxiety, depression, dizziness
EENT: Dry mouth, nasopharyngitis, sinusitis
GI: Abdominal distention or pain, constipation, dyspepsia, elevated bilirubin or liver enzymes, flatulence, gastroenteritis, giardiasis (intestinal parasitic infection), nausea
GU: Frequent daytime urination syndrome, nephrolithiasis, UTI
HEME: **Leukopenia**
MS: Arthralgia: back, extremity, or musculoskeletal pain
RESP: Bronchitis, cough, upper respiratory infection
SKIN: Acne, dermatitis
Other: Herpes zoster

Childbearing Considerations

PREGNANCY

- It is not known if drug can cause fetal harm.
- Because drug is minimally absorbed systemically it is not expected to affect the fetus.

LACTATION

- It is not known if drug is present in breast milk.
- The Centers for Disease Control and Prevention recommends that HIV-1-infected mothers not breastfeed to avoid risking postnatal transmission of HIV-1 infection in HIV-negative infants or developing viral resistance in HIV-positive infants. They also do not recommend breastfeeding because of potential drug-induced adverse reactions in the infant.

Nursing Considerations

- Be aware that crofelemer is used only to treat noninfectious diarrhea in patients with HIV/AIDS on antiretroviral therapy. Infectious etiologies should be ruled out before drug is started because crofelemer is not effective against infectious causes of diarrhea.
- Know that no dosage adjustment is needed related to the patient's CD4 cell count and HIV viral load.

PATIENT TEACHING

- Instruct patient how to administer crofelemer.
- Advise patient to inform prescriber if no improvement in diarrhea is noted.
- Tell mothers that breastfeeding should not be undertaken because of the presence of HIV.

cyclobenzaprine hydrochloride

Amrix

Class and Category

Pharmacologic class: Tricyclic antidepressant-like agent (TCA)
Therapeutic class: Skeletal muscle relaxant

Indications and Dosages

* *As adjunct to rest and physical therapy for relief of muscle spasm associated with acute, painful musculoskeletal conditions*

TABLETS

Adults and adolescents ages 15 and older. 5 mg 3 times daily, increased, as needed, to

7.5 or 10 mg 3 times daily. *Maximum:* 30 mg daily for no more than 3 wk.

±**DOSAGE ADJUSTMENT** For elderly patients and those with hepatic impairment, dosage frequency reduced.

E.R. CAPSULES (AMRIX)

Adults. 15 mg once daily, increased to 30 mg once daily, as needed. *Maximum:* 30 mg once daily for no longer than 3 wk.

Drug Administration

P.O.

- Tablets and E.R. capsules should be swallowed whole and not chewed or crushed. Tablets should not be split.
- If patient is unable to swallow E.R. capsule, contents of capsule may be mixed with applesauce. Have patient swallow mixture immediately after mixing without chewing. Have patient rinse mouth and swallow afterwards.

Route	Onset	Peak	Duration
P.O.	1 hr	4 hr	12–24 hr
P.O./E.R.	1.5 hr	7–8 hr	Unknown

Half-life: 18–31 hr

Mechanism of Action

Acts in the brain stem to reduce or abolish tonic muscle hyperactivity. Because cyclobenzaprine doesn't act at the neuromuscular junction or directly on skeletal muscle, it relieves muscle spasm without disrupting muscle function.

Contraindications

Acute recovery phase of MI; arrhythmias, including heart block and other conduction disturbances; heart failure; hypersensitivity to cyclobenzaprine or its components; hyperthyroidism; MAO inhibitor use within 14 days

Interactions

DRUGS

anticholinergics, antidyskinetics: Possibly potentiated anticholinergic effects of these drugs

bupropion, MAO inhibitors, meperidine, selective serotonin reuptake inhibitors (SSRIs), serotonin norepinephrine reuptake inhibitors (SNRIs), tramadol, tricyclic antidepressants, verapamil: Possibly increased risk of serotonin syndrome

CNS depressants, including barbiturates, tricyclic antidepressants: Possibly additive CNS depressant effects of these drugs; increased risk of adverse effects of antidepressants and cyclobenzaprine

guanadrel, guanethidine: Possibly decreased or blocked antihypertensive effects of these drugs

MAO inhibitors: Possibly hyperpyretic crisis, severe seizures, and death

tramadol: Increased risk of seizures

ACTIVITIES

alcohol use: Possibly additive CNS depression

Adverse Reactions

CNS: Aggression, agitation, anxiety, asthenia, ataxia, confusion, **CVA**, delusions, depression, disorientation, dizziness, drowsiness, EEG alterations, extrapyramidal symptoms, fatigue, fever, hallucinations, headache, hypertonia, insomnia, irritability, malaise, **neuroleptic malignant syndrome**, nervousness, paranoia, paresthesia, psychosis, **seizures**, **serotonin syndrome**, syncope, thirst, tremor, vertigo, weakness

CV: **Arrhythmias**, including tachycardia; **heart block**; hypertension; **hypotension**; **MI**; orthostatic hypotension; palpitations; peripheral neuropathy; vasodilation

EENT: Blurred vision, diplopia, dry mouth, parotid swelling, **tongue** discoloration or edema, stomatitis, tinnitus transient vision loss, unpleasant taste

ENDO: Breast enlargement, galactorrhea, gynecomastia, hyperglycemia, **hypoglycemia**, syndrome of inappropriate ADH syndrome (SIADH)

GI: Anorexia, cholestasis, constipation, diarrhea, elevated liver enzymes, flatulence, gastritis, gastrointestinal pain, **hepatitis**, hiccups, indigestion, jaundice, nausea, paralytic ileus, vomiting

GU: Libido changes, impotence, testicular swelling urinary frequency, urine retention

HEME: **Bone marrow depression**, eosinophilia, **leukopenia**, **thrombocytopenia**

MS: Dysarthria

RESP: Dyspnea

SKIN: Diaphoresis, facial flushing, pruritus, rash, urticaria

Other: **Anaphylaxis**, **angioedema**, weight changes

Childbearing Considerations

PREGNANCY

- It is not known if drug can cause fetal harm.
- Drug should be used with caution during pregnancy only if benefit to mother outweighs potential risk to fetus.

LACTATION

- It is not known if drug is present in breast milk.
- Mothers should check with prescriber before breastfeeding.

Nursing Considerations

- Be aware that drug is not recommended for use in the elderly because higher plasma levels of cyclobenzaprine occur in the elderly, increasing risk of serious adverse reactions.

! **WARNING** Use cyclobenzaprine cautiously in patients with history of low seizure threshold. Institute seizure precautions because drug may cause seizures. Monitor patient closely.

! **WARNING** Monitor patient for a hypersensitivity reaction that could become life-threatening, such as anaphylaxis or angioedema. If present, notify prescriber promptly; expect drug to be discontinued, as ordered; and provide supportive care, as needed and ordered.

! **WARNING** Monitor patient for infection and patient's CBC regularly, as ordered, because drug can cause immunosuppression and other serious hematologic adverse effects.

! **WARNING** Monitor patient closely if cyclobenzaprine is being given with other serotonergic drug, especially when treatment is started and during dosage increases because of the potential for life-threatening serotonin syndrome to develop. Assess patient for autonomic instability, mental status changes, and nervous system abnormalities. If present, withhold both cyclobenzaprine and other serotonergic drugs and notify prescriber immediately. Provide supportive care, as ordered.

- Take safety precautions to prevent falls if patient is confused, dizzy, or weak.

PATIENT TEACHING

- Instruct patient how to administer form of cyclobenzaprine prescribed.

! **WARNING** Alert patient that cyclobenazaprine may cause an allergic reaction. Tell patient to notify prescriber if an allergic reaction occurs and, if severe, to seek immediate medical care.

! **WARNING** Inform patient that drug may cause seizures, especially if patient already has a seizure disorder. Stress importance of alerting prescriber if a seizure occurs and to seek immediate medical attention.

! **WARNING** Review infection control measures with patient and encourage patient to comply with laboratory appointments for blood tests.

- Instruct patient to alert prescriber if persistent, severe, or unusual adverse reactions occur.
- Urge patient to avoid alcohol and other CNS depressants during therapy.
- Inform patient about possible lack of alertness and dexterity.
- Advise patient to avoid driving, or other hazardous activities if he experiences dizziness or weakness.

cyclosporine

Sandimmune

cyclosporine (modified)

Gengraf, Neoral

Class and Category

Pharmacologic class: Polypeptide
Therapeutic class: Antipsoriatic, antirheumatic, immunosuppressant

Indications and Dosages

✱ *To prevent or treat organ rejection in heart, kidney, and liver allogenic transplantation*

CAPSULES, MODIFIED CAPSULES, MODIFIED ORAL SOLUTION, ORAL SOLUTION

Adults and children. *Initial:* 15 mg/kg as a single dose 4 to 12 hr before transplantation, followed by 15 mg/kg once daily postoperatively for 1 to 2 wk and then tapered by 5% per wk to maintenance dose. *Maintenance:* 5 to 10 mg/kg daily in divided doses every 12 hr.

I.V. INFUSION

Adults and children. 5 to 6 mg/kg daily starting 4 to 12 hr before surgery. Postoperatively, 5 to 6 mg/kg once daily until patient can tolerate oral form of drug.

* *To treat severe rheumatoid arthritis in non-immunocompromised patients who have failed to respond to at least one systemic therapy or in patients for whom other systemic therapies are contraindicated or cannot be tolerated*

MODIFIED CAPSULES, MODIFIED ORAL SOLUTION

Adults. 2.5 mg/kg daily in divided doses every 12 hr, increased by 0.5 to 0.75 mg/kg daily after 8 wk, as needed, and again after 12 wk, as needed. *Maximum:* 4 mg/kg daily.

* *To treat severe, recalcitrant plaque psoriasis in non-immunocompromised patients who have failed to respond to at least one systemic therapy or in patients for whom other systemic therapies are contraindicated, or cannot be tolerated*

MODIFIED CAPSULES, MODIFIED ORAL SOLUTION

Adults. *Initial:* 2.5 mg/kg daily in divided doses twice daily, increased after 4 wks in increments of by 0.5 mg/kg daily every 2 wk, as needed. *Maximum:* 4 mg/kg daily.

±**DOSAGE ADJUSTMENT** For patients with severe liver dysfunction, dosage reduced. For patients receiving cyclosporine to treat psoriasis or rheumatoid arthritis and experiencing serious adverse reactions, dosage reduced 25% to 50% in effort to bring adverse reactions under control.

Drug Administration

- Intravenous and oral solutions contain alcohol and shouldn't be administered to patient who drinks heavily or has a history of alcohol dependence. In addition, these forms of cyclosporine should not be used with patients in whom alcohol intake should be avoided or minimized, such as breastfeeding or pregnant females, children, or patients with epilepsy or liver disease. Be aware that for an adult weighing 70 kg or 150 pounds, the maximum daily oral dose would deliver about 6% and a daily intravenous dose would deliver about 15% of the amount of alcohol contained in a standard drink.

P.O.

- Capsules and oral solution aren't interchangeable with modified capsules and modified oral solution. Modified forms have greater bioavailability.
- Be aware that Neoral is not bioequivalent to Sandimmune.
- Administer on a consistent schedule with regard to meals and time of day.
- Avoid giving with grapefruit juice.
- Capsules should not be chewed, crushed, or opened but swallowed whole. Store capsules at 25°C (77°F) in prepackaged foil wrap to protect them from light.
- Administer oral solution doses in oral syringe. Clean outside of dosing syringe with a clean towel and replace protective cover after use. Do not rinse syringe with water or other cleaning agents. However, if syringe must be cleaned, it must be completely dry before reuse.
- To improve taste of Sandimmune oral solution, mix it with chocolate milk, milk, or orange juice. Gengraf or Neoral oral solution may be mixed with apple or orange juice that is at room temperature, but not milk. Don't add water to oral solution because it will alter drug's effectiveness.
- Use a glass container when mixing oral solution with other liquids and have patient drink the mixture at once. Do not let mixture stand before drinking. Rinse glass with more liquid and have patient drink again.
- Oral solution should be kept at room temperature and discarded, once opened, after 2 mo.

I.V.

- Protect drug from light.
- Prepare I.V. infusion immediately before administration by diluting each milliliter of concentrate in 20 to 100 ml of 0.9% Sodium Chloride Injection or 5% Dextrose Injection. Use glass containers because of possible leaching of diethylhexylphthalate from polyvinyl chloride bags into drug solution.
- Administer I.V. infusion slowly over 2 to 6 hr. Avoid rapid I.V. infusion, which may cause acute nephrotoxicity.
- Discard diluted solution after 24 hr.
- *Incompatibilities:* None listed by manufacturer.

Route	Onset	Peak	Duration
P.O.	Unknown	1.5–2 hr	Unknown
I.V.	Unknown	Unknown	Unknown

Half-life: 8.5–27 hr

Mechanism of Action

Causes immunosuppression by inhibiting the proliferation of T lymphocytes, the production and release of lymphokines, and the release of interleukin-2, responsible for organ rejection and in disease processes, such as psoriasis and rheumatoid arthritis.

Contraindications

Abnormal renal function, neoplastic diseases, and uncontrolled hypertension in patients with psoriasis or rheumatoid arthritis (modified capsules and oral solution); hypersensitivity to cyclosporine, its components, or polyoxyethylated castor oil (all indications; I.V. infusion for castor oil)

Interactions

DRUGS

ACE inhibitors, angiotensin II receptor antagonists, potassium-sparing diuretics, potassium supplements: Increased risk of hyperkalemia

aliskiren, ambrisentan, bosentan, colchicine, CYP3A4 substrates, dabigatran, digoxin, daunorubicin, doxorubicin, etoposide, HMG-CoA reductase inhibitors (statins), methotrexate, mitoxantrone, NSAIDs, organic anion transporter protein substrates, P-glycoprotein substrates, prednisolone, repaglinide, sirolimus: Increased blood concentrations of these drugs and possible toxicity

allopurinol, amiodarone, azithromycin, bromocriptine, clarithromycin, colchicine, danazol, diltiazem, erythromycin, fluconazole, HIV protease inhibitors, imatinib, itraconazole, ketoconazole, methylprednisolone, metoclopramide, nefazodone, nicardipine, oral contraceptives, quinupristin and dalfopristin, verapamil, voriconazole: Increased cyclosporine level

amphotericin B, azapropazone, cimetidine, ciprofloxacin, colchicine, co-trimoxazole, diclofenac, fibric acid derivatives (bezafibrate, fenofibrate), gentamicin, ketoconazole, melphalan, naproxen, NSAIDs, sirolimus, sulindac, tacrolimus, tobramycin, vancomycin: Increased risk of nephrotoxicity

atorvastatin, fluvastatin, lovastatin, pravastatin, simvastatin: Risk of myotoxicity

bosentan, carbamazepine, nafcillin, octreotide, orlistat, oxcarbazepine, phenobarbital, phenytoin, rifampin, St. John's wort, sulfinpyrazone, terbinafine, ticlopidine: Decreased blood cyclosporine level and therapeutic response

methotrexate: Increased blood methotrexate level and risk of renal dysfunction

methylprednisolone (high dose): Increased risk of seizures

mycophenolic acid, mycophenolic sodium: Possibly decreased exposure of these drugs with possible decreased effectiveness

nifedipine: Increased risk of gingival hyperplasia

other immunosuppressants: Possibly excessive immunosuppression

repaglinide: Possibly increased repaglinide level and risk of hypoglycemia

vaccines (killed or live virus): Possibly suppressed immune response and increased adverse effects of vaccine

FOODS

grapefruit, grapefruit juice: Increased risk of nephrotoxicity; increased plasma concentration of cyclosporine

potassium-rich foods: Increased risk of hyperkalemia

Adverse Reactions

CNS: Altered level of consciousness, confusion, **encephalopathy**, headache, **intracranial hypertension**, lethargy, loss of motor function, migraine, **neurotoxicity**, paresthesia, **progressive multifocal leukoencephalopathy, posterior reversible encephalopathy syndrome (PRES)**, psychiatric disturbances, **seizures**, tremor

CV: Chest pain, hypertension, **MI**

EENT: Gingival hyperplasia, optic disc edema, oral candidiasis, sinusitis, visual impairment (including blindness)

ENDO: Gynecomastia

GI: Cholestasis, diarrhea, **hepatitis**, **hepatotoxicity**, jaundice, **liver failure**, nausea, **pancreatitis**, vomiting

GU: Albuminuria, elevated serum creatinine and blood urea nitrogen levels, glomerular capillary thrombosis, hematuria, **nephropathy associated with BK virus**, **nephrotoxicity**, proteinuria, **renal failure**

HEME: Anemia, **leukopenia**, **thrombocytopenia**

MS: Lower extremity pain
SKIN: Acne, **cancer**, flushing, hirsutism, pruritus, rash
Other: **Anaphylaxis**; bacterial, fungal, protozoal, and viral infections, including opportunistic infections such as polyomavirus; **hyperkalemia**; **hypomagnesemia**; **life-threatening infections**; **lymphoma and other malignancies**

Childbearing Considerations

PREGNANCY

- Pregnancy exposure registry: 1-877-955-8677 or https://www.transplantpregnancyregistry.org.
- It is not known if drug can cause fetal harm but alcohol content of drug should be taken into account.
- Drug should be used with caution during pregnancy only if benefit to mother outweighs potential risk to fetus.

LACTATION

- Drug is present in breast milk.
- Mothers should check with prescriber before breastfeeding.
- Mothers who are breastfeeding should avoid additional alcohol intake during drug therapy.

Nursing Considerations

- Don't draw blood to measure cyclosporine level through same I.V. tubing used to administer drug, even if line was flushed after administration. Blood level may be falsely elevated.
- Be aware that there is an association between the development of interstitial fibrosis and higher cumulative doses or persistently high circulating trough concentrations of cyclosporine, especially during first 6 months post-transplant, that may increase the risk of chronic nephrotoxicity.

! WARNING Monitor patient closely for hypersensitivity reactions, especially at the beginning of cyclosporine therapy and for at least the first 30 minutes following the start of an intravenous dose, and then frequently thereafter. If anaphylaxis occurs, notify prescriber, stop drug immediately and be prepared to provide supportive care, as needed and ordered.

! WARNING Be aware that although uncommon, cyclosporine may cause neurotoxicity, especially after liver transplantation. Watch for evidence of encephalopathy (impaired consciousness, loss of motor function, psychiatric disturbance, seizures, visual disturbance). Notify prescriber immediately if present and expect cyclosporine dosage to be decreased or drug discontinued to increase possibility of a reversible or improvement of encephalopathy. Also, monitor patients closely for seizures, especially if they are also receiving high-dose methylprednisolone therapy.

! WARNING Watch for evidence of infection (such as cough, fever, malaise, pain) because patients receiving immunosuppressants such as cyclosporine are at increased risk for bacterial, fungal, parasitic, and viral infection. Watch for both generalized and localized infections, including worsening of preexisting infections, and be aware that these infections may become life-threatening. Activation of latent viral infections may also occur and include BK virus–associated nephropathy that can lead to decreased renal function and renal graft loss.

- Monitor blood pressure, especially in patients with a history of hypertension because drug can worsen this condition. Expect to decrease dosage if hypertension develops.
- Monitor liver and renal function tests, as ordered, to detect decreased function. Be aware that it is not unusual for BUN and serum creatinine levels to be elevated during cyclosporine therapy. These elevations warrant investigation but do not always reflect kidney transplant rejection. If not related to rejection, a dosage reduction of cyclosporine often helps to decrease these levels.
- Be aware that cyclosporine use may result in increased serum cholesterol levels.
- Expect about 50% of patients treated for psoriasis to relapse about 4 months after therapy stops. Know that patients with chronic plaque psoriasis may develop erythrodermic psoriasis or generalized pustular psoriasis when cyclosporine dose is reduced, or drug is discontinued.

PATIENT TEACHING

- Instruct patient how to take form of cyclosporine prescribed.
- Advise patient not to stop taking drug without consulting prescriber.
- Inform patient with rheumatoid arthritis that drug effects may not appear for 4 to 6 weeks.

! **WARNING** Tell patient drug may cause an allergic reaction and to notify prescriber if present or to seek immediate emergency treatment, if reaction is severe.

! **WARNING** Review infection control precautions with patient. Caution patient to avoid people who have infections during therapy because cyclosporine causes immunosuppression.

- Stress importance of notifying prescriber of any persistent, servere, or unusual adverse reactions.
- Instruct patient to avoid live or live-attenuated vaccines during therapy and people who have received such vaccines recently. Or suggest wearing a protective mask when he's around them.
- Caution patient to avoid performing hazardous activities such as driving or operating machines until adverse effects are known and resolved.
- Advise good dental hygiene because of risk of gingival hyperplasia.
- Caution patient to avoid excessive exposure to ultraviolet light.
- Instruct mothers who are breastfeeding to avoid alcohol while taking drug.

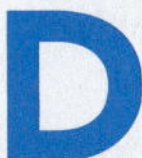

dabigatran etexilate mesylate

Pradaxa

Class and Category

Pharmacologic class: Direct thrombin inhibitor

Therapeutic class: Anticoagulant

Indications and Dosages

* *To reduce the risk of stroke and systemic embolism in patients with nonvalvular atrial fibrillation*

CAPSULES

Adults with creatinine clearance greater than 30 ml/min. 150 mg twice daily.

Adults with creatinine clearance between 15 and 30 ml/min. 75 mg twice daily.

± **DOSAGE ADJUSTMENT** For patients with a creatinine level between 30 and 50 ml/min and taking the P-gp inhibitor, dronedarone or systemic ketoconazole concomitantly, dosage decreased to 75 mg twice daily.

* *To treat deep vein thrombosis and pulmonary emboli in patients who have been treated with a parenteral anticoagulant for 5 to 10 days; to reduce risk of recurrence of deep vein thrombosis and pulmonary emboli in patients who have been previously treated*

CAPSULES

Adults with creatinine clearance greater than 30 ml/min. 150 mg twice daily.

± **DOSAGE ADJUSTMENT** For patients with a creatinine clearance less than 50 ml/min and taking P-gp inhibitors concomitantly, dabigatran should be avoided.

* *To prevent deep vein thrombosis and pulmonary embolism following a hip replacement*

CAPSULES

Adults with creatinine clearance greater than 30 ml/min. 110 mg 1 to 4 hr after surgery and after hemostasis has been achieved on day 1, then 220 mg once daily for 28 to 35 days.

± **DOSAGE ADJUSTMENT** For patients who do not have drug therapy started on the day of surgery, drug initiated at 220 mg once daily after hemostasis has been achieved. For patients with a creatinine clearance less than 50 ml/min and taking P-gp inhibitors concomitantly, dabigatran should be avoided.

* *To treat venous thromboembolic events in children who have been treated with a parenteral anticoagulant for at least 5 days; to reduce risk of recurrence of venous thromboembolic events in children who have been previously treated*

CAPSULES

Children ages 8 to less than 18 weighing 81 kg (178.2 lb) or more with an eGFR greater than 50 ml/min. 260 mg twice daily.

Children ages 8 to less than 18 weighing 61 kg (134.2 lb) to less than 81 kg (178.2 lb) with an eGFR greater than 50 ml/min. 220 mg twice daily.

Children ages 8 to less than 18 weighing 41 kg (90.2 lb) to less than 61 kg (134.2 lb) with an eGFR greater than 50 ml/min. 185 mg twice daily.

Children ages 8 to less than 18 weighing 26 kg (57.2 lb) to less than 41 kg (90.2 lb) with an eGFR greater than 50 ml/min. 150 mg twice daily.

Children ages 8 to less than 18 weighing 16 kg (35.2 lb) to less than 26 kg (57.2 lb) with an eGFR greater than 50 ml/min. 110 mg twice daily.

Children ages 8 to less than 18 weighing 11 kg (24.2 lb) to less than 16 kg (35.2 lb) with an eGFR greater than 50 ml/min. 75 mg twice daily.

ORAL PELLETS

Children ages 2 to less than 12 weighing 41 kg (90.2 lb) or more with an eGFR greater than 50 ml/min. 260 mg twice daily.

Children ages 2 to less than 12 weighing 21 kg (46.2 lb) to less than 41 kg (90.2 lb) with an eGFR greater than 50 ml/min. 220 mg twice daily.

Children ages 2 to less than 12 weighing 16 kg (35.2 lb) to less than 21 kg (46.2 lb) with a eGFR greater than 50 ml/min. 170 mg twice daily.

Children ages 2 to less than 12 weighing 13 kg (28.6 lb) to less than 16 kg (35.2 lb) with an eGFR greater than 50 ml/min. 140 mg twice daily.

Children ages 2 to less than 12 weighing 11 kg (24.2 lb) to less than 13 kg (28.6 lb)

with an eGFR greater than 50 ml/min. 110 mg twice daily.
Children ages 2 to less than 12 weighing 9 kg (19.8 lb) to less than 11 kg (24.2 lb) with an eGFR rate greater than 50 ml/min. 90 mg twice daily.
Children ages 2 to less than 12 weighing 7 kg (15.4 lb) to less than 9 kg (19.8 lb) with an eGFR rate greater than 50 ml/min. 70 mg twice daily.
Children ages 18 months to less than 24 months weighing 21 kg (46.2 lb) to less than 26 kg (57.2 lb) with an eGFR greater than 50 ml/min. 180 mg twice daily.
Children ages 12 months to less than 24 months weighing 16 kg (35.2 lb) to less than 21 kg (46.2 lb) with an eGFR rate greater than 50 ml/min. 140 mg twice daily.
Children and infants ages 11 months to less than 24 months weighing 13 kg (28.6 lb) to less than 16 kg (35.2 lb) with an eGFR rate greater than 50 ml/min. 140 mg twice daily.
Infants ages 10 months to less than 11 months weighing 13 kg (28.6 lb) to less than 16 kg (35.2 lb) with an eGFR rate greater than 50 ml/min. 100 mg twice daily.
Children and infants 18 months to less than 24 months weighing 11 kg (24.2 lb) to less than 13 kg (28.6 lb) with an eGFR greater than 50 ml/min. 110 mg twice daily.
Children and infants 8 months to less than 18 months weighing 11 kg (24.2 lb) to less than 13 kg (28.6 lb) with an eGFR rate greater than 50 ml/min. 100 mg twice daily.
Children and infants 11 months to less than 24 months weighing 9 kg (19.8lb) to less than 11 kg (24.2 lb) with an EGFR rate greater than 50 ml/min. 90 mg twice daily.
Infants 6 months to less than 11 months weighing 9 kg (19.8 lb) to less than 11 kg (24.2 lb) with an eGFR rate greater than 50 ml/min. 80 mg twice daily.
Infants 5 months to less than 6 months weighing 9 kg (19.8 lb) to less than 11 kg (24.2 lb) with an eGFR rate greater than 50 ml/min. 60 mg twice daily.
Children and infants ages 9 months to less than 24 months weighing 7 kg (15.4 lb) to less than 9 kg (19.8 lb) with an eGFR rate greater than 50 ml/min. 70 mg twice daily.
Infants ages 4 months to less than 9 months weighing 7 kg (15.4 lb) to less than 9 kg (19.8 lb) with an eGFR rate greater than 50 ml/min. 60 mg twice daily.
Infants ages 3 months to less than 4 months weighing 7 kg (15.4 lb to less than 9 kg (19.8 lb) with an eGFR rate greater than 50 ml/min. 50 mg twice daily.
Children and infants ages 5 months to less than 24 months weighing 5 kg (11 lb) to less than 7 kg (15.4 lb) with an eGFR rate greater than 50 ml./min. 50 mg twice daily.
Infants ages 3 months to less than 5 months weighing 5 kg (11 lb) to less than 7 kg (15.4 lb) with an eGFR rate greater than 50 ml/min. 40 mg twice daily.
Infants ages 3 months to less than 10 months weighing 4 kg (8.8 lb) to less than 5 kg (11 lb) with an eGFR rate greater than 50 ml/min. 40 mg twice daily.
Infants ages 3 months to less than 6 months weighing 3 kg (6.6 lb) to less than 4 kg (8.8 lb) with an eGFR rate greater than 50 ml/min. 30 mg twice daily.

Drug Administration

P.O.

Capsules

- Capsule should be swallowed whole and not chewed, crushed, or opened. Administer with a full glass of water. Also, administer with food if GI upset occurs.
- If a dose is missed, it should be given when discovered if on the same day of the missed dose, unless it is within 6 hr of the next dose.
- Keep bottle tightly closed when not in use and store in the original package to protect from moisture.
- Discard any remaining drug if not used within 4 mo of initially opening the container.
- When patients convert to dabigatran from warfarin therapy, warfarin should be discontinued, and dabigatran initiated when the INR is below 2.0.
- Expect patients converting from dabigatran to warfarin therapy to do so based on the creatinine clearance level (adults) or eGFR (children). For adult patients who have a creatinine clearance level equal to or greater than 50 ml/min and children who have an eGFR equal to or greater than 50 ml/min, expect warfarin to be started 3 days before dabigatran is discontinued; for adult patients who have a creatinine clearance

level of 30 to 50 ml/min, expect warfarin to be started 2 days before dabigatran is discontinued; for adult patients who have a creatinine clearance level of 15 to 30 ml/min, expect warfarin to be started 1 day before dabigatran is discontinued. No recommendations are available for adult patients who have a creatinine clearance level of less than 15 ml/min. For children who have an eGFR less than 50 ml/min, dabigatran should be avoided.

- For adult patients and children who will begin dabigatran therapy having been receiving a parenteral anticoagulant, expect to start dabigatran therapy up to 2 hr before the time the next dose of the parenteral drug was to have been given or at the time of discontinuation of a continuously administered parenteral drug.
- For adult patients converting from dabigatran to a parenteral anticoagulant, expect to wait 12 hr for patients with a creatinine clearance of 30 ml/min or greater or wait 24 hr for patients with a creatinine clearance of less than 30 ml/min after the last dose of dabigatran and before parenteral anticoagulant is initiated. For children converting from dabigatran to a parenteral anticoagulant, expect to wait 12 hr after the last dose of dabigatran before initiating the parenteral anticoagulant.

Oral pellets

- Twice daily dosing should be as close to 12 hr apart as possible.
- Remove and discard desiccant after opening drug package.
- Administer before meals to be sure patient takes the full dose.
- Spoon oral pellets directly into patient's mouth and have patient swallow with a drink of apple juice or add 1 to 2 ounces of apple juice to the pellets and have patient drink mixture. Drug may also be mixed with 2 teaspooons of applesauce, baby rice cereal prepared with water, mashed banana, or mashed carrots. Do not mix with any other soft foods. Also, do not mix with milk, milk products, or soft foods containing milk products.
- Administer immediately after mixing or no later than 30 min after mixing. If it is not administered within 30 min of mixing, drug should be discarded.
- Do not administer oral pellets via a feeding tube or syringe.
- If a dose is missed it should be administered as soon as possible unless it is less than 6 hr before the next scheduled dose. In that case, the dose should be missed. Never double the dose.
- If only a partial dose has been taken, do not administer a second dose at that time. The next dose should be administered 12 hr later.
- When converting patient from warfarin therapy to dabigatran oral pellets, expect warfarin to be discontinued and oral pellets started when the INR is below 2.0.
- When converting patient from dabigatran oral pellets to warfarin, start warfarin 3 days before discontinuing dabigatran oral pellets if patient's eGFR is 50 ml/min or greater. (oral pellets are not given to patients with a eGFR less than 50 ml/min).
- For pediatric patients currently receiving a parenteral anticoagulant and converting to dabigatran oral pellets, expect to start oral pellets 0 to 2 hr before the time that the next dose of the parenteral drug was to have been given or given at the time of discontinuation of a continuously administered parenteral drug such as intravenous unfractionated hepain.
- For pediatric patients currently receiving dabigatran oral pellets and switching to a parenteral anticoagulant, expect to wait 12 hr after the last dose before switching to the parenteral anticoagulant.
- Expect to throw away oral pellets if not used within 6 mo.

Route	Onset	Peak	Duration
P.O.	Rapid	1–2 hr	Unknown

Half-life: 12–17 hr

Mechanism of Action

Inhibits thrombin from converting fibrinogen into fibrin directly during the coagulation cascade. Inhibition of this activity prevents the development of a blood clot.

Contraindications

Active pathologic bleeding, hypersensitivity to dabigatran or its components, presence of mechanical prosthetic heart valve

Interactions

DRUGS

P-gp inducers, such as rifampin: Decreased exposure to dabigatran
P-gp inhibitors, such as dronedarone, ketoconazole: Increased exposure to dabigatran in patients with renal impairment; possibly increased exposure to dabigatran in children

Adverse Reactions

CNS: **Intracranial or intraspinal hemorrhage**
CV: **Pericardial bleeding**
EENT: Epistaxis, intraocular bleeding
GI: Diarrhea, dyspepsia, esophageal ulcer, gastritis-like symptoms, **gastrointestinal hemorrhage**, nausea, **retroperitoneal bleeding**, upper abdominal pain, vomiting
GU: **Anticoagulant-related nephropathy**, menorrhagia
HEME: **Agranulocytosis**, **bleeding (serious)**, **neutropenia**, **thrombocytopenia**
MS: Intra-articular bleeding, intramuscular bleeding with compartment syndrome
SKIN: Alopecia, pruritus, rash, urticaria
Other: **Anaphylactic reaction or shock**, **angioedema**

Childbearing Considerations

PREGNANCY

- It is not known if drug causes fetal harm, although the use of anticoagulants, such as dabigatran may increase risk of bleeding in the fetus.
- Drug should be used with caution during pregnancy only if benefit to mother outweighs potential risk to fetus.

LABOR AND DELIVERY

- Drug may cause maternal bleeding and hemorrhage if given during labor and delivery.
- Know that drug should be temporarily withheld, or a shorter acting anticoagulant substituted as delivery approaches or if neuraxial anesthesia is expected to be used during delivery.

LACTATION

- It is not known if drug is present in breast milk.
- Breastfeeding is not recommended during drug therapy.

REPRODUCTION

- Females of childbearing age should discuss pregnancy planning with prescriber because significant uterine bleeding, which may require surgical intervention, may occur with drug use.

Nursing Considerations

- Be aware that dabigatran should not be used in patients with triple-positive antiphospholipid syndrome because of increased risk for recurrent thrombosis.
- Assess renal function, as ordered, prior to beginning dabigatran therapy because dose is based on the patient's creatinine level (adults) or eGFR (children). Continue to monitor the patient's serum creatinine level (adults) or eGFR (children) throughout therapy, as ordered, and expect frequency of tests to increase if patient develops a condition that affects renal function because a dosing adjustment may be required. Know that drug should be discontinued if the patient develops acute renal failure.
- Be aware that degree of anticoagulation does not have to be assessed by routine laboratory testing with dabigatran use. However, when necessary, expect the prescriber to use activated partial thromboplastin time (aPTT) or ecarin clotting time (ECT), and not INR, to assess for anticoagulant activity for the patient receiving dabigatran therapy.
- Know that dabigatran can elevate the patient's INR. Therefore, when patients are transitioned, dabigatran must be stopped for at least 2 days before the most accurate effects of warfarin can be known.
- Know that dabigatran therapy should be discontinued, if possible, 1 to 2 days before invasive or surgical procedures for adult patients with a creatinine clearance of 50 ml/min or more, and 3 to 5 days for adult patients whose creatinine clearance is less than 50 ml/min because of the increased risk for bleeding. Longer times may be required for adult patients undergoing major surgery, spinal puncture, or placement of a spinal or epidural catheter or port, in whom complete hemostasis is required. For children with an eGFR greater than 80 ml/min, dabigatran therapy should be discontinued 24 hours before elective surgery; for children with an eGFR of 50 to 80 ml/min, dabigatran therapy should be discontinued 2 days before elective surgery.

If surgery cannot be postponed, monitor patient closely for bleeding. Expect a specific reversal agent such as idarucizumab to be used in adults requiring emergency surgery or an urgent procedure. Know that effectiveness and safety of idarucizumab administration has not been established for children. Expect to restart dabigatran as soon as medically possible.

! **WARNING** Monitor patient closely for bleeding because dabigatran increases risk for bleeding, which can become severe. Bleeding risk increases in patients taking concurrent antiplatelet drugs, fibrinolytic therapy, heparin, or with chronic use of NSAIDs. It also increases during labor and delivery. Monitor patient closely. Promptly report any signs or symptoms of bleeding, such as a drop in hemoglobin and/or hematocrit or the development of hypotension or overt bleeding. Expect to discontinue drug if active bleeding occurs and is persistent or serious. Know that protamine sulfate and vitamin K will not affect the anticoagulant activity of dabigatran. Instead, the prescriber may prescribe platelet concentrates if thrombocytopenia is present or the patient has been exposed to long-acting antiplatelet drugs. If bleeding is life-threatening, expect to administer idarucizumab in adults to reverse the anticoagulant effect of dabigatran.

! **WARNING** Know that premature discontinuation of dabigatran increases the risk of thrombotic events. Assess patient closely for stroke if dabigatran therapy must be discontinued temporarily because of an active bleed, elective surgery, or an invasive procedure. Also, be aware that premature discontinuation of the drug increases risk of other thrombotic events. Know that therapy should be restarted as soon as possible. If the drug must be discontinued for reasons other than pathological bleeding, expect patient to receive coverage with another anticoagulant to decrease the risk of thrombotic events, such as stroke.

! **WARNING** Monitor patient closely for a hypersensitivity reaction, which could become life-threatening, such as anaphylaxis or angioedema. If present, notify prescriber, expect drug to be changed to a different anticoagulant, and provide supportive care, as needed and ordered.

! **WARNING** Be on the alert for an epidural or spinal hematoma formation in patients receiving dabigatran and neuraxial anesthesia or undergoing spinal puncture. This hematoma may result in long-term or permanent paralysis. Assess patient frequently for signs and symptoms of neurological impairment. If present, notify prescriber immediately, as urgent treatment is necessary.

PATIENT TEACHING

! **WARNING** Encourage females of childbearing age to discuss a desire for a pregnancy with prescriber before drug therapy is begun because drug may cause significant uterine bleeding that could require surgical treatment.

- Instruct patient, family, or caregiver how to administer form of dabigatran prescribed. Stress importance of taking dabigatran exactly as prescribed and what to do if a dose is missed.

! **WARNING** Caution patient not to stop taking dabigatran abruptly.

! **WARNING** Review signs and symptoms of an allergic reaction with patient. Tell patient to notify prescriber if present. If signs and symptoms are severe, urge patient to seek immediate medical attention.

! **WARNING** Urge patient to notify prescriber immediately about unusual bleeding and any unexplained symptoms, such as abnormal vaginal bleeding, dizziness, easy bruising, gum bleeding, red or dark brown urine, stools that are black or tarry, vomiting blood, vomit that looks like coffee grounds, and weakness. Urge patient to take precautions against bleeding, such as using an electric shaver and a soft-bristled toothbrush. Caution patient to avoid activities that could cause traumatic injury and bleeding.

- Tell patient to inform all healthcare providers about dabigatran therapy and not to take any medication, including over-the-counter drugs, without first consulting the prescriber.
- Caution mothers not to breastfeed while taking dabigatran.
- Urge patient to carry medical identification that reveals she is taking dabigatran.

dalbavancin hydrochloride

Dalvance

Class and Category

Pharmacologic class: Lipoglycopeptide
Therapeutic class: Antibacterial antibiotic

Indications and Dosages

∗ *To treat acute bacterial skin and skin structure infections caused by* Enterococcus faecalis *(vancomycin-susceptible strains),* Staphylococcus aureus *(including methicillin-susceptible and methicillin-resistant strains),* Streptococcus agalactiae, S. anginosus *group (including* S. anginosus, S. constellatus, *and* S intermedius*),* S. dysgalactiae, *or* S. pyogenes

I.V. INFUSION

Adults with a creatinine clearance of 30 ml/min or more. 1,500 mg infused as a single dose. Alternatively, 1,000 mg followed by 500 mg 1 wk later.

Children ages 6 to less than 18 with a creatinine clearance of 30 ml/min or more. 18 mg/kg (maximum 1,500 mg) infused as a single dose.

Neonates and children less than age 6 with a creatinine clearance of 30 ml/min or more. 22.5 mg/kg (maximum 1,500 mg) infused as a single dose.

± DOSAGE ADJUSTMENT For adult patients with renal impairment (creatinine clearance less than 30 ml/min) and who are not receiving hemodialysis, initial dosage reduced to 1,125 mg as a single dose or 750 mg, followed by 375 mg 1 wk later. There is insufficient information for dosage adjustment in neonates and children with renal impairment (creatinine clearance less than 30 ml/min).

Drug Administration

I.V.

- Reconstitute with 25 ml of either Sterile Water for Injection or 5% Dextrose Injection for each 500-mg vial.
- Avoid foaming by alternating between gently swirling and inverting the vial until contents are completely dissolved. Do not shake. Solution should appear clear and colorless to yellow.
- Once reconstituted, the vial may be refrigerated or stored at room temperature. Do not freeze.
- Further dilute reconstituted solution by transferring the required dose from the vial to an intravenous bag or bottle containing enough solution of 5% Dextrose Injection to provide a final concentration of 1 to 5 mg/ml. Discard any unused portion of the reconstituted solution.
- Once diluted, the intravenous bag or bottle may be refrigerated or stored at room temperature until administration. The total time from the vial being reconstituted until administration ends should not exceed 48 hr. Never freeze the diluted solution.
- Administer as an intravenous infusion over 30 min to minimize infusion reactions. If infusion reaction develops, stop or slow the infusion, as ordered, which may cause reaction to disappear.
- Flush intravenous line with 5% Dextrose Injection before and after administration if the line is used to administer other drugs.
- *Incompatibilities:* Other additives, drugs, or saline-based solutions (including 0.9% Sodium Chloride Injection)

Route	Onset	Peak	Duration
I.V.	Unknown	Unknown	Unknown

Half-life: 14.5 days

Mechanism of Action

Interferes with bacterial cell wall synthesis, which leads to impaired bacterial cell growth or cell death.

Contraindications

Hypersensitivity to dalbavancin or its components

Interactions

None reported by manufacturer.

Adverse Reactions

CNS: Dizziness, fever (children), headache
EENT: Oral candidiasis
ENDO: **Hypoglycemia**
GI: Abdominal pain, ***Clostridioides difficile*-associated colitis**, diarrhea, elevated liver enzymes, **gastrointestinal hemorrhage**, **hepatotoxicity**, **melena**, nausea, passage of bright red blood through anus
GU: Vulvovaginal mycotic infection
HEME: Anemia, **elevated international normalized ratio (INR)**, eosinophilia, **hemorrhagic anemia**, **leukopenia**, **neutropenia**, spontaneous hematoma, thrombocytosis, **thrombocytopenia**
MS: Back pain
RESP: **Bronchospasm**
SKIN: Flushing of upper body, petechiae, pruritus, rash, urticaria
Other: **Anaphylaxis**, infusion reactions (back pain, flushing of upper body, pruritus, rash, urticaria), phlebitis, **wound hemorrhage**

Childbearing Considerations

PREGNANCY

- It is not known if drug causes fetal harm.
- Use with caution only if benefit to mother outweighs potential risk to fetus.

LACTATION

- It is not known if drug is present in breast milk.
- Mothers should check with prescriber before breastfeeding.

Nursing Considerations

- Use cautiously in patients with a history of glycopeptides allergy because of a possibility of cross-sensitivity.
- Use cautiously in patients with a history of hepatic impairment because dosing adjustments for dalbavancin in patients with moderate to severe hepatic impairment are not known. Dosage adjustment is not required for patients with mild hepatic impairment.

! WARNING Monitor patient for hypersensitivity, which could become life-threatening, such as anaphylaxis. If present, discontinue drug and notify prescriber. Provide supportive care, as needed and ordered.

! WARNING Assess patient for signs of secondary infection, such as profuse, watery diarrhea. If such diarrhea develops, contact prescriber and expect to obtain a stool specimen to rule out pseudomembranous colitis caused by *Clostridioides difficile*. It may be mild or become life-threatening. If confirmed, expect to withhold dalbavancin and treat patient with an antibiotic effective against *C. difficile* along with electrolytes, fluids, and protein supplementation, as ordered.

! WARNING Montor patient's bleeding time, CBC, and prothrombin time because drug may have adverse effects on the hematologic system that could become life-threatening. Notify prescriber of any abnormalities.

! WARNING Monitor patient's blood glucose level for hypoglycemia, especially if patient is diabetic. Be prepared to treat a hypoglycemic episode according to institutional protocol. Alert prescriber if hypoglycemia occurs frequently or is serious.

- Montior patient's respiratory status regularly because drug can cause bronchospsasms.

PATIENT TEACHING

- Explain that dalbavancin will be given intravenously in one or two doses. Emphasize importance of obtaining second dose of dalbavancin if patient was prescribed the 2-dose regimen.

! WARNING Tell patient to immediately report any signs and symptoms of an allergic reaction. If reaction is serious, tell patient to seek immediate medical attention.

! WARNING Advise patient to report severe diarrhea to prescriber immediately even up to 2 months after dalbavancin has been discontinued.

! WARNING Inform patient that drug may cause a low blood glucose level, especially if patient is diabetic. Review signs and symptoms of hypoglycemia with patient and how to treat. Tell patient to notify prescriber if frequent episodes occur. If severe, stress importance of calling 911.

- Tell patient to alert prescriber if persistent, severe, or unusual adverse reactions occur.

dalteparin sodium

Fragmin

Class and Category

Pharmacologic class: Low-molecular-weight heparin

Therapeutic class: Anticoagulant

Indications and Dosages

* *To prevent ischemic complications in patients who receive aspirin as part of treatment for unstable angina and non-Q-wave MI*

SUBCUTANEOUS INJECTION

Adults. 120 international units/kg every 12 hr with aspirin (75 to 165 mg daily) until patient is stable, usually 5 to 8 days. *Maximum:* 10,000 international units/dose.

* *To prevent deep vein thrombosis in patients undergoing hip replacement surgery*

SUBCUTANEOUS INJECTION

Adults. *Initial:* 2,500 international units 4 to 8 hr after surgery (or later if hemostasis has not been achieved) and then 5,000 international units once daily for 5 to 10 days postoperatively. Alternatively, 2,500 international units 2 hr before surgery, repeated in 4 to 8 hr after surgery and then 5,000 international units once daily for 5 to 10 days postoperatively or 5,000 international units the evening before surgery followed by 5,000 international units 4 to 8 hr after surgery and then 5,000 international units once daily for 5 to 10 days postoperatively.

* *To prevent deep vein thrombosis in patients undergoing abdominal surgery who are at risk for thromboembolic complications*

SUBCUTANEOUS INJECTION

Adults. 2,500 international units daily, starting 1 to 2 hr before surgery and repeated once daily postoperatively for 5 to 10 days.

±**DOSAGE ADJUSTMENT** For patients at high risk, 5,000 international units the evening before surgery, repeated once daily postoperatively for 5 to 10 days. For patients with cancer, 2,500 international units 1 to 2 hours before surgery followed by 2,500 international units 12 hours later and then 5,000 international units once daily postoperatively for 5 to 10 days.

* *To prevent deep vein thrombosis in patients with severe mobility restrictions during acute illness*

SUBCUTANEOUS INJECTION

Adults. 5,000 international units once daily for 12 to 14 days.

* *To provide extended treatment of symptomatic venous thromboembolism in patients with cancer*

SUBCUTANEOUS INJECTION

Adults. 200 international units/kg once daily for 30 days. Then, 150 international units/kg once daily for 5 more mo. *Maximum:* 18,000 international units daily.

±**DOSAGE ADJUSTMENT** For patients with thrombocytopenia and cancer who experiences a platelet count between 50,000 and 100,000/mm^3, dosage reduced by 2,500 international units until platelet count recovers to or above 100,000 mm^3. For patients with thrombocytopenia and cancer who experience a platelet count less than 50,000 mm^3, dalteparin withheld until platelet count is above 50,000 mm^3. For patients with severely impaired renal function (creatinine clearance below 30 ml/min), anti-Xa levels monitored to determine appropriate dose. Target anti-Xa range is 0.5 to 1.5 international units/ml.

* *To treat symptomatic venous thromboembolism in pediatric patients*

SUBCUTANEOUS INJECTION

Children ages 8 to less than 17. 100 international units/kg twice daily.
Children ages 2 to less than 8. 125 international units/kg twice daily.
Neonates at birth (gestational age at least 35 wk) to children less than 2. 150 international units/kg twice daily.

±**DOSAGE ADJUSTMENT** For neonates from birth (gestational age at least 35 wk) to less than 17 yr, who experience a platelet count between 50,000 and 100,000 mm^3, dosage reduced by 50% until platelet count recovers to or above 100,000 mm^3; platelet count less than 50,000 mm^3, drug withheld until platelet count is above 50,000 mm^3.

Drug Administration

SUBCUTANEOUS

- Don't give drug by I.M. or I.V. injection.
- Needle shield on prefilled syringe may contain natural rubber latex and should not be handled by persons with a latex allergy.
- Administer drug deep into subcutaneous tissue in the abdomen in the U-shaped area

around navel, upper outer thigh, or upper outer quadrant of buttocks with patient seated or lying down. If using area around navel or on thigh, the skin fold must be lifted with thumb and forefinger while giving injection. Insert entire length of needle at a 45- to 90-degree angle.

- Do not expel air bubble from the prefilled syringe with a fixed dose before injection. Hold the syringe assembly by the open sides of the device. After removing the needle shield, insert the needle into the injection area as described above. Depress the plunger of the syringe while holding the finger flange until the entire dose has been given. The needle guard will not be activated unless the entire dose has been given. Remove the needle. Let go of the plunger and allow syringe to move up inside the device until the entire needle is guarded.
- If using a graduated syringe, hold the syringe assembly by the open sides of the device. Remove the needle shield. With the needle pointing up, prepare the syringe by expelling the air bubble and then continuing to push the plunger to the desired dose or volume, discarding the extra solution. Insert the needle into the injection area as described above. Depress the plunger of the syringe while holding the finger flange until the entire dose remaining in the syringe has been given. The needle guard will not be activated unless the entire dose has been given. Remove the needle. Let go of the plunger and allow syringe to move up inside the device until the entire needle is guarded.
- Rotate sites daily.
- After first penetration of rubber stopper, store multiple-dose vials at room temperature for up to 2 weeks.

Route	Onset	Peak	Duration
SubQ	1–2 hr	4 hr	12 hr

Half-life: 2–5 hr

Mechanism of Action

Binds to and accelerates the activity of antithrombin III, thus inhibiting thrombin and blocking the formation of fibrin clots.

Contraindications

Active major bleeding; history of heparin-induced thrombocytopenia or heparin-induced thrombocytopenia with thrombosis; hypersensitivity to dalteparin, heparin, pork products or their components; treatment for unstable angina and non-Q-wave MI or for prolonged venous thromboembolism prophylaxis while undergoing epidural/neuraxial anesthesia

Interactions

DRUGS

NSAIDs, oral anticoagulants, platelet aggregation inhibitors, thrombolytics: Possibly increased risk of hemorrhage and spinal or epidural hematoma

Adverse Reactions

EENT: Epistaxis
GI: Elevated liver enzymes
HEME: **Hemorrhage**, **thrombocytopenia**
MS: Osteoporosis
SKIN: Alopecia, bullous eruption, necrosis, pruritus, rash
Other: **Anaphylaxis**, **hyperkalemia**, injection-site bruising, hematoma, and pain

Childbearing Considerations

PREGNANCY

- It is not known if drug causes fetal harm although it has the potential for adverse effects on preterm infants when used in pregnancy if the 3.8-ml multiple-dose vial of the drug is used because it contains 14 mg/ml of benzyl alcohol.
- Use with caution only if benefit to mother outweighs potential risk to fetus.

LACTATION

- Drug is present in breast milk.
- Mothers should check with prescriber before breastfeeding.

Nursing Considerations

! WARNING Use dalteparin with extreme caution in patients at increased risk for hemorrhage (such as those who use a platelet inhibitor or who have active ulcerative GI disorder, bacterial endocarditis, bleeding disorders, hemorrhagic stroke, or uncontrolled hypertension); and those with recent brain, eye, or spinal surgery.

! WARNING Use drug with extreme caution in patients with bleeding diathesis, diabetic retinopathy, platelet defects, recent GI bleeding, severe hepatic or renal insufficiency, or thrombocytopenia.

D

! **WARNING** Question patient regarding use of aspirin and other NSAIDs, platelet inhibitors, or other anticoagulants prior to dalteparin therapy that may increase risk of bleeding. Be aware that use of aspirin and other NSAIDs may enhance the risk of hemorrhage and should be discontinued prior to dalteparin therapy, if possible. If not, closely monitor patient's clinical and laboratory status throughout therapy.

! **WARNING** Be aware that risk factors for thromboembolic events include age over 40, cancer, history of deep vein thrombosis or pulmonary embolism, obesity, and planned use of anesthesia for more than 30 minutes.

- Inform Jewish or Islamic patients that drug comes from porcine intestine before giving first dose.
- Know that routine coagulation tests and dosage adjustments usually aren't required. Instead, anti-Xa levels are measured, prior to the fourth dose and as needed. Samples should be drawn 4 hours after drug administration. Dosages are then adjusted in increments of 25 international units/kg to achieve a target anti-Xa level between 0.5 and 1 international units/ml. Thereafter anti-Xa levels are measured periodically for adults and children with severe renal impairment or if abnormal coagulation parameters or bleeding occurs during drug therapy.

! **WARNING** Monitor patient for a hypersensitivity reaction that could become life-threatening, such as anaphylaxis. If present, notify prescriber immediately and expect to provide supportive care, as needed and ordered. Expect patient to be given a different anticoagulant.

! **WARNING** Monitor patient closely who are receiving dalteparin and epidural or spinal anesthesia or spinal puncture because spinal hematomas can occur, causing long-term or permanent paralysis. Watch for evidence of neurologic impairment, such as changes in motor or sensory functions. If present, notify prescriber immediately; patient needs urgent care to minimize effect of hematoma. Use of indwelling epidural catheters; concurrent use of other drugs that affect hemostasis such as NSAIDs, platelet inhibitors, and other anticoagulants; a history of traumatic or repeated epidural or spinal punctures; or a history of spinal deformity or spinal surgery increase the risk of spinal or epidural hematoma in patients receiving dalteparin.

PATIENT TEACHING

- Teach patient, family, or caregiver how to administer drug as a subcutaneous injection.

! **WARNING** Alert patient that drug may cause an allergic reaction. If present, tell patient to notify prescriber promptly. If severe, stress importance of seeking immediate medical care.

! **WARNING** Urge patient to report adverse reactions, especially bleeding, and to seek help immediately if signs of blood clots develop, such as severe changes in mental status, difficulty breathing, or motor or sensory abnormalities. Other adverse reactions to report include a rash consisting of dark red spots under the skin. Inform patient that bleeding and/or bruising occur more easily during dalteparin therapy.

! **WARNING** Tell patient who is receiving spinal anesthesia or a spinal puncture to alert medical staff immediately if he experiences muscular weakness, numbness (especially in his legs), or tingling following the procedure.

- Instruct patient to inform all dentists and prescribers of dalteparin therapy.
- Emphasize the importance of follow-up visits.

dapagliflozin propanediol

Farxiga

Class and Category

Pharmacologic class: Sodium glucose co-transporter 2 (SGLT2) inhibitor
Therapeutic class: Antidiabetic

Indications and Dosages

* *As adjunct to diet and exercise to improve glycemic control in patients with type 2 diabetes mellitus*

TABLETS

Adults and children ages 10 and older with an eGFR of 45 ml/min or greater. 5 mg once daily in morning, increased to 10 mg once daily in morning, as needed.

✷ *To reduce risk of hospitalization for heart failure in patients with type 2 diabetes mellitus and established cardiovascular disease or who have multiple cardiovascular risk factors; to reduce risk of cardiovascular death and hospitalization for heart failure, and urgent heart failure visit in patients with heart failure; to reduce the risk of sustained eGFR decline, end-stage kidney disease, cardiovascular death, and hospitalization for heart failure in patients with chronic kidney disease at risk of progression*

TABLETS

Adults with an eGFR of 25 ml/min or greater. 10 mg once daily.

Drug Administration

P.O.

- Administer in morning if being given for glucose control.

Route	Onset	Peak	Duration
P.O.	Unknown	2 hr	Unknown

Half-life: 12.9 hr

Mechanism of Action

Inhibits sodium glucose co-transporter 2 in the kidneys, which prevents glucose reabsorption. This decreases blood glucose levels. Also, reduces sodium reabsorption and increases sodium delivery to the distal tubule in the kidneys, which may influence several physiological functions such as the lowering of both pre- and afterload of the heart, downregulating sympathetic activity, and decreasing intraglomerular pressure. These actions may help reduce severity of heart failure and renal impairment.

Contraindications

Dialysis therapy, hypersensitivity to dapagliflozin or its components

Interactions

DRUGS

insulin, insulin secretagogues: Increased risk of hypoglycemia

lithium: Possibly decreased serum lithium concentrations decreasing its effectiveness

Adverse Reactions

CNS: Syncope

CV: Dyslipidemia, elevated low-density lipoprotein (LDL) cholesterol, **hypotension**

EENT: Nasopharyngitis

ENDO: **Hypoglycemia**, **ketoacidosis**

GI: Constipation, nausea

GU: **Acute kidney injury**, decreased eGFR, dysuria, elevated serum creatinine levels, genital mycotic infections, impaired renal function, increased urination, **necrotizing fasciitis of the perineum (Fournier's gangrene)**, osmotic diuresis, pyelonephritis, **urosepsis**, UTI

HEME: Elevated hematocrit level

MS: Back or extremity pain

SKIN: **Severe cutaneous reactions**, rash, urticaria

Other: **Anaphylaxis**, **angioedema**, flu-like symptoms, **hyperphosphatemia**, volume depletion

Childbearing Considerations

PREGNANCY

- It is not known if drug causes fetal harm.
- Drug is not recommended for use during the second and third trimesters of pregnancy because of potential fetal adverse renal effects as seen in animal studies.

LACTATION

- It is not known if drug is present in breast milk.
- Drug should not be used during breastfeeding because of the potential for adverse renal effects in the breastfed infant since renal maturation continues for up to 2 yr after birth.

Nursing Considerations

- Know that dapagliflozin should not be given to patients with certain genetic forms of polycystic kidney disease, or who are taking or have recently received immunosuppressive therapy to treat kidney disease.

! **WARNING** Use drug cautiously in patients with chronic kidney insufficiency, congestive heart failure, decreased blood volume, and patients taking medications such as ACE inhibitors, angiotensin receptor blockers, diuretics, and NSAIDs because these conditions and treatments may predispose the patient to acute kidney injury while receiving dapagliflozin. Ensure that kidney function has been assessed prior to starting dapagliflozin therapy and then periodically thereafter.

! **WARNING** Assess patient's volume status and correct, if needed and as prescribed, prior to starting dapagliflozin therapy because drug can cause intravascular volume contraction leading to acute kidney injury or symptomatic hypotension. Patients at highest risk include elderly patients, patients receiving loop diuretic therapy or drugs that interfere with the renin–angiotensin–aldosterone system, and patients who have low systolic blood pressure or impaired renal function.

! **WARNING** Know that drug should not be used to treat type 1 diabetes mellitus. Monitor patient closely for ketoacidosis that may occur despite the patient having type 2 diabetes and may be present even if a blood glucose level is less than 250 mg/dl. Patients with pancreatic disorders such as a history of pancreatitis or pancreatic surgery are also at higher risk for ketoacidosis. If signs and symptoms occur such as dehydration, fruity odor to breath, malaise, nausea, shortness of breath, and vomiting, notify prescriber and expect drug to be discontinued. Provide supportive care, as needed and ordered.

! **WARNING** Monitor patient for hypersensitivity reactions. Although rare, anaphylaxis, angioedema, and severe cutaneous adverse reactions have occurred. If present, stop drug immediately and notify prescriber. Provide care, as ordered according to standard of care until signs and symptoms subsides.

! **WARNING** Monitor patient for a rare but serious and life-threatening necrotizing infection of the perineum called Fournier's gangrene. Notify prescriber immediately if patient develops erythema, pain, swelling, or tenderness in the genital or perineal area, along with fever or malaise. Expect treatment with broad-spectrum antibiotics and, if needed, surgical debridement of the area. Expect dapagliflozin to be discontinued and an alternative treatment prescribed for glycemic control. Monitor patient's blood glucose levels closely.

! **WARNING** Be aware that patients receiving insulin or insulin secretagogues may require a lower dose of these agents because combined use with dapagliflozin increases risk of hypoglycemia. Monitor patient closely for hypoglycemia. If present, treat according to standard of care and notify prescriber.

- Expect drug to be temporarily discontinued in patients who experience a reduced oral intake, such as with an acute illness or fasting, or who experience excessive fluid losses because of significant GI illness or heat exposure. Expect drug to be withheld for at least 3 days, if possible, prior to major surgery or procedures associated with prolonged fasting. This will help to reduce risk of acute kidney injury.
- Monitor patient's blood pressure and cholesterol level throughout dapagliflozin therapy. Be aware that patients with diabetes mellitus and renal dysfunction may be at increased risk to experience hypertension.
- Be aware that dapagliflozin interferes with the measurements of 1,5-anhydroglucitol (1,5-AG) assay and is unreliable in assessing glycemic control in patients taking a SGLT2 inhibitor such as dapagliflozin.
- Monitor patients for genital mycotic infections, especially patients with a history of such infections. If present, notify prescriber and treat, as prescribed.

PATIENT TEACHING

- Instruct patient how to administer dapagliflozin and what to do if a dose is missed.
- Inform patient that dapagliflozin therapy is not a replacement for diet and exercise therapy.

! **WARNING** Instruct patient to stop taking drug and seek immediate medical attention if an allergic reaction such as hives or facial or throat swelling occurs while taking dapagliflozin.

! **WARNING** Instruct patient on the signs and symptoms of hyperglycemia and hypoglycemia and how to treat. Inform patient who is also receiving a sulfonylurea or insulin that the risk of hypoglycemia is greater. Tell patient to notify prescriber if hypoglycemia occurs frequently or is severe.

Review signs and symptoms of ketoacidosis with patient and urge him to seek immediate medical attention, if present, even if blood glucose level is less than 250 mg/dl.

! **WARNING** Warn patient to stop dapagliflozin and seek immediate medical attention if pain, redness, swelling, or tenderness occur in the genital or perineal area, along with fever or malaise because, although rare, this cluster of symptoms may become life-threatening.

- Tell patient to monitor the blood glucose level using blood tests instead of urine tests because the drug increases urinary glucose excretion and will lead to positive urine glucose tests.
- Advise patient to maintain adequate fluid intake throughout dapagliflozin therapy. However, tell patient to notify prescriber if he is unable to take a normal amount of daily fluids due to illness or fasting or experiences an excessive loss of fluids from excessive perspiration or GI illnesses, as drug may have to be temporarily withheld
- Advise patient to slowly rise from a lying or sitting position and to notify prescriber if symptoms of light-headedness or feeling faint occur.
- Instruct patient to notify all prescribers of dapagliflozin therapy and not to take any over-the-counter drugs, including herbal products, without alerting prescriber.
- Advise females of childbearing age to notify prescriber if pregnancy occurs.
- Inform mothers breastfeeding should not be done during drug therapy.

daptomycin

Cubicin, Cubicin RF

Class and Category

Pharmacologic class: Cyclic lipopeptide
Therapeutic class: Antibiotic

Indications and Dosages

* *To treat complicated skin and skin structure infections caused by* Enterococcus faecalis *(vancomycin-susceptible isolates only),* Staphylococcus aureus *(including methicillin-resistant isolates),* Streptococcus agalactiae, S. dysgalactiae *subspecies equisimilis, or* S. pyogenes

I.V. INFUSION, I.V. INJECTION (CUBICIN, CUBICIN RF)

Adults. 4 mg/kg once daily for 7 to 14 days.

I.V. INFUSION

Children ages 12 to 17. 5 mg/kg infused over 30 min once every 24 hr for up to 14 days.
Children ages 7 to 11. 7 mg/kg infused over 30 min once every 24 hr for up to 14 days.
Children ages 2 to 6. 9 mg/kg infused over 60 min once every 24 hr for up to 14 days.
Children ages 1 to less than 2. 10 mg/kg infused over 60 min once every 24 hr for up to 14 days.

* *To treat* S. aureus *bloodstream infections (bacteremia), including right-sided infective endocarditis, caused by methicillin-susceptible and methicillin-resistant isolates*

I.V. INFUSION, I.V. INJECTION (CUBICIN, CUBICIN RF)

Adults. 6 mg/kg injected over 2 min or infused over 30 min once daily for 2 to 6 wk.

* *To treat pediatric patients with* S. aureus *bloodstream infections (bacteremia)*

I.V. INFUSION (CUBICIN)

Children ages 12 to 17. 7 mg/kg infused over 30 min once daily for up to 42 days.
Children ages 7 to 11. 9 mg/kg infused over 30 min once daily for up to 42 days.
Children ages 1 to 6. 12 mg/kg infused over 60 min once daily for up to 42 days.

± **DOSAGE ADJUSTMENT** For adult patients with creatinine clearance less than 30 ml/min, including patients on continuous ambulatory peritoneal dialysis or hemodialysis (administered after completion of hemodialysis, if possible), dosage interval increased to every 48 hours. Daptomycin dosage in children with renal impairment is unknown.

Drug Administration

I.V.

- The two formulations of the drug require different storage and methods of reconstitution.
- Reconstitute Cubicin or generic drug by slowly transferring 10 ml of 0.9% Sodium Chloride Injection into 500-mg vial (Cubicin) or 7 ml into 350-mg vial (generic drug) and pointing needle (beveled sterile transfer 21 G needle or smaller or needleless device) toward wall of vial to minimize

foaming. Then, gently rotate vial until all powder is wet. Don't agitate or shake vial. Let vial stand undisturbed for 10 min, then gently rotate or swirl contents for a few minutes, as needed, to obtain a completely reconstituted solution. Remove reconstituted solution from vial slowly using same type of needle used to reconstitute drug.

- Reconstitute Cubicin RF with 10 ml of either Bacteriostatic Water for Injection or Sterile Water for Injection using a beveled sterile transfer needle that is 21 G or smaller in diameter. Saline-based diluents should not be used. Rotate or swirl vial contents for a few minutes, as needed, to obtain a completely reconstituted solution. Remove reconstituted solution from vial slowly using same type of needle used to reconstitute drug.
- For I.V. injection (only for adults), administer either formulation over a period of 2 min.
- For I.V. infusion, further dilute either formulation of reconstituted solution with 50 ml in an I.V. infusion bag containing 0.9% Sodium Chloride for Injection (25 ml for children ages 1 to 6). Infuse over 30 min for adults and children ages 7 and older at a rate of 1.67 ml/min; infuse over 60 min for children ages 6 and under at a rate of 0.42 ml/min.
- Do not use the ReadyMED elastomeric infusion pumps, as drug is not as stable when stored in these pumps.
- Flush I.V. with a compatible intravenous solution before and after infusion of drug if the same I.V. line is being used for sequential infusion of other drugs.
- Refer to manufacturer's guidelines for storage information.
- *Incompatibilities:* Dextrose-containing solutions, other additives, or drugs

Route	Onset	Peak	Duration
I.V.	Rapid	30–60 min	Unknown

Half-life: 8 hr

Mechanism of Action

Binds to bacterial membranes to cause rapid depolarization of membrane potential. This loss of membrane potential inhibits protein, DNA, and RNA synthesis, which results in bacterial cell death.

Contraindications

Hypersensitivity to daptomycin or its components

Interactions

DRUGS

HMG-CoA reductase inhibitors: Possibly increased CPK level and increased risk of myopathy

Adverse Reactions

CNS: Anxiety, asthenia, confusion, dizziness, dyskinesia, fatigue, fever, hallucination, headache, insomnia, mental status changes, paresthesia, peripheral neuropathy, rigors, vertigo, weakness

CV: **Atrial fibrillation or flutter**, **cardiac arrest or failure**, chest pain, hypertension, **hypotension**, peripheral edema, **supraventricular tachycardia**

EENT: Blurred vision, dry mouth, eye irritation, gingival pain, hypoesthesia of mouth, oral candidiasis, pharyngolaryngeal pain, sore throat, stomatitis, taste disturbance, tinnitus, visual disturbances

ENDO: Hyperglycemia, **hypoglycemia**

GI: Abdominal distention or pain, anorexia, ***Clostridioides difficile*–associated diarrhea**, constipation, diarrhea, dyspepsia, dysphagia, elevated liver enzymes, epigastric discomfort, **GI hemorrhage**, jaundice, nausea, vomiting

GU: **Acute kidney injury**, **renal failure or insufficiency**, proteinuria, tubulointerstitial nephritis (TIN), UTI, vaginal candidiasis

HEME: Anemia, **decreased platelet count**, eosinophilia, **increased international normalized ratio (INR)**, leukocytosis, **prolonged prothrombin time**, **thrombocythemia**, **thrombocytopenia**, thrombocytosis

MS: Arthralgia, back or limb pain, elevated myoglobin level, muscle cramps or weakness, myalgia, myopathy, osteomyelitis, **rhabdomyolysis**

RESP: Cough, dyspnea, **eosinophilic or organizing pneumonia**, pleural effusion, pneumonia, pulmonary eosinophilia, shortness of breath

SKIN: Acute generalized exanthematous pustulosis, cellulitis, diaphoresis, eczema, erythema, flushing, pruritus, rash, **Stevens-Johnson syndrome**, **toxic epidermal necrolysis (TEN)**, truncal erythema, urticaria, vesiculobullous rash

Other: **Anaphylaxis**, **angioedema**, **bacteremia**, **drug reaction with eosinophilia and systemic symptoms (DRESS)**, **electrolyte disturbance**, elevated alkaline phosphatase or creatine phosphokinase (CPK) levels, **elevated serum sodium bicarbonate level**, fungal infection, **hyperkalemia**, **hypokalemia**, **hypomagnesemia**, increased serum lactate dehydrogenase (LDH) levels, injection-site reactions, lymphadenopathy, **sepsis**

Childbearing Considerations

PREGNANCY

- It is not known if drug causes fetal harm.
- Use with caution only if benefit to mother outweighs potential risk to fetus.

LACTATION

- Drug is present in breast milk.
- Mothers should check with prescriber before breastfeeding.

Nursing Considerations

- Be aware that concurrent therapy with daptomycin and HMG-CoA reductase inhibitors is not recommended. Expect HMG-CoA reductase inhibitor therapy to be temporarily withheld during daptomycin therapy.
- Obtain blood samples for culture and sensitivity testing before starting daptomycin.

! **WARNING** Monitor patient for serious hypersensitivity reactions such as anaphylaxis and angioedema as well as severe skin reactions accompanied by fever, rash, or swollen lymph nodes that may progress to systemic organ impairment suggesting DRESS. If suspected, notify prescriber and expect drug to be discontinued and provide supportive care given, as needed and ordered.

! **WARNING** Monitor patient closely for diarrhea, which may herald *Clostridioides difficile*-associated diarrhea. Diarrhea may range from being mild to severe causing fatal colitis. Notify prescriber if *C. difficile* is suspected and expect to obtain a stool specimen to confirm diagnosis. If confirmed expect to discontinue drug and administer an antibiotic effective against *C. difficile*, as ordered. In addition, expect to give electrolytes, fluids, and protein supplementation, as ordered and needed.

! **WARNING** Expect to discontinue daptomycin therapy immediately if patient develops signs and symptoms of eosinophilic pneumonia (cough, breathlessness, fever) and prepare to administer systemic steroids, as ordered.

! **WARNING** Monitor patient's bleeding time, CBC, and prothrombin time regularly, as ordered, to detect adverse hematologic reactions, some of which could become life-threatening. Monitor patient closely for bleeding and infections. Be especially aware that daptomycin may cause a significant false increase in INR and PT with some brands of laboratory assays. If this occurs during daptomycin therapy, draw blood sample just before next daptomycin dose and evaluate other causes that could cause such an increase.

- Monitor patient's BUN and serum creatinine levels and patient's response to drug closely. If patient develops renal insufficiency or worsening renal impairment, notify prescriber, expect drug to be discontinued, and provide supportive care, as needed and ordered.
- Assess patient for muscle pain or weakness, especially of distal limbs. Expect to monitor CPK level weekly or more often in patients recently taking an HMG-CoA reductase inhibitor. Expect to stop daptomycin, as ordered, if patient develops myopathy or has a marked rise in CPK level.
- Monitor patient for evidence of superinfection and inform prescriber if present.

PATIENT TEACHING

- Inform patient drug will be given intravenously. Stress importance of completing drug course to prevent decreased drug's effectiveness and increased risk for patient to become resistance to the drug or other antibacterial drugs in the future.

! **WARNING** Review signs and symptoms of an allergic reaction as well as serious skin reactions. Instruct patient to notify prescriber immediately if an allergic reaction or skin reactions occur (initially fever, rash, or swollen lymph nodes for DRESS) because drug may have to be discontinued.

! **WARNING** Inform patient that diarrhea may occur 2 months or more after daptomycin therapy stops. If prolonged or severe, advise patient to notify prescriber as soon as possible; additional treatment may be needed.

! **WARNING** Tell patient that drug may cause adverse blood reactions. Stress importance of complying with ordered laboratory studies. Instruct patient to notify prescriber if bleeding, bruising, or signs of an infection occurs.

! **WARNING** Urge patient to report muscle pain, tenderness, or weakness, and other symptoms of myopathy immediately. Also, tell patient to report breathlessness, cough, or a fever. Also stress importance of notifying prescriber if other adverse reactions occur that are persistent, severe, or unusual.

- Alert patient that drug may cause a superinfection and to report diarrhea, discharge or perineal itching to prescriber. Tell patient to consume buttermilk and yogurt to help prevent occurance.

darbepoetin alfa

Aranesp

Class and Category

Pharmacologic class: Recombinant human erythropoietin

Therapeutic class: Antianemic

Indications and Dosages

∗ *To treat anemia from chronic renal failure*

I.V. OR SUBCUTANEOUS INJECTION

Adults on dialysis. *Initial:* 0.45 mcg/kg as a single dose every wk. Alternatively, 0.75 mcg/kg once every 2 wk. *Maintenance:* Dosage individualized and increased monthly to maintain a hemoglobin level not to exceed 11 g/dl.

Adults not on dialysis. *Initial:* 0.45 mcg/kg as a single dose every 4 wk, as needed.

Children ages 1 mo and older on dialysis. 0.45 mcg/kg once every wk.

Children ages 1 mo and older not on dialysis. 0.75 mcg/kg once every 2 wk.

±**DOSAGE ADJUSTMENT** For all patients, dosage reduced or therapy interrupted if hemoglobin level increases and approaches 12 g/dl for children, 11 g/dl for adults on dialysis, and 10 g/dl for adults not on dialysis. Dosage reduced by about 25% if hemoglobin level increases by more than 1 g/dl in a 2-week period. For all patients, dosage increased by about 25% of previous dose if hemoglobin level increases less than 1 g/dl over 4 weeks. For all patients, dosage increases should be made no sooner than every 4 weeks; dosage decreases can occur sooner than every 4 weeks, but frequent dosing adjustments should be avoided. For patients who are converting from epoetin alfa to darbepoetin alfa and have chronic kidney disease and are on dialysis, the starting weekly dosage is estimated based on the weekly epoetin alfa dosage at the time of substitution and administered every week for patients who previously received epoetin alfa 2 to 3 times/week and once every 2 weeks for patients who previously received epoetin alfa once/week.

∗ *To treat chemotherapy-induced anemia in patients with nonmyeloid malignancies and hemoglobin level less than 10 g/dl providing there is a minimum of 2 additional months of planned chemotherapy*

SUBCUTANEOUS INJECTION

Adults. *Initial:* 2.25 mcg/kg as a single dose every week until completion of a chemotherapy course. Alternatively, 500 mcg every 3 wk until completion of a chemotherapy course. *Maintenance:* Dosage individualized to maintain a target hemoglobin level.

±**DOSAGE ADJUSTMENT** For patients with a hemoglobin level increase less than 1.0 g/dl and hemoglobin remains below 10 g/dl after 6 weeks of therapy, dosage increased to 4.5 mcg/kg/week (no dosage adjustment required if patient is receiving drug every 3 weeks). For patients with a hemoglobin increase of more than 1.0 g/dl over 2 weeks or the hemoglobin level reaches a level needed to avoid a red blood cell (RBC) transfusion, dosage reduced by 40% for both weekly and every 3-week dosage schedule. For patients with a hemoglobin level that exceeds a level needed to avoid RBC transfusion, dose withheld for both weekly and every 3-week dosage schedule until hemoglobin approaches level when RBC transfusion may be required. Then, therapy is restarted at a dose 40% less than last dose given.

Drug Administration

- Don't shake vial during preparation to avoid denaturing drug and rendering it biologically inactive.
- Drug solution should appear clear and colorless.
- Discard drug if discoloration or particulate matter is present.
- Don't dilute drug before giving it.
- Know that needle cover on prefilled syringe contains dry natural rubber and may cause allergic reaction in those with latex sensitivity.
- Discard unused portion of drug because it contains no preservatives.
- Store drug in refrigerator. Don't freeze and do protect from light.

I.V.

- Drug solution should appear clear and colorless.
- Don't shake during preparation and do not dilute drug before injecting it.
- Be aware needle cover on prefilled syringe contains dry natural rubber and may cause an allergic reaction in those with latex sensitivity.
- Inject into a vein.
- *Incompatibilities:* Other drug solutions

SUBCUTANEOUS

- Avoid injecting into an area that is bruised or damaged.

Route	Onset	Peak	Duration
I.V.	Unknown	Unknown	Unknown
SubQ	Slow	24–72 hr	Unknown

Half-life: 21 hr (I.V.); 49 hr (SubQ)

Mechanism of Action

Stimulates release of reticulocytes from the bone marrow into the bloodstream, where they develop into mature RBCs.

Contraindications

History of pure red cell aplasia that began after treatment with darbepoetin alfa or other erythropoietin protein drugs, hypersensitivity to darbepoetin alfa or its components, uncontrolled hypertension

Interactions

DRUGS

None reported by manufacturer.

Adverse Reactions

CNS: Asthenia, **CVA**, dizziness, fatigue, fever, headache, **seizures**, transient ischemic attack
CV: **Acute MI**, angina, **arrhythmias**, **cardiac arrest or death**, chest pain, **congestive heart failure**, edema, hypertension, **hypotension**, peripheral edema, **thromboembolic events**, vascular access thrombosis
GI: Abdominal pain, constipation, diarrhea, nausea, vomiting
HEME: **Low reticulocyte count**, **pure red cell aplasia**, **severe anemia**
MS: Arthralgia, back pain, limb pain, muscle spasm, myalgia
RESP: Bronchitis, **bronchospasm**, cough, dyspnea, pneumonia, **pulmonary embolism**, upper respiratory tract infection
SKIN: **Erythema multiforme**, pruritus, rash, **Stevens-Johnson syndrome**, **toxic epidermal necrolysis**, urticaria
Other: **Anaphylaxis**, **angioedema**, dehydration, infection, flu-like symptoms, injection-site pain, **sepsis**

Childbearing Considerations

PREGNANCY

- It is not known if drug causes fetal harm.
- Use with caution only if benefit to mother outweighs potential risk to fetus.

LACTATION

- It is not known if drug is present in breast milk.
- Mothers should check with prescriber before breastfeeding.

Nursing Considerations

- Ensure that patient has received the medication guide and patient instructions for darbepoetin alfa and that a written acknowledgment of a discussion of the risks involved with this type of therapy has been obtained before first dose is given.
- Be aware that all prescribers and hospitals must enroll in and comply with the ESA APPRISE oncology program to be able to prescribe and dispense the drug.

! **WARNING** Be aware that darbepoetin alfa shouldn't be given to cancer patients when a cure is anticipated because drug may decrease survival rate and increase tumor progression in patients with certain types of cancers, such as breast, cervical, head and neck, lymphoid, and non-small-cell lung cancers. Expect to discontinue darbepoetin in cancer patients if hemoglobin level hasn't increased after 8 weeks or if patient continues to need transfusions despite therapy.

! **WARNING** Use extreme caution with darbepoetin alfa therapy in patients undergoing coronary artery bypass graft surgery because of increased risk of death, and in patients undergoing orthopedic procedures because of increased risk of deep venous thrombosis.

- Know that before starting darbepoetin alfa therapy, expect to correct folic acid or vitamin B_{12} deficiencies because these conditions may interfere with drug's effectiveness.
- Be aware that to ensure effective drug response, expect to obtain serum ferritin level and transferrin saturation before and during therapy, as ordered. If serum ferritin level is less than 100 mcg/L or serum transferrin saturation is less than 20%, expect to begin supplemental iron therapy.
- Monitor hemoglobin level weekly, as ordered, until hemoglobin stabilizes, and maintenance dosage has been achieved. Then, monitor hemoglobin level regularly, as ordered. After each dosage adjustment, expect to check hemoglobin level weekly for 4 weeks until it stabilizes in response to dosage change.

! **WARNING** Know that if hemoglobin level increases more than 1 g/dl during any 2-week period or it exceeds 12 g/dl for children, 11 g/dl for adult patient on dialysis, 10 g/dl for adult patient not on dialysis, or exceeds the target range for cancer patient, the risk for acute MI, cardiac arrest, congestive heart failure, fluid overload with peripheral edema, seizures, shortened survival, stroke, tumor progression, vascular infarction, vascular ischemia, vascular thrombosis, and worsened hypertension increases. Expect to decrease dosage if this occurs.

! **WARNING** Monitor patient for hypersensitivity reactions such as anaphylaxis and angioedema and severe skin reactions that may include blistering and skin exfoliation. Notify prescriber immediately, if noted, and expect darbepoetin therapy to be discontinued. Prepare to provide supportive care, as needed and ordered.

! **WARNING** Monitor patient for seizures, especially during the first 90 days of therapy. Institute seizure precautions according to facility policy.

! **WARNING** Monitor patient for adverse cardiovascular reactions because drug may cause serious reactions such as arrhythmias, acute MI, congestive heart failure, hypotension and thrombus. Notify prescriber immediately if acute cardiovascular signs and symptoms occur and be prepared to provide emergency supportive care, as needed and ordered.

- Monitor patient closely for hypertension during therapy. Expect to reduce dosage or withhold drug if blood pressure is poorly controlled with antihypertensive and dietary measures.
- Monitor renal function and fluid and electrolyte balance for signs of declining renal function in patients with renal impairment. If patient starts dialysis, monitor hemoglobin and blood pressure closely and expect dosage and route of administration to be adjusted, as needed, for the type of dialysis being used.

PATIENT TEACHING

- Instruct patient how to administer drug as a subcutaneous injection, if indicated. Emphasize the importance of complying with the dosage regimen
- Ask patient about latex allergy because needle cover on prefilled syringe contains dry natural rubber and may cause allergic reaction in those with latex sensitivity.
- Encourage patient to eat adequate quantities of iron-rich foods.
- Inform patient that frequent blood tests will be needed and stress importance of complying with laboratory appointments.

! **WARNING** Alert patient that drug may cause serious allergic and skin reactions. If present, tell patient to notify prescriber promptly, and if severe, to seek immediate medical attention.

! **WARNING** Advise patient that the risk of seizures is highest during the first 90 days of therapy. Discourage her from engaging in hazardous activities during this time.

! **WARNING** Stress importance of notifying prescriber immediately of persistent, serious or unusual adverse reactions because drug can adversely affect many body systems. If severe, stress importance of seeking immediate medical care.

- Advise patient to follow up with prescriber for blood pressure monitoring.

daridorexant

Quviviq

Class, Category, and Schedule

Pharmacologic class: Orexin receptor antagonist
Therapeutic class: Hypnotic
Controlled substance schedule: IV

Indications and Dosages

✶ *To treat insomnia, characterized by difficulties with sleep onset and/or sleep maintenance*

TABLETS

Adults. 25 or 50 mg once nightly within 30 min before bedtime.

± **DOSAGE ADJUSTMENT** For patients receiving moderate CYP3A4 inhibitors or who have moderate hepatic impairment, dosage not to exceed 25 mg once nightly.

Drug Administration

P.O.

- Administer 30 min before bedtime with at least 7 hr remaining prior to patient awakening.
- Do not administer with or soon after a meal as time to sleep onset may be delayed.

Route	Onset	Peak	Duration
P.O.	Unknown	1–2 hr	Unknown

Half-life: 8 hr

Mechanism of Action

Blocks the binding of wake-promoting neuropeptides orexin A and B with their respective receptors, which suppresses the wake drive.

Contraindications

Hypersensitivity to daridorexant or its components, narcolepsy

Interactions

DRUGS

moderate and strong CYP3A4 inducers: Decreased exposure to daridorexant, decreasing effectiveness of daridorexant
moderate and strong CYP3A4 inhibitors: Increased exposure to daridorexant, increasing risk of adverse reactions
CYP3A4 substrates: Increased exposure to the CYP3A4 substrates possibly increasing risk of adverse reactions, especially substrates with a narrow therapeutic index
other CNS depressants: Increased risk of additive psychomotor impairment and CNS depression

ACTIVITIES

alcohol use: Increased risk of additive psychomotor impairment and CNS depression

FOODS

meals: Delayed onset of sleep

Adverse Reactions

CNS: Abnormal dreams, cataplexy (mild), complex sleep behaviors (being unaware of driving, food preparation or eating, having sex, making phone calls, or sleepwalking), dizziness, drowsiness, fatigue, hallucinations (hypnagogic, hyponopompic), headache, lethargy, migraine, nightmares, sleep paralysis, somnolence, vertigo, worsening of depression and **suicidal ideation**
EENT: **Labyrinthitis**, **pharyngeal swelling**
GI: Nausea, vomiting
SKIN: Rash, urticaria
Other: **Angioedema and other hypersensitivity reactions**, physical and psychological dependence

Childbearing Considerations

PREGNANCY

- Pregnancy exposure registry: 1-833-400-9611.
- It is not known if drug can cause fetal harm.

D

- Use with caution only if benefit to mother outweighs potential risk to fetus.

LACTATION

- It is not known if drug is present in breast milk.
- Mothers should check with prescriber before breastfeeding.
- If breastfeeding occurs, monitor breastfed infant for excessive sedation.

Nursing Considerations

- Be aware that daridorexant should not be administered to patients receiving strong CYP3A4 inhibitors or strong or moderate CYP3A4 inducers or to patients with severe hepatic impairment.

! **WARNING** Know that daridorexant is a Schedule IV drug. Assess patient for physicial and psychological tendencies before drug therapy begins. Monitor patient for abuse and misuse throughout drug therapy. Have naloxone available if overdose occurs.

! **WARNING** Use cautiously in patients with psychiatric disorders, especially patients with depression and suicidal ideation as these conditions may worsen with drug use. Monitor patient closely and take protective measures, as needed.

! **WARNING** Monitor patient for a hypersensitivity reaction that may become life-threatening, such as angioedema. If present, notify prescriber promptly, expect drug to be discontinued, and provide supportive care, as needed and ordered.

- Monitor patients with compromised respiratory function prescribed daridorexant for decreased respiratory function because drug has not been studied in patients with moderate or severe obstructive sleep apnea.
- Know that sleep paralysis may occur up to several minutes during sleep-wake transitions causing an inability for the patient to move or speak. Likewise, periods of leg weakness can happen either at night or during the day and may last from seconds to a few minutes.
- Be aware that hallucinations, including disturbing and vivid perceptions may occur with daridorexant use.
- Institute fall precautions for elderly patients receiving daridorexant.
- Be aware that if insomnia remains after 7 to 10 days of daridorexant therapy, an unrecognized underlying medical or psychiatric disorder may be present so patient should be evaluated further.

PATIENT TEACHING

- Instruct patient how to administer daridorexant.

! **WARNING** Warn patient that drug can be abused, and dependency and tolerance may occur. Warn patient not to increase the dose of daridorexant without prescriber knowledge and to alert prescriber if drug no longer appears to be effective.

! **WARNING** Caution patient not to consume alcohol during daridorexant therapy.

! **WARNING** Alert patient that daridorexant may cause an allergic reaction. If one occurs, tell patient to notify prescriber promptly. If severe, urge patient to seek immediate medical care.

! **WARNING** Inform patient and family or caregiver that drug may worsen depression to point of causing suicidal ideation. Stress importance to notify prescriber immediately if present. Review suicide precautions with family or caregiver.

! **WARNING** Warn patient and family or caregiver that complex sleep behaviors have occurred with use of hypnotics, including daridorexant. These behaviors may include being unaware of driving, food preparation or eating, having sex, making phone calls, or sleepwalking. If complex sleep behaviors occur, stress importance of notifying prescriber as drug will need to be discontinued.

! **WARNING** Alert patient that next-day somnolence may occur even with proper use of daridorexant and daytime sedation may persist for up to several days after discontinuing daridorexant. Tell patient that increased risk of daytime impairment can occur when drug is taken with less than a full night's sleep or if higher than recommended dose is taken. In addition, taking drug with other CNS depressants, including alcohol, can also increase the risk of daytime sedation. Caution patient to avoid driving and performing any other activities requiring mental alertness if daytime wakefulness is impaired.

- Tell patients to utilize fall precautions while taking daridorexant.
- Inform patient that drug may cause an inability to move or speak for several minutes during sleep-wake transitions and vivid and disturbing perceptions in hallucination may occur during sleep. Also, tell patient that mild symptoms such as leg weakness may occur.
- Tell patient to alert prescriber before taking any medication, including over-the-counter drugs.
- Instruct mother who is breastfeeding to monitor her infant for excessive sedation.

darifenacin hydrobromide

Class and Category

Pharmacologic class: Anticholinergic
Therapeutic class: Bladder antispasmodic

Indications and Dosages

* *To treat overactive bladder with symptoms of frequency, urge incontinence, or urgency*

E.R. TABLETS

Adults. *Initial:* 7.5 mg once daily, increased to 15 mg once daily after 2 wk, as needed.

± **DOSAGE ADJUSTMENT** For patients with moderate hepatic impairment and those taking potent CYP3A4 inhibitors (such as clarithromycin, itraconazole, ketoconazole, nefazodone, nelfinavir, and ritonavir), daily dosage not to exceed 7.5 mg.

Drug Administration

P.O.

- E.R. tablets should be swallowed whole with water and not chewed, crushed, or split.

Route	Onset	Peak	Duration
P.O.	Unknown	7 hr	Unknown

Half-life: 13–19 hr

Mechanism of Action

Antagonizes effect of acetylcholine on muscarinic receptors in detrusor muscle, decreasing muscle spasms that cause inappropriate bladder emptying. This action increases bladder capacity and volume, which relieves sensations of frequency and urgency and enhances bladder control.

Contraindications

Gastric retention, hypersensitivity to darifenacin or its components, uncontrolled narrow-angle glaucoma, urinary retention, and patients at risk for these conditions

Interactions

DRUGS

CYP2D6 substrates such as flecainide, thioridazine, tricyclic antidepressants: Risk of toxicity with these drugs
potent CYP3A4 inhibitors (such as clarithromycin, itraconazole, ketoconazole, nefazodone, nelfinavir, and ritonavir): Decreased metabolism and increased effects of darifenacin, possibly increasing the risk of adverse reactions
other anticholinergics: Increased frequency and severity of anticholinergic adverse reactions

Adverse Reactions

CNS: Asthenia, confusion, dizziness, hallucinations, headache, somnolence
CV: Hypertension, palpitations, peripheral edema
EENT: Abnormal vision, dry eyes or mouth, pharyngitis, rhinitis, sinusitis
GI: Abdominal pain, constipation, diarrhea, indigestion, nausea, vomiting
GU: Urine retention, UTI, vaginitis
MS: Arthralgia, back pain
RESP: **Airway obstruction**, bronchitis
SKIN: Dry skin, **erythema multiforme**, interstitial granuloma annulare, pruritus, rash
Other: **Anaphylaxis**, **angioedema**, flu-like symptoms, **hypersensitivity reactions**, weight gain

Childbearing Considerations

PREGNANCY

- It is not known if drug causes fetal harm.
- Use with caution only if benefit to mother outweighs potential risk to fetus.

D

LACTATION

- It is not known if drug is present in breast milk.
- Mothers should check with prescriber before breastfeeding.

Nursing Considerations

- Use darifenacin cautiously in patients with significant bladder outflow obstruction; they have increased risk of urine retention. Also, use cautiously in patients with controlled narrow-angle glaucoma, as darifenacin therapy may worsen this condition.
- Use darifenacin cautiously in patients with myasthenia gravis, severe constipation, or ulcerative colitis because it may decrease GI motility. Also, use drug cautiously in obstructive GI disorders because it increases the risk of gastric retention.

! **WARNING** Monitor patient closely for hypersensitivity reactions that may become life-threatening, such as anaphylaxis and angioedema of the face, larynx, lips, and/or tongue that may occur even after just 1 dose. If present, withhold drug, notify prescriber immediately, and provide emergency supportive care, as needed and ordered.

- Monitor patient for signs of anticholinergic CNS effects such as confusion, hallucinations, headache, and somnolence, especially at beginning of therapy and when dosage increases.
- Monitor patient for other less serious adverse reactions during drug therapy. Notify prescriber if bothersome, persistent, or serious.

PATIENT TEACHING

- Instruct patient how to administer darifenacin

! **WARNING** Warn patient to seek immediate medical attention if he experiences any signs of a serious drug reaction, including swelling of his face, lips, throat, and/or tongue.

! **WARNING** Advise patient to avoid exercising in hot weather because darifenacin decreases sweating, which increases the risk of heatstroke.

- Caution patient to avoid hazardous activities until drug's CNS effects are known and resolved.

deferoxamine mesylate

Desferal

Class and Category

Pharmacologic class: Iron chelator
Therapeutic class: Heavy metal chelator

Indications and Dosages

✶ *As adjunct to treat acute iron intoxication*

I.M. INJECTION

Adults and children ages 3 and older who are not in shock. *Initial:* 1,000 mg, followed by 500 mg every 4 hr to 12 hr, as needed. *Maximum:* 60 mg/kg/day for adults; 40 mg/kg/day for children and no more than 6,000 mg in 24 hr.

I.V. INFUSION

Adults and children ages 3 and older who are in shock. *Initial:* 1,000 mg at a rate up to 15 mg/kg/hr followed by 500 mg at a rate of 125 mg/hr every 4 hr to 12 hr, as needed. *Maximum:* 60 mg/kg/day for adults; 40 mg/kg/day for children and no more than 6,000 mg in 24 hr.

I.M. INJECTION

Adults and children ages 3 and older. 500 to 1,000 mg daily. *Maximum:* 1,000 mg daily. **Children ages 3 and older.** 20 to 40 mg/kg/day infused over 8 to 12 hr for 5 to 7 days. *Maximum:* 40 mg/kg/day.

✶ *To treat transfusional iron overload in patients with chronic anemia*

I.V. INFUSION

Adults. 40 to 50 mg/kg/day infused at a rate up to 15 mg/kg/hr over 8 to 12 hr for 5 to 7 days/wk. *Maximum:* 60 mg/kg/day.

SUBCUTANEOUS INFUSION

Adults and children ages 3 and older. 20 to 40 mg/kg/day (1,000 to 2,000 mg/day) administered over 8 to 24 hr, 5 to 7 days a wk.

Drug Administration

- Administer immediately after reconstitution. If not possible, reconstituted solution may be stored at room temperature for up to 24 hr. Do not refrigerate.
- Color when reconstituted should be clear to slightly yellowish.
- Discard unused portion.
- *Incompatibilities:* Other solvents, turbid solutions

I.V.

- This route should be used only for patients in a state of cardiovascular collapse.
- Reconstitute by adding 5 ml of Sterile Water for Injection to a 500-mg vial or 20 ml of Sterile Water for Injection to a 2-g vial. Make sure drug is completely dissolved before the solution is withdrawn.
- Dilute reconstituted solution with 0.45% or 0.9% Sodium Chloride Injection, Dextrose for Injection, or Ringer's Lactate solution.
- Administer only by slow infusion at a rate no greater than 15 mg/kg/hr for the first 1,000 mg when treating acute iron intoxication. Subsequent doses, if needed, must be given at a slower rate, not to exceed 125 mg/hr.
- Never give as a rapid infusion.

I.M.

- Preferred route for all patients not in shock.
- Reconstitute by adding 2 ml of Sterile Water for Injection to a 500-mg vial or 8 ml of Sterile Water for Injection to a 2-g vial prior to administration.

SUBCUTANEOUS

- Reconstitute by adding 5 ml of Sterile Water for Injection to a 500-mg vial or 20 ml of Sterile Water for Injection to a 2-g vial. Make sure drug is completely dissolved before the solution is withdrawn.
- Use a portable pump capable of providing continuous mini-infusion when administering drug by subcutaneous infusion.
- Administer over 8 to 24 hr, with rate individualized.

Route	Onset	Peak	Duration
I.V./I.M./SubQ	Unknown	Unknown	Unknown

Half-life: 1–6 hr

Mechanism of Action

Binds iron by forming a stable complex with it. This prevents iron from entering into further chemical reactions. The chelate then passes through the kidneys and out of the body in urine, thereby decreasing the iron level in the body.

Contraindications

Anuria, hypersensitivity to deferoxamine or its components, severe renal disease

Interactions

DRUGS

prochlorperazine: Possibly impaired consciousness
vitamin C: Increased availability of iron for chelation by deferoxamine

Adverse Reactions

CNS: Dizziness, **exacerbation or precipitation of aluminum-related dialysis encephalopathy**, fever, headache, paresthesias, peripheral neuropathy, **seizures**
CV: **Hypotension**, **shock**, tachycardia
EENT: Blurred vision, cataracts, decreased acuity, dyschromatopsia, high-frequency sensorineural hearing loss, loss of vision, night blindness, optic neuritis, retinopathy, scotoma, tinnitus, visual field defects
GI: Abdominal discomfort, diarrhea, **hepatic dysfunction**, increased liver enzymes, nausea, vomiting
GU: **Acute renal failure**, dysuria, increased serum creatinine, renal tubular disorder
HEME: **Leukopenia**, **thrombocytopenia**
MS: Arthralgia, growth retardation, metaphyseal dysplasia, myalgia
RESP: **Acute respiratory distress syndrome**, **asthma**
SKIN: Rash, urticaria
Other: **Anaphylaxis**; **angioedema**; infections with *Yersinia* or *Mucormycosis*; injection-site reactions such as localized irritation, pain, burning, swelling, induration, infiltration, pruritus, erythema, wheal formation, eschar, crust, vesicles, or local edema

Childbearing Considerations

PREGNANCY

- It is not known if drug causes fetal harm.
- Use with caution only if benefit to mother outweighs potential risk to fetus.

LACTATION

- It is not known if drug is present in breast milk.
- Mothers should check with prescriber before breastfeeding.

Nursing Considerations

- Expect to administer vitamin C with deferoxamine therapy because iron overload usually causes a vitamin C deficiency. However, be aware that high doses of vitamin C (more than 500 mg daily in adults, 100 mg in children ages 10 and older, and 50 mg in children under age 10) may cause cardiac dysfunction. Therefore, make sure patient is not receiving vitamin C if he has cardiac dysfunction, expect supplemental vitamin C therapy to begin only after an initial month of regular treatment with deferoxamine, and make sure the daily dose of vitamin C does not exceed the recommended daily allowance (RDA) for vitamin C. Monitor all patients receiving deferoxamine and vitamin C therapy concomitantly for cardiac dysfunction and report any dysfunction immediately to prescriber.

! **WARNING** Expect to administer other supportive measures with deferoxamine therapy, as ordered, when treating acute iron intoxication. Supportive measures include control of shock with blood transfusions, intravenous fluids, oxygen, and vasopressors; correction of acidosis; gastric lavage; induction of emesis with syrup of ipecac; and suction and maintenance of a clear airway.

! **WARNING** Monitor patient for a hypersensitivity reaction that could become life-threatening, such as anaphylaxis or angioedema. If present, notify prescriber promptly, withhold drug as ordered, and provide supportive care, as needed and ordered.

! **WARNING** Be aware that patients with aluminum-related encephalopathy who are receiving dialysis may develop seizures as a result of deferoxamine therapy. Deferoxamine therapy may also precipitate the onset of dialysis dementia in these patients, as well as cause a decrease in the patient's serum calcium levels and aggravate hyperparathyroidism, if present.

! **WARNING** Monitor patient, especially children, closely for signs and symptoms of respiratory distress, particularly following treatment with excessively high intravenous doses of deferoxamine. Also, know that patients with thalassemia inadvertently given a high dose or rapid intravenous infusion of deferoxamine may develop acute respiratory distress syndrome and other life-threatening disorders, such as hypotension, CNS depression, and acute renal failure. There is no specific antidote for deferoxamine, although the drug is readily dialyzable.

! **WARNING** Assess patient regularly for infections because either deferoxamine therapy or iron overload may enhance susceptibility to generalized infections. Some cases of Mucor mycosis have been fatal. If signs and symptoms occur, notify prescriber immediately and expect drug to be discontinued and appropriate treatment instituted.

- Monitor patient closely for changes in hearing or vision, especially in patients receiving. deferoxamine at high doses or over prolonged periods of time, or in patients who have low ferritin levels. If present, notify prescriber immediately and expect drug to be discontinued. Expect audiometry, fundoscopy, slit-lamp examinations, and visual acuity tests to be performed periodically in patients treated for prolonged periods of time. Early detection improves the possibility of reversal of these symptoms and test abnormalities.
- Monitor patient's serum creatinine level and assess patient for symptoms of renal dysfunction because deferoxamine has been associated with renal impairment.
- Assess children regularly for growth retardation, especially if high doses of the drug are being administered in the presence of low ferritin levels. Monitor the child's body weight and growth every 3 months. If abnormalities are detected, notify the prescriber because growth velocity may partially resume to pretreatment rates after a reduction of deferoxamine dosage.
- Discontinue deferoxamine therapy, as ordered, 48 hours prior to scintigraphy because imaging results may be distorted as a result of the rapid urinary excretion of deferoxamine-bound gallium-67.

PATIENT TEACHING

- Tell patient how drug will be administered.
- Inform patient that deferoxamine therapy is an adjunct to, and not a substitute for, standard measures used to treat acute iron intoxication.
- Advise patient not to exceed the recommended dose of daily vitamin C therapy prescribed.

! **WARNING** Alert patient that drug may cause an allergic reaction. Tell patient to notify prescriber promptly if an allergic reaction occurs. If severe, stress importance of seeking immediate medical care.

! **WARNING** Stress importance of seeking immediate medical care if respiratory distress occurs.

- Instruct patient to notify prescriber if persistent, serious, or unusual adverse reactions occur.
- Caution patient not to perform hazardous activities such as driving until CNS, visual, and auditory adverse effects are known and resolved.
- Inform patient that his urine may have a reddish discoloration because of deferoxamine therapy.
- Caution patient to inform all prescribers of deferoxamine therapy and before any radiologic tests are performed.

delafloxacin meglumine

Baxdela

Class and Category

Pharmacologic class: Fluoroquinolone
Therapeutic class: Antibacterial

Indications and Dosages

∗ *To treat acute bacterial skin and skin structure infections (ABSSSI) caused by gram-negative organisms (*Enterobacter cloacae, Escherichia coli, Klebsiella pneumoniae, Pseudomonas aeruginosa*) and gram-positive organisms (*Enterococcus faecalis, Staphylococcus aureus, S. haemolyticus, S. lugdunensis, Streptococcus agalactiae, S. anginosus, S. pyogenes*); to treat community-acquired bacterial pneumonia (CABP) caused by* Chlamydia pneumoniae, E. coli, Haemophilus influenzae, H. parainfluenzae, K. pneumoniae, Legionella pneumophila, Mycoplasma pneumoniae, P. aeruginosa, S.aureus, *or* S. pneumoniae

TABLETS

Adults. 450 mg every 12 hr for 5 to 10 days (CABP) or 5 to 14 days (ABSSSI).

I.V. INFUSION, TABLETS

Adults. 300 mg I.V. every 12 hr for 5 to 10 days (CABP) and 5 to 14 days (ABSSSI). Alternatively, 300 mg I.V. every 12 hr switched to 450 mg P.O. every 12 hr at the discretion of the prescriber for a total of 5 to 10 days (CABP) and 5 to 14 days (ABSSSI).

± **DOSAGE ADJUSTMENT** For patients with a eGFR between 15 and 29 ml/min who are receiving the drug intravenously, dosage reduced to 200 mg every 12 hr or dosage reduced to 200 mg every 12 hr, then switched to 450 mg orally every 12 hr at the discretion of the prescriber.

Drug Administration

P.O.

- Administer tablets at least 2 hr before or 6 hr after antacids containing aluminum or magnesium, didanosine, iron preparations, multivitamins containing iron or zinc, or sucralfate.
- If dose is missed, administer as soon as possible anytime up to 8 hr prior to next scheduled dose. If less than 8 hr remain before next dose, skip missed dose.
- Can be taken with or without food.

I.V.

- Reconstitute drug powder by using 10.5 ml of 0.9% Sodium Chloride Injection or 5% Dextrose Injection for each 300-mg vial. Shake vial vigorously until contents are completely dissolved. Concentration will be 300 mg/12 ml. Solution should appear clear yellow to amber.
- Then dilute reconstituted drug to a total volume of 250 ml, using either 0.9% Sodium Chloride Injection or 5% Dextrose Injection to achieve a concentration of 1.2 mg/ml. To do so, withdraw 12 ml of reconstituted solution for a 300-mg dose and 8 ml of reconstituted solution for a 200-mg dose from vial and transfer to an intravenous bag.
- Discard any unused portion of the reconstituted solution.
- Reconstituted vials or diluted solution already added to an intravenous bag may be stored either in the refrigerator or at room temperature for up to 24 hr. The solution should not be frozen.
- Administer as an infusion over 60 min.
- If a common intravenous line is being used to administer other drugs in addition to

D

delafloxacin, the line should be flushed before and after each delafloxacin infusion with 0.9% Sodium Chloride Injection or 5% Dextrose Injection.

- *Incompatibilities:* Other additives, drugs, or solutions containing multivalent cations such as calcium and magnesium.

Route	Onset	Peak	Duration
P.O.	Unknown	1 hr	Unknown
I.V.	Unknown	1 hr	Unknown

Half-life: 3.7 hr (I.V.); 4.2–8.5 hr (P.O.)

Mechanism of Action

Inhibits both bacterial topoisomerase IV and DNA gyrase enzymes, which are required for bacterial DNA recombination, repair, replication, and transcription.

Contraindications

Hypersensitivity to delafloxacin, other fluoroquinolones, or any of their components

Interactions

DRUGS

antacids containing aluminum or magnesium, didanosine, iron preparations, multivitamins containing iron or zinc, sucralfate: Significantly decreased absorption of oral delafloxacin

Adverse Reactions

CNS: Abnormal dreams, agitation, anxiety, confusion, delirium, depression, disorientation, disturbances in attention, dizziness, hallucinations, headache, hypoesthesia, **increased intracranial pressure**, insomnia, memory impairment, nervousness, nightmares, paresthesia, paranoia, peripheral neuropathy, **seizures**, **suicidal ideation**, syncope, tremors, toxic psychosis, vertigo
CV: **Aortic aneurysm and dissection**, **bradycardia**, hypertension, **hypotension**, palpitations, phlebitis, tachycardia, **ventricular extrasystoles**
EENT: Blurred vision, oral candidiasis, taste alteration, tinnitus
ENDO: Hyperglycemia, **hypoglycemia**
GI: Abdominal pain, ***Clostridioides difficile*–associated diarrhea**, diarrhea, dyspepsia, elevated liver enzymes, nausea, vomiting
GU: Elevated blood creatinine levels, **renal failure**, renal impairment, vulvovaginal candidiasis
HEME: **Agranulocytosis**, anemia, **leukopenia**, **neutropenia**, **pancytopenia**
MS: Myalgia, tendinitis, tendon rupture
RESP: Dyspnea
SKIN: Dermatitis, flushing, pruritus, rash, urticaria
Other: **Anaphylaxis**, **angioedema**, elevated alkaline phosphatase and creatine phosphokinase levels, fungal infection, infusion-site reactions (bruising, discomfort, edema, erythema, irritation, pain, phlebitis, swelling, thrombosis)

Childbearing Considerations

PREGNANCY

- It is not known if drug causes fetal harm.
- Use with caution only if benefit to mother outweighs potential risk to fetus.

LACTATION

- It is not known if drug is present in breast milk.
- Mothers should check with prescriber before breastfeeding.

Nursing Considerations

- Know that fluoroquinolones, including delafloxacin, may exacerbate muscle weakness in patients with myasthenia gravis and should be avoided for patients with a history of myasthenia gravis.

! **WARNING** Be aware that studies have shown an increased risk for aortic aneurysm and dissection within 2 months following use of fluoroquinolones, especially in elderly patients. Drug should only be given to patients with an aortic aneurysm or who are at greater risk for an aortic aneurysm if there are no alternative antibacterial treatments.

! **WARNING** Know that fluoroquinolones like delafloxacin have been associated with disabling and potentially irreversible serious adverse reactions that have occurred together, including central nervous system effects, peripheral neuropathy, tendinitis, and tendon rupture. Fluoroquinolones also have been associated with an increased risk of intracranial pressure and seizures. At the first sign or symptom of any serious adverse reaction, withhold delafloxacin and notify prescriber. Expect delafloxacin to be discontinued.

! **WARNING** Assess patient routinely for signs of a hypersensitivity reaction that could become life-threatening, such as anaphylaxis or angioedema or for a significant skin reactions such as a rash or other hypersensitivity reactions. Know that these reactions may occur even after patient has received multiple doses. Stop drug at first sign of a hypersensitivity or skin reaction, and notify prescriber immediately. Be prepared to provide supportive emergency care, as needed and ordered.

! **WARNING** Monitor patient closely for diarrhea, which may reflect pseudomembranous colitis caused by *Clostridium difficile* infection. It may be mild or become life-threatening. If it occurs, notify prescriber and expect to obtain a stool sample to confirm diagnosis. If confirmed, withhold drug and treat diarrhea with an antibiotic that treats *C. difficile,* as ordered. Also expect to administer electrolytes, fluid, and protein supplementation, as ordered.

! **WARNING** Monitor patient closely for changes in behavior or mood that may be caused by delafloxacin-induced depression or worsening psychotic reactions potentially resulting in self-injurious behavior, such as suicide. Be aware that these reactions may occur even after just 1 dose. Notify prescriber immediately and expect to discontinue delafloxacin therapy, if present, and institute precautions to keep patient safe until adverse effects have disappeared.

! **WARNING** Monitor patient's blood glucose levels, especially in diabetic patients. Also monitor patient for signs and symptoms of symptomatic hyperglycemia and hypoglycemia. If either occurs, alert prescriber and initiate appropriate treatment, as prescribed. Also, be aware that severe hypoglycemia has occurred with other fluoroquinolones. If a severe hypoglycemic reaction occurs, discontinue administration immediately and initiate appropriate treatment for hypoglycemia.

- Monitor patients with severe renal impairment receiving intravenous delafloxacin by obtaining serum creatinine levels and eGFR values, as ordered. Know that if serum creatinine level increases, prescriber should be notified; expect patient to be switched to oral form. Notify prescriber if patient's eGFR decreases to less than 15 ml/min and expect drug to be discontinued.
- Assess patient for evidence of peripheral neuropathy. Notify prescriber and expect to stop drug if patient complains of burning, numbness, pain, tingling, or weakness in extremities or if physical examination reveals deficits in light touch, motor strength, pain, position sense, temperature, or vibratory sensation.
- Monitor patients (especially patients over 60 years of age; patients receiving corticosteroids; and patients who have renal failure or who have had a heart, kidney, or lung transplant) for evidence of tendon rupture, such as inflammation, pain, and swelling at the site. Be aware that tendon rupture may occur within the first 48 hours of therapy, throughout therapy, or months after delafloxacin therapy. Notify prescriber about suspected tendon rupture and have patient rest and refrain from exercise until tendon rupture has been ruled out. If present, expect to provide supportive care, as ordered.

PATIENT TEACHING

- Instruct how to administer oral delafloxacin and what to do if a dose is missed.
- Urge patient to complete the prescribed course of therapy, even if he feels better before it's finished.
- Instruct patient to take tablets at least 2 hours before or 6 hours after antacids containing aluminum or magnesium, didanosine, iron preparations, multivitamins containing iron or zinc, or sucralfate.

! **WARNING** Tell patient to stop taking drug and to notify prescriber at first sign of rash or other hypersensitivity reaction. Tell patient to seek immediate medical care, if severe.

! **WARNING** Urge patient to report bloody, watery stools to prescriber immediately, even up to 2 months after drug therapy has ended.

! **WARNING** Urge family or caregiver to monitor patient closely for suicidal tendencies if patient develops depression or worsening of psychotic behavior during therapy and to notify prescriber.

! **WARNING** Warn patients, especially diabetics, that delafloxacin may alter blood glucose levels. Review signs and symptoms of hyperglycemia and hypoglycemia. Tell patient to immediately report symptomatic changes in blood glucose levels to prescriber and review how to treat hypoglycemia.

- Urge patient to avoid hazardous activities until CNS effects of drug are known and resolved.
- Advise patient to notify prescriber about changes in limb movement or sensation and about inflammation, pain, or swelling over a joint. Urge patient to rest the affected limb at the first sign of discomfort.
- Instruct patient to report any persistent, severe, or unusual signs and symptoms to prescriber.

denosumab

Prolia, Xgeva

denosumab-bbdz

Jubbonti, Wyost

Class and Category

Pharmacologic class: Monoclonal antibody
Therapeutic class: Antiresorptive, antiosteoporotic

Indications and Dosages

✱ *To treat men and postmenopausal women with osteoporosis at high risk for fracture; to treat bone loss in men receiving androgen deprivation therapy for nonmetastatic prostate cancer; to treat bone loss in women receiving adjuvant aromatase inhibitor therapy for breast cancer; to treat glucocorticoid-induced osteoporosis in men and women at high risk of fracture who are either initiating or continuing systemic glucocorticoids in a daily dosage equivalent to 7.5 mg or greater of prednisone and expected to remain on glucocorticoids for at least 6 months*

SUBCUTANEOUS INJECTION (JUBBONTI, PROLIA)

Adult. 60 mg once every 6 mo.

✱ *To prevent skeletal-related events in patients with multiple myeloma and in patients with bone metastasis from solid tumors*

SUBCUTANEOUS INJECTION (WYOST, XGEVA)

Adult. 120 mg every 4 wk.

✱ *To treat giant cell tumor of bone*

SUBCUTANEOUS INJECTION (WYOST, XGEVA)

Adults and skeletally mature adolescents ages 12 to 16. 120 mg every 4 wk with additional 120 mg doses on days 8 and 15 of the first month of therapy.

✱ *To treat hypercalcemia of malignancy refractory to bisphosphonate therapy*

SUBCUTANEOUS INJECTION (WYOST, XGEVA)

Adults. 120 mg every 4 wk with additional 120 mg doses on days 8 and 15 for the first month of therapy.

Drug Administration

SUBCUTANEOUS

- Drug Prolia and Xgeva solutions should appear clear, colorless to pale yellow and may contain trace amounts of translucent to white proteinaceous particles. Jubbonti and Wyost solutions should appear clear to slightly opalescent and colorless to slightly yellowish to slightly brownish. However, do not use if solution is discolored or cloudy, or if solution contains many particles or foreign particulate matter.
- Do not handle the gray needle cap on the prefilled syringe if allergic to latex.
- Remove drug from refrigerator and bring to room temperature, which generally takes 15 to 30 min. Do not warm drug any other way. Once removed from refrigerator, drug should not be exposed to direct light or temperatures above 25°C (77°F).
- When using the single prefilled syringe containing Prolia, do not slide the green safety guard forward over the needle, as it will lock in place and prevent injection. Do so only after the injection to prevent an accidental needle stick.
- When using the single-dose prefilled syringe containing Jubbonti, do not touch the safety guard wings before use because touching them may cause the safety guard to activate too soon. After the injection, confirm that the plunger head is between the safety guard

wings. This ensures that the safety guard has been activated and will cover the needle after the injection is complete.

- When using single-dose vials containing Wyost or Xgeva, withdraw solution using a 27 G needle. Puncture vial only once; do not re-enter vial. Avoid vigorous shaking.
- Administer injection using a 27 G needle. Inject into the abdomen, thigh, or upper arm. Do not administer as an I.M. or I.V. injection.
- Discard if not used within 14 days after being taken from refrigerator.

Route	Onset	Peak	Duration
SubQ	Unknown	10 days	Unknown

Half-life: 25–28 days

Mechanism of Action

Binds to RANKL, a transmembrane or soluble protein required for the formation, function, and survival of osteoclasts, the cells responsible for bone resorption. By preventing RANKL from activating its receptor, RANK, on the surface of osteoclasts, osteoclast formation, function, and survival are inhibited. This action decreases bone resorption and increases bone mass and strength in both cortical and trabecular bone.

Contraindications

Hypersensitivity to denosumab and its components, hypocalcemia, pregnancy

Interactions

DRUGS

other calcium-lowering drugs: Augmentation of calcium-lowering effect with possible severe hypocalcemia

Adverse Reactions

CNS: Asthenia, headache, insomnia, sciatica, vertigo
CV: Angina pectoris, **atrial fibrillation**, **endocarditis**, hypercholesterolemia, peripheral edema, vasculitis
EENT: Ear infection, nasopharyngitis
ENDO: Increased serum parathyroid hormone levels (presence of severe renal impairment or dialysis)
GI: Abdominal pain, constipation, diarrhea, flatulence, gastroesophageal reflux disease, nausea, **pancreatitis**, upper abdominal pain
GU: Cystitis, UTI
HEME: Anemia, **thrombocytopenia**
MS: Arthralgia; atypical subtrochanteric and diaphyseal femoral fractures; back, bone, extremity, including joint, or musculoskeletal pain; jaw osteonecrosis; myalgia; spinal osteoarthritis
RESP: Cough, dyspnea, pneumonia, upper respiratory infection
SKIN: Alopecia, cellulitis, dermatitis, eczema, erysipelas (infection of upper dermis and superficial lymphatics), erythema, lichenoid drug eruptions, pruritus, rash, urticaria
Other: **Anaphylaxis**, **angioedema**, antibodies to denosumab, **drug reaction with eosinophilia and systemic symptoms (DRESS)**, herpes zoster, **hypercalcemia (severe)**, **hypocalcemia**, **hypophosphatemia**, **malignancies (breast**, **gastrointestinal**, **reproductive)**, serious infections

Childbearing Considerations

PREGNANCY

- Pregnancy status of females of childbearing age should be verified before drug therapy is initiated.
- Drug may cause fetal harm.
- Drug is contraindicated during pregnancy.

LACTATION

- It is not known if drug is present in breast milk.
- Mothers should check with prescriber before breastfeeding.

REPRODUCTION

- Females of childbearing age should be advised to use effective contraception during therapy, and for at least 5 months after the last dose of the drug.

Nursing Considerations

! **WARNING** Ensure that a pregnancy test has been performed in females of childbearing age. It must be negative before denosumab therapy is started because drug can be toxic to the fetus.

! **WARNING** Know that preexisting hypocalcemia must be corrected prior to denosumab therapy. Patients with advanced chronic kidney disease (eGFR less than 30 ml/min) should be evaluated for the presence of chronic kidney disease-mineral bone disorder (CKD-MBD) before denosumab therapy is begun because risk of developing servere hypocalcemia increases significantly when CKD-MBD is present. Know that other patients predisposed to severe hypocalcemia or disturbances of mineral metabolism include patients with a history of excision of the small intestine, hypoparathyroidism, malabsorption syndromes, and patients who have had parathyroid or thyroid surgery. Know that severe hypocalcemia has resulted in death in some cases. Monitor patient's calcium levels, as ordered. Monitor patient closely for signs and symptoms of hypocalcemia such as neuromuscular irritability. Notify prescriber immediately, if present. Expect drug to be discontinued, administer calcium replacement therapy, as ordered, and provide supportive care, as needed and ordered.

! **WARNING** Be aware that significant hypercalcemia has also occurred in patients with growing skeletons and patients with a giant cell tumor of the bone weeks to months after drug was discontinued. Monitor patient for signs of hypercalcemia (abdominal or bone pain, confusion, constipation, fatigue, frequent urination, muscle weakness, nausea, thirst, vomiting) and if present, notify prescriber and expect to treat, as prescribed.

! **WARNING** Monitor patient closely for hypersensitivity reactions that may become life-threatening such as anaphylaxis or angioedema. Also, monitor patient for DRESS that may initially present as a rash but may only present with a fever or swollen lymph nodes. If an allergic reaction or a fever, rash, or swollen lymph nodes are present, stop denosumab therapy immediately. Notify prescriber, and provide supportive care, as needed and ordered.

- Monitor patient for signs and symptoms of infection because denosumab increases risk, especially if patient is receiving immunosuppressant therapy or has an impaired immune system. Serious skin infections as well as infections of the abdomen, ear, and urinary tract have occurred. There has also been increased incidence of endocarditis in patients receiving denosumab. Notify prescriber if an infection is suspected.
- Know that fracture risk increases, including the risk of multiple vertebral fractures, when denosumab is discontinued. New vertebral fractures may occur even 7 months after the last dose. If denosumab therapy is discontinued, discuss possibility of patient transitioning to an alternative antiresorptive therapy with prescriber.

PATIENT TEACHING

- Tell patient that if a dose of denosumab is missed, injection should be administered as soon as convenient. Thereafter, future injections should be scheduled from the date of the actual injection.
- Advise patient not to interrupt denosumab therapy without talking with prescriber because of increased risk for multiple vertebral fractures.
- Alert patient that drug is available under different drug names. Stress importance of not receiving any other denosumab products, at the same time as the one prescribed.

! **WARNING** Instruct females of childbearing age to use effective contraception during treatment and for at least 5 months after the last dose of denosumab. Also, tell patient to report pregnancy immediately, as drug may cause fetal harm.

! **WARNING** Instruct patient to take a calcium supplement of 1,000 mg and at least 400 international units of vitamin D daily. Review signs and symptoms of hypocalcemia and instruct patient to seek medical care immediately if present, especially if patient has chronic kidney disease. Also instruct patient on signs and symptoms of hypercalcemia and to notify prescriber if present. Stress importance of complying with blood tests to monitor calcium level.

! **WARNING** Tell patient to stop taking denosumab and seek immediate emergency care if allergic or skin reactions occur. Tell patient to notify prescriber immediately as drug may have to be discontinued and to seek emergency medical care if reactions are severe.

- Advise patient to notify prescriber if signs and symptoms of infection occur, such as drainage, fever, pain, redness, or swelling.

- Inform patient to report bone, joint, and/or muscle pain, as drug may have to be discontinued depending on the severity.
- Instruct patient on proper oral hygiene and on the need to notify dentist of denosumab therapy before invasive dental procedures are performed.
- Advise patient to report new or unusual groin, hip, or thigh pain or tingling or numbness in fingers and toes.
- Advise family or caregiver if caring for an adolescent with growing skeletons to report decreased alertness, headache, nausea, or vomiting following discontinuation of drug, as this could indicate a higher-than-normal calcium level requiring prompt treatment.

desmopressin acetate

DDAVP

Class and Category

Pharmacologic class: Posterior pituitary hormone
Therapeutic class: Antidiuretic, hemostatic

Indications and Dosages

∗ *To manage primary nocturnal enuresis*

TABLETS

Adults and children ages 6 and older. *Initial:* 0.2 mg at bedtime, increased, as needed. *Maximum:* 0.6 mg daily.

∗ *To control symptoms of central diabetes insipidus*

TABLETS

Adults and children ages 4 and older. *Initial:* 0.05 mg twice daily, increased, as needed. *Usual:* 0.1 to 0.8 mg in divided doses 2 or 3 times daily. *Maximum:* 1.2 mg in divided doses 2 to 3 times daily.

I.V. INJECTION, SUBCUTANEOUS INJECTION

Adults and adolescents. *Usual:* 2 to 4 mcg daily in divided doses twice daily. Dosage adjusted, as needed.

∗ *To prevent or manage bleeding episodes in hemophilia A or mild to moderate type I von Willebrand's disease*

I.V. INFUSION

Adults and children ages 3 mo and older. 0.3 mcg/kg (maximum 20 mcg) infused slowly over 15 to 30 min. If used preoperatively, given 30 min before procedure.

Drug Administration

P.O.

- Tablets should be given at bedtime when used to treat primary nocturnal enuresis.

I.V.

- Know that I.V. form is available as either a 4 mcg/ml in a single-dose ampule or as a 40 mcg/10 ml multi-dose vial.
- Gently tap top of ampule to assist the flow of solution from the upper portion of ampule to the lower portion.
- Locate blue dot on upper portion of ampule. Below the dot is a small score on the neck of the ampule. Hold ampule with blue dot facing away.
- Cover ampule with an appropriate wipe. Apply pressure to the top and bottom portions of ampule to snap it open.
- For treatment of central diabetes insipidus, administer as an I.V. injection.
- For treatment of hemophilia A and von Willebrand's disease (Type 1), dilute drug in 0.9% Sodium Chloride. Use 50 ml in adults and children weighing more than 10 kg (22 lb) and 10 ml in children weighing 10 kg (22 lb) or less. Infuse over 15 to 30 min.
- *Incompatibilities:* None reported by manufacturer.

SUBCUTANEOUS

- Do not dilute drug before administration when administered for central diabetes insipidus.
- Do not inject into an area that is damaged.

Route	Onset	Peak	Duration
P.O.	1 hr	4–7 hr	6–14 hr
I.V.	30 min	1.5–2 hr	6–14 hr

Half-life: 1.5–3.5 hr

Mechanism of Action

Exerts an antidiuretic effect similar to that of vasopressin by increasing cellular permeability of renal collecting ducts and distal tubules, thus enhancing water reabsorption, reducing urine flow, and increasing osmolality. As a hemostatic, drug increases blood level of clotting factor VIII (antihemophilic factor) and activity of von

D

Willebrand factor (factor VII_{VWF}). It also may increase platelet aggregation and adhesion at injury sites by directly affecting blood vessel walls.

Contraindications

History or presence of hyponatremia, hypersensitivity to desmopressin or its components, moderate to severe renal impairment (creatinine clearance below 50 ml/min)

Interactions

DRUGS

carbamazepine, chlorpromazine, lamotrigine, NSAIDs, opioid analgesics, selective serotonin reuptake inhibitors, tricyclic antidepressants: Possibly increased risk of water intoxication with hyponatremia

vasopressor drugs: Possibly potentiated vasopressor effect of desmopressin

Adverse Reactions

CNS: Asthenia, chills, **CVA**, dizziness, headache

CV: Hypertension (with high doses), **MI**, **thrombosis**, transient hypotension

EENT: Conjunctivitis, epistaxis, lacrimation, ocular edema, pharyngitis, rhinitis, sore throat

GI: Abdominal cramps, nausea

GU: Vulvar pain (parenteral form)

RESP: Cough, upper respiratory infections

SKIN: Flushing

Other: **Anaphylaxis**, **hyponatremia**, injection-site pain and redness, water intoxication

Childbearing Considerations

PREGNANCY

- It is not known if drug causes fetal harm.
- Nocdurna is not recommended for use during pregnancy.
- Use with caution only if benefit to mother outweighs potential risk to fetus.

LACTATION

- Drug is present in breast milk but is poorly absorbed orally by the breastfed infant.
- Mothers should check with prescriber before breastfeeding.

Nursing Considerations

- Use desmopressin cautiously in patients with conditions associated with fluid and electrolyte imbalance, such as cystic fibrosis, heart failure, and renal disorders; these patients are prone to hyponatremia.
- Use cautiously in patients with habitual or psychogenic polydipsia, as they may be more likely to drink excessive water and raise the risk of hyponatremia.

! WARNING Monitor patient closely for evidence of hyponatremia, such as changes in mental status, depressed reflexes, fatigue, headache, lethargy, nausea, restlessness, and vomiting. If left undetected, coma, respiratory arrest, and seizures may occur. Monitor patient's serum sodium level and notify prescriber of abnormalities.

! WARNING Monitor patient for a hypersensitivity reaction that could become life-threatening, such as anaphylaxis. If a hypersensitivity reaction occurs, notify prescriber promptly, withhold drug as ordered, and provide supportive care, as needed and ordered.

! WARNING Monitor patient's neurologic status regularly because drug may cause neurologic adverse reactions that could become life-threatening, such as a CVA.

- Check blood pressure often during therapy.

PATIENT TEACHING

- Instruct patient taking the tablet form on how to administer it. Instruct patient, family, or caregiver on how to administer the drug as a subcutaneous injection, if appropriate.
- Tell patient and family or caregiver to restrict patient's fluids, as ordered, to prevent hyponatremia and water intoxication, especially in a child or an elderly patient. Patient should empty the bladder immediately before bedtime and limit fluids to a minimum from 1 hour before and until 8 hours after taking drug.

! WARNING Alert patient and family or caregiver that drug may cause an allergic reaction. Tell them to notify prescriber if present. If severe, urge them to seek immediate medical care.

! WARNING Review signs and symptoms of hyponatremia with patient and family or caregiver. Stress importance of complying with laboratory appointments to monitor the sodium level. Tell patient to notify prescriber if signs and symptoms of hyponatremia occur and if severe to seek immediate medical care.

- Urge patient to report adverse reactions that are persistent, serious, or unusual.

deucravacitinib

Sotyktu

Class and Category

Pharmacologic class: Tyrosine kinase 2 (TYK2) inhibitor
Therapeutic class: Immunosuppressant

Indications and Dosages

∗ *To treat moderate to severe plaque psoriasis in patients who are candidates for systemic therapy or phototherapy*

TABLETS

Adults. 6 mg once daily.

Drug Administration

P.O.

- Administer with or without food.
- Tablets should be swallowed whole and not chewed, crushed, or cut.

Route	Onset	Peak	Duration
P.O.	Unknown	2–3 hr	Unknown

Half-life: 10 hr

Mechanism of Action

Unknown although it may selectively inhibit TYK2, a protein found in immune cells and central to what causes psoriasis. This action may be responsible for relieving the signs and symptoms of psoriasis.

Contraindications

Hypersensitivity to deucravacitinib and its components

Interactions

DRUGS

None listed by manufacturer.

Adverse Reactions

CV: Elevated triglyceride levels
EENT: Laryngitis, nasopharyngitis, oral herpes simplex, mouth ulcers, pharyngitis, rhinitis, rhinotracheitis, sinusitis, tonsilitis, tracheitis
GI: Elevated liver enzymes
GU: Decreased glomerular filtration rate, genital herpes simplex
MS: Elevated blood creatine phosphokinase, **rhabdomyolysis**
RESP: Pneumonia
SKIN: Acne, folliculitis
Other: **Angioedema or other hypersensitivity reactions**, herpes viral infections, increased risk for infections including **COVID-19**, **malignancy, including lymphomas**

Childbearing Considerations

PREGNANCY

- Pregnancy exposure registry: 1-800-721-5072.
- It is not known if drug can cause fetal harm.
- Use with caution only if benefit to mother outweighs potential risk to fetus.

LACTATION

- Drug may be present in breast milk.
- Patient should check with prescriber before breastfeeding.

Nursing Considerations

- Know that drug should not be given to patients with severe hepatic impairment.
- Be aware drug should not be given to a patient with an active or serious infection. Monitor patient closely for an infection during and after treatment. Patients at risk include patients who have a chronic or recurrent infection, have been exposed to tuberculosis (TB), have a history of a serious or an opportunistic infection, or have underlying conditions that may predispose patient to infection. If an infection occurs during therapy, notify prescriber, and expect drug to be withheld until the infection is resolved or adequately treated. Monitor patient's response to the antimicrobial therapy.
- Know that deucravacitinib therapy is not recommended for patients with active hepatitis B or C. Expect patient to undergo viral hepatitis screening, if appropriate, before drug therapy is begun because drug may cause viral reactivation.
- Expect patient to be evaluated for active or latent TB before drug therapy is begun. If patient has active TB, expect drug to be withheld; if patient has latent TB, expect patient to be treated for TB before

D

deucravacitinib therapy is begun. Be aware that patients with a past history of TB who cannot confirm an adequate course of treatment was given, should also receive anti-TB treatment before deucravacitinib therapy is begun. Monitor patient for signs and symptoms of active TB throughout drug therapy.

- Ensure that patient's immunizations are up to date before starting deucravacitinib therapy. Do not administer any live vaccines during drug therapy.

! **WARNING** Monitor patient closely for hypersensitivity reactions such as angioedema. Alert prescriber and expect drug to be discontinued. Provide supportive emergency care, as needed and ordered.

! **WARNING** Monitor patient closely for asymptomatic creatine phosphokinase (CPK) elevation as rhadomyolysis has occurred with deucravacitinib therapy.

! **WARNING** Monitor patient closely throughout deucravacitinib therapy for malignancies, including lymphomas, especially in patients with a history of a malignancy in the past (except for non-melanoma skin cancer).

- Monitor patient's liver enzymes and triglyerides periodically, as ordered, because deucravacitinib may increase these levels. If an elevation occurs, notify prescriber and expect to treat the elevation, as ordered. Know that if liver injury is suspected, expect deucravacitinib therapy to be discontinued.

PATIENT TEACHING

- Instruct patient how to administer deucravacitinib.

! **WARNING** Alert patient that an allergic reaction may occur with deucravacitinib therapy. Stress importance of seeking immediate emergency care, if serious, and stop taking drug until prescriber is notified of reaction.

! **WARNING** Advise patients to notify prescriber immediately if they develop muscle tenderness, unexplained muscle pain, or weakness, especially if malaise or fever are present.

! **WARNING** Encourage patient to have regular cancer screenings done and to report any persistent, serious, or unusual adverse reactions to prescriber.

- Review signs and symptoms of an infection, including viral infections such as herpes, and instruct patient to notify prescriber immediately, if an infection is suspected.
- Stress importance of complying with routine blood tests ordered to monitor patient for adverse reactions.
- Instruct patient to avoid immunizations with live vaccines during deucravacitinib therapy.

NEW!

deuruxolitinib phosphate

Leqselvi

Class and Category

Pharmacologic class: Janus kinase (JAK) inhibitor
Therapeutic class: Anti-alopecia agent

Indications and Dosages

✶ *To treat severe alopecia areata*

TABLETS

Adults. 8 mg twice daily.

± **DOSAGE ADJUSTMENT** For patients with an absolute lymphocyte count (ALC) that falls below 500 cells/mm^3, dosage withheld until the ALC returns to 500 cell/mm^3 or higher. For patients with an absolute neutrophil count (ANC) that falls below 1000 cells/mm^3, dosage withheld until the ANC returns to 1000 cells/mm^3 or higher. For patients with a hemoglobin that falls below 8 g/dl, dosage withheld until the hemoglobin returns to 8 g/dl or higher.

Drug Administration

P.O.

- Tablets may be taken with or without food.
- If a dose is missed, the missed dose should be skipped and normal dosing resumed at the next scheduled dose.
- Store at room temperature and in original bottle to protect from moisture.

Route	Onset	Peak	Duration
P.O.	Unknown	1.5 hr	Unknown

Half-life: 4 hr

Mechanism of Action

Blocks the adenosine triphosphate (ATP) binding site, which inhibits Janus kinase 3 and tyrosine kinase activity. Also, inhibits signaling of immune receptors dependent on TEC kinase family members. How the inhibition of specific Janus kinase and tyrosine kinase enzymes causes hair growth is not known.

Contraindications

Concurrent moderate or strong CYP2C9 inhibitor therapy, CYP2C9 poor metabolizers, hypersensitivity to deuruxolitinib or its components

Interactions

DRUGS

CYP3A inducers (strong), CYP2C9 inducers (moderate or strong): Possibly reduced effectiveness of deuruxolitinib

CYP2C9 inhibitors (moderate or strong): Increased concentration of deuruxolitinib leading to possible increased risk of serious adverse reactions, such as thrombosis

Adverse Reactions

CNS: **Central venous sinus thrombosis**, fatigue, headache

CV: **Deep vein thrombosis**, hyperlipidemia, **thrombosis**

EENT: Nasal and oral herpes, oral candidiasis, nasopharyngitis

GI: Elevated lipase levels, **GI perforations**

GU: Candidiasis infection, genital herpes

HEME: Anemia, lymphopenia, **neutropenia**, **thrombocytosis**

RESP: **Pulmonary embolism**

SKIN: Acne, **non-melanoma skin cancer**, skin and soft tissue infections

Other: Elevated blood creatine phosphokinase, herpes simplex or zoster, increased weight, **lymphoproliferative and malignancy disorders, serious infections**

Childbearing Considerations

PREGNANCY

- Drug may cause fetal harm based on animal studies
- Use with caution only if benefit to mother outweighs potential risk to fetus.

LACTATION

- It is not known if drug is present in breast milk.
- Mothers should not breastfeed during drug therapy and for 1 day after last dose because of the possibility of serious adverse reactions in the breastfed infant.

REPRODUCTION

- Females of childbearing age should use effective contraception during drug therapy because drug may cause fetal harm.

Nursing Considerations

D

! **WARNING** Be aware that deuruxolitinib is not recommended for use in combination with biologic immunomodulators, cyclosporine, other JAK inhibitors, or other potent immunosuppressants.

! **WARNING** Expect CYP2C9 genotype determination to be performed before deuruxolitinib therapy is begun because drug is contraindicated in patients who are CYP2C9 poor metabolizers. In addition, question patient about the use of concomitant CYP2C9 inhibitors as drug is also contraindicated in patients taking moderate or strong CYP2C9 inhibitors.

- Ensure that the following screenings/tests are done before deuruxolitinib is given: CBC, hepatitis B screening, tuberculosis (TB) evaluation, and viral hepatitis screening. Know that drug is not recommended for patients with an ALC less than 500 cells/mm^3, an ANC less than 1000 cells/mm^3, and a hemoglobin less than 8 g/dl at the start of therapy. Drug is also not recommended in the presence of an active serious infection, active TB, or viral hepatitis.
- Be aware that TB treatment should be started in patients prior to initiation of deuruxolitinib therapy who are newly diagnosed with latent TB or previously did not receive treatment for latent TB. Also, know that it is recommended to initiate TB treatment in a patient with a negative latent TB test before drug is administered if patient is at high risk for developing TB during treatment with deuruxolitinib.
- Ensure that patient is up to date on recommended immunizations prior to deuruxolitinib therapy, including herpes

zoster vaccinations. Expect live attenuated vaccines to be avoided during drug therapy.

- Expect to obtain a CBC periodically throughout deuruxolitinib therapy because drug will need to be temporarily withheld if the ALC drops below 500/mm^3, ANC drops below 1000/mm^3, or hemoglobin drops below 8 g/dl and not restarted until the ALC is at 500/mm^3 or higher, the ANC is 1000/ mm^3 or higher, and hemoglobin is 8 mg/dl or higher. Also expect to monitor patient's lipid levels as increases in total cholesterol and triglycerides have occurred with deuruxolitinib therapy.

! **WARNING** Monitor patient throughout drug therapy for signs and symptoms of infection. If an opportunistic or serious infection occurs, expect drug to be temporarily withheld, a prompt and complete diagnostic testing appropriate for an immunocompromised patient done, and antimicrobial therapy prescribed. Deuruxolitinib therapy can be resumed once the infection is under control.

! **WARNING** Know that viral reactivation such as hepatitis and herpes zoster, may occur during drug therapy. Know that drug should be temporarily withheld if patient develops herpes zoster during drug therapy until the episode resolves. If non-active hepatitis B infection occurs, expect to monitor for reactivation or provide prophylactic treatment, as ordered. Patient may need to be referred to a liver specialist.

! **WARNING** Be aware that another JAK inhibitor given to patients with rheumatoid arthritis who were 50 years of age and older with at least one cardiovascular risk factor had a higher rate for thromboembolic events such as deep vein thrombosis and pulmonary embolism as well as major cardiovascular events, including sudden cardiovascular death and non-fatal CVA and MI. Deuruxolitinib is also a JAK inhibitor and has caused thrombotic events such as cerebral venous sinus thrombosis, deep vein thrombosis, and pulmonary embolism. Monitor patient closely for thrombotic events.

! **WARNING** Monitor patient closely for a hypersensitivity reaction, which could become life threatening such as anaphylaxis. If present, notify prescriber, expect drug to be discontinued, and provide supportive care, as needed and ordered

! **WARNING** Monitor patients receiving deuruxolitinib for GI perforations, especially patients with a history of diverticulitis.

! **WARNING** Monitor patient for other persistent, serious, or unusual adverse reactions because deuruxolitinib therapy has also caused malignancy and lymphoproliferative disorders. A higher rate of lymphomas and lung cancers has been observed with another JAK inhibitor in patients with rheumatoid arthritis. Periodic skin examinations are recommended for patients at increased risk for skin cancer.

PATIENT TEACHING

- Instruct patient how to take deuruxolitinib, what to do if a dose is missed, and how to properly store drug.

! **WARNING** Alert females of childbearing age to use effective contraception throughout drug therapy because drug may cause fetal harm. If pregnancy occurs, patient should alert prescriber promptly.

! **WARNING** Alert patient that drug may cause an allergic reaction. If present, instruct patient to notify prescriber and, if severe, to seek immediate medical care and to stop taking drug.

! **WARNING** Review infection control measures with patient and family or caregiver. Tell patient and family or caregiver to notify prescriber if any signs and symptoms of an infection occur, including herpes zoster.

! **WARNING** Advise patient that deuruxolitinib therapy increases the risk for a blood clot. Review the signs and symptoms of thrombosis with the patient and family or caregiver and emphasis importance of seeking immediate medical care if any signs and symptoms of a thrombosis occur.

! **WARNING** Warn patient that deuruxolitinib may increase the risk of developing certain cancers. Advise patient to notify prescriber of any persistent, serious, or unusual signs and symptoms. Also, stress importance of having a periodic skin examination while taking deuruxolitinib.

- Inform patient that blood tests will need to be performed before and during deuruxolitinib therapy. Stress importance of compliance with having the tests done.
- Reassure patient that if drug is temporarily interrupted for less than 6 weeks, regrown scalp hair loss is not expected to occur.
- Warn patient not to receive any vaccinations with a live vaccine during deuruxolitinib therapy and to inform all prescribers of deuruxolitinib therapy before any vaccination is done.
- Advise mothers not to breastfeed during deuruxolitinib therapy and for 1 day after the last dose of the drug is taken.

NEW!

deutetrabenazine

Austedo, Austedo XR

Class and Category

Pharmacologic class: Vesicular monoamine transporter 2 (VMAT2) inhibitor
Therapeutic class: Anti chlorea and tardive dyskinesia

Indications and Dosages

✶ *To treat chorea associated with Huntington's disease; to treat tardive dyskinesia*

TABLETS

Adults. *Initial*: 6 mg twice daily, increased weekly by 6 mg daily until there is a reduction of chorea or tardive dyskinesia symptoms or tolerability is reached. *Maximum:* 48 mg daily.

E.R. TABLETS

Adults. *Initial:* 12 mg once daily, increased weekly by 6 mg daily until there is a reduction of chorea or tardive dyskinesia symptoms or tolerability is reached. *Maximum:* 48 mg daily.

±**DOSAGE ADJUSTMENT** For patients receiving strong CYP2D6 inhibitors or who are poor CYP2D6 metabolizers, maximum dosage should not exceed 36 mg daily.

Drug Administration

P.O.

- Immediate-release tablets should be given with food; E.R. tablets can be taken with or without food.
- Immediate-release tablets and E.R. tablets should be swallowed whole and not broken, chewed, or crushed.
- When the patient is being switched from one form of the drug to another, the patient should be given the same total daily dose.
- Be aware that when patient is switched from tetrabenazine to deutetrabenazine, tetrabenazine should be discontinued, as ordered, and manufacturer guidelines followed as a different initial dosing schedule is used.
- If treatment is interrupted for less than 1 week, treatment can be resumed at the previous maintenance dose without titration; if more than 1 week has lapsed, drug needs to be re-titrated when resumed.
- Drug can be discontinued without tapering.

Route	Onset	Peak	Duration
P.O.	Unknown	3-4 hr	Unknown

Half-life: 9-11 hr

Mechanism of Action

Reversibly depletes the levels of monoamines, such as dopamine, histamine, norepinephrine, and serotonin from nerve terminals in the brain, which reduces uptake of these monoamines into synaptic vesicles and depletes monoamine stores. However, how this action improves the symptoms of chlorea associated with Huntington's disease or tardive dyskinesia is unknown.

Contraindications

Concurrent therapy with tetrabenazine or valbenazine, hepatic impairment, hypersensitivity with deutetrabenazine or its components; inadequate or under treated depression or suicidal ideation in patients with Huntington's disease, within 14 days of MAOIs therapy or 20 days with reserpine therapy

Interactions

DRUGS

MAO inhibitors: May cause serious to life-threatening adverse reactions
neuroleptic drugs: Increased risk of akathisia, neuroleptic malignant syndrome, or parkinsonism
reserpine: Inhibits effectiveness of deuterabenazine
sedating drugs: Possible additive effects and worsening of sedation and somnolence

D

strong CYP2D6 inhibitors such as bupropion, fluoxetine, paroxetine, quinidine: Increased systemic exposure of active dihydro-metabolites of deutetrabenazine by about 3-fold
tetrabenazine, valbenazine: Additive effects of deutetrabenazine

Activities

alcohol: Possible additive effects and worsening of sedation and somnolence

Adverse Reactions

CNS: Agitation, akathisia, anxiety, confusion, depression, dizziness, fatigue, insomnia, **neuroleptic malignant syndrome**, parkinsonism, restlessness, sedation, somnolence, **suicidal ideation**
CV: **QTc prolongation**
EENT: Dry mouth, eye abnormalities caused by melanin-containing tissue binding, nasopharyngitis
ENDO: Hyperprolactinemia
GI: Constipation, diarrhea
GU: UTI

Childbearing Considerations

PREGNANCY

- It is not known if drug can cause fetal harm.
- Use with caution only if benefit to mother outweighs potential risk to fetus.

LACTATION

- It is not known if drug is present in breast milk.
- Mothers should check with prescriber before breastfeeding.

Nursing Considerations

! WARNING Know that deutetrabenazine should not be given to patients with congenital long QT syndrome or to patients with a history of cardiac arrhythmias because drug may prolong the QTc interval. Monitor the QTc interval closely in patients with bradycardia, hypokalemia, or hypomagnesemia and in patients who are receiving other drugs that prolong the QTc interval because of an increased risk of torsade de pointes and/or sudden death in patients taking deutetrabenazine.

! WARNING Monitor patient with Huntington's disease closely for new or worsening depression and suicidal ideation because drug increases risk of suicidality in these patients.

! WARNING Monitor patient with a history of breast cancer because drug may cause hyperprolactinemia as about one-third of breast cancers are prolactin driven. Also, know that hyperprolactinemia may increase risk of osteoporosis. If patient develops an elevated prolactin level, know that drug may need to be discontinued.

! WARNING Notify prescriber immediately if patient complains of feeling faint or feeling palpitations or loses consciousness. Expect to obtain an ECG, as ordered, to check patient's QTc interval because drug can cause prolongation.

- Monitor patient with Huntington's disease for worsening of cognition, functional capacity, mood, and rigidity as well as other adverse reactions because it may be difficult to distinguish between progression of the disease and adverse reactions. Alert prescriber of any concerns and expect dosage to be decreased or temporarily discontinued to help prescriber determine underlying cause.
- Monitor patient for signs and symptoms of agitation and restlessness, as these may indicate akathisia is developing. If present, notify prescriber because a dosage reduction of the drug may be needed.
- Be aware that drug may cause parkinsonism exhibited by bradykinesia, gait disturbances and possibly the development of or worsening of tremor. Drug-induced parkinsonism usually occurs within the first two weeks of therapy or when the dose is increased. If parkinsonism is suspected, notify prescriber and expect dosage to be reduced or drug discontinued.
- Be aware that deutetrabenazine or its metabolites bind to melanin-containing tissue and may cause toxicity over time that may cause adverse reactions in the eye. Monitor patient's vision and if abnormalities occur, notify prescriber as an ophthalmologic examination may be warranted.

! **WARNING** Monitor patient for signs of neuroleptic malignant syndrome (NMS), a rare but possibly fatal disorder. While NMS has not been known to occur with deutetrabenazine use, it has occurred with drugs that reduce dopaminergic transmission, so it has the potential to occur during deutetrabenazine administration. Be alert for altered mental status, autonomic instability (arrhythmias, instability of blood pressure or pulse, diaphoresis), fever and increased muscle rigidity in patient. More serious manifestations may include acute renal failure, elevated creatinine phosphokinase, myoglobinuria, or rhabdomyolysis.

PATIENT TEACHING

- Instruct patient, family, or caregiver how to administer form of deutetrabenazine prescribed.
- Advise patient to avoid alcohol intake and other drugs that may cause sleepiness while taking deutetrabenazine.

! **WARNING** Alert patient and family or caregiver for patient with Huntington's disease that drug may increase risk of new or worsening depression or suicidal ideation. Stress importance of reporting concerning behaviors of the patient to prescriber. If patient is expressing suicidal thoughts, urge family or caregiver to seek immediate medical attention for an evaluation.

! **WARNING** Alert patient, especially patients with a history of breast cancer, to notify prescriber if amenorrhea, galactorrhea, gynecomastia, and impotence occurs.

! **WARNING** Advise patient and family or caregiver to seek immediate medical attention if patient feels faint, loses consciousness, or has heart palpitations.

- Instruct patient to avoid hazardous activities until drug's CNS effects are known and resolved, especially sedation and somnolence.
- Review adverse reactions that may occur with deutetrabenazine therapy, especially those that may occur within the first two weeks of therapy or after a dosage increase or if agitation or restlessness occurs. Instruct patient and family or caregiver to notify prescriber of any adverse reactions, especially those involving the nervous and muscular systems as dosage may need to be reduced or drug discontinued.
- Advise patient to notify prescriber of any newly prescribed drugs by other providers and not to take any OTC drugs until prescriber has approved use of the drug (s).

dexamethasone

Dexamethasone Intensol, Hemady

dexamethasone acetate

dexamethasone sodium phosphate

Class and Category

Pharmacologic class: Glucocorticoid
Therapeutic class: Anti-inflammatory, diagnostic aid, immunosuppressant

Indications and Dosages

* *To treat allergic and inflammatory disorders, collagen disorders, dermatologic disease, edematous states, endocrine disorders, GI disorders, hematologic disorders, neoplastic diseases, respiratory diseases, rheumatic disorders, trichinosis with myocardial or neurologic involvement, and tuberculous meningitis*

ELIXIR, ORAL SOLUTION, TABLETS

Adults. Highly individualized dosage based on severity of disorder. *Initial:* 0.75 to 9 mg/day in divided doses and adjusted, as needed.
Children. Highly individualized dosage based on severity of disorder. *Initial:* 0.02 mg to 0.3 mg/kg/day in 3 or 4 divided doses.

I.M. OR I.V. INJECTION

Adults. Highly individualized based on severity of disorder. *Usual:* 0.5 to 9 mg daily in divided doses every 12 hr.

* *To test for Cushing's syndrome*

D

ELIXIR, ORAL SOLUTION, TABLETS

Adults. 0.5 mg every 6 hr for 48 hr, followed by collection of 24-hr urine specimen to determine 17-hydroxycorticosteroid level. Alternatively, 1 mg at 11 p.m., followed by plasma cortisol test performed at 8 a.m. the next day.

* *To distinguish Cushing's syndrome related to pituitary corticotropin excess from Cushing's syndrome from other causes*

ELIXIR, ORAL SOLUTION, TABLETS

Adults. 2 mg every 6 hr for 48 hr, followed by collection of 24-hr urine specimen to determine 17-hydroxycorticosteroid level.

* *To treat cerebral edema*

I.V. AND I.M. INJECTION

Adults. 10 mg I.V. followed by 4 mg I.M. every 6 hr. Decreased after 2 to 4 days, as needed, gradually tapering off over 5 to 7 days.

* *To treat unresponsive shock*

I.V. INFUSION AND INJECTION

Adults. 20 mg as a single dose, followed by 3 mg/kg over 24 hr as a continuous infusion. Alternatively, 40 mg as a single dose, followed by 40 mg every 2 to 6 hr, as needed, or 1 mg/kg to 6 mg/kg as a single dose. All regimens not used more than 3 days.

* *To treat acute exacerbation of multiple sclerosis*

ELIXIR, ORAL SOLUTION, TABLETS

Adults. 30 mg/day for 1 wk, followed by 4 to 12 mg every other day for 1 mo.

* *To decrease localized inflammation*

INTRA-ARTICULAR INJECTION

Adults. *For large joints*: 2 to 4 mg. *For small joints:* 0.8 to 1 mg. *For bursae:* 2 to 3 mg. *For tendon sheaths:* 0.4 to 1 mg.

SOFT-TISSUE INJECTION

Adults. 2 to 6 mg. *For ganglia:* 1 to 2 mg.

INTRALESIONAL INJECTION

Adults. 0.8 to 1.6 mg/injection site. Repeated once every 3 to 5 days to once every 2 to 3 wk, as needed.

* *As adjunct to treat multiple myeloma*

TABLETS (HEMADY)

Adults. 20 mg or 40 mg once daily, on specific days depending on the protocal regimen.

±**DOSAGE ADJUSTMENT** For elderly patients being treated for multiple myeloma, dosage reduced.

Drug Administration

- Do not stop drug therapy abruptly but taper dosage, as prescribed.

P.O.

- Give drug with food to decrease GI distress except for Hemady formulation, which may be taken with or without food.
- Give once-daily dose in the morning.
- For concentrated oral solution, use calibrated dropper that is provided to measure doses. Mix dose well with liquid or semi-solid food, such as applesauce or pudding. Administer immediately after mixing.
- Tablets may be crushed and mixed with semi-solid food except for Hemady formulation. Administer immediately. Do not store mixture.

I.V.

- For I.V. injection, inject undiluted directly into I.V. tubing of an infusing compatible solution over at least 3 min.
- For I.V. infusion, dilute 1 to 50 mg with 50 ml of 0.9% Sodium Chloride Injection or 5% Dextrose Injection and infuse over 15 to 20 min. Dilute 51 to 100 mg with 100 ml and infuse as directed.
- Use within 24 hr.
- *Incompatibilities:* Daunorubicin, doxapam hydrochloride, doxorubicin, glycopyrrolate, vancomycin

I.M.

- Shake I.M. solution before injecting deep into large muscle mass.
- Rotate sites.
- Avoid subcutaneous injection; it may cause atrophy and sterile abscess.

INTRA-ARTICULAR, INTRALESIONAL

- Due to possibility of damage to joint tissues, drug should not be administered frequently.

Route	Onset	Peak	Duration
P.O.	1–2 hr	1–2 hr	2.5 days
I.V.	Rapid	1 hr	Unknown
I.M.	1 hr	1–8 hr	6 days
Intra-articular	Unknown	Unknown	Unknown
Intralesional	Unknown	Unknown	Unknown

Half-life: 36–54 hr

Mechanism of Action

Binds to intracellular glucocorticoid receptors and suppresses inflammatory and immune responses by:

- inhibiting monocyte and neutrophil accumulation at inflammation site and suppressing bactericidal and phagocytic action.
- stabilizing lysosomal membranes.
- suppressing antigen response of helper T cells and macrophages.
- inhibiting synthesis of inflammatory response mediators, such as cytokines, interleukins, and prostaglandins.

Contraindications

Administration of live-virus vaccine to patient or family member, hypersensitivity to dexamethasone or its components (including sulfites), idiopathic thrombocytopenic purpura (I.M. administration), systemic fungal infections

Interactions

DRUGS

aminoglutethimide: Possibly diminished adrenal suppression by dexamethasone
amphotericin B (parenteral), potassium-depleting drugs: Risk of hypokalemia
anticholinesterases: Decreased anticholinesterase effectiveness in myasthenia gravis producing severe weakness
aspirin, NSAIDs: Increased risk of adverse GI effects
cholestyramine: Increased dexamethasone clearance
cyclosporine: Increased activity of both drugs, possibly resulting in seizures
CYP3A4 inducers, such as barbiturates, carbamazepine, phenytoin, rifampin: Possibly enhanced metabolism of dexamethasone requiring dosage increase
CYP3A4 inhibitors, such as clarithromycin, cobicistat-containing drugs, itraconazole, ritonavir: Possibly increased plasma concentrations of dexamethasone with increased adverse reactions
CYP3A4 substrates, such as erythromycin, indinavir: Possibly decreased plasma concentration of these drugs
digoxin: Increased risk of digitalis toxicity related to hypokalemia
ephedrine: Decreased half-life and increased clearance of dexamethasone
isoniazid: Decreased blood isoniazid level
macrolide antibiotics: Decreased dexamethasone clearance and increased dexamethasone effects
oral anticoagulants, such as warfarin: Inhibition of response to oral anticoagulant
oral contraceptives, including estrogens: Increased effect of oral contraceptives
phenytoin: Increased risk of seizures
thalidomide: Increased risk of toxic epidermal necrolysis
toxoids, vaccines: Decreased antibody response

ACTIVITIES

alcohol use: Increased risk of GI bleeding

Adverse Reactions

CNS: Depression, emotional lability, euphoria, fever, headache, **increased intracranial pressure (ICP) with papilledema**, insomnia, light-headedness, malaise, neuritis, neuropathy, paresthesia, psychosis, **seizures**, syncope, tiredness, vertigo, weakness
CV: **Arrhythmias**, **bradycardia**, edema, **fat embolism**, **heart failure**, hypercholesterolemia, hyperlipidemia, hypertension, **myocardial rupture**, tachycardia, **thromboembolism**, thrombophlebitis, vasculitis
EENT: Blurred vision, cataracts, epistaxis, glaucoma, loss of smell and taste, nasal burning and dryness, ocular infections, oral candidiasis, perforated nasal septum, pharyngitis, rebound nasal congestion, rhinorrhea
ENDO: Cushingoid symptoms, decreased iodine uptake, growth suppression in children, hyperglycemia, menstrual irregularities, **secondary adrenocortical and pituitary unresponsiveness**
GI: Abdominal distention, bloody stools, elevated liver enzymes, heartburn, hepatomegaly, increased appetite, indigestion, **intestinal perforation**, **melena**, nausea, **pancreatitis**, peptic ulcer **with possible perforation**, ulcerative esophagitis, vomiting
GU: Glycosuria, increased or decreased number and motility of spermatozoa, perineal irritation, urinary frequency
HEME: Leukocytosis, **leukopenia**
MS: Aseptic necrosis of femoral and humeral heads; muscle atrophy, spasms, or weakness;

myalgia; osteoporosis; pathologic fracture of long bones; tendon rupture (intra-articular injection); vertebral compression fracture
RESP: **Bronchospasm**
SKIN: Acne, allergic dermatitis, diaphoresis, ecchymosis, erythema, hirsutism, necrotizing vasculitis, petechiae, subcutaneous fat atrophy, striae, thin and fragile skin, urticaria
Other: Aggravated or masked signs of infection, **anaphylaxis**, **angioedema**, **hypernatremia**, **hypocalcemia**, **hypokalemia**, **hypokalemic alkalosis**, impaired wound healing, **Kaposi's sarcoma**, **metabolic acidosis**, suppressed skin test reaction, **tumor lysis syndrome**, weight gain

Childbearing Considerations

PREGNANCY

- It is not known if drug causes fetal harm. However, infants born of mothers who have received substantial doses of drug during pregnancy may develop hypoadrenalism.
- Use with caution only if benefit to mother outweighs potential risk to fetus.

LACTATION

- Drug is present in breast milk.
- A decision should be made to discontinue breastfeeding or the drug to avoid potential serious adverse reactions in the breastfed infant.

Nursing Considerations

! **WARNING** Use dexamethasone cautiously in patients with congestive heart failure, hypertension, or renal insufficiency because drug can cause sodium retention, which may lead to edema and hypokalemia. Monitor daily weight and fluid intake and output, and assess for crackles, dyspnea, peripheral edema, and steady weight gain.

! **WARNING** Use cautiously in patients who have had intestinal surgery and in those with diverticulitis, peptic ulcer, or ulcerative colitis because of risk for perforation.

! **WARNING** Monitor patient for hypersensitivity reactions, which could become life-threatening such as anaphylaxis or angioedema, particularly after giving acetate or sodium phosphate form; both may contain bisulfites or parabens, to which some people are allergic. If present, notify prescriber promptly, expect drug to be changed to another corticosteroid, and provide supportive care, as needed and ordered.

! **WARNING** Monitor results of hematology studies and blood glucose, cholesterol, lipid levels, and serum electrolyte levels periodically, as ordered. Dexamethasone may cause hyperglycemia, hypernatremia, hypocalcemia, hypokalemia, or leukopenia, which could become life-threatening. Also, it may increase serum cholesterol and lipid levels, and it may decrease iodine uptake by the thyroid.

- Test stool for occult blood regularly because drug may cause bloody stools.
- Assess patient for evidence of Cushing's syndrome, osteoporosis, and other systemic effects during long-term use.
- Monitor neonate for signs of hypoadrenocorticism if mother received dexamethasone during pregnancy.
- Be aware that the use of corticosteroids, such as dexamethasone, especially for longer than 6 weeks, increases the risk of development of eye disorders, including cataracts and glaucoma, which can possibly damage the optic nerves. It can also lead to ocular infections due to bacteria, fungi, or viruses. Know that patient should be referred to an ophthalmologist if patient develops ocular symptoms while taking dexamethasone.

PATIENT TEACHING

- Instruct patient how to administer oral form of dexamethasone prescribed.
- Advise patient to follow a low-sodium, high-potassium, high-protein diet, if prescribed, to help minimize elevated potassium levels, fluid retention, and weight gain, which is common with dexamethasone therapy. Instruct her to inform prescriber if she's on a special diet.

! **WARNING** Caution against consuming alcohol during dexamethasone therapy because it increases the risk of GI bleeding.

! **WARNING** Instruct patient not to stop drug abruptly, especially if taken long-term as serious adverse reactions may occur. Also, stress importance to notify prescriber about changes in stress, illness, or surgery because dosage may need to be increased to prevent life-threatening condition. Advise patient to notify prescriber if condition recurs or worsens after dosage is reduced or therapy is discontinued.

! **WARNING** Tell patient to watch for allergic reactions. If present, instruct patient to notify prescriber or if serious to seek immediate medical attention.

! **WARNING** Instruct patient to avoid close contact with anyone who has an infection, including people with chickenpox or measles, and to notify prescriber immediately if exposure occurs.

! **WARNING** Stress importance of notifying prescriber promptly if persistent, serious, or unusual adverse reactions occur as drug can affect many body systems.

- Tell patient to notify prescriber about other less serious adverse reactions such as anorexia, depression, light-headedness, malaise, muscle pain, nausea, vomiting, and early hyperadrenocorticism (abdominal distention, amenorrhea, easy bruising, extreme weakness, facial hair, increased appetite, moon face, weight gain). Tell patient and family about possible changes in appearance.
- Urge patient to have regular eye examinations during long-term use and to report any eye abnormalities to prescriber.
- Advise patient, family, or caregiver to check with prescriber before patient receives any immunizations, especially live-virus vaccinations during therapy.
- Inform diabetic patient that drug may affect her blood glucose level.
- Instruct patient having drug injected into a joint about the importance of avoiding putting excessive pressure on the joint afterwards and to notify prescriber if it becomes red or swollen.
- Inform mothers that breastfeeding should not be undertaken.
- Advise patient on long-term therapy to carry medical identification and to notify all healthcare providers that she takes dexamethasone.

dexmedetomidine

Igalmi

Class and Category

Pharmacologic class: Alpha-2 adrenergic receptor agonist
Therapeutic class: Sedative

Indications and Dosages

* *To treat acute agitation associated with schizophrenia or bipolar I or II disorder*

BUCCALLY, SUBLINGUALLY

Adults under age 65. *For patients with mild or moderate agitation:* 120 mcg, followed by 60 mcg 2 hr later, as needed, and an additional 60 mcg 2 hr after second dose, as needed. *Maximum:* 240 mcg/24 hr. *For patients with severe agitation:* 180 mcg followed by 90 mcg 2 hr later, as needed, and an additional 90 mcg 2 hr after second dose, as needed. *Maximum:* 360 mcg/24 hr.
Adults 65 years and older. *Initial for any degree of agitation:* 120 mcg, followed by 60 mcg 2 hr later, as needed, and an additional 60 mcg 2 hr after second dose, as needed. *Maximum:* 240 mcg /24 hr.

± **DOSAGE ADJUSTMENT** For patients with mild or moderate hepatic impairment and mild or moderate agitation, dosage decreased to 90 mcg, followed by 60 mcg 2 hours later, as needed, and an additional 60 mcg 2 hours after second dose, as needed, with maximum dosage in the 24-hr period not to exceed 210 mcg. For patients with mild or moderate hepatic impairment and severe agitation, dosage decreased to 120 mcg, followed by 60 mcg 2 hours later, as needed, and an additional 60 mcg 2 hours after second dose, as needed with maximum dosage in the 24-hr period not to exceed 240 mcg. For patients with severe hepatic impairment and mild or moderate agitation, dosage decreased to 60 mcg, followed by 60 mcg 2 hours later, as needed, and an additional 60 mcg 2 hour after second dose, as needed, with maximum dosage in the 24-hr period not to exceed 180 mcg. For patients with severe hepatic impairment and severe agitation, dosage decreased to 90 mcg, followed by 60 mcg 2 hours later, as needed, and an additional 60 mcg 2 hours after second dose, as needed, with maximum dosage in the 24-hr period not to exceed 210 mcg.

Drug Administration

P.O.

- Ensure patient is adequately hydrated before administering drug and is sitting or lying down during and after drug administration to avoid falls.
- Keep drug in foil pouch until ready to administer. For lower doses, remove film from pouch with clean, dry hands and cut 120 mcg and 180 mcg dosage strengths in half with clean, dry scissors to obtain the 60 mcg and 90 mcg doses. Discard unused half in trash. Then place the other half film for administration back into the pouch.
- Once pouch is opened and film cut, as needed, hand pouch to patient immediately. Have patient remove film from pouch with clean, dry hands.
- For sublingual administration, instruct patient to place film under the tongue.
- For buccal administration instruct patient to place film against the inside of lower lip.
- Have patient close mouth and allow film to dissolve.
- Ensure patient does not chew or swallow the film.
- Patient should not eat or drink for at least 15 min after sublingual administration, or at least 1 hr after buccal administration.
- Monitor alertness and vital signs after each administration of dexmedetomidine to detect adverse reactions such as bradycardia or hypotension.
- Do not administer additional second or third doses in patients with systolic blood pressure less than 90 mm Hg, diastolic blood pressure less than 60 mm Hg, heart rate less than 60 beats/min, or postural decrease in systolic blood pressure of 20 mm Hg or greater or postural decrease in diastolic blood pressure of 10 mm Hg or greater.
- Do not administer drug beyond 24 hr as effectiveness and safety are not known.

Route	Onset	Peak	Duration
P.O.	5–20 min	2 hr	Unknown

Half-life: 2.8 hr

Mechanism of Action

May activate presynaptic alpha-2 adrenergic receptors to provide a sense of calmness.

Contraindications

Hypersensitivity to dexmedetomidine or its components

Interactions

DRUGS

anesthetics, hypnotics, opioids, sedatives: Possibly enhanced CNS depression
drugs that prolong QT interval: Additive risk of QT prolongation

Adverse Reactions

CNS: Agitation, chills, confusion, delirium, dizziness, fever, hallucination, headache, hyperpyrexia, illusion, neuralgia, neuritis, **seizures**, speech disorder, somnolence, thirst
CV: **Arrhythmias (atrial fibrillation, atrioventricular block, extrasystoles, supraventricular tachycardia**, tachycardia, **ventricular arrhythmia, ventricular tachycardia), bradycardia, cardiac arrest or disorder**, hypertension, **hypotension, MI**, orthostatic hypotension, **QT prolongation**, T wave inversion
EENT: Dry mouth, oral hypoesthesia, photopsia, visual impairment
ENDO: **Hypoglycemia**
GI: Abdominal discomfort or pain, diarrhea, elevated blood urea and liver enzymes, hepatic dysfunction, hyperbilirubinemia, nausea, vomiting
GU: Oliguria, polyuria
HEME: Anemia, **hemorrhage**
RESP: **Apnea, bronchospasm**, dyspnea, **hypercapnia, hypoventilation, hypoxia, pulmonary congestion, respiratory acidosis**
SKIN: Hyperhidrosis, pruritus, rash, urticaria
Other: **Acidosis**, elevated blood alkaline phosphatase level, **hyperkalemia, hypernatremia, hypovolemia**, pain

Childbearing Considerations

PREGNANCY

- It is not known if drug can cause fetal harm although drug does cross the placental barrier.
- Use with caution only if benefit to mother outweighs potential risk to fetus.

LACTATION

- It is not known if drug is present in breast milk.
- Mothers should check with prescriber before breastfeeding.
- If breastfeeding occurs, monitor breastfed infant for irritability.

Nursing Considerations

! WARNING Be aware dexmedetomidine should not be given to patients at risk for torsades de pointes or sudden death, especially patients with a history of other arrhythmias; who have hypokalemia or hypomagensemia, QT prolongation, or symptomatic bradycardia; or who are receiving other drugs known to prolong the QT interval. This is because drug may cause QT interval prolongation that could be life-threatening.

! WARNING Know that dexmedetomidine should not be given to patients with advanced heart block, hypotension, orthostatic hypotension, or severe ventricular dysfunction or who have a history of syncope because drug therapy may make these conditions worse.

! WARNING Monitor patient's vital signs, especially for elderly patients or patients with diabetes mellitus, hypertension, or hypovolemia because dexmedetomidine decreases sympathetic nervous system activity, resulting in more pronounced bradycardia or hypotension. Do not allow patient to ambulate until patient is alert and is not experiencing hypotension, including orthostatic hypotension.

- Monitor patient's electrolytes, as ordered because drug cause cause electrolyte disturbances.
- Monitor patient for tachyphylaxis and tolerance or withdrawal reactions because another dexmedetomidine product administered intravenously beyond 24 hours has caused these adverse reactions along with an increased risk for other adverse reactions. Although the film administration of the drug has not be studied for more than 24 hours, keep in mind there may be a risk of physical dependency. Withdrawal syndrome may be experienced if drug is used other than as prescribed.

PATIENT TEACHING

- Instruct patient how to administer form of dexmedetomidine prescribed.
- Advise patient not to eat or drink for at least 15 minutes after taking drug sublingually or at least 1 hour after buccal administration.

! WARNING Instruct patient to alert prescriber immediately if feelings of faintness or heart palpitations occur. Instruct patient to remain lying down or sitting after receiving dexmedetomidine until vital signs are normal to avoid falls. Also, advise the patient to report any symptoms of dizziness or slow heart rate.

- Tell patient to notify prescriber of any persistent, severe, or unusual adverse reactions because drug can affect many body systems and cause serious adverse reactions.
- Inform patient drug can cause somnolence and therefore driving or other activities that require mental alertness should be avoided until effects of drug have worn off.
- Tell mothers who are breastfeeding to monitor their infant for irritability.

dexmethylphenidate hydrochloride

Focalin, Focalin XR

Class, Category, and Schedule

Pharmacologic class: Methylphenidate derivative
Therapeutic class: CNS stimulant
Controlled substance schedule: II

Indications and Dosages

* *To treat attention deficit hyperactivity disorder (ADHD)*

TABLETS (FOCALIN)

Adults and children ages 6 and older who are new to methylphenidate therapy or who are on stimulants other than methylphenidate. 2.5 mg twice daily at least 4 hr apart, increased weekly by 2.5 to 5 mg. *Maximum:* 10 mg twice daily.

Adults and children ages 6 and older who have been receiving methylphenidate. Half of the current daily methylphenidate dose with dose divided and given twice daily at least 4 hr apart. Increased in 2.5 to 5 mg increments weekly, as needed. *Maximum:* 10 mg twice daily at least 4 hr apart.

D

E.R. CAPSULES (FOCALIN XR)

Adults who are new to methylphenidate or who are on stimulants other than methylphenidate. 10 mg daily, increased weekly by 10 mg daily, as needed. *Maximum:* 40 mg daily.

Children ages 6 and older who are new to methylphenidate or who are on stimulants other than methylphenidate. 5 mg daily, increased weekly in 5-mg increments, as needed. *Maximum:* 30 mg daily.

Adults and children ages 6 and older who have been receiving methylphenidate. Half of the current total daily methylphenidate dosage increased weekly in 5-mg increments (children) or 10-mg (adults) increments, as needed. *Maximum:* 40 mg daily (adults) and 30 mg daily (children).

±**DOSAGE ADJUSTMENT** For patients who experience paradoxical aggravation of symptoms or adverse reactions, dosage decreased. For patients currently taking immediate-release tablets, dosage unchanged when switched to extended-release capsules.

Drug Administration

P.O.

- E.R. capsules and tablets should be swallowed whole and not chewed or crushed.
- For patient having difficulty swallowing an E.R. capsule, the capsule may be opened, and contents sprinkled on a small amount of applesauce. However, entire contents from capsule must be ingested at same time; contents should not be divided. Tell patient to consume mixture immediately. Caution patient not to chew mixture or store mixture for future use.

Route	Onset	Peak	Duration
P.O.	Unknown	1–1.5 hr	Unknown
P.O./E.R.	Unknown	1–4 hr	Unknown

Half-life: 2–4.5 hr

Mechanism of Action

May block reuptake of dopamine and norepinephrine into presynaptic neurons in cerebral cortex, which increases availability of dopamine and norepinephrine in extra neuronal space.

Contraindications

Hypersensitivity to dexmethylphenidate, methylphenidate, or their components; use within 14 days of MAO inhibitor

Interactions

DRUGS

antihypertensives: Decreased therapeutic effect of these drugs
halogenated anesthetics: Increased risk of sudden blood pressure and heart rate acceleration during surgery
MAO inhibitors: Increased adverse effects, risk of hypertensive crisis
risperidone: Increased risk of extrapyramidal symptoms when dosage changes for either drug
serotonergic drugs: Increased risk of serotonin syndrome

Adverse Reactions

CNS: Agitation, aggression, anxiety, **cerebral arteritis or occlusion**, **CVA**, depression, dizziness, drowsiness, dyskinesia, fever, headache, insomnia, migraine, motor or vocal tics, nervousness, psychosis, restlessness, **seizures**, tactile or visual hallucinations, Tourette syndrome, toxic psychosis, tremor
CV: Angina, **arrhythmias**, decreased or increased pulse rate, hypertension, **hypotension**, **MI**, palpitations, peripheral vasculopathy, including Raynaud's phenomenon, tachycardia, vasculitis
EENT: Accommodation abnormality, blurred vision, diplopia, dry mouth, increased intraocular pressure, mydriasis, nasopharyngitis
ENDO: Suppression of growth (children)
GI: Abdominal pain, anorexia, dyspepsia, elevated liver enzymes, **hepatic dysfunction (may be severe)**, nausea, vomiting
GU: Libido changes, priapism
HEME: Anemia, **leukopenia**, **thrombocytopenia**, **thrombocytopenic purpura**
MS: Arthralgia, muscle cramps, **rhabdomyolysis**
RESP: Cough
SKIN: Alopecia, **erythema multiforme**, excessive diaphoresis, **exfoliative dermatitis**, necrotizing vasculitis, pruritis, rash, urticaria
Other: **Anaphylaxis**, **angioedema**, physical and psychological dependence, weight loss (prolonged therapy in adults)

Childbearing Considerations

PREGNANCY

- Pregnancy exposure registry: 1-866-961-2388 or visit https://womensmentalhealth.org/adhd -medications/.
- It is not known if drug causes fetal harm, but drug may cause vasoconstriction, which may decrease placental perfusion.
- Use with caution only if benefit to mother outweighs potential risk to fetus.

LACTATION

- Drug is present in breast milk.
- Mothers should check with prescriber before breastfeeding.
- If breastfeeding occurs, infant should be monitored for adverse reactions, such as agitation, anorexia, insomnia, and reduced weight gain.

Nursing Considerations

! **WARNING** Know that dexmethylphenidate should not be given to patients with cardiomyopathy, coronary artery disease, known serious structural cardiac abnormalities, serious heart rhythm abnormalities, and other serious heart problems because of risk of CVA, MI, or sudden death. Notify prescriber if patient develops arrhythmias, exertional chest pain, or unexplained syncope.

! **WARNING** Be aware dexmethylphenidate has a high potential for abuse and misuse, which may lead to a substance use disorder, including addiction. Assess patient for risk before drug therapy is begun and monitor patient closely throughout therapy for physical and psychological dependency on drug.

- Assess patient's family history and patient for presence of tics or Tourette syndrome before drug therapy is begun. Know that drug may cause on onset or exacerbation of motor and verbal tics and worsening of Tourette's syndrome. Alert prescriber, if present, because drug may need to be discontinued.

! **WARNING** Be aware that dexmethylphenidate may induce CNS stimulation, mania, and psychosis, and may worsen behavior disturbances and thought disorders. Use drug cautiously in children with mania or psychosis. Be aware that withdrawal symptoms may occur with long-term use.

! **WARNING** Monitor patient for hypersensitivity reactions, which could become life-threatening such as anaphylaxis or angioedema. If present, notify prescriber, expect drug to be discontinued, and provide supportive care, as needed and ordered.

! **WARNING** Monitor patient for seizures. Institute seizure precautions. Expect to stop drug if seizures occur. Drug may lower seizure threshold, especially in patients with a history of seizures or EEG abnormalities.

! **WARNING** Question male patients, including male children, about painful and prolonged erections, especially after a dosage increase or during a period of drug withdrawal. Know that presence of priapism has sometimes required emergency surgical intervention, so report any findings to prescriber immediately.

- Monitor blood pressure and pulse rate to detect excessive stimulation and hypertension. Notify prescriber if signs appear.
- Monitor CBC and differential and platelet counts, as ordered, during prolonged therapy.
- Assess patient for signs and symptoms of peripheral vasculopathy, including Raynaud's phenomenon. Although mild and intermittent, know that digital ulceration and/or soft-tissue breakdown has occurred. Notify prescriber, if present, as drug dosage may have to be reduced or drug discontinued.
- Encourage patient with open-angle glaucoma to report any changes in vision immediately to prescriber as the drug may elevate intraocular pressure.
- Monitor children on long-term dexmethylphenidate therapy for signs of growth suppression, which has occurred with long-term use of stimulants.

PATIENT TEACHING

- Instruct patient how to administer the oral form of dexmethylphenidate prescribed.
- Teach patient and family or caregiver to watch for improvement in signs and

symptoms of ADHD, such as decreased impulsiveness and increased attention. Stress the need for continued follow-up care and suggest participation in an ADHD program.

! **WARNING** Stress importance of notifying prescriber if chest pain on exertion, fainting, or an irregular pulse develops.

! **WARNING** Warn patient and family or caregiver that drug has a high potential for abuse and misuse. Warn patient not to increase dosage or increase frequency of taking drug without consulting prescriber. Tell patient to alert prescriber if drug no longer seems to be effective. Alert patient and family or caregiver that drug has caused overdose and death. Encourage them to have naloxone on hand and how to use it if an inadvertent overdose occurs. Stress importance of calling 911 as soon as naloxone is administered. Advise storing drug properly in a locked container, if possible, and how to properly dispose of any unused drug.

! **WARNING** Alert patient, family, or caregiver that drug may cause an allergic reaction. If present, tell them to notify prescriber and to seek immediate medical care, if severe.

! **WARNING** Caution patient with seizure disorder that drug may cause seizures and importance of continuing to take seizure precautions.

! **WARNING** Inform male patients and family or caregiver of male children that dexmethylphenidate may cause abnormally sustained or frequent and painful erections, especially when a dosage increase occurs or during a period of drug withdrawal. Advise immediate emergency care if this should occur.

- Urge patient to notify prescriber if she has excessive nervousness, fever, insomnia, nausea, palpitations, or rash while taking dexmethylphenidate.
- Instruct patient to inspect his fingers and toes daily for changes, such as skin breakdown or ulcer formation. Although usually intermittent and mild, patient should contact prescriber if abnormalities occur, as drug may have to be discontinued or dosage reduced.
- Inform mothers who are breastfeeding to monitor infant for adverse reactions, such as agitation, anorexia, insomnia, and reduced weight gain.

diazepam

Diastat, Diastat Acudial, Diazepam Intensol, Libervant, Valium, Valtoco

Class, Category, and Schedule

Pharmacologic class: Benzodiazepine
Therapeutic class: Anticonvulsant, anxiolytic, sedative-hypnotic, skeletal muscle relaxant
Controlled substance schedule: IV

Indications and Dosages

* *To relieve anxiety*

ORAL SOLUTION, TABLETS

Adults. 2 to 10 mg 2 to 4 times daily.
Children ages 6 mo and older. *Initial:* 1 to 2.5 mg 3 or 4 times daily, gradually increased, as needed and tolerated.

I.M. OR I.V. INJECTION

Adults. *For moderate anxiety:* 2 to 5 mg repeated in 3 to 4 hr, as needed. *For severe anxiety:* 5 to 10 mg, repeated in 3 to 4 hr, as needed. I.V. injection given slowly at a rate not exceeding 5 mg/min.

* *To reduce anxiety and tension before cardioversion and to reduce recall of the procedure*

I.V. INJECTION

Adults. 5 to 15 mg slowly at a rate not exceeding 5 mg/min 5 to 10 min before the procedure.

* *To reduce anxiety before endoscopic procedures*

I.V. INJECTION

Adults. Up to 20 mg titrated to desired sedation and given immediately before the procedure and given slowly at a rate not exceeding 5 mg/min.

I.M. INJECTION

Adults. 5 to 10 mg 30 min before the procedure if I.V. route cannot be used.

* *As adjunct to treat convulsive disorders*

ORAL SOLUTION, TABLETS

Adults. 2 to 10 mg 2 to 4 times daily.
Children ages 6 mo and older. *Initial:* 1 to 2.5 mg 3 or 4 times daily. Increased gradually, as needed and tolerated.

∗ To treat status epilepticus and severe recurrent seizures

I.M. OR I.V. INJECTION

Adults. 5 mg to 10 mg I.V. slowly at a rate not exceeding 5 mg/min and repeated every 10 to 15 min, as needed, up to a cumulative dose of 30 mg. Regimen repeated, as needed, in 2 to 4 hr. (Use I.M. route only if I.V. access is unavailable.)

Children ages 3 mo and older. 0.2 mg/kg (maximum 8 mg) slowly over 1 min duration and repeated in 5 min at 0.1 mg/kg (maximum 4 mg) slowly over 1 min duration, as needed. (Use I.M. route only if I.V. access is unavailable.)

∗ As adjunct to treat acute, intermittent, stereotypic episodes of frequent seizure activity such as acute repetitive seizures or seizure clusters that are distinct from patient's usual seizure pattern in patients with epilepsy

NASAL SPRAY (VALTOCO)

Adults and children ages 12 and older weighing 76 kg (167.2 lb) or more. 1 spray (10 mg) in each nostril for a total dose of 20 mg. Dose repeated after 4 hr, as needed. *Maximum:* 2 doses for a single episode; 1 episode treated no more than every 5 days; and no more than 5 episodes treated a month.

Adults and children ages 12 and older weighing 51 kg (112.2 lb) to 75 kg (165 lb). 1 spray (7.5 mg) in each nostril for a total dose of 15 mg. Dose repeated after 4 hr, as needed. *Maximum:* 2 doses for a single episode; 1 episode treated no more than every 5 days; and no more than 5 episodes treated a mo.

Adults and children ages 12 and older weighing 28 kg (61.6 lb) to 50 kg (110 lb). 1 spray (10 mg) in one nostril. Dosage repeated, after 4 hr, as needed. *Maximum:* 2 doses for a single episode; 1 episode treated no more than every 5 days; and no more than 5 episodes treated a mo.

Adults and children ages 12 and older weighing 14 kg (30.8 lb) to 27 kg (59.4 lb). 1 spray (5 mg) in one nostril. Dosage repeated after 4 hr, as needed. *Maximum:* 2 doses for a single episode; 1 episode treated no more than every 5 days; and no more than 5 episodes treated a mo.

Children ages 6 to 11 weighing 56 kg (123.2 lb) to 74 kg (162.8 lb). 1 spray (10 mg) in each nostril for a total dose of 20 mg. Dosage repeated after 4 hr, as needed. *Maximum:* 2 doses for a single episode; 1 episode treated no more than every 5 days; and no more than 5 episodes treated a mo.

Children ages 6 to 11 weighing 38 kg (83.6 lb) to 55 kg (121 lb). 1 spray (7.5 mg) in each nostril for a total dose of 15 mg. Dosage repeated after 4 hr, as needed. *Maximum:* 2 doses for a single episode; 1 episode treated no more than every 5 days; and no more than 5 episodes treated a mo.

Children ages 6 to 11 weighing 19 kg (19.8 lb) to 37 kg (81.4 lb). 1 spray (10 mg) in one nostril. Dosage repeated after 4 hr, as needed. *Maximum:* 2 doses for a single episode; 1 episode treated no more than every 5 days; and no more than 5 episodes treated a month.

Children ages 6 to 11 weighing 10 kg (22 lb) to 18 kg (39.6 lb). 1 spray (5 mg) in 1 nostril. Dosage repeated after 4 hr, as needed. *Maximum:* 2 doses for a single episode; 1 episode treated no more than every 5 days; and no more than 5 episodes treated a mo.

BUCCAL FILM (LIBERVANT)

Children ages 2 to 5 weighing 26 kg (57.2 lb) to 30 kg (66 lb). 15 mg. Dosage repeated after 4 hr, as needed. *Maximum:* 2 doses for a single episode; 1 episode treated no more than every 5 days; and no more than 5 episodes treated a mo.

Children ages 2 to 5 weighing 21 kg (46.2 lb) to 25 kg (55 lb). 12.5 mg. Dosage repeated after 4 hr, as needed. *Maximum:* 2 doses for a single episode: 1 episode treated no more than every 5 days; and no more than 5 episodes treated a mo.

Children ages 2 to 5 weighing 16 kg (35.2 lb) to 20 kg (44 lb). 10 mg. Dosage repeated after 4 hr, as needed. *Maximum:* 2 doses for a single episode: 1 episode treated no more than every 5 days; and no more than 5 episodes treated a mo.

Children ages 2 to 5 weighing 11 kg (24.2 lb) to 15 kg (33 lb). 7.5 mg. Dosage repeated after 4 hr, as needed. *Maximum:* 2 doses for a single episode; 1 episode treated no more than every 5 days; and no more than 5 episodes treated a mo.

Children ages 2 to 5 weighing 6 kg (13.2 lb) to 10 kg (22 lb). 5 mg. Dosage repeated after 4 hr, as needed. *Maximum:* 2 doses for a single episode; 1 episode treated no more than every 5 days; and no more than 5 episodes treated a mo.

RECTAL GEL (DIASTAT ACUDIAL)

Adults and adolescents. 0.2 mg/kg rounded up to next available unit dose (or rounded down for debilitated or elderly patient). Repeated once in 4 to 12 hr, as needed. *Maximum:* 2 doses for a single episode; 1 episode treated no more than every 5 days; and no more than 5 episodes treated a mo.

Children ages 6 to 12. 0.3 mg/kg rounded up to next available unit dose. Repeated once in 4 to 12 hr, as needed. *Maximum:* 2 doses for a single episode; 1 episode treated no more than every 5 days; and no more than 5 episodes treated a mo.

Children ages 2 to 6. 0.5 mg/kg rounded up to next available unit dose. Repeated once in 4 to 12 hr, as needed. *Maximum:* 2 doses for a single episode; 1 episode treated no more than every 5 days; and no more than 5 episodes treated a mo.

✶ *To treat symptoms of acute alcohol withdrawal*

ORAL SOLUTION, TABLETS

Adults. 10 mg 3 or 4 times daily during first 24 hr. Then, 5 mg 3 or 4 times daily, as needed.

I.M. OR I.V. INJECTION

Adults. *Initial:* 10 mg and then 5 to 10 mg in 3 to 4 hr, as needed. I.V. injection given slowly at a rate not exceeding 5 mg/min.

✶ *As adjunct to relieve muscle spasms*

ORAL SOLUTION, TABLETS

Adults. 2 to 10 mg 2 to 4 times daily.

I.M. OR I.V. INJECTION

Adults. *Initial:* 5 to 10 mg; then, repeated in 3 to 4 hr, as needed. I.V. injection given slowly at a rate not exceeding 5 mg/min.

✶ *To treat tetanus*

I.M. OR I.V. INJECTION

Adults. *Initial:* 5 to 10 mg, then 5 to 10 mg in 3 to 4 hr although larger doses may be needed. I.V. injection given slowly at a rate not exceeding 5 mg/min.

Children ages 5 and older. *Initial:* 5 to 10 mg, then 5 to 10 mg repeated every 3 to 4 hr, as needed, to control tetanus spasms. I.V. injection given slowly at a rate not exceeding 5 mg/min.

Children ages 1 mo to 5 yr. 1 to 2 mg, repeated every 3 to 4 hr, as needed, to control tetanus spasms. I.V. injection given slowly at 5 mg/min.

±**DOSAGE ADJUSTMENT** For adult patients who are debilitated and being treated for tetanus with an I.M. or I.V. injection, initial dose reduced to 2 to 5 mg and increased gradually, as needed and tolerated.

✶ *To provide preoperative sedation*

I.M. OR I.V. INJECTION

Adults. 10 mg 30 min before surgery with I.M. route preferred. I.V. rate given slowly at a rate not exceeding 5 mg/min.

±**DOSAGE ADJUSTMENT** For adult patients who are debilitated or elderly, oral dosage reduced to 2 to 2.5 mg once or twice daily and individualized reduction for intranasal or parenteral dosage. Then, for all forms, dosage increased gradually, as needed and tolerated.

Drug Administration

P.O.

- Use the calibrated dropper provided to measure dose of oral solution.
- Mix concentrated oral solution (Intensol) with a liquid, such as juices, soda or soda-like beverages, or water; or semi-solid foods, such as applesauce or pudding. Stir the liquid or food gently for a few seconds after adding drug. Have patient consume immediately. Do not store once mixed.
- Protect oral solution from light. Discard open bottles after 90 days.

I.V.

- Have emergency resuscitation equipment and oxygen at bedside prior to administration.
- Solution should appear colorless to light yellow.
- Protect from light.
- Do not inject into small veins, such as those on the dorsum of the hand or wrist.
- Use extreme care to avoid extravasation or intra-arterial administration.
- Never use the autoinjector to administer drug I.V.
- Inject slowly, at a rate not exceeding 5 mg/min for adults and give over 1 min in children being treated for status epilepticus; other indications give slowly, not exceeding 5 mg/min.
- If not feasible to administer as a direct I.V. injection, it may be injected slowly through the infusion tubing as close as possible to the vein insertion.

- I.V. therapy should be replaced with oral therapy as soon as possible.
- *Incompatibilities:* Other solutions or drugs in same infusion flask or syringe

I.M.

- Inject deeply into the muscle.
- An autoinjector may be used to administer the injection.

INTRANASAL

- No device assembly is required.
- Do not prime or attempt to use for more than one administration per device as it delivers its entire contents upon activation.
- Do not open individual blister packs or test nasal spray devices before use.
- Store at room temperature and protect from light.

P.R.

- Lubricate rectal tip of syringe with lubricating jelly.
- Gently insert syringe tip into rectum. Rim should be snug against rectal opening.
- Slowly count to 3 while gently pushing plunger in until it stops. Then wait 3 sec while holding buttocks together before removing syringe tip.

Route	Onset	Peak	Duration
P.O.	30 min	0.25–2.5 hr	20–80 min
I.V.	1–5 min	1–5 min	15–60 min
I.M.	Unknown	1 hr	Unknown
Intranasal	Unknown	1.5 hr	Unknown
P.R.	2–10 min	90 min	Unknown

Half-life: 20–70 hr

Mechanism of Action

May potentiate effects of gamma-aminobutyric acid (GABA) and other inhibitory neurotransmitters by binding to specific benzodiazepine receptors in cortical and limbic areas of CNS. GABA inhibits excitatory stimulation, which helps control emotional behavior. Limbic system contains a dense area of benzodiazepine receptors, which may explain drug's antianxiety effects. Diazepam suppresses spread of seizure activity caused by seizure-producing foci in cortex, limbic, and thalamus structures.

Contraindications

For all forms: Acute angle-closure glaucoma, hypersensitivity to diazepam or its components, untreated open-angle glaucoma

For oral forms: Children under 6 mo of age, myasthenia gravis, severe hepatic impairment, severe respiratory insufficiency, sleep apnea

Interactions

DRUGS

antacids: Altered rate of diazepam absorption

cimetidine, fluoxetine, fluvoxamine, ketoconazole, omeprazole: Decreased diazepam metabolism, increased blood level and risk of adverse effects, including prolonged sedation

CNS depressants such as anesthetics, anticonvulsants, antipsychotics, anxiolytics, barbiturates, hypnotics, MAO inhibitors, narcotics, other benzodiazepines, phenothiazines, sedatives (including sedative antihistamines), and other antidepressants: Increased CNS depression and risk of falls and fractures

opioids: Increased risk of severe respiratory depression

phenytoin: Decreased metabolic elimination of phenytoin, increased risk of adverse reactions

ACTIVITIES

alcohol use: Increased CNS depression, including severe respiratory depression, significant sedation and somnolence, and increased risk of falls and fractures

Adverse Reactions

CNS: Anterograde amnesia, anxiety, ataxia, confusion, depression, dizziness, drowsiness, fatigue, headache, insomnia, lethargy, light-headedness, paradoxical reactions, psychiatric effects, sedation, sleepiness, slurred speech, **suicidal ideation**, tremor, vertigo

CV: **Hypotension**, palpitations, tachycardia

EENT: Blurred vision, diplopia, dry mouth, increased salivation

GI: Anorexia, constipation, diarrhea, elevated liver enzymes, jaundice, nausea, vomiting

GU: Libido changes, urinary incontinence, urine retention

HEME: **Neutropenia**

MS: Dysarthria, muscle weakness

RESP: **Respiratory depression**

SKIN: Dermatitis

Other: Physical and psychological dependence

Childbearing Considerations

PREGNANCY

- Pregnancy exposure registry: 1-866-961-2388 (Valium) or 1-888-233-2334 (other forms of diazepam) or http://womensmentalhealth.org/pregnancyregistry/ (Valium) or http://www.aedpregnancyregistry.org/ (other forms of diazepam).
- Drug may cause nonteratogenic issues after birth, such as feeding difficulties, neonatal flaccidity, hypothermia, and respiratory problems.
- Drug should not be used during pregnancy, especially in the first and third trimester, unless there is no alternative and the benefit to the mother outweighs the risk to the fetus.

LABOR AND DELIVERY

- Know that if drug is given on a regular basis late in pregnancy, the neonate may experience neonatal sedation and withdrawal symptoms after birth.
- Be aware that high single doses of the drug during labor and delivery may cause fetal heart rate irregularities and after birth hypotonia, hypothermia, poor sucking, and moderate respiratory depression.

LACTATION

- Drug is present in breast milk.
- Breastfeeding is not recommended during drug therapy.

Nursing Considerations

! **WARNING** Use diazepam with extreme caution in patients with a history of alcohol or drug abuse because it can cause physical and psychological dependence. Watch for signs of physical and psychological dependence during drug therapy (strong desire or need to continue taking diazepam, need to increase dose to maintain drug effects, and post-therapy withdrawal symptoms, such as abdominal cramps, insomnia, irritability, nervousness, and tremor).

! **WARNING** Use diazepam cautiously in patients with hepatic or renal impairment. Use extreme caution in patients with hepatic disorders such as hepatic fibrosis and hepatitis because drug's half-life may be significantly increased.

! **WARNING** Expect to give a lower diazepam dose to patient with chronic respiratory insufficiency because of the risk of respiratory depression.

! **WARNING** Be aware that benzodiazepine therapy such as diazepam should only be used concomitantly with opioids in patients for whom other treatment options are inadequate. If prescribed together, expect dosing and duration of the opioid to be limited. Monitor patient closely for signs and symptoms of decrease in consciousness, including coma; profound sedation; and significant respiratory depression. Notify prescriber immediately as death may occur if left untreated and provide emergency supportive care, as needed and ordered.

! **WARNING** Monitor patient closely for increase in frequency or severity of grand mal seizures when diazepam is used with standard anticonvulsant therapy. Dosage of other anticonvulsants may have to be increased. Avoid abrupt withdrawal of diazepam, as ordered, when used as part of the patient's seizure control regimen because a transient increase in frequency or severity of seizures may occur.

! **WARNING** Monitor severely depressed patient or one with depression-related anxiety for suicidal tendencies, particularly when therapy starts and dosage changes; depression may worsen temporarily during these times.

! **WARNING** Be aware that diazepam used late in pregnancy can cause profound sedation with prolonged CNS depression and withdrawal syndrome in the neonate. Monitor neonate closely after birth.

- Monitor patient for adverse reactions, especially if hypoalbuminemia is present, which increases the risk of sedation.
- Watch for paradoxical and psychiatric reactions to diazepam, especially in children and the elderly. If reactions occur, notify prescriber and expect drug to be discontinued.

- Monitor patient for decreased drug effectiveness, especially with prolonged use.
- Check patient's blood counts and liver function periodically, as ordered, because prolonged diazepam therapy rarely causes jaundice and neutropenia.

PATIENT TEACHING

- Instruct patient how to administer the form of diazepam prescribed.
- Advise patient not to take drug to relieve everyday stress.

! **WARNING** Tell patient, family, or caregiver not to administer a second dose of nasal spray if breathing difficulties arise or excessive sedation occurs. If severe, patient will require emergency rescue treatment.

! **WARNING** Warn patient not to increase dosage or take drug more often or for a longer time than prescribed. Warn her that physical and psychological dependence can occur and teach her how to recognize the signs.

! **WARNING** Warn patient not to consume alcohol or take an opioid during diazepam therapy without prescriber knowledge, as severe respiratory depression can occur and may lead to death. Inform patient about potentially fatal additive effects of combining diazepam with an opioid. Instruct patient to inform all prescribers of diazepam use, especially if pain medication may be prescribed. Also tell patient to avoid CNS depressants during therapy.

! **WARNING** Instruct patient not to stop taking drug abruptly without prescriber's supervision. If patient has a history of seizures, warn that abrupt withdrawal may trigger them.

! **WARNING** Urge family or caregiver to watch patient closely for suicidal tendencies, especially when therapy starts or dosage changes.

! **WARNING** Instruct females of childbearing age to notify prescriber immediately if she is or could be pregnant because diazepam therapy will have to be discontinued.

- Instruct patient to avoid hazardous activities until drug's CNS effects are known and resolved. Warn her that risk of falls and fractures increases when diazepam is taken with other sedatives or alcohol and to avoid this combination.
- Inform mothers wishing to breastfeed that breastfeeding is not recommended during drug therapy.

diclofenac

diclofenac epolamine

Flector Patch, Licart

diclofenac potassium

Cambia, Voltaren Rapide (CAN), Zipsor

diclofenac sodium

Voltaren, Voltaren SR (CAN)

D

Class and Category

Pharmacologic class: NSAID
Therapeutic class: Analgesic, anti-inflammatory

Indications and Dosages

✱ *To manage signs and symptoms of rheumatoid arthritis*

TABLETS

Adults. 50 mg 3 or 4 times daily.

D.R. TABLETS

Adults. *Initial:* 50 mg 3 or 4 times daily. Alternatively, 75 mg twice daily. *Maximum:* 200 mg daily.

E.R. TABLETS

Adults. 100 mg once daily. *Maximum:* 100 mg twice daily.

✱ *To manage signs and symptoms of osteoarthritis*

TABLETS

Adults. 50 mg 2 or 3 times daily.

D.R. TABLETS

Adults. 50 mg 2 or 3 times daily. Alternatively, 75 mg twice daily.

E.R. TABLETS

Adults. 100 mg once daily.

✱ *To relieve pain in patients with ankylosing spondylitis*

D.R. TABLETS

Adults. 25 mg 4 times daily, with an extra 25 mg dose at bedtime, as needed.

* *To relieve pain and dysmenorrhea*

TABLETS

Adults. 50 mg 3 times daily, as needed. Alternatively, 100 mg as first dose followed by 50 mg for second and third dose for day 1 and then 50 mg 3 times daily, as needed. *Maximum:* 200 mg for day 1; 150 mg after day 1.

* *To relieve mild to moderate acute pain*

CAPSULES (ZIPSOR)

Adults and children ages 12 and older. 25 mg 4 times daily.

* *To treat acute migraine attacks*

ORAL SOLUTION (CAMBIA)

Adults. 50 mg (1 packet) per attack.

* *To relieve pain due to minor contusions, sprains, or strains*

TOPICAL PATCH 1.3% (FLECTOR PATCH)

Adults and children ages 6 and older. 1 patch to the most painful area twice a day.

TOPICAL PATCH 1.3% (LICART)

Adults. 1 patch to the most painful area once a day.

±**DOSAGE ADJUSTMENT** For patients with hepatic impairment, dosage may be reduced.

Drug Administration

P.O.

- Oral formulations are not interchangeable because they may not be bioequivalent even if the milligram strength is the same.
- Capsules and tablets should be swallowed whole and not chewed, crushed, or opened.
- Empty packet of Cambia into a cup containing 1 to 2 ounces of water, mix well, and have patient drink immediately. Do not use any other liquids to mix drug.
- Drug may be given with food except for Cambia, which should be given on an empty stomach at least 1 hr before or 2 hr after a meal.
- Patient should not lie down for 15 to 30 min after administration of oral drug.

TOPICAL

- Do not apply patch to damaged or nonintact skin.
- If the patch begins to peel off, the edges may be taped down. If problems persist, overlay the patch with a mesh netting sleeve that allows air to pass through, where appropriate, such as ankles, elbows, or knees.
- Wash hands after applying, handling, or removing the patch and avoid eye contact with drug.

Route	Onset	Peak	Duration
P.O.	10 min	1 hr	8 hr
P.O./D.R.	30 min	2–3 hr	8 hr
P.O./E.R.	Unknown	5–6 hr	Unknown
Topical	Unknown	10–20 hr	Unknown

Half-life: 1–2 hr

Mechanism of Action

Blocks the activity of cyclooxygenase, the enzyme needed to synthesize prostaglandins, which mediate inflammatory response and cause local pain, swelling, and vasodilation. By blocking cyclooxygenase and inhibiting prostaglandins, diclofenac reduces inflammatory symptoms. This mechanism also relieves pain because prostaglandins promote pain transmission from periphery to spinal cord.

Contraindications

Active GI bleeding or ulcers; history of asthma attacks, rhinitis, or urticaria from aspirin or other NSAIDs; hypersensitivity to diclofenac, NSAIDs, or their components; pain management following coronary artery bypass graft (CABG) surgery; use on damaged or nonintact skin (topical system)

Interactions

DRUGS

ACE inhibitors, angiotensin receptor blockers (ARBs): Decreased antihypertensive effects of these drugs; decreased renal function in elderly patients or those with existing renal impairment or volume depletion

anticoagulants, antiplatelets, selective serotonin reuptake inhibitors (SSRIs), serotonin norepinephrine reuptake inhibitors (SNRIs), thrombolytics: Prolonged PT, increased risk of bleeding

aspirin, other NSAIDs, salicylates: Increased GI irritability and bleeding, decreased diclofenac effectiveness with aspirin use

beta-blockers: Impaired antihypertensive effect

cyclosporine, nephrotoxic drugs: Increased risk of nephrotoxicity
CYP2C9 inducers, such as rifampin: Decreased effectiveness of diclofenac
CYP2C9 inhibitors, such as voriconazole: Increased risk of diclofenac adverse reactions and toxicity
digoxin: Increased blood digoxin level
lithium: Increased risk of lithium toxicity
loop or thiazide diuretics: Decreased diuretic effects
methotrexate, pemetrexed: Increased risk of methotrexate or pemetrexed toxicity

ACTIVITIES

alcohol use: Increased risk of GI irritability and bleeding

FOODS

any food: Delayed absorption of D.R. tablets

Adverse Reactions

CNS: **Aseptic meningitis**, **cerebral hemorrhage**, **CVA**, dizziness, drowsiness, headache
CV: **Bradycardia and other arrhythmias**, edema, **heart failure**, hypertension, **hypotension**, **MI**, **thrombotic events**, vasculitis
EENT: Glaucoma, hearing loss, tinnitus
ENDO: **Hypoglycemia**
GI: Abdominal pain, constipation, diarrhea, dysphagia, elevated liver enzymes, esophageal ulceration, flatulence, **GI bleeding** or ulceration, **hepatic failure**, **hepatitis**, **hepatotoxicity**, indigestion, jaundice, nausea, **perforation of intestine or stomach**
GU: **Acute renal failure**, interstitial nephritis
HEME: **Agranulocytosis**; anemia, including **aplastic anemia**, **bleeding events**, eosinophilia, leukocytosis, **leukopenia**, **pancytopenia**, porphyria, **thrombocytopenia**
RESP: **Exacerbation of asthma related to aspirin-sensitivity**
SKIN: Acute generalized exanthematous pustulosis, **erythema multiforme**, **exfoliative dermatitis**, pruritus, rash, **Stevens-Johnson syndrome**, **toxic epidermal necrolysis**
Other: **Anaphylaxis**, **angioedema**, **drug reaction with eosinophilia and systemic symptoms (DRESS)**, fixed drug eruptions, **hyperkalemia**, hyperuricemia, **hyponatremia**, lymphadenopathy

Childbearing Considerations

PREGNANCY

- Drug may cause fetal harm if given during the third trimester of pregnancy by increasing the risk of premature closure of the fetal ductus arteriosus. Also, drug can cause oligohydramnios and neonatal renal impairment if given at 20 wk of gestation or later.
- Drug should be avoided in pregnant women starting at 30 wk of gestation. If absolutely needed between 20 and 30 wk of gestation, drug should be given at lowest dose and for shortest time possible.

LACTATION

- Drug may be present in breast milk.
- Mothers should check with prescriber before breastfeeding.

REPRODUCTION

- Drug may affect both female and male fertility.

Nursing Considerations

! **WARNING** Be aware that NSAIDs like diclofenac should be avoided in patients with a recent MI because risk of reinfarction increases with NSAID therapy. If therapy is unavoidable, monitor patient closely for signs of cardiac ischemia.

! **WARNING** Be aware that the risk of heart failure increases with use of NSAIDs, such as diclofenac. Diclofenac should not be given to patients with severe heart failure, but if unavoidable, monitor patient for worsening of heart failure.

! **WARNING** Use diclofenac with extreme caution and for shortest possible time in patients with a history of GI bleeding or ulcer disease because NSAIDs increase risk of GI bleeding and ulceration. Be aware that serious GI bleeding and ulceration, as well as perforation of intestine or stomach, can occur without warning or symptoms. Elderly patients are at greater risk. Monitor patient for signs of GI irritation and ulceration, especially if patient has a predisposing condition (such as a history of GI bleeding); takes an anticoagulant, NSAID (long term), or oral corticosteroid; or has other factors, such as being an alcoholic or smoker, has poor health, is over the age of 60; or tests positive for *Helicobacter pylori.* To minimize risk, give diclofenac with food. If patient develops GI distress, withhold drug and notify prescriber immediately.

! **WARNING** Monitor patient closely for bleeding events that could occur anywhere in the body besides the GI tract and can become life-threatening if hemorrhage occurs. Report signs of bleeding, such as bleeding gums, bloody or cloudy urine, ecchymoses, melena, and petechiae. Know that risk of bleeding is increased when patient is taking certain drugs like anticoagulants, such as warfarin; antiplatelet agents, including aspirin; serotonin norepinephrine reuptake inhibitors; and serotonin reuptake inhibitors.

! **WARNING** Know that use of NSAIDs like diclofenac increases risk of serious cardiovascular thrombotic events, including MI and stroke, which can be life-threatening. These events may occur early in treatment and risk increases with duration of use. Be aware that these events have occurred even in patients who do not have a history of or risk factors for cardiovascular disease. Monitor patient for warning signs, such as chest pain, shortness of breath, slurring of speech, or weakness. If any signs and symptoms develop, withhold diclofenac, alert prescriber immediately, and provide supportive care, as needed and prescribed.

! **WARNING** Monitor patient for a hypersensitivity or skin reaction that could become life-threatening such as anaphylaxis, angioedema or DRESS. At first sign of a hypersensitivity or skin reaction such as DRESS (fever, rash, swollen lymph nodes), stop drug, notify prescriber, and provide supportive care, as needed and ordered.

! **WARNING** Know that because severe hepatic reactions may occur during diclofenac therapy, monitor liver enzymes and serum uric acid level as ordered. Liver enzyme elevations usually occur within 2 months of starting drug and should be reported promptly because dosage may have to be adjusted. Also, monitor patient for evidence of hepatic dysfunction (diarrhea, fatigue, flu-like symptoms, jaundice, lethargy, nausea, pruritus, right upper quadrant tenderness).

- Monitor BUN and serum creatinine levels in elderly patients, patients taking ACE inhibitors, angiotensin II receptor blockers, or diuretics, and patients with heart failure or impaired hepatic or renal function. These patients may have an increased risk of renal failure.
- Monitor patient's blood pressure because drug can cause or worsen hypertension.
- Report weight gain of more than 1 kg (2 lb) in 24 hours because it suggests fluid retention.

PATIENT TEACHING

- Instruct patient how to administer form of diclofenac prescribed.
- Instruct patient not to lie down for 15 to 30 minutes after taking oral form of drug to decrease risk of esophageal ulceration.
- Tell patient prescribed drug to treat migraine headaches not to overuse drug. Explain that this is because overuse, defined as using drug 10 or more days per month, may lead to exacerbation of headache. Inform patient that overuse headache may appear as migraine-like daily headaches or as a marked increase in frequency of migraine attacks. If this occurs, tell patient to notify prescriber, as a withdrawal period may be needed.
- Advise patient not to wear patch form of diclofenac while bathing or showering.
- Advise patient to consult prescriber before taking aspirin or other over-the-counter analgesics. Also, advise patient to avoid alcohol during diclofenac therapy.

! **WARNING** Alert patient about possible serious skin reactions and other signs and symptoms of an allergic reaction. Tell patient to notify prescriber, if present, and to seek immediate medical care, if severe.

! **WARNING** Explain diclofenac may increase risk of serious cardiovascular reactions, including congestive heart failure as well as serious adverse GI reactions. Drug may also cause bleeding that could become severe. Stress importance to notify prescriber of persistent, severe, or unusual adverse reactions. If severe, tell patient to seek immediate medical attention.

! **WARNING** Urge patient to promptly report adverse liver effects (diarrhea, fatigue, flu-like symptoms, jaundice, lethargy, nausea, pruritus, right upper quadrant discomfort).

! WARNING Alert female patients of childbearing age to notify prescriber if pregnancy occurs because drug can cause fetal harm if taken after 20 weeks of gestation. Inform patient that drug should only be taken between 20- and 30-weeks gestation if there is no other alternative. Dosage should be the lowest possible and taken for the shortest period of time. Stress importance of not taking the drug after 30 weeks of gestation.

- Alert female patients of childbearing age and male patients that drug may affect fertility. Instruct patient to discuss any concerns with prescriber.
- Warn patient to avoid hazardous activities until diclofenac's CNS effects are known and resolved.
- Urge patient to notify prescriber about buzzing or ringing in ears, dizziness, edema, impaired hearing, or unexplained weight gain.

dicyclomine hydrochloride

Bentyl

Class and Category

Pharmacologic class: Anticholinergic
Therapeutic class: Antispasmodic

Indications and Dosages

✱ *To treat functional or irritable bowel syndrome*

CAPSULES, SYRUP, TABLETS

Adults. *Initial:* 20 mg 4 times daily, increased, as needed and tolerated, after 1 wk to 40 mg 4 times daily. *Maximum:* 160 mg daily.

I.M. INJECTION

Adults. 10 to 20 mg 4 times daily. Dosage adjusted, as needed and tolerated, but not given longer than 1 or 2 days.

Drug Administration

P.O.

- Administer drug 30 to 60 min before a meal.
- Use calibrated device to measure dosage of syrup.
- Store in a tightly sealed container at room temperature, protected from moisture and direct light. Do not refrigerate syrup.

I.M.

- Aspirate the syringe before injecting drug to avoid intravascular injection, which could cause thrombosis.
- Never administer I.V. or subcutaneously.

Route	Onset	Peak	Duration
P.O./I.M.	1–2 hr	1–1.5 hr	> 4 hr

Half-life: 1.8 hr

Mechanism of Action

Inhibits acetylcholine's muscarinic actions at postganglionic parasympathetic receptors in CNS, secretory glands, and smooth muscles. These actions relax smooth muscles and diminish biliary, GI, and GU tract secretions.

Contraindications

Angle-closure glaucoma; breastfeeding; children less than 6 mo old; GI obstruction; hemorrhagic shock; hypersensitivity to dicyclomine, other anticholinergic, or their components; ileus; myasthenia gravis; obstructive uropathy; reflux esophagitis; severe ulcerative colitis; toxic megacolon

Interactions

DRUGS

adsorbent antidiarrheals, antacids: Decreased dicyclomine absorption
amantadine, antihistamines, antipsychotics, such as phenothiazines, benzodiazepines, class 1 antiarrhythmics, such as quinidine, MAO inhibitors, narcotic analgesics, such as meperidine, nitrates and nitrites, other anticholinergics, sympathomimetic agents, tricyclic antidepressants: Increased dicyclomine effects
digoxin: Increased risk of digitalis toxicity
metoclopramide: Decreased effect of metoclopramide on GI motility
opioid analgesics: Increased risk of ileus, severe constipation, and urine retention

Adverse Reactions

CNS: Agitation, delirium, dizziness, drowsiness, dyskinesia, excitement, fever, insomnia, lethargy, light-headedness (I.M. use), nervousness, paresthesia, psychosis, syncope
CV: Palpitations, tachycardia
EENT: Blurred vision, cycloplegia, dry mouth, loss of taste, mydriasis, nasal congestion, photophobia

D

GI: Constipation, dysphagia, heartburn, ileus, vomiting
GU: Impotence, urine retention
SKIN: Decreased sweating, flushing, pruritus
Other: **Heatstroke**, **hypersensitivity reactions**, injection-site pain, redness, and swelling

Childbearing Considerations

PREGNANCY

- It is not known if drug causes fetal harm.
- Use with caution only if benefit to mother outweighs potential risk to fetus.

LACTATION

- Drug is present in breast milk.
- A decision should be made to discontinue drug or breastfeeding.

Nursing Considerations

- Assess patient for tachycardia before giving dicyclomine; heart rate may increase.

! **WARNING** Watch for symptoms of hypersensitivity. Notify prescriber, if present and expect drug to be discontinued because they usually resolve within 48 hours of stopping drug. Provide supportive care as needed and ordered.

- Monitor patient, especially the elderly and/or patients with mental illness, for delirium and psychosis. If present, notify prescriber and expect drug to be discontinued and symptoms to disappear within 12 to 24 hours.
- Assess patient during long-term use for chronic constipation and fecal impaction, and take corrective measures, as prescribed.

PATIENT TEACHING

- Instruct patient how to take the form of dicyclomine prescribed and what to do if a dose is missed.
- Advise patient not to take an antacid or an antidiarrheal within 2 hours of dicyclomine.
- Inform patient that dicyclomine relieves symptoms but doesn't cure the disorder.

! **WARNING** Instruct patient to notify prescriber if an allergic reaction occurs. If serious, urge patient to seek immediate emergency care.

! **WARNING** Urge patient to avoid getting overheated during exercise or in hot weather because heatstroke may result. Inform patient that hot baths or saunas may cause dizziness or fainting.

- Urge patient and family or caregiver that if delirium or psychosis occurs, stop the drug and notify the prescriber. Inform them that these symptoms usually resolve within 12 to 24 hours after drug is discontinued.
- Tell patient to avoid performing hazardous activities such as driving until CNS effects, such as blurred vision, dizziness, or drowsiness are known and resolved.
- Advise patient to eat high-fiber foods and drink at least eight glasses of water daily to prevent constipation.
- Instruct patient to change position slowly to avoid light-headedness.
- Inform patient that stopping drug abruptly may cause dizziness and vomiting.

difelikefalin

Korsuva

Class and Category

Pharmacologic class: Kappa opioid receptor agonist
Therapeutic class: Antipruritic

Indications and Dosages

✷ *To treat moderate to severe pruritus associated with chronic kidney disease in patients undergoing hemodialysis*

I.V. INJECTION

Adults. 0.5 mcg/kg at the end of each hemodialysis treatment.

Drug Administration

I.V.

- Do not mix or dilute difelikefalin prior to administration.
- Drug is supplied in a single-dose vial. Discard any unused product.
- Inspect solution, which should be clear, colorless, and free of particulate matter.
- Injection volume is based on patient's target dry body weight in kilograms. Use chart in manufacturer's drug package insert to determine injection volume. If patient's target dry body weight falls outside of the ranges given in the chart, use the formula: Total Injection Volume (ml) = Patient

Target Dry Body Weight (kg) × 0.01, rounded to the nearest tenth (0.1 ml).

- Administer within 60 min of syringe preparation.
- Administer as an I.V. bolus into the venous line of the dialysis circuit at the end of the hemodialysis session. The dose may be administered either during or after the rinse back of the dialysis circuit. If the drug is given after rinse back, administer it into the venous line followed by at least a 10 ml normal saline flush. If dose is given during rinse back, no additional normal saline is needed to flush the line.
- *Incompatibilities:* None reported by manufacturer.

Route	Onset	Peak	Duration
I.V.	Unknown	Unknown	Unknown

Half-life: 23–31 hr

Mechanism of Action

Relieves pruritus although mechanism of action is unknown.

Contraindications

Hypersensitivity to difelikefalin or its components

Interactions

None reported by the manufacturer.

Adverse Reactions

CNS: Confusion, dizziness, gait disturbances, headache, mental status changes, somnolence
GI: Diarrhea, nausea
Other: **Hyperkalemia**

Childbearing Considerations

PREGNANCY

- It is not known if drug can cause fetal harm.
- Use with caution only if benefit to mother outweighs potential risk to fetus.

LACTATION

- It is not known if drug is present in breast milk.
- Mothers should check with prescriber before breastfeeding.

Nursing Considerations

- Monitor patient's serum potassium level, as ordered, because difelikefalin may cause hyperkalemia.
- Institute safety precautions because difelikefalin can cause adverse CNS reactions that could lead to patient falling, especially if patient is 65 years of age or older or is taking centrally acting depressants, opioid analgesics, or sedating antihistamines.

PATIENT TEACHING

- Inform patient drug is given as an intravenous injection.
- Alert patient that other drugs, such as those affecting the CNS, opioid analgesics, or sedating antihistamines taken concomitantly with difelikefalin can increase the risk of developing adverse CNS reactions. Patient should consult prescriber before taking these types of drugs.
- Instruct patient on fall precautions, especially if somnolence occurs or patient is 65 years of age or older.
- Caution patient to avoid potentially hazardous activities, such as driving a car or operating heavy machinery until the effects of the drug are known and resolved.

digoxin

Lanoxin, Lanoxin Pediatric

Class and Category

Pharmacologic class: Cardiac glycoside
Therapeutic class: Antiarrhythmic, cardiotonic

Indications and Dosages

✱ *To treat mild to moderate heart failure with rapid digitalization*

I.V. INJECTION

Adults and children over age 10. *Loading:* 8 to 12 mcg/kg in 3 divided doses, with first dose equal to 50% of total dose and 25% of the total loading dose every 6 to 8 hr for 2 doses. *Maintenance:* 2.4 to 3.6 mcg/kg once daily.
Children ages 5 to 10. *Loading:* 15 to 30 mcg/kg in 3 divided doses, with first dose equal to 50% of total dose and 25% of the total loading dose given every 6 to 8 hr for 2 doses. *Maintenance:* 2.3 to 4.5 mcg/kg twice daily.
Children ages 2 to 5. *Loading:* 25 to 35 mcg/kg in 3 divided doses, with first dose equal to 50% of total dose and 25% of the total loading dose given every 6 to 8 hr for 2 doses. *Maintenance:* 3.8 to 5.3 mcg/kg twice daily.

Infants ages 1 to 24 mo. *Loading:* 30 to 50 mcg/kg in 3 divided doses, with first dose equal to 50% of total dose and 25% of the total loading dose given every 6 to 8 hr for 2 doses. *Maintenance:* 4.5 to 7.5 mcg/kg twice daily.
Full-term neonates. *Loading:* 20 to 30 mcg/kg in 3 divided doses, with first dose equal to 50% of total dose and 25% of total loading dose given every 6 to 8 hr for 2 doses. *Maintenance:* 3 to 4.5 mcg/kg twice daily.
Premature neonates. *Loading:* 15 to 25 mcg/kg in 3 divided doses, with first dose equal to 50% of total dose and 25% of the total loading dose given every 6 to 8 hr for 2 doses. *Maintenance:* 1.9 to 3.1 mcg/kg twice daily.

ORAL SOLUTION, TABLETS

Adults and children over age 10. *Loading:* 10 to 15 mcg/kg total given in 3 divided doses every 6 to 8 hr, with first dose equal to 50% of total dose and subsequent 2 doses given each as 25% of the total loading dose. *Maintenance:* 3.4 to 5.1 mcg/kg (tablet) and 3 to 4.5 mcg/kg (oral solution) once daily.
Children ages 5 to 10. *Loading:* 20 to 45 mcg/kg (tablet) and 20 to 35 mcg/kg (oral solution) in 3 divided doses every 6 to 8 hr, with first dose equal to 50% of total dose and remaining 2 doses given each as 25% of the total loading dose. *Maintenance:* 3.2 to 6.4 mcg/kg (tablet) and 2.8 to 5.6 mcg/kg (oral solution) daily in 2 divided doses.

ORAL SOLUTION

Children ages 2 to 5. *Loading:* 30 to 45 mcg/kg in 3 divided doses every 6 to 8 hr, with first dose equal to 50% of total dose and each of remaining 2 doses equal to 25% of total dose. *Maintenance:* 4.7 to 6.6 mcg/kg daily in 2 divided doses.
Infants ages 1 mo to 24 mo. *Loading:* 35 to 60 mcg/kg in 3 divided doses every 6 to 8 hr, with first dose equal to 50% of total dose and each of remaining 2 doses equal to 25% of total dose. *Maintenance:* 5.6 to 9.4 mcg/kg daily in 2 divided doses.
Full-term neonates. *Loading:* 25 to 35 mcg/kg in 3 divided doses every 6 to 8 hr, with first dose equal to 50% of total dose and each of remaining 2 doses equal to 25% of total dose. *Maintenance:* 3.8 to 5.6 mcg/kg daily in 2 divided doses.
Premature neonates. *Loading:* 20 to 30 mcg/kg in 3 divided doses every 6 to 8 hr, with first dose equal to 50% of total dose and each of remaining 2 doses equal to 25% of total dose. *Maintenance:* 2.3 to 3.9 mcg/kg daily in 2 divided doses.

* *To treat mild to moderate heart failure with gradual digitalization*

ORAL SOLUTION, TABLETS

Adults, children, infants, preterm infants. Loading dose eliminated and only maintenance dosage given as listed for rapid digitalization above.

* *To control ventricular response rate in chronic atrial fibrillation with rapid digitalization*

ORAL SOLUTION, TABLETS

Adults. *Loading:* 10 to 15 mcg/kg in 3 divided doses every 6 to 8 hr, with first dose equal to 50% of total loading dose and each of remaining 2 doses given as 25% of total loading dose. *Maintenance:* 3.4 to 5.1 mcg/kg once daily for tablets and 3.0 to 4.5 mcg/kg once daily for oral solution.

I.V. INJECTION

Adults. *Loading:* 8 to 12 mcg/kg every 6 to 8 hr, with first dose equal to 50% of total loading dose and each of remaining 2 doses given as 25% of total loading dose. *Maintenance:* 2.4 to 3.6 mcg/kg once daily.

* *To control ventricular response rate in chronic atrial fibrillation with gradual digitalization*

ORAL SOLUTION, TABLETS

Adults with normal renal function. 3.4 to 5.1 mcg/kg once daily for tablets and 3.0 to 4.5 mcg/kg once daily for oral solution with dosage adjusted every 2 wk, as needed.

I.V. INJECTION

Adults with normal renal function. 2.4 to 3.6 mcg/kg once daily with dosage adjusted every 2 wk, as needed.

± **DOSAGE ADJUSTMENT** For patients who are debilitated or elderly or have implanted pacemakers, dosage carefully adjusted because toxicity may develop at doses tolerated by most patients.

Drug Administration

- Before administering a loading dose, obtain blood pressure, heart rate, and heart rhythm as well as electrolyte levels, as ordered, and question patient about the use of cardiac glycosides within the past 2 to 3 wk.

- Take patient's apical pulse before giving each dose and notify prescriber if it's below 60 beats/min (or other specified level).

P.O.

- Use the calibrated oral dosing syringe supplied by manufacturer to measure dosage of oral solution. However, if dosage is greater than 0.1 ml, use a separate measuring device.

I.V.

- Use I.V. route only if oral administration is not feasible, or a rapid therapeutic effect is necessary.
- Discard if solution is markedly discolored or contains particles.
- Give undiluted or dilute with a 4-fold or greater volume of 0.9% Sodium Chloride for Injection, 5% Dextrose in Water, or Sterile Water for Injection. Diluting with a smaller volume of diluent may cause precipitation of digoxin. Administer immediately, once diluted.
- Administer slowly over 5 min or longer. Rapid administration may cause coronary or systemic vasoconstriction to occur.
- Do not administer as an I.M. injection because of severe local irritation and pain at site of injection.
- *Incompatibilities:* Other I.V. drugs

Route	Onset	Peak	Duration
P.O.	30–120 min	1–3 hr	3–4 days
I.V.	5–30 min	1–4 hr	3–4 days

Half-life: 36–48 hr

Mechanism of Action

Increases the force and velocity of myocardial contraction, resulting in positive inotropic effects. Digoxin produces antiarrhythmic effects by decreasing the conduction rate and increasing the effective refractory period of the AV node.

Contraindications

Hypersensitivity to digoxin or its components, presence of digitalis toxicity, ventricular fibrillation or ventricular tachycardia unless heart failure occurs unrelated to digoxin therapy

Interactions

DRUGS

amiodarone, mirabegron, propafenone, quinine, verapamil: Increased digoxin concentration up to 50%, increasing risk of digitalis toxicity
beta-blockers, calcium channel blockers: Increased additive effects of slowing heart rate, possibly producing bradycardia
calcium supplements given rapidly I.V.: Increased risk of serious arrhythmias
dofetilide: Increased risk for torsades de pointes
dronedarone: Increased risk of sudden death
ivabradine: Increased risk of bradycardia
nephrotoxic drugs: Increased risk of digitalis toxicity
neuromuscular blocking agents, such as succinylcholine: Possibly sudden release of potassium from muscle cells increasing risk of arrhythmias
quinidine, ritonavir: Increased digoxin concentration by more than 50%, significantly increasing risk of digitalis toxicity
sotalol: Increased risk of proarrhythmias
sympathomimetics: Increased risk of arrhythmias
teriparatide: Transiently increases serum calcium which may cause digitalis toxicity
thyroid hormone: Decreased plasma digoxin level, requiring an increase in dosage

FOODS

high-fiber food: Decreased oral digoxin absorption

Adverse Reactions

CNS: Confusion, depression, drowsiness, extreme weakness, headache, syncope
CV: **Arrhythmias**, **heart block**
EENT: Blurred vision, colored halos around objects
GI: Abdominal discomfort or pain, anorexia, diarrhea, nausea, vomiting
Other: **Electrolyte imbalances**

Childbearing Considerations

PREGNANCY

- It is not known if drug causes fetal harm, but drug does cross placenta.
- Use with caution only if benefit to mother outweighs potential risk to fetus.
- Dosage may have to be increased during pregnancy and decreased in the postpartum period.

LABOR AND DELIVERY

- Upon birth, neonates should be monitored for signs and symptoms of digoxin toxicity.

LACTATION

- Drug is present in breast milk.
- Mothers should check with prescriber before breastfeeding.

Nursing Considerations

! **WARNING** Be aware that digoxin therapy is not recommended in patients with acute cor pulmonale involving heart failure associated with amyloid heart disease, constrictive pericarditis, preserved left ventricular ejection fraction, or restrictive cardiomyopathy because of increased susceptibility to digoxin toxicity. The drug is also not recommended in patients with idiopathic hypertrophic subaortic stenosis because outflow obstruction may worsen because of the inotropic effects of digoxin.

- Expect to treat underlying thiamine deficiency in patients with beriberi heart disease because, if left untreated, digoxin therapy may be ineffective.

! **WARNING** Monitor patient closely for signs of digitalis toxicity, such as altered mental status, arrhythmias, heart block, nausea, visual disturbances, and vomiting. If they appear, notify prescriber, check serum digoxin level, as ordered, and expect to withhold drug until level is known. Monitor ECG tracing continuously until toxicity is resolved.

! **WARNING** Obtain an ECG frequently, as ordered, especially in elderly patients because of their reduced renal clearance. Elderly patients, especially those with coronary insufficiency, are more susceptible to arrhythmias—particularly ventricular fibrillation—if digitalis toxicity occurs.

! **WARNING** Monitor patient's serum potassium level regularly because hypokalemia predisposes to digitalis toxicity and serious arrhythmias. Also, monitor potassium level often when giving potassium salts because hyperkalemia in patients receiving digoxin can be fatal.

! **WARNING** Monitor neonates of mothers taking digoxin during pregnancy for signs and symptoms of digoxin toxicity, including arrhythmias and vomiting.

- Assess for drug effectiveness if patient has acute or unstable chronic atrial fibrillation. Ventricular rate may not normalize even when serum drug level falls within therapeutic range. Be aware that the dosage should not be increased in this situation because it probably won't produce a therapeutic effect and may lead to toxicity.
- Be aware that because digoxin has a narrow therapeutic index and interacts with many different drugs, monitoring of serum digoxin levels is important when other drugs are prescribed or discontinued, or dosages adjusted.
- Be aware that digoxin requirements may increase during pregnancy and decrease in the postpartum period. Expect digoxin levels to be monitored closely during pregnancy and the postpartum period. Also, be aware that digoxin does cross the placenta.

PATIENT TEACHING

- Instruct patient, family, or caregiver how to administer the form of digoxin prescribed and what to do if a dose is missed. Emphasize importance of taking digoxin exactly as prescribed.
- Teach patient how to take a pulse and instruct patient to do so before each dose. Urge patient to notify prescriber if pulse falls below 60 beats/min or suddenly increases.

! **WARNING** Warn about possible toxicity from taking too much and decreased effectiveness from taking too little. Urge patient to notify prescriber if she experiences adverse reactions, such as GI distress or pulse changes.

- Advise patient to consult prescriber before using other drugs, including over-the-counter products.
- Instruct patient to carry medical identification that indicates her need for digoxin.
- Inform patient that small, white 0.25-mg tablets can easily be confused with other drugs. Caution against carrying digoxin in anything other than its original labeled container.

digoxin immune Fab (ovine)

Class and Category

Pharmacologic class: Antibody fragment
Therapeutic class: Cardiac glycoside antidote

Indications and Dosages

∗ *To treat acute ingestion of unknown amounts of digoxin and toxicity in the absence of a serum digitalis concentration or estimated ingested amount*

I.V. INFUSION, I.V. INJECTION

Adults and children. *Initial:* 400 mg (10 vials) with a second dose of 400 mg (10 vials) given, as needed.

∗ *To treat acute ingestion of known amounts of digoxin*

I.V. INFUSION, I.V. INJECTION

Adults and children. *Highly individualized based on the following formula:* Amount of digoxin ingested (in mg) divided by 0.5 mg/vial equals dose (in number of vials).

∗ *To treat chronic digoxin toxicity in the absence of a serum digitalis concentration*

I.V. INFUSION, I.V. INJECTION

Adults and children weighing 20 kg (44 lb) or more. 240 mg (6 vials).
Infants and children weighing less than 20 kg (44 lb). 40 mg (1 vial).

∗ *To treat chronic digoxin toxicity with known serum digitalis concentration*

I.V. INFUSION, I.V. INJECTION

Adults and children. *Highly individualized based on the following formula:* Serum digoxin concentration in ng/ml times weight in kg divided by 100 equals dose (in number of vials).

± **DOSAGE ADJUSTMENT** For all patients, a higher dose may need to be administered, if the dose based on ingested amount differs substantially from the dose based on serum digoxin or digitoxin level. Dose repeated after several hours, as needed.

Drug Administration

I.V.

- Expect each 40-mg vial of purified digoxin immune Fab to bind about 0.5 mg of digoxin.

Adults and children (excluding small children)

- Reconstitute by dissolving powder in each vial with 4 ml of Sterile Water for Injection to yield 10 mg/ml. Mix gently.
- Use the reconstituted product immediately. If not used, it can be stored under refrigeration for up to 4 hr.
- Further dilute with 0.9% Sodium Chloride for Injection to proper volume for I.V. infusion.
- Give as an I.V. infusion through a 0.22-micron membrane filter slowly over at least 30 min. Stop the infusion if infusion rate-related anaphylactoid-type reactions occur, such as hypotension, urticaria, or wheezing. Notify prescriber immediately and provide supportive care, as needed and ordered. Know that the infusion may be re-started at a slower rate, as needed. Keep in mind that drug may be given by rapid I.V. injection if cardiac arrest is imminent.

Infants and smaller children

- Reconstitute digoxin immune Fab as ordered and administer undiluted with a tuberculin syringe. For very small doses, reconstituted vial can be diluted with an additional 36 ml of 0.9% Sodium Chloride Injection to achieve a concentration of 1 mg/ml.
- *Incompatibilities:* None reported by manufacturer.

Route	Onset	Peak	Duration
I.V.	15–30 min	Unknown	Unknown

Half-life: 15–20 hr

Mechanism of Action

Binds with digoxin or digitoxin molecules. The resulting complex is excreted through the kidneys. As the free-serum digoxin level declines, tissue-bound digoxin enters the serum and is bound and excreted.

Contraindications

Hypersensitivity to digoxin immune Fab or its components

Interactions

DRUGS

None reported by manufacturer.

Adverse Reactions

CV: **Increased ventricular rate (in atrial fibrillation), worsening of heart failure or low cardiac output**

D

Other: **hypersensitivity reaction**, febrile reaction, **hypokalemia**

Childbearing Considerations

PREGNANCY

- It is not known if drug causes fetal harm.
- Use with caution only if benefit to mother outweighs potential risk to fetus.

LACTATION

- It is not known if drug is present in breast milk.
- Mothers should check with prescriber before breastfeeding.

Nursing Considerations

! **WARNING** Monitor patient for an acute hypersensitivity reaction (angioedema, bronchospasm with cough or wheezing, erythema, hypotension, laryngeal edema, pruritus, stridor, tachycardia, or urticaria). If an anaphylactic reaction occurs during infusion, stop administration, notify prescriber, and provide supportive care, as needed and ordered. Expect to treat all allergic reactions according to protocol. Be aware that patients with a history of hypersensitivity to papaya or papain are at high risk for a hypersensitivity reaction; digoxin immune Fab should be administered to this patient only if the benefits outweigh the risks. Also, know that prior treatment with digoxin-specific Fab might increase the risk of diminished effects of the drug.

! **WARNING** Monitor serum potassium level often, especially during first few hours of therapy. Potassium level may drop rapidly.

! **WARNING** Watch for fluid volume overload when administering drug to an infant or small child.

- Be aware that when giving a large dose, expect a faster onset but watch closely for febrile reaction.

PATIENT TEACHING

- Inform patient of the purpose of digoxin immune Fab and how it will be given.

! **WARNING** Advise patient to immediately report any signs and symptoms associated with an allergic reaction.

diltiazem hydrochloride

Cardizem, Cardizem CD, Cardizem LA, Cartia XT, Dilt-XR, Matzim LA, Taztia XT Tiazac

Class and Category

Pharmacologic class: Calcium channel blocker
Therapeutic class: Antianginal, antiarrhythmic, antihypertensive

Indications and Dosages

✷ *To treat chronic stable angina and angina due to coronary artery spasm*

TABLETS (CARDIZEM)

Adults. *Initial:* 30 mg 4 times daily before meals and at bedtime, increased every 1 or 2 days as needed. *Maximum:* 360 mg daily in divided doses 3 or 4 times daily.

E.R. CAPSULES OR TABLETS

Adults. *Initial:* 120 mg or 180 mg once daily, increased every 7 to 14 days, as needed. *Maximum:* 360 mg daily (Cardizem LA, Matzim LA), 480 mg (Cardizem CD, Cartia XT), and 540 mg (Taztia XT, Tiazac).

✷ *To improve exercise tolerance in patients with chronic stable angina*

E.R. TABLETS (CARDIZEM LA)

Adults. *Initial:* 180 mg once daily, increased in 7 to 14 days, as needed. *Maximum:* 360 mg daily.

✷ *To control hypertension*

E.R. CAPSULES

Adults and adolescents. *Initial:* 120 to 240 mg once daily, increased in 7 to 14 days, as needed. *Maximum:* 480 mg daily (Cardizem CD, Cartia XT) or 540 mg daily (Taztia XT, Tiazac).

E.R. TABLETS (CARDIZEM LA)

Adults. *Initial:* 180 to 240 mg once daily, increased after 14 days, as needed. *Maximum:* 540 mg daily.

✷ *To treat atrial fibrillation, atrial flutter, and paroxysmal supraventricular tachycardia*

I.V. INFUSION OR INJECTION

Adults. 0.25 mg/kg given by bolus over 2 min. If response is inadequate after 15 min, 0.35 mg/kg given by bolus followed by a maintenance continuous infusion at 5 or

10 mg/hr increased by 5 mg/hr, as needed. *Maximum:* 15 mg/hr for up to 24 hr.

Drug Administration

P.O.

- E.R. capsules and tablets must be swallowed whole and not chewed, crushed, opened (except for Tiazac and Taztia XT), or split.
- Administer Cardizem before meals and at bedtime. Administer E.R. tablets (Cardizem LA, Matzim LA), Cardizem CD, and Cartia XT tablets without regards to meals. Administer Cartia XT capsules and Dilt-XR on an empty stomach. Administer Taztia XT and Tiazac without regard to meals. However, for patient unable to swallow Taztia XT or Tiazac capsules, drug capsule may be opened, and entire contents sprinkled on a small amount of cool applesauce immediately prior to administration. The patient should swallow the entire mixture without chewing. Then immediately drink a glass of cool water to ensure the mixture has been completely swallowed. Mixture should not be stored for a later use.

I.V.

- For I.V. injection, administer undiluted and inject slowly over 2 min while monitoring blood pressure and ECG. Be aware that the single-dose ADD-Vantage vial is for continuous I.V. infusion and should not be used to administer an I.V. injection as a bolus.
- For continuous I.V. infusion, diluents to use include 0.9% Sodium Chloride Injection, 5% Dextrose Injection, or 5% Dextrose in Water/0.45% Sodium Chloride Injection.
- For continuous I.V. infusion, dilute 25 ml of drug (5 mg/ml) with 100 ml of diluent for a final concentration of 1 mg/ml; dilute 50 ml of drug (5 mg/ml) with 250 ml of diluent for a final concentration of 0.83 mg/ml; or dilute 50 ml (5 mg/ml) with 500 ml of diluent for a final concentration of 0.45 mg/ml. Infusion rate ranges from 5 to 15 mg/hr.
- Mix thoroughly in a glass bottle or polyvinylchloride bag.
- Diluted solution may be stored in refrigerator or at room temperature for up to 24 hr before use.
- *Incompatibilities:* Diazepam, furosemide, lansoprazole, phenytoin sodium, rifampin, thiopental sodium

Route	Onset	Peak	Duration
P.O.	30–60 min	2–3 hr	6–8 hr
P.O./E.R. cap	2–3 hr	10–14 hr	12–24 hr
P.O./E.R. tab	3–4 hr	11–18 hr	Unknown
I.V.	> 3 min	15 min	0.5–10 hr

Half-life: 3–4.5 hr

Contraindications

Acute MI; cardiogenic shock (I.V. administration); hypersensitivity to diltiazem or its components; Lown-Ganong-Levine

Mechanism of Action

Inhibits calcium movement into coronary and vascular smooth-muscle cells by blocking slow calcium channels in cell membranes, as shown in figure. This action decreases intracellular calcium, which:

- inhibits smooth-muscle cell contractions.
- decreases myocardial oxygen demand by relaxing coronary and vascular smooth muscle, reducing peripheral vascular resistance and systolic and diastolic blood pressures.
- slows AV conduction time and prolongs AV nodal refractoriness.
- interrupts the reentry circuit in AV nodal reentrant tachycardias.

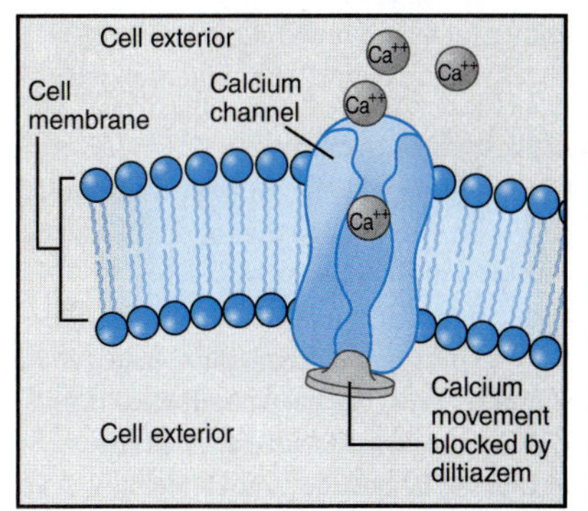

or Wolff-Parkinson-White syndrome (I.V. administration), second- or third-degree AV block, or sick sinus syndrome, unless artificial pacemaker is in place; pulmonary edema; systolic blood pressure below 90 mm Hg; ventricular tachycardia with wide complex (I.V. administration); within a few hours of I.V. beta-blocker therapy (I.V. administration)

Interactions

DRUGS

anesthetic: Additive hypotension; possibly decreased cardiac contractility, conductivity, and automaticity
benzodiazepines: Increased risk of prolonged sedation
beta-blockers: Possibly increased risk of adverse cardiovascular effects, especially AV block and bradycardia
buspirone: Increased effects and risk of buspirone toxicity
carbamazepine, quinidine: Decreased hepatic clearance and increased serum levels of these drugs, leading to toxicity
cimetidine: Decreased diltiazem metabolism, increased blood diltiazem level
clonidine: Increased risk of serious sinus bradycardia
cyclosporine: Possibly increased cyclosporine levels
digoxin: Increased blood digoxin level; increased risk of AV block or bradycardia
ivabradine: Increased ivabradine exposure, which may exacerbate bradycardia and conduction disturbances
rifampin: Decreased blood diltiazem level to undetectable amounts
statins: Increased blood statin level with increased risk of myopathy and rhabdomyolysis

Adverse Reactions

CNS: Abnormal gait, amnesia, asthenia, depression, dizziness, dream disturbances, extrapyramidal reactions, fatigue, hallucinations, headache, insomnia, nervousness, paresthesia, personality change, somnolence, syncope, tremor, weakness
CV: Angina, **atrial flutter**, **AV block**, **bradycardia**, bundle-branch block, **ECG abnormalities**, **heart failure**, **hypotension**, palpitations, peripheral edema, **PVCs**, **sinus arrest**, sinus tachycardia, **ventricular fibrillation**, **ventricular tachycardia**
EENT: Amblyopia, dry mouth, epistaxis, eye irritation, gingival bleeding and hyperplasia, gingivitis, nasal congestion, retinopathy, taste perversion, tinnitus
ENDO: Hyperglycemia
GI: Anorexia, constipation, diarrhea, elevated liver enzymes, indigestion, nausea, thirst, vomiting
GU: **Acute renal failure**, impotence, nocturia, polyuria, sexual dysfunction
HEME: **Hemolytic anemia**, **leukopenia**, **prolonged bleeding time**, **thrombocytopenia**
MS: Arthralgia, muscle spasms, myalgia
RESP: Cough, dyspnea
SKIN: Acute generalized exanthematous pustulosis, alopecia, diaphoresis, **erythema multiforme**, **exfoliative dermatitis**, flushing, leukocytoclastic vasculitis, petechiae, photosensitivity, pruritus, purpura, rash, **Stevens-Johnson syndrome**, **toxic epidermal necrolysis**, urticaria
Other: **Angioedema**, hyperuricemia, weight gain

Childbearing Considerations

PREGNANCY

- It is not known if drug causes fetal harm.
- Use with caution only if benefit to mother outweighs potential risk to fetus.

LACTATION

- Drug is present in breast milk.
- A decision should be made to discontinue breastfeeding or the drug to avoid potential serious adverse reactions in the breastfed infant.

Nursing Considerations

- Use diltiazem cautiously in patients with impaired hepatic or renal function, and monitor liver and renal function, as appropriate; drug is metabolized mainly in the liver and excreted by the kidneys.

! **WARNING** Monitor patient's blood pressure, heart rate and rhythm by continuous ECG, and pulse rate, as appropriate during therapy. Keep emergency equipment and drugs available. Assess patient for signs and symptoms of heart failure. Notify prescriber if any cardiac abnormalities occur.

! **WARNING** Monitor patient for a hypersensitivity or skin reaction, which may become severe such as angioedema or Stevens-Johnson syndrome. If present, notify prescriber promptly, expect to withhold drug as ordered, and provide supportive care, as needed and ordered.

! **WARNING** Watch for digitalis toxicity (nausea, visual color distortion, and vomiting) if patient takes digoxin and has an elevated serum digoxin level.

- Continue sublingual nitroglycerin therapy, as prescribed, during diltiazem therapy.

PATIENT TEACHING

- Advise patient how to take oral drug according to the product prescribed.

! **WARNING** Tell patient that stopping drug suddenly may have life-threatening effects.

! **WARNING** Alert patient that drug may cause an allergic or serious skin reaction. If present, have patient notify prescriber promptly and, if servere, stress importance of seeking immediate medical care.

! **WARNING** Advise patient to monitor blood pressure and pulse rate regularly and to report significant changes to prescriber. Urge patient to notify prescriber of chest pain, difficulty breathing, dizziness, fainting, irregular heartbeat, or swollen ankles.

- Instruct patient to maintain good oral hygiene, perform gum massage, and see a dentist every 6 months to prevent gingival bleeding and hyperplasia and gingivitis.
- Inform all prescribers of diltiazem therapy. Tell patient to consult prescriber before taking any over-the-counter medication.
- Caution mothers not to breastfeed.

diphenhydramine hydrochloride

Banophen, Benadryl, Sominex, Unisom

Class and Category

Pharmacologic class: Antihistamine
Therapeutic class: Antianaphylactic adjunct, antiemetic, antihistamine, antitussive (syrup), sedative-hypnotic

Indications and Dosages

∗ *To treat hypersensitivity reactions, such as allergic conjunctivitis due to food allergies, perennial and seasonal allergic rhinitis, transfusion reactions, uncomplicated allergic skin eruptions, and vasomotor rhinitis*

CAPSULES, CHEWABLE TABLETS, ELIXIR, ORAL SOLUTION, ORALLY DISINTEGRATING TABLETS, TABLETS

Adults and children ages 12 and older. 25 to 50 mg every 4 to 6 hr, as needed. *Maximum:* 300 mg daily.
Children ages 6 to 12. 12.5 to 25 mg every 4 to 6 hr, as needed. *Maximum:* 150 mg daily.

I.V. INJECTION

Adults and children ages 12 and older. 10 to 50 mg up to 100 mg, as needed. I.V. injection not to exceed 25 mg/min. *Maximum:* 400 mg daily.
Children other than premature infants and neonates. 1.25 mg/kg up to 4 times daily, as needed. I.V. injection not to exceed 25 mg/min. *Maximum:* 300 mg daily.

I.M. INJECTION

Adults and children ages 12 and older. 10 to 50 mg up to 100 mg, as needed. *Maximum:* 400 mg daily.
Children other than premature infants and neonates. 1.25 mg/kg 4 times daily.

∗ *To prevent or treat motion sickness*

CAPSULES, CHEWABLE TABLETS, ORAL SOLUTION, ORALLY DISINTEGRATING TABLETS, TABLETS

Adults and children ages 12 and older. 25 to 50 mg, with first dose given 30 min before exposure to motion and before meals and upon retiring for the duration of exposure.

∗ *To treat sleep disorders*

CAPSULES, CHEWABLE TABLETS, ORAL SOLUTION, ORALLY DISINTEGRATING TABLETS, TABLETS

Adults and children ages 12 and older. 50 mg 20 to 30 min before bedtime.

∗ *To provide antitussive effects*

ELIXIR

Adults and children ages 12 and older. 25 mg every 4 hr. *Maximum:* 150 mg/24 hr.

D

Children ages 6 to 11. 12.5 to 25 mg every 4 to 6 hr, as needed. *Maximum:* No more than 6 doses in 24 hr.

Drug Administration

P.O.

- Give with food if drug upsets stomach.
- Chewable tablets should be chewed or allowed to dissolve on the tongue before swallowing.
- Give 30 min before bedtime for insomnia or 30 min before exposure to developing motion sickness.
- Use calibrated device to measure dosages of elixir and oral solution forms.
- Keep elixir container tightly closed.
- Oral solution should not be refrigerated.
- Protect all oral formulations from light and high humidity; film-coated tablets should also be kept from excessive heat.

I.V.

- Available as a prefilled, single-use syringe. Follow manufacturer's instructions on preparing it for administration. All steps must be done sequentially.
- Administer as an injection, not to exceed 25 mg/min.
- Protect from light.
- *Incompatibilities:* Allopurinol, amobarbital, amphotericin B, cefepime, dexamethasone, diatrizoate, foscarnet, furosemide, haloperidol, iodipamide, pentobarbital, phenobarbital, phenytoin, sodium phosphate with lorazepam and metoclopramide, thiopental

I.M.

- Administer as a deep I.M. injection.
- Alternate sites to prevent irritation.
- Protect from light.

Route	Onset	Peak	Duration
P.O.	15–60 min	2–4 hr	4–6 hr
I.V.	Immediate	1–3 hr	4–6 hr
I.M.	15–30 min	1–3 hr	4–6 hr

Half-life: 3.4–9.2 hr

Mechanism of Action

Binds to central and peripheral H_1 receptors, competing with histamine for these sites and preventing it from reaching its site of action. By blocking histamine, diphenhydramine produces antihistamine effects, inhibiting GI, respiratory, and vascular smooth-muscle contraction; decreasing capillary permeability, which reduces flares, itching, and wheals; and decreasing lacrimal and salivary gland secretions. Diphenhydramine produces antitussive effects by directly suppressing the cough center in the medulla oblongata in the brain. Diphenhydramine's antiemetic effect may be related to its ability to bind to CNS muscarinic receptors and depress vestibular stimulation and labyrinthine function. Its sedative effects are related to its CNS depressant action.

Contraindications

Hypersensitivity to diphenhydramine, similar antihistamines or their components; use in newborns or premature infants

Interactions

DRUGS

barbiturates, other CNS depressants: Possibly increased CNS depression
MAO inhibitors: Increased anticholinergic and CNS depressant effects of diphenhydramine

ACTIVITIES

alcohol use: Possibly increased CNS depression

Adverse Reactions

CNS: Confusion, dizziness, drowsiness
CV: **Arrhythmias**, palpitations, tachycardia
EENT: Blurred vision, diplopia
GI: Epigastric distress, nausea
HEME: **Agranulocytosis**, **hemolytic anemia**, **thrombocytopenia**
RESP: Thickened bronchial secretions
SKIN: Photosensitivity

Childbearing Considerations

PREGNANCY

- It is not known if drug causes fetal harm.
- Use with caution only if benefit to mother outweighs potential risk to fetus.

LACTATION

- Drug is present in breast milk.
- Small, occasional doses of drug are not expected to cause adverse effects on breastfed infants. However, larger doses or more prolonged use poses a higher risk of adverse reactions in breastfed infants. Drug also may decrease milk supply.
- Mothers should check with prescriber before breastfeeding.

Nursing Considerations

- Expect to give parenteral form of diphenhydramine only when oral ingestion isn't possible.

! **WARNING** Monitor patient for adverse hematologic reactions, which may become severe and life-threatening. If signs and symptoms appear, notify prescriber and expect blood studies to be done to determine underlying cause.

- Expect to discontinue drug at least 72 hours before skin tests for allergies because drug may inhibit cutaneous histamine response, thus producing false-negative results.

PATIENT TEACHING

- Instruct patient how to take oral form of diphenhydramine prescribed for condition being treated.
- Advise patient to take drug with food if GI distress occurs.
- Caution patient not to take higher than recommended dosage as euphoric highs, hallucinations, and other serious side effects could occur.
- Urge patient to avoid alcohol while taking diphenhydramine.

! **WARNING** Stress importance of notifying prescriber if bleeding, bruising, fatigue, fever or other persistent, serious, or unusual signs and symptoms develop as blood tests may be required to determine the underlying cause and additional treatment needed.

- Caution patient to avoid hazardous activities until drug's CNS effects are known and resolved.
- Instruct patient to use sunscreen to prevent photosensitivity reactions.
- Advise patient to avoid taking other over-the-counter drugs that contain diphenhydramine to prevent additive effects.

dipyridamole

Class and Category

Pharmacologic class: Pyrimidine analogue
Therapeutic class: Antiplatelet

Indications and Dosages

✶ *As adjunct to coumarin anticoagulants to prevent postoperative thromboembolic complications of cardiac valve replacement*

TABLETS

Adults and children ages 12 and older. 75 to 100 mg 4 times daily with warfarin.

✶ *To aid diagnosis during thallium perfusion imaging of myocardium*

I.V. INFUSION

Adults. 0.57 mg/kg infused over 4 min as a single dose. *Maximum:* 60 mg.

Drug Administration

P.O.

- Administer at least 1 hr before or 2 hr after meals. However, if GI distress occurs, give with meals or milk.
- Administer drug at evenly spaced intervals.

I.V.

- Dilute to at least a 1:2 ratio with 0.45% or 0.9% Sodium Chloride Injection or 5% Dextrose Injection for a total volume of 20 to 50 ml.
- When used as a diagnostic drug, infuse over 4 min followed within 5 min by thallium-201 injection.
- Monitor blood pressure, breath sounds, and pulse rate and rhythm, during I.V. infusion.
- Protect from direct light and do not freeze.
- *Incompatibilities:* Other drugs or solutions except for those used to dilute drug

Route	Onset	Peak	Duration
P.O.	Unknown	75 min	3 hr
I.V.	Unknown	Unknown	3 hr

Half-life: 10–12 hr

Mechanism of Action

May increase the intraplatelet level of adenosine, which causes coronary vasodilation and inhibits platelet aggregation. Dipyridamole also may increase the intraplatelet level of cyclic adenosine monophosphate (cAMP) and may inhibit formation of the potent platelet activator stimulant thromboxane A_2, which decreases platelet activation. Vasodilation and increased blood flow occur preferentially in nondiseased coronary vessels, which results in redistribution of blood away from significantly diseased vessels. These changes in perfusion are observed during thallium imaging studies.

Contraindications

Hypersensitivity to dipyridamole or its components

Interactions

DRUGS

adenosinergic agents, such as adenosine, regadenoson: Potentiated cardiovascular effects of adenosine
cholinesterase inhibitors: Decreased anticholinesterase effect, possibly aggravating myasthenia gravis
heparin, NSAIDs, thrombolytics: Possibly increased risk of bleeding
theophylline: Reversal of coronary vasodilation caused by dipyridamole, possibly false-negative thallium imaging result

Adverse Reactions

CNS: Dizziness, headache
CV: Angina, **arrhythmias**, **ECG changes (specifically ST-segment and T-wave changes)**
GI: Abdominal pain, diarrhea, nausea, vomiting
RESP: Dyspnea
SKIN: Flushing, pruritus, rash

Childbearing Considerations

PREGNANCY

- It is not known if drug causes fetal harm.
- Use with caution only if benefit to mother outweighs potential risk to fetus.

LACTATION

- Drug is present in breast milk.
- Mothers should check with prescriber before breastfeeding.

Nursing Considerations

! **WARNING** Be aware that if patients taking oral dipyridamole are scheduled to undergo stress testing using intravenous dipyridamole or other adenosinergic agents, the oral dosage of dipyridamole should be withheld for 48 hours before the test because of increased risk for cardiovascular adverse reactions and possibly impaired sensitivity of the test.

! **WARNING** Monitor patient's cardiac status closely because drug may cause serious to life-threatening adverse effects. Notify prescriber if patient develops chest pain or an irregular and/or fast heartbeat. Expect an ECG to be performed. Provide supportive care, as needed and ordered.

- Expect other adverse reactions to be minimal and transient at therapeutic doses. They typically resolve with long-term use.

PATIENT TEACHING

- Instruct patient how to administer oral dipyridamole. If patient experiences GI distress, advise her to take drug with meals or milk.
- Advise patient to take oral drug at evenly spaced intervals.
- Inform patient that oral drug commonly is taken with warfarin. Tell patient that aspirin should not be administered concomitantly with warfarin. Urge her to keep appointments for coagulation tests.

! **WARNING** Instruct patient to seek immediate emergency treatment if chest pain or an irregular or rapid heartbeat occurs.

- Caution patient to consult prescriber before taking over-the-counter NSAIDs because of the possible increased risk of bleeding.
- Advise patient to notify all healthcare providers about dipyridamole use.

diroximel fumarate

Vumerity

Class and Category

Pharmacologic class: Nuclear factor-like 2 (Nrf2) activator
Therapeutic class: Immunomodulatory agent

Indications and Dosages

* *To treat relapsing forms of multiple sclerosis (MS), to include active secondary progressive disease, clinically isolated syndrome, and relapsing-remitting disease*

D.R. CAPSULES

Adults. *Initial:* 231 mg twice daily followed by dosage increase to 462 mg twice daily after 7 days. *Maintenance:* 462 mg twice daily.

± **DOSAGE ADJUSTMENT** For patients who cannot tolerate maintenance dosage, dosage reduced temporarily to 231 mg twice daily. Within 4 wk, dosage resumed at 462 mg twice daily.

Drug Administration

P.O.

- Administer nonenteric coated aspirin up to a dose of 325 mg 30 min before administering diroximel, as ordered, to reduce the incidence or severity of flushing. Administering with a light snack or meal may also help.
- D. R. capsules should be swallowed whole and not chewed, crushed, or opened.
- A high-fat (more than 30 grams) or a high-calorie (more than 700 calories) meal or snack will interfere with the absorption of the drug.

Route	Onset	Peak	Duration
P.O./D.R.	Unknown	2.5–3 hr	Unknown

Half-life: 1 hr

Mechanism of Action

May activate the nuclear factor (erythroid-derived 2)-like 2 (Nrf2) pathway, which is involved in the cellular response to oxidative stress thought to be a factor in multiple sclerosis.

Contraindications

Concurrent use of dimethyl fumarate; hypersensitivity to diroximel fumarate, dimethyl fumarate, or any of their components

Interactions

DRUGS

dimethyl fumarate: Potentiated effect increasing risk of serious adverse reactions

ACTIVITIES

alcohol use: Possibly may reduce the plasma concentrations of monomethyl fumarate (MMF), the active metabolite of diroximel fumarate

Adverse Reactions

CNS: **Progressive multifocal leukoencephalopathy**

EENT: Rhinorrhea

GI: Abdominal pain; **acute pancreatitis**; diarrhea; dyspepsia; elevated liver enzymes; **GI hemorrhage**, **obstruction**, **perforation**, or **ulceration**; **hepatic injury**; nausea; vomiting

GU: Albumin present in urine

HEME: Eosinophilia, **lymphopenia**

SKIN: Alopecia, erythema, flushing, pruritus, rash

Other: **Anaphylaxis**, **angioedema**, herpes-zoster infections and other opportunistic infections

Childbearing Considerations

PREGNANCY

- Pregnancy exposure registry: 1-833-569-2635 or www.vumeritypregnancyregistry.com.
- It is not known if drug causes fetal harm.
- Use with caution only if benefit to mother outweighs potential risk to fetus.

LACTATION

- It is not known if drug is present in breast milk.
- Mothers should check with prescriber before breastfeeding.

Nursing Considerations

- Expect to obtain laboratory test results for alkaline phosphatase; CBC, including lymphocyte count; serum aminotransferase; and total bilirubin levels prior to starting diroximel.
- Obtain an MRI at baseline and, as clinically indicated and ordered, to assess for signs of progressive multifocal leukoencephalopathy (PML).
- Be aware that diroximel is not recommended for patients with moderate or severe renal impairment.

! **WARNING** Monitor patient closely for hypersensitivity reactions, such as anaphylaxis and angioedema, which have occurred as early as after the first dose and throughout the duration of drug therapy. If present, notify prescriber immediately, expect drug to be discontinued, and provide supportive care, as needed and ordered.

! **WARNING** Monitor patient closely for adverse GI signs and symptoms, which could become life-threatening, such as hemorrhage, obstruction, perforation, and ulceration. Notify prescriber immediately for new or worsening severe GI signs and symptoms, expect drug to be discontinued, and provide supportive care, as needed and ordered.

! **WARNING** Know that liver injury may occur because drug contains the same active metabolite as dimethyl fumarate, which has caused liver injury. Expect to monitor patient's alkaline phosphatase, serum aminotransferase, and total bilirubin levels throughout drug therapy. If abnormalities are noted or patient exhibits signs and symptoms of liver dysfunction, notify prescriber and expect drug to be discontinued.

! **WARNING** Monitor patient for signs and symptoms of PML, such as changes in memory, orientation, or thinking leading to confusion and personality changes, as well as clumsiness of limbs, progressive weakness on one side of the body, and visual disturbances. Although no reports of PML have occurred with diroximel for treating relapsing forms of MS, it is a possibility because it has occurred with dimethyl fumarate, which has the same active metabolite as diroximel. At first sign of PML, notify prescriber, expect drug to be withheld, and ensure that appropriate diagnostic evaluation is done. Know that MRI findings may reveal PML before clinical signs or symptoms are apparent.

! **WARNING** Monitor patient for signs and symptoms of infections, which could become serious because drug decreases the lymphocyte count. Know that drug therapy may have to be interrupted if lymphocyte counts less than 0.5×10^9/L persist for more than 6 months or if serious infections, such as herpes zoster occur.

- Obtain a CBC, including lymphocyte count, 6 months after drug therapy has begun and then every 6 to 12 months thereafter, as indicated and ordered. Also, expect to obtain laboratory results for alkaline phosphatase, serum aminotransferase, and total bilirubin levels during drug therapy, as indicated and ordered.

PATIENT TEACHING

- Instruct patient how to administer diroximel.
- Instruct patient to take a nonenteric coated aspirin, up to a dose of 325 mg, 30 minutes before administering diroximel, if ordered, to reduce the incidence or severity of flushing caused by the drug. Taking drug with food may also help reduce the incidence of flushing.
- Remind patient to avoid taking drug with a high-fat, high-calorie meal/snack; meal or snack should contain no more than 700 calories and no more than 30 g of fat.
- Advise patient to avoid alcohol while taking drug.

! **WARNING** Advise the patient drug may cause an allergic reaction. If one occurs, tell patient to stop taking drug, notify prescriber, and seek emergency medical care, if severe.

! **WARNING** Instruct patient to report any persistent, severe, unexplained, or unusual signs and symptoms to prescriber, including persistent and/or severe GI reactions.

- Review signs and symptoms of an infection and measures to take to decrease risk of infection. If fever or other signs and symptoms of an infection occur, instruct patient to notify prescriber right away.
- Stress importance of being compliant with scheduled laboratory tests.

dobutamine hydrochloride

Class and Category

Pharmacologic class: Sympathomimetic
Therapeutic class: Inotropic

Indications and Dosages

* *To provide short-term inotropic support in patients with cardiac decompensation due to depressed contractility resulting either from organic heart disease or from cardiac surgical procedures*

I.V. INFUSION

Adults. *Initial:* 0.5 to 1 mcg/kg/min adjusted every couple of minutes according to hemodynamic response. *Usual maintenance:* 2 to 20 mcg/kg/min with infusion rate in the range of 2.5 to 15 mcg/kg/min. *Maximum:* 40 mcg/kg/min.

Drug Administration

I.V.

- Expect to administer a digitalis preparation prior to start of therapy if patient has atrial fibrillation with a rapid ventricular response or a suitable volume expander if hypovolemia is present.
- Dilute concentrate with at least 50 ml of a compatible I.V. solution, such as 0.9%

Sodium Chloride Injection or 5% Dextrose Injection (see manufacturer's guidelines for other suitable diluents). Solution should be clear.

- Discard diluted solution after 24 hr.
- Give as a continuous infusion through a central venous line or large peripheral vein using an infusion pump.
- Monitor blood pressure continuously during therapy, preferably by continuous intra-arterial monitoring; systolic increase of 10 to 20 mm Hg may indicate dobutamine-induced increase in cardiac output.
- Monitor infusion site closely because phlebitis and local inflammatory changes, including cutaneous necrosis, have occurred with extravasation. Change I.V. site according to institution protocol.
- Expect to reduce dosage or discontinue drug if hypotension develops.
- *Incompatibilities:* 5% Sodium Bicarbonate Injection or other strongly alkaline solutions, other agents or diluents containing both ethanol and sodium bisulfite, other drugs mixed in same solution

Route	Onset	Peak	Duration
I.V.	1–2 min	10 min	> 5 min

Half-life: 2 min

Mechanism of Action

Stimulates $beta_1$-adrenergic receptors primarily. Also stimulates $beta_2$- and $alpha_1$-adrenergic receptors but to a much lesser degree. $Beta_1$-receptor stimulation produces a positive inotropic effect on the myocardium, increasing cardiac output by boosting myocardial contractility and stroke volume. Increased myocardial contractility raises coronary blood flow and myocardial oxygen consumption. Systolic blood pressure typically rises as a result of increased stroke volume. Other hemodynamic effects include decreased systemic vascular resistance, which reduces afterload and decreased ventricular filling pressure, which reduces preload.

Contraindications

Hypersensitivity to dobutamine or its components, idiopathic hypertrophic subaortic stenosis

Interactions

DRUGS

catechol-O-methyltransferase (COMT) inhibitors, such as entacapone: Possibly increased incidence of arrhythmias, changes in blood pressure, and heart rate

nitroprusside: Increased cardiac output and lowered pulmonary wedge pressure

Adverse Reactions

CNS: Fever, headache, nervousness, restlessness

CV: Angina, **bradycardia**, hypertension, **hypotension**, nonspecific chest pain, palpitations, **PVCs**, **stress cardiomyopathy** (with cardiac stress testing), tachycardia

GI: Nausea, vomiting

RESP: Dyspnea, shortness of breath

SKIN: Extravasation with tissue necrosis and sloughing, rash

Other: **Hypokalemia**

Childbearing Considerations

PREGNANCY

- It is not known if drug causes fetal harm.
- Use with caution only if benefit to mother outweighs potential risk to fetus.

LACTATION

- It is not known if drug is present in breast milk.
- Due to critical nature of situation, breastfeeding would not be done during drug therapy. Mothers should check with prescriber once condition has stabilized before resuming breastfeeding.

Nursing Considerations

! **WARNING** Avoid giving dobutamine to patients with acute MI because it can intensify or extend myocardial ischemia. Also know that dobutamine isn't indicated for long-term treatment of heart failure because it may not be effective and may increase the risk of hospitalization and death.

! **WARNING** Use drug with extreme caution in patients sensitive to sulfite as drug may cause an allergic reaction, including anaphylactic-like signs and symptoms because dobutamine solution contains sodium metabisulfite. If present, notify prescriber immediately, expect drug to be discontinued and another drug substituted,

D

and provide supportive care, as needed and ordered.

! **WARNING** Monitor serum potassium level. Drug can cause hypokalemia, a rare result of $beta_2$ stimulation that causes electrolyte imbalance.

- Use drug cautiously in patients with atrial fibrillation because drug increases AV conduction. Keep in mind that patient should be adequately digitalized before administration.
- Monitor heart rate and rhythm via ECG recordings continuously for premature ventricular contractions (PVCs), which may result from drug's stimulatory effect on heart's conduction system, and sinus tachycardia, which results from positive chronotropic effect of beta stimulation. Heart rate may increase by 5 to 15 beats/min.
- Monitor hemodynamic parameters, such as cardiac output, central venous pressure, and pulmonary artery wedge pressure, as indicated, to assess drug's effectiveness.
- Monitor urine output hourly, as appropriate, to check for improved renal blood flow.

PATIENT TEACHING

- Explain how the drug will be administered and the need for frequent hemodynamic monitoring.
- Reassure patient that he will be under constant supervision.

! **WARNING** Stress importance of patient notifying the staff if he experiences adverse effects such as chest pain, difficulty breathing, palpitations, or any other new signs and symptoms.

dofetilide

Tikosyn

Class and Category

Pharmacologic class: Class III antiarrhythmic
Therapeutic class: Antiarrhythmic

Indications and Dosages

* *To convert symptomatic atrial fibrillation or flutter to normal sinus rhythm or to maintain normal sinus rhythm in patients converted from symptomatic atrial fibrillation or flutter that had lasted 1 wk or longer*

CAPSULES

Adults. Highly individualized based on creatinine clearance and QTc (QT interval used if heart rate is below 60 beats per min). *Usual for patients with creatinine clearance above 60 ml/min:* 500 mcg twice daily. *Maximum:* 500 mcg twice daily.

± **DOSAGE ADJUSTMENT** For patients with renal impairment, initial dose reduced to 250 mcg twice daily if creatinine clearance is 40 to 60 ml/min and to 125 mcg twice daily if creatinine clearance is 20 to 39 ml/min. For all patients with a QTc interval (checked after 2 to 3 hr of initial dose) that has increased by at least 15% or is more than 500 msec (550 msec in patients with ventricular conduction abnormalities), dosage decreased by 50%. For patients receiving lowest initial dose of 125 mcg twice daily, dosage interval reduced to once daily. For patients who experience a QTc interval increase of more than 500 msec (550 msec in patients with ventricular conduction abnormalities) at any time after second dose, drug discontinued.

Drug Administration

P.O.

- Serum potassium level must be in normal range and the QTc or QT must be measured before drug therapy begun. If the QTc or QT is greater than 440 msec (500 msec in patients with ventricular conduction abnormalities), drug therapy should not be initiated.
- Capsules should be swallowed whole with water. Capsules should not be chewed, crushed, or opened.
- Do not administer with grapefruit juice.

Route	Onset	Peak	Duration
P.O.	2 hr	2–3 hr	4 hr

Half-life: 10 hr

Mechanism of Action

Blocks potassium channels selectively in myocardial cell membranes involved in cardiac repolarization. By blocking potassium channels, dofetilide prolongs action potential duration, effective refractory period, and ventricular refractoriness (widens QT interval). These actions terminate or prevent reentrant tachyarrhythmias, such as atrial fibrillation, atrial flutter, and ventricular tachycardia.

Contraindications

Acquired or congenital QT prolongation syndrome; concurrent therapy with cimetidine, dolutegravir, hydrochlorothiazide, ketoconazole, megestrol, prochlorperazine, trimethoprim, or verapamil; hypersensitivity to dofetilide or its components; severe renal impairment (creatinine clearance less than 20 ml/min)

Interactions

DRUGS

amiloride, cimetidine, cotrimoxazole, ketoconazole, megestrol, metformin, sulfamethoxazole-trimethoprim, triamterene, trimethoprim: Possibly increased blood dofetilide level
azole antifungals, cannabinoids, diltiazem, nefazodone, norfloxacin, protease inhibitors, quinine, selective serotonin reuptake inhibitors, zafirlukast: Possibly increased blood dofetilide level and risk of dofetilide toxicity
bepridil, cisapride, macrolide antibiotics, phenothiazines, selected fluoroquinolones, tricyclic antidepressants: Possibly prolonged QT interval
class I and III antiarrhythmics, especially amiodarone: Possibly prolonged QT interval and increased risk of dofetilide-induced proarrhythmias
diuretics (potassium-depleting): Increased risk of torsades de pointes in patients with hypokalemia or hypomagnesemia
hydrochlorothiazide, verapamil: Possibly increased blood dofetilide level and increased risk of torsades de pointes

FOODS

grapefruit juice: Increased dofetilide level

Adverse Reactions

CNS: **Cerebral ischemia**, **CVA**, dizziness, facial or flaccid paralysis, headache, insomnia, paresthesia, slurred speech, syncope
CV: **AV block**, **bradycardia**, **cardiac arrest**, chest pain, edema, **MI**, tachycardia, **ventricular arrhythmias (including torsades de pointes and ventricular tachycardia)**
GI: Abdominal pain, diarrhea, **hepatic dysfunction**, jaundice, nausea
MS: Back pain, muscle weakness
RESP: Cough, dyspnea, respiratory tract infection
SKIN: Rash
Other: **Angioedema**, flu-like symptoms, weight gain

Childbearing Considerations

PREGNANCY

- It is not known if drug causes fetal harm.
- Use with caution only if benefit to mother outweighs potential risk to fetus.

LACTATION

- It is not known if drug is present in breast milk.
- A decision should be made to discontinue breastfeeding during drug therapy.

Nursing Considerations

! WARNING Be aware that dofetilide shouldn't be started if patient has previously received amiodarone until blood amiodarone level is less than 0.3 mcg/ml or until amiodarone has been withdrawn for at least 3 months.

- Evaluate patient's renal function before drug therapy is begun and then periodically during dofetilide therapy, as needed and ordered.
- Place patient on continuous ECG monitoring for at least 3 days, as ordered, when dofetilide therapy is initiated. Monitor continuous ECG for at least 30 hours, as ordered when switching to dofetilide from class I or class III antiarrhythmics, or after withdrawing antiarrhythmic treatment. Know that if patient does not convert to normal sinus rhythm within 24 hours of starting dofetilide, expect possible synchronized electrical cardioversion.
- Evaluate and document QTc interval before and during dofetilide therapy.

! WARNING Monitor patient frequently, especially women, for adverse reactions, including prolonged QTc interval and torsades de pointes. Women have a 12 to 18% lower renal clearance of drug than men and therefore are at a greater risk for developing adverse reactions.

! **WARNING** Monitor laboratory test results for hypokalemia or hypomagnesemia, especially in patients taking diuretics because of the increased risk of dofetilide-induced torsades de pointes.

- Be aware that if patient requires a drug that may interact with dofetilide, expect to discontinue dofetilide, as prescribed, for 2 or more days before starting the other drug. Also, expect a washout period of at least 2 days before other drug(s) are started.

PATIENT TEACHING

- Instruct patient how to administer dofetilide.
- Instruct patient to avoid drinking grapefruit juice while taking this drug.
- Inform patient that she may be hospitalized for at least 3 days when dofetilide is initiated and if and when dosage is increased.
- Teach patient to measure blood pressure and pulse rate during dofetilide therapy.

! **WARNING** Urge patient to report chest discomfort, fluttering, or palpitations immediately. Also, tell patient to notify prescriber immediately if she experiences loss of appetite, severe diarrhea, unusual sweating, vomiting, or if she develops excessive thirst that may occur as a result of certain drug interactions that cause an electrolyte imbalance.

- Advise patient to consult prescriber before using any over-the-counter drugs, herbal products, or nutritional supplements.
- Instruct patient to keep follow-up appointments to monitor heart rhythm.

NEW!

donanemab-azbt

Kisunla

Class and Category

Pharmacologic class: Amyloid beta-directed monoclonal antibody
Therapeutic class: Anti-dementia

Indications and Dosages

∗ *To treat Alzheimer's disease in patients with mild cognitive impairment or mild dementia stage of disease*

I.V. INFUSION

Adults. 700 mg infused over 30 min every 4 wk for 3 doses, then 1400 mg infused over 30 min every 4 wk.

± **DOSAGE ADJUSTMENT** For patients with amyloid-related imaging abnormalities with edema (ARIA-E), dosing adjustments may be needed based on clinical symptoms and radiographic severity. For patients with amyloid-related imaging abnormalities with hemosiderin deposits (ARIA-H,) dosage adjustments is based on presence or absence of symptoms and radiographic severity.

Drug Administration

I.V.

- Store unopened drug vials in refrigerator. Allow drug to reach room temperature before preparing for administration.
- Drug solution should be clear to opalescent, colorless to slightly yellow to slightly brown.
- Drug must be diluted prior to administration with 0.9% Sodium Chloride.
- For a 700 mg dose, withdraw 40 ml of drug from drug vial and add to 30 ml to 135 ml of 0.9% Sodium Chloride to achieve a final concentration of diluted solution of 4 mg/ml to 10 mg/ml. For a 1400 mg dose, withdraw 80 ml of drug from drug vial and add to 60 ml to 270 ml of 0.9% Sodium Chloride to achieve a final concentration of diluted solution of 4 mg/ml to 10 mg/ml.
- Discard any unused portion left in drug vial as each vial is for one-time use only.
- Gently invert the diluted drug solution to mix completely. Do not shake.
- Use immediately after dilution or diluted solution may be stored for up to 72 hr in the refrigerator or for up to 12 hr if stored at room temperature. However, remember that storage time includes the duration of infusion. Do not freeze diluted solution.
- If diluted solution was stored in refrigerator, allow the diluted solution to reach room temperature before administration.
- Infused drug solution as an I.V. infusion over 30 min.
- Discontinue the infusion at the first appearance of any hypersensitivity or infusion reaction and notify prescriber.
- Flush the I.V. line only with 0.9% Sodium Chloride at the end of the infusion per maintenance protocol.

- Observe patient post-infusion for a minimum of 30 min for any evidence of a hypersensitivity or infusion reaction.
- If a dose is missed, expect to resume administration every 4 wk at the same dose as soon as possible.

Route	Onset	Peak	Duration
I.V.	Unknown	Unknown	Unknown

Half-life: 12.1 days

Mechanism of Action

Reduces amyloid beta plaques in the brain that accumulate in Alzheimer's disease to improve cognition.

Contraindications

Hypersensitivity to donanemab-azbt or its components

Interactions

None listed by manufacturer.

Adverse Reactions

CNS: Amyloid-related imaging abnormalities (ARIA) with edema or with hemosiderin deposits (confusion, dizziness, focal neurologic deficits, gait difficulty, headache, **intracerebral hemorrhage**, **seizures**, **status epilepticus**)
EENT: Visual changes
GI: **Intestinal obstruction and perforation**, nausea
Other: **Anaphylaxis**, **angioedema**, anti-donanemab-azbt antibody formation, infusion-related reaction (chest pain, chills, diaphoresis, difficulty breathing, dyspnea, elevated blood pressure, erythema, headache, hypotension, nausea, vomiting)

Childbearing Considerations

PREGNANCY

- It is not known if drug can cause fetal harm.
- Use with caution only if benefit to mother outweighs potential risk to fetus.

LACTATION

- It is not known if drug is present in breast milk.
- Mothers should check with prescriber before breastfeeding.

Nursing Considerations

- Check with prescriber if patient has been enrolled in a voluntary patient registry that collects data on treatments for Alzheimer's disease. Be aware that prescribers can enroll their patient through www.alz-net.org or by contacting alz-net@acr.org.
- Be aware that patients may experience three types of ARIA according to MRI classification criteria: ARIA-E, ARIA-H with microhemorrhage, and ARIA-H with superficial siderosis. Radiographic study of each of these classifications can be further broken down into mild, moderate, or severe.

! WARNING Know that patient should undergo testing to determine risk for ARIA because about 15% of Alzheimer's patients are apolipoprotein E episolon4 homozygotes, which has a higher incidence of ARIA, including symptomatic as well as serious and severe radiographic changes, when compared to heterozygotes and noncarriers. Know that baseline brain MRI and periodic monitoring with MRI are recommended for all patients receiving donanemab-azbt.

! WARNING Monitor patient closely for ARIA because ARIA can occur spontaneously although it most often appears during the first 24 weeks of therapy. Also, know that patients may experience more than 1 episode while receiving the drug and that ARIA E and ARIA-H of any cause can occur together. Notify prescriber if patient demonstrates any of the following signs and symptoms: confusion, dizziness, focal neurologic deficits, gait difficulty, headache, intracranial hemorrhage (can be greater than 1 cm in diameter), nausea, or visual changes. Be aware, that although rare, seizures, or status epilepticus may also occur. Provide supportive care, as needed and ordered knowing that symptoms usually resolve over time.

! WARNING Monitor patient for a hypersensitivity reaction, which can become life-threatening such as anaphylaxis or angioedema. If present, notify prescriber, expect drug to be discontinued and provide supportive care, as needed and ordered.

- Monitor patient for an infusion reaction, especially with the first infusion. Infusion reactions may present with fever, flu-like symptoms (chills, feeling shaky, generalized aches, and joint pain), hypertension, hypotension, nausea, oxygen desaturation, and vomiting. Be aware most infusion reactions are mild or moderate in severity. Notify prescriber if an infusion reaction occurs and expect infusion to be slowed or discontinued depending on the severity of the infusion.

! **WARNING** Use cautiously in patients receiving antithrombotics or a thrombolytic agent such as tissue plasminogen activator during donanemab-azbt therapy because of increased risk for intracerebral hemorrhages.

PATIENT TEACHING

- Inform patient, family, or caregiver donanemab-azbt will be administered by an intravenous infusion given over a half an hour every 4 weeks.

! **WARNING** Alert patient that drug may cause an allergic reaction. Stress importance of notifying staff during infusion or prescriber if a reaction occurs after infusion if patient has difficulty breathing or develops other sudden adverse reactions. Tell patient, family, or caregiver if patient is at home to seek immediate medical care if an allergic reaction is serious.

- Review the signs and symptoms of an infusion reaction with patient, family, or caregiver and stress importance of reporting any, if present. Tell patient reactions can occur even with the first infusion.
- Tell patient, family, or caregiver that MRI scans will be done periodically to detect adverse reactions in the brain.

! **WARNING** Discuss the possibility of ARIA with patient, family, or caregiver and that it commonly causes a temporary swelling in various areas of the brain. Tell patient most patients do not experience symptoms, and condition is usually picked up on an MRI scan. However, review signs and symptoms of ARIA and stress importance of reporting, if present. Reassure patient that ARIA usually resolves over time.

! **WARNING** Review signs and symptoms of an intracranial bleed for the patient also receiving antithrombolytics or a thrombolytic agent. Urge patient, family, or caregiver to seek immediate medical care, if present.

- Advise patient, family, or caregiver that the Alzheimer's network for Treatment and Diagnostics (ALZ-NET) is a voluntary patient registry that collects information on the use of donanemab-azbt for Alzheimer's disease. Encourage patient to ask prescriber to enroll patient.

donepezil hydrochloride

Adiarity, Aricept, Aricept ODT

Class and Category

Pharmacologic class: Acetylcholinesterase inhibitor

Therapeutic class: Antidementia

Indications and Dosages

∗ *To treat mild to moderate Alzheimer's disease*

ORALLY DISINTEGRATING TABLETS, TABLETS

Adults. *Initial:* 5 mg once daily. After 4 to 6 wk, dosage increased to 10 mg once daily, as needed. *Maximum:* 10 mg daily.

TRANSDERMAL SYSTEM

Adults. *Initial:* 5 mg/day patch applied once weekly. After 4 to 6 wk, dosage increased to 10 mg/day patch applied once weekly. *Maximum:* 10 mg/day patch applied once weekly.

∗ *To treat moderate to severe Alzheimer's disease*

ORALLY DISINTEGRATING TABLETS, TABLETS

Adults. *Initial:* 5 mg once daily. After 4 to 6 wk, dosage increased to 10 mg once daily, as needed. Dosage may be further increased, as needed, after 3 mo to 23 mg daily (immediate-release tablets only). *Maximum:* 10 mg daily for orally disintegrating tablets, 23 mg daily for immediate-release tablets.

TRANSDERMAL SYSTEM

Adults. *Initial:* 5 mg/day patch applied once weekly. After 4 to 6 wk, dosage increased to 10 mg/day patch applied once weekly.

Maximum: 10 mg/day patch applied once weekly.

Drug Administration

P.O.

- Administer the once-daily dose at bedtime.
- Immediate-release tablet should not be chewed, crushed, or split.
- When administering oral disintegrating tablets, tell patient not to swallow the tablet whole but to allow it to dissolve on the tongue and follow with a drink of water.

TRANSDERMAL

- Remove 1 transdermal system from refrigerator and allow pouch to reach room temperature before opening the pouch. Do not warm up pouch any other way. Do not apply a cold transdermal system to patient. Transdermal system must be used within 24 hr after being removed from refrigerator.
- Check to be sure pouch seal has not been broken. If the transdermal system is altered in any way, cut or damaged, discard and obtain a new system.
- Do not shave site of application and do not apply to skin that is cut, irritated, or red. Also, do not apply to area that has recently had cream, lotion, or powder applied.
- Apply patch to back but avoid the spine. Other sites include the upper buttocks or the upper outer thigh. Do not apply to an area that will be rubbed by tight clothing. Do not use the same application site for at least 2 wk after removing patch from that site.
- Remove patch from pouch and apply immediately to the patient's skin. Apply to a clean, dry, intact healthy skin area that has no to minimal hair. Press down firmly for 30 sec. Patient may bath while wearing patch.
- If patch falls off or a dose is missed, apply a new patch immediately and then replace the new patch 7 days later.

Route	Onset	Peak	Duration
P.O.	Unknown	3–4 hr	Unknown

Half-life: 70 hr

Mechanism of Action

Inhibits acetylcholinesterase reversibly and improves acetylcholine's concentration at cholinergic synapses. Raising acetylcholine level in the cerebral cortex may improve cognition. Donepezil becomes less effective as Alzheimer's disease progresses and number of intact cholinergic neurons declines.

Contraindications

History of allergic contact dermatitis (transdermal system); hypersensitivity to donepezil, piperidine derivatives, or their components

Interactions

DRUGS

anticholinergics: Possibly interference with activity of these drugs

cholinergic agonists, succinylcholine, and similar neuromuscular blockers: Possibly synergistic effects of these drugs

Adverse Reactions

CNS: Abnormal gait, agitation, aggression, anxiety, asthenia, confusion, depression, dizziness, dream disturbances, fatigue, fever, hallucinations, headache, hostility, insomnia, nervousness, **neuroleptic malignant syndrome**, **seizures**, somnolence, syncope, tremor

CV: **Abnormal ECG**, **AV block**, **bradycardia**, chest pain, edema, **heart failure**, hypertension, **hypotension**, **prolonged QT interval**, **torsades de pointes**

EENT: Pharyngitis

ENDO: Hyperglycemia

GI: Abdominal pain, anorexia, cholecystitis, constipation, diarrhea, dyspepsia, fecal incontinence, gastroenteritis, **hepatitis**, nausea, **pancreatitis**, vomiting

GU: Cystitis, glycosuria, hematuria, urinary frequency or incontinence, UTI

HEME: Anemia, **hemolytic hemorrhage**

MS: Arthralgia, back pain, elevated creatine kinase level, muscle cramps or spasms, **rhabdomyolysis**

RESP: Bronchitis, increased cough, pneumonia

SKIN: Ecchymosis, eczema, pruritus, rash, ulceration

Other: **Angioedema**, application site skin reactions (transdermal system), dehydration, elevated alkaline phosphatase or lactate dehydrogenase level, flu-like syndrome, **hyponatremia**, weight loss

Childbearing Considerations

PREGNANCY

- It is not known if drug causes fetal harm.
- Use with caution only if benefit to mother outweighs potential risk to fetus.

LACTATION

- It is not known if drug is present in breast milk.
- Mothers should check with prescriber before breastfeeding.

Nursing Considerations

- Use donepezil cautiously in patients with bladder obstruction because drug's weak peripheral cholinergic effect could obstruct outflow.
- Use drug cautiously in patients with asthma, COPD, or other pulmonary disorders because it has a weak affinity for peripheral cholinesterase, which may increase bronchoconstriction and bronchial secretions.

! **WARNING** Monitor patient for a hypersensitivity reaction, which may become life-threatening, such as angioedema. If present, notify prescriber promptly, expect drug to be discontinued, and provide supportive care, as needed and ordered.

! **WARNING** Know that if patient has cardiac disease, monitor heart rate and rhythm for bradycardia, which may result from increased vagal tone caused by drug's inhibition of peripheral cholinesterase. Reduced heart rate may be especially significant if patient already has bradycardia, sick sinus syndrome, or other supraventricular arrhythmias. Monitor all patients for cardiac dysfunction, which could become life-threatening, such as heart failure, hypotension, and torsades de pointes.

! **WARNING** Monitor patient for noncardiac persistent, severe, or unusual adverse reactions because drug may cause a variety of adverse effects in different body systems such as hemolytic hemorrhage, hyponatremia, pancreatitis, and rhabdomyolysis.

! **WARNING** Monitor patient for seizure activity because drug may cause seizures, especially in a patient with a seizure history. Institute seizure precautions.

! **WARNING** Monitor patient's blood glucose level, especially if diabetic, because drug may cause hyperglycemia.

- Take safety precautions if patient is dizzy or has other adverse CNS reactions.
- Suspect contact dermatitis when administering the transdermal system if application-site reactions spread beyond the size of the patch, if a more intense local reaction occurs at the site, or if symptoms do not significantly improve within 48 hours after the patch was removed. Notify prescriber if contact dermatitis is suspected and expect the transdermal system to be discontinued.

PATIENT TEACHING

- Instruct patient, family, or caregiver on how to administer form of donepezil prescribed.

! **WARNING** Alert patient that drug may cause an allergic reaction. If present, patient should notify prescriber and if severe, seek immediate medical care.

! **WARNING** Stress importance of notifying prescriber if adverse reactions develop that are persistent, severe, or unusual because drug can affect many different body systems. If chest pain, irregular pulse, muscle weakness or pain, significant abdominal pain, or seizures or any other adverse reaction that is severe, stress importance of seeking immediate medical attention.

! **WARNING** Inform patient with a seizure history to take seizure precautions and a patient with diabetes to monitor blood glucose levels closely.

- Advise patient, family, or caregiver that patient should avoid hazardous activities until drug's CNS effects are known and resolved. Safety precautions should be put in place to prevent patient from falling if adverse reactions such as dizziness occurs.
- Tell patient, family, or caregiver that if patient has a history of gastric irritation or peptic ulcer disease, the drug may aggravate these conditions by increasing gastric acid secretion.

dopamine hydrochloride

Class and Category

Pharmacologic class: Adrenergic
Therapeutic class: Vasopressor

Indications and Dosages

* *To correct hypotension due to inadequate cardiac output; to correct hemodynamic imbalances present in shock syndrome due to chronic cardiac decompensation, endotoxic septicemia, MI, open-heart surgery, renal failure, or trauma*

I.V. INFUSION

Adults. *Initial:* 2 to 5 mcg/kg/min, increased gradually in increments of 5 to 10 mcg/kg/min, as needed. *Usual:* Less than 20 mcg/kg/min.

Adults who are more seriously ill. *Initial:* 5 mcg/kg/min, increased gradually by 5 to 10 mcg/kg/min up to a rate of 50 mcg/kg/min, as needed. *Maximum:* 50 mcg/kg/min.

±**DOSAGE ADJUSTMENT** For patients who have received a MAO inhibitor in the previous 2 to 3 wk, dosage reduced to 10% of usual dosage.

Drug Administration

I.V.

- Ensure adequate fluid resuscitation has been done before giving drug.
- When using the single-dose plastic containers, the solution does not have to be diluted further. Be aware that the overwrap is a moisture and oxygen barrier. Do not remove unit from overwrap until ready to use.
- Visually inspect the container. If the administration port protector is damaged, detached, or not present, discard container because solution's sterility may be impaired. Solution should be clear and almost colorless. If darker or discolored, discard container and obtain a new one.
- Dilute concentrated drug solution with a compatible I.V. solution before administering, such as 0.9% Sodium Chloride Injection or 5% Dextrose Injection (see manufacturer's guidelines for other suitable solutions). When using the 40 mg/ml concentration of the drug, add 5 ml of drug (40 mg/ml) to a 250-ml diluting solution to obtain a concentration of 800 mcg/ml or 10 ml of drug to obtain a concentration of 1,600 mcg/ml; using a 500-ml solution, add 5 ml of drug (40 mg/ml) to obtain a concentration of 400 mcg/ml or 10 ml of drug to obtain a concentration of 800 mcg/ml; or using a 1,000-ml solution, add 5 ml of drug (40 mg/ml) to obtain a concentration of 200 mcg/ml or 10 ml of drug to obtain a concentration of 400 mcg/ml. When using the 80 mg/ml concentration, add 10 ml (80 mg/ml) to 250 ml dilution solution to obtain a concentration of 3,200 mcg/ml; to 500 ml dilution solution to obtain a 1,600 mcg/ml concentration; or to 1,000 ml dilution solution to obtain a 800 mcg/ml concentration,
- Give drug by I.V. infusion using a precision volume control infusion set and an infusion pump. When infusion rate exceeds 20 mcg/kg/min, monitor patient for excessive vasoconstriction and loss of renal vasodilating effects.
- Administer infusion through a central catheter to avoid extravasation and tissue necrosis. If drug must be given via peripheral line, administer through a large vein and inspect site often for signs of extravasation and necrosis. If such signs are detected, start a new I.V. line for the infusion, discontinue previous I.V. line, and notify prescriber immediately.
- Titrate dopamine gradually to minimize hypotension, especially after a high infusion rate.
- Never administer as an I.V. bolus.
- Discard diluted solution after 24 hr.
- *Incompatibilities:* Alkaline solutions, such as sodium bicarbonate, blood products, iron salts, other drugs mixed in same solution

Route	Onset	Peak	Duration
I.V.	> 5 min	Unknown	Up to 10 min

Half-life: 2 min

Mechanism of Action

Stimulates dopamine$_1$ (D_1) and dopamine$_2$ (D_2) postsynaptic receptors. D_1 receptors causing vasodilation in cerebral, coronary, mesenteric, and renal blood vessels. D_2 receptors inhibit norepinephrine release. In higher doses, dopamine also stimulates $alpha_1$ and $alpha_2$ receptors, causing vascular smooth-muscle contraction. It also causes increased renal blood flow, improved GFR, and increased urine output. At doses of 2 to 10 mcg/kg/min, dopamine stimulates $beta_1$-adrenergic receptors, increasing cardiac output while maintaining dopaminergic-induced vasodilation. At doses of 10 mcg/kg/min or more, alpha-adrenergic agonism takes over, causing increased peripheral vascular resistance and renal vasoconstriction.

Contraindications

Hypersensitivity to dopamine or its components, pheochromocytoma, uncorrected ventricular fibrillation, ventricular tachycardia or other tachyarrhythmias

Interactions

DRUGS

alpha-blockers: Antagonized peripheral vasoconstriction with high doses of dopamine
beta-blockers: Antagonized beta receptor–mediated inotropic effects of dopamine
cyclopropane, halogenated hydrocarbon anesthetics: Increased cardiac autonomic irritability with possible increased risk of hypertension and ventricular arrhythmias
diuretics: Possibly increased diuretic effects of dopamine or diuretic
haloperidol: Suppression of dopaminergic mesenteric vasodilation occurs with low rates of dopamine infusion
MAO inhibitors: Prolonged and intensified cardiac stimulation and vasopressor effect
oxytocic drugs, other vasopressors, vasoconstricting agents: Possibly severe persistent hypertension
phenytoin: Possibly sudden bradycardia and hypotension
tricyclic antidepressants: Possibly potentiated pressor response to dopamine

Adverse Reactions

CNS: Anxiety, headache
CV: Angina, **atrial fibrillation**, **bradycardia**, **cardiac conduction abnormalities**, **ectopic beats**, hypertension, **hypotension**, palpitations, peripheral vasoconstriction, sinus tachycardia, **ventricular arrhythmias**, **widened QRS complex**
GI: Nausea, vomiting
GU: **Azotemia**
RESP: Dyspnea
SKIN: Extravasation with tissue necrosis, piloerection

Childbearing Considerations

PREGNANCY

- It is not known if drug causes fetal harm.
- Use with caution only if benefit to mother outweighs potential risk to fetus.

LABOR AND DELIVERY

- Be aware that if a vasopressor drug, such as dopamine, is given during labor and delivery, it may interact with some oxytocic drugs to cause severe hypertension.

LACTATION

- It is not known if drug is present in breast milk.
- Due to the critical nature of situation, breastfeeding would not be done during drug therapy. Mothers should check with prescriber about breastfeeding once condition is stable.

Nursing Considerations

! WARNING Avoid, if possible, giving dopamine to patients with occlusive vascular disease, such as atherosclerosis, Buerger's disease, diabetic endarteritis, or Raynaud's disease because of risk of decreased peripheral circulation. Also, be aware that high doses of dopamine given for a prolonged period of time increases the risk of decreased peripheral circulation and could lead to gangrene in the patient's extremities.

! WARNING Use drug with extreme caution in patients sensitive to sulfites because dopamine may contain a sulfite. Monitor patient closely for a hypersensitivity reaction. If present, notify prescriber immediately and expect to provide supportive care, as needed and prescribed.

- Use drug cautiously in patients with cardiac disease, particularly coronary artery disease, because dopamine increases myocardial oxygen demand.
- Monitor blood pressure continuously with an intra-arterial line, as indicated.

- Place patient on continuous ECG monitoring and assess heart rate and rhythm for arrhythmias.
- Monitor patient's hemodynamic parameters, such as cardiac output, central venous pressure, and pulmonary artery wedge pressure, as indicated, to assess effectiveness of dopamine therapy.
- Monitor urine output hourly as appropriate to assess patient for improved renal blood flow.

PATIENT TEACHING

- Explain patient how the drug will be given and the need for frequent hemodynamic monitoring.
- Reassure patient he will be under constant supervision.
- Stress importance of notifying staff if patient experiences adverse reactions.

doravirine

Pifeltro

Class and Category

Pharmacologic class: Non-nucleoside reverse transcriptase inhibitor (NRTI)
Therapeutic class: Antiretroviral

Indications and Dosages

* *As adjunct to treat human immunodeficiency virus (HIV-1) infection in patients with no prior antiretroviral treatment history; to replace the current antiretroviral regimen in patients who are virologically suppressed (HIV-1 RNA less than 50 copies/ml) on a stable antiretroviral regimen with no history of treatment failure and no known substitutions associated with resistance to doravirine*

TABLETS

Adults and children weighing at least 35 kg (77 lb). 100 mg once daily.

± **DOSAGE ADJUSTMENT** For patients taking rifabutin concomitantly, dosage increased to 100 mg twice daily and given about 12 hours apart.

Drug Administration

P.O.

- Keep bottle tightly closed and do not remove the desiccant.
- Administer at about the same time every day.

Route	Onset	Peak	Duration
P.O.	Unknown	2 hr	Unknown

Half-life: 15 hr

Mechanism of Action

Inhibits HIV-1 replication by noncompetitive inhibition of HIV-1 reverse transcriptase.

Contraindications

Coadministration with carbamazepine, enzalutamide, mitotane, oxcarbazepine, phenobarbital, phenytoin, rifampin, rifapentine, or St. John's wort; hypersensitivity to doravirine or its components

Interactions

DRUGS

CYP3A inducers, such as carbamazepine, efavirenz, etravirine, enzalutamide, mitotane, nevirapine, oxcarbazepine, phenobarbital, phenytoin, rifabutin, rifampin, rifapentine, St. John's wort: Decreased concentration of doravirine with decreased effectiveness
CYP3A inhibitors: Possibly increased concentration of doravirine, increasing risk of adverse reactions

Adverse Reactions

CNS: Abnormal dreams, depression, dizziness, fatigue, headache, insomnia, somnolence, **suicidal ideation**
CV: Elevated lipid levels
GI: Abdominal pain, diarrhea, elevated lipase and liver enzymes, nausea
GU: Elevated bilirubin and creatinine levels
MS: Elevated creatine kinase level
SKIN: Rash **severe skin reactions (Stevens-Johnson syndrome, toxic epidermal necrolysis)**
Other: Elevated alkaline phosphatase, **immune reconstitution syndrome**

Childbearing Considerations

PREGNANCY

- Pregnancy exposure registry: 1-800-258-4263.
- It is not known if drug causes fetal harm.
- Use with caution only if benefit to mother outweighs potential risk to fetus.

LACTATION

- It is not known if drug is present in breast milk.
- The Centers for Disease Control and Prevention recommends that HIV-1 infected mothers not breastfeed to avoid risking

postnatal transmission of HIV-1 infection to infants. They also do not recommend breastfeeding because of potential drug-induced adverse reactions in the infant.

Nursing Considerations

- Obtain cholesterol and triglyceride levels before doravirine therapy is begun and periodically throughout therapy because drug may cause an increase in lipid levels.

! WARNING Monitor patient for severe skin reactions that could become life-threatening such as Stevens-Johnson syndrome or toxic epidermal necrolysis. If skin changes occur, notify prescriber immediately, expect drug to be discontinued, and provide supportive care, as needed and ordered.

! WARNING Monitor patient's mood and emotional status, as doravirine may cause significant depression, mood changes, and suicidal ideation. Report any changes to prescriber.

! WARNING Be aware that immune reconstitution syndrome has occurred in patients treated with combination antiretroviral therapy, including doravirine. The inflammatory response predisposes susceptible patients to opportunistic infections, such as cytomegalovirus, *Mycobacterium avium* infection, *Pneumocystis jiroveci* pneumonia, or tuberculosis. Autoimmune disorders, such as Graves' disease, Guillain-Barré syndrome, or polymyositis have also occurred. Report sudden or unusual adverse reactions to prescriber.

- Monitor patient's renal function throughout therapy, as ordered, because drug can alter renal function.

PATIENT TEACHING

- Instruct patient how to administer doravirine and what to do if a dose is missed.
- Instruct patient to alert prescriber of all medications taken, including over-the-counter drugs and any newly prescribed medication from other prescribers.

! WARNING Alert patient that serious skin reactions may occur with doravirine use. If present, stress importance of notifying prescriber and to seek immediate medical care, if severe.

! WARNING Tell patient, family, or caregiver to report any signs of depression, mood changes, sleep disorders, or suicidal thoughts to prescriber.

! WARNING Alert patient that drug may cause a condition that evokes an inflammatory response in the body making the patient at risk for serious infections. Instruct patient to report any signs of infection. Encourage patient to take infection precautions.

- Tell patient to notify prescriber if persistent, serious, or unusual adverse reactions occur.
- Alert mothers that breastfeeding is not recommended during doravirine therapy.

doxazosin mesylate

Cardura, Cardura XL

Class and Category

Pharmacologic class: Alpha-blocker
Therapeutic class: Antihypertensive, benign prostatic hyperplasia therapeutic agent

Indications and Dosages

* *To manage hypertension*

TABLETS

Adults. *Initial:* 1 mg once daily titrated upward by doubling dose each time to maximum dosage to achieve desired blood pressure, as needed. *Maximum:* 16 mg once daily.

* *To treat benign prostatic hyperplasia (BPH)*

TABLETS

Adults. *Initial:* 1 mg once daily. Doubled every 1 to 2 wk, as needed, based on signs and symptoms. *Maximum:* 8 mg once daily.

E.R. TABLETS

Adults. *Initial:* 4 mg once daily, increased to 8 mg after 3 to 4 wk, as needed.

Drug Administration

P.O.

- Tablets should be swallowed whole and not chewed, crushed, or split.
- Immediate-release tablets to treat BPH can be given in the morning or evening; extended-release tablets should be given with breakfast.
- If therapy is interrupted for either indication for more than several days, dosage should be restarted at 1 mg once daily and then titrated, as needed.

Route	Onset	Peak	Duration
P.O.	1–2 hr	2–3 hr	24 hr

Half-life: 15–22 hr

Mechanism of Action

Inhibits alpha$_1$-adrenergic receptors competitively in the sympathetic nervous system, causing peripheral vasodilation and reduced peripheral vascular resistance. This action decreases blood pressure, especially when the patient stands. Doxazosin also relaxes smooth muscle of the bladder neck, prostate, and prostate capsule, which reduces urethral resistance and pressure and urinary outflow resistance.

Contraindications

Hypersensitivity to doxazosin, other quinazolines (such as prazosin or terazosin), or their components

Interactions

DRUGS

diuretics, phosphodiesterase-5 inhibitors, other antihypertensives, strong CYP3A4 inhibitors: Enhanced hypotensive effects

Adverse Reactions

CNS: Dizziness, drowsiness, headache, nervousness, restlessness, vertigo
CV: **Arrhythmias**, first-dose orthostatic hypotension, palpitations, peripheral edema, sinus tachycardia
EENT: Intraoperative floppy iris syndrome, rhinitis
GI: **GI obstruction**, nausea
GU: Priapism
RESP: Dyspnea

Childbearing Considerations

PREGNANCY

- It is not known if drug causes fetal harm.
- Use with caution for treatment of hypertension only if benefit to mother outweighs potential risk to fetus.

LACTATION

- Drug may be present in breast milk.
- Mothers should check with prescriber before breastfeeding if prescribed for hypertension.

Nursing Considerations

- Be aware that Cardura XL is not for use in female patients and is not to be used to treat hypertension.

! **WARNING** Know that drug should not be given to hypotensive patients.

! **WARNING** Monitor blood pressure for 2 to 6 hours after first dose and with each increase because orthostatic hypotension commonly occurs at this time. Adjust dose as prescribed, based on standing blood pressure. Be aware that hypotensive effects may be more pronounced in elderly patients and in patients with hypovolemia or renal disease. It may be severe enough to cause syncope, especially after exercise.

- Monitor patients with hepatic disease because normal dosage may cause exaggerated effects.
- Monitor patient's pattern of urination, checking for difficulty urinating and urine retention, to assess drug's effects on BPH.

PATIENT TEACHING

- Instruct patient how to take form of doxazosin for condition prescribed.

! **WARNING** Instruct patient to change position slowly to minimize orthostatic hypotension that could cause patient to faint and possibly result in injury. Advise patient to also avoid exercising, going outside in hot weather, standing for long periods, and using alcohol; these activities may worsen orthostatic hypotension.

! **WARNING** Inform the patient taking drug for benign prostatic hyperplasia that he may become dizzy or faint if he takes an oral erectile dysfunction medicine during doxazosin therapy. Therefore, he should not use an oral erectile dysfunction medicine until he has discussed its use with the prescriber. Also, alert him to the rare possibility of developing a painful penile erection caused by doxazosin therapy that could last for hours. He should seek immediate medical attention if it occurs.

- Advise patient to avoid hazardous activities until drug's CNS effects are known and resolved.
- Tell patient to inform surgeon that he is taking doxazosin therapy if cataract surgery is required because drug may cause intraoperative floppy iris syndrome with this procedure.

doxepin hydrochloride

Silenor

Class and Category

Pharmacologic class: Tricyclic antidepressant
Therapeutic class: Antidepressant

Indications and Dosages

∗ *To treat depression or anxiety accompanying organic disease*

CAPSULES, ORAL SOLUTION

Adults. *Initial:* 75 mg daily, decreased or increased according to patient's response. *Usual:* 75 mg to 150 mg/day. *Maximum:* 300 mg daily in divided doses with a single dose not exceeding 150 mg.

∗ *To treat insomnia characterized by difficulty with sleep maintenance*

TABLET (SILENOR)

Adults. 3 to 6 mg once daily within 30 min of bedtime. *Maximum:* 6 mg once daily.

± **DOSAGE ADJUSTMENT** For elderly patients ages 65 and older taking Silenor, dosage initiated with 3 mg but increased to 6 mg daily, as needed.

Drug Administration

P.O.

- When used to treat insomnia, administer within 30 min of bedtime and avoid administering within 3 hr of a meal to minimize next day effects.
- When used to treat anxiety or depression, total daily dose given in a once-a-day dosage or divided dosing schedule. Once-a-day dosing should not exceed 150 mg and should be administered at about the same time daily. It may be administered at bedtime if patient prefers.
- Have patient swallow capsules and tablets whole. Capsules should not be opened.
- Use the dosing syringe provided or a calibrated device to measure dosage of oral solution. Mix oral solution in 120 ml of juice, such as grapefruit, orange, pineapple, or tomato; milk; or water, if desired. Do not mix with a carbonated beverage or grape juice. Stir the mixture and have patient drink it immediately after mixing. Do not save mixture for later use. Store at room temperature.

Route	Onset	Peak	Duration
P.O.	2–3 hr	3.5 hr	Unknown

Half-life: 15 hr

Mechanism of Action

May block norepinephrine and serotonin reuptake by adrenergic nerves. In this way, the tricyclic antidepressant raises norepinephrine and serotonin levels at nerve synapses, which may elevate mood and reduce depression. It is unknown how doxepin maintains sleep but is thought to be due to its antagonism of the H1receptor.

Contraindications

Hypersensitivity to doxepin, other tricyclic antidepressants, or their components; severe urinary retention; untreated narrow-angle glaucoma; use of MAO inhibitor within 14 days

Interactions

DRUGS

cimetidine, flecainide, other tricyclic antidepressants, phenothiazines, propafenone, quinidine, selective serotonin reuptake inhibitors: Increased blood doxepin level from inhibited systemic clearance, resulting in increased risk of toxicity

CNS depressants, sedating antihistamines: Possibly potentiated CNS depression, hypotension, and respiratory depression

MAO inhibitors: Possibly hyperpyrexia, hypertension, seizures, and death
tolazamide: Possibly severe hypoglycemia

ACTIVITIES

alcohol use: Possibly enhanced CNS depression, hypotension, and respiratory depression

Adverse Reactions

CNS: Confusion, delirium, dream disturbances, drowsiness, fatigue, hallucinations, headache, nervousness, parkinsonism, restlessness, sedation, **seizures**, **suicidal ideation**, tremor
CV: **ECG changes**, orthostatic hypotension, palpitations
EENT: Blurred vision, dry mouth, taste perversion
ENDO: Hyperglycemia, **hypoglycemia**
GI: Constipation, diarrhea, heartburn, ileus, increased appetite, jaundice, nausea, vomiting
GU: Decreased libido, ejaculation disorders
SKIN: Diaphoresis
Other: Weight gain

Childbearing Considerations

PREGNANCY

- It is not known if drug causes fetal harm.
- Use with caution only if benefit to mother outweighs potential risk to fetus.

LACTATION

- Drug is present in breast milk.
- Drug use is not recommended during breastfeeding, as it may cause apnea, drowsiness, and hypotonia in the breastfed infant.

REPRODUCTION

- Drug may reduce fertility and it is not known if this effect is reversible.

Nursing Considerations

- Monitor patient within a few hours after giving drug for adverse reactions.
- Evaluate patient for therapeutic response, such as decreased anxiety, apprehension, depression, fear, guilt, somatic symptoms, and worry; increased energy; or more restful sleep.

! **WARNING** Know that for patients with asthma or sulfite sensitivity, doxepin may aggravate asthma or cause allergic reactions because drug contains sulfites.

! **WARNING** Be alert for seizures. Patients with seizure disorder may need increased anticonvulsant dosage to maintain seizure control during drug therapy. Institute seizure precautions.

! **WARNING** Monitor patients, especially young adults, closely for evidence of suicidal thinking and behavior because doxepin increases the risk of suicidal thinking in this group.

- Know that drug should not be discontinued abruptly. Abrupt withdrawal of doxepin after prolonged therapy can cause cholinergic rebound effects, including diarrhea, nausea, and vomiting.
- Plan to withhold drug, as prescribed, several days before elective surgery to avoid significant change in blood pressure.
- Monitor elderly patients for parkinsonism, especially with high-dose therapy.
- Monitor diabetic patient's serum glucose level closely; drug may alter glucose level causing either hyperglycemia or hypoglycemia. Review signs and symptoms of glucose alterations and how to treat.

PATIENT TEACHING

- Instruct patient how to administer form of doxepin prescribed. Tell patient not to stop taking drug abruptly as diarrhea, nausea, and vomiting may occur.
- Instruct patient to avoid alcohol during doxepin therapy because mental alertness may decrease.

! **WARNING** Inform patients with asthma or sulfite sensitivity that doxepin tablets may aggravate asthma or cause allergic reactions because they contain sulfites. Urge patient to notify prescriber if an allergic reaction occurs or to seek immediate emergency care if serious.

! **WARNING** Alert family or caregiver of young adults to watch them closely for abnormal thinking or behavior that may lead to suicidal ideation. Drug may also cause increased aggression or hostility. Emphasize importance of notifying prescriber about unusual changes.

- Advise diabetic patient to measure serum glucose level more often than usual.

doxycycline

Oracea

doxycycline calcium

Vibramycin

doxycycline hyclate

Acticlate, Acticlate CAP, Doryx, Doryx MPC, Morgidox, Vibramycin

doxycycline monohydrate

Monodox, Vibramycin

Class and Category

Pharmacologic class: Tetracycline
Therapeutic class: Antibiotic

∗ *To treat inhalation anthrax post exposure*

CAPSULES, D.R. TABLETS, ORAL SUSPENSION, SYRUP, TABLETS

Adults and children ages 8 and older weighing 45 kg (99 lb) or more. 100 mg (120 mg Doryx MPC) twice daily for 60 days.
Children ages 8 and older weighing less than 45 kg (99 lb). 2.2 mg/kg (2.6 mg/kg Doryx MPC) twice daily for 60 days.

∗ *To treat inflammatory lesions (papules and pustules) of rosacea*

E.R. CAPSULES (ORACEA)

Adults. 40 mg once daily in the morning on an empty stomach.

∗ *To treat endocervical, rectal, and urethral infections caused by* Chlamydia trachomatis

CAPSULES, D.R. TABLETS, ORAL SUSPENSION, SYRUP, TABLETS

Adults. 100 mg (120 mg Doryx MPC) twice daily for 7 days.

∗ *To treat uncomplicated gonococcal infections except anorectal infections in men*

CAPSULES, D.R. TABLETS, ORAL SUSPENSION, SYRUP, TABLETS

Adults. 100 mg (120 mg Doryx MPC) twice a day for 7 days. Alternatively, 300 mg (360 mg Doryx MPC) followed in 1 hr by a second 300 mg (360 mg Doryx MPC) dose.

∗ *To treat epididymo-orchitis caused by C. trachomatis or* Neisseria gonorrhoeae

CAPSULES, D.R. TABLETS, ORAL SUSPENSION, SYRUP, TABLETS

Adults. 100 mg (120 mg Doryx MPC) twice daily for at least 10 days.

∗ *To prevent malaria*

CAPSULES, D.R. TABLETS, ORAL SUSPENSION, SYRUP, TABLETS

Adults. 100 mg (120 mg Doryx MPC) daily starting 1 to 2 days before travel, continued daily during travel, and then daily for 4 wk after travel ends.
Children over age 8. 2 mg/kg (2.4 mg/kg Doryx MPC) daily starting 1 to 2 days before travel, continued daily during travel, and daily for 4 wk after travel ends.

∗ *To treat early syphilis in penicillin-allergic patients*

CAPSULES, D.R. TABLETS, ORAL SUSPENSION, SYRUP, TABLETS

Adults. 100 mg (120 mg Doryx MPC) twice daily for 2 wk.

∗ *To treat syphilis of more than 1-year duration in penicillin-allergic patients*

CAPSULES, D.R. TABLETS, ORAL SUSPENSION, SYRUP, TABLETS

Adults. 100 mg (120 mg Doryx MPC) twice daily for 4 wk.

∗ *To treat all other infections caused by susceptible organisms*

CAPSULES, D.R. TABLETS, ORAL SUSPENSION, SYRUP, TABLETS

Adults and children over age 8 weighing 45 kg (99 lb) or more. 100 mg (120 mg Doryx MPC) every 12 hr on day 1 and then 100 mg (120 mg Doryx MPC) once daily or 50 mg twice daily. *For severe infections:* 100 mg continued every 12 hr.
Children over age 8 weighing less than 45 kg (99 lb). 2.2 mg/kg (2.6 mg/kg Doryx MPC) twice daily on day 1 and then 2.2 mg/kg (2.6 mg/kg Doryx MPC) once daily or 1.1 to 2.2 mg/kg (1.3 mg/kg Doryx MPC) twice daily.

I.V. INFUSION

Adults and children over age 8 weighing more than 45 kg. 200 mg once daily or 100 mg every 12 hr on day 1 and then 100 to 200 mg once daily or 50 to 100 mg every 12 hr.

Children over age 8 weighing 45 kg (99 lb) or less. *For severe or life-threatening infections:* 2.2 mg/kg every 12 hr. *For less severe infections:* 4.4 mg/kg divided into two doses on day 1 and then 2.2 to 4.4 mg/kg once daily or 1.1 to 2.2 mg/kg every 12 hr.

Drug Administration

P.O.

- Doryx and Doryx MPC are not interchangeable. Doryx 100 mg equals 120 mg of Doryx MPC. Also, Doryx MPC cannot be interchanged with other oral doxycycline on a mg-per-mg basis.
- Shake oral liquid container before measuring dose. Use a calibrated device when measuring dosage of oral suspension or syrup.
- Give Oracea 1 hr before or 2 hr after morning meal with a full glass of water. Other products can be taken with food or milk if GI upset occurs.
- Do not administer drug within 1 hr of bedtime because of possible esophageal irritation or ulceration.
- Capsules can be opened and D.R. tablets broken (not crushed) and sprinkled over cold, soft applesauce followed by a cool glass of water. Do not store mixture. Mixture should not be chewed but swallowed.
- Immediate-release capsules and tablets should be swallowed whole followed by a glass of water. However, for emergency administration of doxycycline hyclate for patients unable to swallow pills, do the following: Take one tablet and put in 20 ml of water. Soak at least 10 min. Crush tablet with back of spoon. Stir. Then, measure dose with a calibrated device and squirt it in another container. Mix with 3 teaspoons of milk, formula, chocolate milk, or apple juice that has had 2 to 4 teaspoons of sugar added to it (or add to chocolate pudding). Mix well and administer immediately.

I.V.

- Never administer drug I.M. or subcutaneously.
- Reconstitute with Sterile Water for Injection (see manufacturer's guidelines for other suitable solutions) using 10 ml for a 100-mg vial or 20 ml for a 200-mg vial.
- Dilute (see manufacturer's guidelines for suitable diluents) as follows: Dilute 100 mg of drug with 100 to 1,000 ml of solution; 200 mg of drug with 200 to 2,000 ml of solution. This will result in a concentration of 0.1 to 1.0 mg/ml. Concentrations lower than 0.1 mg/ml or higher than 1.0 mg/ml should not be used.
- Don't expose diluted solution to light. Protect it from direct sunlight during infusion.
- Infusion time varies with dose prescribed, but most range from 1 to 4 hr. Do not infuse rapidly. Check with manufacturer's guidelines for time infusion must be completed because it is dependent on the type of diluent used. Storage times also vary depending on solution used for dilution.
- *Incompatibilities:* None listed by manufacturer.

D

Route	Onset	Peak	Duration
P.O.	Unknown	1.5–4 hr	Unknown
P.O./D.R.	Unknown	2–4 hr	Unknown
I.V.	Immediate	Unknown	Unknown

Half-life: 18–22 hr

Mechanism of Action

Exerts a bacteriostatic effect against a wide variety of gram-positive and gram-negative organisms. Doxycycline is more lipophilic than other tetracyclines, which allows it to pass more easily through the bacterial lipid bilayer, where it binds reversibly to 30S ribosomal subunits. Bound doxycycline blocks the binding of aminoacyl transfer RNA to messenger RNA, thus inhibiting bacterial protein synthesis.

Contraindications

Hypersensitivity to doxycycline, other tetracyclines, or their components

Interactions

DRUGS

antacids that contain aluminum, calcium, magnesium, or zinc; calcium supplements; choline and magnesium salicylates; iron-containing preparations, laxatives that contain magnesium: Decreased doxycycline absorption and effects

barbiturates, carbamazepine, phenytoin: Increased clearance and decreased effects of doxycycline

bismuth subsalicylate: Impaired absorption of oral doxycycline
methoxyflurane: Increased risk of severe or fatal renal toxicity
oral anticoagulants: Possibly increased hypoprothrombinemic effects of these drugs
oral contraceptives: Decreased effectiveness of estrogen-containing oral contraceptives, increased risk of breakthrough bleeding
penicillin: Possibly interference with bactericidal action of penicillin

Adverse Reactions

CNS: Headache, **intracranial hypertension**, paresthesia
CV: **Pericarditis**, phlebitis
EENT: Black "hairy" tongue, glossitis, hoarseness, oral candidiasis, pharyngitis, stomatitis, tooth discoloration, visual disturbances
GI: Anorexia; bulky, loose stools; ***Clostridioides difficile*–associated diarrhea**; diarrhea; dysphagia; enterocolitis; epigastric distress; esophageal ulceration; esophagitis; **hepatotoxicity**, inflammatory lesions in anogenital region; nausea; **pancreatitis**; **pseudomembranous colitis**; rectal candidiasis; vomiting
GU: Anogenital lesions, dark yellow or brown urine, elevated BUN level, vaginal candidiasis
HEME: Eosinophilia, **hemolytic anemia**, **neutropenia**, **thrombocytopenia**, **thrombocytopenic purpura**
MS: Inhibition of bone growth in infants and children
SKIN: Dermatitis, **erythema multiforme**, erythematous and maculopapular rashes, **exfoliative dermatitis**, photosensitivity, rash, skin hyperpigmentation, **Stevens-Johnson syndrome**, **toxic epidermal necrolysis**, urticaria
Other: **Anaphylaxis**, **angioedema**, **drug reaction with eosinophilia and systemic symptoms (DRESS)**, exacerbation of systemic lupus erythematosus, injection-site phlebitis, Jarisch-Herxheimer (systemic inflammatory response) reaction in presence of spirochete infections, serum sickness

Childbearing Considerations

PREGNANCY

- Drug can cause fetal harm, especially retardation of skeleton and permanent discoloration of deciduous teeth if given during second and third trimesters of pregnancy.
- Drug is not recommended for use during pregnancy unless necessary and there is no alternative drug therapy available.

LACTATION

- Drug is present in breast milk.
- Mothers should check with prescriber before breastfeeding.

Nursing Considerations

- Avoid giving drug to children ages 8 and under, if possible; it may cause discoloration and enamel hypoplasia of developing teeth that may be permanent.
- Observe patient often for injection-site phlebitis, a common adverse reaction to I.V. administration.

! WARNING Monitor patient for hypersensitivity reactions and adverse skin reactions which could become life-threatening such as anaphylaxis, angioedema, and DRESS. Notify prescriber as soon as possible; if hypersensitivity or skin adverse reactions occur (especially a rash although sometimes only a fever or swollen lymph nodes are present), provide supportive care, as needed and ordered, and expect drug to be discontinued.

! WARNING Monitor patient closely for diarrhea, which may indicate pseudomembranous colitis caused by *Clostridioides difficile*, which can range from being mild to severe. If diarrhea occurs, notify prescriber and expect to obtain a stool specimen. If confirmed, expect to withhold doxycycline and treat *C. difficile*–associated diarrhea with an antibiotic effective against *C. difficile*, as ordered. Also, expect to treat with electrolytes, fluids, and protein supplementation, as needed and ordered.

! WARNING Monitor patient for signs and symptoms of intracranial hypertension, such as blurred vision, diplopia, headache, and vision loss; papilledema may be seen on fundoscopy. Patients at greater risk include females of childbearing age who are overweight or have a history of intracranial hypertension. If patient complains of visual changes, notify prescriber to obtain an immediate ophthalmologic evaluation because permanent visual loss can occur. Be aware that intracranial pressure may remain elevated for weeks after doxycycline therapy has been discontinued and warrants close follow-up.

! **WARNING** Monitor liver function test results routinely, as ordered, and monitor patient for signs and symptoms of liver dysfunction because drug may cause hepatotoxicity.

- Monitor patient for other persistent, severe, or unusual adverse reactions because drug can affect many body systems adversely.
- Expect doxycycline to increase risk of oral, rectal, or vaginal candidiasis—especially in debilitated or elderly patients and those on prolonged therapy—by changing the normal balance of microbial flora.

PATIENT TEACHING

- Instruct patient how to administer oral form of doxycycline prescribed.
- Tell patient not to take doxycycline just before bed because it may not dissolve properly when patient is recumbent and may cause esophageal burning and ulceration.
- Advise patient to avoid antacids containing aluminum, calcium, or magnesium.
- Instruct patient to drink plenty of fluids while taking doxycycline to reduce the risk of esophageal burning and ulceration.
- Inform patient being treated for a sexually transmitted disease, the importance of discussing with the prescriber the possible need that, the partner may need treatment as well.

! **WARNING** Tell patient to notify prescriber if allergic or skin adverse reactions occur because reactions may become severe, and drug may have to be discontinued. If severe, stress importance of seeking immediate medical care.

! **WARNING** Urge patient to report bloody, watery stools to prescriber immediately, even up to 2 months after drug therapy has ended.

! **WARNING** Advise females of childbearing age who take an oral contraceptive to use an additional contraceptive method during therapy. Also, advise all females of childbearing age to notify prescriber immediately if pregnancy occurs, as drug may cause retardation of skeletal development in the fetus and permanent discoloration of deciduous teeth.

! **WARNING** Tell patient to notify prescriber immediately about anorexia, epigastric distress, nausea, or vomiting during therapy.

! **WARNING** Instruct patient to notify prescriber of persistent, severe, or unusual adverse reactions because drug can adversely affect many body systems.

- Inform patient that her urine may become dark yellow or brown during therapy.
- Urge patient to avoid sun exposure and ultraviolet light as much as possible during therapy and to use sunscreen or sunblock as needed. If patient develops phototoxicity, such as skin eruption, tell her to stop drug and notify prescriber.
- Alert female patients that doxycycline may increase risk of vaginal candidiasis. Tell her to notify prescriber if she develops vaginal discharge or itching.

dronabinol
(delta-9-tetrahydrocannabinol, THC)

Marinol, Syndros

Class, Category, and Schedule

Pharmacologic class: Cannabinoid
Therapeutic class: Antiemetic, appetite stimulant
Controlled substance schedule: II (Syndros), III (Marinol)

Indications and Dosages

✱ *To prevent nausea and vomiting caused by chemotherapy and unresponsive to other antiemetics*

CAPSULES (MARINOL)

Adults and children. 5 mg/m^2 1 to 3 hr before chemotherapy and then every 2 to 4 hr after chemotherapy for a total of 4 to 6 doses daily, increased by 2.5 mg/m^2 increments, as needed. *Maximum:* 15 mg/m^2/dose for a total of 4 to 6 doses daily.

ORAL SOLUTION (SYNDROS)

Adults. 4.2 mg/m^2 1 to 3 hr before chemotherapy and then every 2 to 4 hr after chemotherapy for a total of 4 to 6 doses daily, increased, as needed, in increments of 2.1 mg/m^2. *Maximum:* 12.6 mg/m^2 per dose for 4 to 6 doses daily.

±**DOSAGE ADJUSTMENT** For elderly patients prescribed Marinol, initial dosage may be reduced to 2.5 mg/m^2 1 to 3 hr before chemotherapy to reduce CNS adverse reactions. For elderly patients prescribed Syndros and all patients who experience persistent or severe adverse reactions, dosage reduced to 2.1 mg/m^2 1 to 3 hr before chemotherapy.

✶ *To stimulate appetite in AIDS patients*

CAPSULES (MARINOL)

Adults. *Initial:* 2.5 mg twice daily 1 hr before lunch and dinner, increased, as needed. *Maximum:* 10 mg twice daily.

ORAL SOLUTION (SYNDROS)

Adults. 2.1 mg twice daily 1 hr before lunch and dinner. Increased to 2.1 mg 1 hr before lunch and 4.2 mg 1 hr before dinner, as needed. Then, further increased to 4.2 mg 1 hr before lunch and 4.2 mg 1 hr before dinner, as needed. *Maximum:* 8.4 mg twice daily.

±**DOSAGE ADJUSTMENT** For elderly patients and patients who can't tolerate 5 mg daily, dosage for capsule form (Marinol) reduced to 2.5 mg before dinner or at bedtime. For elderly patients and patients who can't tolerate a twice-daily dosage, dosage maintained for oral solution form (Syndros) at 2.1 mg, but dosage frequency reduced to once daily 1 hour before dinner or bedtime.

Drug Administration

P.O.

- Administer 1 to 3 hr before chemotherapy for the first dose. Although first dose should be given on an empty stomach at least 30 min before patient eats, the remainder of doses can be given without regard to meals. The timing of dosing in relation to mealtimes should be kept consistent for each chemotherapy cycle.
- Administer 1 hr before lunch and dinner if given to treat anorexia and weight loss in patients with AIDS. Administering drug later in the day helps reduce the frequency of CNS adverse reactions.
- Give drug with at least 6 to 8 ounces of water.
- Always use the calibrated oral dosing syringe that comes with drug to measure oral solution doses. If dose is greater than 5 mg, divide the total dose into 2 or more portions using the oral syringe.
- Oral solution may be administered by a feeding tube that is silicone only and equal to or greater than a 14 French. Tubes consisting of polyurethane should not be used. Draw up the prescribed dose of drug using the calibrated dosing syringe packaged with drug. After administering drug via feeding tube, flush feeding tube with 30 ml of water using a catheter-tip syringe.
- Store capsules and oral solution at room temperature. Discard oral solution after 42 days from opening container regardless of any oral solution remaining in container.

Route	Onset	Peak	Duration
P.O.	30–60 min	2–4 hr	6–24 hr

Half-life: 25–36 hr

Mechanism of Action

May exert antiemetic effect by inhibiting the vomiting control mechanism in the medulla oblongata. As the main psychoactive substance in marijuana (*Cannabis sativa L.*), dronabinol's effects may be mediated by cannabinoid receptors in neural tissues.

Contraindications

For Marinol: Hypersensitivity to dronabinol, its components, other cannabinoids, or sesame oil

For Syndros: Hypersensitivity reaction to dronabinol, its components, or alcohol; use of disulfiram- or metronidazole-containing products within past 14 days

Interactions

DRUGS

amitriptyline, amoxapine, amphetamines, antihistamines, atropine, desipramine, other sympathomimetic or tricyclic antidepressants, scopolamine: Increased risk of hemodynamic instability such as hypertension (possible), hypotension, syncope, or tachycardia with risk higher in patients with cardiac disorders

amphotericin B, cyclosporine, warfarin, other drugs highly bound to plasma proteins with a narrow therapeutic index: Possibly increased risk of adverse reactions associated with these drugs

CNS depressants such as antihistamines, barbiturates benzodiazepine, buspirone, lithium, muscle relaxants, opioids, scopolamine, sedatives, tricyclic antidepressants: Additive CNS effects with increased risk of confusion, dizziness, sedation, or somnolence
CYP2C9 inhibitors, such as amiodarone, CYP2C9 and CYP3A4 inducers: Possibly decreased dronabinol exposure and effectiveness of fluconazole
CYP3A4 inhibitors, such as clarithromycin, erythromycin, itraconazole, ketoconazole, ritonavir: Possibly increased dronabinol-related adverse reactions from increased exposure
disulfiram, metronidazole (Syndros only): Possible disulfiram-like reaction

ACTIVITIES

alcohol use: Additive CNS depressant effects

Adverse Reactions

CNS: Altered mental state, amnesia, asthenia, anxiety, ataxia, chills, cognitive impairment, confusion, delirium, delusions, depersonalization, depression, disorientation, dizziness, drowsiness, euphoria, exacerbation of mania or schizophrenia, fatigue, hallucinations, headache, insomnia, irritability, loss of consciousness, malaise, mood changes, movement disorder, nervousness, nightmares, panic attack, paranoid reaction, **seizures**, sleep disturbance, speech difficulties, somnolence, syncope
CV: Orthostatic hypotension, palpitations, sinus tachycardia, vasodilation
EENT: Lip swelling, oral lesions, rhinitis, sinusitis, **throat tightness**, tinnitus, vision difficulties
GI: Abdominal pain, anorexia, diarrhea, elevated liver enzymes, fecal incontinence, nausea, vomiting
MS: Myalgias
RESP: Cough
SKIN: Diaphoresis, disseminated rash, facial flushing, skin burning, urticaria
Other: Physical and psychological dependence

Childbearing Considerations

PREGNANCY

- Drug may cause fetal harm, such as fetal growth restriction, low birth weight, preterm birth, small for gestational age, and stillbirth. Drug contains alcohol, which also may cause fetal harm including behavioral disorders, CNS abnormalities, or impaired intellectual development
- Drug use should be avoided in pregnant women.

LACTATION

- Drug may be present in breast milk.
- The Centers for Disease Control and Prevention recommends that HIV-1 infected mothers not breastfeed to avoid risking postnatal transmission of HIV-1 infection to infants. They also do not recommend breastfeeding because of potential drug-induced adverse reactions in the infant.
- Mothers breastfeeding during treatment for nausea and vomiting related to cancer chemotherapy may adversely affect baby's weight.

Nursing Considerations

- Know that patients under age 45 may tolerate drug better than those over age 45.
- Be aware that oral solution contains alcohol, which can produce disulfiram-like reactions when co-administered with disulfiram or other drugs that produce this reaction. Know that these products should be discontinued at least 14 days before starting oral solution form of dronabinol and not administered for at least 7 days after therapy with dronabinol has ceased.

! WARNING Know that patients with a history of substance abuse or dependence are at higher risk for abusing dronabinol. Assess patient's risk for abuse or misuse prior to dronabinol therapy and monitor patient throughout for evidence of abuse or misuse. Expect tolerance to drug to develop over time, especially if patient has smoked marijuana. Be aware that short-term, low-dose therapy doesn't typically lead to physical and psychological dependence, which may occur with long-term, high-dose therapy. Know that dronabinol shouldn't be discontinued abruptly because withdrawal syndrome may occur.

- Expect patients to be screened for depression, mania, and schizophrenia prior to treatment because dronabinol can exacerbate these conditions. Use with extreme caution, if usage cannot be avoided, in these patients. Monitor patient for new or worsening psychiatric symptoms during therapy. Also, know that concomitant use with other drugs associated with similar psychiatric effects should be avoided
- Anticipate higher risk of cardiovascular reactions, such as blood pressure changes (especially orthostatic hypotension) and increased heart rate, at higher doses and in patients with cardiac conditions. Monitor patient's vital signs closely, especially when drug is initiated or when dosage is increased.

! **WARNING** Monitor patient for a hypersensitivity reaction such as developing a rash, throat tightness, and urticaria. If patient exhibits any signs of hypersensitivity, especially throat tightness that may interfere with respirations, notify prescriber promptly, withhold drug as ordered, and provide supportive care, as needed and ordered.

! **WARNING** Use cautiously in patients with history of seizures because drug may lower seizure threshold. Notify prescriber of seizures immediately and expect to stop drug.

- Alert prescriber if patient experiences changes in mental state or cognitive impairment because dosage will have to be reduced or drug discontinued. Know that elderly patients may be more sensitive to the neurological and psychoactive effects of dronabinol.
- Expect drug to alter rapid eye movement (REM) sleep pattern, even after therapy stops.
- Be aware that paradoxical abdominal pain, nausea, and vomiting can occur with chronic, long-term use of dronabinol.

PATIENT TEACHING

- Instruct patient how to administer form of dronabinol prescribed.
- Urge patient not to use alcohol while taking dronabinol because it may increase CNS depression.

! **WARNING** Alert patient that drug can cause physical and psychological dependence. Warn patient not to increase dose or frequency of drug administration without consulting prescriber. Caution patient not to stop drug abruptly because withdrawal symptoms may occur.

! **WARNING** Inform females of childbearing age to notify prescriber if pregnancy occurs, because dronabinol may cause fetal harm.

! **WARNING** Caution patient that drug may cause an allergic reaction. Tell patient to notify prescriber if hives or a rash occurs. If throat tightness occurs, stress importance of seeking immediate medical care.

! **WARNING** Inform patient drug may cause seizures, especially if patient has a seizure history. Review seizure precautions and seek immediate medical care if a seizure occurs.

- Alert family or caregiver that if patient is elderly and especially if dementia is present, patient may be more sensitive to the neuropsychiatric and postural hypotensive effects of the drug and be at increased risk of falls. Encourage family or caregiver to discuss concerns with prescriber.
- Instruct patient to rise slowly to sitting or standing position to minimize effects of orthostatic hypotension.
- Advise patient to avoid hazardous activities until drug's CNS effects are known and resolved.
- Inform patient that sleep pattern may be adversely affected during therapy and for some time afterward.
- Advise mothers being treated for AIDS not to breastfeed. Tell mothers receiving the drug to treat nausea and vomiting associated with cancer chemotherapy to monitor their breastfed infant's weight.

dronedarone

Multaq

Class and Category

Pharmacologic class: Benzofuran derivative
Therapeutic class: Antiarrhythmic

Indications and Dosages

✱ *To reduce risk of hospitalization for atrial fibrillation in patients in sinus rhythm with a history of paroxysmal or persistent atrial fibrillation*

TABLETS

Adults. 400 mg twice daily.

Drug Administration

P.O.

- Administer drug with breakfast and dinner.
- Do not administer drug with grapefruit juice.

Route	Onset	Peak	Duration
P.O.	Unknown	3–6 hr	Unknown

Half-life: 13–19 hr

Mechanism of Action

Reduces risk of atrial fibrillation although specific effect on heart rhythm is unknown. However, dronedarone possesses properties of all 4 Vaughn–Williams antiarrhythmic classes.

Contraindications

Bradycardia less than 50 beats/min; breastfeeding; concurrent use of drugs or herbal products that prolong QT interval, such as class I and III antiarrhythmics, erythromycin and other selected oral macrolide antibiotics, phenothiazine antipsychotics, and tricyclic antidepressants or strong CYP3A inhibitors, such as clarithromycin, cyclosporine, ketoconazole, itraconazole, nefazodone, ritonavir, telithromycin, and voriconazole; hypersensitivity to dronedarone or its components; liver or lung toxicity related to previous use of amiodarone; pregnancy; PR interval greater than 280 msec or QTc Bazett interval of 500 msec or more; permanent atrial fibrillation; second- or third-degree atrioventricular block or sick sinus syndrome (except when used with a functioning pacemaker); severe hepatic impairment (Child–Pugh class C); symptomatic heart failure with recent decompensation requiring hospitalization or NYHA Class IV symptoms

Interactions

DRUGS

beta-blockers: Increased risk of bradycardia
calcium channel blockers: Possibly increased dronedarone effects on conduction
calcium channel blockers, such as diltiazem, nifedipine, and verapamil; CYP3A substrates with narrow therapeutic range, such as sirolimus and tacrolimus; CYP2D6 substrates, such as beta-blockers, selective serotonin reuptake agents, and tricyclic antidepressant; statins, such as simvastatin: Increased effects of these drugs with possibly increased risk of adverse reactions
class I and III antiarrhythmics, macrolide antibiotics, phenothiazines, tricyclic antidepressants: Possibly increased QT interval
CYP3A inducers, such as carbamazepine, phenobarbital, phenytoin, rifampin, St. John's wort: Decreased dronedarone effects
CYP3A inhibitors, such as clarithromycin, cyclosporine, ketoconazole, itraconazole, nefazodone, ritonavir, telithromycin, voriconazole: Increased dronedarone effects
digoxin and other P-gp substrates, such as dabigatran: Increased effect of these drugs with risk of toxicity
warfarin: Possible increased risk of bleeding and INR

FOODS

grapefruit juice: Increased dronedarone effects

Adverse Reactions

CNS: Asthenia
CV: **Bradycardia**, **heart failure**, **prolonged QT interval**, vasculitis
GI: Abdominal pain, diarrhea, dyspepsia, **liver injury**, nausea, vomiting
GU: Increased serum creatinine levels
RESP: Dyspnea, **interstitial lung disease, such as pneumonitis and pulmonary fibrosis**, nonproductive cough, **pulmonary toxicity**
SKIN: Allergic dermatitis, dermatitis, eczema, photosensitivity, pruritus, rash
Other: **Anaphylaxis**, **angioedema**, **hypokalemia**, **hypomagnesemia**

Childbearing Considerations

PREGNANCY

- Drug may cause fetal harm.
- Females of childbearing age need to have a negative pregnancy test before drug therapy can begin.
- Drug is contraindicated in females of childbearing age who are or who may become pregnant during drug therapy.

LACTATION

- It is not known if drug is present in breast milk.

- Breastfeeding is contraindicated during drug therapy and for 5 days after the last dose because of potential risk of liver injury and pulmonary toxicity to develop in the breastfed infant.

REPRODUCTION

- Females of childbearing age should use an effective contraceptive during drug therapy.

Nursing Considerations

- Check that patient has stopped taking any drug contraindicated with dronedarone, as prescribed, before giving first dose. Also, check that patient is receiving appropriate antithrombotic therapy prior to giving first dose because patients are at increased risk for stroke, especially in the first 2 weeks of therapy. In addition, check patient's serum potassium and magnesium levels prior to initiating therapy and throughout therapy because of increased risk of deficiency and arrhythmias, especially if patient is also taking a potassium-depleting diuretic.

! **WARNING** Ensure females of childbearing age have a negative pregnancy test result before beginning dronedarone therapy because drug can cause fetal harm.

! **WARNING** Obtain an ECG on patient before therapy begins and then regularly as ordered. If patient's QTc becomes 500 ms or greater or heart block is noted, notify prescriber as drug must be discontinued. Also, if atrial fibrillation is found, prepare patient for cardioversion, as ordered.

! **WARNING** Monitor patient for a hypersensitivity reaction, which could become life-threatening, such as anaphylaxis. If present, notify prescriber, expect drug to be discontinued, and provide supportive care, as needed and ordered.

! **WARNING** Assess patient for evidence of heart failure, such as dependent edema, increasing shortness of breath, or weight gain because drug may cause or worsen existing heart failure. If present, notify prescriber; dronedarone may have to be discontinued.

! **WARNING** Monitor patient for dyspnea or nonproductive cough, which could indicate the development of pulmonary toxicity. If confirmed, expect drug to be discontinued.

! **WARNING** Monitor patient's liver function, as ordered, because severe liver injury may occur with dronedarone therapy. If liver enzymes become elevated or the patient develops symptoms of liver dysfunction, such as anorexia, dark urine, fatigue, fever, itching, jaundice, malaise, nausea, right upper quadrant pain, or vomiting, notify prescriber and expect drug to be discontinued immediately.

- Monitor patient's serum creatinine levels, as ordered. Elevation may occur rapidly, then plateau after 7 days, and usually is reversible after therapy stops.

PATIENT TEACHING

- Instruct patient how to administer dronedarone.
- Inform patient that dronedarone should not be taken with grapefruit juice, nor should grapefruit juice be part of patient's diet during drug therapy.

! **WARNING** Alert females of childbearing age that a negative pregnancy test result must be obtained before dronedarone can begin because drug can cause fetal harm. Also, tell patient she should use an effective contraception during drug therapy if sexually active. Stress importance of notifying prescriber if pregnancy occurs as drug will have to be discontinued immediately.

! **WARNING** Alert patient that an allergic reaction can occur with dronedarone therapy. Tell patient to notify prescriber, if present, and to seek immediate medical care, if severe.

! **WARNING** Urge patient to contact prescriber if he develops evidence of heart failure, such as dependent edema, increasing shortness of breath or weight gain because dronedarone may have to be discontinued.

! **WARNING** Review symptoms of liver dysfunction with patient and urge her to seek immediate medical attention, if present, and to stop taking dronedarone.

! **WARNING** Stress importance of notifying prescriber if difficulty breathing or a nonproductive cough develope.

- Stress importance of complying with appointments to obtain an ECG and laboratory appointments. Tell patient to notify prescriber if an irregular or rapid heart beat occurs or patient experiences palpitations.
- Tell patient to inform all prescribers that she is taking dronedarone and to check with prescriber before taking any herbal product with dronedarone, newly prescribed drug, or over-the-counter drugs.

dulaglutide

Trulicity

Class and Category

Pharmacologic class: Glucagon-like peptide-1 receptor agonist
Therapeutic class: Antidiabetic

Indications and Dosages

✱ As adjunct to diet and exercise to improve glycemic control in patients with type 2 diabetes mellitus

SUBCUTANEOUS INJECTION

Adults. *Initial:* 0.75 mg once weekly, then increased to 1.5 mg once weekly, as needed. Then, increased to 3 mg once weekly after 4 wk, as needed, and then increased to 4.5 mg once weekly after 4 wk, as needed. *Maximum:* 4.5 mg once weekly.
Children ages 10 and older. *Initial:* 0.75 mg once weekly, increased after 4 wk to 1.5 mg once weekly, as needed. *Maximum:* 1.5 mg once weekly.

✱ To reduce the risk of major cardiovascular events (cardiovascular death, CVA, or non-fatal MI) in adults with type 2 diabetes mellitus who have established cardiovascular disease or multiple cardiovascular risk factors

SUBCUTANEOUS INJECTION

Adults. 0.75 mg once weekly, then increased to 1.5 mg once weekly, as needed. Then, increased to 3 mg once weekly after 4 wk, as needed, and then increased to 4.5 mg once weekly after 4 wk, as needed. *Maximum:* 4.5 mg once weekly.

Drug Administration

SUBCUTANEOUS

- Solution should appear clear and colorless in the single-dose pen.
- Administer any time of day with or without food.
- Inject into patient's abdomen, thigh, or upper arm following manufacturer's guidelines. It is important when injecting drug to press and hold the green injection button, which should produce a loud click. Continue holding against patient's skin until a second click is heard in about 5 to 10 seconds. The pen can then be removed.
- Rotate injection sites with each dose.
- Never administer as an I.M. or I.V. injection.
- When administering drug with insulin, separate injections and never mix. However, both can be injected into the same body region, but the injections should not be adjacent to each other.
- If a dose is missed and there are at least 3 days (72 hr) until next scheduled dose, drug can be administered. If less than 3 days (72 hr) remains, skip missed dose and administer next dose as scheduled. In either case, a once-weekly dosing schedule can be resumed.
- The day of weekly administration can be changed as long as the last dose was administered 3 or more days before.
- Store drug in refrigerator. If needed, each single-dose pen can be kept at room temperature for up to 2 wk.
- Never freeze drug and protect from light by storing in original carton until time of administration.

Route	Onset	Peak	Duration
SubQ	Unknown	24–72 hr	Unknown

Half-life: 5 days

Mechanism of Action

Activates the GLP-1 receptor to increase intracellular cyclic AMP (cAMP) in beta cells, causing a glucose-dependent insulin release. Insulin lowers blood glucose levels. Dulaglutide also decreases glucagon secretion and slows gastric emptying to further decrease blood glucose levels.

Contraindications

Hypersensitivity to dulaglutide or its components, personal or family history of medullary thyroid carcinoma or multiple endocrine neoplasia syndrome type 2, preexisting severe GI disease

Interactions

DRUGS

insulin, insulin secretagogues: Increased risk of hypoglycemia

orally administered drugs: Possibly decreased absorption of the orally administered drugs

Adverse Reactions

CNS: Asthenia, fatigue, malaise
CV: First-degree AV block, sinus tachycardia
EENT: Diabetic retinopathy occurrence or progression, dysgeusia
GI: Abdominal distention or pain, anorexia, cholecystitis, cholelithiasis, cholestasis, constipation, diarrhea, dyspepsia, elevated liver or pancreatic enzymes, eructation, flatulence, gastroesophageal reflux disease, **hepatitis**, ileus, nausea, **pancreatitis**, **severe GI disturbances**, vomiting
GU: **Acute renal failure**, elevated creatinine level, **worsening chronic renal failure**
SKIN: Pruritus, rash, urticaria
RESP: **Pulmonary aspiration** (during deep sedation or general anesthesia)
Other: **Anaphylactic reactions**, **angioedema**; anti-drug antibody formation; **hypersensitivity reactions**; injection-site reactions, such as erythema and rash

Childbearing Considerations

PREGNANCY

- It is not known if drug causes fetal harm.
- Use with caution only if benefit to mother outweighs potential risk to fetus.

LACTATION

- It is not known if drug is present in breast milk.
- Mothers should check with prescriber before breastfeeding.

Nursing Considerations

- Know that dulaglutide should not be used as first-line therapy for patients who have inadequately controlled their blood glucose levels on diet and exercise alone.

! **WARNING** Use caution when beginning dulaglutide therapy or titrating dose in patients with renal impairment. Monitor renal function closely because drug can induce acute renal failure even in patients with no known renal disease or worsen chronic renal failure. If patient experiences dehydration, diarrhea, or nausea, notify prescriber because the frequency and severity of these symptoms may worsen renal function. Keep patient hydrated throughout drug therapy to help prevent renal impairment.

! **WARNING** Monitor patient for signs of hypersensitivity, which could become life-threatening, such as anaphylaxis and angioedema. If present, withhold drug, notify prescriber. and expect drug to be discontinued. Provide supportive care, as needed and ordered.

! **WARNING** Be aware that dulaglutide may potentially be linked to the development of thyroid C-cell tumors. While elevated serum calcitonin is a biological marker, its value in routine monitoring is unclear. If an elevated serum calcitonin level is found at any time during therapy, expect patient to be referred to an endocrinologist for further evaluation.

! **WARNING** Monitor patient for signs and symptoms of pancreatitis, such as persistent severe abdominal pain, sometimes radiating to the back, which may or may not be accompanied by vomiting. If confirmed, expect dulaglutide to be discontinued. Also, be aware dulaglutide may cause severe GI adverse reactions. Alert prescriber immediately, if present.

! **WARNING** Monitor patient who is also receiving insulin or insulin secretagogue therapy concomitantly for hypoglycemia. The dosage of insulin or insulin secretagogue may have to be lowered to reduce the risk of hypoglycemia. If hypoglycemia occurs, treat it according to institutional protocol and notify prescriber.

! **WARNING** Be aware that because dulaglutide delays gastric emptying, pulmonary aspiration may occur during elective procedures or surgeries if patient receives deep sedation or general anesthesia.

- Monitor patients with hepatic impairment closely because the effect of dulaglutide therapy on the liver is unknown, and in patients with gastroparesis because drug slows gastric emptying.
- Monitor patient for change in vision, as diabetic retinopathy may occur or worsen during drug therapy. Most

patients experience diabetic retinopathy complications if condition was present before drug was started. If visual changes occur, notify prescriber. However, know that a temporary worsening of diabetic retinopathy may occur with rapid improvement in glucose control.

PATIENT TEACHING

! **WARNING** Ensure that patient has been informed of the potential risk for developing thyroid tumors before starting dulaglutide therapy. Tell patient to report any symptoms of thyroid tumors, such as a mass in the neck, difficulty swallowing or breathing, or persistent hoarseness during therapy.

- Instruct patient how to administer dulaglutide as a subcutaneous injection and what to do if a dose is missed.

! **WARNING** Inform patient that dulaglutide may cause an allergic reaction. If present, tell patient to notify prescriber and, if severe, to seek immediate medical care.

! **WARNING** Inform patient who is also receiving an insulin secretagogue or insulin that hypoglycemia may occur. Tell patient to notify prescriber if hypoglycemia occurs frequently or is severe.

! **WARNING** Warn patient that drug can cause acute gallbladder disease or hepatitis. Tell patient to notify prescriber immediately if clay-colored stools, fever, pain in upper abdomen, and yellowing of eyes or skin occurs.

! **WARNING** Also, inform patient that drug can cause severe GI adverse reactions. Tell patient to notify prescriber immediately if persistent or severe GI symptoms occur.

! **WARNING** Alert patient that because drug may cause their stomach to empty more slowly, respiratory complications may develop with anesthesia or deep sedation during planned procedures or surgeries. Stress importance of alerting healthcare providers dulaglutide is being taken.

- Tell patient to notify prescriber if any orally administered drugs appear to be losing their effectiveness, as dulaglutide causes a delay of gastric emptying and has the potential to affect the absorption of drugs taken by mouth. Also, tell prescriber about any new prescribed drugs and tell patient to consult prescriber before taking any over-the-counter drugs.
- Stress importance of reporting visual changes to prescriber.

duloxetine hydrochloride

Cymbalta, Drizalma Sprinkle

D

Class and Category

Pharmacologic class: Selective serotonin and norepinephrine reuptake inhibitor
Therapeutic class: Antidepressant, neuropathic and musculoskeletal pain reliever

Indications and Dosages

* *To treat major depressive disorder*

D.R. CAPSULES (CYMBALTA, DRIZALMA SPRINKLE)

Adults. *Initial:* 20 mg twice daily to 60 mg (given either as 60 mg once daily or as 30 mg twice daily), and then increased, as needed. Alternatively, 30 mg once daily for 1 wk before increasing, as needed. *Maintenance:* 60 mg/day. *Maximum:* 120 mg/day.

* *To relieve neuropathic pain associated with diabetic peripheral neuropathy*

D.R. CAPSULES (CYMBALTA, DRIZALMA SPRINKLE)

Adults. 60 mg once daily.

± **DOSAGE ADJUSTMENT** For adults with renal impairment and patients with lower tolerability, initial dosage reduced, and dosage increases done gradually.

* *To treat generalized anxiety disorder*

D.R. CAPSULES (CYMBALTA, DRIZALMA SPRINKLE)

Adults less than age 65. *Initial:* 60 mg once daily, increased in 30-mg increments weekly, as needed. Alternatively, 30 mg once daily for 1 wk, then increased to 60 mg once daily with further increases in 30-mg increments, as needed. *Maximum:* 120 mg once daily.

Adults ages 65 or older. *Initial:* 30 mg once daily for 2 wk, before dosage increased to 60 mg once daily. Further increases in dosage made in 30-mg increments weekly, as needed. *Maximum:* 120 mg once daily.

D.R. CAPSULES (CYMBALTA, DRIZALMA SPRINKLE)

Children ages 7 to 17. *Initial:* 30 mg once daily for 2 wk, then increased in 30-mg increments weekly, as needed. *Maximum:* 120 mg daily.

✱ *To treat fibromyalgia*

D.R. CAPSULES (CYMBALTA, DRIZALMA SPRINKLE)

Adults. *Initial:* 30 mg once daily for 1 wk; then increased to 60 mg once daily.

D.R. CAPSULES (CYMBALTA)

Adolescents ages 13 to 17. *Initial:* 30 mg once daily, increased to 60 mg once daily, as needed.

✱ *To treat chronic musculoskeletal pain*

D.R. CAPSULES (CYMBALTA, DRIZALMA SPRINKLE)

Adults. *Initial:* 30 mg once daily for 1 wk; then increased to 60 mg once daily.

± **DOSAGE ADJUSTMENT** For patients taking potent CYP1A2 inhibitors or who have hepatic impairment or severe renal impairment, drug therapy should be avoided.

Drug Administration

P.O.

- Cymbalta capsules should be swallowed whole and not chewed, crushed, or opened and given with or without food.
- Drizalma Sprinkle capsules may be swallowed whole without chewing or crushing capsule and given with or without food or opened and sprinkled on applesauce. Have patient swallow mixture immediately and do not store mixture.
- To administer Drizalma Sprinkle capsules via a nasogastric tube, open capsule and add contents to an all-plastic catheter-tip syringe and add 50 ml of water. Gently shake syringe for about 10 sec. Administer promptly through a 12-French or larger nasogastric tube. Check that no pellets are left in the syringe. Rinse syringe with about 15 ml of water, as needed.

Route	Onset	Peak	Duration
P.O.	Unknown	6 hr	Unknown

Half-life: 12 hr

Mechanism of Action

Inhibits dopamine, neuronal serotonin, and norepinephrine reuptake to potentiate noradrenergic and serotonergic activity in the CNS. These activities may elevate mood and inhibit pain signals stemming from peripheral nerves adversely affected by chronically elevated serum glucose level.

Contraindications

Chronic liver disease, including cirrhosis; hypersensitivity to duloxetine or its components; severe renal impairment (glomerular filtration rate less than 30 ml/min); use of linezolid or intravenous methylene blue; use of MAO inhibitors within 5 days of stopping duloxetine or within 14 days of stopping MAO inhibitors

Interactions

DRUGS

amphetamines, buspirone, fentanyl, intravenous methylene blue, lithium, linezolid, MAO inhibitors, opioids, selective serotonin reuptake inhibitors, serotonin norepinephrine reuptake inhibitors, St. John's Wort, tramadol, tricyclic antidepressants, triptans, tryptophan: Increased risk of serotonin syndrome

aspirin, NSAIDs, warfarin: Possibly increased risk of bleeding

cimetidine, fluoxetine, fluvoxamine, paroxetine, quinidine, quinolones: Increased blood duloxetine level

CNS drugs: Increased effect of duloxetine

CYP1A2, CYP2D6 inhibitors: Altered duloxetine metabolism

drugs that raise gastrointestinal pH: Possibly early release of duloxetine

phenothiazines, tricyclic antidepressants (such as amitriptyline, imipramine, nortriptyline), type 1C antiarrhythmics (such as flecainide, propafenone): Increased plasma levels of these drugs with possible increase in adverse reactions

thioridazine: Increased plasma thioridazine levels increasing risk of serious ventricular arrhythmias and sudden death

ACTIVITIES

alcohol use: Increased risk of hepatotoxicity

Adverse Reactions

CNS: Abnormal dreams, aggression, agitation, anger, anxiety, asthenia, chills, dizziness, extrapyramidal disorder, fatigue,

fever, hallucinations, headache, insomnia, migraine, nervousness, **neuroleptic malignant syndrome**, paresthesia, peripheral neuropathy, restless legs syndrome, **seizures**, **serotonin syndrome**, somnolence, **suicidal ideation**, syncope, tremor, vertigo
CV: Hypertension, **hypertensive crisis**, **MI**, orthostatic hypotension, palpitations, paresthesia, peripheral edema or coldness, **supraventricular arrhythmia**, tachycardia, **Takotsubo cardiomyopathy**
EENT: Acute-angle glaucoma, blurred vision, decrease or total loss of sense of smell, dry mouth, glaucoma, nasopharyngitis, oropharyngeal pain, pharyngitis, taste alteration, tinnitus
ENDO: Galactorrhea, hot flashes, hyperglycemia, hyperprolactinemia
GI: **Acute pancreatitis**, abdominal pain, anorexia, cholestatic jaundice, colitis, constipation, diarrhea, dyspepsia, elevated liver enzymes, flatulence, **hepatitis**, **hepatotoxicity**, indigestion, jaundice, nausea, upper abdominal pain, vomiting
GU: Abnormal orgasm; decreased libido; erectile or ejaculatory dysfunction; **gynecological bleeding**; urinary frequency, hesitancy, or retention; UTI
HEME: **Bleeding episodes** (may range from mild to **life-threatening**), **leukopenia**, **thrombocytopenia**
MS: Arthralgia, back or neck pain, extremity pain, muscle cramp or spasm, myalgia
RESP: Cough, upper respiratory tract infection
SKIN: Cutaneous vasculitis, diaphoresis, **erythema multiforme**, flushing, hyperhidrosis, pruritus, rash, **Stevens-Johnson syndrome**, urticaria
Other: **Anaphylaxis**, **angioedema**, discontinuation syndrome, flu-like symptoms, **hyponatremia**, weight gain or loss

Childbearing Considerations

PREGNANCY

- Pregnancy exposure registry: *For Cymbalta:* 1-866-961-2388 or https://womensmentalhealth.org/research/pregnancyregistry/. *For Drizalma Sprinkle:* 1-844-405-6185 or https://womensmentalealth.org/clinical-and-research-programs/pregnancyregistry/antidepressants/.
- It is not known if drug causes fetal harm. However, be aware that neonates exposed to the drug during pregnancy may develop serious and life-threatening adverse reactions, which can arise immediately following birth. These adverse reactions may require prolonged hospitalization, respiratory support, and tube feeding.
- Use with caution only if benefit to mother outweighs potential risk to fetus.
- Exposure to drug in mid to late pregnancy increases risk of preeclampsia.
- Use of drug in the month before delivery may increase risk of postpartum hemorrhage.

LACTATION

- Drug is present in breast milk.
- Mothers should check with prescriber before breastfeeding.
- If breastfeeding occurs, infant should be monitored for drowsiness, poor feeding, and poor weight gain.

Nursing Considerations

! WARNING Know that duloxetine should not be given to patients with severe renal impairment or end-stage renal disease that requires hemodialysis because blood drug levels increase significantly in these patients.

! WARNING Know that duloxetine should be avoided in patients with hepatic insufficiency or who use alcohol excessively because drug is metabolized by the liver. Keep in mind that patients with cirrhosis experience a half-life three times longer than people without liver disease. Expect to monitor patient's hepatic function, throughout therapy as ordered, because drug may increase the risk of hepatotoxicity. Expect duloxetine to be discontinued if patient develops jaundice or other serious liver dysfunction manifestation.

! WARNING Know that treatment with linezolid or I.V. methylene blue is not recommended while patient is taking duloxetine because of increased risk of serotonin syndrome. However, if prescriber feels benefits outweigh the risks, expect duloxetine to be discontinued promptly if serotonin syndrome occurs. Monitor patient closely for serotonin syndrome for 5 days or until 24 hours after the last dose of linezolid or I.V. methylene blue, whichever comes

D

first. Know that therapy with duloxetine may be resumed 24 hours after the last dose of linezolid or I.V. methylene blue.

- Screen patients for a personal or family history of bipolar disorder, mania, or hypomania, which drug may activate.
- Use duloxetine cautiously in patients with delayed gastric emptying because drug's enteric coating resists dissolution until it reaches an area where the pH exceeds 5.5.
- Give cautiously to patients with a seizure disorder because drug effects aren't known in these patients.
- Obtain patient's baseline blood pressure before duloxetine therapy starts and assess it periodically thereafter for changes. If orthostatic hypotension occurs during therapy, notify prescriber and anticipate that drug may have to be discontinued.

! **WARNING** Monitor patient for a hypersensitivity reaction, which could become life-threatening, such as anaphylaxis. If present, notify prescriber promptly, expect drug to be withheld, and provide supportive care, as needed and ordered.

! **WARNING** Inspect patient's skin and mucous membranes often because drug can cause serious skin reactions that could become life-threatening. Notify prescriber immediately if patient develops skin blisters or peeling as well as hives, rash, sores in the mouth, or any other skin reactions.

! **WARNING** Monitor patient for bleeding events because drug increases risk. Bleeding events can range from ecchymoses, epistaxis, hematomas, and petechiae to life-threatening hemorrhages. Know that concomitant use of aspirin, NSAIDs, or other drugs that affect coagulation increases risk.

! **WARNING** Monitor patient for depression that could worsen to point of suicidal ideation. especially at beginning of therapy and when dosage changes. Notify prescriber if abnormal behavior or thinking occurs. Institute suicide precautions.

! **WARNING** Monitor patient for serotonin syndrome, characterized by agitation, chills, confusion, diaphoresis, diarrhea, fever, hyperactive reflexes, poor coordination, restlessness, shaking, talking, or acting with uncontrolled excitement, tremor, and twitching. In its most severe form, serotonin syndrome can resemble neuroleptic malignant syndrome, which includes autonomic instability with possible fluctuations in vital signs, high fever, mental status changes, and muscle rigidity.

- Monitor patient's serum sodium level, as ordered, especially if patient is elderly, is taking a diuretic, or has volume depletion because drug may lower serum sodium level.
- Avoid stopping duloxetine therapy abruptly, if possible, because withdrawal symptoms, such as anxiety, diarrhea, dizziness, fatigue, headache, hyperhidrosis, insomnia, irritability, nausea, nightmares, paresthesia, vertigo, and vomiting may occur. Taper dosage gradually, as ordered.

PATIENT TEACHING

- Instruct patient how to administer form of duloxetine prescribed.
- Inform patient that full effect of duloxetine may take weeks to occur; emphasize the importance of continuing to take the drug as directed.

! **WARNING** Caution patient against excessive alcohol consumption while taking duloxetine because it may increase risk of hepatic dysfunction. Also, tell him to report a yellowing of eyes or skin immediately, as drug may have to be discontinued.

- Advise patient not to stop duloxetine abruptly because adverse reactions may occur.

! **WARNING** Alert patient that duloxetine may cause an allergic reaction. Tell patient to notify prescriber if an allergic reaction occurs and to seek immediate medical care, if severe.

! **WARNING** Stress importance of notifying prescriber if skin blisters or peeling occurs, as well as hives, rash, sores in the mouth, or any other allergic reactions.

! **WARNING** Advise patient that drug may increase risk of bleeding. Tell patient to notify prescriber if mild bleeding occurs or seek immediate medical attention if severe. Tell patient to consult prescriber before taking aspirin or NSAIDs.

! **WARNING** Urge family or caregiver to watch closely for evidence of suicidal tendencies, especially when therapy starts or dosage changes. Concerns should be addressed with prescriber.

! **WARNING** Instruct patient to notify prescriber if any serious or troublesome adverse effects develop, especially if they are persistent, severe, or unusual.

- Advise patient to avoid hazardous activities until drug's CNS effects are known and resolved.
- Instruct patient to rise from a lying or sitting position slowly to minimize drug's effect on lowering blood pressure, which may possibly lead to falls or cause patient to faint.
- Instruct patient with diabetes to monitor blood glucose levels more closely, as duloxetine therapy can alter control.
- Advise patient that drug may cause mild pupillary dilation, which may lead to an episode of acute-angle glaucoma. Encourage him to have an eye exam before starting therapy to see if he is at risk.
- Tell patient to notify prescriber of any new medication, including over-the-counter preparations, before using duloxetine.
- Instruct females of childbearing age to notify prescriber if pregnancy is suspected or occurs.
- Instruct mothers to monitor their breastfed infants for drowsiness, poor feeding, and poor weight gain.
- Advise patient to discuss any sexual dysfunction concerns with prescriber.

dupilumab

Dupixent

Class and Category

Pharmacologic class: Interleukin-4 receptor alpha antagonist
Therapeutic class: Monoclonal antibody

Indications and Dosages

* *To treat atopic dermatitis in patients whose disease is not adequately controlled with topical prescription therapies or when those therapies are not advisable*

SUBCUTANEOUS INJECTION

Adults and children ages 6 to 17 weighing 60 kg (132 lb) or more. *Initial:* 600 mg (two 300 mg injections), followed by 300 mg every other wk.
Children ages 6 to 17 weighing 30 kg (66 lb) to less than 60 kg (132 lb). *Initial:* 400 mg (two 200 mg injections), followed by 200 mg every other wk.
Children ages 6 to 17 weighing 15 kg (33 lb) to less than 30 kg (66 lb). *Initial:* 600 mg (two 300 mg injections), followed by 300 mg every 4 wk.
Infants and children ages 6 mo to 5 yr weighing 15 kg (33 lb) to less than 30 kg (66 lb). 300 mg every 4 wk.
Infants and children ages 6 mo to age 5 yr weighing 5 kg (11 lb) to less than 15 kg (33 lb). 200 mg every 4 wk.

* *As an add-on maintenance treatment for moderate-to-severe asthma characterized by an eosinophilic phenotype or patients with oral corticosteroid dependent-asthma*

SUBCUTANEOUS INJECTION

Adults and children ages 12 and older. *Initial:* 400 mg (two 200-mg injections), followed by 200 mg every 2 wk. Alternatively, initially 600 mg (two 300-mg injections), followed by 300 mg every 2 wk.
Children ages 6 to 11 weighing 30 kg (66 lb) or more. 200 mg every other wk.
Children ages 6 to 11 weighing 15 kg (33 lb) to less than 30 kg (66 lb). 300 mg every 4 wk.

± **DOSAGE ADJUSTMENT** For adults and children ages 12 and older with oral corticosteroid-dependent asthma or with co-morbid moderate-to-severe atopic dermatitis; or adults with co-morbid chronic rhinosinusitis with nasal polyps, dosage increased to 600 mg (two 300-mg injections) initially followed by 300 mg every 2 wk. For children ages 6 to 11 with asthma and co-morbid moderate-to-severe atopic dermatitis, dosage followed for atopic dermatitis, which includes a loading dose.

* *As an add-on maintenance treatment in patients with inadequately controlled chronic rhinosinusitis with nasal polyps (CRSwNP)*

SUBCUTANEOUS INJECTION

Adults and children ages 12 and older. 300 mg every other week.

D

✷ *To treat eosinophilic esophagitis (EoE)*

SUBCUTANEOUS INJECTION

Adults and children ages 1 and older weighing at least 40 kg (88 lb). 300 mg every week.
Children ages 1 and older weighing 30 kg (66 lb) to less than 40 kg (88 lb). 300 mg every other wk.
Children ages 1 and older weighing 15 kg (33 lb) to less than 30 kg (66 lb). 200 mg every other wk.

✷ *To treat prurigo nodularis*

Adults. 600 mg (two 300-mg injections) followed by 300 mg every other wk.

✷ *As an add-on maintenance treatment for inadequately controlled COPD with an eosinophilic phenotype*

Adults. 300 mg every other wk.

Drug Administration

SUBCUTANEOUS

- Remove single-dose prefilled pen or syringe from refrigerator and allow it to reach room temperature (45 min for the 300-mg/2-ml pen or syringe or 30 min for the 200-mg/1.4-ml pen or syringe). Once at room temperature, use within 14 days or discard.
- Inspect solution in pen or syringe. It should appear clear to slightly opalescent, colorless to pale yellow. Do not use if solution appears differently.
- Administer the drug using the prefilled pen on adults and children ages 2 and older; use the prefilled syringe on adults and children ages 6 months and older.
- Do not inject drug into an area that is bruised, damaged, scarred, or tender.
- Administer into the abdomen, thigh, or upper arm. If two injections are required, administer the injections in different sites. Rotate sites.
- Discard any unused solution remaining in the pen or syringe after administration because drug does not contain preservatives.

Route	Onset	Peak	Duration
SubQ	Unknown	1 wk	Unknown

Half-life: Unknown

Mechanism of Action

May inhibit interleukin signaling of IL-4 and IL-13, thought to be responsible for inflammation present in the pathogenesis of asthma, atopic dermatitis, CRSwNP, and EoE although drug's precise mechanism of action is unknown.

Contraindications

Hypersensitivity to dupilumab or its components

Interactions

DRUGS

None reported by manufacturer.

Adverse Reactions

CNS: **CVA**, dizziness, insomnia
CV: **MI**
EENT: Blepharitis, conjunctivitis, dry eye, eye pruritus, keratitis, nasopharyngitis, oral herpes, oropharyngeal pain, toothache
GI: Diarrhea, gastritis
HEME: Eosinophilia
MS: Arthralgia, myalgia
RESP: Upper respiratory tract infections
SKIN: Dermatitis (atopic or exfoliative), erythema nodosum, **erythema multiforme**, facial skin reactions (burning, edema, erythema, pain, papules, pruritus, rash, scaling), urticaria
Other: **Anaphylaxis**, **angioedema**, anti-dupilumab antibodies, helminth infection, herpes simplex viral infection, injection site reactions (bruising, erythema, inflammation, pain, pruritus, swelling), serum sickness like illness

Childbearing Considerations

PREGNANCY

- Pregnancy exposure registry: 1-877-311-8972 or https://mothertobaby.org/ongoing-study/dupixent/.
- It is not known if drug can cause fetal harm although human IgG antibodies are known to cross the placental barrier.
- Use with caution only if benefit to mother outweighs potential risk to fetus.

LACTATION

- It is not known if drug is present in breast milk.
- Mothers should check with prescriber before breastfeeding.

Nursing Considerations

! **WARNING** Know that dupilumab should not be used to treat acute asthma exacerbations or symptoms such as acute bronchospasm or status asthmaticus.

! **WARNING** Be aware that corticosteroid therapy (inhaled, systemic, or topical) should not be discontinued abruptly when dupilumab therapy is begun because systemic withdrawal symptoms or unmasking of conditions previously suppressed may occur.

- Know that patients with a helminth infection should be treated before dupilumab therapy is started because it is unknown if the drug alters the immune response against helminth infections. If patient develops a helminth infection during drug therapy, expect infection to be treated appropriately but, if unresolved, expect dupilumab to be withheld until the infection has been resolved.
- Ensure that patient is up to date on vaccinations prior to initiating dupilumab therapy. Know that administration of live vaccines should be avoided because it is unknown if dupilumab may alter the effectiveness or safety of these vaccines.
- Be aware that topical corticosteroids may be used in conjunction with dupilumab to treat atopic dermatitis.

! **WARNING** Monitor patient for hypersensitivity reactions that may become life-threatening, such as anaphylaxis or angioedema. If present, notify prescriber, expect drug to be discontinued, and provide supportive care as needed and ordered.

! **WARNING** Monitor patient with asthma receiving dupilumab for eosinophilic conditions that may become serious causing eosinophilic pneumonia or vasculitis.

- Monitor patient for conjunctivitis and keratitis, especially in patients being treated for atopic dermatitis. Expect patient to receive an ophthalmological examination if condition does not improve with treatment.

PATIENT TEACHING

- Instruct patient and family or caregiver how to administer dupilumab as a subcutaneous injection and what to do if a dose is missed. However, tell family or caregiver that if patient is younger than 12 years of age, the drug should be administered only by family or caregiver.
- Alert patient and family or caregiver that drug does not contain preservatives so any unused solution remaining in the pen or syringe after administration should be discarded.

! **WARNING** Stress importance of not discontinuing corticosteroid therapy abruptly when starting dupilumab therapy.

! **WARNING** Tell patient not to use dupilumab to treat acute bronchospasms or status asthmaticus and to contact prescriber if asthma remains uncontrolled or worsens after dupilumab therapy is begun. Instruct patient with asthma not to alter or stop asthma treatments while receiving dupilumab therapy without checking with prescriber first.

! **WARNING** Instruct patient that if patient injects too much dupilumab, patient should call prescriber immediately or the Poison Help line at 1-800-222-1222.

! **WARNING** Alert patient that drug may cause an allergic reaction. If present, tell patient to notify prescriber and to seek immediate medical care, if severe.

- Advise patient to report new or worsening eye problems to prescriber.
- Tell patient to alert prescriber if decreased mobility or gait disturbances accompanied with joint symptoms occur.

dutasteride

Avodart

Class and Category

Pharmacologic class: 5-alpha-reductase enzyme inhibitor
Therapeutic class: Benign prostatic hyperplasia agent

Indications and Dosages

∗ *To treat symptomatic benign prostatic hyperplasia (BPH); as adjunct with tamsulosin therapy to treat symptomatic BPH*

CAPSULES

Adult men. 0.5 mg daily.

Drug Administration

P.O.

- Handle drug carefully, as it is a known teratogen. Female medical personnel who

Mechanism of Action

Reduces prostate gland enlargement by inhibiting conversion of testosterone to its active metabolite, 5-alpha dihydrotestosterone (DHT). DHT is the main hormone that stimulates prostate cells to grow. As men age, they may become more sensitive to DHT, resulting in excessive growth of prostatic cells and enlargement of the prostate. This condition, benign prostatic hyperplasia, may cause nocturia, urinary hesitancy, and urinary urgency.

Two forms of the intracellular enzyme 5-alpha-reductase (5α-R types 1 and2) in liver, prostate, and skin, convert testosterone to DHT, as shown below left. Dutasteride, a dual 5α-R inhibitor, deactivates both forms. When 5α-R is inhibited by dutasteride, production of DHT is suppressed, as shown below right. With less circulating DHT, the prostate gland shrinks and symptoms improve.

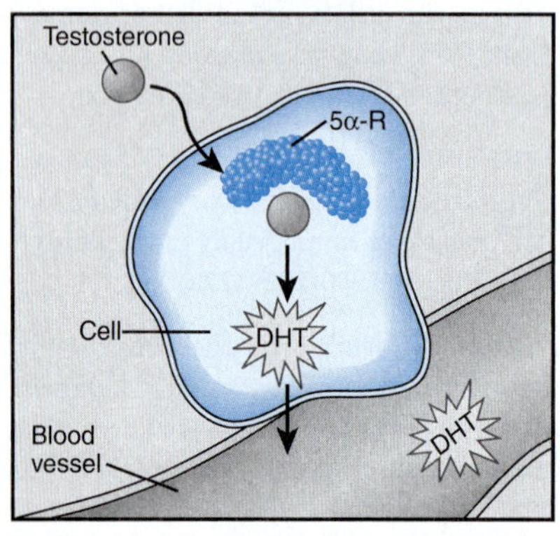

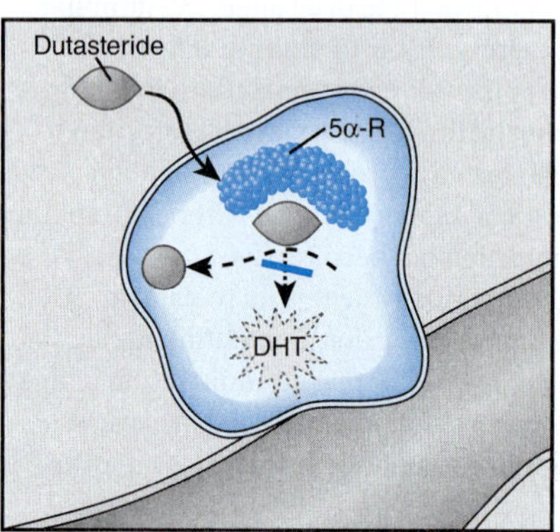

are pregnant or suspect pregnancy should not touch capsules. Follow institutional policies for handling and disposal procedure.

- Capsules should be swallowed whole and not chewed, crushed, or opened.

Route	Onset	Peak	Duration
P.O.	Unknown	2–3 hr	Unknown

Half-life: 5 wk

Contraindications

Children; hypersensitivity to dutasteride, other 5-alpha reductase inhibitors, or their components; pregnancy; females of childbearing age

Interactions

DRUGS

CYP3A4 inhibitors, such as cimetidine, ciprofloxacin, diltiazem, ketoconazole, ritonavir, verapamil: Increased dutasteride exposure and enhanced effects, including increased risk of adverse reactions

Adverse Reactions

CNS: Depression, dizziness
ENDO: Gynecomastia, increased serum testosterone and thyroid-stimulating hormone levels, **male breast cancer**
GU: Decreased ejaculatory volume, decreased libido, **high-grade prostate cancer**, impotence, testicular pain and swelling
SKIN: Localized edema, pruritus, rash, serious skin reactions, urticaria
Other: **Angioedema**, **hypersensitivity reactions**, **male breast cancer**

Childbearing Considerations

PREGNANCY

- Drug may cause fetal harm, such as abnormalities in the genitalia of male fetuses if pregnant women come in contact with drug.
- Drug is not prescribed for women.

LACTATION

- Drug is not prescribed for women.

REPRODUCTION

- Be aware that drug's effect on fertility of male patients is unknown. However, there is some evidence to suggest drug may decrease sperm count.

- Patient or female partner should use an effective contraceptive during drug therapy as drug appears in semen.

Nursing Considerations

! **WARNING** Be aware that dutasteride is absorbed through the skin, so females of childbearing age, including pregnant females who are healthcare workers should not handle dutasteride capsules.

! **WARNING** Know that patient should be evaluated for other urologic conditions, including prostate cancer, before dutasteride therapy starts because dutasteride therapy increases risk of patient developing high-grade prostate cancer.

- Expect patient to undergo a digital rectal examination of the prostate before and periodically during dutasteride therapy.

! **WARNING** Monitor patient for a hypersensitivity reaction, which could become life-threatening, such as angioedema. If present, notify prescriber promptly, expect drug to be discontinued, and provide supportive care, as needed and ordered.

- Anticipate need to obtain a new baseline prostate-specific antigen (PSA) value after 3 to 6 months of dutasteride treatment because drug can decrease PSA concentration by 40% to 50%. Dutasteride also can decrease serum PSA level even in the presence of prostate cancer. Any PSA reading in a patient receiving dutasteride should be doubled for comparison with normal values in untreated men. If value still falls within the normal range for men not taking a 5-alpha-reductase inhibitor, further evaluation should still be done to rule out prostate cancer.

PATIENT TEACHING

! **WARNING** Urge patient and female partners to use reliable contraceptive method during dutasteride therapy because semen of men who take drug can harm male fetuses being carried by female partner. Caution females of childbearing age and children against handling capsules.

- Instruct patient how to administer dutasteride.

! **WARNING** Alert patient that dutasteride may cause an allergic reaction. If present, tell patient to notify prescriber promptly and if severe, to seek immediate medical care.

- Inform patient that drug may decrease ejaculatory volume and libido and may cause impotence.
- Instruct patient to postpone blood donations for 6 months after final dose to avoid transmitting dutasteride to a pregnant woman during a blood transfusion.
- Urge patient to have periodic follow-up appointments.

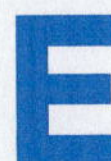

edoxaban tosylate

Savaysa

Class and Category

Pharmacologic class: Factor Xa inhibitor
Therapeutic class: Anticoagulant

Indications and Dosages

✱ To reduce risk of stroke and systemic embolism in nonvalvular atrial fibrillation

TABLETS

Adults. 60 mg once daily.

±**DOSAGE ADJUSTMENT** For patients with impaired renal failure (creatinine clearance between 15 and 50 ml/min), dosage reduced to 30 mg once daily. For patients with a creatinine clearance greater than 95 ml/min, dosage should not be given because of increased risk of ischemic stroke.

✱ To treat deep vein thrombosis and pulmonary embolism

TABLETS

Adults weighing more than 60 kg (132 lb). 60 mg once daily following 5 to 10 days of initial therapy with a parenteral anticoagulant.

±**DOSAGE ADJUSTMENT** For patients with impaired renal failure (creatinine clearance between 15 and 50 ml/min), patients who weigh less than or equal to 60 kg (132 lb), or patients who are taking selected concomitant P-gp inhibitors, dosage reduced to 30 mg once daily.

Drug Administration

P.O.

- Administer with or without food.
- For a patient unable to swallow tablets, crush tablet and mix with 60 to 90 ml of water and immediately administer by mouth or gastric tube. Crushed tablet may also be mixed with applesauce and immediately given by mouth. Do not store mixture.
- If a dose is missed, administer as soon as possible on the same day and then resume dosing on the next day according to the patient's normal dosing schedule. Never double the dose to make up for a missed dose.
- Know that when a patient is being transitioned to edoxaban from warfarin or other vitamin K antagonists, warfarin should be discontinued and edoxaban started when the international normalized ratio (INR) is 2.5 or less. When patient is being transitioned from oral anticoagulants other than warfarin or other vitamin K antagonists, the current oral anticoagulant should be discontinued and edoxaban started at the time of the next scheduled dose of the other oral anticoagulant. When patient is being transitioned from low-molecular-weight heparin, the low-molecular-weight heparin should be discontinued and edoxaban started at the time of the next scheduled administration of the low-molecular-weight heparin. When patient is being transitioned from unfractionated heparin, the unfractionated heparin infusion should be discontinued and edoxaban started 4 hours later.
- Be aware that when a patient is being transitioned from edoxaban (60-mg dose) to warfarin, the dose of edoxaban should be reduced to 30 mg and warfarin begun concomitantly. When a patient is being transitioned from edoxaban (30-mg dose) to warfarin, the dose of edoxaban should be reduced to 15 mg and warfarin begun concomitantly. When a stable INR of 2 or greater is achieved in either situation, edoxaban should be discontinued. When patient is being transitioned from edoxaban to a parenteral anticoagulant and warfarin, edoxaban should be discontinued and a parenteral anticoagulant and warfarin administered, as ordered, at the same time of the next scheduled edoxaban dose. Once a stable INR of 2 or greater is achieved, the parenteral anticoagulant should be discontinued, and warfarin therapy continued. Be aware that when a patient is being transitioned from edoxaban to a non-vitamin K–dependent oral anticoagulant, edoxaban should be discontinued and the other oral anticoagulant started at the time of the next dose of edoxaban. Know that when a patient is being transitioned from edoxaban to a parenteral anticoagulant,

edoxaban should be discontinued and the parenteral anticoagulant should be started at the time of the next dose of edoxaban.

Route	Onset	Peak	Duration
P.O.	Unknown	1–2 hr	Unknown

Half-life: 10–14 hr

Mechanism of Action

Inhibits free FXa and prothrombinase activity and inhibits thrombin-induced platelet aggregation. By inhibiting FXa in the coagulation cascade, thrombin generation and formation is reduced.

Contraindications

Active pathological bleeding, hypersensitivity to edoxaban or its components

Interactions

DRUGS

anticoagulants, antiplatelets, aspirin or aspirin-containing products, NSAIDs (long-term use), selective serotonin reuptake inhibitors, serotonin norepinephrine reuptake inhibitors, thrombolytics: Increased risk of bleeding
quinidine, verapamil, or short-term concomitant administration of azithromycin, clarithromycin, erythromycin, oral itraconazole, or oral ketoconazole: Increased blood level with increased risk of bleeding in patients being treated for deep venous thrombosis or pulmonary embolism
rifampin: Decreased effectiveness of edoxaban

Adverse Reactions

CNS: Dizziness, headache, **intracranial bleeding**
EENT: Epistaxis, intraocular bleeding
GI: Abdominal pain, elevated liver enzymes, **GI bleeding**
GU: Anticoagulant-related nephropathy, hematuria, uterine or vaginal bleeding
HEME: Anemia, **bleeding, thrombocytopenia**
RESP: **Interstitial lung disease**
SKIN: Rash, urticaria
Other: **Angioedema, hypersensitivity reactions**

Childbearing Considerations

PREGNANCY

- Drug may cause fetal harm because use of drug may increase risk of bleeding in the fetus and neonate.
- Use with caution only if benefit to mother outweighs potential risk to fetus.

LABOR AND DELIVERY

- Drug withheld, if possible, and replaced with a shorter-acting anticoagulant as delivery approaches because of increased risk of bleeding.

LACTATION

- It is not known if drug is present in breast milk.
- Breastfeeding is not recommended during drug therapy.

REPRODUCTION

- Females of childbearing age should discuss pregnancy plans with prescriber because drug may cause significant uterine bleeding that may require surgical intervention.

Nursing Considerations

! **WARNING** Keep in mind that edoxaban is not recommended for use in patients with a mechanical heart valve or who have moderate to severe mitral stenosis because the effects of edoxaban in these patients are unknown. Drug is also not recommended for use in patients with triple positive antiphospholipid syndrome because of an increased risk for thrombosis.

! **WARNING** Monitor patient for a hypersensitivity reaction, which could become life-threatening such as angioedema. If present, notify prescriber, expect drug to be discontinued and another anticoagulant drug substituted for edoxaban, and provide supportive care, as needed and ordered.

! **WARNING** Monitor patient closely for bleeding. If present, notify prescriber immediately because there is no antidote to reverse the anticoagulation effects of edoxaban, which may last for up to 24 hours after the last dose. Know that patients who take other drugs that affect hemostasis, such as aspirin and other antiplatelet agents, chronic use of NSAIDs, fibrinolytic therapy, or other antithrombotic drugs, are at increased risk for bleeding.

! **WARNING** Know that the use of anticoagulants, including edoxaban, may increase the risk of bleeding in the fetus and neonate. Monitor neonate for bleeding if mother was taking edoxaban prior to birth.

! **WARNING** Expect to administer another anticoagulant, as ordered, if edoxaban must be discontinued for reasons other than the presence of active bleeding. This is because premature discontinuation of edoxaban increases the risk of ischemic events.

! **WARNING** Be aware that edoxaban should be withheld for at least 24 hours before invasive or surgical procedures are performed to reduce the risk of bleeding. If it is not possible to delay the procedure, monitor patient closely for bleeding. If edoxaban was withheld, know that it may be restarted after the invasive or surgical procedure as soon as the patient has achieved adequate hemostasis. Be prepared to administer a parenteral anticoagulant if oral medication cannot be initially taken and then when oral medication can be taken, the patient may be switched to edoxaban.

! **WARNING** Monitor patient receiving edoxaban and epidural or spinal anesthesia or spinal puncture because spinal hematomas can occur, causing long-term or permanent paralysis. Be aware indwelling epidural or intrathecal catheters should not be removed earlier than 12 hours after the last administration of edoxaban and the next dose of the drug should not be administered earlier than 2 hours after the removal of the catheter. Watch for evidence of neurologic impairment, such as changes in motor or sensory function. If present, notify prescriber immediately; patient needs urgent care to minimize effect of hematoma. Concurrent use of other drugs that affect hemostasis, such as NSAIDs, platelet inhibitors, and other anticoagulants; a history of repeated or traumatic epidural or spinal punctures; a history of spinal deformity or spinal surgery; or use of indwelling epidural catheters increases the risk of epidural or spinal hematoma in patients receiving edoxaban.

PATIENT TEACHING

- Instruct patient how to administer edoxaban and what to do if a dose is missed.
- Caution patient not to stop taking edoxaban without talking to the prescriber first.

! **WARNING** Alert patient that drug may cause an allergic reaction. If present, tell patient to notify prescriber and, if severe, to seek immediate medical care.

! **WARNING** Instruct patient on bleeding precautions. If bleeding occurs, tell her to report any unusual bleeding immediately to the prescriber and seek emergency medical care.

! **WARNING** Stress importance for females of childbearing age to discuss desire for a future pregnancy because drug can cause significant uterine bleeding that may require surgery to stop the bleeding. Also, tell these patients to notify prescriber if pregnancy occurs during therapy. This is because anticoagulants, including edoxaban, may increase the risk of bleeding in the fetus and neonate. Tell mother who took edoxaban during late pregnancy to watch neonate for bleeding.

! **WARNING** Alert patient who is having neuraxial anesthesia or spinal puncture to immediately report signs and symptoms suggestive of epidural or spinal hematomas, such as back pain, muscle weakness, numbness (especially in the lower limbs), stool or urine incontinence, and tingling.

- Advise mothers that breastfeeding is not recommended during edoxaban therapy because of the potential risk of serious adverse reactions.
- Tell patient to alert all healthcare providers and dentists that edoxaban is being taken and to consult the prescriber before taking any new drugs, including over-the-counter drugs.

efavirenz

Sustiva

Class and Category

Pharmacologic class: Non-nucleoside reverse transcriptase inhibitor
Therapeutic class: Antiretroviral

Indications and Dosages

✳ *As adjunct to treat human immunodeficiency virus type 1 (HIV-1) in combination with other antiretroviral agents*

CAPSULES, TABLETS

Adults and children ages 3 mo and older and weighing 40 kg (88 lb) or more. 600 mg once daily.
Children ages 3 mo and older and weighing 32.5 kg (71.5 lb) to less than 40 kg (88 lb). 400 mg once daily.
Children ages 3 mo and older and weighing 25 kg (55 lb) to less than 32.5 kg (71.5 lb). 350 mg once daily.
Children ages 3 mo and older and weighing 20 kg (44 lb) to less than 25 kg (55 lb). 300 mg once daily.
Children ages 3 mo and older and weighing 15 kg (33 lb) to less than 20 kg (44 lb). 250 mg once daily.
Children ages 3 mo and older and weighing 7.5 kg (16.5 lb) to less than 15 kg (33 lb). 200 mg once daily.
Children ages 3 mo and older and weighing 5 kg (11 lb) to less than 7.5 kg (16.5 lb). 150 mg once daily.
Children ages 3 mo and older and weighing 3.5 kg (7.7 lb) to less than 5 kg (11 lb). 100 mg once daily.

±**DOSAGE ADJUSTMENT** For adult patients weighing 50 kg (110 lb) or more and also receiving rifampin, dosage increased to 800 mg once daily. For adult patients receiving voriconazole concurrently, dosage decreased to 300 mg once daily.

Drug Administration

P.O.

- Administer on an empty stomach preferably at bedtime.
- Be prepared to administer an antihistamine, as ordered, before giving drug to a child to reduce the risk of a rash.
- Tablets and capsules should be swallowed whole and not chewed or crushed.
- For adults and children who cannot swallow capsules or tablets, have prescriber order capsule form. Carefully hold capsule horizontally over a small container and carefully twist open. Sprinkle on 1 to 2 teaspoons of soft food (applesauce, grape jelly, or yogurt) and mixed gently. Administer within 30 min.
- For infants, mix contents of capsule (being careful to hold capsule horizontally over a small container and carefully twist open) with 10 ml of reconstituted infant formula that is at room temperature. Draw up mixture in a 10-ml oral dosing syringe and administer. Add 10 ml of formula to cup used to make mixture and stir. Draw up in a 10-ml oral dosing syringe and administer. Use mixture within 30 min.
- Do not give patient any food or formula for 2 hr after administration.

Route	Onset	Peak	Duration
P.O.	Unknown	3–5 hr	Unknown

Half-life: 40–76 hr

Mechanism of Action

Inhibits HIV integrase by binding to the integrase active site and blocking the strand transfer step of retroviral DNA integration, which is needed for the HIV replication cycle.

Contraindications

Concurrent therapy with elbasvir and grazoprevir, hypersensitivity to efavirenz or its components

Interactions

DRUGS

artemether, atazanavir, atorvastatin, atovaquone, boceprevir, bupropion, clarithromycin, cyclosporine, dihydroartemisinin, diltiazem, ethinyl estradiol/norgestimate, etonogestrel implant, felodipine, fosamprenavir, hydroxyitraconazole, immunosuppressants, indinavir, ketoconazole, itraconazole, lopinavir, lumefantrine, maraviroc, methadone, nicardipine, nifedipine, posaconazole, pravastatin, praziquantel, proguanil, rifabutin, saquinavir, sertraline, simeprevir, simvastatin, sirolimus, tacrolimus, velpatasvir/sofosbuvir, velpatasvir/sofosbuvir/voxilaprevir, verapamil: Decreased effectiveness of these drugs
carbamazepine, phenobarbital, phenytoin: Decreased plasma levels of both drugs
CYP3A inducers: Decreased plasma levels of efavirenz with decreased effectiveness
elbasvir/grazoprevir, pibrentasvir/glecaprevir: Possibly loss of virologic response and reduced therapeutic effect
other non-nucleoside reverse transcriptase inhibitors: Decreased or increased plasma levels of both drugs without added efficacy

psychoactive drugs: Possibly additive central nervous system effects
QT prolongation drugs, such as artemether/lumefantrine, clarithromycin: Increased risk of torsades de pointes
rifabutin: Decreased plasma levels of both drugs decreasing effectiveness
rifampin: Decreased plasma efavirenz levels with possible decrease in effectiveness
ritonavir: Increased plasma levels of both efavirenz and ritonavir, possibly leading to elevated liver enzymes and other adverse reactions
voriconazole: Decreased voriconazole level and increased plasma efavirenz
warfarin: Decreased or increased warfarin levels, requiring close monitoring of INR and adjustment of warfarin dosage as needed

ACTIVITIES

alcohol use: Possibly increased additive central nervous system effects

Adverse Reactions

CNS: Abnormal dreams, aggression, agitation, amnesia, anxiety, asthenia, ataxia, catatonia, cerebellar balance and coordination disturbances, confusion, delusions, depersonalization, depression (severe), dizziness, emotional lability, **encephalopathy**, euphoria, fatigue, fever, hallucinations, headache, hypoesthesia, impaired concentration, insomnia, paranoid behavior, manic reactions, nervousness, neuropathy, neurosis, paranoia, paresthesia, psychosis-like behavior, **seizures**, somnolence, stupor, **suicidal ideation**, tremor, vertigo
CV: Elevated cholesterol and triglyceride levels, palpitations, **QT prolongation**
EENT: Abnormal vision, tinnitus
ENDO: Cushingoid appearance, fat redistribution, gynecomastia, hyperglycemia
GI: Abdominal pain, anorexia, constipation, diarrhea, dyspepsia, elevated amylase or liver enzymes, **hepatic failure**, **hepatitis**, **hepatotoxicity**, malabsorption, nausea, **pancreatitis**, vomiting
HEME: **Neutropenia**
MS: Arthralgia, myalgia, myopathy
RESP: Dyspnea
SKIN: Blisters, **erythema multiforme**, flushing, moist desquamation, photoallergic dermatitis, pruritus, rash, **Stevens-Johnson syndrome**, ulcerations
Other: **Hypersensitivity reactions**, nonspecific pain, **immune reconstitution syndrome**

Childbearing Considerations

PREGNANCY

- Pregnancy exposure registry: 1-800-258-4263.
- Be aware pregnancy testing should be done in females of childbearing age prior to initiation of drug therapy.
- It is not known if drug causes fetal harm. However, there are retrospective reports of neural tube defects in infants whose mothers were exposed to an efavirenz-containing regimen in the first trimester of pregnancy.
- Drug should not be given during the first trimester of pregnancy.

LACTATION

- It is not known if drug is present in breast milk.
- The Centers for Disease Control and Prevention recommends that HIV-1 infected mothers not breastfeed to avoid risking postnatal transmission of HIV-1 infection to infants. They also do not recommend breastfeeding because of potential drug-induced adverse reactions in the infant.

REPRODUCTION

- Effective contraceptive measures should be in place prior to beginning drug therapy as well as throughout therapy and for 12 wk after drug is discontinued.
- Barrier contraception should always be used in combination with other methods of contraception.
- Know that hormonal methods of contraception that contain progesterone may not be as effective.

Nursing Considerations

! WARNING Know that drug should not be used in patients taking other medications with a known risk of torsades de pointes or in patients at higher risk of torsades de pointes because efavirenz may cause QT prolongation.

! WARNING Ensure that females of childbearing age have a negative pregnancy

E

test result before efavirenz therapy begins because drug may cause fetal harm if given during the first trimester.

- Be aware that efavirenz should not be used as a single agent in treating HIV infection because resistant virus emerges quickly when drug is used alone.
- Know that efavirenz therapy is not recommended with the combination drug, Atripla, which contains efavirenz, unless needed for dose adjustment when coadministered with rifampin.
- Obtain cholesterol and triglyceride levels, as ordered, before efavirenz is begun and periodically throughout therapy because drug may cause an increase in total cholesterol and triglycerides.

! **WARNING** Obtain liver enzymes, as ordered, before therapy begins in patients with marked transaminase elevations; patients treated with other medications associated with liver toxicity; and patients with underlying hepatic disease, including hepatitis B or C infections. Also, monitor liver enzymes throughout therapy, as ordered, on all patients because efavirenz may cause hepatotoxicity. Know that persistent elevations of serum transaminase levels greater than 5 times the upper limit of the normal range may require efavirenz therapy to be discontinued.

! **WARNING** Use efavirenz cautiously in patients with a history of seizures, as drug may increase risk of seizures. Know that if patient is also taking anticonvulsant medications metabolized by the liver, such as phenobarbital or phenytoin, periodic monitoring of plasma levels of these drugs may be required.

! **WARNING** Monitor patient for a hypersensitivity reaction such as a rash. While usually mild to moderate, occurring within the first 2 weeks of therapy, and resolving within a month, a rash rarely may evolve into more serious skin conditions that could become life-threatening and should be reported. Know that drug may be reinstated after drug therapy is interrupted because of a rash if it was not severe. However, if rash was severe, be aware that drug should be discontinued and antihistamines and/or corticosteroid therapy given to treat rash, as ordered.

! **WARNING** Monitor patient for serious psychiatric adverse reactions, such as aggressive behavior, manic reactions, paranoia, severe depression, or suicidal ideation. Patients at increased risk include patients with drug addiction (injected) or psychiatric history, including the use of psychiatric drugs.

! **WARNING** Monitor patient for nervous system symptoms that commonly occur with efavirenz use. Be especially watchful for abnormal dreams, dizziness, hallucinations, impaired concentration, insomnia, and somnolence. Be aware that these symptoms usually occur within a day or two of starting therapy and usually resolve in the first 2 to 4 weeks. However, know that late-onset neurotoxicity, including ataxia and encephalopathy, may occur months to years after beginning efavirenz therapy.

! **WARNING** Be aware that immune reconstitution syndrome has occurred in patients treated with combination antiretroviral therapy, including efavirenz. The inflammatory response predisposes susceptible patients to opportunistic infections, such as cytomegalovirus, *Mycobacterium avium* infection, *Pneumocystis jiroveci* pneumonia, or tuberculosis. Autoimmune disorders, such as Graves' disease, Guillain-Barré syndrome, or polymyositis have also occurred. Report sudden or unusual adverse reactions to prescriber.

PATIENT TEACHING

- Inform patient that efavirenz is administered with other antiretroviral agents.
- Instruct patient, family, or caregiver how to administer efavirenz and to follow administration instructions as ordered.
- Inform patient, family, or caregiver that neurological adverse reactions, such as drowsiness, dizziness, impaired concentration, and insomnia may occur in the first weeks of efavirenz therapy but taking drug at bedtime will help and symptoms should diminish with continued therapy.

! **WARNING** Warn females of childbearing age that efavirenz may cause fetal harm when administered during the first trimester of pregnancy. Stress importance of using reliable birth control and tell patient to alert prescriber immediately if pregnancy occurs.

! **WARNING** Alert patient, family, or caregiver that drug may cause an allergic reaction such as a rash. Inform patient that although usually mild, an allergic reaction can become severe. If an allergic reaction occurs, especially a rash, tell patient, family, or caregiver to notify prescriber and, if severe, to seek immediate medical care.

! **WARNING** Warn family or caregiver that drug may cause psychiatric symptoms including suicidal thoughts. Stress importance of watching patient closely for evidence of suicidal behavior or thinking and notifying prescriber of any concerns.

! **WARNING** Inform patient drug may cause seizures. If a seizure occurs tell patient to notify prescriber immediately. Also, alert patient to the possibility of late-onset neurotoxicity that may occur months to years after beginning efavirenz therapy. Encourage patient to report any abnormal neurological signs and symptoms regardless of how long efavirenz therapy has been taken.

- Instruct patient, family, or caregiver to notify prescriber of any persistent, severe, or unusual adverse reactions as drug can affect the function of many body systems.
- Alert patient, family, or caregiver that drug may increase risk of an infection. Review signs and symptoms of an infection with patient, family, or caregiver and what infection control measures to take. Tell patient, family, or caregiver to notify prescriber, if an infection occurs.
- Inform patient and family or caregiver that efavirenz therapy may cause changes in his body appearance because of fat redistribution. Prepare him for the possibility of developing breast enlargement, central obesity, dorsocervical fat enlargement (buffalo hump), facial wasting, and peripheral wasting.
- Advise patient, family, or caregiver to contact prescriber before taking any new drugs, including over-the-counter preparations and herbals.
- Caution patient to avoid hazardous activities, such as driving, until nervous system effects are known and resolved.
- Inform mothers that breastfeeding should not be done while taking efavirenz.

eletriptan hydrobromide

Relpax

Class and Category

Pharmacologic class: Triptan
Therapeutic class: Antimigraine agent

Indications and Dosages

∗ *To relieve acute migraine attacks with or without aura*

TABLETS

Adults. *Initial:* 20 or 40 mg as a single dose at first sign of migraine. Repeated in 2 hr, as needed. *Maximum:* 40 mg as single dose, 80 mg daily; and no more than 3 treated migraines in 30-day period.

Drug Administration

P.O.

- Tablets should be swallowed whole and not chewed, crushed, or divided.
- Following administration, have patient drink a full glass of water.

Route	Onset	Peak	Duration
P.O.	0.5 hr	1.5–2 hr	Unknown

Half-life: 4 hr

Mechanism of Action

May stimulate 5-HT_1 receptors, causing selective vasoconstriction of dilated and inflamed cranial blood vessels in carotid circulation, which decreases carotid arterial blood flow and relieves acute migraines.

Contraindications

Bibasilar or hemiplegic migraine, cardiovascular disease (significant), cerebrovascular syndromes (stroke, transient ischemic attack), hepatic impairment (severe), hypersensitivity to eletriptan or components, ischemic bowel disease, ischemic or vasospastic coronary artery disease (CAD), peripheral vascular disease, uncontrolled hypertension, use within 24 hr of another serotonin 5-HT_1 receptor agonist or ergot-type drug, use within 72 hr of a potent CYP3A4 inhibitor (clarithromycin, itraconazole, ketoconazole, nefazodone, nelfinavir, ritonavir, troleandomycin), Wolff-Parkinson-White syndrome or arrhythmias associated with other cardiac accessory conduction pathway disorders.

Interactions

DRUGS

clarithromycin, ketoconazole, itraconazole, nefazodone, nelfinavir, ritonavir, troleandomycin, and other potent CYP3A4 inhibitors: Increase blood eletriptan level significantly

ergot-containing drugs, 5-HT_1 receptor agonists: Possibly additive or prolonged vasoconstrictive effects

MAO inhibitors, selective serotonin norepinephrine reuptake inhibitors, selective serotonin reuptake inhibitors, tricyclic antidepressants: Increased risk of serotonin syndrome

Adverse Reactions

CNS: Asthenia, chills, dizziness, headache, hypertonia, hypesthesia, paresthesia, **seizures**, somnolence, tiredness, weakness, vertigo

CV: Chest tightness, pain, or pressure; **coronary artery vasospasm**; hypertension, **MI**, or myocardial ischemia (transient); palpitations; **shock**; **ventricular fibrillation or tachycardia**

EENT: Dry mouth, pharyngitis, **throat tightness**

GI: Abdominal pain, cramps, discomfort, or pressure; dysphagia; indigestion; nausea, vomiting

MS: Back pain

SKIN: Diaphoresis, flushing

Other: **Hypersensitivity reaction**; **angioedema**; feeling of warmth, pain, or pressure

Childbearing Considerations

PREGNANCY

- It is not known if drug causes fetal harm.
- Use with caution only if benefit to mother outweighs potential risk to fetus.
- Females of childbearing age with migraine may be at increased risk of gestational hypertension and preeclampsia during pregnancy.

LACTATION

- Drug is present in breast milk.
- Mothers should check with prescriber before breastfeeding.
- Infant exposure can be minimized by avoiding breastfeeding for 24 hr after drug has been taken.

Nursing Considerations

- Ensure that patients who are at risk for CAD undergo a satisfactory cardiovascular evaluation before administering the first dose of eletriptan and that they have a periodic reevaluation of their cardiac status during intermittent long-term therapy.

! **WARNING** Obtain an ECG immediately after first dose of drug in patients who have cardiovascular risk factors but who have had a satisfactory cardiovascular evaluation because of the drug's potential to cause coronary vasospasm.

! **WARNING** Evaluate patient for cardiovascular signs and symptoms after administration of eletriptan and notify prescriber if they occur. Expect drug to be withheld, as ordered, while patient undergoes an extensive cardiovascular workup, and discontinued if abnormalities are detected.

! **WARNING** Monitor patient for a hypersensitivity reaction, which could become life-threatening such as angioedema. If present, notify prescriber, expect drug to be discontinued, and provide supportive care, as needed and ordered.

- Monitor patient's blood pressure during therapy because of drug's potential to increase blood pressure.

PATIENT TEACHING

- Advise patient how to administer eletriptan and to take drug as soon as possible after onset of migraine.
- Review maximum dosage for drug with the patient. Advise against exceeding these parameters to avoid medication overuse headache.

! **WARNING** Urge patient to contact prescriber and avoid taking drug if headache symptoms are not typical.

! **WARNING** Instruct patient to seek emergency care for chest, jaw, or neck tightness after taking drug because these may indicate adverse cardiovascular reactions; subsequent doses may require ECG monitoring. Also tell patient to report palpitations.

! **WARNING** Alert patient that an allergic reaction may occur with drug use. Tell patient to notify prescriber if an allergic reaction occurs and to seek immediate medical care, if severe.

- Advise patient to avoid hazardous activities until drug's CNS effects are known and resolved.
- Advise yearly ophthalmic examinations during prolonged eletriptan therapy.
- Instruct patient to inform prescriber of all drugs he's taking, including over-the-counter products and herbal remedies.
- Inform mothers who are breastfeeding that infant exposure can be minimized by avoiding breastfeeding for 24 hr after drug has been taken.

eluxadoline

Viberzi

Class, Category, and Schedule

Pharmacologic class: Mu-opioid receptor agonist
Therapeutic class: Antidiarrheal
Controlled substance schedule: IV

Indications and Dosages

✶ *To treat irritable bowel syndrome with diarrhea (IBS-D)*

TABLETS

Adults. 100 mg twice daily.

± **DOSAGE ADJUSTMENT** For patients who are unable to tolerate the 100-mg dose, who are receiving concomitant OATP1B1 inhibitors, who have an eGFR less than 60 ml/min indicating moderate to severe renal impairment (including end-stage renal disease in patients not yet on dialysis), or who have mild to moderate hepatic impairment, dosage reduced to 75 mg twice daily.

Drug Administration

P.O.

- Administer drug with food.
- If dose is missed, administer the next dose at the regular time and do not double the dose to make up for the missed dose.

Route	Onset	Peak	Duration
P.O.	Unknown	1.5–2 hr	Unknown

Half-life: 3.7–6 hr

Mechanism of Action

Interacts with opioid receptors in the intestines to relieve diarrhea.

Contraindications

Absence of a gallbladder, alcoholism or patients who drink more than 3 alcoholic beverages daily, biliary duct obstruction, history of pancreatitis or structural disease of the pancreas, history of chronic or severe constipation, hypersensitivity to eluxadoline or its components, known or suspected mechanical GI obstruction, severe hepatic impairment, sphincter of Oddi disease, or dysfunction.

Interactions

DRUGS

alosetron, anticholinergics, opioids, or other drugs that cause constipation: Increased risk of constipation and constipation-related adverse reactions
OATP1B1 inhibitors, such as antivirals, cyclosporine, eltrombopag, gemfibrozil, rifampin: Increased exposure to eluxadoline increasing risk of adverse reactions
rosuvastatin: Increased exposure to rosuvastatin with increased risk for myopathy and rhabdomyolysis

ACTIVITIES

alcohol use: Increased risk for acute pancreatitis

Adverse Reactions

CNS: Dizziness, euphoria, fatigue, sedation, sensation of feeling drunk, somnolence
CV: Chest pain or tightness
EENT: Nasopharyngitis, **throat tightness**
GI: Abdominal distention or pain, constipation (which may become severe),

elevated liver enzymes, flatulence, gastroesophageal reflux disease, nausea, **pancreatitis**, sphincter of Oddi spasm, vomiting
RESP: **Asthma**, bronchitis, **bronchospasm**, dyspnea, **respiratory failure**, upper respiratory infection, wheezing
SKIN: Pruritus, rash, urticaria
Other: **Anaphylaxis**, **angioedema**

Childbearing Considerations

PREGNANCY

- It is not known if drug causes fetal harm.
- Use with caution only if benefit to mother outweighs potential risk to fetus.

LACTATION

- It is not known if drug is present in breast milk.
- Mothers should check with prescriber before breastfeeding.

Nursing Considerations

! **WARNING** Assess patient's alcohol intake prior to starting eluxadoline therapy because of increased risk of pancreatitis. Also, question patient about gallbladder removal surgery, as drug is contraindicated in patients without a gallbladder.

! **WARNING** Monitor patient closely for hypersensitivity reactions that could include anaphylaxis, angioedema, difficulty breathing or swallowing, and skin reactions, such as itching, rash, or urticaria. If present, notify prescriber immediately, expect drug to be discontinued, and provide emergency supportive care, as needed and ordered.

! **WARNING** Monitor patient closely for acute abdominal pain, especially during the first few weeks of therapy because mu-opioid receptor agonism increases risk for sphincter of Oddi spasm, which could result in elevated liver enzymes or pancreatitis. If present, notify prescriber and expect eluxadoline to be discontinued.

! **WARNING** Monitor patient's respiratory status closely because drug can have serious to life-threatening effects on the respiratory system. Notify prescriber immediately if patient develops difficulty breathing.

! **WARNING** Notify prescriber if patient develops severe constipation and expect drug to be discontinued. Severe cases of fecal impaction or intestinal obstruction or perforation have occurred with severe constipation, requiring emergency intervention.

- Monitor patient's liver enzymes, as ordered and report any elevations to prescriber.

PATIENT TEACHING

- Instruct patient how to administer eluxadoline and what to do if a dose is missed.

! **WARNING** Warn patient against excessive alcohol intake (more than 3 alcoholic drinks a day) or chronic alcohol intake while taking eluxadoline.

! **WARNING** Instruct patient to stop taking eluxadoline and immediately seek medical attention if she experiences acute epigastric or right, upper quadrant abdominal pain that may radiate to the back or shoulder and may be accompanied by nausea and vomiting. Also, tell patient to seek immediate medical attention if a serious allergic reaction occurs or patient has difficulty breathing.

! **WARNING** Tell patient to notify prescriber immediately if she develops severe constipation and not to use other drugs that may cause constipation during eluxadoline therapy.

- Advise patient to inform all prescribers of eluxadoline therapy.
- Tell patient not to take other drugs to treat diarrheal symptoms unless prescribed, and the prescriber is aware of eluxadoline use.

empagliflozin

Jardiance

Class and Category

Pharmacologic class: Sodium glucose cotransporter 2 inhibitor
Therapeutic class: Antidiabetic, cardiovascular mortality reduction agent

Indications and Dosages

✱ As adjunct to diet and exercise to improve glycemic control in patients with type 2 diabetes mellitus

TABLETS

Adults and children ages 10 and older with an eGFR of 30 ml/min or greater. 10 mg once daily in the morning, increased to 25 mg once daily, as needed.

✱ To reduce risk of cardiovascular death in patients with type 2 diabetes mellitus who have established cardiovascular disease; to reduce the risk of cardiovascular death and hospitalization for heart failure in patients with heart failure; to reduce risk of sustained decline in eGFR, end-stage kidney disease, cardiovascular death, and hospitalization in patients with chronic kidney disease at risk of progression

TABLETS

Adults. 10 mg once daily in the morning.

Drug Administration

P.O.

- Ensure that patient is maintaining an adequate fluid intake before administering drug each day; otherwise, drug may have to be temporarily withheld until volume depletion is resolved.
- Administer drug in the morning with or without food.
- Expect to withhold drug for at least 3 days, if possible, prior to patient having a major procedure or surgery associated with prolonged fasting.

Route	Onset	Peak	Duration
P.O.	Unknown	1.5 hr	3 days

Half-life: 12.4 hr

Mechanism of Action

Inhibits sodium glucose cotransporter 2 in the kidneys, which prevents glucose reabsorption. This decreases blood glucose levels. Also, reduces sodium reabsorption and increases sodium delivery to the distal tubule, which influences several functions such as increasing tubuloglomerular feedback and reducing intraglomerular pressure, lowering both pre- and afterload of the heart and down regulating sympathetic activity. These effects are thought to play a role in reducing the risk of cardiovascular death, heart failure, and sustained decline in renal function.

Contraindications

Hypersensitivity to empagliflozin or its components

Interactions

DRUGS

diuretics: Increased risk of acute kidney injury and renal impairment in presence of dehydration

insulin, insulin secretagogues: Increased risk of hypoglycemia

lithium: Possibly decreased serum lithium concentration with possible decreased lithium effectiveness

Adverse Reactions

CNS: Syncope

CV: Dyslipidemia, elevated low-density lipoprotein (LDL) cholesterol level, **hypotension**

ENDO: **Ketoacidosis**

GI: Constipation, nausea

GU: **Acute kidney injury**, decreased eGFR, dysuria, elevated serum creatinine levels, genital mycotic infections, impaired renal function, increased urination, **necrotizing fasciitis of the perineum (Fournier's gangrene)**, osmotic diuresis, **pyelonephritis**, **urosepsis**, UTI

MS: Arthralgia, increased risk of bone fracture

RESP: Upper respiratory tract infection

SKIN: Rash, urticaria

Other: **Angioedema and other hypersensitivity reactions**, dehydration

Childbearing Considerations

PREGNANCY

- Drug may cause adverse renal effects in the developing fetus.
- Drug is not recommended for use during the second and third trimester of pregnancy.

LACTATION

- It is not known if drug is present in breast milk.
- Mothers should not breastfeed their infant while taking drug because kidney maturation continues through the first 2 yr of life.

REPRODUCTION

- Advise females of childbearing age to use an effective contraception throughout drug therapy.

Nursing Considerations

! **WARNING** Assess patient's volume status and correct, if needed and as prescribed, prior to starting empagliflozin therapy because drug can cause intravascular volume contraction leading to symptomatic hypotension and acute kidney injury. Continue to monitor patient throughout therapy for dehydration and renal dysfunction. Patients at highest risk include the elderly and patients with chronic renal insufficiency, congestive heart failure, hypovolemia, or patients who take diuretics. Notify prescriber immediately if patient has fluid losses or reduced oral intake, as acute kidney injury may occur. Expect that drug may be temporarily withheld until fluid balance can be restored.

! **WARNING** Obtain serum creatinine level, as ordered, prior to starting empagliflozin therapy because empagliflozin can cause adverse renal effects that could become life-threatening such as pyelonephritis and urosepsis. Be aware that the elderly and patients with existing impaired renal function are at higher risk for these adverse effects. Monitor renal function throughout therapy.

! **WARNING** Monitor patient for hypersensitivity reactions that could be serious, such as the development of angioedema. If present, withhold drug, notify prescriber immediately, and be prepared to provide emergency supportive care, as needed and ordered.

- Be aware that patients receiving insulin or insulin secretagogues may require a lower dose of these agents because empagliflozin in combination increases risk of hypoglycemia. Be aware that in children, hypoglycemia may occur regardless of insulin use. Monitor patient closely for hypoglycemia. If present, treat according to standard protocol and notify prescriber.

! **WARNING** Monitor patient closely for ketoacidosis because it has occurred in patients with type 2 diabetes being treated with empagliflozin. Be aware that ketoacidosis can become life-threatening quickly even when blood glucose levels are less than 250 mg/dl. Notify prescriber immediately if ketoacidosis is suspected and expect drug to be discontinued. Be prepared to treat patient's ketoacidosis, as ordered. Be aware that patients at higher risk include patients with an acute febrile illness or having undergone surgery; have a history of alcohol abuse; have a pancreatic insulin deficiency from any cause, including an insulin dose reduction; or have a prolonged reduced caloric intake. Expect drug to be temporarily discontinued as a prophylactic measure if patient must undergo prolonged fasting due to acute illness or surgery.

! **WARNING** Monitor patient for a rare but serious and life-threatening necrotizing infection of the perineum called Fournier's gangrene. Notify prescriber immediately if patient develops erythema, pain, swelling, or tenderness in the genital or perineal area, along with fever or malaise. Expect treatment with broad-spectrum antibiotics and, if needed, surgical debridement of the area. Know that empagliflozin will be discontinued if this occurs. Monitor patient's blood glucose levels closely and expect an alternative treatment for glycemic control.

- Monitor patient's blood pressure and cholesterol level throughout empagliflozin therapy because drug can cause an elevated LDL cholesterol level and hypotension.
- Monitor patients for genital mycotic infections or UTI, especially those with a history of such. If present, notify prescriber and treat, as prescribed.

PATIENT TEACHING

- Instruct patient how to administer empagliflozin.
- Inform patient with diabetes that empagliflozin therapy is not a replacement for diet and exercise therapy.
- Stress importance to maintain adequate fluid intake throughout empagliflozin therapy. However, tell patient to notify prescriber if she is unable to take a normal amount of daily fluids due to fasting or illness or experiences an excessive loss of fluids from excessive perspiration or GI illnesses. Drug may have to be temporarily withheld.

! **WARNING** Tell patient that drug may cause an allergic reaction, such as swelling of the eyes, face, throat, and tongue. It may also cause skin reactions, such as a rash or hives. If present, stress importance of stopping drug, notifying prescriber, and, if severe, to seek immediate medical treatment.

! **WARNING** Instruct patient on the signs and symptoms of hypoglycemia and how to treat it. Inform patient who is also receiving insulin or a sulfonylurea that the risk of hypoglycemia is greater. Tell patient to notify prescriber if hypoglycemia occurs frequently or is severe.

! **WARNING** Review signs and symptoms of ketoacidosis with patient and family or caregiver. Immediate medical attention should be sought, if signs and symptoms are present, even if blood glucose level is less than 250 mg/dl.

! **WARNING** Warn patient to stop empagliflozin and seek immediate medical attention if pain, redness, swelling, or tenderness occurs in the genital or perineal area, along with fever or malaise because, although rare, this cluster of symptoms may become life-threatening.

- Advise females of childbearing age to use an effective contraception throughout drug therapy and to notify prescriber if pregnancy occurs or is suspected.
- Tell mothers that breastfeeding is not recommended while taking empagliflozin.
- Stress importance of notifying prescriber if patient develops dehydration, has onset of hunger or thirst, or notices a sudden change in mental status. Tell patient and family or caregiver not to belittle these symptoms and seek medical attention quickly.
- Caution patient to comply with laboratory appointmnets to check blood glucose levels, electrolytes, and renal function. Also tell patient to notify prescriber if any perisistent, serious, or unusual adverse reactions occur in addition to the ones mentioned above.
- Teach patient to take fall precautions and other safety measures because drug may increase risk of bone fracture as early as 12 weeks after empagliflozin therapy is begun.
- Warn patient that drug may increase risk for urinary tract and yeast infections for both men and women. Review signs and symptoms and advise patient to notify prescriber, if present.
- Tell patient to monitor the blood glucose level using blood tests instead of urine tests because drug increases urinary glucose excretion and will lead to positive urine glucose tests.

emtricitabine

Emtriva

Class and Category

Pharmacologic class: Nucleoside analogue
Therapeutic class: Antiretroviral

Indications and Dosages

✱ *As adjunct to treat human immunodeficiency virus type 1 (HIV-1) infection*

CAPSULES, ORAL SOLUTION

Adults. 200 mg (capsule) or 240 mg (oral solution) once daily.

CAPSULES

Children ages 3 mo to 18 yr weighing more than 33 kg (72.6 lb) and can swallow an intact capsule. 200 mg once daily.

ORAL SOLUTION

Children ages 3 mo to 18 yr. 6 mg/kg once daily and increased, as needed. *Maximum:* 240 mg once daily.

Newborns and infants up to 3 mo. 3 mg/kg once daily.

± **DOSAGE ADJUSTMENT** For adult patients with a creatinine clearance of 30 to 49 ml/min, dosage interval increased to every 48 hours if using capsules or dosage reduced to 120 mg once daily if using oral solution. For adult patients with a creatinine clearance of 15 to 29 ml/min, dosage interval increased to every 72 hours if using capsules or dosage reduced to 80 mg once daily if using oral solution. For adult patients with a creatinine clearance of less than 15 ml/min or who are on hemodialysis, dosage interval increased to every 96 hours if using capsules or dosage reduced to 60 mg once daily if using oral solution. For pediatric patients with renal impairment, there is insufficient data to recommend a specific dose adjustment, but a reduction in dose and/or an increase in dosing interval similar to adults may be considered.

Drug Administration

P.O.

- Keep in original container tightly closed.
- Capsules should be swallowed whole and not chewed, crushed, or opened.
- Use calibrated device to measure oral solution dosage. Solution should be clear but orange to dark orange in color.
- Oral solution should be refrigerated. However, if stored at room temperature, discard after 3 mo.

Route	Onset	Peak	Duration
P.O.	Unknown	1–2 hr	Unknown

Half-life: 10 hr

Mechanism of Action

Phosphorylated by cellular enzymes, emtricitabine then inhibits the activity of the HIV-1 reverse transcriptase by competing with the natural substrate and by being incorporated into the nascent viral DNA, which leads to chain termination of the HIV virus.

Contraindications

Hypersensitivity to emtricitabine or its components

Interactions

DRUGS

None reported by manufacturer.

Adverse Reactions

CNS: Abnormal dreams, asthenia, depression, dizziness, fatigue, fever, headache, insomnia, neuropathy, paresthesia, peripheral neuritis
CV: Elevated cholesterol and triglycerides
EENT: Nasopharyngitis, otitis media, rhinitis, sinusitis
ENDO: Cushingoid appearance, fat redistribution, hyperglycemia
GI: Abdominal pain; diarrhea; dyspepsia; elevated amylase, bilirubin, lipase, and liver enzymes; gastroenteritis; nausea; **severe acute exacerbations of hepatitis B**; **severe hepatomegaly with steatosis**; vomiting
GU: Glycosuria, hematuria, new onset or worsening of renal impairment
HEME: Anemia, decreased hemoglobin, **neutropenia**
MS: Arthralgia, elevated creatine kinase, myalgia
RESP: Increased cough, pneumonia, upper respiratory infections
SKIN: Hyperpigmentation on palms and/or soles, pruritus, rash, urticaria
Other: Elevated alkaline phosphatase, **immune reconstitution syndrome**, infection, **lactic acidosis**

Childbearing Considerations

PREGNANCY

- Pregnancy exposure registry: 1-800-258-4263.
- It is not known if drug causes fetal harm.
- Use with caution only if benefit to mother outweighs potential risk to fetus.

LACTATION

- Drug may be present in breast milk.
- The Centers for Disease Control and Prevention recommends that HIV-1 infected mothers not breastfeed to avoid risking postnatal transmission of HIV-1 infection to infants. They also do not recommend breastfeeding because of potential drug-induced adverse reactions in the infant.

Nursing Considerations

- Perform a complete drug history on patient because combination drugs containing emtricitabine (Atripla, Complera, Truvada) should not be given concurrently with emtricitabine therapy. Also, do not expect to coadminister drugs containing lamivudine (Combivir, Epivir, Epivir-HBV, Epzicom, Trizivir) during emtricitabine therapy because of the similarities between emtricitabine and lamivudine.

! WARNING Expect to test patient for hepatitis B virus (HBV) prior to starting emtricitabine, as ordered. This is because acute severe exacerbations of hepatitis B have occurred after patient has discontinued the drug. Know that in some cases the exacerbation resulted in liver failure.

! WARNING Monitor patient's liver enzymes throughout therapy and for several months after drug is discontinued because lactic acidosis and severe hepatomegaly with steatosis have occurred with emtricitabine therapy, as have acute exacerbations of hepatitis B with patients coinfected. Know that most cases of lactic acidosis and severe hepatomegaly with steatosis have occurred in women with prolonged nucleoside exposure and obesity. Report abnormal liver function signs and symptoms to prescriber, such as abdominal discomfort, jaundice, nausea, vomiting, or weakness.

! **WARNING** Be aware that immune reconstitution syndrome has occurred in patients treated with combination antiretroviral therapy, including emtricitabine. The inflammatory response predisposes susceptible patients to opportunistic infections, such as cytomegalovirus, *Mycobacterium avium* infection, *Pneumocystis jiroveci* pneumonia, or tuberculosis. Autoimmune disorders, such as Graves' disease, Guillain-Barré syndrome, or polymyositis have also occurred. Report sudden or unusual adverse reactions to prescriber.

- Monitor patient's renal function because drug is primarily eliminated by the kidney and dosage alterations are necessary for those with impaired kidney function.

PATIENT TEACHING

- Instruct patient and family or caregiver how to administer emtricitabine.
- Inform patient that emtricitabine will be prescribed along with other antiviral drugs.

! **WARNING** Review signs and symptoms of liver dysfunction (abdominal discomfort, nausea, vomiting, weakness, yellowing of skin or whites of eyes) and stress importance of reporting any occurrence to prescriber.

- Instruct patient to report any persistent, severe, or unusual signs and symptoms.
- Instruct patient to remind all prescribers of emtricitabine therapy.
- Inform patient that emtricitabine therapy may cause changes in his body appearance because of fat redistribution. Prepare him for the possibility of developing breast enlargement, central obesity, dorsocervical fat enlargement (buffalo hump), facial wasting, and peripheral wasting.
- Alert mothers that breastfeeding is not recommended during emtricitabine therapy.

enalapril maleate

Epaned, Vasotec

enalaprilat

E

Class and Category

Pharmacologic class: ACE inhibitor
Therapeutic class: Antihypertensive, vasodilator

Indications and Dosages

∗ *To control hypertension*

ORAL SOLUTION, TABLETS

Adults. *Initial:* 5 mg daily, increased after 1 to 2 wk, as needed. *Maintenance:* 10 to 40 mg once daily or in divided doses twice daily. *Maximum:* 40 mg daily.
Children older than 1 mo. 0.08 mg/kg daily, titrated according to blood pressure response up to 5 mg daily. *Maximum:* 0.58 mg/kg/dose (40 mg).

I.V. INFUSION, I.V. INJECTION

Adults. 1.25 mg every 6 hr. and given slowly over 5 min.

± **DOSAGE ADJUSTMENT** For adult patients who are receiving diuretics or who have a creatinine clearance below 30 ml/min, initial dose reduced to 2.5 mg P.O. and then increased, as needed, to maximum dose of 40 mg daily or dosage decreased to 0.625 mg if given I.V. If response to I.V. dose is inadequate after 1 hr, I.V. dose of 0.625 mg repeated and then therapy continued at 1.25 mg every 6 hours. For adult patients who are sensitive to I.V. dosage, drug may be infused over 1 hour. For children, oral dosage adjustment is not known.

∗ *To convert from I.V. to oral dosage form*

ORAL SOLUTION, TABLETS

Adults. *Initial:* 5 mg once daily, then increased as needed.

± **DOSAGE ADJUSTMENT** For patients with a creatinine clearance of 30 ml/min or less, dosage reduced to 2.5 mg once daily.

∗ *To convert from oral to I.V. dosage form*

I.V. INFUSION, I.V. INJECTION

Adults. *Initial:* 1.25 mg every 6 hr and given slowly over 5 min.

✱ *To treat symptomatic heart failure*

ORAL SOLUTION, TABLETS

Adults. *Initial:* 2.5 mg twice daily, increased after 1 to 2 wk, as needed. *Maintenance:* 5 to 40 mg daily in 2 divided doses. *Maximum:* 40 mg daily in 2 divided doses.

±**DOSAGE ADJUSTMENT** For patients with hyponatremia (serum sodium less than 130 mEq/L) or serum creatinine greater than 1.6 mg/dl, initial dosage interval reduced to once daily.

✱ *To treat asymptomatic left ventricular dysfunction, to decrease the rate of development of overt heart failure and reduce hospitalization for heart failure*

ORAL SOLUTION, TABLETS

Adults. *Initial:* 2.5 mg twice daily, increased, as tolerated, to 20 mg daily in 2 divided doses.

Drug Administration

P.O.

- Tablets are to be swallowed whole and not chewed, crushed, or split.
- Ask for oral solution reconstituted by pharmacist for patient who cannot swallow tablets.
- Use a calibrated device to measure oral solution dosage. No shaking needed prior to measuring each dose.
- Store oral solution at room temperature. Discard oral solution after 60 days.

I.V.

- May be administered undiluted or diluted with up to 50 ml of a compatible diluent, such as 0.9% Sodium Chloride Injection, 5% Dextrose Injection, 0.9% Sodium Chloride Injection with 5% Dextrose, or 5% Dextrose in Lactated Ringer's Injection.
- Solution should be clear and colorless.
- Administer, if undiluted, as an I.V. injection slowly over 5 min or if diluted, administer as an I.V. infusion slowly over 5 min or longer. Administer up to 1 hr for patients at risk of excessive hypotension, as ordered.
- I.V. administration usually not recommended for more than 36 hr up to 7 days.
- *Incompatibilities:* Amphotericin B, cefepime, phenytoin

Route	Onset	Peak	Duration
P.O.	1 hr	4–6 hr	24 hr
I.V.	15 min	1–4 hr	6 hr

Half-life: 11 hr

Mechanism of Action

May reduce blood pressure and development of heart failure by affecting the renin–angiotensin–aldosterone system. By inhibiting angiotensin-converting enzyme (ACE), enalapril:

- prevents conversion of angiotensin I to angiotensin II, a potent vasoconstrictor that also stimulates the adrenal cortex to secrete aldosterone.
- may inhibit renal and vascular production of angiotensin II.
- decreases the serum angiotensin II level and increases serum renin activity, which decreases aldosterone secretion, slightly increases serum potassium level, and causes fluid loss.
- decreases vascular tone and blood pressure.
- inhibits aldosterone release, which reduces sodium and water reabsorption and increases their excretion, further reducing blood pressure, and increasing risk of heart failure.

Contraindications

Concurrent aliskiren therapy in patients with diabetes; concurrent therapy with a neprilysin inhibitor, such as sacubitril; history of hereditary or idiopathic angioedema; hypersensitivity to enalapril, enalaprilat, other ACE inhibitors, or their components; use within 36 hr of sacubitril/valsartan therapy

Interactions

DRUGS

aliskiren, angiotensin receptor blockers, other ACE inhibitors: Increased risk of hyperkalemia, hypotension, and renal dysfunction

diuretics, other antihypertensives: Additive hypotensive effects

lithium: Increased blood lithium level and lithium toxicity

mTOR inhibitors (everolimus, sirolimus, temsirolimus); neprilysin inhibitor (sacubitril): Increased risk of angioedema

NSAIDs, including selective cyclooxygenase-2 inhibitors: Possibly reduced antihypertensive effects of enalapril and enalaprilat; possibly

increased risk of renal dysfunction, especially in the elderly or who are volume-depleted or already have compromised renal function
potassium-sparing diuretics, potassium supplements: Increased risk of hyperkalemia
sodium aurothiomalate: Increased risk of nitritoid reactions, such as facial flushing, nausea, vomiting, and hypotension
thiazide diuretics: Increased loss of potassium

FOODS

potassium-containing salt substitutes: Increased risk of hyperkalemia

Adverse Reactions

CNS: Ataxia, confusion, **CVA**, depression, dizziness, dream disturbances, fatigue, headache, insomnia, nervousness, peripheral neuropathy, somnolence, syncope, vertigo, weakness
CV: Angina, **arrhythmias**, **cardiac arrest**, **hypotension**, **MI**, orthostatic hypotension, palpitations, Raynaud's phenomenon
EENT: Blurred vision, conjunctivitis, dry eyes and mouth, glossitis, hoarseness, lacrimation, loss of smell, pharyngitis, rhinorrhea, stomatitis, taste perversion, tinnitus
ENDO: Gynecomastia
GI: Abdominal pain, anorexia, constipation, diarrhea, **hepatic failure**, **hepatitis**, ileus, indigestion, **melena**, nausea, **pancreatitis**, vomiting
GU: Flank pain, impotence, oliguria, **renal failure**, UTI
MS: Muscle spasms
RESP: Asthma, bronchitis, **bronchospasm**, cough, dyspnea, pneumonia, **pulmonary edema**, **pulmonary embolism and infarction**, **pulmonary infiltrates**, upper respiratory tract infection
SKIN: Alopecia, diaphoresis, **erythema multiforme**, **exfoliative dermatitis**, flushing, pemphigus, photosensitivity, pruritus, rash, **Stevens-Johnson syndrome**, **toxic epidermal necrolysis**, urticaria
Other: **Anaphylaxis**, **angioedema**, herpes zoster, **hyperkalemia**

Childbearing Considerations

PREGNANCY

- Drug may cause adverse renal effects to the developing fetus, especially in the second and third trimester.
- Drug should be discontinued when pregnancy is known.

LACTATION

- Drug is present in breast milk.
- Mothers should not breastfeed their infant while taking drug because kidney maturation continues through the first 2 yr of life.

REPRODUCTION

- Females of childbearing age should use effective contraception throughout drug therapy.

Nursing Considerations

- Use enalapril and enalaprilat cautiously in patients with impaired renal function.

! WARNING Measure patient's blood pressure immediately after first dose and frequently for at least 2 hours thereafter. If hypotension develops, place patient in a supine position and expect to give I.V. 0.9% Sodium Chloride Injection or other volume expander, as prescribed. If hypotension requires a dosage reduction, monitor blood pressure frequently for 2 hours after reduced dosage is administered and for another hour after blood pressure has stabilized.

- Monitor patient's heart rate and rhythm. Expect to obtain repeated 12-lead ECG tracings, as ordered.

! WARNING Monitor patient closely for a hypersensitivity reaction, which could become life-threatening such as angioedema. If present, notify prescriber, expect drug to be discontinued, and provide supportive care, as needed and ordered.

! WARNING Monitor laboratory test results to check hepatic and renal function, and serum potassium level. Also, monitor patient's CBC, as ordered, for abnormalities because other ACE inhibitors have caused agranulocytosis, leukopenia with myeloid hypoplasia, and neutropenia.

PATIENT TEACHING

- Instruct patient how to administer oral form of drug prescribed.

! WARNING Alert patient that drug may cause an allergic reaction. Tell patient to notify prescriber if an allergic reaction occurs. If severe, stress importance of seeking immediate medical care.

E

! **WARNING** Inform patient that fainting and light-headedness may occur, especially during first few days of therapy. Advise him to change position slowly and avoid hazardous activities until drug's CNS effects are known and resolved.

! **WARNING** Inform patient that diarrhea, excessive sweating, vomiting, and other conditions may cause dehydration, which can lead to dizziness, fainting, and very low blood pressure during therapy. Urge sufficient fluid intake to prevent dehydration and related adverse reactions. If diarrhea or vomiting is severe or prolonged, instruct patient to notify prescriber.

! **WARNING** Caution females of childbearing age that they should use a reliable form of contraception and should notify prescriber immediately if pregnancy occurs.

- Instruct patient to notify prescriber if persistent, severe, or unusual adverse reactions such as a persistent dry cough. Explain that drug can affect many body systems and not to make light of any symptom.
- Advise patient to consult prescriber before using potassium supplements, salt substitutes, or other drugs (including over-the-counter drugs) while taking drug.
- Tell mothers not to breastfeed their infant during drug therapy.

enfuvirtide

Fuzeon

Class and Category

Pharmacologic class: Fusion inhibitor
Therapeutic class: Antiretroviral

Indications and Dosages

∗ *As adjunct to treat human immunodeficiency virus type 1 (HIV-1) infection in treatment-experienced patients with HIV-1 replication despite ongoing antiretroviral therapy*

SUBCUTANEOUS INJECTION

Adults. *Initial:* 90 mg twice daily.
Children weighing at least 11 kg (24.2 lb). 2 mg/kg twice daily. *Maximum:* 90 mg twice daily.

Drug Administration

SUBCUTANEOUS

- Reconstitute with 1 ml of Sterile Water for Injection provided in the convenience kit. Then, gently tap vial for 10 sec, followed by gently rolling vial between hands to avoid foaming and to ensure that all particles of drug are in contact with the liquid. Let vial stand until powder is completely dissolved, which may take up to 45 min. If the solution is foamy or jelled, allow more time for it to dissolve.
- Once reconstituted, use immediately or keep refrigerated in the original vial for up to 24 hr. If refrigerated, allow reconstituted solution to come to room temperature before administration and recheck that drug is still fully dissolved and appears clear, colorless, and without bubbles or particulate matter.
- Administer into patient's abdomen, anterior thigh, or upper arm.
- Rotate site of injections, avoiding injecting into any anatomical areas where large nerves course close to the skin; directly over a blood vessel; or into skin abnormalities, such as bruises, burn sites, moles, near the navel, scar tissue, surgical scars, or tattoos.

Route	Onset	Peak	Duration
SubQ	Unknown	4–8 hr	Unknown

Half-life: 3.8 hr

Mechanism of Action

Interferes with the entry of HIV-1 into cells to inhibit fusion of cellular membranes with the virus. It does this by binding to the viral envelope glycoprotein and preventing the conformational changes required for the fusion.

Contraindications

Hypersensitivity to enfuvirtide or its components

Interactions

DRUGS

None reported by manufacturer.

Adverse Reactions

CNS: Anxiety, asthenia, chills, depression, fatigue, fever, **Guillain-Barré syndrome**, insomnia, peripheral neuropathy, rigors, sixth nerve palsy, **suicidal ideation**

CV: Elevated triglycerides, **hypotension**, **unstable angina pectoris**
EENT: Conjunctivitis, dry mouth, sinusitis, taste disturbance
ENDO: Hyperglycemia
GI: Anorexia; constipation; diarrhea; elevated amylase, lipase, and liver enzymes; hepatic steatosis; nausea; **pancreatitis**; **toxic hepatitis**; upper abdominal pain; vomiting
GU: **Glomerulonephritis**, **renal failure or insufficiency**, **tubular necrosis**
HEME: Eosinophilia, **neutropenia**, **thrombocytopenia**
MS: Elevated creatine phosphokinase, extremity pain, myalgia
RESP: Cough, pneumonia (bacterial), respiratory distress
SKIN: Cutaneous amyloidosis at injection site, folliculitis, pruritus, rash
Other: Formation of anti-enfuvirtide antibodies, flu-like symptoms, herpes simplex infection, **immune reconstitution syndrome**, local injection-site reactions (bruising, cyst formation, discomfort, ecchymosis, erythema, hematomas, **hypersensitivity reaction**, induration, infection, neuralgia, nodule formation, pain, paresthesia, pruritus), lymphadenopathy, post-injection bleeding, **sepsis**, weight loss

Childbearing Considerations

PREGNANCY

- Pregnancy exposure registry: 1-800-258-4263.
- It is not known if drug causes fetal harm.
- Use with caution only if benefit to mother outweighs potential risk to fetus.

LACTATION

- It is not known if drug is present in breast milk.
- The Centers for Disease Control and Prevention recommends that HIV-1 infected mothers not breastfeed to avoid risking postnatal transmission of HIV-1 infection to infants. They also do not recommend breastfeeding because of potential drug-induced adverse reactions in the infant.

Nursing Considerations

- Assess patient's injection site for local adverse reactions because most patients experience at least one local injection-site reaction. Be especially alert for infection, such as cellulitis or a local infection. Provide supportive care, as needed and ordered, to manage injection-site reactions.

! **WARNING** Monitor patient for hypersensitivity reactions, which may become life-threatening. Be alert for systemic hypersensitivity reactions associated with enfuvirtide therapy, which may include chills, fever, hypotension, nausea, rash, rigors, and vomiting. If present, notify prescriber, expect drug to be discontinued, and provide emergency medical care, as needed and ordered.

! **WARNING** Monitor patient's respiratory status closely, as bacterial pneumonia may occur and be serious enough to warrant hospitalization. Be especially alert for pneumonia in patients with a high initial viral load, history of intravenous drug use, low initial CD4 lymphocyte count, prior history of lung disease, or who are smokers.

! **WARNING** Be aware that immune reconstitution syndrome has occurred in patients treated with combination antiretroviral therapy, including enfuvirtide. The inflammatory response predisposes susceptible patients to opportunistic infections, such as cytomegalovirus, *Mycobacterium avium* infection, *Pneumocystis jiroveci* pneumonia, or tuberculosis. Autoimmune disorders, such as Graves' disease, Guillain-Barré syndrome, or polymyositis have also occurred. Report sudden or unusual adverse reactions to prescriber.

! **WARNING** Watch patient closely for suicidal ideation.

PATIENT TEACHING

- Inform patient that enfuvirtide therapy will be used in conjunction with other antiretroviral agents.
- Instruct patient, family, or caregiver how to administer enfuvirtide, including giving a subcutaneous injection.
- Advise patient to alert prescriber to persistent or severe local injection-site adverse reactions, including any signs or symptoms of infection. Inform her that almost all patients experience at least one injection-site reaction.

! **WARNING** Review signs and symptoms of an allergic reaction with patient. Tell patient to notify prescriber and stress importance of seeking immediate medical attention, if severe.

! **WARNING** Tell patient to seek medical attention if she develops signs or symptoms suggestive of pneumonia, such as cough with fever, rapid breathing, or shortness of breath. Also, instruct patient to report any persistent, severe, or unusual signs and symptoms.

! **WARNING** Alert family or caregiver that drug may cause patient to have suicidal thoughts. If present, prescriber should be notified.

- Alert mothers that breastfeeding is not recommended during enfuvirtide therapy.

enoxaparin sodium

Lovenox

Class and Category

Pharmacologic class: Low-molecular-weight heparin

Therapeutic class: Anticoagulant

Indications and Dosages

∗ *To prevent deep vein thrombosis (DVT) after hip or knee replacement and for continued prophylaxis after hospitalization for hip replacement*

SUBCUTANEOUS INJECTION

Adults. 30 mg every 12 hr, starting 12 to 24 hr after surgery for 7 to 10 days. Alternatively for hip replacement surgery, 40 mg once daily, starting 9 to 15 hr before surgery and then once daily for up to 3 wk.

± **DOSAGE ADJUSTMENT** For patients with severe renal impairment (creatinine clearance less than 30 ml/min), dosage interval changed from twice daily to once daily or dosage reduced from 40 mg once daily to 30 mg once daily.

∗ *To prevent DVT after abdominal surgery for patients at risk for thromboembolic complications*

SUBCUTANEOUS INJECTION

Adults. *Initial:* 40 mg once daily, starting 2 hr before surgery with subsequent dose of 40 mg given 24 hr after initial dose and then continued once daily for 7 to 10 days.

± **DOSAGE ADJUSTMENT** For patients with severe renal impairment (creatinine clearance less than 30 ml/min), dosage reduced to 30 mg once daily.

∗ *To prevent DVT in medical patients who are at risk for thromboembolic complications due to severely restricted mobility during acute illness*

SUBCUTANEOUS INJECTION

Adults. 40 mg once daily for 6 to 11 days.

± **DOSAGE ADJUSTMENT** For patients with severe renal impairment (creatinine clearance less than 30 ml/min), dosage reduced to 30 mg once daily.

∗ *To treat acute DVT for inpatients with or without pulmonary embolism*

SUBCUTANEOUS INJECTION

Adults. 1 mg/kg every 12 hr or 1.5 mg/kg once daily for a minimum of 5 days after warfarin therapy has been initiated and a therapeutic oral anticoagulant effect has been achieved. *Usual duration:* 7 days.

± **DOSAGE ADJUSTMENT** For patients with severe renal impairment (creatinine clearance less than 30 ml/min) and taking warfarin concomitantly, dosage reduced or kept at 1 mg/kg and dosage interval increased to once daily.

∗ *To treat acute DVT as outpatient without pulmonary embolism*

SUBCUTANEOUS INJECTION

Adults. 1 mg/kg every 12 hr for a minimum of 5 days after warfarin therapy has been initiated and a therapeutic oral anticoagulant effect has been achieved. *Usual duration:* 7 days.

± **DOSAGE ADJUSTMENT** For patients with severe renal impairment (creatinine clearance less than 30 ml/min) and taking warfarin concomitantly, dosage interval increased to once daily.

∗ *As adjunct to prevent ischemic complications of unstable angina and non-Q-wave MI*

SUBCUTANEOUS INJECTION

Adults. 1 mg/kg every 12 hr with 100 to 325 mg of aspirin P.O. daily for 2 to 8 days or until condition is stable.

± **DOSAGE ADJUSTMENT** For patients with severe renal impairment (serum creatinine less than 30 ml/min) when administered in conjunction with aspirin, dosage interval increased to once daily.

∗ *To treat acute ST-segment–elevation MI (STEMI)*

I.V. INJECTION, THEN SUBCUTANEOUS INJECTION

Adults. 30 mg I.V. as a single dose plus 1 mg/kg subcutaneously. Then, 1 mg/kg subcutaneously every 12 hr (maximum 100 mg for first 2 doses) with aspirin 75 to 325 mg P.O. once daily.

±**DOSAGE ADJUSTMENT** For patients with STEMI also receiving a thrombolytic, enoxaparin should be given between 15 minutes before and 30 minutes after fibrinolytic therapy starts. If STEMI patients have percutaneous coronary intervention, expect to give 0.3-mg/kg I.V. bolus if last enoxaparin dose was given more than 8 hours before balloon inflation. For patients less than 75 years of age with STEMI and severe renal impairment (less than 30 ml/min) when administered in conjunction with aspirin, 30 mg as a single I.V. bolus plus a 1 mg subcutaneous dose followed by 1 mg/kg subcutaneously once daily. For elderly patients with STEMI who are 75 years of age and older, initial I.V. bolus eliminated and initial subcutaneous injection dosage reduced to 0.75 mg/kg every 12 hours (maximum 75 mg for the first 2 doses only), followed by 0.75 mg/kg for remaining doses. For elderly patients ages 75 and older who also have severe renal impairment (creatinine clearance less than 30 ml/min) and concurrent aspirin therapy is taken, dosage interval increased to once daily.

Drug Administration

- Use of multidose vials should be avoided, if at all possible, in pregnant women because benzyl alcohol may cross the placenta and cause fetal harm.
- Use a tuberculin syringe or equivalent when using multiple-dose vials to ensure correct dose is withdrawn.

I.V.

- Solution should appear clear, colorless to pale yellow.
- Always flush I.V. access with 0.9% Sodium Chloride Injection or 5% Dextrose Injection before and after administration.
- Administer bolus as an I.V. injection.
- Don't give drug by I.M. injection.
- *Incompatibilities:* Other drugs and solutions (except for 0.9% Sodium Chloride Injection or 5% Dextrose Injection)

SUBCUTANEOUS

- Administer by first putting patient in a supine position.
- Do not expel the air bubble from prefilled syringes before the injection, to avoid the loss of drug.
- Administer as a deep subcutaneous injection by introducing the whole length of needle into a skin fold held between the thumb and forefinger; hold the skin fold throughout the injection.
- Do not rub the injection site after injection, to minimize bruising.
- The prefilled syringe safety system will only be activated once the syringe is empty and removed from patient. Activation may cause a minimal splatter of fluid, so activate the system while holding syringe downward and away from people.
- Rotate sites by alternating injection sites between the left and right anterolateral and left and right posterolateral abdominal wall.
- Monitor for site bleeding.

Route	Onset	Peak	Duration
SubQ	Unknown	3–5 hr	24 hr
I.V.	Unknown	Unknown	Unknown

Half-life: 4.5–7 hr

Mechanism of Action

Potentiates the action of antithrombin III, a coagulation inhibitor. By binding with antithrombin III, enoxaparin rapidly binds with and inactivates clotting factors (primarily factor Xa and thrombin). Without thrombin, fibrinogen can't convert to fibrin and thrombus can't form.

Contraindications

Active major bleeding; history of immune-mediated heparin-induced thrombocytopenia (HIT) within past 100 days or in the presence of circulating antibodies, which may persist for several years; hypersensitivity to benzyl alcohol (multidose vial), enoxaparin, heparin (including low-molecular-weight heparins), pork products or their components

Interactions

DRUGS

NSAIDs; oral anticoagulants; platelet aggregation inhibitors, such as aspirin, dipyridamole, salicylates, sulfinpyrazone, and ticlopidine; thrombolytics, such as alteplase, anistreplase, streptokinase, and urokinase: Possibly increased risk of bleeding

Adverse Reactions

CNS: Confusion, **CVA**, epidural or spinal hematoma, fever, headache, paralysis
CV: **Atrial fibrillation**, **congestive heart failure**, hyperlipidemia, peripheral edema, **thrombosis**
EENT: Epistaxis
GI: Bloody stools, **cholestatic and hepatocellular liver injury**, diarrhea, elevated liver enzymes, **hematemesis**, **melena**, nausea, vomiting
GU: Hematuria, menstrual irregularities
HEME: Anemia, eosinophilia, **hemorrhage**, **heparin-induced thrombocytopenia (HIT) or immune-mediated thrombocytopenia**, **purpura**, **thrombocytopenia purpura**, **thrombocytopenia**, thrombocytosis
MS: Osteoporosis (with long-term therapy)
RESP: Dyspnea, pneumonia, **pulmonary edema or embolism**
SKIN: Alopecia, cutaneous vasculitis, ecchymosis, persistent bleeding or oozing from mucous membranes or surgical wounds, pruritus, skin necrosis at injection site or distant from injection site, urticaria, vesiculobullous rash
Other: **Anaphylaxis, including shock**, **hyperkalemia**; injection-site erythema; hematoma; inflammation; irritation; nodules; oozing; and pain

Childbearing Considerations

PREGNANCY

- It is not known if drug causes fetal harm.
- Use with caution only if benefit to mother outweighs potential risk to fetus.
- Be aware that all patients receiving anticoagulants, including pregnant women, are at risk for bleeding.
- Know that the multiple-dose vial of the drug contains 15 mg benzyl alcohol per 1 ml as a preservative. Cases of gasping syndrome have occurred in premature infants when large amounts of benzyl alcohol have been administered (99 to 405 mg/kg/day) to the mother.

LABOR AND DELIVERY

- Be aware that drug therapy may be changed to a shorter-acting anticoagulant as delivery approaches to decrease bleeding risk for both mother and fetus.

LACTATION

- It is not known if drug is present in breast milk.
- Mothers should check with prescriber before breastfeeding.

Nursing Considerations

! **WARNING** Be aware that drug isn't recommended for patients with prosthetic heart valves, especially pregnant women because of risk of prosthetic valve thrombosis. If enoxaparin is needed, monitor peak and trough antifactor Xa levels often and adjust dosage, as needed and ordered.

! **WARNING** Use enoxaparin with extreme caution in patients with a history of HIT. Know that enoxaparin should only be used in these patients if more than 100 days have elapsed since the prior HIT episode and no circulating antibodies are present.

! **WARNING** Use extreme caution in patients with an increased risk of hemorrhage, as from active ulcerative or angiodysplastic GI disease; bacterial endocarditis; acquired or congenital bleeding disorder; concurrent treatment with a platelet inhibitor; hemorrhagic stroke; or recent brain, ophthalmologic, or spinal surgery.

! **WARNING** Use cautiously in patients with bleeding diathesis, diabetic retinopathy, hepatic or renal impairment, recent GI hemorrhage or ulceration, or uncontrolled hypertension. Expect delayed elimination in elderly patients and those with renal insufficiency.

! **WARNING** Watch closely for bleeding. Notify prescriber immediately if platelet count falls below 100,000/mm^3. Expect to stop drug and start treatment if patient has a thromboembolic event, such as a stroke.

- Expect to give drug with aspirin to patient with unstable angina, STEMI, and non-Q-wave MI. To minimize risk of bleeding after vascular procedures, give enoxaparin at recommended intervals.

- Know that after a percutaneous revascularization procedure, it is important to achieve hemostasis at the puncture site. A closure device may be removed right away; however, if a manual compression method is used, the sheath should be removed 6 hours after last enoxaparin dose. If enoxaparin therapy will continue, give next scheduled dose no sooner than 6 to 8 hours after sheath removal.

! **WARNING** Monitor patient for a hypersensitivity reaction, which could become life-threatening such as anaphylaxis. If present, notify prescriber, expect drug to be switched to a different anticoagulant, and provide supportive care, as needed and ordered.

! **WARNING** Know that if patient is receiving enoxaparin with epidural or spinal anesthesia or spinal puncture, watch closely for development of spinal hematoma, which may cause long-term or permanent paralysis. If evidence of neurologic impairment, such as changes in sensory or motor function, occurs, notify prescriber immediately because urgent care is needed to minimize hematoma's effect. Risk of epidural or spinal hematoma during enoxaparin therapy is increased by concurrent use of other drugs that affect hemostasis, a history of repeated or traumatic epidural or spinal punctures, a history of spinal deformity or spinal surgery, or presence of indwelling epidural catheters. Know that placement or removal of a catheter should be delayed for at least 12 hours after administration of lower doses of enoxaparin (30 mg once or twice daily or 40 mg once daily) and at least 24 hours after the administration of higher doses (0.75 mg/kg twice daily, 1 mg/kg twice daily, or 1.5 mg/kg once daily). However, for patients with creatinine clearance of less than 30 ml/min, timing of removal should be doubled because enoxaparin elimination is more prolonged in renal dysfunction.

- Test stool for occult blood, as ordered.
- Keep protamine sulfate nearby in case of accidental overdose.
- Check serum potassium level for elevation, especially in patients with renal impairment or who are currently using potassium-sparing diuretics.

PATIENT TEACHING

- Teach patient, family, or caregiver how to give enoxaparin subcutaneously if it will be given at home.

! **WARNING** Alert patient that drug may cause an allergic reaction. If present, tell patient to notify prescriber, and, if severe, to seek immediate medical care.

! **WARNING** Inform patient that he may bruise and/or bleed more easily and that it may take longer than usual to stop bleeding while taking enoxaparin. Review bleeding precautions with patient. Inform patient that taking aspirin or other NSAIDs may increase risk for bleeding and to use aspirin only if prescribed and avoid use of NSAIDs. Advise patient to notify prescriber about adverse reactions, especially significant or unusual bleeding, bruising, or rash consisting of dark red spots under the skin.

! **WARNING** Tell females of childbearing age to notify prescriber if pregnancy occurs as bleeding is a risk during pregnancy.

! **WARNING** Instruct patient to seek immediate help for evidence of thromboembolism, such as neurologic changes and severe shortness of breath. Also, tell patient to report any unusual bleeding, bruising, or rash of dark red spots under the skin to prescriber.

! **WARNING** Instruct patient to alert all healthcare providers, but especially those administering anesthesia, about enoxaparin therapy. If neuraxial anesthesia or spinal puncture is necessary, and especially if patient is taking other drugs that could affect bleeding, tell patient to watch for signs and symptoms of epidural or spinal bleeding, such as muscle numbness or weakness or tingling in lower extremities.

- Emphasize the importance of complying with follow-up visits with prescriber.

ensifentrine

NEW!

Ohtuvayre

Class and Category

Pharmacologic class: Phosphodiesterase 3 (PDE3) and phosphodiesterase 4 (PDE4) inhibitors

Therapeutic class: Anti-inflammatory, bronchodilator

Indications and Dosages

∗ *To maintain treatment of chronic obstructive pulmonary disease (COPD)*

ORAL INHALATION SUSPENSION

Adults. 3 mg (1 ampule) twice daily, once in the morning and once in the evening.

Drug Administration

P.O.

- Do not physically mix with other drugs or add to solutions containing other drugs.
- Remove unit-dose ampule from foil pouch immediately before use.
- Shake ampule vigorously.
- Squeeze and completely empty contents of the ampule into the nebulizer cup for administration. Discard ampule.
- Administer by oral inhalation using a standard jet nebulizer equipped with a mouthpiece and connected to an air compressor.

Route	Onset	Peak	Duration
Oral Inhalation	Unknown.	0.6 to 1.5 hr.	Unknown

Half-life: 10.6 to 12.6 hr

Mechanism of Action

Inhibits PDE3 and PDE4, which results in accumulation of intracellular levels of cAMP and/or cGMP. By blocking PDE3 action, muscle relaxation around the airways occurs, which helps to relieve COPD symptoms such as coughing, shortness of breath, and wheezing. By blocking PDE4 action, inflammation in the lungs is reduced.

Contraindications

Hypersensitivity to ensifentrine or its components

Interactions

DRUGS

None listed by manufacturer.

Adverse Reactions

CNS: Adjustment disorder, anxiety, depression, insomnia, mood changes, **suicidal ideation**

CV: Hypertension

GI: Diarrhea

GU: UTI

MS: Back pain

RESP: **Paradoxical bronchospasm**

Childbearing Considerations

PREGNANCY

- It is not known if drug can cause fetal harm.
- Use with caution only if benefit to mother outweighs potential risk to fetus.

LACTATION

- It is not known if drug is present in breast milk.
- Mothers should check with prescriber before breastfeeding.

Nursing Considerations

! **WARNING** Know that ensifentrine should not be used to provide relief of acute symptoms. Rescue therapy such as an inhaled, short-acting bronchodilator should be used instead.

! **WARNING** Monitor patient closely for paradoxical bronchospasm, which could become life-threatening. If present, notify prescriber, administer an inhaled, short-acting bronchodilator, as ordered, and expect drug to be discontinued.

! **WARNING** Monitor patient closely for psychiatric adverse reactions, especially suicidal ideation.

PATIENT TEACHING

- Instruct patient and family or caregiver how to administer ensifentrine using a standard jet nebulizer with a mouthpiece. Stress that drug should never be swallowed or injected.

! **WARNING** Warn patient that drug should not be used to relieve acute symptoms of COPD and extra doses should not be taken for that purpose.

! **WARNING** Instruct patient to stop ensifentrine therapy and notify prescriber immediately if paradoxical bronchospasms occur.

! **WARNING** Tell patient to seek medical care immediately if he experiences decreased effectiveness of inhaled, short-acting $beta_2$ agonists, needs more inhalations than usual of his rescue inhaler, or experiences worsening symptoms.

! **WARNING** Alert patient and family or caregiver that drug may cause psychiatric adverse reactions such as anxiety, depression, insomnia, mood changes, and suicidal ideation. Tell patient, family, or caregiver to notify prescriber if present.

entecavir

Baraclude

Class and Category

Pharmacologic class: Nucleoside analogue
Therapeutic class: Antiviral

Indications and Dosages

* *To treat chronic hepatitis B virus infection in patients with evidence of active viral replication and either evidence of persistent elevations in serum aminotransferases (ALT or AST) or histologically active disease*

ORAL SOLUTION, TABLETS

Adults and adolescents ages 16 and older with compensated liver disease who are nucleoside-inhibitor-treatment-naïve. 0.5 mg once daily.
Adults and adolescents ages 16 and older with compensated liver disease who have a history of hepatitis B viremia while receiving lamivudine or have experienced known lamivudine or telbivudine resistance substitutions. 1 mg once daily.
Adults with decompensated liver disease. 1 mg once daily.
Children ages 2 and older weighing more than 30 kg (66 lb). 0.5 mg (tablet) or 10 ml (oral solution) once daily if treatment-naïve or 1 mg (tablet) or 20 ml (oral solution) once daily if lamivudine-experienced.

ORAL SOLUTION

Children ages 2 and older weighing more than 26 kg (57.2 lb) but less than 30 kg (66 lb). 9 ml once daily if treatment-naïve or 18 ml once daily if lamivudine-experienced.
Children ages 2 and older weighing more than 23 kg (50.6 lb) but less than 26 kg (57.2 lb). 8 ml once daily if treatment-naïve or 16 ml once daily if lamivudine-experienced.
Children ages 2 and older weighing more than 20 kg (44 lb) but less than 23 kg (50.6 lb). 7 ml once daily if treatment-naïve or 14 ml once daily if lamivudine-experienced.
Children ages 2 and older weighing more than 17 kg (37.4 lb) but less than 20 kg (44 lb). 6 ml once daily if treatment-naïve or 12 ml once daily if lamivudine-experienced.
Children ages 2 and older weighing more than 14 kg (30.8 lb) but less than 17 kg (37.4 lb). 5 ml once daily if treatment-naïve or 10 ml once daily if lamivudine-experienced.
Children ages 2 and older weighing more than 11 kg (24.2 lb) but less than 14 kg (30.8 lb). 4 ml once daily if treatment-naïve or 8 ml once daily if lamivudine-experienced.
Children ages 2 and older weighing at least 10 kg (22 lb) but less than 11 kg (24.2 lb). 3 ml once daily if treatment-naïve or 6 ml once daily if lamivudine-experienced.

± **DOSAGE ADJUSTMENT** For adult patients with a creatinine clearance between 30 and less than 50 ml/min, dosage reduced to 0.25 mg once daily or 0.5 mg every 48 hours, and dosage reduced to 0.5 mg once daily or 1 mg every 48 hours if lamivudine-refractory or decompensated liver disease is present. For adult patients with a creatinine clearance between 10 and less than 30 ml/min, dosage reduced to 0.15 mg once daily or 0.5 mg every 72 hours, and dosage reduced to 0.3 mg once daily or 1 mg every 72 hours if lamivudine-refractory or decompensated liver disease is present. For adult patients with a creatinine clearance less than 10 ml/min or on dialysis, dosage reduced to 0.05 mg once daily or 0.5 mg every 7 days (given after hemodialysis), and dosage reduced to 0.1 mg once daily or 1 mg every 7 days (given after hemodialysis) if lamivudine-refractory or decompensated liver disease is present. For pediatric patients with renal impairment, there is insufficient data to recommend a specific dose adjustment but a reduction in dose and/or an increase in dosing interval similar to adults may be considered.

E

Drug Administration

P.O.

- Administer on an empty stomach 2 hr before or after a meal.
- Tablets should be swallowed whole and not chewed, crushed, or split.
- To measure oral solution dosage, hold the dosing spoon in a vertical position and fill it gradually to the mark corresponding to the prescribed dose.
- Administer oral solution for doses less than 0.5 mg and for children weighing less than 30 kg (66 lb).
- Rinse dosing spoon after each use with water.

Route	Onset	Peak	Duration
P.O.	Unknown	0.5–1.5 hr	Unknown

Half-life: 5–6 hr

Mechanism of Action

Inhibits all 3 activities of the hepatitis B virus (HBV) reverse transcriptase: base priming, reverse transcription of the negative strand from the pregenomic messenger RNA, and synthesis of the positive strand of HBV DNA. This lowers the ability of HBV to multiply and infect new liver cells.

Contraindications

Hypersensitivity to entecavir or its components

Interactions

DRUGS

drugs that reduce renal function or compete for active tubular secretion: Possibly increased serum concentrations of either entecavir or the coadministered drug, increasing risk of adverse reactions

Adverse Reactions

CNS: Dizziness, **encephalopathy** (hepatic-induced), fatigue, fever, headache, insomnia, somnolence
CV: Peripheral edema
EENT: Taste abnormality
ENDO: Hyperglycemia
GI: Abdominal pain, ascites, diarrhea, dyspepsia, elevated liver and pancreatic enzymes, **exacerbation of hepatitis** (after discontinuation of therapy), **GI hemorrhage**, **hepatic failure**, **hepatorenal syndrome**, hyperalbuminemia, hyperbilirubinemia, nausea, **severe hepatomegaly with steatosis**, vomiting
GU: Elevated creatinine level, glycosuria, hematuria, **renal failure**
HEME: **Decreased platelet count**
RESP: Upper respiratory infection
SKIN: Alopecia, rash
Other: **Anaphylaxis**, **decreased serum bicarbonate level**, **lactic acidosis**

Childbearing Considerations

PREGNANCY

- Pregnancy exposure registry: 1-800-258-4263.
- It is not known if drug causes fetal harm.
- Use with caution only if benefit to mother outweighs potential risk to fetus.

LACTATION

- It is not known if drug is present in breast milk.
- Mothers should check with prescriber before breastfeeding.

Nursing Considerations

- Ensure that patient has been tested for HIV infection before entecavir therapy begins because resistance to HIV therapy may develop when entecavir is administered to treat chronic hepatitis B virus infection in patients who also have an HIV infection that is not being treated. Know that entecavir therapy is not recommended for coinfected patients who are not receiving treatment.

! WARNING Monitor patient for signs and symptoms of a hypersensitivity reaction, which could become life-threatening such as anaphylaxis. If present, notify prescriber, expect drug to be discontinued, and provide supportive care, as needed and ordered.

! WARNING Know that lactic acidosis and severe hepatomegaly with steatosis have occurred with entecavir therapy and death has occurred in some patients. Risk factors include being a woman, being obese, or having a prolonged nucleoside exposure. However, know that lactic acidosis and severe hepatomegaly with steatosis have also occurred in patients with no known risk factors. Monitor patient's liver enzymes, as ordered. Expect entecavir to be discontinued in any patient who develops clinical or laboratory findings suggestive of lactic acidosis or pronounced hepatotoxicity, even in the absence of marked transaminase elevations.

! **WARNING** Expect patient to be closely monitored for at least several months after entecavir has been discontinued because severe acute exacerbation of hepatitis may occur.

PATIENT TEACHING

- Instruct patient with hepatitis B on the importance of testing for HIV before therapy begins and then periodically throughout therapy to avoid development of resistance to HIV treatment.
- Instruct patient, family, or caregiver how to administer entecavir and what to do if a dose is missed.
- Tell patient that entecavir therapy does not reduce the transmission of HBV to others through blood contamination or sexual contact.

! **WARNING** Inform patient that drug may cause an allergic reaction. If present, instruct patient to notify prescriber and, if severe, to seek immediate medical care.

! **WARNING** Alert patient that severe conditions may develop while taking entecavir. If patient experiences persistent, severe, or unusual signs and symptoms, encourage him to notify prescriber and stop taking drug, if advised to do so, and seek medical attention immediately if in acute distress.

! **WARNING** Warn patient with hepatitis B that acute severe exacerbations of hepatitis B may occur following discontinuation of entecavir. He should not discontinue drug without prescriber knowledge. Tell patient to report any reappearance of signs and symptoms of hepatitis B immediately to prescriber.

epinephrine

(adrenaline)

Adrenaclick, Adrenalin, Auvi-Q, EpiPen, EpiPen Jr, Neffy, Symjepi

Class and Category

Pharmacologic class: Sympathomimetic
Therapeutic class: Antianaphylactic, bronchodilator, cardiac stimulant, vasopressor

Indications and Dosages

✻ *To provide emergency treatment of allergic reactions (type I), including anaphylaxis to allergen immunotherapy, biting and stinging insects, diagnostic testing substances, drugs, foods, and other allergens, as well as exercise-induced or idiopathic anaphylaxis*

I.M. OR SUBCUTANEOUS INJECTION (ADRENALIN)

Adults and children weighing 30 kg (66 lb) or more. 0.3 to 0.5 mg, repeated every 5 to 10 min, as needed. *Maximum:* 0.5 mg/injection
Children weighing less than 30 kg (66 lb). 0.01 mg/kg, repeated every 5 to 10 min, as needed. *Maximum:* 0.3 mg/injection.

I.M. INJECTION, SUBCUTANEOUS INJECTION (ADRENACLICK, AUVI-Q, EPIPEN, SYMJEPI)

Adults and children weighing 30 kg (66 lb) or more who are at increased risk for anaphylaxis. 0.3 mg immediately upon exposure and repeated 1 time, as needed.

I.M. INJECTION, SUBCUTANEOUS INJECTION (ADRENACLICK, AUVI-Q, EPIPEN JR, SYMJEPI)

Adults and children weighing 15 to 30 kg (33 to 66 lb) who are at increased risk of anaphylaxis. 0.15 mg immediately upon exposure and repeated 1 time, as needed.

I.M. INJECTION, SUBCUTANEOUS INJECTION (AUVI-Q)

Children weighing 7.5 to 15 kg (16.5 to 33 lb) who are at increased risk of anaphylaxis. 0.1 mg immediately upon exposure and repeated 1 time, as needed.

NASAL SPRAY (NEFFY)

Adults and children weighing 30 kg (66 lb) or more. 2 mg (1 spray) in one nostril followed by 2 mg (1 spray) in the same nostril 5 min or later after the first dose, as needed.

✻ *To treat hypotension associated with septic shock*

I.V. INFUSION (ADRENALIN)

Adults. 0.05 mcg/kg/min to 2 mcg/kg/min, titrated to achieve desired mean arterial pressure by adjusting dose every 10 to 15 min, in increments of 0.05 to 0.2 mcg/kg/min.

✻ *To induce and maintain mydriasis during intraocular surgery*

INTRAOCULAR (ADRENALIN)

Adults. 10 mcg/ml to 1 mcg/ml used as an irrigating solution during eye surgery.

Drug Administration

- Some preparations contain sulfites, which may cause allergic-type reactions. However, the presence of sulfites in epinephrine should not deter its use in a patient with anaphylaxis, even if patient is sensitive to sulfites.
- Protect solution from light.

I.V.

- Prepare I.V. infusion by diluting 1 mg of epinephrine to 1,000 ml of a 5% Dextrose or 5% Dextrose and 0.9% Sodium Chloride Injection solution to produce a 1 mcg/ml dilution. Administration in 0.9% Sodium Chloride Injection alone is not recommended.
- Administer as a continuous infusion only to treat hypotension associated with septic shock. Do not use autoinjectors I.V.
- When possible, administer I.V. infusion through a central line or, if not possible, a large vein. Avoid using a catheter tie-in technique because the obstruction to blood flow around the tubing may cause stasis and increased local concentration of drug.
- Avoid injecting into the veins of the leg in elderly patients or in those suffering from occlusive vascular diseases.
- Avoid extravasation of epinephrine into the tissues to prevent local necrosis. Assess infusion site frequently for free flow and look for blanching along the course of the infused vein, which may indicate some leakage from the vein wall. If blanching occurs, change infusion site. To prevent sloughing and necrosis in areas in which extravasation has taken place, obtain an order to infiltrate the area with 10 to 15 ml of saline solution containing 5 to 10 mg phentolamine. Using a syringe with a fine hypodermic needle, infiltrate the area liberally, which is easily identified by its cold, hard, and pallid appearance.
- The diluted solution may be stored up to 4 hr at room temperature and 24 hr if refrigerated.
- *Incompatibilities:* Alkaline solutions, aminophylline, hyaluronidase, sodium bicarbonate, mephentermine, thiopental

I.M. AND SUBCUTANEOUS

- When given by these routes, the drug is intended for use as emergency supportive therapy only and is not a substitute for immediate medical care.
- Inspect epinephrine solution before use. If it is pink or brown, air has entered a multidose vial. If it is discolored or contains particles, discard it. Also, discard unused portions.
- Do not administer by intra-arterial injection because marked vasoconstriction may cause gangrene. Also, accidental injection of drug into patient's feet, fingers, or hands may result in loss of blood flow to the affected area.
- NEVER inject drug into the buttocks or use the deltoid muscle for injection.
- Inject drug only into the anterolateral aspect of the thigh, through clothing, if necessary.
- When administering drug to a child, hold the leg firmly in place and limit movement prior to and during an injection to minimize the risk of injury related to the injection or inadvertently injecting drug into the buttocks.
- Remember to rotate sites because repeated injections in the same site may cause vasoconstriction and localized necrosis.
- Assess injection site periodically after administration of drug for signs of infection, such as persistent redness, swelling, tenderness, or warmth because, although rare, serious skin and soft-tissue infections, including myonecrosis and necrotizing fasciitis caused by *Clostridia* (gas gangrene), have been reported at the injection site, especially if drug was inadvertently injected into buttocks. Cleaning the site with alcohol before injecting drug does not kill bacterial spores and therefore does not reduce the risk.
- Store drug at room temperature and protect from light.

NASAL SPRAY

- Know that each nasal spray device is for single use. Deliver the entire dose upon activation.
- Do not prime or attempt to reuse drug device for more than 1 administration.

- Use right hand to administer drug to right nostril and left hand to administer drug to the left nostril.
- Insert nozzle of nasal spray fully into 1 nostril until your fingers touch the nose. Hold the nasal spray straight into the nose; do not angle the spray to the inside septum or outer wall of the nose as some of the drug may be lost. Press the plunger firmly to activate.
- Tell patient to avoid sniffing during and after administration.

INTRAOCULAR

- If the Adrenalin brand of epinephrine is used during intraocular surgery to induce and maintain mydriasis, the 30-ml multiple-dose vial of the drug should not be used because it contains chlorobutanol, which may be harmful to the corneal endothelium.
- The Adrenalin 1-ml single-use vial must be diluted before intraocular use. Dilute in 100 ml to 1,000 ml of an ophthalmic irrigation fluid to obtain a concentration of 1:100,000 to 1:1,000,000 (10 mcg/ml to 1 mcg/ml).

Route	Onset	Peak	Duration
I.V.	Immediate	5 min	Short
I.M.	Rapid	Unknown	Short
SubQ	5–15 min	30 min	Short
Nasal Spray.	Rapid	5-10 min	Short

Half-life: < 2 min

Mechanism of Action

Acts on alpha and beta receptors. This nonselective adrenergic agonist stimulates:

- $alpha_1$ receptors, which constricts arteries and may decrease bronchial secretions
- presynaptic $alpha_2$ receptors, which inhibits norepinephrine release by way of negative feedback
- postsynaptic $alpha_2$ receptors, which constricts arteries
- $beta_1$ receptors, which induces positive chronotropic and inotropic responses
- $beta_2$ receptors, which dilates arteries, relaxes bronchial smooth muscles, increases glycogenolysis, and prevents mast cells from secreting histamine and other substances, thus reversing bronchoconstriction and edema.

Contraindications

Angle-closure glaucoma, cerebral arteriosclerosis, coronary insufficiency, dilated cardiomyopathy, during labor, general anesthesia with halogenated hydrocarbons or cyclopropane, hypersensitivity to epinephrine or its components, organic brain damage, shock (nonanaphylactic)

Interactions

DRUGS

alpha-blockers, such as phentolamine: Antagonized pressor effects of epinephrine
antiarrhythmics, cardiac glycosides, diuretics: Increased risk of cardiac arrhythmias
antihistamines (chlorpheniramine, diphenhydramine, tripelennamine), levothyroxine, MAO inhibitors, tricyclic antidepressants: Increased risk of potentiated effect of epinephrine
beta-adrenergic blockers, such as propranolol: Antagonized bronchodilating and cardiostimulating effects of epinephrine
ergot alkaloids: Possibly reverse pressor effects of epinephrine

Adverse Reactions

CNS: Anxiety, apprehensiveness, chills, **CVA**, disorientation, dizziness, drowsiness, excitability, fever, hallucinations, headache, impaired memory, insomnia, lightheadedness, nervousness, panic, psychomotor agitation, restlessness, **seizures**, sleepiness, temporary worsening of Parkinson's disease, tingling, tremor, weakness
CV: Angina (in presence of coronary artery disease); **arrhythmias, including ventricular fibrillation**; chest discomfort or pain; fast, irregular, or slow heartbeat; increased cardiac output; **myocardial ischemia**; palpitations; peripheral vasoconstriction; **severe hypertension**; **stress cardiomyopathy**; tachycardia; vasoconstriction; **ventricular ectopy**
EENT: Blurred vision, dry mouth or throat, miosis *For nasal spray:* gingival pain; hypoesthesia (oral); nasal congestion, discomfort, or itching; rhinorrhea; sneezing; throat irritation
ENDO: Hyperglycemia in diabetics
GI: Abdominal pain, anorexia, heartburn, nausea, vomiting
GU: Dysuria, oliguria, renal impairment
MS: Muscle twitching, severe muscle spasms
RESP: Dyspnea, **pulmonary edema**
SKIN: Cold skin, diaphoresis, ecchymosis, flushed or red face or skin, pallor, tissue necrosis

Other: **Hyperkalemia**; **hypokalemia**; injection-site coldness, hypoesthesia, infections (*Clostridia*), pain, pallor, and stinging

Childbearing Considerations

PREGNANCY

- It is not known if drug causes fetal harm.
- Use with caution only if benefit to mother outweighs potential risk to fetus.

LABOR AND DELIVERY

- May delay second stage of labor because drug usually inhibits spontaneous or oxytocin-induced contractions. It may also cause a prolonged period of uterine atony with hemorrhage.
- Drug should be avoided during second stage of labor and in patients with a blood pressure that exceeds 130/80 mm Hg.
- While drug may improve maternal hypotension associated with anaphylaxis and septic shock, it may cause decreased uterine blood flow, fetal anoxia, and uterine vasoconstriction.

LACTATION

- It is not known if drug is present in breast milk.
- Mothers should check with prescriber before breastfeeding after receiving epinephrine.

Nursing Considerations

! **WARNING** Use epinephrine with extreme caution in patients with angina, arrhythmias, asthma, degenerative heart disease, or emphysema. Epinephrine's inotropic effect equals that of dopamine and dobutamine; its chronotropic effect exceeds that of both.

- Use drug cautiously in elderly patients and those with cardiovascular disease, diabetes mellitus, hypertension, hyperthyroidism, prostatic hypertrophy, and psychoneurologic disorders.

! **WARNING** Do not administer epinephrine in the buttocks or deltoid muscle. Inject only into the anteriolateral aspect of the thigh. Monitor injection site after administering epinepherine I.M. or subcutaneously. Although rare, serious skin and soft tissue infections, including necrotizing fasciitis and myonecrosis caused by *Clostridia* (gas gangrene) have occurred at the injection site. Notify prescriber immediately if signs and symptoms of infection, such as persistent redness, warmth, and swelling, or tenderness occurs at the injection site.

! **WARNING** Be aware that nasal spray form of epinephrine may alter nasal mucosa for up to 2 weeks after administration and may increase systemic absorption of nasal products possibly leading to increase in adverse reactions.

- Monitor patient's blood pressure frequently and titrate I.V. dosages to avoid excessive increases in blood pressure.
- Monitor patient for cardiac arrhythmias and myocardial ischemia.
- Monitor patient for potassium imbalances. Hyperkalemia may occur first followed quickly by hypokalemia.

PATIENT TEACHING

- Teach patient and family how to administer epinephrine by nasal spray or subcutaneously with the product prescribed.
- Teach patient, family, or caregiver how to administer drug subcutaneously, if prescribed, using the specific autoclick device prescribed and importance of following the manufacturer guidelines. Inform them they may request an "Autoclick Trainer" device to practice using an autoclick device (has no drug or needle) so injecting epinephrine in an emergency can be more familiar. Stress importance of placing the blue safety release back on the Trainer and reset it after practicing. This small piece poses a choking hazard for children.
- Tell them to inject drug subcutaneously only into anterolateral aspect of the thigh, through the clothing if necessary. If injecting drug into a child, stress importance of holding the leg firmly in place and limiting movement prior to and during the injection to prevent injury.

! **WARNING** Instruct patient, family, or caregiver never to give epinephrine in the buttocks, as absorption may be hindered. Also, a serious infection (gas gangrene) may occur if injected in the buttocks. In addition, tell patient, family, or caregiver to inspect the thigh for signs of infection at the injection site and report if persistent redness, swelling, tenderness, and warmth develop.

! **WARNING** Caution patient to avoid accidentally injecting drug into his fingers, hands, toes, or feet because epinephrine is a strong vasoconstrictor and could cause loss of blood flow to the area, resulting in gangrene. Instruct patient using an EpiPen to never put fingers, hand, or thumb over the orange tip and not to press or push the orange tip with fingers, hand, or thumb because the needle comes out of the orange tip. If accidental injection occurs in any of these areas, instruct patient to go immediately to nearest emergency room.

! **WARNING** Tell patient using an EpiPen or EpiPen Jr to always check to make sure the blue safety release is not raised. If blue safety release is raised this means it has been activated and is useless. Tell him to never flip the blue safety release off using a thumb, pull it sideways, or bend and twist the blue safety release. This may cause the device to activate by accident: a "click" is heard, the orange tip is extended, and the window is blocked. Once activated, the device cannot be used in an emergency. A new pen should be obtained in either case. Also, stress importance of throwing away the blue safety release immediately after using because it can pose a choking hazard for children.

! **WARNING** Inform patient that if nasal spray form of epinephrine is used, the nasal mucosa in the nostril the drug was given in may increase absorption of other nasal products for up to 2 weeks increasing risk of adverse reactions.

! **WARNING** Stress importance to patient, family, or caregiver to keep drug away from young children.

! **WARNING** Remind patient, family, or caregiver that drug used in an emergency situation to treat anaphylaxis is intended for emergency supportive therapy only. Stress importance of seeking immediate care after drug is administered.

! **WARNING** Inform patient that epinephrine may cause anxiety, apprehension, difficulty breathing, dizziness, headache, increase in heart rate or sensation of a more forceful heartbeat, nausea, nervousness, palpitations, shakiness, sweating, vomiting, or weakness. Reassure patient these signs and symptoms usually subside rapidly, especially with being quiet, lying down, and resting. If signs and symptoms continue or get worse, advise patient to notify prescriber immediately.

- Inform patient with diabetes that epinephrine may cause hyperglycemia. Inform patient with Parkinson's disease that symptoms may temporarily worsen. Tell patient with hypertension or hyperthyroidism, more severe or persistent effects may be experienced. Tell these patients this should not deter use of drug as it is used in an emergency.
- Explain that solution is light sensitive and should be stored in the carrying case and at room temperature. Tell them not to refrigerate drug or keep it in overheated areas such as a closed car and to replace solution if it discolors.
- Instruct patient never to throw away expired, unwanted, or unused epinephrine injections into household trash. Instead, drug should be disposed of in an FDA-cleared sharps disposal container or a container made of heavy-duty plastic, leak-resistant, able to stand upright during use, closed with a tight-fitting, puncture-resistant lid, without sharps being able to protrude out and properly labeled to warn of hazardous waste inside the container. Dispose of container when almost full according to state regulations. If not sure, tell patient to go to the FDA's website at: http://fda.gov/safesharpsdisposal.
- Remind patient, family, or caregiver using the EpiPen or EpiPen Jr that the pen delivers a fixed dose of epinephrine and the autoinjectors cannot be reused. Offer reassurance that it is normal for some of the drug to remain in the autoinjector after the dose has been injected. The dose has been injected if the orange tip is extended and the window is blocked.

eplerenone

Inspra

Class and Category

Pharmacologic class: Aldosterone receptor blocker

Therapeutic class: Antihypertensive

Indications and Dosages

∗ *As adjunct to standard treatment to reduce risk of cardiovascular mortality and hospitalization for heart failure in patients with NYHA class II systolic chronic heart failure and left ventricular systolic dysfunction; as adjunct to standard treatment to reduce risk of mortality and hospitalization for heart failure following MI in clinically stable patients who have evidence of heart failure and left ventricular systolic dysfunction (ejection fraction equal to or less than 40%)*

TABLETS

Adults with eGFR equal to or greater than 50 ml/min. *Initial:* 25 mg once daily, increased to 50 mg once daily within 4 wk, as needed. Then, dosage adjusted based on the serum potassium level. *Maximum:* 50 mg once daily.

Adults with an eGFR between 30 and 49 ml/min. *Initial:* 25 mg once every other day, increased to 25 mg once daily within 4 wk, as needed. Then, dosage adjusted based on the serum potassium level. *Maximum:* 25 mg once daily.

±**DOSAGE ADJUSTMENT** For patients taking a mild to moderate CYP3A4 inhibitor, maximum dosage reduced to 25 mg once daily. For patients with a potassium level less than 5.0 mEq/L taking 25 mg every other day, dosage interval increased to daily; for patient taking 25 mg once daily, dosage increased to 50 mg once daily. For patients with a potassium level of 5.0 to 5.4 mEq/L, no adjustment needed. For patients with a potassium level between 5.5 and 5.9 mEq/L and taking 50 mg once daily, dosage reduced to 25 mg once daily; if patients are taking 25 mg once daily, dosage interval increased to 25 mg every other day; or if patients were taking 25 mg every other day, drug withheld, until potassium level returns to acceptable level and then restarted only after potassium level falls below 5 mEq/L. For patients with a potassium level 6.0 mEq/L or higher, drug withheld until potassium level returns to acceptable level and then restarted at 25 mg every other day.

∗ *To treat mild to moderate hypertension alone or with other antihypertensive drugs*

TABLETS

Adults. *Initial:* 50 mg once daily, increased to 50 mg twice daily after 4 wk, as needed.

±**DOSAGE ADJUSTMENT** For patients taking mild to moderate CYP3A4 inhibitors, such as erythromycin, fluconazole, saquinavir, and verapamil, initial dosage reduced to 25 mg once daily.

Drug Administration

P.O.

- Drug may be given without regard to meals.

Route	Onset	Peak	Duration
P.O.	Unknown	1.5–2 hr	Unknown

Half-life: 4–6 hr

Mechanism of Action

Blocks the binding of aldosterone at its mineralocorticoid receptor sites located in the blood vessels, brain, heart, and kidneys. This action decreases blood pressure by preventing aldosterone from inducing sodium reabsorption and possibly other mechanisms that contribute to raising blood pressure.

Contraindications

For all patients: Concurrent therapy with strong CYP3A inhibitors (clarithromycin, ketoconazole, itraconazole, nefazodone, nelfinavir, ritonavir, telithromycin); potassium-sparing diuretics; potassium supplements; hypersenstivity to eplerenone or its components; serum potassium level greater than 5 mEq/L at initiation of therapy or presence of clinically significant hyperkalemia; severe hepatic or renal impairment

For patients with hypertension: Moderate to severe renal impairment (eGFR less than 50 ml/min), serum creatinine greater than 132 µmol/L or 115 µmol/L in females, type 2 diabetes with microalbuminuria

Interactions

DRUGS

ACE inhibitors, angiotensin II receptor antagonists: Increased risk of hyperkalemia
strong CYP3A4 inducers (carbamazepine, phenobarbital, phenytoin, rifampicin, St. John's wort): Significant decreased exposure and increased clearance of eplerenone decreasing effectiveness
CYP3A inhibitors: Increased blood level and effect of eplerenone
herbal preparations: Possibly increased risk of hypotension or hypertension; possibly increased risk of hyperkalemia
lithium: Possibly lithium toxicity
NSAIDs: Possibly reduced antihypertensive effect of eplerenone; severe hyperkalemia in patients with impaired renal function

FOODS

salt substitutes: Possibly increased risk of hypotension or hypertension; possibly increased risk of hyperkalemia

Adverse Reactions

CNS: Asthenia, cerebrovascular disorder, dizziness, fatigue, fever, headache, syncope
CV: Angina pectoris, hypercholesterolemia, hypertriglyceridemia, **hypotension**, **MI** non-cardiac chest pain, palpitations, peripheral edema, **ventricular tachycardia**
EENT: Nasopharyngitis, sinusitis, coronary artery disorder
ENDO: Gynecomastia, hyperglycemia, mastodynia
GI: Abdominal pain, constipation, diarrhea, dyspepsia, increased liver enzymes, nausea, vomiting
GU: Albuminuria, elevated BUN and serum creatinine levels, hematuria, **renal impairment**, vaginal bleeding
Heme: Anemia
MS: Extremity pain
RESP: Bronchitis, cough, upper respiratory tract infection
SKIN: Pruritus
Other: Elevated creatine phosphokinase levels, flu-like symptoms, **hyperkalemia**, **hypokalemia**, **hyponatremia**, increased uric acid level

Childbearing Considerations

PREGNANCY

- It is not known if drug causes fetal harm.
- Use with caution only if benefit to mother outweighs potential risk to fetus.

LACTATION

- It is not known if drug is present in breast milk.
- Mothers should check with prescriber before breastfeeding.

REPRODUCTION

- Male fertility may become compromised with drug therapy based on animal studies.

Nursing Considerations

- Monitor patient's serum potassium level before start of therapy, within the first week of therapy, at 1 month, and periodically thereafter, as ordered. Notify prescriber of abnormalities, as dosage will have to be adjusted.

! **WARNING** Be aware that patients with diabetes, impaired renal function, proteinuria, or who take an ACE inhibitor or an angiotensin II receptor antagonist during eplerenone therapy have an increased risk of hyperkalemia. Monitor patients over age 65 closely because the risk of hyperkalemia may be increased because of age-related decreases in creatinine clearance.

- Monitor patient's blood pressure regularly to evaluate eplerenone effectiveness.

PATIENT TEACHING

- Instruct patient how to administer eplerenone.

! **WARNING** Caution patient not to use potassium salt substitutes or potassium-containing supplements because increased potassium levels can lead to serious adverse reactions to eplerenone.

! **WARNING** Advise patient to alert prescriber if persistent, serious, or unusual adverse reactions occur. Stress importance of seeking immediate medical care if patient is experiencing signs and symptoms of a heart attack.

- Urge patient to tell all prescribers about eplerenone use because of possible interactions.
- Caution patient to comply with scheduled laboratory appointments to monitor potassium level.

epoetin alfa
(EPO, erythropoietin alfa, recombinant erythropoietin, r-HuEPO)

Epogen, Eprex (CAN), Procrit

epoetin alfa-epbx

Retacrit

Class and Category

Pharmacologic class: Erythropoietin
Therapeutic class: Antianemic

Indications and Dosages

* *To treat anemia due to chronic kidney disease for patients on dialysis and who have a hemoglobin less than 10 g/dl; to treat anemia due to chronic kidney disease for patients not on dialysis but have a hemoglobin less than 10 g/dl with the rate of decline of hemoglobin level indicating patient will need an RBC transfusion, and the treatment goal is to reduce the risk of alloimmunization and other RBC transfusion-related risks*

I.V. OR SUBCUTANEOUS INJECTION

Adults. *Initial:* 50 to 100 units/kg 3 times/wk, increased, as needed, by 25% at 4-wk intervals or longer. *Maintenance:* Dosage highly individualized to lowest dose that keeps hemoglobin below 11 g/dl.
Neonates ages 1 mo and older and children. 50 units/kg 3 times/wk; increased, as needed, by 25% at 4-wk intervals or longer. *Maintenance:* Dosage highly individualized to lowest dose that keeps hemoglobin below 12 g/dl.

±DOSAGE ADJUSTMENT For patients with anemia from renal failure on dialysis, dosage temporarily reduced or drug discontinued if hemoglobin approaches or exceeds 11 g/dl (12 g/dl for children). For patients with anemia from renal failure not on dialysis, dosage temporarily reduced or drug discontinued if hemoglobin exceeds 10 g/dl (12 g/dl for children). For patients with anemia from renal failure with or without dialysis, dosage reduced 25% or more if hemoglobin rises rapidly (more than 1 g/dl in any 2-week period).

* *To treat anemia in HIV-infected patients due to zidovudine administered at 4,200 mg or more each week and patient's endogenous serum erythropoietin level is 500 mU/ml or less.*

I.V. OR SUBCUTANEOUS INJECTION

Adults. *Initial:* 100 units/kg 3 times/wk, increased by 50 to 100 units/kg every 4 to 8 wk after 8 wk of therapy. *Maintenance:* Dosage gradually titrated to maintain desired response, based on such factors as variations in zidovudine dosage and occurrence of infection or inflammation. *Maximum:* 300 units/kg 3 times/wk or hemoglobin has reached a level needed to avoid RBC transfusions.

±DOSAGE ADJUSTMENT For patients with a hemoglobin that exceeds 12 g/dl, drug withheld and resumed at a dose 25% below the previous dose when hemoglobin has declined to less than 11 g/dl.

* *To treat anemia from chemotherapy*

SUBCUTANEOUS INJECTION

Adults with a hemoglobin less than 10 g/dl, and there is a minimum of 2 additional months of planned chemotherapy. *Initial:* 150 units/kg 3 times/wk until completion of a chemotherapy course. Alternatively, 40,000 units weekly until completion of a chemotherapy course. Dosage increased to 300 units/kg 3 times/wk or 60,000 units weekly after 4 wk, as needed. *Maximum:* 300 units/kg 3 times/wk or 60,000 units weekly.

I.V. INJECTION

Children ages 5 to 18 with a hemoglobin less than 10 g/dl, and if there is a minimum of 2 additional months of planned chemotherapy. 600 units/kg once weekly until completion of a chemotherapy course. Dosage increased to 900 units/kg weekly after initial 4 wk of therapy if hemoglobin increases by less than 1 g/dl and remains below 10 g/dl. *Maximum:* 900 units/kg (60,000 units) weekly.

±DOSAGE ADJUSTMENT For adults and children, dosage decreased by 25% if hemoglobin level approaches a level needed to avoid RBC transfusion or increases more than 1 g/dl in any 2-week period. For adults and children, dose withheld if hemoglobin exceeds a level needed to avoid RBC transfusion and resumed at 25% less than previous dose when hemoglobin approaches a level where RBC transfusions may be required.

✶ *To reduce need for allogeneic red blood cell transfusions in patients undergoing elective, noncardiac, nonvascular surgery*

SUBCUTANEOUS INJECTION

Adults. 300 units/kg daily for 10 days before surgery, on day of surgery, and 4 days after surgery. Alternatively, 600 units/kg/wk on 21, 14, and 7 days before surgery and a fourth dose on the day of surgery.

Drug Administration

- Don't shake vial while preparing, to avoid inactivating drug.
- Discard unused portion of single-dose vial because it contains no preservatives. Store multidose vial in refrigerator and discard unused portion after 21 days.
- Do not use multidose vials, which contain benzyl alcohol, for pregnant or breastfeeding patients, neonates, or infants.
- Protect drug vials from light.
- Do not use if drug vial has been frozen or shaken. Also, do not use if the green area of the freeze strip indicator on Retacrit vials appears cloudy or white.

I.V.

- Administer as an injection undiluted. Manufacturer does not specify rate of administration.
- I.V. is the preferred route for patients on hemodialysis. Inject into the venous port of the hemodialysis tubing.
- *Incompatibilities:* Other I.V. drugs

SUBCUTANEOUS

- Injection sites that can be used include abdomen (except for 2-inch area around the navel), front of thighs, outer area of upper arms, and upper outer area of buttocks.
- Administer as an injection undiluted while pinching a fold of skin. Do not inject into an area that is bruised, hard, red, tender, or has scars or stretch marks.
- Know that preservative-free drug from a single-dose vial may be mixed in a syringe with Bacteriostatic 0.9% Sodium Chloride Injection with benzyl alcohol 0.9% (bacteriostatic saline) in a 1:1 ratio for administration. Do not use this mixture in pregnant or breastfeeding women, neonates, or infants.
- Rotate sites.

Route	Onset	Peak	Duration
I.V.	Immediate	15 min	2 wk
SubQ	Unknown	5–24 hr	2 wk

Half-life: 4–13 hr

Mechanism of Action

Stimulates the release of reticulocytes from the bone marrow into the bloodstream, where they develop into mature RBCs.

Contraindications

Hypersensitivity to epoetin alfa, epoetin alfa-epbx, or their components; pure red cell aplasia that began after treatment with epoetin alfa, epoetin alfa-epbx, or other erythropoietin protein drugs; uncontrolled hypertension; use of multidose vials in infants, neonates, or females of childbearing age who are breastfeeding or pregnant

Interactions

DRUGS

None reported by manufacturer.

Adverse Reactions

CNS: Anxiety, asthenia, **CVA**, dizziness, fatigue, fever, headache, insomnia, paresthesia, **seizures**
CV: Chest pain, **congestive heart failure**, **deep vein thrombosis**, edema, hypertension, **MI**, tachycardia, **thromboembolic events**
GI: Constipation, diarrhea, indigestion, nausea, vomiting
GU: UTI
HEME: Polycythemia
MS: Arthralgia, bone pain, muscle weakness
RESP: Cough, dyspnea, **pulmonary congestion**, upper respiratory tract infection
SKIN: **Erythema multiforme**, rash, pruritus, **Stevens-Johnson syndrome**, **toxic epidermal necrolysis**, urticaria
Other: Anti-epoetin alfa antibodies, flu-like symptoms, **hyperkalemia**, injection-site reaction, trunk pain

Childbearing Considerations

PREGNANCY

- It is not known if drug causes fetal harm.
- Use with caution only if benefit to mother outweighs potential risk to fetus.
- Know that use of the multiple-dose vials of the drug are contraindicated for use in pregnant women because it contains benzyl alcohol. A benzyl alcohol-free formulation

should be used instead, such as the single-dose vial.

- Do not mix drug with bacteriostatic saline containing benzyl alcohol when administering to pregnant women.

LACTATION

- It is not known if drug is present in breast milk.
- Advise mothers to check with prescriber before breastfeeding if drug will be administered from a single-dose vial.
- Use of the multiple-dose vial of the drug is contraindicated in mothers who are breastfeeding.
- Do not mix drug with bacteriostatic saline containing benzyl alcohol being administering to mothers who are breastfeeding.
- Inform breastfeeding mothers that if drug is administered using a multiple-dose vial, breastfeeding should be withheld for at least 2 wk after the last dose.

Nursing Considerations

! **WARNING** Be aware that epoetin alfa shouldn't be given to cancer patients when a cure is anticipated because drug may decrease survival rate and increase tumor progression in patients with certain types of cancers, such as breast, cervical, head and neck, lymphoid, or non-small-cell lung cancers. Know that lowest possible dose should be used. Cancer patient should only receive drug to treat anemia caused by myelosuppressive chemotherapy.

- Know that all prescribers and hospitals must enroll and comply with the ESA APPRISE Oncology program to be able to prescribe and dispense the drug.
- Ensure that patient has received the medication guide and patient instructions for epoetin alfa and that a written acknowledgment of a discussion of the risks involved with this type of therapy has been obtained before first dose is given.
- Evaluate the patient's serum iron level before and during treatment, as ordered. Expect to give an iron supplement (I.V. iron dextran), as needed, because iron requirements rise when erythropoiesis consumes existing iron stores.
- Use epoetin alfa cautiously in patients who have conditions that could decrease or delay response to drug, such as aluminum intoxication, folic acid deficiency, hemolysis, infection, inflammation, iron deficiency, malignant neoplasm, osteitis (fibrosa cystica), or vitamin B_{12} deficiency.
- Use drug cautiously in patients with cardiovascular disorders caused by a variety of conditions such as hematologic disorders (hypercoagulation, myelodysplastic syndrome, or sickle cell disease), hypertension, porphyria or seizure disorders, or vascular disease.
- Check hemoglobin levels, as ordered, with twice-weekly measurements recommended for chronic renal failure patients, until stable and then monthly thereafter and weekly measurements recommended for zidovudine-treated HIV-infected and cancer patients.

! **WARNING** Be aware that baseline hemoglobin level should be above 10 g/dl but below 13 g/dl if drug is given to patient scheduled for surgery. Watch closely throughout surgical period for deep vein thrombosis, especially in patients not receiving prophylactic anticoagulation.

! **WARNING** Know that hemoglobin shouldn't exceed 11 g/dl when treating anemia in patients with chronic renal failure on dialysis and 10 g/dl for patients not on dialysis. Exceeding these parameters increases risk of life-threatening adverse cardiovascular effects.

! **WARNING** Monitor patient throughout therapy for skin reactions, which may include blistering and skin exfoliation that could be severe. If present, notify prescriber at once and expect drug to be discontinued.

! **WARNING** Monitor patient for hypertensive or thrombotic complications, especially if hemoglobin is approaching target goal.

! **WARNING** Expect to increase heparin dose if patient receives hemodialysis because epoetin alfa can increase the RBC volume, which could cause clots to form in the dialyzer, hemodialysis vascular access, or both.

PATIENT TEACHING

- Ensure that patient has been instructed on the serious adverse effects related to epoetin alfa therapy before therapy begins.
- Teach patient how to administer epoetin alfa as a subcutaneous injection, if drug will be given at home.
- Emphasize the importance of complying with the dosage regimen and keeping follow-up medical appointments and laboratory test appointments.
- Encourage patient to eat iron-rich foods.

! **WARNING** Instruct patient to notify prescriber if he experiences chest pain, headache, hives, rapid heartbeat, rash, seizures, shortness of breath, swelling, or other persistent, serious, or unusual adverse reactions. Also, inform patient of the possibility of severe skin reactions, such as blistering and exfoliation. Stress importance of stopping drug and alerting prescriber immediately, if present.

eptifibatide

Class and Category

Pharmacologic class: Glycoprotein IIb/IIIa inhibitor
Therapeutic class: Antiplatelet

Indications and Dosages

∗ *To treat acute coronary syndrome managed medically or through use of percutaneous coronary intervention (PCI)*

I.V. INFUSION, I.V. INJECTION

Adults. *Initial:* 180 mcg/kg as soon as possible after diagnosis, followed by continuous infusion at 2 mcg/kg/min immediately after initial dose and continued until discharge or coronary artery bypass grafting (CABG), up to 72 hr. If patient is to undergo PCI, infusion continued until hospital discharge or up to 18 to 24 hr after the procedure, whichever comes first, allowing for up to 96 hr of therapy.

±**DOSAGE ADJUSTMENT** For patients with serum creatinine level less than 50 ml/min, initial bolus remains unchanged at 180 mcg/kg but continuous infusion rate decreased to 1.0 mcg/kg/min.

∗ *To provide urgent intervention in patients undergoing PCI, including need for intracoronary stenting*

I.V. INFUSION, I.V. INJECTION

Adults. *Initial:* 180 mcg/kg immediately before procedure, immediately followed by continuous infusion at 2 mcg/kg/min, and a second 180 mcg/kg bolus administered 10 min after the first bolus. The continuous infusion continued until hospital discharge, or for up to 18 to 24 hr, whichever comes first. A minimum of 12 hr of infusion recommended. For patient undergoing CABG surgery, infusion discontinued prior to surgery.

±**DOSAGE ADJUSTMENT** For patients with serum creatinine level less than 50 ml/min, initial and subsequent bolus remains unchanged at 180 mcg/kg, but continuous infusion rate decreased to 1.0 mcg/kg/min.

Drug Administration

I.V.

- Expect to administer concurrent aspirin therapy (160–325 mg) daily when giving drug to treat acute coronary syndrome. Expect to administer concurrent aspirin therapy (160–325 mg) 1 to 24 hr prior to PCI and then daily afterwards.
- Protect drug from light before administration.
- May administer in the same I.V. line as alteplase, atropine, dobutamine, heparin, lidocaine, meperidine, metoprolol, midazolam, morphine, nitroglycerin, or verapamil.
- May also administer drug in same I.V. line with 0.9% Sodium Chloride Injection or 0.9% Sodium Chloride Injection and 5% Dextrose Injection solution. These solutions may contain up to 60 mEq/L of potassium chloride during drug administration.
- Withdraw bolus dose from a 10-ml (2-mg/ml) vial into a syringe.
- Administer I.V. injection as a bolus over 1 to 2 min.
- Administer continuous infusion immediately following I.V. bolus. When administering drug undiluted directly from the 100-ml (0.75 mg/ml) vial, use an infusion pump. Be sure to spike the vial with the vented infusion set centering the spike in the circle on top of vial stopper. Administer infusion rate according to the patient's weight (see manufacturer's guidelines). Discard any unused portion left in the vial.

- Drug should be given concomitantly with heparin with medical management or PCI for acute coronary syndrome. Be aware that heparin should not be continued after PCI is completed.
- If patient requires thrombolytic therapy, drug should be discontinued.
- Vials should be stored in refrigerator. Vials may be stored at room temperature but must be discarded if not used within 2 mo.
- *Incompatibilities:* Furosemide

Route	Onset	Peak	Duration
I.V.	Immediate	5 min	4 hr

Half-life: 2.5–2.8 hr

Mechanism of Action

Inhibits platelet aggregation reversibly by preventing fibrinogen, von Willebrand factor, and other adhesive ligands from binding to glycoprotein IIb/IIIa receptors on activated platelets. As a result, eptifibatide disrupts final cross-linking stage of platelet aggregation—and thrombus formation.

Contraindications

Active bleeding, bleeding diathesis, or stroke during prior 30 days, current or planned administration of another parenteral GP IIb/IIIa inhibitor, dependency on dialysis, history of hemorrhagic stroke, hypersensitivity to eptifibatide or its components, major surgery during previous 6 wk, severe uncontrolled hypertension (systolic pressure above 200 mm Hg, diastolic pressure above 110 mm Hg)

Interactions

DRUGS

anticoagulants, other antiplatelet agents, other platelet aggregation inhibitors (especially inhibitors of platelet receptor glycoprotein IIb/IIIa, such as abciximab) thrombolytics: Increased risk of additive pharmacologic effects, increased risk of bleeding

Adverse Reactions

CNS: **Intracranial hemorrhage**
CV: **Hypotension**
GI: **GI hemorrhage, hematemesis**
GU: Hematuria
HEME: **Bleeding that may be severe**, decreased hemoglobin level, **immune-mediated thrombocytopenia, thrombocytopenia**
RESP: **Pulmonary hemorrhage**
Other: **Anaphylaxis**

Childbearing Considerations

PREGNANCY

- It is not known if drug causes fetal harm.
- Use with caution only if benefit to mother outweighs potential risk to fetus.

LACTATION

- It is not known if drug is present in breast milk.
- Mothers should check with prescriber before breastfeeding.

Nursing Considerations

- Expect to obtain aPTT and PT, hematocrit and hemoglobin, platelet count, and serum creatinine as a baseline before drug therapy begins. Also, expect to obtain a baseline for activated clotting time (ACT) if patient is undergoing PCI.
- Know that bleeding can be minimized in patients also receiving heparin by monitoring ACT and aPTT. Expect to keep aPTT between 50 and 70 seconds during therapy unless patient has PCI. If patient has PCI, expect to maintain ACT between 200 and 300 seconds during the procedure.
- Avoid arterial and venous punctures, I.M. injections, nasotracheal or nasogastric intubation, urinary catheters, and noncompressible I.V. sites (jugular and subclavian veins) during therapy.

! WARNING Monitor patient for bleeding. Notify prescriber immediately if present because bleeding can become severe rapidly.

! WARNING Monitor patient for hypersensitivity, which can become life-threatening such as anaphylaxis. If present, notify prescriber, expect drug to be discontinued and another drug substituted, and provide supportive care, as needed and ordered.

- Expect to discontinue eptifibatide and heparin at least 4 hours before discharge for patient who has undergone PCI. Ensure sheath hemostasis has occurred before discharge.
- Plan to stop drug, as prescribed, if patient undergoes coronary artery bypass surgery.

PATIENT TEACHING

- Inform patient drug will be given intravenously.

- Reassure patient that he'll be monitored closely throughout therapy.

! **WARNING** Instruct patient to immediately report bleeding during eptifibatide therapy.

! **WARNING** Alert patient that drug may cause an allergic reaction. If present, tell patient to notify prescriber and seek immediate medical care, if severe.

- Advise patient to avoid activities that may lead to bleeding and bruising when discharged to home.

eptinezumab-jjmr

Vyepti

Class and Category

Pharmacologic class: Monoclonal antibody (calcitonin gene-related peptide antagonist)
Therapeutic class: Antimigraine

Indications and Dosages

✳ *To prevent migraine*

I.V. INFUSION

Adults. 100 mg infused over 30 min every 3 mo; dosage increased to 300 mg every 3 mo, as needed.

Drug Administration

I.V.

- Must be diluted before administration. Dilute with 100 ml of 0.9% Sodium Chloride Injection using an infusion bag made of polyvinyl chloride (PVC), polyethylene (PE), or polyolefin (PO).
- Discard any unused portion because it contains no preservative.
- Gently invert the drug solution to mix completely. Do not shake.
- Must be infused within 8 hr after being mixed.
- Infuse over approximately 30 min using an intravenous infusion set with a 0.2-micron or 0.22-micron inline or add-on sterile filter.
- After infusion is complete, flush the line with 20 ml of 0.9% Sodium Chloride Injection.
- Never administer as a bolus injection or intravenous push.
- May be stored at room temperature. Do not freeze.
- *Incompatibilities:* Other drugs or solutions other than 0.9% Sodium Chloride Injection

Route	Onset	Peak	Duration
I.V.	Unknown	30 min	Unknown

Half-life: 27 days

Mechanism of Action

Binds to calcitonin gene-related peptide ligand and blocks its binding to the receptor, which interferes with pain mechanism in migraine headaches.

Contraindications

Hypersensitivity to eptinezumab-jjmr or its components

Interactions

DRUGS

None reported by manufacturer.

Adverse Reactions

CNS: Fatigue
EENT: Nasopharyngitis
ENDO: Hot flashes
RESP: Dyspnea
SKIN: Facial flushing, pruritus, rash, urticaria
Other: **Anaphylaxis**, **angioedema**, anti-eptinezumab-jjmr antibodies, **hypersensitivity reactions**

Childbearing Considerations

PREGNANCY

- It is not known if drug can cause fetal harm.
- Use with caution only if benefit to mother outweighs potential risk to fetus.
- Females of childbearing age with migraine may be at increased risk of gestational hypertension and preeclampsia during pregnancy.

LACTATION

- It is not known if drug is present in breast milk.
- Mothers should check with prescriber before breastfeeding.

Nursing Considerations

! **WARNING** Monitor patient for hypersensitivity reactions that may become serious. Reactions such as angioedema, dyspnea, facial flushing, rash, and urticaria may occur. Hypersensitivity reactions usually occur during the infusion of eptinezumab-jjmr rather than after drug administration. If a reaction occurs, notify prescriber, expect drug to be discontinued, and institute supportive therapy, as needed and ordered.

- Be aware that, as with all therapeutic proteins, there is a potential for the development of anti-eptinezumab-jjmr antibodies. Alert prescriber if drug seems less effective.

PATIENT TEACHING

! **WARNING** Review signs and symptoms of an allergic reaction. Explain that an allergic reaction usually occurs during the infusion of the drug rather than afterwards and is usually not serious. However, advise patient to alert medical staff if he suddenly doesn't feel well or is experiencing difficulty breathing, itching, or other signs of an allergic reaction.

- Review other signs and symptoms of adverse reactions associated with the drug.
- Tell patient to alert prescriber if drug seems less effective as time goes on.

erenumab-aooe

Aimovig

Class and Category

Pharmacologic class: Human monoclonal antibody
Therapeutic class: Antimigraine

Indications and Dosages

* *To prevent migraine headaches*

SUBCUTANEOUS INJECTION

Adults. 70 mg monthly. Increased to 140 mg (given as two 70-mg consecutive injections) monthly, as needed.

Drug Administration

SUBCUTANEOUS

- Needle shield within the white cap of the prefilled autoinjector and the gray needle cap of the prefilled syringe contain dry natural rubber, a derivative of latex. Handling the caps may cause allergic reactions in individuals sensitive to latex.
- Store in refrigerator in original container until ready to use, protecting from light. However, if original container is removed from refrigerator, drug may be kept at room temperature but must be used within 7 days or discarded.
- Allow erenumab-aooe to sit at room temperature for at least 30 min protected from direct sunlight prior to administration. Drug should not be warmed by using a heat source, such as hot water or a microwave.
- Do not shake solution.
- Inspect solution and do not use if solution is cloudy or discolored or contains flakes or particles.
- Both prefilled autoinjector and prefilled syringe are single dose devices; give entire contents. If patient is prescribed a 140-mg dose, give two 70-mg consecutive injections.
- Administer in the abdomen, thigh, or upper arm. Do not inject into areas where the skin is bruised, hard, red, or tender.
- If a dose is missed, give as soon as possible and then reschedule monthly dose from that dose.

Route	Onset	Peak	Duration
SubQ	Unknown	4–6 days	Unknown

Half-life: 28 days

Mechanism of Action

Binds to the calcitonin gene-related peptide (CGRP) receptor. The CGRP receptor is thought to be responsible for transmitting signals that can cause incapacitating pain. By binding to the CGRP receptor, the drug antagonizes its function, preventing pain signals from being transmitted.

Contraindications

Hypersensitivity to erenumab-aooe or its components

Interactions

DRUGS

None reported by manufacturer.

Adverse Reactions

CV: Hypertension
EENT: Mucosal ulceration
GI: Constipation (may become severe)
MS: Muscle cramps or spasms
SKIN: Alopecia, rash
Other: **Anaphylaxis**, **angioedema**, erenumab-aooe antibody formation, injection-site reactions (erythema, pain, pruritus)

Childbearing Considerations

PREGNANCY

- It is not known if drug causes fetal harm.
- Use with caution only if benefit to mother outweighs potential risk to fetus.
- Know that females of childbearing age with migraine may be at increased risk of gestational hypertension and preeclampsia during pregnancy.

LACTATION

- It is not known if drug is present in breast milk.
- Mothers should check with prescriber before breastfeeding.

Nursing Considerations

- Monitor effectiveness of drug to relieve migraine headaches.

! **WARNING** Monitor patient for hypersensitivity reactions, which usually are not serious and occur within hours of administration. However, some have occurred more than 1 week after drug administration, and some have been serious or severe such as anaphylaxis or angioedema. If present, notify prescriber, expect drug to be discontinued and be prepared to initiate supportive treatment, as needed and ordered.

! **WARNING** Monitor patient for constipation, which could become severe with serious complications requiring hospitalization. Patients who are taking drugs that decrease GI motility are at increased risk.

! **WARNING** Monitor patient's blood pressure because hypertension may develop or worsen, if preexisting. Hypertension may occur at any time, but most commonly occurs within 7 days of dose administration. Notify prescriber, as drug may have to be discontinued.

PATIENT TEACHING

- Instruct patient how to administer erenumab-aooe as a subcutaneous injection and what to do if a dose is missed.
- Warn patient that the needle shield within the white cap of the prefilled autoinjector and the gray needle cap of the prefilled syringe contain dry natural rubber, a derivative of latex. Handling the caps may cause allergic reactions if patient is sensitive to latex. If latex allergy exists, tell patient to alert prescriber before handling drug device.
- Inform patient prescribed the 140-mg dose to administer the drug once a month as 2 separate but consecutive subcutaneous injections of 70 mg each.
- Inform patient that drug may cause injection-site reactions, such as itching, pain, or redness.

! **WARNING** Alert patient that hypersensitivity reactions may occur even as late as 1 week after administration. Although most are not serious, stress importance of notifying prescriber and seeking immediate medical attention, if severe.

! **WARNING** Inform patient that constipation is one of the most common adverse reactions related to drug use. However, tell patient to report constipation that is prolonged or severe because a bowel obstruction could occur, if left untreated.

- Tell patient that blood pressure may become elevated at any time during therapy, but most commonly occurs within 7 days of dosage administration. Have patient monitor blood pressure, if possible, and notify prescriber if blood pressure becomes elevated.

E

ertapenem sodium

Invanz

Class and Category

Pharmacologic class: Carbapenem
Therapeutic class: Antibiotic

Indications and Dosages

∗ *To treat moderate to severe infections, such as acute pelvic infections (including postpartum endomyometritis, postsurgical gynecologic infections, or septic abortion) due to* Bacteroides fragilis, Escherichia coli, Peptostreptococcus *species,* Prevotella bivia, Porphyromonas asaccharolytica, *or* Streptococcus agalactiae; *community-acquired pneumonia due to* Haemophilus influenzae *(beta-lactamase-negative strains only),* Moraxella catarrhalis, *or* Streptococcus pneumoniae *(penicillin-susceptible strains only, including cases with concurrent bacteremia); complicated intra-abdominal infections due to* B. distasonis, B. fragilis, B.ovatus, B. thetaiotaomicron, B. uniformis, Clostridium clostridioforme, E. coli, Eubacterium lentum, *or* Peptostreptococcus *species; complicated skin and skin structure infections, including diabetic foot infections without osteomyelitis, due to* B. fragilis, E. coli, Klebsiella pneumoniae, Peptostreptococcus *species,* Porphyromonas asaccharolytica, P. bivia, Proteus mirabilis, Staphylococcus aureus, S. agalactiae, *or* S. pyogenes; *and complicated UTI (including pyelonephritis) due to* E. coli *(including cases with concurrent bacteremia), or* K. pneumoniae

I.V. INFUSION

Adults and adolescents. 1 g once daily, 3 to 10 days for acute pelvic infections, 10 to 14 days for community-acquired pneumonia or complicated UTIs, 5 to 14 days for complicated intra-abdominal infections, and 7 to 14 days for complicated skin and skin structure infections (diabetic foot infections may require up to 28 days).

Children ages 3 mo to 12 yr. 15 mg/kg every 12 hr, for 3 to 10 days for acute pelvic infections, 10 to 14 days for community-acquired pneumonia or complicated UTIs, 5 to 14 days for complicated intra-abdominal infections, and 7 to 14 days for complicated skin and skin structure infections (diabetic foot infections may require up to 28 days). *Maximum:* 1 g daily.

I.M. INJECTION

Adults and adolescents. 1 g daily for up to 7 days.

Children ages 3 mo to 12 yr. 15 mg/kg every 12 hr for 3 to 10 days for acute pelvic infections, 10 to 14 days for community-acquired pneumonia or complicated UTIs, 5 to 14 days for complicated intra-abdominal infections, and 7 to 14 days for complicated skin and skin structure infections (diabetic foot infections may require up to 28 days). *Maximum:* 15 mg/kg twice daily.

∗ *To provide prophylaxis of surgical site infection following elective colorectal surgery*

I.V. INFUSION

Adults. 1 g given 1 hr prior to surgical incision.

±**DOSAGE ADJUSTMENT** For adult patients with advanced renal insufficiency (creatinine clearance less than or equal to 30 ml/min) or end-stage renal insufficiency (creatinine clearance less than or equal to 10 ml/min), dosage decreased to 500 mg daily. For adult patients on hemodialysis who have received 500 mg of ertapenem within 6 hours of hemodialysis, supplemental dose of 150 mg given after hemodialysis. For children, there is no information on dosage adjustments.

Drug Administration

I.V.

- Reconstitute 1 g with 10 ml 0.9% of Sodium Chloride Injection, Bacteriostatic Water for Injection, or Sterile Water for Injection using a syringe equipped with a 21 G or smaller needle. Do not use a needleless I.V. system. Don't use solutions that contain dextrose.
- Shake well to dissolve.
- For adults, immediately transfer reconstituted drug to 50 ml of 0.9% Sodium Chloride Injection solution. For children ages 3 mo to 12 yr, immediately withdraw a reconstituted volume equal to 15 mg/kg (not to exceed 1 g/day) and dilute in 0.9% Sodium Chloride Injection to a final concentration of 20 mg/ml or less.
- Solution should appear colorless to pale yellow but variations of color within this range do not affect the potency of the drug.
- Infuse over 30 min.
- Complete infusion within 6 hr of reconstitution and dilution or store in refrigerator for up to 24 hr and use within 4 hr after removal from refrigerator. Do not freeze.
- *Incompatibilities:* Dextrose solutions, other drugs

I.M.

- Reconstitute 1 g of drug with 3.2 ml of 1% Lidocaine Hydrochloride Injection (without epinephrine). Shake thoroughly.
- Use within 1 hr after preparation.
- For adults, withdraw contents of vial and inject deep into a large muscle mass, such as the gluteal muscles or lateral part of thigh. For children ages 3 mo to 13 yr, withdraw a reconstituted volume equal to 15 mg/kg (not to exceed 1 g/day) and inject deep into a large muscle mass, such as the gluteal muscles or lateral part of the thigh.
- Don't give reconstituted I.M. solution by I.V. route because of possible adverse reaction

to lidocaine hydrochloride injection used to reconstitute drug.

Route	Onset	Peak	Duration
I.V.	Immediate	30 min	24 hr
I.M.	Unknown	2 hr	24 hr

Half-life: 4 hr

Mechanism of Action

Inhibits bacterial cell wall synthesis by binding to specific penicillin-binding proteins inside the cell wall. Penicillin-binding proteins are responsible for various steps in bacterial cell wall synthesis. By binding to these proteins, ertapenem leads to bacterial cell wall lysis.

Contraindications

Hypersensitivity to ertapenem, beta-lactams, other drugs in the same class, or their components; hypersensitivity to local anesthetics of the amide type (I.M. injection)

Interactions

DRUGS

divalproex sodium, valproic acid: Possibly decreased serum valproic acid level and increased risk of breakthrough seizures
probenecid: Increased ertapenem half-life, increased and prolonged blood ertapenem level

Adverse Reactions

CNS: Abnormal coordination, aggression, agitation, altered mental status, anxiety, asthenia, confusion, delirium, depressed level of consciousness, disorientation, dizziness, dyskinesia, **encephalopathy**, fatigue, fever, gait disturbance, hallucinations, headache, hypothermia, insomnia, mental changes, myoclonus, **seizures**, somnolence, stupor, tremor
CV: Chest pain, edema, hypersensitivity vasculitis, hypertension, **hypotension**, tachycardia, thrombophlebitis
EENT: Nasopharyngitis, oral candidiasis, rhinitis, rhinorrhea, teeth staining, viral pharyngitis
ENDO: Hyperglycemia
GI: Abdominal pain, acid regurgitation, anorexia, ***Clostridioides difficile*–associated diarrhea**, constipation, diarrhea, elevated liver enzymes, indigestion, nausea, **small intestinal obstruction**, vomiting
GU: Dysuria, elevated serum creatinine level, genital rash, proteinuria, RBCs and WBCs in urine, UTI, vaginitis
HEME: Anemia, decreased hematocrit, eosinophilia, leukocytosis, **leukopenia**, **neutropenia**, **prolonged PT**, **thrombocytopenia**, thrombocytosis
MS: Arthralgia, leg pain, muscle weakness
RESP: **Atelectasis**, cough, crackles, dyspnea, pleural effusion, pneumonia, **respiratory distress**, upper respiratory tract infection, wheezing
SKIN: Acute generalized exanthematous pustulosis, cellulitis, dermatitis, erythema, extravasation, pruritus, rash
Other: **Anaphylaxis**; **death**; **drug reaction with eosinophilia and systemic symptoms (DRESS)**; **hyperkalemia**; **hypokalemia**; infusion-site induration, pain, phlebitis, pruritus, redness, swelling, or warmth

Childbearing Considerations

PREGNANCY

- It is not known if drug causes fetal harm.
- Use with caution only if benefit to mother outweighs potential risk to fetus.

LACTATION

- Drug is present in breast milk.
- Mothers should check with prescriber before breastfeeding.

Nursing Considerations

- Obtain sputum, urine, or other specimens for culture and sensitivity testing, as ordered, before giving ertapenem. Expect to start therapy before results are available.

! WARNING Monitor patient closely for a life-threatening anaphylactic reaction. Patients with a history of hypersensitivity to cephalosporins, penicillin, other allergens or other beta-lactams are at increased risk. Know that if drug triggers an anaphylactic reaction, stop drug, notify prescriber immediately, and provide supportive therapy, as needed and ordered.

! WARNING Monitor patient for diarrhea during and for at least 2 months after drug therapy; diarrhea may signal pseudomembranous colitis caused by *C. difficile* and may range from mild to fatal colitis. If diarrhea occurs, notify prescriber and expect to obtain a stool sample. If confirmed, expect ertapenem to be discontinued, and treatment with an antibiotic effective against *C. difficile* ordered, as well as electrolytes, fluids, and protein supplementation, as needed and ordered.

! **WARNING** Monitor patient's hematologic status closely because adverse reactions can become serious and life-threatening.

! **WARNING** Be aware that patients at increased risk for seizures include a history of seizures or presence of other CNS disorders that predispose them to seizures such as brain lesions or compromised renal function. Institute seizure precautions with these patients.

! **WARNING** Know that patients with renal impairment who develop ertapenem-induced encephalopathy usually experience a prolonged recovery.

PATIENT TEACHING

! **WARNING** Alert patient taking divalproex or valproic acid for seizure control to notify prescriber of this type of concurrent therapy before therapy begins because ertapenem may interfere with these drugs' effectiveness to control seizures.

- Inform patient ertapenem will be administered by an I.M. injection or intravenously.

! **WARNING** Alert patient that drug may cause an allergic reaction. If present, tell patient to notify prescriber and, if severe, to seek immediate medical care.

! **WARNING** Urge patient to tell prescriber about diarrhea that is severe or lasts longer than 3 days. Remind patient that watery or bloody stools can occur 2 or more months after antibiotic therapy and can be serious, requiring prompt treatment.

! **WARNING** Monitor patient for seizures, especially a patient with a seizure history.

! **WARNING** Tell patient to alert prescriber if bleeding, bruising, or infection occurs as well as any other persistent, serious, or unusual adverse reactions.

ertugliflozin

Steglatro

Class and Category

Pharmacologic class: Sodium glucose-dependent cotransporter inhibitor
Therapeutic class: Antidiabetic

Indications and Dosages

* *As adjunct to improve glycemic control in patients with type 2 diabetes mellitus*

TABLETS

Adults. *Initial:* 5 mg once daily in the morning, increased as needed. *Maximum:* 15 mg once daily.

Drug Administration

P.O.

- Administer in the morning.
- Drug may have to be temporarily discontinued if dehydration occurs.

Route	Onset	Peak	Duration
P.O.	Unknown	1 hr	Unknown

Half-life: 16.6 hr

Mechanism of Action

Inhibits sodium glucose link transporter-2 to reduce renal reabsorption of filtered glucose and lower the renal threshold for glucose. These actions increase urinary glucose excretion and lower blood glucose levels.

Contraindications

Dialysis, end-stage renal disease, hypersensitivity to ertugliflozin or its components, severe renal impairment

Interactions

DRUGS

insulin, insulin secretagogues: Increased risk of hypoglycemia
lithium: Possibly decreased lithium concentrations with possible decreased lithium effectiveness

Adverse Reactions

CNS: Headache, thirst
CV: Elevated low-density lipoprotein cholesterol, **hypotension**
EENT: Nasopharyngitis
ENDO: **Ketoacidosis**

GU: **Acute kidney injury and impairment, acute prerenal failure**, decreased estimated glomerular filtration rate, elevated serum creatinine levels, genital mycotic infections, increased urination, **necrotizing fasciitis of the perineum (Fournier's gangrene), pyelonephritis, urosepsis**, UTI, vaginal pruritus
HEME: Increased hemoglobin level
MS: Back pain, lower limb amputation
SKIN: Rash
Other: **Angioedema**, dehydration, **hyperphosphatemia**, weight loss

Childbearing Considerations

PREGNANCY

- Drug may cause fetal harm, especially on the renal system.
- Drug is not recommended during the second and third trimesters of pregnancy.

LACTATION

- It is not known if drug is present in breast milk.
- Breastfeeding is not recommended because kidney maturation continues through the first 2 yr of life.

Nursing Considerations

- Know that volume depletion should be corrected before ertugliflozin therapy is begun.

! WARNING Assess patient for factors that may predispose patient to acute kidney injury before ertugliflozin therapy is begun. Risk factors may include presence of chronic renal insufficiency, congestive heart failure, and hypovolemia and use of drugs, such as ACE inhibitors, ARBs, diuretics, and NSAIDs. Be aware that ertugliflozin should not be initiated in patients who have an eGFR below 45 ml/min. Assess renal function before ertugliflozin is initiated and periodically throughout drug therapy, as ordered.

! WARNING Monitor patient's blood pressure closely because ertugliflozin causes intravascular volume contraction. Those at greater risk include the elderly and patients with impaired renal function or low systolic blood pressure or with concomitant use of diuretics.

! WARNING Monitor patient for signs and symptoms of metabolic acidosis. If present, also assess patient for ketoacidosis. Know that patient may have ketoacidosis even if her blood glucose level is less than 250 mg/dl. If ketoacidosis is suspected, notify prescriber. If confirmed, expect ertugliflozin to be discontinued and treatment with carbohydrates, fluid, and insulin replacement to be given.

! WARNING Monitor patient for a rare but serious and life-threatening necrotizing infection of the perineum called Fournier's gangrene. Notify prescriber immediately if patient develops erythema, pain, swelling, or tenderness in the genital or perineal area, along with fever or malaise. Expect treatment with broad-spectrum antibiotics and, if needed, surgical debridement of the area. Know that ertugliflozin will be discontinued if this occurs.

! WARNING Expect ertugliflozin to be withheld when oral intake is reduced, such as in acute illness or fasting, or when fluid losses occur, such as excessive heat exposure or GI illness. This is because dehydration increases risk of kidney impairment that could be quite serious.

! WARNING Monitor patients also receiving insulin or an insulin secretagogue, such as a sulfonylurea for hypoglycemia. Dosage of these drugs may have to be reduced to minimize the risk of hypoglycemia.

- Assess both men and women for genital mycotic infections, which may occur with ertugliflozin therapy. Patients at higher risk include those with a history of genital mycotic infections or men who are uncircumcised.
- Assess patient's lower legs for signs and symptoms of infection (including osteomyelitis), new pain or tenderness, sores, or ulcers. If present, notify prescriber immediately, expect drug to be discontinued, and provide supportive care, as needed and ordered.

PATIENT TEACHING

! WARNING Advise females of childbearing age to notify prescriber if pregnant and what trimester she is in before ertugliflozin therapy begins because ertugliflozin therapy is not recommended during the second and third trimesters of pregnancy. Also, stress importance of using effective contraception throughout drug therapy. If pregnancy occurs, during drug therapy, prescriber should be notified immediately.

- Instruct patient how to administer ertugliflozin and what to do if a dose is missed.

! **WARNING** Instruct patient to maintain adequate fluid intake, as dehydration increases the risk of the blood pressure dropping and renal impairment. Advise patient to notify prescriber if patient is unable to take in adequate fluids, experiences excessive fluid loss though diarrhea or vomiting, or is exposed to excessive heat resulting in dehydration. Drug may need to be temporarily discontinued until fluid balance is restored.

- Remind patient with diabetes to test blood for glucose, not urine, because ertugliflozin causes glucose to be eliminated in urine making urine testing an inaccurate measurement for blood glucose control.

! **WARNING** Teach patient how to check urine for ketones and review signs and symptoms of ketoacidosis with patient. Remind patient that ketoacidosis may occur even when her blood glucose is not elevated. Tell patient to seek immediate medical attention if she experiences abdominal pain, labored breathing, nausea, tiredness, and vomiting and ketones are present in urine.

! **WARNING** Inform patients also prescribed insulin or antidiabetic agents known to cause hypoglycemia to monitor blood glucose level closely, as hypoglycemia may occur. Also, review the signs and symptoms of hypoglycemia and how to treat it in the event it occurs.

! **WARNING** Warn patient to stop ertugliflozin and seek immediate medical attention if pain, redness, swelling, or tenderness occurs in the genital or perineal area along with fever or malaise because, although rare, this cluster of symptoms may become life-threatening.

- Review signs and symptoms of genital mycotic infection. Tell patient to notify prescriber if present.
- Advise patient about the importance of routine foot care to prevent complications. Tell patient to notify prescriber immediately if signs and symptoms of an infection occur or new pain or tenderness, sores, or ulcers develop on the lower legs as drug will need to be discontinued and additional medical treatment given.
- Instruct patient to report any persistent, severe, or unusual signs and symptoms to prescriber, especially if changes in kidney function occur.
- Tell patient to seek medical care if a UTI occurs because it can become serious if left untreated.
- Tell mothers considering breastfeeding that it is not recommended during ertugliflozin therapy.

erythromycin base

ERY-C, Ery-Tab

erythromycin ethylsuccinate

E.E.S., EryPed

erythromycin lactobionate

Erythrocin

erythromycin stearate

Erythrocin Stearate

Class and Category

Pharmacologic class: Macrolide
Therapeutic class: Antibiotic

Indications and Dosages

∗ *To treat mild to moderate respiratory tract infections caused by* Haemophilus influenzae,

Streptococcus pneumoniae, *or* S. pyogenes *(group A beta-hemolytic streptococcus)*

CAPSULES, CHEWABLE TABLETS, D.R. CAPSULES, D.R. TABLETS, ORAL SUSPENSION, TABLETS

Adults. 250 (base) or 400 mg (ethylsuccinate) every 6 hr for 10 days. Alternatively, 500 mg (base) every 12 hr.
Children. 30 to 50 mg/kg daily in divided doses every 6 hr for 10 days. For more severe infection, dosage may be doubled.

✶ *To treat severe respiratory tract infections caused by* H. influenzae, S. pneumoniae, *or* S. pyogenes *(group A beta-hemolytic streptococcus)*

I.V. INFUSION (ERYTHROMYCIN LACTOBIONATE)

Adults. 15 to 20 mg/kg daily continuously or in divided doses every 6 hr for 10 days.
Children. 15 to 20 mg/kg daily in divided doses every 6 hr for 10 days.

✶ *To treat respiratory tract infections caused by* Mycoplasma pneumoniae

CAPSULES, CHEWABLE TABLETS, D.R. CAPSULES, D.R. TABLETS, ORAL SUSPENSION, TABLETS

Adults with mild to moderate infection. 250 mg (base) every 6 hr to 500 mg (base) every 12 hr or 400 mg (ethylsuccinate) every 6 hr for up to 3 wk.
Children. 30 to 50 mg/kg given in equally divided doses every 6 hr.

I.V. INFUSION (ERYTHROMYCIN LACTOBIONATE)

Adults with severe infection. 1 to 4 g daily continuously or in divided doses every 6 hr.
Children with severe infection. 15 to 20 mg/kg continuously or in divided doses no more than every 6 hr.

✶ *To treat skin and soft-tissue infections caused by* S. pyogenes *or* Staphylococcus aureus

CAPSULES, CHEWABLE TABLETS, D.R. CAPSULES, D.R. TABLETS, ORAL SUSPENSION, TABLETS

Adults with mild to moderate infection. 250 mg (base) every 6 hr to 500 mg (base) every 12 hr or 400 mg (ethylsuccinate) every 6 hr.

I.V. INFUSION (ERYTHROMYCIN LACTOBIONATE)

Adults with severe infection. 1 to 4 g (lactobionate) daily continuously or in divided doses every 6 hr for up to 3 wk.

✶ *To treat pertussis (whooping cough) caused by* Bordetella pertussis

CAPSULES, CHEWABLE TABLETS, D.R. CAPSULES, D.R. TABLETS, ORAL SUSPENSION, TABLETS

Adults and children. 40 to 50 mg/kg (base) daily in divided doses for 5 to 14 days.

✶ *To treat intestinal amebiasis caused by* Entamoeba histolytica

CAPSULES, CHEWABLE TABLETS, D.R. CAPSULES, D.R. TABLETS, ORAL SUSPENSION, TABLETS

Adults. 250 mg (base or stearate) or 400 mg (ethylsuccinate) every 6 hr or 500 mg (base, stearate) every 12 hr for 10 to 14 days.
Children. 30 to 50 mg/kg (base or ethylsuccinate) daily in divided doses for 10 to 14 days.

✶ *To treat pelvic inflammatory disease caused by* Neisseria gonorrhoeae

CAPSULES, CHEWABLE TABLETS, D.R. CAPSULES, D.R. TABLETS, ORAL SUSPENSION, TABLETS, I.V. INFUSION

Adults. 500 mg I.V. (lactobionate) every 6 hr for 3 days and then 250 mg (base) P.O. every 6 hr or 500 mg (base) every 12 hr for 7 days.

✶ *To treat conjunctivitis in newborns*

ORAL SUSPENSION

Neonates. 50 mg/kg (base) daily in 4 divided doses for 14 days.

✶ *To treat pneumonia in neonates caused by* Chlamydia trachomatis

I.V. INFUSION (ERYTHROMYCIN LACTOBIONATE)

Neonates. 15 to 20 mg/kg daily continuously or in divided doses every 6 hr.

ORAL SUSPENSION

Neonates. 50 mg/kg (base, stearate) daily in 4 divided doses for at least 3 wk.

✶ *To treat urogenital infections caused by* C. trachomatis *during pregnancy*

CAPSULES, CHEWABLE TABLETS, D.R. CAPSULES, D.R. TABLETS, ORAL SUSPENSION, TABLETS

Adults. 500 mg (base, stearate) every 6 hr for 7 days; or 250 mg (base, stearate) every 6 hr for at least 14 days.

∗ *To treat nongonococcal urethritis or uncomplicated urethral, endocervical, or rectal infections caused by* C. trachomatis

CAPSULES, CHEWABLE TABLETS, D.R. CAPSULES, D.R. TABLETS, ORAL SUSPENSION, TABLETS

Adults. 500 mg (base, stearate) every 6 hr for 7 days. If patient can't tolerate high doses, 250 mg (base, stearate) every 6 hr for 14 days. Alternatively, 800 mg (ethylsuccinate) 3 times daily for at least 7 days.

∗ *To treat Legionnaire's disease*

CAPSULES, CHEWABLE TABLETS, D.R. CAPSULES, D.R. TABLETS, ORAL SUSPENSION, TABLETS, I.V. INFUSION

Adults. 1 to 4 g (base, stearate) daily in divided doses for 10 to 14 days. I.V. (lactobionate) dosage infused continuously or dosage divided and given every 6 hr.

∗ *To prevent initial or recurrent attacks of rheumatic fever*

CAPSULES, CHEWABLE TABLETS, D.R. CAPSULES, D.R. TABLETS, ORAL SUSPENSION, TABLETS

Adults. 250 mg (base, stearate) or 400 mg (ethylsuccinate) every 12 hr.

Children. 250 mg (base, stearate) twice daily.

Drug Administration

P.O.

- Chewable tablets should be thoroughly chewed before swallowing. They are not to be swallowed whole.
- Capsules or tablets should be swallowed whole and not chewed, crushed, split, or opened.
- For oral suspension, use the calibrated measuring device provided to ensure accurate doses. Shake the suspension before measuring a dose.
- Administer with a full glass of water and on an empty stomach. However, if patient experiences GI upset, give with food or milk.

I.V.

- Don't use diluent with benzyl alcohol if drug is being given to a neonate.
- Reconstitute by adding 10 ml of preservative-free Sterile Water for Injection to each 500-mg vial. Do not use other diluents. Each ml contains 50 mg. Reconstituted solution is stable for 24 hr if stored at room temperature or 2 wk if refrigerated.
- Dilute the reconstituted solution to a concentration of 1 to 5 mg/ml for intermittent infusion and 1 mg/ml for continuous infusion using 0.9% Sodium Chloride Solution, Lactated Ringer's solution, or other solutions recommended by manufacturer. Diluted solution must be administered within 8 hr.
- Dextrose solutions should only be used if they are first buffered with 4% Sodium Bicarbonate.
- Infuse intermittent infusions over 20 to 60 min.
- Don't store infusions prepared in the ADD-Vantage system.
- Do not use flexible containers in series connections.
- *Incompatibilities:* None listed by manufacturer.

Route	Onset	Peak	Duration
P.O.	Unknown	2.5–4 hr	Unknown
I.V.	Unknown	Immediate	Unknown

Half-life: 1.5–2 hr

Mechanism of Action

Binds with the 50S ribosomal subunit of the 70S ribosome in many types of aerobic, anaerobic, gram-negative, and gram-positive organisms. This action inhibits RNA-dependent protein synthesis in bacterial cells, causing them to die.

Contraindications

Astemizole, cisapride, dihydroergotamine, ergotamine, lovastatin, pimozide, simvastatin, or terfenadine therapy; hypersensitivity to erythromycin, other macrolide antibiotics, or their components

Interactions

DRUGS

alfentanil: Decreased alfentanil clearance, prolonged alfentanil action

amiodarone, dofetilide, procainamide, quinidine, sotalol: Increased risk of prolonged QT interval

astemizole, cisapride, pimozide, terfenadine: Increased risk of cardiotoxicity, prolonged QT interval, torsades de pointes, ventricular tachycardia, and death

calcium channel blockers, such as amlodipine, diltiazem, verapamil: Increased risk of hypotension
carbamazepine, valproic acid: Possibly inhibited metabolism of these drugs, increasing their blood levels and risk of toxicity
clindamycin: Antagonized effects of these drugs
colchicine: Possible life-threatening colchicine toxicity
cyclosporine: Increased risk of nephrotoxicity
digoxin: Increased serum digoxin level and risk of digitalis toxicity
dihydroergotamine, ergotamine: Decreased ergotamine metabolism, increased risk of ergot toxicity with ischemia and vasospasm
HMG-CoA reductase inhibitors, such as atorvastatin, lovastatin, simvastatin: Possibly increased risk of rhabdomyolysis
midazolam, triazolam, and other related benzodiazepines: Increased pharmacologic effects of these drugs
oral anticoagulants: Increased anticoagulant effects, especially in the elderly
oral contraceptives: Decrease or loss of effectiveness of oral contraceptive
sildenafil: Increased effects of sildenafil
verapamil: Increased risk of bradyarrhythmias, hypotension, and lactic acidosis
xanthines (except dyphylline): Increased serum theophylline level with high doses and risk of theophylline toxicity

ACTIVITIES

alcohol use: Increased alcohol level (by 40%) with I.V. erythromycin

Adverse Reactions

CNS: Fatigue, fever, malaise, weakness
CV: **Prolonged QT interval**, **torsades de pointes**, **ventricular arrhythmias**
EENT: Hearing loss, oral candidiasis
GI: Abdominal cramps and pain, ***Clostridioides difficile*–associated diarrhea**, diarrhea, **hepatotoxicity**, infantile hypertrophic pyloric stenosis, jaundice, nausea, vomiting
GU: Interstitial nephritis, vaginal candidiasis
MS: New or aggravated myasthenia gravis syndrome
SKIN: Erythema, pruritus, rash
Other: Fluid overload (from I.V. infusion), **hypersensitivity reaction** (rare), injection-site inflammation and phlebitis

Childbearing Considerations

PREGNANCY

- It is not known if drug causes fetal harm.
- Use with caution only if benefit to mother outweighs potential risk to fetus.

LACTATION

- Drug is present in breast milk.
- Mothers should check with prescriber before breastfeeding.

Nursing Considerations

! WARNING Be aware that erythromycin should not be used in patients with history of QT interval prolongation or in patients with ongoing proarrhythmic conditions such as uncorrected hypokalemia or hypomagnesemia, serious bradycardia, and in patients receiving class IA or class III antiarrhythmic agents.

! WARNING Use erythromycin cautiously in elderly patients, especially those with renal or hepatic dysfunction because these patients are at increased risk of hearing loss and prolonged QT interval, which could possibly lead to the development of torsades de pointes. They're also at increased risk of bleeding if taking an oral anticoagulant.

- Use erythromycin cautiously in patients with impaired hepatic function because drug is metabolized by the liver. Monitor liver enzymes periodically to detect hepatotoxicity, which is most common with erythromycin estolate. Signs typically appear within 2 weeks after continuous therapy starts and resolve when it is discontinued.
- Expect to obtain body fluid or tissue sample for culture and sensitivity testing before giving first erythromycin dose.

! WARNING Know that erythromycin rarely causes a hypersensitivity reaction. However, if present, notify prescriber, withhold drug, and provide supportive care, as needed and ordered.

! WARNING Watch for evidence of fluid overload, such as acute dyspnea and crackles, during I.V. therapy.

! **WARNING** Monitor patient for diarrhea during and for at least 2 months after erythromycin therapy; diarrhea may signal pseudomembranous colitis caused by *Clostridioides difficile*. Severity ranges from being mild to severe possibly causing fatal colitis. If diarrhea occurs, notify prescriber and expect to obtain a stool sample. If confirmed, withhold drug, and expect to treat with an antibiotic effective against *C. difficile*, as ordered. In addition, expect to administer electrolytes, fluids, and protein supplementation, as needed and ordered.

- Assess hearing regularly, especially in elderly patients and those who receive 4 g or more daily or have hepatic or renal disease. Hearing impairment begins 36 hours to 8 days after treatment starts and usually begins to improve 1 to 14 days after it stops.
- Monitor infants for irritability with feeding or vomiting because infantile hypertrophic pyloric stenosis has been reported with erythromycin use.
- Assess myasthenia gravis patients for weakness because drug may aggravate it. Keep in mind that myasthenic syndrome may arise in patients previously undiagnosed with myasthenia gravis.
- Watch closely for signs and symptoms of superinfection. If they occur, notify prescriber and expect to stop drug and provide appropriate therapy.
- Know that if patient receives an order for urine catecholamine analysis, notify prescriber because erythromycin interferes with fluorometric measurement of urine catecholamines.

PATIENT TEACHING

- Instruct patient how to administer form of erythromycin prescribed.
- Urge patient to complete prescribed therapy, even if he feels better before it is finished.
- Tell patient to notify prescriber if symptoms worsen or don't improve after a few days.

! **WARNING** Instruct patient to promptly notify prescriber if an allergic reaction develops. If severe, stress importance of seeking immediate medical care.

! **WARNING** Urge patient to tell prescriber about diarrhea that's severe or lasts longer than 3 days. Remind patient that watery or bloody stools can occur 2 or more months after antibiotic therapy and can be serious, requiring prompt treatment.

! **WARNING** Review signs and symptoms of liver dysfunction such as fatigue, loss of appetite, and yellowing of skin. Tell patient to notify prescriber immediately, if present.

- Instruct patient to alert prescriber if hearing changes occur.

escitalopram oxalate

Lexapro

Class and Category

Pharmacologic class: Selective serotonin reuptake inhibitor (SSRI)
Therapeutic class: Antidepressant

Indications and Dosages

∗ *To treat acute generalized anxiety disorder*

ORAL SOLUTION, TABLETS

Adults. *Initial:* 10 mg once daily increased to 20 mg once daily after 1 or more wk, as needed. **Children ages 7 and older.** 10 mg once daily increased to 20 mg once daily after 2 or more wk, as needed.

∗ *To provide treatment and maintenance for major depression*

ORAL SOLUTION, TABLETS

Adults. *Initial:* 10 mg once daily, increased to 20 mg once daily after 1 wk, as needed. **Adolescents ages 12 to 17.** *Initial:* 10 mg once daily, increased to 20 mg once daily after 3 wk, as needed.

± **DOSAGE ADJUSTMENT** For elderly patients and those with hepatic impairment, dosage shouldn't exceed 10 mg daily.

Drug Administration

P.O.

- Administer drug in the morning or evening.
- Administer with or without food.

Route	Onset	Peak	Duration
P.O.	Unknown	5 hr	Unknown

Half-life: 27–32 hr

Mechanism of Action

Inhibits reuptake of the neurotransmitter serotonin by CNS neurons, thereby increasing the amount of serotonin available in nerve synapses. An elevated serotonin level may result in elevated mood and reduced anxiety or depression.

Contraindications

Concomitant therapy with pimozide; hypersensitivity to escitalopram, citalopram or its components; use within 14 days of MAO inhibitor therapy, including intravenous methylene blue or linezolid

Interactions

DRUGS

amphetamines, buspirone, fentanyl, lithium, St. John's wort, tramadol, tricyclic antidepressants, triptans, tryptophan: Increased risk of serotonin syndrome
aspirin, NSAIDs, warfarin: Possibly increased risk of bleeding
carbamazepine: Possibly increased clearance of escitalopram
cimetidine: Possibly increased plasma escitalopram level
CNS drugs: Additive CNS effects
lithium: Possible enhancement of the serotonergic effects of escitalopram
MAO inhibitors: Possibly hyperpyretic episodes, hypertensive crisis, serotonin syndrome, and severe seizures
metoprolol: Increased plasma metoprolol levels with decreased cardioselectivity of metoprolol
pimozide: Increased risk of QT prolongation
sumatriptan: Increased risk of hyperreflexia, incoordination, and weakness
triptans: Increased risk of serotonin syndrome

ACTIVITIES

alcohol use: Possibly increased cognitive and motor effects of alcohol

Adverse Reactions

CNS: Abnormal gait, acute psychosis, aggression, agitation, akathisia, amnesia, anger, anxiety, apathy, asthenia, ataxia, choreoathetosis, confusion, **CVA**, delirium, depersonalization, depression (aggravated), delirium, delusion, disorientation, dizziness, dyskinesia, dystonia, extrapyramidal effects, fatigue, feeling unreal, headache, hypoaesthesia, hypomania, insomnia, irritability, lethargy, malaise, mania, myoclonus, **neuroleptic malignant syndrome**, paresthesia, paranoia, parkinsonism, restless legs, restlessness, **seizures**, **serotonin syndrome**, somnolence, syncope, **suicidal ideation**, tardive dyskinesia, tremor, vertigo
CV: **Atrial fibrillation**, **bradycardia**, **cardiac failure**, **deep vein thrombosis**, edema, hypercholesterolemia, **hypotension**, **MI**, **prolonged QT interval**, tacycardia, **torsades de pointes**, **ventricular arrhythmias**
EENT: Acute-angle glaucoma, decreased or loss of smell, diplopia, dry mouth, epistaxis, mydriasis, nasal congestion, nasopharyngitis, nystagmus, rhinitis, sinusitis, toothache, visual disturbances and hallucinations
ENDO: Diabetes mellitus, hyperglycemia, hyperprolactinemia, **hypoglycemia**, syndrome of inappropriate ADH secretion
GI: Abdominal discomfort or pain, constipation, decreased appetite, diarrhea, dysphagia, elevated bilirubin and liver enzymes, flatulence, **fulminant hepatitis**, gastroesophageal reflux, **GI bleeding or hemorrhage**, **hepatic failure or necrosis**, **hepatitis**, indigestion, nausea, **pancreatitis**, **rectal hemorrhage**, vomiting
GU: **Acute renal failure**, anorgasmia, decreased libido, dysuria, ejaculation disorders, impotence, menorrhagia, priapism, urinary retention, UTI
HEME: Anemia, **agranulocytosis**, **aplastic anemia**, **bleeding**, **decreased prothrombin time**, **elevated international normalized ratio (INR)**, **hemolytic anemia**, **idiopathic thrombocytopenia purpura**, **leukopenia**, **thrombocytopenia**
MS: Back pain; dysarthria; muscle cramps, stiffness, or weakness; neck or shoulder pain; **rhabdomyolysis**
RESP: Dyspnea, **pulmonary embolism**, **pulmonary hypertension of the newborn**
SKIN: Alopecia, dermatitis, ecchymosis, **erythema multiforme**, increased sweating, photosensitivity, **Stevens-Johnson syndrome**, **toxic epidermal necrolysis**, urticaria
Other: **Anaphylaxis**, **angioedema**, discontinuation syndrome, **drug reaction with eosinophilia and systemic symptoms (DRESS)**, flu-like symptoms, **hypokalemia**, **hyponatremia**, weight loss

Childbearing Considerations

PREGNANCY

- Pregnancy exposure registry: 1-844-405-6185 or https://womensmentalhealth.org/research/pregnancyregistry/antidepressants.
- It is not known if drug causes fetal harm. However, be aware that neonates exposed to the drug late in the third trimester of pregnancy may develop serious and life-threatening adverse reactions, which can arise immediately following birth. These adverse reactions may require prolonged hospitalization, respiratory support, and tube feeding.
- Use with caution only if benefit to mother outweighs potential risk to fetus.

LABOR AND DELIVERY

- Use in the month before delivery may increase risk of postpartum hemorrhage.

LACTATION

- Drug is present in breast milk.
- Mothers should check with prescriber before breastfeeding.
- If breastfeeding occurs, infant should be monitored for agitation, excessive drowsiness, poor feeding, restlessness, and weight loss.

Nursing Considerations

! **WARNING** Be aware that escitalopram should not be given to patients with bradycardia, congenital long QT syndrome, hypokalemia or hypomagnesemia, recent acute MI, or uncompensated heart failure because of increased risk of prolonged QT interval and torsades de pointes. It should also not be given to patients who are taking other drugs that prolong the QT interval. Expect hypokalemia and hypomagnesemia to be corrected before escitalopram therapy is begun.

- Be aware that patients should be assessed for bipolar disorder before escitalopram therapy begins because its use in treating depression may precipitate a mixed/manic episode
- Use escitalopram cautiously in patients with history of mania or seizures, patients with severe renal impairment, and those with conditions or diseases that produce altered metabolism or hemodynamic responses.

! **WARNING** Monitor patient for a hypersensitivity reaction that may include a skin reaction, both of which could become severe and life-threatening. If a hypersensitivity reaction or skin reaction such as a rash occurs, (although with DRESS the only initial signs may be a fever or swollen lymph nodes) notify prescriber immediately, expect drug to be discontinued, and provide supportive care, as needed and ordered.

! **WARNING** Monitor patient for bleeding, especially if patient is also taking an anticoagulant, aspirin, or an NSAID or is receiving other anticoagulants or antiplatelet drugs, or warfarin. Know that drugs that interfere with serotonin reuptake increases risk of GI bleeding. Bleeding can range from ecchymoses, epistaxis, hematomas, and petechiae to life-threatening hemorrhages. Monitor patient's INR closely, if patient is taking warfarin.

! **WARNING** Know that if patient (particularly an adolescent) takes escitalopram for depression, watch closely for suicidal tendencies, especially when therapy starts or dosage changes because depression may worsen temporarily.

! **WARNING** Know that when escitalopram dosage increases, monitor patient for possible serotonin syndrome, which may include agitation, chills, confusion, diaphoresis, diarrhea, fever, hyperactive reflexes, poor coordination, restlessness, shaking, talking or acting with uncontrolled excitement, tremor, and twitching. In its most severe form, serotonin syndrome can resemble neuroleptic malignant syndrome, which includes autonomic instability with possible changes in vital signs, a high fever, muscle rigidity, and mental status changes.

! **WARNING** Monitor patient for any other persistent, severe, or unusual adverse reactions because drug can adversely affect many body systems and cause multiple adverse reactions, including life-threatening reactions.

- Monitor patient—especially elderly patient—for hypo-osmolarity of serum and urine and for hyponatremia (headache, impaired memory, trouble concentrating, unsteadiness, weakness) because they may indicate escitalopram-induced syndrome of inappropriate ADH secretion.
- Watch for signs of abuse or misuse in patient's receiving drug long term; drug's potential for psychological dependence may occur.
- Expect prescriber to reassess patient periodically to determine the continued need for therapy and evaluate dosage.
- Expect to taper dosage to avoid serious adverse reactions caused by withdrawal syndrome when therapy is no longer needed.

PATIENT TEACHING

- Instruct patient how to take escitalopram.
- Inform patient that alcohol use isn't recommended during escitalopram therapy because it may decrease his ability to think clearly and perform motor skills.
- Tell patient that improvement may not be noticed for 1 to 4 weeks after therapy begins. Emphasize the importance of continuing therapy as prescribed.
- Advise patient not to stop taking drug abruptly. Explain that gradual tapering helps to avoid withdrawal symptoms.

! **WARNING** Alert patient and family or caregiver that drug can cause an allergic reaction. If present, patient should notify prescriber, and, if severe, to seek immediate medical attention.

! **WARNING** Warn patient that escitalopram increases bleeding risk if taken with an anticoagulant, aspirin, or an NSAID and that bleeding events could range from mild to severe. Tell patient to seek emergency care for serious or prolonged bleeding.

! **WARNING** Urge family or caregiver to watch closely for suicidal tendencies, especially in adolescents and young adults and when therapy starts or dosage changes.

! **WARNING** Instruct patient to notify prescriber immediately if patient develops persistent, severe, or unusual adverse reactions besides those mentioned above.

- Review signs and symptoms of hyponatremia and instruct patient to report them to prescriber.
- Advise patient to avoid hazardous activities until drug's CNS effects are known and resolved.
- Advise patient that drug may cause mild pupillary dilation, which may lead to an episode of acute-angle glaucoma. Encourage patient to have an eye exam before starting therapy to see if he is at risk.
- Urge patient to inform prescriber of any over-the-counter drugs or other newly prescribed prescription drugs taken because of potential for interaction.
- Stress importance to females of childbearing age to notify prescriber if pregnancy occurs.
- Tell mothers who are breastfeeding to monitor their infant for agitation, excessive drowsiness, poor feeding, restlessness, and weight loss.

E

esketamine

Spravato

Class, Category, and Schedule

Pharmacologic class: Ionotropic glutamate receptor
Therapeutic class: Antidepressant
Controlled substance schedule: III

Indications and Dosages

* *As adjunct with an oral antidepressive agent or as monotherapy for treatment-resistant depression*

NASAL SPRAY

Adults. *Induction phase (wk 1–4):* 56 or 84 mg twice a wk. *Maintenance phase (wk 5–8):* 56 mg or 84 mg once a wk. *Maintenance phase (wk 9 and thereafter):* 56 mg or 84 mg every 2 wk unless weekly dosing is needed.

* *As adjunct to treat depressive symptoms in patients with major depressive disorder with acute suicidal ideation or behavior*

NASAL SPRAY

Adults. 84 mg twice a wk for 4 wk.

± **DOSAGE ADJUSTMENT** For patients unable to tolerate 84-mg dosage, dosage reduced to 56 mg twice a week for 4 weeks.

Drug Administration

NASAL SPRAY

- Administration of esketamine should be at least 2 hr after patient ate and at least 30 min after patient had something to drink because drug may cause nausea and vomiting after administration.
- Assess patient's blood pressure prior to administration because drug can elevate blood pressure. If baseline blood pressure is elevated (greater than 140 mm Hg systolic, greater than 90 mm Hg diastolic), drug should not be administered if the increase in blood pressure poses a serious risk.
- Do not prime nasal spray before use. Expect to use 2 devices for a 56-mg dose or 3 devices for an 84-mg dose, with a 5-min rest period between use of each device. Each device delivers 2 sprays (1 spray for each nostril) for a total amount of 28 mg of esketamine.
- Administer drug by first having patient blow their nose. Peel blister and remove device. Check that indicator shows 2 green dots. If not, dispose of device and get a new one.
- Hand device to patient. Instruct patient to hold device with thumb gently supporting the plunger. Patient should not press the plunger yet. Instruct patient to recline head at about 45 degrees during administration to keep drug inside nose. Then, have patient insert the device tip straight into the first nostril. The device nose rest should touch the skin between the nostrils. Instruct patient to close opposite nostril and breathe through nose while pushing plunger all the way up until it stops.
- Encourage patient to sniff gently after spraying to keep drug inside nose. Then, instruct patient to switch hands to insert tip into the second nostril and repeat the same procedure.
- After administration, take device from patient and check that indicator shows no green dots. If a green dot is visible, have patient spray again into the second nostril. Check again to confirm that device is empty.
- Have patient rest in a comfortable position (preferably semi-reclined) for 5 min before using next device. If liquid drips out, have patient dab nose with a tissue.
- Warn patient not to blow nose.
- Discard used devices per facility procedure for a schedule III drug.
- After the drug has been administered, monitor patient for the mandatory 2 hr observation period. Reassess blood pressure often during the 2 hr. If blood pressure remains high, notify prescriber immediately as patient may need treatment to avert a hypertensive crisis. If blood pressure is decreasing after drug is administered and patient appears stable for at least 2 hr, patient may be discharged at the end of the post-dose monitoring period; if not, continue to monitor patient.
- Expect that if patient misses treatment sessions and there is worsening of depression, prescriber may consider returning to patient's previous dosing schedule, such as from every 2 weeks to weekly or weekly to twice weekly.
- Administer a prescribed nasal corticosteroid or nasal decongestant at least 1 hour before administering esketamine.

Route	Onset	Peak	Duration
Intranasal	2–24 hr	20–40 min*	Unknown

Half-life: 7–12 hr

*After last nasal spray dose

Mechanism of Action

Exerts its antidepressant effect through an unknown mechanism.

Contraindications

Aneurysmal vascular disease (including abdominal and thoracic aorta, intracranial, and peripheral arterial vessels) or arteriovenous malformation; history of intracerebral hemorrhage; hypersensitivity to esketamine, ketamine, or any of their components

Interactions

DRUGS

CNS depressants (benzodiazepines, opioids): Increased sedation

MAOIs, psychostimulants (amphetamines, armodafinil, methylphenidate, modafinil): Possibly increased blood pressure

ACTIVITIES

alcohol use: Increased sedation

Adverse Reactions

CNS: Anxiety, cognitive impairment, depersonalization, depression, derealization, dissociation, dizziness, euphoria, feeling intoxicated, headache, hypoesthesia, insomnia, lethargy, loss of consciousness, mental impairment, panic attacks, sedation, **suicidal ideation**, tremor, vertigo
CV: Hypertension, **hypotension**, tachycardia
EENT: Dry mouth, nasal discomfort, oropharyngeal pain, taste alteration, throat irritation
GI: Constipation, diarrhea, nausea, vomiting
GU: Interstitial or ulcerative cystitis, pollakiuria
MS: Dysarthria, muscular weakness
RESP: **Respiratory arrest or depression**
SKIN: Diaphoresis
Other: Physical and psychological dependence

Childbearing Considerations

PREGNANCY

- Pregnancy exposure registry: 1-844-405-6185 or https://womensmentalhealth.org/clinical-and-research-programs/pregnancyregistry/antidepressants.
- Drug may cause fetal harm, based on animal studies.
- Drug therapy is not recommended during pregnancy.

LACTATION

- Drug is present in breast milk.
- Breastfeeding is not recommended during drug therapy because of the potential for neurotoxicity in infant.

REPRODUCTION

- Females of childbearing age should use effective contraception throughout drug therapy.

Nursing Considerations

- Know that esketamine is available only through a restricted program called the Spravato REMS. To receive drug, patient must be enrolled in the Spravato REMS program prior to administration.

! **WARNING** Assess patient for psychosis before drug administration because of the potential for dissociation and perceptual changes to occur after administration. Also, assess patient for a history of drug abuse or dependency because drug is a schedule III–controlled substance. Monitor patient for signs of abuse or dependence after esketamine therapy is started.

! **WARNING** Monitor patient at least 2 hours after each treatment is given for dissociation, respiratory depression (including pulse oximetry readings), and sedation. Know that some patients may lose consciousness. Some patients may also display diminished respirations or even go into a respiratory arrest. Patient should not be allowed to leave the facility until he is considered clinically stable.

- Be aware that esketamine must be administered with an oral antidepressant.
- Be aware that long-term cognitive and memory impairment may occur with drug abuse or misuse.

! **WARNING** Know that concomitant use with psychostimulants or MAOIs increases risk of blood pressure elevation. Promptly seek emergency assistance if patient displays symptoms of a hypertensive crisis or hypertensive encephalopathy after drug administration. Also, be aware that up to 19% of patients in clinical studies experienced an increase of greater than or equal to 40 mm Hg in systolic blood pressure and/or 25 mm Hg in diastolic blood pressure in the first 1.5 hour after administration at least once during the first 4 weeks of therapy.

! **WARNING** Monitor patient for suicidal tendencies, particularly when therapy starts and when dosage changes are made.

- Monitor patient for signs and symptoms of cystitis because esketamine use may increase risk of adverse urinary tract symptoms.

PATIENT TEACHING

- Inform patient that esketamine is available only through a restricted program called the Spravato REMS. Review the program requirements with patient.
- Tell patient that drug will be prepared for administration by a healthcare professional. Drug cannot be self-administered at home.

! **WARNING** Alert patient that because of the potential for serious adverse reactions, patient will need to remain in the facility for at least 2 hours after every treatment and will only be released when stable.

! **WARNING** Inform patient that drug use may increase risk of physical or psychological dependency. Instruct patient to discuss concerns with prescriber.

! **WARNING** Urge family or caregiver to watch patient closely for suicidal tendencies, especially when therapy starts or dosage changes.

- Caution patient to avoid performing activities that are considered hazardous (such as driving or operating machinery) until sedation has resolved, which usually is the next day after a restful night of sleep.
- Alert females of childbearing age to use effective contraception during drug therapy. Explain importance of notifying prescriber if pregnancy occurs while taking esketamine.
- Inform mothers that breastfeeding is not recommended during drug therapy.

esmolol hydrochloride

Brevibloc

Class and Category

Pharmacologic class: Beta-blocker
Therapeutic class: Antiarrhythmic, antihypertensive

Indications and Dosages

* *To treat supraventricular tachycardia, including atrial fibrillation and atrial flutter; to control heart rate in noncompensatory sinus tachycardia*

I.V. INFUSION

Adults. The dosage is titrated in a stepwise fashion as follows: *Step 1:* Optional loading dose of 500 mcg/kg infused over 1 min, followed by a maintenance infusion of 50 mcg/kg/min infused over 4 min. If response occurs, infusion continued at 50 mcg/kg/min for up to 48 hr, as needed. If response does not occur within 5 min, step 2 initiated. *Step 2:* Optional loading dose of 500 mcg/kg infused over 1 min followed by a maintenance infusion of 100 mcg/kg/min infused over 4 min. If response occurs, infusion continued at 100 mcg/kg/min for up to 48 hr, as needed. If response is not adequate, step 3 initiated. *Step 3:* Optional loading dose of 500 mcg/kg infused over 1 min followed by a maintenance dose of 150 mcg/kg/min infused over 4 min. If response occurs, infusion continued at 150 mcg/kg/min for up to 48 hr, as needed. If response is not adequate, step 4 initiated. *Step 4:* Maintenance dose increased to a continuous infusion of 200 mcg/kg/min and continued for up to 48 hr, as needed.

* *To treat intraoperative and postoperative hypertension and tachycardia*

I.V. INJECTION, I.V. INFUSION

Adults. *For immediate control:* 1,000 mcg/kg given as a bolus over 30 sec, followed by an infusion of 150 mcg/kg/min. Infusion adjusted, as needed, to maintain desired blood pressure and heart rate but not exceeding maximum dosage. *For gradual control*: 500 mcg/kg given as a bolus over 1 min, followed by a maintenance infusion of 50 mcg/kg/min given over 4 min. If response is inadequate, a second bolus of 500 mcg/kg given over 1 min followed by a maintenance infusion of 100 mcg/kg/min given over 4 min. If response is still inadequate, a third bolus of 500 mcg/kg given over 1 min followed by a maintenance infusion of 150 mcg/kg/min given over 4 min. If response remains inadequate, maintenance dose increased to a continuous infusion of 200 mcg/kg/min and continued until maximum dose reached, as needed. *Maximum:* 200 mcg/kg/min for tachycardia; 300 mcg/kg/min for hypertension.

± **DOSAGE ADJUSTMENT** For patients transitioning from esmolol infusion to alternative drugs, esmolol infusion rate reduced by 50% 30 minutes following the first dose of the alternative drug. After administration of the second dose of the alternative drug, if patient's response is satisfactory and maintained for the first hour, esmolol infusion discontinued.

Drug Administration

I.V.

- Drug is available in a premixed bag and ready-to-use vial; don't dilute either one.
- The ready-to-use vial may be used to administer a loading dose by handheld syringe while the maintenance infusion is being prepared.
- Do not remove premixed bag from overwrap until ready to use. Tear overwrap at notch and remove premixed bag. Some opacity of the plastic due to moisture absorption during the sterilization process may be observed and will diminish gradually. This is normal and does not affect the solution quality or safety.
- Check for minute leaks by squeezing the inner premixed bag firmly. If a leak is present, discard. Solution should be colorless to light yellow and the seal intact.
- Use the medication port solely for withdrawing an initial bolus from the premixed bag. Do not add any additional drugs to the bag.
- Once drug has been withdrawn from the premixed bag, the bag should be used within 24 hr with any unused portion discarded.
- Do not use plastic containers in series connections when administering drug.
- Don't infuse into a small vein or through a butterfly catheter.
- Administer loading or bolus doses of 1,000 mcg/kg dose over 30 sec and 500 mcg/kg over 1 min using an infusion-control device.
- Inspect site often for thrombophlebitis (pain, redness, swelling at site). Infusion of 20 mg/ml is more likely to cause serious vein irritation than 10 mg/ml. Extravasation of 20 mg/ml may cause a serious local reaction and skin necrosis and so should be administered through a central line.
- *Incompatibilities:* Furosemide, 5% Sodium Bicarbonate Injection

Route	Onset	Peak	Duration
I.V.	Immediate	2–6 min	10–20 min

Half-life: 9 min

Mechanism of Action

Inhibits stimulation of $beta_1$ receptors mainly in the heart, which decreases cardiac excitability, cardiac output, and myocardial oxygen demand. Esmolol also decreases renin release from kidneys, which helps reduce blood pressure.

Contraindications

Cardiogenic shock; concomitant use of IV cardiodepressant calcium-channel antagonists (verapamil); decompensated heart failure; hypersensitivity to esmolol, other beta-blockers and their components; pulmonary hypertension; second- or third-degree heart block; severe sinus bradycardia; sick sinus syndrome

Interactions

DRUGS

anticholinesterases, such as mivacurium, succinylcholine: Prolonged clinical duration and recovery of mivacurium and prolonged duration of succinylcholine-induced neuromuscular blockage
calcium channel antagonists: Increased risk of fatal cardiac arrest in patients with depressed myocardial function
clonidine, guanfacine, moxonidine: Increased risk of withdrawal rebound hypertension
digitalis glycosides: Increased risk of bradycardia
positive inotropic and vasoconstrictive agents, such as dopamine, epinephrine, or norepinephrine: Increased risk of reducing cardiac contractility in presence of high systemic resistance
sympathomimetics that have beta-adrenergic agonist activity: May counter effects of esmolol

Adverse Reactions

CNS: Anxiety, confusion, depression, dizziness, fatigue, fever, headache, light-headedness, paresthesia, **seizures**, speech disorder, somnolence, syncope
CV: **Bradycardia**, **cardiac arrest or failure, cardiogenic shock, coronary arteriospasm** chest pain, decreased peripheral circulation, **heart block**, **hypotension** peripheral ischemia
EENT: Dry mouth
ENDO: **Hypoglycemia**
GI: Abdominal discomfort, constipation, dyspepsia, nausea, vomiting

E

GU: Urinary retention
RESP: Dyspnea, wheezing
SKIN: Diaphoresis, flushing, pallor, psoriasis, urticaria
Other: **Angioedema**; infusion-site pain, redness, and swelling

Childbearing Considerations

PREGNANCY

- Drug may cause fetal bradycardia if given during the last trimester of pregnancy.
- Use with caution only if benefit to mother outweighs potential risk to fetus.

LABOR AND DELIVERY

- Drug may cause fetal bradycardia if given during labor and delivery, which may continue after drug is discontinued.
- Use with caution only if benefit to mother outweighs potential risk to fetus.

LACTATION

- It is not known if drug is present in breast milk.
- A decision should be made to discontinue breastfeeding or the drug to avoid potential serious adverse reactions in the breastfed infant.

Nursing Considerations

! **WARNING** Be aware that esmolol should not be given for intraoperative or postoperative hypertension caused by hypothermia-induced vasoconstriction.

! **WARNING** Use esmolol cautiously if patient has supraventricular arrhythmias with decreased cardiac output, hypotension, or other hemodynamic compromise or is taking drugs that decrease contractility, impulse generation, myocardial filling, or peripheral resistance.

- Use drug cautiously in patients with impaired renal function because drug is excreted by the kidneys. Patients with end-stage renal disease have an increased risk of adverse reactions.

! **WARNING** Expect to give lowest possible dose to patients with allergies, asthma, bronchitis, or emphysema. If patient develops wheezing, expect to discontinue infusion immediately and give a beta$_2$-stimulating drug, as ordered.

! **WARNING** Monitor patient for a hypersensitivity reaction which could become life-threatening such as angioedema. If present, notify prescriber, expect drug to be discontinued and replaced with a different drug, and provide supportive care, as needed and ordered.

! **WARNING** Monitor patient's blood pressure for hypotension, heart rate for bradycardia, and ECG for evidence of heart block. Also, monitor patient for signs and symptoms of heart failure because beta-blockers such as esmolol can depress myocardial contractility and precipitate cardiogenic shock and heart failure. If changes in cardiovascular function occur, notify prescriber immediately, expect esmolol therapy to be discontinued, and provide supportive care, as needed and ordered.

! **WARNING** Monitor patient for seizure activity and institute seizure precautions.

! **WARNING** Know that esmolol may prevent early warnings of hypoglycemia, such as tachycardia. This could increase the risk for severe or prolonged hypoglycemia at any time during treatment, especially in patients with diabetes mellitus or children and patients who are fasting because of surgery, not eating regularly, or are vomiting. Monitor patient's blood glucose level closely. If present, notify prescriber and treat according to institutional protocol.

PATIENT TEACHING

- Inform patient that drug will be given intravenously.
- Reassure patient that blood pressure, heart rate, and response to therapy will be monitored throughout esmolol therapy.

! **WARNING** Alert patient that drug may cause an allergic reaction. Tell patient to notify staff immediately if swelling occurs (especially of face and throat) or hives appear.

- Urge patient to report any persistent, serious, or unsual adverse reactions immediately.
- Tell patient to expect blood glucose monitoring during esmolol therapy.

esomeprazole magnesium

Nexium, Nexium 24 HR

esomeprazole sodium

Nexium I.V.

Class and Category

Pharmacologic class: Proton pump inhibitor
Therapeutic class: Antiulcerative

Indications and Dosages

✱ *To treat symptomatic gastroesophageal reflux disease (GERD)*

D.R. CAPSULES, D.R. SUSPENSION (NEXIUM)

Adults. 20 mg daily for 4 wk, with cycle repeated once more, as needed.
Adolescents ages 12 to 17. 20 mg once daily for 4 wk.

D.R. SUSPENSION (NEXIUM)

Children ages 1 to 11. 10 mg once daily for up to 8 wk.

✱ *To promote healing of erosive esophagitis in patient with GERD*

D.R. CAPSULES, D.R. SUSPENSION (NEXIUM)

Adults. 20 or 40 mg once daily for 4 to 8 wk, with cycle repeated once more if healing has not taken place after first 8 wk. *Maintenance:* 20 mg once daily for up to 6 months.
Adolescents ages 12 to 17. 20 or 40 mg once daily for 4 to 8 wk.

D.R. SUSPENSION (NEXIUM)

Children ages 1 to 11 weighing 20 kg (44 lb) or more. 10 or 20 mg once daily for 8 wk.
Children ages 1 to 11 weighing less than 20 kg (44 lb). 10 mg once daily for 8 wk.

✱ *To treat erosive esophagitis due to acid-mediated GERD*

D.R. SUSPENSION

Infants ages 1 mo to less than 1 yr weighing 7.5 kg (16.5 lb) to 12 kg (26.4 lb). 10 mg once daily for up to 6 wk.
Infants ages 1 mo to less than 1 yr weighing 5 kg (11 lb) to 7.5 kg (16.5 lb). 5 mg once daily for up to 6 wk.
Infants ages 1 mo to less than 1 yr weighing 3 kg (6.6 lb) to 5 kg (11 lb). 2.5 mg once daily for up to 6 wk.

✱ *To treat GERD in a patient with erosive esophagitis who can't take drug by mouth*

I.V. INJECTION

Adults. 20 or 40 mg injected over 3 min once daily up to 10 days with switch to oral therapy as soon as possible.

I.V. INFUSION

Adults. 20 or 40 mg infused over 10 to 30 min once daily up to 10 days with switch to oral therapy as soon as possible.
Children ages 1 to 17 weighing 55 kg (121 lb) or more. 20 mg daily infused over 10 to 30 min up to 10 days with switch to oral therapy as soon as possible.
Children ages 1 to 17 weighing less than 55 kg (121 lb). 10 mg infused over 10 to 30 min daily up to 10 days with switch to oral therapy as soon as possible.
Children ages 1 mo to less than 1 yr. 0.5 mg/kg infused over 10 to 30 min daily up to 10 days with switch to oral therapy as soon as possible.

± **DOSAGE ADJUSTMENT** For adult patients with severe liver impairment, dosage should not exceed 20 mg once daily.

✱ *As adjunct to treat duodenal ulcer associated with* Helicobacter pylori

D.R. CAPSULES (NEXIUM), D.R. SUSPENSION (NEXIUM)

Adults. 40 mg daily with amoxicillin 1,000 mg twice a day and clarithromycin 500 mg twice a day for 10 days.

✱ *To reduce the risk of gastric ulcer formation in patients who are receiving continuous NSAID therapy and who either are 60 and older or have a history of gastric ulcer*

D.R. CAPSULES (NEXIUM), D.R. SUSPENSION (NEXIUM)

Adults. 20 or 40 mg daily for up to 6 mo.

✱ *To treat pathological hypersecretory conditions, including Zollinger-Ellison syndrome*

D.R. CAPSULES, D.R. SUSPENSION

Adults. *Initial:* 40 mg twice daily, increased as needed. *Maximum:* 240 mg daily.

± **DOSAGE ADJUSTMENT** For patients with severe hepatic insufficiency, maximum dose of 20 mg daily.

E

∗ *To reduce risk of rebleeding of duodenal or gastric ulcers following therapeutic endoscopy for acute-bleeding duodenal or gastric ulcers*

I.V. INFUSION

Adults. *Initial:* 80 mg infused over 30 min followed by continuous infusion of 8 mg/hr for 71.5 hr after initial dose is completed.

±**DOSAGE ADJUSTMENT** For patients with mild to moderate liver impairment, maximum continuous infusion should not exceed 6 mg/hr; for patients with severe liver impairment, maximum continuous infusion should not exceed 4 mg/hr.

Drug Administration

P.O.

- Give oral drug at least 1 hr before meals because food decreases bioavailability.
- Use D.R. capsules or oral suspension specific for nasogastric tube administration and D.R. oral suspension specific for nasogastric or gastric tube administration when administering to a patient with a nasogastric or gastric tube. Follow manufacturer's directions for administration.
- D.R. capsules or tablets should be swallowed whole and not chewed, crushed, or split/opened. However, if patient has difficulty swallowing capsules, tell patient to open the D.R. capsules and sprinkle contents onto 1 tablespoon of cool applesauce and mix. Caution him not to use any other food and not to chew or crush the granules.
- Mix oral suspension by adding 5 ml of water to the contents of a 2.5- or 5-mg packet or 15 ml of water to 10-, 20-, or 40-mg packet. Let mixture sit for 2 to 3 min to thicken. Stir and give to patient to drink within 30 min.

I.V.

- Always flush I.V. line with 0.9% Sodium Chloride Injection, 5% Dextrose Injection, or Lactated Ringer's Injection before and after giving drug.
- For I.V. injection, reconstitute each vial with 5 ml of 0.9% Sodium Chloride Injection. Administer I.V. injection over at least 3 min.
- For intermittent I.V. infusion, reconstitute each vial with 5 ml of 0.9% Sodium Chloride Injection, 5% Dextrose Injection, or Lactated Ringer's Injection, then further dilute reconstituted solution with 45 ml of 0.9% Sodium Chloride Injection, 5% Dextrose Injection, or Lactated Ringer's Injection. Administer over 10 to 30 min. For continuous infusion, prepare infusion in the same manner but administer over 71.5 hr at a rate of 8 mg/hr or decrease rate to 6 mg/hr for mild to moderate liver impairment and to 4 mg/hr for severe liver impairment, as ordered.
- Reconstituted drug may be stored at room temperature up to 6 hr if mixed with 5% Dextrose Injection or up to 12 hr if mixed with 0.9% Sodium Chloride Injection or Lactated Ringer's Injection.
- I.V. therapy should be switched to oral form as soon as possible.
- *Incompatibilities:* Other I.V. drugs

Route	Onset	Peak	Duration
P.O.	Immediate	1.5 hr	13–17 hr
I.V.	Unknown	Unknown	Unknown

Half-life: 1–1.5 hr

Mechanism of Action

Interferes with gastric acid secretion by inhibiting the hydrogen–potassium–adenosine triphosphatase (H^+–K^+–ATPase) enzyme system, or proton pump, in gastric parietal cells. Normally, the proton pump uses energy from hydrolysis of ATPase to drive H^+ and chloride (Cl^-) out of parietal cells and into the stomach lumen in exchange for potassium (K^+), which leaves the stomach lumen and enters parietal cells. After this exchange, H^+ and Cl^- combine in the stomach to form hydrochloric acid (HCl). Esomeprazole irreversibly inhibits the final step in gastric acid production by blocking exchange of intracellular H^+ and extracellular K^+, thus preventing H^+ from entering the stomach and additional HCl from forming.

Contraindications

Concurrent therapy with rilpivirine-containing products, hypersensitivity to esomeprazole, substituted benzimidazoles, or their components

Interactions

DRUGS

atazanavir, dasatinib, erlotinib, ketoconazole, iron salts, itraconazole, mycophenolate mofetil, nelfinavir nilotinib, rilpivirine: Decreased blood levels of these drugs

cilostazol: Possibly increased blood cilostazol levels
citalopram: Increased exposure of citalopram leading to an increased risk of QT prolongation
clopidogrel: Reduced effectiveness of clopidogrel
digoxin: Possibly increased risk of digoxin toxicity
methotrexate: Increased risk of methotrexate toxicities
rifampin, St. John's wort: Decreased blood esomeprazole level
saquinavir: Increased plasma saquinavir level with increased toxicity
tacrolimus: Increased serum tacrolimus level
voriconazole: Increased esomeprazole exposure and risk of adverse effects
warfarin: Possibly increased INR and PT leading to abnormal bleeding

FOODS

all foods: Decreased bioavailability of esomeprazole

Adverse Reactions

CNS: Agitation, aggression, depression, dizziness, fever, headache, hallucinations, **encephalopathy** (hepatic), vertigo
EENT: Blurred vision, dry mouth, mucosal discoloration, sinusitis, stomatitis, taste disturbance
ENDO: Gynecomastia
GI: Abdominal pain; Barrett's esophagus; benign polyps or nodules; candidiasis; ***Clostridioides difficile*-associated diarrhea**; constipation; diarrhea; duodenitis; dyspepsia; esophagitis; esophageal stricture, ulceration, or varices; flatulence; fundic gland polyps; gastric ulcer; gastritis; **hepatic failure**; **hepatitis**; jaundice; microscopic colitis; nausea; **pancreatitis**
GU: Acute tubulointerstitial nephritis, erectile dysfunction
HEME: **Agranulocytosis**, **pancytopenia**
MS: Bone fracture, muscle weakness, myalgia
RESP: **Bronchospasm**, cough, respiratory tract infection
SKIN: Acute generalized exanthematous pustulosis, alopecia, cutaneous lupus erythematosus, diaphoresis, **erythema multiforme**, hyperhidrosis, photosensitivity, pruritus, **Stevens-Johnson syndrome**, **toxic epidermal necrolysis**
Other: **Anaphylaxis**, cyanocobalamin deficiency (prolonged use), **drug reaction with eosinophilia and systemic symptoms (DRESS)**, **hypocalcemia**, **hypokalemia**, **hypomagnesemia**, **hyponatremia**, infusion-site reactions (erythema, inflammation, phlebitis, pruritus, swelling), systemic lupus erythematosus, vitamin B_{12} deficiency

Childbearing Considerations

PREGNANCY

- It is not known if drug causes fetal harm.
- Use with caution only if benefit to mother outweighs potential risk to fetus.

LACTATION

- Drug may be present in breast milk.
- Mothers should check with prescriber before breastfeeding.

E

Nursing Considerations

! **WARNING** Monitor patient closely for hypersensitivity reactions, including severe cutaneous adverse reactions such as a rash that may cause bleeding, blistering, or peeling on any skin area. The rash also may be accompanied by body aches, chills, enlarged lymph nodes, fever, or shortness of breath although DRESS may only initially present with a fever or swollen lymph nodes. Notify prescriber immediately if a rash or other hypersensitivity reactions occur. Expect drug to be discontinued and provide supportive care, as needed and ordered.

! **WARNING** Know that hypomagnesemia may lead to hypocalcemia and/or hypokalemia and may exacerbate underlying hypocalcemia for patients at risk. Obtain levels, as ordered, before esomeprazole begins and periodically throughout drug therapy if patient is at risk because of a preexisting condition such as hypoparathyroidism. Hypomagnesemia may occur when esomeprazole therapy has been administered longer than 3 months, although most cases have occurred after therapy had been given for more than a year. Notify prescriber immediately if magnesium level drops below normal as hypomagnesemia may cause tetany, arrhythmias, and seizures. Also, notify prescriber if calcium or potassium levels decrease. Expect patient to receive calcium, potassium, and magnesium replacement, as needed, and esomeprazole to be discontinued, if warranted.

! **WARNING** Monitor patient for diarrhea throughout therapy because drug may increase the risk of *Clostridioides difficile*–associated diarrhea. Know that the lowest dose possible for the shortest amount of time should be used to decrease this risk. If diarrhea occurs, expect to obtain a stool specimen to determine if diarrhea is caused by *C. difficile*. If it is, expect esomeprazole to be discontinued and an antibiotic effective against *C. difficile* to be given, as ordered. Also, expect to administer electrolytes, fluids, and protein supplementation, as needed and ordered.

- Monitor patients for bone fractures, especially in patients who are receiving multiple daily doses for a year or longer, as proton pump inhibitors such as esomeprazole have been associated with an increased risk for osteoporosis-related fractures of the hip, spine, or wrist.
- Be aware that esomeprazole therapy may have to be temporarily halted for at least 14 days if patient is undergoing testing for neuroendocrine tumors because drug may cause false positive results in diagnostic testing.
- Monitor patient for signs and symptoms of cutaneous and systemic lupus erythematosus or exacerbation of these conditions, if already present. Notify prescriber, if present, and expect serological testing to be done. If results are positive, expect drug to be discontinued. Symptoms are usually relieved in most patients within 4 to 12 weeks.
- Be aware that patients who take esomeprazole long term, especially after 1 year, are at increased risk for developing fundic gland polyps.

PATIENT TEACHING

- Instruct patient how to administer form of esomeprazole prescribed.
- Tell patient that drug should be taken at the lowest dose possible and for the shortest time to decrease risk of adverse effects. Tell patient never to increase dosage or take it long term without consulting prescriber.
- Urge patient to tell prescriber if antacids or any other over-the-counter or prescription drugs are taken.
- Remind patient that esomeprazole, including the over-the-counter preparation, is not intended for immediate relief of heartburn; the drug may take up to 4 days before the full effect is experienced.

! **WARNING** Instruct patient to notify prescriber if an allergic reaction occurs. Urge patient to seek immediate medical attention if he experiences a serious allergic reaction to esomeprazole, especially a rash that may cause bleeding, blistering or peeling on any skin area.

! **WARNING** Advise patient to contact prescriber if he develops abdominal pain, diarrhea (could be severe and bloody), and fever that does not improve, especially if he has recently taken or is taking an antibiotic. Also, advise patient to report any other persistent or serious signs and symptoms that occur while taking esomeprazole. Instruct patient to stop taking drug if he develops joint pain and to see his doctor for an evaluation of these symptoms.

! **WARNING** Review the signs and symptoms of hypomagnesemia if taking drug longer than 3 months or vitamin B_{12} deficiency if taking drug longer than 3 years.

- Advise patient that drug may increase risk for osteoporosis-related fractures of the hip, spine, or wrist. Instruct him to take fall precautions and have bone health evaluated regularly.

estazolam

Class, Category, and Schedule

Pharmacologic class: Benzodiazepine
Therapeutic class: Sedative-hypnotic
Controlled substance schedule: IV

Indications and Dosages

✶ To treat insomnia short-term

TABLETS

Adults. 1 to 2 mg once daily.
Elderly adults. 1 mg once daily.

± **DOSAGE ADJUSTMENT** For small or debilitated elderly patients, starting dose reduced to 0.5 mg.

Drug Administration

P.O.

- Administer drug at bedtime.

Route	Onset	Peak	Duration
P.O.	Unknown	2 hr	Variable

Half-life: 10–24 hr

Mechanism of Action

May potentiate effects of gamma-aminobutyric acid (GABA) and other inhibitory neurotransmitters by binding to specific benzodiazepine receptors in cortical and limbic areas of CNS. By binding to these receptors, estazolam increases GABA's inhibitory effects and blocks cortical and limbic arousal.

Contraindications

Concurrent therapy with itraconazole or ketoconazole; hypersensitivity to estazolam, other benzodiazepines, or their components; pregnancy

Interactions

DRUGS

anticonvulsants, antihistamines, barbiturates, CNS depressants, MAO inhibitors, narcotics, phenothiazines, psychotropics: Possibly potentiated action of estazolam
barbiturates, carbamazepine, phenytoin, rifampin: Possibly decreased estazolam level
cimetidine, diltiazem, fluvoxamine, isoniazid, itraconazole, ketoconazole, nefazodone, selected macrolide antibiotics: Possibly increased blood level and impaired hepatic metabolism of estazolam
opioids: Possibly significant respiratory depression and sedation

ACTIVITIES

alcohol use: Possibly potentiated CNS depression, including respiratory depression and sedation
smoking: Increased clearance of estazolam

Adverse Reactions

CNS: Amnesia, anxiety, ataxia, confusion, delusions, depression, dizziness, drowsiness, euphoria, headache, hypokinesia, irritability, malaise, nervousness, slurred speech, tremor
CV: Chest pain, palpitations, tachycardia
EENT: Blurred vision, dry mouth, increased salivation, photophobia
GI: Abdominal pain, constipation, diarrhea, nausea, thirst, vomiting
GU: Libido changes
RESP: **Respiratory depression**
SKIN: Diaphoresis
Other: **Anaphylaxis**, **angioedema**, physical or psychological dependence

Childbearing Considerations

PREGNANCY

- Drug may cause fetal harm.
- Drug is contraindicated in pregnant women.
- Be aware that if mother takes drug prior to delivery, neonate may experience withdrawal symptoms during the postnatal period.

LACTATION

- It is not known if drug is present in breast milk.
- Breastfeeding should not be undertaken during drug therapy.

Nursing Considerations

! **WARNING** Use estazolam with extreme caution in patients with a history of alcohol or drug abuse because of risk of addiction. Expect to give drug for no more than 12 weeks.

- Use cautiously in debilitated or elderly patients and those with depression or impaired hepatic, renal, or respiratory function.

! **WARNING** Monitor patient for hypersensitivity reactions, which could become life-threatening although rare such as anaphylaxis or angioedema. If present, notify prescriber immediately, expect drug to be discontinued, and provide supportive care, as needed and ordered.

! **WARNING** Monitor respiratory status, especially in patients with respiratory compromise, who are at increased risk for respiratory depression.

! **WARNING** Expect to stop drug gradually to prevent withdrawal symptoms. Avoid stopping abruptly if patient has history of seizures.

PATIENT TEACHING

! **WARNING** Advise females of childbearing age to notify prescriber if pregnant before estazolam therapy is begun and immediately during drug therapy if pregnancy occurs because drug is contraindicated during pregnancy.

- Instruct patient how to administer estazolam.

! **WARNING** Advise patient not to drink alcohol or take other CNS depressants during therapy because of the risk of additive effects.

- Warn patient not to exceed prescribed time because of risk of addiction.
- Tell patient not to stop taking drug abruptly as withdrawal symptoms may occur.

! **WARNING** Alert patient that although rare, drug may cause an allergic reaction. If present, tell patient to notify prescriber immediately and, if severe, to seek immediate medical care.

- Warn debilitated or elderly patients and those with impaired hepatic or renal function about risk of excessive sedation or mental impairment and the need to report them.
- Advise patient to avoid hazardous activities until CNS effects of the drug are known and resolved.
- Inform mothers breastfeeding should not be undertaken during drug therapy.

estradiol

Divigel 1%, Elestrin, Estrace, Estrasorb, Estring, Estrogel, Evamist, Imvexxy, Vagifem, Yuvafem

estradiol acetate

Femring

estradiol cypionate

Depo-Estradiol

estradiol transdermal system

Alora, Climara, Dotti, Menostar, Minivelle, Vivelle, Vivelle-Dot

estradiol valerate

Delestrogen

Class and Category

Pharmacologic class: Estrogen
Therapeutic class: Hormone

Indications and Dosages

✱ To treat menopausal symptoms

TABLETS (ESTRADIOL)

Adult menopausal and postmenopausal women. *Initial:* 0.5 to 2 mg once daily and then adjusted to control symptoms.

VAGINAL RING (ESTRADIOL ACETATE [FEMRING])

Adult females. One ring (0.05 or 0.1 mg of estradiol/24 hr) inserted into upper third of vaginal vault and replaced every 3 mo.

I.M. INJECTION (ESTRADIOL CYPIONATE IN OIL)

Adult females. 1 to 5 mg as a single dose every 3 to 4 wk, as needed.

I.M. INJECTION (ESTRADIOL VALERATE INOIL)

Adult females. 10 to 20 mg every 4 wk, as needed.

TRANSDERMAL (ALORA)

Adult menopausal and postmenopausal females. *Initial:* 0.05 mg continuously with one patch replaced twice/wk if uterus is not present or in cycles of 3 wk on (patch replaced twice/wk), 1 wk off (no patch applied) if uterus is intact. Dosage adjusted to control symptoms, as needed.

TRANSDERMAL (VIVELLE, VIVELLE-DOT)

Adult menopausal and postmenopausal females. *Initial:* 0.0375 mg/day with one patch applied to trunk or buttocks and replaced twice/wk (every 3 to 4 days). Dosage adjusted to control symptoms, as needed.

TRANSDERMAL (CLIMARA)

Adult females. *Initial:* 0.025 mg daily. One patch applied to trunk or buttocks, replaced every week. Dosage titrated to control symptoms, as needed.

TRANSDERMAL (ESTROGEL)

Adult females. 1.25 g daily applied in thin layer from wrist to shoulder on inside and outside of one arm.

∗ *To treat postmenopausal moderate to severe symptoms of vulvar and vaginal atrophy*

TABLETS (ESTRADIOL)

Adult women. 0.5 to 2 mg once daily. Dosage adjusted to control symptoms, as needed.

VAGINAL CREAM (ESTRACE)

Adult females. *Initial:* 2 to 4 g daily for 1 to 2 wk. Then, dosage gradually reduced to half of initial dose, for 1 to 2 wk. *Maintenance:* 1 g daily 1 to 3 times/wk.

VAGINAL RING (ESTRING)

Adult females. One ring (7.5 mcg of estradiol/24 hr) inserted into upper third of vaginal vault and replaced every 3 mo.

VAGINAL RING (FEMRING)

Adult females. One ring (0.05 or 0.1 mg of estradiol/24 hr) inserted into upper third of vaginal vault and replaced every 3 mo.

∗ *To treat atrophic vaginitis due to menopause*

VAGINAL INSERT (VAGIFEM)

Adult females. *Initial:* 10-mcg insert daily for 2 wk, followed by 1 insert twice/wk.

∗ *To treat moderate to severe dyspareunia*

VAGINAL INSERT (IMVEXXY)

Adult females. *Initial:* 4 mcg (1 insert) daily for 2 wk, followed by 4 mcg (1 insert) twice weekly. Dosage increased to 10 mcg (1 insert), as needed.

∗ *To treat moderate to severe vasomotor symptoms due to menopause*

TRANSDERMAL (MINIVELLE)

Adult females. 0.0375 mg daily with patch replaced twice/wk. Dosage adjusted, as needed.

GEL (DIVIGEL 0.1%)

Adult females. *Initial:* 0.25 mg once daily to skin of left or right upper thigh and then dosage increased, as needed.

GEL (ELESTRIN 0.06%)

Adult females. 1 pump of gel (0.52 mg) once per day applied to the upper arm. Dosage increased to 2 pumps of gel (1.04 mg) once per day applied to the upper arm, as needed.

TRANSDERMAL SPRAY (EVAMIST)

Adult females. *Initial:* 1.53 mg (1 spray) daily to the inner surface of the forearm, starting near the elbow, increased to 2 sprays (3.06 mg), as needed and further increased to 3 sprays (4.59 mg), as needed.

∗ *To prevent osteoporosis secondary to estrogen deficiency due to either natural or surgical menopause*

TRANSDERMAL (ALORA)

Adult females. Initial: 0.025 mg daily with one patch applied to lower abdomen or buttocks and replaced twice/wk if uterus is not present or in cycles of 3 wk on (patch replaced twice/wk), 1 wk off (no patch applied) if uterus is intact. Dosage adjusted to control symptoms, as needed.

TRANSDERMAL (MINIVELLE, VIVELLE-DOT)

Adult females. 0.025 mg daily.

TRANSDERMAL (CLIMARA)

Adult females. *Initial:* 0.025 mg daily. One patch applied to trunk or buttocks and replaced every wk. Dosage adjusted to control symptoms, as needed.

TRANSDERMAL (MENOSTAR)

Adult females. *Initial:* 0.014 mg daily. One patch applied to lower abdomen and replaced every wk.

∗ *To treat estrogen deficiency due to oophorectomy, primary ovarian failure, or female hypogonadism*

TABLETS (ESTRADIOL)

Adult females. 1 to 2 mg daily.

EMULSION POUCH (ESTRASORB)

Adult females. 1 pouch (2.5 mg) applied to left calf and thigh and 1 pouch (2.5 mg) applied to right calf and thigh each morning.

I.M. INJECTION (ESTRADIOL CYPIONATE IN OIL)

Adult females. 1.5 to 2 mg every mo (for female hypogonadism only).

I.M. INJECTION (ESTRADIOL VALERATE INOIL)

Adult females. 10 to 20 mg every mo, as needed.

TRANSDERMAL (ALORA, ESTRADERM)

Adult females. *Initial:* 0.05 mg daily with one patch applied to trunk or buttocks and replaced twice/wk. Dosage titrated to control symptoms, as needed. A cyclic schedule is followed unless patient has had a hysterectomy.

TRANSDERMAL (VIVELLE)

Adult females. 0.0375 mg daily with one patch applied to trunk or buttocks and replaced twice/wk. Dosage titrated to control symptoms, as needed. A cyclic schedule is followed unless patient has had a hysterectomy.

TRANSDERMAL (CLIMARA)

Adult females. *Initial:* 0.025 mg daily. One patch applied to trunk or buttocks and replaced every wk. Dosage adjusted to control symptoms, as needed.

✶ *To provide palliative treatment for inoperable, progressive breast cancer in selected men and postmenopausal women*

TABLETS (ESTRADIOL)

Adults. 10 mg 3 times daily for at least 3 mo.

✶ *To treat advancing, inoperable prostate cancer*

TABLETS (ESTRADIOL)

Adult males. 1 to 2 mg or 3 times daily, adjusted or continued, as needed, according to patient response.

I.M. INJECTION (ESTRADIOL VALERATE)

Adult males. 30 mg every 1 to 2 wk, adjusted or continued, as needed, according to patient response.

Drug Administration

P.O.

- Administer oral preparations with or immediately after food to decrease nausea.
- Avoid administering with grapefruit juice.

I.M.

- Roll vial and syringe between palms of hands to evenly disperse drug. Use at least a 21 G needle (estradiol cypionate) or a 20 G needle (estradiol valerate).
- Inject deep into upper outer quadrant of gluteal muscle.
- Rotate sites.
- Never administer I.V.

TRANSDERMAL

- If patient is converting from oral estrogen to transdermal system, oral estrogen should be stopped 1 wk before skin patches are applied.
- Apply patch to the area designated by product being used. Apply patch to clear, dry, intact skin that is hairless on abdomen or buttock. Hold in place for at least 10 sec.
- Do not apply patch to breasts, waistline, or other areas where it may not adhere properly.
- Rotate application sites at least weekly and remove old patch before applying new one.
- If patch falls off, reapply it to another area or apply a new patch and continue the original treatment schedule. Patient may bathe while wearing the patch. Discard used patch according to institutional protocol.
- Prime spray pump by holding pump upright and vertical and spraying 3 sprays with cover on before initial use. Apply spray in the morning to adjacent, nonoverlapping areas on the inner surfacer of the forearm, starting near the elbow. Do not apply anywhere else. Allow area to dry for at least 2 min before covering area with clothing. Do not wash site for at least an hour after application.

TOPICAL

- Apply to clean, dry skin in area designated by product being used. Wash hands with soap and water afterward.
- Never apply gel to breasts.
- Rotate Divigel gel to the opposite site on alternating days. Application surface area should be about 5 to 7 inches (about the size of 2 palm prints). The entire contents of a unit-dose packet should be applied each day. Gel should never be applied to the breasts, face, irritated skin, or in or around vagina. After application, let gel dry before patient gets dressed. Do not wash the site for 1 hr after application. Wash hands after application.

VAGINAL

- Patient should remain recumbent for at least 30 min after applying estradiol vaginal cream. A sanitary napkin (but not a tampon) may be used to protect clothing after application.
- Imvexxy vaginal inserts are inserted with the smaller end first for a depth of about 2 inches into the vaginal canal. Each insert should be inserted at about the same time every day.
- When a vaginal ring is to be inserted, have patient squeeze sides of ring together and insert into upper third of her vagina where it will stay for 90 days, and then removed and a new ring inserted. If it is removed during the 90-day dosage period, patient should rinse it with lukewarm (not hot or boiling) water, and reinsert it, as needed for personal hygiene. Patient shouldn't be able to feel the ring when it's in place. If she does, she should use a finger to push the ring farther into her vagina.

Route	Onset	Peak	Duration
All routes	Unknown	Unknown	Unknown

Half-life: Unknown

Mechanism of Action

Increases the rate of DNA and RNA synthesis in cells of female reproductive organs, pituitary gland, hypothalamus, and other target organs. In the hypothalamus, estrogens reduce release of gonadotropin-releasing hormone, which decreases pituitary release of follicle-stimulating hormone and luteinizing hormone. In women, these hormones are required for normal genitourinary and other essential body functions.

At the cellular level, estrogens increase cervical secretions, cause endometrial cell proliferation, and improve uterine tone.

Estrogen replacement helps maintain genitourinary function and reduces vasomotor symptoms when estrogen production declines as a result of menopause, surgical removal of ovaries, or other estrogen deficiency states.

Estrogen replacement also helps prevent osteoporosis by inhibiting bone resorption.

In men, estrogens inhibit pituitary secretion of luteinizing hormone and decrease testicular secretion of testosterone. These actions may decrease prostate tumor growth and lower the level of prostate-specific antigen (PSA).

Contraindications

Active deep vein thrombosis, pulmonary embolism, or history of these conditions; active or recent (within past year) arterial thromboembolic disease, such as MI or stroke; hepatic dysfunction or disease; history of anaphylactic reaction or angioedema to estradiol; history of jaundice with previous oral contraceptive use; hypersensitivity to estradiol, ethinyl estradiol, or their components; hypersensitivity to tartrazine dye (contained in 0.02-mg estradiol and ethinyl estradiol tablets); known or suspected breast cancer or history of breast cancer except in appropriately selected patients being treated for metastatic disease; known or suspected estrogen-dependent cancer; known protein C, protein S, or antithrombin deficiency, or other known thrombophilic disorders; pregnancy; liver tumors; uncontrolled diabetes mellitus with hypertension or vascular involvement; undiagnosed abnormal genital bleeding

Interactions

DRUGS

aromatase inhibitors: Possible interference with aromatase inhibitor's effectiveness

corticosteroids: Increased therapeutic and toxic effects of corticosteroids

cyclosporine: Increased risk of hepatotoxicity and nephrotoxicity

CYP3A4 inducers, such as carbamazepine, phenobarbital, rifampin, St. John's wort: Possibly reduced plasma concentration of estradiol affecting therapeutic effects

CYP3A4 inhibitors, such as clarithromycin, erythromycin, itraconazole, ketoconazole, ritonavir: Possibly increased plasma concentration of estradiol increasing risk of adverse effects

hepatotoxic drugs, such as isoniazid: Increased risk of hepatitis and hepatotoxicity

insulin, oral antidiabetic drugs: Decreased therapeutic effects of these drugs

tamoxifen: Possibly decreased therapeutic effects of tamoxifen

thyroid hormone replacement: Decreased effectiveness

warfarin: Decreased anticoagulant effect

ACTIVITIES

smoking: Increased risk of pulmonary embolism, stroke, thrombophlebitis, and transient ischemic attack

FOODS

grapefruit juice: Decreased estradiol metabolism and possibly increased adverse effects

Adverse Reactions

CNS: Affect liability, chorea, **CVA**, dementia, depression, dizziness, emotional lability, fatigue, headache, insomnia, irritability, malaise, migraine headache, mood swings, nervousness, paresthesia

CV: **Deep venous thrombosis**, hypertension, **MI**, palpitations, peripheral edema, **thromboembolism**, thrombophlebitis, **unstable angina**

EENT: Intolerance of contact lenses, oral paresthesia, **pharyngeal edema**, retinal vascular thrombosis, swollen lip or tongue, vision changes

ENDO: Breast enlargement, pain, tenderness, or **tumors**; **breast cancer**, elevated estrogen levels, exacerbation of hypothyroidism, fibrocystic breast changes; gynecomastia;

hyperglycemia; nipple discharge or nipple and areola discoloration
GI: Abdominal cramps or pain, anorexia, bloating, **bowel obstruction** (vaginal ring), cholelithiasis, constipation, diarrhea, elevated liver enzymes, enlargement of abdomen or hepatic hemangiomas, gallbladder disease, **gallbladder obstruction, GI hemorrhage, hepatitis**, increased appetite, jaundice, nausea, **pancreatitis, portal vein thrombosis**, vomiting
GU: Amenorrhea, breakthrough bleeding, cervical or vaginal erosion, clear vaginal discharge, decreased libido, dysmenorrhea, **endometrial hyperplasia or cancer**, genital edema or itching, impotence, increased libido (females), **ovarian cancer**, pelvic pain, prolonged or heavy menstrual bleeding, ring adherence to vaginal wall, testicular atrophy, urinary frequency, uterine leiomyomata, vaginismus, vaginitis, vaginal abrasion or ulceration (ring), vaginal candidiasis or discharge, vulvovaginal discomfort (burning sensation, pain, rash, swelling), worsening of endometriosis
MS: Arthralgia, leg cramps, muscle spasms
RESP: Dyspnea, **pulmonary embolism**
SKIN: Acne, alopecia, diaphoresis, discoloration or dry skin, **erythema multiforme**, erythema nodosum, facial pigmentation, hirsutism, melasma, oily skin, pruritus, purpura, rash, seborrhea, urticaria
Other: Angioedema, application-site reactions (transdermal), folic acid deficiency, **hypercalcemia** (in metastatic bone disease), **hypersensitivity reactions, hypocalcemia (in presence of hypoparathyroidism), toxic shock syndrome** (vaginal ring), weight gain or loss

Childbearing Considerations

PREGNANCY

- Drug is not known to cause fetal harm if inadvertently taken during early pregnancy.
- Drug has no therapeutic use during pregnancy and is contraindicated in pregnancy.

LACTATION

- Drug is present in breast milk and decreases the quality and quantity of breast milk but is less likely to do so once breastfeeding is well established.
- Mothers should check with prescriber before breastfeeding.

Nursing Considerations

! WARNING Use estradiol cautiously in patients with asthma, chorea, diabetes mellitus, epilepsy, hepatic hemangiomas, migraine headaches, porphyria, or systemic lupus erythematosus because estradiol may worsen these disorders.

- Expect to begin prophylaxis treatment against osteoporosis at the start of menopause.
- Be aware that estradiol, which is an estrogen, should be given cyclically or combined with a progestin for 10 to 14 days per month in women with an intact uterus to minimize the risk of endometrial hyperplasia.

! WARNING Monitor patient closely for hypersensitivity reactions which could become life-threatening such as angioedema. Monitor patient with history of hereditary angioedema closely because estradiol may exacerbate symptoms of angioedema. If present, notify prescriber immediately, expect drug to be discontinued, and provide supportive care, as needed and ordered.

! WARNING Closely monitor patient's blood pressure. Patients may experience a substantial increase in blood pressure as an idiosyncratic reaction to estrogen. Monitor patients who already have hypertension for increases in blood pressure because estrogens like estradiol may cause fluid retention. Also, monitor patients with asthma, heart disease, migraines, renal disease, or seizure disorder for exacerbation of these conditions.

! WARNING Be aware that severe hypercalcemia may occur in patients with bone metastasis due to breast cancer because estrogens influence the metabolism of calcium and phosphorus. Monitor for toxic effects of increased calcium absorption in patients who are predisposed to hypercalcemia or nephrolithiasis. Also, monitor patient with hypoparathyroidism for hypocalcemia.

! WARNING Check patient's triglyceride level routinely because in patients with hypertriglyceridemia, estradiol therapy may increase serum triglyceride level enough to cause pancreatitis and other complications.

! WARNING Expect to stop estradiol therapy in any woman who develops signs or symptoms of cancer; cardiovascular disease, such as MI or stroke; dementia; pulmonary embolism; or venous thrombosis.

! WARNING Be aware that women at risk for arterial vascular disease include patients who smoke and those with diabetes mellitus, hypercholesterolemia, hypertension, obesity, or venous thromboembolism. Know that these factors, if present, should be addressed and brought under control.

! WARNING Monitor PT test results of patients receiving warfarin for loss of anticoagulant effect because estradiol, as an estrogen, increases production of clotting factors VII, VIII, IX, and X and promotes platelet aggregation.

! WARNING Expect to stop estradiol therapy several weeks before patient undergoes major surgery, as ordered, because certain procedures are associated with prolonged immobilization and therefore pose a risk of thromboembolism.

! WARNING Watch for elevated liver enzymes because estrogens like estradiol may worsen such conditions as acute intermittent or variegate hepatic porphyria.

! WARNING Assess patient for possible contact lens intolerance or changes in vision or visual acuity because estradiol can cause keratoconus, leading to increased curvature of the cornea. Be prepared to discontinue drug immediately, as prescribed, if patient experiences sudden partial or complete loss of vision or sudden onset of diplopia, migraine, or proptosis.

- Monitor serum PSA level in patients with inoperable prostate cancer to determine if patient is responding to hormone therapy. If patient responds (usually within 3 months), expect therapy to continue until disease is significantly advanced.
- Watch for peripheral edema or mild weight gain because estradiol can cause sodium and fluid retention.
- Monitor serum glucose level frequently in patients who have diabetes mellitus because estradiol may decrease insulin sensitivity and alter glucose tolerance.
- Be aware that exogenous estradiol and progestins may worsen mood disorders, including depression. Monitor patient for anxiety, depression, dizziness, fatigue, insomnia, or mood changes.
- Assess skin for melasma (tan or brown patches), which may develop on forehead, cheeks, temples, and upper lip. These patches may persist after drug is stopped.
- Be aware that if patient takes thyroid hormone replacement therapy, monitor her for increased signs and symptoms of hypothyroidism because estradiol may increase thyroid-binding globulin levels, which may make the patient's current dose of thyroid hormone insufficient.

PATIENT TEACHING

! WARNING Inform patient of risks involved in estradiol therapy, which is an estrogen drug, before therapy starts. These risks may include increased risk of breast, endometrial, or ovarian cancer; cardiovascular disease; dementia (if age 65 or over); gallbladder disease; and vision abnormalities. Encourage patient to discuss concerns with prescriber before estradiol therapy is initiated.

- Instruct patient how to administer form of estradiol prescribed.
- Tell patient who has an intact uterus and is prescribed transdermal Menostar that she will need to receive progestin for 14 days every 6 to 12 months and have an endometrial biopsy done yearly.

! WARNING Instruct patient using estradiol vaginal ring to remove ring immediately and to seek immediate medical care if she develops dizziness, diarrhea, faintness, fever, muscle pain, nausea, a sunburn rash on face or body, or vomiting. These symptoms may suggest a rare but serious bacterial infection called toxic shock syndrome. Also, urge patient to seek prompt medical care if ring becomes attached to vaginal wall (rare), making removal difficult.

! WARNING Alert patient that estradiol therapy may cause an allergic reaction. If present, tell patient to notify prescriber and, if severe, to seek immediate medical care.

- Tell patient using Elestrin not to apply sunscreen to the application site for at least 25 minutes. Alert patients prescribed Etrasorb that absorption of the drug increases when sunscreen is applied 10 to 25 minutes before drug is applied.

! **WARNING** Urge patient to report any vaginal bleeding to prescriber as well as any persistent, severe, or unusual adverse reactions.

! **WARNING** Inform patient receiving estradiol treatment that she should have an annual pelvic examination to screen for cervical dysplasia and be followed closely for other types of cancers and disorders associated with estradiol use.

- Advise patient that less serious but common side effects of estradiol therapy include abdominal or stomach cramps, bloating, breast pain or tenderness, fluid retention, hair loss, irregular vaginal bleeding or spotting, nausea and vomiting, and vaginal yeast infection.

estrogens (conjugated)

Premarin

Class and Category

Pharmacologic class: Estrogen
Therapeutic class: Hormone

Indications and Dosages

* *To treat moderate to severe vasomotor menopausal symptoms; to treat vaginal and vulvar atrophy*

TABLETS

Adult females. 0.3 mg daily or cyclically 25 days on, 5 days off. Dosage increased, as needed, to control symptoms.

* *To treat atrophic vaginitis and kraurosis*

VAGINAL CREAM

Adult females. 0.5 to 2 g once daily in cycles of 3 wk on, 1 wk off.

* *To treat moderate to severe dyspareunia, a symptom of vulvar and vaginal atrophy in menopause*

VAGINAL CREAM

Adult females. 0.5 g twice/wk. Otherwise, 0.5 g daily for 21 days followed by 7 days off, with cycle repeated every 28 days.

* *To prevent postmenopausal osteoporosis*

TABLETS

Adult females. 0.3 mg daily continuously or in cycles of 25 days on, 5 days off. Dosage increased, as needed, to control symptoms.

* *To provide palliative treatment for advanced androgen-dependent prostate cancer*

TABLETS

Adult males. 1.25 to 2 mg 3 times daily.

* *To provide palliative treatment for metastatic breast cancer*

TABLETS

Adult females. 10 mg 3 times daily for 3 mo or longer.

* *To treat dysfunctional uterine bleeding*

I.V. INJECTION, I.M. INJECTION

Adult females. 25 mg, repeated in 6 to 12 hr, as needed. I.V. injection given slowly.

* *To treat estrogen deficiency from oophorectomy or primary ovarian failure*

TABLETS

Adult females. 1.25 mg daily in cycles of 3 wk on, 1 wk off. Dosage adjusted, as needed.

* *To treat female hypogonadism*

TABLETS

Adult females. 0.3 to 0.625 mg daily in cycles of 3 wk on, 1 wk off. Dosage adjusted, as needed.

Drug Administration

P.O.

- Administer drug at the same time every day.

I.V.

- I.V. is preferred route over I.M. route.
- Keep drug refrigerated before reconstituting.
- Reconstitute by adding 5 ml of Sterile Water for Injection to drug vial by directing stream slowly against the side of the vial and agitate gently. Do not shake.
- Administer immediately after reconstitution. Inject drug slowly as an I.V. injection to prevent a flushing reaction.
- Compatible with 0.9% Sodium Chloride Injection, 5% Dextrose Injection, and invert sugar solutions.
- *Incompatibilities:* Ascorbic acid, protein hydrolysate, or any solution with an acid pH

I.M.

- Follow manufacturer's guidelines for preparing drug for I.M. injection.

- Inject deeply into a large muscle, such as in the buttocks or thigh.
- Rotate sites.

VAGINAL

- Place patient in a supine position.
- Clean vaginal area with soap and water.
- Insert applicator into the vagina about two-thirds the length of the applicator.
- Push plunger to release drug.
- Have patient remain supine for 30 min after administration.
- Store at room temperature.

Route	Onset	Peak	Duration
P.O.	Unknown	7 hr	Unknown
I.V./I.M.	Unknown	Unknown	Unknown
Vaginal	Unknown	7 hr	Unknown

Half-life: 17 hr

Mechanism of Action

Increases the rate of DNA and RNA synthesis in the cells of female reproductive organs, hypothalamus, pituitary glands, and other target organs. In the hypothalamus, estrogens reduce the release of gonadotropin-releasing hormone, which decreases pituitary release of follicle-stimulating hormone and luteinizing hormone. In women, these hormones are required for normal genitourinary and other essential body functions. At the cellular level, estrogens increase cervical secretions, cause endometrial cell proliferation, and increase uterine tone. Estrogen replacement helps maintain genitourinary function and reduce vasomotor symptoms when estrogen production declines from menopause, surgical removal of ovaries, or other estrogen deficiency. Estrogen also helps prevent osteoporosis by keeping bone resorption from exceeding bone formation. In men, estrogens inhibit pituitary secretion of luteinizing hormone and decrease testicular secretion of testosterone. These actions may decrease prostate tumor growth and lower the level of prostate-specific antigen.

Contraindications

Active deep vein thrombosis, pulmonary embolism, or history of these conditions; active or recent (within past year) arterial thromboembolic disease, such as MI or stroke; hypersensitivity to estrogens or their components; known or suspected breast cancer or history of breast cancer; known or suspected estrogen-dependent cancer; known protein C, protein S, or antithrombin deficiency or other known thrombophilic disorders; pregnancy; liver impairment or disease; undiagnosed abnormal genital bleeding

Interactions

DRUGS

aromatase inhibitors: Possibly interference with aromatase inhibitor's effectiveness
barbiturates, carbamazepine, hydantoins, rifabutin, rifampin: Possibly reduced activity of estrogen and medroxyprogesterone
corticosteroids: Increased therapeutic and toxic effects of corticosteroids
cyclosporine: Increased risk of hepatotoxicity and nephrotoxicity
hepatotoxic drugs (such as isoniazid): Increased risk of hepatitis and hepatotoxicity
insulin, oral antidiabetic drugs: Decreased therapeutic effects of these drugs
tamoxifen: Possibly interference with tamoxifen's therapeutic effects
thyroid hormone replacement: Decreased effectiveness
warfarin: Decreased anticoagulant effect

ACTIVITIES

smoking: Increased risk of pulmonary embolism, stroke, thrombophlebitis, and transient ischemic attack

Adverse Reactions

CNS: Asthenia, CVA, dementia, depression, dizziness, growth benign meningioma, headache, insomnia, migraine headache, mood disturbance, nervousness, paresthesia
CV: **Deep vein thrombosis**, hypertension, **MI**, peripheral edema, **thromboembolism**, thrombophlebitis, vasodilation
EENT: Intolerance of contact lenses, pharyngitis, retinal vascular thrombosis, rhinitis, sinusitis
ENDO: Breast enlargement, pain, tenderness, or **tumors**; gynecomastia (men); hot flashes; hyperglycemia
GI: Abdominal cramps or pain, abdominal distention, anorexia, cholestatic jaundice, constipation, diarrhea, flatulence, gallbladder disease, **gallbladder obstruction**, hepatic hemangioma enlargement, **hepatitis**, increased appetite, **ischemic colitis**, nausea, **pancreatitis**, vomiting

GU: Amenorrhea, breakthrough bleeding, cervical erosion, clear vaginal discharge, decreased libido (men), dysmenorrhea, **endometrial cancer** or hyperplasia, impotence, increased libido (women), leukorrhea, **ovarian cancer**, prolonged or heavy menstrual bleeding, testicular atrophy, uterine leiomyomata enlargement, vaginal candidiasis, vaginitis, vaginal-site reactions (vaginal administration only, such as burning, irritation, and genital pruritus)
MS: Arthralgias, back pain, muscle spasms
RESP: Bronchitis, increased cough, **pulmonary embolism**
SKIN: Acne, alopecia, chloasma, **erythema multiforme**, erythema nodosum, hemorrhagic eruption, hirsutism, melasma, oily skin, pruritus, purpura, rash, seborrhea, urticaria
Other: **Anaphylaxis**, **angioedema**, flu-like syndrome, folic acid deficiency, **hypercalcemia** (in metastatic bone disease), weight gain

Childbearing Considerations

PREGNANCY

- Drug is not known to cause fetal harm if inadvertently taken during early pregnancy.
- Drug is contraindicated in pregnancy.

LACTATION

- Drug decreases the quality and quantity of breast milk.
- Breastfeeding should not be undertaken during drug therapy.

Nursing Considerations

! **WARNING** Monitor patient closely for a hypersensitivity reaction, especially within minutes to hours of taking first dose, as anaphylaxis may occur, requiring emergency intervention. Be aware that estrogen therapy may exacerbate symptoms of angioedema in women with hereditary angioedema. Monitor for signs of swelling of the face, lips, throat, or tongue. If present, notify prescriber immediately, expect drug to be discontinued, and provide supportive care, as needed and ordered.

! **WARNING** Monitor serum calcium level to detect severe hypercalcemia in patients with bone metastasis from breast cancer. Use conjugated estrogens cautiously in patients with severe hypocalcemia because a sudden increase in serum calcium level may cause adverse reactions.

! **WARNING** Watch for elevated liver enzymes because estrogen and progestins may worsen such conditions as acute intermittent or variegate hepatic porphyria.

! **WARNING** Check triglyceride level routinely because in hypertriglyceridemia, estrogen therapy may increase triglycerides enough to cause pancreatitis and other complications.

! **WARNING** Monitor patients with asthma, diabetes mellitus, endometriosis, heart disease, lupus erythematosus, migraine headaches, renal disease, or seizure disorder for worsening of these conditions.

! **WARNING** Assess PT for loss of anticoagulant effects if patient takes warfarin because estrogens increase production of clotting factors and promote platelet aggregation.

! **WARNING** Expect to stop estrogen therapy in any woman who develops signs or symptoms of cancer; cardiovascular disease, such as MI, stroke, or venous thrombosis; dementia; or pulmonary embolism.

- Assess hypertensive patients for increases in blood pressure because estrogens may cause fluid retention.
- Expect drug to be withheld during periods of immobilization, 4 weeks before elective surgery, and if jaundice develops.
- Know that if patient takes thyroid hormone replacement therapy, monitor her for increased signs and symptoms of hypothyroidism because estrogen may increase thyroid-binding globulin level, which may make the patient's current dose of thyroid hormone insufficient.
- Be aware that estrogen may worsen mood disorders, including depression. Monitor patient for depression, fatigue, insomnia, or mood changes.

PATIENT TEACHING

! **WARNING** Explain the risks of estrogen therapy, including increased risk of breast, endometrial, or ovarian cancer;

cardiovascular disease; dementia; and gallbladder disease, especially with long term use. Tell patient to discuss any concerns about risks with prescriber before taking estrogen.

- Instruct patient how to take form of estrogen prescribed.

! WARNING Review signs and symptoms of an allergic reaction that could become severe. Urge patient to stop drug, notify prescriber, or seek immediate medical help if serious. Inform patients with a history of hereditary angioedema that estrogen therapy may exacerbate symptoms of angioedema.

! WARNING Urge patient to immediately report breakthrough bleeding to prescribe and instruct patient to notify prescriber if persistent, severe, or unusal adverse reactions occur.

! WARNING Inform patient that she should have an annual pelvic examination to screen for cervical dysplasia and be followed closely for other types of cancers and disorders associated with estradiol use. Urge patient to perform monthly breast self-examination.

- Inform patient that estrogen vaginal cream may alter effectiveness of cervical caps, condoms, or diaphragms made of latex or rubber.
- Instruct patient to notify prescriber if she sees something that resembles a tablet in her stool.

eszopiclone

Lunesta

Class, Category, and Schedule

Pharmacologic class: Pyrrolopyrazine derivative
Therapeutic class: Sedative-hypnotic
Controlled substance schedule: IV

Indications and Dosages

✻ *To treat insomnia when at least 7 or 8 hours are remaining before the planned time of awakening*

TABLETS

Adults. *Initial:* 1 mg at bedtime. May be increased to 2 or 3 mg, as needed. *Maximum:* 3 mg.

±**DOSAGE ADJUSTMENT** For patients with severe hepatic impairment, patients taking potent CYP3A4 inhibitors, or debilitated or elderly patients, dosage should not exceed 2 mg. Dosage adjustment may be needed if other CNS depressants are also being taken.

Drug Administration

P.O.

- Administer immediately before bedtime.
- Avoid administering after a heavy, high-fat meal.

Route	Onset	Peak	Duration
P.O.	Unknown	1 hr	Unknown

Half-life: 6–9 hr

Mechanism of Action

May potentiate effects of the inhibitory neurotransmitter gamma-aminobutyric acid (GABA) by binding close to or with benzodiazepine receptors in cortical and limbic areas of the CNS. By binding to these receptor sites and areas, eszopiclone increases GABA's inhibitory effects and blocks cortical and limbic arousal, thereby inducing and maintaining sleep.

Contraindications

Complex sleep behaviors with past administration of eszopiclone, hypersensitivity to eszopiclone or its components

Interactions

DRUGS

CYP3A inducers, such as rifampin: Decreased eszopiclone level
CYP3A inhibitors, such as clarithromycin, itraconazole, ketoconazole, nefazodone, nelfinavir, ritonavir, troleandomycin: Increased eszopiclone level
other CNS depressants: Possibly additive effects

ACTIVITIES

alcohol use: Additive effect on psychomotor performance

E

FOOD

heavy, high-fat meal: Possibly reduced effectiveness of eszopiclone

Adverse Reactions

CNS: Aggressiveness that seems out of character, agitation, anxiety, bizarre behavior, such as sleep driving or walking, confusion, decreased level of consciousness, depersonalization, depression with possible **suicidal ideation**, dizziness, drowsiness, hallucinations, headache (including migraine), nervousness, neuralgia, next day psychomotor impairment, somnolence, unusual dreams
CV: Chest pain, peripheral edema
EENT: Dry mouth; smell distortion; **swelling of glottis**, **larynx**, **or tongue**; taste perversion
ENDO: Gynecomastia
GI: Diarrhea, **hepatitis**, indigestion, nausea, vomiting
GU: Decreased libido, dysmenorrhea, UTI
RESP: **Asthma**, respiratory tract infection
SKIN: Pruritus, rash
Other: **Angioedema**, generalized pain, **heatstroke**, viral infection

Childbearing Considerations

PREGNANCY

- It is not known if drug causes fetal harm.
- Use with caution only if benefit to mother outweighs potential risk to fetus.

LACTATION

- It is not known if drug is present in breast milk.
- Mothers should check with prescriber before breastfeeding.

Nursing Considerations

! **WARNING** Monitor patient for a hypersensitivity reaction, which could become life-threatening such as angioedema. If present, notify prescriber, expect drug to be discontinued, and provide supportive care, as needed and ordered.

! **WARNING** Use eszopiclone cautiously in patients with severe mental depression or reduced respiratory function; drug may intensify mental depression leading to suicidal ideation and reduced respiratory function could lead to respiratory depression.

- Monitor patient's liver function and patient for signs and symptoms of liver dysfunction.
- Institute safety and prevention of fall measures because of the adverse CNS effects of the drug.

PATIENT TEACHING

- Instruct patient how to administer eszopiclone.
- Tell patient not to exceed prescribed eszopiclone dosage and not to stop drug abruptly because withdrawal symptoms may occur.

! **WARNING** Urge patient to avoid alcohol and CNS depressants because of additive effects.

! **WARNING** Alert patient that drug may cause an allergic reaction. If present, tell patient to notify prescriber promptly and, if severe, to seek immediate medical care.

! **WARNING** Instruct family or caregiver to monitor patient for mood changes or suicidal behavior or thoughts. Notify prescriber immediately, if present.

! **WARNING** Warn patient, family, or caregiver that some patients have performed bizarre activities after taking drug, such as driving the car, having sex, making phone calls, or preparing and eating food while not fully awake and often with no memory of the event. These episodes usually occur in patients who have taken the drug with alcohol or other CNS depressants, who have taken the drug with less than a full night of sleep remaining (7 to 8 hours), or who have exceeded the recommended dose. If such an episode occurs, the prescriber should be notified and eszopiclone therapy discontinued immediately.

- Alert patient, especially if debilitated or elderly, that drug may impair motor and/or cognitive performance increasing risk of falls. Advise patient to avoid potentially hazardous activities until drug's CNS effects are known and resolved.
- Explain that sleep may be disturbed for the first few nights after therapy stops.

etanercept

Enbrel

etanercept-szzs

Erelzi

etanercept-ykro

Eticovo

Class and Category

Pharmacologic class: Tumor necrosis factor (TNF) blocker
Therapeutic class: Immunosuppressant

Indications and Dosages

∗ *To treat rheumatoid arthritis alone or in combination with methotrexate; to treat psoriatic arthritis alone or in combination with methotrexate; to treat active ankylosing spondylitis*

SUBCUTANEOUS INJECTION

Adults. 50 mg once/wk on same day each wk. *Maximum:* 50 mg/wk.

∗ *To treat juvenile psoriatic arthritis*

SUBCUTANEOUS INJECTION (ENBREL)

Children ages 2 and older weighing 63 kg (138 lb) or more. 50 mg once/wk on same day each wk.
Children ages 2 and older weighing less than 63 kg (138 lb). 0.8 mg/kg/wk. *Maximum:* 50 mg/wk.

∗ *To treat chronic moderate to severe plaque psoriasis in candidates for systemic therapy or phototherapy*

SUBCUTANEOUS INJECTION

Adults. *Initial:* 50 mg twice/wk 3 to 4 days apart for 3 mo; then reduced to 50 mg/wk. Alternatively, 25 mg or 50 mg/wk for 3 mo; then 50 mg once/wk.
Children ages 4 and older weighing 63 kg (138 lb) or more. 50 mg once/wk on same day each week.

SUBCUTANEOUS INJECTION (ENBREL, ERELZI)

Children ages 4 and older weighing less than 63 kg (138 lb). 0.8 mg/kg/wk. *Maximum:* 50 mg/wk.

∗ *To reduce signs and symptoms of moderately to severely active polyarticular juvenile idiopathic arthritis*

SUBCUTANEOUS INJECTION

Children ages 2 and older weighing 63 kg (138 lb) or more. 50 mg once/wk on same day each week.

SUBCUTANEOUS INJECTION (ENBREL, ERELZI)

Children ages 2 and older weighing less than 63 kg (138 lb). 0.8 mg/kg/wk. *Maximum:* 50 mg/wk.

Drug Administration

SUBCUTANEOUS

- Follow manufacturer's guidelines for storage as it varies from trade name to trade name and with products of same trade name.
- It is normal for small white particles of protein to be present in the solution, but the solution should not be cloudy, discolored, or contain foreign particulate matter. If solution doesn't appear normal, discard.
- If drug was refrigerated, leave at room temperature for time specified in manufacturer's guidelines (between 15 and 30 min). Do not return product to the refrigerator once placed at room temperature.
- Rotate injection sites among abdomen, middle front of thigh, and upper back of arms and avoid areas that are bruised, hard, red, or tender. Keep each site at least 1 inch away from a previous site.
- Injection site should not be rubbed after drug is administered.

Enbrel

- When using the Enbrel single-dose prefilled syringe, check to see if the amount of liquid falls between the 2 purple fill level indicator lines on the syringe. If not, discard and obtain a new syringe. Allow syringe to warm to room temperature for about 15 to 30 minutes before administering drug. Do not remove the needle cover while allowing syringe to reach room temperature and only allow needle cover to be off for no more than 5 minutes prior to injection because this can dry out the drug. When ready to inject drug, tap syringe with finger until air bubbles rise to the top. Slowly push the plunger up to force the air bubbles out of the syringe. Inject subcutaneously using standard technique.

- If using a single-dose vial, allow vial contents to warm to room temperature for at least 30 min before injecting. Use a 1-ml Luer-Lock syringe and a withdrawal needle with a Luer-Lock connection that is a 22 G 1 ½-inch size needle to withdraw solution and then change to a 27 G, ½-inch needle for administration. Two vials may be required to administer the total dose. If so, use a new syringe for each vial. Discard unused portions in vial. Inject drug subcutaneously using standard technique.
- If preparing dose from a multidose vial, leave the dose tray at room temperature for about 15 to 30 min before injecting drug. Reconstitute with 1 ml of supplied Bacteriostatic Water for Injection. Inject the solution slowly into vial. Use a 25 G needle rather than the supplied vial adapter if the vial will be used for multiple doses. (If using the vial adapter, twist the vial adapter onto the diluent syringe. Then, place the vial adapter over the drug vial and insert the vial adapter into the vial stopper. Push down on the plunger to inject the diluent into the drug vial.) Gently swirl during dissolution rather than shaking vial. If syringe was used to add diluent to vial, keep syringe in place while gently swirling during dissolution. It will take less than 10 minutes for the powder to be dissolved. Do not shake or vigorously agitate vial. Resulting solution contains 25 mg/1 ml. Withdraw dose into the syringe. Expect to see some bubbles or foam. Remove the syringe from the vial. Remove 25 G needle from the syringe, if used instead of the vial adaptor. Attach a 27 G needle to syringe to inject drug. Use drug as soon as possible after dissolving powder. Inject subcutaneously using standard technique. When injection is delayed, the dissolved powder must be kept in refrigerator for up to 14 days. Discard if not used within that time frame. Do not mix one vial of drug solution with another vial of drug solution. Also, do not add any other drugs to the solutions or use other diluents. Do not filter reconstituted solution during preparation.
- When using the SureClick autoinjector, leave the autoinjector at room temperature for at least 30 min before injecting. Do not remove the needle cover while allowing syringe to reach room temperature. When injecting drug, expect the window to turn yellow when the injection is complete. If after removing the autoinjector, the window has not turned yellow or it appears drug is still injecting, patient has not received the full dose. Notify prescriber for further instructions.
- When using the AutoTouch reusable autoinjector, leave the prefilled cartridge at room temperature for at least 30 min before injecting. Do not remove the purple cap while allowing drug to reach room temperature. Open the door by pushing the door button and inserting the mini single-dose prefilled cartridge into AutoTouch. It should slide freely and completely into the door. Close the door and inject drug. The AutoTouch will make sounds to help guide the injection. To turn sound off, slide the sound switch up (red bar visible). However, even when the sound is turned off, it still will produce the noise of the motor during the injection and will provide error alerts. Follow manufacturer's guidelines on what to do if an error alert occurs and how to reset the AutoTouch.

Erelzi

- Avoid handling the needle cap of the prefilled syringe and the internal needle cover within the cap of the Sensoready Pen, if allergic to latex.
- Leave drug at room temperature for about 15 to 30 min before injecting. Do not remove the needle cover while allowing the prefilled syringe to reach room temperature.
- Reconstitute drug using a multiple-dose vial with 1 ml of the supplied Sterile Bacterostatic Water for Injection. Inject solution very slowly into the vial to avoid excessive foaming using a syringe with a 25 G needle or the supplied vial adapter. If using the vial adapter, twist the vial adapter onto the diluent syringe. Then, place the vial adapter over the drug vial and insert the vial adapter into the vial stopper. Push down on the plunger to inject the diluent into the drug vial. Use a 25 G needle rather than the vial adapter if the vial will be used for multiple doses. Gently swirl during dissolution. If syringe was used to add diluent to vial, keep syringe in place while gently swirling during dissolution. It takes up to less than 10 minutes for the powder to be dissolved. Do not shake or vigorously agitate vial. Resulting solution contains 25 mg/1 ml. Withdraw dose into the syringe. Expect to see some bubbles or

foam. Remove the syringe from the vial adapter or remove the syringe from the vial (and 25 G needle) and attach a 27 G needle to inject drug. Use drug as soon as possible after dissolving powder. Dissolved powder must be kept in refrigerator if not used immediately for up to 14 days. Discard if not used within that time frame. Do not mix one vial of drug solution with another vial of drug solution. Also, do not add any other drugs to the solution or use other diluents. Do not filter reconstituted solution during preparation.

- When using the single-dose prefilled Sensoready Pen, the window will turn green when injection is complete. If window has not turned green, or if it looks like drug is still injecting, patient has not received the full dose. Notify prescriber for further instructions.
- Inject subcutneously using standard technique.

Eticovo

- Allow the single-dose prefilled syringe to come to room temperature for at least 30 min before administering drug.
- When removing needle cover there may be a drop of liquid at the end of the needle, which is normal.
- Do not shake the prefilled syringe. Do not use if the prefilled syringe has been dropped onto a hard surface as parts of the prefilled syringe may be broken.
- Be careful not to touch or bump plunger before injection as doing so could cause the liquid to leak out.
- Slowly inject drug subcutaneously using standard technique.

Route	Onset	Peak	Duration
SubQ	1–2 wk	72 hr	Unknown

Half-life: 4–5 days

Contraindications

Hypersensitivity to etanercept or its components, sepsis

Interactions

DRUGS

abatacept anakinra: Increased risk of adverse reactions, especially infections

Mechanism of Action

Reduces inflammation by binding with tumor necrosis factor (TNF), a cytokine, or protein that plays an important role in normal inflammatory and immune responses.

The immune and inflammatory process triggers release of TNF, mainly from macrophages. TNF then binds to TNF receptors on cell membranes, as shown below left. This action renders TNF biologically active and triggers a cascade of inflammatory events that results in increased inflammation, release of destructive lysosomal enzymes, and joint destruction.

Etanercept binds to TNF and prevents it from binding with TNF receptors on the cell membranes, as shown below right. This action renders bound TNF biologically inactive, prevents TNF-mediated cellular responses, and significantly reduces inflammatory activity.

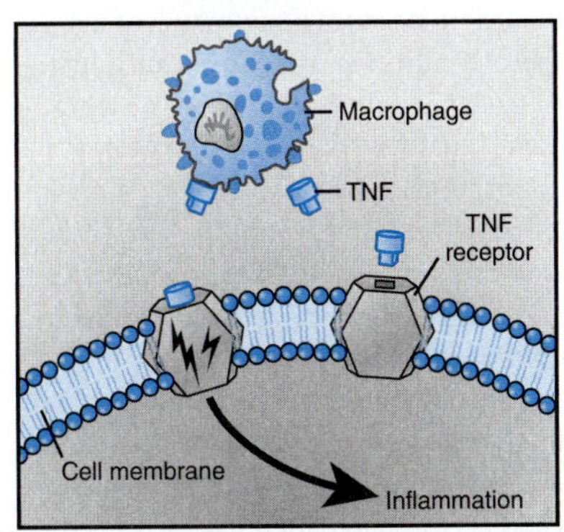

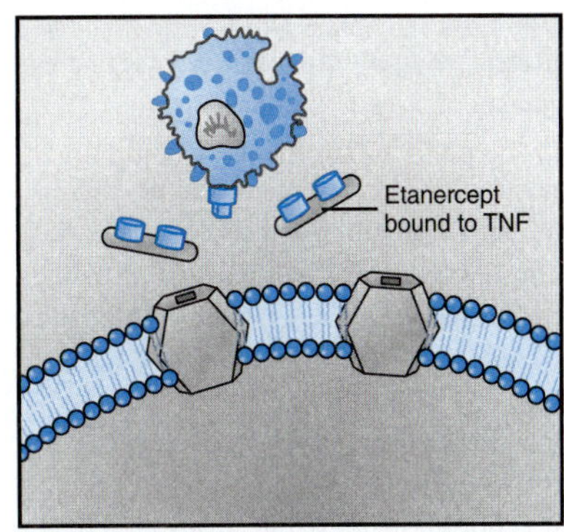

cyclophosphamide: Possibly increased risk of malignancy
live vaccines: Possibly increased risk of secondary transmission of infection from live vaccine
sulfasalazine: Possibly decreased neutrophil count

Adverse Reactions

CNS: Asthenia; chills; demyelination, including both central and peripheral nervous systems; dizziness; fever; headache; multiple sclerosis; paresthesias; **seizures**
CV: Chest pain, **congestive heart failure**, hypertension, **hypotension**, peripheral edema, systemic vasculitis
EENT: Optic neuritis, pharyngitis, rhinitis, scleritis, sinusitis, uveitis
GI: Abdominal abscess or pain, **autoimmune hepatitis**, cholecystitis, diarrhea, elevated liver enzymes, gastroenteritis, indigestion, inflammatory bowel disease, nausea, **noninfectious hepatitis**, **reactivation of hepatitis B**, vomiting
GU: **Glomerulonephritis**, **pyelonehpritis**
HEME: Anemia, **aplastic anemia**, **leukemia**, **leukopenia**, **macrophage activation syndrome**, **neutropenia**, **pancytopenia**, **thrombocytopenia**
MS: Osteomyelitis, septic arthritis, transverse myelitis
RESP: Bronchitis, cough, **interstitial lung disease**, pneumonia, upper respiratory tract infection
SKIN: Cellulitis, cutaneous lupus erythematosus or vasculitis, **erythema multiforme**, foot abscess, leg ulceration, **melanoma and nonmelanoma skin cancers**, **Merkel cell carcinoma**, new or worsening psoriasis, pruritus, rash, **Stevens-Johnson syndrome**, **toxic epidermal necrolysis**, urticaria
Other: **Angioedema**; antibody formation against etanercept; bacterial, fungal, mycobacterial, parasitic, and viral infections; injection-site bruising, edema, erythema, itching, and pain; etanercept-induced antibodies; lymphadenopathy; lupus-like syndrome; **malignancy**, **such as lymphoma**; sarcoidosis; **sepsis**

Childbearing Considerations

PREGNANCY

- It is not known if drug causes fetal harm.
- Use with caution only if benefit to mother outweighs potential risk to fetus.
- Safety of administering live or live attenuated vaccines in infants exposed to drug in utero is unknown.

LACTATION

- Drug is present in breast milk in low levels.
- Mothers should check with prescriber before breastfeeding.

Nursing Considerations

! **WARNING** Be aware that etanercept should not be given to patients with granulomatosis with polyangiitis who are receiving other immunosuppressants because of a higher incidence of noncutaneous solid malignancies and because etanercept therapy does not offer any more improvement for this condition.

- Screen patient for latent tuberculosis (TB) with a tuberculin skin test before starting etanercept therapy. If test is positive, expect to give treatment, as ordered, before starting etanercept. Know that TB may develop during therapy even though the test was negative for latent TB prior to beginning etanercept therapy. Monitor patient closely. Also, screen patient for hepatitis B. If present, expect etanercept therapy to be withdrawn because antirheumatic therapies like etanercept may reactivate hepatitis B.
- Use cautiously in patients with COPD and monitor respiratory status closely because etanercept therapy may increase patient's risk of adverse respiratory reactions.
- Use cautiously in patients with preexisting or recent onset CNS demyelinating disorders because drug may worsen these conditions. Also, use cautiously in patients with heart failure or who have a history of serious hematologic abnormalities because drug also may worsen these conditions.
- Continue giving corticosteroids, NSAIDs, and other analgesics, as prescribed, during etanercept therapy.
- Ensure patients, especially children, are up to date on immunizations prior to etanercept therapy. Avoid giving live-virus vaccines to patients who are taking

etanercept because drug decreases immune response and increases risk of secondary transmission of vaccine virus.

! WARNING Monitor patient for a hypersensitivity reaction, which could become life-threatening such as angioedema. If present, notify prescriber, expect drug to be discontinued, and provide supportive care, as needed and ordered.

! WARNING Be aware that etanercept increases risk for developing serious infections due to bacterial (including *Legionella* and *Listeria*), fungal, mycobacterial, parasitic, and viral pathogens. These infections can become life-threatening and involve multiple organ systems. Be aware that use of abatacept or anakinra concurrently is not recommended because of increased incidence of serious infections. Monitor patient closely throughout therapy. Use cautiously in patients with a history of recurrent infection, underlying conditions that may predispose patients to infections, or if patients have an existing chronic, latent, or localized infection because etanercept increases the risk of infection. Expect to stop etanercept if patient develops sepsis.

! WARNING Be aware that malignancies, especially leukemias and lymphomas, although rare, have been reported in patients taking tumor necrosis factor blockers, such as etanercept. Children, adolescents, and patients with rheumatoid arthritis, especially those with very active disease, are at greatest risk. Monitor closely.

! WARNING Monitor patient for signs and symptoms suggestive of autoimmune hepatitis or lupus-like syndrome. If suspected, notify prescriber and expect tests to be done to determine if these conditions are present. If confirmed, expect drug to be discontinued.

! WARNING Monitor patient's CBC regularly, as ordered because drug can cause serious to life-threatening adverse reactions in the patient's hematological system.

PATIENT TEACHING

- Reassure patient, family, or caregiver that other medications, such as analgesics, NSAIDs, and steroid therapy may be continued while patient is receiving etanercept.
- Instruct patient, family, or caregiver how to administer etanercept as a subcutaneous injection. Inform them that the first injection will need to be given by a healthcare professional.

! WARNING Alert patient that drug may cause an allergic reaction. If present, tell patient to notify prescriber and, if severe, to seek immediate medical care.

! WARNING Review signs and symptoms of an infection and infection control measures to take while receiving etanercept. Urge patient to consult prescriber immediately if he develops an infection because drug may decrease the body's infection-fighting ability. Tell patient who hasn't had chickenpox to contact prescriber right away if he's exposed because he may develop a more serious infection.

! WARNING Caution patient that the risk of malignancies such as leukemia and lymphoma may be higher in those who take etanercept, especially children and adolescents. Tell him to seek medical attention promptly for any suspicious signs and symptoms.

! WARNING Urge patient to notify prescriber if persistent, severe, or unusual adverse reactions occur.

- Advise mothers who received drug while pregnant to alert pediatrician before live or live attenuated vaccines are given to infant.

ethacrynic acid

Edecrin

ethacrynate sodium

Edecrin

Class and Category

Pharmacologic class: Loop diuretic
Therapeutic class: Diuretic

Indications and Dosages

✱ *To promote diuresis in heart failure, hepatic cirrhosis, or renal disease; to provide short-term management of ascites caused by cancer, idiopathic edema, or lymphedema; to provide short-term management of edema in hospitalized children other than infants, with congenital heart disease or nephrotic syndrome*

TABLETS

Adults. *Initial:* 50 to 100 mg daily as a single dose in the morning or in divided doses. Dosage increased by 25 to 50 mg daily, as needed. *Maintenance:* 50 to 200 mg daily and given continuously or on an intermittent schedule after effective diuresis is obtained. *For patients with severe refractory edema:* 200 mg twice daily for both initial and maintenance dosage *Maximum:* 200 mg twice daily.

Children (except infants). *Initial:* 25 mg daily in the morning. Dosage increased in 25-mg increments daily, as needed and then decreased once dry weight has been achieved.

± **DOSAGE ADJUSTMENT** For patients who are sensitive to diuretic therapy, the following schedule may be used: Day 1, 50 mg once daily in the morning after a meal; day 2, 50 mg twice daily after meals, as needed; and day 3, 100 mg in morning after a meal and 50 to 100 mg following the afternoon or evening meal, depending on the response of the morning dose.

∗ *To provide rapid onset of diuresis, when needed, in acute pulmonary edema or when GI absorption is impaired or oral medication is not practicable.*

I.V. INJECTION

Adults. *Initial:* 50 mg or 0.5 to 1 mg/kg. Dose repeated in 2 to 4 hr, as needed. *Maximum:* 100 mg as single dose.

Drug Administration

P.O.

- Administer once-daily dosing in the morning or last dose of the day several hours before bedtime.
- Administer after meals.

I.V.

- Reconstitute with 50 ml of 0.9% Sodium Chloride Injection or 5% Dextrose Injection. Be aware that some 5% Dextrose solutions may have a low pH resulting in a hazy or opalescent appearance. If this occurs, do not use.
- Administer slowly through the tubing of a running infusion or by direct intravenous injection over several min.
- If second injection is needed, choose a new injection site to avoid possible thrombophlebitis.
- Do not give drug subcutaneously or intramuscularly.
- Discard unused portion after 24 hr.
- *Incompatibilities:* Whole blood, or its derivatives

Route	Onset	Peak	Duration
P.O.	30 min	2 hr	6–8 hr
I.V.	5 min	15–30 min	2 hr

Half-life: 1–4 hr

Mechanism of Action

May inhibit the sulfhydryl-catalyzed enzyme systems that cause sodium and chloride resorption in the proximal and distal tubules and the ascending limb of the loop of Henle. These inhibitory effects increase urinary excretion of sodium, chloride, and water, causing profound diuresis. Drug also increases the ammonium, bicarbonate, calcium, excretion of potassium, hydrogen, magnesium, and phosphate.

Contraindications

Anuria; hypersensitivity to ethacrynic acid, ethacrynate sodium, or their components; infancy; severe diarrhea

Interactions

DRUGS

aminoglycosides, some cephalosporins: Increased risk of ototoxicity
digoxin: Increased risk of digitalis toxicity
lithium: Increased risk of lithium toxicity
NSAIDs: Possibly decreased effects of ethacrynic acid
warfarin: Increased risk of bleeding

Adverse Reactions

CNS: Confusion, fatigue, headache, malaise, nervousness
CV: Orthostatic hypotension
EENT: Blurred vision, hearing loss, ototoxicity (ringing or buzzing in ears), sensation of fullness in ears, yellow vision
ENDO: Hyperglycemia, **hypoglycemia**
GI: Abdominal pain, anorexia, diarrhea, dysphagia, **GI bleeding (I.V.)**, nausea, vomiting

GU: Hematuria (I.V. form), interstitial nephritis, polyuria
HEME: **Agranulocytosis**, **severe neutropenia**, **thrombocytopenia**
SKIN: Rash
Other: Hyperuricemia, **hypochloremic alkalosis**, **hypokalemia**, **hypomagnesemia**, **hyponatremia**, hypovolemia, infusion-site irritation and pain

Childbearing Considerations

PREGNANCY

- It is not known if drug causes fetal harm.
- Use with caution only if benefit to mother outweighs potential risk to fetus.

LACTATION

- It is not known if drug is present in breast milk.
- A decision should be made to discontinue breastfeeding or the drug to avoid potential serious adverse reactions in the breastfed infant.

Nursing Considerations

! WARNING Give ethacrynic acid and ethacrynate sodium cautiously in patients with advanced hepatic cirrhosis, especially those with a history of electrolyte imbalance or hepatic encephalopathy because drug may lead to lethal hepatic coma.

- Weigh patient daily and assess for signs and symptoms of dehydration and electrolyte imbalances. Monitor blood pressure and fluid intake and output and check laboratory test results. Report significant changes. Prescriber may reduce dosage or temporarily stop drug.

! WARNING Monitor patient for signs and symptoms of electrolyte imbalances. Know that if hypokalemia develops, administer replacement potassium, as ordered.

! WARNING Monitor serum glucose level frequently, especially if patient has diabetes mellitus; drug may cause hyperglycemia or hypoglycemia.

- Notify prescriber if patient experiences buzzing, ringing in his ears, or a sense of fullness; hearing loss; or vertigo. Drug may have to be discontinued.

PATIENT TEACHING

- Instruct patient how to administer ethacrynic acid.
- Urge patient to eat more high-potassium foods, unless contraindicated, and to take a potassium supplement, if prescribed, to prevent hypokalemia.

! WARNING Caution patient not to drink alcohol, stand for prolonged periods, or exercise during hot weather because these activities may exacerbate orthostatic hypotension.

- Advise patient to change position slowly to minimize effects of orthostatic hypotension, especially if he also takes an antihypertensive.
- Instruct patient to notify prescriber if he has buzzing, fullness, or ringing in his ears; diarrhea; hearing loss; severe nausea; vertigo; or vomiting. Drug may have to be discontinued.
- Remind diabetic patients to check their blood glucose levels often for changes.
- Inform mothers breastfeeding should not be undertaken during ethacrynic acid therapy.

ethambutol hydrochloride

Etibi (CAN), Myambutol

Class and Category

Pharmacologic class: Synthetic antituberculotic
Therapeutic class: Antituberculotic

Indications and Dosages

✷ *As adjunct to treat pulmonary tuberculosis (TB) caused by Mycobacterium tuberculosis*

TABLETS

Adults and adolescents who have not received previous antituberculotic therapy. 15 mg/kg once daily.
Adults and adolescents who have received previous antituberculotic therapy. 25 mg/kg once daily for 60 days or until bacteriologic tests results come back negative; after 60 days, then decreased to 15 mg/kg once daily.

Drug Administration

P.O.

- Administer with food if GI distress occurs.

Route	Onset	Peak	Duration
P.O.	Unknown	2–4 hr	Unknown

Half-life: 2.5–3.5 hr

Mechanism of Action

May suppress bacterial multiplication by interfering with RNA synthesis in susceptible bacteria that are actively dividing.

Contraindications

Hypersensitivity to ethambutol or its components, inability to report changes in vision, optic neuritis

Interactions

DRUGS

antacids that contain aluminum hydroxide: Decreased absorption of ethambutol

Adverse Reactions

CNS: Burning sensation or weakness in arms and legs, confusion, disorientation, dizziness, fever, headache, malaise, paresthesia, peripheral neuritis
EENT: Blurred vision, decreased visual acuity, eye pain, optic neuritis, red-green color blindness
GI: Abdominal pain, anorexia, **hepatic dysfunction**, nausea, vomiting
HEME: **Leukopenia**, **neutropenia**, **thrombocytopenia**
MS: Arthralgia, gouty arthritis, joint pain
RESP: **Pulmonary infiltrates**
SKIN: Dermatitis, **erythema multiforme**, **exfoliative dermatitis**, pruritus, rash
Other: **Anaphylaxis**, **hypersensitivity syndrome**, lymphadenopathy

Childbearing Considerations

PREGNANCY

- It is not known if drug causes fetal harm. However, there are reports of neonatal ophthalmic abnormalities born to women who took drug during pregnancy.
- Use with caution only if benefit to mother outweighs potential risk to fetus.

LACTATION

- Drug is present in breast milk.
- Mothers should check with prescriber before breastfeeding.

Nursing Considerations

- Expect prescriber to refer patient for an ophthalmologic examination that includes tests for acuity, red-green color blindness, and visual fields before taking ethambutol and monthly thereafter. This is especially important if therapy is prolonged, or dosage exceeds 15 mg/kg daily.
- Expect to give patient at least one other antituberculotic with ethambutol, as prescribed, because bacteria may become resistant quickly to a single drug.

! WARNING Monitor patient for hypersensitivity reactions, which may become life-threatening such as anaphylaxis. If present, notify prescriber immediately, expect drug to be discontinued, and provide supportive care, as needed and ordered.

- Monitor patient for vision changes and, if present, notify prescriber immediately.
- Monitor laboratory test results for changes in liver function or for increased serum uric acid level if patient has gouty arthritis or impaired renal function. Notify prescriber of any abnormalities.
- Obtain a monthly sputum specimen, as ordered, to check bacteriologic response in sputum-positive patient.
- Know that successful ethambutol therapy typically takes 6 to 12 months but may take years.

PATIENT TEACHING

- Instruct patient how to administer ethambutol and what to do if a dose is missed.
- Explain that ethambutol therapy may last months or years and that compliance is essential.

! WARNING Tell patient to notify prescriber immediately if an allergic reaction or vision changes occur. If allergic reaction is serious, urge patient to seek immediate medical care.

- Advise patient to notify prescriber if persistent, serious, or unusual adverse reactions occur.

etrasimod arginine

Velsipity

Class and Category

Pharmacologic class: Sphingosine 1-phosphate receptor modulator
Therapeutic class: Intestinal anti-inflammatory

Indications and Dosages

✶ *To treat moderately to severely active ulcerative colitis*

TABLETS

Adults. 2 mg once daily.

Drug Administration

P.O.

- Tablets should be swallowed whole.
- Tablets may be taken with or without food.
- If a dose is missed, do not administer but follow the next scheduled administration time; never double the next dose to make up for a missed dose.

Route	Onset	Peak	Duration
P.O.	Unknown	2–8 hr	Unknown

Half-life: 30 hr

Mechanism of Action

Binds with high affinity to sphingosine 1-phosphate (SIP) receptors to partially and reversibly block the capacity of lymphocytes to leave lymphoid organs, thereby reducing the number of lymphocytes in the peripheral bloodstream. Although exactly how the drug improves ulcerative colitis is unknown, it may involve reduced lymphocyte movement into the intestines thereby decreasing inflammation associated with ulcerative colitis.

Contraindications

Experienced within last 6 mo decompensated heart failure requiring hospitalization or class III or IV heart failure, MI, stroke, transient ischemic attack, or unstable angina pectoris; history or presence of Mobitz type II second-degree or third-degree AV block, sick sinus syndrome, or sino-artial block, unless functioning pacemaker is in place; hypersensitivity to etrasimod or its components

Interactions

DRUGS

antineoplastics, immune-modulating drugs, noncorticosteroid immunosuppressants: Possible risk of additive immune effects
beta blockers, calcium channel blockers: Possibly transient decrease in heart rate and AV conduction delays when estrasimod therapy initiated
class IA and class III antiarrhythmic drugs, QT prolonging drugs: Possibly increased risk of QT prolongation and torsades de pointes
CYP2C9 and CYP3A4 moderate to strong inhibitors: Increased exposure to etrasimod increasing risk of adverse reactions
CYP2C9 and CYP3A4 inducers (rifampin): Decreased exposure to etrasimod decreasing effectiveness

Adverse Reactions

CNS: Dizziness, headache, **posterior reversible encephalopathy syndrome**
CV: **AV conduction delays**, **bradyarrhythmia**, **bradycardia**, hypercholesterolemia, hypertension
EENT: Decreased visual acuity, macular edema
GI: Elevated liver enzymes, nausea
GU: UTI
MS: Arthralgia
RESP: Decreased absolute forced expiratory volume over 1 second (FEV_1)
SKIN: **Skin cancer**
Other: **Herpes viral infections**, **immunosuppression**, **life-threatening infections**

Childbearing Considerations

PREGNANCY

- Pregnancy exposure registry: 1-800-616-3791.
- Drug may cause fetal harm based on animal studies.
- Use with caution only if benefit to mother outweighs potential risk to fetus.

LACTATION

- It is not known if drug is present in breast milk.
- Mothers should check with prescriber before breastfeeding.

REPRODUCTION

- Females of childbearing age should use effective contraception during drug treatment and for one week following the last dose.

E

Nursing Considerations

- Ensure the following has been assessed before etrasimod therapy is begun: CBC within last 6 months, including lymphocyte count; ECG to determine preexisting conduction abnormalities and, if present, a cardiologist evaluation; liver function studies (bilirubin, transaminase) within the last 6 months; ophthalmic with baseline evaluation of the fundus, including the macula; past or current medication history of drugs that slow AV conduction or heart rate and drugs that affect the immune system such as antineoplastics drugs, immune-modulating drugs, and noncorticosteroid immunosuppressants; and a skin evaluation.
- Ascertain that immunizations are up to date. If needed, live attenuated vaccine immunizations should be administered at least 4 weeks prior to starting etrasimod therapy.

! **WARNING** Determine need to test patient for varicella zoster virus (no history of chickenpox or no documentation of a full course of vaccination against varicella zoster virus) and, if negative, ensure patient is vaccinated prior to starting etrasimod therapy. This is because drugs in the same class as etrasimod have been associated with the development of herpes simplex encephalitis, varicella zoster meningitis, and localized herpes viral infections.

! **WARNING** Expect etrasimod therapy to be delayed in any patient with an active infection until the infection is resolved. Monitor patient throughout drug therapy and for at least 5 weeks after therapy is stopped for signs and symptoms of infection because the drug can reduce peripheral blood lymphocyte count as much as 45%. Know that life-threatening infections have occurred with other drugs in the same class as etrasimod. If an infection occurs notify prescriber and expect etrasimod therapy to be temporarily withheld. Monitor patient for cryptococcal infection because cases of fatal cryptococcal meningitis and disseminated cryptococcal infections have occurred with use of other drugs in the same class as etrasimod. If suspected, notify prescriber, expect diagnostic evaluation to be done, and if confirmed treatment given including temporarily withholding etrasimod therapy until infection has been resolved.

! **WARNING** Be aware that although rare, patients taking other drugs in the same class as etrasimod have developed posterior reversible encephalopathy syndrome (PRES), which can be life-threatening. Monitor patient for neurological or psychiatric signs and symptoms. If noted, alert prescriber immediately as a delay in diagnosis and treatment may cause permanent neurological deficits. Expect etrasimod to be discontinued if even PRES is suspected.

! **WARNING** Monitor patient closely for additive immune suppression if patient is switching from drugs with prolonged immune effects. Also, monitor patient receiving concomitant immunosuppressants for infectious complications up to 5 weeks after the last dose of etrasimod.

! **WARNING** Monitor patient's heart rate for a reduction and ECG for a slowing of AV conduction at the start of etrasimod therapy. Report any abnormalities to prescriber. Be aware that a cardiology consult is recommended before starting etrasimod therapy for patients with arrhythmias requiring treatment with class 1A or class III antiarrhythmic drugs or QT prolonging drugs; class I or II heart failure; history of cardiac arrest, cerebrovascular disease or uncontrolled hypertension; history of Mobitz type I second-degree AV block unless functioning pacemaker in place, recurrent cardiogenic syncope, severe untreated sleep apnea, or symptomatic bradycardia; resting heart rate less than 50 beats per minutes; significant QT prolongation, or unstable ischemic heart disease.

! **WARNING** Monitor patient's liver function throughout therapy because drug may adversely affect liver function. Notify prescriber if patient develops symptoms of hepatic dysfunction such as abdominal pain, anorexia, dark urine, fatigue, jaundice, and unexplained nausea and vomiting. Expect drug to be discontinued if significant liver dysfunction occurs.

! **WARNING** Perform a skin examination on the patient regularly because cases of skin cancer have occurred with drugs in the same class as etrasimod.

- Monitor patient's blood pressure regularly because etrasimod may cause hypertension. Report any significant rise in blood pressure and expect it to be treated.
- Expect patient to have regular eye examination for the evaluation of the fundus, including the macula, while receiving etrasimod therapy and any time there is a change in vision because drug may cause macular edema, which can lead to permanent visual loss if it is present for 6 months or more. Notify prescriber of any visual changes and know that drug may need to be discontinued if macular edema occurs.
- Monitor the patient's respiratory function throughout etrasimod therapy because drug may decrease respiratory function as soon as 3 months after drug therapy is begun. Expect a spirometric evaluation to be done if respiratory abnormalities occur.
- Know that therapy with drugs that suppress the immune system should be avoided during etrasimod therapy and in the weeks following administration of etrasimod because of an additive suppressant effect.

PATIENT TEACHING

- Instruct patient how to administer etrasimod.

! **WARNING** Review infection control measures patient should take while receiving etrasimod therapy. Stress importance of notifying prescriber promptly if an infection occurs. Also inform patient that immunosuppressive effects may last for up to 5 weeks after the drug is continued.

! **WARNING** Stress importance of seeking immediate medical care if a seizure occurs or patient experiences a sudden onset of an altered mental status, severe headache, or visual changes.

! **WARNING** Advise patient that etrasimod therapy may have an adverse effect on liver function and to notify prescriber if patient develops abdominal pain, anorexia, dark urine, fatigue, jaundice, nausea, or vomiting.

! **WARNING** Inform patient that a new onset or worsening dyspnea should be reported to prescriber.

! **WARNING** Advise females of childbearing age to use effective contraception during etrasimod therapy and for 1 week after the drug is discontinued. Stress importance of reporting pregnancy immediately to prescriber.

- Tell patient to avoid immunizations with live attenuated vaccines during etrasimod therapy and for 5 weeks after therapy is discontinued.
- Alert patient that etrasimod therapy may initially cause a transient decrease in heart rate. Advise patient to notify prescriber if symptomatic.
- Instruct patient to have an eye examination early on and then periodically while taking etrasimod and to notify prescriber if visual changes occur.
- Tell patient to limit sun and ultraviolet light exposure during etrasimod therapy and to wear protective clothing and use a sunscreen with a high protection faction. If a suspicious skin lesion occurs, stress importance of notifying prescriber immediately.
- Stress importance of complying with tests ordered throughout etrasimod therapy used to monitor for adverse effects of etrasimod therapy.

etravirine

Intelence

Class and Category

Pharmacologic class: Non-nucleoside reverse transcriptase inhibitor (NNRTI)
Therapeutic class: Antiretroviral

Indications and Dosages

∗ *As adjunct to treat HIV-1 infection in patients who are antiretroviral treatment-experienced*

TABLETS

Adults, pregnant women, and children ages 2 to 18 weighing 30 kg (66 lb) or more. 200 mg twice daily.

Children ages 2 to 18 weighing 25 kg (55 lb) to less than 30 kg (66 lb). 150 mg twice daily.
Children ages 2 to 18 weighing 20 kg (44 lb) to less than 25 kg (55 lb). 125 mg twice daily.
Children ages 2 to 18 weighing 10 kg (22 lb) to less than 20 kg (44 lb). 100 mg twice daily.

Drug Administration

P.O.

- Administer drug after meals.
- Tablet should be swallowed whole with a liquid and not chewed, crushed, or split.
- For patient unable to swallow tablets, dissolve tablet in 5 ml of water and stir well until the water looks milky. Then, add 15 ml of milk, orange juice, or water (not carbonated beverages, grapefruit juice, or warm liquids). Have patient drink mixture immediately and then add more milk, orange juice, or water to glass and have patient drink it. Do this several times to ensure that patient has received the entire dose.

Route	Onset	Peak	Duration
P.O.	Unknown	2.5–4 hr	Unknown

Half-life: 21–61 hr

Mechanism of Action

Binds directly to reverse transcriptase and blocks the RNA-dependent and DNA-dependent DNA polymerase activities by causing a disruption of the enzyme's catalyticsite.

Contraindications

Hypersensitivity to etravirine or its components

Interactions

DRUGS

amiodarone, artemether, atazanavir, atazanavir/ritonavir, atorvastatin, bepridil, buprenorphine, clopidogrel, cyclosporine, dihydroartemisinin, disopyramide, dolutegravir, dolutegravir/darunavir/ritonavir, dolutegravir/lopinavir/ritonavir, flecainide, indinavir, lidocaine (systemic), lovastatin, lumefantrine, maraviroc, mexiletine, propafenone, quinidine, rilpivirine, sildenafil, simvastatin, sirolimus, tacrolimus, telaprevir, warfarin: Decreased plasma concentrations of these drugs with possible decreased effectiveness
boceprevir: Decreased plasma concentration of etravirine with possible decreased effectiveness; increased plasma concentration of boceprevir with possible increased risk of adverse reactions
carbamazepine, darunavir/ritonavir, dexamethasone (systemic), efavirenz, lopinavir/ritonavir, nevirapine, phenobarbital, phenytoin, rifampin, rifapentine, ritonavir, St. John's wort, saquinavir/ritonavir, tipranavir/ritonavir: Decreased plasma concentration of etravirine and its effectiveness
clarithromycin, itraconazole, ketoconazole: Decreased plasma concentrations of these drugs with possible decreased effectiveness; increased plasma concentration of etravirine
delavirdine: Increased plasma concentration of etravirine with possible increased risk of serious adverse reactions
diazepam, digoxin, fluvastatin, fosamprenavir, fosamprenavir/ritonavir, maraviroc/darunavir/ritonavir, nelfinavir, pitavastatin: Increased plasma concentration of these drugs with possible increased risk of serious adverse reactions
rifabutin: Decreased plasma concentration of both etravirine and rifabutin with possible decreased effectiveness of both drugs
voriconazole: Increased plasma concentrations of both etravirine and voriconazole with possible increased risk of serious adverse reactions

Adverse Reactions

CNS: Abnormal dreams, amnesia, anxiety, confusion, **CVA**, difficulty concentrating, disorientation, fatigue, fever, general malaise, hypoesthesia, nervousness, nightmares, paresthesia, peripheral neuropathy, **seizures**, sleep disorders, sluggishness, somnolence, syncope, tremor, vertigo
CV: Angina pectoris, **atrial fibrillation**, dyslipidemia, elevated cholesterol and triglyceride levels, **MI**
EENT: Blurred vision, conjunctivitis, dry mouth, oral lesions, stomatitis
ENDO: Cushingoid appearance, diabetes mellitus, fat redistribution, gynecomastia, hyperglycemia
GI: Abdominal distention, anorexia, constipation, elevated liver or pancreatic enzymes, flatulence, gastroesophageal

reflux disease, gastritis, hematemesis, **hepatic failure**, hepatic steatosis, **hepatitis**, hepatomegaly, **pancreatitis**, vomiting
GU: **Acute renal failure**, elevated creatinine level
HEME: Decreased hemoglobin eosinophilia, **hemolytic anemia**, **leukopenia**, **neutropenia**, **thrombocytopenia**
MS: Joint or muscle aches, **rhabdomyolysis**
RESP: **Bronchospasm**, exertional dyspnea
SKIN: Blisters, diaphoresis, dry skin, **erythema multiforme**, lipohypertrophy, night sweats, **Stevens-Johnson syndrome**, **toxic epidermal necrolysis**
Other: **Angioedema**, **drug reaction with eosinophilia and systemic symptoms (DRESS)**, **immune reconstitution syndrome**, lipodystrophy

Childbearing Considerations

PREGNANCY

- Pregnancy exposure registry: 1-800-258-4263.
- It is not known if drug causes fetal harm.
- Use with caution only if benefit to mother outweighs potential risk to fetus.

LACTATION

- Drug is present in breast milk.
- The Centers for Disease Control and Prevention recommends that HIV-1 infected mothers not breastfeed to avoid risking postnatal transmission of HIV-1 infection to infants. They also do not recommend breastfeeding because of potential drug-induced adverse reactions in the infant.

Nursing Considerations

! WARNING Assess patient for hypersensitivity reactions, including skin changes, especially a rash (DRESS may only initially exhibit with a fever or swollen lymph nodes) that may occur anytime but most commonly within the first 6 weeks of treatment. Notify prescriber immediately, expect drug to be discontinued as symptoms can evolve into a life-threatening reaction if not discontinued, and provide supportive care, as needed and ordered.

! WARNING Monitor patient for seizures. Expect liver and kidney function tests to be performed regularly to assess drug-induced dysfunction because drug can cause acute renal failure or hepatitis.

! WARNING Be aware that immune reconstitution syndrome has occurred in patients treated with combination antiretroviral therapy, including etravirine. The inflammatory response predisposes susceptible patients to opportunistic infections, such as cytomegalovirus, *Mycobacterium avium* infection, *Pneumocystis jiroveci* pneumonia, or tuberculosis. Autoimmune disorders, such as Graves' disease, Guillain-Barré syndrome, or polymyositis have also occurred. Report sudden or unusual adverse reactions to prescriber.

! WARNING Monitor patient for persistent, serious, or unusual adverse reactions because etravirine may adversely affect many body systems and may cause life-threatening reactions such as bronchospasms, MI, and pancreatitis.

- Observe patient for redistribution of body fat, including breast enlargement, central obesity, development of buffalo hump, facial wasting, and peripheral wasting, which may produce a cushingoid-type appearance.

PATIENT TEACHING

- Instruct patient, family, or caregiver how to administer etravirine and what to do if a dose is missed.

! WARNING Tell patient to notify prescriber immediately of any allergic reactions or skin changes, especially a fever, rash, or swollen lymph nodes that may be associated with other symptoms. Drug will have to be discontinued if serious.

! WARNING Alert patient, family, or caregiver that drug can cause serious adverse reactions affecting various body systems. Stress importance of notifying prescriber of any persistent, severe, or unusual adverse reactions, including serious infections, kidney or liver dysfunction, and seizures.

- Alert patient to the possibility of fat distribution with the appearance of a buffalo hump, thin extremities and face, and breast enlargement.

- Instruct patient to inform all prescribers of etravirine therapy and not to take any drugs, including over-the-counter drugs and herbal medicines, without prescriber consent, because etravirine interacts with many drugs.
- Tell mothers not to breastfeed their infants while receiving etravirine.

everolimus

Afinitor, Afinitor Disperz, Zortress

Class and Category

Pharmacologic class: mTOR kinase inhibitor
Therapeutic class: Immunosuppressant

Indications and Dosages

* *As adjunct to prevent organ rejection in renal transplantation in patients at low-moderate immunologic risk*

TABLETS (ZORTRESS)

Adults. *Initial:* 0.75 mg twice daily administered as soon as possible after transplantation in combination with basiliximab induction, reduced-dose cyclosporine, and corticosteroids. Dosage adjusted at 4- to 5-day intervals, as needed.

* *As adjunct to prevent organ rejection in liver transplantation*

TABLETS (ZORTRESS)

Adults. *Initial*: 1 mg twice daily in combination with corticosteroids and reduced-dose tacrolimus begun 30 days post-transplant.

± **DOSAGE ADJUSTMENT** For patients taking Zortress for kidney or liver transplantation, dosage adjusted at 4- to 5-day intervals, as needed, according to everolimus blood concentrations. For patients with a trough concentration below 3 ng/ml total daily dose doubled; if trough concentration is greater than 8 ng/ml on 2 consecutive measures, the dose is decreased by 0.25 mg twice daily. For patients with mild hepatic impairment, initial daily dose reduced by one-third, and for patients with moderate or severe hepatic impairment, initial daily dose is reduced by 50% with further adjustments made according to everolimus blood concentration levels. For patients taking concomitant cannabidiol, dosage may need to be reduced. For all patients, dosage also adjusted according to tolerability, change in concomitant medications, the clinical situation, and individual response.

* *To treat advanced hormone receptor-positive, HER2-negative breast cancer in postmenopausal women in combination with exemestane after failure of treatment with anastrozole or letrozole; to treat progressive neuroendocrine tumors of pancreatic origin with unresectable, locally advanced or metastatic disease; to treat progressive, well-differentiated, nonfunctional tumors of GI or lung origin with unresectable, locally advanced or metastatic disease; to treat renal cell carcinoma after failure of treatment with sorafenib or sunitinib; to treat renal angiomyolipoma and tuberous sclerosis complex that does not require immediate surgery*

TABLETS (AFINITOR)

Adults. 10 mg once daily. Treatment continued until disease progression or unacceptable toxicity occurs.

* *To treat tuberous sclerosis complex-associated subependymal giant cell astrocytoma (SEGA) that cannot be curatively resected*

ORAL SUSPENSION (AFINITOR DISPERZ), TABLETS (AFINITOR)

Adults and children ages 1 and older. 4.5 mg/m^2 once daily until disease progresses or unacceptable toxicity occurs.

* *As adjunct to treat tuberous sclerosis complex-associated partial-onset seizures*

ORAL SUSPENSION (AFINITOR DISPERZ)

Adults and children ages 2 and older. 5 mg/m^2 once daily until disease progresses or unacceptable toxicity occurs.

± **DOSAGE ADJUSTMENT** For patients taking Afinitor or Afinitor Disperz, dosage adjusted according to degree of adverse reactions present. For patients with breast cancer, neuroendocrine tumors, renal cell carcinoma, or tuberous sclerosis complex-associated renal angiomyolipoma and who have mild hepatic impairment, dosage reduced to 7.5 mg once daily or 5 mg once daily if 7.5 mg is not tolerated; for moderate hepatic impairment, dosage reduced to 5 mg once daily or 2.5 mg once daily if 5 mg is not tolerated; and for patients with severe hepatic impairment, dosage reduced to 2.5 mg once daily. For patients with tuberous sclerosis complex-associated subependymal giant cell astrocytoma or tuberous sclerosis complex-associated partial-onset seizures and who have severe hepatic impairment, dosage reduced to 2.5 mg/m^2 once daily. For patients taking a P-gp and moderate CYP3A inhibitors and who have breast cancer, neuroendocrine tumor, renal cell carcinoma, or tuberous sclerosis complex-associated renal angiomyolipoma, dosage reduced to 2.5 mg once daily, with dosage then increased to 5 mg once daily, if tolerated. For patients taking P-gp and moderate CYP3A inhibitors and who have tuberous sclerosis complex-associated subependymal giant cell astrocytoma or tuberous sclerosis complex-associated partial-onset seizures, daily dosage reduced by 50%. For patients taking a P-gp and strong CYP3A4 inducers and who have any indication treated by everolimus, dosage doubled using increments of 5 mg or less.

Drug Administration

P.O.

- Zortress brand of everolimus isn't recommended in transplants other than kidney or liver transplantation. Everolimus therapy should not begin until 30 days after liver transplant because of patient's increased risk of developing hepatic artery thrombosis, which may lead to graft loss or death.
- Another form of everolimus under the trade names of Afinitor and Afinitor Disperz are used only to treat certain cancers. The 3 brands are not interchangeable. To avoid a medication error, make sure the right brand is being used for indication being treated.
- Tablets should be swallowed whole and given with a glass of water and not chewed or crushed before ingesting.
- Administer drug at the same time each day and consistently either with or without food. Twice-daily dosages should be consistently taken approximately 12 hr apart and at the same time as cyclosporine or tacrolimus dose, if prescribed.
- Wear gloves when preparing and administering oral suspension (Afinitor Disperz). Prepare suspension with only water using an oral syringe or small drinking glass according to manufacturer's guidelines.
- Use a calibrated device to measure oral suspension dose. Administer immediately after preparation. Discard within 60 min if not administered.
- Do not administer with grapefruit juice or products.
- If a dose of Afinitor or Afinitor Disperz is missed, administer it up to 6 hr after the time it was to be administered. If more than 6 hr has passed, skip missed dose and resume normal dosing schedule the following day. Never double doses to make up for a missed dose.

Route	Onset	Peak	Duration
P.O.	Unknown	1–2 hr	Unknown

Half-life: 30 hr

Mechanism of Action

Causes immunosuppression by inhibiting antigenic and interleukin (IL-2 and IL-15) stimulated activation and proliferation of B and T lymphocytes.

Contraindications

Hypersensitivity to everolimus, other rapamycin derivatives, or their components

Interactions

DRUGS

ACE inhibitors: Possibly increased risk of angioedema

amprenavir, aprepitant, atazanavir, clarithromycin, cyclosporine, digoxin, diltiazem, erythromycin, fluconazole, fosamprenavir, indinavir, itraconazole, ketoconazole, macrolide antibiotics, nefazodone, nelfinavir, nicardipine, ritonavir, saquinavir, telithromycin, verapamil, voriconazole: Possible increased blood everolimus level

anticonvulsants, carbamazepine, efavirenz, nevirapine, phenobarbital, phenytoin, rifabutin, rifampin, rifapentine, St. John's wort: Possibly decreased blood everolimus level

cannabidiol: Increased everolimus blood levels possibly causing everolimus toxicity

lovastatin, simvastatin: Possible development of rhabdomyolysis and other adverse reactions

octreotide (depot): Increased octreotide levels

live vaccines: Possibly increased risk of contracting disease from live virus; decreased therapeutic effect of vaccine

FOODS

grapefruit, grapefruit juice: Possibly decreased metabolism of everolimus increasing everolimus level

Adverse Reactions

CNS: Aggression, agitation, anxiety, asthenia, chills, dizziness, fatigue, fever,

headache, insomnia, **progressive multiple leukoencephalopathy (PML)**, multiple, paresthesia, reflex sympathetic dystrophy
CV: **Arterial thrombotic events**, chest pain, **congestive heart failure**, **deep vein thrombosis**, hyperlipidemia, hypertension, **pericardial effusion**, peripheral edema, tachycardia, **thrombotic microangiopathy**
EENT: Conjunctivitis, dry mouth, epistaxis, eyelid pain, oropharyngeal pain, rhinorrhea, stomatitis
ENDO: Hot flashes, hyperglycemia, new-onset diabetes mellitus
GI: Abdominal pain, anorexia, ascites, cholecystitis, cholelithiasis, constipation, diarrhea, elevated bilirubin or liver enzymes, gastroenteritis, **hepatic artery thrombosis** (liver transplant), nausea, **pancreatitis**
GU: **Acute renal failure**, amenorrhea, azoospermia, **BK virus-associated nephropathy**, elevated creatinine level, **kidney graft thrombosis**, **nephrotoxicity**, oligospermia, proteinuria, UTI
HEME: Anemia, **bleeding**, **elevated partial thromboplastin time**, **elevated prothrombin time**, **leukopenia**, **lymphopenia**, **neutropenia**, **thrombocytopenia**
MS: Arthralgia; back, extremity, or jaw pain; muscle spasm; myalgia
RESP: Cough, dyspnea, **interstitial lung disease**, noninfectious pneumonitis, pleural effusion, **pulmonary embolism**, upper respiratory infection
SKIN: Acne, alopecia, dermatitis, erythema, nail disorders, pruritus, rash, **skin cancer**
Other: **Angioedema or other hypersensitivity reactions**; **decreased bicarbonate level**; delayed wound healing; elevated alkaline phosphatase; **hyperkalemia**; **hypocalcemia**; **hypokalemia**; **hyponatremia**; **hypophosphatemia**; infections, such as bacterial, fungal, protozoal, and viral; lymphedema; **lymphomas and other malignancies**; opportunistic infections, including polyoma virus; radiation sensitization and radiation recall (cancer treatment); **sepsis**; **septic shock**; weight loss

Childbearing Considerations

PREGNANCY

- A negative pregnancy test result is required before starting drug therapy.
- Drug may cause fetal harm based on animal studies.
- Use with caution only if benefit to mother outweighs potential risk to fetus.

LACTATION

- It is not known if drug is present in breast milk.
- Breastfeeding should not occur during drug therapy.

REPRODUCTION

- Advise females of childbearing age to use highly effective contraception methods while receiving drug and up to 8 wk after drug is discontinued.
- Advise male patients with female partners of childbearing age to use highly effective contraception during treatment and for 4 wk after the last dose.
- Drug therapy may cause both female and male infertility.

Nursing Considerations

- Know that patients with galactose intolerance, glucose–galactose malabsorption, or Lapp lactase deficiency should not receive everolimus therapy because this may result in diarrhea and malabsorption.

> **! WARNING** Expect females of childbearing age to undergo a pregnancy test prior to initiating everolimus therapy because drug can cause fetal harm.

- Assess patient's renal function before therapy with Afinitor or Afinitor Disperz brand of everolimus is begun, and annually thereafter unless patient has underlying risk factors for renal failure. Renal evaluation in these patients should be done every 6 months.
- Measure whole blood trough concentrations of both cyclosporine and everolimus, as ordered, in patient with kidney transplant or tacrolimus and everolimus in liver transplant because of increased risk of nephrotoxicity when either combination of drugs are used or when drug is used to treat malignancies or tuberous sclerosis complex-associated partial-onset seizures. Everolimus levels, ideally drawn 4 to 5 days after a previous dosing change, will also reveal if the therapeutic range has been achieved (3 to 8 ng/ml).
- Know that everolimus levels should be obtained during concomitant

administration of CYP3A4 inducers or inhibitors, when switching cyclosporine formulations, and/or when cyclosporine dosing is reduced as well as in patients with hepatic impairment.

- Know that there is little to no pharmacokinetic interaction of tacrolimus on everolimus. Therefore, there is no need to alter everolimus dosing if tacrolimus dosing is altered.

! **WARNING** Monitor patient closely for hypersensitivity reactions, which could become life-threatening such as angioedema. If present, notify prescriber, expect drug to be discontinued and another drug substituted, and provide supportive care, as needed and ordered.

! **WARNING** Monitor patient, especially within the first 30 days post-transplantation, for evidence of kidney arterial and venous thrombosis (kidney transplant) or hepatic artery thrombosis (liver transplant) resulting in graft loss.

! **WARNING** Watch for evidence of infection (such as cough, fever, pain, malaise) because patients receiving immunosuppressants, such as everolimus are at increased risk for bacterial, fungal, parasitic, or viral infection. Watch for both generalized and localized infections, including worsening of preexisting infections, and be aware that these infections may become life-threatening. Activation of latent viral infections may also occur and include BK-virus-associated nephropathy that can lead to decreased renal function and renal graft loss.

! **WARNING** Monitor patient's CBC and platelet count, as ordered, routinely because of increased risk of hemolytic uremic syndrome, thrombotic microangiopathy, or thrombotic thrombocytopenic purpura that may occur with combined everolimus and cyclosporine therapy used with kidney transplantation. Also, know that drug causes myelosuppression, which may lead to hematologic disorders, such as anemia, lymphopenia, neutropenia, and thrombocytopenia.

! **WARNING** Monitor cancer patient receiving radiation during or sequentially with everolimus therapy as radiation sensitization and recall involving cutaneous and visceral organs may occur, resulting in worsening adverse effects of radiation therapy. Adverse effects may become severe.

- Be aware that interstitial lung disease may occur in patients with symptoms consistent with infectious pneumonia but usually only becomes apparent when patient does not respond to antibiotic therapy and other causes have been ruled out. If this occurs, expect everolimus therapy to be interrupted until the noninfectious pneumonitis has been resolved. Know that glucocorticoid therapy may also be prescribed to help resolve it.
- Monitor patient's lipid levels routinely because hyperlipidemia may occur as a result of everolimus therapy. If hyperlipidemia drug therapy is required, be aware that lovastatin or simvastatin should not be used to treat it for patient with a kidney transplant because of a potential interaction with cyclosporine.
- Monitor patient for persistent, serious, or unusual adverse reactions because drug can adversely affect multiple systems. Report abnormalities promptly to prescriber.
- Monitor patient's blood glucose levels regularly because everolimus therapy may increase the risk of new-onset diabetes mellitus after transplant or alter blood glucose control in patients with diabetes mellitus.
- Monitor patient's incision, as everolimus delays wound healing and increases the occurrence of wound-related complications, such as wound dehiscence, wound infection, incisional hernia, lymphocele, and seroma.

PATIENT TEACHING

- Instruct patient how to administer form of everolimus prescribed.
- Emphasize importance of avoiding grapefruit and grapefruit juice while receiving concomitant therapy with everolimus and cyclosporine.
- Advise patient to avoid immunizations that use live vaccines, such as BCG, intranasal influenza, measles, mumps, rubella, oral polio, TY21a typhoid, varicella, and yellow fever during drug therapy.

- Alert both men and women that drug may affect fertility. Encourage patient to discuss any concerns with prescriber before drug therapy begins.

! WARNING Urge females of childbearing age to use a highly effective birth control method throughout everolimus therapy and for 8 weeks after the drug has been discontinued. Advise male patients with female partners of childbearing age to use a highly effective contraception during treatment and for 4 weeks after the last dose. If pregnancy occurs, prescriber should be notified immediately.

! WARNING Advise patient to report an allergic reaction or signs and symptoms of an infection to prescriber, but if serious tell patient to seek immediate medical attention.

- Instruct patient to report any persistent, severe, or unusual symptoms to prescriber.
- Caution patient to avoid excessive exposure to ultraviolet light, to wear protective clothing when outdoors, and use a sunscreen with a high protection factor.
- Inform patient that stomatitis most often occurs within the first 8 weeks of treatment. Instruct patient that he will be prescribed a dexamethasone alcohol-free oral solution and to use it as a swish-and-spit mouthwash. Caution him to avoid alcohol-, hydrogen peroxide-, iodine-, or thyme-containing products.
- Stress importance of alerting all prescribers of everolimus therapy because some drugs can increase everolimus blood levels increasing risk of adverse reactions or even toxicity or decrease blood levels making everolimus less effective. Tell patient not to take any over-the-counter drugs such as herbal or dietary supplements without consulting prescriber.
- Inform mothers that they should not breastfeed while taking everolimus.

evinacumab-dgnb

Evkeeza

Class and Category

Pharmacologic class: Angiopoietin-like 3 (ANGPTL3) inhibitor
Therapeutic class: Antilipemic

Indications and Dosages

∗ *As adjunct to other low-density lipoprotein-cholesterol (LDL-C) lowering therapies for patients with homozygous familial hypercholesterolemia (HoFH)*

I.V. INFUSION

Adults and children ages 5 and older. 15 mg/kg infused over 60 min once every 4 wk.

Drug Administration

I.V.

- Calculate the dose in mg, total volume required in ml, and the number of vials required based on the patient's current weight.
- Drug solution should appear clear to slightly opalescent, colorless to pale yellow. Do not use if solution is cloudy or discolored or contains particulate matter.
- Know that the drug vials are single-dose containers and do not contain a preservative.
- Do not shake the vial. Withdraw the required volume from the vial(s) and transfer into an I.V. infusion bag containing a maximum volume of 250 ml of 0.9% Sodium Chloride Injection or 5% Dextrose injection. Mix diluted solution by gently inverting container. Do not shake.
- Final concentration of diluted solution should be between 0.5 mg/ml and 20 mg/ml depending on the patient's current body weight.
- Administer immediately after mixing. If not able to be used immediately, store the diluted solution in the refrigerator for no more than 24 hr or at room temperature up to 25 degrees C (77 degrees F) for no more than 6 hr from the time of infusion preparation to the end of the infusion. Never freeze the diluted solution.
- If diluted solution has been refrigerated, allow the drug solution to come to room temperature before administration.
- Administer the drug solution as an IV infusion over 60 min through an IV line containing a sterile, in-line or add-on, 0.2-micron to 5-micron filter.
- Monitor patient for any signs of adverse reactions, including hypersensitivity or infusion reactions. Notify prescriber if adverse reactions occur as the infusion rate may need to be slowed, interrupted, or discontinued.

- If a dose is missed, expect to administer it as soon as possible and dosing schedule changed to occur 1 mo after missed dose administered.
- *Incompatibilities:* Other drugs

Route	Onset	Peak	Duration
I.V.	Unknown	Unknown	Unknown

Half-life: Not constant

Mechanism of Action

Binds to and inhibits angiopoietin-like 3 protein which leads to a reduction in LDL-C, high-density lipoprotein cholesterol (HDL-C), and triglycerides (TG).

Contraindications

Hypersensitivity to evinacumab-dgnb or its components

Interactions

None reported by manufacturer.

Adverse Reactions

CNS: Asthenia, dizziness, fatigue
EENT: Nasal congestion, nasopharyngitis, rhinorrhea
GI: Abdominal pain, constipation, nausea
MS: Extremity pain
RESP: Upper respiratory infection
OTHER: **Anaphylaxis**, flu-like illness, infusion reactions (infusion site pruritus, muscular weakness, nasal congestion, nausea, pyrexia)

Childbearing Considerations

PREGNANCY

- Pregnancy exposure registry: 1-833-385-3392.
- Drug may cause fetal harm according to animal studies.
- Females of childbearing age should have a negative pregnancy test before drug therapy begins.
- Drug should not be given during pregnancy and for 5 mo following last dose.

LACTATION

- It is not known if drug is present in breast milk.
- Mothers should check with prescriber before breastfeeding.

REPRODUCTION

- Females of childbearing age should use effective contraception during drug therapy and for 5 mo following last dose.

Nursing Considerations

- Be aware evinacumab-dgnb should not be prescribed for patients with other types of hypercholesterolemia, including heterozygous familial hypercholesterolemia (HeFH)

! **WARNING** Expect females of childbearing age to have a negative pregnancy test result prior to the initiation of evinacumab-dgnb because drug may cause fetal harm.

- Monitor patient's LDL-C, as ordered throughout evinacumab-dgnb therapy. Know that its LDL lowering effects can be seen as early as 2 weeks after drug is initiated.

! **WARNING** Monitor patient for hypersensitivity reactions, which could be life-threatening such as anaphylaxis. Notify prescriber immediately if a hypersensitivity reaction occurs and expect drug to be discontinued. Provide supportive care, as needed and ordered.

PATIENT TEACHING

- Review with patient how drug will be administered and importance of adhering to dosage schedule.

! **WARNING** Inform females of childbearing age that a negative pregnancy test is recommended prior to evinacumab-dgnb therapy being initiated. Advise her to use effective contraception throughout drug therapy and for a minimum of 5 months after the last dose. Instruct her to notify prescriber if pregnancy occurs during drug therapy and encourage her to report pregnancy, if confirmed, to manufacturer.

! **WARNING** Alert patient that evinacumab-dgnb may cause an allergic reaction. If present, tell patient to notify prescriber and, if severe, to seek immediate medical care.

- Instruct patient about the importance of complying to periodic blood studies ordered to determine the effectiveness of the drug.

E

exenatide

Bydureon BCise, Byetta

Class and Category

Pharmacologic class: Glucagon-like peptide-1 (GLP-1) receptor agonist
Therapeutic class: Antidiabetic

Indications and Dosages

∗ *As adjunct treatment to diet and exercise to improve blood glucose levels in patients with type 2 diabetes mellitus*

SUBCUTANEOUS INJECTION (BYETTA)

Adults. *Initial:* 5 mcg twice daily. After 1 mo, increased, as needed, to 10 mcg twice daily.

SUBCUTANEOUS INJECTION (BYDUREON BCISE)

Adults and children ages 10 and older. 2 mg once every 7 days.

Drug Administration

SUBCUTANEOUS

- Administer drug into patient's abdomen, thigh, or upper arm. Rotate sites.
- Prior to first use, store in refrigerator, protected from light.
- Monitor injection site for serious reactions, which, rarely, may require surgical intervention.

Byetta

- Administer within 60 min before morning and evening meals or before 2 main meals that are about 6 hr or more apart.
- Drug should not be administered after a meal.
- If a dose is missed, do not administer but resume with next scheduled dose.
- Once pen is used, it can be kept at room temperature protected from light.
- Discard pen after 30 days from first use, even if some drug remains in the pen.

Bydureon BCise

- Expect to discontinue any other exenatide product before Bydureon BCise is begun.
- Store flat in original package in refrigerator protected from light. Or it can be kept at room temperature for no more than 4 wk total.
- Remove from refrigerator, if stored there, and let autoinjector come to room temperature for 15 min.
- Mix drug by shaking the autoinjector hard until drug is mixed evenly and no white powder is seen. It will appear cloudy. Shake at least 15 sec but shake longer if it was not stored flat.
- Hold the autoinjector straight up with the orange cap toward the ceiling. Unlock the autoinjector by turning knob from the lock to unlock position until a click is heard.
- While holding the autoinjector straight up, firmly unscrew the orange cap. The cap may have to be turned a few times before it loosens. If a clicking sound is heard, it is being turned in the wrong direction. A green shield will pop up after the cap is removed.
- Inject at the selected site. A click will be heard when the injection begins. Keep holding the autoinjector against the skin for 15 sec to ensure that the total dose has been given. An orange rod should be seen in the window after the injection.
- If a dose is missed, administer as soon as possible as long as the next regularly schedule dose is at least 3 days later. Thereafter, subsequent dose given once every 7 days. However, if missed dose is only 1 to 2 days from the next scheduled dose, do not administer the missed dose and instead continue with regularly scheduled dose.

Route	Onset	Peak	Duration
SubQ	Immediate	2.1 hr	Unknown
SubQ/E.R.	Unknown	6–7 wk	10 wk

Half-life: 2.5 hr; E.R. unknown

Contraindications

History of drug-induced immune-mediated thrombocytopenia, hypersensitivity to exenatide or its components, personal or family history of medullary thyroid carcinoma or multiple endocrine neoplasia syndrome type 2 (Bydureon BCise)

Interactions

DRUGS

oral antidiabetics, such as meglitinides or sulfonylureas, insulin: Increased risk of hypoglycemia
oral drugs: May decrease rate and extent of absorption of these drugs
warfarin: Possibly increased INR with increased risk of bleeding

Adverse Reactions

CNS: Asthenia, dizziness, fatigue, headache, jitteriness, somnolence
CV: Chest pain
EENT: Decreased taste
ENDO: **Hypoglycemia**,
GI: Abdominal distention or pain, acute gallbladder disease, anorexia, cholecystitis, cholelithiasis, constipation, diarrhea, dyspepsia, flatulence, gastroesophageal reflux, indigestion, nausea, **pancreatitis (including life-threatening hemorrhagic or necrotizing)**, vomiting
GU: **Acute renal failure**, decreased renal function, elevated serum creatinine level, **kidney transplant dysfunction**, **worsening chronic renal failure**
HEME: **Drug-induced thrombocytopenia**
RESP: **Chronic hypersensitivity pneumonitis**
SKIN: Alopecia, diaphoresis, hyperhidrosis, macular or papular rash, pruritus, rash, urticaria
Other: **Anaphylaxis**, **angioedema**, dehydration, elevated anti-exanatide antibody level, hematoma, injection-site reactions (abscess, cellulitis, hematoma, necrosis, pruritus, redness, subcutaneous nodules), weight loss

Childbearing Considerations

PREGNANCY

- It is not known if drug causes fetal harm. However, animal studies suggest drug may increase risk for fetal harm.
- Use with caution only if benefit to mother outweighs potential risk to fetus.

LACTATION

- It is not known if drug is present in breast milk.
- Mothers should check with prescriber before breastfeeding.

Nursing Considerations

- Know that exenatide isn't recommended for patients with severe GI disease, patients with creatinine clearance less than 30 ml/min, patients with an estimated glomerular filtration rate less than 45 ml/min, or patients receiving dialysis because of adverse GI or renal effects.
- Monitor patient's blood glucose level. If control decreases despite the patient's best efforts, drug may have to be discontinued because of the possibility that anti-exenatide antibodies have formed. Be aware that if patient is already taking the rapid-release form of exenatide (Byetta) and is switching to the extended-release form of exenatide (Bydureon BCise), Byetta must be discontinued first. Also, know that he may experience a transient elevation in his blood glucose levels for about 2 wk as his body adjusts to the extended-release form.
- Know that the immediate-release form of exenatide (Byetta) may be used concomitantly with insulin glargine (Lantus), which is a long-acting insulin to help improve the patient's blood glucose control. Byetta should not be used with any other type of insulin. If the patient is susceptible to hypoglycemia, expect the insulin glargine dosage to be decreased when used with Byetta.

Mechanism of Action

Restores the first-phase insulin response that normally occurs within 10 min when serum glucose level rises but is absent in type 2 diabetes and improves the second-phase response that immediately follows. It does so by promoting incretins that spur insulin synthesis and release from beta cells by binding and activating human GLP-1 receptors to reduce fasting and postprandial serum glucose levels. Suppresses inappropriately elevated glucagon secretion also. Lower serum glucagon level leads to decreased hepatic glucose output and decreased insulin demand. It also slows gastric emptying and thus the rise of serum glucose level.

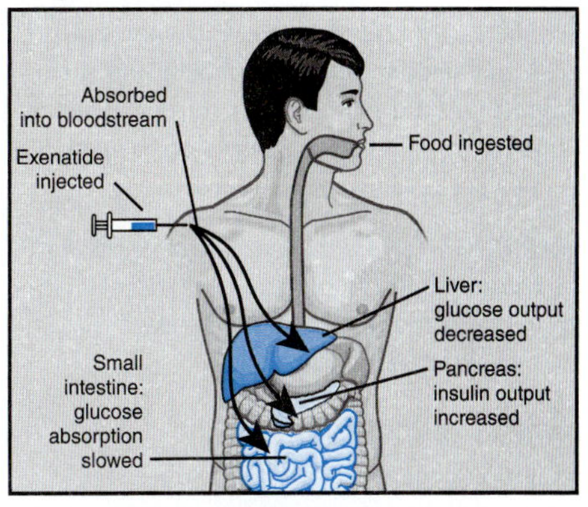

E

! **WARNING** Use exenatide cautiously in a renal transplant patient or patient with moderate renal disease when dosage of Byetta is increased from 5 to 10 mcg or the E.R. formulation, Bydureon BCise, is used. Monitor renal function throughout therapy, especially in the elderly, and notify prescriber of abnormalities because drug can cause acute kidney injury, especially if patient becomes hypovolemic from nausea and vomiting.

! **WARNING** Monitor patient for hypersensitivity reactions, which could become life-threathening such as anaphylaxis or angioedema. If present, notify precriber, expect drug to be discontinued, and provide supportive care, as needed and ordered.

! **WARNING** Monitor patient for bleeding because drug can induce immune-mediated thrombocytopenia, which can be fatal. If suspected, notify prescriber immediately and expect drug to be discontinued.

! **WARNING** Be aware that if patient also takes a sulfonylurea or insulin, patient may be at higher risk for hypoglycemia, which could become severe and may require the insulin or sulfonylurea dosage to be decreased to reduce the risk of hypoglycemia. Usually, no dosage adjustment is needed for a patient taking metformin.

! **WARNING** Monitor patient for evidence of acute pancreatitis, such as persistent, severe abdominal pain accompanied by vomiting, especially when drug is started, or dosage increased. Notify prescriber, expect to stop exenatide, and give supportive care, as needed and ordered.

! **WARNING** Be aware that exenatide may induce acute gallbladder disease. If cholelithiasis is suspected, expect gallbladder studies to be ordered and appropriate follow-up to occur. A cholecystectomy may be needed.

! **WARNING** Be aware that because drug delays gastric emptying, pulmonary aspiration may occur in patients undergoing elective procedures or surgeries.

PATIENT TEACHING

- Caution patient that exenatide doesn't replace diet and exercise measures.
- Instruct patient on how to prepare the type of exenatide product prescribed. Also, teach patient how to give a subcutaneous injection and what to do if a dose is missed.
- Caution patient not to share his pen or needles with anyone else.
- Warn patient that nausea may occur at the beginning of therapy but usually subsides over time.

! **WARNING** Alert patient that drug may cause an allergic reaction. If present, tell patient to notify prescriber and, if severe, to seek immediate medical care.

! **WARNING** Inform patient taking a sulfonylurea or insulin glargine to be alert for hypoglycemic reactions because risk increases with both drugs. Review ways to treat such reactions and tell patient to alert prescriber if they occur often or are severe.

! **WARNING** Stress importance of notifying prescriber if bleeding occurs and stop taking drug. If bleeding is serious, tell patient to seek immediate emergency care. Also, tell patient to seek emergency care for persistent, severe abdominal pain and vomiting.

! **WARNING** Inform patient that gallbladder problems may occur when exenatide therapy is given. Tell patient to report to prescriber right away if patient experiences clay-colored stools, fever, pain in the upper abdomen, or yellowing of eyes or skin.

- Tell patient to maintain adequate hydration throughout therapy. If unable to do so or dehydration occurs, stress importance of notifying prescriber promptly because kidney function may become impaired.
- Stress importance of alerting any prescriber of exenatide therapy but especially if preparing for an elective procedure or surgery.

ezetimibe

Zetia

Class and Category

Pharmacologic class: Cholesterol absorption inhibitor
Therapeutic class: Antilipemic

Indications and Dosages

As adjunct to diet to reduce elevated LDL-C in patients with primary hyperlipidemia, including heterozygous familial hypercholesterolemia (HeFH) in combination with a statin or as monotherapy; as adjunct to diet to reduce elevated LDL-C in patients with mixed hyperlipidemia in combination with fenofibrate

TABLETS

Adults. 10 mg once daily.

As adjunct to diet in combination with a statin and other LDL-C lowering therapies to reduce elevated LDL-C levels in patients with homozygous familial hypercholesterolemia (HoFH); as adjunct to diet in combination with a statin to reduce elevated LDL-C levels in pediatric patients with heterozygous familial hypercholesterolema (HeFH)

TABLETS

Children ages 10 and older. 10 mg once daily.

As adjunct to diet to reduce elevated sitosterol and campesterol levels in patients with homozygous sitosterolemia

TABLETS

Adults and children ages 9 and older. 10 mg once daily.

Drug Administration

P.O.

- Administer with or without food.
- Administer 2 hr before or 4 hr after giving bile acid sequestrant or cholestyramine.
- Can be administered at the same time as fenofibrate or an HMG-CoA reductase inhibitor.
- If a dose is missed, give as soon as possible. However do not double the next dose.

Route	Onset	Peak	Duration
P.O.	< 1 wk	4–12 hr	Unknown

Half-life: 22 hr

Contraindications

Active liver disease or unexplained persistent elevations in hepatic transaminase levels (with concurrent statin use), breastfeeding (with concurrent statin use), hypersensitivity to ezetimibe or its components, pregnancy (with concurrent statin use)

Interactions

DRUGS

cholestyramine: Reduced effects of ezetimibe
cyclosporine: Increased blood cyclosporine and ezetimibe levels
fibrates: Increased cholesterol excretion into the bile, leading possibly to cholelithiasis
warfarin: Possibly altered international normalized ratio (INR)

Adverse Reactions

CNS: Depression, dizziness, fatigue, headache, paresthesia
CV: Chest pain
EENT: Pharyngitis, sinusitis
GI: Abdominal pain, cholelithiasis, cholecystitis, diarrhea, elevated liver enzymes, **hepatitis**, nausea, **pancreatitis**
HEME: **Thrombocytopenia**
MS: Arthralgia, back or limb pain, elevated creatinine kinase level, myalgia, myopathy, **rhabdomyolysis**
RESP: Cough, upper respiratory tract infection
SKIN: **Erythema multiforme**, rash, urticaria
Other: **Anaphylaxis**, **angioedema**, flu-like symptoms, viral infection

Childbearing Considerations

PREGNANCY

- It is not known if drug causes fetal harm.
- Use with caution only if benefit to mother outweighs potential risk to fetus.
- Know that all statins are contraindicated in pregnancy. If a statin is combined with ezetimibe, the resulting combination is a contraindication for use during pregnancy.

LACTATION

- It is not known if drug is present in breast milk.
- Breastfeeding is not recommended with ezetimibe therapy and is contraindicated if a statin is given concurrently.

Nursing Considerations

! **WARNING** Know that when fenofibrate, a statin, or other LDL-C lowering therapy are contraindicated, use in combination with ezetimibe therapy is also contraindicated.

E

Mechanism of Action

Reduces blood cholesterol by inhibiting its absorption through the small intestine.

Normally, in the intestinal lumen, lipids break down to cholesterol and other substances that create smaller droplets called micelles, as shown below left. The micelles enter intestinal epithelial cells called enterocytes, where they combine with cholesterol, triglycerides, and other substances to form chylomicrons. Chylomicrons then pass through to the lymphatic system to be carried to the blood.

Blocks cholesterol absorption into enterocytes and keeps cholesterol from moving through the intestinal wall, as shown below right. Reduced cholesterol absorption from the intestine decreases chylomicron and LDL cholesterol content.

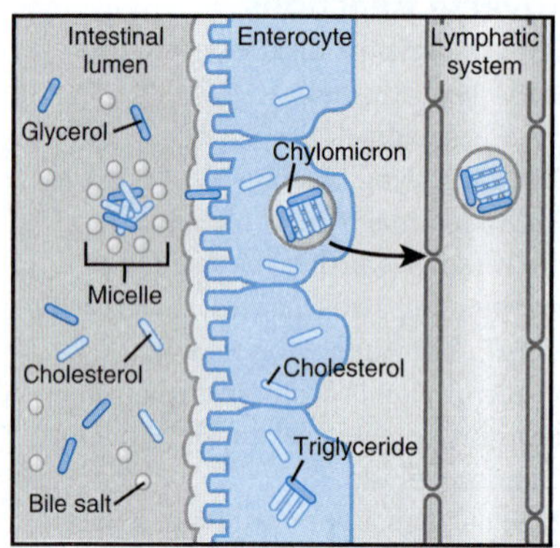

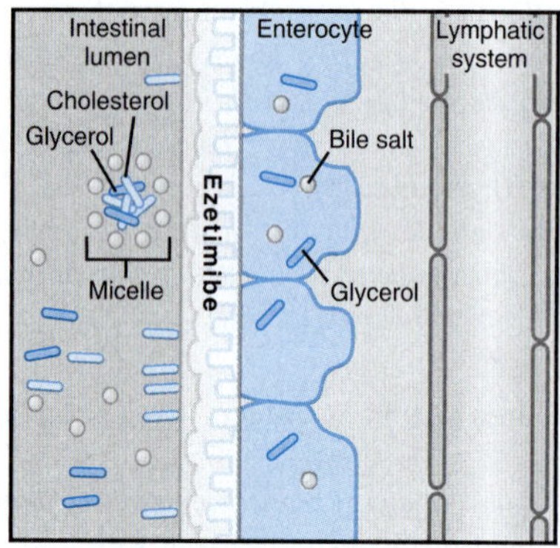

- Obtain a baseline of patient's lipid profile, as ordered, before therapy is begun and periodically throughout therapy to assess effectiveness of ezetimibe therapy.

! WARNING Monitor patient for a hypersensitivity reactions, which could become life-threatening such as anaphylaxis and angioedema. If present, notify prescriber, expect drug to be discontinued, and provide supportive care, as needed and ordered.

! WARNING Monitor patient for signs and symptoms of myopathy such as muscle pain, tenderness, or weakness in conjunction with an elevated creatine kinase. Because drug can cause rhabdomyolysis, expect drug to be discontinued if myopathy is suspected.

- Monitor liver enzymes before and during ezetimibe therapy, as ordered. Expect drug to be discontinued if liver enzyme elevations are equal to or greater than three times the upper normal limit.

PATIENT TEACHING

- Direct patient to follow a low-cholesterol diet as an adjunct to ezetimibe therapy. Recommend weight loss and exercise programs, as appropriate.
- Instruct patient, family, or caregiver how to administer ezetimibe and what to do if a dose is missed.

! WARNING Inform patient an allergic reaction may occur with drug use. Tell patient to notify prescriber if present and, if severe, to seek immediate medical care.

! WARNING Advise patient to report unexplained muscle pain, tenderness, or weakness.

- Stress importance to females of childbearing age to notify prescriber if pregnancy occurs as drug might need to be discontinued. If patient is also taking a statin, drug will have to be discontinued.
- Inform mothers wishing to breastfeed that breastfeeding is not recommended during ezetimibe therapy and is contraindicated if patient is also taking a statin.

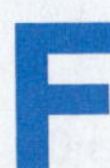

famciclovir

Class and Category

Pharmacologic class: Nucleoside analogue
Therapeutic class: Antiviral

Indications and Dosages

✷ *To treat recurrent episodes of herpes labialis*

TABLETS

Immunocompetent adults. 1,500 mg as a single dose at first sign of burning, itching, lesion formation, pain, or tingling.

✷ *To treat recurrent episodes of genital herpes*

TABLETS

Immunocompetent adult. 1,000 mg twice a day for 1 day beginning at the first sign of a recurrent episode (burning, itching, lesion formation, pain, or tingling).

✷ *To suppress chronic recurrent episodes of genital herpes*

TABLETS

Immunocompetent adults. 250 mg twice daily.

✷ *To treat herpes zoster*

TABLETS

Immunocompetent adults. 500 mg every 8 hr for 7 days and initiated as soon as herpes zoster is diagnosed.

✷ *To treat recurrent episodes of genital or orolabial herpes in HIV-infected patients*

TABLETS

Adults. 500 mg twice daily for 7 days beginning at the first sign of a recurrent episode (burning, itching, lesion formation, pain, tingling).

± **DOSAGE ADJUSTMENT** For patients with renal impairment, dosage decreased and/or dosage interval increased depending on the creatinine clearance level at the time of treatment and the herpes condition being treated.

Drug Administration

P.O.

- Administer drug without regard to meals.

Route	Onset	Peak	Duration
P.O.	Unknown	1 hr	Unknown

Half-life: 2.4 hr as penciclovir

Mechanism of Action

Inhibits herpes viral DNA synthesis and replication selectively.

Contraindications

Hypersensitivity to famciclovir or its components, use of penciclovir cream

Interactions

DRUGS

drugs eliminated by active renal tubular secretion, such as probenecid: Possibly increased plasma concentration of famciclovir, with increased risk of adverse reactions

Adverse Reactions

CNS: Confusion, dizziness, fatigue, hallucinations, headache, migraine, paresthesia, **seizures**, somnolence
CV: **Hypersensitivity vasculitis**, palpitations
GI: Abdominal pain, cholestatic jaundice, diarrhea, elevated bilirubin levels, elevated liver or pancreatic enzymes, flatulence, nausea, vomiting
GU: **Acute renal failure**, dysmenorrhea, elevated serum creatinine
HEME: Anemia, **leukopenia**, **neutropenia**, **thrombocytopenia**
SKIN: **Erythema multiforme**, pruritus, rash, **Stevens-Johnson syndrome**, **toxic epidermal necrolysis**, urticaria
Other: **Anaphylaxis**, **angioedema**

Childbearing Considerations

PREGNANCY

- Pregnancy exposure registry: 1-888-669-6682.
- It is not known if drug causes fetal harm.
- Use with caution only if benefit to mother outweighs potential risk to fetus.

LACTATION

- It is not known if drug is present in breast milk.
- Patient should check with prescriber before breastfeeding.
- Mothers with HIV infection should not breastfeed.

F

Nursing Considerations

! **WARNING** Determine patient's level of renal function prior to initiating famciclovir therapy, as ordered. Be aware that dosage adjustment must be made in patients with renal impairment. Acute renal failure has occurred in patients with underlying renal disease who have received inappropriately high doses of famciclovir for their level of renal function. Monitor renal function closely throughout therapy.

- Use cautiously in patients with hepatic impairment because conversion of famciclovir to its active metabolite may be impaired, resulting in a lower plasma concentration and possibly decreased effectiveness of the drug.

! **WARNING** Monitor patient for a hypersensitivity reaction, which could become life threatening such as anaphylaxis and angioedema. If present, notify prescriber, expect drug to be discontinued, and provide supportive care, as needed and ordered.

! **WARNING** Monitor patient for seizures that may be drug induced.

! **WARNING** Monitor patient's CBC regularly, as ordered, because famciclovir may cause serious adverse hematological reactions. Monitor patient for bleeding, bruising, or infections. Alert prescriber, if present.

PATIENT TEACHING

- Instruct patient how to administer famciclovir.
- Alert patient that famciclovir contains lactose and to alert prescriber if lactose intolerant before taking the drug.
- Remind patient that famciclovir should be initiated as soon as possible after a recurrent onset of a herpes-related condition exhibited by sensations of burning, itching, pain, tingling, or when a lesion has appeared.
- Inform patient that famciclovir is not a cure for herpes. Because genital herpes is a sexually transmitted disease, instruct patient to avoid intercourse when lesions and/or symptoms are present, to avoid infecting partners. Remind patient, however, that genital herpes is frequently transmitted in the absence of symptoms and therefore patient should always engage in safe sex practices.

! **WARNING** Tell patient that drug may cause an allergic reaction. If present, tell patient to notify prescriber and, if severe, to seek immediate medical care.

- Instruct patient to notify prescriber at once if she experiences serious adverse reactions, such as bleeding, bruising, confusion, feeling short of breath, increased thirst, infections, pounding heartbeats, swelling, urinating less than usual or not at all, weakness, or weight gain.
- Advise patient to avoid hazardous activities such as driving until the CNS effects of the drug are known and resolved.
- Tell mothers with HIV not to breastfeed their infant.

famotidine

Pepcid, Pepcid AC, Zantac 360

Class and Category

Pharmacologic class: Histamine-2 blocker
Therapeutic class: Antiulcer agent

Indications and Dosages

∗ *To provide short-term treatment of active duodenal ulcer*

ORAL SUSPENSION

Adults. 40 mg once daily or 20 mg twice daily up to 8 wk.

CHEWABLE TABLETS, TABLETS

Adults and children weighing 40 kg (88 lb) or more. 40 mg once daily or 20 mg twice daily up to 8 wk.

∗ *To prevent recurrence of duodenal ulcer*

CHEWABLE TABLETS, ORAL SUSPENSION, TABLETS

Adults. 20 mg once daily up to 1 yr.

∗ *To provide short-term treatment for active, benign gastric ulcer*

ORAL SUSPENSION

Adults. 40 mg once daily up to 8 wk.

CHEWABLE TABLETS, TABLETS

Adults and children weighing 40 kg (88 lb) or more. 40 mg once daily up to 8 wk.

✱ *To treat gastroesophageal reflux disease (GERD)*

ORAL SUSPENSION

Adults. 20 mg twice daily for up to 6 wk.
Children ages 1 to 17. 0.5 mg/kg twice daily for 6 to 12 wk. *Maximum:* 40 mg twice daily.
Infants ages 3 mo to 1 yr. *Initial:* 0.5 mg/kg twice daily for up to 8 wk, increased to 1 mg/kg twice daily, as needed. *Maximum:* 40 mg/day.
Infants ages less than 3 mo. 0.5 mg/kg once daily for up to 8 wk, increased to 1 mg/kg once daily, as needed.

✱ *To treat symptomatic nonerosive GERD*

CHEWABLE TABLETS, ORAL SUSPENSION, TABLETS

Adults and children weighing 40 kg (88 lb) or more. 20 mg twice daily up to 6 wk.

✱ *To treat erosive esophagitis due to GERD diagnosed by endoscopy*

ORAL SUSPENSION

Adults. 20 or 40 mg twice daily for up to 12 wk.

CHEWABLE TABLETS, TABLETS

Adults and children weighing 40 kg (88 lb) or more. 20 or 40 mg twice daily for up to 12 wk.

✱ *To treat pediatric peptic ulcer disease*

CHEWABLE TABLETS, ORAL SUSPENSION, TABLETS

Children ages 1 to 17. *Initial:* 0.5 mg/kg once daily or 0.25 mg/kg twice daily for 8 wk, increased to 1 mg/kg once daily or 0.5 mg/kg twice daily, as needed. *Maximum:* 40 mg/day.

✱ *To treat gastric hypersecretory conditions, such as Zollinger-Ellison syndrome*

CHEWABLE TABLETS, ORAL SUSPENSION, TABLETS

Adults. *Initial:* 20 mg every 6 hr. Dosage adjusted, as needed, based on patient response. *Maximum:* 160 mg every 6 hr.

✱ *To treat hospitalized patients with intractable ulcers or pathological hypersecretory conditions; to treat patients who are unable to take oral medication*

I.V. INFUSION OR INJECTION

Adults. 20 mg every 12 hr.
Children ages 1 to 16. *Initial:* 0.25 mg/kg every 12 hr. *Maximum:* 40 mg daily.

✱ *To prevent heartburn and indigestion*

CHEWABLE TABLETS, TABLETS

Adults. 10 mg 1 hr before eating. *Maximum:* 20 mg every 24 hr for up to 2 wk.

✱ *To treat heartburn and indigestion*

CHEWABLE TABLETS, TABLETS

Adults. 10 mg at onset of symptoms. *Maximum:* 20 mg every 24 hr for up to 2 wk unless prescribed otherwise.

± **DOSAGE ADJUSTMENT** For patients with renal insufficiency and creatinine clearance less than 60 ml/min, oral or parenteral dosage reduced or dosing interval increased to 48 hours, as needed.

F

Drug Administration

P.O.

- Drug should be taken once daily at bedtime or twice daily in the morning and before bedtime.
- Reconstitute oral suspension by slowly adding 46 ml of Purified Water. Shake vigorously for 5 to 10 sec immediately after adding the water and immediately before use. Store at room temperature. Discard after 30 days.
- Chewable tablets should be chewed thoroughly before swallowing.
- Tablets should be swallowed whole and not chewed, crushed, or split.

I.V.

- Store drug in refrigerator until ready to administer.
- For I.V. injection, dilute 2 ml (20 mg) of drug with 0.9 Sodium Chloride for Injection, 5% or 10% Dextrose Injection, 5% Sodium Bicarbonate Injection, Lactated Ringer's Injection, or Sterile Water for Injection to a total volume of either 5 or 10 ml. Inject over no less than 2 min.
- For I.V. infusion, dilute 2 ml (20 mg) of drug with 100 ml of 5% Dextrose Injection or other compatible intravenous solution mentioned above. Infuse over 15 to 30 min. Although manufacturer's guidelines state diluted solution may be

stored for 7 days at room temperature there is a concern about the maintenance of sterility after dilution. Therefore, it is recommended that diluted solutions be refrigerated, if not used immediately and used within 48 hr. If diluted solution is stored in refrigerator, allow solution to warm to room temperature before infusing drug.

- Drug also comes as a premixed solution ready for infusion administration. Check container for minute leaks prior to use by squeezing the bag firmly. Solution must be clear and seal intact to use. Do not administer with plastic containers in series connections.
- *Incompatibilities:* Amphotericin B, azithromycin, cefepime, furosemide (at 2 mg/ml), piperacillin-tazobactam

Route	Onset	Peak	Duration
P.O.	< 1 hr	1–4 hr	10–12 hr
I.V.	< 30 min	20 min	10–12 hr

Half-life: 2.5–3.5 hr

Contraindications

Hypersensitivity to famotidine, other H_2-receptor antagonists, or their components

Interactions

DRUGS

drugs dependent on gastric pH for absorption: Reduced absorption of these drugs
tizanidine: Possibly substantial increase in blood tizanidine levels with increased risk of adverse reactions

Adverse Reactions

CNS: Agitation (infants), anxiety, asthenia, confusion, delirium, depression, dizziness, fatigue, fever, hallucinations, headache, insomnia, lethargy, mental or mood changes, paresthesia, **seizures**, somnolence
CV: **Arrhythmias**, **AV block**, palpitations, **prolonged QT interval**
EENT: Dry mouth, **laryngeal edema**, taste alteration, tinnitus
GI: Abdominal pain, anorexia, cholestatic jaundice, constipation, diarrhea, elevated liver enzymes, **hepatitis**, jaundice, nausea, vomiting
GU: Decreased libido, impotence
HEME: **Agranulocytosis**, **aplastic anemia**, **leukopenia**, **neutropenia**, **pancytopenia**, **thrombocytopenia**
MS: Arthralgia, muscle cramps, musculoskeletal pain, **rhabdomyolysis**
RESP: **Bronchospasm**, dyspnea, **interstitial pneumonia**, wheezing

Mechanism of Action

Know that with normal digestion, parietal cells in the gastric epithelium secrete hydrogen (H^+) ions, which combine with chloride ions (Cl^-) to form hydrochloric acid (HCl), as shown below left. However, HCl can inflame, ulcerate, and perforate gastric and intestinal mucosa normally protected by mucus. Famotidine, an H_2-receptor antagonist, reduces HCl formation by preventing histamine from binding with H_2 receptors on the surface of parietal cells, as shown below right. By doing so, the drug helps prevent peptic ulcers from forming and helps heal existing ones.

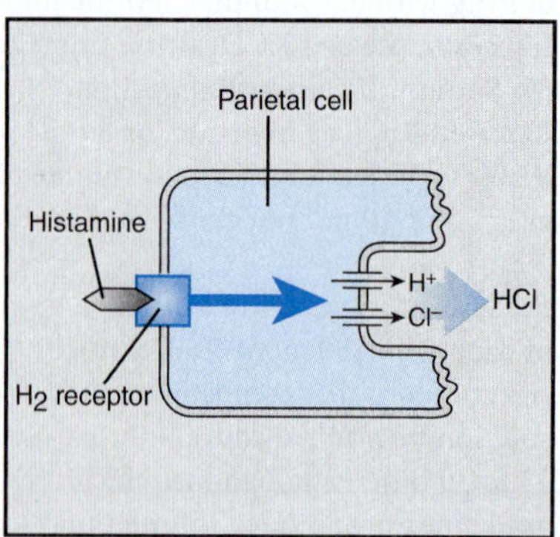

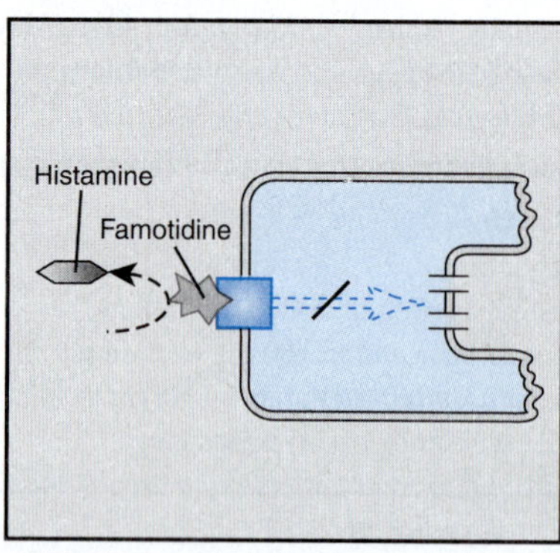

SKIN: Acne, alopecia, dry skin, **erythema multiforme**, **exfoliative dermatitis**, flushing, pruritus, rash, **Stevens-Johnson syndrome**, **toxic epidermal necrolysis**, urticaria
Other: **Anaphylaxis**, **angioedema**, hyperuricemia

Childbearing Considerations

PREGNANCY

- It is not known if drug causes fetal harm.
- Use with caution only if benefit to mother outweighs potential risk to fetus.

LACTATION

- Drug is present in breast milk.
- Mothers should check with prescriber before breastfeeding.

Nursing Considerations

! **WARNING** Be aware that Pepcid AC chewable tablets contain aspartame, and should not be given to patients who have phenylketonuria.

! **WARNING** Monitor patient for hypersensitivity reactions, which could be life-threatening such as anaphylaxis and angioedema. Notify prescriber, if present, expect drug to be discontinued, and provide supportive care, as needed and ordered.

! **WARNING** Know that adult patients who have a suboptimal response, or an early symptomatic relapse after completing famotidine therapy, should be evaluated for gastric malignancy.

! **WARNING** Know that, although rare, drug may cause serious to life threatening hematologic adverse reactions. Monitor patient's CBC regularly throughout drug therapy, as ordered, and report any abnormal findings.

PATIENT TEACHING

- Instruct patient how to administer form of famotidine prescribed.
- Caution patient to avoid alcohol and smoking during famotidine therapy because they irritate the stomach and can delay ulcer healing.
- Caution patient not to take famotidine with other acid-reducing products.

! **WARNING** Advise patient drug may cause allergic reactions that could be quite serious. If present, tell patient to notify prescriber and to seek immediate medical care, if serious. Also, have patient report signs of bleeding, including GI bleeding such as bloody vomit or black stools to prescriber, which could become life-threatening.

- Caution patient, especially the elderly and patients with renal impairment, to avoid hazardous activities until drug's CNS effects are known and resolved.

febuxostat

Uloric

Class and Category

Pharmacologic class: Xanthine oxidase inhibitor
Therapeutic class: Antigout

Indications and Dosages

* *To treat chronic hyperuricemia in patients with gout, in patients who have an inadequate response to a maximally titrated dose of allopurinol, who are intolerant to allopurinol, or for whom treatment with allopurinol is not advisable*

TABLETS

Adults. *Initial:* 40 mg once daily, increased after 2 wk to 80 mg once daily, as needed.

± **DOSAGE ADJUSTMENT** For patients with severe renal impairment (creatinine clearance less than 30 ml/min), dosage limited to 40 mg once daily.

Drug Administration

P.O.

- Tablets can be taken with or without food.

Route	Onset	Peak	Duration
P.O.	Unknown	1–1.5 hr	Unknown

Half-life: 5–8 hr

Mechanism of Action

Inhibits the action of xanthine oxidase, the key enzyme responsible for purine breakdown. Xanthine oxidase catalyzes conversion of xanthine to uric acid, thereby increasing uric acid levels. High uric acid levels cause gout attacks. Inhibiting xanthine oxidase causes uric acid levels to drop, decreasing the risk of gout attack.

Contraindications

Concurrent use of azathioprine or mercaptopurine, hypersensitivity to febuxostat or its components

Interactions

DRUGS

azathioprine, mercaptopurine, theophylline: Possibly increased serum levels of these drugs, leading to toxicity

Adverse Reactions

CNS: Aggression, **CVA**, dizziness, hemiparesis, **lacunar infarction**, psychotic behavior, transient ischemic attack
CV: Angina, chest pain or discomfort, **ECG abnormalities**, **MI**
EENT: Blurred vision, deafness, epistaxis, nasal dryness, paranasal sinus hypersecretion, **pharyngeal edema**, sneezing, taste disturbance, throat irritation, tinnitus
ENDO: Breast pain, gynecomastia, hot flashes, **hypoglycemia**
GI: Diarrhea, dyspepsia, elevated liver enzymes, GI discomfort, **hepatic failure**, hepatomegaly, jaundice, nausea, vomiting
GU: Decreased libido, erectile dysfunction, hematuria, nephrolithiasis, pollakiuria, proteinuria, **renal failure or insufficiency**, tubulointerstitial nephritis, urgency
HEME: **Agranulocytosis**, anemia, eosinophilia, **idiopathic thrombocytopenic purpura**, leukocytosis, **leukopenia**, **neutropenia**, **pancytopenia**, splenomegaly, **thrombocytopenia**
MS: Arthralgia, joint stiffness or swelling, **rhabdomyolysis**
RESP: Upper respiratory tract infection
SKIN: Dermatitis, eczema, **erythema multiforme**, flushing, hair color or growth changes, hyperhidrosis, peeling skin, petechiae, photosensitivity, pruritis, rash, **Stevens-Johnson syndrome**, **toxic epidermal necrolysis**, urticaria
Other: **Anaphylaxis and other hypersensitivity reactions**, **drug reaction with eosinophilia and systemic symptoms (DRESS)**, gout flares

Childbearing Considerations

PREGNANCY

- It is not known if drug causes fetal harm.
- Use with caution only if benefit to mother outweighs potential risk to fetus.

LACTATION

- It is not known if drug is present in breast milk.
- Mothers should check with prescriber before breastfeeding.

Nursing Considerations

- Know that febuxostat therapy is not recommended for patients in whom rate of urate formation is greatly increased, as in malignancy and its treatment or Lesch-Nyhan syndrome.
- Obtain a liver test panel, as ordered, prior to initiating febuxostat therapy and then periodically thereafter. Monitor patient for signs and symptoms of liver dysfunction, such as anorexia, dark urine, fatigue, jaundice, or right upper abdominal discomfort throughout therapy. If signs and symptoms occur or if abnormal liver tests occur, especially an elevated serum alanine aminotransferase (ALT) level greater than 3 times the upper normal limit, notify prescriber and expect drug to be withheld until underlying cause is determined. If no other cause can be found other than febuxostat therapy, expect drug to be discontinued permanently.
- Monitor patient's serum uric acid level, as prescribed, to determine drug effectiveness. Expect it to take about 2 weeks for uric acid level to be therapeutically altered. Dose may be increased from 40 to 80 mg daily if target serum uric acid level fails to fall below 6 mg/dl.
- Monitor patient for gout flares, which may occur after therapy is started because of changing serum uric acid levels that result in mobilization of urate from tissue deposits. Expect prescriber to order colchicine or an NSAID when febuxostat therapy starts. If patient has a gout flare-up during treatment, notify prescriber and expect symptoms to be managed. Know that febuxostat therapy usually isn't discontinued during this time.

! WARNING Assess patient for hypersensitivity reactions and skin for abnormalities. At first sign of hypersensitivity or rash (DRESS may only initially present with fever or swollen lymph nodes) notify prescriber and expect drug to be discontinued because febuxostat may cause severe reactions. Also, know that patients who have experienced hypersensitivity reactions to allopurinol may be at increased risk of developing serious skin reactions to febuxostat. Provide supportive care, as needed and ordered.

! WARNING Monitor patient with established cardiovascular disease because use of febuxostat increases the risk of death from cardiovascular conditions. Also, monitor patient for evidence of cardiovascular thrombosis, such as acute MI or stroke, because drug may increase patient's risk of developing these disorders, which may result in death.

PATIENT TEACHING

- Instruct patient how to administer febuxostat.
- Inform patient that a gout attack may occur when febuxostat therapy starts and that colchicine or a NSAID may be prescribed, usually along with febuxostat, to treat it.

! WARNING Advise patient to notify prescriber at first sign of an allergic reaction or skin reactions such as a fever, rash, or swollen lymph nodes. If serious, urge patient to seek immediate medical care.

! WARNING Instruct patient to seek immediate emergency care for signs or symptoms of a heart attack or stroke.

! WARNING Tell patient to alert prescriber if persistent, serious, or unusual adverse reactions occur, especially anorexia, dark urine, fatigue, jaundice, or right upper abdominal discomfort.

- Tell patient that periodic blood tests will be needed to determine drug's effectiveness and to detect adverse effects.

felodipine

Class and Category

Pharmacologic class: Calcium channel blocker
Therapeutic class: Antihypertensive

Indications and Dosages

∗ *To manage mild to moderate hypertension alone or with other antihypertensives*

E.R. TABLETS

Adults. *Initial:* 5 mg daily. Dosage adjusted no sooner than every 2 wk, as needed. *Maintenance:* 2.5 to 10 mg daily based on patient response.

±**DOSAGE ADJUSTMENT** For patients over age 65, initial dosage reduced to 2.5 mg daily. For patients with impaired liver function, dosage may have to be reduced based on blood pressure.

Drug Administration

P.O.

- Administer on an empty stomach or with a light meal (low in carbohydrates and fat).
- Do not administer with grapefruit juice.
- Tablets should be swallowed whole and not chewed, crushed, or split.
- Store drug at room temperature and protect it from light.

Route	Onset	Peak	Duration
P.O.	2–5 hr	2.5–5 hr	24 hr

Half-life: 11–16 hr

Mechanism of Action

May slow the movement of extracellular calcium into myocardial and vascular smooth-muscle cells by deforming calcium channels in cell membranes, inhibiting ion-controlled gating mechanisms, and interfering with calcium release from the sarcoplasmic reticulum. The effect of these actions is a decrease in intracellular calcium ions, which inhibits contraction of smooth-muscle cells and dilates coronary and systemic arteries. As with other calcium channel blockers, felodipine's actions result in increased oxygen to the myocardium and reduced afterload, blood pressure, and peripheral resistance.

Contraindications

Hypersensitivity to felodipine, other dihydropyridine calcium channel blockers, or their components

Interactions

DRUGS

antihypertensives: Increased risk of hypotension
cimetidine, erythromycin itraconazole, ketoconazole: Increased felodipine level and effects

clarithromycin: Increased risk of acute kidney injury in elderly patients
CYP3A4 inducers (long term), such as carbamazepine, phenobarbital, phenytoin: Decreased felodipine levels
CYP3A4 substrates, such as benzodiazepines, flecainide, imipramine, propafenone, terfenadine, theophylline: Increased felodipine plasma concentrations
metoprolol: Possible altered pharmacokinetics of metoprolol
tacrolimus: Possibly increased blood tacrolimus level and risk of adverse effects

ACTIVITIES

alcohol use: Induced vasodilation enhancing the effects of felodipine and increasing risk of hypotension

FOODS

grapefruit juice: Significant increase in felodipine levels, increasing risk of hypotension
high carbohydrate or fat diet: Significantly increased felodipine bioavailability with increased risk of hypotension

Adverse Reactions

CNS: Asthenia, dizziness, drowsiness, fatigue, headache, paresthesia, syncope, weakness
CV: Chest pain, **hypotension**, palpitations, peripheral edema, tachycardia
EENT: Gingival hyperplasia, pharyngitis, rhinitis
GI: Abdominal cramps, constipation, diarrhea, indigestion, nausea
HEME: **Agranulocytosis**
MS: Back pain
RESP: Cough
SKIN: Flushing, rash

Childbearing Considerations

PREGNANCY

- It is not known if drug causes fetal harm. However, animal studies have shown the possibility of digital anomalies.
- While manufacturer makes no recommendations regarding use during pregnancy, some authorities recommend not to use the drug during pregnancy.

LACTATION

- It is not known if drug is present in breast milk.
- Drug or breastfeeding should be discontinued.

REPRODUCTION

- Females of childbearing age should use effective contraception throughout drug therapy.

Nursing Considerations

! **WARNING** Use felodipine cautiously in patients with heart failure or reduced ventricular function.

! **WARNING** Monitor blood pressure during dosage titration and throughout felodipine therapy for effectiveness of drug or detection of hypotension, especially in elderly patients. Be aware that felodipine may cause severe hypotension with syncope, which may lead to reflex tachycardia. This can precipitate angina in patients with coronary artery disease or a history of angina.

! **WARNING** Watch for signs of overdose, such as excessive peripheral vasodilation, marked hypotension, and, possibly, bradycardia. If they appear, place patient in supine position with legs elevated and give I.V. fluids, as ordered. Expect to give I.V. atropine for bradycardia, if ordered.

PATIENT TEACHING

- Instruct patient how to administer felodipine.
- Caution patient not to drink grapefruit juice during therapy.

! **WARNING** Instruct patient to monitor pulse rate and blood pressure. Advise patient to notify prescriber immediately if palpitations, pronounced dizziness, or swelling of hands or feet occur.

- Teach patient how to minimize gingival hyperplasia.
- Instruct females of childbearing age to use effective contraception thoughout drug therapy and to notify prescriber if pregnancy occurs.
- Tell mothers not to breastfeed during drug therapy.

fenofibrate

Antara (micronized), Fenoglide, Lipofen, Tricor, Triglide

fenofibrate choline

Trilipix

fenofibric acid

Fibricor

Class and Category

Pharmacologic class: Fibrate
Therapeutic class: Antilipemic

Indications and Dosages

✻ *To treat primary hypercholesterolemia or mixed hyperlipidemia*

CAPSULES (LIPOFEN)

Adults. 150 mg daily.

CAPSULES (ANTARA)

Adults. 130 mg daily.

D.R. CAPSULES (TRILIPIX)

Adults. 135 mg daily.

TABLETS (TRICOR)

Adults. 145 mg daily.

TABLETS (FIBRICOR)

Adults. 105 mg daily.

TABLETS (TRIGLIDE)

Adults. 160 mg daily.

TABLETS (FENOGLIDE)

Adults. 120 mg daily.

✻ *As adjunct to diet to treat severe hypertriglyceridemia*

CAPSULES (ANTARA)

Adults. *Initial:* 43 mg or 130 mg once daily, adjusted as needed, at 4- to 8-wk intervals.

CAPSULES (LIPOFEN)

Adults. *Initial:* 50 to 150 mg daily, increased, as needed, at 4- to 8-wk intervals. *Maximum:* 150 mg daily.

D.R. CAPSULES (TRILIPIX)

Adults. *Initial:* 45 to 135 mg once daily, increased, as needed, at 4- to 8-wk intervals. *Maximum:* 135 mg daily.

TABLETS (FIBRICOR)

Adults. *Initial:* 35 to 105 mg daily, increased, as needed, at 4- to 8-wk intervals. *Maximum:* 105 mg daily.

TABLETS (TRICOR)

Adults. *Initial:* 48 to 145 mg daily, increased, as needed, at 4- to 8-wk intervals. *Maximum:* 145 mg daily.

TABLETS (TRIGLIDE)

Adults. 160 mg daily, *Maximum:* 160 mg daily.

TABLETS (FENOGLIDE)

Adults. 40 to 120 mg daily, increased, as needed, at 4- to 8-wk intervals. *Maximum:* 120 mg daily.

± **DOSAGE ADJUSTMENT** For patients with mild to moderate renal impairment or elderly patients, dosage limited for all indications to lowest dosage prescribed with increase only after drug's therapeutic and renal effects are known. For patients with mild to moderate renal impairment,Triglide should not be used because it does not come in the lower dosages needed by these patients.

Drug Administration

P.O.

- Administer drug consistently with or without food except for Fenoglide and Lipofen, which have to be given with food to enhance absorption.
- Administer drug 1 hr before or 4 hr after bile acid sequestrants.
- Capsules and tablets must be swallowed whole and not chewed, crushed, or split/opened. Do not administer broken or chipped tablets.
- Protect from moisture. Fibricor, Lipofen, and Triglide should also be protected from light.
- Follow specific manufacturer's instructions if a dose is missed.

Route	Onset	Peak	Duration
P.O.	2 wk	6–8 wk	Unknown

Half-life: 20 hr

Mechanism of Action

May increase the lipolysis of triglyceride-rich lipoproteins and decrease the synthesis of fatty acids and triglycerides by enhancing the activation of lipoprotein lipase and acyl-coenzyme A synthetase. Fenofibrate also may:

- increase hepatic elimination of cholesterol as bile salts.

F

- promote the catabolism of larger, less dense LDLs with a high-binding affinity for cellular LDL receptors.

Contraindications

Active liver disease (Triglide); gallbladder disease; dialysis; hypersensitivity to fenofibrate, fenofibric acid, or their components; severe hepatic impairment, including primary biliary cirrhosis, and unexplained persistently elevated liver enzymes; severe renal impairment (eGFR less than 30 ml/min including end-stage renal disease)

Interactions

DRUGS

bile acid sequestrants: Decreased fenofibrate absorption
colchicine: Increased risk of myopathy and rhabdomyolysis
coumarin anticoagulants: Increased risk of bleeding
immunosuppressants, such as cyclosporine and tacrolimus: Increased risk of nephrotoxicity

FOODS

all foods: Increased fenofibrate bioavailability when given in capsule form

Adverse Reactions

CNS: Asthenia, fatigue, headache
CV: **Deep vein thrombosis**, severely depressed HDL cholesterol levels
EENT: Rhinitis
GI: Abdominal pain, cholelithiasis, **cirrhosis**, constipation, diarrhea, elevated bilirubin or liver enzymes, **hepatitis**, **hepatotoxicity**, nausea, **pancreatitis**
GU: **Acute renal failure**, increased serum creatinine level
HEME: **Agranulocytosis**, anemia, **leukopenia**, **thrombocytopenia**
MS: Arthralgia, back pain, elevated creatinine phosphokinase, muscle spasms, myalgia, myopathy, myositis, **rhabdomyolysis**
RESP: **Interstitial lung disease**, **pulmonary embolus**
SKIN: Photosensitivity, rash, **Stevens-Johnson syndrome**, **toxic epidermal necrolysis**, urticaria
Other: **Anaphylaxis**, **angioedema**, **delayed hypersensitivity reactions**, **drug reaction with eosinophilia and systemic symptoms (DRESS)**, flu-like symptoms

Childbearing Considerations

PREGNANCY

- It is not known if drug causes fetal harm.
- Use with caution only if benefit to mother outweighs potential risk to fetus.

LACTATION

- It is not known if drug is present in breast milk.
- Mothers should not breastfeed during drug therapy; some manufacturers recommend to also avoid breastfeeding for 5 days after final dose.

Nursing Considerations

- Be aware that all drugs that increase serum triglycerides, such as beta-blockers, estrogens, and thiazides, should be stopped, and baseline lipid levels obtained before starting fenofibrate.
- Monitor results of liver function tests. If liver enzyme levels rise to more than 3 times the upper limit of normal and persist, or if the patient develops gallstones, expect to stop drug.
- Monitor patient's renal function, as elevations in serum creatinine levels have occurred with fenofibrate therapy. Know that if eGFR drops below 30 ml/min, the drug will have to be discontinued.
- Monitor serum cholesterol and triglyceride levels at 4- to 8-week intervals, as ordered. If levels don't decrease after 2 months at maximum dosage, expect therapy to be discontinued.

! **WARNING** Monitor patient closely for hypersensitivity reactions, including severe skin reactions often initially seen as a rash although DRESS may initially only present with a fever or swollen lymph nodes. Also, monitor patient for delayed cutaneous hypersensitivity reactions that may be severe and can occur days to weeks after fenofibrate therapy is initiated. Notify prescriber, if present, expect drug to be discontinued, and provide supportive care, as needed and ordered.

! **WARNING** Assess blood counts periodically, as ordered, during first 12 months of therapy to detect adverse hematologic effects that could become life-threatening.

! **WARNING** Watch closely for evidence of deep vein thrombosis (pain, redness in extremity, or swelling) or pulmonary embolus (sudden onset of anxiety, restlessness, or shortness of breath) because risk is higher in patients taking fenofibrate. Notify prescriber immediately, and start emergency treatment, as prescribed.

! **WARNING** Monitor patient for myopathy (muscle pain, tenderness, or weakness) associated with an elevated creatine kinase. Risk factors for myopathy include being 65 years of age or older, concomitant use of certain drugs, or presence of renal impairment, or uncontrolled hypothyroidism. The life-threatening complications of rhabdomyolysis may occur. Expect to monitor patient's creatine kinase levels, as ordered and notify prescriber if markedly elevated because drug will need to be discontinued.

PATIENT TEACHING

- Instruct patient how to administer form of drug prescribed and what to do if a dose is missed.
- Emphasize importance of carefully following prescriber's instructions about diet and exercise as drug is not a substitute for diet and exercise.
- Advise patient to comply with ordered laboratory tests, as directed, to determine drug's effectiveness and to detect certain adverse drug reactions. Tell patient tests typically include a lipid profile periodically throughout therapy, liver function tests after 3 to 6 months, hematocrit and hemoglobin levels, and WBC counts periodically during first year.

! **WARNING** Tell patient drug may cause an allergic reaction or severe skin reaction. Advise patient to notify prescriber immediately at the first sign of an allergic reaction, including a fever, rash, or swollen lymph nodes and, if serious, to seek immediate medical care.

! **WARNING** Urge patient to notify prescriber immediately about chills, fever, or sore throat. Also, urge her to tell prescriber about unexplained muscle pain, tenderness, or weakness, especially if accompanied by fatigue or fever and signs and symptoms of liver injury, such as abdominal pain, abnormal stool, dark urine, itching, malaise, or yellowing of skin or white portion of eyes.

! **WARNING** Tell patient to seek emergency treatment if he develops pain, swelling, and redness in his limb or sudden shortness of breath, anxiety, and restlessness.

- Instruct patient to use sunscreen and protective clothing while in sun and to limit time spent in sun because photosensitivity may occur weeks to months after drug is initiated.
- Tell mothers breastfeeding should not be undertaken during drug therapy and for possibly 5 days after drug is discontinued.

F

fentanyl citrate

Actiq, Fentora

fentanyl transdermal system

Class, Category, and Schedule

Pharmacologic class: Opioid
Therapeutic class: Opioid analgesic
Controlled substance schedule: II

Indications and Dosages

* *To provide surgical premedication*

I.M. INJECTION

Adults. 0.05 to 0.1 mg 30 to 60 min before surgery.

* *As adjunct to regional anesthesia*

I.V. OR I.M. INJECTION

Adults. 0.05 to 0.1 mg, as needed. I.V. injection given slowly over 1 to 2 min.

* *To induce and maintain anesthesia*

I.V. OR I.M. INJECTION

Children ages 2 to 12. 2 to 3 mcg/kg. I.V. injection given slowly.

* *To manage postoperative emergence delirium, pain, or tachypnea in postanesthesia care unit*

I.M. INJECTION

Adults. 0.05 to 0.1 mg. Repeated in 1 to 2 hr, as needed.

✱ *As adjunct to general anesthesia*

I.V. INJECTION

Adults. *For low-dose therapy:* 0.002 mg/kg followed by 0.002 mg/kg, as needed. *For moderate-dose therapy:* 0.002 to 0.02 mg/kg, followed by 0.025 to 0.1 mg, as needed. *For high-dose therapy:* 0.02 to 0.05 mg/kg followed by 0.025 mg to one-half initial loading dose, as needed. I.V. injection given slowly.

✱ *To treat breakthrough pain in cancer patients who are receiving around-the-clock opioid therapy and have developed tolerance to it*

TRANSMUCOSAL LOZENGE (ACTIQ)

Adults and adolescents ages 16 and older. *Initial:* 200 mcg and allowed to dissolve, followed by second dose 15 min after first dose is dissolved, as needed. Dosage increased according to patient's needs. *Maximum:* 2 doses of same strength per episode with at least 4 hr between episodes treated; once successful dosage has occurred, no more than 4 lozenges/day.

BUCCAL TABLETS (FENTORA)

Adults. *Initial:* 100 mcg, followed by second dose 30 min after first dose, as needed. Dosage increased to 200 mcg, as needed. Further increased to 400 mcg, as needed. Further titration done in multiples of 200 mcg, as needed, until maximum dose of 800 mcg per dose is reached. *Maximum:* 800 mcg given twice 30 min apart 4 times daily with at least 4 hr between each episode treated.

✱ *To relieve severe chronic pain in opioid-tolerant patient who doesn't respond to less potent drugs and requires around-the-clock opioid administration for an extended time*

TRANSDERMAL SYSTEM

Adults and children ages 2 and older. *Initial:* Highly individualized and based on current opioid therapy. Each patch may be worn for 48 to 72 hr. Dosage increased after first 72 hr and then every 6 days, as needed. For more than 100 mcg/hr, more than one patch required.

± **DOSAGE ADJUSTMENT** For cachectic, debilitated, or elderly patients, initial transdermal system dosage should not exceed 25 mcg/hr, unless patient is already receiving more of an equivalent dose of another opioid. For patients receiving long-term opioid therapy regardless of product used, dosage adjusted based on previous day's drug requirement. For patients with mild to moderate hepatic or renal failure regardless of product used, initial dosage reduced.

Drug Administration

- Do not substitute one form of fentanyl for another. Do not convert dosage to or from other products on a microgram-per-microgram basis because doing so may result in a fatal overdose.

P.O.

- For Actiq transmucosal form, open package just before use and save plastic cap for discarding the unused part of the lozenge. Have patient place lozenge between the cheek and gum and suck, not chew, on it for 15 min. Show her how to move lozenge from one side of her mouth to the other using the handle provided separately.
- For Fentora buccal tablets, have patient place tablet between the upper cheek and gum or under the tongue and allow to dissolve, which may take from 14 to 25 min. Tablet should not be chewed, crushed, sucked on, or swallowed. Do not have patient eat or drink anything until tablet is completely dissolved. However, if after 30 min, some remnants of the tablet(s) remain, the patient may swallow some water. If 2 tablets are needed, place one tablet on each side of mouth in buccal cavity. If 4 tablets are needed, place 2 tablets on each side of mouth in buccal cavity.

I.V.

- Administered only by persons specifically trained in the use of intravenous anesthetics.
- Have emergency resuscitative equipment and naloxone close at hand.
- As an I.V. injection, administer slowly (for regional anesthesia give over 1 to 2 min) directly into a vein or into the tubing of a freely flowing I.V. solution. If injected too rapidly, apnea may occur.
- *Incompatibilities:* None reported by manufacturer.

I.M.

- Administered only by persons specifically trained in the use of anesthetics.
- Inject into a large muscle.

TRANSDERMAL

- Choose a site with intact (not irritated or irradiated) skin on a flat surface, such as the chest, back, flank, or upper arm.
- If needed, clip, not shave, hair from the site and clean site with water (no soaps, lotions, oils, or alcohol). Dry area completely before applying patch.
- Do not apply transdermal patch if seal has been broken or the patch has been cut, damaged, or changed in any way because drug may be released too rapidly.
- Put on gloves and remove patch from package. Apply by pressing patch firmly in place with palm of hand for 30 sec, making sure edges are sealed. If applying more than one patch, the edges shouldn't touch or overlap.
- Remove gloves and wash hands immediately after application with soap and water.
- If patch loosens, tape edges down but do not cover the entire patch. If problems with adhesion still exists, overlay patch with a transparent adhesive film dressing.
- Avoid exposing patch to external heat sources such a a heating pad or electric blanket while patch is worn.
- When removing patch after 72 hr, fold it in half with adhesive sides together, and discard according to institutional guidelines.
- Do not reuse a site for at least 3 days.

Route	Onset	Peak	Duration
P.O.	1–3 min	Unknown	15–45 min
I.V.	1–2 min	3–5 min	30–60 min
I.M.	7–15 min	20–30 min	1–2 hr
Transdermal	12–24 hr	24–72 hr	1–4 days
Transmucosal	3–5 min	20–30 min	2–3 hr

Half-life: 7–18 hr

Mechanism of Action

Binds to opioid receptor sites in the CNS, altering perception of and emotional response to pain by inhibiting ascending pain pathways. Fentanyl may alter neurotransmitter release from afferent nerves responsive to painful stimuli, and it causes respiratory depression by acting directly on respiratory centers in the brainstem.

Contraindications

All forms: Hypersensitivity to fentanyl, alfentanil, sufentanil, or their components; intermittent pain; opioid nontolerance; significant respiratory depression; treatment of mild to moderate pain responsive to nonopioid drugs; upper airway obstruction
Buccal or transdermal form: Management of acute or postoperative pain including headache/migraine, opioid non-tolerant patients
Transdermal form: Hypersensitivity to adhesives; management of postoperative pain or pain that may be acute, intermittent, or mild, or pain in patients requiring opioid therapy for a short period of time; opioid non-tolerant patients

Interactions

DRUGS

anticholinergics: Increased risk of severe constipation and urinary retention
antimigraine agents; cyclobenzaprine; dextromethorphan; dolasetron; granisetron; linezolid; MAO inhibitors; metaxalone; methylene blue (I.V.); ondansetron; palonosetron; selected psychiatric drugs, such as amoxapine, buspirone, lithium, mirtazapine, nefazodone, trazodone, vilazodone; selective serotonin reuptake inhibitors; serotonin norepinephrine reuptake inhibitors; St. John's wort; tramadol; tricyclic antidepressants; triptans; tryptophan: Increased risk of serotonin syndrome
benzodiazepines, CNS depressants, muscle relaxants, other opioids, sedating antihistamines, tricyclic antidepressants: Increased risk of sedation and somnolence and severe respiratory depression
buprenorphine, butorphanol, nalbuphine, pentazocine: Decreased analgesic effect of fentanyl and possibly precipitation of withdrawal symptoms
CYP3A4 inducers, such as barbiturates, carbamazepine, efavirenz, glucocorticoids, modafinil, nevirapine, oxcarbazepine, phenytoin, pioglitazone, rifabutin, rifampin, St. John's wort, troglitazone: Possibly induced metabolism and increased clearance of fentanyl with decreased effectiveness and potential development of withdrawal syndrome in dependent patients

CYP3A4 inhibitors, such as amiodarone, amprenavir, aprepitant, cimetidine, clarithromycin, diltiazem, erythromycin, fluconazole, fosamprenavir, indinavir, itraconazole, ketoconazole, nefazodone, nelfinavir, ritonavir, saquinavir, telithromycin, troleandomycin, verapamil: Possibly increased opioid effect, leading to increased or prolonged adverse effects, including severe respiratory depression
diuretics: Possibly decreased efficacy of diuretics
MAO inhibitors: Possibly unpredictable or fatal effects if taken within 14 days

ACTIVITIES

alcohol use: Increased serum fentanyl level, possibly resulting in fatal overdose from CNS and respiratory depression and hypotension

FOODS

grapefruit juice: Increased blood fentanyl level

Adverse Reactions

CNS: Agitation, amnesia, anxiety, asthenia, ataxia, confusion, delusions, depression, dizziness, drowsiness, euphoria, fever, hallucinations, headache, lack of coordination, light-headedness, nervousness, paranoia, sedation, **seizures**, sleep disturbance, slurred speech, syncope, tremor, weakness, yawning
CV: **Asystole**, **bradycardia**, chest pain, edema, **hypotension**, orthostatic hypotension, tachycardia
EENT: Blurred vision, dental caries, dry mouth, gum-line erosion, **laryngospasm**, rhinitis, sneezing, tooth loss
ENDO: **Adrenal insufficiency (rare)**, androgen deficiency, **hypoglycemia**
GI: Anorexia, constipation, elevated serum amylase levels, ileus, indigestion, nausea, spasm of the sphincter of Oddi, vomiting
GU: Anorgasmia, decreased libido, ejaculatory difficulty, impotence, infertility, lack of menstruation, urinary hesitancy, urine retention
RESP: **Apnea**, **depressed cough reflex**, dyspnea, **hypoventilation**, **respiratory depression**
SKIN: Diaphoresis, **exfoliative dermatitis**, localized skin redness and swelling (with transdermal form), pruritus, rash
Other: **Anaphylaxis**, drug tolerance, drug withdrawal syndrome, physical or psychological dependence with long-term use, opioid-induced hyperalgesia (increase pain) and allodynia (increase in sensitivity to pain), weight loss

Childbearing Considerations

PREGNANCY

- It is not known if drug causes fetal harm. However, prolonged use during pregnancy may cause neonatal opioid withdrawal syndrome.
- Use with caution only if benefit to mother outweighs potential risk to fetus.

LABOR AND DELIVERY

- Drug may prolong labor.
- Drug crosses the placental barrier and may produce excessive sedation and respiratory depression in the neonate.
- Drug should not be used during labor and delivery.

LACTATION

- Drug is present in breast milk.
- Breastfeeding is not recommended during drug therapy.

REPRODUCTION

- Use of opioids for an extended period of time may reduce fertility in patient, both female and male patients. It is not known if effects on fertility are reversible.

Nursing Considerations

- Be aware that fentanyl is now only available through a restricted program called Risk Evaluation and Mitigation Strategy (REMS) because of the risk of accidental exposure, abuse, addiction, misuse, and overdose. In addition, under the Transmucosal Immediate-Release Fentanyl (TIRF) REMS program, healthcare professionals, outpatient departments, and pharmacies must enroll in the program to prescribe the drug to outpatients. Inpatient pharmacies must have policies and procedures in place to verify opioid tolerance for inpatients who require an immediate-release type of fentanyl while hospitalized.

! WARNING Monitor patients at risk for opioid abuse, such as those with mental illness or personal or family history of substance abuse. Monitor patient throughout therapy for fentanyl abuse or addiction. Monitor patient's intake of drug closely. Be aware that excessive use of fentanyl may lead to abuse, addiction, misuse, overdose, and possibly death.

! **WARNING** Monitor patient closely for evidence of an overdose, which may include cardiopulmonary arrest, hypoventilation, pupil constriction, respiratory and CNS depression, seizures, and shock. Give naloxone (possibly in repeated doses), as prescribed. Be prepared to assist with endotracheal intubation and mechanical ventilation and provide fluids and additional supportive care, as needed and ordered.

- Know that to achieve optimum pain control with the lowest possible fentanyl dose, also plan to give a nonopioid analgesic, such as acetaminophen, as prescribed.

! **WARNING** Know that fentanyl buccal or transmucosal form as well as the transdermal system should be used only in patients already receiving opioid therapy and with demonstrated opioid tolerance (taking for a week or longer of at least 60 mg of morphine daily, 30 mg of oral oxycodone daily, 8 mg of oral hydromorphone daily, or an equianalgesic dose of another opioid), and require at least a fentanyl dosage of 25 mcg/hour to manage their pain.

! **WARNING** Use with extreme caution in patients who may be susceptible to the intracranial effects of carbon dioxide retention, such as those with brain tumors, head injury, increased intracranial pressure, or impaired consciousness. Monitor these patients closely for signs of sedation and respiratory depression.

! **WARNING** Use with extreme caution in patients with significant chronic obstructive pulmonary disease or cor pulmonale and in patients having a substantially decreased respiratory reserve, hypoxia, hypercapnia, or preexisting respiratory depression because even therapeutic doses of fentanyl may decrease respiratory drive in these patients to the point of apnea. Monitor these patients closely when titrating fentanyl dosage, especially when using I.V. route because these patients are more sensitive to the drug's effects.

! **WARNING** Monitor patient's respiratory status closely, especially during the first 24 to 72 hours after therapy starts or with dosage increases because severe hypoventilation may occur without warning at any time during therapy. Patients at increased risk include cachectic, debilitated, or elderly patients. Respiratory depression can occur in patients even if the drug is not misused or abused. Be aware that significant amounts of fentanyl can be absorbed from the skin for 24 hours or more after a transdermal patch is removed. Monitor patient for at least 72 hours after patch has been removed for respiratory depression. Have emergency equipment available, including an opioid antagonist.

! **WARNING** Expect respiratory depressant effects to last longer than analgesic effects. Also, be prepared for residual drug to potentiate effects of subsequent doses. Residual drug can be detected for at least 6 hours after I.V. dose and 17 hours after other forms. Monitor patient closely for at least 24 hours after therapy ends.

! **WARNING** Monitor patient's blood pressure closely, especially after initiating or titrating dosage of fentanyl because drug may cause severe hypotension, including orthostatic hypotension and syncope in ambulatory patients. Patients at increased risk include patients with decreased blood volume or who receive concurrent administration of certain CNS depressant drugs such as general anesthetics or phenothiazine.

! **WARNING** Monitor patient for a hypersensitivity reaction, which could become life-threatening such as anaphylaxis. If present, notify prescriber immediately and expect to substitute drug for another analgesic, as ordered. Provide supportive care, as needed and ordered.

! **WARNING** Montior patient with a seizure disorder closely because fentanyl may increase frequency of seizures in these patients. Notify prescriber if patient experiences worsening of seizure control.

! **WARNING** Monitor patient for adrenal insufficiency. Although rare, it can be life-threatening. Monitor patient for anorexia, dizziness, fatigue, hypotension, nausea, vomiting, or weakness. Notify prescriber if adrenal insufficiency is suspected and expect diagnostic testing to be done. If diagnosis is confirmed, expect to administer corticosteroids and wean patient off fentanyl, if possible.

! **WARNING** Monitor patient's blood glucose level because hypoglycemia can occur, especially in patients with at least one predisposing risk factor such as diabetes.

! **WARNING** Be aware that if pregnant or breastfeeding mothers take fentanyl for an extended perioid of time, the newborn or breastfed infant may experience neonatal opioid withdrawal syndrome (NOWS). NOWS may be life-threatening and is exhibited in the neonate or infant as excessive or high-pitched crying, poor feeding, rapid breathing, and trembling,

! **WARNING** Be aware that fentanyl should only be used concomitantly with benzodiazepines or other CNS depressants in patients for whom other treatment options are inadequate. If prescribed together, expect dosing and duration of opioid to be limited. Monitor patient closely for signs and symptoms of a decrease in consciousness, including coma, profound sedation, and significant respiratory depression. Notify prescriber immediately and provide emergency supportive care, as death may occur.

! **WARNING** Monitor patient closely who is receiving concurrent CYP3A4 inhibitor therapy along with fentanyl because these drugs may result in an increase in plasma fentanyl concentrations, which could increase or prolong adverse drug effects and may cause sedation and potentially fatal respiratory depression. Notify prescriber immediately, if present. Be aware that discontinuation of CYP3A4 inducers can result in a fatal overdose of fentanyl. Monitor patients closely when CYP3A4 inducers are discontinued and expect fentanyl dosage to be adjusted.

! **WARNING** Know that many drugs may interact with opioids like fentanyl to cause serotonin syndrome. Monitor patient closely for signs and symptoms, such as agitation, diaphoresis, diarrhea, fever, hallucinations, labile blood pressure, muscle twitching or stiffness, nausea, shakiness, shivering, tachycardia, trouble with coordination, or vomiting. Notify prescriber at once because serotonin syndrome may be life-threatening. Be prepared to discontinue drug, if possible and ordered, and provide supportive care.

- Monitor patient who is receiving the drug via a transdermal system and who develops a fever for opioid adverse effects because a fever may increase fentanyl release from the system and increase skin permeability. If symptoms occur, notify prescriber and anticipate dosage may be decreased.
- Monitor patient for a paradoxical increase in pain or increased sensitivity to pain. Notify prescriber because dose may need to be decreased or opioid rotation prescribed.
- Be aware that for a patient with bradycardia, implement cardiac monitoring, as ordered, and assess heart rate and rhythm frequently during fentanyl therapy because drug may further slow heart rate.
- Monitor blood glucose level of diabetic patient receiving transdermal fentanyl because each unit contains about 2 g of sugar.
- Monitor patient for constipation that could become severe. Encourage fluid intake, if not contraindicated, and encourage increasing fiber in diet. If constipation occurs, alert prescriber as patient may need a stool softner or laxative.
- Monitor patients with biliary tract disease, including acute pancreatitis because fentanyl may worsen symptoms.
- Know that to prevent withdrawal symptoms after long-term use, expect to taper drug dosage gradually, as prescribed. Assess patient for withdrawal symptoms after dosage reduction or conversion to another opioid analgesic.

PATIENT TEACHING

- Instruct patient, family, or caregiver on the proper use of the fentanyl product prescribed and what safety guidelines to follow with administration.

! **WARNING** Warn patient not to take more drug than prescribed and not to take it longer than absolutely needed because excessive or prolonged use can lead to abuse, addiction, misuse, overdose, and possibly death. Instruct family or caregiver in the event of an overdose to keep naloxone in the home and how to use naloxone. Stress importance to call 911 if administered.

- Tell patient to inform prescriber if pain acutally increases with fentanyl administration or patient experiences increased sensitivity to pain.
- Instruct patient to avoid alcohol and other CNS depressants, including benzodiazepines during fentanyl therapy, unless prescribed.
- Tell patient not to stop drug abruptly, as dosage must be tapered to prevent return of pain or withdrawal symptoms.

! **WARNING** Alert patient that drug may cause an allergic reaction. If an allergic reaction occurs, tell patient to notify prescriber immediately and, if severe, to seek immediate medical care.

! **WARNING** Inform pregnant females or breastfeeding mothers that prolonged use of fentanyl during pregnancy or while breastfeeding may cause the neonate or infant to experience life-threatening withdrawal symptoms. Stress importance of avoiding fentanyl use as much as possible during prepnancy and not to breastfeed once baby is born.

! **WARNING** Remind patient to keep used and unused dosage units out of reach of children and to dispose of drug properly. For buccal tablets, patient should flush leftover drug down the toilet when no longer needed. For sublingual spray, remind patient to dispose of any used or unneeded units immediately in the disposal bottle provided with every dispensed carton. For transdermal patch, patient should fold in half and flush down toilet.

! **WARNING** Caution patient that accidentally exposing others to transdermal fentanyl could cause serious adverse reactions that may become life-threatening, especially in children, even with one dose. If accidental exposure occurs, the person should remove the patch, wash the area well with water, and seek medical attention.

! **WARNING** Alert patient with a seizure disorder that fentanyl may worsen seizure control. Stress importance of patient notifying prescriber if an increase in seizures occurs during drug therapy.

! **WARNING** Instruct patient to inform prescriber if persistent, serious (such as hypoglycemia), or unusual adverse reactions occur.

- Tell patient to increase fiber and fluid intake, unless contraindicated, because drug may cause severe constipation. If it persists or becomes severe, urge patient to notify prescriber.
- Tell patient to inform all prescribers of fentanyl use.
- Caution patient to avoid hazardous activities until drug's CNS effects are known and resolved.
- Inform patient that long-term use of opioids like fentanyl may decrease sex hormone levels, causing decreased libido, erectile dysfunction, impotence, infertility, or lack of menstruation. Lont-term use may also reduce fertility and that it is not known if it can be reversed. Encourage patient to discuss concerns with prescriber.

ferric carboxymaltose

Injectafer

Class and Category

Pharmacologic class: Hematinic
Therapeutic class: Antianemic

Indications and Dosages

✱ *To treat iron-deficiency anemia in patients who are intolerant to oral iron or have had an unsatisfactory response to oral iron*

I.V. INFUSION, I.V. INJECTION

Adults weighing 50 kg (110 lb) or more. 750 mg followed by a second dose of 750 mg given no sooner than 7 days later.

F

Alternatively, 15 mg/kg up to 1,000 mg given as a single-dose treatment course.

Children ages 1 and older weighing 50 kg (110 lb) or more. 750 mg followed by a second dose of 750 mg given no sooner than 7 days later.

Adults and children ages 1 and older weighing less than 50 kg (110 lb). 15 mg/kg followed by a second dose of 15 mg/kg given no sooner than 7 days later.

✶ *To treat iron-deficiency anemia in patients who have nondialysis-dependent chronic kidney disease*

I.V. INFUSION, I.V. INJECTION

Adults weighing 50 kg (110 lb) or more. 750 mg followed by a second dose of 750 mg given no sooner than 7 days later. Alternatively, 15 mg/kg up to 1,000 mg given as a single-dose treatment course.

Adults weighing less than 50 kg (110 lb). 15 mg/kg followed by a second dose of 15 mg/kg given no sooner than 7 days later.

✶ *To treat iron deficiency in patients with heart failure and New York Heart Association class II and III to improve exercise capacity*

IV. INFUSION, I.V. INJECTION

Adults weighing 70 kg (154 lb) or more and hemoglobin is greater than 14 g/dl but less than 15 g/dl. *Initial:* 500 mg. *Maintenance:* 500 mg at wks 12, 24, and 36 if serum ferritin is less than 100 ng/ml or serum ferritin is 100 to 300 ng/ml with transferrin saturation less than 20%.

Adults weighing 70 kg (154 lb) or more and hemoblobin is between 10 g/dl and 14 g/dl. *Initial:* 1,000 mg followed by a second dose of 500 mg 6 wk later. *Maintenance:* 500 mg at wks 12, 24, and 36 if serum ferritin is less than 100 ng/ml or serum ferritin is 100 to 300 ng/ml with transferrin saturation less than 20%.

Adults weighing 70 kg (154 lb) or more and hemoglobin is less than 10 g/dl. *Initial:* 1,000 mg followed by a second dose of 1,000 mg 6 wk later. *Maintenance:* 500 mg at wks 12, 24, and 36 if serum ferritin is less than 100 ng/ml or serum ferritin is 100 to 300 ng/ml with transferrin saturation less than 20%.

Adults weighing less than 70 kg (154 lb) with a hemoglobin greater than 14 g/dl but less than 15 g/dl. *Initial:* 500 mg. *Maintenance:* 500 mg at wks 12, 24, and 36 if serum ferritin is less than 100 ng/ml or serum ferritin is 100 to 300 ng/ml with transferrin saturation less than 20%.

Adults weighing less than 70 kg (154 lb) with a hemoglobin of 10 to 14 g/dl. *Initial:* 1,000 mg. *Maintenance:* 500 mg at wks 12, 24, and 36 if serum ferritin is less than 100 ng/ml or serum ferritin is100 to 300 ng/ml with transferrin saturation less than 20%.

Adults weighing less than 70 kg with a hemoglobin less than 10 g/dl. *Initial:* 1,000 mg followed by a second dose of 500 mg 6 wk later. *Maintenance:* 500 mg at wks 12, 24, and 36 if serum ferritin is less than 100 ng/ml or serum ferritin is 100 to 300 ng/ml with transferrin saturation less than 20%.

Drug Administration

I.V.

- For I.V. injection, administer undiluted. For dosage of 500 or 750 mg, inject slowly by slow intravenous push given at a rate of 100 mg (2 ml)/min. For 1,000 mg dosage, give slowly as an I.V. push over 15 min.
- For I.V. infusion, dilute up to 1,000 mg of iron in no more than 250 ml of 0.9% Sodium Chloride Injection, so that the concentration of the infusion is not less than 2 mg of iron per ml. Infuse over at least 15 min.
- Monitor injection site closely. Avoid extravasation, if at all possible, because a brown discoloration at the extravasation site may be long lasting. If extravasation occurs, discontinue administration of the drug at that site.
- Infusion solution at concentrations ranging from 2 mg to 4 mg of iron per ml can be stored at room temperature for 72 hr.
- *Incompatibilities:* None reported by manufacturer.

Route	Onset	Peak	Duration
I.V.	Unknown	15 min–1.21 hr	Unknown

Half-life: 7–12 hr

Mechanism of Action

Releases iron as a colloidal iron (III) hydroxide in complex with carboxymaltose, a carbohydrate polymer to increase hemoglobin formation.

Contraindications

Hypersensitivity to ferric carboxymaltose or its components

Interactions

DRUGS

None reported by manufacturer.

Adverse Reactions

CNS: Chills, dizziness, fever, headache, paresthesia, syncope
CV: Chest pain, hypertension, **hypotension**, tachycardia
EENT: Nasopharyngitis, sneezing, taste distortion
GI: Abdominal pain, constipation, diarrhea, elevated liver enzymes, nausea, vomiting
HEME: **Decreased platelet and WBC counts**
MS: Arthralgia, back pain
RESP: Dyspnea
SKIN: Erythema, flushing, hot flash, pruritus, rash, urticaria
Other: **Anaphylaxis (including shock), angioedema, or other hypersensitivity reactions**; **hypophosphatemia**; injection-site discoloration or irritation

Childbearing Considerations

PREGNANCY

- It is not known if drug can cause fetal harm but maternal hypersensitivity reactions to the drug may cause fetal bradycardia, especially in the second and third trimesters.
- Use with caution only if benefit to mother outweighs potential risk to fetus.

LACTATION

- Drug is present in breast milk.
- Mothers should check with prescriber before breastfeeding.
- If breastfeeding occurs, infant should be monitored for constipation or diarrhea.

Nursing Considerations

! **WARNING** Monitor patient for hypersensitivity reactions that may become life-threatening, such as anaphylaxis or angioedema. Monitor patient during and for at least 30 minutes after completion of infusion or until patient is clinically stable. If hypersensitivity occurs, stop infusion or injection if still being administered, notify prescriber, and provide supportive care, as needed and ordered.

! **WARNING** Monitor serum phosphate levels, as ordered in patients at risk for low serum phosphate who require a repeat course of treatment. Possible risk factors for hypophosphatemia include concurrent or prior use of medications that affect proximal renal tubular function; a history of GI disorders associated with malabsorption of fat-soluble vitamins or phosphate; or the presence of hyperparathyroidism, malnutrition, or vitamin D deficiency.

- Monitor patient for transient hypertension following each administration of ferric carboxymaltose. Assess patient's blood pressure and monitor patient for accompanying signs and symptoms of dizziness, facial flushing, or nausea that usually occur immediately after dosing and resolve within 30 minutes.
- Be aware that in the 24 hours after administration of drug, laboratory assays may overestimate serum iron and transferring bound iron.

PATIENT TEACHING

- Urge patient to inform prescriber if patient had experienced a prior history of allergies to parenteral iron products.
- Inform patient ferric carboxymaltose will be given intravenously.
- Reassure patient that he will be monitored throughout drug administration.

! **WARNING** Stress importance of reporting any signs and symptoms of an allergic reaction to staff if experiencing a reaction during drug administration, such as breathing problems, dizziness, itching, light-headedness, rash, or swelling. Urge patient to seek immediate medical care after returning home, if severe.

- Alert patient that a long-lasting brown discoloration may occur at the site of injection. Tell patient to alert staff immediately if pain or swelling occurs at the injection site.
- Instruct mother breastfeeding to monitor infant for constipation or diarrhea.

ferric citrate

Auryxia

Class and Category

Pharmacologic class: Ferric iron-based phosphate binder
Therapeutic class: Phosphate binder

Indications and Dosages

✱ *To control serum phosphorus levels in patients with chronic kidney disease on dialysis*

TABLETS

Adults. *Initial:* 2 tablets (420 mg ferric iron), 3 times daily with meals, increased or decreased by 1 to 2 tablets per day at 1-wk intervals or longer, as needed. *Maximum:* 12 tablets (2,520 mg ferric iron).

✱ *To treat iron-deficiency anemia in patients with chronic kidney disease not on dialysis*

TABLETS

Adults. 1 tablet (210 ferric iron), 3 times daily with meals, titrated to achieve and maintain hemoglobin at target levels. *Maximum:* 12 tablets (2,520 mg ferric iron) daily.

Drug Administration

P.O.

- Administer with meals.
- Tablets should be swallowed whole, and not chewed, crushed, or split.
- Protect from moisture during storage.

Route	Onset	Peak	Duration
P.O.	Unknown	Unknown	Unknown

Half-life: Unknown

Mechanism of Action

Binds dietary phosphate in the gastrointestinal (GI) tract and precipitates as ferric phosphate, which is then excreted in the stool. By binding phosphate in the GI tract and decreasing absorption, serum phosphate levels are reduced. Also, replaces iron stores in body.

Contraindications

Hypersensitivity to ferric citrate or its components, iron overload syndromes

Interactions

DRUGS

ciprofloxacin, doxycycline: Decreased effectiveness of these drugs

Adverse Reactions

GI: Abdominal pain, constipation, diarrhea, discolored stools, nausea, vomiting
HEME: Increased serum ferritin and transferrin saturation levels
RESP: Cough
Other: **Hyperkalemia**

Childbearing Considerations

PREGNANCY

- It is not known if drug causes fetal harm. However, an overdose of iron in pregnant females may carry a risk for fetal malformation or spontaneous abortion.
- Use with caution only if benefit to mother outweighs potential risk to fetus.

LACTATION

- Drug is present in breast milk.
- Mothers should check with prescriber before breastfeeding.

Nursing Considerations

- Be aware that ferric citrate produces dark stools because of its iron content, but this effect does not affect laboratory tests for occult bleeding.
- Know that iron absorption from ferric citrate therapy may cause an excessive elevation in iron stores. Assess patients' serum ferritin and transferrin saturation levels before initiating ferric citrate therapy, as ordered, and monitor throughout therapy.
- Expect that patients also receiving iron intravenously may need a reduction in dose or discontinuation of I.V. iron therapy.

! WARNING Monitor patient's potassium level, as ordered, and patient for signs and symptoms of hyperkalemia.

Patient Teaching

- Instruct patient how to administer ferric citrate.
- Stress importance to take drug exactly as ordered.

! WARNING Review signs and symptoms of hyperkalemia with patient and, if present, urge patient to notify prescriber.

! WARNING Remind patient that accidental overdose of iron-containing products is a leading cause of death in children under age

6. Stress the importance of keeping ferric citrate tablets out of the reach of children. If accidental overdose occurs, poison control center should be called, and immediate emergency treatment sought for the child.

ferric derisomaltose

Monoferric

Class and Category

Pharmacologic class: Hematinic
Therapeutic class: Antianemic

Indications and Dosages

∗ *To treat iron-deficiency anemia in patients who are intolerant to oral iron or have had unsatisfactory response to oral iron; to treat iron-deficiency anemia in patients who have nonhemodialysis-dependent chronic kidney disease*

I.V. INFUSION

Adults weighing 50 kg (110 lb) or more. 1,000 mg infused as a single dose. Dose repeated, if iron-deficiency anemia reoccurs.
Adults weighing less than 50 kg (110 lb). 20 mg/kg infused over at least 20 min as a single dose. Dose repeated, if iron-deficiency anemia reoccurs.

Drug Administration

I.V.

- To dilute, withdraw the appropriate volume of drug and inject into 100 ml to 500 ml of 0.9% Sodium Chloride Injection solution. Final diluted concentration should be more than 1 mg iron/ml.
- Infuse over at least 20 min.
- Monitor injection site closely. Avoid extravasation, if at all possible, because a brown discoloration at the extravasation site may be long lasting. If extravasation occurs, discontinue administration of the drug at that site.
- Following dilution, drug solution may be stored at room temperature for up to 8 hr.
- *Incompatibilities:* Other drugs

Route	Onset	Peak	Duration
I.V.	Unknown	7 days	Unknown

Half-life: 1–4 days

Mechanism of Action

Releases iron, which then binds to transferrin for transport to erythroid precursor cells to be incorporated into hemoglobin.

Contraindications

Hypersensitivity to ferric derisomaltose or its components

Interactions

DRUGS

None reported by manufacturer.

Adverse Reactions

CNS: Anxiety, chills, dizziness, fatigue, fever, headache, loss of consciousness, malaise, paresthesia, **seizures**, syncope
CV: Chest pain, hypertension, **hypotension**, tachycardia
EENT: Taste distortion
GI: Abnormal pain, constipation, diarrhea, elevated liver enzymes, nausea, vomiting
HEME: **Iron overload**
MS: Arthralgia, back pain, muscle spasms, myalgia
RESP: **Bronchospasm**, cough, dyspnea, mediastinal and thoracic disorders
SKIN: Diaphoresis, discoloration of skin, erythema, flushing, pruritus, rash, skin exfoliation, urticaria
Other: **Anaphylactic reaction (including shock), angioedema, or other hypersensitivity reactions (may be severe)**; extravasation (long-lasting brown discoloration, irritation); Fishban reaction (chest tightness, facial flushing, truncal myalgia, and/or joint pains); flu-like symptoms; **hypophosphatemia**; injection site reactions (phlebitis, pain)

Childbearing Considerations

PREGNANCY

- It is not known if drug can cause fetal harm. However, maternal hypersensitivity reaction may cause fetal bradycardia, especially in the second and third trimesters.
- Use with caution only if benefit to mother outweighs potential risk to fetus.

LACTATION

- Drug is present in breast milk.
- Mothers should check with prescriber before breastfeeding.

F

- If breastfeeding occurs, infant should be monitored for constipation or diarrhea.

Nursing Considerations

! **WARNING** Know that ferric derisomaltose should not be given to patients with iron overload. Iron overload can lead to life-threatening conditions such as cardiac problems and liver disease.

! **WARNING** Expect to monitor the hematologic response to ferric derisomaltose, such as hemoglobin and hematocrit and iron parameters (serum ferritin, transferring saturation). Excessive therapy with parenteral iron can lead to excess iron storage and possibly iatrogenic hemosiderosis or hemochromatosis.

! **WARNING** Monitor patient for hypersensitivity reactions that may become life-threatening, such as anaphylaxis or angioedema. Monitor patient closely during and for at least 30 minutes after infusion or until patient is clinically stable. If present, stop infusion if still being administered, notify prescriber, and provide supportive care, as needed and ordered.

PATIENT TEACHING

- Urge patient to inform prescriber if patient had experienced a prior history of allergies to parenteral iron products.
- Inform patient that drug will be administered intravenously.
- Reassure patient that he will be monitored during administration.

! **WARNING** Stress importance of reporting any signs and symptoms of an allergic reaction to staff, such as breathing problems, dizziness, itching, light-headedness, rash, or swelling. If severe, urge patient to seek immediate medical care if patient has returned home.

- Alert patient that a long-lasting brown discoloration may occur at the site of injection. Tell patient to alert staff immediately if pain or swelling occurs at the injection site.
- Instruct mother breastfeeding to monitor infant for constipation or diarrhea.

ferric maltol

Accrufer

Class and Category

Pharmacologic class: Iron agent
Therapeutic class: Hematinic

Indications and Dosages

✶ *To treat iron deficiency*

CAPSULES

Adults. 30 mg twice daily on an empty stomach until iron stores are replenished.

Drug Administration

P.O.

- Administer on an empty stomach at least 1 hr before or 2 hr after meals.
- Capsules should be swallowed whole and not chewed, crushed, or opened.
- Separate drug administration from other oral drugs by at least 4 hr to prevent decreased bioavailability of other oral drugs.

Route	Onset	Peak	Duration
P.O.	Unknown	1.5–3 hr	Unknown

Half-life: 0.7 hr

Mechanism of Action

Delivers iron for uptake across the intestinal wall and transfer to transferrin and ferritin.

Contraindications

Hemochromatosis and other iron overload syndromes, hypersensitivity to ferric maltol or its components, repeated blood transfusions

Interactions

DRUGS

dimercaprol: Possibly increased risk of nephrotoxicity
oral administration of ciprofloxacin, doxycycline, ethynyl estradiol, mycophenolate: Possibly decreased absorption of these drugs and decreased bioavailability

Adverse Reactions

GI: Abdominal discomfort, distension, pain; constipation; diarrhea; discolored feces; flatulence; increased risk of inflammation in GI tract; nausea, vomiting
HEME: **Iron overload**

Childbearing Considerations

PREGNANCY

- Drug is not absorbed systemically, and maternal use is not expected to result in fetal exposure.
- Overdose of iron in pregnant females may carry a risk for fetal malformation, gestational diabetes, or spontaneous abortion.
- Use with caution only if benefit to mother outweighs potential risk to fetus

LACTATION

- It is not known if drug is present in breast milk, but presence is not expected because drug is not absorbed systemically.
- Mothers should check with prescriber before breastfeeding.

Nursing Considerations

- Know that ferric maltol should be avoided in patients with an active inflammatory bowel disease flare because drug has the potential to increase inflammation in the GI tract.

! **WARNING** Be aware that ferric maltol should not be given to patients with evidence of iron overload or patients also receiving intravenous iron to avoid excess storage of iron. Iron overload can lead to life-threatening conditions such as cardiac problems and liver disease

- Expect to monitor iron parameters, as ordered, during therapy.

Patient Teaching

- Instruct patient how to administer ferric maltol.
- Inform patient that treatment duration will depend on the severity of iron deficiency but that generally at least 12 weeks of therapy is required. However, treatment will continue as long as necessary until ferritin levels are within normal range.
- Tell patient to alert prescriber of other drugs being taken, including over-the-counter products, to determine if ferric maltol should be taken 4 hours before or after other drugs.

! **WARNING** Urge patient to keep ferric maltol out of reach of children, as accidental overdose of iron-containing products is a leading cause of fatal poisoning in children under age 6.

ferrous salts

ferrous fumarate

Ferretts, Ferrocite, Fumerin, Hemocyte, Iron Fumarate, Neo-Fer (CAN), Novofumar (CAN), Palafer (CAN)

ferrous gluconate

Ferate, Fergon, Ferralet, Ferralet Slow Release, Fertinic (CAN), Novo-Ferrogluc (CAN), Simron

ferrous sulfate

iron, carbonyl

Feosol Natural Release, Ferra-Cap, Icar

Class and Category

Pharmacologic class: Hematinic
Therapeutic class: Antianemic, nutritional supplement

Indications and Dosages

✶ *To prevent iron deficiency based on recommended daily allowances*

CAPLETS, CAPSULES, CHEWABLE TABLETS, DRIED CAPSULES, DRIED E.R. CAPSULES, DRIED E.R. TABLETS, DRIED TABLETS, ELIXIR, ENTERIC-COATED TABLETS, E.R. CAPSULES, E.R. TABLETS, ORAL SOLUTION, ORAL SUSPENSION, SYRUP, TABLETS

Adults ages 51 and older. 8 mg daily.
Adult females ages 19 to 50. 18 mg daily.
Adult males ages 19 to 50. 8 mg daily.
Pregnant females. 27 mg daily.
Breastfeeding mothers. 9 to 10 mg daily.
Boys ages 14 to 18. 11 mg daily.
Girls ages 14 to 18. 15 mg daily.
Children ages 9 to 13. 8 mg daily.
Children ages 4 to 8. 10 mg daily.
Children ages 1 to 3. 7 mg daily.
Infants ages 7 mo to 12 mo. 11 mg daily.
Newborns to age 6 mo. 0.27 mg daily.

✶ *To replace iron in deficiency states*

CAPLETS, CAPSULES, CHEWABLE TABLETS, DRIED CAPSULES, DRIED E.R. CAPSULES, DRIED E.R. TABLETS, DRIED TABLETS, ELIXIR, ENTERIC-COATED TABLETS, E.R. CAPSULES, E.R. TABLETS, ORAL SOLUTION, ORAL SUSPENSION, SYRUP, TABLETS

Adults and adolescents. 300 to 325 mg daily. Alternatively, 100 to 200 mg of elemental iron daily and divided into 3 equal doses and given every other day. *Maintenance:* 325 mg daily or 60 mg up to 3 times daily or every other day for several wk or mo.

Infants and children. *For mild to moderate iron-deficiency anemia:* 3 mg elemental iron/kg/day in 1 to 2 divided doses. *For severe iron-deficiency anemia:* 4 to 6 mg elemental iron/kg/day in 3 divided doses.

Premature neonates. 2 to 4 mg elemental iron/kg/day divided every 12 to 24 hr. *Maximum:* 15 mg daily.

* *To provide iron supplementation during pregnancy*

CAPLETS, CAPSULES, CHEWABLE TABLETS, DRIED CAPSULES, DRIED E.R. CAPSULES, DRIED E.R. TABLETS, DRIED TABLETS, ELIXIR, ENTERIC-COATED TABLETS, E.R. CAPSULES, E.R. TABLETS, ORAL SOLUTION, ORAL SUSPENSION, SYRUP, TABLETS

Pregnant women. 30 mg elemental iron daily.

± **DOSAGE ADJUSTMENT** For elderly patients, who may not absorb iron as easily as younger adults do, dosage increased, as needed.

Drug Administration

P.O.

- Administer iron salts 1 hr before or 2 hr after meals. If GI irritation occurs, give with or just after meals.
- Don't give antacids, coffee, dairy products, eggs, tea, or whole-grain breads or cereals within 1 hr before or 2 hr after iron.
- Tablets and capsules should be given with a full glass of juice or water. Don't crush enteric-coated tablets or open capsules.
- Chewable tablets should be chewed thoroughly before swallowing.
- Dilute and administer drops with a straw or place drops in back of patient's throat because iron solutions may stain teeth.
- Mix elixir form in water.
- Use a measuring device to measure dosage of liquid forms.
- Protect liquid form from freezing.

Route	Onset	Peak	Duration
P.O.	4–7 days	5–8 days	Unknown

Half-life: Variable

Mechanism of Action

Acts to normalize RBC production by binding with hemoglobin or by being oxidized and stored as hemosiderin or aggregated ferritin in reticuloendothelial cells of the bone marrow, liver, and spleen. Iron is an essential component of hemoglobin, myoglobin, and several enzymes, including catalase, cytochromes, and peroxidase. Iron is needed for catecholamine metabolism and normal neutrophil function.

Contraindications

Hemochromatosis, hemolytic anemias, hemosiderosis, hypersensitivity to iron salts or their components, other anemic conditions unless accompanied by iron deficiency

Interactions

DRUGS

antacids: Possibly decreased absorption of iron salts
bisphosphonates, dolutegravir, integrase inhibitors: Decreased absorption of these drugs
dimercaprol: Increased risk of nephrotoxic effect of iron salts
levodopa: Possibly chelation with iron, decreasing levodopa absorption and blood level
levothyroxine: Decreased levothyroxine effectiveness and, possibly, hypothyroidism
methyldopa: Decreased methyldopa absorption and efficacy
quinolones, tetracyclines: Decreased effectiveness of these antibiotics

ACTIVITIES

alcohol abuse (acute or chronic): Increased serum iron level

FOODS

coffee; eggs; foods that contain bicarbonates, carbonates, oxalates, or phosphates; milk and milk products; tea that contains tannic acid; whole grain breads, cereals, and other high-fiber foods: Decreased iron absorption and effectiveness

Adverse Reactions

CNS: Chills, dizziness, fever, headache, paresthesia, syncope
CV: Chest pain, hypertension, **hypotension**, tachycardia
EENT: Metallic taste, tooth discoloration
GI: Abdominal cramps, constipation, epigastric pain, nausea, stool discoloration, vomiting
HEME: Hemochromatosis, **hemolysis**, hemosiderosis
MS: Arthralgia, back pain, hypophosphatemic osteomalacia (rare)
RESP: Dyspnea, wheezing
SKIN: Diaphoresis, erythema, flushing, pruritus, rash, urticaria
Other: **Angioedema**

Childbearing Considerations

PREGNANCY

- It is not known if drug causes fetal harm.
- Use with caution only if benefit to mother outweighs potential risk to fetus.

LACTATION

- Drug is present in breast milk.
- Mothers should check with prescriber before breastfeeding.

Nursing Considerations

- Be aware that at usual dosages, serum hemoglobin level usually normalizes in about 2 months unless blood loss continues. Treatment may last for 3 to 6 months to help replenish iron stores.

! **WARNING** Monitor patient for signs of iron overdose, which may include abdominal pain, diarrhea (possibly bloody), nausea, severe vomiting, and sharp abdominal cramps. In case of iron toxicity or accidental iron overdose (a leading cause of fatal poisoning in children under age 6), give deferoxamine, as prescribed. As few as 3 adult iron tablets can cause serious poisoning in young children.

! **WARNING** Monitor patient for a hypersensitivity reaction, which could become life-threatening such as angioedema. If present, notify prescriber, expect drug to be discontinued, and provide supportive care, as needed and ordered.

- Remember that unabsorbed iron turns stool black or green and can mask blood in stool. Check stool for occult blood, as ordered.

PATIENT TEACHING

- Instruct patient how to administer form of iron prescribed.
- Tell patient to minimize tooth stains from liquid iron, by mixing dose with fruit juice, tomato juice, or water, and to drink it with a straw. If patient must take liquid iron by dropper, direct her to place drops well back on the tongue and to follow with water or juice. Tell her that iron stains can be removed by brushing with baking soda (sodium bicarbonate).
- Urge patient to eat chicken, fish, lean red meat, and turkey, as well as foods rich in vitamin C (such as citrus fruits and fresh vegetables) to improve iron absorption.
- Urge patient to avoid foods that impair iron absorption, including dairy products, eggs, spinach, and high-fiber foods, such as whole grain breads, cereals, and bran. Also advise her to avoid drinking coffee or tea within 1 hour of iron intake.
- Caution patient not to take antacids or calcium supplements within 1 hour before and 2 hours after taking iron supplement.

! **WARNING** Alert patient drug can cause an allergic reaction. If present, tell patient to notify prescriber, stop taking drug, and, if severe, to seek immediate medical care.

! **WARNING** Warn patient about high risk of accidental poisoning in children and urge patient to keep iron preparations out of the reach of children.

- Inform patient that stool should become dark green or black during therapy. Advise her to notify prescriber if it doesn't.
- Advise patient to consult prescriber before taking large amounts of iron for longer than 6 months.

NEW!

fezolinetant

Veozah

Class and Category

Pharmacologic class: Neurokinin 3 (NK3) receptor antagonist
Therapeutic class: antimenopausal agent

Indications and Dosages

✱ To treat moderate to severe vasomotor symptoms due to menopause

TABLETS

Adult women. 45 mg once daily.

Drug Administration

P.O.

- Tablets may be administered with or without food.
- Tablets should be taken with liquids and swallowed whole.
- Tablets should not be chewed, crushed, or cut before being administered.
- Administer tablets at the same time every day.
- Administer a missed dose as soon as possible, unless there is less than 12 hr before the next dose.

Route	Onset	Peak	Duration
P.O.	Unknown	1-4 hr	Unknown

Half-life: 9.6 hr

Mechanism of Action

Blocks neurokinin B binding on the kisspeptin/neurokinin B/dynorphin neuron to regulate neuronal activity in the thermoregulatory center to relieve vasomotor symptoms caused by menopause.

Contraindications

Concomitant use with CYP1A2 inhibitors, end-stage renal disease or severe renal impairment, hypersensitivity to fezolinetant or its components, known cirrhosis

Interactions

DRUGS

CYP1A2 inhibitors: Increased plasma concentrations of fezolinetant with possible increase in adverse reactions

Adverse Reactions

CNS: Insomnia

ENDO: Hot flashes

GI: Abdominal pain, diarrhea, elevated transaminase levels and total bilirubin, **hepatotoxicity**

MS: Back pain

Childbearing Considerations

PREGNANCY

- It is not known if drug can cause fetal harm.
- Use with caution only if benefit to mother outweighs potential risk to fetus.

LACTATION

- It is not known if drug is present in breast milk.
- Mothers should check with prescriber before breastfeeding.

Nursing Considerations

! WARNING Expect to obtain liver function tests, as ordered, prior to administering fezolinetant because drug can cause hepatic dysfunction. Know that drug should not be started in a patient with an aminotransferase level 2 or more times the upper level of normal (ULN) or the total bilirubin is 2 or more times greater than the ULN.

! WARNING Expect to review liver function tests, as ordered, monthly for the first 3 months of therapy, then at 6 and 9 months and any time transaminase elevations occur. Know that drug should be discontinued if transaminase elevations become greater than 5 times the ULN or the transaminase elevations are greater than 3 times ULN and the total bilirubin levels exceeds 2 times ULN.

! WARNING Notify prescriber immediately and stop drug therapy, as ordered, if patient experiences adverse reactions associated with hepatic dysfunction such as abdominal pain, dark urine, decreased appetite, nausea, new onset fatigue, pale feces, pruritus, or vomiting.

PATIENT TEACHING

- Instruct patient how to take fezolinetant and what to do if a dose is missed.

! WARNING Stress importance of complying with ordered laboratory tests to monitor liver function. Review signs and symptoms of liver dysfunction and urge patient to notify prescriber if any develops and to stop taking drug.

- Advise patient to notify prescriber of any newly prescribed drugs by other providers and not to take any OTC drugs until prescriber has approved use of the drug(s).

fidaxomicin

Dificid

Class and Category

Pharmacologic class: Macrolide
Therapeutic class: Antibiotic

Indications and Dosages

∗ *To treat* Clostridioides difficile*–associated diarrhea*

TABLET

Adults and children weighing at least 12.5 kg (27.5 lb) and more and able to swallow tablets. 200 mg twice daily for 10 days.

ORAL SUSPENSION

Children weighing at least 12.5 kg (27.5 lb) or more and unable to swallow tablets. 200 mg (5 ml) twice daily for 10 days.
Children ages 6 mo and older weighing 9 kg (19.8 lb) to less than 12.5 kg (27.5 lb). 160 mg (4 ml) twice daily for 10 days.
Children ages 6 mo and older weighing 7 kg (15.4 lb) to less than 9 kg (19.8 lb). 120 mg (3 ml) twice daily for 10 days.
Children ages 6 mo and older weighing 4 kg (8.8 lb) to less than 7 kg (15.4 lb). 80 mg (2 ml) twice daily for 10 days.

Drug Administration

P.O.

- Tablets should be swallowed whole and not chewed, crushed, or split.
- Oral suspension and tablets may be administered with or without food.
- To reconstitute oral suspension, shake bottle to loosen powder. Measure 130 ml of Purified Water, add to the glass bottle, and cap tightly. Hold bottle in a horizontal position and shake vigorously for at least 2 min. Verify that a homogeneous suspension is obtained. If not, repeat shaking. Once homogeneous suspension is visually confirmed, shake an additional 30 sec. Let bottle stand for 1 min. Verify that suspension is still homogeneous. If not, shake for at least 2 min, then 30 sec and let bottle stand again for 1 min. Once reconstituted, oral suspension appears white to yellowish white in color.
- Remove oral suspension from refrigerator 15 min before each administration. Shake vigorously until suspension has an even consistency. Use an oral dosing syringe to measure dose.
- Store in refrigerator and discard after 12 days.

Route	Onset	Peak	Duration
P.O.	<1 hr	1–5 hr	Unknown

Half-life: 12 hr

Mechanism of Action

Inhibits RNA synthesis in *Clostridioides-difficile* bacterial cells by RNA polymerases, causing the cells to die.

Contraindications

Hypersensitivity to fidaxomicin or its components

Interactions

DRUGS

cyclosporine: Possible increased blood fidaxomicin level

Adverse Reactions

CNS: Fever
ENDO: Hyperglycemia
GI: Abdominal distention or pain, constipation, diarrhea, dyspepsia, dysphagia, elevated liver enzymes, flatulence, **GI hemorrhage**, **intestinal obstruction**, **megacolon**, nausea, vomiting
HEME: Anemia, **neutropenia**, **thrombocytopenia**
RESP: Dyspnea
SKIN: Drug eruption, pruritus, rash, urticaria
Other: **Angioedema and other acute hypersensitivity reactions**, **decreased blood bicarbonate**, elevated blood alkaline phosphatase, **metabolic acidosis**

Childbearing Considerations

PREGNANCY

- It is not known if drug causes fetal harm.
- Use with caution only if benefit to mother outweighs potential risk to fetus.

LACTATION

- It is not known if drug is present in breast milk.
- Mothers should check with prescriber before breastfeeding.

Nursing Considerations

- Be aware that fidaxomicin should only be used to treat infections that are caused or strongly suspected to be caused by *Clostridioides difficile*.

- Know that fidaxomicin is most effective when patients are not taking other antibiotics. If other antibiotics can be stopped safely, expect them to be withheld during the 10 days of fidaxomicin therapy.

! **WARNING** Monitor patient for hypersensitivity reactions that may include angioedema, dyspnea, pruritus, or rash. Patients with a history of allergy to other macrolides are at increased risk. If a severe reaction occurs, discontinue fidaxomicin immediately and notify prescriber. Provide supportive care, as needed and ordered.

- Monitor patient for other adverse effects and notify prescriber, if present.

PATIENT TEACHING

- Instruct patient how to administer the form of fidaxomicin prescribed.
- Tell patient to take drug exactly as prescribed and for the full 10 days, regardless of how he is feeling.

! **WARNING** Alert patient that an allergic reaction may occur. If present, tell patient to notify prescriber, stop taking drug and, if serious, to seek immediate medical care.

- Tell patient to notify prescriber if symptoms worsen at any time or don't improve after a few days.

filgrastim (granulocyte colony-stimulating factor, G-CSF)

Grastofil (CAN), Neupogen

filgrastim-aafi

Nivestym

filgrastim-ayow (granulocyte colony-stimulating actor, rG-CSF)

Releuko

filgrastim-sndz (granulocyte colony-stimulating factor, G-CSF)

Zarxio

filgrastim-txid

Nypoz

tbo-filgrastim

Granix

Class and Category

Pharmacologic class: Colony-stimulating factor

Therapeutic class: Hematopoietic

Indications and Dosages

∗ *To reduce infection in patients with nonmyelid malignancies after myelosuppressive chemotherapy associated with a significant incidence of severe neutropenia with fever; to reduce neutrophil recovery time and duration of fever following induction or consolidation chemotherapy in patients with acute myeloid leukemia*

I.V. INFUSION, SUBCUTANEOUS INJECTION (GRASTOFIL, NEUPOGEN, NIVESTYM, NYPOZI, RELEUKO, ZARXIO)

Adults and children. *Initial:* 5 mcg/kg daily for up to 2 wk or until absolute neutrophil count (ANC) has reached 10,000/mm^3 following the expected chemotherapy-induced neutrophil nadir beginning 24 hr or more after cytotoxic chemotherapy. Increased, as needed, by 5 mcg/kg with each chemotherapy cycle. I.V. infused over 15 to 30 min or infused as a continuous infusion.

SUBCUTANEOUS INJECTION (GRASTOFIL, NEUPOGEN, NIVESTYM, RELEUKO, ZARXIO)

Adults and children. *Initial:* 5 mcg/kg daily for up to 2 wk or until ANC has reached 10,000/mm^3 following the expected chemotherapy-induced neutrophil nadir beginning 24 hr or more after cytotoxic chemotherapy. Increased, as needed, by 5 mcg/kg with each chemotherapy cycle.

∗ *To reduce the duration of severe neutropenia in patients with nonmyeloid malignancies after receiving myelosuppressive chemotherapy associated with a significant incidence of febrile neutropenia*

SUBCUTANEOUS INJECTION (GRANIX)

Adults and children ages 1 mo and older. 5 mcg/kg daily starting no earlier than 24 hr after myelosuppressive chemotherapy and continued until the neutrophil count has recovered to normal.

∗ *To reduce duration of neutropenia in patients with nonmyeloid malignancies undergoing myeloablative chemotherapy followed by bone marrow transplantation*

I.V. INFUSION (GRASTOFIL, NEUPOGEN, NIVESTYM, NYPOZI, RELEUKO, ZARXIO)

Adults. *Initial:* 10 mcg/kg daily as a continuous infusion for no longer than 24 hr beginning at least 24 hr after bone marrow infusion and cytotoxic chemotherapy. Dosage adjusted according to ANC response.

∗ *To mobilize autologous hematopoietic progenitor cells into the peripheral blood for collection by leukapheresis*

SUBCUTANEOUS INJECTION (GRASTOFIL, NEUPOGEN, NIVESTYM, NYPOZI, ZARXIO)

Adults. 10 mcg/kg daily starting at least 4 days before first leukapheresis and continuing until last day of leukapheresis.

∗ *To reduce occurrence and duration of severe chronic neutropenia in congenital neutropenia*

SUBCUTANEOUS INJECTION (GRASTOFIL, NEUPOGEN, NIVESTYM, NYPOZI, RELEUKO, ZARXIO)

Adults and children. *Initial:* 6 mcg/kg twice daily. Dosage adjusted, as needed.

∗ *To reduce the occurrence and duration of severe neutropenia in idiopathic or cyclic neutropenia*

SUBCUTANEOUS INJECTION (GRASTOFIL, NEUPOGEN, NIVESTYM, NYPOZI, RELEUKO, ZARXIO)

Adults and children. *Initial:* 5 mcg/kg daily. Dosage adjusted, as needed.

∗ *To treat patients acutely exposed to myelosuppressive doses of radiation*

SUBCUTANEOUS INJECTION (NEUPOGEN, NYPOZI, ZARXIO)

Adults and children. 10 mcg/kg daily beginning as soon as possible after exposure to radiation doses greater than 2 gray and continued until ANC remains greater than 1,000/mm^3 for 3 consecutive CBCs or exceeds 10,000/mm^3 after a radiation-induced nadir.

∗ *To prevent and treat neutropenia in patients with HIV infection*

SUBCUTANEOUS INJECTION (GRASTOFIL)

Adults. *Initial:* 1 mcg/kg/day or 300 mcg 3 times weekly and continued with dosage adjustment, as needed, until a normal neutrophil count is reached, and ANC is maintained at or greater than 2 × 10^9/L.

±**DOSAGE ADJUSTMENT** For all patients, dosage adjusted according to CBC with differential and platelet count response.

Drug Administration

- Remove drug from refrigeration and allow drug to come to room temperature (minimum 30 min, maximum 24 hr) before administering. Discard drug if stored longer than 24 hr at room temperature. Solution should be clear and colorless.
- Withdraw only one dose from a vial; don't repuncture the vial.
- Don't shake the solution.
- Be aware that needle cover on single-use prefilled syringe contains dry natural rubber (for Neupogen and Zarxio) and may cause sensitivity reaction. It shouldn't be handled by people allergic to latex.
- Don't give within 24 hr before or after cytotoxic chemotherapy.

I.V.

- Dilute with 5% Dextrose Injection to a concentration between 5 and 15 mcg/ml depending on the product. Never dilute with 0.9% Sodium Chloride Injection and do not dilute to less than 5 mcg/ml.
- Administer by continuous infusion over 24 hr or by intermittent infusion over 15 to 30 min daily.
- Protect absorption in plastic materials by the addition of albumin (human) at a concentration of 2 mg/ml making solution compatible with PVC or polyolefin intravenous bags. If albumin is not added to solution, a glass bottle must be used.
- Diluted solution can be stored at room temperature for up to 4 hr (Releuko), 14 hr (Nypozi), or 24 hr (other forms), which includes infusion and storage time.

- *Incompatibilities:* 0.9% Sodium Chloride solutions

SUBCUTANEOUS

- For subcutaneous dose larger than 1 ml, divide and give in more than one site.
- For direct administration of doses less than 0.3 ml, the single-dose vial should be used to ensure accuracy.
- Inject in abdomen, outer upper arms or outer areas of buttock, or thighs.
- Inject only in normal-appearing skin.
- Rotate injection sites.
- Nivestym, Nypozi, Releuko, and Zarxio prefilled syringes with BD UltraSafe Plus Passive Needle Guard cannot be used for doses less than 0.3 ml (180 mcg) because the spring mechanism of the needle guard apparatus affixed to the prefilled syringe interferes with the visibility of the graduation markings on the syringe barrel corresponding to 0.1 ml and 0.2 ml.
- Be aware that the brand Granix's prefilled syringe has a safety needle guard device for use by healthcare professionals only. To safely use the device, hold the syringe assembly by the open sides of the device and remove the needle shield. Expel any extra volume depending on dose needed. Inject Granix into site and push plunger as far as it will go to inject all of the drug. Injection of the entire prefilled syringe contents is needed to activate the needle guard. With the plunger still pressed all the way down, remove the needle from the skin. Slowly let go of the plunger and allow the empty syringe to move up inside the device until the entire needle is guarded. Discard the syringe assembly in an approved container.
- Follow manufacturer guidelines for storage instructions for specific product.

Route	Onset	Peak	Duration
I.V.	1–2 days	Unknown	4 days
SubQ	1–2 days	2–8 hr	4 days
SubQ (tbo-filgrastim)	3–5 days	4–6 hr	21 days

Half-life: 3–3.5 hr

Mechanism of Action

Is pharmacologically identical to human granulocyte colony-stimulating factor, an endogenous hormone synthesized by endothelial cells, fibroblasts, and monocytes. Filgrastim induces formation of neutrophil progenitor cells by binding directly to receptors on the surface of granulocytes, which then divide and differentiate. It also potentiates the effects of mature neutrophils, which reduces fever and the risk of infection raised by severe neutropenia.

Contraindications

Hypersensitivity to filgrastim, other human granulocyte colony-stimulating factors, such as pegfilgrastim or their components

Interactions

DRUGS

None reported by manufacturer.

Adverse Reactions

CNS: Fever, headache
CV: **Aortitis**, **capillary leak syndrome**, transient **supraventricular tachycardia**
GI: **Splenic rupture**, splenomegaly
GU: **Glomerulonephritis**
HEME: **Acute myeloid leukemia**, **extramedullary hematopoiesis**, leukocytosis, **myelodysplastic syndrome** (patients with congenital neutropenia), **thrombocytopenia**
MS: Arthralgia; decreased bone density (children with chronic treatment); myalgia; pain in arms, legs, lower back, or pelvis: osteoporosis (children with chronic therapy)
RESP: **Acute respiratory distress syndrome (ARDS)**, **alveolar hemorrhage**, dyspnea, **hemoptysis**, wheezing
SKIN: Cutaneous vasculitis, pruritus, rash, Sweet's syndrome (acute febrile neutrophilic dermatosis)
Other: **Anaphylaxis**, **angioedema**, injection-site pain and redness, sickle cell crisis

Childbearing Considerations

PREGNANCY

- Pregnancy exposure registry: Enroll women prescribed Neupogen in Amgen's Pregnancy Surveillance Program by calling 1-800-77-AMGEN.
- It is not known if drug causes fetal harm.
- Use with caution only if benefit to mother outweighs potential risk to fetus.

LACTATION

- Drug is present in breast milk.
- Patient should check with prescriber before breastfeeding. Filgrastim products are

generally secreted poorly into breast milk and are not absorbed orally by neonates, However, the manufactuer of Granix does not recommend breastfeeding and for 2 weeks after the last dose.

Nursing Considerations

- Expect to monitor CBC and platelet count 2 or 3 times weekly.
- Inform prescriber and expect to stop drug if leukocytosis develops or absolute neutrophil count consistently exceeds 10,000/mm^3.
- Anticipate decreased response to drug if patient has received extensive radiation therapy or long-term chemotherapy.

! **WARNING** Monitor patient for hypersensitivity reactions, which could become life-threatening such as anaphylaxis or angioedema. If present, stop drug therapy, notify prescriber, and provide supportive care, as needed and ordered.

! **WARNING** Know that aortitis has occurred in patients receiving filgrastim, occurring as early as the first week after start of therapy. Monitor patient for generalized signs and symptoms, such as abdominal pain, back pain, fever, and malaise. Increased inflammatory markers (e.g., C-reactive protein and WBC count) help to confirm the diagnosis. Expect drug to be discontinued if aortitis is suspected.

! **WARNING** Monitor patient's renal function, as ordered, because drug may cause glomerulonephritis. If abnormalities occur, expect dosage to be reduced or drug discontinued.

! **WARNING** Monitor patients with chronic congenital neutropenia for signs and symptoms of myelodysplastic syndrome (MDS) and acute myeloid leukemia (AML). Also, know that patients with breast or lung cancer who are receiving chemotherapy and/or radiotherapy are at higher risk for developing MDS and AML.

! **WARNING** Monitor patients with sickle cell anemia receiving filgrastim, as sickle cell crisis can occur that can be life-threatening. Notify prescriber immediately if sickle cell crisis occurs and expect drug to be discontinued.

PATIENT TEACHING

- Instruct patient, family, or caregiver how to administer the filgrastim product prescribed as a subcutaneous injection and what to do if a dose is missed.
- Alert patient with a latex allergy to request a brand of filgrastim that does not have latex in the needle cover.

! **WARNING** Alert patient that drug may cause an allergic reaction. If present, tell patient to notify prescriber and, if severe, to seek immediate medical care.

! **WARNING** Review possible serious side effects (capillary leak syndrome, hematological abnormalities, inflammation of blood vessels, kidney injury, respiratory distress syndrome, and sickle cell crises) with patient before drug is given and determine patient's understanding. Tell her the most common side effect is aching in the bones and muscles.

! **WARNING** Advise patient to promptly report pain in left upper quadrant of abdomen or shoulder-tip pain. Also, tell patient to report any persistent, severe, or unusual signs and symptoms to prescriber and, if severe, to seek emergency medical attention.

- Emphasize the importance of returning for follow-up laboratory tests.
- Instruct patient to inform all prescribers of filgrastim use. Patient should alert prescriber before taking any new drugs, including over-the-counter drugs.
- Alert mothers wishing to breastfeed to request a brand of filgrastim that allows breastfeeding and to avoid Granix brand of filgrastim, which does not recommend breastfeeding throughout filgrastim therapy and for 2 weeks after Granix is discontinued.

finasteride

Propecia, Proscar

Class and Category

Pharmacologic class: 5-alpha reductase inhibitor
Therapeutic class: Benign prostatic hyperplasia agent, hair growth stimulant

F

Indications and Dosages

* *To treat symptomatic benign prostatic hyperplasia; to reduce the risk of symptomatic progression of benign prostatic hyperplasia when given with doxazocin*

TABLETS (PROSCAR)

Men. 5 mg daily.

* *To treat male-pattern baldness*

TABLETS (PROPECIA)

Men. 1 mg daily.

Drug Administration

P.O.

- Drug is a potential teratogen. Handle and dispose of drug according to institutional protocol.
- Do not handle broken or crushed tablets if pregnant or suspect pregnancy because of drug's adverse effects on male fetus.

Route	Onset	Peak	Duration
P.O.*	Unknown	2–6 hr	Unknown
P.O.†	3 mo	Unknown	12 mo

Half-life: 6 hr

*For benign prostatic hyperplasia
†For male-pattern baldness

Mechanism of Action

Inhibits 5-alpha reductase, an intracellular enzyme that converts testosterone to its metabolite (5-alpha dihydrotestosterone) in liver, prostate, and skin. The metabolite is a potent androgen partially responsible for benign prostatic hyperplasia and hair loss.

Contraindications

Females, hypersensitivity to finasteride or its components

Interactions

DRUGS

None reported by manufacturer.

Adverse Reactions

CNS: Asthenia, depression, dizziness, headache, **progressive multifocal leukoencephalopathy** (extremely rare), **suicidal ideation**
CV: **Hypotension**, peripheral edema
EENT: Lip swelling, rhinitis
ENDO: Breast enlargement and tenderness, gynecomastia, **male breast cancer**
GI: Abdominal pain, diarrhea
GU: Altered prostate-specific antigen level, blood in semen, decreased ejaculatory volume, decreased libido, erectile dysfunction, hematospermia, **high-grade prostate cancer**, impotence, male infertility, testicular pain
MS: Back pain
RESP: Dyspnea
SKIN: Pruritus, rash, urticaria
Other: **Angioedema**

Childbearing Considerations

PREGNANCY

- Drug is known to cause fetal harm in the male fetus by preventing normal development of male genitalia.
- Drug is not indicated for use in females and is contraindicated in females.
- Females of childbearing age or females who are pregnant should not handle crushed or broken tablets because of the possibility of absorption and subsequent potential risk to a male fetus.

LACTATION

- It is not known if drug is present in breast milk.
- Drug is not indicated for use in females.

REPRODUCTION

- Patient and female partner of childbearing age should use an effective contraceptive during drug therapy.

Nursing Considerations

! **WARNING** Be aware that females of childbearing age who may not know pregnancy status or pregnant female healthcare workers should not handle broken finasteride tablets because of potential adverse effect on male fetus.

! **WARNING** Be aware that patient should have a urologic evaluation prior to starting finasteride therapy and periodically throughout therapy because drug can increase the risk of prostate cancer, especially high-grade prostate cancer.

- Expect patient to have a digital rectal examination of the prostate before and periodically during finasteride therapy.

! **WARNING** Monitor patient for a hypersensitivity reaction, which could become life-threatening such as angioedema.

If present, notify prescriber, expect drug to be discontinued, and provide supportive care, as needed and ordered.

! **WARNING** Monitor patient for depression that may become severe causing suicidal ideation.

- Be aware that finasteride therapy affects PSA levels. For example, drug may decrease levels even in the presence of prostate cancer. Any increases, no matter how slight or even if increase is still within normal limits, warrant further evaluation because of finasteride's risk of high-grade prostate cancer.

PATIENT TEACHING

! **WARNING** Urge patient and female partners to use reliable contraception during therapy because semen of men who take drug can harm male fetuses. Caution females of childbearing age, including pregnant females and children not to handle broken tablets.

- Instruct patient how to administer finasteride.

! **WARNING** Alert patient drug may cause an allergic reaction. If present, tell patient to notify prescriber and stop taking drug. If severe, stress importance of seeking immediate medical care.

! **WARNING** Instruct family or caregiver to monitor patient for depression. If severe, notify prescriber because drug can cause suicidal ideation.

- Inform patient that drug may cause a variety of sexual dysfunction problems, including decreased libido, ejaculation disorder, erectile dysfunction, and male infertility, which may continue after drug is discontinued. Advise patient to discuss concerns with prescriber.
- Urge patient to have periodic follow-up to determine drug effectiveness.

finerenone

Kerendia

Class and Category

Pharmacologic class: Nonsteroidal mineralocorticoid receptor (MR) antagonist
Therapeutic class: Selected steroid blocker

Indications and Dosages

* *To reduce the risk of cardiovascular death, end-stage kidney disease, hospitalization for heart failure, nonfatal MI, and sustained eGFR decline in patients with chronic kidney disease associated with type 2 diabetes*

TABLETS

Adults with an eGFR greater than 60 ml/min. *Initial:* 20 mg once daily. *Maintenance:* 20 mg once daily.
Adults with an eGFR greater than 25 but less than 60 ml/min. *Initial:* 10 mg once daily. *Target dose:* 20 mg once daily.

± **DOSAGE ADJUSTMENT** For patients with a serum potassium level greater than 5.5 mEq/L, drug withheld until serum potassium drops to 5.0 mEq/L or less, then drug restarted at 10 mg once daily. For patients with a serum potassium level 4.8 mEq/L or less and patient is taking 10 mg once daily, dosage increased to 20 mg once daily; for patients taking 20 mg once daily, no dosage adjustment needed.

Drug Administration

P.O.

- Administer drug once daily at about the same time each day.
- For patient unable to swallow tablets, crush tablet and mix with water or soft foods such as applesauce immediately before administration.
- Do not administer with grapefruit juice.

Route	Onset	Peak	Duration
P.O.	Unknown	0.5 to 1.25 hr	Unknown

Half-life: 2–3 hr

Mechanism of Action

Blocks MR-mediated sodium reabsorption and MR overactivation in both epithelial tissues such as the kidney and nonepithelial tissues, including the heart and blood vessels, thereby reducing MR overactivation believed to help cause fibrosis and inflammation.

Contraindications

Adrenal insufficiency, concomitant therapy with strong CYP3A4 inhibitors, hypersensitivity to finerenone or its components

Interactions

DRUGS

CYP3A4 inducers: Decreased finerenone exposure, decreasing effectiveness of drug

CYP3A4 inhibitors: Increased finerenone exposure; increasing risk of adverse reactions
drugs and supplements affecting serum potassium: Possibly increased serum potassium level

FOODS

grapefruit, grapefruit juice: Increased finerenone exposure, increasing risk of adverse reactions

Adverse Reactions

CV: **Hypotension**
GU: Mild decrease in eGFR
Other: **Hyperkalemia**, **hyponatremia**

Childbearing Considerations

PREGNANCY

- It is not known if drug can cause fetal harm. However, animal studies suggest a fetal risk.
- Use with caution only if benefit to mother outweighs potential risk to fetus.

LACTATION

- It is not known if drug is present in breast milk.
- Mothers should avoid breastfeeding during drug therapy and for 1 day after drug is discontinued.

Nursing Considerations

- Be aware finerenone should be avoided in patients with severe hepatic impairment. Patients with moderate hepatic impairment may require increased serum potassium monitoring during drug therapy.

! **WARNING** Check serum potassium level before finerenone therapy is started and periodically during drug therapy because drug may cause hyperkalemia. Know that drug should not be initiated if serum potassium is greater than 5.0 mEq/L until level decreases below 5.0 mEq/L. Also, know that during drug therapy, notify prescriber if serum potassium level becomes greater than 5.5 mEq/L, as drug will have to be withheld and dosage restarted at 10 mg once daily when serum potassium is 5.0 mEq/L or less. Patients at risk for hyperkalemia are those with decreasing kidney function. Risk is greater in patients who have higher baseline serum potassium levels or other risk factors for hyperkalemia such as patients on concomitant drugs that impair potassium excretion or increase serum potassium levels. These patients may require increased monitoring. Also monitor patient's sodium levels, as ordered because drug can cause hyponatremia.

! **WARNING** Monitor patient's blood pressure regularly because drug may cause hypotension.

PATIENT TEACHING

- Instruct patient how to administer finerenone.
- Advise patient to avoid using potassium supplements or salt substitutes containing potassium without consulting prescriber first.
- Instruct patient not to eat grapefruit or drink grapefruit juice during finerenone therapy.
- Stress importance of being compliant for required periodic blood work to measure serum electrolyte levels.

! **WARNING** Review signs and symptoms of hyperkalemia and hyponatremia with patient. If present, urge patient to contact prescriber. Know that patient's serum potassium and sodium levels must be checked, and possible medical intervention may be required.

- Inform mothers that breastfeeding is not recommended during finerenone therapy and for 1 day after drug is discontinued.

fingolimod hydrochloride

Gilenya

fingolimod lauryl sulfate

Tascenso ODT

Class and Category

Pharmacologic class: Sphingosine 1-phosphate receptor modulator
Therapeutic class: Antimultiple sclerotic

Indications and Dosages

∗ *To treat relapsing forms of multiple sclerosis (MS), including active secondary progressive disease, clinically isolated syndrome, and relapsing-remitting disease*

CAPSULES (GILENYA), ORALLY DISINTEGRATING TABLETS (TASCENSO ODT)

Adults and children ages 10 and older weighing more than 40 kg (88 lb). 0.5 mg once daily.
Children ages 10 and older weighing 40 kg (88 lb) or less. 0.25 mg once daily.

Drug Administration

P.O.

- Capsules should be swallowed whole and not chewed, crushed, or opened.
- When administering ODT form, use dry gloved hands to open blister pack. Peel back the foil covering of one blister and gently remove the tablet. Do not push the tablet through the foil. Immediately have patient place tablet on tongue and allow it to dissolve before swallowing. Tablet may be taken with or without water. Do not store the tablet outside of blister pack for future use.
- After first dose, monitor patient for 6 hr for symptomatic bradycardia. Obtain hourly blood pressure and pulse checks and, if warranted, ECG monitoring. If an abnormality occurs, monitor for an additional 6 hr. Patient may need to stay overnight for additional monitoring. If abnormalities occurred with first dose, monitoring repeated for second dose.
- When restarting drug after treatment interrupted, perform first-dose monitoring again because of potential effects on heart rate and AV conduction.

Route	Onset	Peak	Duration
P.O.	Unknown	12–16 hr	Unknown

Half-life: 6–9 days

Mechanism of Action

May reduce lymphocyte migration into the central nervous system to produce improved physical mobility.

Contraindications

Baseline QTc interval equal to or greater than 500 msec; experience within past 6 mo of class III or IV heart failure, decompensated heart failure requiring hospitalization, MI, stroke, TIA, or unstable angina; history or presence of Mobitz Type II second-degree or third-degree atrioventricular block or sick sinus syndrome unless patient has functioning pacemaker in place; hypersensitivity to fingolimod or its components; presence of arrhythmias requiring the use of class IA or class III antiarrhythmic drugs

Interactions

DRUGS

antineoplastics, immunosuppressives, immunomodulators: Increased immunosuppression
beta-blockers, calcium channel blockers, such as diltiazem or verapamil, digoxin: Possibly increased severity of bradycardia or slowing of atrioventricular conduction
chlorpromazine, citalopram, erythromycin, haloperidol, methadone: Possibly increased risk for prolonged QT interval, which may lead to torsades de pointes
ketoconazole: Increased fingolimod levels
live attenuated vaccines: Increased risk of contracting disease from live virus
vaccines: Decreased effectiveness of vaccines during and up to 2 mo after fingolimod therapy

Adverse Reactions

CNS: Asthenia, depression, dizziness, headache, migraine, paresthesia, **posterior reversible encephalopathy syndrome**, **progressive multifocal leukoencephalopathy**, **seizures**, **status epilepticus**, syncope, tumefactive demyelinating lesions
CV: **Atrioventricular blocks**, **bradycardia**, elevated blood triglycerides, hypertension, **transient asystole**
EENT: Blurred vision, eye pain, macular edema, sinusitis
GI: Diarrhea, elevated liver enzymes, gastroenteritis, **liver injury**
HEME: **Hemolytic anemia**, **leukopenia**, lymphopenia, **thrombocytopenia**
MS: Arthralgia, back pain, myalgia, severe increase in disability with discontinuation of therapy
RESP: Bronchitis, cough, dyspnea, pulmonary dysfunction
SKIN: Alopecia, **basal cell carcinoma**, eczema, **melanoma**, **Merkel cell carcinoma**, pruritus, rash, **squamous cell carcinoma**, tinea infections, urticaria

Other: **Angioedema**; flu-like symptoms; increased severity of herpes viral infections, including human papilloma viral infections; infections such as bacterial, fungi, and viral; **Kaposi sarcoma**; lymphomas; weight loss

Childbearing Considerations

PREGNANCY

- Pregnancy exposure registry: 1-877-598-7237; email: gpr@quintiles.com, or website: www.gilenyapregnancyregistry.com.
- Drug may cause fetal harm. Animal studies suggest an increased risk of developmental toxicity.
- Pregnancy status of females of childbearing age should be determined before drug therapy is started.
- Drug is not recommended during pregnancy.

LACTATION

- It is not known if drug is present in breast milk.
- Mothers should check with prescriber before breastfeeding.

REPRODUCTION

- Females of childbearing age should use effective contraception during drug therapy and for 2 mo after drug is discontinued.
- Females of childbearing age who plan to become pregnant need to have drug discontinued 2 mo before planned conception.

Nursing Considerations

! **WARNING** Ensure females of childbearing age have a negative pregnancy test result before fingolimod therapy is begun.

! **WARNING** Be aware that fingolimod therapy should not begin in a patient with an active acute or chronic infection until the infection is resolved because drug causes a dose-dependent reduction in peripheral lymphocyte count up to 30% of baseline values. Obtain results of a recent CBC (within past 6 months) prior to starting therapy, as ordered, because drug increases risk of infection, especially bacterial, fungi, and viral, which may become serious and life-threatening. Monitor patient throughout drug therapy for signs and symptoms of infection. If present, notify prescriber, expect drug to be discontinued if serious, and therapy given to eradicate the infection.

- Obtain a recent liver enzyme evaluation (within past 6 months) prior to initiating fingolimod therapy, as ordered, because drug may cause elevation of liver enzymes. Monitor periodically throughout therapy and expect drug to be discontinued if liver enzymes exceed 5 times the upper limit of normal. Also, monitor patients for symptoms suggestive of hepatic dysfunction, such as unexplained abdominal pain, anorexia, dark urine, fatigue, jaundice, nausea, and vomiting. Know that patients with preexisting liver disease may be at increased risk for further elevation in liver enzymes during fingolimod therapy.
- Immunize patient against the varicella-zoster virus if he is antibody negative, as ordered. Be aware that fingolimod therapy will have to be postponed for 1 month to allow the full effect of vaccination to occur.
- Expect patient to be vaccinated against human papilloma virus (HPV) prior to fingolimod therapy taking into account vaccination recommendations because infections caused by HPV have occurred during drug therapy. Cancer screening, including Papanicolaou test, should be done routinely.

! **WARNING** Obtain an ECG on patients receiving antiarrhythmic therapy, including beta-blockers and calcium channel blockers, those with cardiac risk factors, and those who have an irregular or slow heartbeat prior to beginning fingolimod therapy because drug may cause bradycardia and increased risk for atrioventricular block, especially in the first 24 hours of therapy.

- Expect patient to have an ophthalmologic evaluation prior to beginning drug therapy and then again 3 to 4 months after therapy has begun to assess for macular edema. Patients with diabetes mellitus or a history of uveitis should have ongoing evaluations because they are at increased risk for macular edema. Report any visual disturbances to prescriber during drug therapy and expect additional ophthalmologic evaluation to be performed. If abnormalities are detected, expect drug to be discontinued. Visual acuity loss may persist even after resolution of macular edema in some patients.

! **WARNING** Observe patient for 24 hours after the first dose of fingolimod for signs and symptoms of bradycardia. Heart rate usually begins to decrease within an hour of the first dose. The maximal decline in heart rate usually occurs within 6 hours and recovers level within 10 hours after the first dose. A second decline may occur within the first 24 hours after the first dose of the drug has been given. Monitor patient closely because the second decline may be more pronounced than the first. If patient develops chest pain, dizziness, fatigue, hypotension, or palpitations, notify prescriber, initiate appropriate management, as ordered, and continue observation until the symptoms have resolved. Know that with continued drug use, the heart rate returns to baseline within 1 month. Also, observe patient closely for cardiac effects after dosage increases or when drug is reinitiated if treatment was discontinued or interrupted for a period of time.

! **WARNING** Monitor patient for hypersensitivity reactions which could become life-threatening such as angioedema. If present, notify prescriber, expect drug to be discontinued, and provide supportive care, as needed and ordered.

! **WARNING** Be aware that tumefactive demyelinating lesions may occur within the first 9 months after fingolimod has begun and may also occur within 4 months after drug is discontinued. Expect prompt imaging evaluation and initiation of appropriate treatment in patients who develop a severe multiple sclerosis relapse during fingolimod therapy.

- Monitor patient for dyspnea throughout fingolimod therapy because drug may reduce diffusion lung capacity for carbon monoxide (DLCO) and forced expiratory volume over 1 second. Expect to monitor spirometric evaluations of respiratory function and evaluation of DLCO during therapy, if clinically indicated.
- Monitor patient's blood pressure regularly to detect development of hypertension.

! **WARNING** Assess patient's skin for abnormalities, as drug may increase risk of basal cell carcinoma, melanoma, and Merkel cell carcinoma. Promptly report any suspicious looking lesions.

- Monitor patient for up to 2 months after therapy has been discontinued because effects of drugs may continue that long. Also, be aware that severe increase in disability may occur after discontinuation of drug and can occur up to 24 weeks after drug is stopped. Assess patient's level of function during this time and expect appropriate treatment to be given, as needed.

PATIENT TEACHING

! **WARNING** Inform females of childbearing age that a negative pregnancy test result must be obtained before drug therapy can begin. Instruct these patients to use effective contraception to avoid pregnancy during and for 2 months after fingolimod therapy is discontinued because of potential fetal harm. Stress importance of notifying prescriber immediately if pregnancy occurs during drug therapy. Advise females of childbearing age contemplating a pregnancy that drug will have to be discontinued for 2 months before conception.

- Instruct patient how to administer form of fingolimod prescribed.
- Inform patient that patient will need to be observed for at least 6 hours after the first dose. Inform patient of the need to repeat this observation period again for 6 hours if treatment is interrupted for more than 1 day within the first 2 weeks of therapy, if treatment is interrupted for more than 7 days during week 3 and 4 of therapy, or if treatment is discontinued for more than 14 days and then treatment is reinitiated. Also, tell patient an observation period for 6 hours will be required any time dosage is increased.

! **WARNING** Alert patient fingolimod may cause an allergic reaction. If present, tell patient to notify prescriber. If severe, stress importance of seeking immediate medical care.

! **WARNING** Tell patient to report any adverse signs and symptoms of infection or any other persistent or serious abnormalities to prescriber promptly, even up to 2 months after drug has been discontinued.

! **WARNING** Advise patient to examine his skin regularly for skin abnormalities because drug may increase risk of skin cancer, including melanoma. Tell patient to report any suspicious skin lesion to prescriber for evaluation. Remind patient to limit exposure to sunlight and ultraviolet light, wear protective clothing, and use a sunscreen with a high protection factor when going outdoors.

- Instruct patient how to check his pulse and tell him to notify prescriber if his pulse rate drops below 60 beats/min or becomes irregular.
- Advise patient to notify prescriber immediately if patient experiences visual changes.
- Tell patient to notify prescriber if he notices symptoms suggestive of liver dysfunction, such as unexplained abdominal pain, anorexia, dark urine, fatigue, jaundice, nausea, or vomiting.
- Alert patient of the need to have periodic blood work done during fingolimod therapy and urge him to be compliant with these evaluations.
- Inform patient that adverse effects of the drug may occur as long as 2 months after the drug has been discontinued. Also, inform patient that a severe increase in disability may occur after drug is discontinued for up to 24 weeks after the drug has been discontinued. If present, tell patient to notify prescriber.

flecainide acetate

Class and Category

Pharmacologic class: Benzamide derivative
Therapeutic class: Class IC antiarrhythmic

Indications and Dosages

✶ *To prevent life-threatening ventricular arrhythmias such as sustained ventricular tachycardia*

TABLETS

Adults. *Initial:* 100 mg every 12 hr. Increased by 50 mg twice daily no more frequently than once every 4 days, as needed, until response occurs. *Usual:* Up to 150 mg every 12 hr. *Maximum:* 400 mg daily.
Children over age 6 mo. *Initial:* 100 mg/m²/day in divided doses 2 to 3 times daily. *Maximum:* 200 mg/m²/day.
Children ages 6 mo and younger. *Initial:* 50 mg/m²/day in divided doses 2 to 3 times daily. *Maximum:* 200 mg/m²/day.

✶ *To prevent paroxysmal supraventricular tachycardias (PSVT), including atrioventricular nodal reentrant tachycardia, atrioventricular reentrant tachycardia and other supraventricular tachycardias associated with disabling symptoms in patients without structural heart disease; to prevent paroxysmal atrial fibrillation or flutter associated with disabling symptoms*

TABLETS

Adults. *Initial:* 50 mg every 12 hr. Increased by 50 mg twice daily no more frequently than once every 4 days, as needed, until response occurs. *Maximum:* 300 mg daily.

± **DOSAGE ADJUSTMENT** For adult patients with a creatinine clearance less than 35 ml/min, initial dose reduced to 100 mg once daily or 50 mg every 12 hours. For adult patients taking amiodarone concurrently, dosage reduced by 50%. While administration of drug has not been deemed safe in children, dosage may be prescribed by a cardiologist, if deemed absolutely necessary. The cardiologist will prescribe a dosage for children over ages 6 months that is different from children ages 6 months and younger. For example, children over age 6 month, initial dose is usually 100 mg/m² daily in 2 to 3 evenly divided doses; for children ages 6 month and younger initial dose is usually 50 mg/m² daily in 2 to 3 evenly divided doses.

Drug Administration

P.O.

- Take patient's pulse before each dose.
- Heart rate may have to be monitored with an ECG during the first few doses.
- Give drug with or without food.

Route	Onset	Peak	Duration
P.O.	Unknown	1–6 hr	Unknown

Half-life: 12–27 hr

Mechanism of Action

Achieves antiarrhythmic effect by inhibiting fast sodium channels of myocardial cell membranes, which increase myocardial recovery after repolarization, and by depressing the upstroke of the action potential. Flecainide also produces its antiarrhythmic effect by:

- slowing intracardiac conduction, which slightly increases the duration of the action potential in atrial and ventricular muscle, thus prolonging the PR interval, QRS complex, and QT interval.
- shortening the action potential of Purkinje fibers without affecting surrounding myocardial tissue.
- inhibiting extracellular calcium influx (at high doses).
- stopping paroxysmal reentrant supraventricular tachycardias by acting on antegrade pathways of dysfunctional AV conduction.
- decreasing conduction in accessory pathways in those with Wolff-Parkinson-White syndrome.

Contraindications

Cardiogenic shock, hypersensitivity to flecainide or its components, recent MI, right bundle-branch block associated with left hemiblock or second- or third-degree AV block unless pacemaker is present

Interactions

DRUGS

amiodarone: Increased blood flecainide level
antiretrovirals: Possibly increased flecainide levels
beta-blockers, such as propranolol: Possibly myocardial depression and increased blood levels of both drugs
digoxin: Possibly increased blood digoxin level
quinidine: Possibly increased plasma flecainide concentrations in patients on chronic flecainide therapy, especially if these patients are extensive metabolizers

ACTIVITIES

smoking: Increased flecainide clearance

FOODS

acidic juices, foods that decrease urine pH below 5.0: Increased flecainide elimination and decreased therapeutic effects
foods that increase urine pH above 7.0, strict vegetarian diet: Decreased flecainide elimination and increased therapeutic effects

Adverse Reactions

CNS: Anxiety, depression, dizziness, drowsiness, fatigue, headache, lightheadedness, tremor, weakness
CV: **Arrhythmias**, chest pain, **heart failure**, **hypotension**
EENT: Blurred vision
GI: Abdominal pain, anorexia, constipation, **hepatic dysfunction**, nausea, vomiting
RESP: Dyspnea
SKIN: Rash

Childbearing Considerations

PREGNANCY

- It is not known if drug causes fetal harm.
- Use with caution only if benefit to mother outweighs potential risk to fetus.

LACTATION

- Drug is present in breast milk.
- A decision may be made to discontinue breastfeeding or the drug to avoid potential serious adverse reactions in the breastfed infant.

Nursing Considerations

! WARNING Be aware that drug use in children has not been established as being safe and effective. Children with structural heart disease may experience cardiac arrest and sudden death. Although drug may sometimes be used in children, it is not generally a preferred antiarrhythmic drug in pediatric patients. If it is used at all, it must be under the direct supervision of a cardiologist experienced in the treatment of arrhythmias in children with therapy initiated in a hospital setting that is equipped with ECG monitoring.

! WARNING Be aware flecainide has a negative inotropic effect and may cause or worsen congestive heart failure, especially in patients with cardiomyopathy or low ejection fractions (less than 30%) or who have preexisting severe heart failure (NYHA functional class III or IV).

- Monitor trough flecainide level periodically; therapeutic level is 0.2 to 1 mcg/ml.

! **WARNING** Know that because hypokalemia or hyperkalemia may interfere with flecainide's therapeutic effects, serum potassium level must be monitored before and during therapy as ordered and notify prescriber immediately if potassium imbalance develops. Also, monitor for and notify prescriber about prolonged PR interval, QRS complex, or QT interval; chest pain; or hypotension. Keep in mind that drug can cause fatal proarrhythmias, which is why it isn't considered a first-line antiarrhythmic.

- Monitor patient's ECG for arrhythmias.
- Check blood pressure, fluid intake and output, and weight regularly during therapy.

PATIENT TEACHING

- Instruct patient how to administer flecainide and to take drug at regular intervals to keep a constant blood level.
- Teach patient how to take pulse, and to record it daily, along with patient's weight. Advise patient to bring record to follow-up visits.
- Advise patient to notify prescriber if pulse is rapid or irregular or a weight gain of more than 2 lbs/day occurs.
- Advise patient to notify prescriber if persistent, serious, or unusual adverse reactions occur.
- Inform mothers wishing to breastfeed their infant that breastfeeding or the drug must be discontinued.
- Caution patient not to stop taking flecainide suddenly but to taper dosage gradually according to prescriber's instructions.

fluconazole

Diflucan

Class and Category

Pharmacologic class: Azole antifungal
Therapeutic class: Antifungal

Indications and Dosages

* *To treat oropharyngeal candidiasis*

ORAL SUSPENSION, TABLETS, I.V. INFUSION

Adults. *Initial:* 200 mg on day 1 followed by 100 mg once daily for at least 2 wk.
Children ages 6 mo and older. *Initial:* 6 mg/kg on day 1, followed by 3 mg/kg once daily for at least 2 wk.

* *To treat esophageal candidiasis*

ORAL SUSPENSION, TABLETS, I.V. INFUSION

Adults. *Initial:* 200 mg on day 1 followed by 100 mg once daily and given for a minimum of 3 wk and for at least 2 wk following resolution of symptoms. Dosage increased, as needed. *Maximum:* 400 mg/day.
Children ages 6 mo and older. *Initial:* 6 mg/kg on day 1, followed by 3 mg/kg once daily and increased, as needed, and given for a minimum of 3 wk and for at least 2 wk after esophageal symptoms resolve. *Maximum:* 12 mg/day.

* *To treat systemic Candida infections, including candidemia, disseminated candidiasis, and pneumonia*

ORAL SUSPENSION, TABLETS, I.V. INFUSION

Adults. Therapeutic dosages have not been established but doses up to 400 mg once daily have been given.

ORAL SUSPENSION

Children ages 3 mo and older. *Initial*: 25 mg/kg on day 1 (not to exceed 800 mg), followed by 12 mg/kg once daily (not to exceed 400 mg) and given for a minimum of 3 wk and for at least 2 wk after resolution of symptoms.
Infants from birth to 3 mo postnatal age and gestational age 30 wk and over. *Initial*: 25 mg/kg on day 1, followed by 12 mg/kg once daily and given for a minimum of 3 wk and for at lest 2 wk after resolution of symptoms.
Infants from birth to 3 mo postnatal age and gestational age less than 30 wk. *Initial*: 25 mg/kg on day 1, followed by 9 mg/kg once daily and given for a minimum of 3 wk and for at least 2 wk after resolution of symptoms.

± **DOSAGE ADJUSTMENT** For children ages 3 months and older on extracorporeal membrane oxygenation (EMCO), initial dosage increased to 35 mg/kg on day 1 (not to exceed 800 mg), For infants from birth to 3 months on EMCO, initial dosage increased to 35 mg/kg on day 1.

∗ *To treat peritonitis and UTIs*

ORAL SUSPENSION, TABLETS, I.V. INFUSION

Adults. 50 to 200 mg once daily.

∗ *To treat acute cryptococcal meningitis*

ORAL SUSPENSION, TABLETS, I.V. INFUSION

Adults. *Initial:* 400 mg on day 1, followed by 200 to 400 mg once daily based on patient's response, and continued for 10 to 12 wk after cerebrospinal fluid (CSF) culture is negative. **Children ages 6 mo and older.** *Initial:* 12 mg/kg on day 1, followed by 6 to 12 mg/kg once daily and continued for 10 to 12 wk after CSF culture is negative.

∗ *To prevent relapse of cryptococcal meningitis in patients with AIDs*

ORAL SUSPENSION, TABLETS, I.V. INFUSION

Adults. 200 mg once daily.
Children ages 6 mo and older. 6 mg/kg once daily.

∗ *To prevent candidiasis after bone marrow transplantation in patients who receive cytotoxic chemotherapy and/or radiation*

ORAL SUSPENSION, TABLETS, I.V. INFUSION

Adults. 400 mg once daily starting several days before procedure if severe neutropenia is expected and continued for 7 days after absolute neutrophil count exceeds 1,000/mm^3.

∗ *To treat vaginal candidiasis*

ORAL SUSPENSION, TABLETS

Adults. 150 mg as a single dose.

±**DOSAGE ADJUSTMENT** For all adult patients except female patients being treated for vaginal candidiasis and after initial loading dose, dosage reduced by 50% for patients with creatinine clearance of 50 ml/min or less. For adult patients on hemodialysis, usual dosage given after each hemodialysis; on nondialysis days, dosage reduced according to the patient's creatinine clearance. For pediatric patients, dosage adjustment for renal impairment has not been studied but is expected to parallel that recommended for adults.

Drug Administration

P.O.

- Tablets should be swallowed whole.
- Prepare oral suspension by first tapping bottle until all the powder flows freely. Reconstitute by adding 24 ml of Distilled Water or Purified Water to bottle and shake vigorously.
- Shake suspension well before administering. Use a measuring device for determining dosage.
- Store suspension at room temperature and discard after 2 wk.
- Protect drug from freezing.

I.V.

- Know that the drug is available in glass bottles or in Viaflex Plus plastic containers.
- Discard I.V. solution that's cloudy or contains precipitate.
- For use of Viaflex Plus plastic containers, do not remove unit from overwrap until ready for use. Tear overwrap down the side at slit and remove solution container. Some opacity of the plastic may occur but does not affect solution quality or safety. The opacity will diminish gradually. Check for minute leaks by squeezing inner bag firmly. If leaks are found, discard.
- Do not use plastic containers in series connections.
- Infuse continuously at rate that does not exceed 200 mg/hr.
- Use an infusion pump for administration.
- *Incompatibilities:* Other I.V. drugs

Route	Onset	Peak	Duration
P.O./I.V.	Unknown	1–2 hr	Unknown

Half-life: 20–50 hr

Mechanism of Action

Damages fungal cells by interfering with a cytochrome P-450 enzyme needed to convert lanosterol to ergosterol, an essential part of the fungal cell membrane. Decreased ergosterol synthesis causes increased cell permeability, which allows cell contents to leak. Fluconazole also may inhibit endogenous respiration, interact with membrane phospholipids, inhibit transformation of yeasts to mycelial forms, inhibit purine uptake, and impair biosynthesis of triglycerides and phospholipids.

Contraindications

Coadministration of drugs known to prolong QT interval and which are metabolized via the enzyme CYP3A4 (erythromycin, pimozide, or quinidine), hypersensitivity to fluconazole or its components

Interactions

DRUGS

abrocitinib: Increased systemic exposure of abrocitinib and its active metabolites increasing risk of adverse reactions
alfentanil, amitriptyline, astemizole, celecoxib, cyclosporine, halofantrine, methadone, nortriptyline, olaparib, phenytoin, rifabutin, saquinavir, sirolimus, theophylline, tofacitinib, triazolam, zidovudine: Increased blood levels of these drugs with possible increase in adverse reactions
amiodarone, astemizole, cisapride, erythromycin, pimozide, quinidine: Increased risk of QT interval prolongation possibly leading to torsades de pointes
benzodiazepines (short-acting): Possibly increased benzodiazepine level and psychomotor effects
calcium channel blockers: Possibly increased systemic exposure of calcium channel blockers causing adverse effects
carbamazepine: Possibly increased risk of carbamazepine toxicity
cyclophosphamide: Increased serum bilirubin and creatinine levels
fentanyl: Possibly elevated fentanyl concentration that may lead to respiratory depression
glipizide, glyburide, tolbutamide and other sulfonylurea oral hypoglycemic agents: Increased risk of hypoglycemia
HMG-CoA reductase inhibitors: Increased risk of myopathy and rhabdomyolysis
hydrochlorothiazide: Increased fluconazole level from decreased excretion
ibrutinib: Possibly increased plasma ibrutinib concentrations and increased risk of adverse reactions from ibrutinib administration
ivacaftor, ivacaftor fixed dose combinations (ivacaftor/tezacaftor/elexacaftor, tezacaftor/vacaftor): Increased ivacaftor exposure increasing risk of adverse reactions
lemborexant: Increased plasma concentration of lemborexant increasing risk of adverse reactions
losartan: Possibly decreased hypotensive effect of losartan
lurasidone: Increased lurasidone exposure increasing risk of adverse reactions
NSAIDs: Increased systemic exposure of NSAIDs
oral anticoagulants: Increased anticoagulant effects
prednisone: Possibly increased risk of acute adrenal cortex insufficiency
rifampin: Decreased serum fluconazole level
tacrolimus: Increased tacrolimus levels, possibly leading to nephrotoxicity
terfenadine: Increased risk of serious cardiac arrhythmias; increased terfenadine levels when dosage of terfenadine is 400 mg/day or greater
theophylline: Increased serum theophylline concentrations increasing risk of adverse reactions
tolvaptan: Increased plasma exposure to tolvaptan with possible significant increase in risk of tolvaptan-induced adverse reactions
vinca alkaloids: Possibly increased plasma vinca alkaloids, which may lead to neurotoxicity
vitamin A: Possible adverse CNS effects
voriconazole: Increased risk of toxicity

Adverse Reactions

CNS: Chills, dizziness, drowsiness, fever, headache, **seizures**
CV: **Prolonged QT interval**, **torsades de pointes**
EENT: Change in taste
ENDO: **Adrenal insufficiency**
GI: Abdominal pain, anorexia, constipation, diarrhea, **hepatic failure**, **intestinal perforation** (premature infants weighing less than 750 g at birth), nausea, vomiting
HEME: **Agranulocytosis**, **leukopenia**, **thrombocytopenia**
SKIN: Acute generalized exanthematous pustulosis, alopecia, diaphoresis, drug eruption, **exfoliative dermatitis**, photosensitivity, pruritus, rash, **Stevens-Johnson syndrome**, **toxic epidermal necrolysis**
Other: **Anaphylaxis**, **angioedema**, **drug reaction with eosinophilia and systemic symptoms (DRESS)**

Childbearing Considerations

PREGNANCY

- Drug can cause fetal harm such as distinct congenital anomalies in infants exposed in utero to high doses of the drug (400 to 800 mg per day) during most or all of the first trimester. Spontaneous abortions and congenital abnormalities may be potential risks even with 150 mg of the drug given as a single or repeated dose during the first trimester.

- Drug should be avoided in pregnancy except in patients with severe or potentially life-threatening fungal infections in whom the beneficial use of the drug outweighs the potential risk to the fetus.

LACTATION

- Drug is present in breast milk.
- Mothers should check with prescriber before breastfeeding.

REPRODUCTION

- Advise females of childbearing age to use effective contraceptive measures during drug therapy and for 1 wk after the final dose.

Nursing Considerations

! WARNING Use fluconazole cautiously in patients with potentially proarrhythmic conditions because drug may prolong the QT interval, which can lead to life-threatening torsades de pointes.

- Obtain a specimen for culture and sensitivity before drug therapy begins, as ordered, but know that drug therapy may begin before results are known.
- Expect to obtain BUN and serum creatinine levels, and liver enzymes, as ordered, before therapy starts. Monitor hepatic and renal function periodically during therapy, as ordered, and notify prescriber if signs of dysfunction are present.

! WARNING Know that oral suspension form contains sucrose and should not be administered to patients with glucose/galactose malabsorption, hereditary fructose, or sucrase-isomaltase deficiency.

! WARNING Assess patient for hypersensitivity reactions, including rash during therapy, and notify prescriber if present because drug can cause severe allergic reactions, including skin reactions that could become life-threatening. If hypersensitivity is present, notify prescriber, expect drug to be discontinued, and provide supportive care, as needed and ordered.

! WARNING Monitor patient for signs and symptoms of adrenal insufficiency, which may be reversible when drug is discontinued.

- Monitor coagulation test results and assess patient for bleeding if patient is receiving an oral anticoagulant.

PATIENT TEACHING

! WARNING Urge females of childbearing age to alert prescriber if pregnancy could be a possibility before fluconazole is administered and if pregnancy occurs during drug therapy. To prevent pregnancy, tell females of childbearing age to use an effective contraception during drug therapy and for 1 week after drug is discontinued.

- Instruct patient, family, or caregiver how to administer oral form of fluconazole. Alert patient that drug may need to be given intravenously.
- Advise patient to complete entire course of therapy, even if she feels better.

! WARNING Inform patient drug may cause an allergic reaction that may involve the skin. Tell patient to notify prescriber if signs and symptoms of an allergic reaction occur, including a rash. Urge patient to seek immediate medical care, if serious.

- Tell patient to inform all prescribers of fluconazole use and not to take any over-the-counter preparations, including herbal preparations, without consulting prescriber first, as drug can interact with many other drugs and substances.
- Alert patient that fluconazole may change the taste of food.
- Encourage patient to notify prescriber of persistent, severe, or unusual adverse reactions.
- Tell patient not to perform hazardous activities such as driving until effects of drug are known and resolved.
- Urge patient to monitor blood glucose level often if she takes an oral antidiabetic drug because of increased risk of hypoglycemia.

flumazenil

Class and Category

Pharmacologic class: Imidazobenzodiazepine derivative

Therapeutic class: Benzodiazepine antidote

Indications and Dosages

✷ To reverse conscious sedation or general anesthesia from benzodiazepine therapy

I.V. INJECTION

Adults. *Initial:* 0.2 mg given over 15 sec. If response is inadequate after 45 sec dose repeated. Repeated every 1 min thereafter, as needed, up to maximum total dose of 1 mg (first dose plus 4 more doses). If sedation recurs, dosage regimen repeated every 20 min or longer, as needed not exceeding maximum dosage. *Maximum:* 1 mg/episode; 20 min separating each episode; and no more than 3 mg given in a 1-hour period.

✷ To reverse conscious sedation in children from benzodiazepine therapy

I.V. INJECTION

Children ages 1 and older. *Initial:* 0.01 mg/kg (up to 0.2 mg) given over 15 sec. If response is inadequate after 45 sec, dose repeated. Repeated every 1 min thereafter, as needed, up to maximum total dose of 0.05 mg/kg or 1 mg, whichever is lower (first dose plus 4 more doses). *Maximum:* 5 doses total, not exceeding accumulative dosage of 0.05 mg/kg or 1 mg, whichever is lower.

✷ To reverse benzodiazepine toxicity or suspected overdose

I.V. INJECTION

Adults. *Initial:* 0.2 mg given over 30 sec. If response is inadequate after 30 sec, 0.3 mg given over 30 sec. Then 0.5 mg given over 30 sec at 1-min intervals thereafter, as needed, to maximum total dose of 3 mg in 1-hr period. If sedation recurs after 20 min or more, dosage regimen repeated with maximum dosage of 3 mg in 1-hr period not exceeded. *Maximum:* 3 mg/episode; 20 min between episodes; 3 mg in 1-hr period.

Drug Administration

I.V.

- Do not remove drug from drug vial until ready for administration.
- Give undiluted or diluted in a syringe with 0.9% Sodium Chloride Injection, 5% Dextrose Injection, or Lactated Ringer's solution.
- Avoid aerosol generation when preparing syringes for injection. If drug splatters onto skin, wash area with cool water.
- Administer over 15 sec to reverse conscious sedation or general anesthesia and over 30 sec to reverse benzodiazepine toxicity or suspected overdose. Inject directly into tubing of a free-flowing compatible I.V. solution.
- Use a large vein, if possible, to minimize pain at site. Avoid extravasation because drug may irritate tissue.
- Once drug is drawn into a syringe discard after 24 hr, if not used.
- *Incompatibilities:* None reported by manufacturer.

Route	Onset	Peak	Duration
I.V.	1–2 min	6–10 min	Variable

Half-life: 40–80 min

Mechanism of Action

Antagonizes CNS effects of benzodiazepines by competing for their binding sites.

Contraindications

Evidence of tricyclic antidepressant overdose; hypersensitivity to flumazenil, benzodiazepines, or their components; use of benzodiazepine to control a potentially life-threatening condition such as increased intracranial pressure or status epilepticus

Interactions

DRUGS

benzodiazepines: Benzodiazepine withdrawal symptoms, including seizures

nonbenzodiazepine agonists: Loss of effectiveness of these drugs

tetracyclic or tricyclic antidepressant overdose: High risk of seizures

Adverse Reactions

CNS: Agitation, anxiety, ataxia, confusion, dizziness, drowsiness, emotional lability, fatigue, headache, hypoesthesia, insomnia, paresthesia, resedation, **seizures**, tremor, vertigo

CV: Hypertension, palpitations

EENT: Blurred vision, diplopia, dry mouth

GI: Nausea, vomiting
RESP: Dyspnea, hyperventilation, **hypoventilation**
SKIN: Diaphoresis, flushing, rash
Other: Injection-site pain and thrombophlebitis

Childbearing Considerations

PREGNANCY

- It is not known if drug causes fetal harm.
- Use with caution only if benefit to mother outweighs potential risk to fetus.

LABOR AND DELIVERY

- Not recommended for use during labor and delivery.

LACTATION

- It is not known if drug is present in breast milk.
- Mothers should check with prescriber before breastfeeding.

Nursing Considerations

- Use flumazenil cautiously in patients with cardiac disease. Assess for increased anxiety or stress from benzodiazepine withdrawal because patient's blood pressure may rise.

! **WARNING** Monitor patient for signs of hypoventilation or resedation for at least 2 hours after giving flumazenil because drug has a short half-life. Be aware that patient shouldn't be discharged until the risk of resedation has resolved.

! **WARNING** Monitor patient for seizures.

- Be aware that drug may cause signs of benzodiazepine withdrawal in drug-dependent patient. Also, abrupt awakening from benzodiazepine overdose can cause agitation, dysphoria, and increased adverse reactions.
- Be aware that benzodiazepine reversal may cause an anxiety or a panic attack for patient with a history of these episodes. Expect to adjust dosage carefully.

PATIENT TEACHING

- Caution patient to avoid alcohol and over-the-counter drugs for 10 to 24 hours after receiving drug.
- Advise patient to avoid hazardous activities for 18 to 24 hours after discharge.
- Inform patient and family that agitation, emotional lability, fear, and panic attack (if patient has a history of them) may occur. Tell them to notify prescriber if patient develops adverse reactions.
- Provide written instructions and give instructions to family or caregiver even if patient is alert because drug doesn't always reverse postprocedure amnesia immediately.

fluoxetine hydrochloride

Prozac

Class and Category

Pharmacologic class: Selective serotonin reuptake inhibitor (SSRI)
Therapeutic class: Antidepressant

Indications and Dosages

✱ *To treat acute major depressive disorder (MDD); to provide maintenance therapy for MDD*

CAPSULES, ORAL SOLUTION, TABLETS (PROZAC)

Adults. *Initial:* 20 mg once daily in the morning. Dosage increased every couple of weeks, as needed. Doses above 20 mg daily given once daily in the morning or divided and given in morning and at noon. *Maximum:* 80 mg daily.
Children ages 8 and older. *Initial:* 10 or 20 mg once daily. Initial dosage of 10 mg increased after 1 wk or longer to 20 mg daily, as needed.

✱ *To treat acute obsessive–compulsive disorder (OCD); to provide maintenance therapy for OCD*

CAPSULES, ORAL SOLUTION, TABLETS (PROZAC)

Adults. *Initial:* 20 mg once daily in the morning. Dosage increased every couple of wk, as needed. Doses above 20 mg daily given once daily in the morning or divided and given in morning and at noon. *Maximum:* 80 mg daily.
Children ages 7 and older. *Initial:* 10 mg once daily in the morning. Dosage increased after 2 wk to 20 mg daily. Subsequent dosage increased, as needed, at intervals of at least several wk. *Maintenance:* 20 to 60 mg daily. for adolescents and higher weight children; 20 to 30 mg daily

F

for lower weight children. *Maximum*: 60 mg daily.

✱ *To treat moderate to severe bulimia nervosa; to provide maintenance therapy for bulimia nervosa*

CAPSULES, ORAL SOLUTION, TABLETS (PROZAC)

Adults. 60 mg once daily in the morning. Alternatively, dosage titrated up to 60 mg once daily over several days.

✱ *To treat acute panic disorder with or without agoraphobia*

CAPSULES, ORAL SOLUTION, TABLETS (PROZAC)

Adults. *Initial:* 10 mg daily. Dosage increased in 1 wk to 20 mg daily, as needed. Dosage further increased after several wk, as needed. *Maximum:* 60 mg daily.

✱ *As adjunct to treat acute depressive episodes associated with bipolar I disorder*

CAPSULES, ORAL SOLUTION, TABLETS (PROZAC)

Adults. *Initial:* 20 mg given with 5 mg olanzapine once daily in the evening. Dosage adjusted, as needed. *Usual:* 20 to 50 mg with 5 to 12.5 mg olanzapine.

Children ages 10 and older. *Initial:* 20 mg given with 2.5 mg olanzapine once daily in the evening. Dosage adjusted, as needed. *Maximum:* 50 mg given with 12 mg of olanzapine once daily in the evening.

✱ *As adjunct to treat resistant depression*

CAPSULES, ORAL SOLUTION, TABLETS (PROZAC)

Adults. *Initial:* 20 mg with 5 mg olanzapine once daily in the evening. Dosage adjusted, as needed. *Usual:* 20 to 50 mg with 5 to 20 mg olanzapine once daily in the evening.

± **DOSAGE ADJUSTMENT** For adult patients who are taking Prozac and have concurrent illness or hepatic impairment, those who take multiple medications, or are elderly, dose reduced or dosing interval increased. For lower-weight children taking drug for depression, dosage increased to 20 mg daily only if improvement insufficient after several weeks. For lower-weight children taking drug for OCD, dosage increased above 10 mg daily only if clinical improvement remains insufficient after several weeks. Maintenance dosage for such children is 20 to 30 mg daily.

✱ *To treat premenstrual dysmorphic disorder*

TABLETS (FLUOXETINE HYDROCHLORIDE)

Adults. 20 mg once daily given continuously (every day of menstrual cycle) or intermittently (starting 14 days prior to the anticipated onset of menstruation through the first full day of menses and repeated with each new cycle). Dosage increased as needed. *Maximum:* 80 mg daily.

± **DOSAGE ADJUSTMENT** For elderly patients or patients with hepatic impairment, dose reduced or dosing interval increased. For patients with concurrent disease or those who take multiple medications, individualized dose adjustments may be required.

Drug Administration

P.O.

- Capsules and tablets should be swallowed whole and not chewed, crushed, or opened/split.
- Use calibrated device when measuring dose using Prozac oral solution. Store oral solution at room temperature and protect from light.

Route	Onset	Peak	Duration
P.O.	2–4 wk	6–8 hr	Unknown

Half-life: 1–6 days

Mechanism of Action

Selectively inhibits reuptake of the neurotransmitter serotonin by CNS neurons and increases the amount of serotonin available in nerve synapses. An elevated serotonin level may result in elevated mood and, consequently, reduce depression, lessen obsessive–compulsive behavior, and diminish panic symptoms, as well as relieve premenstrual dysmorphic discomfort.

Contraindications

Concurrent therapy with pimozide or thioridazine; hypersensitivity to fluoxetine, other selective serotonin reuptake inhibitors or their components; use within 14 days of MAO inhibitor therapy, including linezolid or intravenous methylene blue.

Interactions

DRUGS

alprazolam, diazepam: Possibly prolonged half-life of these drugs

anticonvulsants: Increased anticonvulsant levels with potential for toxicity
aspirin, NSAIDs, warfarin: Increased anticoagulant activity and risk of bleeding
benzodiazepines, CNS depressants: Increased CNS effect and development of adverse effects
CYP2D6-metabolized drugs, such as antiarrhythmics (especially flecainide, propafenone), antidepressants (tricyclics), antipsychotics (phenothiazines and most atypicals), thioridazine, and vinblastine: Increased plasma levels of these drugs and increased risk of serious adverse reactions
buspirone, fentanyl, intravenous methylene blue, linezolid, serotonergics (such as amphetamines and other psychostimulants, antidepressants, and dopamine agonists), St. John's wort, tramadol, tricyclic antidepressants, triptans, tryptophan: Increased risk of serotonin syndrome
highly protein-bound drugs: Possibly increased risk of elevated plasma levels of drugs increasing risk of adverse effects
lithium: Decreased or increased lithium levels; potential for serotonergic effects
MAO inhibitors: Possibly severe and life-threatening adverse effects; increased risk of serotonin syndrome
olanzapine: Increased blood olanzapine levels with decreased clearance resulting in possible increased risk for adverse reactions
phenytoin: Increased blood phenytoin level and risk of toxicity
pimozide, thioridazine, or other drugs that may prolong QT interval: Increased blood levels of these drugs; possibly increased risk of prolonged QT interval

Adverse Reactions

CNS: Akathisia, anxiety, ataxia, balance disorder, chills, **CVA**, depersonalization, dream disturbances, drowsiness, dyskinesia, emotional lability, euphoria, fatigue, fever, headache, hypertonia, hypomania, insomnia, mania, memory impairment, movement disorders, myoclonus, nervousness, **neuroleptic malignant syndrome**, paranoid reaction, restlessness, **seizures**, **serotonin syndrome**, somnolence, **suicidal ideation**, tremor, vertigo, violent behaviors, weakness, yawning
CV: **Arrhythmias**, **atrial fibrillation**, **cardiac arrest**, **hypotension**, palpitations, **prolonged QT interval**, **torsades de pointes**, **ventricular arrhythmias**
EENT: Abnormal vision, angle-closure glaucoma, cataracts, dry mouth, mydriasis, optic neuritis, partial or complete loss of smell, pharyngitis, sinusitis, taste perversion, teeth grinding
ENDO: Galactorrhea, gynecomastia, hyperprolactinemia, **hypoglycemia**, syndrome of inappropriate antidiuretic hormone secretion (SIADH)
GI: Anorexia, cholestatic jaundice, diarrhea, dysphagia, gastritis, gastroenteritis, **hepatic failure or necrosis**, indigestion, **melena**, nausea, **pancreatitis**, stomach ulcer
GU: Decreased or increased libido, delayed or absent orgasm (females), dysuria, ejaculation disorders, erectile dysfunction, **gynecological bleeding**, impotence, micturition disorder, **renal failure**, **vaginal bleeding**
HEME: **Altered platelet function**, **aplastic anemia**, **immune-related hemolytic anemia**, **pancytopenia**, **thrombocytopenia**, **thrombocytopenic purpura**, **unusual bleeding (mild to severe)**
MS: Arthralgia, myalgia
RESP: Dyspnea, **pulmonary embolism**, **pulmonary hypertension**
SKIN: Alopecia, diaphoresis, ecchymosis, **eosinophilic pneumonia**, epidermal necrolysis, **erythema multiforme**, erythema nodosum, **exfoliative dermatitis**, pruritus, rash, **Stevens-Johnson syndrome**, urticaria
Other: **Drug reaction with eosinophilia and systemic symptoms (DRESS)**, flu-like symptoms, **hyponatremia**, weight loss

Childbearing Considerations

PREGNANCY

- Pregnancy exposure registry: 1-844-405-6185 or https://womenshealth.org/clinical-and-research-programs/pregnancyregistry/antidepressants/.
- Neonates exposed to drug late in the third trimester may develop serious complications after birth requiring prolonged hospitalization, respiratory support, and tube feeding.
- Use with extreme caution only if benefit to mother outweighs potential risk to fetus.

LACTATION

- Drug is present in breast milk.

F

- Patient should check with prescriber before breastfeeding.
- If breastfeeding occurs, infant should be monitored for agitation, irritability, poor feeding, and poor weight gain.

Nursing Considerations

! **WARNING** Avoid giving fluoxetine within 14 days of an MAO inhibitor or starting MAO inhibitor therapy within 5 weeks of discontinuing fluoxetine.

- Know that patients with depression should be screened for bipolar disorder before fluoxetine therapy is started because treating depression alone in these patients may precipitate a manic or mixed episode.

! **WARNING** Use fluoxetine with extreme caution in patients with congenital long QT syndrome, previous history of QT prolongation, or family history of long QT syndrome or sudden cardiac death. In addition, use caution in presence of other conditions that increase risk of QT prolongation and ventricular arrhythmia, such as concurrent drug therapy with drugs known to prolong the QT interval, hypokalemia, hypomagnesemia, recent MI, significant arrhythmias, uncompensated heart failure and conditions that predispose patient to increased fluoxetine exposure, such as hepatic impairment or concurrent use of drugs known to increase blood fluoxetine levels, such as CYP2D6 inhibitors, CYP2D6 poor metabolizer status, or use of other highly protein-bound drugs. Obtain an ECG recording, as ordered, before fluoxetine begins in these patients and periodically throughout therapy. Expect fluoxetine to be discontinued if the QT interval becomes prolonged or patient develops a ventricular arrhythmia.

! **WARNING** Monitor patient for a rash that could signal a life threatening cutaneous hypersensitivity reaction. Other symptoms that may accompany rash include arthralgias, edema, fever, lymphadenopathy, and respiratory distress. However, know that although rash is a common sign of DRESS, it sometimes only initially presents with a fever or swollen lymph nodes. If patient develops a rash, notify prescriber immediately, expect drug to be discontinued, and provide supportive care, as needed and tolerated.

! **WARNING** Monitor patient's serum sodium level regularly, as ordered and patient for signs and symptoms of hyponatremia such as confusion, difficulty concentrating, headache, memory impairment, unsteadiness, and weakness. Be alert for more severe signs and symptoms such as coma, hallucinations, seizures, and syncope. Know that if left untreated, hyponatremia can cause respiratory arrest and death. Monitor patient—especially an elderly patient—for hypoosmolarity of serum and urine and for hyponatremia, which may indicate fluoxetine-induced SIADH.

! **WARNING** Monitor patient closely for evidence of bleeding, especially if patient takes another drug known to increase the risk, such as aspirin, NSAIDs, or warfarin and other anticoagulants. Bleeding can range from ecchymoses, epistaxis, hematomas, and petechiae to life-threatening hemorrhages. If bleeding occurs and is significant, notify prescriber and provide supportive care, as needed and ordered.

! **WARNING** Monitor patient for seizures, especially if patient has a history of seizures.

! **WARNING** Monitor patient with depression (especially children, adolescents, and young adults) and watch closely for suicidal tendencies, particularly when therapy starts and dosage changes because depression may worsen temporarily during those times.

! **WARNING** Monitor patient for possible serotonin syndrome, characterized by agitation, chills, confusion, diaphoresis, diarrhea, fever, hyperactive reflexes, poor coordination, restlessness, shaking, talking or acting with uncontrolled excitement, tremor, and twitching, especially if patient is receiving another drug that raises serotonin level (such as amphetamine, dopamine agonist, MAO inhibitor, tryptophan, or other antidepressant or psychostimulant). In its most severe form, serotonin syndrome can resemble neuroleptic malignant syndrome, which includes autonomic instability, high fever, muscle rigidity, and possible fluctuations in vital signs and mental status.

! WARNING Monitor patient for any persistent, serious, or unusual adverse reactions because drug can affect many body systems and cause symptoms that range from mild to life-threatening.

- Monitor patient with diabetes mellitus for altered blood glucose level because drug may cause hypoglycemia during therapy and hyperglycemia when it stops. Expect to adjust dosage of antidiabetic drug, as prescribed.
- Expect patient to be reevaluated periodically to determine continued need for therapy.
- Expect to taper drug when being discontinued, as ordered, to minimize adverse reactions.

PATIENT TEACHING

- Instruct patient how to administer form of fluoxetine prescribed.
- Inform patient that drug may take several weeks to achieve full effects.
- Caution against stopping fluoxetine abruptly because serious adverse effects may result.

! WARNING Urge females of childbearing age to notify prescriber if pregnancy occurs because fluoxetine therapy may increase risk of serious adverse effects in the newborn.

! WARNING Stress importance of notifying prescriber immediately if a rash or other skin reactions develop that may be accompanied with other systemic symptoms. Also tell patient to notify prescriber of any persistent, serious, or unusual adverse reactions as drug can adversely affect many systems that may range from mild to severe.

! WARNING Review signs and symptoms of low sodium and urge patient to notify prescriber immediately, if present.

! WARNING Alert patient that drug may increase risk of bleeding, especially if patient is taking aspirin, NSAIDs, warfarin, and other anticoagulants.

! WARNING Urge family or caregiver to watch patient closely for suicidal tendencies, especially when therapy starts or dosage changes, and particularly if patient is a child, teenager, or young adult.

! WARNING Caution patient that fluoxetine may cause seizures, especially if a patient has a history of seizures. If a seizure occurs or seizure activity increases, tell patient to alert prescriber.

! WARNING Tell patient that drug increases risk of serotonin syndrome, a rare but serious complication, especially when taken with certain other drugs. Teach patient to recognize its signs and symptoms and advise her to notify prescriber immediately if they occur.

- Caution patient to avoid hazardous activities until CNS effects of drug are known and resolved.
- Inform patient that drug may cause mild pupillary dilation, which may lead to an episode of acute-angle glaucoma. Encourage patient to have an eye exam prior to starting fluoxetine therapy to see if she is at risk.
- Advise patient to consult prescriber before taking any new over-the-counter or prescription drugs.
- Alert patient that drug may cause sexual dysfunction. Advise patient to discuss sexual dysfunction with prescriber.
- Tell mothers breastfeeding to monitor their breastfed infant for agitation, irritability, poor feeding, and poor weight gain.

fluticasone propionate

Flonase, Flonase Allergy Relief, Xhance

fluticasone furoate

Arnuity Ellipta, Flonase Sensimist

Class and Category

Pharmacologic class: Corticosteroid
Therapeutic class: Antiasthmatic, anti-inflammatory

F

Indications and Dosages

To prevent asthma attacks, alone or with oral corticosteroids as maintenance therapy

INHALATION AEROSOL (FLUTICASONE PROPIONATE HFA)

Adults and children ages 12 and older not on an inhaled corticosteroid. *Initial:* 88 mcg twice daily. After 2 wk, dosage may be increased, as needed. *Maximum:* 880 mcg twice daily.

Adults and children ages 12 and older previously taking other corticosteroids. Initial dosage highly individualized and based on previous asthma therapy and severity. After 2 wk, dosage may be increased, as needed. *Maximum:* 880 mcg twice daily.

Children ages 4 to 11 regardless of previous therapy. 88 mcg inhaled twice daily. *Maximum:* 88 mcg twice daily.

INHALATION AEROSOL (ARNUITY ELLIPTA)

Adults and children ages 12 and older not on inhaled corticosteroid therapy. 100 mcg inhaled once daily, increased after 2 wk to 200 mcg once daily, as needed. *Maximum:* 200 mcg once daily.

Adults and children ages 12 and older receiving other drug treatments for asthma. Highly individualized based on patient's previous asthma drug therapy and disease severity.

Children ages 5 to 11. 50 mcg inhaled once daily.

To manage nasal symptoms of perennial nonallergic rhinitis

NASAL SUSPENSION (FLONASE, FLONASE ALLERGY RELIEF)

Adults. *Initial:* 100 mcg (2 sprays) in each nostril once daily or 50 mcg (1 spray) in each nostril twice daily. *Maximum:* 100 mcg (2 sprays) in each nostril daily.

Children ages 4 and older. 50 mcg (1 spray) in each nostril daily, increased, as needed, to 100 mcg (2 sprays) in each nostril daily. *Maximum:* 100 mcg (2 sprays) in each nostril daily.

To treat perennial and seasonal allergic rhinitis

NASAL SUSPENSION (FLONASE SENSIMIST)

Adults and children ages 12 and older. *Initial:* 55 mcg (2 sprays) in each nostril once daily for 1 wk. Beginning wk 2 through 6 mo, 27.5 or 55 mcg (1 to 2 sprays) in each nostril once daily.

Children ages 2 to 11. 27.5 mcg (1 spray) in each nostril.

To treat chronic rhinosinusitis with or without nasal polyps

NASAL SPRAY (XHANCE)

Adults. 93 mcg (1 spray) in each nostril twice daily, increased to 186 mcg (2 sprays) in each nostril twice daily, as needed. *Maximum:* 186 mcg (2 sprays) in each nostril twice daily for total daily dose of 744 mcg.

Drug Administration

- If 2 doses are prescribed daily, space doses about 12 hr apart and administer at the same time every day.
- Avoid exposing inhalers and nasal sprays to extreme cold, heat, and humidity.

INHALATION

- Follow manufacturer's guidelines for administering product prescribed. Check to see if product has to be primed before first use and if not used for a period of time.
- Do not use spacer or volume holding chamber with Armonair Digihaler.
- If patient is prescribed 2 inhalations, wait at least 1 min between them.
- If patient is prescribed more than 1 inhaler, use fluticasone last, at least 5 min after other inhaler.
- Have patient gargle and rinse mouth after each dose of an oral inhaler to help prevent dry mouth and throat, oropharyngeal yeast infection, and throat irritation.
- Clean inhaler according to manufacturer's guidelines at least once a week after evening dose. However, when using Armonair Digihaler brand, never wash or put any part of inhaler in water, as routine maintenance is not required. If the mouthpiece is cleaned, do so by gently wiping mouthpiece with a dry cloth or tissue.
- When counter reaches 000 or 0, discard the inhaler.

INTRANASAL

- Shake container well before each use.
- Prime the container before using for the first time by pressing the bottle 6 times (Flonase, Flonase Sensimist) or 7 times (Xhance) or until a fine mist appears. If the container is not used for 7 days or more (Flonase, Xhance) or

30 days or if cap has been left off for 5 or more days (Flonase Sensimist), container will have to be reprimed with 6 sprays for Flonase and Flonase Sensimist and 2 sprays for Xhance.

- To administer Flonase or Flonase Sensimist, have patient blow nose. Then, have patient close 1 nostril while tilting head slightly forward and keeping bottle upright. Then, have patient carefully insert the nasal applicator into the other nostril. Tell patient to press firmly and quickly down 1 time on the Flonase applicator while breathing in through the nose. For Flonase Sensimist, have patient sniff gently and while sniffing press the button all the way in twice. A light mist may be felt in the nose. Have the patient breath out through their mouth and then repeat in other nostril. Repeat steps with other nostril if 2 sprays are needed.
- Wipe nasal applicator with a clean tissue and replace cover.
- To administer Xhance, have patient insert the tip of the nosepiece deep into one nostril and form a tight seal between the nosepiece and nostril. Next, have patient place the mouthpiece into mouth, bending it, if needed, to maintain a tight seal. Have patient blow hard into the mouthpiece, and while continuing to blow, have patient push the bottle up to actuate the spray pump. Repeat the process in the other nostril.
- Although Xhance container does not have to be cleaned, it can be wiped after each use with a clean, dry, lint-free cloth.
- Protect Xhance from light and discard after using 120 sprays after initial priming.

Route	Onset	Peak	Duration
Inhalation	24 hr	Unknown	Unknown
Nasal	< 12 hr	Unknown	24 hr

Half-life: 11–12 hr

Mechanism of Action

Inhibits cells involved in the inflammatory response of asthma, such as basophils, eosinophils, lymphocytes, macrophages, mast cells, and neutrophils. Fluticasone also inhibits production or secretion of chemical mediators, such as cytokines eicosanoids, histamine, and leukotrienes. These actions also relieve nasal symptoms of rhinitis.

Contraindications

Hypersensitivity to fluticasone or its components, or to milk proteins; primary treatment of status asthmaticus or other acute asthma episodes that require intensive measures (inhalation form); untreated nasal mucosal infection (nasal suspension)

Interactions

DRUGS

strong CYP3A4 inhibitors, such as atazanavir, clarithromycin, indinavir, itraconazole, ketoconazole, nefazodone, nelfinavir, ritonavir, saquinavir, telithromycin: Possibly increased fluticasone level with increased risk of corticosteroid adverse effects

Adverse Reactions

CNS: Aggressiveness, agitation, anxiety, depression, difficulty speaking, dizziness, fatigue, fever, headache, insomnia, irritability, malaise, restlessness
CV: **Hypotension** (as part of hypersenstiivity reaction)
EENT: Allergic rhinitis, blurred vision, cataracts, central serous chorioretinopathy, conjunctivitis, dental caries, difficulty speaking, dry mouth and throat, ear infection, elevated intraocular pressure, epistaxis, esophageal or pharyngeal candidiasis, eye irritation, **facial and oropharyngeal edema**, glaucoma, hoarseness, impaired nasal wound healing, laryngitis, loss of voice, nasal *Candida* infection, nasal congestion or discharge, nasal discomfort (burning, dryness, erythema, irritation, soreness), nasal erosion, nasal sinus pain, nasal septal perforation or ulceration, nasopharyngitis, oropharyngeal candidiasis, otitis media, pharyngitis, rhinitis, sinusitis, throat irritation, tonsillitis, tooth discoloration
ENDO: **Adrenal insufficiency**, cushingoid symptoms, hypercorticism, hyperglycemia, slower growth in children
GI: Abdominal pain, diarrhea, indigestion, intestinal candidiasis, nausea, vomiting
GU: Dysmenorrhea
HEME: **Churg-Strauss syndrome**, easy bruising, eosinophilia
MS: Arthralgia, back pain, bone mineral density reduction (long-term use), myalgia, osteoporosis

RESP: **Asthma exacerbation**, bronchitis, **bronchospasm**, chest congestion and tightness, cough, dyspnea, pneumonia, upper respiratory tract infection, wheezing
SKIN: Dermatitis, ecchymosis, pruritus, rash, urticaria
Other: **Anaphylaxis**, **angioedema**, flu-like symptoms, immunosuppression, infections, weight gain

Childbearing Considerations

PREGNANCY

- It is not known if drug causes fetal harm.
- Use with caution only if benefit to mother outweighs potential risk to fetus.

LACTATION

- It is not known if drug is present in breast milk.
- Mothers should check with prescriber before breastfeeding.

Nursing Considerations

- Use fluticasone cautiously in patients with ocular herpes simplex, pulmonary tuberculosis, or untreated systemic bacterial, fungal, parasitic, or viral infection. Monitor patient throughout therapy for signs and symptoms of infection, as drug causes immunosuppression and increased risk of infections. Also, use cautiously in patients with moderate or severe hepatic impairment.

! WARNING Be aware that fluticasone should not be given to a patient with a severe allergy to milk. Monitor patient closely at start of therapy for a hypersensitivity reaction to the drug which could become life-threatening such as anaphylaxis or angioedema. If hypersensitivity reaction occurs, notify prescriber, expect drug to be discontinued, and provide supportive care, as needed and ordered.

- Know that if patient takes a systemic corticosteroid, expect to taper dosage by no more than 2.5 mg daily at weekly intervals, starting 1 week after fluticasone therapy begins.

! WARNING Be aware that if patient is switched from systemic corticosteroid to fluticasone, assess for adrenal insufficiency (fatigue, hypotension, lassitude, nausea, vomiting, weakness) early in therapy and when patient has an infection, stress, surgery, trauma, or develops other electrolyte-depleting conditions or procedures. Notify prescriber immediately if signs or symptoms develop.

! WARNING Administer a fast-acting inhaled bronchodilator, as ordered, if bronchospasm occurs immediately after oral inhalation form of fluticasone use. Expect to stop fluticasone and start another drug therapy, as ordered.

- Expect to titrate fluticasone to lowest effective dosage after asthma has stabilized.
- Inspect patient's nasal cavity regularly if patient prescribed nasal form of drug, If abnormalities are noted such as nasal erosion or ulceration and nasal septal perforation or patient shows evidence of a *Candida* infection, notify prescriber and expect drug to be discontinued.
- Expect nasal form of drug to be withheld in a patient who has experienced recent nasal surgery or trauma or has developed nasal ulceration until healing has been complete.
- Notify prescriber if patient develops ocular adverse reactions because fluticasone therapy may cause many such as cataracts, increased intraocular pressure, and glaucoma that should be checked by an ophthalmologist.

PATIENT TEACHING

! WARNING Warn patient to alert prescriber if patient has an allegy to milk protein before taking first dose as a milk allergy is a contraindication for fluticasone use.

- Instruct patient how to administer the form of fluticasone prescribed.
- Urge patient to use fluticasone regularly, as prescribed.
- Explain that symptoms may improve within 2 days, but that full improvement may not occur for 1 to 2 weeks or longer. However, tell patient it may take up to 16 weeks or longer to experience improvement if patient is being treated for chronic rhinosinusitis with or without nasal polyps.
- Caution patient not to increase dosage but to contact prescriber if symptoms continue or worsen.

! WARNING Stress to patient prescribed drug to manage asthma that drug cannot be used to treat acute bronchospasm. Instruct her to have a rescue inhaler accessible if acute bronchospasm occurs.

! **WARNING** Urge patient to tell prescriber immediately if asthma attacks don't respond to bronchodilators during inhaled fluticasone therapy.

! **WARNING** Alert patient that drug may cause an allergic reaction. Tell patient to notify prescriber. If reaction is severe, tell patient to seek immediate medical care.

- Know that if patient is switching from an oral corticosteroid to inhaled fluticasone, urge her to carry medical identification indicating the need for supplemental systemic corticosteroids during stress or severe asthma attack.
- Instruct patient prescribed the nasal form to inspect the inside of his nose regularly for abnormalities. Tell patient to notify prescriber if nasal erosion or ulcers occur or the nasal spectrum becomes perforated and to stop taking drug until healing is complete.
- Caution patient to avoid people who have infections because fluticasone suppresses the immune system, increasing the risk of infection. Instruct patient to notify prescriber about exposure to chickenpox, measles, or other infections because additional treatment may be needed.
- Instruct patient to report ocular adverse reactions to prescriber.

fluvastatin sodium

Lescol XL

Class and Category

Pharmacologic class: HMG-CoA reductase inhibitor
Therapeutic class: Antilipemic

Indications and Dosages

✱ *As adjunct to diet to lower cholesterol level in primary hypercholesterolemia (heterozygous familial and nonfamilial) and mixed dyslipidemia (Fredrickson Type IIa and II b); to decrease progression of coronary atherosclerosis; to reduce risk in patients with coronary artery disease undergoing coronary revascularization*

CAPSULES

Adults. *Initial:* 20 to 40 daily in evening, dependent on target goal of LDL-C reduction. Increased up to 40 mg twice daily, as needed. *Maximum:* 40 mg twice daily.

E.R. TABLETS

Adults. 80 mg once daily. *Maximum:* 80 mg daily.

✱ *As adjunct to diet to lower cholesterol level in children with heterozygous familial hypercholesterolemia whose LDL-C remains 190 ml/dl or greater or whose LDL-C remains 160 mg/dl or greater combined with a positive family history of premature cardiovascular disease or two or more other cardiovascular disease risk factors are present*

CAPSULES

Boys and girls (who are at least 1 yr past menarche) ages 10 to 16. *Initial:* 20 mg once daily in evening increased every 6 wk, as needed. *Maximum:* 40 mg twice daily

E.R. TABLETS

Boys and girls (who are at least 1 yr past menarche) ages 10 to 16. 80 mg once daily after being stabilized on 40 mg twice daily on immediate-release form. *Maximum:* 80 mg once daily.

± **DOSAGE ADJUSTMENT** For patients taking cyclosporine or fluconazole, dosage not to exceed 20 mg twice daily.

Drug Administration

P.O.

- Capsules and tablets should be swallowed whole and not chewed, crushed, or split/opened.
- Administer immediate-release capsules in the evening. Do not administer two 40-mg capsules at the same time.
- Administer E.R. tablets at any time of day but be consistent.

Route	Onset	Peak	Duration
P.O.	Unknown	1 hr	Unknown
P.O. (E.R.)	Unknown	3 hr	Unknown

Half-life: 3–9 hr

Mechanism of Action

Interferes with the hepatic enzyme hydroxymethylglutaryl-coenzyme A reductase, reducing formation of mevalonic acid (a cholesterol precursor)

F

and interrupting the pathway by which cholesterol is synthesized. When cholesterol level declines in hepatic cells, LDLs are consumed, which reduces circulating total cholesterol and serum triglycerides.

Contraindications

Acute hepatic disease or decompensated cirrhosis, females of childbearing age who may become pregnant, hypersensitivity to fluvastatin or its components, pregnancy, unexplained persistently elevated liver enzyme levels

Interactions

DRUGS

colchicine, cyclosporine, erythromycin, gemfibrozil, niacin, other fibrates: Increased risk of severe myopathy and rhabdomyolysis
cyclosporine, fluconazole, glyburide, phenytoin: Increased drug levels of these drugs
protease inhibitors: Possible increased blood fluvastatin level; possible increased risk of myopathy and rhabdomyolysis
rifampin: Significantly decreased blood fluvastatin level, increased plasma clearance
warfarin: Possibly increased bleeding and/or increased prothrombin times

ACTIVITIES

alcohol use: Increased risk of liver dysfunction

Adverse Reactions

CNS: Anxiety, asthenia, chills, cranial nerve dysfunction, cognitive impairment, depression, dizziness, fatigue, fever, headache, hypoesthesia, insomnia, memory loss, malaise, myasthenia gravis (new onset or exacerbation), paresthesia, peripheral nerve palsy, peripheral neuropathy, psychic disturbances, syncope, tremor, vertigo, weakness
CV: **Atrial fibrillation**, hypertension, intermittent claudication, peripheral edema, vasculitis
EENT: Cataract progression, nasopharyngitis, ocular myasthenia, pharyngitis, rhinitis, sinusitis
ENDO: **Adrenal insufficiency**, decreased gonadal steroid hormone production, elevated hemoglobin A1C levels, gynecomastia, hyperglycemia, thyroid function abnormalities
GI: Abdominal cramps and pain, anorexia, cholesatic jaundice, **cirrhosis**, constipation, diarrhea, dyspepsia, elevated liver enzymes, fatty liver changes, flatulence, **fulminant hepatic necrosis**, **hepatic failure**, **hepatitis**, **hepatoma**, hyperbilirubinemia, indigestion, jaundice, nausea, **pancreatitis**, vomiting
GU: Elevated bilirubin, erectile dysfunction, loss of libido, UTI
HEMA: **Hemolytic anemia**, elevated erythrocyte sedimentation rate, eosinophilia, **leukopenia**, positive ANA, **thrombocytopenia**
MS: Arthropathy; back or extremity pain; **immune-mediated necrotizing myopathy**; muscle pain, spasm, or weakness; myalgia; myopathy; myositis; polymyalgia rheumatica, **rhabdomyolysis**
RESP: Bronchitis, cough, dyspnea, exertional dyspnea, **interstitial lung disease**, upper respiratory tract infection
SKIN: Alopecia, **erythema multiforme**, dermatitis, eczema, flushing, lichen planus, nail and skin alterations, purpura, photosensitivity, pruritus, rash, **Stevens-Johnson syndrome**, **toxic epidermal necrolysis**, urticaria
Other: **Anaphylaxis**, **angioedema**, elevated alkaline phosphatase, flu-like symptoms, lupus erythematosus-like syndrome

Childbearing Considerations

PREGNANCY

- Drug may cause fetal harm because cholesterol and cholesterol derivatives are needed for normal fetal development.
- Drug is not recommended in pregnancy and should be discontinued if pregnancy occurs.

LACTATION

- Drug is present in breast milk.
- Breastfeeding is not recommended during drug therapy.

Nursing Considerations

- Administer fluvastatin with caution in patients with predisposing factors for myopathy such as advanced age (greater than 65 years of age), inadequately treated hypothyroidism, and renal impairment. Also, know risk is increased with concurrent therapy with colchicine, cyclosporine, erythromycin, fibrates, or niacin (1 g/day). Notify prescriber if patient develops unexplained muscle pain, tenderness, or weakness, especially if fever or malaise is present. Expect to stop drug if CPK level rises sharply, or myopathy is suspected.

! **WARNING** Expect liver enzymes to be checked before fluvastatin therapy starts and then thereafter as clinically necessary. Assess patient for signs and symptoms of hepatic dysfunction throughout drug therapy such as dark urine or jaundice, fatigue, and/or elevation in liver enzymes to more than 3 times the upper limit of normal. Also, look for hyperbilirubinemia. Be aware that liver dysfunction could become life-threatening. If present, notify prescriber and expect fluvastatin to be discontinued until cause of liver dysfunction has been identified. If no cause can be found, expect the drug to be discontinued permanently.

! **WARNING** Monitor patient for a hypersensivity reaction, which may become life-threatening such as anaphylaxis or angioedema or skin abnormalites such as Stevens-Johnson syndrome. If any sign of hypersensitivity is present, notify prescriber, expect drug to be discontinued, and provide supportive care, as needed and ordered.

! **WARNING** Know that fluvastatin can cause many different types of adverse reactions, some of which are life-threatening. Notify prescriber if patient experiences persistent, serious, or unusual adverse reactions.

- Be aware that fluvastatin can increase fasting blood glucose levels and HbA1C. Monitor patient for hyperglycemia, especially diabetic patients, and for other endocrine signs and symptoms. If present, notify prescriber.

PATIENT TEACHING

- Instruct patient how to administer form of fluvastatin prescribed.
- Tell patient to follow prescribed low-fat diet.

! **WARNING** Alert patient that fluvastatin may cause an allergic reaction that may include skin reactions. If an allergic reaction, including a rash occurs, tell patient to notify prescriber and to stop taking drug. If reaction is severe, tell patient to seek immediate medical care.

! **WARNING** Encourage patient to notify prescriber if persistent, severe, or unusual adverse effects occur because drug affects many body systems and can cause reactions that could become quite serious.

- Encourage patient to notify prescriber promptly about muscle pain or unexplained weakness, even after drug has been discontinued.
- Instruct patient with diabetes to monitor his blood glucose level more closely.
- Inform females of childbearing age drug is not recommended in pregnancy. Tell these patients to alert prescriber if pregnancy occurs as drug will need to be discontinued.
- Tell mothers breastfeeding should not be undertaken while taking fluvastatin.
- Urge patient to comply with monthly laboratory tests early in treatment.

fluvoxamine maleate

Class and Category

Pharmacologic class: Selective serotonin reuptake inhibitor (SSRI)
Therapeutic class: Antidepressant

Indications and Dosages

✷ *To treat obsessive–compulsive disorder (OCD)*

TABLETS

Adults. *Initial:* 50 mg daily at bedtime, increased by 50 mg every 4 to 7 days, as needed. *Maximum:* 300 mg daily, with doses greater than 100 mg daily given as 2 divided doses.
Children ages 8 to 17. *Initial:* 25 mg daily at bedtime, increased by 25 mg every 4 to 7 days, as needed. *Maximum:* 200 mg daily (children ages 8 to 11) and 300 mg daily (children ages 11 to 17), with doses greater than 50 mg daily divided into 2 doses.

E.R. CAPSULES

Adults. *Initial:* 100 mg daily at bedtime, increased by 50 mg weekly, as needed. *Maximum:* 300 mg daily.

± **DOSAGE ADJUSTMENT** For elderly patients or those with hepatic impairment, initial dosage decreased for immediate-release form; dosage increases made more slowly for both immediate-release tablets and E.R.capsules.

Drug Administration

P.O.

- Administer once-daily dosage at bedtime; twice-daily dosage, once in the morning and once at bedtime.
- E.R. capsules and immediate-release tablets should be swallowed whole and not chewed, crushed, or opened.

Route	Onset	Peak	Duration
P.O.	Unknown	3–8 hr	Unknown
P.O./E.R.	Unknown	Unknown	Unknown

Half-life: 9–28 hr

Mechanism of Action

May potentiate serotonin's action by blocking its reuptake at neuronal membranes. An elevated serotonin level may elevate mood and decrease depression and anxiety, which often accompany obsessive–compulsive disorder.

Contraindications

Concurrent therapy with alosetron, pimozide, thioridazine, or tizanidine therapy; hypersensitivity to fluvoxamine maleate or its components; use within 14 days of MAO inhibitor, including intravenous methylene blue and linezolid

Interactions

DRUGS

alosetron, antipsychotics, benzodiazepines, ramelteon, tacrine, tricyclic antidepressants: Elevated plasma levels of these drugs with increased risk of adverse reactions
amphetamines, buspirone, fentanyl, linezolid, lithium, methylene blue (intravenous), other serotonergic drugs, St. John's wort, tramadol, tricyclic antidepressants, triptans, tryptophan: Increased risk of serotonin syndrome
aspirin, NSAIDs, warfarin: Risk of bleeding
astemizole, cisapride, pimozide, terfenadine, thioridazine: Possibly fatal QT prolongation
carbamazepine: Increased risk of carbamazepine toxicity
clozapine: Increased blood clozapine level increasing risk of orthostatic hypotension and seizures
diltiazem: Increased risk of bradycardia
lithium: Possibly increased serotonin reuptake action of fluvoxamine and increased risk of seizures
MAO inhibitors: Possibly serious or fatal reactions (such as agitation, autonomic instability, coma, delirium, fluctuating vital signs, hyperthermia, myoclonus, and rigidity); increased risk of serotonin syndrome
methadone: Possibly significantly increased blood methadone level; increased risk of methadone toxicity
metoprolol, propranolol, and other beta-blockers: Increased blood levels of these drugs; possibly reduced diastolic blood pressure and heart rate induced by these drugs
mexiletine: Possibly decreased clearance of mexiletine
pimozide, thioridazine: Increased plasma levels of these drugs with increased risk of QT interval associated with serious ventricular arrhythmias
sumatriptan: Increased risk of hyperreflexia, incoordination, and weakness
theophylline: Decreased theophylline clearance; increased risk of theophylline toxicity
tizanidine: Increased risk of serious adverse effects, such as hypotension and profound sedation
tryptophan: Enhanced effect of tryptophan and possibly induced severe vomiting
warfarin: Significant increased plasma level of warfarin with prolonged prothrombin time

ACTIVITIES

alcohol: Possibly increased CNS effects
smoking: Increased fluvoxamine metabolism

Adverse Reactions

CNS: Agitation, anxiety, apathy, chills, confusion, depression, dizziness, drowsiness, fatigue, headache, hypomania, insomnia, malaise, mania, nervousness, **neuroleptic malignant syndrome**, sedation, **serotonin syndrome**, **suicidal ideation**, tremor, vertigo, yawning
CV: Palpitations, tachycardia, **torsades de pointes**, vasculitis, **ventricular tachycardia**
EENT: Acute-angle glaucoma, altered taste, blurred vision, dry mouth, partial or complete loss of smell
GI: Anorexia, constipation, diarrhea, flatulence, **hepatitis**, **ileus**, indigestion, nausea, **pancreatitis**, **upper GI bleeding**, vomiting
GU: **Acute renal failure**, amenorrhea, decreased libido, delayed or absent orgasm

(females), erectile dysfunction, ejaculation disorders, impotence, urinary frequency, urine retention
HEME: **Agranulocytosis**, **aplastic anemia**, **bleeding events**
MS: Muscle twitching
RESP: Dyspnea, upper respiratory tract infection
SKIN: Bullous eruption, diaphoresis, Henoch-Schoenlein purpura, rash, **Stevens-Johnson syndrome**, **toxic epidermal necrolysis**
Other: **Anaphylaxis**, **angioedema**, flu-like symptoms, porphyria, weight gain

Childbearing Considerations

PREGNANCY

- Pregnancy exposure registry: 1-844-405-6185 or https://womensmentalhealth.org/clinical-and-research-programs/pregnancyregistry/antidepressants/.
- It is not known if drug causes fetal harm but may have adverse effects if given late in third trimester.
- Use with caution only if benefit to mother outweighs potential risk to fetus.

LABOR AND DELIVERY

- Fetal exposure to drug late in third trimester may cause neonatal complications as soon as birth. Complications such as persistent pulmonary hypertension of the newborn may require prolonged hospitalization, respiratory support, and tube feeding.
- Drug administered in the month before delivery increases risk of postpartum hemorrhage.

LACTATION

- Drug is present in breast milk.
- Mothers should check with prescriber before breastfeeding.
- If breastfeeding occurs, infant should be monitored for agitation, decreased sleep, diarrhea, and vomiting.

REPRODUCTION

- Fertility may be impaired while taking drug according to animal studies.

Nursing Considerations

! WARNING Use fluvoxamine cautiously in patients with cardiovascular disease, impaired hepatic or renal function, mania, seizures, or suicidal tendencies.

! WARNING Be aware that fluvoxamine shouldn't be given within 14 days of an MAO inhibitor.

! WARNING Monitor patient for a hypersensitivity reaction, which may become life-threatening such as anaphylaxis or angioedema. If present, notify prescriber, withhold drug, and provide supportive care, as needed and ordered. Also, monitor patient for persistent, serious, or unusual adverse reactions because drug can cause a variety of adverse reactions, some of which could be quite serious or even life-threatening.

! WARNING Watch patient closely (especially children, adolescents, and young adults) for suicidal tendencies, particularly when therapy starts and dosage changes because depression may worsen temporarily during these times and lead to suicidal ideation.

! WARNING Monitor patient for bleeding, especially if patient also takes aspirin, an anticoagulant, or NSAIDs. Bleeding can range from ecchymoses, epistaxis, hematomas, and petechiae to life-threatening hemorrhage.

! WARNING Monitor patient for possible serotonin syndrome, characterized by agitation, chills, confusion, diaphoresis, diarrhea, fever, hyperactive reflexes, poor coordination, restlessness, shaking, talking, or acting with uncontrolled excitement, tremor, and twitching, especially if patient is receiving another drug that raises serotonin level (such as amphetamine, dopamine agonist, MAO inhibitor, tryptophan, or other antidepressant or psychostimulant). In its most severe form, serotonin syndrome can resemble neuroleptic malignant syndrome, which includes autonomic instability, a high fever, muscle rigidity, and possible fluctuations in vital signs and mental status.

- Discontinue fluvoxamine therapy gradually, as ordered, to prevent unpleasant adverse reactions.

PATIENT TEACHING

- Instruct patient how to administer form of fluvoxamine prescribed.
- Caution patient not to drink alcohol during fluvoxamine therapy.

- Instruct patient not to stop taking drug abruptly. Explain that gradual tapering helps avoid withdrawal symptoms.

! **WARNING** Advise pregnant patient to consult with prescriber before her third trimester about ongoing fluvoxamine therapy because of an increased risk to her unborn child and potential for postpartum hemorrhage.

! **WARNING** Alert patient that drug may cause an allergic reaction. If present, tell patient to stop taking drug, notify prescriber, and if severe, to seek immediate medical attention. Also tell patient to notify prescriber if persistent, serious, or unusual adverse reactions occur because drug can affect many body systems and cause, in some cases, serious adverse reactions.

! **WARNING** Urge family or caregiver to watch patient closely for suicidal tendencies, especially when therapy starts or dosage changes and particularly if patient is a child, teenager, or young adult.

! **WARNING** Warn patient that fluvoxamine increases bleeding risk if taken with an anticoagulant, aspirin, or NSAIDs, and that bleeding events could range from mild to severe. Tell patient to seek emergency care for serious or prolonged bleeding.

! **WARNING** Inform patient that fluvoxamine increases the risk of a rare but serious problem called serotonin syndrome. Review signs and symptoms with patient and encourage her to notify prescriber immediately if signs and symptoms develop.

- Urge patient to avoid potentially hazardous activities until drug's CNS effects are known and resolved.
- Advise patient that drug may cause mild pupillary dilation, which may lead to an episode of acute-angle glaucoma. Encourage patient to have an eye exam before starting therapy to see if she is at risk.
- Alert patient that drug may cause sexual dysfunction and to discuss concerns with prescriber.
- Instruct mother who is breastfeeding during drug therapy to monitor breastfed infant for agitation, decreased sleep, diarrhea, and vomiting.

fondaparinux sodium

Arixtra

Class and Category

Pharmacologic class: Activated factor X inhibitor
Therapeutic class: Anticoagulant

Indications and Dosages

∗ *To provide prophylaxis against deep vein thrombosis, which may lead to pulmonary embolism in patients undergoing abdominal surgery, hip fracture surgery, hip replacement surgery, or knee replacement surgery in patients at risk for thromboembolic complications*

SUBCUTANEOUS INJECTION

Adults. *Initial:* After hemostasis has been established, 2.5 mg 6 to 8 hr after surgery, followed by 2.5 mg daily for 5 to 9 days, except for hip fracture surgery, which may be given up to 24 additional days for a total of 32 days.

∗ *To treat acute deep vein thrombosis (with warfarin); to treat acute pulmonary embolism (with warfarin) in a hospital setting*

SUBCUTANEOUS INJECTION

Adults weighing more than 100 kg (220 lb). 10 mg once daily for at least 5 days and until INR is between 2.0 and 3.0 (usually in 5 to 9 days).
Adults weighing 50 kg (110 lb) to 100 kg (220 lb). 7.5 mg once daily for at least 5 days and until INR is between 2.0 and 3.0 (usually in 5 to 9 days).
Adults weighing less than 50 kg (110 lb). 5 mg once daily for at least 5 days and until INR is between 2.0 and 3.0 (usually in 5 to 9 days).

∗ *To treat venous thromboembolism in pediatric patients*

SUBCUTANEOUS INJECTION

Children ages 1 and older weighing at least 10 kg (22 lb). 0.1 mg/kg once daily. with dosage rounded to nearest 0.1 mg for children weighing between 10 kg (22 lb) and 20 kg (44 lb) and dosage rounded to the nearest prefilled syringe dose as follows: for children weighing more than 60 kg (132 lb), 7.5 mg/0.6 ml; for children weighing more than 40 kg (88 lb) but less than 60 kg (132 lb),

5 mg/0.4 ml; and for children weighing more than 20 kg (44 lb) but less than 40 kg (88 lb), 2.5 mg/0.5 ml.

± **DOSAGE ADJUSTMENT** For patients who do not fall within the therapeutic range of 0.5 mg/L to 1 mg/L, a dosage adjustment made as follows: if fondaparinux-based anti-Xa Level is less than 0.3 mg/L, dosage increased by 0.03 mg/kg; if 0.3 mg/L to 0.49 mg/L, dosage increased by 0.01 mg/kg; if 1.01 mg/L to 1.2 mg/L, dosage decreased by 0.01 mg/kg, and if greater than 1.2 mg/L, dosage decreased by 0.03 mg/kg with any dosage adjustment rounded to the nearest 0.1 mg.

Drug Administration

SUBCUTANEOUS

- For children weighing 10 kg (22 lb) to 20 kg (44 lb), a patient-specific dose may be prepared by a pharmacist.
- Do not handle needle guard on prefilled syringe if latex sensitive because it contains dry natural latex rubber.
- Never administer as an I.M. injection.
- Don't give initial dose less than 6 hr after surgery.
- Don't expel air bubble from prefilled syringe before injection, to prevent expelling drug from syringe.
- Alternate injection sites using left and right anterolateral or left and right posterolateral abdominal wall.
- After injecting drug, the plunger should be released. The plunger will then rise automatically while the needle is withdrawn from the skin and retracted into the security sleeve. To be certain the syringe safety feature has worked, listen or feel for a soft click when the plunger rod is released fully. When the needle is pulled back into the security sleeve, the white safety indicator will appear above the upper body.
- If a dose is missed, administer the dose as soon as possible but never inject 2 doses at the same time.
- Store drug at a controlled room temperature.

Route	Onset	Peak	Duration
SubQ	Unknown	2–3 hr	Unknown

Half-life: 17–21 hr

Mechanism of Action

Binds selectively to antithrombin III, which enhances the inactivation of clotting factor Xa by antithrombin III. Inactivation of factor Xa interrupts the blood coagulation pathway, which then inhibits thrombin formation. Without thrombin, fibrinogen can't convert to fibrin and clots can't form.

Contraindications

Active major bleeding; bacterial endocarditis; body weight less than 50 kg (110 lb) for venous thromboembolism prophylaxis; fondaparinux-induced thrombocytopenia associated with a positive in vitro test for antiplatelet antibodies; hypersensitivity to fondaparinux or its components; severe renal impairment (creatinine clearance less than 30 ml/min)

Interactions

DRUGS

drugs that increase risk of bleeding: Increased risk of hemorrhage and epidural or spinal hematoma

Adverse Reactions

CNS: Confusion, dizziness, fever, headache, insomnia

CV: Edema, **hypotension**

GI: Constipation, diarrhea, elevated liver enzymes, indigestion, nausea, vomiting

GU: Urine retention, UTI

HEME: Anemia, **bleeding**, **elevated activated partial thromboplastin time**, hematoma, **hemorrhage**, **thrombocytopenia**, **thrombocytopenia with thrombosis**

SKIN: Bullous eruption, increased wound drainage, purpura, rash

Other: **Anaphylaxis**; **angioedema**; generalized pain; **hypokalemia**; injection-site bleeding, pruritus, and rash

Childbearing Considerations

PREGNANCY

- It is not known if drug causes fetal harm but drug does cross the placental barrier, which may increase risk of bleeding in the fetus and neonate.
- Use with caution only if benefit to mother outweighs potential risk to fetus.

LABOR AND DELIVERY

- Increased risk of bleeding during labor and delivery and epidural or spinal hematoma formation if neuraxial anesthesia is used.

- A shorter-acting anticoagulant may be substituted as delivery approaches.

LACTATION

- It is not known if drug is present in breast milk.
- Patient should check with prescriber before breastfeeding.

Nursing Considerations

! **WARNING** Use fondaparinux cautiously in elderly patients, especially those weighing less than 50 kg (110 lb) and are receiving the drug for pulmonary embolism or deep vein thrombosis because the risk of drug-induced bleeding increases with age.

- Perform periodic CBC, including platelet count, as ordered. Expect prescriber to discontinue drug if platelet count falls below 100,000/mm^3. Be aware that routine coagulation tests such as INR and PT are not used to monitor fondaparinux therapy; an anti-Xa assay may be used instead. However, an INR and PT are used to monitor warfarin, which is given in conjunction with fondaparinux to treat deep venous thrombosis or pulmonary embolus. Also, test stools for occult blood, as ordered.

! **WARNING** Monitor patient for a hypersensitivity reaction, which could become life-threatening such as anaphylaxis or angioedema. If present, notify prescriber, expect drug to be withheld and different anticoagulant substituted, and provide supportive care, as needed and ordered.

! **WARNING** Closely monitor patient for bleeding (such as ecchymosis, epistaxis, hematemesis, hematuria, and melena), especially those at risk for decreased drug elimination (such as elderly patients and patients with mild to moderate renal impairment) and those at increased risk for bleeding (such as adult patients with acquired or congenital bleeding disorders; active ulcerative and angiodysplastic GI disease; diabetic retinopathy; hemorrhagic stroke; uncontrolled arterial hypertension; recent brain, spinal, or ophthalmologic surgery; history of heparin-induced thrombocytopenia; and those being treated concomitantly with platelet inhibitors; for children with antiphospholipid syndrome, antithrombin III deficiency, Factor V Leiden, hypertensive encephalpathy, indwelling chest tubes, intestinal lymphangiectasia, invasive infections, malignancy, pancytopenia, systemic lupus erythematosus, thoracotomy, von Willebrand disease, or Wilms tumor). Also, monitor neonates born to mothers taking fondaparinux for bleeding because drug does cross the placenta.

! **WARNING** Monitor patient with thrombocytopenia for evidence of thrombosis that may appear similar to heparin-induced thrombocytopenia even when no exposure to heparin has taken place. If patient's platelet count falls below 100,000/mm^3, fondaparinux should be discontinued.

! **WARNING** Monitor renal function test results, as ordered. Expect to discontinue drug if labile renal function or severe renal impairment occurs during fondaparinux therapy because the risk of hemorrhage increases as renal function decreases.

! **WARNING** Be aware that elevations of heaptic transaminases have occurred in children with elevations greater than 10x the upper limit of normal. Monitor patient closely for any signs and symptoms of hepatic dysfunction and alert prescriber if present.

! **WARNING** Know that if patient is receiving fondaparinux with epidural or spinal anesthesia or spinal puncture, patient must be watched closely for development of spinal hematoma, which may cause long-term or permanent paralysis. If evidence of neurologic impairment, such as changes in motor or sensory function occurs, notify prescriber immediately because urgent care is needed to minimize hematoma's effect. Risk of spinal or epidural hematoma during fondaparinux therapy is increased by concurrent use of other drugs that affect hemostasis, a history of traumatic or repeated epidural or spinal punctures, or a history of spinal deformity or spinal surgery as well as the presence of indwelling epidural catheters. Be aware that optimal timing between the administration of fondaparinux and neuraxial procedures is unknown.

- Monitor patient's electrolytes, as ordered and monitor patient for hypokalemia.

PATIENT TEACHING

- Inform patient that fondaparinux can't be taken orally.
- Teach patient, family, or caregiver how to administer fondaparinux by subcutaneous injection, if needed and what to do if a dose is missed.
- Advise patient to alert prescriber about any new drugs being taken, including over-the-counter drugs and especially drugs that affect clotting, such as aspirin or NSAIDs.

! **WARNING** Alert patient that drug may cause an allergic reaction. If present, tell patient to not take another injection of the drug until prescriber notified and, if reaction is severe, to seek immediate emergency care.

! **WARNING** Inform patient about the increased risk of bleeding. Instruct patient, family, or caregiver to watch for and report immediately abdominal or lower back pain, black stools, bleeding gums, bloody urine, or severe headaches.

! **WARNING** Instruct patient to seek immediate help if signs of thromboembolism are experienced. These could include pain, redness of the skin, swelling, or tenderness in the leg, pelvis or thigh; or chest pain, coughing up blood, difficulty breathing, fainting, faster-than-normal or irregular heartbeat, or light-headedness.

! **WARNING** Tell patient receiving fondaparinux with epidural or spinal anesthesia or spinal puncture to alert staff immediately if changes in motor or sensory function occur.

- Tell patient that fondaparinux may cause other serious side effects and to report any persistent, severe, or unusual signs and symptoms to prescriber.
- Advise patient to comply with follow-up appointments and prescribed laboratory tests.

formoterol fumarate

Oxeze Turbuhaler (CAN), Perforomist

Class and Category

Pharmacologic class: Selective $beta_2$-adrenergic agonist
Therapeutic class: Bronchodilator

Indications and Dosages

* *To prevent exercise-induced bronchospasm*

POWDER FOR ORAL INHALATION (OXEZE TURBUHALER)

Adults and children ages 6 and older. 6 or 12 mcg at least 15 min before exercise every 12 hr, as needed. *Maximum:* 24 mcg daily (children) and 48 mcg daily (adults).

* *To provide long-term maintenance treatment of bronchospasm in patients with chronic obstructive pulmonary disease (COPD), including chronic bronchitis and emphysema*

POWDER FOR ORAL INHALATION (OXEZE TURBUHALER)

Adults. 6 or 12 mcg every 12 hr through inhaler device, dosage increased, as needed. *Maximum:* 48 mcg daily in 2 divided doses.

SOLUTION FOR ORAL INHALATION (PERFOROMIST)

Adults. 20 mcg twice daily by nebulization. *Maximum:* 40 mcg daily.

Drug Administration

INHALATION

Perforomist

- Administer solution only by oral inhalation using a standard jet nebulizer and air compressor.
- Store drug in its original packaging, and open immediately before use.
- Solution should be colorless; if not, discard.
- Avoid diluting drug before administration and do not mix any other drug with formoterol solution.

Oxeze Turbuhaler

- If using for the first time, prime inhaler. Hold the inhaler upright and turn the greenish-blue grip as far as it will go in one direction, then turn in the opposite direction. Repeat turning process one more time. At some point in the process, a click will be heard; this is part of the process. After initial priming, inhaler need not be reprimed even if the inhaler is not used regularly.
- To load a dose, hold container in an upright position. Turn the greenish-blue grip as far as it will go in one direction and then turn in the opposite direction. A dose has now been loaded. At some point, a clicking sound will be heard; this is part of the process. Do not interrupt the turning process. If inhaler is dropped or shaken or if patient breathes out into the turbuhaler, the

dose will be lost, and the loading steps will have to be repeated.

- To administer, hand the loaded inhaler to patient and have patient breathe out away from mouthpiece, then close the mouthpiece gently between the teeth, and close lips over the mouthpiece. The mouthpiece should not be bitten or chewed. Tell patient to inhale as deeply and strongly as possible. Remove mouthpiece before exhalation. Repeat loading and administration steps if more than one dose has been prescribed.
- Mouthpiece should be cleaned once a week with a dry tissue. Never use water or any other fluid.
- For the last 10 doses, the background of the indicator will turn red. When the 0 appears, discard.

Route	Onset	Peak	Duration
Oral inhalation	< 15 min	1–3 hr	12 hr

Half-life: 7–10 hr

Mechanism of Action

Attaches selectively to beta$_2$ receptors on bronchial membranes, stimulating the intracellular enzyme adenyl cyclase to convert adenosine triphosphate to cAMP. The resulting increase in the intracellular cAMP level inhibits histamine release, relaxes bronchial smooth-muscle cells, and stabilizes mast cells.

Contraindications

Hypersensitivity to formoterol fumarate or its components, patients who also have asthma and are not taking an inhaled corticosteroid, treatment of asthma as monotherapy

Interactions

DRUGS

adrenergics: Possibly increased sympathetic effects of formoterol
beta-blockers: Decreased effects of both beta-blockers and formoterol
corticosteroids, diuretics, xanthine derivatives: Possibly increased hypokalemic effect of formoterol
disopyramide, macrolides, MAO inhibitors, phenothiazines, procainamide, quinidine, tricyclic antidepressants: Possibly prolonged QT interval, increasing risk of ventricular arrhythmias

Adverse Reactions

CNS: Anxiety, dizziness, fatigue, fever, headache, insomnia, malaise, tremor
CV: Angina, **arrhythmias**, chest pain, hypertension, **hypotension**, palpitations, **prolonged QT interval**, tachycardia
EENT: Dry mouth, laryngeal irritation, **laryngeal spasm or swelling**, hoarseness, pharyngitis, rhinitis and tonsillitis (in children), sinusitis
ENDO: Hyperglycemia
GI: Abdominal pain, gastroenteritis, indigestion (in children); nausea
MS: Back pain, leg cramps, muscle spasms
RESP: **Asthma exacerbation**, bronchitis, **bronchospasm**, cough, dyspnea, increased sputum production, **paradoxical bronchospasm**, upper respiratory tract infection
SKIN: Dermatitis, pruritus, rash, urticaria
Other: **Anaphylaxis**, **angioedema**, **hypokalemia**, **metabolic acidosis**

Childbearing Considerations

PREGNANCY

- It is not known if drug causes fetal harm.
- Use with caution only if benefit to mother outweighs potential risk to fetus.

LABOR AND DELIVERY

- It is not known if drug affects a pregnant woman or fetus during labor and delivery. However, other beta-agonists may interfere with uterine contractility.
- Use of drug should be restricted to patients during labor and delivery only if benefits outweighs the risks.

LACTATION

- It is not known if drug is present in breast milk.
- Mothers should check with prescriber before breastfeeding.

Nursing Considerations

! **WARNING** Know that formoterol therapy should not be used in patients as monotherapy to treat asthma. If asthma is present, patient must be on an inhaled corticosteroid before receiving formoterol because of an increased risk of hospitalization and death. There does not appear to be an increased risk of death with use of formoterol in patients with COPD.

! WARNING Be aware that formoterol therapy should not be initiated in patients with acutely deteriorating COPD, which may be a life-threatening condition, nor should it be administered for the relief of acute symptoms.

- Use caution when administering formoterol to patients with cardiovascular disorders, such as aneurysm, arrhythmias, coronary insufficiency, or hypertension; in patients with pheochromocytoma, seizure disorders or thyrotoxicosis; and in patients who are unusually responsive to sympathomimetic amines.
- Expect inhaled, short-acting beta$_2$-agonists taken by the patient on a regular basis to be discontinued and used only for symptomatic relief of acute respiratory symptoms when formoterol therapy is begun. If an inhaled, short-acting beta$_2$-agonist has not been prescribed for symptomatic relief of acute respiratory symptoms, expect one to be prescribed.

! WARNING Monitor patient for a hypersensitivity reaction, which could become life-threatening such as anaphylaxis or angioedema. If present, notify prescriber, expect drug to be switched to a different drug, and provide supportive care, as needed and ordered.

! WARNING Watch closely for paradoxical bronchospasm; if this occurs, discontinue formoterol immediately and notify prescriber. Also, monitor patient for hypersensitivity reactions. If hypersensitivity reactions are present, notify prescriber, expect drug to be discontinued, and supportive care given, as needed and ordered.

! WARNING Notify prescriber of any significant increases in blood pressure or pulse rate or worsening of chronic conditions because formoterol may produce cardiovascular reactions, including angina, arrhythmias, hypertension or hypotension, palpitations, and tachycardia. Drug may have to be discontinued if such reactions occur.

PATIENT TEACHING

! WARNING Ensure that patient has been informed that long-acting beta-agonists, such as formoterol, increase the risk of asthma-related death and should not be used without a long-term asthma control drug prior to starting formoterol therapy.

- Advise patient, especially if she has a significant cardiac history, to inform prescriber of any other drugs she takes before beginning formoterol therapy to prevent harmful drug interactions.
- Teach patient how to use form of formoterol prescribed.
- Teach patient using solution form how to use, clean, and store nebulizer equipment.
- Instruct patient who currently uses inhaled or oral corticosteroids to continue using them, as prescribed, even if she feels better after starting formoterol.
- Caution patient not to increase formoterol dosage or frequency without consulting prescriber because she may need a rapid-acting bronchodilator and excessive use may result in an overdose.
- Urge patient to notify prescriber if her symptoms worsen, if formoterol becomes less effective, or if she needs more inhalations of short-acting beta$_2$-agonist than usual. This may indicate that her asthma is worsening.

! WARNING Instruct patient to notify prescriber immediately if she experiences chest pain, nervousness, palpitations, rapid heart rate, or tremor while taking formoterol because dosage may have to be adjusted. Also, alert patient to stop drug and seek immediate emergency care if allergic reaction occurs, such as the presence of difficulty breathing or swallowing, hives, itching, rash, or swelling.

foscarnet sodium

Foscavir

Class and Category

Pharmacologic class: Pyrophosphate analogue
Therapeutic class: Antiviral

F

Indications and Dosages

∗ *To treat cytomegalovirus (CMV) retinitis in patients with acquired immunodeficiency syndrome (AIDS)*

I.V. INFUSION

Adults. *Initial:* 90 mg/kg infused over 90 to 120 min every 12 hr or 60 mg/kg infused over 60 min every 8 hr for 2 to 3 wk, depending on clinical response. *Maintenance:* 90 mg/kg/day to 120 mg/kg/day infused over 120 min.

∗ *To treat acyclovir-resistant mucocutaneous herpes simplex virus (HSV) infections in immunocompromised patients*

I.V. INFUSION

Adults. 40 mg/kg infused over 60 min every 8 or 12 hr for 2 to 3 wk or until healing has taken place.

± **DOSAGE ADJUSTMENT** For patients with renal impairment (creatinine clearance 1.4 ml/min/kg or less), dosage reduction and possibly dosage interval increase is based on patient's creatinine clearance level.

Drug Administration

I.V.

- Calculate each dose, before administration, even in the presence of a normal serum creatinine, to reduce risk of nephrotoxicity.
- Maintain adequate hydration of patient to reduce the risk of nephrotoxicity. Expect to administer 750 to 1,000 ml of 0.9% Sodium Chloride Injection or 5% Dextrose Injection prior to the first infusion to establish diuresis. With subsequent infusions, expect to infuse 750 to 1,000 ml of hydration fluid with a dose of 90 to 120 mg/kg of foscarnet and 500 ml of hydration fluid with a dose of 40 to 60 mg/kg. Oral hydration may be used instead if patient is able to drink the required amount of fluid.
- Do not administer drug by bolus or rapid intravenous injection.
- The standard 24-mg/ml solution may be used with or without dilution when using a central venous catheter for infusion. If a peripheral vein catheter is used, the standard 24-mg/ml solution must be diluted to a 12-mg/ml concentration with 0.9% Sodium Chloride Injection or 5% Dextrose Injection prior to administration to avoid local irritation of peripheral veins.
- Use an infusion pump to control the rate of infusion.
- Administer at a rate not exceeding 1 mg/kg/min.
- Discard diluted solution within 24 hr.
- Flush eyes or skin with water if accidental contact with drug occurs because a burning sensation and local irritation may occur.
- *Incompatibilities:* Other drugs, including 30% dextrose, acyclovir sodium, amphotericin, diazepam, digoxin, divalent cations, ganciclovir, leucovorin, midazolam, pentamidine isethionate, phenytoin, prochlorperazine, trimethoprim/sulfamethoxazole, trimetrexate glucuronate, vancomycin; other solutions other than 0.9% Sodium Chloride Injection or 5% Dextrose in Water, including solutions containing calcium, such as Ringer's Lactate and total parenteral nutrition

Route	Onset	Peak	Duration
I.V.	Unknown	Unknown	Unknown

Half-life: 2–4 hr

Mechanism of Action

Inhibits selectively the pyrophosphate binding site on virus-specific DNA polymerases, which inhibits herpes virus replication.

Contraindications

Hypersensitivity to foscarnet sodium or its components

Interactions

DRUGS

acyclovir, aminoglycosides, amphotericin B, cyclosporine, loop diuretics, methotrexate, pentamidine (intravenous), ritonavir, ritonavir and saquinavir, tacrolimus: Increased risk of renal dysfunction

class IA antiarrhythmics (procainamide, quinidine), class III antiarrhythmics (amiodarone, dofetilide, sotalol), phenothiazines, selected fluoroquinolones and macrolides, tricyclic antidepressants: Increased risk of QT prolongation and possible torsades de pointes

pentamidine (intravenous) and other drugs known to influence serum calcium levels: Possibly hypocalcemia

Adverse Reactions

CNS: Abnormal coordination, aggressive reaction, agitation, amnesia, anxiety, aphasia, asthenia, ataxia, **coma**, confusion, dementia,

depression, dizziness, EEG abnormalities, fatigue, fever, hallucination, headache, hypoesthesia, insomnia, malaise, **meningitis**, nervousness, neuropathy, paresthesia, rigors, **seizures, including grand mal**, sensory disturbances, somnolence, **status epilepticus**, stupor, thirst, tremors
CV: **Cardiac arrest**, chest pain, nonacute ECG abnormalities (first-degree AV block, nonspecific ST-T segment changes, sinus tachycardia), edema, elevated gamma GT level, hypertension, **hypotension**, palpitations, **prolonged QT interval**, **torsades de pointes**, **thrombosis**, **ventricular arrhythmia**
EENT: Conjunctivitis, dry mouth, eye abnormalities or pain, pharyngitis, rhinitis, sinusitis, **stridor**, taste perversions, vision abnormalities, ulcerative stomatitis
ENDO: Diabetes insipidus (usually nephrogenic), syndrome of inappropriate antidiuretic hormone secretion
GI: Abdominal pain, abnormal albumin-to-globulin ratio, anorexia, cachexia, constipation, diarrhea, dyspepsia, dysphagia, elevated liver or pancreatic enzymes, esophageal ulceration, flatulence, **GI hemorrhage**, **hepatic dysfunction**, **melena**, nausea, **pancreatitis**, **rectal hemorrhage**, vomiting
GU: **Acute renal failure**, **acquired Fanconi syndrome**, albuminuria, crystal-induced nephropathy, decreased creatinine clearance, dysuria, elevated BUN or serum creatinine level, **glomerulonephritis**, hematuria, **nephrotic syndrome**, **nephrotoxicity**, nocturia, polyuria, renal calculus or impairment, **renal tubular acidosis or necrosis**, urethral disorder, urinary retention, UTI
HEME: Anemia, **granulocytopenia**, **leukopenia**, **neutropenia**, **pancytopenia**, **thrombocytopenia**
MS: Arthralgia, back pain, generalized spasms, involuntary muscle contractions, leg cramps, muscle weakness, myalgia, myositis, **rhabdomyolysis**
RESP: **Bronchospasm**, coughing, dyspnea, **hemoptysis**, pneumonia, **pneumothorax**, **pulmonary infiltration**, **respiratory insufficiency**
SKIN: Diaphoresis, **erythema multiforme**, erythematous or maculopapular rash, flushing, pruritus, rash, seborrhea, skin discoloration or ulceration, **Stevens-Johnson syndrome**, **toxic epidermal necrolysis**, urticaria
Other: **Acidosis**, **anaphylaxis**, **angioedema**, dehydration, elevated alkaline phosphatase or LDH, flu-like symptoms, generalized pain, **hypercalcemia**, **hypernatremia**, hyperphosphatemia, **hypocalcemia**, **hypokalemia**, **hypomagnesemia**, **hypophosphatemia**, hypoproteinemia, infections (bacterial, fungal, moniliasis), injection-site inflammation or pain, localized edema, lymphadenopathy, **lymphoma-like disorder**, **sarcoma**, **sepsis**, weight loss

Childbearing Considerations

PREGNANCY

- It is not known if drug causes fetal harm.
- Use with caution only if benefit to mother outweighs potential risk to fetus.

LACTATION

- It is not known if drug is present in breast milk.
- The Centers for Disease Control and Prevention recommends that HIV-1 infected mothers not breastfeed to avoid risking postnatal transmission of HIV-1 infection to infants. They also do not recommend breastfeeding because of potential drug-induced adverse reactions in the infant.
- For mothers with HSV, breastfeeding or the drug should be discontinued.

Nursing Considerations

- Know that foscarnet therapy should not be used in patients on a controlled sodium diet because of the sodium content of the drug.
- Assess patient's estimated or measured creatinine clearance before foscarnet therapy is begun, 2 to 3 times a week during initial therapy, and once weekly during maintenance therapy, as ordered, because most patients will experience some decrease in renal function as a result of foscarnet therapy. Know also that a 24-hour creatinine clearance should be determined before therapy is begun and periodically thereafter to ensure correct dosing. Expect foscarnet to be discontinued if creatinine clearance drops below 0.4 ml/min/kg.
- Determine patient's serum calcium, magnesium, phosphorus, and potassium levels before foscarnet therapy is begun,

F

2 to 3 times a week during initial therapy, and once weekly during maintenance therapy, as ordered, because foscarnet can chelate divalent metal ions and alter levels of serum electrolytes. Monitor patient for symptoms of electrolyte abnormalities (mild: perioral numbness or paresthesias; severe: seizures) regularly. If present, notify prescriber and expect serum electrolyte and mineral levels to be assessed as soon as possible and treatment initiated if abnormalities are present.

! **WARNING** Assess patient closely for hypersensitivity reactions, which could become life-threatening such as anaphylaxis or angioedema. If present, notify prescriber immediately, expect foscarnet to be discontinued, and provide supportive care, as needed and ordered.

! **WARNING** Monitor patients closely who have a history of prolonged QT interval, in patients taking drugs known to prolong the QT interval, in patients with electrolyte disturbances, or in patients who have other risk factors for QT prolongation, as QT prolongation and torsades de pointes have occurred with foscarnet therapy. Expect prescriber to order routine ECGs and measure patient's electrolytes before foscarnet therapy is begun and periodically throughout therapy.

! **WARNING** Monitor patients with neurologic abnormalities (especially seizure disorders). Institute seizure precautions, if needed. If seizures occur, notify prescriber.

- Know that combination therapy with foscarnet and ganciclovir is indicated for patients who have relapsed after monotherapy with either drug used to treat CMV retinitis.

PATIENT TEACHING

- Inform patient that drug will be administered intravenously.
- Reassure patient that he will be monitored closely throughout drug administration.
- Advise patient that foscarnet is not a cure for either CMV retinitis or mucocutaneous acyclovir-resistant HSV infection.
- Tell patient that it is important to maintain hydration during foscarnet therapy.

! **WARNING** Advise patient to alert staff immediately or get immediate emergency medical treatment if home if any signs of an allergic reaction, such as difficulty breathing, hives, or swelling of face, lips, tongue, or throat occurs.

! **WARNING** Inform patient that the major adverse reactions related to foscarnet therapy are electrolyte abnormalities, kidney dysfunction, and seizures. Stress importance of reporting any persistent, severe, or unusual signs and symptoms to staff or prescriber, as dosage may have to be adjusted for next administration or drug discontinued.

! **WARNING** Instruct patient to notify staff or prescriber at once if she experiences serious adverse reactions such as confusion, feeling short of breath, increased thirst, pounding heartbeats, swelling, urinating less than usual or not at all, weakness, or weight gain.

- Caution patient to avoid performing hazardous activities such as driving until the effects of the drug on her nervous system are known and resolved.
- Inform mothers that breastfeeding is not recommended during foscarnet therapy.
- Encourage patient being treated for CMV retinitis to have regular ophthalmologic examinations.

fosinopril sodium

Class and Category

Pharmacologic class: ACE inhibitor
Therapeutic class: Antihypertensive, vasodilator

Indications and Dosages

∗ *To treat hypertension as monotherapy or with thiazide diuretics*

TABLETS

Adults. *Initial:* 10 mg once daily. *Maintenance:* 20 to 40 mg once daily or in divided doses. *Maximum:* 80 mg once daily or in divided doses.
Children ages 6 and older weighing more than 50 kg (110 lb). 5 to 10 mg once daily as monotherapy.

∗ *As adjunct to treat heart failure*

TABLETS

Adults. 10 mg once daily with dosage increased over several weeks, as needed. *Maintenance:* 20 to 40 mg once daily. *Maximum:* 40 mg once daily.

±**DOSAGE ADJUSTMENT** For patients with heart failure who have moderate to severe renal failure or recent aggressive diuresis, initial dosage reduced to 5 mg daily, as needed.

Drug Administration

P.O.

- Administer with or without food.
- Observe patient being treated for heart failure for at least 2 hr after giving drug, to detect hypotension or orthostatic hypotension. If either develops, notify prescriber and monitor patient until blood pressure stabilizes. Keep in mind that orthostatic hypotension is unlikely to develop in patient with a systolic blood pressure over 100 mm Hg who has received a 10-mg dose.
- Separate administration times between antacids and fosinopril by at least 2 hr.

Route	Onset	Peak	Duration
P.O.	1 hr	2–6 hr	24 hr

Half-life: 12 hr

Mechanism of Action

May reduce blood pressure by affecting renin–angiotensin–aldosterone system. By inhibiting angiotensin-converting enzyme, fosinopril:

- prevents conversion of angiotensin I to angiotensin II, a potent vasoconstrictor that also stimulates the adrenal cortex to secrete aldosterone.
- may inhibit renal and vascular production of angiotensin II.
- decreases serum angiotensin II level and increases serum renin activity, which decreases aldosterone secretion, slightly increasing the serum potassium level and fluid loss.
- decreases vascular tone and blood pressure.
- inhibits aldosterone release, which reduces sodium and water reabsorption and increases their excretion, further reducing blood pressure and symptoms of heart failure.

Contraindications

Hypersensitivity to fosinopril, other ACE inhibitors, or their components

Interactions

DRUGS

antacids: Impaired fosinopril absorption
diuretics, other antihypertensives: Possibly additive hypotension
lithium: Increased blood lithium level and risk of lithium toxicity
potassium-sparing diuretics, potassium supplements: Increased risk of hyperkalemia
sodium aurothiomalate: Nitritoid reactions, including facial flushing, hypotension, nausea, and vomiting

FOODS

salt substitutes: Increased risk of hyperkalemia

Adverse Reactions

CNS: Confusion, depression, dizziness, drowsiness, fatigue, fever, headache, insomnia, mood changes, sleep disturbance, syncope, tremor, vertigo, weakness
CV: **Angina**, **arrhythmias (including AV conduction disorders**, **bradycardia**, and tachycardia), claudication, **hypotension**, **MI**, orthostatic hypotension, palpitations
EENT: Dry mouth, epistaxis, eye irritation, hoarseness, rhinitis, sinus problems, taste perversion, tinnitus, vision changes
GI: Abdominal distention and pain, anorexia, constipation, diarrhea, flatulence, **hepatic failure**, **hepatitis**, hepatomegaly, jaundice, nausea, **pancreatitis**, vomiting
GU: Decreased libido, flank pain, **renal insufficiency**, sexual dysfunction, urinary frequency
MS: Arthralgia, gout, myalgia
RESP: **Asthma**; bronchitis; **bronchospasm**; dry, persistent, tickling cough; dyspnea; tracheobronchitis; upper respiratory tract infection
SKIN: Diaphoresis, photosensitivity, pruritus, rash, urticaria
Other: **Anaphylaxis**, **angioedema**, **hyperkalemia**, weight gain

Childbearing Considerations

PREGNANCY

- Drug may cause fetal harm during second and third trimester. Anuria, hypotension, neonatal skull hypoplasia, oligohydramnios, and reversible and irreversible renal failure have occurred along with fetal demise.

- Drug should be discontinued as soon as pregnancy is known.

LACTATION

- Drug is present in breast milk.
- A decision should be made to discontinue breastfeeding or the drug to avoid potential serious adverse reactions in the breastfed infant.

Nursing Considerations

- Monitor serum potassium level before and during fosinopril therapy, as ordered.
- Know that if patient also receives a diuretic or another antihypertensive, expect to reduce its dosage over 2 to 3 days before starting fosinopril.
- Monitor blood pressure for effectiveness of drug. If blood pressure isn't controlled with fosinopril alone, other antihypertensive therapy may be added, as prescribed.

! **WARNING** Monitor patient for hypotension, especially if other antihypertensive drugs are being administered because excessive hypotension can occur.

! **WARNING** Monitor patient for hypersensitivity reactions, which could become life-threatening such as anaphylaxis or angioedema. If present, notify prescriber immediately, expect fosinopril to be discontinued, and provide supportive care, as needed and ordered.

! **WARNING** Monitor patient for persistent, serious, or unusual adverse reactions because fosinopril can affect many body systems and has the potential to cause serious to life-threatening adverse reactions such as arrhythmias, bronchospasms, MI, and pancreatitis.

PATIENT TEACHING

- Instruct patient how to administer fosinopril.
- Stress importance of taking the drug at same time each day to improve compliance and maintain drug's therapeutic effect.
- Emphasize the importance of taking fosinopril, as prescribed, even if patient feels well. Caution her not to stop taking drug without consulting prescriber.
- Advise patient not to take other drugs or use salt substitutes without consulting prescriber.

! **WARNING** Urge females of childbearing age to use contraception during therapy because drug may harm fetus. Also, advise her to notify prescriber immediately if pregnancy occurs.

! **WARNING** Alert patient that drug may cause an allergic reaction. If present, tell patient to notify prescriber and, if severe, to seek immediate medical care.

! **WARNING** Advise patient to use caution during exercise and hot weather because of the increased risk of dehydration from excessive sweating. Also, instruct patient to notify prescriber about persistent, severe diarrhea, nausea, and vomiting; resulting dehydration may lead to hypotension.

- Caution patient about possible dizziness or other CNS adverse reactions. Advise patient not to perform hazardous activities such as driving until effects are known and resolved.
- Advise patient to rise slowly from a lying or sitting position and to dangle legs over bed for several minutes before standing to minimize effects of orthostatic hypotension.
- Reinforce prescriber's recommendations for lifestyle changes, such as alcohol avoidance, dietary improvements, smoking cessation, regular exercise, and stress reduction.
- Inform mothers breastfeeding should not be undertaken or the drug will need to be discontinued.
- Encourage patient to keep scheduled appointments with prescriber to monitor blood pressure, blood test results, and effects of therapy.

fosphenytoin sodium

Cerebyx

Class and Category

Pharmacologic class: Hydantoin derivative
Therapeutic class: Anticonvulsant

Indications and Dosages

∗ *To treat generalized tonic-clonic status epilepticus*

I.V. INFUSION, I.M. INJECTION

Adults. *Emergent loading dose:* 15 to 20 mg of phenytoin equivalent (PE)/kg

I.V. infused at a rate of 100 to 150 PE/min. *Non-emergent loading dose*: 10 to 20 mg PE/kg with infusion rate not to exceed 150 mg PE/min. *Maintenance:* 4 to 6 mg PE/kg daily in divided doses and infused at a rate no greater than 150 mg PE/min. I.M. injection given only if I.V. route is impossible.

I.V. INFUSION

Neonates, infants, children, and adolescents to age 17. *Emergent loading dose:* 15 to 20 mg PE/kg infused at a rate of 2 mg PE/kg/min or 150 mg PE/min, whichever is slower. *Non-emergent loading dose:* 10 to 15 mg PE/kg with infusion rate not to exceed 1 to 2 mg PE/kg/min or 150 mg PE/min, whichever is slower. *Maintenance:* Initial maintenance dose of 2 to 4 mg PE/kg given 12 hr after initial loading dose infused at a rate of 1 to 2 mg PE/kg/min, or 100 mg PE/min, whichever is slower. Maintenance dosage then continued at a rate of 4 to 8 mg PE/kg/min in 2 divided doses (every 12 hr) infused at a rate of 1 to 2 mg PE/kg/min or 100 mg PE/min, whichever is slower.

* *To prevent or treat seizures during neurosurgery*

I.V. INFUSION, I.M. INJECTION

Adults. *Nonemergent loading dose:* 10 to 20 mg PE/kg, infused at an I.V. rate not exceeding 150 mg PE/min or given I.M. *Maintenance:* 4 to 6 mg PE/kg in divided doses infused at an I.V. rate not exceeding 150 mg/PE/min or given I.M.

I.V. INFUSION

Neonates, infants, children, and adolescents to age 17. *Nonemergent loading dose:* 10 to 15 mg PE/kg infused at a rate of 1 to 2 mg PE/kg/min or 150 mg PE/min, whichever is slower. *Maintenance:* 2 to 4 mg PE/kg given 12 hr after initial dose and then continued every 12 hr infused at a rate of 1 to 2 mg PE/kg/min or 100 mg PE/min, whichever is slower.

* *To substitute for oral phenytoin therapy when administration of oral phenytoin is not possible*

I.V. INFUSION, I.M. INJECTION

Adults. Same total daily phenytoin sodium equivalents (PE) dose. I.V. infusion rate should not exceed 150 mg PE/min.

I.V. INFUSION

Neonates, infants, children, and adolescents to age 17. Same total daily phenytoin sodium equivalents (PE) dose. I.V. infusion rate should not exceed 2 mg PE/kg/min or 150 mg PE/min, whichever is slower.

±**DOSAGE ADJUSTMENT** For elderly patients, dosage reduced or dosing interval increased.

Drug Administration

- Usually stored in refrigerator. If stored at room temperature, discard after 48 hr.
- Injection vials are single dose only. Discard any unused drug left in vial. Inspect drug solution. It should be clear, colorless to pale yellow. If not, or particles are present, discard.
- The dosage, concentration, and infusion rate of drug are expressed in phenytoin sodium equivalents (PE) units. Do not confuse the concentration of drug with the total amount of drug in the vial. Misreading an order or a label could result in massive overdose.

I.V.

- For status epilepticus, I.V. route should be used rather than I.M. route because therapeutic drug level occurs more rapidly.
- Dilute drug in 0.9% Sodium Chloride Injection or 5% Dextrose in Water to a concentration of 1.5 to 25 mg PE/ml.
- Follow manufacturer guidelines for infusion rate administration. Do not exceed these rates because of the risk of cardiac arrhythmias and severe hypotension.
- Expect to give an I.V. benzodiazepine (such as diazepam or lorazepam), as prescribed, with fosphenytoin to control status epilepticus; otherwise, drug's full antiepileptic effect won't be immediate.
- Monitor patient throughout the infusion for adverse signs and symptoms of cardiovascular toxicity. If present, notify prescriber and expect infusion rate to be slowed or drug discontinued.
- Monitor blood pressure, ECG, and respiratory function during infusion and for 10 to 20 min after infusion ends.
- Monitor patient for signs of sensory disturbances during the infusion, such as severe burning, itching, and/or paresthesia, especially in the groin. Know that the intensity of discomfort can be lessened by slowing or temporarily stopping the infusion.

- Expect to obtain blood fosphenytoin (phenytoin) level 2 hr after I.V. infusion. Therapeutic level generally ranges from 10 to 20 mcg/ml; steady state may take several days to several weeks to reach.
- Patient should be switched to oral phenytoin as soon as possible because of the risks of cardiac and local toxicity associated with I.V. administration.
- *Incompatibilities:* Other I.V. drugs

I.M.

- Be aware that loading doses shouldn't be given I.M. because I.V. route allows faster onset and peak. Use only if I.V. access is impossible.
- Do not administer I.M. injection in children unless I.V. access is impossible.
- Expect to obtain blood fosphenytoin (phenytoin) level 4 hr after I.M. injection.

Route	Onset	Peak	Duration
I.V.	Unknown	End of infusion	Unknown
I.M.	Unknown	30 min	Unknown

Half-life: 15 min to convert to phenytoin

Mechanism of Action

Converted from fosphenytoin (a prodrug) to phenytoin, which limits the spread of seizure activity and the start of new seizures. Phenytoin does so by regulating voltage-dependent sodium and calcium channels in neurons, inhibiting calcium movement across neuronal membranes, and enhancing the sodium–potassium–adenosine triphosphatase activity in glial cells and neurons. These actions may stem from phenytoin's ability to slow the recovery rate of inactivated sodium channels.

Contraindications

Adams-Stokes syndrome; concurrent delavirdine use; history of prior acute hepatotoxicity caused by fosphenytoin or phenytoin: hypersensitivity to fosphenytoin, phenytoin, other hydantoins, or their components; second- or third-degree AV block; sinoatrial block; sinus bradycardia

Interactions

DRUGS

acyclovir: Decreased blood phenytoin level, loss of seizure control
alfentanil: Increased clearance and decreased effectiveness of alfentanil
albendazole, anticoagulants (apixaban, dabigatran, edoxaban, rivaroxaban), antiepileptics (carbamazepine, felbamate, lacosamide, lamotrigine, topiramate, oxcarbazepine), antilipidemics (atorvastatin, fluvastatin, simvastatin), antivirals (efavirenz, fosamprenavir, lopinavir/ritonavir, indinavir, nelfinavir, ritonavir, saquinavir), calcium channel blockers (nifedipine, nimodipine, nisoldipine, verapamil), chlorpropamide, clozapine, cyclosporine, digoxin, disopyramide, folic acid, methadone, mexiletine, praziquantel, quetiapine, ticagrelor: Decreased blood levels of these drugs
amiodarone, calcium channel blockers, capecitabine, chloramphenicol, chlordiazepoxide, cimetidine, disulfiram, estrogen, ethosuximide, felbamate, fluconazole, fluorouracil, fluoxetine, fluvastatin, fluvoxamine, isoniazid, itraconazole, ketoconazole, methylphenidate, miconazole, omeprazole, oxcarbazepine, phenothiazines, salicylates, sertraline, sulfadiazine, sulfamethizole, sulfamethoxazole-trimethoprim, sulfaphenazole, ticlopidine, tolbutamide, topiramate, trimethoprim, voriconazole, warfarin: Possibly increased blood phenytoin level and risk of toxicity
antineoplastics, carbamazepine, diazepam, diazoxide, folic acid, fosamprenavir, nelfinavir, reserpine, rifampin, ritonavir, St. John's wort, theophylline, vigabatrin: Increased phenytoin metabolism and decreased phenytoin level
antineoplastic agents (irinotecan, paclitaxel, teniposide), azoles (fluconazole, ketoconazole, itraconazole, posaconazole, voriconazole), corticosteroids, delavirdine, doxycycline, estrogens, furosemide, neuromuscular blocking agents (cisatracurium, pancuronium, rocuronium, vecuronium), oral contraceptives, paroxetine, quinidine, rifampin, sertraline, theophylline, vitamin D, warfarin: Decreased effectiveness of these drugs
fosamprenavir/ritonavir: Possibly increased amprenavir concentration, the active metabolite of fosamprenavir
lithium: Increased risk of lithium toxicity
methadone: Possibly increased methadone
phenobarbital, valproate sodium, valproic acid: Possible decrease or increase in phenytoin serum levels
tricyclic antidepressants: Possibly lowered seizure threshold and decreased therapeutic

effects of phenytoin; possibly decreased blood antidepressant level
valproic acid: Increased blood valproic acid level

ACTIVITIES

alcohol use: Possibly decreased or increased phenytoin effectiveness

Adverse Reactions

CNS: Agitation, amnesia, asthenia, ataxia, **cerebral edema**, chills, **coma**, confusion, **CVA**, decreased or increased reflexes, delusions, depression, dizziness, dyskinesia, emotional lability, **encephalitis**, **encephalopathy**, extrapyramidal reactions, fever, headache, hemiplegia, hostility, hypoesthesia, lack of coordination, malaise, **meningitis**, nervousness, neurosis, paralysis, paresthesia, personality disorder, positive Babinski's sign, **seizures**, somnolence, speech disorders, stupor, **subdural hematoma**, syncope, transient paresthesia, tremor, vertigo
CV: **Atrial flutter**, **bradycardia**, bundle-branch block, **cardiac arrest**, **cardiomegaly**, edema, **heart failure**, hypertension, **hypotension**, orthostatic hypotension, palpitations, **PVCs**, **serious arrhythmias**, **shock**, tachycardia, thrombophlebitis, vasodilation
EENT: Amblyopia, conjunctivitis, diplopia, dry mouth, earache, epistaxis, eye pain, gingival hyperplasia, hearing loss, hyperacusis, increased salivation, loss of taste, mydriasis, nystagmus, pharyngitis, photophobia, rhinitis, sinusitis, taste perversion, tinnitus, **tongue swelling**, visual field defects
ENDO: Decreased dexamethasone, metyrapone, or T4 levels; diabetes insipidus; hyperglycemia; **ketosis**
GI: Anorexia, constipation, diarrhea, dysphagia, elevated liver enzymes, flatulence, gastritis, **GI bleeding**, **hepatic necrosis**, **hepatitis**, ileus, indigestion, nausea, vomiting
GU: Albuminuria, dysuria, incontinence, oliguria, polyuria, **renal failure**, urine retention, vaginal candidiasis
HEME: **Agranulocytosis**, anemia, easy bruising, **granulocytopenia**, **leukopenia**, macrocytosis, megaloblastic anemia, **pancytopenia**, **pure red cell aplasia**, **thrombocytopenia**
MS: Arthralgia, back or pelvic pain, dysarthria, leg cramps, muscle twitching, myalgia, myasthenia, myoclonus, myopathy
RESP: **Apnea**, **asthma**, **atelectasis**, bronchitis, dyspnea, **hemoptysis**, hyperventilation, **hypoxia**, increased cough, increased sputum production, pneumonia, **pneumothorax**
SKIN: Acute generalized exanthematous pustulosis (AGEP), contact dermatitis, diaphoresis, maculopapular or pustular rash, photosensitivity, pruritus, skin discoloration, skin nodule, **Stevens-Johnson syndrome**, **toxic epidermal necrolysis**, urticaria
Other: **Anaphylaxis**; **angioedema**; cachexia; **cryptococcosis**; dehydration; **drug reaction with eosinophilia and systemic symptoms (DRESS)**; elevated alkaline phosphatase; flu-like symptoms; **hyperkalemia**; **hypokalemia**; **hypophosphatemia**; infection; injection-site reaction such as edema, discoloration, and pain distal to the site of injection; lymphadenopathy; porphyria; **sepsis**

Childbearing Considerations

PREGNANCY

- Pregnancy exposure registry: 1-888-233-2334 or http://www.aedpregnancyregistry.org/.
- Drug may cause fetal harm increasing risk for congenital malformations and other adverse developmental outcomes, including hydantoin syndrome. In addition, malignancies, including neuroblastoma have been reported in children whose mothers received drug during pregnancy.
- A potentially life-threatening bleeding disorder may occur in neonates exposed to drug in utero.
- Drug is not recommended during pregnancy unless absolutely necessary and no other alternative is available.

LACTATION

- It is not known if drug is present in breast milk, but the active metabolite of the drug is present in human milk.
- Mothers should check with prescriber before breastfeeding.

REPRODUCTION

- Females of childbearing age should use effective contraception throughout drug therapy.

Nursing Considerations

! **WARNING** Know that patients of Asian ancestry who have the genetic allelic variant HLA-B 1502 or CYP2C9*3 variant develop

F

serious and sometimes fatal dermatologic reactions 10 times more often than people without this variant when given carbamazepine, another antiepileptic drug. Because early data suggest a similar effect with fosphenytoin, this drug shouldn't be used as a substitute for carbamazepine in these patients.

! **WARNING** Monitor patient for a hypersensitivity or skin reaction, which may become life-threatening such as anaphylaxis, angioedema, or DRESS. Know that while a rash is usually the first sign of DRESS, it may only present with a fever or swollen lymph nodes. If a hypersensitivity reaction or fever, rash, or swollen lymph nodes are present, notify prescriber, expect drug to be discontinued and another drug substituted. Provide supportive care, as needed and ordered.

! **WARNING** Know that antiepileptic drugs such as fosphenytoin should not be discontinued abruptly because of the possibility of increased seizure frequency, including status epilepticus. If drug must be discontinued because of a hypersensitivity reaction including a skin reaction or toxicity signs and symptoms appear, expect to rapidly substitute drug with alternative therapy not belonging to the hydantoin chemical class to avoid increased risk of seizures, including status epilepticus.

! **WARNING** Know that if serious adverse reactions occur such as acute hepatotoxicity (hepatic necrosis and hepatitis), during first 2 months of therapy, drug will need to be discontinued and an alternative nonhydantoin drug rapidly substituted. Provide supportive care, as needed and ordered. Also monitor patient for other adverse reactions that are persistent, serious, or unusual because drug can affect many body systems and cause very serious to life-threatening adverse reactions such as electrolyte imbalance, hepatic dysfunction, ketosis, and shock.

- Anticipate increased frequency and severity of adverse reactions after I.V. administration in patients with hepatic or renal impairment or hypoalbuminemia. Know that the phosphate load contained in fosphenytoin should be kept in mind when patients with severe renal impairment are treated.

! **WARNING** Monitor phenytoin level to detect early signs of toxicity, such as diplopia, nausea, severe confusion, slurred speech, and vomiting. Remember that when switching between phenytoin and fosphenytoin, small differences in phenytoin bioavailability can lead to significant changes in blood phenytoin level and an increased risk of toxicity. Monitor patient closely. If toxicity occurs, expect to reduce dosage or rapidly substitute drug with alternative nonhydantoin as ordered to avoid increased risk of seizures, including status epilepticus.

! **WARNING** Monitor patient for seizures; at toxic levels, phenytoin is excitatory. Document onset, characteristics, and type of seizures and response to treatment. Notify prescriber immediately if a seizure occurs and institute seizure precautions.

! **WARNING** Know that if patient has bradycardia or heart block rhythm, notify prescriber and expect to withhold drug; severe cardiovascular reactions and death have occurred.

- Monitor serum albumin level and results of liver and renal function tests.
- Monitor patient for injection-site reactions such as local toxicity known as Purple Glove syndrome, exhibited by discoloration, edema, and pain distal to the site of injection. Know that this may occur without extravasation being present and up to several days after injection. If present, notify prescriber and expect drug to be discontinued.
- Monitor CBC for leukopenia or thrombocytopenia—signs of hematologic toxicity. Be aware that drug may cause macrocytosis and megaloblastic anemia but that these conditions usually respond well to folic acid therapy.
- Expect to provide vitamin D supplement if patient has inadequate dietary intake and is receiving long-term anticonvulsant treatment.

PATIENT TEACHING

! **WARNING** Stress importance for females of childbearing age to alert prescriber if pregnant before drug is administered. Advise patient to use effective contraceptive throughout drug therapy and to notify prescriber immediately if pregnancy occurs.

- Inform patient that fosphenytoin typically is used for short-term treatment and is given usually as an intravenous infusion. An intramuscular injection may be used but only if drug cannot be administered intravenously.
- Inform patient that some sensory discomfort may be felt during fosphenytoin intravenous administration. Advise patient to alert the nurse, if discomfort is felt, as slowing the infusion can decrease the discomfort.

! **WARNING** Urge patient to notify staff or seek immediate medical care if home if allergic reactions occur, especially if severe or patient develops a fever, rash, or swollen lymph nodes.

! **WARNING** Instruct patient to notify staff or prescriber immediately about bothersome symptoms, especially a local reaction at injection site, including discoloration, edema, and pain distal to the site, and swelling. Also, tell patient to notify staff or prescriber immediately if persistent, severe, or unusual signs and symptoms occur.

- Tell patient to inform prescriber of any new drugs being used, including over-the-counter preparations and alcohol products prior to taking them.
- Emphasize need for good oral hygiene and gum massage because gingival hyperplasia may develop during long-term therapy.
- Urge patient to consume adequate amounts of vitamin D.

fremanezumab-vfrm

Ajovy

Class and Category

Pharmacologic class: Calcitonin gene-related peptide antagonist
Therapeutic class: Antimigraine

Indications and Dosages

∗ *To prevent migraine headaches*

SUBCUTANEOUS INJECTION

Adults. 225 mg monthly. Alternatively, 675 mg every 3 mo given as 3 consecutive injections of 225 mg each.

Drug Administration

SUBCUTANEOUS

- Remove drug from refrigerator and allow it to sit at room temperature for 30 min protected from direct sunlight prior to administration. Do not warm drug using a heat source, such as hot water or a microwave. Discard if drug (kept in original carton) has been left at room temperature for 7 days or longer.
- Do not use if solution appears to be cloudy, discolored, or contains particles.
- Inject drug using autoinjector into the abdomen, thigh, or upper arm in an area that is not bruised, indurated, red, or tender. If giving 3 consecutive injections, the same body site may be used, but not the exact location.
- When injecting drug, press down on the prefilled autoinjector and keep holding it against the skin for about 30 sec. Do not remove pressure until a click is heard and the blue plunger starts to move, a second click is heard about 15 sec after first click and the plunger continues to move to the bottom of the viewing window, and then wait another 10 sec making sure blue plunger has filled the viewing window before lifting autoinjector from the skin.
- Do not rub injection site afterwards but gently press on the injection site with a clean, dry cotton ball or gauze pad for a few sec.
- Do not coadminister drug with other injectable drugs at the same injection site.

Route	Onset	Peak	Duration
SubQ	Unknown	5–7 days	Unknown

Half-life: 31 days

Mechanism of Action

Binds to the calcitonin gene-related peptide (CGRP) receptor. The CGRP receptor is thought to be responsible for transmitting signals that can cause incapacitating pain.

F

By binding to the CGRP receptor, drug antagonizes its function, preventing pain signals from being transmitted.

Contraindications

Hypersensitivity to fremanezumab-vfrm or its components

Interactions

DRUGS

None reported by manufacturer.

Adverse Reactions

SKIN: Pruritus, rash, urticaria
Other: **Anaphylaxis**, **angioedema**, fremanezumab-vfrm antibody formation, injection-site reactions (induration, pain, redness)

Childbearing Considerations

PREGNANCY

- Pregnancy exposure registry: 1-833-927-2605 or www.tevamigrainepregnancyregistry.com.
- It is not known if drug causes fetal harm.
- Use with caution only if benefit to mother outweighs potential risk to fetus.
- Know that females of childbearing age with migraine may be at increased risk of gestational hypertension and preeclampsia during pregnancy.

LACTATION

- It is not known if drug may be present in breast milk.
- Mothers should check with prescriber before breastfeeding.

Nursing Considerations

! **WARNING** Monitor patient for a hypersensitivity reaction, which could become life-threatening such as anaphylaxis or angioedema occur. Be aware that most hypersensitivity reactions occur within hours to 1 month after administration. Know that if a hypersensitivity reaction occurs, notify prescriber, expect drug to be discontinued, and provide supportive care, as needed and ordered.

- Know that when switching dosage options, the first dose of the new regimen should be administered on the next scheduled date of administration.

PATIENT TEACHING

- Teach patient how to prepare and administer fremanezumab-vfrm subcutaneously and what to do if a dose is missed.
- Inform patient that when switching dosage options, first dose of the new regimen should be administered on the next scheduled date of administration.

! **WARNING** Advise patient that drug may cause an allergic reaction within hours to up to 1 month following administration. If present, tell patient to notify prescriber immediately, because more serious reactions may develop requiring drug to be discontinued. If reaction is serious, urge patient to seek immediate medical care.

- Tell patient to notify prescriber if a local reaction occurs at the injection site.

! **WARNING** Stress importance of keeping drug out of the reach of small children.

frovatriptan succinate

Frova

Class and Category

Pharmacologic class: Serotonin 5-HT_1 receptor agonist
Therapeutic class: Antimigraine

Indications and Dosages

✱ *To treat acute migraine headache*

TABLETS

Adults. 2.5 mg, as needed. If migraine returns, 2.5-mg dose repeated providing there is at least a 2-hr interval between the 2 doses. *Maximum:* 7.5 mg (three 2.5-mg doses) per 24 hr; treatment of more than 4 migraines within 30 days.

Drug Administration

P.O.

- Do not exceed maximum dosage.

Route	Onset	Peak	Duration
P.O.	Unknown	2–4 hr	Unknown

Half-life: 26 hr

Mechanism of Action

Binds to 5-HT_1 receptors on intracranial blood vessels and sensory nerves of the trigeminal system to produce cranial vessel constriction and inhibition of proinflammatory neuropeptide release, which causes pain relief.

Contraindications

Arrhythmias associated with cardiac accessory conduction pathway disorders such as Wolff-Parkinson-White syndrome; history of basilar or hemiplegic migraine, stroke, or transient ischemic attack; hypersensitivity to frovatriptan or its components; ischemic coronary artery disease or coronary artery vasospasm; ischemic bowel disease; peripheral vascular disease; uncontrolled hypertension; use within 24 hr of another 5-HT_1 agonist or an ergotamine-containing or ergot-type drug, such as dihydroergotamine or methysergide

Interactions

DRUGS

ergot-containing or ergot-type drugs, such as dihydroergotamine, methysergide: Increased risk of prolonged vasospastic reaction
MAO inhibitors, selective serotonin reuptake inhibitors, serotonin norepinephrine reuptake inhibitors, tricyclic antidepressants: Possible development of serotonin syndrome
other 5-HT_1 agonists: Potential additive effects increasing risk of serious adverse reactions

Adverse Reactions

CNS: Anxiety; **cerebral hemorrhage**, **CVA, and other cerebrovascular events**; dizziness; dysesthesia; exacerbation of headache; fatigue; hypoesthesia; insomnia; palpitations; paresthesia; **seizure**; **serotonin syndrome**; **subarachnoid hemorrhage**
CV: **Arrhythmias**, **including ventricular fibrillation or tachycardia**; chest, jaw, neck, or **throat** pain, pressure, or **tightness**; **MI**; **myocardial ischemia**; peripheral vascular ischemia; Prinzmetal's angina; Raynaud's syndrome
EENT: Abnormal vision, blindness (transient or permanent), dry mouth, partial vision loss, rhinitis, sinusitis, tinnitus
GI: Abdominal pain, bloody diarrhea, diarrhea, dyspepsia, **GI vascular infarction or ischemia**, splenic infarction, vomiting
RESP: Bone pain
SKIN: Diaphoresis, flushing
Other: **Anaphylaxis**, **angioedema**, generalized pain, sensation of being cold or hot

Childbearing Considerations

PREGNANCY

- It is not known if drug causes fetal harm.
- Use with caution only if benefit to mother outweighs potential risk to fetus.
- Know that females of childbearing age with migraine may be at increased risk of gestational hypertension and preeclampsia during pregnancy.

LACTATION

- It is not known if drug is present in breast milk.
- Mothers should check with prescriber before breastfeeding.

Nursing Considerations

! **WARNING** Expect triptan-naïve patient with multiple cardiovascular risk factors such as diabetes, increased age, hypertension, obesity, smoking, or strong family history of coronary artery disease to have a cardiovascular evaluation prior to frovatriptan being prescribed because drug can cause serious cardiovascular disorders, such as MI or ischemia and Prinzmetal's angina. In patients who have a negative cardiovascular evaluation, know that the first dose of frovatriptan may be administered in a medically supervised setting with an ECG performed immediately following administration to detect adverse effects. Expect periodic cardiovascular evaluations to be performed throughout frovatriptan therapy. Also, expect drug to be immediately discontinued if patient develops arrhythmias because of potential life-threatening consequences.

! **WARNING** Know that if patient complains of chest, jaw, neck, or throat pain, pressure, or tightness, an immediate cardiovascular evaluation should be performed even though these symptoms are usually noncardiac in nature.

! **WARNING** Monitor patient for hypersensitivity reactions to frovatriptan. These reactions may be life-threatening and include anaphylaxis and angioedema. Stop drug therapy immediately and notify prescriber if a hypersensitivity reaction occurs. Provide supportive care, as needed and ordered.

! **WARNING** Monitor patient for signs and symptoms of cerebrovascular events because drug use increases risk of CVAs and cerebrovascular hemorrhage.

! **WARNING** Monitor patient for noncardiovascular vasospasm events, such as GI vascular infarction and ischemia (abdominal pain, bloody diarrhea), peripheral vascular ischemia, Raynaud's syndrome, or splenic infarction. If suspected, notify prescriber immediately, stop frovatriptan therapy, and be prepared to provide emergency supportive care according to institutional protocol.

! **WARNING** Monitor patient for evidence of serotonin syndrome, such as agitation, chills, confusion, diaphoresis, diarrhea, fever, hyperactive reflexes, poor coordination, restlessness, shaking, talking or acting with uncontrolled excitement, tremor, and twitching. Be aware that risk is greater during coadministration with monoamine oxidase inhibitors, selective serotonin reuptake inhibitors, serotonin norepinephrine reuptake inhibitors, and tricyclic antidepressants. Onset of symptoms usually occurs within minutes to hours of receiving a new or a greater dose of a serotonergic medication. If serotonin syndrome is suspected, notify prescriber immediately, expect drug to be discontinued, and provide symptomatic supportive care, as prescribed.

! **WARNING** Monitor patient's blood pressure because significant elevation in blood pressure, including hypertensive crisis, has been reported in patients treated with other 5-HT_1 agonists.

PATIENT TEACHING

- Instruct patient how to administer frovatriptan.
- Tell patient to take drug exactly as prescribed and not to overuse drug by exceeding maximum dosages in a month because medication-overuse headache may develop. If patient begins to experience daily migraine-like headaches or a marked increase in frequency of headaches, tell him to notify prescriber. Inform him that a period of detoxification may be necessary.

! **WARNING** Alert patient that frovatriptan therapy may cause allergic reactions that may become severe. Tell patient to notify prescriber at the first sign of an allergic reaction and to seek immediate medical attention if severe.

! **WARNING** Inform patient that drug has the potential to cause a heart attack or stroke or other forms of vasospastic disorders. Instruct patient to seek immediate emergency treatment if chest pain, shortness of breath, slurring of speech, or weakness, is experienced or if persistent, severe, or unusual signs and symptoms develop.

- Advise patient to notify all prescribers of frovatriptan therapy because serious drug interactions can occur with certain medications when taken concomitantly with frovatriptan.

furosemide

Furoscix, Lasix, Lasix Special (CAN)

Class and Category

Pharmacologic class: Loop diuretic
Therapeutic class: Antihypertensive, diuretic

Indications and Dosages

∗ *To reduce edema caused by cirrhosis, heart failure, and renal disease, including nephrotic syndrome*

ORAL SOLUTION, TABLETS

Adults. 20 to 80 mg as a single dose, increased by 20 to 40 mg every 6 to 8 hr until desired response occurs. *Maintenance:* Effective dose given once or divided and given twice daily (8 a.m. and 2 p.m.). *Maximum:* 600 mg daily.
Children. 2 mg/kg as a single dose, increased by 1 to 2 mg/kg every 6 to 8 hr until desired response occurs. *Maximum:* 6 mg/kg/dose.

I.V. INFUSION, I.V. OR I.M. INJECTION

Adults. 20 to 40 mg as a single dose, increased by 20 mg every 2 hr until desired response occurs.

I.V. OR I.M. INJECTION

Children. 1 mg/kg as a single dose, increased by 1 mg/kg every 2 hr until desired response occurs. *Maximum:* 6 mg/kg/dose (children), 1 mg/kg/day (premature infants).

∗ *To treat edema in patients with chronic heart failure or chronic kidney disease, including the nephrotic syndrome*

SUBCUTANEOUS INFUSION (FUROSCIX)

Adults. 30 mg over first hr followed by 12.5 mg/hr over subsequent 4 hr. *Maximum:* 80 mg over 5 hr.

∗ *To treat acute pulmonary edema*

I.V. INJECTION

Adults. 40 mg injected over 1 to 2 min with dosage repeated but increased to 80 mg after 1 hr, as needed.

∗ *To manage hypertension*

ORAL SOLUTION, TABLETS

Adults. *Initial:* 20 to 40 mg twice daily, adjusted until desired response occurs.

±**DOSAGE ADJUSTMENT** For elderly patients dosing started at the low end of dosing range.

Drug Administration

P.O.

- Administer once-daily doses in morning and twice-daily doses in morning and early afternoon 6 hr apart (e.g., 8 a.m. and 2 p.m.).
- Protect from light, which may cause a slight discoloration. Do not administer discolored tablets.
- Use a calibrated measuring device to obtain accurate dosing of oral solution.

I.M.

- Use only if oral or I.V. administration is not feasible.
- Do not administer drug I.M. for treatment of pulmonary edema or if solution is discolored.

I.V.

- Use only when patient is unable to take oral medication or in emergency situations. Replace with oral therapy as soon as possible.
- Do not use solution if discolored.
- For I.V. injection, inject undiluted directly or into tubing of actively running I.V. slowly over 1 to 2 min to prevent ototoxicity.
- For I.V. infusion, prepare drug for infusion with 0.9% Sodium Chloride Injection, 5% Dextrose Injection, or Lactated Ringer's solution after pH has been adjusted to above 5.5. Administer with an infusion pump at a rate not to exceed 4 mg/min in adults as an intermittent infusion. Use prepared solution within 24 hr.
- *Incompatibilities:* Other I.V. drugs except for cimetidine, epinephrine, heparin, nitroglycerin, potassium chloride, verapamil; for Y-site: other I.V. drugs except for epinephrine, fentanyl, heparin, norepinephrine, nitroglycerin, potassium chloride, vitamins B and C

SUBCUTANEOUS (FUROSCIX)

- Do not use in an emergency situation or in patients with acute pulmonary edema.
- Use only in a setting where patient can limit their activity for the duration of administration.
- On-body infusor is not for chronic use and should be replaced with oral diuretics as soon as possible.
- Ensure device is not on patient going for an MRI; it is incompatible with use in an MRI setting.
- Remove cartridge from carton only when ready to use. Inspect prefilled cartridge prior to administration. Solution should be clear to slightly yellow. Do not use if solution is cloudy or discolored.
- Load the prefilled cartridge into the on-body infusor and close the cartridge holder.
- Peel away the adhesive liner on the infusor and apply to a clean, dry area on the abdomen between the top of the beltline and the bottom of the rib cage that is not tender, bruised, red, or indurated. Keep the distance from the top of the beltline to the bottom of the ribcage at least 2 ½ inches.
- Start the injection by firmly pressing and releasing the blue start button. Do not remove the infusor until the injection is complete, which will be indicated with a solid green status light, beeping sound, and the white plunger rod filling the cartridge window.
- Rotate the site for each subcutaneous administration.
- Store cartridges at room temperature. Do not refrigerate or freeze. Protect from light. Protect on-body infusor from water.

Route	Onset	Peak	Duration
P.O.	20–60 min	1–2 hr	6–8 hr
I.V.	5 min	30 min	2 hr
I.M.	30 min	Unknown	Unknown
SubQ	Unknown	4 hr	Unknown

Half-life: 0.5–2 hr; 2 hr (SubQ)

F

Mechanism of Action

Inhibits sodium and water reabsorption in the loop of Henle and increases urine formation. As the body's plasma volume decreases, aldosterone production increases, which promotes sodium reabsorption and the loss of potassium and hydrogen ions. Furosemide also increases the excretion of ammonium, bicarbonate, calcium, magnesium, and phosphate. By reducing intracellular and extracellular fluid volume, the drug reduces blood pressure and decreases cardiac output. Over time, cardiac output returns to normal.

Contraindications

Anuria, hepatic ascites or cirrhosis (Furoscix), hypersensitivity to furosemide or its components; medical ahesives (Furoscix)

Interactions

DRUGS

ACE inhibitors, angiotensin II receptor blockers: Possibly first-dose hypotension, severe hypotension, deterioration in renal function
aminoglycosides, cisplatin, ethacrynic acid: Increased risk of ototoxicity
cephalosporins: Increased risk of cephalosporin-induced nephrotoxicity
chloral hydrate: Possibly diaphoresis, hot flashes, and hypertension
cyclosporine: Increased risk of gouty arthritis
ganglionic or peripheral adrenergic blocking agents: Increased furosemide effects
indomethacin: Possibly reduced natriuretic and antihypertensive effects of furosemide
lithium: Increased risk of lithium toxicity
methotrexate and other drugs that undergo significant renal tubular secretion: Possibly decreased therapeutic effects of furosemide
norepinephrine: Possibly decreased arterial response to norepinephrine
NSAIDs: Possibly increased BUN, serum creatinine and serum potassium levels; weight gain
phenytoin: Possibly decreased therapeutic effects of furosemide
succinylcholine: Increased action of succinylcholine
sucralfate: Possibly reduced natriuretic and antihypertensive effects of furosemide
thiazide diuretics: Possibly profound diuresis and electrolyte imbalances
thyroid hormones: Possibly overall decrease in total thyroid hormone levels with high doses (greater than 80 mg) of furosemide
tubocurarine: Antagonized skeletal muscle relaxing effect of tubocurarine

Adverse Reactions

CNS: Dizziness, drowsiness, fever, headache, lethargy, paresthesia, restlessness, vertigo, weakness
CV: **Arrhythmias**, elevated cholesterol and triglyceride levels, orthostatic hypotension, shock, tachycardia, **thromboembolism**, thrombophlebitis, vertigo
EENT: Blurred vision, deafness, dry mouth, oral irritation, ototoxicity, stomatitis, tinnitus, hearing loss (rapid I.V. injection), yellow vision
ENDO: Hyperglycemia
GI: Abdominal cramps, anorexia, constipation, diarrhea, elevated liver enzymes, gastric irritation, **hepatocellular insufficiency**, indigestion, jaundice, nausea, **pancreatitis**, vomiting
GU: **Anuria**, **azotemia**, bladder spasms, glycosuria, oliguria
HEME: **Agranulocytosis (rare)**, anemia, **aplastic anemia (rare)**, eosinophilia, **hemolytic anemia**, **leukopenia**, **thrombocytopenia**
MS: Muscle pain or spasms
SKIN: Acute generalized exanthematous pustulosis, bullous pemphigoid, **erythema multiforme**, **exfoliative dermatitis**, photosensitivity, pruritus, purpura, rash, **Stevens-Johnson syndrome**, **toxic epidermal necrolysis**, urticaria
Other: **Anaphylaxis and other hypersensitivity reactions**, dehydration, **drug reaction with eosinophilia and systemic symptoms (DRESS)**, hyperuricemia, **hypocalcemia**, hypochloremia, **hypokalemia**, **hypomagnesemia**, **hyponatremia**, hypovolemia, subcutaneous injection site reactions (bruising, edema, erythema, pain), thirst

Childbearing Considerations

PREGNANCY

- It is not known if drug causes fetal harm.
- Use with caution only if benefit to mother outweighs potential risk to fetus.
- If drug is used during pregnancy, fetal growth should be monitored.

LACTATION

- Drug is present in breast milk and as a diuretic partially inhibits lactation.
- Mothers should check with prescriber before breastfeeding.

Nursing Considerations

! **WARNING** Use furosemide (except Furoscix brand which is contraindicated in patients with ascites or cirrhosis) with extreme caution in patients with advanced hepatic cirrhosis, especially those who also have a history of electrolyte imbalance or hepatic encephalopathy; drug may lead to lethal hepatic coma.

- Obtain patient's weight before and periodically during furosemide therapy to monitor fluid loss.

! **WARNING** Be aware that patients who are allergic to sulfonamides may also be allergic to furosemide. Monitor patient closely for a hypersensitivity reaction that may include skin reactions such as DRESS. Know that although a rash is the usual initial sign of DRESS it may only initially present with a fever or swollen lymph nodes. If present, notify prescriber, expect drug to be discontinued and an alternative drug substituted, and provide supportive care, as needed and ordered.

! **WARNING** Monitor patient for hypokalemia, which may occur with brisk diuresis, inadequate oral electrolyte intake, or when cirrhosis is present. It may also occur during concomitant use of ACTH or corticosteroid therapy, intake of large amounts of licorice, or prolonged use of laxatives. Digoxin may exaggerate the metabolic effects of hypokalemia, especially cardiac effects. If patient is at high risk for hypokalemia, give potassium supplements along with furosemide, as prescribed.

! **WARNING** Monitor elderly patients closely because they are more susceptible to hypotensive and electrolyte-altering effects and thus are at greater risk for shock and thromboembolism.

- Monitor premature infants through the first year of life receiving furosemide because drug may precipitate nephrocalcinosis/nephrolithiasis. Premature infants less than 31 weeks exposed to more than 1 mg/kg/24 hr increases the risk of toxic effects, including ototoxicity. Drug may also increase the risk of persistence of patent ductus arteriosus in premature infants.
- Know that in patients with nephrotic syndrome who are hypoproteinemic, furosemide therapy may be less effective, and its ototoxicity potentiated.
- Expect patient to have periodic hearing tests during prolonged or high-dose I.V. therapy. Be aware that concomitant therapy with aminoglycoside antibiotics, ethacrynic acid, or other ototoxic drugs increases risk of ototoxicity. Be aware that patients with hypoproteinemia, such as occurs with nephrotic syndrome, may weaken effect of furosemide and increase its ototoxicity potential. Notify prescriber if patient experiences buzzing, ringing, or sense of fullness in her ears as well as hearing loss or vertigo. Drug may have to be discontinued.
- Monitor blood pressure and hepatic and renal function as well as BUN, blood glucose, and serum creatinine, electrolyte, and uric acid levels, as ordered.
- Be aware that furosemide may worsen left ventricular hypertrophy, systemic lupus erythematosus, or renal retention and adversely affect glucose tolerance and lipid metabolism. Drug also may increase risk of decreased renal function in patients at high risk for radiocontrast nephropathy after a procedure.
- Expect to discontinue furosemide at maximum dosage if oliguria persists for more than 24 hours.

PATIENT TEACHING

- Instruct patient how to take oral form of furosemide, if prescribed.
- Instruct patient prescribed the drug by subcutaneous injection using the on-body infusor how to administer and store the drug. Family or caregiver may also need instructions, if patient will not be self-administering the drug. Warn patient that device should not get wet. Also, remind patient to check device for alarms to ensure a complete dose is given.

F

- Tell patient to take drug at the same time each day to maintain therapeutic effects. Urge her to take it as prescribed, even if she feels well.
- Emphasize the importance of weight and diet control, especially limiting sodium intake.
- Urge patient (unless contraindicated) to eat more high-potassium foods and to take a potassium supplement, if prescribed, to prevent hypokalemia.

! **WARNING** Alert patient that drug may cause an allergic reaction, including skin reactions such as a fever, rash, or swollen lymph nodes. If present, tell patient to notify prescriber and, if severe, to seek immediate medical attention.

! **WARNING** Caution patient about drinking alcoholic beverages, standing for prolonged periods, and exercising in hot weather because these actions increase the hypotensive effect of furosemide.

! **WARNING** Urge patient to notify prescriber about persistent, severe nausea, vomiting, and diarrhea because they may cause dehydration.

- Advise patient to change position slowly to minimize effects of orthostatic hypotension.
- Inform diabetic patient that furosemide may increase blood glucose level and advise her to check her blood glucose level frequently.
- Tell patient with hypertension to avoid drugs that may increase blood pressure, including over-the-counter products for appetite suppression and treatment of cold symptoms.
- Advise patient to avoid direct sunlight or if in sunlight to protect skin from burning by using sunscreen and wearing long sleeved clothing and a hat.
- Instruct patient to keep follow-up appointments with prescriber to monitor progress.

G H I

gabapentin

Gralise, Neurontin

gabapentin enacarbil

Horizant

Class and Category

Pharmacologic class: 1-amino-methyl cyclohexaneacetic acid
Therapeutic class: Anticonvulsant

Indications and Dosages

* *To manage postherpetic neuralgia*

CAPSULES, ORAL SOLUTION, TABLETS (NEURONTIN)

Adults. *Initial:* 300 mg on day 1, increased to 300 mg twice daily on day 2, increased to 300 mg 3 times daily on day 3, and increased gradually thereafter according to pain response, up to 600 mg 3 times daily. *Maximum:* 1,800 mg daily in divided doses.

TABLETS (GRALISE)

Adults. *Initial:* 300 mg once daily on day 1, 600 mg once daily on day 2, 900 mg once daily on days 3 through 6, 1,200 mg once daily on days 7 through 10, 1,500 mg once daily on days 11 through 14, and 1,800 mg once daily on day 15 and thereafter. Administer all doses with evening meal.

E.R. TABLETS (HORIZANT)

Adults. *Initial:* 600 mg once daily with morning meal for 3 days, followed by 600 mg twice daily with morning and evening meal. *Maximum:* 600 mg twice daily.

± **DOSAGE ADJUSTMENT** For elderly patients, dosage may need adjustment based upon the creatinine clearance values. For patients taking Gralise who have a reduced creatinine clearance of 30 to 60 ml/min, dosage must be individualized and may have to be reduced after initial dose of 300 mg on day 1. Patients with a creatinine clearance less than 30 ml/min or who are receiving hemodialysis should not receive Gralise. For patients taking Neurontin who have a reduced creatinine clearance, including patients on hemodialysis, dosage reduced but reduction is highly individualized as follows: for creatinine clearance between 30 and 59 ml/min, total daily doses range from 400 to 1,400 mg; for creatinine clearance between 15 and 29 ml/min, total daily doses range from 200 to 700 mg; and for creatinine clearance less than 15 ml/min, total daily doses range from 100 to 300 mg. For patients taking Horizant with a creatinine clearance between 30 and 59 ml/min, dosage reduced to 300 mg once daily for 3 days, followed by 300 mg twice daily with further increase to 600 mg twice daily, as needed. For patients taking Horizant with a creatinine clearance between 15 and 29 ml/min, dosage reduced to 300 mg once daily on days 1 and 3, followed by 300 mg once daily with further increase to 300 mg twice daily, as needed. For patients taking Horizant with a creatinine clearance less than 15 ml/min and not on dialysis, dosage reduced to 300 mg once daily every other day, followed by 300 mg once daily, as needed. For patient with a creatinine clearance less than 15 ml/min and on hemodialysis, 300 mg following every dialysis with further increase to 600 mg following every dialysis, as needed.

* *As adjunct to treat partial seizures with epilepsy*

CAPSULES, ORAL SOLUTION, TABLETS (NEURONTIN)

Adults and children ages 12 yr and older. *Initial:* 300 mg 3 times daily, increased gradually according to clinical response. *Maintenance:* 300 to 600 mg 3 times daily. *Maximum:* 3,600 mg daily with maximum time between doses not to exceed 12 hr.
Children ages 3 to 11 yr: *Initial:* 10 to 15 mg/kg/day in 3 divided doses, increased, as needed, over a period of 3 days. *Maintenance for ages 5 to 11:* 25 to 35 mg/kg/day, given in 3 divided doses. *Maintenance for ages 3 to 4:* 40 mg/kg/day, given in 3 divided doses. *Maximum:* 50 mg/kg/day, given in 3 divided doses with maximum time between doses not to exceed 12 hr.

± **DOSAGE ADJUSTMENT** For elderly patients, dosage may need adjustment based upon the creatinine clearance values. For adult patients and children ages 12 and older who have a reduced creatinine clearance, including patients on hemodialysis, dosage reduced but reduction is highly individualized as follows:

for creatinine clearance between 30 and 59 ml/min, total daily doses range from 400 to 1,400 mg; for creatinine clearance between 15 and 29 ml/min, total daily doses range from 200 to 700 mg; and for creatinine clearance less than 15 ml/min, total daily doses range from 100 to 300 mg.

✶ *To treat moderate to severe primary restless leg syndrome*

E.R. TABLETS (HORIZANT)

Adults. 600 mg once daily at about 5 p.m.

± **DOSAGE ADJUSTMENT** For elderly patients, dosage may need to be adjusted based upon the creatinine clearance values. For patients with a creatinine clearance between 30 and 59 ml/min, dosage reduced to 300 mg daily and then increased to 600 mg, as needed. For patients with a creatinine clearance between 15 and 29 ml/min, dosage reduced to 300 mg daily and not increased. For patients with a creatinine clearance of less than 15 ml/min and not on hemodialysis, dosage reduced to 300 mg every other day. For patients with a creatinine clearance of less than 15 ml/min and receiving hemodialysis Horizant should not be given.

Drug Administration

P.O.

- Brands of gabapentin aren't interchangeable.
- Capsules and E.R. tablets should be swallowed whole with water and not chewed, crushed, or split/opened.
- Immediate-release tablets should be swallowed whole with water and not chewed or crushed. However, the 600- and 800-mg Neurontin immediate-release tablets are scored and may be divided. Administer the unused half-tablet as the next dose. Half-tablets not used within 28 days of dividing should be discarded.
- Oral solution should be refrigerated. Use a calibrated measuring device for dosing to ensure an accurate dose.
- Administer Gralise brand with evening meal.
- Administer Horizant once daily dose with morning meal and twice daily doses with morning and evening meals except for treatment of restless leg syndrome, which requires administration at about 5 p.m. with food.
- Give drug at least 2 hr after an antacid.
- Don't exceed 12 hr between doses on a 3-times-a-day schedule.

Route	Onset	Peak	Duration
P.O.	Unknown	2–4 hr	Unknown
P.O./E.R.	Unknown	8 hr	Unknown

Half-life: 5–7 hr

Mechanism of Action

Gabapentin is structurally like gamma-aminobutyric acid (GABA), the main inhibitory neurotransmitter in the brain. Although gabapentin's exact mechanism of action is unknown, GABA inhibits the rapid firing of neurons associated with seizures. It also may prevent exaggerated responses to painful stimuli and pain-related responses to a normally innocuous stimulus to account for its effectiveness in relieving postherpetic neuralgia and restless leg syndrome symptoms.

Contraindications

Hypersensitivity to gabapentin or its components

Interactions

DRUGS

aluminum- and magnesium-containing antacids: Decreased gabapentin bioavailability
CNS depressants: Increased CNS depression
hydrocodone: Decreased hydrocodone exposure
morphine: Increased CNS depression
opioids, such as buprenorphine, hydrocodone, morphine, oxycodone: Increased risk of decreased awareness, respiratory depression, and severe sleepiness

ACTIVITIES

alcohol: Increased risk of CNS and respiratory depression, which may become severe

Adverse Reactions

CNS: Agitation, altered proprioception, amnesia, anxiety, apathy, aphasia, asthenia, ataxia, cerebellar dysfunction, chills, **CNS tumors**, delusions, depersonalization, depression, disappearance of aura, dizziness, dream disturbances, dysesthesia, dystonia, emotional lability, euphoria, facial paralysis, fatigue, fever, hallucinations, headache,

hemiplegia, hostility, hyperkinesia, hyperreflexia, hypoesthesia, hypotonia, **intracranial hemorrhage**, lack of coordination, malaise, migraine headache, movement disorder, nervousness, occipital neuralgia, paranoia, paresis, paresthesia, positive Babinski's sign, psychosis, reflexes (absent or decreased), sedation, **seizures**, somnolence, **status epilepticus**, stupor, **subdural hematoma**, **suicidal ideation**, syncope, tremor, vertigo, **withdrawal precipitated seizure**
CV: Angina, hypertension, **hypotension**, murmur, palpitations, peripheral edema, peripheral vascular insufficiency, tachycardia, vasodilation
EENT: Abnormal vision, amblyopia, blepharospasm, cataracts, conjunctivitis, diplopia, dry eyes and mouth, earache, epistaxis, eye hemorrhage, eye pain, gingival bleeding, gingivitis, glossitis, hearing loss, hoarseness, increased salivation, inner ear infection, loss of taste, nystagmus, pharyngitis, photophobia, ptosis (bilateral or unilateral), rhinitis, sensation of fullness in ears, stomatitis, taste perversion, tinnitus, tooth discoloration, visual field defects
ENDO: Breast hypertrophy, hyperglycemia, **hypoglycemia**
GI: Abdominal pain, anorexia, constipation, diarrhea, elevated liver enzymes, fecal incontinence, flatulence, gastroenteritis, hemorrhoids, **hepatitis**, hepatomegaly, increased appetite, indigestion, jaundice, **melena**, nausea, thirst, vomiting
GU: **Acute renal failure**, anorgasmia, decreased libido, ejaculation disorders, impotence
HEME: Anemia, **coagulation defect**, **leukopenia**, **thrombocytopenia**
MS: Arthralgia, arthritis, back pain, bone fractures, dysarthria, elevated creatine kinase level, joint stiffness or swelling, muscle twitching, myalgia, positive Romberg test, **rhabdomyolysis**, tendinitis
RESP: **Apnea**, cough, dyspnea, pneumonia, pseudocroup, **respiratory depression**
SKIN: Acne, alopecia, bullous pemphigoid, cyst, diaphoresis, dry skin, eczema, **erythema multiforme**, hirsutism, pruritus, purpura, rash, seborrhea, **Stevens-Johnson syndrome**, urticaria
Other: **Anaphylaxis**, **angioedema**, dehydration, **drug reaction with eosinophilia and systemic symptoms (DRESS)**, **hyponatremia**, increased risk of viral infection, lymphadenopathy, weight gain or loss

Childbearing Considerations

PREGNANCY

- Pregnancy exposure registry: 1-888-233-2334 or http://www.aedpregnancyregistry.org/.
- It is not known if drug causes fetal harm.
- Use with caution only if benefit to mother outweighs potential risk to fetus.

LACTATION

- Drug is present in breast milk except for Horizant, which is unknown.
- Mothers should check with prescriber before breastfeeding.

Nursing Considerations

- Be aware that routine monitoring of blood gabapentin level isn't needed.
- Obtain renal function test results, as ordered before gabapentin therapy begins and then periodically throughout therapy, as ordered. Expect to adjust dosage, as needed.

! **WARNING** Monitor patient for hypersensitivity, such as anaphylaxis and angioedema or a cluster of reactions that may include fever, lymphadenopathy, and rash suggestive of DRESS. Although rare, DRESS may be life-threatening because it can involve many organs. If hypersensitivity occurs, notify prescriber immediately, expect gabapentin to be discontinued, and supportive care given, as needed and ordered.

! **WARNING** Monitor patient being treated for seizures for effectiveness of gabapentin. Alert prescriber if seizure activity occurs or increases. Know that to discontinue drug used to treat seizures or switch to a different anticonvulsant, expect to change gradually over at least 1 week, as prescribed, to avoid loss of seizure control. When gabapentin is discontinued after treating other indications, expect to reduce dosage, as ordered, over 1 week.

! **WARNING** Monitor patient who is receiving concomitant therapy with CNS depressants, including opioids, for respiratory depression and sedation, which may become life-threatening or even fatal because gabapentin enhances the effects of CNS depressants. Patients at higher risk are those who have an underlying respiratory impairment. Expect CNS depressant dosage to be reduced and if prescribed with Neurontin brand, expect Neurontin dosage to be started at a lower dose.

! **WARNING** Monitor patient closely for evidence of suicidal thinking or behavior, especially when therapy starts or dosage changes.

- Monitor patient's blood pressure as drug may cause hypotension. Also, monitor patient's blood glucose level, especially diabetic patients, because drug may cause hypoglycemia.
- Monitor patient for other persistent, serious or unusual adverse reactions as drug affects many body sytems and has the potential to cause a variety of adverse reactions.

PATIENT TEACHING

- Tell patient, family, or caregiver how to administer form of gabapentin prescribed and what to do if a dose is missed.
- Instruct patient not to take drug within 2 hours after taking an antacid.

! **WARNING** Inform patient that an allergic reaction may occur after the first dose, but it may also occur at any time. Tell patient serious skin reactions such as DRESS may occur that initially presents with a rash (DRESS may only present with a fever or swollen lymph nodes initially) as well as possible other signs and symptoms. If present, prescriber should be notified immediately, and drug discontinued. If severe, patient should seek immediate medical care.

! **WARNING** Caution patient not to stop drug abruptly, especially if taking drug for a seizure disorder.

! **WARNING** Urge patient to seek immediate medical care if breathing problems, decreased awareness, and severe sleepiness occur.

Tell the patient to inform all prescribers of over-the-counter and prescribed drugs being taken, especially drugs that affect the CNS such as depressants like opioids.

! **WARNING** Urge family or caregiver to watch patient closely for evidence of suicidal tendencies, especially when therapy starts or dosage changes, and to report concerns immediately.

- Inform patient about possible ataxia, dizziness, drowsiness, and nystagmus. Advise the patient to avoid hazardous activities until drug's CNS effects are known and resolved.
- Instruct patient how to prevent complications from adverse oral reactions (such as gingivitis) by encouraging patient to use good oral hygiene and to seek routine dental care.
- Explain that adverse effects usually are mild to moderate and decline with time. However, stress importance of notifying prescriber if adverse ractions occur that are persistent, serious, or unusual.
- Urge patient to keep follow-up appointments with prescriber to check progress.

galcanezumab-gnlm

Emgality

Class and Category

Pharmacologic class: Calcitonin gene-related peptide (CGRP) humanized monoclonal antibody
Therapeutic class: Antimigraine

Indications and Dosages

✱ *To prevent migraine headaches*

SUBCUTANEOUS INJECTION

Adults. *Loading*: 240 mg given as 2 consecutive injections of 120 mg each, followed by 120 mg monthly.

✱ *To treat episodic cluster headache*

SUBCUTANEOUS INJECTION

Adults. 300 mg (administered as 3 consecutive injections of 100 mg each) at the onset of the cluster period, and then monthly until the end of the cluster period.

Drug Administration

SUBCUTANEOUS

- Use the single-dose prefilled pen or single-dose prefilled syringe.
- Protect drug from direct sunlight.
- Prior to injection, remove from refrigerator and allow drug to sit at room temperature for 30 min. Do not warm drug by using a heat source such as hot water or a microwave. Also, do not shake the pen or syringe.
- Do not use if solution looks cloudy or has visible particles.
- Inject drug into patient's abdomen, back of the upper arm, buttocks, or thigh.
- Do not inject into areas where the skin is bruised, hard, red, or tender.
- Store pen or syringe in refrigerator.

Route	Onset	Peak	Duration
SubQ	Unknown	5 days	Unknown

Half-life: 27 days

Mechanism of Action

Binds to calcitonin gene-related peptide ligand to block its binding to the receptor as a means of pain relief.

Contraindications

Hypersensitivity to galcanezumab-gnlm or its components

Interactions

DRUGS

None reported by manufacturer.

Adverse Reactions

RESP: Dyspnea
SKIN: Rash, urticaria
Other: **Anaphylaxis**, **angioedema**, antibody formation to galcanezumab-gnlm, injection-site reactions (erythema, pain, pruritus)

Childbearing Considerations

PREGNANCY

- Pregnancy exposure registry: 1-833-464-4724 or https://migrainepregnancyregistry.com.
- It is not known if drug causes fetal harm.
- Use with caution only if benefit to mother outweighs potential risk to fetus.
- Know that women with migraines may be at increased risk of preeclampsia during pregnancy.

LACTATION

- It is not known if drug is present in breast milk.
- Mothers should check with prescriber before breastfeeding.

Nursing Considerations

! **WARNING** Monitor patient for hypersensitivity reactions, which could become life-threatening such as anaphylaxis or angioedema. If present, notify prescriber, expect drug to be discontinued, and initiate supportive therapy, as needed and ordered. Know that a hypersensitivity reaction may occur days after administration and may be prolonged.

PATIENT TEACHING

- Instruct patient on how to administer galcanezumab-gnlm as a subcutaneous injection and what to do if a dose is missed.

! **WARNING** Alert patient that drug may cause an allergic reaction. If present, tell patient to notify prescriber, stop taking drug, and, if severe, to seek immediate medical attention.

- Instruct patient to inform prescriber if drug becomes less effective over time.

ganciclovir sodium

Class and Category

Pharmacologic class: Nucleoside analogue
Therapeutic class: Antiviral

Indications and Dosages

∗ *To treat cytomegalovirus (CMV) retinitis in immunocompromised patients, including patients with acquired immunodeficiency syndrome (AIDS)*

I.V. INFUSION

Adults with normal renal function. *Induction:* 5 mg/kg infused over 1 hr every 12 hr for 14 to 21 days. *Maintenance:* 5 mg/kg once daily for 7 days per wk. Alternatively, 6 mg/kg once daily for 5 days every wk.

∗ *To prevent CMV disease in transplant recipients at risk for CMV disease*

I.V. INFUSION

Adults with normal renal function. *Induction:* 5 mg/kg infused over 1 hr every 12 hr for 7 to 14 days. *Maintenance:*

5 mg/kg once daily for 7 days per wk for 100 to 120 days post-transplantation. Alternatively, 6 mg/kg once daily for 5 days every wk for 100 to 120 days post-transplantation.

±**DOSAGE ADJUSTMENT** For patients with a creatinine clearance between 50 and 69 ml/min, dosage for induction and maintenance reduced by 50%. For patients with a creatinine clearance between 25 and 49 ml/min, dosage for induction reduced by half and dosage interval increased to every 24 hours while maintenance dosage reduced to 1.25 mg/kg every 24 hours. For patients with a creatinine clearance between 10 and 24 ml/min, induction dosage reduced to 1.25 mg/kg and dosage interval increased to every 24 hours while maintenance dosage reduced to 0.625 mg/kg every 24 hours. For patients with a creatinine clearance of less than 10 ml/min, induction dosage reduced to 1.25 mg/kg with dosage interval increased to only 3 times per week following hemodialysis while maintenance dosage decreased to 0.625 mg/kg with dosage interval increased to only 3 times per week following hemodialysis.

Drug Administration

I.V.

- Ensure patient is adequately hydrated before administering drug.
- Wear disposable gloves during reconstitution and dilution and when wiping the outer surface of vial and table after reconstitution. Avoid direct contact of the skin or mucous membranes with drug. If contact occurs, wash thoroughly with soap and water, rinse eyes thoroughly with plain water. Guidelines issued for antineoplastic drugs should be considered in the handling and disposal of drug because it shares some of the properties of antitumor agents.
- Reconstitute by injecting 10 ml of Sterile Water for Injection into the 500 mg vial to obtain a concentration of 50 mg/ml. Do not use Bacteriostatic Water for Injection containing parabens as it is incompatible with the drug. Gently swirl until a clear solution is obtained. Reconstituted solution is stable at room temperature for 12 hr.
- Using patient's weight determine how much reconstituted solution should be used. Add to 50 to 250 ml (usually 100 ml) of 0.9% Sodium Chloride Injection, 5% Dextrose, Lactated Ringer's Injection, or Ringer's Injection.
- Diluted infusion solution should be refrigerated if not used immediately. Use within 24 hr.
- Administer as an intravenous infusion slowly over 1 hr, using an infusion pump and preferably via a plastic cannula.
- Do not administer drug by rapid or bolus injection, which may increase toxicity; do not administer drug intramuscularly or subcutaneously because it may cause severe tissue irritation.
- Do not exceed the recommended dosage and infusion rate.
- *Incompatibilities:* Bacteriostatic Water for Injection containing parabens

Route	Onset	Peak	Duration
I.V.	Unknown	Unknown	Unknown

Half-life: 3.5 hr

Mechanism of Action

Initially, drug is phosphorylated and then slowly metabolized intracellularly into virus-infected cells. There it inhibits the viral DNA polymerase pUL54 to prevent replication of human CMV.

Contraindications

Hypersensitivity to ganciclovir, valganciclovir, or their components

Interactions

DRUGS

amphotericin B, cyclosporine: Increased risk of renal dysfunction
dapsone, doxorubicin, flucytosine, hydroxyurea, pentamidine, tacrolimus, trimethoprim/sulfamethoxazole, vinblastine, vincristine, zidovudine: Increased risk of myelosuppression or nephrotoxicity
didanosine: Increased risk of didanosine toxicity
imipenem-cilastatin: Increased risk of generalized seizures
mycophenolate mofetil: Increased risk for hematologic and renal toxicity
probenecid: Increased serum ganciclovir concentration with increased risk of ganciclovir toxicity

Adverse Reactions

CNS: Agitation, amnesia, anxiety, aphasia, asthenia, chills, confusion, **CVA**, depression, dizziness, dream abnormality, dysesthesia, **encephalopathy**, extrapyramidal disorder, facial paralysis, fatigue, fever, hallucinations, headache, hypoesthesia, insomnia, **intracranial hypertension**, irritability, malaise, paresthesia, peripheral neuropathy, psychotic disorder, **seizures**, somnolence, thinking abnormality, third cranial nerve paralysis, tremor
CV: **Arrhythmias**, **cardiac arrest**, chest pain, **conduction disorder**, edema, elevated triglycerides, hypertension, **hypotension**, peripheral ischemia, phlebitis, **torsades de pointes**, vasculitis, vasodilation, **ventricular tachycardia**
EENT: Cataracts, conjunctivitis, deafness, dry eyes or mouth, ear pain, loss of smell, macular edema, mouth ulceration, retinal detachment, taste disturbance, tinnitus, visual impairment, vitreous disorders
ENDO: Inappropriate antidiuretic hormone secretion
GI: Abdominal distention or pain, anorexia, cholelithiasis, cholestasis, constipation, diarrhea, dyspepsia, dysphagia, elevated liver enzymes, eructation, flatulence, **GI perforation**, **hepatic dysfunction or failure**, **hepatitis**, intestinal ulcer, nausea, **pancreatitis**, vomiting
GU: Abnormal kidney function, decreased creatinine clearance, elevated serum creatinine, hematuria, **hemolytic uremic syndrome**, infertility, **kidney failure**, renal tubular disorder, testicular hypotrophy, urinary frequency
HEME: **Agranulocytosis**; **anemia, including hemolytic**, **bone marrow failure**, **decreased platelet count**; **granulocytopenia**; **leukopenia**; **pancytopenia**; **thrombocytopenia**
MS: Arthralgia, arthritis, back pain, leg cramps, muscle spasms, myalgia, myasthenia, myelopathy, **rhabdomyolysis**
RESP: **Bronchospasm**, cough, dyspnea, **pulmonary fibrosis**
SKIN: Alopecia, dermatitis, diaphoresis, dry skin, **exfoliative dermatitis**, pruritus, rash, **Stevens-Johnson syndrome**, urticaria
Other: **Acidosis**, **anaphylaxis**, elevated blood alkaline phosphatase, generalized pain, **hypercalcemia**, **hyponatremia**, infection including *Candida*, injection-site inflammation, **multiple organ failure**, **sepsis**, weight loss

Childbearing Considerations

PREGNANCY

- Drug may cause fetal harm such as mutagenic and teratogenic effects based on animal studies.
- A negative pregnancy test in females of childbearing age should be obtained before starting drug therapy.
- Use with extreme caution only if benefit to mother outweighs potential risk to fetus.

LACTATION

- It is not known if drug is present in breast milk.
- Breastfeeding is not recommended.

REPRODUCTION

- Females of childbearing age should use effective contraception during drug therapy and for at least 30 days following the last dose of the drug.
- Men should use condoms during drug therapy and for at least 90 days after the last dose of the drug when engaging in sexual activity.
- Drug may cause permanent or temporary female and male infertility.

Nursing Considerations

! WARNING Be aware that ganciclovir therapy is not recommended if the absolute neutrophil count is less than 500 cells/µl, hemoglobin is less than 8 g/dl, or the platelet count is less than 25,000 cells/µl.

! WARNING Expect females of childbearing age to have a pregnancy test done prior to receiving ganciclovir because drug can cause fetal harm.

! WARNING Administer ganciclovir with extreme caution in patients with preexisting cytopenias and in patients receiving myelosuppressive drugs or irradiation because ganciclovir can cause hematologic toxicities.

! WARNING Obtain patient's CBC with differential and platelet counts before therapy begins and then frequently throughout therapy, as ordered, especially in patients in whom ganciclovir therapy or other nucleoside analogues have previously caused cytopenias, or in whom absolute neutrophil counts are less than 1,000 cells/µl at the beginning of treatment. Granulocytopenia usually occurs during the first or second week of treatment but may occur at any time during treatment. Notify prescriber of hematologic abnormalities and expect possibility that drug will be discontinued. Cell counts usually begin to recover within 3 to 7 days after drug is discontinued. Colony-stimulating factors may be helpful in increasing neutrophil and WBC counts.

- Obtain a serum creatinine or creatinine clearance prior to starting ganciclovir therapy, as ordered, to establish a baseline for renal function, and then frequently throughout therapy to determine need for and degree of dosage adjustment. Ensure that patient has adequate hydration while receiving ganciclovir to reduce adverse effects on renal function. Assess patient for signs and symptoms of renal dysfunction, especially elderly patients and those patients receiving concurrent therapy with nephrotoxic drugs, such as amphotericin B or cyclosporine.

! WARNING Monitor patient for a hypersensitivity or skin reaction that could become life-threatening. If present, notify prescriber, expect drug to be discontinued, and provide supportive care, as needed and ordered. Also monitor patient for other persistent, serious, or unusual adverse reactions because ganciclovir can cause many types of adverse reactions, some of which could be life-threatening.

! WARNING Be aware that ganciclovir has the potential to cause cancer.

- Expect patient to have frequent ophthalmologic examinations during treatment to monitor ganciclovir effectiveness.

PATIENT TEACHING

- Tell patient that ganciclovir will be given intravenously.
- Remind patient with CMV retinitis that ganciclovir is not a cure and that it is important to comply with ophthalmologic follow-up examinations.
- Stress importance of maintaining adequate hydration throughout ganciclovir therapy because of potential adverse effect of drug on the kidneys.

! WARNING Alert patient that drug may cause an allergic reaction. If present, tell patient to notify prescriber and, if severe, to seek immediate medical attention.

! WARNING Instruct patient to notify prescriber of other persistent, severe, or unusual adverse effects because drug can cause many adverse reactions, some of which could be serious or even life-threatening.

! WARNING Instruct females of childbearing age to use effective contraception during treatment and for at least 30 days following treatment because drug may cause fetal toxicity. Instruct men to practice barrier contraception during and for at least 90 days following treatment.

- Inform patient that drug may cause temporary or permanent infertility. Encourage patient to discuss this with prescriber, if concerned.
- Inform patient that frequent blood tests will have to be done throughout ganciclovir therapy because drug may cause blood toxicities. Stress importance of not missing any appointments. In addition, review signs and symptoms of anemia and infections and instruct patient to notify prescriber, if present.
- Tell patient to inform all prescribers of ganciclovir therapy because drug can interact with other drugs.
- Advise patient not to perform any hazardous activities, such as driving, if cognitive impairment is present until CNS effects are known and resolved.
- Advise mothers not to breastfeed infant while taking ganciclovir.

gemfibrozil

Lopid

Class and Category

Pharmacologic class: Fibric acid derivative
Therapeutic class: Antilipemic

Indications and Dosages

∗ *As adjunct (with diet) to treat hyperlipidemia types IV and V in patients at high risk for pancreatitis; to reduce risk of coronary artery disease (CAD) in patients with type IIb hyperlipidemia who do not have a history of or symptoms of existing CAD, who have had an inadequate response to lifestyle changes or other pharmacologic agents, and have the following triad of lipid abnormalities: low-HDL-cholesterol levels, elevated LDL-cholesterol levels, and elevated triglycerides*

TABLETS

Adults. 600 mg twice daily before morning and evening meals.

Drug Administration

P.O.

- Administer 30 min before morning and evening meals.
- Protect from light and humidity.

Route	Onset	Peak	Duration
P.O.	2–5 days	1–2 hr	Unknown

Half-life: 5–9 hr

Mechanism of Action

May decrease hepatic triglyceride production by decreasing hepatic extraction of free fatty acids, inhibiting peripheral lipolysis, and reducing VLDL synthesis. Gemfibrozil also may inhibit synthesis and increase clearance of apolipoprotein B, a carrier molecule for VLDL. In addition, it may accelerate turnover and removal of total cholesterol from the liver while increasing cholesterol excretion in the feces. As a result, total cholesterol, triglyceride, and VLDL levels decrease; the HDL level increases; and the LDL level is unaffected.

Contraindications

Concurrent therapy with dasabuvir, repaglinide, selexipag, or simvastatin; gallbladder disease; hepatic or severe renal dysfunction, including primary biliary cirrhosis; hypersensitivity to gemfibrozil or its components

Interactions

DRUGS

colchicine: Increased toxicity of either drug; risk of myopathy, including rhabdomyolysis

CYP2 c8 substrates, such as dabrafenib, loperamide, montelukast, paclitaxel, pioglitazone, rosiglitazone, selexipag: Increased plasma concentration of these drugs

dasabuvir: Increased dasabuvir plasma concentration increasing risk of QT prolongation

enzalutamide: Increased enzalutamide plasma concentration increasing risk of seizures

HMG-CoA reductase inhibitors: Increased risk of acute renal failure and rhabdomyolysis

OATP1B1 substrates, such as atrasentan, atorvastatin, bosentan, ezetimibe, fluvastatin, glyburide, olmesartan, pitavastatin, pravastatin, rifampin, rosuvastatin, SN-38 (active metabolite of irinotecan), simvastatin, valsartan: Increased plasma concentrations of these drugs

oral anticoagulants, such as warfarin: Increased anticoagulation

repaglinide: Increased serum repaglinide level and risk of severe hypoglycemia

resin-granule drugs, such as colestipol: Decreased blood gemfibrozil levels

Adverse Reactions

CNS: Chills, fatigue, headache, hypoesthesia, paresthesia, **seizures**, somnolence, syncope, vertigo

CV: Vasculitis

EENT: Blurred vision, cataracts, hoarseness, retinal edema, taste perversion

GI: Abdominal or epigastric pain, cholelithiasis, colitis, diarrhea, flatulence, heartburn, **hepatoma**, jaundice, nausea, **pancreatitis**, vomiting

GU: Decreased male fertility, dysuria, impotence

HEME: Anemia, **bone marrow hypoplasia**, eosinophilia, **leukopenia**, **thrombocytopenia**

MS: Arthralgia, back pain, myalgia, myasthenia, myopathy, myositis, **rhabdomyolysis**, synovitis

RESP: Cough

SKIN: Eczema, pruritus, rash

Other: **Anaphylaxis**, **angioedema**, increased risk of bacterial and viral infections, lupus-like symptoms, weight loss

Childbearing Considerations

PREGNANCY

- It is not known if drug causes fetal harm.
- Use with caution only if benefit to mother outweighs potential risk to fetus.

LACTATION

- It is not known if drug is present in breast milk.
- A decision should be made to discontinue breastfeeding or the drug to avoid potential serious adverse reactions in the breastfed infant.

Nursing Considerations

! **WARNING** Monitor patient for a hypersensitivity reaction, which could become life-threatening such as anaphylaxis or angioedema. If present, notify prescriber, expect drug to be discontinued, and supportive care given, as needed and ordered.

- Monitor serum triglyceride and cholesterol levels, as ordered. Know that if serum cholesterol and triglyceride levels don't improve within 3 months, expect patient to be switched to a different drug, as prescribed.
- Review CBC and liver enzymes during therapy periodically, as ordered. Monitor patient for signs and symptoms of hematologic or liver dysfunction.
- Monitor patient's PT, as ordered, if patient is also receiving warfarin therapy because gemfibrozil therapy may cause a drug interaction with warfarin. Warfarin dosage may have to be decreased to maintain PT at a level needed to prevent adverse bleeding effects.

PATIENT TEACHING

- Instruct patient how to administer gemfibrozil and what to do if a dose is missed.
- Emphasize importance of alcohol avoidance, a low-fat diet, regular exercise, and smoking cessation, as appropriate.

! **WARNING** Alert patient that gemfibrozil may cause an allergic reaction. If present, tell patient to notify prescriber and, if severe, to seek immediate medical care.

! **WARNING** If patient also takes an oral anticoagulant, urge the patient to report unusual bleeding or bruising; anticoagulant dosage may have to be reduced.

- Instruct patient to notify prescriber if he experiences other adverse reactions such as chills; cough; fever; hoarseness; lower back, side, or muscle pain; painful or difficult urination; severe abdominal pain with nausea and vomiting; tiredness; or weakness.
- Caution patient to avoid hazardous activities until drug's CNS effects are known and resolved.
- Advise patient to keep scheduled appointments with prescriber to check progress.

gentamicin sulfate

Class and Category

Pharmacologic class: Aminoglycoside
Therapeutic class: Antibiotic

Indications and Dosages

* *To treat serious bacterial infections caused by* Citrobacter *species,* Escherichia coli, Klebsiella-Enterobacter-Serratia *species,* Proteus *species (indole negative and indole positive),* Pseudomonas aeruginosa, *or* Staphylococcus *species*

I.M. INJECTION, I.V. INFUSION

Adults and adolescents. 3 mg/kg/day in 3 divided doses every 8 hr for 7 to 10 days. *For life-threatening infections:* Up to 5 mg/kg/day in 3 or 4 divided doses for 7 to 10 days or longer with dosage reduced as soon as possible to 3 mg/kg/day.
Children. 2 to 2.5 mg/kg every 8 hr for 7 to 10 days.
Infants and neonates over age 1 wk. 2.5 mg/kg every 8 hr for 7 to 10 days.
Premature or full-term neonates up to 1 wk of age. 2.5 mg/kg every 12 hr for 7 to 10 days.

± **DOSAGE ADJUSTMENT** For adults with impaired renal function, highly individualized and dependent on degree of renal function and drug level. For adult patients receiving dialysis, 1 to 1.7 mg/kg at the end of each dialysis period has been suggested. For children receiving dialysis, a dose of 2 mg/kg at the end of each dialysis period has been suggested.

Drug Administration

I.V.

- May be the preferred route for patients with bacterial septicemia or those in shock. It may also be the preferred route for patients with congestive heart failure, hematologic disorders, severe burns, or those with reduced muscle mass.

- Dilute each dose with 50 to 200 ml of 0.9% Sodium Chloride Injection or 5% Dextrose in Water. In children, infants, and neonates, the volume of diluent should be less.
- Administer as an intermittent infusion slowly over 30 min to 2 hr.
- Flush I.V. line before and after I.V. infusion with either 0.9% Sodium Chloride Injection or 5% Dextrose in Water.
- Expect to adjust dosage based on peak and trough blood drug levels.
- *Incompatibilities:* Other drugs

I.M.

- Inject deeply into a large muscle.
- Rotate sites.

Route	Onset	Peak	Duration
I.V.	Immediate	30–60 min	Unknown
I.M.	Unknown	30–90 min	Unknown

Half-life: 2–3 hr

Mechanism of Action

Binds to negatively charged sites on the outer cell membrane of bacteria, thereby disrupting the membrane's integrity. Gentamicin also binds to bacterial ribosomal subunits and inhibits protein synthesis. Both actions lead to cell death.

Contraindications

Hypersensitivity to gentamicin, other aminoglycosides, or their components

Interactions

DRUGS

loop diuretics (ethacrynic acid, furosemide), other aminoglycosides (kanamycin, neomycin, streptomycin): Increased risk of nephrotoxicity and ototoxicity
neuromuscular blockers: Prolonged respiratory depression, increased neuromuscular blockade
other nephrotoxic drugs: Increased risk of nephrotoxicity
penicillins: Inactivation of gentamicin by certain penicillins, increased risk of nephrotoxicity

Adverse Reactions

CNS: Acute organic mental syndrome, confusion, depression, fever, headache, increased protein in cerebrospinal fluid, lethargy, myasthenia gravis-like syndrome, **neurotoxicity**, peripheral neuropathy or **encephalopathy**, **pseudotumor cerebri**, **seizures**
CV: Hypertension, **hypotension**, palpitations
EENT: Blurred vision, increased salivation, **laryngeal edema**, ototoxicity, stomatitis, vision changes
GI: Anorexia, nausea, splenomegaly, transient hepatomegaly, vomiting
GU: **Nephrotoxicity**
HEME: Anemia, eosinophilia, **granulocytopenia**, increased or decreased reticulocyte count, **leukopenia**, **thrombocytopenia**
MS: Arthralgia, leg cramps
RESP: **Pulmonary fibrosis**, **respiratory depression**
SKIN: Alopecia, generalized burning sensation, pruritus, purpura, rash, urticaria
Other: **Anaphylaxis**, injection-site pain, superinfection, weight loss

Childbearing Considerations

PREGNANCY

- Aminoglycosides, such as gentamicin, may cause fetal harm as they cross the placental barrier and may cause irreversible deafness and severe muscle weakness in the neonate.
- Drug is usually not recommended during pregnancy except in life-threatening situations.

LACTATION

- Drug is present in breast milk.
- A decision should be made to discontinue breastfeeding or the drug to avoid potential serious adverse reactions in the breastfed infant.

Nursing Considerations

- Expect to obtain a body fluid or tissue specimen for culture and sensitivity testing, as ordered, before gentamicin therapy begins, or check test results, if available.

! **WARNING** Know that drug should not be given to a pregnant patient because it can cause irreversible deafness and severe muscle weakness in the neonate.

! **WARNING** Be aware that premature infants, neonates, and elderly patients have an increased risk of nephrotoxicity.

! **WARNING** Monitor patient for a hypersensitivity reaction, which may become life-threatening such as anaphylaxis. If present, notify prescriber, expect to discontinue drug, and provide supportive care, as needed and ordered.

- Know that any report of dizziness, hearing loss, or ringing in the ears should be taken very seriously. Withhold drug and notify prescriber of these problems.
- Assess patient for evidence of other infections because gentamicin may cause overgrowth of nonsusceptible organisms.

PATIENT TEACHING

- Inform patient that gentamicin is given intravenously or as an I.M. injection.
- Emphasize importance of completing full course of gentamicin therapy.

! **WARNING** Inform females of childbearing age to notify prescriber if pregnancy occurs because drug will need to be discontinued.

! **WARNING** Review signs and symptoms of an allergic reaction and emphasize importance of reporting an allergic reaction to the prescriber and seeking immediate emergency care, if severe.

- Instruct patient to immediately report adverse reactions, such as hearing loss, to avoid permanent effects.
- Inform mothers breastfeeding should not be undertaken during gentamicin therapy; otherwise the drug will need to be discontinued.

gepirone

Exxua

Class and Category

Pharmacologic class: Azapirone
Therapeutic class: Antidepressant

Indications and Dosages

∗ *To treat major depressive disorder*

E.R. TABLETS

Adults. *Initial*: 18.2 mg once daily increased to 36.3 mg once daily on day 4, if tolerated, and further increased to 54.5 mg once daily after day 7 and to 72.6 once daily after an additional week, as needed and tolerated. *Maximum:* 72.6 mg once daily.

± **DOSAGE ADJUSTMENT** For elderly patients, patients with a creatinine clearance level less than 50 ml/min, and patients with moderate hepatic impairment, initial dose started at 18.2 mg once daily but maximum dose kept at 36.3 mg once daily after day 7. For patients taking concomitant moderate CYP3A4 inhibitors, dosage reduced by 50%.

Drug Administration

P.O.

- Administer with food at about the same time each day.
- Tablets should be swallowed whole and not chewed, crushed, or split.

Route	Onset	Peak	Duration
P.O.	Unknown	6 hr	Unknown

Half-life: 5 hr

Mechanism of Action

May act to modulate serotonergic activity in the central nervous system by selective agonist activity at serotonin 5-hydroxytrptamine$_{1A}$ receptors in the brain, which elevates mood.

Contraindications

Concomitant therapy with strong CYP34A inhibitors, linezolid, or I.V. methylene blue therapy; congenital long QT syndrome; hypersensitivity to gepirone or its components; prolonged QTc interval greater than 450 msec at baseline; severe hepatic impairment; use of a MAOI within 14 days

Interactions

DRUGS

CYP3A4 inducers (strong): Decreased gepirone exposure with possible decreased effectiveness

CYP3A4 inhibitors: Increased gepirone exposure with possible increased adverse reactions

drugs that prolong QTc interval: Additive QTc prolongation effects increasing risk of cardiac arrhythmias

MAOIs including linezolid and IV methylene blue, other serotonergic drugs: Increased risk of serotonin syndrome

Adverse Reactions

CNS: Abnormal feelings or thinking, activation of hypomania or mania, agitation, confusion, dizziness, fatigue, feeling jittery, headache, hypoesthesia, increased energy, insomnia, lethargy, paresthesia, poor sleep quality, **suicidal ideation**
CV: Increased heart rate, palpitations, peripheral edema, **QT prolongation**
EENT: Dry mouth, nasal congestion, nasopharyngitis
ENDO: Breast tenderness
GI: Abdominal pain, constipation, diarrhea, dyspepsia, increased appetite, nausea, vomiting
RESP: Dyspnea, upper respiratory infection
SKIN: Hyperhidrosis, pruritus, rash, urticaria
Other: Weight gain

Childbearing Considerations

PREGNANCY

- Pregnancy exposure registry: 1-866-961-2388 or https://womensmentalhealth.org/research/pregnancyregistry/antidepressants/.
- Drug may cause fetal harm according to animal studies especially if exposed in the third trimester. Complications possible immediately upon birth include apnea, constant crying, cyanosis, feeding difficulties, hyperreflexia, hypertonia, hypotonia, hypoglycemia, irritability, jitteriness, seizures, temperature instability, tremors, and vomiting. Exposure to drug late in pregnancy increases risk for persistent pulmonary hypertension with potential for substantial neonatal morbidity and mortality.
- Drug is not recommended during pregnancy.

LACTATION

- It is not known if drug is present in breast milk.
- Mother should check with prescriber before breastfeeding.
- If breastfeeding occurs, infant should be monitored for decreased feeding, excessive sleepiness, irritability, restlessness, and weight loss.

Nursing Considerations

- Expect to correct any electrolyte abnormalities, as ordered, before gepirone is started. Also, expect to continue monitoring electrolytes during dose titration and periodically during therapy with gepirone in patients with electrolyte abnormalities or who have a history of hypokalemia or hypomagnesemia, and in patients who are receiving diuretics or glucocorticoids.

! WARNING Obtain an electrocardiogram (ECG) before gepirone is started, during dosage titration, and periodically during gepirone therapy. Know that drug should not be started if the QTc is greater than 450 msec at baseline. Expect to monitor ECGs more frequently in patients with a significant risk of developing torsade de pointes, patients who develop QTc of 450 msec or greater during gepirone therapy, and in patients who are taking drugs known to prolong the QT interval. Know that during titration, dosage should not be increased if patient develops a QTcF greater than 450 msec.

- Screen patient for a family or personal history of bipolar disorder, hypomania, or mania before gepirone therapy is begun. This is because gepirone therapy can precipitate a manic, mixed, or hypomanic episode. Risk is higher in patients with a family history of bipolar disorder, depression, or suicide.

! WARNING Monitor patient for suicidal thinking and behavior, especially in young adults and when therapy is begun, and dosage changes are made because gepirone therapy may cause suicidal ideation.

! WARNING Know that many drugs may interact with gepirone to cause serotonin syndrome. Monitor patient closely for signs and symptoms, such as agitation, diaphoresis, diarrhea, fever, hallucinations, labile blood pressure, muscle twitching or stiffness, nausea, shakiness, shivering, tachycardia, trouble with coordination, or vomiting. Notify prescriber at once because serotonin syndrome may be life-threatening. Be prepared to discontinue drug, if possible and ordered, and provide supportive care.

PATIENT TEACHING

- Instruct patient how to administer gepirone.

! **WARNING** Urge family or caregiver to watch patient closely for suicidal tendencies, especially when therapy starts or dosage changes.

! **WARNING** Tell patient and family or caregiver to notify prescriber immediately if persistent, serious, or unusual adverse effects occur such as fainting, heart palpations, or loss of consciousness and to seek emergency care immediately.

! **WARNING** Advise females of childbearing age to notify prescriber if pregnancy occurs. Inform pregnant patients that if drug is taken late in pregnancy, neonatal complications requiring prolonged hospitalization may occur.

- Alert patient and family that drug may cause hypomania or mania. If significant behavior changes occur, have family notify prescriber.
- Advise mothers who choose to breastfeed during drug therapy to monitor their infant for agitation, excess sedation, poor feeding and weight gain, and restlessness.

glimepiride

Amaryl

Class and Category

Pharmacologic class: Sulfonylurea
Therapeutic class: Antidiabetic

Indications and Dosages

∗ *As adjunct to control blood glucose level in type 2 diabetes mellitus*

TABLETS

Adults. *Initial:* 1 or 2 mg once daily with first meal of the day. Dosage increased by 1 to 2 mg every 1 to 2 wk, as needed for blood glucose control. *Maximum:* 8 mg once daily with first meal of the day.

± **DOSAGE ADJUSTMENT** For the elderly, patients at risk for hypoglycemia, and patients with renal impairment, initial dosage reduced to or kept at 1 mg once daily and dosage titrated more slowly.

Drug Administration

P.O.

- Administer with first meal of the day.

Route	Onset	Peak	Duration
P.O.	1 hr	2–3 hr	>24 hr

Half-life: 5–9 hr

Mechanism of Action

Stimulates insulin release from beta cells in pancreas. Glimepiride also increases peripheral tissue sensitivity to insulin, either by enhancing insulin binding to cellular receptors or by increasing the number of insulin receptors.

Contraindications

Hypersensitivity to glimepiride, sulfonamide derivatives, or their components

Interactions

DRUGS

ACE inhibitors, anabolic steroids, androgens, azole antifungals, bromocriptine, chloramphenicol, clarithromycin, clonidine, cyclophosphamide, disopyramide, fibric acid derivatives, fluconazole, fluoxetine, guanethidine, H_2-receptor antagonists, insulin, magnesium salts, MAO inhibitors, methyldopa, NSAIDs, octreotide, oral anticoagulants, other oral hypoglycemic agents, oxyphenbutazone, pentoxifylline, phenylbutazone, phenyramidol, pramlintide, probenecid, propoxyphene, quinidine, quinolones, reserpine, salicylates, somatostatin analogs, sulfonamides, tetracyclines, theophylline, tricyclic antidepressants, urinary acidifiers: Increased risk of hypoglycemia

asparaginase, barbiturates, calcium channel blockers, cholestyramine, clonidine, clozapine, colesevelam, corticosteroids, danazol, diazoxide, estrogens, glucagon, hydantoins, isoniazid, laxatives, lithium, morphine, nicotinic acid, olanzapine, oral contraceptives, phenothiazines, phenytoin, protease inhibitors, reserpine, rifabutin, rifampin, somatropin, sympathomimetics, thiazide and other diuretics, thyroid hormones, urinary alkalinizers: Increased risk of hyperglycemia

beta-blockers, clonidine, reserpine: Possibly hyperglycemia or masking of hypoglycemia signs

miconazole (oral): Increased risk of severe hypoglycemia
sympatholytic drugs, such as beta-blockers, clonidine, guanethidine, reserpine: Reduced or absent hypoglycemic signs and symptoms

ACTIVITIES

alcohol use: Altered blood glucose control (usually hypoglycemia)

Adverse Reactions

CNS: Abnormal gait, anxiety, asthenia, chills, depression, dizziness, fatigue, headache, hypertonia, hypoesthesia, insomnia, malaise, migraine headache, nervousness, paresthesia, somnolence, syncope, tremor, vertigo
CV: **Arrhythmias**, edema, hypertension, vasculitis
EENT: Blurred vision, conjunctivitis, eye pain, pharyngitis, retinal hemorrhage, rhinitis, taste perversion, tinnitus
ENDO: **Hypoglycemia**, increased release of antidiuretic hormone secretion (SIADH)
GI: Anorexia, cholestasis, constipation, diarrhea, elevated liver enzymes, epigastric discomfort or fullness, flatulence, heartburn, hepatic porphyria, **hepatotoxicity**, hunger, jaundice, **liver failure**, nausea, proctocolitis, trace blood in stool, vomiting
GU: Darkened urine, decreased libido, dysuria, polyuria
HEME: **Agranulocytosis**, **aplastic anemia**, eosinophilia, **hemolytic anemia**, **leukopenia**, **pancytopenia**, **thrombocytopenia**, **thrombocytopenic purpura**
MS: Arthralgia, leg cramps, myalgia
RESP: Dyspnea
SKIN: Allergic skin reactions, alopecia, diaphoresis, eczema, **erythema multiforme**, **exfoliative dermatitis**, flushing, lichenoid reactions, maculopapular or morbilliform rash, photosensitivity, pruritus, **Stevens-Johnson syndrome**, urticaria
Other: **Anaphylaxis**, **angioedema**, disulfiram-like reaction, **hyponatremia**

Childbearing Considerations

PREGNANCY

- It is not known if drug can cause fetal harm. However, it may cause neonatal hypoglycemia.
- Drug is not recommended during pregnancy because abnormal blood glucose levels during pregnancy are associated with a higher incidence of congenital abnormalities, making insulin the preferred drug of choice during pregnancy.

LABOR AND DELIVERY

- At birth, neonate may experience birth injury, respiratory distress, and prolonged severe hypoglycemia lasting 4 to 10 days if mother receives drug at time of delivery.
- If drug is used during pregnancy, expect it to be discontinued at least 2 wk before expected delivery.

LACTATION

- It is not known if drug is present in breast milk.
- Mothers should check with prescriber before breastfeeding.
- If breastfeeding occurs, infant should be monitored for signs and symptoms of hypoglycemia.

Nursing Considerations

! **WARNING** Use cautiously in patients with glucose 6-phosphate dehydrogenase (G6PD) deficiency because glimepiride is a sulfonylurea, and sulfonylureas can cause hemolytic anemia in these patients.

- Give glimepiride at least 4 hours before administering colesevelam, if prescribed, because colesevelam decreases exposure to glimepiride.

! **WARNING** Monitor patient closely for hypersensitivity reactions that could become life-threatening such as anaphylaxis or angioedema. If present, stop drug immediately and notify prescriber. Provide supportive care, as needed and ordered.

! **WARNING** Expect a higher risk of hypoglycemia when giving glimepiride to a debilitated or malnourished patient or one with adrenal, hepatic, pituitary, or renal insufficiency. Also, be aware that hypoglycemia may be more difficult to recognize in patients with autonomic neuropathy, the elderly, and patients taking beta-blockers or other sympatholytic agents. Monitor blood glucose level closely and treat, as needed, according to institutional protocol. Notify prescriber if hypoglycemia occurs frequently or is severe.

! **WARNING** Monitor patient's CBC, as ordered, because glimepiride may cause serious to life-threatening adverse reactions.

- Monitor fasting blood glucose level to determine response to glimepiride. Expect to check glycosylated hemoglobin level every 3 to 6 months to evaluate long-term blood glucose control, as ordered.
- Expect to switch patient to insulin therapy, as needed and ordered, during physical stress, such as infection, surgery, and trauma or if pregnancy occurs.

PATIENT TEACHING

- Instruct patient how to administer glimepiride.
- Urge patient not to skip doses or increase dosage without consulting prescriber.
- Advise patient to avoid alcohol during glimepiride therapy because alcohol can alter blood glucose control.
- Alert patient prescribed both glimepiride and colesevelam of the need to take glimepiride 4 hours before colesevelam.

! **WARNING** Alert patient that drug may cause an allergic reaction. If present, tell patient to stop taking drug, notify prescriber, and, if severe, to seek immediate medical care. Also, tell patient to notify prescriber of any other persistent, serious, or unusual adverse reactions.

- Teach patient how to monitor his blood glucose level.

! **WARNING** Instruct patient on signs and symptoms of hypoglycemia such as anxiety, confusion, dizziness, excessive sweating, headache, and nausea. Teach patient how to treat hypoglycemia in the event it should occur. Advise patient to notify prescriber if hypoglycemia frequently occurs or is severe. Ensure family or caregiver knows how to administer glucagon for a severe episode of hypoglycemia.

! **WARNING** Tell females of childbearing age to notify prescriber if pregnancy occurs.

- Advise patient to consult prescriber before taking any over-the-counter drug.
- Urge patient to carry identification indicating that he has diabetes.
- Instruct patient to avoid direct sunlight and to wear sunscreen.
- Have mothers who are breastfeeding while taking glimepiride monitor their infant for signs of low blood sugar. If present, ensure mother knows how to treat it, including reporting infant hypoglycemia to pediatrician. Breastfeeding or drug may have to be discontinued.

glipizide

Glucotrol XL

Class and Category

Pharmacologic class: Sulfonylurea
Therapeutic class: Antidiabetic

Indications and Dosages

∗ *As adjunct to control blood glucose level in type 2 diabetes mellitus*

E.R. TABLETS (GLUCOTROL XL)

Adults. *Initial:* 2.5 to 5 mg once daily with first main meal of the day. Dosage increased, as needed, based on patient's glucose response. *Maximum:* 20 mg daily.

TABLETS

Adults. *Initial:* 5 mg once daily 30 min before morning meal. Dosage adjusted by 2.5 to 5 mg every 2 to 3 days and given as a single dose, if dosage is 15 mg or less, or given in 2 divided doses, if dosage exceeds 15 mg daily. *Maximum:* 40 mg daily in divided doses 30 min before meals.

± **DOSAGE ADJUSTMENT** For patients over age 65, patients who are debilitated or malnourished, patients with impaired hepatic function or patients at risk for hypoglycemia, initial dosage reduced to 2.5 mg daily, as needed. For patients converting from insulin and receiving 20 units of insulin or less, insulin discontinued and 5 mg given once daily 30 min before morning meal. Dosage adjusted by 2.5 to 5 mg, as needed every 3 to 4 days. For patients converting from insulin and receiving more than 20 units of insulin daily, 5 mg once daily given initially 30 min before morning meal while insulin dosage decreased by one-half. Dosage adjusted by 2.5 to 5 mg, as needed, every 3 to 4 days. Further insulin reductions are made based on clinical response.

Drug Administration

P.O.

- Give immediate-acting tablets as a single dose if dosage is 15 mg or less; give twice daily if dosage exceeds 15 mg daily.
- Administer immediate-acting tablets 30 min before the first meal of the day if given once daily and 30 min before meals if given in divided doses.
- Administer X.L. tablets with the first main meal of the day. X.L. tablets should be swallowed whole and not chewed, crushed, or split.

Route	Onset	Peak	Duration
P.O.	30 min	1–3 hr	12–24 hr
P.O./X.L.	2–3 hr	6–12 hr	24 hr

Half-life: 2–5 hr

Mechanism of Action

Stimulates insulin release from beta cells in pancreas. Glipizide also increases peripheral tissue sensitivity to insulin, either by increasing insulin binding to cellular receptors or by increasing number of insulin receptors.

Contraindications

Hypersensitivity to glipizide, sulfonylureas, or their components; ketoacidosis; type 1 diabetes mellitus

Interactions

DRUGS

ACE inhibitors, anabolic steroids, androgens, angiotensin II receptor blocking agents, azole antifungals (selected), beta-blockers, bromocriptine, chloramphenicol, coumarins, disopyramide, fibric acid derivatives, fluconazole, fluoxetine, guanethidine, H_2-receptor antagonists, insulin and other antidiabetic drugs, magnesium salts, MAO inhibitors, methyldopa, NSAIDs, octreotide, oral anticoagulants, oxyphenbutazone, pentoxifylline, phenylbutazone, pramlintide, probenecid, propoxyphene, quinidine, quinolones, salicylates, sulfonamide antibiotics, tetracycline, theophylline, tricyclic antidepressants, urinary acidifiers, voriconazole: Increased risk of hypoglycemia

asparaginase, atypical antipsychotics, calcium channel blockers, cholestyramine, clonidine, colesevelam, corticosteroids, danazol, diazoxide, estrogen, glucagon, hydantoins, isoniazid, lithium, morphine, niacin, nicotinic acid, oral contraceptives, phenothiazines, phenytoin, protease inhibitors, rifabutin, rifampin, somatropin, sympathomimetics, thiazides and other diuretics, thyroid drugs, urinary alkalinizers: Increased risk of hyperglycemia

beta-blockers, clonidine, reserpine: Possibly hyperglycemia or hypoglycemia

miconazole (oral): Possibly severe hypoglycemia

sympatholytic drugs, such as beta-blockers, clonidine, guanethidine, reserpine: Possible masking of hypoglycemia signs

ACTIVITIES

alcohol use: Altered blood glucose control (usually hypoglycemia)

FOODS

all foods: Possibly delayed absorption of immediate-release tablets if taken within 30 min of meal

Adverse Reactions

CNS: Abnormal gait, anxiety, asthenia, chills, depression, dizziness, fatigue, headache, hypertonia, hypoesthesia, insomnia, malaise, migraine headache, nervousness, paresthesia, somnolence, syncope, tremor, vertigo
CV: **Arrhythmias**, edema, hypertension, vasculitis
EENT: Blurred vision, conjunctivitis, eye pain, pharyngitis, retinal hemorrhage, rhinitis, taste perversion, tinnitus
ENDO: **Hypoglycemia**
GI: Abdominal pain, anorexia, cholestatic jaundice, constipation, diarrhea, elevated liver, enzymes, epigastric discomfort or fullness, flatulence, heartburn, hepatic porphyria, **hepatitis**, hunger, jaundice, nausea, proctocolitis, trace blood in stool, vomiting
GU: Darkened urine, decreased libido, dysuria, polyuria
HEME: **Agranulocytosis**, **aplastic anemia**, eosinophilia, **hemolytic anemia**, **leukopenia**, **pancytopenia**
MS: Arthralgia, leg cramps, myalgia
RESP: Dyspnea
SKIN: Allergic skin reactions, diaphoresis, eczema, **erythema multiforme**, **exfoliative dermatitis**, flushing, lichenoid reactions, maculopapular or morbilliform rash, photosensitivity, urticaria

Other: Disulfiram-like reaction

Childbearing Considerations

PREGNANCY

- It is not known if drug can cause fetal harm. However, it may cause neonatal hypoglycemia.
- Drug is not recommended during pregnancy because abnormal blood glucose levels during pregnancy are associated with a higher incidence of congenital abnormalities, making insulin the preferred drug of choice during pregnancy.

LABOR AND DELIVERY

- At birth, neonate may experience birth injury, respiratory distress, and prolonged severe hypoglycemia, lasting 4 to 10 days if mother receives drug at time of delivery.
- If drug is used during pregnancy, expect it to be discontinued at least 4 wk before expected delivery.

LACTATION

- It is not known if drug is present in breast milk.
- Drug or breastfeeding should be discontinued because of risk for infant hypoglycemia.

Nursing Considerations

! WARNING Use cautiously in patients with glucose 6-phosphate dehydrogenase deficiency because hemolytic anemia may develop. Monitor patient's CBC closely.

- Check blood glucose level at least 3 times daily for a patient switching from insulin to glipizide. Patients who take more than 40 units of insulin daily may need hospitalization during transition.
- Monitor blood glucose levels to determine response to drug. Expect to check glycosylated hemoglobin every 3 to 6 months or as ordered to evaluate long-term blood glucose control.
- Expect to switch patient to insulin therapy, as prescribed, during physical stress, such as infection, surgery, or trauma or if pregnancy occurs.

! WARNING Expect a higher risk of hypoglycemia when giving drug to a debilitated or malnourished patient or one with adrenal or pituitary insufficiency. Also, be aware that hypoglycemia may be more difficult to recognize in patients with autonomic neuropathy, the elderly, and patients who are taking beta-blockers or other sympatholytic agents. Monitor blood glucose level closely. Treat hypoglycemia according to institutional protocol. Notify prescriber if hypoglycemia occurs frequently or is severe.

! WARNING Monitor patient's CBC, as ordered, because glimepiride may cause serious to life-threatening adverse reactions.

! WARNING Assess patient's skin regularly as drug may cause skin reactions, which may become severe. Notify prescriber immediately, if present.

PATIENT TEACHING

- Instruct patient how to take form of glipizide prescribed.
- Caution the patient not to skip the meal after taking drug.
- Advise patient not to skip doses or increase the dosage without consulting prescriber.
- Advise patient to avoid alcohol during glipizide therapy because alcohol can alter blood glucose control.
- Alert patient prescribed both extended-release form of glipizide and colesevelam of the need to take glipizide extended-release 4 hours before colesevelam.
- Teach patient how to monitor his blood glucose level.

! WARNING Instruct patient on signs and symptoms of hypoglycemia such as anxiety, confusion, dizziness, excessive sweating, headache, and nausea. Teach patient how to treat hypoglycemia in the event it should occur. Advise patient to notify prescriber if hypoglycemia frequently occurs or is severe. Ensure family or caregiver knows how to administer glucagon for a severe episode of hypoglycemia. Be aware that the risk of hypoglycemia is higher when giving glipizide to a debilitated or malnourished patient or to a patient with adrenal or pituitary insufficiency.

! WARNING Tell patient to notify prescriber of any other persistent, serious, or unusual adverse reactions.

> **! WARNING** Advise females of childbearing age to notify prescriber if pregnancy occurs. Be aware that if a pregnant patient is not switched to insulin during pregnancy that glipizide will have to be temporarily withheld for about 4 weeks before expected delivery to prevent infant hypoglycemia, which could be severe.

- Caution patient to consult prescriber before taking any over-the-counter drugs.
- Urge patient to carry identification indicating that he has diabetes.
- Instruct patient to avoid direct sunlight and to wear sunscreen.
- Tell mothers to discontinue breastfeeding or the drug will have to be discontinued because of the risk for infant hypoglycemia.

glucagon

Baqsimi, Gvoke HypoPen, Gvoke PFS

glucagon hydrochloride

GlucaGen, Glucagon Diagnostic Kit

Class and Category

Pharmacologic class: Pancreatic hormone
Therapeutic class: Antihypoglycemic, diagnostic aid adjunct

Indications and Dosages

* *To provide emergency treatment of severe hypoglycemia*

I.V., I.M., OR SUBCUTANEOUS INJECTION (GLUCAGEN, GLUCAGON)

Adults and children weighing more than 20 kg (44 lb) or, with GlucaGen, more than 25 kg (55 lb) and for children ages 6 yr and older of unknown weight. 1 mg, repeated in 15 min as needed.
Children weighing 20 kg (44 lb) or less or, with GlucaGen, 25 kg (55 lb) or less or for children who are less than 6 yr of unknown weight. 0.5 mg repeated in 15 min, as needed.

SUBCUTANEOUS INJECTION (GVOKE)

Adults and children ages 12 yr and older. 1 mg, repeated in 15 min, if needed.
Children ages 2 to less than 12 yr weighing 45 kg (99 lb) or more. 1 mg, repeated in 15 min, if needed.
Children ages 2 to less than 12 yr weighing less than 45 kg (99 lb). 0.5 mg, repeated in 15 min, if needed.

NASAL SPRAY (BAQSIMI)

Adults and children ages 4 and older. 3 mg (1 spray) into 1 nostril. If no response after 15 min, dosage repeated.

* *To provide diagnostic assistance by inhibiting bowel peristalsis in radiologic examination of GI tract*

I.M. INJECTION (GLUCAGEN, GLUCAGON)

Adults. *For relaxing duodenum, small bowel, or stomach:* 1 mg before procedure. *For relaxing colon:* 1 to 2 mg before procedure.

I.V. INJECTION (GLUCAGEN, GLUCAGON)

Adults. *For relaxing duodenum, small bowel, or stomach:* 0.2 to 0.5 mg before procedure. *For relaxing colon:* 0.5 to 0.75 mg before procedure.

Drug Administration

- Don't mix parenteral preparations of glucagon with 0.9% Sodium Chloride Injection or solutions that have a pH of 3.0 to 9.5; use with dextrose solutions instead.
- Store drug in its original package for up to 24 mo at room temperature and protected from light. Do not freeze.

I.V. (GLUCAGEN, GLUCAGON)

- Reconstitute 1-mg vial with 1 ml of diluent, either supplied or Sterile Water for Injection. Shake vial gently until powder is completely dissolved. Reconstituted fluid should be clear and colorless. Concentration should be 1 mg/ml.
- Use drug immediately after reconstitution.
- Place unconscious patient on his side before injecting drug, to prevent aspiration of vomitus when he regains consciousness.
- Administer by slow I.V. injection over 1 min to decrease risk of adverse reactions, such as tachycardia and vomiting.
- Give I.V. dextrose, as ordered, if patient doesn't respond to drug or oral carbohydrates once responsive.
- *Incompatibilities:* Electrolyte-containing solutions, such as Sodium Chloride or Potassium Chloride

I.M. (GLUCAGEN, GLUCAGON)

- Reconstitute 1-mg vial of drug with 1 ml of supplied diluent or Sterile Water for Injection. Shake vial gently until powder is completely dissolved. Solution should be clear and colorless. Concentration should be 1 mg/ml. Use immediately.
- Place unconscious patient on his side before injecting drug, to prevent aspiration of vomitus when he regains consciousness.
- Inject into buttocks, outer thigh, or outer upper arm.
- Give I.V. dextrose, as ordered, if patient doesn't respond to glucagon or oral carbohydrates once responsive.

SUBCUTANEOUS (GLUCAGEN, GLUCAGON, GVOKE)

GlucaGen or Glucagon

- Same instructions as for I.M. injection.

Gvoke

- Gvoke comes as either an autoinjector or prefilled syringe. Do not open foil pouch until ready to administer. Follow instructions printed on foil pouch label, carton, or the Instructions for Use. Solution should be clear and colorless to pale yellow.
- Place unconscious patient on his side before injecting drug to prevent aspiration of vomitus when he regains consciousness.
- Inject into the lower abdomen, outer thigh, or outer upper arm.
- Each autoinjector or prefilled syringe contains 1 dose of glucagon and cannot be reused. If a repeat dose is needed, a new device must be used.
- Give I.V. dextrose, as ordered, if patient doesn't respond to drug or oral carbohydrates once responsive.

INTRANASAL (BAQSIMI)

- The plunger should not be pushed or tested prior to use.
- Administer dose by inserting the device tip into one nostril and pressing the device plunger all the way in until the green line is no longer showing. The dose does not have to be inhaled.
- Each device contains 1 dose of glucagon and cannot be reused. If a repeat dose is needed, a new device must be used.

Route	Onset	Peak	Duration
I.V.	Immediate	5–20 min	1–2 hr
I.M.	8–10 min	30 min	1–2 hr
SubQ	<10 min	30 min	1–2 hr
Intranasal	Unknown	15 min	Unknown

Half-life: < 35 min

Mechanism of Action

Increases production of adenylate cyclase, which catalyzes conversion of adenosine triphosphate to cAMP, a process that in turn activates phosphorylase. Phosphorylase promotes breakdown of glycogen to glucose (glycogenolysis) in the liver. As a result, blood glucose level increases and GI smooth muscles relax.

Contraindications

Glucagonoma (when used as a diagnostic aid), hypersensitivity to glucagon or its components, insulinoma, pheochromocytoma

Interactions

DRUGS

anticholinergic drugs: Increased gastrointestinal adverse reactions
beta-blockers: Transient increase in blood pressure and pulse
indomethacin: Possibly loss of effectiveness to raise blood glucose; possibly even produce hypoglycemia
insulin: Antagonistic toward glucagon
oral anticoagulants: Possibly increased anticoagulant effects

Adverse Reactions

CNS: Asthenia, dizziness, headache, somnolence
CV: Hypertension, **hypotension**, tachycardia
EENT: *Nasal form:* Altered taste, eye itchiness or redness, itchy ears or throat, nasal congestion or itching, running nose, sneezing, watery eyes
ENDO: **Hyperglycemia** (presence of diabetes mellitus during diagnostic testing), **hypoglycemia** (presence of glucagonoma or insulinoma)
GI: Abdominal pain, diarrhea, nausea, vomiting
RESP: **Bronchospasm**, **respiratory distress**, upper respiratory irritation (nasal form)

SKIN: Necrolytic migratory erythema, pallor, pruritus (nasal form), urticaria
Other: Hypersensitivity reactions (**anaphylactic shock**, **breathing difficulties**, generalized rash, **hypotension**), injection-site reactions (discomfort, redness, swelling)

Childbearing Considerations

PREGNANCY

- It is not known if drug causes fetal harm.
- Use with caution only if benefit to mother outweighs potential risk to fetus.

LACTATION

- It is not known if drug is present in breast milk.
- Mothers should check with prescriber before breastfeeding.

Nursing Considerations

! WARNING Do not administer glucagon in patients with depleted hepatic glycogen stores caused by such conditions as adrenal insufficiency, chronic hypoglycemia, and starvation because the drug is ineffective. Another form of treatment will need to be prescribed in these patients.

! WARNING Identify and treat hypoglycemia as quickly as possible because prolonged hypoglycemia can cause cerebral damage.

! WARNING Prepare patient for cardiac monitoring when glucagon is used as a diagnostic aid because glucagon may increase blood pressure, myocardial oxygen demand, and pulse rate, which may become life-threatening in patients with cardiac disease. Also, monitor patients with diabetes mellitus receiving glucagon for diagnostic purposes for hyperglycemia and, if present, treat according to institutional protocol.

! WARNING Be aware hypersensitivity reactions have occurred with glucagon use. Although a generalized rash has occurred, anaphylactic shock with breathing difficulties and hypotension have also occurred. Monitor patient closely and alert prescriber, if present. Expect to provide supportive care, as needed and ordered.

- Expect to administer 5 to 10 mg of phentolamine mesylate intravenously, as ordered, if glucagon is administered to a patient with undiagnosed pheochromocytoma and substantial increase in blood pressure occurs.
- Monitor patient for necrolytic migratory erythema, a skin rash common with glucagonomas that may present with bullae, erosions, and scaly, pruritic erythematous plaques following glucagon administration. These lesions may appear on patient's face, groin, legs, or perineum, and may become more widespread. Notify prescriber and expect glucagon to be discontinued. Know that treatment with corticosteroids is not effective in treating necrolytic migratory erythema.

PATIENT TEACHING

- Teach patient and family or caregiver how to recognize signs and symptoms of hypoglycemia, when to notify prescriber, and when and how to administer form of glucagon prescribed.

! WARNING Instruct family or caregiver to keep patient on his side and give the patient both a fast-acting and long-acting carbohydrate when he awakens. Advise against giving fluids by mouth until patient is fully conscious. Instruct family or caregiver to call for emergency medical assistance after glucagon treatment, especially if patient can't ingest oral glucose or is not responding. Have family or caregiver repeat dose after 15 minutes, if patient does not respond, while waiting for emergency medical help.

! WARNING Alert patient, family, or caregiver that drug may cause an allergic reaction. If present, tell patient to notify prescriber, and, if severe, to seek immediate medical care.

glyburide (glibenclamide)

Glynase

Class and Category

Pharmacologic class: Sulfonylurea
Therapeutic class: Antidiabetic

Indications and Dosages

∗ As adjunct to control blood glucose level in type 2 diabetes mellitus

TABLETS (MICRONIZED)

Adults. *Initial:* 1.5 to 3 mg daily with morning meal, increased by up to 1.5 mg at weekly intervals, if needed. *Maintenance:* 0.75 to 12 mg as a single dose or in divided doses. *Maximum:* 12 mg daily.

TABLETS (NONMICRONIZED)

Adults. *Initial:* 2.5 to 5 mg daily with morning meal, increased by up to 2.5 mg at weekly intervals, if needed. *Maintenance:* 1.25 to 20 mg daily as a single dose or in divided doses. *Maximum:* 20 mg daily.

±**DOSAGE ADJUSTMENT** For elderly patients or patients more sensitive to hypoglycemic drugs, initial glyburide dosage possibly reduced to 1.25 mg (nonmicronized) daily, gradually increased by 2.5 mg/wk, as needed; or reduced to 0.75 mg (micronized) daily, gradually increased by 1.5 mg/wk, as needed. For patients converting from insulin to glyburide using more than 40 units of insulin daily, glyburide started at 5 mg (nonmicronized) or 3 mg (microized) as a single dose with 50% of usual insulin dose; glyburide dosage increased gradually, as needed, while insulin dosage is tapered off. For patients converting from insulin to glyburide and using less than 40 units but more than 20 units of insulin, glyburide started at 5 mg (nonmicronized) or 3 mg (micronized) daily as a single dose and insulin discontinued. For patients taking less than 20 units of insulin daily, usual glyburide dosage is used, and insulin discontinued.

Drug Administration

P.O.

- Give as a single dose before first meal of the day. If patient takes more than 10 mg of glyburide (nonmicronized) or more than 6 mg of glyburide (micronized) or develops severe GI distress, give in 2 divided doses before meals.
- Ensure patient eats after drug has been administered.
- Nonmicronized tablets aren't equal to micronized tablets; they contain smaller particles, which affects drug bioavailability.
- Do not administer nonmicronized glyburide with a high-fat meal because it may reduce glyburide bioavailability.

Route	Onset	Peak	Duration
P.O.*	1 hr	2–3 hr	24 hr
P.O.†	2 hr	3–4 hr	24 hr

Half-life: 4–10 hr

* Micronized
† Nonmicronized

Mechanism of Action

Stimulates insulin release from beta cells in the pancreas. Glyburide also increases peripheral tissue sensitivity to insulin either by enhancing insulin binding to cellular receptors or by increasing the number of insulin receptors.

Contraindications

Concurrent therapy with bosentan; diabetic ketoacidosis; hypersensitivity to glyburide, sulfonylureas, or their components; type 1 diabetes mellitus

Interactions

DRUGS

ACE inhibitors, anabolic steroids, azole antifungals, chloramphenicol, clarithromycin, disopyramide, drugs highly protein bound, fluoxetine, guanethidine, MAO inhibitors, NSAIDs, oxyphenbutazone, phenylbutazone, probenecid, quinolones, salicylates, sulfonamides: Increased risk of hypoglycemia

calcium channel blockers, colesevelam, corticosteroids, estrogens, isoniazid, nicotinic acid, oral contraceptives, phenothiazines, phenytoin, sympathomimetics, thiazide diuretics and other diuretics, thyroid drugs: Increased risk of hyperglycemia

beta-blockers: Possibly hyperglycemia or masking of hypoglycemia signs

bosentan: Increased risk of elevated liver enzymes

cyclosporine: Increased cyclosporine plasma level and toxicity

CYP2 c9 and CYP3A4 inducers or inhibitors: Possibly altered blood glucose levels

miconazole (oral): Possibly severe hypoglycemia

oral anticoagulants: Possibly potentiated or weakened anticoagulant effects; increased risk of hypoglycemia

rifampin: Decreased glyburide effectiveness

ACTIVITIES

alcohol use: Altered blood glucose control (usually hypoglycemia)

FOODS

high-fat foods: Reduced bioavailability of nonmicronized glyburide

Adverse Reactions

CNS: Abnormal gait, anxiety, asthenia, chills, depression, dizziness, fatigue, headache, hypertonia, hypoesthesia, insomnia, malaise, migraine headache, nervousness, paresthesia, somnolence, syncope, tremor, vertigo
CV: **Arrhythmias**, edema, hypertension, vasculitis
EENT: Blurred vision, changes in accommodation, conjunctivitis, eye pain, pharyngitis, retinal hemorrhage, rhinitis, taste perversion, tinnitus
ENDO: **Hypoglycemia**
GI: Anorexia, constipation, cholestatic jaundice, diarrhea, elevated liver enzymes, epigastric discomfort or fullness, flatulence, heartburn, **hepatic failure** or porphyria, **hepatitis**, hunger, jaundice, nausea, proctocolitis, trace blood in stool, vomiting
GU: Decreased libido, dysuria, polyuria
HEME: **Agranulocytosis**, **aplastic anemia**, eosinophilia, **hemolytic anemia**, **leukopenia**, **pancytopenia**, purpura, **thrombocytopenia**
MS: Arthralgia, leg cramps, myalgia
RESP: Dyspnea
SKIN: Allergic skin reactions, bullous reactions, diaphoresis, eczema, erythema, **erythema multiforme**, **exfoliative dermatitis**, flushing, lichenoid reactions, maculopapular or morbilliform rash, photosensitivity, porphyria cutanea tarda, pruritus, urticaria
Other: **Angioedema**, disulfiram-like reaction, **hyponatremia**, weight gain

Childbearing Considerations

PREGNANCY

- It is not known if drug can cause fetal harm. However, it may cause neonatal hypoglycemia.
- Drug is not recommended during pregnancy because abnormal blood glucose levels during pregnancy are associated with a higher incidence of congenital abnormalities, making insulin the preferred drug of choice during pregnancy.

LABOR AND DELIVERY

- At birth, neonate may experience birth injury, respiratory distress, and prolonged severe hypoglycemia, lasting 4 to 10 days if mother receives drug at time of delivery.
- If drug is used during pregnancy, expect it to be discontinued at least 2 wk before expected delivery.

LACTATION

- It is not known if drug is present in breast milk.
- Drug or breastfeeding should be discontinued.

Nursing Considerations

! **WARNING** Use cautiously in patients with glucose 6-phosphate dehydrogenase deficiency because hemolytic anemia may develop.

- Monitor blood glucose levels to determine patient's response to glyburide. Expect to check glycosylated hemoglobin every 3 to 6 months or as ordered to evaluate long-term blood glucose control.

! **WARNING** Monitor patient for a hypersensitivity reaction, especially patients with a history of allergies to other sulfonamide derivatives. Know that a hypersensitivity reaction may become life-threatening, such as angioedema. If a hypersensitivity reaction occurs, notify prescriber, expect drug to be discontinued, and provide supportive care, as needed and ordered.

! **WARNING** Expect a higher risk of hypoglycemia when giving drug to a debilitated or malnourished patient or one with adrenal or pituitary insufficiency. Also, be aware that hypoglycemia may be more difficult to recognize in patients with autonomic neuropathy, the elderly, and patients who are taking beta-blockers or other sympatholytic agents. Monitor blood glucose level closely and treat according to institution protocol, if present. Notify prescriber if hypoglycemia occurs frequently or is severe.

! **WARNING** Monitor patient's CBC closely because drug can cause serious to life-threatening adverse reactions.

- Administer insulin as needed and prescribed during periods of increased stress, such as infection, surgery, and trauma or during pregnancy.

PATIENT TEACHING

- Instruct patient how to administer form of glyburide prescribed.
- Advise patient not to take nonmicronized glyburide with a high-fat meal because it may reduce glyburide bioavailability.
- Caution patient to avoid skipping doses, discontinuing glyburide, or taking over-the-counter drugs without first consulting prescriber.
- Advise patient to avoid alcohol while taking glyburide because alcohol can affect glucose control.
- Teach patient how to monitor his blood glucose level and when to notify prescriber about changes.

! **WARNING** Alert patient that drug may cause an allergic reaction. Tell patient to notify prescriber if an allergic reaction occurs and to seek immediate medical care, if severe.

! **WARNING** Instruct patient on signs and symptoms of hypoglycemia such as anxiety, confusion, dizziness, excessive sweating, headache, and nausea. Teach patient how to treat hypoglycemia in the event it should occur. Advise patient to notify prescriber if hypoglycemia frequently occurs or is severe. Ensure family or caregiver knows how to administer glucagon for a severe episode of hypoglycemia and to call for emergency medical help.

! **WARNING** Tell patient to notify prescriber if other persistent, serious, or unusual adverse reactions occur.

! **WARNING** Advise females of childbearing age to notify prescriber if pregnancy occurs. However, if drug is continued during pregnancy, alert patient that drug will need to be discontinued 2 weeks before delivery to prevent hypoglycemia in the newborn.

- Instruct patient to avoid direct sunlight and to wear sunscreen.
- Advise patient to carry identification indicating that he has diabetes.

golimumab

Simponi, Simponi Aria

Class and Category

Pharmacologic class: Tumor necrosis factor (TNF) blocker

Therapeutic class: Biologic disease-modifying antirheumatic drug (DMARD)

Indications and Dosages

✱ *To treat active psoriatic arthritis; to treat ankylosing spondylitis with or without methotrexate or other nonbiologic disease-modifying antirheumatic drugs (DMARDs); to treat moderate to severe rheumatoid arthritis with methotrexate*

SUBCUTANEOUS INJECTION (SIMPONI)

Adults. 50 mg monthly.

I.V. INFUSION (SIMPONI ARIA)

Adults. 2 mg/kg infused over 30 min at wk 0 and 4, then every 8 wk thereafter.

✱ *To treat polyarticular juvenile idiopathic arthritis and psoriatic arthritis*

I.V. INFUSION (SIMPONI ARIA)

Children ages 2 and older. 80 mg/m^2 infused over 30 min at wks 0 and 4, and every 8 wks thereafter.

✱ *To treat moderate to severe active ulcerative colitis in patients who have demonstrated corticosteroid dependence or who have had an inadequate response to or failed to tolerate 6-mercaptopurine, azathioprine, oral aminosalicylates, or oral corticosteroid*

SUBCUTANEOUS INJECTION (SIMPONI)

Adults. *Initial:* 200 mg at wk 0, followed by 100 mg at wk 2. *Maintenance:* 100 mg every 4 wk.

Drug Administration

I.V.

- Each 4-ml vial contains 50 mg of golimumab. Solution should appear colorless to light yellow. Dilute the total volume of the drug solution with 0.45% or 0.9% Sodium Chloride Injection to a final volume of 100 ml. Gently mix.
- Discard any unused solution remaining in the vials.
- Use within 4 hr, keeping diluted solution at room temperature.

- Inspect diluted solution prior to infusion for particulate matter or discoloration. Do not use if present.
- Use only an infusion set with an in-line, low-protein-binding, nonpyrogenic, sterile filter (pore size 0.22 micrometer or less).
- Infuse the diluted solution over 30 min.
- Do not infuse concomitantly in the same intravenous line with other drugs.
- *Incompatibilities:* Other drugs

SUBCUTANEOUS

- Needle cover of syringe contains dry rubber and should not be handled by anyone with a latex allergy.
- Take prefilled syringe or autoinjector out of the refrigerator 30 min before giving injection to allow time for drug to warm up to room temperature. Never warm drug in any other way.
- Solution should be clear to slightly opalescent to light yellow.
- Do not inject drug into areas that are bruised, hard, red, or tender.
- When using autoinjector, do not pull the device away from the skin until a first "click" and then a second "click" is heard, indicating the injection is finished. It may take up to 15 sec before second click is heard. If device is pulled away from the skin before the second click, a full dose may not have been given.
- Rotate injection sites. If more than 1 subcutaneous injection is required, administer the injections at different sites on the body.
- Discard any leftover product remaining in the prefilled syringe or autoinjector.

Route	Onset	Peak	Duration
I.V.	Unknown	Unknown	Unknown
SubQ	Unknown	2–6 days	Unknown

Half-life: 12–14 days

Mechanism of Action

Binds to a cytokine protein, tumor necrosis factor-alpha (TNF-alpha), to block interaction with its receptors, which prevents biological activity of TNF-alpha. Elevated TNF-alpha levels in the blood, joints, and synovium may play an important role in pathophysiology of inflammatory diseases, such as ankylosing spondylitis, psoriatic arthritis, rheumatoid arthritis, and ulcerative colitis. Reduced TNF-alpha activity in these disorders improves signs and symptoms.

Contraindications

Hypersensitivity to golimumab or its components

Interactions

DRUGS

abatacept, anakinra, rituximab: Possibly increased risk of serious infection
cytochrome P-450 substrates, such as cyclosporine, theophylline, warfarin: Effects or blood levels of these drugs may change when golimumab therapy starts or stops
live vaccines, therapeutic infectious agents, such as BCG bladder instillation for treatment of cancer: Increased risk of adverse vaccine effects
methotrexate: Decreased clearance of golimumab

Adverse Reactions

CNS: Demyelinating disorders both central and peripheral, dizziness, fever, paresthesia
CV: **Congestive heart failure**, hypertension
EENT: Nasopharyngitis, oral herpes, pharyngitis, rhinitis, sinusitis
GI: Elevated liver enzymes, nausea
HEME: **Agranulocytosis**, **aplastic anemia**, **leukemia**, **leukopenia**, **neutropenia**, **thrombocytopenia**
RESP: Bronchitis, dyspnea, **interstitial lung disease**, pneumonia, tuberculosis, upper respiratory tract infection
SKIN: Bullous skin reactions, cellulitis, lichenoid reactions, **melanoma**, **Merkel cell carcinoma**, new or worsening psoriasis, pruritus, rash, skin exfoliation, urticaria
Other: Abscess; **anaphylaxis**; antibody formation to golimumab; bacterial (including *Legionella* and *Listeria*), fungal (including invasive), mycobacterial, parasitic, or viral infections (including **reactivation of hepatitis B infection** in chronic carriers); injection-site erythema; lupus-like syndrome; **malignancies, such as lymphomas**; sarcoidosis; **sepsis**

Childbearing Considerations

PREGNANCY

- It is not known if drug causes fetal harm. However, it does cross the placenta during the third trimester of pregnancy and may affect immune response of the infant after birth.
- If drug is given during pregnancy, know that infant is at increased risk for

infection. Administration of live vaccines to infants exposed to drug in utero is not recommended for 6 mo following the mother's last dose during pregnancy.

LACTATION

- It is not known if drug is present in breast milk.
- Mothers should check with prescriber before breastfeeding.

Nursing Considerations

- Ensure that patient is current on immunizations before therapy is begun.
- Make sure patient has a tuberculin skin test before therapy starts. If skin test is positive, treatment of latent tuberculosis (TB) must start before golimumab therapy starts, as prescribed. Also, antituberculosis therapy may be started if patient has a history of active or latent TB if adequate therapy can't be confirmed, or if patient has a negative test for latent TB but also has risk factors for TB.

! **WARNING** Know that patients with a history of cancer, except those successfully treated for nonmelanoma skin cancer, should be thoroughly evaluated before golimumab therapy starts because treatment may pose more risks than benefits. Patients with rheumatoid arthritis may have a higher risk than the general population for developing leukemia while taking a TNF blocker, such as golimumab.

! **WARNING** Know that if patient has evidence of an active infection when drug is prescribed, golimumab therapy shouldn't start until infection has been treated. Use golimumab cautiously in patients with recurrent infection or who are at increased risk for infection, patients who live in regions where histoplasmosis and TB are endemic, and patients with a history of hepatitis B infection because drug increases risk of infection. Monitor all patients for bacterial (including *Legionella* and *Listeria*), fungal, mycobacterial, parasitic, or viral infections during therapy, especially those receiving immunosuppressants. Know that the infection could become life-threatening and affect multiple organs. If a serious infection, an opportunistic infection, or sepsis develops, expect prescriber to stop drug and start appropriate antimicrobial therapy. Monitor patient closely for TB throughout golimumab therapy because active TB has occurred in patients during and after treatment of latent TB.

- Use golimumab cautiously in patients with congestive heart failure; demyelinating disorders, such as multiple sclerosis; and hematologic cytopenias because these disorders may develop or become worse with golimumab therapy.

! **WARNING** Monitor patient for a hypersensitivity reaction, which may become life-threatening, such as anaphylaxis. If present, notify prescriber, expect drug to be discontinued, and provide supportive care, as needed and ordered.

! **WARNING** Monitor patient, especially young adult males, for signs and symptoms of malignancies throughout drug therapy. Although lymphomas account for about half of all malignancies associated with golimumab therapy, leukemia and rare malignancies, including melanomas and Merkel cell carcinoma, have also occurred. Report any persistent, severe, or unusual signs and symptoms to prescriber.

! **WARNING** Monitor patient's CBC regularly, as ordered and patient for evidence of hematologic disorders, which could become life-threatening. Notify prescriber if patient experiences unusual bruising or bleeding.

PATIENT TEACHING

- Inform family or caregiver drug will be given to the child intravenously. Tell adult patients that drug may be given intravenously or as a subcutaneous injection.
- Explain that first injection of golimumab given subcutaneously must be administered with a healthcare professional present.
- Teach patient, family, or caregiver how to give golimumab as a subcutaneous injection at home, if applicable, including the use of the autoinjector, if prescribed.
- Alert patient, family, or caregiver that needle cover contains natural dry rubber and should not be handled by anyone with a latex allergy.

! **WARNING** Alert patient that golimumab may cause an allergic reaction. If present, tell patient to notify prescriber, If severe, urge patient to seek immediate medical care.

! **WARNING** Teach patient how to recognize evidence of bleeding disorders and infection and to tell prescriber if they occur; drug may have to be stopped. Advise patient to take infection control precautions, such as avoiding people with infections and bleeding precautions such as using a soft bristle toothbrush and a safety razor.

! **WARNING** Inform patient that golimumab therapy increases the risk of certain kinds of cancer, especially leukemias and lymphomas. Emphasize the importance of having follow-up visits and reporting to prescriber any sudden onset, persistent or unusual signs or symptoms. Also, encourage patient to have regular skin examinations.

- Explain that TB may occur during golimumab therapy. Instruct the patient to report low-grade fever, persistent cough, and wasting or weight loss to prescriber.
- Instruct patient to check with prescriber before receiving any vaccines. Live vaccines should be avoided.
- Tell patient to report lupus-like signs and symptoms that, although rare, may occur during therapy, such as chest pain that doesn't go away, joint pain, a rash on arms or cheeks that's sensitive to the sun, or shortness of breath. Explain that drug may have to be discontinued if these occur.
- Advise patient to tell all healthcare providers about golimumab therapy and to tell prescriber about any over-the-counter drugs, herbal remedies, and mineral or vitamin supplements being taken.
- Inform mothers who received golimumab therapy during pregnancy to monitor their infant for infections and not to have their infant receive live vaccines for 6 months following the mother's last golimumab dose during the pregnancy.
- Stress importance of complying with all ordered laboratory tests.

granisetron

Sancuso, Sustol

granisetron hydrochloride

Class and Category

Pharmacologic class: Serotonin blocker ($5\text{-}HT_3$ receptor antagonist)
Therapeutic class: Antiemetic

Indications and Dosages

To prevent nausea and vomiting caused by emetogenic chemotherapy, including high-dose cisplatin

TABLETS

Adults. 1 mg up to 1 hr before chemotherapy, repeated 12 hr later. Alternatively, 2 mg up to 1 hr before chemotherapy.

I.V. INFUSION, I.V. INJECTION

Adults and children ages 2 and older. 10 mcg/kg starting 30 min before chemotherapy. I.V. injection given undiluted over 30 sec; I.V. infusion given diluted over 5 min.

To prevent nausea and vomiting associated with moderately and/or highly emetogenic chemotherapy regimens of up to 5 consecutive days duration

TRANSDERMAL (SANCUSO)

Adults. 3.1-mg/24-hr patch 24 to 48 hr before chemotherapy and worn up to 7 days. Patch removed no sooner than 24 hr after chemotherapy is completed.

As adjunct with other antiemetics to prevent acute and delayed nausea and vomiting associated with initial and repeat course of moderately emetogenic chemotherapy (MEC) or anthracycline and cyclophosphamide (CP) combination chemotherapy regimens

E.R. SUBCUTANEOUS INJECTION (SUSTOL)

Adults. 10 mg in combination with dexamethasone at least 30 min before chemotherapy on day 1. *Maximum:* 10 mg no more frequently than once every 7 days.

± **DOSAGE ADJUSTMENT** For patients with a creatinine clearance of between 30 to 59 ml/min, Sustol brand dosage interval should not be more than once every 14 days.

G H I

∗ *To prevent nausea and vomiting caused by radiation therapy, including fractionated abdominal radiation and total body irradiation*

TABLETS

Adults. 2 mg daily given 1 hr before radiation therapy.

Drug Administration

P.O.

- May give drug on an empty stomach, if preferred.
- Give tablets up to 1 hr before chemotherapy or 1 hr before radiation.

I.V.

- For I.V. injection, administer undiluted over 30 sec, 30 min before chemotherapy.
- For I.V. infusion, dilute with 0.9% Sodium Chloride or 5% Dextrose Injection to total volume of 20 to 50 ml. Infuse over 5 min, 30 min before chemotherapy. Mixture may be stored up to 24 hr. Use only on days when chemotherapy is given.
- *Incompatibilities:* Other drugs

SUBCUTANEOUS

- Know that the Sustol brand is the only granisetron that can be administered subcutaneously and comes as a refrigerated kit. Do not substitute nonkit components for any of the components from the kit.
- Remove kit at least 60 min prior to administration. Unpack kit to allow the syringe containing drug as well as all other contents to warm to room temperature. Activate 1 of the syringe warming pouches, and wrap the warming pouch around the syringe containing the drug for 5 to 6 min.
- Inspect the syringe containing drug prior to administration for particulate matter and discoloration. Know that the syringe is amber-colored glass. Do not use if particulate matter or discoloration is seen, the tip cap is missing or has been tampered with, or if the Luer fitting is missing or dislodged.
- A topical anesthetic may be applied to the injection site prior to administration.
- Administer at least 30 min before chemotherapy on day 1.
- To administer, inject into abdomen at least 1 inch away from the umbilicus or into the back of the upper arm. Avoid injecting drug into areas that are burned, hardened, inflamed, swollen, or otherwise compromised.
- Inject as a slow, sustained injection that may take up to 30 sec. Pressing the plunger harder will not expel the drug faster.
- Once drug has been removed from refrigerator, it can remain at room temperature for up to 7 days. Otherwise, store in refrigerator and protect from light. Do not freeze.

TRANSDERMAL

- Apply immediately after opening pouch containing the patch.
- Do not cut the patch.
- Apply transdermal patch to patient's upper outer arm 24 to 48 hr before chemotherapy, and don't remove it until at least 24 hr after chemotherapy is completed although it can remain in place for up to 7 days.
- Remove each transdermal system by peeling off gently from the skin. After removal, fold the transdermal system in half with the sticky side together and discard.

Route	Onset	Peak	Duration
P.O.	Unknown	Unknown	24 hr
I.V.	< 30 min	Unknown	< 24 hr
SubQ	Unknown	24 hr	7 days
Transdermal	Unknown	48 hr	Unknown

Half-life: 5–24 hr

Mechanism of Action

Has a high affinity for serotonin receptors along vagal nerve endings in intestines. Because of this affinity, granisetron prevents nausea and vomiting that usually result when serotonin is released by damaged enterochromaffin cells.

Contraindications

Hypersensitivity to granisetron, its components, or any other 5-HT_3 receptor antagonists

Interactions

DRUGS

drugs that prolong the QT interval: Increased risk of QT interval prolongation

serotonin and nonadrenaline reuptake inhibitors (SNRIs), selective serotonin reuptake inhibitors (SSRIs): Increased risk of serotonin syndrome

Adverse Reactions

CNS: Asthenia, chills, CNS stimulation, drowsiness, fever, headache, insomnia, **serotonin syndrome**, somnolence
CV: **Bradycardia**, chest pain, hypertension, palpitations, **prolonged QT interval**, **sick sinus syndrome**
EENT: Taste perversion
GI: Abdominal pain, anorexia, constipation, diarrhea, elevated liver enzymes, gastric distention, nausea, progressive ileus, vomiting
HEME: Anemia, **leukopenia**, **thrombocytopenia**
SKIN: Alopecia, reactions at patch application site (burns, discoloration, irritation, pruritus, rash, redness, vesicles, urticaria)
Other: **Anaphylaxis**; subcutaneous injection-site reactions (bleeding, bruising, hematomas, infections, nodules, pain, or tenderness)

Childbearing Considerations

PREGNANCY

- It is not known if drug causes fetal harm.
- Use with caution only if benefit to mother outweighs potential risk to fetus.

LACTATION

- It is not known if drug is present in breast milk.
- Mothers should check with prescriber before breastfeeding.

Nursing Considerations

- Assess patient receiving subcutaneous granisetron for injection-site reactions following administration. Know that some of the reactions, such as bruising, hematoma, and infection, may develop up to 2 weeks or more after the injection. Monitor patients receiving anticoagulants or antiplatelet agents closely, as bruising or hematoma formation may be more severe.

! **WARNING** Monitor patient for hypersensitivity reactions. Know that because the Sustol brand has extended-release properties, a reaction may not occur until 7 days or longer following administration and may take longer to resolve. If hypersensitivity is present, notify prescriber and provide supportive care, as needed and ordered.

! **WARNING** Monitor patient's ECG, as ordered for patients with arrhythmias or cardiac conduction disorders because granisetron may prolong the QT interval. Patients especially at risk include those with cardiac disease or electrolyte abnormalities and those receiving cardiotoxic chemotherapy or therapy with another drug that prolongs QT interval.

! **WARNING** Monitor patient for serotonin syndrome, characterized by agitation, chills, confusion, diaphoresis, diarrhea, fever, hyperactive reflexes, poor coordination, restlessness, shaking, talking tremor, twitching, or uncontrolled excitement behavior.

- Monitor patient for persistent or severe GI effects such as constipation, gastric distention, or progressive ileus that may become severe and require hospitalization. Monitor patient closely, especially if patient is also receiving opioid medications. Consult with prescriber about using a bowel regimen, if needed. Know that the drug may mask gastric distention and/or a progressive ileus, especially in patients with recent abdominal surgery. Assess patient for decreased bowel sounds regularly.

PATIENT TEACHING

- Instruct how to administer form of granisetron prescribed or inform patient that drug will be given intravenously if that is the form ordered for the patient.
- Inform patient receiving drug subcutaneously about possible injection-site reactions that can occur and that these reactions may occur up to 2 weeks or more after the injection. Instruct patient to seek immediate medical care if bleeding occurs and is severe or lasts for longer than 1 day or the site looks infected. Tell the patient to notify prescriber if he experiences bruising, hematoma, persistent nodule at the injection site, or pain or tenderness severe enough to interfere with activities of daily living or for the patient to take pain medication.
- Instruct patient prescribed the transdermal system to be sure to cover the application site with clothing, if there is a risk of it being exposed to direct artificial or natural sunlight throughout the period of wear

and for 10 days following its removal. Remind patient to discard removed patch in a way that would prevent accidental contact or ingestion by children, pets, or others.

! **WARNING** Review signs and symptoms of an allergic reaction. Tell patient to seek immediate emergency care if present. Inform patient receiving drug subcutaneously to watch for allergic reactions for 7 days or longer after administration because of length of time drug can stay in the body.

! **WARNING** Instruct patient to seek immediate medical attention if the following symptoms occur: radical changes in blood pressure or pulse, changes in mental status, or neuromuscular symptoms with or without GI symptoms. Also, tell patient to contact prescriber immediately if he experiences other persistent, severe, or unusual symptoms.

- Advise patient to report constipation, fever, severe diarrhea, or severe headache. Also, caution about possible drowsiness and need to take safety measures until effects of drug are known and resolved.

guselkumab

Tremfya

Class and Category

Pharmacologic class: Monoclonal antibody
Therapeutic class: Antipsoriatic

Indications and Dosages

∗ *To treat moderate to severe plaque psoriasis in patients who are candidates for systemic therapy or phototherapy; to treat active psoriatic arthritis*

SUBCUTANEOUS INJECTION

Adults. 100 mg at wk 0, wk 4, and every 8 wk thereafter.

∗ *To treat moderate to severe active ulcerative colitis*

I.V. INFUSION FOLLOWED BY SUBCUTANEOUS INJECTION

Adults. *Induction:* 200 mg I.V. infused over at least 1 hr at wk 0, 4, and 8. *Maintenance:* 100 mg subcutaneously at wk 16 and every 8 wk thereafter or 200 mg subcutaneously at wk 12 and every 4 wk thereafter.

Drug Administration

SUBCUTANEOUS

- Remove prefilled pen, prefilled syringe or single-dose One-Press injector from refrigerator and allow to warm to room temperature, keeping needle cap in place until ready to use.
- Inspect solution. It should be clear and colorless to light yellow and may contain small translucent particles. Do not use if the liquid contains large particles, is discolored, or is cloudy.
- Inject the full amount of solution in the prefilled pen, prefilled syringe or injector into the lower abdominal area (except for 2 inches around the navel), front of the thighs, upper area of the buttock, or upper outer area of the arms.
- Do not inject into an area where the skin is bruised, hard, scaly, tender, thick, or affected by psoriasis.
- Discard any unused product remaining in the prefilled pen, prefilled syringe or injector because it does not contain preservatives.

I.V.

- Withdraw and discard 20 ml of 0.9% Sodium Chloride Injection from a 250 ml infusion bag, which is equal to the volume of the drug to be added.
- Withdraw 20 ml of drug from vial and add to the 250 ml infusion bag of 0.9% Sodium Chloride Injection for a final concentration of 0.8 mg/ml. Gently mix the diluted solution. Discard the vial with any remaining solution.
- Infuse the diluted solution over at least one hour using an infusion set with an in-line, sterile, nonpyrogenic, low protein binding filter (pore size 0.2 micrometer).
- Do infuse drug concomitantly in the same IV line with other drugs.
- Store diluted infusion solution at room temperature for up to 10 hr, which begins once the diluted solution has been prepared.
- Infusion should be completed within 10 hr after the drug is diluted.

Incompatibilities: Other drugs

Route	Onset	Peak	Duration
SubQ	Unknown	5.5 days	Unknown

Half-life: 15–18 days

Mechanism of Action

Selectively binds to the p19 subunit of interleukin 23 (IL-23) and inhibits its interaction with the IL-23 receptor, which prevents the release of proinflammatory chemokines and cytokines.

Contraindications

Hypersensitivity to guselkumab or its components

Interactions

DRUGS

CYP450 substrates: Possibly decreased effectiveness of these drugs
live vaccines: Possible decreased response to vaccine

Adverse Reactions

CNS: Headache, migraine
EENT: Nasopharyngitis, oral herpes, pharyngitis
GI: Diarrhea, elevated liver enzymes, gastroenteritis
GU: Genital herpes
MS: Arthralgia
RESP: Upper respiratory infections
SKIN: Rash, tinea infections, urticaria
Other: Antibody formation to guselkumab; candidal infections; herpes simplex infections and other infections; **hypersensitivity reactions** (**angioedema**, chest or **throat tightness**, **difficulty breathing**, hives, rash), injection-site reactions (bruising, discoloration, edema, erythema, hematoma, hemorrhage, induration, inflammation, pain, pruritus, swelling, urticaria)

Childbearing Considerations

PREGNANCY

- Pregnancy exposure registry: 1-877-311-8972, www.mothertobaby.org/ongoing-study/tremfya-guselkumab, or email: MotherToBaby@health.ucsd.edu.
- It is not known if drug causes fetal harm. However, human IgG antibodies are known to cross the placental barrier and therefore may be transmitted to the fetus.
- Use with caution only if benefit to mother outweighs potential risk to fetus.

LACTATION

- It is not known if drug is present in breast milk.
- Mothers should check with prescriber before breastfeeding.

Nursing Considerations

- Assess patient for tuberculosis (TB) before guselkumab therapy is begun. Expect treatment for latent TB to be given prior to starting guselkumab therapy.
- Know that all age-appropriate immunizations should be done before guselkumab therapy begins.

! **WARNING** Monitor patient closely for hypersensitivity reactions, which could become life-threatening such as anaphylaxis. If present, notify prescriber, expect drug to be discontinued if serious, and provide supportive emergency care, as needed and ordered.

- Monitor patient for infections throughout drug therapy, as guselkumab increases risk. Institute infection precautions. Be aware that if infection occurs and is severe or does not respond to appropriate treatment, guselkumab may need to be discontinued.

PATIENT TEACHING

- Instruct patient on how to administer guselkumab as a subcutaneous injection and what to do if a dose is missed.

! **WARNING** Urge patient that if an allergic reaction occurs to stop taking drug and seek immediate emergency care, as reactions can become serious enough to warrant hospitalization.

- Review infection prevention practices with patient. Emphasize importance of notifying prescriber if an infection should occur.
- Inform patient that immunizations, especially live vaccines, should not be given during guselkumab therapy.

haloperidol

haloperidol decanoate

Haldol Decanoate

haloperidol lactate

Haldol Concentrate

Class and Category

Pharmacologic class: Butyrophenone derivative
Therapeutic class: Antipsychotic

Indications and Dosages

* *To treat psychosis and schizophrenia*

ORAL SOLUTION, TABLETS

Adults and adolescents. *Initial:* 0.5 to 2 mg every 8 to 12 hr. *For severe symptoms:* 3 to 5 mg every 8 to 12 hr, as needed. *Maximum:* 100 mg/day.

Children ages 3 to 12 weighing 15 kg (33 lb) to 40 kg (88 lb). *Initial:* 0.5 mg daily in divided doses twice daily or 3 times daily. Increased by 0.5 mg every 5 to 7 days, as needed. *Maintenance:* 0.05 to 0.15 mg/kg/day given in 2 to 3 divided doses.

± **DOSAGE ADJUSTMENT** For debilitated or elderly patients, initial dosage kept at 0.5 to 2 mg every 8 to 12 hr but increased gradually, as needed.

* *To treat nonpsychotic behavior disorders*

ORAL SOLUTION, TABLETS

Children ages 3 to 12 weighing 15 kg (33 lb) to 40 kg (88 lb). *Initial:* 0.5 mg daily in divided doses twice daily or 3 times daily. Increased by 0.5 mg every 5 to 7 days, as needed and then reduced to lowest effective maintenance dose. *Maintenance:* 0.05 to 0.075 mg/kg daily in 2 or 3 divided doses. *Maximum:* 6 mg/day in divided doses.

* *To treat Tourette's syndrome*

ORAL SOLUTION, TABLETS

Adults and adolescents weighing more than 40 kg (88 lb). *Moderate symptomology:* 0.5 to 2 mg every 8 to 12 hr. *Severe symptomology:* 3to 5 mg every 8 to 12 hr. *Maximum:* 100 mg daily in divided doses.

Children ages 3 to 12 weighing 15 kg (33 lb) to 40 kg (88 lb). *Initial:* 0.5 mg daily divided in 2 or 3 doses, increased by 0.5 mg every 5 to 7 days, as needed. *Maintenance:* 0.05 to 0.075 mg/kg daily in 2 or 3 divided doses.

± **DOSAGE ADJUSTMENT** For patients who are debilitated or elderly, dosage kept at 0.5 to 2 mg twice daily or three times daily regardless of severity of symptoms. For patients with chronic symptoms or resistant to treatment, dosage given as 3 mg to 5 mg twice daily or three times daily regardless of severity of symptoms.

* *To treat acutely agitated schizophrenic patient*

PROMPT-ACTING I.M. INJECTION (LACTATE)

Adults and adolescents. *Initial:* 2 to 5 mg, with subsequent doses every 60 min, as needed. Or, if symptoms are controlled, dose may be repeated every 4 to 8 hr. First oral dose may be given 12 to 24 hr after last parenteral dose. *Maximum:* 20 mg daily.

* *To provide long-term antipsychotic therapy for patients with schizophrenia who require conversion from oral therapy to parenteral therapy*

LONG-ACTING I.M. (DECANOATE) INJECTION

Adults. Highly individualized with titration based on response. *If stabilized on low daily oral doses (up to 10 mg/day):* 10 to 15 times daily oral dose given once, followed one month later by monthly doses of 10 to 15 times previous daily oral dose. *If stabilized on a high dose or at risk of relapse:* 20 times daily oral dose given once, followed one month later by monthly doses of 10 to 15 times previous daily oral dose.

± **DOSAGE ADJUSTMENT** For patients with a variation in response, dosage and/or dosing interval adjusted.

Drug Administration

P.O.

- Tablets may be administered with or without food.
- Protect concentrate from light. Slight yellowing is common and doesn't affect potency. Discard very discolored solution.
- Measure oral solution dosage with the dropper that comes with the bottle. Do not

use other droppers, as dosage may not be accurate.

- Dilute oral solution with a beverage, such as apple, orange, or tomato juice; cola; or water. Administer immediately.

I.M.

- Be sure right parenteral formulation is being used; there is a prompt-acting one and a long-acting one.
- Know that a slight yellow discoloration of injection solution doesn't affect
- potency.
- Do not administer parenteral form intravenously.
- Administer by deep I.M. injection into gluteal muscle using Z-track technique and 21 G needle.
- Don't give more than 3 ml per site.

Route	Onset	Peak	Duration
P.O.	Unknown	2–6 hr	Unknown
I.M. (lactate)	30–60 min	10–20 min	Unknown
I.M. (decanoate)	Unknown	6 days	2–4 wk

Half-life: 18 hr; 3 wk (decanoate)

Mechanism of Action

May block postsynaptic dopamine receptors in the limbic system and increase brain turnover of dopamine, producing an antipsychotic effect.

Contraindications

Dementia with Lewy bodies, hypersensitivity to haloperidol or its components, Parkinson's disease, severe toxic CNS comatose states, or depression

Interactions

DRUGS

anticholinergics: Increased anticholinergic effects
buspirone, CYP2 d6 inhibitors (chlorpromazine, promethazine, quinidine, paroxetine, sertraline, venlafaxine), CYP3A4 inhibitors (alprazolam, itraconazole, ketoconazole, nefazodone, ritonavir), combined CYP2 d6 and CYP3A4 inhibitors (fluoxetine, fluvoxamine, ritonavir): Increased haloperidol plasma concentrations and increased risk of adverse events, including prolonged QT interval
carbamazepine, phenobarbital, phenytoin, rifampin, St. John's wort: Decreased plasma haloperidol levels
citalopram, class IA and 3 antiarrhythmics, corticosteroids, diuretics, erythromycin, ketoconazole, levofloxacin, methadone, paroxetine, ziprasidone: Possibly increased risk of QT prolongation
CNS depressants, such as anesthetics and opiates: Increased CNS depression and risk of respiratory depression and hypotension
levodopa and other dopamine agonists: Possibly decreased therapeutic effects of these drugs
tricyclic antidepressants, such as desipramine, imipramine: Increased plasma concentrations of these drugs with increased risk of adverse reactions

ACTIVITIES

alcohol use: Increased CNS depression and risk of hypotension and respiratory depression

Adverse Reactions

CNS: Agitation, akinesia, anxiety, cogwheel rigidity, confusion, depression, dizziness, drowsiness, dystonia, euphoria, extrapyramidal reactions that may be irreversible, **hypothermia**, insomnia, masked facies, **neuroleptic malignant syndrome**, opisthotonus, parkinsonism, restlessness, **seizures**, slurred speech, somnolence, tremor, vertigo
CV: **Cardiac arrest**, edema, **extrasystoles**, hypertension, hypersensitivity vasculitis, orthostatic hypotension, **QT interval prolongation**, **ventricular arrhythmias**, tachycardia, **torsades de pointes**
EENT: Blurred vision, dry mouth, increased salivation (all drug forms), **laryngeal edema**, **laryngospasm**, nystagmus, oculogyric crisis, stomatitis (oral solution)
ENDO: Breast discomfort and engorgement, galactorrhea, gynecomastia, hyperprolactinemia, inappropriate antidiuretic hormone secretion
GI: **Acute hepatic failure**, cholestasis, constipation, elevated liver enzymes, **hepatitis**, jaundice, nausea, vomiting
GU: Decreased or loss of libido, difficult ejaculation, impotence, menstrual irregularities, priapism, urinary retention
HEME: **Agranulocytosis**, anemia, leukocytosis, **leukopenia**, **neutropenia**, **pancytopenia**, **thrombocytopenia**

MS: Muscle rigidity or twitching, **rhabdomyolysis**, torticollis, trismus
RESP: **Bronchospasm**, dyspnea
SKIN: Acneiform skin reactions, diaphoresis, **exfoliative dermatitis**, photosensitivity, pruritus, rash, urticaria
Other: **Anaphylaxis**, **angioedema**, **heatstroke**, other **hypersensitivity reactions**, weight gain or loss

Childbearing Considerations

PREGNANCY

- Drug may cause fetal harm with a potential increase risk for limb malformations when given during the first trimester of pregnancy.
- Neonates exposed to antipsychotic drugs such as haloperidol during the third trimester of pregnancy are at risk for extrapyramidal and/or withdrawal symptoms at birth.
- Use with caution only if benefit to mother outweighs potential risk to fetus.

LACTATION

- Drug is present in breast milk.
- Breastfeeding is not recommended during drug therapy.

Nursing Considerations

! **WARNING** Be aware that haloperidol shouldn't be used to treat dementia-related psychosis in the elderly because of an increased mortality risk.

! **WARNING** Use haloperidol cautiously in patients with a history of prolonged QT interval, patients with uncorrected electrolyte disturbances, and patients receiving class IA or III antiarrhythmics because of an increased risk of prolonged QT interval. Monitor elderly patients closely because they may have an increased risk of prolonged QT interval. Know that QT interval prolongation, sudden death, and torsades de pointes, although uncommon, may occur in patients receiving haloperidol despite the lack of predisposing factors.

- Be aware that haloperidol concentrations may increase in hepatically impaired patients. Monitor closely for adverse reactions.
- Know that if extrapyramidal reactions occur during the first few days of treatment, dosage should be reduced as prescribed. If symptoms persist, drug may need to be discontinued. Dystonia also may occur during first few days of treatment, especially in patients receiving higher doses and in males and younger age groups. Notify prescriber, if present.

! **WARNING** Monitor patient for a hypersensitivity reaction, which could become life-threatening, such as anaphylaxis or angioedema. If present, notify prescriber, expect drug to be discontinued, and provide supportive care as needed and ordered.

- Monitor CBC often during the first few months of therapy, as ordered, especially if patient has a low WBC count or history of drug-induced leukopenia or neutropenia. If WBC count drops, especially if neutrophil count drops below 1,000/mm^3, expect haloperidol to be discontinued. If neutropenia is significant, also monitor patient for fever or other symptoms of infection and provide appropriate treatment, as needed and ordered.

! **WARNING** Monitor for signs of neuroleptic malignant syndrome, a rare but possibly fatal disorder linked to antipsychotic drugs. Signs include altered mental status, arrhythmias, fever, and muscle rigidity.

! **WARNING** Be aware that if patient develops hypotension while receiving haloperidol therapy, and a vasopressor is required, epinephrine must not be used because haloperidol may block its vasopressor activity and paradoxically cause hypotension to worsen.

- Assess patient for fall risks, such those who are elderly and those with conditions or diseases or who are taking drugs that exacerbate CNS adverse effects, such as motor instability, orthostatic hypotension, and somnolence. Use fall precautions in patients at risk.
- Watch for tardive dyskinesia (potentially irreversible involuntary movements) in patients receiving long-term therapy, especially elderly women who take large doses.
- Avoid stopping haloperidol abruptly unless severe adverse reactions occur because withdrawal emergent dyskinesia may occur.

PATIENT TEACHING

- Instruct patient how to administer the form of haloperidol prescribed.
- Advise patient to take haloperidol exactly as prescribed and not to stop taking drug abruptly because withdrawal symptoms may occur.

! **WARNING** Alert patient that haloperidol may cause an allergic reaction. If present, patient should notify prescriber and, if severe, seek immediate medical care.

! **WARNING** Tell patient to notify prescriber of any persistent, serious, or unusual adverse reactions.

! **WARNING** Alert females of childbearing age to notify prescriber immediately if pregnancy occurs.

- Instruct patient to consume adequate fluids and to take precautions against heatstroke.
- Urge patient not to drink alcohol during therapy.
- Caution patient to avoid driving and other hazardous activities if sedation occurs until resolved. Also, warn patient to take measures to avoid falls because of adverse effects.
- Instruct patient to report repetitive movements, tremor, and vision changes.
- Inform mothers that breastfeeding should not be undertaken during drug therapy.

heparin sodium

Heparin Lock Flush, Heparin Sodium Injection

Class and Category

Pharmacologic class: Anticoagulant
Therapeutic class: Anticoagulant

Indications and Dosages

∗ *To prevent and treat pulmonary embolism and venous thrombosis; to prevent postoperative deep venous thrombosis and pulmonary embolism in patients undergoing major abdominothoracic surgery or who, for other reasons, are at risk of developing thromboembolic disease; to treat atrial fibrillation with embolization; to treat acute and chronic consumptive coagulopathies (disseminated intravascular coagulation)*

FULL-DOSE I.V. INJECTION, FULL-DOSE I.V. INFUSION

Adults receiving continuous intravenous therapy. *Initial:* 5,000 units by I.V. injection followed by 20,000 to 40,000 units infused per 24 hr.
Children ages 1 yr and older. *Initial:* 75 to 100 units/kg by I.V. injection over 10 min followed by infusion of 18 to 20 units/kg/hr.
Infants ages 2 mo to 1 yr. *Initial:* 75 to 100 units/kg by I.V. injection given over 10 min followed by infusion of 25 to 30 units/kg/hr.
Infants less than 2 mo. *Initial:* 75 to 100 mg/kg by I.V. injection given over 10 min followed by individualized infusion with average of 28 units/kg/hr.
Adults receiving intermittent intravenous therapy. *Initial:* 10,000 units followed by 5,000 to 10,000 units every 4 to 6 hr.

FULL-DOSE SUBCUTANEOUS INJECTION

Adults. *Initial:* 5,000 units by I.V. injection and 10,000 to 20,000 units subcutaneously with a concentrated solution; then 8,000 to 10,000 units subcutaneously with a concentrated solution every 8 hr or 15,000 to 20,000 units subcutaneously with a concentrated solution every 12 hr.

∗ *To prevent postoperative thromboembolism*

LOW-DOSE SUBCUTANEOUS INJECTION

Adults. 5,000 units 2 hr before surgery and then 5,000 units every 8 to 12 hr for 7 days or until patient is fully ambulatory, whichever is longer.

∗ *To prevent clots in patients undergoing cardiovascular surgery*

I.V. INFUSION OR INJECTION

Adults. Undergoing total body perfusion for open-heart surgery. *Initial:* Not less than 150 units/kg. *Usual:* 300 units/kg for procedures that last less than 60 min; 400 units/kg for procedures that last longer than 60 min.

∗ *To provide anticoagulation with blood transfusions*

I.V. INFUSION

Adults. 400 to 600 units/100 ml of whole blood.

∗ *To provide anticoagulation with extracorporeal dialysis*

I.V. INFUSION, I.V. INJECTION

Adults. *Loading:* 25 to 30 units/kg by I.V. injection followed by infusion of 1,500 to 2,000 units/hr.

∗ *To maintain heparin lock patency*

I.V. INJECTION

Adults. 10 or 100 units/ml heparin flush solution (enough to fill device) after each use of device.

±**DOSAGE ADJUSTMENT** For patients over age 60, especially women, because of an increased risk of bleeding, dosage possibly decreased.

Drug Administration

- Know that vial of heparin must state the strength of the entire container of heparin, followed by how much heparin is in 1 ml. To lessen risk of a drug error, look for the red cautionary label that extends above the main label. Read and confirm that the correct medication and strength have been selected. Remove red cautionary label prior to removing the flip-off cap.
- Never administer heparin by I.M. route.
- Don't use heparin sodium injection as a catheter-lock flush because fatal errors have occurred. Do not confuse 1-ml heparin sodium injection vials with 1-ml catheter-lock flush vials. Always examine vial labels closely to ensure that correct product is being used.
- Some heparin products contain benzyl alcohol and should not be used in pregnant women, neonates, infants, or mothers who are breastfeeding; instead use preservative-free Heparin Sodium Injection.

I.V.

Heparin Sodium Injection

- Concentrated heparin solutions contain more than 100 units/ml, which can irritate blood vessels.
- For continuous infusion, invert container at least 6 times to ensure adequate mixing and to prevent drug from pooling. Solution should appear clear and the seal intact.
- Use an infusion pump.
- During continuous I.V. therapy, expect to obtain APTT before therapy begins to obtain a baseline and then every 4 hr, or as ordered after therapy begins. Use the arm opposite the infusion site.
- For I.V. injection, expect to adjust dose based on coagulation test results performed 30 min before each injection during initiation and then at ordered intervals. Therapeutic range is typically 1.5 to 2.5 times the control.
- Expect to adjust the heparin dose based on frequent blood coagulation tests, as ordered, when patient is receiving a full-dose heparin regimen. If coagulation test is unduly prolonged or hemorrhage occurs, heparin should be discontinued immediately.
- Do not piggyback other drugs while heparin infusion is being administered and do not mix other drugs with heparin in the same syringe when giving heparin as an I.V. injection.

Heparin Lock Flush

- Make sure product being used is heparin lock flush and not heparin sodium injection.
- Use enough flush to fill entire device.
- If a drug is known to be incompatible with heparin, the entire device should be flushed with 0.9% Sodium Chloride Injection before and after the medication is given; followed by a second saline flush. Then, a heparin lock flush should be reinstalled into the device.
- Clear heparin solution from device before withdrawing blood sample if heparin may interfere with test results.
- *Incompatibilities:* Alteplase, amikacin sulfate, atracurium besylate, ciprofloxacin, cytarabine, daunorubicin, droperidol, erythromycin lactobionate, gentamicin sulfate, idarubicin, kanamycin sulfate, mitoxantrone HCl, polymyxin B sulfate, promethazine HCl, streptomycin sulfate, tobramycin sulfate

SUBCUTANEOUS

- Inject into anterior abdominal wall, above the iliac crest, and 5 cm (2 in) or more away from the umbilicus.
- To minimize subcutaneous tissue trauma, lift adipose tissue away from deep tissues; don't aspirate for blood before injecting drug; don't move needle while injecting drug; and don't massage injection site before or after injection. Apply gentle pressure to the site after withdrawing needle.
- Alternate injection sites and watch for signs of bleeding and hematomas.
- Expect blood samples to be drawn 4 to 6 hr after each injection to determine adequacy of dosage.

Route	Onset	Peak	Duration
I.V.	Immediate	Immediate	2–6 hr
SubQ	20–60 min	2–4 hr	8–12 hr

Half-life: 60–90 min

Mechanism of Action

Binds with antithrombin III, enhancing antithrombin III's inactivation of the coagulation enzymes thrombin (factor IIa) and factors Xa and XIa. At low doses, heparin inhibits factor Xa and prevents conversion of prothrombin to thrombin. Thrombin is needed for conversion of fibrinogen to fibrin; without fibrin, clots can't form. At high doses, heparin inactivates thrombin, preventing fibrin formation and existing clot extension.

Contraindications

Breastfeeding, infants, neonates, or pregnant woman (heparin sodium injection, USP, preserved with benzyl alcohol); history of heparin-induced thrombocytopenia or heparin-induced thrombocytopenia and thrombosis, or thrombocytopenia with pentosan polysulfate; hypersensitivity to heparin, pork, or its components; inability to monitor coagulation parameters when full-dose heparin is used; uncontrolled active bleeding, except in disseminated intravascular coagulation (DIC)

Interactions

DRUGS

antihistamines, digoxin, nicotine, nitroglycerin (I.V.), tetracyclines: Decreased anticoagulant effect of heparin
antithrombin III (human): Increased risk of bleeding
aspirin, dextran, dipyridamole, glycoprotein IIb/IIIa antagonists, hydroxychloroquine, NSAIDs, phenylbutazone, platelet aggregation inhibitors, thienopyridines: Increased platelet inhibition and risk of bleeding
dicumarol, warfarin: Possibly invalid PT if blood drawn sooner than 5 hr after last intravenous dose or 24 hr after last subcutaneous dose of heparin
ethacrynic acid, glucocorticoids, salicylates: Increased risk of bleeding

ACTIVITIES

smoking: Decreased anticoagulant effect

Adverse Reactions

CNS: Chills, dizziness, fever, headache, peripheral neuropathy
CV: Chest pain, rebound hyperlipemia on discontinuation of heparin, **thrombosis**, vasospastic reactions including episodes of painful, ischemic, and cyanosed extremities
EENT: Epistaxis, gingival bleeding, rhinitis
ENDO: **Adrenal hemorrhage causing acute adrenal insufficiency**
GI: Abdominal distention and pain, elevated liver enzymes, **hematemesis**, **melena**, nausea, **retroperitoneal hemorrhage**, vomiting
GU: Hematuria, hypermenorrhea, **ovarian hemorrhage**, priapism
HEME: **Delayed onset of heparin-induced thrombocytopenia**, easy bruising, **excessive bleeding from wounds**, **hemorrhage**, **heparin-induced thrombocytopenia**, **heparin-induced thrombocytopenia and thrombosis**, **thrombocytopenia**
MS: Back pain, myalgia, osteoporosis (long-term use of high doses)
RESP: **Asthma**, dyspnea, wheezing
SKIN: Alopecia, cutaneous necrosis following subcutaneous injection, cyanosis, erythema, petechiae, pruritus, urticaria
Other: **Anaphylaxis and other hypersensitivity reactions** (**asthma**, chills, fever, rhinitis, urticaria); **heparin resistance**; histamine-like reactions at injection site, including necrosis and ulceration of the skin; **hyperkalemia**; injection-site hematoma, irritation, pain, redness, and ulceration

Childbearing Considerations

PREGNANCY

- It is not known if drug causes fetal harm.
- Use with caution only if benefit to mother outweighs potential risk to fetus.
- Use preservative-free Heparin Sodium Injection during pregnancy.

LACTATION

- It is not known if drug is present in breast milk.
- Mothers should check with prescriber before breastfeeding.
- If mother is breastfeeding, use preservative-free Heparin Sodium Injection.

Nursing Considerations

- Expect to obtain platelet counts before heparin therapy begins and then periodically monitor patient's hematocrit, platelet counts, and occult blood in stool, as ordered, during the entire course of heparin therapy, regardless of the route of administration. Also, monitor patient's blood coagulation test results frequently because the heparin dosage in a full dose heparin regimen is based on these results. Notify prescriber if the coagulation test is abnormal as dosage may need to be adjusted or heparin will need to be discontinued.

! **WARNING** Obtain a plasma potassium level before heparin therapy begins and periodically thereafter in all patients, as ordered, especially if heparin therapy lasts for more than 5 days. This is because heparin may suppress the adrenal secretion of aldosterone, which can result in hyperkalemia. Patients at higher risk include patients with chronic renal failure or diabetes mellitus as well as patients with preexisting metabolic acidosis or an elevated plasma potassium level, or in patients who are taking potassium sparing drugs, Be aware that the risk of hyperkalemia increases the longer heparin therapy is needed but is usually reversible when heparin is discontinued.

! **WARNING** Use only heparin lock flush to maintain heparin lock patency as use of any other heparin product can result in a fatal medication error. Carefully examine the heparin product to confirm the correct one is being used prior to administration.

- Keep protamine sulfate on hand to use as an antidote for heparin. Be aware that each milligram of protamine sulfate neutralizes 100 units of heparin.

! **WARNING** Monitor patient for a hypersensitivity reaction to heparin, which could become life-threatening, such as anaphylaxis. Patients at higher risk for a life-threatening reaction are those with asthma because heparin contains a sulfite which can induce an asthmatic episode. However, an allergic reaction to sulfite also may occur in a patient who does not have asthma. Know that chills, fever, and urticaria are the most usual allergic manifestations with anaphylactoid reactions (including shock), asthma, headache, lacrimation, nausea, rhinitis, and vomiting occurring less often. Burning and itching, especially on the plantar site of the feet may occur. If a hypersensitivity reaction is present, notify prescriber immediately, expect a different anticoagulant to be ordered, and provide supportive care, as needed and ordered.

! **WARNING** Know that bleeding is a major adverse effect of heparin therapy. Take safety precautions to prevent bleeding, such as having patient use a soft-bristled toothbrush and an electric razor. Bleeding may occur at any site and also may indicate an underlying problem, such as GI or urinary tract bleeding. Other sites of bleeding that could be fatal and require immediate attention include adrenal, ovarian, and retroperitoneal hemorrhage. Report an unexplained fall in blood pressure or hematocrit immediately to prescriber as these are potential warning signs that a hemorrhagic condition may be present.

! **WARNING** Be aware that patients with a higher risk of bleeding include alcoholics; menstruating women; patients over age 60, especially women; and patients with conditions that increase risk of hemorrhage, such as certain cardiovascular conditions (severe hypertension, subacute bacterial endocarditis), GI conditions (continuous tube drainage of small intestine or stomach, ulcerative lesions), hematologic conditions that increase risk of bleeding (hemophilia, thrombocytopenia, some vascular purpuras), liver disease with impaired hemostasis, presence of hereditary antithrombin III deficiency in patients receiving concurrent antithrombin III therapy, or presence of indwelling catheters, severe renal disease, and during or immediately following major surgery (especially involving the brain, eye, or spinal cord) or following spinal anesthesia or spinal tap.

- Watch closely if patient is receiving heparin therapy and nitroglycerin I.V. because partial thromboplastin time (PTT) may decrease and then rebound after nitroglycerin is discontinued. Monitor PTT closely, and be prepared to adjust heparin dose, as prescribed.

! **WARNING** Be aware that heparin-induced thrombocytopenia (HIT) can occur in patients exposed to heparin, including delayed onset, and is due to the development of antibodies to a platelet factor 4-heparin complex. A drop in patelet count that is more than 50% from baseline indicates the presence of HIT. It may progress to the development of arterial and venous thromboses. Monitor blood test results, and observe for signs of bleeding, such as ecchymosis, epistaxis, hematemesis, hematuria, melena, and petechiae. Thrombocytopenia of any degree can occur 2 to 20 days following the onset of heparin therapy, so patient should be monitored closely. If platelet count drops below 100,000/mm^3 or recurrent thrombosis develops, notify prescriber and expect heparin to be discontinued.

- Avoid injecting any drugs by I.M. route during heparin therapy to decrease risk of bleeding and hematoma.
- Be aware that heparin resistance may occur, especially in patients with antithrombin III deficiency, cancer, fever, infections with thrombosing tendencies, MI, thrombophlebitis, or thrombosis and post-surgery. Monitor coagulation tests closely in these patients and expect an adjustment in the heparin dose, as needed. If heparin resistance is suspected, expect the prescriber to measure antithrombin levels to confirm diagnosis.
- Make sure all healthcare providers know that patient is receiving heparin.
- Be aware that prescriber may order oral anticoagulants before discontinuing heparin to avoid increased coagulation caused by heparin withdrawal. Heparin may be discontinued when full therapeutic effect of oral anticoagulant is achieved.

PATIENT TEACHING

- Explain that heparin can't be taken orally. Inform patient how heparin will be administered.

! **WARNING** Alert patient that heparin may cause an allergic reaction or if patient has asthma, an asthmatic attack may occur. Tell patient to notify staff immediately if an allergic reaction or an asthmatic attack occurs after beginning heparin therapy.

! **WARNING** Instruct patient, family, or caregiver to watch for and report abdominal or lower back pain, black stools, bleeding gums, bloody urine, excessive menstrual bleeding, nosebleeds, and severe headaches. Also, tell patient to report any persistent, severe, or unusual signs and symptoms to prescriber immediately. Alert patient receiving heparin subcutaneously that necrosis of the skin has been reported following subcutaneous administration of heparin and to alert prescriber if any abnormalities occur at injection sites.

- Review bleeding precautions with patient such as avoiding injuries and to use a soft-bristled toothbrush and an electric razor. Also, advise patient to avoid drugs that increase risk of bleeding, such as aspirin and ibuprofen.

! **WARNING** Review signs and symptoms of hyperkalemia with patient and to notify prescriber if present.

- Inform patient that delayed adverse reactions may occur, even weeks after heparin has been discontinued and to notify prescriber if any occur.
- Stress importance of complying with frequent laboratory tests, as ordered.
- Explain that temporary hair loss may occur.

hydralazine hydrochloride

Apresoline (CAN)

Class and Category

Pharmacologic class: Vasodilator
Therapeutic class: Antihypertensive

Indications and Dosages

∗ *To manage essential hypertension, alone or with other antihypertensives*

TABLETS

Adults. *Initial:* 10 mg 4 times daily for first 2 to 4 days and then increased to 25 mg 4 times daily for remainder of first wk. Further increased to 50 mg 4 times daily beginning wk 2 and thereafter. *Maintenance:* 50 to 200 mg daily in divided doses. *Maximum:* 300 mg daily.

∗ *To manage severe essential hypertension when drug can't be taken orally or when need to reduce blood pressure is urgent*

I.V. INJECTION

Adults. 10 to 20 mg and repeated every 4 to 6 hr, as needed. Alternatively, 20 to 40 mg repeated as needed.

I.M. INJECTION

Adults. 20 to 40 mg repeated as needed.

±**DOSAGE ADJUSTMENT** For adult patients with marked renal impairment, dosage may have to be reduced. For slow acetylators, dosage may have to be reduced or dosage frequency changed.

Drug Administration

P.O.

- Do not use if blister is torn or broken.
- Administer with or without food but be consistent.

I.V.

- I.V. route used only if oral administration is not feasible.
- Solution may become discolored if in contact with metal. If solution is discolored, discard.
- Administer immediately after vial is opened. Inject undiluted rapidly.
- *Incompatibilities:* None reported by manufacturer

I.M.

- Administer undiluted.
- Rotate sites.

Route	Onset	Peak	Duration
P.O.	20–30 min	1–2 hr	3–8 hr
I.V.	5–20 min	10–80 min	1–4 hr
I.M.	10–30 min	1 hr	2–6 hr

Half-life: 3–7 hr

Mechanism of Action

May act in a manner that resembles organic nitrates and sodium nitroprusside, except that hydralazine is selective for arteries. It:

- exerts a direct vasodilating effect on vascular smooth muscle.
- interferes with calcium movement in vascular smooth muscle by altering cellular calcium metabolism.
- dilates arteries, not veins, which minimizes orthostatic hypotension and increases cardiac output and cerebral blood flow.
- causes reflex autonomic response that increases, cardiac output, heart rate, and left ventricular ejection fraction.
- has a positive inotropic effect on the heart.

Contraindications

Coronary artery disease, hypersensitivity to hydralazine or its components, mitral valvular rheumatic heart disease

Interactions

DRUGS

diazoxide, MAO inhibitors, other antihypertensives: Risk of severe hypotension
NSAIDs: Decreased hydralazine effects

FOODS

all foods: Possibly increased bioavailability of hydralazine

Adverse Reactions

CNS: Chills, fever, headache, peripheral neuritis
CV: Angina, edema, orthostatic hypotension, palpitations, tachycardia
EENT: Lacrimation, nasal congestion
GI: Anorexia, constipation, diarrhea, nausea, vomiting
RESP: Dyspnea
SKIN: Blisters, flushing, pruritus, rash, urticaria
Other: Lupus-like symptoms, especially with high doses; lymphadenopathy

Childbearing Considerations

PREGNANCY

- It is not known if drug causes fetal harm.
- Use with caution only if benefit to mother outweighs potential risk to fetus.

LACTATION

- Drug is present in breast milk.
- Mothers should check with prescriber before breastfeeding.

Nursing Considerations

- Evaluate ANA titer, CBC, and lupus erythematosus cell preparation results before therapy begins and monitor periodically, as ordered, during long-term treatment.

! WARNING Expect to discontinue drug immediately if patient has lupus-like symptoms, such as arthralgia, fever, myalgia, pharyngitis, and splenomegaly.

- Monitor blood pressure and pulse rate regularly and weigh patient daily during therapy. Check blood pressure with patient in lying, sitting, and standing positions, and watch for signs of orthostatic hypotension. Expect orthostatic hypotension to be most common in the morning, during hot weather, and with exercise.

! **WARNING** Expect prescriber to withdraw hydralazine gradually to avoid a rapid increase in blood pressure.

PATIENT TEACHING

- Instruct patient how to administer hydralazine.

! **WARNING** Caution patient against stopping drug abruptly because doing so may cause severe hypertension.

! **WARNING** Instruct patient to immediately notify prescriber about fever, joint and muscle aches, and sore throat.

- Advise patient to change position slowly, especially in the morning. Caution that hot showers may increase orthostatic hypotension.
- Urge patient to report numbness and tingling in limbs, which may require treatment with another drug.

hydrochlorothiazide

Microzide, Urozide (CAN)

Class and Category

Pharmacologic class: Thiazide diuretic
Therapeutic class: Diuretic

Indications and Dosages

∗ *To manage hypertension as monotherapy or as adjunct with other antihypertensive drugs in more severe forms of hypertension*

CAPSULES

Adults. *Initial:* 12.5 to 25 mg daily increased, as needed, to 50 mg daily given as a single dose or 2 divided doses. *Maximum:* 50 mg daily.

TABLETS

Adults. *Initial:* 25 mg once daily, increased to 50 mg daily, as needed, and given as a single dose or in divided doses twice daily.
Children ages 2 to 12. 100 mg daily.
Children ages 6 mo to 2 yr. 1 to 2 mg/kg daily as a single dose or 2 divided doses. *Maximum:* 37.5 mg daily.
Infants less than 6 mo of age. Up to 3 mg/kg daily in 2 divided doses. *Maximum:* 37.5 mg daily.

∗ *As adjunct to treat edema caused by cirrhosis, corticosteroids, estrogen, heart failure, or renal disorders*

TABLETS

Adults. 25 to 100 mg daily given as a single dose or divided and given twice daily. Alternatively, dosage given intermittently on alternate days or given 3 to 5 days each wk.
Children ages 2 to 12. 100 mg daily.
Children ages 6 mo to 2 yr. 1 to 2 mg/kg daily as a single dose or 2 divided doses. *Maximum:* 37.5 mg daily.
Infants less than 6 mo of age. Up to 3 mg/kg daily in 2 divided doses. *Maximum:* 37.5 mg daily.

Drug Administration

P.O.

- Capsules and tablets should be swallowed whole and not chewed, crushed, or opened.
- Administer once-daily dose in morning; twice-daily dose in morning and late afternoon.
- Administer with food or milk if GI upset occurs.

Route	Onset	Peak	Duration
P.O.	2 hr	4 hr	6–12 hr

Half-life: 6–15 hr

Contraindications

Anuria; hypersensitivity to hydrochlorothiazide, other thiazides, sulfonamide derivatives, or their components

Interactions

DRUGS

ACTH, corticosteroids: Increased electrolyte depletion, especially potassium
antihypertensives: Increased antihypertensive effects
barbiturates, opioids: Possibly orthostatic hypotension
cholestyramine, colestipol: Reduced GI absorption of hydrochlorothiazide
insulin, oral antidiabetic drugs: Possibly increased blood glucose level
lithium: Decreased lithium clearance, increased risk of lithium toxicity
nondepolarizing skeletal muscle relaxants: Possibly increased response to muscle relaxants

GHI

Mechanism of Action

A thiazide diuretic, hydrochlorothiazide promotes movement of sodium (Na^+), chloride (Cl^-), and water (H_2O) from blood in peritubular capillaries into nephron's distal convoluted tubule, as shown. Initially, it may decrease cardiac output, extracellular fluid volume, or plasma volume, which helps explain blood pressure reduction. It also may reduce blood pressure by direct arterial dilation. After several weeks, cardiac output, extracellular fluid volume, and plasma volume return to normal, and peripheral vascular resistance remains decreased.

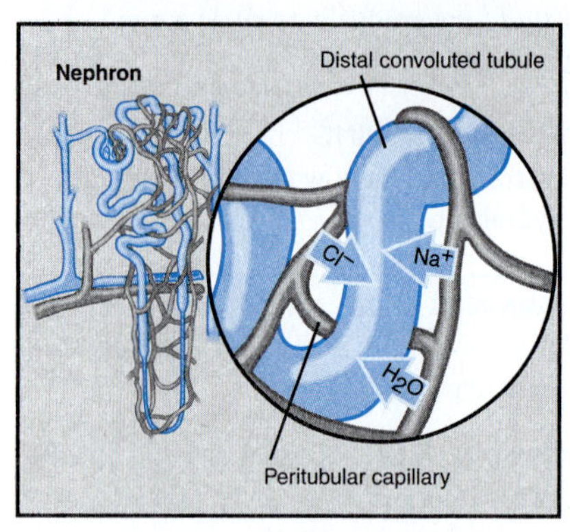

NSAIDs: Decreased diuretic effect of hydrochlorothiazide, increased risk of renal failure

ACTIVITIES

alcohol use: Possibly orthostatic hypotension

Adverse Reactions

CNS: Asthenia, dizziness, fever, headache, insomnia, paresthesia, restlessness, vertigo, weakness

CV: Elevated cholesterol and triglycerides levels, **hypotension**, orthostatic hypotension, vasculitis

EENT: Acute myopia, acute angle-closure glaucoma, blurred vision, dry mouth

ENDO: Hyperglycemia

GI: Abdominal cramps, anorexia, constipation, diarrhea, indigestion, jaundice, nausea, **pancreatitis**, vomiting

GU: Decreased libido, impotence, interstitial nephritis, nocturia, polyuria, **renal failure**

HEME: **Agranulocytosis**, **aplastic anemia**, **bone marrow failure**, **hemolytic anemia**, **leukopenia**, **neutropenia**, **thrombocytopenia**

MS: Muscle spasms and weakness

RESP: **Pneumonitis**, **pulmonary edema**

SKIN: Alopecia, cutaneous vasculitis, **erythema multiforme**, **exfoliative dermatitis**, **nonmelanoma skin cancer**, photosensitivity, purpura, rash, **Stevens-Johnson syndrome**, **toxic epidermal necrolysis**, urticaria

Other: **Anaphylaxis**, dehydration, **hypercalcemia**, hyperuricemia, hypochloremia, **hypokalemia**, **hypomagnesemia**, **hyponatremia**, hypovolemia, **metabolic alkalosis**, weight loss

Childbearing Considerations

PREGNANCY

- It is not known if drug causes fetal harm but because it crosses the placental barrier, there is a risk of fetal or neonatal jaundice, thrombocytopenia, and possibly other adverse reactions.
- Use with caution only if benefit to mother outweighs potential risk to fetus.

LACTATION

- Drug is present in breast milk.
- A decision should be made to discontinue breastfeeding or the drug to avoid potential serious adverse reactions in the breastfed infant.

Nursing Considerations

! **WARNING** Monitor patient for a hypersensitivity reaction, which could become life-threatening, such as anaphylaxis. If present, notify prescriber, expect drug to be discontinued, and provide supportive care, as needed and ordered.

! **WARNING** Monitor patient's electrolytes regularly as ordered because drug can cause electrolyte disturbances. Also, assess patient regularly for signs and symptoms of an electrolyte imbalance, especially hypokalemia exhibited by muscle spasms and weakness.

! WARNING Be aware that even minor alterations in fluid and electrolyte balance may precipitate hepatic coma in patients with impaired hepatic function.

! WARNING Monitor BUN and serum creatinine levels, as ordered, especially in patients with chronic kidney disease, renal artery stenosis, severe congestive heart failure, or volume depletion because of increased risk of acute renal failure with hydrochlorothiazide therapy. Notify prescriber if serum creatinine levels become elevated, as drug may have to be withheld or discontinued.

- Monitor blood pressure, weight, and fluid intake and output daily.
- Monitor patient for decreased visual acuity or ocular pain, especially within hours to weeks of beginning drug therapy and in patients with a history of penicillin or sulfonamide allergy, as acute myopia and acute angle-closure glaucoma may develop. If left untreated, permanent blindness may occur. If present, notify prescriber immediately, expect to discontinue hydrochlorothiazide, and assist with prompt medical or surgical intervention, as indicated.
- Check blood glucose level often, as ordered, in diabetic patients, and expect to increase antidiabetic dosage, as needed and prescribed.
- Know that if patient has gouty arthritis, expect increased risk of gout attacks during therapy.

PATIENT TEACHING

- Advise patient how to administer hydrochlorothiazide.
- Tell patient to weigh herself at the same time each day wearing the same amount of clothing and to notify prescriber if she gains more than 0.9 kg (2 lb) per day or 2.3 kg (5 lb) per week.
- Instruct patient to eat a diet high in potassium-rich food, including bananas, citrus fruits, dates, and tomatoes to avoid a low potassium level.

! WARNING Alert patient that drug may cause an allergic reaction. If present, tell patient to notify prescriber and, if severe, to seek immediate medical attention.

! WARNING Urge patient to report any persistent, serious, or unusual adverse reactions such as decreased urination, muscle cramps and weakness, and unusual bleeding or bruising.

- Advise patient to change position slowly to minimize effects of orthostatic hypotension.
- Advise patient to protect skin from the sun and undergo regular skin cancer screening.
- Stress importance of complying with laboratory appointments.
- Inform mothers that breastfeeding should not be undertaken during hydrochlorothiazide therapy or drug will need to be discontinued.

hydrocodone bitartrate

Hysingla ER

Class, Category, and Schedule

Pharmacologic class: Opioid
Therapeutic class: Opioid analgesic
Controlled substance schedule: II

Indications and Dosages

✷ *To manage severe pain in patients requiring continuous, around-the-clock opioid analgesia for an extended period of time and for which alternative treatment options are inadequate*

E.R. CAPSULES

Adults who are opioid naïve or opioid nontolerant. *Initial:* 10 mg every 12 hr, increased, as needed, in increments of 10 mg every 12 hr every 3 to 7 days to effective and tolerable dose. *Maximum:* 40 mg/dose or 80 mg total daily dose.
Adults who are opioid tolerant and converting from another opioid. Highly individualized.

± **DOSAGE ADJUSTMENT** For patients with severe hepatic impairment, a single dose of 10 mg given, followed by close monitoring for respiratory depression and sedation. If single dose tolerated, 10 mg every 12 hr, as needed, and titrated carefully.

E.R. TABLETS (HYSINGLA ER)

Adults who are opioid naïve or opioid nontolerant. *Initial:* 20 mg every 24 hr, increased, as needed, in increments of 10 to 20 mg daily every 3 to 5 days to effective and tolerable dose. *Maximum:* 80 mg every 24 hr. **Adults who are opioid tolerant and converting from another opioid.** Highly individualized.

±DOSAGE ADJUSTMENT For patients with moderate or severe renal impairment, including end-stage renal disease or severe hepatic impairment, initial dosage decreased by half.

Drug Administration

P.O.

- Tablets and capsules should be swallowed whole and not chewed, crushed, dissolved, or split/opened.
- Administer with enough water to ensure complete swallowing immediately after patient places drug in mouth.
- Have patient take capsules and tablets one at a time.
- Naloxone should always be readily available with hydrocodone administration.

Route	Onset	Peak	Duration
P.O./E.R. tab	Unknown	6–30 hr	Unknown
P.O./E.R. cap	Unknown	5 hr	Unknown

Half-life: 7–12 hr

Mechanism of Action

Binds to and activates opioid receptors at sites in the periaqueductal and periventricular gray matter, the ventromedial medulla, and the spinal cord to produce pain relief.

Contraindications

Acute or severe bronchial asthma (in an unmonitored setting or in the absence of resuscitative equipment); hypersensitivity to hydrocodone bitartrate or any of its components; known or suspected GI obstruction, including paralytic ileus; significant respiratory depression

Interactions

DRUGS

5-HT$_3$ receptor antagonists, drugs that affect the serotonin neurotransmitter system (mirtazapine, trazodone, tramadol), linezolid, methylene blue (I.V.), selective serotonin reuptake inhibitors, serotonin and norepinephrine reuptake inhibitors, tricyclic antidepressants triptans, tryptophan: Increased risk of serotonin syndrome

anticholinergics: Increased risk of urinary retention or severe constipation, which may lead to paralytic ileus

antipsychotics, anxiolytics, benzodiazepines and other CNS depressants, general anesthetics, muscle relaxants, other opioids and sedatives/hypnotics, sedating antihistamines, tranquilizers, tricyclic antidepressants: Increased risk of coma, hypotension, profound sedation, and severe respiratory depression

CYP3A4 inducers: Increased clearance of hydrocodone with decreased effectiveness

CYP3A4 inhibitors: Decreased clearance of hydrocodone resulting in increased or prolonged opioid effects

diuretics: Possible reduction of the effectiveness of diuretics

MAO inhibitors: Increased risk of serotonin syndrome or opioid toxicity

mixed agonist/antagonist analgesics such as buprenorphine, butorphanol, nalbuphine, pentazocine: Possible reduced hydrocodone effectiveness or precipitation of withdrawal symptoms

muscle relaxants: Enhanced neuromuscular blocking action of skeletal muscle relaxants producing increased degree of respiratory depression

ACTIVITIES

alcohol use: Possibly increased hydrocodone plasma levels with potentially fatal overdose

Adverse Reactions

CNS: Anxiety, **CNS depression**, **coma**, depression, dizziness, fatigue, fever, headache, insomnia, lethargy, migraine, paresthesia, **seizures**, somnolence, syncope, tremor

CV: Hypercholesterolemia, **hypotension**, peripheral edema

EENT: Dry mouth

ENDO: **Adrenal insufficiency** (rare), hot flashes, **hypoglycemia**

GI: Abdominal discomfort or pain, constipation (may be severe), elevated liver enzymes, gastroesophageal reflux disease,

nausea, spasm of the Sphincter of Oddi, vomiting
GU: Decreased libido, erectile dysfunction, impotence, infertility, lack of menstruation, UTI
MS: Arthralgia; back, extremity, musculoskeletal, or neck pain; muscle spasms
RESP: Cough, dyspnea, **respiratory depression**
SKIN: Pruritus, rash, sweating (night sweats)
Other: Dehydration, **hypokalemia**, noncardiac chest pain, opioid-induced allodynia and hyperalgesia, physical and psychological dependence

Childbearing Considerations

PREGNANCY

- Drug may cause fetal harm.
- Prolonged use of drug during pregnancy can result in neonatal opioid withdrawal syndrome (NOWS) after birth, which may be life-threatening if not recognized and treated.
- Prolonged use during pregnancy should be avoided. Use with caution only if benefit to mother outweighs potential risk to fetus.

LABOR AND DELIVERY

- Drug is not recommended for use in pregnant women immediately before or during labor. Opioids may alter length of time of labor.
- Opioids cross the placental barrier and may produce respiratory depression and psychophysiologic effects in the newborn. Monitor newborn closely for signs of excess sedation and respiratory depression.
- An opioid antagonist, such as naloxone, must be available at the time of delivery in the event it is needed to reverse opioid-induced respiratory depression in the neonate.

LACTATION

- Drug is present in breast milk.
- Breastfeeding should not be undertaken during drug therapy. However, if mother does breastfeed, monitor infant for excess sedation and respiratory depression. Know that when mother stops drug or breastfeeding, infant may experience withdrawal symptoms.

REPRODUCTION

- Chronic use of opioids may reduce fertility in females and males.

Nursing Considerations

! WARNING Be aware that opioids like hydrocodone should not be given to women during pregnancy for an extended period of time and, while in labor as the newborn or infant may experience neonatal opioid withdrawal syndrome (NOWS), which could be life-threatening. This syndrome may exhibit as excessive or high-pitched crying, poor feeding, rapid breathing, or trembling. If not recognized and treated appropriately, it can become life-threatening.

! WARNING Know that hydrocodone should not be given to a patient with impaired consciousness, nor should the drug be administered on an as-needed basis.

! WARNING Be aware that hydrocodone increases the risk of abuse, addiction, and misuse. Know that to ensure that the benefits of hydrocodone therapy outweigh the risks, a Risk Evaluation and Mitigation Strategy (REMS) is required. Monitor patient for evidence of physical dependence or abuse. Know that addiction can occur not only in those who obtain the drug illicitly but also in patients who are appropriately prescribed the drug at recommended doses. Be aware that excessive use of hydrocodone may not only lead to abuse, addiction, and misuse, it can lead to overdose, and possibly death. Monitor patient's intake of drug closely.

- Be aware that patients who are considered opioid tolerant are those who have received for 1 week or longer, at least 8 mg of oral hydromorphone per day, 60 mg of oral morphine daily, 30 mg of oral oxycodone per day, 25 mg of oral oxymorphone per day, 25 mcg transdermal fentanyl per hour, or an equianalgesic dose of another opioid.

! WARNING Do not administer hydrocodone to a patient wearing a transdermal fentanyl patch until the patch has been removed for 18 hours. Also, know that close monitoring is especially important for a patient converting from methadone because methadone has a long half-life and tends to accumulate in the blood.

! **WARNING** Be aware that hydrocodone available as an extended-release formulation increases risk of overdose and death because of larger amount of drug present in this form. Also, know that crushing, chewing, snorting, or injecting the contents of the Hysingla E.R. tablet dissolved in a liquid base will result in the uncontrolled delivery of hydrocodone and can result in overdose and death. Be aware that E.R. capsules are made with a formulation that deters abuse because it forms an immediate inactive viscous gel when crushed or dissolved in liquids or solvents.

- Monitor effectiveness of hydrocodone in relieving pain; consult prescriber as needed.
- Monitor patient for a paradoxic increase in pain known as opioid-induced hyperalgesia or an increase in sensitivity to pain known as opioid-induced allodynia, especially when hydrocodone dosage increases. Do not confuse this with tolerance, which is the need for increasing doses of opioids to maintain an effect. If opioid-induced allodynia and hyperalgesia is suspected, notify prescriber and expect dosage to be decreased or opioid rotation to be prescribed.

! **WARNING** Use extreme caution when administering hydrocodone to patients with significant chronic obstructive pulmonary disease or cor pulmonale, and in patients having a substantially decreased respiratory reserve, hypoxia, hypercapnia, or preexisting respiratory depression, especially when initiating or titrating therapy. These patients may develop respiratory depression, even with usual therapeutic doses because hydrocodone may decrease the patient's respiratory drive to the point of apnea.

! **WARNING** Use hydrocodone cautiously in cachectic, debilitated or elderly patients, especially when initiating and titrating therapy, as they are at increased risk for adverse effects, especially respiratory depression.

! **WARNING** Be aware that opioid therapy like hydrocodone should only be used concomitantly with benzodiazepines and other CNS depressants in patients for whom other treatment options are inadequate. If prescribed together, expect dosing and duration of hydrocodone to be limited. Monitor patient closely for signs and symptoms of decrease in consciousness, including coma, profound sedation, and significant respiratory depression. Notify prescriber immediately and provide emergency supportive care, as death may occur.

! **WARNING** Monitor patient's vital signs closely, especially after initiating or titrating dose of hydrocodone. Know that in addition to respiratory depression, hydrocodone may cause severe hypotension, especially in patients whose blood pressure is already compromised by a depleted blood volume or after concurrent administration of drugs that decrease blood pressure.

! **WARNING** Monitor patient for respiratory depression, especially when initiating therapy or when increasing dosage, even when the drug has been used as prescribed and not abused or misused. Be aware that overestimating hydrocodone dose when converting patients from another opioid medication can result in fatal overdose with the first dose. To avoid this, know that it is recommended to underestimate a patient's 24-hour oral hydrocodone requirement and provide rescue medication, as needed, until the right dose is determined. Keep resuscitation equipment nearby.

! **WARNING** Monitor patients closely who may be susceptible to the intracranial effects of carbon dioxide retention from respiratory depression caused by hydrocodone therapy, such as patients with head injuries or those who have a preexisting elevation in intracranial pressure.

! **WARNING** Monitor patient's blood glucose level, especially if diabetic, because opioids may cause hypoglycemia. Monitor patients with a seizure history or disorder because hydrocodone may cause or worsen seizures.

! WARNING Be aware that concomitant use with CYP3A4 inhibitors or discontinuation of CYP3A inducers can result in a fatal overdose of hydrocodone.

! WARNING Know that many drugs may interact with opioids like hydrocodone to cause serotonin syndrome. Monitor patient closely for signs and symptoms, such as agitation, diaphoresis, diarrhea, fever, hallucinations, labile blood pressure, muscle twitching or stiffness, nausea, shakiness, shivering, tachycardia, trouble with coordination, or vomiting. Notify prescriber at once because serotonin syndrome may be life-threatening. Be prepared to discontinue drug, if possible and ordered, and provide supportive care.

! WARNING Monitor patient for adrenal insufficiency. Although rare, it can be life-threatening. Monitor patient for anorexia, dizziness, fatigue, hypotension, nausea, vomiting, or weakness. Notify prescriber if adrenal insufficiency is suspected and expect diagnostic testing to be done. If diagnosis is confirmed, expect to administer corticosteroids and wean patient off of hydrocodone, if possible.

- Notify prescriber if serious adverse reactions occur with hydrocodone therapy and expect dosage to be reduced.
- Be aware that drug can cause sleep-related breathing disorders, including central sleep apnea and sleep-related hypoxemia, that may require a dosage decrease, if present.
- Assess patient for constipation and provide a high-fiber diet and adequate fluid intake, if not contraindicated, because constipation can become severe.
- Monitor patient for decreased bowel motility in postoperative patients receiving hydrocodone, as drug may obscure the development of acute abdominal conditions.
- Expect to taper hydrocodone dosage gradually every 2 to 4 days when patient no longer requires therapy, to prevent withdrawal symptoms in the physically dependent patient. Know that hydrocodone should not be discontinued abruptly.

PATIENT TEACHING

- Instruct patient how to take form of hydrocodone prescribed.

! WARNING Advise females of childbearing age to notify prescriber immediately if pregnancy occurs.

! WARNING Warn patient of possibility of addiction even when taken as prescribed. Inform the patient that excessive or prolonged use can also lead to addiction, misuse, overdose, and possibly death. Instruct family or caregiver on how to use naloxone and to have it readily available while patient is taking hydrocodone in the event an overdose occurs. Stress importance of calling 911 if naloxone is administered. Advise patient not to increase dosage but to notify prescriber if hydrocodone becomes ineffective or pain increases when dosage increases.

! WARNING Caution patient to avoid ingesting alcohol, including medications containing alcohol, as the combination increases the risk of overdose, respiratory depression, and death, as does taking other types of depressants, including benzodiazepines, together with hydrocodone therapy. Patient should notify all prescribers of hydrocodone use.

! WARNING Warn patient to keep hydrocodone away from the reach of children, as accidental consumption of even one capsule or tablet can cause significant respiratory depression and death.

! WARNING Tell patient to alert prescriber of any persistent, serious, or unusual adverse reactions.

! WARNING Tell patient not to abruptly stop taking hydrocodone, especially if drug has been taken long-term but to consult prescriber with questions or concerns.

- Tell mothers not to breastfeed while taking oxycodone. However, if mother insists, tell her to monitor infant for excess sedation and respiratory depression. Alert her that when she stops drug or breastfeeding, infant may experience withdrawal symptoms and, if present, immediate medical care should be sought for infant.

- Caution patient to avoid hazardous activities until drug's CNS effects are known and resolved.
- Instruct patient to rise slowly from a lying or sitting position and to lie or sit down if he experiences light-headedness. If effect is frequent or severe, tell the patient to notify prescriber.
- Urge patient to consume plenty of fluids and high-fiber foods, if not contraindicated, to prevent constipation.
- Inform patient that long-term use of opioids like hydrocodone may decrease sex hormone levels, causing decreased libido, erectile dysfunction, impotence, infertility, or lack of menstruation. Encourage patient to report any such symptoms.
- Advise patients to take unused drug to a proper disposal place when drug is no longer needed.

hydrocortisone (cortisol)

Alkindi Sprinkle, Cortef, Cortenema

hydrocortisone acetate

Cortifoam

hydrocortisone sodium succinate

Solu-Cortef

Class and Category

Pharmacologic class: Glucocorticoid
Therapeutic class: Adrenocorticoid replacement, anti-inflammatory

Indications and Dosages

∗ *To treat severe inflammation related to collagen and dermatologic diseases, endocrine dysfunction, hematologic disorders, hypersensitivity states, nervous system disorders, palliative care of certain cancers, respiratory conditions, rheumatic disorders, selective GI diseases (regional enteritis, ulcerative colitis), trichinosis with myocardial or neurologic involvement, or tuberculous meningitis with subarachnoid block*

TABLETS (CORTEF)

Adults. 20 to 240 mg daily as a single dose or in divided doses.

±**DOSAGE ADJUSTMENT** For patients with acute disease, dosage increased to more than 240 mg.

I.V. INFUSION; I.M. OR I.V. INJECTION (SOLU-CORTEF)

Adults. 100 to 500 mg every 2, 4, or 6 hr.
Children. 0.56 to 8 mg/kg daily in 3 or 4 divided doses.

∗ *To treat pediatric adrenocortical insufficiency*

ORAL GRANULES (ALKINDI SPRINKLE)

Children. *Initial:* 8 to 10 mg/m^2 daily and in 3 equally divided doses for younger children and 2 or 3 equally divided doses for older children. Dosage rounded to nearest 0.5 or 1 mg and increases individualized.

∗ *As adjunct to treat ulcerative proctitis of the distal portion of the rectum in patients who can't retain hydrocortisone or other corticosteroid enemas*

RECTAL AEROSOL (CORTIFOAM)

Adult males. *Initial:* 1 applicatorful (90 mg) once or twice daily for 2 to 3 wk; then every other day thereafter. *Maintenance:* Highly individualized.

∗ *As adjunct to treat nonspecific inflammatory diseases involving the rectum, sigmoid, and left colon, such as idiopathic ulcerative colitis, ulcerative proctitis, regional enteritis with left side involvement, proctitis, proctocolitis, and radiation proctitis*

ENEMA (CORTENEMA)

Adults. 100 mg every night for 21 days or until remission occurs. If therapy extends beyond 21 days, dosage interval increased to every other evening over 2 to 3 wk when drug being discontinued.

Drug Administration

P.O.

- Administer drug in the morning.
- Give drug with food or milk to prevent GI upset.
- To administer oral granules, hold the capsule so that the printed strength is at the top and tap to ensure that all the granules are in the lower half of the capsule. Squeeze the bottom of the capsule gently and twist

off the top of the capsule. Pour directly onto child's tongue or pour onto a spoon and place in child's mouth, or sprinkle onto a spoonful of cold or room temperature soft food (such as fruit puree or yogurt). Administer granules and have child swallow them within 5 min after capsule is opened to avoid a bitter taste. Do not wet the capsule on the tongue or soft food prior to administration but immediately follow administration with a beverage to ensure all the granules have been swallowed. Capsules should not be chewed or crushed, nor should the contents be administered in a gastric or nasogastric tube.

I.M.

- Reconstitute with no more than 2 ml of Bacteriostatic Water or Bacteriostatic Saline solution for each vial or use the ACT-O-VIAL system as previously described.
- Administer undiluted injecting as an I.M. injection deep into gluteal muscle.
- Rotate injection sites to prevent muscle atrophy.

I.V.

- Reconstitute with no more than 2 ml of Bacteriostatic Water or Bacteriostatic Saline solution for each drug vial to be given by I.V. injection; use only Bacteriostatic Water for Injection if giving as an infusion.
- The ACT-O-VIAL system does not contain any preservative. To use the ACT-O-VIAL system, press down on plastic activator to force diluent into the lower compartment. Gently agitate. Remove plastic tab covering center of stopper. Sterilize top of stopper and insert needle squarely through center of stopper until tip is just visible. Invert vial and withdraw dose. Administer as an I.V. injection undiluted or as an I.V. infusion as described below.
- For I.V. injection, rate of administration is dependent on dosage. For example, administer as rapidly as over 30 sec for doses up to 100 mg or as long as 10 min for doses of 500 mg or more.
- For intermittent I.V. infusion after reconstitution, dilute with 0.9% Sodium Chloride Injection, 5% Dextrose Injection, or 5% Dextrose/0.9% Sodium Chloride Injection. The 100-mg reconstituted solution may be added to 100 to 1,000 ml of diluent, 250-mg solution may be added to 250 to 1,000 ml; 500-mg solution may be added to 500 to 1,000 ml; and 1,000-mg solution may be added to 1,000 ml of diluent. If patient requires fluid restriction, 100 to 3,000 mg of drug may be added to 50 ml of the above diluents. Diluted solution is stable for at least 4 hr. Rate of administration is dependent on dosage.
- *Incompatibilities:* Solutions other than 0.9% Sodium Chloride Injection, 5% Dextrose in Water, or 5% Dextrose in Water/0.9% Sodium Chloride Injection; other drugs

P.R.

- For rectal foam administration, shake foam container vigorously for 5 to 10 sec before each use. Do not remove container cap during use of product. Gently place tip of the applicator onto the nose of the container cap while container is upright on a level surface. Pull plunger past the fill line on the applicator barrel. Press firmly down on cap flanges, hold for 1–2 sec and release. Pause 5 to 10 sec to allow foam to expand in applicator barrel. Repeat until foam reaches fill line. Remove applicator from cap. Allow some foam to remain on the applicator tip. Hold applicator firmly by barrel, making sure thumb and middle finger are positioned securely underneath and resting against barrel wings. Place index finger over the plunger. Gently insert tip into anus. Once in place, push plunger to expel foam, then withdraw applicator. Never insert any part of the aerosol container directly into the anus. After each use, wash applicator, container cap, and underlying tip with warm water.
- For enema administration, have patient lie on the left side for administration and for 30 min afterward. Administer enema using normal procedure. Encourage patient to retain enema for at least an hour, and preferably all night.

Route	Onset	Peak	Duration
P.O.	Unknown	1–2 hr	Unknown
I.V.	1 hr	1–2 hr	Unknown
I.M./P.R.	Variable	Variable	Variable

Half-life: 1–3 hr

Mechanism of Action

Binds to intracellular glucocorticoid receptors and suppresses inflammatory and immune responses by:

- inhibiting monocyte and neutrophil accumulation at inflammation site and suppressing their bactericidal and phagocytic activity.
- stabilizing lysosomal membranes.
- suppressing antigen response of helper T cells and macrophages.
- inhibiting synthesis of cellular mediators of inflammatory response, such as cytokines, interleukins, and prostaglandins.

Contraindications

Hypersensitivity to hydrocortisone or its components, idiopathic thrombocytopenic purpura (I.M.), intestinal conditions prohibiting intrarectal steroids (P.R.), systemic fungal infection

Interactions

DRUGS

aspirin, NSAIDs: Increased risk of GI distress and bleeding; increased risk of salicylate toxicity with chronic high doses of aspirin
phenobarbital, phenytoin, rifampin: Decreased blood hydrocortisone level
insulin, oral antidiabetic drugs: Possibly increased blood glucose level
ketoconazole, troleandomycin: Decreased clearance of hydrocortisone with increased plasma levels and higher risk of adverse reactions
oral anticoagulants: May decrease or increase anticoagulant effect
vaccines (live attenuated): Decreased antibody response and increased risk of neurologic complications

ACTIVITIES

alcohol use: Increased risk of GI distress and bleeding

Adverse Reactions

CNS: Ataxia, behavioral changes, delirium, depression, dizziness, epidural lipomatosis, euphoria, fatigue, headache, **increased intracranial pressure with papilledema**, insomnia, malaise, mania, mood changes, paresthesia, **seizures**, steroid psychosis with hallucinations, syncope, vertigo
CV: **Arrhythmias**, **fat embolism**, **heart failure**, hypertension, **hypertrophic cardiomyopathy**, **hypotension**, **thromboembolism**, thrombophlebitis
EENT: Blurred vision, central serous chorioretinopathy, exophthalmos, glaucoma, increased intraocular pressure, nystagmus, posterior subcapsular cataracts, secondary ocular infections
ENDO: **Adrenal insufficiency during stress**, cushingoid symptoms (buffalo hump, central obesity, moon face, supraclavicular fat pad enlargement), diabetes mellitus, growth suppression in children, hyperglycemia, negative nitrogen balance from protein catabolism
GI: Abdominal distention; **GI perforation**; hiccups; increased appetite; nausea; **pancreatitis**; peptic ulcer; rectal abnormalities, such as **bleeding**, blistering, burning, itching, or pain (rectal form); ulcerative esophagitis; vomiting
GU: Amenorrhea, glycosuria, menstrual irregularities, perineal burning or tingling
HEME: Easy bruising, leukocytosis
MS: Arthralgia; aseptic necrosis of femoral and humeral heads; compression fractures; muscle atrophy, twitching, or weakness; myalgia; osteoporosis; spontaneous fractures; steroid myopathy; tendon rupture
SKIN: Acne; altered skin pigmentation; diaphoresis; erythema; hirsutism; necrotizing vasculitis; petechiae; purpura; rash; scarring; sterile abscess; striae; subcutaneous fat atrophy; thin, fragile skin; urticaria
Other: **Anaphylaxis**, **hypocalcemia**, **hypokalemia**, **hypokalemic alkalosis**, impaired wound healing, **immunosuppression and increased risk of infection** (with dosage greater than used for replacement), **Kaposi's sarcoma**, masking of signs of infection, **metabolic alkalosis**, **pheochromocytoma crisis** (in presence of pheochromocytoma), suppressed skin test reaction, **tumor lysis syndrome**, weight gain

Childbearing Considerations

PREGNANCY

- Drug has the potential to cause fetal harm, as it does cross the placental barrier.
- Infants born of mothers who have received substantial doses of corticosteroids during pregnancy must be observed for signs of

adrenal insufficiency. Cataracts have also been observed in mothers undergoing long-term treatment with corticosteroids during pregnancy.
- Use with caution only if benefit to mother outweighs potential risk to fetus.

LACTATION
- Drug is present in breast milk and could suppress infant growth.
- Mothers should check with prescriber before breastfeeding.

REPRODUCTION
- Drug may alter male fertility.

Nursing Considerations

- Know that systemic hydrocortisone shouldn't be given to immunocompromised patients, such as those with fungal and other infections, including amebiasis, hepatitis B, tuberculosis, vaccinia, and varicella. Expect hydrocortisone to worsen infections or mask signs and symptoms. Monitor patient closely.
- Be aware that high-dose therapy shouldn't be given for longer than 48 hours. Be alert for depression and psychotic episodes.

! **WARNING** Monitor patient for hypersensitivity reactions, which could become life-threatening, such as anaphylaxis. If present, notify prescriber, expect patient to be switched to a different glucocorticoid, and provide supportive care, as needed and ordered.

! **WARNING** Know that abrupt withdrawal of hydrocortisone or switching between oral hydrocortisone formulations, if the other oral hydrocortisone product had been altered through crushing or splitting a tablet or was compounded in anyway, may cause adrenocortical insufficiency, adrenal crisis, or death. Avoid withdrawing drug suddenly after long-term therapy. Instead, expect to reduce dosage gradually and monitor response when hydrocortisone is being discontinued. Monitor patient closely for several days if patient is switched to a different oral hydrocortisone product. Adrenal crisis may also be induced by stressful events such as infections or surgery. Expect dose to be increased during periods of stress. Also, expect to switch patients to a parenteral form if patient is severely ill, unable to take oral hydrocortisone, or is vomiting.

! **WARNING** Monitor tumor lysis syndrome (TLS) in patients with malignancies, including hematological malignancies and solid tumors, following the use of systemic corticosteroids such as hydrocortisone alone or in combination with other chemotherapeutic agents. Patients who are at high risk include patients with tumors that have a high proliferative rate, high tumor burden, and high sensitivity to cytotoxic agents. Monitor patient closely.

! **WARNING** Know that patients receiving chronic corticosteroid therapy such as hydrocortisone at a dosage greater than for replacement are increased risk of developing Kaposi's sarcoma.

- Monitor blood pressure, electrolyte levels, and weight regularly during therapy.
- Monitor blood glucose level in diabetic patients, and increase insulin or oral antidiabetic drug dosage, as needed and ordered.
- Know that elderly patients are at high risk for osteoporosis during long-term therapy.
- Know that when Alkindi Sprinkle form is given at the recommended dosage, immunosuppression or increase in the risk of infection is not expected. Therefore, administration of live vaccines may be acceptable in children with adrenocortical insufficiency receiving replacement corticosteroids if prescribed Alkindi Sprinkle form of hydrocortisone.

PATIENT TEACHING
- Instruct patient how to take oral form of hydrocortisone, if prescribed.
- Teach patient how to use enema or foam form of hydrocortisone, if prescribed.

! **WARNING** Alert patient that drug may cause an allergic reaction. If present, tell patient to notify prescriber and to seek immediate medical care, if severe.

! **WARNING** Caution patient not to stop taking long-term hydrocortisone therapy abruptly. Inform patient and family or caregiver that abrupt withdrawal of drug or switching between oral hydrocortisone formulations may cause adrenocortical insufficiency, adrenal crisis, and even death. Tell patient and family or caregiver to be alert for signs and symptoms of adrenal crisis for several days after an oral product has been switched to a different oral product. Instruct patient and family or caregiver to report early evidence of adrenal insufficiency: anorexia, difficulty breathing, dizziness, fainting, fatigue, joint pain, muscle weakness, and nausea. Alert patient that adrenal crisis may also be induced by stressful events such as infections or surgery. Tell patient, family, or caregiver to notify prescriber immediately if patient becomes severely ill, unable to take oral hydrocortisone, or is vomiting.

- Caution patient to avoid people with infections because drug can suppress immune system, increasing risk of infection. If patient comes into contact with chickenpox or measles, instruct the patient to call prescriber because he may need prophylactic care.
- Inform patient that he may bruise easily.
- Advise patient on long-term therapy to have periodic eye examinations. Stress importance of notifying prescriber if blurred vision or other visual disturbances occur. Know that drug should not be used in active ocular herpes simplex.
- If patient receives long-term therapy, urge the patient to carry or wear medical identification.

hydromorphone hydrochloride (dihydromorphinone)

Dilaudid

Class, Category, and Schedule

Pharmacologic class: Opioid
Therapeutic class: Opioid analgesic
Controlled substance schedule: II

Indications and Dosages

✱ *To relieve pain severe enough to require opioid treatment and for which alternative treatment options such as nonopioid analgesics or opioid combination products are inadequate or not tolerated*

ORAL SOLUTION (DILAUDID)

Adults. 2.5 to 10 mg every 3 to 6 hr, as needed.

TABLETS (DILAUDID)

Adults. 2 to 4 mg every 4 to 6 hr, as needed.

I.V. INJECTION (DILAUDID)

Adults. 0.2 to 1 mg given slowly over at least 2 to 3 min every 2 to 3 hr, as needed.

I.M. OR SUBCUTANEOUS INJECTION (DILAUDID)

Adults. 1 or 2 mg every 2 to 3 hr, as needed.

SUPPOSITORIES (DILAUDID)

Adults. 3 mg every 6 to 8 hr, as needed.

±**DOSAGE ADJUSTMENT** For patients with hepatic or renal impairment, initial dosage is given at 25 to 50% of normal dosage. For debilitated or elderly patients, initial dosage of I.V. injection reduced to 0.2 mg.

✱ *To treat opioid-tolerant patients who require higher doses of opioids for the management of pain severe enough to require an opioid analgesic and for which alternate treatments are inadequate*

I.M., OR SUBCUTANEOUS INJECTION (DILAUDID-HP) (HIGH POTENCY FORMULATION)

Adults who are opioid tolerant. *Initial:* 1 to 2 mg every 2 to 3 hr, as needed. Dosage titrated based on patient's response to initial dose.

I.V. INJECTION

Adults who are opioid tolerant. 0.2 mg to 1 mg injected slowly over at least 2 to 3 min every 2 to 3 hr.

±**DOSAGE ADJUSTMENT** For debilitated or elderly patients, initial dosage of I.V. injection kept at or reduced to 0.2 mg. For other patients with hepatic or renal impairment, initial dosage given at 25 to 50% of normal dosage.

✱ *To manage severe and persistent pain in opioid-tolerant patients requiring an extended treatment period with a daily opioid analgesic and for which alternative treatment options are inadequate*

E.R. TABLETS

Adults. Highly individualized and dependent on patient's previous total 24-hr opioid use and risk factors for abuse, addiction, and misuse. Once dosage is determined, drug is given once daily. Dosage may be increased by 4 to 8 mg every 3 to 4 days, as needed.

±**DOSAGE ADJUSTMENT** For patients taking extended-release tablets, dosage started at 25% of normal dosage for moderate hepatic impairment or for severe renal impairment; dosage started at 50% of normal dosage for moderate renal impairment.

Drug Administration

- Administer before pain becomes intense.
- Have naloxone readily available.

P.O.

- Use a calibrated device when measuring oral solution dosage.
- Tablets should be swallowed whole and not chewed, crushed, or split.
- Administer with food if GI upset occurs.

I.V.

- Parenteral form of hydromorphone comes in two strengths. Do not confuse immediate-release formulation with the high potency formulation.
- Inspect solution. A slight yellowish discoloration may develop in ampuls, but potency is not affected.
- Administer as an injection slowly over at least 2 to 3 min.
- *Incompatibilities:* None reported by manufacturer

I.M.

- Rotate sites.

SUBCUTANEOUS

- Rotate sites.

P.R.

- Keep suppositories in refrigerator until ready to administer.

Route	Onset	Peak	Duration
P.O.	15–30 min	30–60 min	3–4 hr
P.O./E.R.	6 hr	12–16 hr	13 hr
I.V.	5 min	10–20 min	3–4 hr
I.M.	15 min	30–60 min	4–5 hr
SubQ	15 min	30–90 min	4 hr

Half-life: 2–3 hr; 11 hr E.R.

Mechanism of Action

May bind with opioid receptors in the spinal cord and higher levels in the CNS. In this way, hydromorphone is believed to stimulate kappa and mu receptors, thus altering the perception of and emotional response to pain.

Contraindications

Acute or severe bronchial asthma (in an unmonitored setting or in the absence of resuscitative equipment); hypersensitivity to hydromorphone, hydromorphone salts, sulfite-containing drugs, or their components; known or suspected GI obstruction, including paralytic ileus; narrowing of GI tract, including blind loops (E.R. tablets); opioid nontolerant patients (E.R. tablets); significant respiratory depression

Interactions

DRUGS

5-HT_3 receptor antagonists, drugs that affect the serotonin neurotransmitter system (mirtazapine, trazodone, tramadol), linezolid, methylene blue (I.V.), selective serotonin reuptake inhibitors, serotonin and norepinephrine reuptake inhibitors, tricyclic antidepressants, triptans, tryptophan: Increased risk of serotonin syndrome

anticholinergics: Increased risk of ileus, severe constipation, or urine retention

anxiolytics, antipsychotics, benzodiazepines and other CNS depressants, general anesthetics, muscle relaxants, other opioids and sedative/hypnotics, sedating antihistamines, tranquilizers, tricyclic antidepressants: Increased risk of coma, hypotension, profound sedation, and severe respiratory depression

diuretics: Reduced effects of diuretics

mixed agonist/antagonist, partial agonist opioid analgesics, such as buprenorphine, butorphanol, nalbuphine, pentazocine: Possibly reduced analgesic effect of hydromorphone; may precipitate withdrawal symptoms

MAO inhibitors: Increased risk of serotonin toxicity; increased risk of opioid toxicity

muscle relaxants: Possibly enhanced neuromuscular blocking action of skeletal muscle relaxants producing increased degree of respiratory depression

ACTIVITIES

alcohol use: Increased CNS and respiratory depression, which may become severe

Adverse Reactions

CNS: Anxiety, **CNS depression**, confusion, dizziness, drowsiness, dysphoria, euphoria, hallucinations, headache, light-headedness, nervousness, restlessness, sedation, somnolence, tremor, weakness
CV: Hypertension, orthostatic hypotension, palpitations, tachycardia
EENT: Blurred vision, diplopia, dry mouth, **laryngeal edema**, **laryngeal spasms**, nystagmus, tinnitus
ENDO: **Adrenal insufficiency**, **hypoglycemia**
GI: Abdominal cramps, anorexia, biliary tract spasm, constipation, **hepatotoxicity**, nausea, vomiting
GU: Decreased libido, dysuria, erectile dysfunction, impotence, infertility, lack of menstruation, urine retention
RESP: Dyspnea, **respiratory depression**, wheezing
SKIN: Diaphoresis, flushing, pruritus
Other: Injection-site pain, redness, and swelling; opioid-induced allodynia and hyperalgesia; physical and psychological dependence

Childbearing Considerations

PREGNANCY

- Drug may cause fetal harm.
- Prolonged use of drug during pregnancy can result in neonatal opioid withdrawal syndrome (NOWS), which may be life-threatening if not recognized and treated.
- Avoid prolonged use during pregnancy. Use with caution only if benefit to mother outweighs potential risk to fetus.

LABOR AND DELIVERY

- Drug is not recommended for use in pregnant women immediately before or during labor. Opioids may alter length of time of labor.
- Opioids cross the placental barrier and may produce respiratory depression and psycho-physiologic effects in the newborn. Monitor newborn closely for signs of excess sedation and respiratory depression.
- An opioid antagonist, such as naloxone, must be available at the time of delivery in the event it is needed to reverse opioid-induced respiratory depression in the neonate.

LACTATION

- Drug is present in breast milk.
- Mothers should check with prescriber before breastfeeding.
- If breastfeeding occurs, infant should be monitored for excess drowsiness and respiratory depression. Be aware that when mother stops drug or breastfeeding, infant may experience withdrawal symptoms.

REPRODUCTION

- Chronic use of opioids may reduce fertility.

Nursing Considerations

- Be aware that hydromorphone therapy increases risk of abuse, addiction, and misuse. A Risk Evaluation and Mitigation Strategy (REMS) is required. Monitor patient closely throughout therapy for abuse, addiction, or misuse. Monitor patient for evidence of physical dependence or abuse. Know that addiction can occur not only in those who obtain the drug illicitly but also in patients who are appropriately prescribed the drug at recommended doses. Be aware that excessive use of hydromorphone may not only lead to abuse, addiction, and misuse, it can lead to overdose, and possibly death. Monitor patient's intake of drug closely.
- Be aware that all other around-the-clock opioid analgesics should be stopped when E.R. tablets are prescribed.
- Be aware that opioids like hydromorphone should not be given to pregnant women for an extended period of time because chronic maternal use of hydromorphone during pregnancy can result in neonatal opioid withdrawal syndrome (NOWS), which may be life-threatening, if not recognized and treated appropriately. NOWS occurs when a newborn has been exposed to opioid drugs for a prolonged period while in utero.

> ! **WARNING** Monitor patient for coma, hypotension, profound sedation, or respiratory depression when administering hydromorphone around-the-clock; these reactions can occur if alcohol or illicit drugs are being used without the prescriber's knowledge.

- Monitor effectiveness of hydromorphone in relieving pain; consult prescriber as needed.

Anticipate that drug may mask or worsen gallbladder pain.

- Monitor patient for paradoxic increase in pain known as opioid-induced hyperalgesia or an increase in sensitivity to pain known as allodynia, especially when hydromorphone dosage increases. Do not confuse this with tolerance, which is the need for increasing doses of opioids to maintain an effect. If opioid-induced allodynia or hyperalgesia is suspected, notify prescriber and expect dosage to be decreased or opioid rotation to be prescribed.

! **WARNING** Monitor patient for respiratory depression even when administering oral form of drug such as oral solution or tablets, especially within the first 72 hours of initiating therapy or when increasing dosage, even when the drug has been used as prescribed and not abused or misused. Patients who are especially vulnerable include the elderly and those who are cachectic or debilitated. Be aware that overestimating hydromorphone dose when converting patients from another opioid medication can result in fatal overdose with the first dose. To avoid this, know that it is recommended to underestimate a patient's 24-hour oral hydromorphone requirement and provide rescue medication, as needed, until the right dose is determined. Keep resuscitation equipment and naloxone nearby.

! **WARNING** Monitor patient very closely when administering hydromorphone to patients with cor pulmonale or significant chronic obstructive pulmonary disease, and in patients having a substantially decreased respiratory reserve, hypercapnia, hypoxia, or preexisting respiratory depression, especially when initiating and titrating therapy. These patients may develop respiratory depression, even with usual therapeutic doses because hydromorphone may decrease the patient's respiratory drive to the point of apnea.

! **WARNING** Be aware that hydromorphone should only be used concomitantly with benzodiazepines and other CNS depressants in patients for whom other treatment options are inadequate. If prescribed together, expect dosing and duration of hydromorphone to be limited. Monitor patient closely for signs and symptoms of decrease in consciousness, including coma, profound sedation, and significant respiratory depression. Notify prescriber immediately, expect drug to be discontinued, and provide emergency supportive care, as death may occur.

! **WARNING** Monitor patients closely who may be susceptible to the intracranial effects of carbon dioxide retention from respiratory depression caused by hydromorphone therapy, such as patients with head injuries or those who have a preexisting elevation in intracranial pressure.

! **WARNING** Monitor patients closely whose ability to maintain a normal blood pressure is already compromised by a reduced blood volume or concurrent administration of certain CNS depressant drugs; the drug may cause severe hypotension in these patients, especially when initiating or titrating the dose of hydromorphone. Assess blood pressure frequently.

! **WARNING** Monitor patient's blood glucose level, especially if patient is a diabetic because opioids like hydromorphone may cause hypoglcyemia. Monitor patients with seizure disorders because hydromorphone therapy may aggravate or induce convulsions.

! **WARNING** Know that many drugs may interact with opioids like hydromorphone to cause serotonin syndrome. Monitor patient closely for signs and symptoms, such as agitation, diaphoresis, diarrhea, fever, hallucinations, labile blood pressure, muscle twitching or stiffness, nausea, shakiness, shivering, tachycardia, trouble with coordination, or vomiting. Notify prescriber at once because serotonin syndrome may be life-threatening. Be prepared to discontinue drug, if possible and ordered, and provide supportive care.

! **WARNING** Monitor patient for adrenal insufficiency. Although rare, it can be life-threatening. Monitor patient for anorexia, dizziness, fatigue, hypotension, nausea, vomiting, or weakness. Notify prescriber if adrenal insufficiency is suspected and expect to do diagnostic testing. If diagnosis is confirmed, expect to administer corticosteroids and wean patient off hydromorphone, if possible.

- Be aware that drug can cause sleep-related breathing disorders, including central sleep apnea and sleep-related hypoxemia that may require a dosage decrease, if present.
- Monitor patient for other adverse reactions, especially adverse reactions that are persistent, serious, or unusual. Know that the most common adverse reactions to hydromorphone are dizzinesss, dry mouth, dysphoria, euphoria, flushing, light-headedness, nausea, pruritus, sedation, sweating, and vomiting.
- Assess patient for constipation.
- Know that E.R. tablets may be visible on abdominal X-rays under certain circumstances, especially when digital enhancing techniques are utilized because the tablet is nondeformable and does not change much in shape in the GI tract.
- Expect to taper dosages of hydromorphone that have been administered for an extended period of time to the opioid-tolerant patient gradually by 25 to 50% every 2 to 3 days before the drug is discontinued. This will help prevent signs and symptoms of withdrawal.

PATIENT TEACHING

- Instruct patient how to administer form of hydromorphone prescribed. Caution patient, family, or caregiver administering oral solution to use a calibrated device to ensure correct dose is being given as dosing errors causing serious to lethal adverse reactions have occurred.
- Stress importance of taking drug exactly as prescribed and before pain is severe. Also, tell her not to take more drug than prescribed and not to take it longer than absolutely needed because excessive or prolonged use can lead to abuse, addiction, misuse, overdose, and possibly death. However, advise patient that if pain increases when dose is increased to alert prescriber.

! **WARNING** Instruct family or caregiver on use of naloxone and importance of having drug available in case of an overdose. Stress importance of calling 911 if naloxone is administered.

! **WARNING** Inform patient about potentially fatal additive effects of combining hydromorphone with a benzodiazepine or other CNS depressants. In addition, other serious drug reactions can occur. Instruct patient to inform all prescribers of hydromorphone use before taking any other drug.

! **WARNING** Caution patient to avoid alcohol while taking hydromorphone.

! **WARNING** Warn patient to keep drug out of reach of children, as accidental ingestion may cause death. Also, remind patient that drug is a controlled substance. She should take steps to protect drug from theft.

! **WARNING** Advise mothers who are breastfeeding to monitor infant for drowsiness and respiratory depression. Alert mother that when drug or breastfeeding is stopped, infant may experience withdrawal symptoms and will need immediate medical care.

! **WARNING** Tell patient not to abruptly stop taking hydromorphone especially if drug taken long-term.

- Instruct patient to report persistent, serious, or unusual adverse reactions to prescriber.
- Inform patient that drug may cause drowsiness and sedation. Advise her to avoid hazardous activities until drug's CNS effects are known and resolved.
- Tell patient to change position slowly to minimize orthostatic hypotension.
- Advise females of childbearing age to notify prescriber if pregnancy occurs.
- Inform patient that long-term use of opioids like hydromorphone may decrease sex hormone levels, causing decreased libido, erectile dysfunction, impotence, infertility, or lack of menstruation. Encourage patient to report any such symptoms.
- Advise patients when hydromorphone tablets or solution are no longer needed to remit to authorities at a certified drug take-back program.

hydroxychloroquine sulfate

Plaquenil, Sovuna

Class and Category

Pharmacologic class: Aminoquinoline
Therapeutic class: Antimalarial, antirheumatic, lupus erythematosus suppressant

Indications and Dosages

✱ *To prevent malaria*

TABLETS (PLAQUENIL)

Adults. 400 mg once a wk on the same day of each wk starting 2 wk before entering endemic area and continued for 4 wk after departure from endemic area.
Children weighing 31 kg (68.2 lb) or more. 6.5 mg/kg (maximum 400 mg) once a wk on the same day of each wk, starting 2 wk before entering endemic area and continued for 4 wk after departure from endemic area. *Maximum:* 400 mg once weekly.

TABLETS (SOVUNA)

Adults. 400 mg once a wk on the same day of each wk starting 2 wk before entering endemic area and continued for 4 wk after departure from endemic area.
Children weighing 23 kg (50.6 lb) or more. 6.5 mg/kg (maximum 400 mg) once a wk on the same day of each wk starting 2 wk before entering endemic area and continued for 4 wk after departure from endemic area.

✱ *To treat uncomplicated malaria caused by* Plasmodium falciparum, P. malariae, P. ovale, *or* P. vivax

TABLETS (PLAQUENIL)

Adults. *Initial:* 800 mg, followed by 400 mg in 6 hr, 24 hr, and 48 hr after initial dose.
Children weighing 31 kg (68.2 lb) or more. *Initial*: 13 mg/kg (up to 800 mg), then 6.5 mg/kg (up to 400 mg) at 6 hr, 24 hr, and 48 hr after initial dose.

TABLETS (SOVUNA)

Adults. *Initial:* 800 mg, followed by 400 mg in 6 hr, 24 hr, and 48 hr after initial dose.
Children weighing 23 kg (50.6 lb) or more. *Initial:* 13 mg/kg (up to 800 mg), then 6.5 mg/kg (up to 400 mg) at 6 hr, 24 hr, and 48 hr after initial dose.

✱ *To treat chronic discoid lupus erythematosus*

TABLETS (PLAQUENIL, SOVUNA)

Adults. 200 mg once daily or 400 mg daily in 2 divided doses. *Maximum:* 400 mg daily.

✱ *To treat systemic lupus erythematosus*

TABLETS (PLAQUENIL)

Adults. 200 mg once daily or 400 mg daily in 2 divided doses. *Maximum*: 400 mg daily.

TABLETS (SOVUNA)

Adults. 200 mg, 300 mg, or 400 mg daily as a single dose or 2 divided doses.

✱ *To treat acute or chronic rheumatoid arthritis*

TABLETS (PLAQUENIL, SOVUNA)

Adults. *Initial:* 400 to 600 mg daily as a single dose or in 2 divided doses. Following a good response, dosage reduced by 50%. *Maintenance:* 200 mg daily to 400 mg daily as a single dose or in 2 divided doses.

Drug Administration

P.O.

- Administer with a meal or a glass of milk.
- Tablets should not be chewed, crushed, or split.

Route	Onset	Peak	Duration
P.O.	Unknown	3–4 hr	Unknown

Half-life: 40–50 days

Mechanism of Action

May mildly suppress the immune system, inhibiting production of rheumatoid factor and acute phase reactants. Hydroxychloroquine accumulates in WBCs, stabilizing lysosomal membranes and inhibiting enzymes such as collagenase and proteases that cause cartilage breakdown. These actions may decrease symptoms of rheumatoid arthritis and lupus erythematosus. Hydroxychloroquine also binds to and alters DNA of malaria parasite to prevent it from reproducing. It also may increase the pH of acid vesicles, which interferes with vesicle function and may inhibit parasitic phospholipid metabolism in erythrocytes, thereby halting plasmodial activity.

Contraindications

Hypersensitivity to hydroxychloroquine, other 4-aminoquinoline compounds, or their components

Interactions

DRUGS

ampicillin: Possibly significant decrease in bioavailability of ampicillin, decreasing its effectiveness
antacids, kaolin: Possibly reduced absorption of hydroxychloroquine
antidiabetic drugs, insulin: Possibly increased risk of hypoglycemia
antiepileptics, mefloquine, other drugs that lower seizure threshold: Increased risk of seizures
cimetidine: Possibly increased plasma hydroxychloroquine levels
cyclosporin: Increased plasma cyclosporin levels
digoxin: Increased digoxin concentrations
drugs that prolong QT interval, including other arrhythmogenic drugs: Increased risk of arrhythmias
hepatotoxic or nephrotoxic drugs: Possibly increased risk of kidney or liver toxicity
methotrexate: Possibly increased risk of adverse reactions
praziquantel: Possibly reduced bioavailability of praziquantel affecting its effectiveness

Adverse Reactions

CNS: Abnormal nerve conduction, agitation, anxiety, ataxia, confusion, delusions, depression, dizziness, emotional lability, extrapyramidal disorders, fatigue, hallucinations, headache, insomnia, irritability, lassitude, mania, nervousness, neuromuscular sensory abnormalities, neuropathy, nightmares, paranoia, psychosis, **seizures, suicidal ideation**, vertigo
CV: Atrioventricular blocks, bundle branch block, **cardiac failure, cardiomyopathy** (prolonged high doses), **cardiotoxicity, prolonged QT interval, sick sinus syndrome, torsades de pointes, ventricular arrhythmias**
EENT: Abnormal pigmentation (bullseye appearance) or colored vision, blurred vision, central scotoma with decreased visual acuity, corneal deposits or edema, decreased corneal sensitivity, decreased dark adaptation, diplopia, irreversible retinal damage, halo vision, lassitude, macular atrophy or edema, macular degeneration, nerve-related hearing loss, nystagmus, paracentral or pericentral scotoma, photophobia, retinal fundus changes, retinal toxicity, retinopathy, sensorineural hearing loss, tinnitus, visual abnormalities including visual fields
ENDO: Hypoglycemia
GI: Abdominal cramps or pain, **acute or fulminant hepatic failure**, anorexia, diarrhea, elevated liver enzymes, nausea, vomiting
GU: Renal toxicity
HEME: Agranulocytosis, anemia, **aplastic anemia, bone marrow depression, hemolysis** (in patients with glucose-6 phosphate dehydrogenase [G6PD] deficiency), **leukopenia**, porphyria, **thrombocytopenia**
MS: Atrophy of proximal skeletal muscle groups, depressed tendon reflexes, muscle weakness, myopathy
RESP: Bronchospasm, pulmonary hypertension
SKIN: Acute generalized exanthematous pustulosis, alopecia, altered mucosal and skin pigmentation, bleaching of hair, dermatitis (including bullous and **exfoliative dermatitis**), **erythema multiforme**, hyperpigmentation, non-light-sensitive psoriasis, photosensitivity, pruritus, psoriasis exacerbation, rash, **Stevens-Johnson syndrome, toxic epidermal necrolysis**, urticaria
Other: Angioedema; drug reaction with eosinophilia and systemic symptoms (DRESS); porphyria, including worsening, weight loss

Childbearing Considerations

PREGNANCY

- Pregnancy exposure registry: 1-877-311-8972.
- It is not known if drug may cause fetal harm.
- Use with caution only if benefit to mother outweighs potential risk to fetus.

LACTATION

- Drug is present in breast milk.
- Mothers should check with prescriber before breastfeeding.

Nursing Considerations

! WARNING Be aware hydroxychloroquine should be avoided in patients at risk for prolonged QT interval because of potential to cause life-threatening ventricular arrhythmias, including torsades de pointes. Drug is not recommended in patients taking other drugs that have the potential to prolong the QT interval as well as if patient has a history of acquired or congenital QT prolongation or ventricular arrhythmias, presence of cardiac disease or proarrhythmic conditions (e.g., bradycardia with heart beat below 50), or uncorrected hypokalemia and/or hypomagnesemia. Maximum dose should not be exceeded because the magnitude of QT prolongation increases as concentration of the drug increases. Expect electrolyte imbalances to be corrected before drug is initiated.

! **WARNING** Be aware that drug should not be given to patients with porphyria or psoriasis unless benefit outweighs risk. If drug is given, observe patients with psoriasis closely because hydroxychloroquine may lead to a severe psoriasis attack. Monitor patients with porphyria closely because hydroxychloroquine may worsen condition.

! **WARNING** Be aware that drug has not been approved for use by the FDA to treat the COVID-19 virus.

- Use hydroxychloroquine cautiously in patients with G6PD deficiency, patients with alcoholism or hepatic disease, and patients taking hepatotoxic drugs. Also, use cautiously in patients with blood, GI, or neurological disorders and in patients who are sensitive to quinine.

! **WARNING** Monitor patient for hypersensitivity reactions, that could become life-threatening, such as angioedema or severe cutaneous reactions such as DRESS. If present or at first sign of a rash (DRESS may only present initially as a fever or swollen lymph nodes), notify prescriber, expect drug to be discontinued, and provide supportive care, as needed and ordered.

! **WARNING** Monitor patients' renal function throughout drug therapy because drug can cause renal toxicity. Proteinuria with or without moderate reduction in glomerular filtration rate has occurred with hydroxychloroquine use. Expect drug to be discontinued if renal toxicity is suspected.

! **WARNING** Monitor patient for neuropsychiatric adverse reactions, which typically occurs within the first month of hydroxychloroquine therapy. Know that patients with and without a prior history of psychiatric disorders may develop this type of adverse reaction. Monitor patient closely as suicidal ideation may occur.

! **WARNING** Monitor patient for abnormal signs and symptoms of cardiac compromise because drug may cause cardiotoxicity, which could be life-threatening. Patient may exhibit conduction disorders, including sick sinus syndrome; pulmonary hypertension; or ventricular hypertrophy. The patient's ECG may reveal left or right atrioventricular bundle branch block. Notify prescriber and expect drug to be discontinued if cardiotoxicity is suspected. Prepare patient for a tissue biopsy to confirm cardiotoxcity, if ordered.

! **WARNING** Monitor patient's blood glucose level because drug can cause severe and potentially life-threatening hypoglycemia. Be prepared to treat hypoglycemia according to institutional protocol and alert prescriber. Also, obtain periodic blood cell counts, as ordered, during prolonged therapy to detect adverse hematologic effects. Expect to stop drug if severe adverse effects occur.

! **WARNING** Monitor patient's vision when giving hydroxychloroquine because irreversible retinal damage may occur in some patients during high-dose or long-term therapy. Ask regularly about vision abnormalities, such as light flashes or streaks that may indicate retinopathy. Expect patient to have an initial ophthalmologic examination, followed by examinations every 3 months. Be aware that in patients of Asian descent, retinal toxicity may first be noticed outside the macula. Report changes to prescriber immediately and expect drug to be stopped. Retinal changes may progress even after therapy stops.

- Assess patient on long-term therapy for neuropathy or skeletal myopathy, which can lead to abnormal nerve conduction, atrophy of proximal muscle groups, depressed tendon reflexes and progressive muscle weakness. Assess these patient's deep tendon reflexes and muscle strength periodically. If present, notify prescriber and expect drug to be discontinued.

! **WARNING** Notify prescriber immediately if other persistent, serious, or unusual adverse reactions occur. Monitor children closely for adverse reactions because they're especially sensitive to 4-aminoquinoline compounds.

- Expect drug to be stopped if patient with rheumatoid arthritis shows no improvement, such as reduced joint swelling or increased mobility, in 6 months.

PATIENT TEACHING

- Instruct patient how to administer hydroxychloroquine.
- Tell patient to take hydroxychloroquine exactly as prescribed because taking too much may cause serious adverse reactions and taking too little or skipping doses decreases effectiveness.

! **WARNING** Inform patients that drug has not been approved by the FDA for treatment of COVID-19 virus.

! **WARNING** Alert patient that drug may cause an allergic reaction, including skin reactions that could become severe. Tell patient to notify prescriber, if present or at the first sign of a fever, rash, or swollen lymph nodes and to seek immediate medical care, if severe.

! **WARNING** Alert patient, family, or caregiver that drug may cause neuropsychiatric adverse reactions within the first month of drug therapy such as depression, mood swings, and suicidal ideation. If present, stress importance of notifying prescriber.

! **WARNING** Review signs and symptoms of hypoglycemia with patient and family or caregiver and how to treat. Stress importance of seeking immediate medical care if hypoglycemia occurs as it quickly can become life-threatening.

! **WARNING** Review early signs and symptoms of toxicity with patient, family, or caregiver. Caution patient to notify prescribe about other troublesome adverse reactions, especially if persistent, severe, or unusual. Inform family or caregiver that children are more sensitive to the drug requiring immediate notification of any adverse reactions to the prescriber. Hydroxychloroquine dosage may have to be adjusted or drug stopped.

! **WARNING** Warn patient to keep drug out of reach of children, as fatalities have occurred when drug has been accidentally ingested, even in small amounts.

- Caution patient about possible visual reactions and the need for periodic eye examinations. Tell patient to notify prescriber about abnormal visual changes, including blurred vision, halos around lights, and light flashes or streaks; explain that drug will have to be stopped.
- Tell patient receiving prolonged therapy about the need for periodic blood tests to detect adverse effects. Urge compliance.
- Advise patient to notify prescriber if muscle weakness develops.

hydroxyzine hydrochloride

Atarax (CAN)

hydroxyzine pamoate

Class and Category

Pharmacologic class: Piperazine derivative
Therapeutic class: Anxiolytic, antiemetic, antihistamine, sedative-hypnotic

Indications and Dosages

* *To relieve anxiety and tension associated with psychoneurosis; as adjunct in organic disease states in which anxiety is manifested*

CAPSULES, ORAL SUSPENSION, SYRUP, TABLETS

Adults. 50 to 100 mg 4 times daily.
Children ages 6 and older. 50 to 100 mg daily in divided doses.
Children under 6 yr of age. 50 mg daily in divided doses.

I.M. INJECTION

Adults. 50 to 100 mg every 4 to 6 hr, as needed.

∗ To treat pruritus due to allergic conditions

CAPSULES, ORAL SUSPENSION, SYRUP, TABLETS

Adults. 25 mg 3 times daily or 4 times daily, as needed.
Children ages 6 and older. 50 to 100 mg daily in divided doses.
Children under 6 yr of age. 50 mg daily in divided doses.

∗ To treat nausea and vomiting excluding nausea and vomiting of pregnancy

I.M. INJECTION

Adults. 25 to 100 mg given only once.
Children. 1.1 mg/kg dose given only once.

∗ As a sedative when used as premedication and following general anesthesia

CAPSULES, ORAL SUSPENSION, SYRUP, TABLETS

Adults. 50 to 100 mg given only once.
Children. 0.6 mg/kg given only once.

I.M. INJECTION

Adults. 25 to 100 mg given only once.
Children. 1.1 mg/kg dose given only once

±**DOSAGE ADJUSTMENT** For elderly patients, treatment started at lowest possible dosage.

Drug Administration

P.O.

- Capsules and tablets should be swallowed whole and not chewed, crushed, or split/opened.
- Use a calibrated device when measuring oral suspension or syrup, to ensure an accurate dose.
- Shake suspension well before measuring dose.

I.M.

- Do not dilute before administration.
- Never administer intra-arterially, I.V., or subcutaneously.
- Aspirate carefully before pushing plunger to avoid an inadvertent I.V. injection.
- Inject deeply into a large muscle (gluteus maximus or mid-lateral thigh for adults; mid-lateral thigh for children) using the Z-track method.

Route	Onset	Peak	Duration
P.O.	15–60 min	2 hr	4–6 hr
I.M.	Rapid	Unknown	4–6 hr

Half-life: 20 hr

Mechanism of Action

Competes with histamine for histamine$_1$ receptor sites on surfaces of effector cells. This suppresses results of histaminic activity, including edema, flare, and pruritus. Sedative actions occur at subcortical level of CNS and are dose-related.

Contraindications

Early pregnancy; hypersensitivity to cetirizine, hydroxyzine, levocetirizine or their components; prolonged QT interval

Interactions

DRUGS

antibiotics, such as azithromycin, erythromycin, clarithromycin, gatifloxacin, or moxifloxacin; antidepressants, such as citalopram or fluoxetine; antipsychotics, such as chlorpromazine, clozapine, iloperidone, quetiapine, or ziprasidone; class IA, such as procainamide or quinidine; class III antiarrhythmics, such as amiodarone or sotalol; droperidol; methadone; ondansetron; pentamidine: Increased risk of QT prolongation
CNS depressants: Increased CNS depression

ACTIVITIES

alcohol use: Increased CNS depression

Adverse Reactions

CNS: Drowsiness, hallucinations, headache, involuntary motor activity, **seizures**, tremor
CV: **Prolonged QT interval**, **torsades de pointes**
EENT: Dry mouth
SKIN: Fixed drug eruptions, pruritus, rash, urticaria
Other: **Hypersensitivity reactions**, injection-site pain

Childbearing Considerations

PREGNANCY

- Drug may cause fetal harm.
- Drug is contraindicated in early pregnancy.

LACTATION

- It is not known if drug is present in breast milk.
- Breastfeeding should not be undertaken during drug therapy.

Nursing Considerations

! **WARNING** Determine pregnancy status of females of childbearing age before drug is administered because its use is contraindicated in early pregnancy.

G H I

! **WARNING** Use hydroxyzine cautiously in patients with risk factors for QT prolongation, such as concomitant arrhythmogenic drug use, electrolyte imbalance, or preexisting heart disease. Also, use cautiously in patients with bradyarrhythmias, congenital or family history of long QT syndrome, other conditions that predispose patient to QT prolongation and ventricular arrhythmia, recent MI, or uncompensated heart failure. Monitor patient closely for QT prolongation throughout therapy, which could lead to torsades de pointes.

! **WARNING** Monitor patient for hypersensitivity reactions. If present, notify prescriber, expect drug to be discontinued, and provide supportive care, as needed and ordered.

! **WARNING** Monitor patient for seizure activity. Institute seizure precautions, as needed.

- Observe for oversedation if patient takes another CNS depressant.

PATIENT TEACHING

! **WARNING** Instruct females of child bearing age to tell prescriber if she is or could be pregnant because drug is contraindicated in early pregnancy. Tell her a pregnancy test may be performed before drug therapy is begun.

- Instruct patient how to take the form of hydroxyzine prescribed.

! **WARNING** Alert patient that drug may cause an allergic reaction. If present, tell patient to notify prescriber and, if severe, to seek immediate medical care.

- Urge patient to avoid alcohol.
- Caution patient about drowsiness; tell her to avoid hazardous activities until drug's CNS effects are known and resolved.
- Inform mothers breastfeeding is not recommended during therapy.

ibalizumab-uiyk

Trogarzo

Class and Category

Pharmacologic class: CD4-directed post-attachment HIV-1 inhibitor
Therapeutic class: Antiretroviral

Indications and Dosages

* *As adjunct to treat human immunodeficiency virus (HIV) type 1 infection in heavily treatment-experienced patients with multidrug-resistant HIV-1 infection who are failing their current antiretroviral regimen*

I.V. INFUSION, I.V. INJECTION

Adults. *Loading:* 2,000 mg infused diluted over at least 30 min or injected undiluted over at least 90 sec. *Maintenance:* 800 mg every 2 wk starting 2 wk after loading dose and infused diluted over at least 15 min (providing there were no infusion-associated reactions with loading dose) or injected undiluted over at least 30 sec.

± **DOSAGE ADJUSTMENT** For patients who miss a maintenance dose by 3 days or longer beyond the scheduled dosing day, a loading dose of 2,000 mg administered as early as possible, and the maintenance dosing of 800 mg resumed 2 wk later.

Drug Administration

I.V.

- Use 10 vials to prepare the loading dose of 2,000 mg and 4 vials to prepare each maintenance dose of 800 mg.
- Administer in the cephalic vein of patient's left or right arm. If this vein is not accessible, know that an appropriate vein located elsewhere can be used.
- To prepare for I.V. infusion, withdraw 1.33 ml of drug from each of the 10 vials and transfer into a 250-ml intravenous bag of 0.9% Sodium Chloride Injection. Do not use any other diluent solutions.
- Once diluted, administer I.V. infusion immediately or store at room temperature for up to 4 hr or refrigerated for up to 24 hr. If refrigerated, allow diluted drug solution to stand at room temperature for at least 30 min but no more than 4 hr prior to administration.

- Infuse loading dose over at least 30 min or more. After infusion is complete, flush intravenous line with 30 ml of 0.9% Sodium Chloride Injection.
- For I.V. injection, allow vials to stand at room temperature for about 5 min. Withdraw 1.33 ml from each of the 4 vials. Administer undiluted immediately over at least 90 sec for loading dose and over at least 30 sec for maintenance dose. After injection is complete, flush the intravenous line with 2 to 5 ml of 0.9% Sodium Chloride Injection.
- After the I.V. infusion or injection, observe patient for 1 hr after loading dose is complete. If no infusion-associated adverse reactions occur, time of observation can be decreased to 15 min for subsequent maintenance intravenous administration.
- *Incompatibilities:* I.V. solutions other than 0.9% Sodium Chloride Injection.

Route	Onset	Peak	Duration
I.V.	Unknown	Unknown	Unknown

Half-life: 2.7–64 hr (dose-dependent)

Mechanism of Action

Blocks HIV-1 from infecting CD4 T cells by binding to domain 2 of CD4 and interfering with post-attachment steps required for entry of HIV-1 virus particles into host cells. Also, prevents the viral transmission that occurs via cell–cell infusion.

Contraindications

Hypersensitivity to ibalizumab-uiyk or its components

Interactions

DRUGS

None reported by manufacturer.

Adverse Reactions

CNS: Dizziness
ENDO: Hyperglycemia
GI: Diarrhea, elevated bilirubin and lipase levels, nausea
GU: Elevated creatinine level
HEME: Anemia, **decreased platelet count**, **leukopenia**, **neutropenia**
SKIN: Pruritus, rash
Other: Antibody formation to ibalizumab-uiyk, elevated uric acid level, **hypersensitivity reactions** (**anaphylaxis**, **angioedema**, chest pain or tightness, cough, dyspnea, hot flush, nausea, vomiting), **immune reconstitution inflammatory syndrome**, infusion reactions

Childbearing Considerations

PREGNANCY

- Pregnancy exposure registry: 1-800-258-4263.
- Drug may cause fetal harm based on animal studies because drug does cross placental barrier increasingly as pregnancy progresses and may cause reversible immunosuppression in infants exposed to drug in utero.
- Use with caution only if benefit to mother outweighs potential risk to fetus.

LACTATION

- It is not known if drug is present in breast milk.
- The Centers for Disease Control and Prevention recommends that HIV-1 infected mothers not breastfeed to avoid risking postnatal transmission of HIV-1 infection to infants. They also do not recommend breastfeeding because of potential drug-induced adverse reactions in the infant.

Nursing Considerations

! WARNING Monitor patient for an infusion-related reaction or hypersensitivity reactions, which could become life-threatening such as anaphylaxis. If present, notify prescriber, discontinue drug immediately, and provide supportive care, as needed and ordered.

! WARNING Monitor patient for signs and symptoms of infection, which could be caused by immune reconstitution inflammatory syndrome and may become life-threatening. Although rare, this syndrome may occur in combination with other antiretroviral therapy in patients whose immune systems respond during the initial phase causing an inflammatory reaction to indolent or residual opportunistic infections. If present, further evaluation and treatment will be needed.

- Know that the safety of administering live or live-attenuated vaccines in infants exposed to drug in utero is unknown.

PATIENT TEACHING

- Inform patient drug must be administered intravenously. Tell patient to alert staff immediately if a reaction occurs. Stress importance of compliance with dosage schedule of every 2 weeks. Remind patient that if dose is missed for 3 days or longer, a loading dosage will have to be repeated before maintenance dosing can be reestablished.
- Advise patient not to change the dosing schedule of any other antriretroviral medication without consulting prescriber as it may affect effectiveness of ibalizumab-uiyk. Tell patient to immediately notify prescriber if they stop taking ibalizumab-uiyk or any other drug in their antiretroviral regimen.

! **WARNING** Alert patient to possibility of an allergic reaction that could be severe. If an allergic reaction occurs, tell patient to inform healthcare staff immediately.

! **WARNING** Instruct patient to immediately report any signs and symptoms of an infection to prescriber.

- Advise mothers not to breastfeed their infant while receiving ibalizumab-uiyk and to alert pediatrician if she received drug during her pregnancy.

ibandronate sodium

Class and Category

Pharmacologic class: Bisphosphonate
Therapeutic class: Antiosteoporotic

Indications and Dosages

∗ *To prevent osteoporosis in postmenopausal women*

TABLETS

Adult females. 150 mg once monthly.

∗ *To treat osteoporosis in postmenopausal women*

TABLETS

Adult females. 150 mg once monthly.

I.V. INJECTION

Adult females. 3 mg every 3 mo.

Drug Administration

P.O.

- Tablet should be swallowed whole and not chewed, crushed, split, or sucked on.
- Administer at least 60 min before the first food, beverage, or medication of the day with 6 to 8 ounces of plain water.
- Ensure that patient does not lie down for at least 60 min after drug is administered.
- Do not administer with any other medication and ensure that patient does not drink anything except water for 60 min after drug is administered.
- Administer tablets same day of each month.

I.V.

- Administer undiluted over 15 to 30 sec as an I.V. injection using the prefilled syringe and needle supplied by manufacturer.
- Take care not to administer drug intra-arterially or paravenously, as this can lead to tissue damage.
- Do not administer by I.M. or subcutaneously.
- Administer a missed dose as soon as possible when realized and schedule future doses from that date, not the original date.
- *Incompatibilities:* Calcium-containing solutions or other I.V. drugs

Route	Onset	Peak	Duration
P.O.	Unknown	0.5–2 hr	Unknown
I.V.	Rapid	Unknown	Unknown

Half-life: 4.5–25.5 hr

Mechanism of Action

Based on its affinity for hydroxyapatite, which is part of the mineral matrix of bone, osteoclast activity is inhibited, and bone resorption and turnover are reduced. In postmenopausal women, the elevated rate of bone turnover is reduced leading to, on average, a net gain in bone mass.

Contraindications

Esophageal abnormalities that delay esophageal emptying, such as achalasia or stricture (oral form); hypersensitivity to ibandronate or its components; inability to stand or sit upright for at least 60 min (oral form); uncorrected hypocalcemia

Interactions

DRUGS

aspirin, NSAIDs: Increased risk of GI irritation

products containing calcium and other multivalent cations, such as aluminum, magnesium, iron: Impaired absorption of ibandronate

FOODS

all foods: Decreased ibandronate bioavailability

Adverse Reactions

CNS: Asthenia, depression, dizziness, fatigue, headache, insomnia, nerve root lesion, vertigo

CV: Hypercholesterolemia, hypertension

EENT: Nasopharyngitis, pharyngitis, tooth disorder

GI: Abdominal pain, constipation, diarrhea, dyspepsia, gastritis, gastroenteritis, nausea, vomiting

GU: Cystitis, UTI

MS: Arthralgia; arthritis; atypical subtrochanteric and diaphyseal femoral fractures; back, bone, extremity, joint, or muscle pain; joint disorder; localized osteoarthritis; myalgia; osteonecrosis of jaw and other orofacial sites

RESP: **Asthma exacerbations**, bronchitis, **bronchospasm**, pneumonia, upper respiratory infection

SKIN: Dermatitis bullous, **erythema multiforme**, rash, **Stevens-Johnson syndrome**

Other: **Anaphylaxis**, **angioedema**, **and other hypersensitivity reactions**; flu-like symptoms; **hypocalcemia**; infection; injection-site reactions, such as redness or swelling

Childbearing Considerations

PREGNANCY

- It is not known if drug causes fetal harm.
- Drug is not indicated for use in females of childbearing age.

LACTATION

- It is not known if drug is present in breast milk.
- Drug is not indicated for use in breastfeeding mothers.

Nursing Considerations

- Be aware that hypocalcemia, hypovitaminosis D, and other disturbances of bone and mineral metabolism must be effectively treated before starting ibandronate therapy.
- Know that ibandronate should not be administered to patients with severe renal impairment.
- Use cautiously in patients with active upper GI problems (such as known Barrett's esophagus, dysphagia, other esophageal diseases, duodenitis, gastritis, ulcers) because drug may cause local irritation of the upper GI mucosa.

! WARNING Obtain serum creatinine level in patients receiving injection form of ibandronate prior to administering each dose because other bisphosphonates have been associated with serious renal toxicity. If renal deterioration occurs, expect drug to be discontinued.

! WARNING Monitor patient for a hypersensitivity reaction, which could become life-threatening, such as anaphylaxis or angioedema. If present, notify prescriber, expect drug to be discontinued, and provide supportive care, as needed and ordered.

! WARNING Monitor patient's respiratory status for bronchospasms or asthma exacerbation. Notify prescriber immediately, if present, expect drug to be discontinued, and provide supportive care, as needed and ordered.

- Make sure patient has had a dental checkup before having invasive dental procedures during ibandronate therapy, especially if patient has cancer; is receiving chemotherapy, head or neck radiation, or a corticosteroid; or has poor oral hygiene because the risk of jaw osteonecrosis is increased in patients who have taken other bisphosphonates, a class of drugs of which ibandronate is a member.

PATIENT TEACHING

- Instruct patient how to administer oral ibandronate prescribed and what to do if a dose is missed. Caution against lying down for at least 60 minutes after taking drug to keep it from lodging in esophagus and causing irritation.
- Alert patient receiving drug intravenously that injection site reactions may occur such

as redness or swelling and to alert staff if present.

- Inform patient of need for and importance of taking supplemental calcium and vitamin D on daily basis. Instruct patient to take calcium supplements at least 2 hours before or after oral ibandronate.

! **WARNING** Alert patient that drug may cause an allergic reaction. Also warn patient that drug can cause asthma exacerbation or bronchospasms. If present, tell patient to notify prescriber and stop taking ibandronate. If severe, urge patient to seek immediate medical care.

! **WARNING** Advise patient to stop taking drug and to notify prescriber if GI symptoms appear or become worse. Also, tell patient to stop taking drug and notify prescriber if she develops dysphagia, pain while swallowing, retrosternal pain, or new or worsening heartburn.

- Alert patient that drugs in the same class as ibandronate have caused severe bone, joint, or muscle pain. If such symptoms appear while taking ibandronate, advise patient to contact prescriber. Also, tell her to report new or worsening groin or thigh pain.
- Instruct patient on proper oral hygiene and on the need to notify prescriber about invasive dental procedures because risk of developing osteonecrosis of the jaw decreases in the absence of bisphosphonate therapy.

ibrexafungerp

Brexafemme

Class and Category

Pharmacologic class: Triterpenoid antifungal
Therapeutic class: Azole antifungal

Indications and Dosages

∗ *To treat vulvovaginal candidiasis*

TABLETS

Adult females and postmenarchal pediatric females. 300 mg (two 150-mg tablets) given twice (12 hr apart) in one 24-hr period. *Maximum:* 600 mg in one 24-hr period.

∗ *To reduce incidence of recurrent vulvovaginal candidiasis*

TABLETS

Adult females and postmenarchal pediatric females. 300 mg (two 150 mg tablets) given twice (12 apart) in one 24-hr period monthly for 6 mo.

±**DOSAGE ADJUSTMENT** For patients taking a strong CYP3A inhibitor, dosage decreased to 150 mg and given twice (12 hr apart) in one 24-hr period.

Drug Administration

P.O.

- Verify pregnancy status prior to administering drug.
- Administer the 2 doses of drug about 12 hr apart, preferably in the morning and evening. However, if first dose is administered in the afternoon or evening, the second dose should be taken the following morning.

Route	Onset	Peak	Duration
P.O.	Unknown	4–6 hr	Unknown

Half-life: 20 hr

Mechanism of Action

Inhibits glucan synthase, an essential component for the development of the fungal cell wall, causing fungicidal activity against *Candida* species.

Contraindications

Hypersensitivity to ibrexafungerp or its components, pregnancy

Interactions

DRUGS

CYP3A strong and moderate inducers, such as bosentan, carbamazepine, efavirenz, etravirine, long-acting barbiturates, phenytoin, rifampin, St. John's wort: Possibly significant reduction in plasma concentration of ibrexafungerp, thereby reducing effectiveness

CYP3A strong inhibitors, such as itraconazole, ketoconazole: Significantly increases plasma concentration of ibrexafungerp, which increases risk of adverse reactions

Adverse Reactions

CNS: Dizziness
GI: Abdominal pain, diarrhea, elevated liver enzymes, flatulence, nausea, vomiting
GU: Dysmenorrhea, vaginal bleeding
MS: Back pain

SKIN: Rash
Other: **Hypersensitivity reaction**

Childbearing Considerations

PREGNANCY

- Pregnancy exposure registry: 1-888-982-7299.
- Drug may cause fetal harm based on animal studies.
- Drug is contraindicated in pregnancy.

LACTATION

- It is not known if drug is present in breast milk.
- Mothers should check with prescriber before breastfeeding.

REPRODUCTION

- A negative pregnancy test must be obtained before drug is initiated and before each monthly dose, if applicable.
- Females of childbearing age must use effective contraception throughout drug treatment, including the 6-month treatment period, if applicable, and for 4 days after last dose.

NURSING CONSIDERATIONS

! **WARNING** Be aware that ibrexafungerp should not be given to premenarchal pediatric females. Ensure that a negative pregnancy test has been obtained before drug is administered because drug is contraindicated in pregnant females

! **WARNING** Monitor patient for a hypersensitivity reaction. If present, notify prescriber, expect drug to be discontinued, and provide supportive care, as needed and ordered.

PATIENT TEACHING

- Review with patient how tablets are to be taken.
- Tell patient to inform prescriber if she is taking any other drugs, including over-the-counter drugs such as St. John's wort, before taking ibrexafungerp.
- Instruct females of child bearing age that a pregnancy test will be required before drug can be given because drug may cause fetal harm. Tell patient prescribed the 6-month treatment regimen that a negative pregnancy test must be reconfirmed every month during the 6-month treatment regimen.

! **WARNING** Advise females of childbearing age to use effective contraception while taking drug, including throughout 6-month treatment period, if applicable, and for 4 days after the last dose.

! **WARNING** Instruct patient to notify prescriber if an allergic reaction occurs. If reaction is serious, instruct patient to seek immediate medical attention.

ibuprofen

Advil, Advil Migraine, Caldolor, Children's Advil, Children's Motrin, Excedrin, Motrin

ibuprofen lysine

NeoProfen

Class and Category

Pharmacologic class: NSAID
Therapeutic class: Analgesic, anti-inflammatory, antipyretic

Indications and Dosages

✱ *To relieve pain in rheumatoid arthritis and osteoarthritis*

CAPSULES, CHEWABLE TABLETS, ORAL SUSPENSION, TABLETS

Adults. 300 mg 4 times daily; or 400, 600, or 800 mg 3 times daily or 4 times daily. *Usual:* 1.2 to 3.2 g daily. *Maximum:* 3.2 g daily.

✱ *To relieve pain in juvenile arthritis*

CAPSULES, CHEWABLE TABLETS, ORAL SUSPENSION, TABLETS

Children. 20 to 40 mg/kg daily in 3 or 4 divided doses.
Maximum: 50 mg/kg daily.

✱ *To relieve mild to moderate pain*

CAPSULES, CHEWABLE TABLETS, ORAL SUSPENSION, TABLETS

Adults. 200 to 400 mg every 4 to 6 hr, as needed.
Children ages 12 and older. 200 to 400 mg every 4 to 6 hr, as needed. *Maximum:* 1.2 g.

CHEWABLE TABLETS, ORAL SUSPENSION

Children age 11 weighing 33 kg (72 lb) to 43 kg (95 lb). 300 mg every 6 to 8 hr, as needed.

Children ages 9 and 10 weighing 27 kg (59 lb) to 32 kg (70 lb). 250 mg every 6 to 8 hr, as needed.
Children ages 6 to 8 weighing 22 kg (48 lb) to 27 kg (59 lb). 200 mg every 6 to 8 hr, as needed.
Children ages 4 and 5 weighing 16 kg (35 lb) to 21 kg (46 lb). 150 mg every 6 to 8 hr, as needed.
Children ages 2 and 3 weighing 11 kg (24 lb) to 16 kg (35 lb). 100 mg every 6 to 8 hr, as needed.

ORAL DROPS

Children ages 12 to 23 mo weighing 8.18 kg (18 lb) to 10.45 kg (23 lb). 75 mg every 6 to 8 hr, as needed.
Children ages 6 to 11 mo weighing 5.45 kg (12 lb) to 7.73 kg (17 lb). 50 mg every 6 to 8 hr, as needed.

I.V. INFUSION (CALDOLOR)

Adults. 400 to 800 mg infused over at least 30 min every 6 hr, as needed. *Maximum:* 3,200 mg daily.
Adolescents. 400 mg infused over at least 10 min every 4 to 6 hr, as needed. *Maximum:* 2,400 mg daily.
Children ages 6 mo to 12 yr. 10 mg/kg (400 mg maximum) infused over at least 10 min every 4 to 6 hr, as needed. *Maximum:* 400 mg/single dose; 40 mg/kg or 2,400 mg daily, whichever is less.
Infants ages 3 mo to less than 6 mo. 10 mg/kg (100 mg maximum) as a single dose infused over at least 10 min.

* *As adjunct with opioid analgesics to relieve moderate to severe pain*

I.V. INFUSION (CALDOLOR)

Adults. 400 to 800 mg infused over at least 30 min every 6 hr, as needed. *Maximum:* 3,200 mg daily.
Adolescents. 400 mg infused over at least 10 min every 4 to 6 hr, as needed. *Maximum:* 2,400 mg daily.
Children ages 6 mo to 12 yr. 10 mg/kg (400 mg maximum) infused over at least 10 min every 4 to 6 hr, as needed. *Maximum:* 400 mg/single dose; 40 mg/kg or 2,400 mg daily, whichever is less.
Infants ages 3 mo to less than 6 mo. 10 mg/kg (100 mg maximum) as a single dose infused over at least 10 min.

* *To reduce fever*

CAPSULES, CHEWABLE TABLETS, ORAL SUSPENSION, TABLETS

Adults and adolescents. 200 to 400 mg every 4 to 6 hr, as needed.

CHEWABLE TABLETS, ORAL SUSPENSION

Children age 11 weighing 33 kg (72 lb) to 43 kg (95 lb). 300 mg every 6 to 8 hr, as needed.
Children ages 9 and 10 weighing 27 kg (59 lb) to 32 kg (70 lb). 250 mg every 6 to 8 hr, as needed.
Children ages 6 to 8 weighing 22 kg (48 lb) to 27 kg (59 lb). 200 mg every 6 to 8 hr, as needed.
Children ages 4 and 5 weighing 16 kg (35 lb) to 21 kg (46 lb). 150 mg every 6 to 8 hr, as needed.
Children ages 2 and 3 weighing 11 kg (24 lb) to 16 kg (35 lb). 100 mg every 6 to 8 hr, as needed.

ORAL DROPS

Children ages 12 to 23 mo weighing 8.18 kg (18 lb) to 10.45 kg (23 lb). 75 mg every 6 to 8 hr, as needed.
Children ages 6 to 11 mo weighing 5.45 kg (12 lb) to 7.73 kg (17 lb). 50 mg every 6 to 8 hr, as needed.

I.V. INFUSION (CALDOLOR)

Adults. 400 mg infused over at least 30 min, followed by 400 mg every 4 to 6 hr or 100 to 200 mg every 4 hr, as needed. *Maximum:* 3,200 mg daily.
Adolescents. 400 mg infused over at least 10 min every 4 to 6 hr, as needed. *Maximum:* 2,400 mg daily.
Children ages 6 mo to 12 yr. 10 mg/kg (400 mg maximum) infused over at least 10 min every 4 to 6 hr, as needed. *Maximum:* 400 mg/single dose; 40 mg/kg or 2,400 mg daily, whichever is less.
Infants ages 3 mo to less than 6 mo. 10 mg/kg (100 mg maximum) as a single dose infused over at least 10 min.

* *To treat patent ductus arteriosus*

I.V. INFUSION (NEOPROFEN)

Gestational age 32 wk or less and weighing between 500 and 1,500 g. *Initial:* 10 mg/kg (based on birth weight) followed by 5 mg/kg 24 hr later and 5 mg/kg 24 hr after second dose. Each dose infused over 15 min.

* *To relieve migraine pain and related symptoms, like nausea and sensitivity to light and sound.*

CAPSULES (ADVIL MIGRAINE)

Adults. 400 mg as a single dose at onset of symptoms. *Maximum:* 400 mg/24 hr.

Drug Administration

P.O.

- Administer with food or after meals to reduce GI distress.
- Give drug with a full glass of water.
- Ensure that patient does not lie down for 15 to 30 min, to prevent esophageal irritation.
- Shake oral suspension and drops well before measuring dosage. Use a calibrated measuring device to measure dosage.

I.V.

Caldolor

- Dilute to final concentration of 4 mg/ml or less using 0.9% Sodium Chloride Injection, 5% Dextrose Injection, or Lactated Ringer's solution. For an 800-mg dose, dilute 8 ml in at least 200 ml of diluent; for a 400-mg dose, dilute 4 ml in at least 100 ml of diluent; for a 200-mg dose, dilute 2 ml in at least 100 ml of diluent; and for a 100-mg dose, dilute 1 ml in at least 100 ml of diluent.
- Diluted solutions may be kept at room temperature up to 24 hr.
- Infuse over at least 30 min for adults and 10 min for children and infants.

NeoProfen

- Withdraw drug from vial and discard any remaining drug in vial because it does not contain a preservative. Dilute to an appropriate volume with 0.9% Sodium Chloride Injection or 5% Dextrose Injection.
- Administer within 30 min of preparation.
- Administer via the I.V. port that is nearest the insertion site. Infuse over 15 min.
- Total Parenteral Nutriton (TPN) should be interrupted for a 15-min period prior to and after drug administration.
- *Incompatibilities:* TPN simultaneously through the same I.V. line

Route	Onset	Peak	Duration
P.O.	30–60 min	1–2 hr	4–6 hr
I.V.	Unknown	Unknown	Unknown

Half-life: 2–4 hr

Mechanism of Action

Blocks activity of cyclooxygenase, the enzyme needed to synthesize prostaglandins, which mediate inflammatory response and cause local pain, swelling, and vasodilation. By inhibiting prostaglandins, this NSAID reduces inflammatory symptoms and relieves pain. Ibuprofen's antipyretic action probably stems from its effect on the hypothalamus, which increases peripheral blood flow, causing vasodilation and encouraging heat dissipation.

Contraindications

For all forms except ibuprofen lysine: Angioedema, asthma, bronchospasm, nasal polyps, rhinitis, or urticaria caused by hypersensitivity to aspirin or other NSAIDs; hypersensitivity to ibuprofen or its components; pain with coronary artery bypass graft (CABG) surgery; previous history of serious skin reactions

For ibuprofen lysine: Bleeding (especially active intracranial hemorrhage or GI bleeding), coagulation defects, congenital heart disease where patency of the patent ductus arteriosus is necessary for satisfactory pulmonary or systemic blood flow (pulmonary atresia, severe coarctation of the aorta, severe tetralogy of Fallot), hypersensitivity to ibuprofen or its components, known or suspected infection or necrotizing enterocolitis, significant renal impairment, thrombocytopenia

Interactions

DRUGS

ACE inhibitors, angiotensin receptor blockers (ARBs), beta-blockers (including propranolol): Possibly diminished antihypertensive effect of these drugs

aspirin: Possibly decreased cardioprotective and stroke-preventive effects of aspirin; increased risk of bleeding and adverse GI effects

cyclosporine: Increased risk of nephrotoxicity

digoxin: Increased blood digoxin level and risk of digitalis toxicity

diuretics (loop, potassium-sparing, and thiazide): Decreased diuretic and antihypertensive effects

heparin, oral anticoagulants, selective serotonin reuptake inhibitors, serotonin norepinephrine reuptake inhibitors, thrombolytics: Increased anticoagulant effects, increased risk of hemorrhage

lithium: Increased blood lithium level

methotrexate: Decreased methotrexate clearance and increased risk of toxicity
other NSAIDs, salicylates: Increased risk of GI toxicity
pemetrexed: Increased risk of GI and renal toxicity; myelosuppression

ACTIVITIES

alcohol use: Increased risk of adverse GI effects

Adverse Reactions

CNS: **Aseptic meningitis**, **CVA**, dizziness, headache, nervousness, **seizures**
CV: Fluid retention, **heart failure**, hypertension, **MI**, peripheral edema, tachycardia
EENT: Amblyopia, epistaxis, stomatitis, tinnitus
GI: Abdominal cramps, distention, or pain; anorexia; constipation; diarrhea; diverticulitis; dyspepsia; dysphagia; elevated liver enzymes; epigastric discomfort; esophagitis; flatulence; gastritis; gastroenteritis; gastroesophageal reflux disease; **GI bleeding**, **hemorrhage**, **perforation**, or ulceration; heartburn; hemorrhoids; **hepatic failure**; **hepatitis**; hiatal hernia; indigestion; **melena**; nausea; **necrotizing enterocolitis**; vomiting
GU: Cystitis, hematuria, **renal failure (acute)**
HEME: **Agranulocytosis**, anemia, **aplastic anemia**, eosinophilia, **hemolytic anemia**, **leukopenia**, **neutropenia**, **pancytopenia**, **prolonged bleeding time**, **thrombocytopenia**
RESP: **Bronchospasm**, dyspnea, **pulmonary hypertension (neonates)**, wheezing
SKIN: Acute generalized exanthematous pustulosis, blisters, **erythema multiforme**, **exfoliative dermatitis**, fixed drug eruption, **generalized bullous fixed drug eruption**, photosensitivity, pruritus, rash, **Stevens-Johnson syndrome**, **toxic epidermal necrolysis**, urticaria
Other: **Anaphylaxis**, **angioedema**, **drug reaction with eosinophilia and systemic symptoms (DRESS)**, flu-like symptoms, **hypokalemia**, weight gain

Childbearing Considerations

PREGNANCY

- Drug increases risk of premature closure of the fetal ductus arteriosus if given at 30 wk or later during pregnancy. Neonatal renal impairment and oligohydramnios may occur if drug is given at 20 wk gestation or later.
- Drug is contraindicated at 30 wk or later during pregnancy and should be avoided beginning at 20 wk of pregnancy.

LACTATION

- Drug is present in breast milk.
- Breastfeeding is not recommended because maturation of renal system in infant may take up to 2 yr.

REPRODUCTION

- Drug may delay or prevent rupture of ovarian follicles, which may cause reversible infertility in some women.

Nursing Considerations

! **WARNING** Be aware that NSAIDs, such as ibuprofen, should be avoided in patients with a recent MI because increased risk of reinfarction. If therapy is unavoidable, monitor patient closely for signs of cardiac ischemia. Be aware that the risk of serious cardiovascular thrombotic events such as MI or stroke increases the longer ibuprofen is used. Expect to give drug for shortest time possible. These events may occur early in treatment and happen even in patients who do not have a history of or risk factors for cardiovascular disease. Monitor patient for warning signs, such as chest pain, slurring of speech, shortness of breath, or weakness. If any signs and symptoms develop, withhold ibuprofen, alert prescriber immediately, and provide supportive care as needed and ordered.

! **WARNING** Know that the risk of heart failure increases with use of NSAIDs, such as ibuprofen. Ibuprofen should not be used in patients with severe heart failure but, if unavoidable, monitor patient for worsening of heart failure.

! **WARNING** Use ibuprofen with extreme caution in patients with a history of GI bleeding or ulcer disease because NSAIDs, such as ibuprofen, increase risk of GI bleeding and ulceration. Expect to use ibuprofen for shortest time possible in these patients.

- Expect higher doses for rheumatoid arthritis than for osteoarthritis.

- Be aware that ibuprofen oral suspension may contain sucrose, which may affect blood glucose level in diabetic patients.

! **WARNING** Monitor patient for a hypersensitivity reaction, which could become life-threatening such as anaphylaxis or angioedema and serious skin reactions such as DRESS. Assess patient's skin regularly for signs of rash or other hypersensitivity reactions because ibuprofen is a NSAID and may cause severe skin reactions without warning, even in patients with no history of NSAID sensitivity. At first sign of reaction including a rash (DRESS may only initially present with a fever or swollen lymph nodes), stop drug, notify prescriber, and provide supportive care, as needed and ordered.

! **WARNING** Keep in mind that serious GI tract bleeding, perforation, and ulceration may occur without warning symptoms. Elderly patients are at greater risk. To minimize risk, give oral drug with food. If GI distress occurs, withhold drug and notify prescriber immediately.

- Monitor patient—especially if he is elderly or receiving long-term oral ibuprofen therapy—for less common but serious adverse GI reactions, including anorexia, constipation, diverticulitis, dysphagia, esophagitis, gastritis, gastroenteritis, gastroesophageal reflux disease, hemorrhoids, hiatal hernia, melena, stomatitis, and vomiting.

! **WARNING** Monitor BUN and serum creatinine levels in elderly patients, patients taking ACE inhibitors or diuretics, and patients with heart failure, hepatic dysfunction, or impaired renal function; drug may cause renal failure. Also monitor liver enzymes, as ordered, because, in rare cases, elevations may progress to severe hepatic reactions, including fatal hepatitis, hepatic failure, or liver necrosis.

! **WARNING** Be aware that if patient has bone marrow suppression or is receiving an antineoplastic drug, monitor laboratory results (including WBC count), and watch for evidence of infection. Be aware that ibuprofen's anti-inflammatory and antipyretic actions may mask signs and symptoms, such as fever and pain.

- Monitor patients with hypertension and assess blood pressure closely throughout therapy. Drug may cause hypertension or worsen it.
- Monitor CBC for decreased hemoglobin and hematocrit. Drug may worsen anemia.

PATIENT TEACHING

! **WARNING** Tell patient to alert prescriber before taking ibuprofen if he has ever had an allergic reaction to any other analgesic or fever-reducing drug or has a history of asthma or previous serious skin reactions.

! **WARNING** Advise family or caregiver to consult prescriber before giving over-the-counter ibuprofen to a child if the child has any of the following: asthma; bleeding problems; heart or kidney disease; high blood pressure; need for diuretic therapy; persistent stomach problems, such as heartburn, stomach pain, or upset stomach; serious adverse effects from previous use of fever reducers or pain relievers; or GI ulcers.

- Instruct patient how to administer form of ibuprofen prescribed.
- Urge patient not to take higher doses of drug or for a longer time than prescribed because stomach bleeding may occur, and risk of heart attack or stroke may increase.

! **WARNING** Instruct patient, especially if elderly, to consult prescriber if he needs to take drug for more than 3 days for fever or 10 days for pain or if persistent, severe, or unusual signs and symptoms occur.

! **WARNING** Inform patient with phenylketonuria that Motrin chewable tablets contain aspartame.

- Inform patient that full therapeutic effect for arthritis may take 2 weeks or longer.
- Urge patient to avoid taking 2 different NSAIDs at the same time, unless directed.

! **WARNING** Caution pregnant patient not to take oral ibuprofen at 20 weeks of gestation or more unless directed to do so by prescriber because of adverse effects on fetal renal system and potential for premature closure of the ductus arteriosus after 30 weeks' gestation.

! WARNING Alert patient that drug may cause an allergic reaction, including severe skin reactions. Urge the patient to stop taking ibuprofen and to seek immediate medical attention for blisters, fever, itching, rash, swollen lymph nodes, or other indications of hypersensitivity.

! WARNING Explain that ibuprofen may increase risk of serious adverse cardiovascular reactions; urge patient to seek immediate medical attention if signs or symptoms arise, such as chest pain, edema, shortness of breath, slurring of speech, swelling in legs, unexplained weight gain, or weakness.

! WARNING Urge family or caregiver to seek medical care and to tell prescriber promptly if child receiving drug develops headache, high fever, nausea, persistent diarrhea, severe and persistent sore throat, or vomiting, or hasn't been drinking fluids.

! WARNING All ibuprofen products should be kept out of reach of children. If an overdose occurs, instruct family or caregiver to get immediate medical help or contact a Poison Control Center immediately.

- Urge patient to avoid alcohol or taking aspirin or corticosteroids while taking ibuprofen, unless prescribed. If patient takes aspirin as prevention of MI or stroke, explain that ibuprofen may interfere with this effect.
- Suggest that patient wear sunscreen and protective clothing when outdoors.
- Inform mothers breastfeeding is not recommended.

ibutilide fumarate

Corvert

Class and Category

Pharmacologic class: Methane sulfonanilide derivative

Therapeutic class: Class III antiarrhythmic

Indications and Dosages

∗ *To rapidly convert recent-onset atrial flutter or fibrillation to sinus rhythm*

I.V. INFUSION

Adults weighing 60 kg (132 lb) or more. 1 mg infused over 10 min. Dose repeated 10 min after first dose is finished if arrhythmia persists.

Adults weighing less than 60 kg (132 lb). 0.01 mg/kg infused over 10 min. Dose repeated 10 min after first dose is completed if arrhythmia persists.

Drug Administration

I.V.

- Give drug undiluted or diluted in 50 ml of 0.9% Sodium Chloride Injection or 5% Dextrose Injection by adding contents of one 10-ml vial (0.1 mg/ml) to form a concentration of about 0.017 mg/ml.
- Use polyvinyl chloride plastic bags or polyolefin bags.
- Give drug within 24 hr if stored at room temperature or 48 hr if refrigerated.
- Infuse over 10 min.
- Immediately stop infusion if conversion occurs or patient develops marked prolongation of QT interval or ventricular tachycardia.
- *Incompatibilities:* None reported by manufacturer

Route	Onset	Peak	Duration
I.V.	< 90 min	Unknown	24 hr

Half-life: 6 hr

Mechanism of Action

May promote sodium movement through slow, inward sodium channels in myocardial cell membranes. Ibutilide also may inhibit potassium channels in myocardial cell membranes involved in cardiac repolarization. These actions prolong cardiac action potential by delaying repolarization and increasing atrial and ventricular refractoriness. As a result, sinus rate slows, and AV conduction is delayed.

Contraindications

Hypersensitivity to ibutilide or components

Interactions

DRUGS

antihistamine drugs (selective), such as H1 receptor antagonists, class IA antiarrhythmics

(disopyramide, procainamide, quinidine), class III antiarrhythmics (amiodarone, sotalol), phenothiazines, tetracyclic or tricyclic antidepressants: Possibly increased risk of prolonged QT interval, leading to increased risk of proarrhythmias
digoxin: Possibly masking cardiotoxicity associated with excessive digoxin levels

Adverse Reactions

CNS: Headache, syncope
CV: **AV block**, **bradycardia**, bundle branch block, **heart failure**, hypertension, **hypotension**, **idioventricular rhythm**, orthostatic hypotension, palpitations, **prolonged QT interval**, sinus tachycardia, **supraventricular arrhythmias**, **ventricular arrhythmias**
GI: Nausea
GU: **Renal failure**

Childbearing Considerations

PREGNANCY

- Drug may cause fetal harm, according to animal studies.
- Use with caution only if benefit to mother outweighs potential risk to fetus.

LACTATION

- It is not known if drug is present in breast milk.
- The seriousness of the situation would not allow breastfeeding to take place during drug administration. However, have mothers check with prescriber when breastfeeding can be resumed following administration of the drug.

Nursing Considerations

- Check serum electrolyte levels and expect to correct abnormalities, as prescribed, before ibutilide therapy is initiated. Be especially alert for hypokalemia and hypomagnesemia, which can lead to arrhythmias.

! **WARNING** As ordered, monitor patient's cardiac rhythm continuously during infusion and for at least 4 hours afterward—longer if arrhythmias appear or if patient has abnormal hepatic function. Observe patient for ventricular ectopy.

! **WARNING** Make sure defibrillator and drugs to treat sustained ventricular tachycardia are available during therapy and when monitoring patient after therapy.

PATIENT TEACHING

- Inform patient that ibutilide will be given by I.V. infusion and that his heart rhythm will be monitored continuously.

! **WARNING** Ask patient to report chest pain, faintness, numbness, palpitations, shortness of breath, and tingling immediately to staff.

- Advise patient to keep follow-up appointments to monitor heart rhythm.
- Know that while the seriousness of the situation would not allow breastfeeding to take place during drug administration, have mothers check with prescriber when breastfeeding can be resumed following administration of the drug.

idarucizumab

Praxbind

Class and Category

Pharmacologic class: Humanized monoclonal antibody fragment
Therapeutic class: Antidote

Indications and Dosages

* *To reverse anticoagulant effects of dabigatran needed for emergency surgery, life-threatening bleeding, urgent procedures, or uncontrolled bleeding*

I.V. INFUSION, I.V. INJECTION

Adults. 5 g given in two 2.5-g doses consecutively, and repeated 1 time, as needed.

Drug Administration

I.V.

- Administer drug solution undiluted immediately after it is removed from vial. Solution should be clear and colorless to slightly yellow. Do not shake vials.
- Using two 2.5-g/50-ml vials, administer drug as two 2.5-g doses back-to-back either as an intravenous infusion or injection.

- Flush intravenous line with 0.9% Sodium Chloride Injection prior to administering drug.
- Administration should take no longer than 5 to 10 min.
- Drug vial solution should be stored in refrigerator in original carton protected from light. It may be stored at room temperature for up to 48 hr in original carton protected from light but must be used within 6 hr if stored out of the carton and exposed to light.
- *Incompatibilities:* Other drugs in the same intravenous line

Route	Onset	Peak	Duration
I.V.	Rapid	Unknown	24 hr

Half-life: 10.3 hr

Mechanism of Action

Binds to dabigatran and its acyl-glucuronide metabolites with higher affinity than the binding of dabigatran to thrombin, thereby neutralizing their anticoagulant effect and reversing the effects of dabigatran.

Contraindications

Hypersensitivity to idarucizumab or its components

Interactions

DRUGS

None reported by manufacturer.

Adverse Reactions

CNS: Delirium, fever
CV: **Thrombotic events**
GI: Constipation
RESP: **Bronchospasm**, hyperventilation, pneumonia
SKIN: Pruritus, rash
Other: **Anaphylaxis**, formation of idarucizumab antibodies, **hypokalemia**

Childbearing Considerations

PREGNANCY

- It is not known if drug causes fetal harm.
- Use with caution only if benefit to mother outweighs potential risk to fetus.

LACTATION

- Drug is present in breast milk.
- Mothers should check with prescriber before breastfeeding.

Nursing Considerations

! **WARNING** Use extreme caution when administering idarucizumab to a patient with hereditary fructose intolerance because idarucizumab contains 4 g of sorbitol. The amount of sorbitol that may cause serious or even fatal adverse reactions is not known.

- Provide standard supportive measures to control dabigatran-induced bleeding, as needed and ordered, in conjunction with idarucizumab treatment.
- Monitor patient's coagulation parameters such as activated partial thromboplastin time (aPTT) or ecarin clotting time (ECT), as ordered.

! **WARNING** Monitor patient for a hypersensitivity reaction to idarucizumab, which could become life-threatening, such as anaphylaxis. If present, stop administration immediately, notify prescriber, and provide emergency supportive care, as needed and ordered.

! **WARNING** Monitor patient closely for thrombotic events because reversing dabigatran with idarucizumab increases the risk of such events. Know that resumption of anticoagulant therapy should be done as soon as possible. For example, dabigatran may be resumed 24 hours after the administration of idarucizumab.

PATIENT TEACHING

! **WARNING** Instruct patient to alert staff immediately if difficulty breathing or skin reactions such as itchiness or a rash develop during or after idarucizumab has been administered.

- Alert patient that anticoagulant therapy will be needed once the bleeding episode has been resolved to prevent future blood clots. Patient may be able to resume dabigatran therapy 24 hours after idarucizumab therapy is given, if ordered.
- Tell patient that blood tests will be needed to monitor effectiveness of idarucizumab therapy and that a second dose of idarucizumab may be required, if needed.

iloperidone

Fanapt

Class and Category

Pharmacologic class: Atypical antipsychotic
Therapeutic class: Second-generation antipsychotic

Indications and Dosages

✱ *To treat schizophrenia*

TABLETS

Adults. *Initial:* 1 mg twice daily, adjusted to target dosage range as follows: 2 mg twice daily on day 2, 4 mg twice daily on day 3, and 6 mg twice daily on day 4. Dosage may be further increased, as needed, as follows: 8 mg twice daily on day 5, 10 mg twice daily on day 6, and 12 mg twice daily on day 7. *Maximum:* 12 mg twice daily.

✱ *To treat acute manic or mixed episodes associated with bipolar I disorder*

TABLETS

Adults. *Initial:* 1 mg twice day, adjusted to target dosage range as follows: 3 mg twice daily on day 2, 6 mg twice daily on day 3, 9 mg twice daily on day 4, 12 mg twice daily on day 5 and thereafter. *Maximum:* 12 mg twice daily.

± **DOSAGE ADJUSTMENT** For patients taking strong CYP2D6 inhibitors, including fluoxetine and paroxetine, CYP3A4 inhibitors, such as clarithromycin and ketoconazole, or are poor metabolizers of CYP2D6, dosage reduced by half. For patients with moderate hepatic impairment, dose reduced, as needed.

Drug Administration

P.O.

- Expect to restart dosage adjustment schedule in patients who have been off drug for more than 3 days.
- Protect from light and moisture when stored.

Route	Onset	Peak	Duration
P.O.	Unknown	2–4 hr	Unknown

Half-life: 18–33 hr

Mechanism of Action

Selectively blocks dopamine type 2 (D_2) and serotonin type 2 (5-HT_2) receptors in CNS, thereby suppressing psychotic symptoms.

Contraindications

Hypersensitivity to iloperidone or its components

Interactions

DRUGS

alpha-adrenergic blocking agents: Increased risk of symptomatic hypotension
antibiotics, such as fluoroquinolones or macrolides, class IA antiarrhythmics, such as procainamide or quinidine, class III antiarrhythmics, such as amiodarone or sotalol, other antipsychotic drugs, such as chlorpromazine or thioridazine, or any other drug that affects the QT interval, such as methadone or pentamidine: Possibly prolonged QT interval
antihypertensive drugs: Increased antihypertensive effects
CNS depressants: Possibly additive CNS effects
CYP2D6 inhibitors, such as fluoxetine or paroxetine, CYP3A4 inhibitors, such as clarithromycin or ketoconazole: Increased plasma iloperidone level
dextromethorphan: Increased blood dextromethorphan level

ACTIVITIES

alcohol: Possibly increased CNS effects

Adverse Reactions

CNS: Aggression, akathisia, delusion, dizziness, extrapyramidal effects, fatigue, headache, impaired cognitive and motor impairment, lethargy, **neuroleptic malignant syndrome**, restlessness, **seizures**, somnolence, **suicidal ideation**, tardive dyskinesia, syncope, tremor
CV: **Congestive heart failure**, dyslipidemia, **hypotension**, orthostatic hypotension, palpitations, **QT interval prolongation**, tachycardia
EENT: Blurred vision, conjunctivitis, dry mouth, intraoperative floppy iris syndrome, nasal congestion, nasopharyngitis, **oropharyngeal swelling**, **throat tightness**, upper respiratory tract infection
ENDO: **Diabetic ketoacidosis**, elevated prolactin levels, hyperglycemia, **hyperosmolar coma**
GI: Abdominal discomfort, diarrhea, elevated liver enzymes, nausea, vomiting
GU: Ejaculation failure, erectile dysfunction, polyuria, priapism, urinary incontinence and urgency

HEME: **Leukopenia**
MS: Arthralgia, musculoskeletal stiffness, muscle spasms, myalgia
RESP: Dyspnea, upper respiratory infections
SKIN: Pruritus, rash, urticaria
Other: **Anaphylaxis, angioedema,** weight gain

Childbearing Considerations

PREGNANCY

- Pregnancy exposure registry: 1-866-961-2388 or http://womensmentalhealth.org/clinical-and-research-programs/pregnancyregistry/.
- Drug may cause fetal harm.
- Exposure during third trimester increases risk of fetus developing extrapyramidal and/or withdrawal symptoms following delivery.
- Use with caution only if benefit to mother outweighs potential risk to fetus.

LACTATION

- It is not known if drug is present in breast milk.
- Breastfeeding is not recommended during drug therapy.

Nursing Considerations

! WARNING Know that iloperidone shouldn't be used in patients with a history of cardiovascular disease, such as cardiac arrhythmias, QT interval prolongation, recent MI, or uncompensated heart failure. It also shouldn't be used in patients taking other drugs known to prolong the QT interval and in patients with hepatic impairment.

! WARNING Be aware that iloperidone shouldn't be used to treat patients with dementia-related psychosis, especially elderly patients, because of an increased risk of death.

! WARNING Obtain baseline serum magnesium and potassium levels in patients at risk for electrolyte imbalances, and then monitor periodically throughout therapy, as ordered, because electrolyte imbalances increase risk of arrhythmias or prolonged QT interval. If patient reports dizziness, palpitations, or syncope, notify prescriber and expect further evaluation to be done.

! WARNING Monitor patient for a hypersensitivity reaction, which may become life-threatening such as anaphylaxis or angioedema. If present, notify prescriber, expect drug to be discontinued, and provide supportive care, as needed and ordered.

! WARNING Monitor patient closely for abnormal behavior or thinking that may suggest suicidal thinking, especially when iloperidone therapy starts or dosage is changed.

! WARNING Monitor patients who have a history of seizures or who have conditions that lower the seizure threshold, such as Alzheimer's dementia because drug increases risk of seizures in these patients. Also, use cautiously in patients who are at risk for aspiration pneumonia or who have moderate hepatic impairment (not recommended for use in patients with severe hepatic impairment).

! WARNING Monitor patient's CBC periodically, as ordered, especially during first few months of therapy because iloperidone may cause leukopenia. Also, be aware that other antipsychotic drugs sometimes have caused fatal agranulocytosis and leukopenia. If patient's WBC count decreases, expect drug to be discontinued.

! WARNING Know that neuroleptic malignant syndrome has occurred in patients taking other antipsychotic drugs. Monitor patient for altered mental status, autonomic instability, hyperpyrexia, and muscle rigidity. If present, notify prescriber immediately, expect drug to be discontinued, and start intensive treatment, as prescribed. Watch for recurrence if patient resumes antipsychotic therapy.

! WARNING Monitor blood glucose level, especially in patients with diabetes mellitus, because iloperidone may alter blood glucose enough to induce life-threatening hyperosmolar coma or ketoacidosis.

- Monitor patient for tardive dyskinesia, which has occurred with other antipsychotic drugs. If patient develops involuntary, dyskinetic movements, notify prescriber and expect to discontinue drug.

PATIENT TEACHING

- Instruct patient how to administer iloperidone.
- Inform patient that when iloperidone therapy starts, dosage must be adjusted for up to a week to reach target level. Also, explain that adjustment process will have to be repeated if drug is skipped for more than 3 days.

! **WARNING** Alert patient that drug may cause an allergic reaction. Tell patient to notify prescriber if an allergic reaction is present and to seek immediate medical care if severe.

! **WARNING** Urge family or caregiver to monitor patient for suicidal behavior or thoughts, especially when therapy starts or dosage changes.

! **WARNING** Advise patient, family, or caregiver to notify prescriber about persistent, severe, or unusual adverse reactions because drug may have to be discontinued.

- Tell patient drug may increase blood glucose levels, especially if patient is a diabetic. Review signs and symptoms of hyperglycemia and have patients with diabetes mellitus monitor blood glucose levels closely. Tell patient to report signs and symptoms of hyperglycemia or persistent elevations immediately to prescriber.
- Caution patient to avoid hazardous activities until CNS effects of drug are known and resolved. Tell patient to avoid alcohol.
- Instruct patient to avoid activities that might raise body temperature, such as being exposed to extreme heat, being subjected to dehydration, doing strenuous exercise, or taking other drugs with anticholinergic activity.
- Tell patient to rise slowly from lying to sitting position and from sitting position to standing to avoid dizziness or light-headedness during therapy.
- Advise female patient of childbearing age to notify prescriber if she becomes pregnant.
- Inform mothers that breastfeeding is not recommended during drug therapy.
- Emphasize the need to comply with follow-up appointments and laboratory tests.

immune globulin intramuscular (human)

(gamma globulin, IG)

GamaSTAN S/D 5%

immune globulin intravenous (human)

(IGIV)

Alyglo 10%, Asceniv 10%, Bivigam Liquid 10%, Flebogamma DIF 5% and 10%, Gammagard Liquid 10%, Gammagard S/D 5%, Gammaplex 5% and 10%, Gamunex-C 10%, Octagam 5%, Panzyga 10%, Privigen 10%, Yimmugo 10%

immune globulin subcutaneous (human)

Cutaquig 16.5%, Cuvitru 20%, Gammagard Liquid 10%, Gamunex-C 10%, Hizentra 20%, HyQvia 10%, Xembify 20%

Class and Category

Pharmacologic class: Immune serum
Therapeutic class: Antibody production stimulator

Indications and Dosages

∗ *To treat primary immunodeficiency*

I.V. INFUSION (GAMMAGARD S/D 5%)

Adults. 300 to 600 mg/kg every 3 to 4 wk. If response is inadequate, dose or frequency may be adjusted. Initially infused at 0.5 ml/kg/hr, then gradually increased as tolerated to maximum rate of 4 ml/kg/hr.

SUBCUTANEOUS INFUSION (HYQVIA 10%)

Adults and children ages 2 and older. Highly individualized. Consult manufacturer's guidelines for initial ramp-up schedule given for first 7 wk. *For adults naïve to IgG therapy or switching from another IgG* *subcutaneous therapy*: After initial ramp-up schedule given over 7 wk, 300 to 600 mg/kg every 3 to 4 wk. *For adults switching from IGIV therapy*: After initial ramp-up schedule given over 7 wk, same dose and frequency given as the previous IGIV therapy every 3 to 4 wk. Consult manufacturer's guidelines for subsequent dose adjustments.

I.V. INFUSION (YIMMUGO)

Adults and children ages 2 and older. *First infusion:* 300 to 800 mg/kg infused at a rate of 0.5 mg/kg/min for 30 min followed by gradual increase in infusion rate every 30 min up to 3 mg/kg/min. *Second infusion:* 300 to 800 mg/kg infused at a rate of 0.5 mg/kg/min for 30 min followed by gradual increase in infusion rate every 30 min up to 13 mg/kg/min. First and second infusions given every 3 to 4 wk. Dosage adjusted over time based on response.

* *To treat primary immunodeficiency disorders associated with defects in humoral immunity*

I.V. INFUSION (FLEBOGAMMA DIF 5%, GAMMAGARD LIQUID 10%)

Adults and children ages 2 and older. 300 to 600 mg/kg every 3 to 4 wk. Initially infused at 0.5 mg/kg/min and gradually increased to 5 mg/kg/min for maintenance rate for Flebogamma DIF 5% and initially infused at 0.8 mg/kg/min for 30 min, then increased every 30 min up to 8 mg/kg/min for maintenance rate for Gammagard Liquid 10%.

I.V. INFUSION (FLEBOGAMMA DIF 10%)

Adults. 300 to 600 mg/kg every 3 to 4 wk. Initially infused at 1 mg/kg/min and gradually increased to 8 mg/kg/min.

I.V. INFUSION (GAMUNEX-C 10%)

Adults and children ages 2 and older. 300 to 600 mg/kg every 3 or 4 wk. Initially infused at 1 mg/kg/min and increased as tolerated to maintenance infusion rate of 8 mg/kg/min.

I.V. INFUSION (OCTAGAM 5%)

Adults. *Initial:* 300 to 600 mg/kg every 3 to 4 wk and adjusted as needed. Initially infused at 0.5 mg/kg/min for first 30 min; increased, if tolerated, to 1 mg/kg/min for second 30 min and, if tolerated, to 2 mg/kg/min for another 30 min. Maintenance infused up to 3.33 mg/kg/min.

±**DOSAGE ADJUSTMENT** For patients with risk of developing renal dysfunction, infusion rate should not exceed 3.33 mg/kg/min.

I.V. INFUSION (PANZYGA 10%)

Adults and children ages 2 and older. 300 to 600 mg/kg every 3 to 4 wk. Initially infused for first 30 min at 1 mg/kg/min and then adjusted. Infusion rate should not exceed 14 mg/kg/min.

I.V. INFUSION (PRIVIGEN 10%)

Adults. 200 to 800 mg/kg every 3 to 4 wk. Initially infused at 0.5 mg/kg/min and gradually increased, as tolerated, to 8 mg/kg/min for maintenance infusion rate.

I.V. INFUSION (BIVIGAM LIQUID 10%)

Adults and children ages 2 and older. 300 to 800 mg/kg every 3 to 4 wk. Infused at 0.5 mg/kg/min for the first 10 min, then infusion rate increased every 20 min, if tolerated, by 0.8 mg/kg/min up to 6 mg/kg/min.

I.V. INFUSION (ASCENIV 10%)

Adults and adolescents. 300 to 800 mg/kg every 3 to 4 wk. Infused at 0.5 mg/kg/min for the first 15 min, then increased gradually every 15 min up to 8 mg/kg/min, if tolerated.

I.V. INFUSION (GAMMAPLEX 5% AND 10%)

Adults and children ages 2 and older. 300 to 800 mg/kg once every 3 to 4 wk. *For 5% solution*: Initially infused at 0.5 mg/kg/min for 15 min and then gradually increased every 15 min, if tolerated, to final infusion rate of 4 mg/kg/min. *For 10% solution*: Initially infused at 0.5 mg/kg/min for 15 min followed by gradual rate increase every 15 min, if tolerated, to maintenance infusion rate of 8 mg/kg/min.

I.V. INFUSION (ALYGLO 10%)

Adults. *First infusion:* 300 to 800 mg/kg infused initially at 1 mg/kg/min and then infusion rate doubled every 30 min (if tolerated) up to an infusion rate of 8 mg/kg/min followed by second infusion. *Second infusion:* 300 to 800 mg/kg infused initially at 2 mg/kg/min and then infusion rate doubled every 15 min (if tolerated) up to an infusion rate of 8 mg/kg/min. First and second infusion given every 21 to 28 days.

SUBCUTANEOUS INFUSION (HIZENTRA 20%)

Adults and children ages 2 and older. Highly individualized and administered at regular intervals from daily up to every 2 wk. *For patients switching from IGIV*: Initial weekly dosage started 1 wk after patient's last IGIV infusion. Initial weekly dosage obtained by dividing the previous IGIV dose in grams by the number of wk between doses during the patient's previous IGIV treatment, followed by multiplying the result by 1.37. To calculate dose in grams to milliliters, multiply the calculated dose by 5.

SUBCUTANEOUS INFUSION (XEMBIFY 20%)

Adults and children ages 2 and older. Highly individualized. *For patients switching from IGIV*: Initial weekly dosage started 1 wk after patient's last IGIV infusion. Initial weekly dosage obtained by dividing the previous IGIV dose in grams by the number of wk between doses during the patient's previous IGIV treatment. Then, multiply the result by 1.37. To convert dose in grams to milliliters, multiply the calculated dose by 5.

SUBCUTANEOUS INFUSION (GAMMAGARD LIQUID 10%, GAMUNEX-C 10%)

Adults and children ages 2 and older. Highly individualized. *For patients switching from IGIV*: Initial weekly dosage started 1 wk after patient's IGIV infusion.

SUBCUTANEOUS INFUSION (CUTAQUIG 16.5%)

Adults and children ages 2 and older. Highly individualized and started 1 wk after patient's last IGIV infusion, with initial weekly dosage obtained by dividing the previous IGIV dose in grams by the number of wk between intravenous doses. Then, multiply this number by 1.30. Multiply the calculated dose by 6 to convert the dose calculated in grams to milliliters.

±**DOSAGE ADJUSTMENT** For all patients, consult manufacturer's guidelines for dosage interval adjustment, if needed, and infusion administration rate to use, which is based on patient's age.

SUBCUTANEOUS INJECTION (CUVITRU 20%)

Adults and children ages 2 and older. Highly individualized and administered at regular intervals from daily up to every 2 wk. *For patient switching from IGIV or adult patients switching from HyQvia:* First dosage administered 1 wk after patient's last IGIV infusion or adult's last dose of HyQvia. Initial weekly dosage obtained by dividing the previous IGIV or HyQvia dose in grams by the number of weeks between intravenous doses. Then, multiply this number by 1.30. Multiply the calculated dose by 5 to convert the dose calculated in grams to milliliters.

∗ *To treat thrombocytopenic purpura (ITP)*

I.V. INFUSION (GAMMAPLEX 5% AND 10%)

Adults. 1 g/kg for 2 consecutive days. *For 5% solution*: Initially infused at 0.5 mg/kg/min for 15 min and then gradually increased every 15 min, if tolerated, to final infusion rate of 4 mg/kg/min. *For 10% solution*: Initially infused at 0.5 mg/kg/min for 15 min followed by gradual rate increase every 15 min, if tolerated, to maintenance infusion rate of 8 mg/kg/min.

I.V. INFUSION (PRIVIGEN 10%)

Adults and adolescents ages 15 and older. 1 g/kg daily for 2 consecutive days. Initially infused at 0.5 mg/kg/min and then gradually increased to 4 mg/kg/min for maintenance infusion rate.

I.V. INFUSION (FLEBOGAMMA DIF 10%)

Adults and children ages 2 and older. 1 g/kg daily for 2 consecutive days infused at a rate of 1 mg/kg/min. Subsequent maintenance infusions infused at a rate adjusted, as tolerated, to 8 mg/kg/min.

I.V. INFUSION (OCTAGAM 10%)

Adults. 1 g/kg (10 ml/kg) daily for 2 consecutive days. Initially infuse at 1 mg/kg/min for 30 min. If tolerated, increase infusion rate to 2 mg/kg/min for next 30 min. If tolerated, further increase infusion rate to 4 mg/kg/min for 30 min. If tolerated, further increase infusion rate to 8 mg/kg/min for 30 min. If tolerated, infusion rate may be increased up to 12 mg/kg/min for remainder of infusion.

I.V. INFUSION (GAMUNEX-C 10%)

Adults. 2 g/kg in 2 divided doses of 1 g/kg and given on 2 consecutive days or 5 divided doses of 0.4 g/kg each and given on 5 consecutive days. Initially infused at 1 mg/kg/min and increased gradually, as tolerated, to maintenance infusion rate of 8 mg/kg/min.

I.V. INFUSION (GAMMAGARD S/D 5%)

Adults. 1 g/kg as a single dose. If response is inadequate, up to 3 separate doses may be administered on alternate days. Initially infused at 0.5 ml/kg/hr and then gradually increased, as tolerated, up to a maximum of 4 ml/kg/hr.

I.V. INFUSION (PANZYGA 10%)

Adults. 2 g/kg in 2 divided doses of 1 g/kg and given on 2 consecutive days. Initially infused at 1 mg/kg/min over first 30 min and then rate adjusted. Maximum infusion rate should not exceed 8 mg/kg/min.

I.V. INFUSION (GAMMAPLEX LIQUID 5%)

Adults. 1 g/kg on 2 consecutive days, initially infused at 0.5 mg/kg/min and then gradually rate increased every 15 min, if tolerated, to final infusion rate of 4 mg/kg/min.

±**DOSAGE ADJUSTMENT** In chronic ITP, dosage of Gammaplex 5% liquid may have to be reduced in patients at risk for thrombosis, hemolysis, acute kidney injury, or volume overload.

* *To prevent coronary artery aneurysms associated with Kawasaki syndrome*

I.V. INFUSION (GAMMAGARD S/D 5%)

Children. 1 g/kg as a single dose or 400 mg/kg daily for 4 consecutive days and started within 7 days of onset of fever. Administered with aspirin 80 to 100 mg/kg/day in 4 divided doses. Initially infused at a rate of 0.5 ml/kg/hr and then gradually increased to maximum of 4 ml/kg/hr, as tolerated.

* *To treat chronic inflammatory demyelinating polyneuropathy (CIDP)*

I.V. INFUSION (GAMUNEX-C 10%)

Adults. *Loading dose:* 2 g/kg given in divided doses over 2 to 4 consecutive days with infusion rate of 2 mg/kg/min. *Maintenance dose:* 1 g/kg every 3 wk infused over 1 day or 2 divided doses of 0.5 g/kg and given on 2 consecutive days with infusion rate gradually increased to 8 mg/kg/min, as tolerated.

I.V. INFUSION (PRIVIGEN 10%)

Adults. *Loading dose:* 2 g/kg given in divided doses over 2 to 5 consecutive days. Initially infused at 0.5 mg/kg/min and, if tolerated, rate gradually increased up to a maximum of 8 mg/kg/min. *Maintenance:* 1 g/kg as a single infusion or 2 divided doses given on 2 consecutive days, every 3 wk for up to 6 mo. Minimum infusion rate is 0.5 mg/kg/min and maximum infusion rate is 8 mg/kg/min.

I.V. INFUSION (PANZYGA 10%)

Adults. *Loading dose:* 1 g/kg twice daily on 2 consecutive days. Initially infused at 1 mg/kg/min over first 30 min and then adjusted. Infusion rate should not exceed 12 mg/kg/min. *Maintenance:* 0.5 to 1 g/kg twice daily on 2 consecutive days every 3 wk.

SUBCUTANEOUS INFUSION (HIZENTRA 20%)

Adults. 0.2 g/kg/wk administered in 1 or 2 sessions over 1 or 2 consecutive days, increased to 0.4 g/kg/wk administered in 2 sessions over 1 or 2 consecutive days. Dosage increased to 0.4 g/kg/wk, as needed, given in 2 sessions per wk over 1 or 2 consecutive days.

SUBCUTANEOUS INFUSION (HYQVIA 10%)

Adults. Highly individualized. Consult manufacturer's guidelines for initial ramp-up schedule given for first 9 wk. Alternatively, 0.4 g/kg or less given without a ramp-up schedule providing patient can tolerate it. *For patients switching from IGIV therapy:* The starting dose and dosing frequency is the same as the patient's previous IGIV treatment.

I.V. INFUSION (GAMMAGARD LIQUID 10%)

Adults. *Loading dose:* 2 g/kg infused at 0.8 mg/kg/min in divided doses over 2 to 5 consecutive days. *Maintenance:* 1 g/kg infused up to 9 mg/kg/min in divided doses over 1 to 4 consecutive days, every 3 wk.

* *To prevent bacterial infections in hypogammaglobulinemia and/or recurrent bacterial infections associated with B-cell chronic lymphocytic leukemia*

I.V. INFUSION (GAMMAGARD S/D 5%)

Adults. 400 mg/kg every 3 to 4 wk. Initially infused at 0.5 ml/kg/hr and then gradually increased to maximum of 4 ml/kg/hr, as tolerated.

* *To improve muscle strength and disability as maintenance therapy in patients with multifocal motor neuropathy*

I.V. INFUSION (GAMMAGARD LIQUID 10%)

Adults. 0.5 to 2.4 g/kg/mo, based on clinical response. Initially infused at 0.8 mg/kg/min with rate increased, as needed, up to 9 mg/kg/min.

* *To treat dermatomyositis*

I.V. INFUSION (OCTAGAM 10%)

Adults. 2 g/kg divided in equal doses given over 2 to 5 consecutive days every 4 wk.

Initially infused at 1 mg/kg/min and then increased as tolerated to maintenance infusion rate up to 4 mg/kg/min.

∗ *To prevent hepatitis A within 2 wk of exposure*

I.M. INJECTION (GAMASTAN S/D 5%)

Adults and children. 0.01 ml/kg as a single dose for household and institutional hepatitis A contact, as soon as possible after exposure.

∗ *To prevent hepatitis A when traveling in areas where hepatitis A is common*

I.M. INJECTION (GAMASTAN S/D 5%)

Adults and children staying in area up to 1 mo. 0.01 ml/kg as a single dose.
Adults and children staying in area up to 2 mo. 0.2 ml/kg as a single dose.
Adults and children staying in area 2 mo or longer. 0.06 ml/kg as a single dose and repeated every 2 mo while in the area.

∗ *To prevent or modify measles in a susceptible person exposed fewer than 6 days previously*

I.M. INJECTION (GAMASTAN S/D 5%)

Adults and children. 0.25 ml/kg as a single dose as soon as possible after exposure.
Immunocompromised children. 0.5 ml/kg (maximum dose 15 ml) as a single dose as soon as possible after exposure.

SUBCUTANEOUS INFUSION (HYQVIA 10%)

Adults. 400 mg/kg as a single dose as soon as possible after exposure. *For patients at risk of future measles exposure and receives a dose for primary immunodeficiency of less than 530 mg/kg every 3 to 4 wk:* Dose increased to at least 530 mg/kg.

I.V. INFUSION (OCTAGAM 5%)

Adults. 400 mg as a single dose as soon as possible after exposure. *For patients at risk of future measles exposure and receives a dose for primary immunodeficiency of less than 530 mg/kg every 3 to 4 wk:* Dose increased to at least 530 mg/kg.

∗ *To modify varicella infection when Varicella-Zoster Immune Globulin is unavailable*

I.M. INJECTION (GAMASTAN S/D 5%)

Adults and children. 0.6 to 1.2 ml/kg as a single dose given as soon as possible after exposure only if Varicella-Zoster Immune Globulin (Human) is unavailable.

∗ *To lessen effects of rubella exposure*

I.M. INJECTION (GAMASTAN S/D 5%)

Women in first trimester of pregnancy. 0.55 ml/kg as a single dose as soon as possible after exposure.

Drug Administration

- When preparing immune globulin, verify that appropriate form is being used—either immune globulin intramuscular for I.M. injection, immune globulin intravenous for I.V. infusion, or immune globulin subcutaneous for subcutaneous infusion.
- To reconstitute drug, if required, follow manufacturer's guidelines and use only diluent recommended by manufacturer. Don't shake solution because excessive shaking causes foaming. If drug or diluent is cold, drug may take up to 20 min to dissolve.
- Know that if drug is reconstituted outside of sterile laminar airflow conditions, administer it immediately and discard unused portions.

I.V.

- An in-line filter may be required for intravenous infusion of drug. Check manufacturer's guidelines for specific product being used.
- Consult manufacturer's guidelines to determine appropriate flow rate for infusion.
- *Incompatibilities:* Check manufacturer's guidelines for specific product being used

I.M.

- Inject only into deltoid muscle of upper arm or anterolateral aspect of upper thigh.
- If giving a dose larger than 5 ml, divide it and administer at separate sites.

SUBCUTANEOUS

- Use an infusion pump to administer drug.
- Infusion sites should be at least 2 inches apart and sites changed each week.
- Consult manufacturer's guidelines to determine number of sites that can be used simultaneously and infusion flow rate.

Route	Onset	Peak	Duration
I.V.	Immediate	< 30 min	Unknown
I.M.	Unknown	2 days	Unknown
SubQ	Unknown	Unknown	Unknown

Half-life: 16–31 days

Mechanism of Action

Releases antibody-specific globulins to produce an antibody–antigen reaction that results in bacterial lysis and facilitates bacterial phagocytosis. In treatment of ITP, immune globulin blocks iron receptors on macrophages to increase immunoglobulin action. Immune globulin also increases cytokine production and improves B-cell immune function by regulating macrophage and T-cell activity. Newly formed antigen–antibody complexes produce split complement components that cause bacterial lysis.

In Kawasaki disease and bacterial infections with B-cell chronic lymphocytic leukemia, immune globulin neutralizes bacterial and viral toxins that harm immune and inflammatory responses.

Contraindications

Hypersensitivity to immune globulin (human) or its components; IgA deficiency in patients with known antibody to IgA

Interactions

DRUGS

live-virus vaccines: Possibly decreased response to vaccine

Adverse Reactions

CNS: **Aseptic meningitis** (rare), headache, malaise

CV: Chest discomfort, hypertension, tachycardia, **thrombotic events**, **volume overload**

EENT: Blurred vision, oropharyngeal pain

GI: Nausea, vomiting

GU: **Acute renal dysfunction or failure**, osmotic nephrosis

HEME: **Acute hemolysis**, **delayed hemolytic anemia**, **disseminated intravascular coagulation (DIC)**, positive Coombs test

MS: Arthralgia, back or extremity pain, muscle spasms or weakness, myalgia

RESP: Dyspnea, **pulmonary edema or embolism**

Other: Acute inflammatory reaction, hyperproteinemia, **hyponatremia**, increased serum viscosity

Childbearing Considerations

PREGNANCY

- It is not known if drug causes fetal harm although immune globulins increasingly cross the placental barrier after 30 wk gestation.
- Use with caution only if benefit to mother outweighs potential risk to fetus.

LACTATION

- Drug may be present in breast milk.
- Mothers should check with prescriber before breastfeeding.

Nursing Considerations

! WARNING Know that before giving immune globulin, assess patient's fluid volume and BUN and serum creatinine levels, as ordered, to determine risk for acute renal failure. Those at increased risk include patients with diabetes mellitus, paraproteinemia, renal insufficiency, sepsis, or volume depletion; those taking nephrotoxic drugs; and those over age 65. Expect drug to be discontinued if renal function deteriorates.

! WARNING Use caution when administering immune globulin, regardless of the route of administration, because of risk for thrombosis. Monitor closely patients with increased risk of thrombosis, such as advanced age, coagulation disorders, a history of atherosclerosis, impaired cardiac output, multiple cardiovascular risk factors, or prolonged periods of immobilization, and/or hyperviscosity. In such patients, obtain a baseline assessment of blood viscosity, as ordered. Ensure patient is adequately hydrated prior to administration. When administering drug intravenously, expect to infuse at the lowest rate possible. Report any signs and symptoms suggestive of a thrombotic event immediately to prescriber and be prepared to administer treatment, as ordered.

! WARNING Watch for an acute inflammatory reaction in patients who have never received immune globulin therapy before, in those whose last treatment was more than 8 weeks before, and in those whose initial infusion rate exceeded 1 ml/min. Within 30 minutes to 1 hour after beginning infusion, assess for chills, diaphoresis, dizziness, facial flushing, feeling of tightness in chest, fever, hypotension, nausea, and vomiting. Notify prescriber immediately if such symptoms occur and be prepared to stop infusion until symptoms have subsided.

! WARNING Monitor patient closely for signs and symptoms of hemolysis, especially patients with risk factors. For patients at increased risk, expect to obtain a baseline measurement of hematocrit or hemoglobin prior to infusion and within 36 to 96 hours post-infusion. Notify prescriber of any abnormalities.

! WARNING Be aware that after immune globulin administration, monitor patient closely for aseptic meningitis. Notify prescriber if patient develops drowsiness, fever, nausea, nuchal rigidity, painful eye movements, photophobia, severe headache, or vomiting.

- Be aware that immune globulin intravenous is made from human plasma and therefore may contain infectious agents, such as viruses. Risk of transmitting a virus by infusion has been reduced by inactivating or removing certain viruses from the product, screening blood donors, and testing donated blood.

PATIENT TEACHING

- Review with patient how immune globulin will be administered.

! WARNING Instruct patient to report immediately any symptoms experienced during or after receiving immune globulin.

- Inform patient to postpone live-virus vaccinations for up to 11 months after receiving immune globulin because drug may delay or inhibit response to vaccine.

inclisiran

Leqvio

Class and Category

Pharmacologic class: Small interfering ribonucleic acid (siRNA)
Therapeutic class: Antilipemic

Indications and Dosages

✱ *As adjunct to diet and statin therapy in patients with primary hyperlipidemia, including heterozygous familial hypercholesterolemia, to reduce low-density lipoprotein cholesterol (LDL-C)*

SUBCUTANEOUS INJECTION

Adults. *Initial:* 284 mg as a single dose, repeated in 3 mo and then every 6 mo. *Maintenance:* 284 mg every 6 mo.

Drug Administration

SUBCUTANEOUS INJECTION

- Inspect solution before injecting. Solution should be clear, colorless to pale yellow with no particulate matter.
- Inject into abdomen, thigh, or upper arm. Do not inject into areas of skin disease or injury.
- If a planned dose is missed by less than 3 mo, administer missed dose and maintain dosing schedule.
- If a planned dose is missed longer than 3 mo, restart dosing schedule with an initial dose followed by a dose in 3 mo and then every 6 mo thereafter.

Route	Onset	Peak	Duration
SubQ	Unknown	4 hr	Unknown

Half-life: 9 hr

Mechanism of Action

After entering hepatocytes, breakdown of mRNA for PCSK9 occurs resulting in an increase in LDL-C uptake. This lowers LDL-C levels in circulation.

Contraindications

Hypersensitivity to inclisiran or its components

Interactions

DRUGS

None reported by manufacturer.

Adverse Reactions

MS: Arthralgia
RESP: Bronchitis
SKIN: Rash, urticaria
Other: Angioedema, injection-site reaction (redness, pain, and rash)

Childbearing Considerations

PREGNANCY

- Drug may cause fetal harm.
- Drug should not be given during pregnancy.

LACTATION

- It is not known if drug is present in breast milk.
- Mothers should check with prescriber before breastfeeding.

Nursing Considerations

- Be aware that inclisiran should only be given by a healthcare professional.

! WARNING Monitor patient for hypersensitivity reactions, which could be become life-threatening such as angioedema.

If present, notify prescriber, expect drug to be discontinued, and provide supportive care, as needed and ordered.

- Monitor patient's lipid levels, as ordered, to assess effectiveness of the drug. Know that drug effectiveness may be seen as early as 30 days after drug therapy is initiated.
- Assess injection site for redness or rash and determine if pain is present at the injection site.

PATIENT TEACHING

- Inform patient that the subcutaneous injection must be administered by a healthcare professional.

! **WARNING** Alert patient that drug may cause an allergic reaction. If present, tell patient to notify prescriber and, if severe, to seek immediate medical care.

- Instruct patient to inform prescriber if pain, rash, or redness occurs at the injection site.
- Tell women of childbearing age to notify prescriber if pregnancy occurs, as drug is generally not necessary during pregnancy and should be discontinued.

indomethacin

Indocin

indomethacin sodium trihydrate

Class and Category

Pharmacologic class: NSAID
Therapeutic class: Analgesic

Indications and Dosages

* *To relieve moderate to severe symptoms of ankylosing spondylitis, osteoarthritis, and rheumatoid arthritis*

CAPSULES, ORAL SUSPENSION

Adults and adolescents ages 15 and older. 25 mg 2 times daily or 3 times daily, increased by 25 or 50 mg daily every wk, as needed. *Maximum:* 200 mg daily. After adequate response, dosage reduced as low as possible.

E.R. CAPSULES

Adults and adolescents ages 15 and older. 75 mg daily, increased to 75 mg twice daily, as needed.

SUPPOSITORIES

Adults and adolescents ages 15 and older. 50 mg up to 3 times daily.

* *To relieve symptoms of acute gouty arthritis*

CAPSULES, ORAL SUSPENSION, SUPPOSITORIES (INDOCIN)

Adults. 50 mg 3 times daily until gout attack relieved, and then drug rapidly reduced to complete cessation.

* *To treat inflammation and relieve acute shoulder pain from bursitis or tendinitis*

CAPSULES, ORAL SUSPENSION

Adults and adolescents ages 15 and older. 75 to 150 mg daily in divided doses 3 times daily or 4 times daily for 7 to 14 days.

E.R. CAPSULES

Adults and adolescents ages 15 and older. 75 mg once or twice daily for 7 to 14 days.

SUPPOSITORIES

Adults and adolescents ages 15 and older. 50 mg up to 4 times daily for 7 to 14 days. *Maximum:* 200 mg daily.

* *To treat hemodynamically significant patent ductus arteriosus in premature infants weighing 500 to 1,750 g (1 to 3.9 lb)*

I.V. INFUSION

Infants over age 7 days. *Initial:* 200 mcg/kg (0.2 mg/kg) over 20 to 30 min; 2 additional doses of 250 mcg/kg (0.25 mg/kg) given at 12- to 24-hr intervals. A second course maybe repeated if ductus arteriosus reopens.
Neonates ages 2 to 7 days. *Initial:* 200 mcg/kg (0.2 mg/kg) over 20 to 30 min; 2 additional doses of 200 mcg/kg (0.2 mg/kg) given at 12- to 24-hr intervals. A second course may be repeated if ductus arteriosus reopens.
Neonates under age 48 hr. *Initial:* 200 mcg/kg (0.2 mg/kg) over 20 to 30 min; 2 additional doses of 100 mcg/kg (0.1 mg/kg) given at 12- to 24-hr intervals. A second course may be repeated if ductus arteriosus reopens.

±**DOSAGE ADJUSTMENT** For the neonate experiencing anuria or a significant decrease in urine output (less than 0.6 ml/kg/hr) at the second or third I.V. dose, the dose withheld until renal function returns to normal.

Drug Administration

P.O.

- Administer drug immediately after meals or with food.
- Capsules should be swallowed whole without chewing, crushing, or opening. Administer capsules with a full glass of water.
- Shake suspension well before giving it. Use a calibrated device to measure dosage.
- Ensure that patient does not lie down for at least 15 min after drug has been administered.

I.V.

- To reconstitute, add 1 to 2 ml of preservative-free 0.9% Sodium Chloride Injection or preservative-free Sterile Water Solution to drug vial. Do not dilute further.
- Use solution immediately because it contains no preservatives. Discard unused portion.
- Infuse over 20 to 30 min.
- Avoid extravasation to protect surrounding tissue.
- Anticipate a second course (3 more doses) if patent ductus arteriosus reopens. After 2 courses, surgery may be performed.
- *Incompatibilities:* Other I.V. infusion solutions except for preservative-free 0.9% Sodium Chloride Injection or preservative-free Sterile Water for Injection

P.R.

- If suppository is too soft, put in refrigerator for 15 min or run it under cold water while still wrapped.
- Make sure suppository stays in rectum at least 1 hr to improve absorption.
- Be aware that suppositories can be substituted for capsule administration in the treatment of ankylosing spondylitis, osteoarthritis, and rheumatoid arthritis but only if necessary because there is a significant difference in blood levels between the 2 dosage forms.

Route	Onset	Peak	Duration
P.O.	30 min	2 hr	4–6 hr
P.O./E.R.	30 min	2 hr	Unknown
I.V.	Unknown	Unknown	Unknown
P.R.	Unknown	Unknown	4–6 hr

Half-life: 2.6–11.2 hr

Mechanism of Action

Blocks activity of cyclooxygenase, the enzyme needed to synthesize prostaglandins, which mediate inflammatory response and cause local pain, swelling, and vasodilation. By blocking cyclooxygenase and inhibiting prostaglandins, this NSAID reduces inflammatory symptoms and helps relieve pain.

Contraindications

History of asthma, urticaria, or other allergic-type reactions after taking aspirin or other NSAIDs; hypersensitivity to indomethacin, other NSAIDs, or their components; history of proctitis or recent rectal bleeding (suppositories); postoperative pain with coronary artery bypass graft (CABG) surgery

Interactions

DRUGS

Note: All effects listed are for oral forms and suppositories unless indicated.

ACE inhibitors, angiotensin receptor blockers (ARBs), or beta-blockers (including propranolol): Decreased antihypertensive effects of these drugs; in the elderly or patients with renal impairment or who are volume-depleted, increased risk of acute renal failure

anticoagulants, such as warfarin; antiplatelets, such as aspirin; selective serotonin reuptake inhibitors; serotonin norepinephrine reuptake inhibitors: Increased risk of serious bleeding

aspirin, other NSAIDs, other salicylates: Increased risk of adverse GI effects and non-GI bleeding

cyclosporine: Increased risk of nephrotoxicity

digoxin: Increased blood digoxin level and risk of digitalis toxicity (all forms)

diuretics (loop, potassium-sparing, and thiazide): Decreased antihypertensive and diuretic effects; increased risk of hyperkalemia with potassium-sparing diuretics

lithium: Increased blood lithium level and risk of toxicity
methotrexate: Increased risk of methotrexate toxicity
pemetrexed: Increased risk of myelosuppression; increased risk of GI and renal toxicity
probenecid: Increased blood level and effectiveness of indomethacin, increased risk of indomethacin toxicity

ACTIVITIES

alcohol use: Increased risk of adverse GI effects

Adverse Reactions

Note: All reactions are for oral forms and suppositories unless indicated.

CNS: Confusion, **CVA**, depression, dizziness, drowsiness, fatigue, hallucinations, headache, **intraventricular hemorrhage (I.V.)**, peripheral neuropathy, **seizures**, syncope, vertigo
CV: **Arrhythmias**, chest pain, edema, fluid retention (all forms), **heart failure**, hypertension, **MI**, **pulmonary hypertension (I.V.)**, tachycardia
EENT: Blurred vision, corneal and retinal damage, epistaxis, hearing loss, stomatitis, tinnitus
ENDO: **Hypoglycemia (I.V.)**
GI: Abdominal cramps or pain, abdominal distention (I.V.), anorexia, constipation, diarrhea, diverticulitis, dyspepsia, dysphagia, elevated liver enzymes, epigastric discomfort, esophagitis, gastritis, gastroenteritis, gastroesophageal reflux disease, **GI bleeding** and ulceration (all forms), hemorrhoids, **hepatic dysfunction (I.V.)**, **hepatic failure**, hiatal hernia, ileus (I.V.), indigestion, **melena**, nausea, **necrotizing enterocolitis (I.V.)**, **pancreatitis**, peptic ulcer, **perforation of intestine or stomach**, vomiting (all forms)
GU: **Acute renal failure**, hematuria, interstitial nephritis, **nephrotic syndrome**, oliguria (I.V.), proteinuria, renal dysfunction (I.V.), vaginal bleeding
HEME: **Agranulocytosis**, anemia, **aplastic anemia**, **bone marrow depression**, **decreased platelet aggregation (I.V.)**, **disseminated intravascular coagulation (DIC)**, **hemolytic anemia**, iron deficiency anemia, **leukopenia**, **neutropenia**, **pancytopenia**, **thrombocytopenia**, **unusual bleeding** or bruising (all forms)
RESP: **Asthma**, **respiratory depression**
SKIN: Acute generalized exanthematous, ecchymosis, **erythema multiforme**, erythema nodosum, **exfoliative dermatitis**, fixed drug eruptions, photosensitivity, pruritus, rash, **Stevens-Johnson syndrome**, **toxic epidermal necrolysis**, urticaria
Other: **Anaphylaxis**, **angioedema**, **drug reaction with eosinophilia and systemic symptoms (DRESS)**, **hyperkalemia (I.V.)**, **hyponatremia (I.V.)**, injection-site irritation

Childbearing Considerations

PREGNANCY

- Drug increases risk of premature closure of the fetal ductus arteriosus if given during the third trimester of pregnancy and may cause fetal renal dysfunction, leading to oligohydramnios and neonatal renal impairment if given at 20 wk or thereafter.
- Drug should be avoided in pregnant women starting at 30 wk of gestation and onward and the lowest dose for the shortest period of time should be used between 20 and 30 wk gestation only if absolutely necessary.

LACTATION

- Drug may be present in breast milk.
- Mothers should check with prescriber before breastfeeding because many manufacturers do not recommend drug use during breastfeeding.

REPRODUCTION

- Drug may delay or prevent rupture of ovarian follicles, which has been associated with reversible infertility in some women.

Nursing Considerations

! WARNING Be aware that NSAIDs like indomethacin should be avoided in patients with a recent MI because risk of reinfarction increases with NSAID therapy. If therapy is unavoidable, monitor patient closely for signs of cardiac ischemia.

! WARNING Know that the risk of heart failure increases with indomethacin use because it is an NSAID. This class of drugs should not be used in patients with severe heart failure but, if unavoidable, monitor patient for worsening of heart failure.

! **WARNING** Monitor patient for a hypersensitivity reaction such as anaphylaxis or angioedema as well as serious skin reactions (including DRESS) that may occur without warning, even in patients with no history of sensitivity to indomethacin or other NSAIDs. These reactions could become life-threatening. At first sign of a hypersensitivity reaction, including a rash (DRESS may only initially present with a fever or swollen lymph nodes), stop drug, notify prescriber, and provide supportive care, as needed and ordered.

! **WARNING** Know that patients with history of GI bleeding or ulcer disease should be monitored very closely because NSAIDs, such as indomethacin, increase risk of GI bleeding and ulceration. Expect to use drug for shortest time possible in these patients. Also, be aware that serious GI tract bleeding, perforation, and ulceration may occur without warning symptoms. Elderly patients are at greater risk. To minimize risk, give oral indomethacin with an antacid, food, or a full glass of water to reduce GI distress. If GI distress occurs, withhold drug and notify prescriber.

- Monitor patient—especially if he's elderly or receiving long-term indomethacin therapy—for less common but serious adverse GI reactions, including anorexia, constipation, diverticulitis, dysphagia, esophagitis, gastritis, gastroenteritis, gastroesophageal reflux disease, hemorrhoids, hiatal hernia, melena, stomatitis, and vomiting.

! **WARNING** Monitor patient closely for thrombotic events, including MI and stroke because NSAIDs increase the risk. These events may occur early in treatment and risk increases with duration of use. Be aware that these events have occurred even in patients who do not have a history or risk factors for cardiovascular disease. Monitor patient for warning signs, such as chest pain, slurring of speech, shortness of breath, or weakness. If any signs and symptoms develop, withhold indomethacin, alert prescriber immediately, and provide supportive care as prescribed.

! **WARNING** Monitor liver enzymes because, rarely, elevations may progress to severe hepatic reactions, including fatal hepatitis, hepatic failure, and liver necrosis. Also, monitor BUN and creatinine levels, especially in elderly patients, those taking ACE inhibitors or diuretics, and those with heart failure, hepatic dysfunction, or impaired renal function; drug may cause renal failure.

! **WARNING** Know that if patient has bone marrow suppression or is receiving an antineoplastic drug, monitor laboratory results (including WBC count), and watch for evidence of infection because anti-inflammatory and antipyretic actions of indomethacin may mask signs and symptoms, such as fever and pain. Also, monitor CBC for decreased hemoglobin and hematocrit. Drug may worsen anemia.

- Monitor weight and blood pressure, especially if patient has hypertension or heart failure, because indomethacin causes sodium retention and may worsen hypertension or heart failure.
- Keep in mind that when drug is used to treat gouty arthritis, significant swelling will gradually disappear over 3 to 5 days.
- Assess for improved joint mobility and reduced pain and inflammation to evaluate drug effectiveness.
- Expect patient to have intermittent checkups during long-term therapy and an ophthalmologic examination if vision changes.

PATIENT TEACHING

- Instruct patient, family, or caregiver how to administer form of indomethacin prescribed.
- Urge patient to avoid alcohol during indomethacin therapy.
- Remind patient that improvement may not occur for 2 to 4 weeks after starting indomethacin to treat arthritis or ankylosing spondylitis and that he should continue taking drug, as prescribed.

! **WARNING** Alert patient that drug may cause an allergic reaction and serious skin reactions. If present, tell patient to notify prescriber, stop taking drug, and, if severe, to seek immediate medical care.

! **WARNING** Explain that indomethacin may increase risk of serious adverse GI reactions; emphasize need to seek immediate medical attention for such signs and symptoms as abdominal or epigastric pain, black or tarry stools, indigestion, or vomiting blood or material that looks like coffee grounds.

! **WARNING** Explain that indomethacin may increase risk of serious adverse cardiovascular reactions; urge patient to seek immediate medical attention if signs or symptoms arise, such as chest pain, edema, shortness of breath, slurring of speech, unexplained weight gain, or weakness.

! **WARNING** Instruct patient to immediately report any other persistent, serious, or unusual adverse reactions because drug can affect many body systems.

! **WARNING** Caution pregnant patient not to take NSAIDs, such as indomethacin from 30 weeks gestation and on because they may cause premature closure of the ductus arteriosus and to avoid drug between 20- and 30-weeks gestation unless directed to do so by prescriber.

- Alert breastfeeding mothers that some manufacturer's of indomethacin do not recommend breastfeeding while using indomethacin. Tell her to check with prescriber before taking drug.
- Review infection control measures with patient who has bone marrow suppression or who is receiving an antineoplastic drug. Urge patient to notify prescriber if she suspects an infection even if it appears mild as drug may mask symptoms of fever and pain.
- Caution against prolonged sun exposure during therapy.
- Emphasize importance of having ordered laboratory tests and eye examinations during long-term therapy.

infliximab
Remicade

infliximab-abda
Renflexis

infliximab-axxq
Avsola

infliximab-dyyb
Inflectra, Zymfentra

infliximab-qbtx
Ixifi

Class and Category

Pharmacologic class: Monoclonal antibody (tumor necrosis factor [TNF] blocker)
Therapeutic class: Anti-inflammatory

Indications and Dosages

✱ *To control moderate to severe Crohn's disease long term; to reduce number of draining enterocutaneous and rectovaginal fistulas; to maintain fistula closure in patients with fistulizing Crohn's disease; to treat active ankylosing spondylitis; to treat psoriatic arthritis with or without methotrexate; to treat moderate to severe active ulcerative colitis in patients who have had an inadequate response to conventional therapy; to treat chronic severe plaque psoriasis in patients who are candidates for systemic therapy and when other systemic therapies are medically less appropriate*

I.V. INFUSION

Adults. *Initial:* 5 mg/kg infused over at least 2 hr, repeated 2 and 6 wk after first infusion. *Maintenance:* 5 mg/kg every 6 wk (active ankylosing spondylitis) or 8 wk (other indications).

± **DOSAGE ADJUSTMENT** For adult patients responding to treatment for Crohn's disease and then lose response, dosage may be increased to 10 mg/kg.

∗ *To provide maintenance treatment for patients with moderate to severe active Crohn's disease or moderate to severe active ulcerative colitis*

SUBCUTANEOUS INJECTION (ZYMFENTRA)

Adults following treatment with an infliximab product administered intravenously. 120 mg once every 2 wk starting at wk 10 and thereafter.

±**DOSAGE ADJUSTMENT** For adult patients responding to maintenance therapy with an infliximab product administered I.V, first subcutaneous dose of Zymfentra administered in place of the next scheduled I.V. infusion and continued every 2 wk thereafter.

∗ *To treat moderate to severe pediatric Crohn's disease; to treat moderate to severe pediatric active ulcerative colitis*

I.V. INFUSION

Children ages 6 and older. 5 mg/kg infused over at least 2 hr, repeated 2 and 6 wk after first infusion. *Maintenance:* 5 mg/kg every 8 wk.

∗ *As adjunct to treat moderate to severe active rheumatoid arthritis along with methotrexate*

I.V. INFUSION

Adults. *Initial:* 3 mg/kg infused over at least 2 hr, repeated 2 and 6 wk after first infusion. *Maintenance:* 3 mg/kg every 8 wk.

±**DOSAGE ADJUSTMENT** For adult patients who have an incomplete response for treatment of rheumatoid arthritis, dosage increased up to 10 mg/kg per infusion or treatment frequency increased to every 4 weeks.

Drug Administration

I.V.

- Store unopened drug vials in a refrigerator. If needed, unopened drug vials may be stored at room temperature for a single period of up to 6 mo but not exceeding expiration date. Once removed from refrigerator, do not return to refrigerator.
- Expect to premedicate patient, as prescribed, with acetaminophen, antihistamines, and/or corticosteroids to decrease an infusion reaction.
- Calculate dose, total volume of reconstituted drug solution required, and the number of vials needed. More than 1 vial may be needed for a full dose.
- Reconstitute drug by using a 21 G (or smaller) needle to add 10 ml Sterile Water for Injection to each 100-mg drug vial. Concentration will be 10 mg/ml.
- Swirl to mix; don't shake. Let reconstituted solution stand for 5 min. Solution may foam and should be clear or light brown or yellow.
- Do not store reconstituted solution.
- Withdraw volume equal to amount of reconstituted drug from a 250-ml bottle or bag of 0.9% Sodium Chloride Injection. Then, slowly add reconstituted drug to the 250-ml bottle or bag. Gently invert bag to mix. Infusion concentration should range between 0.4 mg/ml (minimum concentration) and 4 mg/ml (maximum concentration). For volumes greater than 250 ml, either use a larger infusion bag (e.g., 500 ml) or multiple 250-ml infusion bags to ensure that the concentration of the infusion solution does not exceed 4 mg/ml.
- Use within 3 hr of reconstitution and dilution.
- Infuse over at least 2 hr using infusion set and in-line, sterile, nonpyrogenic, low-protein-binding filter with pores 1.2 microns or less.
- If a mild to moderate infusion reaction occurs, notify prescriber and expect to slow or suspend infusion. If infusion was suspended, know that once the reaction has been resolved, the infusion may be restarted at a lower infusion rate and patient premedicated if not done before.
- If a severe infusion reaction occurs (anaphylaxis, erythematous rash, hypotension, seizures), know that infusion should be stopped, and drug permanently discontinued. Be prepared to provide supportive emergency care according to protocol.
- *Incompatibilities:* Diluents except for 0.9% Sodium Chloride Injection; other I.V. drugs infused in the same I.V. line

SUBCUTANEOUS INJECTION

- Know that all patients must complete an I.V. induction regimen with an infliximab product before starting subcutaneous therapy.
- Available as a prefilled syringe, prefilled syringe with needle shield, and prefilled pen.

- Solution in syringe should be clear, colorless to pale brown.
- Do not use the syringe or pen if it has been dropped or is visibly damaged as it may not function properly.
- Do not reuse or shake the syringe or pen at any time.
- Inject subcutaneously into abdomen (except for 2 inches around the navel), front of the thighs, or outer area of upper arms.
- Never inject into area where the skin is bruised, indurated, red, or tender. Rotate sites.
- Allow at least 1.2 inches between the new injection site and the previous injection site.
- If a dose is missed, inject the next dose as soon as possible and then every 2 wk thereafter.

Route	Onset	Peak	Duration
I.V., SubQ	Unknown	Unknown	Unknown

Half-life: 7.7–9.5 days

Mechanism of Action

Binds with cytokine tumor necrosis factor-alpha (TNF-alpha), preventing it from binding with its receptors. As a result, TNF-alpha can't produce proinflammatory cytokines and endothelial permeability. Infiltration of inflammatory cells declines.

Contraindications

Doses greater than 5 mg/kg in patients with moderate to severe heart failure; hypersensitivity to infliximab, murine proteins, or their components

Interactions

DRUGS

abatacept, anakinra, etanercept, tocilizumab: Increased risk of neutropenia and serious infections
CYP450 substrates, such as cyclosporine, theophylline, warfarin: May normalize formation of CYP450 enzymes which could affect dosage requirements of these drugs
immunosuppressants: Fewer infusion reactions in patients treated for Crohn's disease
live vaccines, therapeutic infectious agents, such as BCG in bladder instillation: Increased risk of adverse vaccine effects
methotrexate: Decreased incidence of anti-infliximab antibody production and increased infliximab product concentrations

Adverse Reactions

CNS: Chills, **CVA**, central nervous system demyelinating disorders, dizziness, fatigue, fever, headache, **meningitis**, neuritis, neuropathies, numbness, paresthesia, peripheral demyelinating disorders, **seizures**, syncope, tingling
CV: **Arrhythmias**, **bradycardia**, chest pain, edema, **heart failure**, hypertension, **hypotension**, **MI**, myocardial ischemia, myelitis, neuropathies, **pericardial effusion**, systemic vasculitis, thrombophlebitis
EENT: **Laryngeal/pharyngeal edema**, oral candidiasis, pharyngitis, rhinitis, sinusitis, transient vision loss, visual changes
GI: Abdominal hernia; abdominal pain; **acute hepatic failure**; cholecystitis; cholestasis; constipation; diarrhea; dyspepsia; elevated liver enzymes; **GI hemorrhage**; **hepatitis**; **hepatotoxicity**; ileus; **intestinal obstruction**, **perforation**, or stenosis; jaundice; **melena**; nausea; **pancreatitis**; splenic infarction; splenomegaly; vomiting
GU: **Cervical cancer**, kidney infection, **renal failure**, ureteral obstruction, UTI, vaginal candidiasis, vaginitis
HEME: **Agranulocytosis**, anemia, **aplastic anemia**, **hemolytic anemia**, **leukemia**, **leukopenia**, **neutropenia**, **pancytopenia**, **thrombocytopenia**, **thrombocytopenic purpura**, **thrombotic thrombocytopenic purpura**
MS: Ankylosing spondylitis, arthralgia, back pain, limb weakness, myalgia, psoriatic arthritis, transverse myelitis
RESP: **Adult respiratory distress syndrome**, bronchitis, **bronchospasms (severe)**, cough, dyspnea, **interstitial lung disease**, pleurisy, pneumonia, **pulmonary edema**, tuberculosis, respiratory tract infection, **severe bronchospasm**, wheezing
SKIN: Acute generalized exanthematous pustulosis, cellulitis, cutaneous vasculitis, diaphoresis, **erythema multiforme**, facial flushing, lichenoid reactions, linear IgA bullous dermatosis, **melanoma**, **Merkel cell cancer**, pruritus, psoriasis (new or worsening), rash, **Stevens-Johnson syndrome**, **toxic epidermal necrolysis**, urticaria
Other: **Anaphylaxis**; antibody formation to infliximab; bacterial (including *Legionella* and *Listeria*), fungal, mycobacterial, parasitic, or viral infections; dehydration;

infusion reaction; lupus-like symptoms; lymphadenopathy; **malignancies, such as lymphomas, including hepatosplenic T-cell lymphoma**; sarcoidosis; **sepsis**; serum sickness; vaccine breakthrough infection

Childbearing Considerations

PREGNANCY

- It is not known if drug causes fetal harm, but it does cross the placental barrier and cases of agranulocytosis in infants exposed to drug in utero have been reported as well as an increased risk of infection that can become fatal.
- Use with caution only if benefit to mother outweighs potential risk to fetus.
- Know that a 6-month waiting period following birth is recommended before live vaccines should be administered to the infant because these infants are at increased risk for secondary transmission of infection by live vaccines, which could become quite serious.

LACTATION

- Drug may be present in breast milk at low levels.
- Mothers should check with prescriber before breastfeeding.

Nursing Considerations

- Update patient's vaccinations with current vaccination guidelines prior to initiating infliximab.
- Know that because drug increases risk of developing tuberculosis (TB) or reactivating latent TB, expect prescriber to evaluate patient's risk and start TB treatment, as needed, before starting infliximab.
- Be aware that use of TNF-blocking therapy, including infliximab, may reactivate hepatitis B virus in patients who are chronic carriers of this virus. Ensure that patient has been tested for hepatitis B infection before infliximab therapy is begun. For patients who develop reactivation of hepatitis B, know that therapy should be stopped and antiviral therapy with appropriate supportive treatment begun.

! **WARNING** Know that infliximab therapy shouldn't be started in a patient with an active infection, including serious localized infection. Use with extreme caution if patient has a history of chronic or recurrent infection, known exposure to TB, an underlying condition that predisposes to infection, or residence or travel to areas of endemic tuberculosis or mycoses, such as blastomycosis, coccidioidomycosis, or histoplasmosis. Use cautiously in elderly patients because they have a higher risk of infection than younger patients taking infliximab.

! **WARNING** Be aware that infliximab increases risk of serious or fatal opportunistic infections, including invasive fungal infections, as well as bacterial (including *Legionella* and *Listeria*), mycobacterial, parasitic, and viral infections. The most common ones include aspergillosis, blastomycosis, candidiasis, coccidioidomycosis, cryptococcosis, histoplasmosis, legionellosis, listeriosis, pneumocystis, salmonellosis, and tuberculosis. Watch for other infections, especially if patient receives immunosuppressant therapy or has a chronic infection. Upper respiratory tract infections and UTIs are most common, but sepsis and fatal infections have occurred. If infection is suspected, notify prescriber, and if a serious infection is confirmed, expect drug to be discontinued.

! **WARNING** Use with extreme caution in patients with heart failure because drug can worsen heart failure and increase mortality in these patients. Also, know that new heart failure can develop in patients without known preexisting cardiovascular disease. Closely monitor patient throughout infliximab therapy for signs and symptoms of heart failure. If new or worsening symptoms of heart failure occur, expect drug to be discontinued.

! **WARNING** Use with extreme caution in patients with previous or ongoing hematologic abnormalities because infliximab may cause serious or even life-threatening adverse hematologic effects. Monitor patient's CBC regularly, as ordered. If adverse effects occur, expect drug to be discontinued.

! **WARNING** Monitor patient for a hypersensitivity or infusion reaction, which usually occurs during or within 2 hours of infliximab infusion. However, a reaction may occur 2 hours to 12 days after infusion. Reactions may include anaphylaxis, chest pain, chills, dypsnea, erythematous rash, facial edema, fever, hypertension, hypotension, pruritus, seizures, or urticaria. Patients are at a two-to three-fold risk of developing an infusion reaction if they become positive for antibodies to infliximab and have a higher risk for infusion reactions following re-administration. If present, notify prescriber and expect drug to be discontinued for severe hypersensitivity reactions. Provide supportive care, as needed and ordered.

! **WARNING** Monitor patient closely for the first 24 hours after the initial drug infusion because serious cardiovascular and cerebrovascular reactions, such as CVA, MI, seizures, or severe bronchospasms, may occur during and after infusion. Also, monitor patient for transient visual loss during or within 2 hours of infusion.

! **WARNING** Monitor liver function because severe hepatic reactions may occur. Expect to stop drug if jaundice develops or liver enzymes are 5 times or more the upper limit of normal.

! **WARNING** Be aware that infliximab is a tumor necrosis factor (TNF) blocker. Malignancies, especially leukemia and such rare lymphomas as hepatosplenic T-cell lymphoma, have been reported in patients, particularly children and adolescents, receiving TNF blockers. Patients at increased risk of leukemia are those with rheumatoid arthritis. Patients at increased risk of lymphomas are those with ankylosing spondylitis, Crohn's disease, plaque psoriasis, psoriatic arthritis, and rheumatoid arthritis, especially those with long-term or very active disease. However, the majority of malignancies developed in the head, lungs, or neck. Other malignancies, such as cervical cancer and skin cancer, have also occurred. Monitor patient closely for persistent, severe, or unusual signs and symptoms.

- Monitor patients with CNS demyelinating disorders, such as multiple sclerosis and optic neuritis and in patients with peripheral demyelinating disorders, such as Guillain-Barré syndrome. If these disorders develop or worsen, expect drug to be discontinued.

PATIENT TEACHING

- Inform patient that infliximab must be given I.V. initially but then may then be followed by subcutaneous injections for some conditions.

! **WARNING** Tell patient infusion reactions may occur up to 12 days after infusion is given. Urge patient to report infusion reaction (chest pain, chills, dyspnea, facial flushing, fever, itching, headache, rash) immediately.

- Instruct patient, family, or caregiver how to administer drug subcutaneously, if prescribed, after intravenous therapy has initially been given.

! **WARNING** Alert patient that drug may cause an allergic reaction. If present, tell patient to notify prescriber and, if severe, to seek immediate medical care.

! **WARNING** Review signs and symptoms of heart failure, hepatotoxicity, and hematologic reactions as well as neurologic abnormalities that may occur, and instruct patient to notify prescriber if any develops. Stress importance of seeking immediate medical attention if patient experiences heart or stroke signs and symptoms within 24 hours of drug administration.

! **WARNING** Review infection control measures. Urge patient to report evidence of infection, such as cough, painful urination, or sore throat immediately to prescriber.

! **WARNING** Explain that infliximab increases the risk of lymphoma and other malignancies; urge prompt medical attention for suspicious signs or symptoms. Also, advise patient to have regular skin examinations because drug increases risk of skin cancer and for female patients to have periodic screening for cervical cancer.

! **WARNING** Advise patient not to receive vaccinations using live vaccines or infectious agents during drug therapy. Also, advise family or caregiver not to have infant exposed to live vaccines for up to 6 months after birth if the mother was taking infliximab during the pregnancy.

ipratropium bromide

Atrovent HFA, Atrovent Nasal Spray 0.03%, Ipravent (CAN)

Class and Category

Pharmacologic class: Anticholinergic
Therapeutic class: Bronchodilator

Indications and Dosages

* *To provide maintenance treatment for bronchospasm associated with chronic obstructive pulmonary disease (COPD), including chronic bronchitis and emphysema*

INHALATION AEROSOL (ATROVENT HFA)

Adults. *Initial:* 2 inhalations (17 mcg each inhalation) 4 times daily, increased, as needed. *Maximum:* Up to 12 inhalations/24 hr.

INHALATION SOLUTION FOR NEBULIZER (IPRAVENT)

Adults and adolescents. 250 to 500 mcg dissolved in preservative-free sterile normal saline solution every 6 hr.

* *To treat rhinorrhea associated with allergic and nonallergic perennial rhinitis*

NASAL SPRAY (ATROVENT NASAL SPRAY 0.03%)

Adults and children ages 6 and older. 2 sprays of 0.03% (21 mcg/spray) per nostril twice daily or 3 times daily. *Maximum:* 12 sprays (252 mcg)/24 hr.

Drug Administration

INTRANASAL

- Before using for first time, prime nasal spray by pumping bottle 7 times or until a fine spray comes out.
- Have patient blow his nose.
- Have patient insert tip into one nostril pointing the tip toward the back and outer side of the nose. Have patient hold opposite nostril closed and lean head slightly forward.
- Have patient spray by firmly and quickly pressing upwards with the thumb at the base while holding the white shoulder portion of the pump between the index and middle fingers and sniff deeply, then breathe out through mouth. After administration, have patient lean head backward for a few seconds. Then, repeat in the other nostril.
- If spray pump gets clogged, hold tip of bottle under warm running water for about 1 minute. Dry the pump and prime again.
- If spray bottle is not used for more than 24 hr, prime it again by releasing 2 sprays. If bottle is not used for more than 7 days, prime bottle again by releasing 7 sprays.

INHALATION

Nebulizer

- Inhalation solution is for use with an oral nebulizer. See manufacturer's guidelines for administration. When using the nebulizer, apply a mouthpiece to prevent drug from leaking out around mask and causing blurred vision or eye pain.
- Dilute to 2 to 3 ml with normal saline and nebulize until the entire volume of solution is inhaled. 1 ml of solution usually takes over 3 min and 2 ml usually takes over 8 to 10 min.
- Protect vials from light and keep unused vials in foil pouch until ready to use.

Mechanism of Action

After acetylcholine is released from cholinergic fibers, ipratropium prevents it from attaching to muscarinic receptors on membranes of smooth muscle cells, as shown here. By blocking acetylcholine's effects in bronchi and bronchioles, ipratropium relaxes smooth muscles and causes bronchodilation.

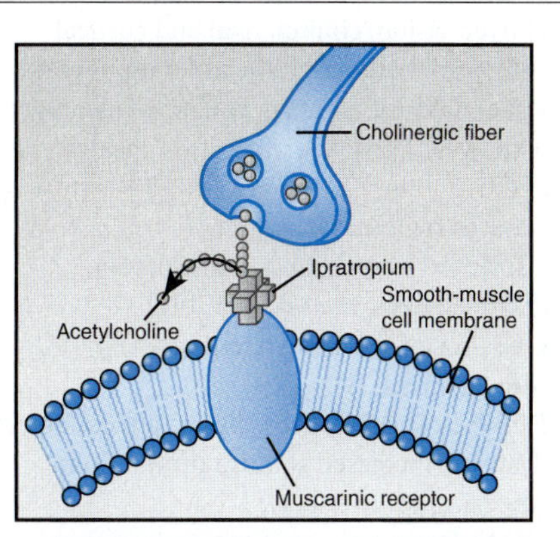

Inhaler

- Inhaler should be initially primed with 2 test sprays; if not used for more than 3 days, repeat priming. There is no need to shake inhaler before administration. Wait 15 sec between inhalations. Attach spacer device to inhaler to improve delivery, if needed. Have patient rinse mouth after inhaling drug. Wash mouthpiece once a wk for 30 sec in warm water and let air-dry. Discard inhaler after the labeled number of actuations has been used, which is usually 200 actuations. The canister may not be completely empty but should be discarded.

Route	Onset	Peak	Duration
Inhalation	15 min	1–2 hr	2–8 hr
Nasal	15 min	Unknown	Unknown

Half-life: 1.6–2 hr

Contraindications

Hypersensitivity to atropine, ipratropium bromide, or their components

Interactions

DRUGS

anticholinergics: Increased anticholinergic effects

Adverse Reactions

CNS: Dizziness, insomnia
CV: **Atrial fibrillation** (oral inhalation), **bradycardia** (nasal spray), edema, hypertension, palpitations, **supraventricular tachycardia** (oral inhalation), tachycardia
EENT: Acute eye pain, dry mouth or pharyngeal area, increased intraocular pressure, **laryngospasm**, taste perversion, **oropharyngeal edema** (all drug forms); blurred vision, conjunctival and corneal congestion, eye irritation and pain, mydriasis, visual halos (if nasal spray comes in contact with eyes); epistaxis, mydriasis, nasal dryness and irritation, pharyngitis, rhinitis, sinusitis, tinnitus (with nasal spray)
GI: **Bowel obstruction**, constipation, diarrhea, ileus, nausea, vomiting
GU: Prostatitis, urine retention
MS: Arthritis
RESP: Bronchitis, **bronchospasm**, cough, dyspnea, increased sputum production, wheezing
SKIN: Dermatitis, pruritus, rash, urticaria
Other: **Anaphylaxis**, **angioedema**, flu-like symptoms

Childbearing Considerations

PREGNANCY

- It is not known if drug causes fetal harm.
- Use with caution only if benefit to mother outweighs potential risk to fetus.

LACTATION

- It is not known if drug is present in breast milk.
- Mothers should check with prescriber before breastfeeding.

Nursing Considerations

- Use ipratropium cautiously in patients with angle-closure glaucoma, benign prostatic hyperplasia, or bladder neck obstruction and in patients with hepatic or renal dysfunction.

! **WARNING** Monitor patient for hypersensitivity reactions that could be life-threatening, such as anaphylaxis or angioedema. If present, stop drug use immediately, notify prescriber, and provide supportive care, as needed and ordered.

! **WARNING** Notify prescriber if patient experiences persistent, serious, or unusual adverse reactions because ipratropium has the potential to cause serious adverse effects such as bronchospasms and bowel obstruction.

PATIENT TEACHING

! **WARNING** Caution patient not to use ipratropium inhaler to treat acute bronchospasm.

- Teach patient how to use inhaler, nasal spray, or nebulizer, whichever is prescribed.
- Advise patient to keep spray out of his eyes because it may irritate them or blur his vision. If spray comes in contact with eyes, instruct patient to flush them with cool tap water for several minutes and to contact prescriber.
- Instruct patient to rinse mouth after each nebulizer or inhaler treatment to help minimize throat dryness and irritation.

! **WARNING** Warn patient that an allergic reaction, which could become severe, may occur after using drug. If present, tell patient to immediately discontinue use of drug and notify prescriber if not severe, or seek immediate emergency attention if difficulty breathing or swelling occurs.

! **WARNING** Tell patient to notify prescriber if persistent, serious, or unusual adverse reactions occur.

- Advise patient to report decreased response to ipratropium.

irbesartan

Avapro

Class and Category

Pharmacologic class: Angiotensin II receptor antagonist
Therapeutic class: Antihypertensive

Indications and Dosages

∗ *To manage hypertension, alone or with other antihypertensives*

TABLETS

Adults and adolescents. *Initial:* 150 mg once daily, and increased, as needed. *Maximum:* 300 mg daily.

∗ *To treat nephropathy in type 2 diabetes mellitus in patients with hypertension, an elevated serum creatinine, and proteinuria*

TABLETS

Adults. 300 mg once daily.

± **DOSAGE ADJUSTMENT** For patients with hyponatremia or hypovolemia from such causes as hemodialysis or vigorous diuretic therapy, initial dosage reduced to 75 mg daily.

Drug Administration

P.O.

- Administer drug at the same time each day to maintain its therapeutic effect.

Route	Onset	Peak	Duration
P.O.	Unknown	1.5–2 hr	24 hr

Half-life: 11–15 hr

Mechanism of Action

Selectively blocks binding of the potent vasoconstrictor angiotensin (AT) II to AT_1 receptor sites in many tissues, including adrenal glands and vascular smooth muscle. This inhibits the aldosterone-secreting and vasoconstrictive effects of AT II, which reduces blood pressure.

Contraindications

Concurrent aliskiren use in patients with diabetes, hypersensitivity to irbesartan or its components

Interactions

DRUGS

aliskiren (patients with diabetes or renal impairment), angiotensin-converting enzyme (ACE) inhibitors, other angiotensin receptor blockers: Increased risk of hyperkalemia, hypotension, and renal dysfunction
lithium: Possibly increased serum lithium level
NSAIDs: Possible decreased renal function in patients who are elderly, volume-depleted, or have a compromised renal function
potassium-sparing diuretics, potassium supplements, or salt substitutes containing potassium: Possible hyperkalemia

Adverse Reactions

CNS: Anxiety, dizziness, fatigue, headache, nervousness
CV: Chest pain, **hypotension**, peripheral edema, tachycardia
EENT: Pharyngitis, rhinitis, tinnitus
ENDO: **Hypoglycemia** (in diabetic patients)
GI: Abdominal pain, diarrhea, elevated liver enzymes, heartburn, **hepatitis**, indigestion, jaundice, nausea, vomiting
GU: Impaired renal function, **renal failure**, UTI
HEME: Anemia, **thrombocytopenia**
MS: Increased CPK level, musculoskeletal pain, **rhabdomyolysis**
RESP: Upper respiratory tract infection
SKIN: Rash, urticaria
Other: **Anaphylaxis**, **including angioedema**, **hyperkalemia**, **shock**

Childbearing Considerations

PREGNANCY

- Drug can cause fetal harm, especially if exposure occurs during the second or third trimester.
- Drug reduces fetal renal function leading to anuria and renal failure and increases fetal and neonatal morbidity and death. It can also cause fetal lung hypoplasia, hypotension, and skeletal deformations, such as skull hypoplasia.

- Drug is contraindicated in pregnant women and should be discontinued as soon as possible when pregnancy is known.

LACTATION

- It is not known if drug is present in breast milk.
- A decision should be made to discontinue breastfeeding or the drug to avoid potential serious adverse reactions, including hyperkalemia, hypotension, and renal impairment in the breastfed infant.

Nursing Considerations

- Know that if patient has known or suspected hypovolemia, provide treatment, such as I.V. 0.9% Sodium Chloride Injection, as ordered, to correct this condition before beginning irbesartan therapy. Or, expect to begin therapy with a lower dosage.
- Check blood pressure often to evaluate drug's effectiveness to treat hypertension. Be aware that if blood pressure isn't controlled with irbesartan alone, expect to also give a diuretic, such as hydrochlorothiazide, as prescribed. Also, monitor patient's renal function to evaluate drug's effectiveness to treat nephropathy.

! WARNING Monitor patient for a hypersensitivity reaction, which could become life-threatening, such as anaphylaxis or angioedema. If present, notify prescriber, expect drug to be discontinued, and provide supportive care, as needed and ordered.

! WARNING Monitor patient for increased BUN and serum creatinine levels if patient has heart failure or impaired renal function because drug may cause acute renal failure. If increases are significant or persistent, notify prescriber immediately.

! WARNING Be alert for hypotension in a patient who receives a diuretic or another antihypertensive during irbesartan therapy. Frequently monitor blood pressure. If patient experiences symptomatic hypotension, expect to stop drug temporarily. Immediately place the patient in supine position and prepare to give I.V. normal saline solution, as ordered. Expect to resume drug therapy after blood pressure stabilizes.

! WARNING Monitor patients with diabetes mellitus for hypoglycemia. If present, treat according to institutional protocol and notify prescriber.

- Be aware that if patient receives a diuretic, provide adequate hydration, as appropriate, to help prevent hypovolemia. Also, monitor patient for signs and symptoms of hypovolemia, such as dizziness, fainting, and hypotension.

PATIENT TEACHING

- Instruct patient how to administer irbesartan.

! WARNING Alert patient that drug may cause an allergic reaction. Tell patient to notify prescriber if an allergic reaction occurs and to seek immediate medical care, if severe.

! WARNING Advise females of child bearing age to notify prescriber immediately if pregnancy occurs. Explain that if she becomes pregnant, prescriber may replace irbesartan with another antihypertensive that's safe to use during pregnancy.

! WARNING Advise patients with diabetes mellitus to be alert for signs and symptoms of hypoglycemia and to treat immediately. If hypoglycemia occurs frequently or is severe, tell patient to notify prescriber.

! WARNING Stress importance of notifying prescriber of any persistent, serious, or unusual adverse reactions as drug has the potential to affect many body systems, especially the kidneys.

- Caution patient to avoid hazardous activities until drug's CNS effects are known and resolved.
- Instruct patient to consult prescriber before taking any new drug.
- To reduce risk of dehydration and hypotension, advise patient to drink adequate fluids during hot weather and exercise. Also, instruct patient to contact prescriber if diarrhea, severe nausea, or vomiting occurs because of the risk of dehydration and hypotension.
- Inform mothers that breastfeeding should not be undertaken during drug therapy or the drug must be discontinued.

- Urge patient to keep follow-up appointments with prescriber to monitor progress.

iron dextran

(contains 50 mg of elemental iron per milliliter)
InFeD

Class and Category

Pharmacologic class: Iron mineral
Therapeutic class: Hematinic

Indications and Dosages

✶ *To treat iron deficiency anemia in patients who have an intolerance to oral iron or an unsatisfactory response to oral iron*

I.M. OR I.V. INJECTION

Adults and children ages 4 mo and older weighing more than 15 kg (33 lb). Calculated using following formula: Dose (ml) = 0.0442 (desired hemoglobin − observed hemoglobin) × lean body weight (LBW) in kg (Males = 50 kg + 2.3 kg for each inch of patient's height over 5 feet. Females = 45.5 kg + 2.3 kg for each inch of patient's height over 5 feet) + (0.26 × LBW). Or, consult dosage table in manufacturer's guideline. *Test dose on day 1:* 0.5 ml injected I.M. or I.V. slowly over at least 30 sec followed in 1 hr or more with remainder of dose, if no reaction occurs. Total dosage repeated once daily thereafter. *Maximum:* 100 mg daily.

Children ages 4 mo and older weighing 5 to 15 kg (11 to 33 lb). Calculated using following formula: Dose (ml) = 0.0442 (desired hemoglobin − observed hemoglobin) × weight in kg + (0.26 × weight in kg). Or, consult dosage table in manufacturer's guidelines. *Test dose on day 1:* 0.5 ml injected I.M. or I.V. slowly over at least 30 sec followed in 1 hr or more with remainder of dose, if no reaction occurs. Total dosage repeated once daily thereafter. *Maximum daily dosage:* 2 ml (100 mg) for heavier children; 1 ml (50 mg) for children weighing less than 10 kg but more than 5 kg.

✶ *To replace iron lost in blood loss*

I.V. INJECTION

Adults. Replacement iron (mg) = Blood loss (ml) × hematocrit divided by 50 mg/ml.

Drug Administration

I.M.

- Change needle after drawing up iron dextran into syringe.
- Administer using Z-track method using a 2- to 3-inch, 19 G or 20 G needle with patient lying in a lateral position with injection site uppermost. Injection can also be given with patient standing with patient bearing weight on the leg opposite the injection site.
- Inject deep into the upper outer quadrant of patient's buttock. Do not inject drug into any other site.

I.V.

- Infuse undiluted slowly, at no more than 1 ml/min (50 mg/minute). Avoid rapid injection because flushing and hypotension may occur.
- Flush with 10 ml of 0.9% Sodium Chloride Injection after administration.
- *Incompatibilities:* Other drugs, or parenteral nutrition solutions for I.V. infusion

Route	Onset	Peak	Duration
I.V./I.M.	1–2 days	7–9 days	Unknown

Half-life: 6 hr

Mechanism of Action

Restores hemoglobin and replenishes iron stores. Iron, an essential component of hemoglobin, myoglobin, and several enzymes (including catalase, cytochromes, and peroxidase), is needed for catecholamine metabolism and normal neutrophil function.

In iron dextran therapy, iron binds to available protein parts after the drug has been split into dextran and iron by cells of the reticuloendothelial system. The bound iron forms hemosiderin or ferritin, physiologic forms of iron, and transferrin, which replenish hemoglobin and deplete iron stores. Dextran is metabolized or excreted.

Contraindications

Anemia other than iron deficiency, hypersensitivity to iron dextran or its components

Interactions

DRUGS

angiotensin-converting enzyme inhibitors: Possibly increased risk for anaphylactic-type reaction

Adverse Reactions

CNS: Chills, disorientation, dizziness, fever, headache, malaise, paresthesia, **seizures**, syncope, unconsciousness, weakness
CV: **Acute myocardial ischemia with or without MI or in-stent thrombosis (hypersensitivity reaction)**, **arrhythmias**, **bradycardia**, **cardiac arrest**, chest pain, hypertension, **hypotension**, **shock**, tachycardia
EENT: Altered taste
GI: Abdominal pain, diarrhea, nausea, vomiting
GU: Hematuria
HEME: Leukocytosis
MS: Arthralgia, arthritis, backache, myalgia, **rhabdomyolysis**
RESP: **Bronchospasm**, **cyanosis**, dyspnea, **respiratory arrest**, wheezing
SKIN: **Diaphoresis**, flushing, rash, pruritus, purpura, urticaria
Other: **Anaphylaxis**, infusion-site phlebitis, **iron overload**

Childbearing Considerations

PREGNANCY

- It is not known if drug causes fetal harm. However, fetal bradycardia may occur, especially in the second and third trimester, if mother develops a severe hypersensitivity reaction to the drug.
- Use with caution only if benefit to mother outweighs potential risk to fetus.

LACTATION

- Drug is present in breast milk in trace amounts.
- Mothers should check with prescriber before breastfeeding.

Nursing Considerations

- Be aware that iron dextran is given only when oral therapy isn't feasible.
- Expect to monitor hematocrit, hemoglobin level, serum ferritin level, and transferrin saturation, as ordered, before, during, and after iron dextran therapy.

! WARNING Expect with first dose to administer a test dose as prescribed and monitor patient closely for anaphylactic reaction. Expect to wait 1 or more hours before giving remainder of dose if no reaction occurs.

! WARNING Monitor patient after test dose closely for signs and symptoms of anaphylaxis (such as collapse, dyspnea, loss of consciousness, seizures, and severe hypotension) during and after drug administration. Patients with a history of allergies or asthma or who take ACE inhibitors are at increased risk for anaphylaxis, possibly death. Institute emergency resuscitation measures, as needed and ordered.

! WARNING Assess blood pressure often after iron dextran administration, especially if given intravenously because hypotension is a common adverse effect that may be related to infusion rate; avoid rapid infusion.

! WARNING Monitor patient for iron overload, characterized by bleeding in GI tract and lungs, decreased activity, pale eyes, and sedation. If present, notify prescriber immediately, expect iron dextran to be discontinued and provide supportive care, as needed and ordered.

! WARNING Know that if patient has cardiovascular disease, condition may worsen because of drug's adverse effects. Notify prescriber immediately of any change.

- Be aware that patient may have adverse reactions, including arthralgia, backache, chills, and vomiting, 1 to 2 days after drug therapy. Symptoms should resolve within 3 to 4 days.
- Assess patients with a history of rheumatoid arthritis for exacerbation of joint pain and swelling.
- Be aware iron dextran may give a brown color to serum from a blood sample drawn 4 hours after administration and may cause falsely elevated serum bilirubin and falsely decreased values of serum calcium. Serum iron determinations may not be accurate for 23 weeks following iron dextran administration, especially if done by colorimetric assays.

PATIENT TEACHING

- Tell patient iron dextran is administered either by intramuscular or intravenous injection
- Inform patient that a test dose will be given prior to initiating iron dextran therapy because drug may cause an allergic reaction.

! **WARNING** Instruct patient to immediately report signs and symptoms of an allergic reaction with test dose as well as during iron dextran therapy, such as appearance of a rash, shortness of breath or wheezing. Also, tell patient to report feelings of light-headedness or fainting because low blood pressure may occur after drug is administered, especially if given intravenously.

! **WARNING** Review signs and symptoms of iron overload with patient. Advise patient not to take any oral iron without first consulting prescriber. Stress importance of contacting prescriber if patient experiences any such effects.

! **WARNING** Alert patient with cardiovascular disease that iron dextran has the potential to make the disease worse. Tell patient to notify prescriber if he experiences increased cardiovascular signs and symptoms.

- Urge patient to plan periods of activity and rest to avoid excessive fatigue.
- Emphasize need to keep follow-up medical and laboratory appointments.

iron sucrose

(contains 100 mg of elemental iron per 5 ml)
Venofer

Class and Category

Pharmacologic class: Iron mineral
Therapeutic class: Hematinic

Indications and Dosages

* *To treat iron deficiency anemia in patients with hemodialysis-dependent chronic kidney disease*

I.V. INJECTION, I.V. INFUSION

Adults. *Initial:* 100 mg injected undiluted over 2 to 5 min within first hr during dialysis. Alternatively, 100 mg infused diluted and infused over at least 15 min within first hr during dialysis. *Usual:* 1,000 mg for total treatment course. Dosage repeated as needed to maintain target levels of hemoglobin and hematocrit and acceptable blood iron level.

* *To treat iron deficiency anemia patients with peritoneal dialysis-dependent chronic kidney disease*

I.V. INFUSION

Adults. *Initial:* 300 mg infused diluted over 1.5 hr on days 1 and 14, followed by 400 mg infused diluted over 2.5 hr on day 28. Dosage repeated as needed to maintain target levels of hemoglobin and hematocrit and acceptable blood iron level.

* *To maintain iron therapy in children with chronic kidney disease who are nondialysis-dependent receiving erythropoietin or who are peritoneal dialysis-dependent receiving erythropoietin; to maintain iron therapy in children with hemodialysis-dependent chronic kidney disease (HDD-CKD)*

I.V. INJECTION, I.V. INFUSION

Children ages 2 yr and older. 0.5 mg/kg, not to exceed 100 mg/dose, every 2 wk (HDD-CKD) or 4 wk (other indications) for 12 wk given undiluted over 5 min as an I.V. injection or diluted and infused over 5 to 60 min as an I.V. infusion. Treatment repeated, as needed.

* *To treat iron deficiency anemia in nondialysis patients with chronic renal disease (NDD-CKD).*

I.V. INJECTION, I.V. INFUSION

Adults. *Initial:* 200 mg injected undiluted over 2 to 5 min and repeated 4 more times over a 14-day period. Alternatively, 200 mg infused diluted over at least 15 min and repeated 4 more times over a 14-day period. *Maximum:* 1,000 mg/14 days.

Drug Administration

I.V.

- Follow guidelines given under each indication for administration times for both injection and infusion, as there are differences based on indication.
- If given during hemodialysis, administer early during the dialysis session (usually within the first hour).
- For I.V. injection, administer undiluted.
- For I.V. infusion in adults, dilute 100 mg or 200 mg in maximum of 100 ml 0.9% Sodium Chloride Injection; 300 or 400 mg in maximum of 250 ml of 0.9% Sodium Chloride Injection. Dilute immediately before infusion.
- For I.V. infusion in children, dilute with 0.9% Sodium Chloride Injection to a concentration of 1 to 2 mg/ml. Do not dilute to concentrations below 1 mg/ml. Dilute immediately before infusion.

G H I

- Discard any unused diluted solution.
- Store in original carton at controlled room temperature.
- Drug diluted or undiluted can be stored in a plastic syringe or mixed in I.V. infusion bags (PVC or non-PVC) containing 0.9% Sodium Chloride Injection for 7 days at controlled room temperature. Drug in plastic syringe can also be stored in refrigerator.
- *Incompatibilities:* Other I.V. drugs, parenteral nutrition solutions

Route	Onset	Peak	Duration
I.V.	Unknown	Unknown	Unknown

Half-life: 6 hr

Mechanism of Action

Acts to replenish iron stores lost during dialysis because of increased erythropoiesis and insufficient absorption of iron from GI tract. Iron is an essential component of hemoglobin, myoglobin, and several enzymes, including catalase, cytochromes, and peroxidase, and is needed for catecholamine metabolism and normal neutrophil function. Iron sucrose also normalizes RBC production by binding with hemoglobin or being stored as ferritin in reticuloendothelial cells of the bone marrow, liver, or spleen.

Contraindications

Anemia other than iron deficiency, hypersensitivity to iron components, iron overload

Interactions

DRUGS

oral iron preparations: Possibly reduced absorption of oral iron supplements

Adverse Reactions

CNS: Asthenia, **collapse**, confusion, dizziness, fatigue, fever, headache, hypoesthesia, light-headedness, loss of consciousness, malaise, **seizures**

CV: **Acute myocardial ischemia with or without MI or with in-stent thrombosis (hypersensitivity reaction), bradycardia**, chest pain, edema, **heart failure**, hypertension, **hypotension**, peripheral edema, **shock**

EENT: Conjunctivitis, ear pain, nasal congestion, nasopharyngitis, rhinitis, sinusitis, taste perversion

ENDO: Hyperglycemia, **hypoglycemia**

GI: Abdominal pain, constipation, diarrhea, elevated liver enzymes, nausea, occult-positive feces, peritoneal infection, vomiting

GU: Chromaturia, UTI

MS: Arthralgia, arthritis, back pain, joint swelling, leg cramps, muscle pain or weakness, myalgia

RESP: **Bronchospasm**, cough, dyspnea, pneumonia, upper respiratory tract infection

SKIN: Hyperhidrosis, pruritus, rash

Other: **Anaphylaxis**; **angioedema**; **iron overload**; gout; infusion or injection-site burning, pain, redness, or skin discoloration (with extravasation); **sepsis**

Childbearing Considerations

PREGNANCY

- It is not known if drug causes fetal harm. However, fetal bradycardia may occur, especially in the second and third trimester, if mother develops a severe hypersensitivity reaction to drug.
- Use with caution only if benefit to mother outweighs potential risk to fetus.

LACTATION

- Drug is present in breast milk.
- Mothers should check with prescriber before breastfeeding.
- If breastfeeding occurs, infant should be monitored for GI toxicity (constipation, diarrhea).

Nursing Considerations

- Expect to monitor hematocrit, hemoglobin, serum ferritin, and transferrin saturation, as ordered, before, during, and after iron sucrose therapy.

> **! WARNING** Monitor patient closely for evidence of a hypersensitivity reaction which could become life-threatening such as anaphylaxis (collapse, dyspnea, loss of consciousness, seizures, or severe hypotension) or angioedema (swelling) during and for at least 30 minutes after therapy. Institute emergency resuscitation measures, as needed.

! **WARNING** Assess blood pressure often after drug administration because hypotension is a common adverse reaction that may be related to infusion rate (avoid rapid infusion) or total cumulative dose.

! **WARNING** Watch for evidence of iron overload, such as bleeding in GI tract and lungs, decreased activity, pale eyes, and sedation. Notify prescriber and expect to stop therapy if blood iron levels are normal or elevated, to prevent iron toxicity. If evidence of iron overload is present, notify prescriber immediately, expect iron dextran to be discontinued and provide supportive care, as needed and ordered.

- Test serum iron level 48 hours after last dose, as ordered.

PATIENT TEACHING

! **WARNING** Tell patient to inform prescriber if she has a prior history of reactions to parenteral iron products before drug is given.

! **WARNING** Instruct patient to report any of the following signs and symptoms of an allergic reaction that may develop during and following the infusion of iron sucrose: breathing problems, dizziness, itching, light-headedness, rash, and swelling. If severe and already back home, tell patient to seek immediate emergency care.

! **WARNING** Review signs and symptoms of iron overload with patient. Advise patient not to take any oral iron without first consulting prescriber. Stress importance of contacting prescriber if patient experience any such effects.

! **WARNING** Tell mothers who are breastfeeding while receiving iron sucrose to monitor their infant for constipation or diarrhea. If present, pediatrician should be notified, as this may indicate GI toxicity.

- Urge patient to plan periods of activity and rest to avoid excessive fatigue.
- Emphasize need to keep follow-up medical and laboratory appointments.

isoniazid (isonicotinic acid hydrazide, INH)

Isotamine (CAN), PDP-Isoniazid (CAN)

Class and Category

Pharmacologic class: Isonicotinic acid derivatives
Therapeutic class: Antitubercular agent

Indications and Dosages

✷ *To prevent tuberculosis (TB)*

ORAL SOLUTION, TABLETS I.M. INJECTION

Adults weighing more than 30 kg (66 lb). 300 mg daily for 6 to 12 mo.
Infants and children. 10 mg/kg once daily (up to 300 mg) for up to 1 yr. Alternatively, when daily compliance is uncertain, 20 to 30 mg/kg (not to exceed 900 mg) twice weekly under direct observation of a healthcare worker.

✷ *As adjunct to treat active TB*

ORAL SOLUTION, TABLETS, I.M. INJECTION

Adults. 5 mg/kg up to 300 mg once daily. Alternatively, 15 mg/kg (up to 900 mg) 2 or 3 times/wk.
Children. 10 to 15 mg/kg (up to 300 mg) once daily. Alternatively, 20 to 40 mg/kg (up to 900 mg) 2 or 3 times/wk.

Drug Administration

- Expect to administer drug with other antitubercular drugs to prevent development of resistant organisms.

P.O.

- Give oral drug 1 hr before or 2 hr after meals to promote absorption.
- If patient has trouble swallowing tablets, obtain oral solution.
- Use a calibrated device, such as a dropper or syringe, to measure dosage of oral solution.

I.M.

- Use reserved for when patient cannot take oral form of drug.
- Solution may crystallize at low temperatures. If this occurs, warm vial to room temperature before administering to redissolve the crystals.
- Inject deeply into a large muscle mass.

Route	Onset	Peak	Duration
P.O./I.M.	Unknown	1–2 hr	Unknown

Half-life: 0.5–5 hr

Mechanism of Action

Interferes with lipid and nucleic acid synthesis in actively growing tubercule bacilli cells. Isoniazid also disrupts bacterial cell wall synthesis and may interfere with mycolic acid synthesis in mycobacterial cells.

Contraindications

History of severe adverse reactions (acute liver disease of any etiology, including drug-induced hepatitis; arthritis; chills; drug fever); hypersensitivity to isoniazid or its components

Interactions

DRUGS

acetaminophen: Increased risk of hepatotoxicity
carbamazepine: Increased blood carbamazepine level and toxicity
hepatotoxic drugs, rifampin: Increased risk of hepatotoxicity
ketoconazole: Possibly decreased blood ketoconazole level and resistance to antifungal treatment
phenytoin: Increased blood phenytoin level, increased risk of phenytoin toxicity
theophylline, valproate: Increased levels of these drugs

ACTIVITIES

alcohol use: Increased risk of hepatotoxicity

FOODS

all food: Decreased absorption of isoniazid
histamine-containing foods, such as tuna, skipjack, and other tropical fish: Inhibited action of the enzyme diamine oxidase in foods, possibly resulting in flushing, headache, hypotension, palpitations, and sweating.
tyramine-containing foods, such as cheese and fish: Increased response to tyramine in foods, possibly resulting in chills; diaphoresis; headache; light-headedness; and red, itchy, clammy skin

Adverse Reactions

CNS: Clumsiness, confusion, dizziness, **encephalopathy**, fatigue, fever, hallucinations, **neurotoxicity**, paresthesia, peripheral neuritis, psychosis, **seizures**, weakness
CV: Vasculitis
EENT: Optic neuritis
ENDO: Gynecomastia, hyperglycemia
GI: Abdominal pain, anorexia, elevated liver enzymes, epigastric distress, **hepatitis**, jaundice, nausea, **pancreatitis**, vomiting
GU: Glycosuria
HEME: **Agranulocytosis**, **aplastic anemia**, eosinophilia, **hemolytic anemia**, sideroblastic anemia, **thrombocytopenia**
MS: Arthralgia, joint stiffness
SKIN: **Pruritus**, rash, **Stevens-Johnson syndrome**, **toxic epidermal necrolysis**
Other: **Anaphylaxis**, **drug reaction with eosinophilia and systemic symptoms (DRESS)**, **hypocalcemia**, **hypophosphatemia**, injection-site irritation, lupus-like symptoms, lymphadenopathy

Childbearing Considerations

PREGNANCY

- Drug may be used to treat active TB in pregnant women.
- Drug should be deferred to treat latent TB until after delivery to avoid risk to fetus.
- Be aware that risk of fatal maternal isoniazid-associated hepatitis may be increased, especially during the postpartum period.

LACTATION

- Drug is present in breast milk.
- Breastfeeding may take place during drug therapy.

Nursing Considerations

- Administer isoniazid cautiously to alcoholic, diabetic, or malnourished patients and those at risk for peripheral neuritis.

! **WARNING** Monitor patient for a hypersensitivity reaction, which may become life-threatening, such as anaphylaxis or severe skin reactions such as DRESS. Notify prescriber at first sign of a hypersensitivity reaction including a rash (DRESS may initially only present with fever or swollen lymph nodes), expect drug to be discontinued, and provide supportive care, as needed and ordered.

! **WARNING** Know that about 50% of patients metabolize isoniazid slowly, which may lead to increased toxic effects. Watch for adverse reactions, such as peripheral neuritis; if they occur, expect to decrease dosage.

! **WARNING** Monitor liver enzyme studies, which may be ordered monthly, because isoniazid can cause severe (possibly fatal) hepatitis.

! **WARNING** Be aware that patients with advanced HIV infection may experience more severe adverse reactions in greater numbers. Monitor these patients closely.

- Follow patient compliance with the Potts-Cozart test, which is a simple colorimetric method of checking drug in the urine. Additionally, isoniazid test strips are also available to check compliance.

PATIENT TEACHING

- Instruct patient how to administer oral form of isoniazid prescribed.
- Tell patient to take drug exactly as prescribed and not to stop without first consulting prescriber. Explain that treatment may take months or years.

! **WARNING** Alert patient that drug may cause an allergic reaction. If present, tell patient to notify prescriber and, if severe, to seek immediate medical care.

! **WARNING** Advise patient to report signs of hepatic dysfunction, including dark urine, decreased appetite, fatigue, and jaundice. Caution patient not to drink alcohol while taking isoniazid because alcohol increases the risk of hepatotoxicity.

! **WARNING** Urge patient to report any persistent, severe, or unusual adverse effects, including fever, nausea, numbness and tingling in arms and legs, rash, vision changes, vomiting, and yellowing skin.

! **WARNING** Tell females of child bearing age to notify prescriber if pregnant because drug for latent TB should be delayed until after delivery takes place.

- Give patient a list of tyramine-containing foods to avoid when taking isoniazid, such as cheese, fish, red wine, salami, and yeast extracts. Explain that consuming these foods during isoniazid therapy may cause unpleasant adverse reactions, such as chills, pounding heartbeat, and sweating.
- Tell patient to avoid histamine-containing foods, such as tuna, skipjack, and other tropical fish during therapy to avoid such adverse reactions as flushing, headache, low blood pressure, rapid heartbeat, and sweating.
- Tell patient that he'll need periodic laboratory tests and physical examinations.

isosorbide dinitrate

Isordil Titradose

isosorbide mononitrate

Monoket

Class and Category

Pharmacologic class: Nitrate
Therapeutic class: Antianginal

Indications and Dosages

✱ *To prevent angina due to coronary artery disease*

TABLETS

Adults. *Initial:* 5 to 20 mg (dinitrate) 2 or 3 times daily. *Maintenance:* 10 to 40 mg 2 or 3 times daily. Alternatively, 5 to 20 mg (mononitrate) twice daily 7 hr apart.

E.R. TABLETS

Adults. *Initial:* 30 to 60 mg (mononitrate) once daily, increased after several days to 120 mg once daily and then after several more days to 240 mg once daily, as needed.

✱ *To treat angina due to coronary artery disease*

TABLETS

Adults. *Initial:* 5 to 20 mg (mononitrate) twice daily 7 hr apart.

Drug Administration

P.O.

- Give immediate-acting drug 30 min before or 2 hr after meals.

Mechanism of Action

Isosorbide may interact with nitrate receptors in vascular smooth muscle cell membranes. By interacting with receptors' sulfhydryl groups, drug is reduced to nitric oxide. Nitric oxide activates the enzyme guanylate cyclase, increasing intracellular formation of cyclic guanosine monophosphate (cGMP). An increased cGMP level may relax vascular smooth muscle by forcing calcium out of muscle cells, causing vasodilation. This improves cardiac output by reducing mainly preload but also afterload.

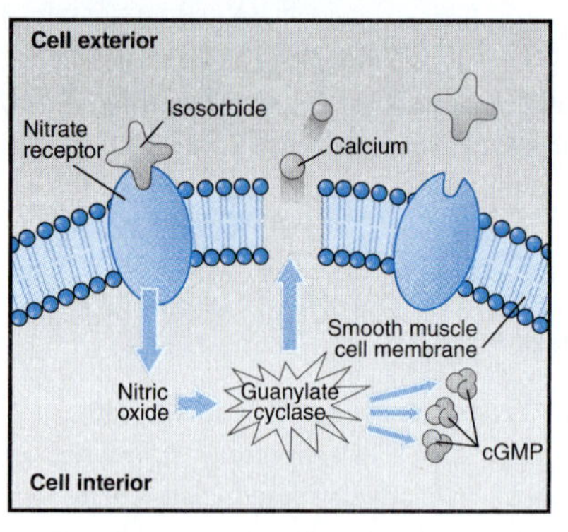

- E.R. tablets should be swallowed whole and not chewed, crushed, or split. E.R. tablets are administered once daily in the morning.
- Drug requires a drug-free interval daily. Expect a nitrate-free interval of at least 14 hr for immediate-release form and greater than 18 hr for extended-release form.
- Protect drug from heat and light.

Route	Onset	Peak	Duration
P.O.	7.5–45 min	30–60 min	2–6 hr
P.O. (E.R.)	60–90 min	3–4.5 hr	10–14 hr

Half-life: 5 hr

Contraindications

Concurrent use of phosphodiesterase inhibitors (sildenafil, tadalafil, vardenafil) or riociguat; hypersensitivity to isosorbide, other nitrates, or their components

Interactions

DRUGS

phosphodiesterase inhibitors, such as sildenafil, tadalafil, vardenafil: Increased risk of hypotension, myocardial ischemia, syncope, and possibly death
riociguat: Increased risk of hypotension
vasodilators: Additive effects

ACTIVITIES

alcohol use: Increased risk of orthostatic hypotension

Adverse Reactions

CNS: Agitation, confusion, dizziness, headache, insomnia, restlessness, syncope, vertigo, weakness
CV: **Arrhythmias**, orthostatic hypotension, palpitations, peripheral edema, tachycardia
EENT: Blurred vision, diplopia (all forms); sublingual burning (S.L. form)
GI: Abdominal pain, diarrhea, indigestion, nausea, vomiting
GU: Dysuria, impotence, urinary frequency
HEME: **Hemolytic anemia**
MS: Arthralgia, muscle twitching
RESP: Bronchitis, pneumonia, upper respiratory tract infection
SKIN: Diaphoresis, flushing, rash

Childbearing Considerations

PREGNANCY

- It is not known if drug causes fetal harm.
- Use with caution only if benefit to mother outweighs potential risk to fetus.

LACTATION

- It is not known if drug is present in breast milk.
- Mothers should check with prescriber before breastfeeding.

Nursing Considerations

- Use isosorbide cautiously in patients with hypovolemia or mild hypotension.
- Know that patient may experience daily headaches from isosorbide's vasodilating effects. Give acetaminophen, as prescribed, to relieve pain.

! **WARNING** Do not stop drug abruptly because angina may occur and increase the risk of MI.

! **WARNING** Monitor blood pressure often during isosorbide therapy, especially in elderly patients; drug may cause severe hypotension.

! **WARNING** Notify prescriber if patient experiences blurred vision, fainting, increased angina attacks, persistent or severe headaches, and rash.

PATIENT TEACHING

- Instruct patient how to administer the form of isosorbide prescribed.
- Advise patient on length of time to follow between doses if drug is to be taken more than once daily.
- Inform patient that drug commonly causes headache, which typically resolves after a few days of continuous therapy. Suggest that patient take acetaminophen, as needed and ordered.
- Urge patient to avoid alcohol consumption.

! **WARNING** Caution patient not to abruptly stop taking drug because doing so may cause angina and increase the risk of MI.

! **WARNING** Instruct patient to notify prescriber about blurred vision, fainting, increased angina attacks, persistent or severe headaches, and rash.

! **WARNING** Advise male patient with erectile dysfunction to alert prescriber that he is taking isosorbide because sildenafil, tadalafil, and vardenafil can cause fatal reactions when taken with isosorbide.

- Teach patient to reduce the effects of orthostatic hypotension by changing position slowly. Advise the patient to lie down if he becomes dizzy.
- Advise patient to avoid potentially hazardous activities until drug's CNS effects are known and resolved.

isotretinoin

Absorica, Absorica LD, Amnesteem, Claravis, Myorisan, Zenatane

Class and Category

Pharmacologic class: Retinoid
Therapeutic class: Acne inhibitor

Indications and Dosages

∗ *To treat severe recalcitrant nodular acne unresponsive to conventional therapy*

CAPSULES (AMNESTEEM, CLARAVIS, MYORISAN, ZENATANE)

Adults and adolescents ages 12 and older. *Initial:* 0.5 mg to 1 mg/kg daily in 2 divided doses, increased as needed up to 2 mg/kg daily given in 2 divided doses. *Maximum:* 2 mg/kg daily. Course of therapy given for 15 to 20 wk with second course given, as needed, after a period of 2 mo or more off therapy.

CAPSULES (ABSORICA)

Adults and adolescents ages 12 and older. 0.5 to 1 mg/kg daily in 2 divided doses for 15 to 20 wk. Second course of therapy given, as needed, after a period of 2 mo or more off therapy.
Adults with severe scarring or primarily manifested on the trunk. Up to 2 mg/kg/day in 2 divided doses for 15 to 20 wk. Second course of therapy given, as needed, after a period of 2 mo or more off therapy.

CAPSULES (ABSORICA LD)

Adults and adolescents age 12 and older. 0.4 to 0.8 mg/kg daily in 2 divided doses for 15 to 20 wk. Second course of therapy may be given, as needed, after a period of 2 mo or more off therapy.
Adults with severe scarring or primarily manifested on the trunk. Up to 1.6 mg/kg/day in 2 divided doses for 15 to 20 wk. Second course of therapy given, as needed, after a period of 2 mo or more off therapy.

Drug Administration

P.O.

- Administer drug with food or milk except for Absorica or Absorica LD brands, which may be taken with or without food.
- Capsules should be swallowed whole and not chewed, crushed, or opened. Capsules should also be taken with a full glass of liquid to avoid esophageal irritation.
- The brands Absorica and Absorica LD are not interchangeable.

Route	Onset	Peak	Duration
P.O.	Unknown	3–5 hr	Unknown

Half-life: 22 hr

Mechanism of Action

Inhibits sebaceous gland function and keratinization, which results in diminished nodular formation associated with recalcitrant nodular acne.

Contraindications

Hypersensitivity to isotretinoin parabens, vitamin A, or any of their components, pregnancy

Interactions

DRUGS

corticosteroids (systemic): Possibly increased risk of osteoporosis
hormonal contraceptives, including levonorgestrel implants, medroxyprogesterone injection, microdosed progesterone preparations: Possibly decreased effectiveness of contraceptive
phenytoin: Possibly increased risk of osteomalacia
tetracyclines: Increased risk of benign intracranial hypertension
vitamin A supplements: Increased risk of additive toxic effects

Adverse Reactions

CNS: Aggressive or **violent** behavior, anger, anxiety, **CVA**, depression, dizziness, drowsiness, emotional instability, euphoria, fatigue, hallucinations, headache, insomnia, irritability, lethargy, malaise, nervousness, panic attack, paresthesias, **pseudotumor cerebri**, psychosis, **seizures**, **suicidal ideation**, syncope, weakness
CV: Chest pain, decreased high-density lipoprotein level, edema, hypercholesteremia, hypertriglyceridemia, palpitation, tachycardia, **vascular thrombotic disease**, vasculitis
ENDO: Abnormal menses, hyperglycemia, **hypoglycemia**
EENT: Bleeding and inflammation of gums, blurred vision, cataracts, color vision disorder, conjunctivitis, corneal opacities, decreased night vision, dry eyes, dry mouth or nose, epistaxis, eye irritation or pruritus, eye strain, eyelid inflammation, hearing impairment, keratitis, nasal dryness, nasopharyngitis, optic neuritis, photophobia, reduced visual acuity, stye, tinnitus, visual disturbances, voice alteration
GI: Colitis, **hepatitis**, ileitis, inflammatory bowel disease, elevated liver enzymes, nausea, **pancreatitis**
GU: Abnormal menses, decreased libido, erectile dysfunction, **glomerulonephritis**, hematuria, proteinuria, sexual dysfunction, vaginal dryness, WBCs in urine
HEME: Anemia, **agranulocytosis**, **elevated platelet count**, **leukopenia**, **neutropenia**, sedimentation rate elevation, **thrombocytopenia**, thrombocytosis
MS: Arthralgia, arthritis, back or musculoskeletal pain, bone abnormalities, calcification of ligaments and tendons, musculoskeletal stiffness, myalgia, premature epiphyseal closure, **rhabdomyolysis**, skeletal hyperostosis, tendinitis
RESP: **Bronchospasms**, respiratory infection
SKIN: Alopecia, bruising, contact dermatitis, diaphoresis, disseminated herpes simplex, dry lips or skin, eczema, eruptive xanthomas, **erythema multiforme**, facial erythema, flushing, fulminant acne, hair abnormalities, hirsutism, hyperpigmentation, hypopigmentation, increased sunburn susceptibility, infections, nail dystrophy, paronychia, peeling of palms and soles, photoallergic or photosensitizing reactions, pruritus, pyogenic granuloma, rash, seborrhea, skin fragility, **Stevens-Johnson syndrome**, **toxic epidermal necrolysis**, urticaria
Other: Abnormal wound healing, alkaline phosphatase increase, **disseminated herpes simplex**, elevated creatine phosphokinase levels, **hypersensitivity reactions (may become severe)**, hyperuricemia, lymphadenopathy, weight loss

Childbearing Considerations

PREGNANCY

- Pregnancy exposure registry: 1-866-495-0654; www.ipledgeprogam.com; or MedWatch at 1-800-FDA-1088.
- Drug causes fetal harm, especially severe congenital defects, spontaneous abortions, and premature births. Drug must be discontinued immediately if pregnancy occurs. Pregnancy registry should also be notified.
- It is contraindicated in pregnant women and females of childbearing age who are not using reliable contraception during drug therapy and for at least 1 mo following drug discontinuation.
- Females of childbearing age must meet all of the following conditions before drug can be prescribed:
  - Patient agrees to participate in the "iPLEDGE" program.

- Patient understands that no more than a 30-day supply of the drug will be given at any 1 time.
- Patient agrees to talk about effective birth control methods with healthcare provider and agrees to use 2 separate methods of effective birth control at the same time 1 mo before, while taking the drug, and for 1 mo after drug is discontinued.
- Patient has a negative monthly pregnancy test before prescription is refilled.
- Patient agrees to have a pregnancy test done 30 days after drug is discontinued.
- Patient understands drug may interfere with the contraceptive effect of microdosed progestin preparations and knows that microdosed "minipill" is not recommended for use with the drug.
- Patient expresses an understanding that it is not known if there is an interaction between the drug and combined oral contraceptives.
- Patient agrees not to use St. John's wort during drug therapy because it may make hormonal birth control pills less effective.
- Patient agrees not to donate blood during and for at least 1 mo following the completion of therapy because females of childbearing potential must not receive blood from patients being treated with drug.

LACTATION

- It is not known if drug is present in breast milk.
- A decision should be made to discontinue breastfeeding or the drug to avoid potential serious adverse reactions in infant.

Nursing Considerations

! WARNING Ensure that females of childbearing age have met the iPLEDGE restricted program requirements before drug therapy begins because drug can cause severe fetal harm. Ensure these patients have a negative pregnancy test before drug is given. If pregnancy occurs during or 1 month after drug initiated, pregnancy must be reported to the FDA (Medwatch) and the iPLEDGE pregnancy registry.

- Obtain serum lipid level before therapy and periodically thereafter, as ordered, to detect elevated lipid levels that may result from isotretinoin therapy.

! WARNING Alert prescriber immediately if patient develops bronchospasms after isotretinoin is administered.

! WARNING Monitor patient for hypersensivity reactions. If present, notify prescriber, expect drug to be discontinued, and provide supportive care, as needed and ordered.

! WARNING Notify prescriber if elevated serum triglyceride levels can't be controlled or if symptoms of pancreatitis occur (abdominal pain, nausea, vomiting). Drug may have to be discontinued because fatal hemorrhagic pancreatitis has occurred with drug use.

! WARNING Monitor liver enzyme levels periodically, as ordered, because drug can cause hepatitis.

! WARNING Monitor patient's CBC results and patient for signs and symptoms of bleeding, bruising, or infection, as ordered, because drug may cause serious to life-threatening hematological adverse reactions.

! WARNING Monitor patient for abnormal behavior or thinking as drug may cause suicidal ideation.

- Assess patient frequently for other adverse reactions and report to prescriber any that occur; drug may have serious adverse effects that require discontinuation.

PATIENT TEACHING

- Inform patient that drug is available only through a restricted program. Review criteria and question patient regarding understanding and willingness to comply.
- Instruct patient how to take isotretinoin.

! WARNING Advise females of childbearing age that 2 forms of contraceptives must be used simultaneously (unless absolute abstinence is the chosen method) 1 month before therapy and for 1 month after therapy has stopped because of potential for fetal harm. Inform females of childbearing age who use oral contraceptives that drug may lessen effectiveness of oral contraceptives. Urge patient to notify prescriber immediately if pregnancy occurs.

! **WARNING** Stress importance of stopping isotretinoin therapy and seeking immediate medical care if bronchospasms occur after taking drug.

! **WARNING** Alert patient that drug may cause an allerigic reaction. For example, tell patient Absorica brand of isotretinoin contains the color additive FD&C Yellow No. 5 (tartrazine), which may cause allergic reactions, especially in patients with an allergy to aspirin or who have asthma. Tell patient that if an allergic reaction occurs, regardless of brand taken, to notify prescriber, stop taking isotretinoin, and to seek immediate medical attention, if severe.

! **WARNING** Review bleeding and infection control precautions with patient. If patient experiences bleeding or signs and symptoms of an infection, tell patient to stop taking drug, notify prescriber immediately, and if serious, to seek immediate medical care.

! **WARNING** Urge patient to report headache, nausea, vomiting and visual disturbances immediately to prescriber because drug will have to be discontinued immediately and patient referred to a neurologist.

! **WARNING** Caution patient and family or caregiver that isotretinoin may cause aggressive or violent behavior, depression, psychosis, and suicidal ideation. Instruct patient to notify prescriber immediately if changes in mood occur.

! **WARNING** Advise patient not to take vitamin A supplements while on isotretinoin therapy because of potentially additive toxic effects. Also, advise female patients of childbearing age not to self-treat depression with the herbal St. John's wort because it may interfere with hormonal contraceptives being used.

! **WARNING** Tell patient to report any other persistent, severe, or unusual adverse reaction to prescriber as drug has the potential to cause serious adverse reactions.

- Advise patient to avoid hazardous activities until drug's CNS effects are known and resolved. Caution that changes in night vision may occur suddenly.
- Caution patient not to donate blood during therapy and for 1 month after therapy has stopped because blood might be given to a pregnant woman.
- Warn patient that transient exacerbation of acne may occur, especially during initial therapy and to notify prescriber if this occurs.
- Instruct patient to avoid wax epilation and skin resurfacing procedures during therapy and for at least 6 months thereafter because of scarring potential.
- Caution patient to avoid exposure to direct sunlight or UV light and to wear sunscreen when outdoors.
- Inform patient that contact lens tolerance may decrease during and after isotretinoin therapy and night vision may decrease as well.
- Alert patient to the potential for mild musculoskeletal adverse reactions, which usually clear rapidly after drug is discontinued. Urge patient to notify prescriber if symptoms become bothersome or serious because drug may have to be discontinued. Inform adolescents and their family or caregiver that participation in sports with repetitive impact may increase their risk of hip growth plate injuries or spondylolisthesis.
- Inform mothers breastfeeding should not be undertaken during drug therapy or drug will need to be discontinued.
- Instruct patient to notify all prescribers of isotretinoin use because of the risk of interactions.
- Inform patient of need for frequent laboratory tests and importance of complying with scheduled appointments.

istradefylline

Nourianz

Class and Category

Pharmacologic class: Adenosine A_{2A} receptor antagonist
Therapeutic class: Antiparkinson agent, central nervous system agent

Indications and Dosages

∗ *As adjunct to treat patients with Parkinson's disease on levodopa/carbidopa experiencing "off" episodes*

TABLETS

Adults. 20 mg once daily, increased to 40 mg if needed. *Maximum:* 40 mg once daily.

±**DOSAGE ADJUSTMENT** For patients taking strong CYP3A4 inhibitors or patients with moderate hepatic impairment, maximum dosage should not exceed 20 mg once daily. For patients who smoke 20 or more cigarettes per day (or use the equivalent of another tobacco product), dosage is initiated and maintained at 40 mg once daily.

Drug Administration

P.O.

- Store drug at room temperature.

Route	Onset	Peak	Duration
P.O.	Unknown	4 hr	Unknown

Half-life: 83 hr

Mechanism of Action

The precise mechanism in which a therapeutic effect is exerted in Parkinson's disease is unknown, although it is thought to be related to its adenosine A_{2A} receptor antagonist action.

Contraindications

Hypersensitivity to istradefylline or its components

Interactions

DRUGS

drugs to treat Parkinson's disease: May cause impulse control issues

strong CYP3A4 inducers, such as carbamazepine, phenytoin, rifampin, St. John's wort: Decreased istradefylline levels and effectiveness

strong CYP3A4 inhibitors, such as clarithromycin, itraconazole, ketoconazole: Increased istradefylline levels with increased risk of adverse reactions

CYP3A4 substrates, such as atorvastatin, P-gp substrates such as digoxin: Increased CYP3A4 substrate level with increased risk of adverse reactions

ACTIVITIES

smoking 20 cigarettes a day or more (or equivalent use of another tobacco product): Decreased effectiveness of istradefylline

Adverse Reactions

CNS: Dizziness, dyskinesia, hallucination, insomnia

ENDO: Hyperglycemia

GI: Constipation, decreased appetite, diarrhea, nausea

GU: Elevated blood urea, increased libido

RESP: Upper respiratory tract inflammation

SKIN: Rash

Childbearing Considerations

PREGNANCY

- It is not known if drug causes fetal harm. However, animal studies suggest it might cause fetal harm.
- Use is not recommended during pregnancy.

LACTATION

- It is not known if drug may be present in breast milk.
- Mothers should check with prescriber before breastfeeding.

REPRODUCTION

- Females of childbearing potential should use contraception during treatment.

Nursing Considerations

- Confirm smoking status in patients before istradefylline is begun as dosage adjustment will be needed.

! **WARNING** Know that patient with a major psychotic disorder should not be administered istradefylline because of the potential risk of exacerbating psychosis. Monitor patient who does not have a major psychotic disorder for hallucinations or psychotic behavior. If present, expect dosage to be decreased or drug discontinued.

- Monitor patient for a rash during istradefylline. If present, notify prescriber and determine if drug should be discontinued.
- Expect to monitor liver function tests. Dosage may require adjustment.
- Monitor patient for adverse reactions, especially CNS adverse effects. The most common effect leading to discontinuation of drug is dyskinesia.
- Be aware that patients taking istradefylline and 1 or more medications for the treatment of Parkinson's disease (including levodopa) may develop intense urges to binge eat, gamble, have sex, or spend money excessively. If patient develops an impulse control disorder, notify prescriber. Dosage may have to be reduced or drug discontinued.

PATIENT TEACHING

- Instruct patient and family or caregiver how to administer istradefylline.
- Advise patient and family or caregiver that when istradefylline is taken with 1 or more drugs to treat Parkinson's disease (including levodopa), impulse control problems or compulsive behaviors may develop, such as intense urges to binge eat, gamble, have sex, or spend money excessively. Prescriber should be notified if an impulse control disorder occurs.
- Tell females of childbearing age that contraception should be used while taking istradefylline because use is not recommended in pregnancy. Stress importance of notifying prescriber if pregnancy occurs as drug will need to be discontinued.
- Inform patient that drug may cause dyskinesia or exacerbate preexisting dyskinesia and to notify prescriber, if present.
- Warn patient that istradefylline may cause hallucinations or psychotic behavior. If present, advise patient, family, or caregiver to notify prescriber.
- Tell patient to inform prescribers of all medications taken, including over-the-counter drugs and herbal products, such as St. John's wort.

itraconazole

Sporanox, Tolsura

Class and Category

Pharmacologic class: Triazole derivative
Therapeutic class: Antifungal

Indications and Dosages

✱ *To treat blastomycosis caused by* Blastomyces dermatitidis *and histoplasmosis caused by* Histoplasma capsulatum

CAPSULES (SPORANOX)

Adults. *Initial:* 200 mg daily, increased, in 100-mg increments, as needed. *Maximum:* 400 mg daily, with dosage greater than 200 mg given in divided doses twice daily.

CAPSULES (TOLSURA)

Adults. *Initial:* 130 mg once daily, increased in increments of 65 mg to maximum of 130 mg twice daily. *Maximum:* 260 mg daily in 2 divided doses.

✱ *To treat aspergillosis unresponsive to amphotericin B*

CAPSULES (SPORANOX)

Adults. 200 to 400 mg daily, with dosage greater than 200 mg daily given in divided doses twice daily.

CAPSULES (TOLSURA)

Adults. *Initial:* 130 mg once daily. *Maximum:* 260 mg daily in 2 divided doses.

✱ *To treat life-threatening aspergillosis, blastomycosis, or histoplasmosis infections*

CAPSULES (SPORANOX)

Adults. *Loading dose:* 200 mg given 3 times daily for 3 days followed by usual dosage for specific fungal infection and continued for a minimum of 3 mo and until clinical parameters and laboratory tests indicate the active fungal infection has subsided.

CAPSULES (TOLSURA)

Adults. *Loading dose:* 130 mg 3 times daily for first 3 days, followed by usual dosage for specific fungal infection and continued for a minimum of 3 mo and until clinical parameters and laboratory tests indicate the active fungal infection has subsided.

✱ *To treat oropharyngeal candidiasis*

ORAL SOLUTION (SPORANOX)

Adults and adolescents. 200 mg once a day for 7 to 14 days.

✱ *To treat fluconazole-resistant oropharyngeal candidiasis*

ORAL SOLUTION (SPORANOX)

Adults and adolescents. 100 mg twice daily for 2 to 4 wk.

✱ *To treat esophageal candidiasis*

ORAL SOLUTION (SPORANOX)

Adults. 100 mg daily increased to 200 mg daily, if needed, for a minimum of 3 wk, with treatment continued for 2 wk following resolution of symptoms.

✱ *To treat onychomycosis of toenails and fingernails in non-immunocompromised patients*

CAPSULES (SPORANOX)

Adults. 200 mg once daily for 12 wk.

✱ *To treat onychomycosis of fingernails only in non-immunocompromised patients*

CAPSULES (SPORANOX)

Adults. 200 mg twice daily for 7 days; then repeated after 3 wk.

* *To treat onychomycosis of toenails only in non-immunocompromised patients*

CAPSULES (SPORANOX)

Adults. 200 mg once daily for 12 wk.

±**DOSAGE ADJUSTMENT** For some immunocompromised patients taking capsule form of drug, dosage may have to be increased because oral bioavailability of capsule form may be decreased.

Drug Administration

P.O.

- Administer drug for the first time to females of childbearing age on day 2 or 3 following the onset of menses for the treatment of onychomycosis.
- Capsules should be swallowed whole with a full meal and not chewed, crushed, or split/opened. Oral solution should be given on an empty stomach, if possible.
- Capsules are not interchangeable with oral solution.
- Use a calibrated device when measuring dosage of oral solution. Oral solution concentration is 10 mg/ml. Have patient vigorously swish oral solution 10 ml at a time for several seconds in the mouth and then swallow.

Route	Onset	Peak	Duration
P.O.	Unknown	3–7 hr	Unknown

Half-life: 20–30 hr

Mechanism of Action

Inhibits the synthesis of ergosterol, an essential component of fungal cell membranes, by binding with a cytochrome P-450 enzyme needed to convert lanosterol to ergosterol. Lack of ergosterol results in increased cellular permeability and leakage of cell contents. Itraconazole also may lead to fungal cell death by inhibiting fungal respiration under aerobic conditions.

Contraindications

Concurrent therapy with CYP3A4 substrates such as avanafil, cisapride, disopyramide, dofetilide, dronedarone, eplerenone, ergot alkaloids, felodipine, finerenone, HMG-CoA inhibitors (lovastatin and simvastatin), irinotecan, isavuconazole, ivabradine, levomethadyl, lomitapide, lovastatin, lurasidone, methadone, naloxegol, nisoldipine, oral midazolam, pimozide, quinidine, ranolazine, simvastatin, ticagrelor, triazolam or voclospoirn; concurrent therapy with colchicine, fesoterodine, or solifenacin in patients with hepatic or renal impairment; concurrent therapy with eliglustat in patients who are poor or intermediate metabolizers of CYP2D6 or are taking moderate or strong CYP2D6 inhibitors; concurrent therapy with venetoclax in patients with chronic lymphocytic leukemia/small lymphocytic lymphoma; evidence of ventricular dysfunction, as in congestive heart failure (CHF) or a history of it (onychomycosis treatment); hypersensitivity to itraconazole or its components; pregnancy or contemplating pregnancy during onychomycosis treatment

Interactions

DRUGS

alfentanil, budesonide, buspirone, busulfan, carbamazepine, cyclosporine, dexamethasone, digoxin, docetaxel, felodipine, fluticasone, indinavir, methylprednisolone, phenytoin, pimozide, rifabutin, ritonavir, saquinavir, sirolimus, tacrolimus, trimetrexate, vinca alkaloids: Possibly increased blood levels of these drugs and serious adverse effects

alprazolam, diazepam, oral midazolam, triazolam: Elevated blood levels and possibly prolonged sedative effects of these drugs

atorvastatin, lovastatin, simvastatin: Increased blood levels of these drugs; possibly rhabdomyolysis

avanafil, cisapride, colchicine, dofetilide, dronedarone, eplerenone,entrectinib, ergot alkaloids, felodipine, fesoterodine, finerenone, halofantrine, irinotecan, isavuconazole, ivabradine, levomethadyl, lovastatin, lurasidone, methadone, midazolam (oral), naloxegol,pemigatinib, pimozide, quinidine, ranolazine, simvastatin, solifenacin, talazoparib, ticagrelor, triazolam, voclosporin: Possibly increased plasma levels of these drugs leading to potentially life-threatening adverse reactions, especially affecting cardiovascular system

calcium channel blockers: Possibly edema and increased risk of CHF; increased blood levels of these drugs

carbamazepine, isoniazid, nevirapine, phenobarbital, phenytoin, rifabutin, rifampin: Possibly decreased blood itraconazole level

cilostazol; eletriptan; glucocorticosteroids, such as budesonide, dexamethasone, fluticasone, and methylprednisolone; trimetrexate: Possibly inhibited metabolism increasing concentrations of these drugs
clarithromycin, erythromycin, indinavir, ritonavir: Possibly increased blood itraconazole level
ergot alkaloids: Possibly increased plasma ergot alkaloid elevation, leading to cerebral ischemia and ischemia of the extremities
fentanyl: Possibly increased plasma fentanyl level, causing potentially fatal respiratory depression
mobocertinib: Increased QT interval
oral antidiabetic drugs, such as repaglinide, saxagliptin: Possibly increased blood levels of these drugs and risk of hypoglycemia
systemic contraceptive hormones: Increased concentrations of these contraceptives
venetoclax: Increased risk of tumor lysis syndrome
warfarin: Increased anticoagulant effect of warfarin

Adverse Reactions

CNS: Chills, confusion, dizziness, drowsiness, fatigue, fever, headache, hypoesthesia, paresthesia, peripheral neuropathy, tremor, vertigo
CV: **Bradycardia, cardiac failure**, chest pain, **congestive heart failure**, hypertension, hypertriglyceridemia, **hypotension, left ventricular failure**, peripheral edema, tachycardia
EENT: Altered sense of taste, blurred vision, diplopia, dysphonia, transient or permanent hearing loss, tinnitus
ENDO: Hyperglycemia, pseudoaldosteronism
GI: Abdominal pain, anorexia, constipation, diarrhea, elevated liver enzymes, flatulence, **hepatic failure, hepatitis, hepatotoxicity**, hyperbilirubinemia, indigestion, jaundice, nausea, **pancreatitis**, vomiting
GU: Erectile dysfunction, menstrual irregularities, pollakiuria, renal impairment, urinary incontinence
HEME: **Leukopenia, neutropenia, thrombocytopenia**
MS: Arthralgia, myalgia
RESP: Cough, dyspnea, **pulmonary edema**
SKIN: Acute generalized exanthematous pustulosis, alopecia, diaphoresis, **erythema multiforme, exfoliative dermatitis**, leukocytoclastic vasculitis, photosensitivity, pruritus, rash, **Stevens-Johnson syndrome, toxic epidermal necrolysis**, urticaria
Other: **Anaphylaxis, angioedema, hyperkalemia, hypokalemia, hypomagnesemia**, serum sickness

Childbearing Considerations

PREGNANCY

- Drug may cause fetal harm such as congenital abnormalities.
- Drug should be used to treat systemic fungal infections in pregnancy only if the benefit to mother outweighs the potential risk to fetus.
- Drug should not be used to treat onychomycosis in pregnant females or in females of childbearing age contemplating pregnancy.

LACTATION

- Drug is present in breast milk.
- Mother who is HIV negative should check with prescriber before breastfeeding.
- The Centers for Disease Control and Prevention recommends that HIV-1 infected mothers not breastfeed to avoid risking postnatal transmission of HIV-1 infection to infants. They also do not recommend breastfeeding because of potential drug-induced adverse reactions in the infant.

REPRODUCTION

- Drug should not be used in females of childbearing age for treatment of onychomycosis unless they are using effective measures to prevent pregnancy and they begin therapy on the second or third day following the onset of menses.
- Highly effective contraception should be continued throughout drug therapy and for 2 mo following drug discontinuation.

Nursing Considerations

! WARNING Know that itraconazole should not be used for the treatment of onychomycosis in patients with evidence of ventricular dysfunction, such as congestive heart failure (CHF) or a history of CHF. Determine if patient has risk factors for CHF, such as ischemic or valvular heart disease, renal failure and other edematous disorders before itraconazole therapy begins. If so, monitor these patients closely. If signs and symptoms of CHF develops during therapy, notify prescriber immediately and expect drug to be discontinued.

! **WARNING** Be aware that itraconazole should not be used in females of childbearing age for treatment of onychomycosis unless they are using effective measures to prevent pregnancy.

- Know that because itraconazole has been linked to serious adverse cardiac and hepatic effects, expect to send appropriate nail specimens for laboratory testing to confirm onychomycosis before beginning therapy.

! **WARNING** Use itraconazole with extreme caution in patients with, or significant pulmonary disease, such as chronic obstructive pulmonary disease because of increased risk of developing CHF during itraconazole treatment.

- Keep in mind that a patient with a compromised immune system may have hypochlorhydria, which reduces drug absorption. For such a patient, expect to administer higher doses of itraconazole.

! **WARNING** Monitor patient for a hypersensitivity reaction, especially patients with hypersensitivity to other azole antifungals (cross-hypersensitivity unknown) because severe or life-threatening adverse reactions may occur, such as anaphylaxis or angioedema. If a hypersensitivity occurs notify prescriber, expect drug to be discontinued, and provide supportive care, as needed and ordered.

! **WARNING** Monitor patient for serious skin reactions. At first sign of a rash or other skin abnormalities, notify prescriber, expect drug to be discontinued, and provide supportive care, as needed and ordered.

! **WARNING** Keep in mind that itraconazole is a potent inhibitor of the cytochrome P-450 3A4 (CYP3A4) isoenzyme system, which may increase blood levels of drugs metabolized by this system. Patients taking such drugs as cisapride with itraconazole or other CYP3A4 inhibitors have experienced life-threatening cardiovascular complications, such as prolonged QT interval, torsades de pointes, and ventricular tachycardia, as well as sudden death.

! **WARNING** Know that if patient also receives warfarin, monitor PT and assess patient for signs and symptoms of bleeding.

! **WARNING** Keep in mind that if patient also receives digoxin, monitor blood digoxin level as appropriate to detect toxic level, and assess patient for signs and symptoms of digitalis toxicity, such as nausea and yellow vision.

! **WARNING** Monitor liver enzymes in patients with impaired hepatic function and those who have experienced hepatotoxicity with other drugs. Also, monitor renal function, as ordered, because drug may cause renal impairment.

- Monitor patient's blood pressure and serum potassium levels, as ordered, because drug may cause pseudoaldosteronism, which presents with onset of hypertension or worsening of hypertension and hypokalemia. If confirmed, drug may need to be discontinued.
- Be aware that if patient develops signs and symptoms of peripheral neuropathy, expect to discontinue drug.
- Know that if a patient with cystic fibrosis does not respond to itraconazole therapy, alternative therapy should be considered.

PATIENT TEACHING

- Instruct patient how to administer form of itraconazole prescribed.
- Advise patient to avoid taking antacids with oral itraconazole.

! **WARNING** Tell females of childbearing age to begin therapy for onychomycosis on the second or third day following the onset of menses. Also, advise these patients to use effective contraception to prevent pregnancy during itraconazole therapy and for 2 months following the end of treatment. Tell patient to notify prescriber immediately if pregnancy occurs. Explain that itraconazole should not be given to treat onychomycosis in pregnant females or females of childbearing age contemplating pregnancy.

! **WARNING** Instruct patient to stop itraconazole and notify prescriber immediately if he experiences an allergic reaction. Tell the patient to seek immediate emergency care, if severe.

! **WARNING** Stress importance of notifying prescriber of any persistent, severe, or unusual adverse reactions because drug has the potential to affect many body systems and cause serious adverse effects.

! **WARNING** Tell patient with diabetes who takes an oral antidiabetic drug to check his blood glucose level often and monitor self for signs and symptoms of hypoglycemia because of the increased risk of hypoglycemia. Review appropriate treatment for hypoglycemia with patient and family or caregiver.

- Advise patient to notify prescriber immediately of changes in other drugs being taken, such as new drugs being prescribed or dosage changes.
- Caution patient to avoid performing hazardous activities such as driving until CNS effects such as dizziness or change in vision are not present.

ivabradine

Corlanor

Class and Category

Pharmacologic class: Nucleotide-gated channel blocker

Therapeutic class: Cardiac pacemaker regulator

Indications and Dosages

∗ *To reduce risk of hospitalization for worsening heart failure in patients with stable, symptomatic chronic heart failure who have a left ventricular ejection fraction of 35% or less, who are in sinus rhythm with a resting heart rate of 70 beats/min or more and either are on maximally tolerated doses of beta-blockers or have a contraindication to beta-blocker use*

ORAL SOLUTION, TABLETS

Adults. *Initial:* 5 mg twice daily followed by a dosage adjustment in 2 wk to achieve a resting heart rate between 50 and 60 beats/min. *Maximum:* 7.5 mg twice daily.

±**DOSAGE ADJUSTMENT** For patients with a history of conduction defects or patients in whom bradycardia could lead to hemodynamic compromise, dose initiated at 2.5 mg twice daily before increasing dose based on heart rate. For patients with a resting heart rate greater than 60 beats/min, dosage increased by 2.5 mg given twice daily up to a maximum dose of 7.5 mg twice daily, as needed. For patients with a heart rate between 50 and 60 beats/min, dose maintained. For patients with a resting heart rate below 50 beats/min or who experience signs and symptoms of bradycardia, dosage decreased by 2.5 mg given twice daily; if current dose is already 2.5 mg twice daily, drug discontinued.

∗ *To treat stable symptomatic heart failure due to dilated cardiomyopathy in children who are in sinus rhythm with an elevated heart rate*

ORAL SOLUTION, TABLETS

Children weighing 40 kg (88 lb) or greater. *Initial:* 2.5 mg twice daily. Dose adjusted at 2-wk intervals by 2.5 mg to target a heart rate reduction of at least 20%, if tolerated. *Maximum:* 7.5 mg twice daily.

ORAL SOLUTION

Children ages 6 mo and older weighing less than 40 kg (88 lb). *Initial:* 0.05 mg/kg twice daily. Dose adjusted at 2-wk intervals by 0.05 mg/kg to target a heart rate reduction of at least 20%, if tolerated. *Maximum:* 0.3 mg/kg twice daily (patients 1 yr and older) up to 7.5 mg twice daily; 0.2 mg/kg twice daily (patients 6 mo to less than 1 yr).

±**DOSAGE ADJUSTMENT** For children who develop bradycardia, dosage reduced to previous titration step. If child is at the recommended initial dosage, dosage reduced to 0.02 mg/kg twice daily.

Drug Administration

P.O.

- Instruct patient to take drug with meals.
- Give oral solution to younger children and patients who have difficulty swallowing tablets.
- Empty entire contents of the ampule(s) into a medication cup. Use a calibrated oral syringe to draw up drug dosage from medicine cup to avoid dosing errors and administer using the syringe.

- Drug dose should not be doubled up if child spits out the drug.

Route	Onset	Peak	Duration
P.O.	Unknown	1–2 hr	Unknown

Half-life: 6 hr

Mechanism of Action

Blocks the hyperpolarization-activated cyclic nucleotide-gated (HCN) channel responsible for the cardiac pacemaker, which regulates heart rate. This results in a reduction in heart rate.

Contraindications

Acute decompensated heart failure; clinically significant bradycardia or hypotension; concomitant use of strong cytochrome P-450 3A4 (CYP3A4) inhibitors; hypersensitivity to ivabradine or its components; pacemaker dependence; severe hepatic impairment; sick sinus syndrome, sinoatrial block, or third-degree AV block, unless a functioning demand pacemaker is present

Interactions

DRUGS

CYP3A4 inducers, such as barbiturates, phenytoin, rifampicin, St. John's wort: Decreased ivabradine plasma concentrations decreasing effectiveness

moderate and strong CYP3A4 inhibitors, such as azole antifungals, diltiazem, HIV protease inhibitors, macrolide antibiotics, nefazodone, verapamil: Increased ivabradine plasma concentrations, which may exacerbate bradycardia and conduction disturbances

negative chronotropes, such as amiodarone, beta-blockers, digoxin: Increased risk of bradycardia

FOODS

grapefruit juice: Increased ivabradine plasma concentrations, which may exacerbate bradycardia and conduction disturbances

Adverse Reactions

CNS: Syncope, vertigo

CV: **Atrial fibrillation**, **bradycardia**, conduction disturbances, hypertension, **hypotension**, **sinus arrest**, **torsades de pointes**, **ventricular fibrillation and tachycardia**

EENT: Colored bright lights, diplopia, halos, image decomposition such as kaleidoscopic or stroboscopic effects, multiple images, transiently enhanced brightness in a limited area of the visual field, visual impairment

SKIN: Erythema, pruritus, rash, urticaria

Other: **Angioedema**

Childbearing Considerations

PREGNANCY

- Drug may cause fetal harm based on animal studies.
- Use with caution only if benefit to mother outweighs potential risk to fetus.
- Be aware that pregnant females with congestive heart failure, who are started on drug, especially during the first trimester, should be followed closely for destabilization that could result from a decreased heart rate.
- Monitor pregnant females with chronic heart failure in third trimester for preterm birth.

LACTATION

- It is not known if drug is present in breast milk.
- Breastfeeding is not recommended during drug therapy.

REPRODUCTION

- Advise females of childbearing age to use effective contraception during drug therapy.

Nursing Considerations

- Be aware that ivabradine should not be given to patients with demand pacemakers set to a rate of 60 beats/min or greater because these patients will not be able to achieve a target heart rate of less than 60 beats/min.
- Know that although drug is not contraindicated, it is not recommended for use in patients with a second-degree heart block unless a functioning demand pacemaker is in place.

! **WARNING** Monitor patient for hypersensitivity reactions, which could be life-threatening, such as angioedema. If present, notify prescriber, expect drug to be discontinued, and provide supportive care, as needed and ordered.

! **WARNING** Monitor patient's cardiac rhythm regularly because ivabradine increases the risk of atrial fibrillation and conduction disturbances. Also, monitor patient's heart rate because drug may cause bradycardia.

Risk factors for bradycardia include conduction defects, sinus node dysfunction, ventricular dysfunction, and use of other negative chronotropic drugs, such as amiodarone, digoxin, diltiazem, or verapamil. Be aware that bradycardia may increase risk of prolonged QT interval, which may lead to life-threatening ventricular arrhythmias. Notify prescriber if arrhythmias such as atrial fibrillation or conduction disturbances occurs, or the patient's heart rate drops below 50 beats/min. Expect drug to be discontinued in these situations.

! **WARNING** Monitor closely pregnant females with congestive heart failure, who are started on drug, especially during the first trimester, for destabilization that could result from a decreased heart rate.

PATIENT TEACHING

- Instruct patient how to administer form of ivabradine prescribed.

! **WARNING** Alert patient that drug may cause an allergic reaction. If present, tell patient to notify prescriber and stop taking drug. If severe, urge patient to seek immediate medical care.

! **WARNING** Tell patient to notify prescriber if pulse becomes irregular or less than 50 beats/min or visual disturbances occur.

- Advise females of childbearing age to use an effective contraceptive during therapy. Tell patient to notify prescriber if pregnancy occurs as drug may need to be discontinued.
- Instruct patient to notify all prescribers of ivabradine therapy.

ixekizumab

Taltz

Class and Category

Pharmacologic class: Interleukin-17 A antagonist
Therapeutic class: Immunomodulator

Indications and Dosages

∗ *To treat moderate to severe plaque psoriasis in patients who are candidates for phototherapy or systemic therapy*

SUBCUTANEOUS INJECTION

Adults. *Initial:* 160 mg (two 80-mg injections) at wk 0, followed by 80 mg at wk 2, 4, 6, 8, 10, and 12; then 80 mg every 4 wk. **Children ages 6 and older weighing more than 50 kg (110 lb).** 160 mg (two 80-mg injections) and then 80 mg every 4 wk. **Children ages 6 and older weighing 25 kg (55 lb) up to and including 50 kg (110 lb).** 80 mg and then 40 mg every 4 wk. **Children ages 6 and older weighing less than 25 kg (55 lb).** 40 mg and then 20 mg every 4 wk.

∗ *To treat active psoriatic arthritis; to treat active ankylosing spondylitis*

SUBCUTANEOUS INJECTION

Adults. *Initial:* 160 mg (two 80-mg injections), followed by 80 mg every 4 wk.

± **DOSAGE ADJUSTMENT** For patients with psoriatic arthritis with coexistent moderate to severe plaque psoriasis, the dosing regimen for plaque psoriasis should be used.

∗ *To treat active non-radiographic axial spondyloarthritis with objective signs of inflammation*

SUBCUTANEOUS INJECTION

Adults. 80 mg every 4 wk.

Drug Administration

SUBCUTANEOUS

- Remove autoinjector or prefilled syringe from refrigerator and allow about 30 min for drug to reach room temperature. Don't remove the needle cap during this time.
- Inspect solution for particulate matter or discoloration. Solution should appear clear and colorless to slightly yellow.
- Administer drug using either the autoinjector or prefilled syringe for 80 mg dosage. Don't shake. Inject the full amount (1 ml), which provides 80 mg, into any quadrant of the abdomen or the thighs, or upper arms.
- Administer 20 mg or 40 mg doses of drug by expelling the entire contents of the prefilled syringe into the sterile vial. Do not shake or swirl the vial. No other medications should be added. Using a 0.5-ml or 1-ml disposable syringe and sterile needle, withdraw the prescribed dose from the vial (0.25 ml for a 20-mg dose; 0.5 ml for a 40-mg dose). Remove the needle from the syringe and replace it with a 27 G needle prior to administering. Prepared solution

may be stored at room temperature for up to 4 hr from first puncturing the sterile vial.

- Discard any unused solution because the solution does not contain a preservative.
- Rotate injection sites and do not inject into areas where the skin is affected by psoriasis or is bruised, erythematous, or indurated.

Route	Onset	Peak	Duration
SubQ	Unknown	4 days	Unknown

Half-life: 13 days

Mechanism of Action

Selectively binds with the interleukin 17A cytokine and inhibits its interaction with the IL-17 receptor. This inhibits the release of proinflammatory cytokines and chemokines involved in normal inflammatory and immune responses. Binding of IL-17 receptors prevents inflammation-related signals from being relayed, which reduces the inflammatory response and relieves signs and symptoms of inflammatory disorders.

Contraindications

Hypersensitivity to ixekizumab or its components

Interactions

DRUGS

CYP450 substrates with a narrow therapeutic index, such as cyclosporine, warfarin: Possibly decreased plasma levels of these drugs with decreased effectiveness

live vaccines: Increased risk of adverse vaccine effects

Adverse Reactions

EENT: Conjunctivitis, oral candidiasis, rhinitis
GI: Crohn's disease (new onset or exacerbation), nausea, ulcerative colitis (new onset or exacerbation)
HEME: **Neutropenia**, **thrombocytopenia**
RESP: Upper respiratory infections
SKIN: Eczematous eruptions, tinea infections, urticaria
Other: **Anaphylaxis**; **angioedema**; anti-ixekizumab antibodies; flu-like symptoms; infections, including bacterial, fungal, and viral opportunistic infections and activation of latent infections such as tuberculosis; injection-site reactions, such as erythema and pain

Childbearing Considerations

PREGNANCY

- Pregnancy exposure registry: 1-800-284-1695 or http://www.pregnancyregistry.lilly.com
- It is not known if drug causes fetal harm although human IgG is known to cross the placental barrier so drug may be transmitted from mother to fetus.
- Use with caution only if benefit to mother outweighs potential risk to fetus.

LACTATION

- It is not known if drug is present in breast milk.
- Mothers should check with prescriber before breastfeeding.

Nursing Considerations

- Check patient's immunization history and make sure all age-appropriate immunizations according to current guidelines have been administered prior to initiating ixekizumab therapy. Live vaccines should be avoided during ixekizumab therapy.
- Make sure patient has a tuberculin skin test before therapy starts. If skin test is positive, tuberculosis (TB) treatment will have to be started before ixekizumab therapy can begin. Even patients who have tested negative for TB may develop TB during therapy. Monitor patient for low-grade fever, persistent cough, and wasting or weight loss; report such findings to prescriber.

! WARNING Know that if patient has evidence of an active infection when drug is prescribed, therapy shouldn't start until infection has been treated. Monitor patients for the development of infections, such as conjunctivitis, oral candidiasis, tinea infections, and upper respiratory tract infections during therapy; report such findings to prescriber. Know that if a patient develops a serious infection or does not respond to treatment prescribed for the infection, ixekizumab may have to be temporarily withheld until the infection is resolved.

! WARNING Monitor patient closely for hypersensitivity. If a serious reaction occurs, such as angioedema or urticaria, discontinue drug immediately, notify prescriber, and provide supportive care, as needed and ordered.

- Monitor patient for abnormal skin changes because cases of severe eczematous eruptions have occurred with ixekizumab use, some of which required hospitalization. Onset may occur any time from days to months after the first dose. If present, notify prescriber as drug may need to be discontinued.
- Monitor patient closely for evidence of inflammatory bowel disease. Know that Crohn's disease and ulcerative colitis may occur. During treatment, monitor patient for onset or exacerbation of inflammatory bowel disease.

PATIENT TEACHING

- Instruct patient, family, or caregiver on how to administer drug subcutaneously. Children who weigh less than 50 kg will need to have drug administered by a healthcare provider.
- Alert patient to the possibility of experiencing redness or pain at injection site but advise the patient that these are not usually severe.

! **WARNING** Alert patient, family, or caregiver that drug may cause an allergic reaction. If present, tell patient to notify prescriber and, if severe, to seek immediate medical care.

! **WARNING** Warn patient not to receive immunizations that contain live vaccines while taking ixekizumab.

- Inform patient that infections, including activation of latent infections such as TB, may occur during ixekizumab therapy. Instruct the patient to report persistent, severe, or unusual signs and symptoms to prescriber. Advise patient to avoid people with infections.
- Tell patient to notify prescriber of any skin changes because some may become serious.
- Alert patient that irritable bowel syndrome may occur or be aggravated by ixekizumab therapy. Tell him to notify prescriber of adverse reactions such as abdominal distention or pain or diarrhea that is persistent or severe.

J K L

ketorolac tromethamine

Sprix, Toradol (CAN)

Class and Category

Pharmacologic class: NSAID
Therapeutic class: Analgesic

Indications and Dosages

✱ *To provide short-term management (up to 5 days) of moderate to severe acute pain that requires analgesia at the opioid level, usually in a postoperative setting*

TABLETS

Adults younger than 65 and adolescents ages 17 and older weighing 50 kg (110 lb) or more following parenteral therapy. *Initial:* 20 mg as single dose, followed by 10 mg every 4 to 6 hr, as needed, up to 4 times a day. *Maximum:* 40 mg daily for no more than 5 days, including parenteral dosage.

±DOSAGE ADJUSTMENT For elderly patients (65 years or older), patients with impaired renal function, or patients weighing less than 50 kg (110 lb), initial dose reduced to 10 mg and given after receiving parenteral therapy followed by 10 mg every 4 to 6 hours, as needed, up to 4 times daily. Maximum: 40 mg daily for no more than 5 days, including parenteral dosage.

I.M. INJECTION

Adults younger than 65 and adolescents ages 17 and older weighing 50 kg (110 lb) or more. *Initial for single-dose therapy:* 60 mg, followed by oral ketorolac, as needed. *For multiple-dose therapy:* 30 mg every 6 hr, as needed. *Maximum:* 120 mg daily for no more than 5 days for combined oral and intramuscular therapy.

±DOSAGE ADJUSTMENT For elderly patients (65 years and older), patients with impaired renal function, or patients weighing less than 50 kg (110 lb), initial dose reduced to 30 mg as a single dose, followed by oral ketorolac as needed; or 15 mg every 6 hours, as needed. Maximum: 60 mg daily for no more than 5 days for combined oral and intramuscular therapy.

I.V. INJECTION

Adults younger than 65 and adolescents ages 17 and older weighing 50 kg (110 lb) or more. *Initial for single-dose therapy:* 30 mg, followed by oral ketorolac, as needed. *For multiple-dose therapy:* 30 mg every 6 hr, as needed. *Maximum:* 120 mg daily for no more than 5 days for combined oral and intravenous therapy.

±DOSAGE ADJUSTMENT For elderly patients (65 years and older), patients with impaired renal function, or patients weighing less than 50 kg (110 lb), initial dose reduced to 15 mg as a single dose, followed by oral ketorolac, as needed; or 15 mg every 6 hours, as needed. Maximum: 60 mg daily for no more than 5 days for combined oral and intravenous therapy.

NASAL SPRAY (SPRIX)

Adults younger than 65 yr of age. 31.5 mg (one 15.75 mg spray in each nostril) every 6 to 8 hr. *Maximum:* 126 mg (4 doses) daily for no more than 5 days.

±DOSAGE ADJUSTMENT For elderly patients (65 years and older), patients with impaired renal function, or patients weighing less than 50 kg (110 lb), 15.75 mg in only one nostril every 6 to 8 hours with maximum dose of 63 mg (4 doses) daily for no more than 5 days.

Drug Administration

P.O.

- Oral drug only given after a parenteral dose of drug has been administered first.
- Administer with an antacid, food, or milk to lessen GI upset, and give with a full glass of water.
- Patient should not lie down for at least 15 min after administration.

I.V.

- Administer as an I.V. injection over more than 15 sec.
- Store at room temperature and protect from light.
- *Incompatibilities:* Hydroxyzine hydrochloride, meperidine hydrochloride, morphine sulfate, promethazine hydrochloride

I.M.

- Administer slowly and deeply into the muscle.
- Store at room temperature and protect from light.

INTRANASAL

- Activate container prior to first use by pressing down evenly and releasing pump 5 times.
- Have patient blow nose before administration and sit up straight or stand with head tilting slightly forward.
- Give container to patient and have patient insert tip of container into one nostril, pointing container away from the center of the nose.
- Tell patient to hold breath and spray once by pressing down evenly on both sides. Immediately after administration, patient should resume breathing through mouth to reduce expelling the product. The nose can also be pinched to help retain spray if it starts to drip.
- Repeat procedure using other nostril to administer second spray, if ordered.
- Replace clear plastic cover and store bottle in cool, dry place out of direct sunlight. Unopened bottles should be refrigerated.
- After initial priming, discard after 24 hr regardless of what is remaining in the bottle (each bottle contains dosage for 8 sprays).

Route	Onset	Peak	Duration
P.O.	30–60 min	1–2 hr	4–6 hr
I.M., I.V.	< 30 min	1–2 hr	4–6 hr
Nasal	Unknown	45 min	Unknown

Half-life: 2–6 hr

Mechanism of Action

Blocks cyclooxygenase, an enzyme needed to synthesize prostaglandins. Prostaglandins mediate inflammatory response and cause local vasodilation, pain, and swelling. They also promote pain transmission from periphery to spinal cord. By blocking cyclooxygenase and inhibiting prostaglandins, this NSAID reduces inflammation and relieves pain.

Contraindications

Active peptic ulcer disease or recent GI bleeding or perforation or history of GI bleeding or peptic ulcer disease; advanced renal impairment or risk of renal impairment due to volume depletion; cerebrovascular bleeding, hemorrhagic diathesis, incomplete hemostasis, or high risk of bleeding; concurrent therapy with aspirin, other NSAIDs, or probenecid; history of asthma, urticaria, or other allergic-type reactions after taking aspirin or other NSAIDs; hypersensitivity to ketorolac tromethamine or its components; labor and delivery; postoperative pain after coronary artery bypass graft (CABG) surgery; use as a prophylactic analgesic before any major surgery

Interactions

DRUGS

ACE inhibitors, angiotensin II receptor antagonists: Decreased antihypertensive effect of these drugs; increased risk of decreased renal function in patients who are elderly, volume depleted, or have existing renal impairment
anticoagulants, such as warfarin; platelet aggregation inhibitors, such as aspirin, pentoxifylline; selective serotonin reuptake inhibitors; serotonin–norepinephrine reuptake inhibitors: Increased risk of serious bleeding
antiepileptic drugs, such as carbamazepine, phenytoin: Increased risk of seizures
aspirin and other salicylates, other NSAIDs: Increased risk of GI adverse reactions and bleeding, including GI toxicity
cyclosporine: Increased risk of cyclosporine-induced nephrotoxicity
digoxin: Increased digoxin levels with risk of digoxin toxicity
diuretics: Reduced effects of loop and thiazide diuretics in some patients
lithium: Possibly increased blood lithium level and increased risk of lithium toxicity
methotrexate: Possibly methotrexate toxicity
pemetrexed: Increased risk of pemetrexed-associated myelosuppression and GI and renal toxicity
probenecid: Decreased elimination of ketorolac, increased risk of adverse effects

ACTIVITIES

alcohol use: Increased risk of adverse GI effects

Adverse Reactions

CNS: **Aseptic meningitis**, **cerebral hemorrhage**, **coma**, **CVA**, dizziness, drowsiness, headache, psychosis, **seizures**
CV: Edema, hypertension
EENT: **Laryngeal edema**, stomatitis
ENDO: Hyperglycemia
GI: Abdominal pain; **acute pancreatitis**; bloating; constipation; diarrhea; diverticulitis; elevated liver enzymes; flatulence; **GI bleeding**, **perforation**, or ulceration;

hepatitis; **hepatic failure**; jaundice; indigestion; nausea; vomiting; worsening of inflammatory bowel disease
GU: Interstitial nephritis, **renal failure**, urine retention
HEME: **Agranulocytosis**, anemia, **aplastic or hemolytic anemia**, eosinophilia, **leukopenia**, **pancytopenia**, **thrombocytopenia**
RESP: **Bronchospasm**, pneumonia, **respiratory depression**
SKIN: Acute generalized exanthematous pustulosis, diaphoresis, **erythema multiforme**, **exfoliative dermatitis**, fixed skin eruptions, photosensitivity, pruritus, rash, **Stevens-Johnson syndrome**, **toxic epidermal necrolysis**, urticaria
Other: **Anaphylaxis**, **angioedema**, **drug reaction with eosinophilia and systemic symptoms (DRESS)**, **hyperkalemia**, **hyponatremia**, injection-site pain, lymphadenopathy, **sepsis**, unusual weight gain

Childbearing Considerations

PREGNANCY

- Drug increases risk of premature closure of the fetal ductus arteriosus if given at 30 wk gestation and beyond and fetal renal dysfunction if given after 20 wk of gestation.
- Drug should be avoided in pregnant women starting at 20 wk of gestation and beyond. If drug must be used between 20 and 30 wk of gestation, drug should be administered in the smallest dose and for shortest period of time. Drug should not be administered at 30 wk of gestation and beyond.

LABOR AND DELIVERY

- Drug may affect fetal circulation and inhibit uterine contractions.
- Use of drug is contraindicated during labor and delivery.

LACTATION

- Drug is present in breast milk.
- Mothers should check with prescriber before breastfeeding.

REPRODUCTION

- Drug may affect fertility by delaying or preventing rupture of ovarian follicles.
- Drug should not be given to females of childbearing age who plan to become pregnant or who are having difficulty conceiving.

Nursing Considerations

! **WARNING** Be aware that NSAIDs like ketorolac should be avoided in patients with a recent MI because risk of reinfarction increases with NSAID therapy. If therapy is unavoidable, monitor patient closely for signs of cardiac ischemia.

! **WARNING** Know that the risk of heart failure increases with ketorolac use because drug is an NSAID. This class of drugs should not be used in patients with severe heart failure but, if unavoidable, monitor patient for worsening of heart failure. Assess patient for decreased activity tolerance, dyspnea, edema, and unexplained rapid weight gain. Notify prescriber if such symptoms develop

- Notify prescriber if pain relief is inadequate or if breakthrough pain occurs between doses because supplemental doses of an opioid analgesic may be required.

! **WARNING** Assess patient for hypersensitivity reactions, which may become life-threatening such as anaphylaxis or angioedema. Also, assess patient's skin routinely for serious skin reactions because ketorolac is an NSAID and may cause serious skin reactions without warning, even in patients with no history of NSAID hypersensitivity, including serious skin reactions. Stop drug at first sign of a hypersensitivity reaction, including a rash (DRESS may only initially present with a fever or swollen lymph nodes), notify prescriber, and provide supportive care, as needed and ordered.

! **WARNING** Monitor patient closely for thrombotic events, including MI and stroke because NSAIDs, such as ketorolac increase risk. These events may occur early in treatment and risk increases with duration of use. Be aware that these events have occurred even in patients who do not have a history of or risk factors for cardiovascular disease. Monitor patient for warning signs, such as chest pain, shortness of breath, slurring of speech, or weakness. If any signs and symptoms develop, withhold ketorolac, alert prescriber immediately, and provide supportive care, as needed and ordered.

! **WARNING** Monitor BUN and serum creatinine levels in the elderly; patients with heart failure, hepatic impairment, or impaired renal function; and those who are taking ACE inhibitors or diuretics because drug may cause renal failure.

! **WARNING** Know that in a patient who has bone marrow suppression or is receiving antineoplastic drug therapy, monitor CBC (including WBC) and assess for evidence of infection because ketorolac has anti-inflammatory and antipyretic actions that may mask signs and symptoms, such as fever and pain. Also monitor CBC for decreased hemoglobin and hematocrit because drug may worsen anemia.

! **WARNING** Monitor patients with history of GI bleeding or ulcer disease very closely because NSAIDs like ketorolac increase risk of GI bleeding and ulceration. Use ketorolac in these patients for shortest length of time possible. Know that serious GI tract bleeding, ulceration, and perforation of intestine or stomach can occur without warning and without symptoms. Elderly patients are at greater risk. To minimize risk, give drug with food. If GI distress occurs, withhold drug and notify prescriber immediately.

- Monitor patient—especially if elderly—for less common but serious adverse GI reactions, including anorexia, constipation, diverticulitis, dysphagia, esophagitis, gastritis, gastroenteritis, gastroesophageal reflux disease, hemorrhoids, hiatal hernia, melena, stomatitis, and vomiting.
- Monitor blood pressure closely throughout therapy because drug can lead to onset of hypertension or worsen existing hypertension.
- Monitor liver enzymes, as ordered. If elevated levels persist or worsen, notify prescriber and expect to stop drug, as ordered, to prevent hepatic impairment.
- Monitor patient with history of inflammatory bowel disease, such as Crohn's disease or ulcerative colitis, because ketorolac may worsen these conditions.

PATIENT TEACHING

- Instruct patient how to administer the form of ketorolac prescribed. If taking tablet form, tell patient he will need to receive the drug by an intramuscular or intravenous injection before tablets can be administered.
- Advise the patient to stay upright for at least 15 minutes after taking oral form.
- Caution patient not to use ketorolac for more than 5 days, as serious adverse effects may occur.
- Advise patient not to take aspirin, other NSAIDs, or other salicylates while taking ketorolac without consulting prescriber. Urge patient to limit use of acetaminophen to only a few days during ketorolac therapy and to notify prescriber of use. Also urge patient to avoid alcohol while taking ketorolac.

! **WARNING** Caution pregnant females that NSAIDs like ketorolac shouldn't be taken from 30 weeks, gestation onward because drug may cause premature closure of the ductus arteriosus. It also should be avoided between 20 and 30 wk of gestation because of risk of fetal renal dysfunction. However, if there are no other alternatives it must be taken only under direction of prescriber for smallest dose and shortest period of time.

! **WARNING** Alert patient drug may cause an allergic or skin reaction that could become serious. If present, tell patient to notify prescriber and, if severe, to seek immediate medical care.

! **WARNING** Explain that ketorolac may increase risk of serious adverse cardiovascular reactions; urge patient to seek immediate medical attention if signs or symptoms arise, such as chest pain, edema, shortness of breath, slurring of speech, unexplained weight gain, or weakness.

! **WARNING** Tell patient that ketorolac also may increase risk of serious adverse GI reactions; stress importance of seeking immediate medical attention if signs or symptoms occur, such as abdominal or epigastric pain, black tarry stools, indigestion, and vomiting blood or coffee-ground material.

! **WARNING** Stress importance of alerting prescriber of any other adverse reactions, especially if they are persistent, serious, or unusual.

- Caution patient to avoid hazardous activities until drug's CNS effects are known and resolved.
- Encourage patient to have dental procedures performed before starting drug therapy because of increased risk of bleeding. Also teach patient proper oral hygiene measures and encourage the patient to use a soft-bristled toothbrush while taking ketorolac.

labetalol hydrochloride

Class and Category

Pharmacologic class: Noncardioselective beta-blocker/alpha[1]-blocker
Therapeutic class: Antihypertensive

Indications and Dosages

✱ *To manage hypertension*

TABLETS

Adults. *Initial:* 100 mg twice daily, increased by 100 mg twice daily every 2 to 3 days, as needed and tolerated. *Maintenance:* 200 to 400 mg twice daily. *Maximum:* 2,400 mg daily in 2 divided doses.

✱ *To manage severe hypertension*

TABLETS

Inpatient adults after receiving drug parenterally. *Initial:* May require from 1,200 to 2,400 mg per day in 2 divided doses. Titrated in increments not to exceed 200 mg twice daily, as needed. *Maximum:* 2,400 mg daily in 2 divided doses.

I.V. INFUSION

Adults. 2 mg/min continuously until desired response occurs.

I.V. INJECTION

Adults. 0.25 mg/kg (maximum 20 mg) given over 2 min; additional doses given in increments of 40 to 80 mg every 10 min as indicated until desired response occurs. *Maximum:* 300 mg.

± **DOSAGE ADJUSTMENT** For elderly patients, lower maintenance dosages to between 100 and 200 mg twice daily may be required. For patients experiencing dizziness, daily dosage may need to be split into 3 times daily.

Drug Administration

P.O.

- Administer tablets with or without food but in a consistent manner.
- If dizziness occurs, check with prescriber about dividing the daily dosage into 3 times daily rather than 2 times daily.

I.V.

- Keep patient in a supine position during I.V. administration and for up to 3 hr afterward.
- Before using prefilled syringe for I.V. injection, know that glass syringes may break, clog, or malfunction when connected to some needleless luer access devices (NLADs) and needles. Spontaneous disconnection of glass syringe from needles and NLADs may cause leakage to occur. Check the needle or NLAD is securely attached before beginning the injection and also during administration. Push plunger rod slightly to break the stopper loose from tip cap, then remove tip cap by twisting it off. Connect the syringe to an appropriate injection connection.
- For I.V. injection, administer slowly over a 2-min period. Take patient's blood pressure immediately before injection and at 5 and 10 min after injection.
- For I.V. infusion, know that labetalol in Dextrose Injection or Sodium Chloride Injection come in ready to use solutions and do not require further dilution. Check for leaks by squeezing the bag firmly. If leaks are found, discard solution. Administer continuously at 2 mg/min with rate of infusion adjusted according to blood pressure. Administer drug with an infusion control device.
- Monitor patient's blood pressure throughout administration and after infusion is discontinued according to facility protocol, which is usually every 5 min for 30 min, then every 30 min for 2 hr, and then every hour for 6 hr.
- *Incompatibilities:* Alkaline solutions, such as 5% Sodium Bicarbonate Injection, alkaline drugs, such as furosemide

Route	Onset	Peak	Duration
P.O.	20–120 min	1–2 hr	8–24 hr
I.V.	< 5 min	5–15 min	2–4 hr

Half-life: 5.5–8 hr

Mechanism of Action

Blocks $alpha_1$ and $beta_2$ receptors selectively in vascular smooth muscle and $beta_1$ receptors in heart to reduce blood pressure and peripheral vascular resistance. Potent beta-blockade prevents reflex tachycardia, which commonly occurs when alpha-blockers reduce cardiac output, resting heart rate, or stroke volume.

Contraindications

Bronchial asthma, cardiogenic shock, hypersensitivity to labetalol or its components, obstructive airway disease, other conditions associated with severe and prolonged hypotension, overt heart failure, second- or third-degree heart block, severe bradycardia

Interactions

DRUGS

calcium antagonist of verapamil type: Increased risk of adverse reactions
cimetidine: Possibly increased labetalol concentration and effects
epinephrine: Possibly unresponsiveness to usual doses of epinephrine
halothane anesthesia: Increased risk of hypotension
nitroglycerin: Blunted reflex tachycardia
other beta-blocker agonists: Possibly blunted bronchodilator effect of these drugs in patients with bronchospasm
tricyclic antidepressants: Increased risk of tremor

Adverse Reactions

CNS: Anxiety, confusion, depression, dizziness, drowsiness, fatigue, paresthesia, syncope, vertigo, weakness, yawning
CV: **Bradycardia**, chest pain, edema, **heart block**, **heart failure**, **hypotension**, orthostatic hypotension, **ventricular arrhythmias**
EENT: Nasal congestion, taste perversion
ENDO: Hypoglycemia
GI: Elevated liver enzymes, **hepatic necrosis**, **hepatitis**, indigestion, jaundice, nausea, vomiting
GU: Ejaculation failure, impotence
RESP: Dyspnea, wheezing
SKIN: Pruritus, rash, scalp tingling

Childbearing Considerations

PREGNANCY

- It is not known if drug causes fetal harm. However, drug does cross the placental barrier and may cause bradycardia, hypoglycemia, hypotension, and respiratory depression in newborns of mothers who were treated with the drug for hypertension during late pregnancy.
- Use with caution only if benefit to mother outweighs potential risk to fetus.

LACTATION

- Drug is present in breast milk.
- Mothers should check with prescriber before breastfeeding.

Nursing Considerations

- Monitor blood pressure to determine effectiveness of drug and when dosage should be altered.

! WARNING Monitor patient for a hypersensitivity reaction such as rash or pruritus. Notify prescriber, if present, and expect drug to be discontinued.

! WARNING Be aware that labetalol masks common signs of shock. Monitor acutely ill patient closely.

! WARNING Monitor blood glucose level in patients, especially in children, patients with diabetes mellitus, and patients who are fasting (not eating regularly, having surgery, or are vomiting) because beta blockers such as labetalol may mask early signs of hypoglycemia such as tachycardia and increase the risk of prolonged or severe hpoglycemia that may occur any time during treatment. If hypoglycemia occurs, treat according to institutional protocol, and notify prescriber.

! WARNING Be aware that stopping labetalol tablets abruptly after long-term therapy could result in angina, MI, or ventricular arrhythmias. Expect to taper dosage over 2 weeks while monitoring response.

PATIENT TEACHING

- Instruct patient how to administer oral form of labetalol prescribed.
- Inform patient receiving drug intravenously that he must remain lying down throughout administration and for up to 3 hours afterward. Tell the patient to report feelings of light-headedness or if fainting occurs.
- Suggest that patient minimize effects of orthostatic hypotension by avoiding sudden

position changes, rising to a sitting or standing position slowly, and dividing daily dosage into 3 times a day rather than 2 times a day if approved by prescriber.

- Urge patient to avoid alcohol during labetalol therapy.

! **WARNING** Alert patient that drug may cause an allergic reaction such as itching and a rash. If present, tell patient to notify prescriber as drug will need to be discontinued and patient switched to a different drug.

! **WARNING** Advise patient to report other adverse reactions such as confusion, difficulty breathing, slow pulse, and swelling in arms or legs.

! **WARNING** Instruct all patients and family or caregiver to be alert for signs and symptoms of hypoglycemia, especially when not eating enough, not able to eat because of surgery, or vomiting. Also, teach them how to treat hypoglycemia. Tell patient to notify prescriber if a hypoglycemic episode occurs and to seek immediate medical attention if severe.

- Inform patient that scalp tingling may occur early in treatment but is transient.
- Advise patient to inform eye healthcare provider if he needs cataract surgery because intraoperative floppy iris syndrome has occurred during cataract surgery in some patients treated with the class of drugs of which labetalol is a member.

! **WARNING** Caution patient not to stop drug abruptly after long-term therapy because doing so could cause angina and rebound hypertension.

lacosamide

Motpoly XR, Vimpat

Class, Category, and Schedule

Pharmacologic class: Functionalized aminoacid

Therapeutic class: Anticonvulsant

Controlled substance schedule: V

Indications and Dosages

∗ *To treat partial-onset seizures as monotherapy or adjunctive therapy*

I.V. INFUSION, ORAL SOLUTION, TABLETS

Adults and adolescents ages 17 and older. *Initial for monotherapy:* 100 mg twice daily, increased by 50 mg twice daily every wk to recommended maintenance dose. Alternatively, 200 mg given as single loading dose, followed 12 hr later by 100 mg twice daily for 1 wk. Then increased by 50 mg twice daily each wk, as needed to recommended maintenance dose. *Initial for adjunctive therapy:* 50 mg twice daily. Dosage increased by 50 mg twice daily, as needed, up to recommended maintenance dose. *Maintenance:* 150 to 200 mg twice daily for monotherapy; 100 to 200 mg twice daily for adjunctive therapy.

Children weighing 50 kg (110 lb) or more. *Initial:* 50 mg twice daily, increased by 50 mg twice daily every wk to recommended maintenance dose. Alternatively, 200 mg given as single loading dose, followed 12 hr later by 100 mg twice daily for 1 wk, then increased by 50 mg twice daily each wk, as needed to recommended maintenance dose. *Maintenance:* 150 to 200 mg twice daily as monotherapy; 100 to 200 mg twice daily as adjunctive therapy.

Children weighing 30 kg (66 lb) to less than 50 kg (110 lb). *Initial:* 1 mg/kg twice daily, increased by 1 mg/kg twice daily every wk to recommended maintenance dose. Alternatively 4 mg/kg as a single loading dose, followed 12 hr later by 2 mg/kg twice daily for 1 wk, then increased by 1 mg/kg twice daily each wk, as needed, to recommended maintenance dose. *Maintenance:* 2 to 4 mg/kg twice daily.

Infants ages 1 mo and older and children weighing 6 kg (13.2 lb) to less than 30 kg (66 lb). *Initial:* 1 mg/kg twice daily, increased by 1 mg/kg twice daily every wk to recommended maintenance dose. Alternatively, 4.5 mg/kg as a single loading dose, followed 12 hr later by 3 mg/kg twice daily for 1 wk, then increased by 1 mg/kg twice daily each wk, as needed, to recommended maintenance dose. *Maintenance:* 3 to 6 mg/kg twice daily.

ORAL SOLUTION

Infants weighing less than 6 kg (13.2 lb). *Initial:* 1 mg/kg twice daily, increased by 1 mg/kg twice daily every wk to recommended maintenance dose.

J K L

Alternatively, 3.75 mg/kg twice daily for 1 wk, then increased by 1 mg/kg twice daily every wk, as needed, to recommended maintenance dose. *Maintenance:* 3.75 to 7.5 mg/kg twice daily.

I.V. INFUSION

Infants weighing less than 6 kg (13.2 lb). *Initial:* 0.66 mg/kg 3 times daily, increased by 0.66 mg/kg 3 times daily every wk to recommended maintenance dose. Alternatively, 2.5 mg/kg 3 times daily for 1 wk, then increased by 0.66 mg/kg 3 times daily every wk, as needed, to recommended maintenance dose. *Maintenance:* 2.5 to 5 mg/kg 3 times daily.

E.R. CAPSULES (MOTPOLY XR)

Adults and adolescents ages 17 and older. *Initial for monotherapy:* 200 mg once daily, increased by 100 mg once daily every wk. *Maximum:* 300 to 400 mg once daily. *Initial for adjunctive therapy:* 100 mg once daily, increased by 100 mg once daily every wk. *Maximum:* 200 to 400 mg once daily.

Children weighing at least 50 kg (110 lb). *Initial for monotherapy:* 100 mg once daily, increased by 100 once daily every wk. *Maximum:* 300 to 400 mg once daily. *Initial for adjunctive therapy:* 100 mg once daily, increased by 100 mg once daily every wk. *Maintenance:* 200 to 400 mg once daily.

* *As adjunct to treat primary generalized tonic–clonic seizures*

I.V. INFUSION, ORAL SOLUTION, TABLETS

Adults and adolescents ages 17 and older. *Initial:* 50 mg twice daily, increased by 50 mg twice daily at weekly intervals based on response and tolerance. Dosage increased at weekly intervals by 50 mg twice daily, as needed, up to recommended maintenance dose. Alternatively, 200 mg given as a single loading dose, followed 12 hr later by 100 mg twice daily for 1 wk, then increased by 50 mg twice daily each wk, as needed, to recommended maintenance dose. *Maintenance:* 100 to 200 mg twice daily.

Children ages 4 to 17 weighing 50 kg (110 lb) or more. 50 mg twice daily, increased by 50 mg twice daily every wk to recommended maintenance dose. Alternatively, 200 mg given as a single loading dose, followed 12 hr later by 100 mg twice daily for 1 wk, then increased by 50 mg twice daily each wk, as needed, to recommended maintenance dose. *Maintenance:* 100 mg to 200 mg twice daily.

Children ages 4 to 17 weighing 30 kg (66 lb) to less than 50 kg (110 lb). 1 mg/kg twice daily, increased by 1 mg/kg twice daily every wk to recommended maintenance dose. Alternatively, 4 mg/kg as a single loading dose, followed 12 hr later by 2 mg/kg twice daily for 1 wk, then increased by 1 mg/kg twice daily each wk, as needed, to recommended maintenance dose. *Maintenance:* 2 mg/kg to 4 mg/kg twice daily.

Children ages 4 to 17 weighing 11 kg (24.2 lb) to less than 30 kg (66 lb). 1 mg/kg twice daily, increased by 1 mg/kg twice daily every wk to recommended maintenance dose. Alternatively, 4.5 mg/kg as a single loading dose, followed 12 hr later by 3 mg/kg twice daily for 1 wk, then increased by 1 mg/kg twice daily each wk, as needed, to recommended maintenance dose. *Maintenance:* 3 mg/kg to 6 mg/kg twice daily.

± **DOSAGE ADJUSTMENT** For patients with mild to moderate hepatic impairment or severe renal impairment (creatinine clearance less than 30 ml/min), including end-stage renal disease, dosage reduced by 25% (300 mg for E.R. capsules) of maximum dosage recommended. Following a 4-hour hemodialysis treatment, dosage supplementation of up to 50% may be required. For patients with hepatic or renal impairment taking strong CYP2C9 or CYP3A4 inhibitors concurrently, dosage may have to be reduced. For patients already on a single antieplieptic drug and converting to monotherapy, withdrawal of the concomitant antieplileptic drug should not occur until the therapeutic dosage of lacosamide is achieved and has been administered for at least 3 days (4 days for E.R. capsules). A gradual withdrawal of the concomitant antiepileptic drug over at least 6 weeks is recommended.

Drug Administration

- Know that if a loading dose is required it will need to be administered with supervision and patient monitored for increased development of adverse reactions, especially cardiovascular and CNS adverse reactions such as ataxia and dizziness.

P.O.

- E.R. capsules and tablets should be swallowed whole with a beverage and not chewed, crushed, or split.

- Use a calibrated device to measure oral solution dosage. Discard after 6 mo of first opening the bottle.
- Oral solution may be administered through a gastrostomy or nasogastric tube.

I.V.

- Drug may be administered without further dilution or may be mixed with 0.9% Sodium Chloride Injection, 5% Dextrose Injection, or Lactated Ringer's Injection. If diluted, do not store diluted solution for more than 4 hr at room temperature.
- Administer over 30 to 60 min, although more rapid infusion of 15 min may be used in adults, if needed, but not in children.
- *Incompatibilities:* None reported by manufacturer

Route	Onset	Peak	Duration
P.O.	Unknown	1–4 hr	Unknown
I.V.	Unknown	30–60 min	Unknown

Half-life: 13 hr

Mechanism of Action

May inactivate voltage-gated sodium channels selectively, which prevents seizure activity by inhibiting repetitive neuronal firing in the brain and stabilizing hyperexcitable neuronal membranes.

Contraindications

Hypersensitivity to lacosamide and its components

Interactions

DRUGS

beta-blockers, calcium channel blockers, potassium channel blockers, sodium channel blockers, including those that prolong PR interval, such as sodium channel blocking antiepileptic drugs: Increased risk of AV block, bradycardia, or ventricular tachyarrhythmias

strong CYP2C9 inhibitors or CYP3A4 inhibitors (in presence of hepatic or renal impairment): Possibly significant increase in lacosamide exposure and adverse effects

Adverse Reactions

CNS: Aggression, agitation, asthenia, ataxia, attention deficit, cerebellar syndrome, confusion, depression, dizziness, dyskinesia, fatigue, feeling drunk, fever, hallucinations, headache, hypoesthesia, impaired balance, insomnia, irritability, memory impairment, mood alteration, paresthesia, psychotic disorder, **seizures** (new or worsening), somnolence, **suicidal ideation**, tremor, vertigo

CV: **Atrial fibrillation or flutter**, **AV block**, **bradycardia**, **conduction disturbances**, palpitations, prolonged PR interval, **prolonged QT interval**

EENT: Blurred vision, diplopia, dry mouth, nystagmus, oral hypoesthesia, tinnitus

GI: Constipation, diarrhea, dyspepsia, nausea, vomiting

HEME: **Agranulocytosis**, anemia, **neutropenia**

MS: Dysarthria, muscle spasms

SKIN: Pruritus, rash, **Stevens-Johnson syndrome**, **toxic epidermal necrolysis**, urticaria

Other: **Angioedema**; **drug reaction with eosinophilia and systemic symptoms (DRESS)**; injection-site erythema, irritation, and pain

Childbearing Considerations

PREGNANCY

- Pregnancy exposure registry: 1-888-233-2334 or http://www.aedpregnancyregistry.org/.
- It is not known if drug may cause fetal harm.
- Use with caution only if benefit to mother outweighs potential risk to fetus.

LACTATION

- Drug is present in breast milk.
- Mothers should check with prescriber before breastfeeding. If breastfeeding occurs, infants should be monitored for excess sedation.

Nursing Considerations

! **WARNING** Monitor patients closely receiving concomitant drug therapy that prolong the PR interval, conduction disorders (such as AV block, sick sinus syndrome, and no pacemaker in place) or in patients who have severe cardiac disease (such as heart failure, myocardial ischemia), or sodium channel disorders, such as Brugada syndrome, because lacosamide may affect conduction. For these patients, ensure that an ECG has been done, as ordered, prior to starting therapy and after dosage titration. Also,

JKL

be aware that patients with cardiovascular disease or diabetic neuropathy may be at increased risk for atrial fibrillation or flutter.

! **WARNING** Monitor patient closely for hypersensitivity reactions, including serious skin reactions. Know that DRESS, while commonly presents as a rash initially may only present with a fever or swollen lymph nodes. If signs and symptoms are present to suggest a hypersensitivity reaction or DRESS, notify prescriber immediately and expect drug to be discontinued. Provide supportive care, as needed and ordered. Know that the incidence of rash occurring within 30 days after I.V. administration was discontinued was higher in patients reaching the maintenance dose in a shorter time span having received a loading dose and/or a higher initial dose compared to patients who received a lower initial dosage regimen.

! **WARNING** Watch patient closely for suicidal tendencies, particularly when therapy starts and dosage changes because depression may worsen temporarily during these times and lead to suicidal ideation.

! **WARNING** Monitor patient for seizure activity. Institute seizure precautions, as needed. Be aware that lacosamide therapy should be discontinued gradually over at least 1 week to minimize seizure frequency.

- Monitor effectiveness of lacosamide to treat seizures.

PATIENT TEACHING

- Instruct patient and family or caretaker how to administer oral form of lacosamide prescribed.

! **WARNING** Alert patient that the oral solution of lacosamide contains aspartame, a source of phenylalanine that could be harmful to patients with phenylketonuria (PKU).

- Tell patient to notify prescriber if seizure activity remains unchanged or increases after lacosamide is initated.

! **WARNING** Alert patient that drug may cause an allergic or skin reaction that could become quite serious and affect other body organs. Tell patient to notify prescriber if an allergic reaction occurs or at the first sign of a rash. If severe, urge patient to seek immediate medical attention.

! **WARNING** Urge family or caregiver to watch patient closely for suicidal tendencies, especially when therapy starts or dosage changes.

! **WARNING** Instruct patient to report any persistent, severe, or unusual signs and symptoms to prescriber immediately.

- Caution patient to avoid hazardous activities until drug's CNS effects are known and resolved.
- Advise mothers who are breastfeeding while taking lacosamide to monitor infant for excessive drowsiness.
- Encourage patient to carry medical identification that indicates her diagnosis and drug therapy.

lactitol

Class and Category

Pharmacologic class: Simple monosaccharide sugar alcohol
Therapeutic class: Osmotic laxative

Indications and Dosages

✷ *To treat chronic idiopathic constipation*

POWDER FOR ORAL SOLUTION

Adults. 20 g once daily.

± **DOSAGE ADJUSTMENT** For patients with persistent loose stools, dosage reduced to 10 grams once daily.

Drug Administration

P.O.

- Administration with meals is preferable.
- To mix using multidose bottle: Bottle top is a measuring cap marked to contain 10 grams of powder. For a 20-gram dose, fill the measuring cap twice to the top of the white section in cap marked by the arrow. For a 10-gram dose, fill the measuring cap once to the top of the white section in cap marked by the arrow. Pour the measured dose into an empty 8-ounce glass. Add 4 to 8 ounces of common beverages (coffee, soda, tea), juice, or water and stir to dissolve. Have patient drink entire contents of the glass.

- To use unit-dose packets: Pour the contents of 1 or 2 unit-dose packets, as prescribed, into an empty 8-ounce glass. Add 4 to 8 ounces of common beverages (coffee, soda, tea), juice, or water and stir thoroughly to dissolve. Have patient drink entire contents of the glass.
- Administer other oral drugs at least 2 hr before or after administration of drug.

Route	Onset	Peak	Duration
P.O.	Unknown	2.4–4.8 hr	Unknown

Half-life: 2.4 hr

Mechanism of Action

Exerts an osmotic effect, causing the influx of water into the small intestine leading to a laxative effect in the colon.

Contraindications

Galactosemia, hypersensitivity to lactitol or its components, mechanical GI obstruction

Interactions

DRUGS

other oral drugs: Possibly decreased absorption

Adverse Reactions

CV: Hypertension
EENT: Nasopharyngitis
GI: Abdominal distention or pain, diarrhea (may be severe), flatulence
GU: UTI
RESP: Upper respiratory infection
SKIN: Pruritus, rash
Other: Elevated blood creatinine phosphokinase, **hypersensitivity reactions**

Childbearing Considerations

PREGNANCY

- It is not known if drug can cause fetal harm.
- Although drug is minimally absorbed systemically, use with caution in pregnant women.

LACTATION

- It is not known if drug is present in breast milk.
- Mothers should check with prescriber before breastfeeding.

Nursing Considerations

! WARNING Monitor patient for hypersensitivity reactions, such as pruritus and rash, after administration. If present, notify prescriber, expect drug to be discontinued, and provide supportive care, as needed and ordered.

- Monitor patient's bowel movements to determine effectiveness of drug.
- Monitor patient's blood pressure for evidence of drug-induced hypertension.

PATIENT TEACHING

- Instruct patient how to mix and administer lactitol.
- Tell patient to take any other oral drugs 2 hours before or 2 hours after taking lactitol.

! WARNING Instruct patient to notify prescriber if itching or a rash appears after taking lactitol.

- Advise patient to notify prescriber if persistent loose stools occur as dosage will need to be reduced.

lactulose

JKL

Class and Category

Pharmacologic class: Disaccharide
Therapeutic class: Colonic acidifier

Indications and Dosages

✱ *To treat constipation*

POWDER, ORAL SOLUTION

Adults. *Initial:* 10 to 20 g daily, increased, as needed. *Maximum:* 40 g daily.

✱ *To treat portal-systemic (hepatic) encephalopathy*

POWDER, ORAL SOLUTION

Adults. *Initial:* 20 to 30 g 3 times daily or 4 times daily with dosage adjustment made every day or 2, as needed, until 2 or 3 soft stools occur daily. *Usual:* 60 to 100 g daily in divided doses. *Rapid laxation:* 20 to 30 g every hr initially and then reduced to usual dosage.

RETENTION ENEMA

Adults. 200 g (300 ml); if evacuated too promptly, repeated immediately. Dosage given every 4 to 6 hr, as needed.

✱ *To prevent portal-systemic (hepatic) encephalopathy*

ORAL SOLUTION

Adults. 20 g (30 ml) to 30 g (45 ml) 3 or 4 times daily, adjusted every day or 2 to produce 2 to 3 soft stools daily.
Children ages 1 and older. 26.7 g (40 ml) to 60 g (90 ml) daily in divided doses with dosage adjusted every day or 2, as needed, to produce 2 to 3 soft stools daily.
Infants up to 1 yr. 1.7 (2.5 ml) to 6.8 g (10 ml) daily in divided doses with dosage adjusted every day or 2, as needed, to produce 2 to 3 soft stools daily.

Drug Administration

P.O.

- For powder form, dissolve contents of packet in 4 ounces of fruit juice, milk, or water. Shake well before using.
- Use calibrated device to measure dosage of oral solution.

P.R.

- Retention enema used for impending coma or when coma has already occurred.
- Dilute 300 ml of drug in 700 ml of water or normal saline solution and administer as an enema. Use a rectal tube with a balloon to help with retention.
- Patient should retain enema for 30 to 60 min. If retention is less than 30 min, enema repeated.

Route	Onset	Peak	Duration
P.O.	24–48 hr	Unknown	Unknown
P.R.	Unknown	Unknown	Unknown

Half-life: 1.7–2 hr

Mechanism of Action

Arrives unchanged in the colon, where it breaks down into lactic acid and small amounts of acetic and formic acids, acidifying fecal contents. Acidification leads to increased osmotic pressure in the colon, which, in turn, increases stool water content and softens stool.
Makes intestinal contents more acidic than blood. This prevents ammonia diffusion from intestine into blood, as occurs in hepatic encephalopathy. The trapped ammonia is converted into ammonia ions and, by lactulose's cathartic effect, is expelled in feces with other nitrogenous wastes.

Contraindications

Hypersensitivity to lactulose or its components, low-galactose diet

Interactions

DRUGS

antacids (nonabsorbable), antibiotics (especially oral neomycin): Decreased effectiveness of lactulose
other laxatives: Possibly falsely indicating adequate lactulose dosage when used to treat hepatic encephalopathy

Adverse Reactions

ENDO: Hyperglycemia
GI: Abdominal cramps and distention, diarrhea, flatulence
Other: **Hypernatremia**, **hypokalemia**, hypovolemia

Childbearing Considerations

PREGNANCY

- It is not known if drug causes fetal harm.
- Use with caution only if benefit to mother outweighs potential risk to fetus.

LACTATION

- It is not known if drug is present in breast milk.
- Mothers should check with prescriber before breastfeeding.

Nursing Considerations

- Monitor number of stools patient passes daily to determine effectiveness of therapy and need for dosage adjustment.

! WARNING Monitor blood ammonia level in patient with hepatic encephalopathy. Also, watch for dehydration, hypernatremia, and hypokalemia when giving higher lactulose doses to treat this condition.

- Monitor diabetic patient for hyperglycemia because lactulose contains galactose and lactose.
- Plan to replace fluids if frequent bowel movements cause hypovolemia.
- Expect to periodically check serum electrolyte levels of debilitated or elderly patient who uses oral drug longer than 6 months.

PATIENT TEACHING

- Instruct patient how to administer lactulose.
- Inform patient that because oral lactulose must reach the colon to work, bowel

movement may not occur for 24 to 48 hours after taking drug.
- Direct patient not to use other laxatives while taking lactulose.

! **WARNING** Review with patient and family or caregiver signs and symptoms of electrolyte imbalance if patient has encephalopathy and to report to prescriber, if present.

- Instruct patient to report abdominal distention or severe diarrhea.
- Advise diabetic patient to check blood glucose level often and to report hyperglycemia.
- Instruct patient to increase fluid intake if frequent bowel movements occur.
- Teach patient with chronic constipation the importance of exercising, increasing fiber in diet, and increasing fluid intake.

lamivudine

Epivir, Epivir-HBV, Heptovir (CAN)

Class and Category

Pharmacologic class: Synthetic nucleoside analogue
Therapeutic class: Antiviral

Indications and Dosages

∗ *To treat chronic hepatitis B virus (HBV) infection associated with active liver inflammation and evidence of hepatitis B viral replication*

ORAL SOLUTION, TABLETS (EPIVIR-HBV)

Adults. 100 mg once daily.
Children ages 2 to 17. 3 mg/kg once daily. *Maximum:* 100 mg once daily.

±**DOSAGE ADJUSTMENT** For adult patients with renal impairment receiving Epivir-HBV, dosage adjustment is as follows: Adults with creatinine clearance between 30 and 49 ml/min, 100 mg first dose, then reduced to 50 mg once daily thereafter. For adults with creatinine clearance between 15 and 29 ml/min, 100 mg first dose, then reduced to 25 mg once daily thereafter. For adults with creatinine clearance between 5 and 14 ml/min, first dose reduced to 35 mg, then reduced to 15 mg once daily thereafter. For adults with creatinine clearance less than 5 ml/min, first dose reduced to 35 mg, then reduced to 10 mg once daily thereafter. There is no recommendation for pediatric patients with renal impairment for Epivir-HBV.

∗ *As adjunct to treat human immunodeficiency virus type 1 (HIV-1) infection*

ORAL SOLUTION, TABLETS (EPIVIR)

Adults. 300 mg once daily or 150 mg twice daily.

TABLETS

Children weighing 25 kg (55 lb) or more. 300 mg once daily or 150 mg in a.m. and 150 mg in p.m. *Maximum:* 300 mg daily.
Children weighing 20 kg (44 lb) to less than 25 kg (55 lb). 225 mg once daily or 75 mg in a.m. and 150 mg in p.m. *Maximum:* 225 mg daily.
Children weighing 14 kg (30.8 lb) to less than 20 kg (44 lb). 150 mg once daily or 75 mg in a.m. and 75 mg in p.m. *Maximum:* 150 mg daily.

ORAL SOLUTION (EPIVIR)

Infants ages 3 mo and older. 10 mg/kg once daily or 5 mg/kg twice daily. *Maximum:* 300 mg daily.

±**DOSAGE ADJUSTMENT** For adults and adolescents weighing 25 kg (55 lb) or more with renal impairment receiving Epivir, dosage adjustment is as follows: Adults with creatinine clearance between 30 and 49 ml/min, dosage reduced to 150 mg once daily. For adults with creatinine clearance between 15 and 29 ml/min, 150 mg first dose, then reduced to 100 mg once daily thereafter. For adults with creatinine clearance between 5 and 14 ml/min, 150 mg first dose, then reduced to 50 mg once daily thereafter. For adults with creatinine clearance less than 5 ml/min, 50 mg first dose, then reduced to 25 mg once daily. For pediatric patients with renal impairment taking Epivir, dosage may be reduced or dosing interval increased.

Drug Administration

P.O.

- Do not confuse Epivir with Epivir-HBV. They are not interchangeable.
- The tablets and oral solution of Epivir-HBV are interchangeable and may be administered with or without food. Oral solution of Epivir-HBV should be used for doses less than 100 mg.
- Do not administer with other drugs that contain emtricitabine or lamivudine.

Route	Onset	Peak	Duration
P.O.	Unknown	1–3 hr	Unknown

Half-life: 5–7 hr

Mechanism of Action

Phosphorylated to its active metabolite occurs first then inhibition of the DNA- and RNA-dependent polymerase activities of HBV and HIV-1 reverse transcriptases occurs via DNA chain termination after incorporation of the nucleotide analogue into viral DNA. This destroys the activity of the hepatitis B and HIV-1 viruses.

Contraindications

Hypersensitivity to lamivudine or its components

Interactions

DRUGS

drugs inhibiting organic cation transporters, such as trimethoprim: Possibly altered excretion of lamivudine
sorbitol: Reduced lamivudine exposure and effectiveness

Adverse Reactions

CNS: Chills, depression, dizziness, fatigue, fever, headache, insomnia, malaise, neuropathy, paresthesia, peripheral neuropathy, sleep disorders, weakness
EENT: Ear, nose, throat infections; nasal congestion or discharge; sore throat; stomatitis
ENDO: Cushingoid appearance, fat redistribution, hyperglycemia
GI: Abdominal pain, anorexia, bilirubin increase, diarrhea, dyspepsia, elevated lipase and liver enzyme levels, **exacerbation of hepatitis posttreatment**, **hepatic decompensation in patient co-infected with HIV-1 and hepatitis C**, **hepatomegaly with steatosis**, nausea, **pancreatitis**, vomiting
HEME: Anemia; **severe anemias, including pure red cell aplasia and neutropenia**; splenomegaly; **thrombocytopenia**
MS: Abdominal cramps, arthralgia, elevated CPK level, musculoskeletal pain, myalgia, **rhabdomyolysis**
RESP: Abnormal breath sounds, cough, wheezing
SKIN: Alopecia, pruritus, rash, urticaria
Other: **Anaphylaxis**, **emergence of resistant HBV infection or HIV-1 infection**, **immune reconstitution syndrome**, **lactic acidosis**, lymphadenopathy

Childbearing Considerations

PREGNANCY

- Pregnancy exposure registry: 1-800-258-4263.
- It is not known if drug causes fetal harm.
- Use with caution only if benefit to mother outweighs potential risk to fetus.

LACTATION

- Drug is present in breast milk.
- The Centers for Disease Control and Prevention recommends that HIV-1 infected mothers not breastfeed to avoid risking postnatal transmission of HIV-1 infection to infants. They also do not recommend breastfeeding because of potential drug-induced adverse reactions in the infant.
- Mothers who are not HIV-1 positive should check with prescriber before breastfeeding.

Nursing Considerations

- Be aware that Epivir-HBV oral solution and tablets contain a lower dose of lamivudine than used to treat HIV-1 infection and should not be used to treat patients co-infected with HBV and HIV-1 infections. Patients with unrecognized or untreated HIV infection exposed to Epivir-HBV may develop a rapid emergence of HIV-1 resistance. Make sure appropriate HIV counseling and testing have been done before treatment and periodically during treatment with lamivudine to ensure this does not happen.

! WARNING Use extreme caution when administering lamivudine to patient with known risk factors for liver disease. Know that lactic acidosis and severe hepatomegaly with steatosis have occurred with lamivudine therapy, and death has occurred in some patients. Risk factors include presence of obesity, prolonged nucleoside exposure, and being a woman. However, know that lactic acidosis and severe hepatomegaly with steatosis have also occurred in patients with no known risk factors. Expect lamivudine to be discontinued in any patient who develops clinical or laboratory findings suggestive of lactic acidosis or pronounced hepatotoxicity, even in the absence of marked transaminase elevations.

! **WARNING** Monitor patient for a hypersensitivity reaction, which may become life-threatening, such as anaphylaxis. If present, notify prescriber, expect drug to be switched to another drug, and provide supportive care, as needed and ordered.

! **WARNING** Monitor patients co-infected with HIV-1 and hepatitis C closely for signs and symptoms of liver dysfunction because hepatic decompensations, some of which resulted in death, have occurred in patients receiving combination antiretroviral therapy for HIV-1 that included interferon alfa.

! **WARNING** Be aware that immune reconstitution syndrome has occurred in patients treated with combination antiretroviral therapy, including lamivudine. The inflammatory response predisposes susceptible patients to opportunistic infections, such as cytomegalovirus, *Mycobacterium avium* infection, *Pneumocystis jiroveci* pneumonia, or tuberculosis. Autoimmune disorders, such as Graves' disease, Guillain-Barré syndrome, or polymyositis have also occurred. Report sudden or unusual adverse reactions to prescriber.

- Monitor patient throughout treatment for evidence of loss of therapeutic response. Indicators include increasing levels of HBV DNA over time after an initial decline below assay limit, progression of clinical signs or symptoms of hepatic disease and/or worsening of hepatic necroinflammatory findings or return of persistently elevated alanine transaminase (ALT) levels. These findings may require drug to be discontinued.
- Be aware that a switch to an alternative regimen may be needed for patients in whom serum HBV DNA remains detectable after 24 weeks of treatment, to reduce the risk of resistance in patients receiving monotherapy with Epivir-HBV.
- Monitor patient's ALT and HBV DNA levels during treatment to determine treatment options if viral mutants emerge.
- Observe patient for redistribution of body fat, including breast enlargement, central obesity, development of buffalo hump, facial wasting, and peripheral wasting, which may produce a cushingoid-type appearance.

! **WARNING** Expect patient to be closely monitored for at least several months after lamivudine has been discontinued because exacerbation of hepatitis may occur.

PATIENT TEACHING

- Instruct patient with hepatitis B on the importance of testing for HIV before therapy begins and then periodically throughout therapy to avoid development of resistance to HIV treatment if HIV occurs.
- Instruct patient how to administer oral form of lamivudine prescribed and what to do if a dose is missed.
- Inform diabetic patient using oral solution that each 15-ml dose of Epivir contains 3 g of sucrose; 20-ml dose of Epivir-HBV contains 4 g of sucrose.
- Advise patient that treatment with lamivudine does not reduce the risk of transmission of HBV or HIV to others through blood contamination or sexual contact.

! **WARNING** Alert patient that an allergic reaction may occur. If present, tell patient to notify prescriber. If severe, urge patient to seek immediate medical care.

! **WARNING** Warn patient with hepatitis B not to discontinue drug without prescriber knowledge because acute severe exacerbations of hepatitis B may occur following discontinuation of lamivudine. Tell patient to immediately report any reappearance of signs and symptoms of hepatitis B or new or worsening symptoms because emergence of resistant hepatitis B virus may occur, or disease may worsen during treatment.

! **WARNING** Alert patient that severe conditions may develop while taking lamivudine. Encourage the patient to seek medical attention immediately if he experiences any persistent, severe, or unusual symptoms.

- Warn patient that fat distribution may occur with lamivudine therapy and may alter his appearance.
- Advise patient to alert all prescribers of lamivudine therapy and to tell the prescriber if patient is taking any other prescription or over-the-counter drugs.

Instruct patient to avoid chronic use of sorbitol-containing drugs, when possible, as drug may become less effective.
- Advise mothers with HIV not to breastfeed.

lamotrigine

Lamictal, Lamictal CD, Lamictal ODT, Lamictal XR, Subvenite

Class and Category

Pharmacologic class: Phenyltriazine
Therapeutic class: Anticonvulsant

Indications and Dosages

∗ *As adjunct to treat partial seizures; to treat generalized seizures of Lennox-Gastaut syndrome; to treat primary generalized tonic–clonic seizures*

CHEWABLE DISPERSIBLE TABLETS, ORAL SUSPENSION, ORALLY DISINTEGRATING TABLETS, TABLETS

Adults and children over the age of 12 taking valproate. 25 mg every other day for 2 wk, followed by 25 mg once daily for 2 wk. Increased by 25 to 50 mg every 1 to 2 wk, as needed. *Maintenance:* 100 to 200 mg daily.

Children ages 2 to 12 weighing 6.7 kg (14.74 lb) to 40 kg (88 lb) taking valproate. 0.15 mg/kg/day (rounded down to nearest whole tablet) as a single dose or in divided doses twice daily for 2 wk and then 0.3 mg/kg/day (rounded down to nearest whole tablet) as single dose or in divided doses twice daily for next 2 wk. Increased by 0.3 mg/kg/day (rounded down to the nearest whole tablet and amount added to previously administered daily dose), every 1 to 2 wk, as needed, to reach maintenance dosage. *Maintenance:* 1 to 5 mg/kg/day as single dose or in divided doses twice daily. *Maximum:* 200 mg/day.

Adults and children over the age of 12 NOT taking carbamazepine, phenobarbital, phenytoin, primidone, or valproate. 25 mg once daily for 2 wk, followed by 50 mg once daily for 2 wk. Increased by 50 mg every 1 to 2 wk, as needed. *Maintenance:* 225 to 375 mg daily in 2 divided doses.

Children ages 2 to 12 weighing 6.7 kg (14,74 lb) to 40 (88 lb) NOT taking carbamazepine, phenobarbital, phenytoin, primidone, or valproate. 0.3 mg/kg/day (rounded down to the nearest whole tablet) in 1 or 2 divided doses for 2 wk; followed by 0.6 mg/kg/day (rounded down to the nearest whole tablet) in 2 divided doses for 2 wk. Increased by 0.6 mg/kg/day (rounded down to the nearest whole tablet and added to the previously administered daily dose) every 1 to 2 wk, as needed. *Maintenance:* 4.5 to 7.5 mg/kg/day in 2 divided doses. *Maximum:* 300 mg daily in 2 divided doses.

Adults and children over the age of 12 taking carbamazepine, phenobarbital, phenytoin, or primidone but NOT valproate. 50 mg once daily for 2 wk and then 100 mg daily in 2 divided doses for 2 wk. Increased by 100 mg/day every 1 to 2 wk, as needed. *Maintenance:* 300 to 500 mg daily in 2 divided doses.

Children ages 2 to 12 weighing 6.7 kg (14.74 lb) to 40 kg (88 lb) taking carbamazepine, phenobarbital, phenytoin, or primidone but NOT valproate. 0.6 mg/kg/day (rounded down to the nearest whole tablet) in 2 divided doses for 2 wk and then 1.2 mg/kg/day (rounded down to the nearest whole tablet) in 2 divided doses for 2 wk. Increased by 1.2 mg/kg/day (rounded down to the nearest whole tablet and this amount added to the previously administered daily dose) every 1 to 2 wk, as needed to reach maintenance dosage. *Maintenance:* 5 to 15 mg/kg/day (rounded down to the nearest whole tablet) in 2 divided doses. *Maximum:* 400 mg daily in 2 divided doses.

±**DOSAGE ADJUSTMENT** For children ages 2 to 12 weighing less than 30 kg (66 lb), maintenance dosage, regardless of what drugs are or are not taken adjunctively, may have to be increased by 50%, based on clinical response.

∗ *To treat partial seizures as monotherapy with conversion from carbamazepine, phenobarbital, phenytoin, primidone, or valproate*

CHEWABLE DISPERSIBLE TABLETS, ORAL SUSPENSION, ORALLY DISINTEGRATING TABLETS, TABLETS

Adults and adolescents ages 16 and older converting from carbamazepine, phenytoin, phenobarbital, or primidone. 50 mg once daily for 2 wk, followed by

50 mg twice daily for next 2 wk. Increased by 100 mg daily every 1 to 2 wk (while continuing to take carbamazepine, phenobarbital, phenytoin, or primidone), until usual maintenance dosage—500 mg daily in 2 divided doses—is achieved. Then, carbamazepine, phenobarbital, phenytoin, or primidone dosage tapered in 20% decrements weekly over 4 wk and then discontinued.

Adults and adolescents ages 16 and older converting from valproate. 25 mg every other day for 2 wk followed by 25 mg once daily for 2 wk. Then, increased by 25 to 50 mg daily every 1 to 2 wk until maintenance dosage of 200 mg daily is achieved. Then, valproate dosage decreased to 500 mg daily by decrements no greater than 500 mg daily every wk and then maintained at 500 mg daily for 1 wk. After valproate dosage has been at 500 mg for 1 wk, lamotrigine dosage increased to 300 mg daily while valproate dosage decreased to 250 mg daily for 1 wk. Then, lamotrigine dosage increased by 100 mg daily every wk until maintenance dose of 500 mg daily is reached (given in 2 divided doses). Valproate therapy is then discontinued.

E.R. TABLETS

Adults and adolescents ages 13 and older converting from carbamazepine, phenobarbital, phenytoin, or primidone. 50 mg once daily for first 2 wk, then increased as follows: 100 mg once daily for wk 3 and 4, then 200 mg once daily for wk 5, then 300 mg once daily for wk 6, then 400 mg once daily for wk 7, and 500 mg once daily for wk 8. Once maintenance dosage of 500 mg daily has been reached, carbamazepine, phenobarbital, phenytoin, or primidone dosage tapered in 20% decrements weekly over 4 wk and then discontinued. Two weeks after carbamazepine, phenobarbital, phenytoin, or primidone has been discontinued, lamotrigine dosage decreased no more than 100 mg/day each week until monotherapy maintenance dosage of 250 to 300 mg daily has been reached.

Adults and adolescents ages 13 and older converting from valproate. 25 mg every other day for 2 wk, then increased as follows: 25 mg once daily for wk 3 and 4, then 50 mg once daily for wk 5, then 100 mg once daily for wk 6, then 150 mg once daily for wk 7. Once lamotrigine dosage has reached 150 mg once daily, valproate dosage decreased by decrements no more than 500 mg/day/wk to 500 mg/day and then maintained for 1 wk. Then, lamotrigine dosage increased to 200 mg daily with valproate dosage decreased to 250 mg/day for 1 wk. This is followed by lamotrigine dosage increased to 250 to 300 mg daily and valproate discontinued.

* *To treat partial seizures with conversion from a single antiepileptic drug other than carbamazepine, phenobarbital, phenytoin, primidone, or valproate*

E.R. TABLETS

Adults and adolescents ages 13 and older converting from an antiepileptic drug other than carbamazepine, phenobarbital, phenytoin, primidone, or valproate. 25 mg once daily for 2 wk, followed by 50 mg once daily for next 2 wk. Increased to 100 mg once daily for wk 5, followed by 150 mg once daily for wk 6 and 200 mg once daily for wk 7. Once dosage has reached 250 to 300 mg once daily, antiepileptic drug tapered in 20% decrements weekly over 4 wk and then discontinued.

* *As adjunct to treat primary generalized tonic-clonic seizures and partial-onset seizures*

E.R. TABLETS

Adults and children ages 13 and older taking valproate. 25 mg every other day for 2 wk, followed by 25 mg once daily for 2 wk, followed by 50 mg once daily for 1 wk. Then, 100 mg once daily for 1 wk, then 150 mg once daily. Dosage increased further, as needed, but increased no more than 100 mg/day on a weekly basis. *Maintenance:* 200 to 250 mg once daily.

Adults and children ages 13 and older NOT taking carbamazepine, phenobarbital, phenytoin, primidone, or valproate. 25 mg once daily for 2 wk, followed by 50 mg once daily for 2 wk, followed by 100 mg once daily for 1 wk. Then, 150 mg once daily for 1 wk, followed by 200 mg once daily. Dosage increased further, as needed, but increased no more than 100 mg/daily on a weekly basis. *Maintenance:* 300 to 400 mg once daily.

Adults and children ages 13 and older taking carbamazepine, phenobarbital,

phenytoin, or primidone and NOT taking valproate. 50 mg once daily for 2 wk, followed by 100 mg once daily for 2 wk, followed by 200 mg once daily for 1 wk. Then, 300 mg once daily for 1 wk, followed by 400 mg once daily. Dosage increased further, as needed, but increased no more than 100 mg/daily on a weekly basis. *Maintenance:* 400 to 600 mg once daily.

∗ *As maintenance therapy for bipolar 1 disorder to delay occurrence of mood episodes (depression, mania, hypomania, mixed episodes) in patients being treated for acute mood episodes with standard therapy*

CHEWABLE DISPERSIBLE TABLETS, ORAL SUSPENSION, ORALLY DISINTEGRATING TABLETS, TABLETS

Adults NOT taking carbamazepine, phenobarbital, phenytoin, primidone, rifampin, or valproate. 25 mg once daily for 2 wk, followed by 50 mg once daily for 2 wk, followed by 100 mg once daily for 1 wk, and then increased to 200 mg once daily as maintenance dose. *Maximum:* 200 mg daily.

Adults taking valproate. 25 mg every other day for 2 wk, followed by 25 mg once daily for 2 wk, followed by 50 mg once daily for 1 wk, and then increased to 100 mg once daily as maintenance dose.

Adults taking carbamazepine, lopinavir/ritonavir, phenobarbital, phenytoin, primidone, or rifampin, but NOT valproate. 50 mg once daily for 2 wk, followed by 100 mg once daily in divided doses for 2 wk, followed by 200 mg once daily in divided doses for 1 wk, then increased to 300 mg daily in divided doses for 1 wk, and then increased to 400 mg daily in divided doses as maintenance dose.

± **DOSAGE ADJUSTMENT** *For all indications:* For females of childbearing age taking estrogen-containing oral contraceptives and NOT taking carbamazepine, phenobarbital, phenytoin, primidone, or other drugs, such as rifampin and protease inhibitors, including atazanavir/ritonavir or lopinavir/ritonavir, maintenance dose may have to be increased gradually by as much as 2-fold over recommended target maintenance dose. For females of childbearing age discontinuing estrogen-containing oral contraceptives who have been stabilized on lamotrigine prior to discontinuation and NOT taking carbamazepine, phenobarbital, phenytoin, primidone, or other drugs, such as rifampin and protease inhibitors, including atazanavir/ritonavir or lopinavir/ritonavir, maintenance dose may have to be decreased gradually by as much as half. For patients with moderate to severe hepatic impairment without ascites, all dosages decreased by 25%, and for patients with severe hepatic impairment with ascites, all dosages decreased by 50%. For patients with significant renal impairment, maintenance dosage may have to be reduced on individual basis. Dosage may have to be increased during pregnancy.

Drug Administration

P.O.

- Starter and titration kits can be used for the first 5 wk of treatment, based upon concomitant medications, for patients with epilepsy (older than age 12) and bipolar I disorder (adults). The kits are recommended for use in appropriate patients who are starting or restarting drug.
- E.R. tablets should be swallowed whole and not chewed, crushed, or split.
- Chewable dispersible tablets may be swallowed whole, chewed, or dispersed in water or diluted with fruit juice. If the tablets are chewed, administer a small amount of water or diluted fruit juice to aid in swallowing. To disperse tablets for oral suspension, add tablets to a small amount of liquid (1 teaspoon or enough to cover drug). Wait 1 min for dispersion to take place, swirl solution, and administer immediately. Never attempt to administer partial quantities of the dispersed tablets.
- Have patient place oral disintegrating tablets onto tongue and move around in mouth. The orally disintegrating tablets can be swallowed with or without water.

Route	Onset	Peak	Duration
P.O.	Unknown	1–5 hr	Unknown
P.O./E.R.	Unknown	4–11 hr	Unknown

Half-life: Variable

Mechanism of Action

May stabilize neuron membranes by blocking their sodium channels and inhibiting release of excitatory neurotransmitters, such as aspartate and glutamate, through these channels. By blocking the release of neurotransmitters, lamotrigine inhibits the spread of seizure activity in the brain, reduces seizure frequency, and diminishes mood swings.

Contraindications

Hypersensitivity to lamotrigine or its components

Interactions

DRUGS

atazanavir/ritonavir, carbamazepine, lopinavir/ritonavir, phenobarbital, phenytoin, primidone, rifampin: Decreased blood lamotrigine level
estrogen-containing oral contraceptive preparations containing 30 mcg ethinylestradiol and 150 mcg levonorgestrel: Decreased blood levels of both drugs
organic cationic transporter 2 (OCT2) substrates, such as dofetilide: Possibly increased plasma levels of these drugs
valproic acid: Increased lamotrigine level

Adverse Reactions

CNS: Aggression, amnesia, anxiety, **aseptic meningitis**, ataxia, confusion, depression, dizziness, drowsiness, emotional lability, exacerbation of parkinsonian symptoms, fever, headache, **increased seizure activity**, lack of coordination, **suicidal ideation**, tics
CV: Chest pain, **conduction abnormalities**, **proarrhythmias**, vasculitis
EENT: Blurred vision, diplopia, dry mouth, nystagmus
GI: Abdominal pain, anorexia, constipation, diarrhea, esophagitis, **hepatic failure**, **pancreatitis**, vomiting
HEME: **Agranulocytosis**, anemia, **aplastic or hemolytic anemia**, **disseminated intravascular coagulation (DIC)**, eosinophilia, **hemophagocytic lymphohistiocytosis**, **leukopenia**, **neutropenia**, **pancytopenia**, **severe anemia (such as pure red cell aplasia)**, **thrombocytopenia**
MS: **Rhabdomyolysis**
RESP: **Apnea**
SKIN: **Petechiae**, photosensitivity, pruritus, rash, **Stevens-Johnson syndrome**, **toxic epidermal necrolysis**
Other: **Angioedema**, **drug reaction with eosinophilia and systemic symptoms (DRESS)**, flu-like symptoms, hypogammaglobulinemia lupus-like reaction, lymphadenopathy, **progressive immunosuppression**

Childbearing Considerations

PREGNANCY

- Pregnancy exposure registry: 1-888-233-2334 or http://www.aedpregnancyregistry.org/.
- It is not known if drug causes fetal harm, but animal studies suggest developmental toxicity may occur.
- Use with caution only if benefit to mother outweighs potential risk to fetus.
- Dosage may have to be adjusted during pregnancy.

LACTATION

- Drug is present in breast milk.
- Mothers should check with prescriber before breastfeeding.
- If breastfeeding occurs, infant should be monitored for lamotrigine toxicity; if present, breastfeeding should be discontinued.

REPRODUCTION

- Females of childbearing age taking estrogen-containing oral contraceptive preparations containing 30 mcg ethinyl estradiol and 150 mcg levonorgestrel should use a different contraceptive method because of decreased blood levels of both drugs.

Nursing Considerations

! WARNING Know that lamotrigine is not recommended for patients with functional or structural heart disease because drug could widen QRS interval and induce proarrhythmias (severe enough to cause death). Also, know that concomitant use of other sodium channel blockers may further increase the risk for proarrhythmias in these patients.

- Use cautiously in patients with illnesses that could affect elimination or metabolism of lamotrigine, such as cardiac, hepatic, or renal functional impairment.
- Be aware that the patient may be converted directly from immediate-release lamotrigine to extended-release lamotrigine with the initial dose of extended-release matching the total daily dose of immediate-release lamotrigine. However, monitor effects

closely, especially for patient who is receiving an enzyme-inducing agent that may lower plasma levels of lamotrigine on conversion. If drug effectiveness appears to be altered, notify prescriber and expect a dosage adjustment.

! **WARNING** Monitor patient for hypersensitivity, which may become life threatening; such as angioedema and for fever, rash, or lymphadenopathy in association with other organ system dysfunction that may be suggestive of DRESS. Although rare, DRESS may be life-threatening. If hypersensitivity occurs, including a rash or DRESS is suspected, notify prescriber immediately and expect lamotrigine to be discontinued. Provide supportive care, as needed and ordered.

! **WARNING** Monitor patient for adverse reactions, especially suicidal thoughts, at start of therapy and with each dosage increase.

! **WARNING** Monitor patient closely for signs and symptoms of aseptic meningitis, such as fever, headache, nausea, nuchal rigidity, or vomiting. Additional signs and symptoms may include altered consciousness, chills, myalgia, photophobia, rash, and somnolence. These symptoms may occur within 1 day to 1.5 months following the initiation of lamotrigine therapy. Notify prescriber immediately, if suspected, and expect drug to be discontinued.

! **WARNING** Monitor patient for seizure activity during lamotrigine therapy. Institute seizure precautions.

! **WARNING** Monitor patient closely for signs and symptoms of hemophagocytic lymphohistiocytosis, such as coagulation abnormalities, cytopenias, fever, hepatosplenomegaly, liver dysfunction, lymphadenopathy, neurologic symptoms, and rash that may occur within 8 to 24 days from start of lamotrigine therapy. Be aware that this is a life-threatening condition of extreme systemic inflammation.

- Expect to taper dosage over at least 2 weeks, even for treatment of bipolar disorder, to avoid stopping lamotrigine abruptly, which may increase seizure activity.

PATIENT TEACHING

- Instruct patient how to take the form of lamotrigine prescribed.
- Advise patient to take lamotrigine exactly as prescribed and not to stop drug abruptly because seizure activity may increase.

! **WARNING** Instruct patient to seek immediate emergency help or call local poison control center if too much lamotrigine is taken.

! **WARNING** Tell family or caregiver to monitor patient for suicidal behavior or thoughts, especially when therapy begins or dosage changes and to report any occurrence to prescriber.

! **WARNING** Alert patient that drug may cause an allergic reaction or serious skin reactions. If present, tell patient to notify prescriber and, if severe, to seek immediate medical care.

! **WARNING** Inform patient that excessive immune activation may occur with lamotrigine therapy and to immediately report fever, rash, or swollen lymph nodes.

! **WARNING** Advise patient to notify prescriber immediately if she develops any combination of an abnormal sensitivity to light, chills, confusion, drowsiness, fever, headache, myalgia, nausea, rash, stiff neck, or vomiting while taking lamotrigine. Also, instruct patient to report increased seizure activity, irregular pulse, vision changes, and vomiting.

! **WARNING** Review with mothers who are breastfeeding signs and symptoms of drug toxicity to watch for in their infant. If present, instruct the mother to seek immediate medical attention for the infant and discontinue breastfeeding.

- Caution patient to avoid hazardous activities until drug's CNS effects are known and resolved.
- Advise patient to avoid direct sunlight and to wear protective clothing to minimize risk of photosensitivity.
- Advise patient that if syncope occurs, to lie down with legs raised and contact prescriber.
- Tell females of childbearing age to notify prescriber if she becomes pregnant

as dosage may need to be adjusted. Also, instruct females of childbearing age taking estrogen-containing oral contraceptive preparations containing 30 mcg ethinyl estradiol and 150 mcg levonorgestrel to use a different contraceptive method because of decreased blood levels of both drugs.

- Instruct patient to wear or carry medical identification stating that she takes lamotrigine.

NEW!

landiolol

Rapiblyk

Class and Category

Pharmacologic class: Beta adrenergic blocker

Therapeutic class: Antiarrhythmic

Indications and Dosages

∗ *To reduce ventricular rate short-term in patients with supraventricular tachycardia including atrial fibrillation and atrial flutter*

I.V. INFUSION

Adults with normal cardiac function. *Initial:* 9 mcg/kg/min titrated every 10 min by 9 mcg/kg/min, as needed. *Maximum:* 36 mcg/kg/min.

Adults with impaired cardiac function. *Initial:* 1 mcg/kg/min titrated every 15 min by 1 mcg/kg/min, as needed. *Maximum:* 36 mcg/kg/min.

±**DOSAGE ADJUSTMENT** For patients transitioning from landiolol to an oral beta-blocker, landiolol infusion rate reduced 10 min after administration of the oral beta-blocker. If satisfactory control is maintained for at least 1 hr, landiolol infusion discontinued. For patients with mild hepatic impairment, titration rate is done more conservatively.

Drug Administration

I.V.

- Reconstitute each 280 mg drug vial with 50 ml of 0.9% Sodium Chloride Injection or 5% Dextrose Injection. Gently swirl to dissolve contents. Reconstituted solution should be clear and colorless.
- Avoid infusing drug into small veins or through a butterfly catheter.
- Administer drug immediately but, if not possible, and drug was reconstituted with 0.9% Sodium Chloride Injection, store at room temperature and use within 4 hr or if drug was reconstituted with 5% Dextrose Injection, store at room temperature and use within 48 hr.
- Following reconstitution, the solution contains 280 mg landiolol/50 ml which equals 5.6 mg/ml. Calculate infusion rate using the following formula. Infusion rate (ml/hr) = target dose (mcg/kg/min) x body weight (kg)/93.
- Monitor patient for a local infusion site reaction throughout the infusion. If a reaction occurs, change infusion site. Avoid extravasation.
- Monitor patient's blood pressure, heart rate, and heart rhythm during infusion. Expect to reduce or stop infusion if bradycardia or hypotension occurs. Know that blood pressure should return to pre-infusion level within 30 min.
- Monitor patients with reactive airway disease for bronchospasms during infusion. These patients may be titrated to the lowest possible effective dose. If bronchospasms still occur, notify prescriber immediately, expect infusion to be stopped and be prepared to administer a beta-2 stimulating agent, as ordered.
- Do not abruptly discontinue drug in patients with coronary artery disease because severe exacerbations of angina, MI, or ventricular arrhythmias may occur.

Route	Onset	Peak	Duration
I.V.	Unknown	15 min	Unknown

Half-life: 4.5 min

Mechanism of Action

Reduces heart rate by inhibiting the positive chronotropic effects of catecholamines, epinephrine and norepinephrine, on the heart, where beta-1-receptors are predominantly located.

Contraindications

Cardiogenic shock, decompensated heart failure, heart block greater than first degree, hypersensitivity to landiolol or its components, pulmonary hypertension, severe sinus bradycardia, sick sinus syndrome

Interactions

DRUGS

catecholamine depleting drugs such as MAO inhibitors, reserpine: Possibly additive effects, which may increase risk of hypotension or marked bradycardia leading to postural hypotension, syncope, or vertigo
chronotropes, negative inotropes: Possibly increased depression of myocardial contractility increasing risk of bradycardia or heart block
positive inotropes, sympathomimetics, vasoconstrictors: Antagonizes effects of landiolol, which may reduce the ability of the drug to lower heart rate and blood pressure

Adverse Reactions

CV: Anginal attacks exacerbated (Prinzmetal's angina), **bradycardia**, **cardiogenic shock**, **hypotension**, **heart failure**, peripheral circulatory disorders exacebated (peripheral occlusive vascular disease, Raynaud's disease)
ENDO: **Prolonged or severe hypoglycemia**
GU: **Hyperkalemic renal tubular acidosis**
RESP: **Bronchospasm**
Other: **Anaphylaxis**, **hyperkalemia**, infusion reactions (erythema, pain, swelling)

Childbearing Considerations

PREGNANCY

- Drug may cause fetal harm increasing risk of bradycardia, hypoglycemia, hypotension, and respiratory depression to occur at birth.
- Use with caution only if benefit to mother outweighs potential risk to fetus.

LACTATION

- It is not known if drug is present in breast milk.
- While breastfeeding is unlikely to occur during drug therapy, mothers should check with prescriber before resuming breastfeeding.
- The breastfed infant should be monitored for bradycardia and other symptoms of beta blockage, such as lethargy caused by hypoglycemia.

Nursing Considerations

! **WARNING** Be aware landiolol is not recommended in patients with moderate or severe hepatic impairment.

! **WARNING** Monitor patient for hypersensitivity reactions that may become life-threatening, such as anaphylaxis. If present, notify prescriber immediately, expect drug to be discontinued, and provide supportive care, as needed and ordered. Be aware that beta blocker use may make patient unresponsive to the usual doses of epinephrine used to treat anaphylactoid reactions.

- Know that patients at higher risk for developing hypotension include patients with hemodynamic compromise, hypovolemia, or are on interacting drugs, especially if blood pressure is low before infusion starts. Also know that patients at greater risk for developing bradycardia, including cardiac arrest, heart block, severe bradycardia, and sinus pause include patients with conduction disorders, first-degree atrioventricular block, or sinus node dysfunction. Monitor patient's blood pressure and heart rate and rhythm closely.

! **WARNING** Monitor patient for cardiogenic shock or heart failure because beta-blockers such as landiolol can depress myocardial contractility. Notify prescriber immediately at the first sign of heart failure, expect landiolol therapy to be discontinued, and provide supportive therapy, as needed and ordered.

! **WARNING** Monitor patients for hypoglycemia, especially patients with diabetes mellitus or patients who are fasting because of surgery, not eating regularly or are vomiting. Be aware that beta-blockers may hide early warning signs of hypoglycemia, such as tachycardia, and increase the risk for prolonged or severe hypoglycemia that may occur at any time during treatment.

! **WARNING** Monitor patient's serum potassium levels, as ordered and patient for signs and symptoms of hyperkalemia, especially in patients with risk factors such as renal impairment. Know that I.V. administration of beta-blockers such as landiolol may cause life-threatening hyperkalemia in hemodialysis patients. In addition, know that drug may cause hyperkalemic renal tubular acidosis.

! **WARNING** Monitor patients with hyperthyroidism because drug may hide certain signs of hyperthyroidism such as tachycardia. Be aware that abrupt withdrawal of beta blockade might precipitate thyroid storm. Monitor patients for signs of thyrotoxicosis when landiolol therapy is discontinued.

- Monitor patients with Prinzmetal's angina for increased anginal attacks because beta-blockers cause unopposed alpha receptor-mediated coronary artery vasoconstriction.
- Be prepared to administer an alpha-blocker, as ordered, in combination with landiolol therapy in patients with pheochromocytoma to prevent a paradoxical increase in the patient's blood pressure.
- Monitor patients with peripheral occlusive vascular disease or Raynaud's disease for increase in signs and symptoms because landiolol therapy may exacerbate peripheral circulatory disorders.
- Monitor patient for myocardial ischemia when landiolol therapy is discontinued.

PATIENT TEACHING

- Inform patient that drug will be administered as an intravenous infusion.

! **WARNING** Alert patient that drug may cause an allergic reaction and to notify staff immediately if signs and symptoms of an allergic reaction occurs.

- Tell patient that frequent vital signs will be taken to assess patient's reaction to drug. Stress importance of reporting any sudden or unusual adverse effects to the staff immediately.

! **WARNING** Inform patient that blood glucose levels will be monitored during drug therapy, especially if patient is a diabetic or is in a fasting state because of surgery, unable to eat, or vomiting. Review signs and symptoms of hypoglycemia and to report any such effects immediately to the staff.

lansoprazole

Prevacid, Prevacid-24 Hour, Prevacid SoluTab

dexlansoprazole

Dexilant

Class and Category

Pharmacologic class: Proton pump inhibitor
Therapeutic class: Antiulcer

Indications and Dosages

∗ *To treat duodenal ulcers short-term and maintain healed duodenal ulcers*

D.R. CAPSULES, D.R. SUSPENSION, D.R. ORALLY DISINTEGRATING TABLETS (LANSOPRAZOLE)

Adults. 15 mg daily for 4 wk. *Maintenance:* 15 mg daily.

∗ *To treat benign gastric ulcers short-term*

D.R. CAPSULES, D.R. SUSPENSION, D.R. ORALLY DISINTEGRATING TABLETS (LANSOPRAZOLE)

Adults. 30 mg daily for up to 8 wk.

∗ *To treat NSAID-associated gastric ulcer and risk reduction for NSAID-associated gastric ulcer in patients who need to continue NSAID therapy*

D.R. CAPSULES, D.R. SUSPENSION, D.R. ORALLY DISINTEGRATING TABLETS (LANSOPRAZOLE)

Adults. 30 mg daily for 8 wk. *Risk reduction:* 15 mg daily for up to 12 wk.

∗ *To treat symptomatic gastroesophageal reflux disease (GERD) short-term*

D.R. CAPSULES, D.R. SUSPENSION, D.R. ORALLY DISINTEGRATING TABLETS (LANSOPRAZOLE)

Adults and children ages 12 to 17. 15 mg daily for up to 8 wk.
Children ages 1 to 11 weighing more than 30 kg (66 lb). 30 mg once daily for up to 12 wk.
Children ages 1 to 11 weighing 30 kg (66 lb) or less. 15 mg once daily for up to 12 wk.

∗ *To treat symptomatic nonerosive gastroesophageal reflux disease*

JKL

D.R. CAPSULES (DEXLANSOPRAZOLE)

Adults and children ages 12 and older. 30 mg once daily for 4 wk.

∗ *To heal all grades of erosive esophagitis*

D.R. CAPSULES (DEXLANSOPRAZOLE)

Adults and children ages 12 and older. 60 mg once daily for up to 8 wk.

∗ *To treat erosive esophagitis short-term*

D.R. CAPSULES, D.R. SUSPENSION, D.R. ORALLY DISINTEGRATING TABLETS (LANSOPRAZOLE)

Adults and children ages 12 and older. 30 mg once daily for up to 8 wk. Course may be repeated an additional 8 wk, as needed (adults).

Children ages 1 to 11 weighing more than 30 kg (66 lb). 30 mg once daily for up to 12 wk.

Children ages 1 to 11 weighing 30 kg (66 lb) or less. 15 mg once daily for up to 12 wk.

∗ *To maintain healed erosive esophagitis*

D.R. CAPSULES, D.R. SUSPENSION, D.R. ORALLY DISINTEGRATING TABLETS (LANSOPRAZOLE)

Adults and children ages 12 and older. 15 mg once daily.

D.R. CAPSULES (DEXLANSOPRAZOLE)

Adults and children ages 12 and older. 30 mg once daily.

∗ *To treat pathological hypersecretory conditions, such as Zollinger-Ellison syndrome*

D.R. CAPSULES, D.R. SUSPENSION, D.R. ORALLY DISINTEGRATING TABLETS (LANSOPRAZOLE)

Adults. *Initial:* 60 mg daily, increased, as needed, according to patient's condition. Doses exceeding 120 mg/day administered in divided doses.

∗ *To eradicate* Helicobacter pylori *to reduce risk of duodenal ulcer recurrence*

D.R. CAPSULES, D.R. SUSPENSION, D.R. ORALLY DISINTEGRATING TABLETS (LANSOPRAZOLE)

Adults. 30 mg plus 1 g amoxicillin and 500 mg clarithromycin every 12 hr for 10 to 14 days or 30 mg plus 1 g amoxicillin 3 times daily for 14 days.

∗ *To treat frequent heartburn*

E.R. CAPSULES (PREVACID 24-HR)

Adults. 15 mg daily for 14 days. May repeat course every 4 mo.

±**DOSAGE ADJUSTMENT** For patients with severe hepatic impairment prescribed lansoprazole, dosage not to exceed 15 mg daily regardless of condition being treated. For patients with moderate hepatic impairment prescribed dexlansoprazole for the healing of erosive esophagitis, dosage not to exceed 30 mg once daily.

Drug Administration

P.O.

- Antacids may be administered with drug.
- Drug should be administered at least 30 min before taking sucralfate, if prescribed.
- D.R. capsules (lansoprazole) should be administered before meals and not chewed or crushed. D.R. capsules (dexlansoprazole) may be administered with or without food but should be swallowed whole, without chewing.
- For patient who has difficulty swallowing D. R. lansoprazole capsules, open and sprinkle on 60 ml of apple, orange, or tomato juice. Mix briefly and have patient swallow immediately. Rinse glass with 60 ml of juice and have patient swallow immediately to ensure entire contents have been given. Alternatively, D. R. lansoprazole capsule may be opened and sprinkled on 1 tablespoon of either applesauce, cottage cheese, ENSURE, pudding, or strained pears. Have patient swallow mixture immediately.
- For patient who has difficulty swallowing capsules and is taking dexlansoprazole brand, place one tablespoon of applesauce into a clean container and sprinkle capsule contents on applesauce. Administer immediately, making sure patient does not chew granules. Do not save mixture. Alternatively, dexlansoprazole granules may be mixed with 20 ml of water, gently swirled, withdrawn into a syringe, and administered. After administration, syringe should be refilled with 10 ml of water, swirled gently, and administered.
- D.R. capsules may be opened and administered through a nasogastric tube (16 French or greater) by opening and sprinkling contents into 40 ml of apple juice (lansoprazole) or mixed with 20 ml of water (dexlansoprazole). Mix briefly and draw up mixture using a catheter-tipped syringe. Inject drug mixture through the nasogastric

tube. Flush with additional fluid used to mix drug to clear the tube.

- D.R. suspension should be administered before meals. Shake well before use. Use the calibrated device that comes with drug to measure dose. May be given through feeding tubes; flush the tube afterward.
- To administer D.R. orally disintegrating tablets, place tablet on patient's tongue with gloved hand without breaking or cutting it. Tablet should disintegrate in less than 1 min.
- For patient who has difficulty using orally disintegrating tablets, place a 15-mg tablet in oral syringe and draw up 4 ml of water or place a 30-mg tablet in oral syringe and draw up 10 ml of water. Shake gently. After tablet has been dispersed, administer contents into patient's mouth within 15 min of mixing. Refill syringe with about 2 ml (for 15-mg tablet) or 5 ml (for 30-mg tablet) of water, shake gently, and administer any remaining contents.
- For patient with a nasogastric tube 8 French or greater who is prescribed orally disintegrating tablets, place tablet in catheter-tip syringe and draw up 4 ml of water (for 15-mg tablet) or 10 ml of water (for 30-mg tablet). Shake gently. After tablet has dispersed, shake syringe gently again to keep granules from settling and immediately inject mixture through the nasogastric tube within 15 min of mixing. Refill syringe with about 5 ml of water, shake gently, and flush tube.

Route	Onset	Peak	Duration
P.O./D.R.	1–3 hr	1.7 hr	> 24 hr

Half-life: < 2 hr

Mechanism of Action

Binds to and inactivates the hydrogen-potassium adenosine triphosphate enzyme system (also called the proton pump) in gastric parietal cells. This action blocks the final step of gastric acid production.

Contraindications

Concurrent therapy with rilpivirine-containing products, hypersensitivity to lansoprazole or its components

Interactions

DRUGS

antiretrovirals, such as atazanavir, nelfinavir, rilpivirine: Possible decreased antiviral effect and increased risk of drug resistance to antiretroviral
dasatinib, erlotinib, iron salts, itraconazole, ketoconazole, mycophenolate mofetil, nilotinib, other drugs that depend on low gastric pH for bioavailability: Inhibited absorption of these drugs
digoxin: Increased digoxin absorption with possible toxicity
methotrexate: Possibly elevated methotrexate levels, which may cause toxicity
rifampin, St. John's wort, and other strong CYP2C19 or CYP3A4 inducers: Decreased plasma levels of dexlansoprazole
saquinavir: Possibly increased toxicity of saquinavir
sucralfate: Decreased and delayed lansoprazole absorption
tacrolimus: Possibly increased blood tacrolimus levels
theophylline: Increased clearance of theophylline reducing effectiveness
voriconazole and other strong CYP2C19 or CYP3A4 inhibitors: Increased exposure of lansoprazole possibly causing toxicity
warfarin: Increased INR and PT with possibly increased risk of serious bleeding

Adverse Reactions

CNS: **CVA**, dizziness, headache, transient ischemic attack
EENT: Blurred vision, deafness, oral edema oropharyngeal pain, **pharyngeal edema**, **throat tightness**
GI: Abdominal pain, anorexia, ***Clostridioides difficile*–associated diarrhea**, diarrhea, elevated liver enzymes, flatulence, fundic gland polyps, **hepatitis**, **hepatotoxicity**, increased appetite, nausea, **pancreatitis**, vomiting
GU: **Acute renal failure**, acute tubulointerstitial nephritis, erectile dysfunction, urine retention
HEME: **Agranulocytosis**, **aplastic anemia**, decreased hemoglobin, **hemolytic anemia**, **idiopathic thrombocytopenic purpura**, **leukopenia**, **neutropenia**, **pancytopenia**, **thrombocytopenia**, **thrombotic thrombocytopenic purpura**

MS: Arthralgia, bone fracture, bursitis, myositis
RESP: Upper respiratory tract infection
SKIN: Acute generalized exanthematous pustulosis, cutaneous lupus erythematosus, **erythema multiforme**, **exfoliative dermatitis**, leukocytoclastic vasculitis, pruritus, rash, **Stevens-Johnson syndrome**, **toxic epidermal necrolysis**
Other: **Anaphylactic shock**, **hyperkalemia**, **drug reaction with eosinophilia and systemic symptoms (DRESS)**, **hypersensitivity reactions (acute tubulointerstitial nephritis**, **anaphylaxis**, **angioedema**, **bronchospasm**, urticaria), **hypocalcemia**, **hypokalemia**, **hypomagnesemia**, **hyponatremia**, injection-site reaction, systemic lupus erythematosus, vitamin B_{12} deficiency

Childbearing Considerations

PREGNANCY

- It is not known if drug causes fetal harm.
- Use with caution only if benefit to mother outweighs potential risk to fetus.

LACTATION

- It is not known if drug is present in breast milk.
- Mothers should check with prescriber before breastfeeding.

Nursing Considerations

! **WARNING** Know that drug should not be given to children under 1 year of age because of the potential risk of heart valve thickening.

! **WARNING** Expect to obtain calcium, magnesium, and potassium levels prior to initiating lansoprazole therapy and then periodically during drug therapy, as ordered. Also, monitor patient for hypomagnesemia, especially high-risk patients (e.g., presence of hypoparathyroidism) or who takes lansoprazole with other drugs such as digoxin or drugs that may cause hypomagnesemia such as diuretics. Hypomagnesemia may cause arrhythmias, seizures, and tetany because hypomagnesemia may lead to hypocalcemia and/or hypokalemia and may exacerbate underlying hypocalcemia in patients at risk. If patient is to remain on lansoprazole long term, expect to monitor patient's serum magnesium level, as ordered, and if level becomes low, anticipate that magnesium replacement therapy will need to be started, and lansoprazole discontinued.

! **WARNING** Monitor patient closely for hypersensitivity reactions and serious skin reactions that may become life-threatening. If present, notify prescriber, expect drug to be discontinued at first sign of a hypersensitivity reaction or severe cutaneous adverse reactions. DRESS usually exhibits a rash as the first sign but may only present with a fever or swollen lymph nodes. Provide supportive measures, as needed and ordered.

! **WARNING** Be aware that diarrhea from *Clostridioides difficile* infection can occur with or without concurrent antibiotics when lansoprazole is used. *C. difficile*–associated diarrhea may be mild or become life-threatening. If *C. difficile*–associated diarrhea is suspected, notify prescriber and expect to obtain a stool specimen to confirm. If confirmed, expect drug to be withheld and provide treatment with an antibiotic effective against *C. difficile*, electrolytes, fluids, and protein supplementation, as ordered.

! **WARNING** Monitor patient for renal dysfunction because drug may cause acute renal failure at any point during lansoprazole therapy. Expect drug to be discontinued if it occurs.

- Monitor patient for cutaneous and systemic lupus erythematosus either as new onset or exacerbation of existing disorder. Know that cutaneous lupus erythematosus occurs more commonly. Expect lansoprazole to be discontinued if present.
- Monitor patient for bone fracture, especially in patients receiving multiple daily doses for more than a year because proton pump inhibitors, such as lansoprazole, increase risk for osteoporosis-related fractures of the hip, spine, or wrist.
- Be aware that long-term use (especially more than one year) of lansoprazole increases risk for the development of fundic

gland polyps. Be aware that drug should be given for the shortest duration possible for the condition being treated.

- Be aware that drug may cause false-positive results in diagnostic investigations for neuroendocrine tumors. Expect drug to be temporarily discontinued for at least 14 days before testing is done. Also, know that drug can cause a hyper-response in gastrin secretion in response to secretin stimulation test. Expect lansoprazole to be temporarily withheld at least 30 days before assessment is done. Be aware that false-positive urine screening tests for tetrahydrocannabinol may occur during lansoprazole therapy.

PATIENT TEACHING

- Instruct patient how to administer form of drug prescribed. Urge patient to take drug exactly as prescribed.
- Inform patient antacids may be taken with lansoprazole or dexlansoprazole. But also tell patient to inform all prescribers of lansoprazole therapy.

! **WARNING** Alert patient that drug may cause an allergic reaction, including serious skin reactions. Tell patient to notify prescriber if an allergic or serious skin reaction occurs such as fever, rash, or swollen lymph nodes. If severe, urge patient to seek immediate medical care.

! **WARNING** Urge patient to tell prescriber about diarrhea that's severe or lasts longer than 3 days. Remind patient that bloody or watery stools can occur 2 or more months after therapy and can be serious, requiring prompt treatment.

! **WARNING** Instruct patient to notify prescriber of any persistent, serious, or unusual adverse reactions. If severe, urge patient to seek immediate medical care.

lanthanum carbonate

Fosrenol

Class and Category

Pharmacologic class: Rare earth element
Therapeutic class: Phosphate binder

Indications and Dosages

✱ *To reduce serum phosphate levels in patients with end-stage renal disease*

ORAL POWDER, TABLETS (CHEWABLE)

Adults. *Initial:* 500 mg 3 times daily with or immediately after meals, increased, as needed, by 750 mg daily every 2 to 3 wk until acceptable serum phosphate level is reached. *Usual:* 1,500 to 3,000 mg daily in divided doses.

Drug Administration

P.O.

- Administer drug with or immediately after meals.
- Chewable tablets should be chewed thoroughly before swallowing or, if patient has trouble chewing tablets, they can be crushed.
- Sprinkle oral powder form on a small quantity of applesauce or other similar foods and administer immediately. Do not store mixture once powder is mixed with food. Do not dissolve in liquid for administration because the powder is insoluble.
- Administer drugs with a narrow therapeutic range at least 1 hr before or 3 hr after lanthanum administration; quinolone antibiotics at least 1 hr before or 4 hr after lanthanum administration; and drugs which bind to cationic antacids (i.e., aluminum-calcium,-magnesium based) such as ACE inhibitors, antimalarials, ampicillin, statin lipid regulators, tetracyclines, and thyroid hormones) at least 2 hr before or 2 hr after lanthanum administration.

Route	Onset	Peak	Duration
P.O.	Unknown	0.5–3 hr	Unknown

Half-life: 53 hr

Contraindications

Bowel obstruction, fecal impaction, hypersensitivity to lanthanum carbonate or any of its components, hypophosphatemia, ileus

Interactions

DRUGS

ACE inhibitors; antibiotics, such as ampicillin, fluoroquinolones or tetracyclines; antimalarials; drugs with narrow therapeutic

Mechanism of Action

Releases phosphate during digestion into the upper GI tract (below left) and absorbed into the bloodstream, increasing serum phosphate levels. In patients with end-stage renal disease, however, inefficient phosphate clearance from the blood leads to abnormally elevated levels.

Lanthanum dissociates in the upper GI tract, releasing ions that attach to unbound phosphate to form an insoluble complex (below right). Unabsorbed into the bloodstream, these altered phosphate molecules can't elevate the patient's serum phosphate level.

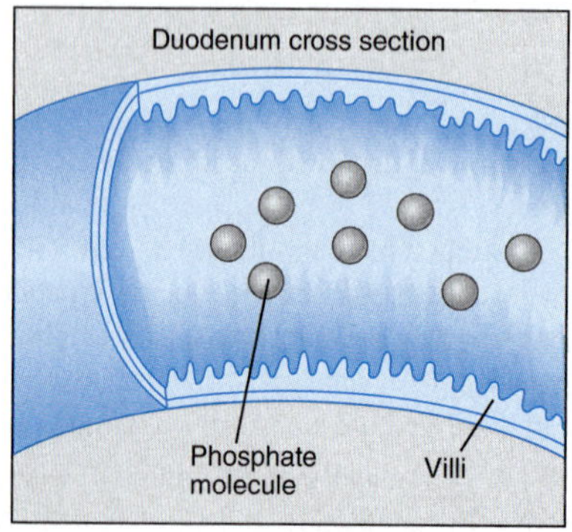

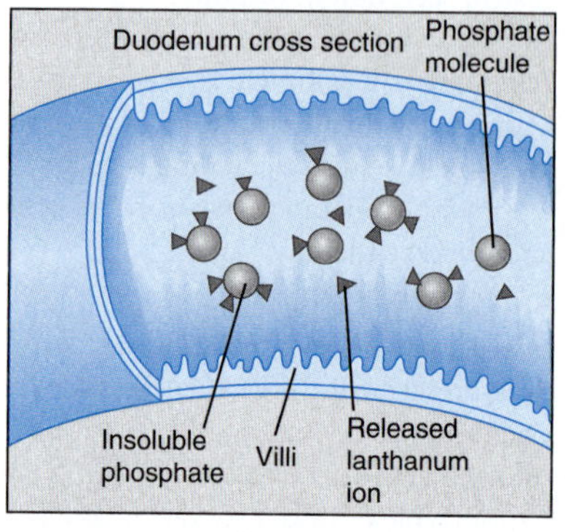

range; statins; thyroid hormones: Possibly reduced bioavailability with these drugs

Adverse Reactions

CNS: Headache
CV: **Hypotension**
EENT: Rhinitis, tooth injury while chewing tablet
GI: Abdominal pain, constipation, diarrhea, dyspepsia, fecal impaction, **GI obstruction or perforation**, ileus, nausea, subileus, vomiting
GU: Dialysis graft occlusion
RESP: Bronchitis
SKIN: Pruritus, rash, urticaria
Other: **Hypercalcemia**, **hypocalcemia**, **hypophosphatemia**

Childbearing Considerations

PREGNANCY

- It is not known if drug causes fetal harm.
- Drug is not recommended for use during pregnancy.

LACTATION

- It is not known if drug is present in breast milk.
- Drug is not recommended during breastfeeding.

Nursing Considerations

- Use lanthanum carbonate cautiously in patients with acute peptic ulcer, Crohn's disease, or ulcerative colitis because drug effects are unknown in these patients.
- Monitor the patient's serum phosphate levels, as ordered, especially during dosage adjustment, to determine effectiveness of lanthanum carbonate therapy. Serum phosphate levels should fall below 6 mg/dl.

! WARNING Monitor patient closely for signs and symptoms of bowel obstruction, fecal impaction, or ileus, especially the patient with a history of colon cancer, GI surgery, or hypomotility disorders, as well as patient receiving calcium channel blockers. Notify prescriber, if present, because these GI adverse effects may become serious enough to require hospitalization or surgery. Expect drug to be discontinued in patients with adverse GI effects if there is no other identifiable cause for the GI dysfunction.

- Be aware that drug may show product residue during endoscopic imaging.

PATIENT TEACHING

- Instruct patient how to administer form of lanthanum carbonate prescribed.

- Urge patient to take drug exactly as prescribed and explain that it may take weeks to reach a desired serum phosphate level.

! **WARNING** Advise patient to notify prescriber if she experiences GI discomfort that becomes prolonged or severe.

- Tell females of childbearing age to notify prescriber if pregnancy occurs as drug will need to be discontinued.
- Instruct mothers that breastfeeding should not be undertaken during lanthanum therapy.

NEW!

lebrikizumab-lbkz

Ebglyss

Class and Category

Pharmacologic class: Interleukin-13 antagonist
Therapeutic class: Anti-inflammatory

Indications and Dosages

∗ *To treat moderate-to-severe atopic dermatitis in patients not adequately controlled with topical prescription therapies or when those therapies are not advisable.*

SUBCUTANEOUS INJECTION

Adults and children ages 12 and older weighing at least 40 kg (88 lb). *Initial:* 500 mg (two 250 mg injections) and repeated at wk 2, followed by 250 mg once every 2 wk until wk 16 or later, whenever adequate clinical response is achieved. *Maintenance:* 250 mg every 4 wk.

Drug Administration

SUBCUTANEOUS

- Remove prefilled pen or syringe from refrigerator. Pen can be used immediately. Syringe must be left at room temperature for 45 min before use with needle cap in place. Do not warm syringe any other way.
- Do not shake pen or syringe at any time.
- Protect pen or syringe from light until administration.
- Do not use if pen or syringe is dropped on a hard surface because of glass parts. Handle with care.
- Drug solution should appear opalescent, colorless to slightly yellow to slightly brown. Do not use if solution appears frozen or appears cloudy, discolored, or has particles.
- Choose site for administration, which includes abdomen, back of upper arm, or thigh. Do not inject within 2 in (5 cm) of the navel or into areas where skin is bruised, hard, red, or tender, or in an area of skin affected by atopic dermatitis or a skin lesion. Rotate sites.
- If using pen, prepare it for use by twisting off the gray base cap (do not put gray base cap back on as this may damage the needle). Place and hold the clear base flat and firmly against the skin. While keeping base on skin, turn the lock ring to the unlock position. Press and hold the purple injection button and listen for 2 loud clicks. The second click indicates the injection is finished, which may take up to 15 sec. The gray plunger should then be visible. Be aware that a soft click may be heard right before the second loud click. This is normal. Do not remove the pen from the skin until a second loud click is heard. Once pen is removed, do not rub the injection site.
- If using syringe, prepare it for use by first holding it in the middle of the syringe body and pull the needle cap straight off. Do not put the needle cap back on as this could damage the needle. Gently pinch a fold of skin at the injection site with other hand. Insert the needle completely into the fold of skin at about a 45-degree angle. Gently relax the pinch while keeping needle in place. Push the plunger rod all the way down as far as it will go to inject all the drug. Know that it is normal to feel some resistance. Also, know that a full dose must be given to activate the needle shield. Once injection is done, lift thumb to release plunger rod until needle is covered by the needle shield. Remove needle from skin. Do not rub the skin after the injection.
- Store unused pens or syringes in refrigerator although they can be stored at room temperature for up to 7 days if left in the original carton. Throw away if left at room temperature longer than 7 days.
- Administer a missed dose as soon as possible and then resume dosing at the regular scheduled time.

Route	Onset	Peak	Duration
SubQ	Unknown	7-8 days	Unknown

Half-life: 24.5 days

Mechanism of Action

Binds to human interleukin-13 (IL-13) to inhibit its interaction with selected IL-13 receptors. This action inhibits the release of proinflammatory cytokines, chemokines, and IgE to reduce inflammation found with atopic dermatitis.

Contraindications

Hypersensitivity to lebrikizumab-lbkz or its components

Interactions

DRUGS

live vaccines: Possibly increased risk of infection

Adverse Reactions

EENT: Conjunctivitis, keratitis
HEME: Eosinophilia
SKIN: Urticaria
Other: **Angioedema**, injection site reactions (dermatitis, erythema, pain, pruritus, rash, swelling)

Childbearing Considerations

PREGNANCY

- Pregnancy exposure registry: 1-800-545-5979.
- It is not known if drug can cause fetal harm.
- Use with caution only if benefit to mother outweighs potential risk to fetus.

LACTATION

- It is not known if drug is present in breast milk.
- Mothers should check with prescriber before breastfeeding.

Nursing Considerations

- Expect patients with preexisting helminth infections to be treated for the infection before lebrikizumab-lbkz is begun. Be aware that if patient develops a helminth infection during drug therapy and does not respond to treatment, drug will need to be withheld until the infection is eradicated.
- Ensure that all appropriate vaccinations have been completed before lebrikizumab-lbkz therapy begins because drug alters patient's immune response.
- Know that lebrikizumab-lbkz can be used with or without topical corticosteroids. However, while calcineurin topical treatment may be used, it should only be used on sensitive areas, such as face, genital and intertriginous areas, and neck.

! **WARNING** Monitor patient closely for a hypersensitivity reaction such as angioedema. If present, notify prescriber immediately, expect drug to be discontinued, and provide supportive care, as needed and ordered.

PATIENT TEACHING

- Train patient, family, or caregiver how to administer drug by a subcutaneous injection using the pen or syringe method and what injection sites to use. Tell patient with a hearing or visual problem to have help in giving the injection from family or a caregiver.

! **WARNING** Alert patient that drug may cause an allergic reaction. If an allergic reaction is present, tell patient to notify prescriber and, if severe, to seek immediate medical care.

- Alert patient to report new or worsening eye symptoms.
- Advise patient not to receive vaccinations using live vaccines during lebrikizumab-lbkz therapy. Also, tell patient to inform prescriber of lebrikizumab-lbkz therapy before non-live vaccines are administered.

lecanemab-irmb

Leqembi

Class and Category

Pharmacologic class: Amyloid beta-directed monoclonal antibody
Therapeutic class: antidementia

Indications and Dosages

* *To treat Alzheimer's disease in patients with mild cognitive impairment or mild dementia stage of disease*

I.V. INFUSION

Adults. 10 mg/kg infused over 1 hr, once every 2 wk for 18 months then continued at same dose given every 2 wk or transitioned to maintenance dose. *Maintenance:* 10 mg/kg once every 4 wks.

± **DOSAGE ADJUSTMENT** For patients with amyloid-related imaging abnormalities with edema (ARIA-E), of any degree and moderate to severe symptoms, drug may be suspended for a time (usually 2 to 4 months), For patients who have mild ARIA-E severity on MRI and are either asymptomatic or have mild symptoms, dosing may continue while moderate ARIA-E severity on MRI even if patient is asymptomatic or mild, dosing suspended for a time (usually 2 to 4 months). For patients with mild amyloid-related imaging abnormalities with hemosiderin deposits (ARIA-H and the patient is asymptomatic, dosing may continue or if ARIA-H severity is moderate to severe, dosing suspended for about 2 to 4 months while patient who is symptomatic with any degree of ARIA-H severity, dosing suspended for about 2 to 4 months.

Drug Administration

I.V.

- Store unopened vials of drug in refrigerator in the original carton to protect from light.
- Expect to premedicate patient with antihistamines, NSAIDs, or corticosteroids, as ordered, to reduce risk of infusion reactions.
- Calculate the dose in mg, the total volume of solution required in ml, and number of vials needed based on patient's actual body weight and the recommended dose of 10 mg/kg. Each vial contains a lecanemab-irmb concentration of 100 mg/ml.
- Withdraw the required volume of drug from the vial(s) and dilute drug in 250 ml of 0.9% Sodium Chloride Injection. Solution should be clear to opalescent and colorless to pale yellow. Discard if solution is discolored or contains opaque or other foreign particles. Also, discard any unused portion left in drug vial as it is for a one-time use only.
- Gently invert infusion bag to mix drug completely in solution. Do not shake.
- Infuse immediately after dilution, if possible. If not, refrigerate or store diluted drug at room temperature for no more than 4 hours. Never freeze drug solution.
- Allow refrigerated drug solution to warm to room temperature prior to beginning infusion.
- Infuse over 1 hr using a terminal low-protein binding 0.2 micron in-line filter. After infusion, flush infusion line to be sure entire dose has been administered.
- Monitor patient for infusion reactions during and after administration. If present, notify prescriber as infusion rate may need to be reduced or the infusion discontinued and appropriate supportive care given, as needed and ordered.
- If a dose is missed, administer the next dose as soon as possible.

Route	Onset	Peak	Duration
I.V.	Unknown	Unknown	Unknown

Half-life: 5 to 7 days

Mechanism of Action

Reduces amyloid beta plaques in the brain that accumulate in Alzheimer's disease to improve cognition.

Contraindications

Hypersensitivity to lecanemab-irmb or its components

Interactions

DRUGS

None listed by manufacturer.

Adverse Reactions

CNS: Amyloid-related imaging abnormalities (ARIA) with edema (ARIA-E) or with hemosiderin deposits (ARIA-H) possibly causing confusion, dizziness, focal neurologic deficits, gait difficulty, headache, **seizures**, **status epilepticus**; **intracerebral hemorrhage**
CV: **Atrial fibrillation**
EENT: Visual changes if ARIA present
GI: Diarrhea, nausea if ARIA present
HEME: Lymphopenia
RESP: **Bronchospasm**, cough
Other: **Anaphylaxis**; **angioedema**; infusion-related reactions such as fever, flu-like symptoms (chills, feeling shaky, generalized aches, joint pain), **hypotension**, hypertension, nausea, **oxygen desaturation**, and vomiting

Childbearing Considerations

PREGNANCY

- It is not known if drug can cause fetal harm.
- Use with caution only if benefit to mother outweighs potential risk to fetus.

LACTATION

- It is not known if drug is present in breast milk.
- Mothers should check with prescriber before breastfeeding.

Nursing Considerations

- Check with prescriber if patient has been enrolled in a voluntary patient registry that collects data on treatments for Alzheimer's disease. Be aware that prescribers can enroll their patient through www.alz-net.org or by contacting alz-net@acr.org.
- Be aware that patients may experience three types of ARIA according to MRI classification criteria: ARIA-E, ARIA-H with microhemorrhage, and ARIA-H with superficial siderosis. Radiographic study of each of these classifications can be further broken down into mild, moderate, or severe.
- Know that drug should be used cautiously in patients with factors that may suggest increased risk for intracerebral hemorrhage, especially patients on anticoagulant therapy or patients with findings on MRI suggestive of cerebral amyloid angiopathy.
- Be aware drug should be used cautiously in patients who may be candidates for antithrombotic therapy or a thrombolytic agent such as tissue plasminogen activator.

! **WARNING** Know that patient should undergo testing to determine risk for ARIA because about 15% of Alzheimer's patients are apolipoprotein E4 (Apo4) homozygotes, which has a higher incidence of ARIA, including symptomatic as well as serious and severe radiographic changes, when compared to heterozygotes and noncarriers. Know that baseline brain MRI and periodic monitoring with MRI are recommended for all patients receiving lecanemab-irmb.

! **WARNING** Monitor patient closely for adverse signs and symptoms of ARIA because ARIA can occur spontaneously although it most often appears during the first 14 weeks of therapy. Also, know that patients may experience more than 1 episode while receiving lecanemab-irmb and that ARIA-E and ARIA-H of any cause can occur together. Notify prescriber if patient demonstrates any of the following signs and symptoms: confusion, dizziness, focal neurologic deficits, gait difficulty, headache, intracranial hemorrhage (can be greater than 1 cm in diameter), nausea, or visual changes. Know that because ARIA-E may cause focal neurologic deficits that mimic an ischemic stroke, ARIA-E should be considered as the possible cause before patient is treated with thrombolytic therapy. Be aware that although rare, seizures and status epilepticus may also occur. Provide supportive care, as needed and ordered knowing that symptoms usually resolve over time.

! **WARNING** Monitor patient for a hypersensivity reaction, which can become life threatening such as anaphylaxis, angioedema and/or bronchospasms. If present, notify prescriber, expect drug to be discontinued, and provide supportive care, as needed and ordered.

- Monitor patient for an infusion reaction, especially with the first infusion. Infusion reactions may present with fever, flu-like symptoms (chills, feeling shaky, generalized aches, and joint pain), hypertension, hypotension, nausea, oxygen desaturation, and vomiting. Be aware most infusion reactions are mild or moderate in severity. Notify prescriber if an infusion reaction occurs and expect infusion to be slowed or discontinued depending on the severity of the infusion.

! **WARNING** Use cautiously in patients receiving antithrombotics or a thrombolytic agent such as tissue plasminogen activator during lecanemab-irmb because of increased risk for intracerebral hemorrhages.

PATIENT TEACHING

- Inform patient, family, or caregiver lecanemab-irmb is administered by an intravenous infusion given over 1 hour every 2 weeks for 18 months and then either continued every 2 or 4 wk.

! **WARNING** Alert patient, family, or caregiver that drug may cause an allergic reaction. Stress importance of notifying staff during infusion and prescriber after infusion if patient has difficulty breathing or develops other sudden allergic adverse reactions. Tell patient who is at home to seek immediate medical care if an allergic reaction is severe.

- Review the signs and symptoms of an infusion reaction with patient, family, or caregiver and stress importance of reporting any, if present. Tell patient reactions can occur even with the first infusion.
- Tell patient, family, or caregiver that MRI scans will be done periodically to detect adverse reactions in the brain.

! **WARNING** Discuss the possibility of ARIA with patient family, or caregiver and that it commonly causes a temporary swelling in various areas of the brain. Tell patient most patients do not experience symptoms and condition is usually picked up on an MRI scan. However, review signs and symptoms of ARIA and stress importance of reporting, if present. Reassure patient that ARIA usually resolves over time.

! **WARNING** Review signs and symptoms of an intracranial bleed for the patient family, or caregiver also receiving antithrombolytics or a thrombolytic agent. Urge them to seek immediate medical care, if present.

- Advise patient, family, or caregiver that the Alzheimer's network for Treatment and Diagnostics (ALZ-NET) is a voluntary patient registry that collects information on the use of lecanemab-irmb for Alzheimer's disease. Encourage patient to ask prescriber to enroll patient.

lefamulin

Xenleta

Class and Category

Pharmacologic class: Pleuromutilin derivative
Therapeutic class: Antibacterial

Indications and Dosages

∗ *To treat community-acquired bacterial pneumonia caused by* Chlamydophila pneumoniae, Haemophilus influenzae, Legionella pneumophila, Mycoplasma pneumoniae, Staphylococcus aureus *(methicillin-susceptible isolates), or* Streptococcus pneumoniae

TABLETS

Adults. 600 mg at least 1 hr before or 2 hr after a meal every 12 hr for 5 days.

I.V. INFUSION

Adults. 150 mg infused over 60 min every 12 hr for 5 to 7 days with option to switch to oral therapy to complete course of therapy.

±**DOSAGE ADJUSTMENT** For patients with severe hepatic impairment, dosing interval increased to every 24 hours when administering drug intravenously. Oral dosage is not recommended for patients with moderate or severe hepatic impairment.

Drug Administration

P.O.

- Administer tablets at least 1 hr before a meal or 2 hr after a meal with 6 to 8 ounces of water.
- Tablets should be swallowed whole and not chewed, crushed, or split.
- If a dose is missed, administer as soon as possible and anytime up to 8 hr prior to the next scheduled dose. If less than 8 hr remain before the next scheduled dose, do not administer the missed dose and resume dosing at the next scheduled time.

I.V.

- Dilute 15 ml drug vial contents with 250-ml solution of 10-mM citrate buffered 0.9% Sodium Chloride for Injection supplied with drug. Mix thoroughly. Solution should be clear.
- After drug is diluted, it may be stored for up to 24 hr at room temperature or 48 hr if refrigerated.
- Do not use the diluent bag in series connections.
- Infuse over 60 min. Do not exceed the recommended rate of infusion of 60 min or increase the concentration of drug because the magnitude of QT prolongation may be increased.
- *Incompatibilities:* Other I.V. drugs or solutions

Route	Onset	Peak	Duration
P.O.	Unknown	0.88–2 hr	Unknown
I.V.	Unknown	Unknown	Unknown

Half-life: 8 hr

Mechanism of Action

Inhibits bacterial protein synthesis through interactions with the A- and P-sites of the peptidyl transferase center (PTC) in the V domain of the 23S rRNA of the 50S subunit.

Contraindications

Concurrent use with sensitive CYP3A4 substrates that prolong QT interval, such as pimozide; hypersensitivity to lefamulin, other pleuromutilin-class drugs, or their components

Interactions

DRUGS

drugs that prolong QT interval, such as class IA antiarrhythmics (procainamide, quinidine), class III antiarrhythmics (amiodarone, sotalol), antipsychotics, erythromycin, moxifloxacin, pimozide, tricyclic antidepressants: Increased risk of prolonged QT interval and life-threatening arrhythmias

moderate and strong CYP3A inducers, P-gp inducers: Decreased lefamulin concentration and effectiveness

moderate and strong CYP3A inhibitors, P-gp inhibitors: Increased lefamulin concentration and risk of adverse reactions

sensitive CYP3A4 substrates (alprazolam, diltiazem, pimozide, verapamil, simvastatin, vardenafil): Increased risk of cardiac conduction toxicities

Adverse Reactions

CNS: Anxiety, headache, insomnia, somnolence

CV: **Atrial fibrillation**, palpitations, **prolonged QT interval**

EENT: Oropharyngeal candidiasis

GI: Abdominal pain, ***Clostridioides difficile*-associated colitis**, constipation, diarrhea, dyspepsia, elevated liver enzymes, epigastric discomfort, erosive gastritis, nausea, vomiting

GU: Urine retention, vulvovaginal candidiasis

HEME: Anemia, **thrombocytopenia**

Other: Elevated alkaline phosphatase and creatine phosphokinase, **hypersensitivity reactions**, **hypokalemia**, injection-site reactions (pain, phlebitis, reactions)

Childbearing Considerations

PREGNANCY

- Pregnancy exposure registry: 1-855-5NABRIVA.
- Pregnancy status of females of childbearing age should be verified before drug therapy is initiated.
- Drug may cause fetal harm based on animal studies.
- Drug is not recommended for use during pregnancy and should be discontinued as soon as pregnancy is known.

LACTATION

- It is not known if drug is present in breast milk.
- Breastfeeding mothers should pump and discard breast milk for the duration of treatment with drug and for 2 days after final dose.

REPRODUCTION

- Females of childbearing age should use effective contraception during treatment with drug and for 2 days after final dose.

Nursing Considerations

! WARNING Know that lefamulin should not be given to patients with known prolongation of the QT interval or ventricular arrhythmias (including torsades de pointes), or in patients receiving class IA or class III antiarrhythmics or other drugs that prolong the QT interval. Lefamulin should also not be given to patients with hepatic impairment or renal failure (if dialysis is required) because metabolic disturbances associated with these conditions may lead to QT prolongation.

! WARNING Ensure that female patients of childbearing age have a pregnancy test performed and it is negative before lefamulin therapy is begun.

- Expect ECG monitoring in patients who are predisposed to QT prolongation for whom use of lefamulin cannot be avoided.
- Be aware that patient may be switched to the oral form of lefamulin to complete the treatment.

! WARNING Monitor patient for hypersensitivity reactions. If present, notify prescriber, expect drug to be discontinued, and provide supportive care, as needed and ordered.

! WARNING Assess patients for signs of secondary infection, such as profuse, watery diarrhea. If such diarrhea develops, contact prescriber and expect to obtain a stool specimen to rule out pseudomembranous colitis caused by *Clostridioides difficile*. Know that *C. difficile* diarrhea may be mild or become life-threatening. If confirmed, expect to discontinue lefamulin and treat with an antibiotic effective against *C. difficile*. Also, expect to administer electrolytes, fluids, and protein supplementation, as needed and ordered.

- Monitor patient with hepatic impairment for adverse reactions throughout lefamulin therapy.

PATIENT TEACHING

- Instruct patient how to administer oral form of lefamulin and what to do if a dose is missed.

! **WARNING** Warn females of childbearing age that pregnancy should be avoided during drug therapy. Tell female patients of childbearing age that a pregnancy test will be performed before lefamulin therapy is begun. Instruct these patients to use effective contraception throughout drug therapy and for 2 days after the last dose.

! **WARNING** Inform patient that allergic reactions may occur. Tell patient, if present, to notify prescriber and, if severe, to seek immediate medical care.

! **WARNING** Urge patient to tell prescriber if diarrhea develops, even 2 months or more after lefamulin therapy ends.

- Inform patient that nausea and vomiting are common adverse reactions.
- Advise patient to tell prescriber of all drugs taken, including over-the-counter drugs and herbal products because lefamulin can interact with other drugs.
- Instruct mothers who are breastfeeding to pump and discard breast milk throughout lefamulin therapy and for 2 days after the last dose.

leflunomide

Arava

Class and Category

Pharmacologic class: Pyrimidine synthesis inhibitor

Therapeutic class: Antirheumatic

Indications and Dosages

∗ *To treat active rheumatoid arthritis*

TABLETS

Adults who are at low risk for hepatotoxicity and myelosuppression. *Loading:* 100 mg daily for 3 days, followed by 20 mg daily. *Maximum:* 20 mg/day (after loading dose).

Adults at high risk for hepatotoxicity or myelosuppression. 20 mg daily without a loading dose. *Maximum:* 20 mg/day.

±**DOSAGE ADJUSTMENT** For patients for whom the drug is poorly tolerated, dosage reduced to 10 mg daily.

Drug Administration

P.O.

- Tablets given with or without food.
- Store at room temperature and protect from light.
- Be prepared to assist with an accelerated drug elimination procedure when drug is discontinued; without such a procedure it may take up to 2 yr for undetectable plasma concentrations to occur.

Route	Onset	Peak	Duration
P.O.	Unknown	6–12 hr	Unknown

Half-life: 2 wk

Mechanism of Action

Inhibits dihydroorotate dehydrogenase, the enzyme in autoimmune process that leads to rheumatoid arthritis. With this action, leflunomide relieves inflammation and prevents alteration of the autoimmune process.

Contraindications

Hypersensitivity to leflunomide, teriflunomide, or their components; pregnancy; severe hepatic impairment

Interactions

DRUGS

BCRP and organic anion transporting polypeptide B1 and B3 (AOTP1B1) substrates, such as HMG-Co reductase inhibitors (atorvastatin, nateglinide, pravastatin, repaglinide, rosuvastatin, simvastatin), methotrexate, mitoxantrone, rifampin: Elevated blood levels of these drugs

CYP1A2 substrates, such as alosetron, duloxetine, theophylline, tizanidine: Possibly decreased exposure with decreased effectiveness of these drugs

CYP2C8 substrates, such as paclitaxel, pioglitazone, repaglinide, rosiglitazone: Possibly increased levels of these drugs with increased risk of adverse reactions
oral contraceptives organic anion transporter 3 (OAT3) substrates, such as cefaclor, cimetidine, ciprofloxacin, furosemide, ketoprofen, methotrexate, penicillin G, zidovudine: Possibly increased exposure of these drugs with increased risk of adverse reactions
rifampin: Increased blood leflunomide level
warfarin: Possibly decreased peak INR by about 25%

Adverse Reactions

CNS: Anxiety, dizziness, drowsiness, fatigue, fever, headache, paresthesia, peripheral neuropathy
CV: Chest pain, hypertension, palpitations, tachycardia, vasculitis
EENT: Blurred vision, conjunctivitis, dry mouth, epistaxis, mouth ulcers, pharyngitis, rhinitis, sinusitis
GI: Abdominal pain, **acute hepatic necrosis**, cholestasis, colitis, constipation, diarrhea, elevated liver enzymes, flatulence, gastritis, gastroenteritis, **hepatic injury or failure**, **hepatitis**, **hepatotoxicity**, jaundice, nausea, **pancreatitis**, vomiting
GU: Hypophosphaturia, UTI
HEME: **Agranulocytosis**, anemia, **leukopenia**, **neutropenia**, **pancytopenia**, **thrombocytopenia**
MS: Back pain, synovitis, tendinitis
RESP: **Asthma**, bronchitis, dyspnea, **interstitial lung disease**, **pulmonary fibrosis or hypertension**, respiratory tract infection
SKIN: Alopecia (transient), cutaneous lupus erythematosus, cutaneous necrotizing vasculitis, **erythema multiforme**, erythematous rash, pruritus, pustular psoriasis, skin ulcers, **Stevens-Johnson syndrome**, **toxic epidermal necrolysis**, urticaria, worsening psoriasis
Other: **Angioedema**, **drug reaction with eosinophilia and systemic symptoms (DRESS)**, **immunosuppression including bone marrow suppression**, opportunistic infections, **sepsis**, weight loss

Childbearing Considerations

PREGNANCY

- Pregnancy exposure registry: 1-877-311-8972 or http://www.pregnancystudies.org/participate-in-a-study/.
- Drug can cause fetal harm.
- Drug is contraindicated during pregnancy.
- A negative pregnancy test must be obtained before drug therapy is begun.
- If pregnancy occurs, drug must be discontinued immediately, and an accelerated drug elimination procedure done to reduce the risk to the fetus.

LACTATION

- It is not known if drug is present in breast milk.
- Breastfeeding should be discontinued during drug therapy.

REPRODUCTION

- Females of childbearing age and female partners of men not wishing to father a child need to use an effective contraception during drug therapy and also when drug is discontinued while undergoing the drug elimination procedure until verification that the plasma teriflunomide concentration is less than 0.02 mg/L.

Nursing Considerations

! **WARNING** Know that leflunomide isn't recommended for patients with severe immunodeficiency, or severe, uncontrolled infections because of its immunosuppressant effect. Patients are at higher risk for myelosuppression if taking concomitant immunosuppressants.

! **WARNING** Be aware that drug is not recommended for patients with liver disease or those with a serum alanine aminotransferase level greater than 2 times the upper level normal prior to initiation of therapy because drug may worsen liver dysfunction. Know that patients at high risk for drug-associated hepatotoxicity are those who are taking concomitant methotrexate. Assess liver enzyme (ALT and AST) levels at start of therapy, monthly during first 6 months, and if stable, every 6 to 8 weeks thereafter, as ordered. If levels become elevated greater than 3-fold upper-level normal, notify prescriber and expect leflunomide therapy to be withheld until underlying cause is determined. If the elevation is thought to be leflunomide-induced, expect to start cholestyramine washout, as ordered, and monitor liver test weekly until normalized. If another cause is found for the elevation, expect to resume leflunomide therapy.

! **WARNING** Ensure females of childbearing age have a negative pregnancy test result before administering drug.

! **WARNING** Obtain platelet count, hemoglobin or hematocrit, and WBC count at start of therapy and every 4 to 8 weeks thereafter, as ordered because drug can cause life-threatening adverse hematological reactions.

- Test patient for latent tuberculosis before starting leflunomide, as ordered. If positive, expect standard medical treatment to be given before leflunomide therapy starts.
- Obtain baseline blood pressure before starting leflunomide and monitor periodically thereafter because drug may cause hypertension.

! **WARNING** Monitor patient for a hypersensivity reaction which may become life-threatening, such as angioedema. Notify prescriber at first sign of a hypersensitivity reaction. Expect drug to be discontinued, be prepared to administer charcoal or cholestyramine to eliminate drug rapidly, and provide supportive care, as needed and ordered.

! **WARNING** Monitor patient for skin reactions such as skin ulcers or reactions that may become severe such as DRESS. Assess patient's skin regularly. If a rash or other skin abnormalities occur (DRESS may only initially present with a fever or swollen lymph nodes), notify prescriber, expect drug to be discontinued if severe or reaction persists, and provide supportive care, as needed and ordered that may include an accelerated drug elimination procedure.

! **WARNING** Notify prescriber if patient develops a serious infection because drug may have to be interrupted and charcoal or cholestyramine given to eliminate drug rapidly.

! **WARNING** Monitor patient's respiratory function closely because drug may cause interstitial lung disease that could become life-threatening. If patient develops a cough and dyspnea, notify prescriber. Drug will have to be stopped and patient may need charcoal or cholestyramine to eliminate drug rapidly.

- Monitor patients who are over age 60, in patients taking concomitant neurotoxic drugs, or in patients with diabetes because of an increased risk of developing peripheral neuropathy. If peripheral neuropathy occurs during leflunomide therapy, notify prescriber, expect drug to be discontinued, and possibly cholestyramine washout ordered.

PATIENT TEACHING

- Advise patient that leflunomide doesn't cure arthritis but may relieve its symptoms and improve physical function.
- Instruct patient how to administer leflunomide.

! **WARNING** Alert females of childbearing age that a negative pregnancy test must be obtained before drug therapy begins because of the high risk of birth defects. Instruct patient as well as female partners of male patient to use an effective contraception during drug therapy and during drug elimination procedure after drug is discontinued. Stress importance of notifying prescriber immediately if pregnancy occurs as drug will need to be discontinued if confirmed.

! **WARNING** Inform patient that drug may cause an allergic reaction, including serious skin reactions. Advise patient to notify prescriber at first sign of an allergic or skin reaction, and to stop taking drug. If the allergic reaction is serious, urge patient to seek immediate medical care.

! **WARNING** Instruct patient to report signs of hepatotoxicity, such as unusual bleeding or bruising and yellow skin or eyes immediately to prescriber.

! **WARNING** Tell patient to report signs of respiratory dysfunction, such as cough and dyspnea, immediately to prescriber.

! **WARNING** Review signs and symptoms of an infection with patient and infection control measures to take. If present, tell patient to notify prescriber immediately as further treatment may be needed and drug discontinued.

! **WARNING** Advise patient that drug may lower their blood counts and to be compliant with frequent hematologic tests ordered. Also tell patient to immediately report easy bruising or bleeding, fever, paleness, recurrent infections, or unusual tiredness to prescriber.

- Tell mothers that breastfeeding should be discontinued during drug therapy.
- Inform patient that reversible hair loss may occur.
- Advise patient to avoid live vaccines during leflunomide therapy.

lenacapavir

Sunlenca

Class and Category

Pharmacologic class: Human immunodeficiency virus type 1 (HIV-1) inhibitor
Therapeutic class: Antiretroviral

Indications and Dosages

* *As adjunct with other antiretroviral(s) to treat HIV-1 infection in heavily treatment-experienced adults with multidrug resistant HIV-infection failing their current antiretroviral regimen due to resistance, intolerance, or safety considerations*

SUBCUTANEOUS INJECTION, TABLETS

Adults. 927 mg by subcutaneous injection and 600 mg PO on day 1 followed by 600 mg PO on day 2. Alternatively, 600 mg PO on day 1 and 2; 300 mg on day 8; and 927 mg by subcutaneous injection on day 15. *Maintenance:* 927 mg by subcutaneous injection every 6 months.

± **DOSAGE ADJUSTMENT** For patients planning to miss a scheduled 6-month injection visit by more than 2 weeks, tablets may be taken for up to 6 months until injection resumes as follows: 300 mg taken once every 7 days for up to 6 months followed by the maintenance injection dosage within 7 days after the last oral dose. For patients who miss a scheduled injection visit and more than 28 weeks have passed since the last injection and tablet form has not been taken, the dosage regimen is reinitiated using either option.

Drug Administration

P.O.

- May be taken with or without food.
- Administer from and store only in original blister pack.

SUBCUTANEOUS

- Be aware there are 2 available injection kits, which differ only how the injection is prepared.
- The injection kit components are to be used only once and two 1.5 ml injections are required for a complete dose.
- Inject subcutaneously at a preferred 90 degree angle, although a 45 degree angle is acceptable.

Vial access device kit

- Inspect vial solution; it should be yellow and contain no particles.
- Prepare vial by removing cap and cleaning vial stopper with alcohol wipe, then prepare vial access device by pushing down onto vial and twisting white cap off of device.
- Attach syringe and inject 1.5 ml of air into vial. Flip vial upside down and withdraw all contents.
- Attach a 22 G needle to syringe, expel air bubbles, and prime to 1.5 ml.
- Inject ONLY in the patient's abdomen (an accidental intradermal injection can cause necrosis and skin ulcer) keeping at least 2 inches away from the navel.
- Repeat steps to administer second injection.

Withdrawal needle injection kit

- Inspect drug solution. It should be yellow and contain no particles.
- Remove cap from vial and clean vial stopper with alcohol wipe.
- Attach an 18 G withdrawal needle to syringe. Inject 1.5 ml of air into the vial, then withdraw all contents from vial. Remove needle.
- Attach a 22 G needle to syringe, expel air bubbles and prime to 1.5 ml.
- Inject ONLY in the abdomen (an accidental intradermal injection can cause necrosis and skin ulcer) keeping at least 2 inches away from navel.
- Repeat steps to administer second injection.

Route	Onset	Peak	Duration
P.O.	Unknown	4 hr	Unknown
SubQ	Unknown	77–84 days	Unknown

Half-life: 10–12 days (PO); 8–12 wk (SubQ)

Mechanism of Action

Inhibits HIV integrase by binding to the integrase active site and blocking the strand transfer step of retroviral DNA integration, which is needed for the HIV replication cycle.

Contraindications

Hypersensitivity to lenacapavir or its components, strong CYP3A inducers

Interactions

DRUGS

anticonvulsants (carbamazepine, oxcarbazepine, phenobarbital, phenytoin), antimycobacterials (rifabutin, rifampin, rifapentine), antiretroviral agents (efavirenz, nevirapine, tipranavir/ritonavir), St. John's wort: Decreased lenacapavir level, decreasing drug's effectiveness

antiretroviral agents (atazanavir/cobicistt, atazanavir/ritonavir); combined P-gp, UGT1A1, and strong CYP3A inhibitors: Possibly significant increased lenacapavir plasma concentrations, which may increase risk of adverse reactions

corticosteroids (systemic: cortisone, dexamethasone, hydrocortisone), digoxin, direct oral anticoagulants (dabigatran, edoxaban, rivaroxaban), ergot derivatives (dihydroergotamine, ergotamine, methylergonovine), HMG-CoA reductase inhibitors (lovastatin, simvastatin), opioid antagonist (naloxegol), phosphodiesterase-5 inhibitors (sildenafil, tadalafil, vardenafil), sedatives/hypnotics (oral midazolam, triazolam): Increased plasma concentrations of these drugs, which may increase risk of adverse reactions

drugs primarily metabolized by CYP3A: Possibly increased exposure of these drugs, which may increase risk of adverse reactions

strong CYP3A inducers: Decreased lenacapavir plasma concentrations, which may decrease therapeutic effect; may cause resistance to lenacapavir

Adverse Reactions

ENDO: Hyperglycemia

GI: Elevated bilirubin and liver enzymes, nausea

GU: Elevated creatinine level, glycosuria, proteinuria

Other: **Immune reconstitution syndrome**, injection site reactions (discomfort, edema, erythema, extravasation, hematoma, induration, mass or nodule, pain, pruritus, swelling, ulceration or necrosis and skin ulcer with accidental intradermal injection)

Childbearing Considerations

PREGNANCY

- Pregnancy exposure registry: 1-800-258-4263.
- It is not known if drug can cause fetal harm.
- Use with caution only if benefit to mother outweighs potential risk to fetus.

LACTATION

- It is not known if drug is present in breast milk.
- The Centers for Disease Control and Prevention recommends that HIV-1 infected mothers not breastfeed to avoid risking postnatal transmission of HIV-1 infection in HIV-negative infants or developing vial resistance in HIV-positive infants. They also do not recommend breastfeeding because of potential drug-induced adverse reactions in the infant.

Nursing Considerations

- Ensure patient has agreed to comply with the every 6 month dosing schedule to help maintain viral suppression and reduce risk of viral rebound and potential development of resistance with missed doses.
- Monitor patient closely for injection site reactions. Notify prescriber, if present. If clinically significant, also expect to provide appropriate care, as needed and ordered

! WARNING Be aware that immune reconstitution syndrome has occurred in patients treated with combination antiretroviral therapy, including lenacapavir. The inflammatory response predisposes susceptible patients to opportunistic infections, such as cytomegalovirus, *Mycobacterium avium* infection, *Pneumocystis jiroveci* pneumonia, or tuberculosis. Autoimmune disorders such as Graves' disease, Guillain-Barré syndrome, or polymyositis have also occurred. Report sudden or unusual adverse reactions to prescriber.

- Know that if lencapavir is discontinued in order to minimize a risk of viral resistance, expect patient to receive an alternative, fully suppressive antiretroviral regimen, when possible and no later than 28 weeks after the final injection of lenacapavir. Know that if virologic failure occurs during lenacapavir therapy, expect patient to be switched to an alternative regimen, when possible.
- Be aware that residual concentrations of lenacapavir may remain in the systemic circulation of patients for up to 12 months or longer after the last injection.
- Monitor patient for at least 9 months after last lenacapavir injection if patient is receiving drugs primarily metabolized by CYP3A because of increased risk of adverse reactions.

PATIENT TEACHING

- Inform patient that drug will be administered as a subcutaneous injection by a healthcare provider.

! **WARNING** Stress importance of adhering to administration schedule for lenacapavir, which requires treatment with the drug every 6 months. Warn patient that noncompliance could lead to decreased effectiveness of the drug or the development of resistance to the drug.

- Review injection site reactions with patient and advise to notify prescriber, if present.

! **WARNING** Tell patient to notify prescriber of any persistent, serious, or unusual adverse reactions, especially signs and symptoms of an infection.

- Advise mothers breastfeeding should be avoided during lenacapavir therapy.
- Tell patient to notify prescriber of any drugs taken, including over-the-counter drugs because lenacapavir can interfere with the action of many drugs.

leuprolide acetate

Eligard, Fensolvi, Lupron, Lupron Depot 3.75 mg, Lupron Depot-3 Month 11.25 mg, Lupron Depot-3 Month 22.5 mg, Lupron Depot-4 Month 30 mg, Lupron Depot-6 Month 45 mg, Lupron Depot-Ped-1 Month, Lupron Depot-Ped-3 Month

leuprolide mesylate

Camcevi

Class and Category

Pharmacologic class: Gonadotropin-releasing hormone analogue
Therapeutic class: Antineoplastic, gonadotropin inhibitor

Indications and Dosages

∗ *To provide palliative treatment of advanced prostate cancer*

SUBCUTANEOUS INJECTION (ELIGARD)

Adults. 7.5 mg/mo, 22.5 mg every 3 mo, 30 mg every 4 mo, or 45 mg every 6 mo.

SUBCUTANEOUS INJECTION (LUPRON)

Adults. 1 mg daily.

SUBUTANEOUS INJECTION (CARCEVI)

Adults. 42 mg every 6 mo.

I.M. INJECTION (LUPRON DEPOT, LUPRON DEPOT-3 MONTH, LUPRON DEPOT-4 MONTH, LUPRON DEPOT-6 MONTH)

Adults. 7.5 mg every mo, 22.5 mg every 3 mo, 30 mg every 4 mo, or 45 mg every 6 mo.

∗ *To treat central precocious puberty*

I.M. INJECTION (LUPRON DEPOT-PED-1 MONTH)

Children ages 1 and older weighing more than 37.5 kg (83 lb). 15 mg once a mo. *Maximum:* 15 mg once a mo.
Children ages 1 and older weighing more than 25 kg (55 lb) but less than 37.5 kg (83 lb). *Initial:* 11.25 mg once a mo. Dosage increased to next available dose at next monthly injection, as needed. *Maximum:* 15 mg once a mo.
Children ages 1 and older weighing 25 kg (55 lb) or less. *Initial:* 7.5 mg once a mo. Dosage increased to next available dose at next monthly injection, as needed. *Maximum:* 15 mg once a mo.

I.M. INJECTION (LUPRON DEPOT-PED 3 MONTH)

Children ages 1 and older. 11.25 or 30 mg once every 3 mo (dose not based on weight).

I.M. INJECTION (LUPRON DEPOT-PED 6 MONTH)

Children ages 1 and older. 45 mg once every 6 mo.

SUBCUTANEOUS INJECTION (FENSOLVI)

Children ages 2 and older. 45 mg once every 6 mo.

∗ *To treat endometriosis as monotherapy or as adjunctive therapy in combination with norethindrone acetate*

I.M. INJECTION (LUPRON DEPOT 3.75 MG, LUPRON DEPOT-3 MONTH)

Adults. 3.75 mg every mo for up to 6 mo. Retreated for up to an another 6 mo, as needed. Alternatively, 11.25 mg every 3 mo for up to 6 mo. Retreated for another 6 mo, as needed.

∗ *As adjunct to treat anemia due to uterine leiomyomas in combination with iron therapy*

I.M. INJECTION (LUPRON DEPOT 3.75 MG, LUPRON DEPOT-3 MONTH)

Adults. 3.75 mg every consecutive mo up to 3 mo. Alternatively, 11.25 mg as a single dose. *Maximum:* 11.25 mg total dose.

Drug Administration

- Never administer by I.V. route.
- Do not substitute one product for another. Be sure the product prescribed is the one to be administered.
- Do not substitute one strength for another by giving a lesser amount, administering more often in place of another product, or increasing dose to achieve dosage of another product.
- Do not administer longer than product indicates.

I.M.

- Let drug come to room temperature before using.
- Do not use syringe if clumping or caking is evident. A thin layer of powder on the wall of the syringe is normal prior to mixing with the provided diluent. Diluent should appear clear.
- To prepare for injection, screw the white plunger into the end stopper until the stopper begins to turn.
- Hold syringe upright. Release the diluent by slowly pushing the plunger for 6 to 8 sec until the first middle stopper is at the blue line in the middle of the barrel.
- Keeping the syringe upright, mix the powder thoroughly by gently shaking the syringe until the powder forms a uniform suspension. The suspension should appear milky. If powder adheres to the stopper or caking/clumping occurs, tap the syringe with a finger to disperse. Do not use if powder has not gone into a suspension.
- Keeping syringe upright, remove needle cap and expel the air from the syringe.
- Administer within 2 hr after mixing and discard any unused portion.
- Insert I.M. needle into the anterior thigh, deltoid, or gluteal area. Aspirate to ensure blood vessel is not accidentally penetrated. If no blood is seen through the transparent safety device, injection can be given. If blood is present, do not inject the drug.
- After injection, withdraw the needle. Immediately activate the Lupro Loc safety device by pushing the arrow on the lock upward towards the needle tip with finger or thumb until the needle cover of the safety device over the needle is fully extended and a click is felt or heard.
- Rotate sites within the same region from 1 injection to the next.

SUBCUTANEOUS

- No dilution or reconstitution is needed for leuprolide acetate injection (Lupron).
- Leuprolide acetate for injectable suspension (Camcevi and Eligard) is approved only for use in men for palliative treatment of prostate cancer. Fensolvi is approved only for use in children ages 2 and older with central precocious puberty.
- Allow drug to reach room temperature before using. Follow manufacturer directions carefully in preparing product prescribed. Camcevi comes as an off-white to pale yellow, viscous, and opalescent emulsion in a single-dose, prefilled syringe. Eligard and Fensolvi require reconstitution and come as a pre-connected syringe system consisting of Syringe A (contains the in situ polymeric extended release technology) and syringe B (contains drug powder) connected using a coupling device.
- Inject into abdomen for Camcevi injection; inject into abdomen, upper buttocks, or another location with adequate amounts of subcutaneous tissue for Elligard or Fensolvi injection. Do not inject drug into areas that have excessive pigment, hair, lesions, or nodules. Also do not inject into an area that has been used recently.
- Rotate sites.

J K L

Route	Onset	Peak	Duration
I.M./SubQ	2–4 wk	1–2 mo	60–90 days

Half-life: 3 hr

Mechanism of Action

Suppresses secretion of gonadotropin-releasing hormone, after stimulating follicle-stimulating hormone (FSH) and luteinizing hormone (LH) through continuous leuprolide therapy. Decreased estradiol and testosterone levels then occurs. Stops menses and reproductive organ development in children with central precocious puberty.

Suppression in a continuous manner in adult males decreases testosterone levels and causes pharmacologic castration, which slows the activity of prostatic neoplastic cells. Suppresses ovarian function in women with endometriosis or uterine leiomyomas thereby inactivating endometrial tissues and causing amenorrhea.

Contraindications

For all forms: Hypersensitivity to leuprolide, other gonadotropin-releasing hormone analogues,
For leuprolide acetate for depot: Breastfeeding, pregnancy, undiagnosed abnormal uterine bleeding
For injectable suspension (Fensolvi): Pregnancy

Interactions

DRUGS

None reported by manufacturer.

Adverse Reactions

CNS: Aggression, anger, anxiety, asthenia, **CVA**, delusions, depression, dizziness, emotional lability, fatigue, fever, headache (including migraine), hyperkinesia, insomnia, irritability, lethargy, malaise, memory loss, mood changes, nervousness (adult female), paresthesia, paralysis (from spinal fracture), peripheral neuropathy, personality disorder, **pseudotumor cerebri (idiopathic intracranial hypertension [children])**, rigors, **seizures**, somnolence, **suicidal ideation**, syncope, thirst, transient ischemic attacks, vertigo, weakness
CV: **Angina**, **arrhythmias**, **bradycardia**, **chest pain**, **deep vein thrombosis**, edema, elevated cholesterol and triglyceride levels, hypertension, **hypotension**, **MI** (higher risk in men), palpitations, peripheral vascular disorder, **prolonged QT interval**, **sudden cardiac death**, tachycardia, vasodilation
EENT: Blurred vision, conjunctivitis, decreased vision, dry mouth, epistaxis, gingivitis, hearing disorder, pharyngitis, rhinitis, sinusitis
ENDO: Amenorrhea, androgenic effects in women, breast tenderness or swelling, decreased testicle size, diabetes mellitus, goiter, growth retardation, gynecomastia, hot flashes, hyperglycemia, increased signs and symptoms of puberty (children), **pituitary apoplexy**
GI: Anorexia, **cirrhosis**, colitis, constipation, diarrhea, dyspepsia, dysphagia, elevated liver enzymes, flatulence, gastroenteritis, **hepatic dysfunction**, increased appetite, **liver injury**, nausea, non-alcoholic fatty liver disease, vomiting
GU: Bladder spasm, cervix disorder, **cervical neoplasm**, decreased libido, decreased penis size, dysmenorrhea and other menstrual disorders, dysuria, endometriosis flare-up, impotence, incontinence, nocturia, **prostate cancer flare-up**, prostate pain, renal calculus, urinary incontinence, uterine bleeding, vaginal bleeding or discharge in girls, vaginitis
HEME: **Leukopenia**, purpura
MS: Arthralgia, back pain, bone density loss, bone or limb pain, epiphysiolysis, fibromyalgia, joint disorder, leg cramps, ligament sprain, myalgia, myopathy, severe muscle pain or spasms (children), spinal fracture, tenosynovitis-like symptoms
RESP: **Asthmatic attack**, dyspnea, **interstitial lung disease**, pneumonitis, **pulmonary embolism**
SKIN: Acne, acute generalized exanthematous pustulosis (AGEP), alopecia, bullous dermatitis, clamminess, ecchymosis, **erythema multiforme**, **exfoliative dermatitis**, flushing, hirsutism, hyperhidrosis, leukoderma, nail disorder, night sweats, photosensitivity, pruritus, rash, seborrhea, skin hypertrophy, **Stevens-Johnson syndrome, toxic epidermal necrolysis,** urticaria
Other: **Aggravation of preexisting tumor**; **anaphylaxis**; **angioedema (face)**; body pain (children); **drug reaction with eosinophilia**

and systemic symptoms (DRESS); elevated uric acid; flu-like symptoms; infection; injection-site abscess, burning, edema, induration, itching, pain, redness, or swelling; **tumor flare**; weight gain or loss

Childbearing Considerations

PREGNANCY

- Drug may cause fetal harm such as major fetal abnormalities and increases risk for pregnancy loss.
- Drug is contraindicated in pregnant females and in females of childbearing age who may become pregnant.
- Females of childbearing age should have a negative pregnancy test before starting drug therapy.

LACTATION

- It is not known if drug is present in breast milk.
- Mothers should check with prescriber before breastfeeding. Drug is contraindicated with breastfeeding for leuprolide acetate for depot.

REPRODUCTION

- Females of childbearing age should use a nonhormonal method of contraception throughout drug therapy.
- Drug may impair fertility.

Nursing Considerations

! **WARNING** Ensure females of childbearing age have a negative pregnancy test result before administering drug.

- Monitor patient for possible injection site reactions (erythema and induration) because leuprolide injections contain benzyl alcohol.
- Be aware that during the first weeks of leuprolide therapy, patient being treated for prostate cancer should be monitored for initial worsening of symptoms, such as difficulty urinating, increased bone pain, and paralysis or paresthesia (in patients with vertebral metastasis). Also, be aware that following the first dose of leuprolide depot form used to treat endometriosis, an increase in symptoms may occur during the initial days of therapy because of a temporary rise in the hormone levels. These symptoms usually abate with time. Monitor patient's PSA and serum testosterone levels periodically, as ordered, to determine response to leuprolide therapy used to treat prostate cancer.

! **WARNING** Be aware that life-threatening hypersensitivity reactions such as anaphylaxis and asthmatic attacks have occurred with leuprolide therapy. Patients at higher risk for an asthma attack include those with a preexisting history of asthma, drug and environmental allergies, and sinusitis. If present, alert prescriber, expect drug to be discontinued, and provide supportive emergency care, as needed and ordered.

! **WARNING** Monitor patient for severe cutaneous adverse reactions, including DRESS that may become life-threatening. Notify prescriber at the first sign of rash (DRESS may only initially present with fever or swollen lymph nodes), expect drug to be discontinued, and provide supportive care, as needed and ordered.

! **WARNING** Monitor patients at risk for prolonged QT interval, such as in the presence of congenital long QT syndrome, congestive heart failure, or frequent electrolyte abnormalities, and in patients taking drugs that may prolong the QT interval. Know that electrolyte abnormalities should be corrected, as ordered, prior to therapy beginning. Monitor patient's ECG and electrolytes regularly throughout therapy, as ordered. Notify prescriber of any abnormalities.

! **WARNING** Watch patient closely for signs and symptoms of cardiovascular disease because leuprolide therapy increases risk of MI, stroke, and sudden cardiac death.

! **WARNING** Monitor patient for changes in behavior or thinking suggestive of suicidal ideation. Alert prescriber at once, if present, and institute suicidal precautions.

! **WARNING** Monitor children for pseudotumor cerebri. Assess child for signs and symptoms such as blurred vision, diplopia, dizziness, headache, loss of vision, nausea, pain behind the eye or pain with eye movement, papilledema, or tinnitus. Alert prescriber immediately, if present.

! **WARNING** Monitor patient for evidence of pituitary apoplexy, such as altered mental status, and possibly cardiovascular collapse, ophthalmoplegia, sudden headache, visual changes, and vomiting. Although rare, it may occur within 2 weeks of first dose, sometimes within the first hour. Notify prescriber immediately and provide supportive care, as needed and ordered.

! **WARNING** Institute seizure precautions, especially in patients with a history of central nervous system dysfunction or tumors, cerebrovascular disorders, epilepsy, or history of seizures or in patients who are taking medications that may cause seizures.

! **WARNING** Be aware that therapeutic doses of leuprolide suppress the pituitary–gonadal system and that normal function doesn't return for 4 to 12 weeks after drug is stopped.

- Monitor patient's blood glucose level and lipid levels, as ordered, because leuprolide therapy may elevate blood glucose and lipid levels, leading to a diagnosis of metabolic syndrome, Drug may adversely affect glycemic control in patients with diabetes.
- Monitor bone density test results, as ordered, for women at risk for osteoporosis who are receiving leuprolide because of possible drug-induced estrogen loss, which may result in decreased bone density.
- Expect to stop drug before onset of puberty in patients treated for precocious central puberty.

PATIENT TEACHING

- Instruct patient, family, or caregiver how to administer leuprolide subcutaneously.
- Alert patient for possible injection-site reactions and to notify prescriber if present.
- Caution patient being treated for prostate cancer that drug may initially worsen such symptoms as bone pain and that it may cause new signs or symptoms to occur during first few weeks of treatment. Also, inform women receiving drug for treatment of endometriosis that an increase in symptoms may occur during the initial days of therapy. Reassure these patients that these reactions are transient.

! **WARNING** Alert patient that drug can cause an allergic reaction or serious skin reactions. Tell patient to notify prescriber, if present, and to seek immediate medical attention, if severe.

! **WARNING** Advise females of childbearing age to notify prescriber immediately if pregnancy occurs. Instruct her to use a nonhormonal form of contraception during leuprolide therapy to prevent pregnancy. Advise patient to report monthly menses or breakthrough bleeding to prescriber immediately.

! **WARNING** Emphasize importance of seeking immediate emergency care if patient develops signs and symptoms suggestive of a heart attack or stroke.

! **WARNING** Inform family or caregiver to watch for emotional lability, such as aggression, anger, crying, depression, impatience, or irritability. Also, warn family or caregiver that although rare, suicidal behaviors and thoughts have occurred during leuprolide therapy. If present, tell family or caregiver to notify prescriber.

! **WARNING** Review seizure precautions with patient, family, or caregiver.

! **WARNING** Instruct family or caregiver to notify prescriber immediately if child complains of blurred vision, diplopia, dizziness, headache, loss of vision, nausea, pain behind the eye or pain with eye movement, papilledema, or tinnitus.

! **WARNING** Instruct patient to report to prescriber any other symptoms that are persistent, serious, or unusual.

- Inform family or caregiver of child being treated for central precocious puberty that they should expect normal gonadal-pituitary function to return 4 to 12 weeks after therapy ends. Also, tell family member or caregiver to notify prescriber if an increase in signs and symptoms of puberty, including vaginal bleeding, occurs during the first weeks of therapy or after subsequent doses.
- Inform patient with osteoporosis or at risk for developing it that drug may increase bone density loss.

- Be aware that mothers should check with prescriber before breastfeeding because it may be contraindicated depending on product used.
- Stress importance of compliance with routine laboratory studies because drug can increase blood glucose and lipid levels as well as adversely affect the liver. Also advise patient with diabetes to monitor his blood glucose level closely.

levalbuterol hydrochloride

Xopenex

levalbuterol tartrate

Xopenex HFA

Class and Category

Pharmacologic class: Beta$_2$ agonist
Therapeutic class: Bronchodilator

Indications and Dosages

To prevent or treat bronchospasm in reversible obstructive airway disease

INHALATION AEROSOL (XOPENEX HFA)

Adults and children ages 4 and older. 45 or 90 mcg (1 or 2 inhalations) every 4 to 6 hr.

INHALATION SOLUTION (XOPENEX)

Adults and children ages 12 and older. *Initial:* 0.63 mg 3 times daily every 6 to 8 hr, increased to 1.25 mg 3 times daily every 6 to 8 hr, as needed. *Maximum:* 1.25 mg 3 times daily.

Children ages 6 to 11. *Initial:* 0.31 mg 3 times daily, increased to 0.63 mg 3 times daily, as needed. *Maximum:* 0.63 mg 3 times daily.

±**DOSAGE ADJUSTMENT** For elderly patients using Xopenex, dosage limited to 0.63 mg 3 times daily every 6 to 8 hours and only increased, as needed.

Drug Administration

INHALATION

Xopenex

- Administer solution by nebulization. Once pouch is opened, vial immediately but if not used immediately, protect from light and use within 1 wk. Solution should be colorless; if not, discard.
- Monitor blood pressure and pulse rate before and after nebulizer treatment.
- Twist the body of the vial to open the vial. Squeeze entire contents of vial into the reservoir. Do not add any other drugs to reservoir. Connect the nebulizer reservoir to the face mask or mouthpiece.
- Connect the nebulizer to an air compressor.
- Have patient sit in an upright, comfortable position. Have patient breathe as calmly, deeply, and evenly as possible until no more mist is seen in the nebulizer reservoir, which will take about 5 to 15 min.
- Do not exceed recommended dose. Monitor patients receiving the highest dose for adverse systemic effects.
- Store unused vials in the protective foil pouch at room temperature and protect from excessive heat and light. Once pouch is opened, the remaining vials should be used within 2 wk.

Xopenex HFA

- Prime inhaler before using it for the first time or when it hasn't been used for more than 3 days by releasing 4 test sprays into the air, aiming inhaler away from face.
- Shake inhaler well for 5 sec before each use, including when priming.
- A spacer device may be used, if recommended.
- To administer, have patient hold inhaler upright with mouthpiece pointing towards them. Have patient breathe out through their mouth pushing as much air as possible out, then put mouthpiece into their mouth closing their lips around it. Then while breathing in deeply and slowly, have patient push down on the center of the targeting rings until a spray is released. The patient can then stop pressing the dose indicator.
- For a second dose, have patient wait 1 min, then shake the inhaler and repeat steps for the second spray, if ordered.
- Clean inhaler at least weekly by washing actuator with warm water and let it air-dry. If it becomes clogged, wash the actuator to remove blockage.
- The inhaler will deliver 200 actuations. When nearing the end of the usable inhalations, the color behind the number in the dose indicator window will change to red. Discard when display window shows 0. Never immerse canister in water to determine how full the canister is.

Route	Onset	Peak	Duration
Inhalation	5–15 min	1 hr	3–4 hr

Half-life: 3–4 hr

Mechanism of Action

Attaches to $beta_2$ receptors on bronchial cell membranes, which stimulates the intracellular enzyme adenyl cyclase to convert adenosine triphosphate to cAMP. Increased intracellular cAMP level relaxes bronchial smooth muscle and inhibits histamine release from mast cells.

Contraindications

Hypersensitivity to levalbuterol, racemic albuterol, or their components

Interactions

DRUGS

beta-blockers: Possibly block pulmonary effects of levalbuterol; may cause severe bronchospasms

digoxin: Decreased blood digoxin level and effectiveness

loop or thiazide diuretics: Increased risk of hypokalemia

MAO inhibitors, sympathomimetics, tricyclic antidepressants: Increased risk of adverse cardiovascular effects

Adverse Reactions

CNS: Anxiety, chills, dizziness, dysphonia, hypertonia, insomnia, migraine headache, nervousness, paresthesia, syncope, tremor

CV: **Arrhythmias**, chest pain, hypertension, **hypotension**, tachycardia

EENT: Dry mouth and throat, rhinitis, sinusitis

GI: Diarrhea, gastroesophageal reflux disease (GERD), indigestion, nausea, vomiting

MS: Leg cramps, myalgia

RESP: **Asthma exacerbation**, cough, dyspnea, **paradoxical bronchospasm**

SKIN: Rash, urticaria

Other: **Anaphylaxis**, **angioedema**, flu-like symptoms, lymphadenopathy, **metabolic acidosis**

Childbearing Considerations

PREGNANCY

- Pregnancy exposure registry: 1-877-311-8972 or www.mothertobaby.org/ongoing-study/asthma.
- It is not known if drug causes fetal harm.
- Use with caution only if benefit to mother outweighs potential risk to fetus.

LABOR AND DELIVERY

- Drug should not be used during labor and delivery unless there are no other alternatives because drug may interfere with uterine contractility.
- Be aware drug has not been approved for management of preterm labor. Serious adverse reactions, including maternal pulmonary edema, have occurred during or following treatment of premature labor.

LACTATION

- It is not known if drug is present in breast milk.
- Mothers should check with prescriber before breastfeeding.

Nursing Considerations

- Use levalbuterol cautiously in patients with arrhythmias, diabetes mellitus, hypertension, hyperthyroidism, or a history of seizures.

! WARNING Monitor patient for a hypsersensitivity reaction that could become life threatening such as anaphylaxis or angioedema. If present, notify prescriber, expect drug to be discontinued, and provide supportive care, as needed and ordered.

! WARNING Observe patient for dyspnea, increased coughing, and wheezing because drug may provoke paradoxical bronchospasm. Notify prescriber immediately if patient develops bronchospasms, expect drug to be discontinued, and provide supportive care, as needed and ordered.

! WARNING Monitor patient for persistent, serious, or unusual adverse reactions.

PATIENT TEACHING

- Teach patient how to administer the product of levalbuterol prescribed.
- Instruct patient not to increase dosage or frequency unless told by prescriber.

! WARNING Alert patient that drug may cause an allergic reaction. If present, tell patient to notify prescriber and, if severe, to seek immediate medical care.

! WARNING Urge patient to stop drug and call prescriber if she has paradoxical bronchospasm. Also tell patient to notify prescriber if persistent, serious, or unusual adverse reactions occur.

- Instruct patient to notify prescriber if drug fails to work or if she needs more treatments because asthma is worsening.
- Urge patient to consult prescriber before using over-the counter or other drugs.

levamlodipine

Class and Category

Pharmacologic class: Dihydropyridine calcium channel blocker
Therapeutic class: Antihypertensive

Indications and Dosages

∗ *To treat hypertension*

TABLETS

Adults. *Initial:* 2.5 mg once daily increased after 7 to 14 days to 5 mg once daily, as needed. *Maximum:* 5 mg once daily.
Children ages 6 to 17. *Initial:* 1.25 to 2.5 mg once daily. *Maximum:* 2.5 mg once daily.

±**DOSAGE ADJUSTMENT** For elderly or frail patients and patients with hepatic insufficiency, initial dose decreased to 1.25 mg once daily and titrated slowly.

Drug Administration

P.O.

- Administer once daily keeping time of day consistent.
- Keep in tight, light-resistant containers.

Route	Onset	Peak	Duration
P.O.	Unknown	6–12 hr	Unknown

Half-life: 30–50 hr

Mechanism of Action

Inhibits the transmembrane influx of calcium ions into vascular smooth muscle to produce peripheral vasodilation, which reduces peripheral vascular resistance and thus reduces blood pressure.

Contraindications

Hypersensitivity to levamlodipine, amlodipine, or their components

Interactions

DRUGS

immunosuppressants (cyclosporine, tacrolimus), simvastatin: Increased systemic exposure of these drugs with increased risk of adverse reactions
moderate and strong CYP3A inducers: Decreased concentration of levamlodipine
moderate and strong CYP3A inhibitors: Increased exposure of levamlodipine and risk of adverse reactions
sildenafil: Increased risk of hypotension

Adverse Reactions

CNS: Abnormal dreams, anxiety, asthenia, depersonalization, depression, dizziness, extrapyramidal disorder, fatigue, hypoesthesia, insomnia, malaise, nervousness, paresthesia, peripheral neuropathy, rigors, somnolence, syncope, thirst, tremor, vertigo
CV: **Arrhythmias (including atrial fibrillation, ventricular tachycardia), bradycardia**, chest pain, edema, palpitation, peripheral ischemia, tachycardia, vasculitis
EENT: Abnormal vision, conjunctivitis, diplopia, dry mouth, epistaxis, eye pain, gingival hyperplasia, tinnitus
ENDO: Hot flashes, hyperglycemia
GI: Abdominal pain, anorexia, cholestasis, constipation, diarrhea, dysphagia, elevated liver enzymes, flatulence, **hepatitis**, jaundice, nausea, **pancreatitis**, vomiting
GU: Female and male sexual dysfunction, nocturia, urinary frequency or other micturition disorders
HEME: **Leukopenia, purpura, thrombocytopenia**
MS: Arthralgia, arthrosis, back pain, muscle cramps, myalgia
RESP: Dyspnea
SKIN: Diaphoresis, **erythema multiforme**, flushing, pruritus, rash
Other: **Angioedema**, generalized pain, **hypersensitivity reactions**, weight gain or loss

Childbearing Considerations

PREGNANCY

- It is not known if drug causes fetal harm.
- Use with caution only if benefit to mother outweighs potential risk to fetus.

LACTATION

- Drug is present in breast milk.
- Mothers should check with prescriber before breastfeeding.

Nursing Considerations

- Monitor patient's blood pressure to determine effectiveness. Know that symptomatic hypotension is possible, particularly in patients with severe aortic stenosis but acute hypotension is not expected to occur.

> ! **WARNING** Monitor patient closely after levamlodipine is initiated or dosage is increased, especially in patients with severe obstructive coronary artery disease, because drug may cause an acute MI or worsen angina.

> ! **WARNING** Monitor patient for hypersensitivity reactions. Although uncommon, hypersensitivity reactions may become life-threatening such as angioedema. Notify prescriber and expect drug to be discontinued and provide supportive care, as needed and ordered.

PATIENT TEACHING

- Instruct patient how to administer levamlopidine.

> ! **WARNING** Tell patient to notify prescriber if an allergy or other serious adverse reactions occur. Urge patient to seek immediate emergency care if serious allergic reactions occur or heart disorders worsen.

- Tell patient to inform prescriber of all medications taken, including over-the-counter and herbal products.

levetiracetam

Elepsia XR, Keppra, Keppra XR, Spritam

Class and Category

Pharmacologic class: Pyrrolidine derivative
Therapeutic class: Anticonvulsant

Indications and Dosages

* *To treat partial seizures as monotherapy or adjunctive therapy*

I.V. INFUSION, ORAL SOLUTION

Adults and adolescents ages 16 and older. *Initial:* 500 mg twice daily, increased by 500 mg twice daily every 2 wk until the recommended daily dose of 3,000 mg given in 2 divided doses is reached. *Maximum:* 3,000 mg daily in 2 divided doses.
Children ages 4 to 16. *Initial:* 10 mg/kg twice daily, increased by 10 mg/kg twice daily every 2 wk until recommended daily dose of 60 mg/kg given in 2 divided doses is reached.
Children ages 6 mo to 4 yr. *Initial:* 10 mg/kg twice daily, increased by 10 mg/kg twice daily every 2 wk until the recommended daily dose of 50 mg/kg given in 2 divided doses is reached.
Infants ages 1 to 6 mo. *Initial:* 7 mg/kg twice daily, increased by 7 mg/kg twice daily every 2 wk until recommended daily dose of 42 mg/kg given in 2 divided doses is reached.

TABLETS (KEPPRA)

Adults and adolescents ages 16 and older. *Initial:* 500 mg twice daily, increased by 500 mg twice daily every 2 wk until the recommended daily dose of 3,000 mg given in 2 divided doses is reached. *Maximum:* 1,500 mg twice daily.
Children ages 4 to 16 weighing more than 40 kg (88 lb). *Initial:* 500 mg twice daily, increased by 500 mg twice daily, to a maximum recommended daily dose. *Maximum:* 1,500 mg twice daily.
Children ages 4 to 16 weighing 20 to 40 kg (44 to 88 lb). *Initial:* 250 mg twice daily, increased by 250 mg twice daily every 2 wk to a maximum recommended daily dose. *Maximum:* 750 mg twice daily. *Maximum:* 750 mg twice daily.

TABLETS (SPRITAM)

Adults and children ages 4 and older weighing more than 40 kg (88 lb). *Initial:* 500 mg twice daily, increased by 500 mg twice daily every 2 wk to a maximum recommended daily dose. *Maximum:* 1,500 mg twice daily.
Children ages 4 and older weighing 20 to 40 kg (44 to 88 lb). *Initial:* 250 mg twice daily, increased by 250 mg twice daily every 2 wk until maximum recommended daily dose is reached. *Maximum:* 750 mg twice daily.

XR TABLETS (KEPPRA XR)

Adults and children ages 12 and older. 1,000 mg once daily, increased by 1,000 mg daily every 2 wk until maximum recommended daily dose is reached. *Maximum:* 3,000 mg once daily.

∗ *As adjunctive therapy to treat partial-onset seizures*

XR TABLETS (ELEPSIA XR)

Adults and children ages 12 and older. *Initial:* 1,000 mg once daily, increased by 1,000 mg daily every 2 wk until maximum recommended daily dose is reached. *Maximum:* 3,000 mg once daily.

∗ *As adjunct to treat myoclonic seizures in patients with juvenile myoclonic epilepsy*

I.V. INFUSION, ORAL SOLUTION, TABLETS

Adults and children ages 12 and older. *Initial:* 500 mg twice daily, increased by 500 mg twice daily every 2 wk to maximum recommended dose. *Maximum:* 1,500 mg twice daily.

∗ *As adjunct to treat primary generalized tonic–clonic seizures in patients with idiopathic generalized epilepsy*

I.V. INFUSION, ORAL SOLUTION, TABLETS

Adults and children ages 16 and older. *Initial:* 500 mg twice daily, increased by 500 mg twice daily every 2 wk to the maximum recommended dose given in 2 divided doses. *Maximum:* 1,500 mg twice daily.

Children ages 6 to 16. *Initial:* 10 mg/kg twice daily, increased by 10 mg/kg twice daily every 2 wk to the maximum recommended daily dose. *Maximum:* 30 mg/kg twice daily.

TABLETS (SPRITAM)

Adults and children ages 6 and older weighing more than 40 kg (88 lb). *Initial:* 500 mg twice daily, increased by 500 mg twice daily every 2 wk to recommended daily dose. *Maximum:* 1,500 mg twice daily.

Children ages 6 and older weighing 20 (44 lb) to 40 kg (88 lb). *Initial:* 250 mg twice daily, increased by 250 twice daily every 2 wk to the recommended daily dose of 750 mg twice daily.

±**DOSAGE ADJUSTMENT** For adult patients with creatinine clearance of 50 to 80 ml/min, maximum dosage reduced to no more than 2,000 mg daily; to no more than 1,500 mg daily for clearance of 30 to 50 ml/min; and to no more than 1,000 mg daily for clearance less than 30 ml/min. For adult patients with end-stage renal disease who are having dialysis, expect to give another 250 to 500 mg, as prescribed, after each dialysis session. For children, manufacturer does not provide renal impairment dosage adjustments. For children who can't tolerate maximum daily dose, dosage reduced to point of tolerance.

Drug Administration

- Keep in mind that when switching patient from oral dosing to intravenous dosing and from intravenous dosing to oral dosing, no dosage or frequency changes are needed.

P.O.

- Tablets and X.R. tablets should be swallowed whole and not chewed, crushed, or split.
- Know that children not old enough to swallow tablets or patients who can not swallow tablets should be given only the oral solution form.
- Do not push Spritam tablet through the foil; peel foil from blister. Administer tablet by having patient place tablet on tongue with a dry hand and immediately follow with a sip of water, as it is intended to disintegrate in the mouth. Alternatively, add whole tablet(s) to about 1 tablespoon of liquid to cover tablet(s) in a cup. Allow tablet(s) to disperse prior to administering the entire contents to patient immediately. After administration, resuspend any residue by adding an additional small volume of liquid to cup and have patient swallow the full amount. Do not administer partial quantities of the dispersed tablets.
- For solution administered orally, shake bottle well before using and use a calibrated measuring device to measure dose.

I.V.

- Intravenous form should be used only as an alternative for patients when oral administration is temporarily not possible.
- Do not dilute if drug is already premixed in a single-dose I.V. bag.
- For vials, dilute in 100 ml of compatible diluent, such as 0.9% Sodium Chloride Injection, 5% Dextrose Injection, or Lactated Ringer's solution. If a smaller volume is needed (fluid restriction or for children), the amount of diluent should be calculated to not exceed maximum concentration of 15 mg/ml of diluted solution.
- Use within 4 hr of dilution.
- Infuse each dose over 15 min.

- Store drug at room temperature.
- *Incompatibilities:* Other drugs except for diazepam, lorazepam, and valproate sodium; other solutions except for 0.9% Sodium Chloride Injection, 5% Dextrose Injection, and Lactated Ringer's solution.

Route	Onset	Peak	Duration
P.O.	1 hr	1 hr	12 hr
P.O./X.R.	Unknown	4 hr	Unknown
I.V.	Unknown	5–30 min	Unknown

Half-life: 6–8 hr

Mechanism of Action

May protect against secondary generalized seizure activity by preventing coordination of epileptiform burst firing. Levetiracetam doesn't seem to involve inhibitory and excitatory neurotransmission.

Contraindications

Hypersensitivity to levetiracetam or its components

Interactions

DRUGS

None reported by manufacturer.

Adverse Reactions

CNS: Abnormal gait, affect lability, aggression, agitation, altered mood, amnesia, anger, anxiety, apathy, asthenia, ataxia, behavioral difficulties (children), choreoathetosis (movement disorder), confusion, coordination difficulties, depersonalization, depression, dizziness, dyskinesia, emotional lability, fatigue, hallucinations, headache, hostility, hypersomnia, increased reflexes, insomnia, involuntary movements, irritability, lethargy, mental or mood changes, nervousness, neurosis, obsessive-compulsive disorders, panic attacks, paranoia, paresthesia, personality disorder, psychosis, **seizures** (worsening), somnolence, **suicidal ideation**, vertigo
CV: Elevated diastolic blood pressure (children up to 4 years of age), **hypotension**
EENT: Amblyopia, conjunctivitis, diplopia, ear pain, nasal congestion, nasopharyngitis, pharyngitis, rhinitis, sinusitis
GI: Abdominal pain (upper), anorexia, constipation, diarrhea, elevated liver enzymes, gastroenteritis, **hepatic failure**, **hepatitis**, **pancreatitis**, vomiting
GU: **Acute kidney injury**, albuminuria
HEME: **Agranulocytosis**; decreased hematocrit, hemoglobin, and red blood cell counts; elevated eosinophil count; **leukopenia**; **neutropenia**; **pancytopenia**; **thrombocytopenia**
MS: Arthralgia, joint sprain, muscle weakness, neck pain
RESP: **Asthma**, cough, dyspnea
SKIN: Alopecia, ecchymosis, **erythema multiforme**, pruritus, rash, skin discoloration, **Stevens-Johnson syndrome**, **toxic epidermal necrolysis**, vesiculobullous rash, urticaria
Other: **Anaphylaxis**, **angioedema**, dehydration, **drug reaction with eosinophilia and systemic symptoms (DRESS)**, flu-like symptoms, **hyponatremia**, infection, weight loss

Childbearing Considerations

PREGNANCY

- Pregnancy exposure registry: 1-888-233-2334 or http://www.aedpregnancyregistry.org/.
- It is not known if drug causes fetal harm.
- Use with caution only if benefit to mother outweighs potential risk to fetus.
- Drug levels may decrease during pregnancy, requiring dosage adjustments.

LACTATION

- Drug is present in breast milk.
- Mothers should check with prescriber before breastfeeding.

Nursing Considerations

- Assess compliance, especially during the first 4 weeks of therapy, when certain adverse effects, including abnormal behaviors, coordination problems, fatigue, and somnolence may be more likely to occur.

! **WARNING** Monitor patient closely for evidence of suicidal thinking or behavior, especially when therapy starts or dosage changes.

! **WARNING** Monitor patient for hypersensitivity and skin reactions. Know that anaphylaxis or angioedema have occurred with levetiracetam therapy as early as after the first dose, but also at other times during treatment. Monitor patient for difficulty breathing, hives, hypotension, and swelling. Also, monitor patient for a rash and other adverse skin reactions (DRESS may only initially present with fever or swollen lymph nodes.) because serious dermatological reactions have occurred with levetiracetam therapy. Although these adverse skin reactions usually appear within 14 to 17 days after therapy has begun, some have occurred as late as 4 months later. Notify prescriber immediately at the first sign of a hypersensitivity reaction or fever, rash, swollen lymph nodes or other skin abnormalities and expect drug to be discontinued. Provide emergency supportive care, as needed and ordered.

! **WARNING** Monitor patient for seizure activity during therapy. As appropriate, implement seizure precautions according to facility policy. Avoid stopping drug abruptly because doing so may increase seizure activity. Expect to taper dosage gradually.

! **WARNING** Monitor patient for bleeding, fever, recurrent infections, or significant weakness. If present, notify prescriber and expect to obtain a CBC to assess patient's hematological status. Also monitor patient for persistent, serious, or unusual adverse reactions and notify prescriber, if present.

- Monitor blood pressure in children because increased diastolic blood pressure may occur in patients up to 4 years old.

PATIENT TEACHING

- Instruct patient how to administer form of levetiracetam prescribed and urge compliance with drug therapy.

! **WARNING** Urge family or caregiver to watch patient closely for evidence of suicidal tendencies, especially when therapy starts or dosage changes, and to report concerns immediately.

! **WARNING** Alert patient that drug may cause an allergic reaction and serious skin reactions. If present, tell patient to notify prescriber and, if severe, to seek immediate medical care. Also instruct patient to notify prescriber of any other persistent, serious, or unusual adverse reactions.

! **WARNING** Caution patient not to stop taking levetiracetam abruptly; inform her that drug dosage should be tapered under prescriber's direction to reduce the risk of breakthrough seizures.

- Caution patient that levetiracetam may cause dizziness and drowsiness, especially during first 4 weeks of therapy. Advise patient to avoid hazardous activities until drug's CNS effects are known and resolved.
- Explain to patient, family, or caregiver that levetiracetam may cause mental and behavioral changes, such as aggression, depression, irritability, and rarely psychotic symptoms. The prescriber should be contacted about any bothersome changes.
- Advise patient to keep taking other anticonvulsants, as ordered, while taking levetiracetam.
- Instruct patient to see prescriber regularly so that her progress can be monitored.

levocetirizine

Xyzal, Xyzal 24-HR

Class and Category

Pharmacologic class: H_1-receptor antagonist
Therapeutic class: Antihistamine

Indications and Dosages

✶ *To treat uncomplicated skin manifestations of chronic idiopathic urticaria*

TABLETS, ORAL SOLUTION

Adults and children ages 12 and older. 2.5 or 5 mg once daily in evening. *Maximum:* 5 mg daily.
Children ages 6 to 11. 2.5 mg once daily in evening. *Maximum:* 2.5 mg daily.

ORAL SOLUTION

Children ages 6 mo to age 5. 1.25 mg once daily in evening. *Maximum:* 1.25 mg daily.

✶ *To relieve symptoms associated with seasonal and perennial allergic rhinitis*

ORAL SOLUTION, TABLETS

Adults and children ages 12 and older. 2.5 or 5 mg once daily in evening. *Maximum:* 5 mg daily.
Children ages 6 to 11. 2.5 mg once daily. *Maximum:* 2.5 mg daily in evening

Children ages 2 to 5. 1.25 mg once daily. Maximum: 1.25 mg daily in evening.

∗ *To relieve symptoms associated with pediatric perennial allergic rhinitis*

ORAL SOLUTION

Children ages 6 mo to 2 yr. 1.25 mg once daily in evening. *Maximum:* 1.25 mg daily.

±**DOSAGE ADJUSTMENT** For children, maximum dosage should not be exceeded because systemic exposure in children is about twice that of adults. For adult patients and children ages 12 or older with mild renal impairment (creatinine clearance 50 to 80 ml/min), dosage should not exceed 2.5 mg daily. For adult patients and children ages 12 and older with moderate renal impairment (creatinine clearance 30 to 50 ml/min), dosage should not exceed 2.5 mg once every other day. For adult patients and children ages 12 and older with severe renal impairment (creatinine clearance 10 to 30 ml/min), dosage should not exceed 2.5 mg once every 3 to 4 days. For children under the age of 12, drug should not be used in the presence of renal impairment. For adult patients with both hepatic and renal impairment, dosage adjusted.

Drug Administration

P.O.

- Administer drug in evening.
- Use calibrated device to measure dosage of oral solution.

Route	Onset	Peak	Duration
P.O.	< 1 hr	0.5–1 hr	24 hr

Half-life: 8–9 hr

Mechanism of Action

Binds to central and peripheral H_1 receptors, competing with histamine for these sites and preventing it from reaching its site of action. By blocking histamine, levocetirizine produces antihistamine effects, inhibiting respiratory, vascular, and GI smooth-muscle contraction; decreasing capillary permeability, which reduces wheals, flares, and itching; and decreasing salivary and lacrimal gland secretions to relieve chronic urticaria and signs and symptoms of allergic rhinitis.

Contraindications

Children under the age of 12 with impaired renal function; creatinine clearance less than 10 ml/min (end-stage renal disease): hemodialysis; hypersensitivity to levocetirizine, cetirizine, or their components

Interactions

DRUGS

CNS depressants: Possibly increased CNS depression

ritonavir: Possibly increased risk of adverse effects of levocetirizine

theophylline: Possibly decreased clearance of levocetirizine

ACTIVITIES

alcohol use: Possibly increased CNS depression

Adverse Reactions

CNS: Aggression, agitation, asthenia, depression, dizziness, fatigue, fever, hallucinations, insomnia, movement disorders, myoclonus and extrapyramidal symptoms, paresthesia, **seizures**, somnolence, **suicidal ideation**, syncope, tic, tremor, vertigo

CV: Edema, palpitations, tachycardia

EENT: Blurred vision, dry mouth, epistaxis, nasopharyngitis, pharyngitis, visual disturbances

GI: **Hepatitis**, increased appetite, nausea, vomiting

GU: Dysuria, urinary retention

MS: Arthralgia, myalgia

RESP: Cough, dyspnea

SKIN: Acute generalized exanthematous pustulosis, fixed drug eruption, pruritus, rash, urticaria

Other: **Anaphylaxis**, **angioedema**, weight gain

Childbearing Considerations

PREGNANCY

- It is not known if drug causes fetal harm.
- Use with caution only if benefit to mother outweighs potential risk to fetus.

LACTATION

- It is not known if levocetirizine is present in breast milk although cetirizine is present.
- Mothers should check with prescriber before breastfeeding.

Nursing Considerations

- Use levocetirizine cautiously in patients with predisposing risk factors for urinary retention, such as prostatic hyperplasia or spinal cord lesion. Monitor patient's intake and output closely. If urinary retention is suspected, notify prescriber and expect drug to be discontinued if confirmed.

! WARNING Monitor patient for a hypersensivity reaction, which could become life threatening such as anaphylaxis or angioedema. If present, notify prescriber, expect drug to be discontinued, and provide supportive care, as needed and ordered.

! WARNING Monitor patient for suicidal behavior or thinkings. If present, notify prescriber immediately and institute suicide precautions.

- Expect to stop drug at least 72 hours before skin tests for allergies because drug may inhibit cutaneous histamine response, thus producing false-negative results.

PATIENT TEACHING

- Instruct patient how to administer levocetirizine.
- Stress importance to take drug exactly as prescribed.
- Urge patient to avoid alcohol while taking levocetirizine.

! WARNING Alert patient that drug can cause an allergic reaction. Tell patient to notify prescriber, if present, and to seek immediate medical care, if severe.

! WARNING Instruct family or caregiver that if patient develops abnormal thoughts, especially thoughts of harming oneself the prescriber should be notified immediately and safety measures put in place.

- Advise patient to avoid hazardous activities until drug's CNS effects are known and resolved.
- Tell patient to notify prescriber if he is feeling bladder fullness or notices that his urine output is significantly less than his intake.
- Alert patient taking levocetirizine long-term that rebound itching may occur within days after drug is discontinued.

levofloxacin

Class and Category

Pharmacologic class: Fluoroquinolone
Therapeutic class: Antibiotic

Indications and Dosages

* *To reduce incidence or progression of inhalation anthrax after exposure to aerosolized* Bacillus anthracis; *to treat plague, including pneumonic and septicemic plague, caused by* Yersinia pestis; *to provide prophylaxis for plague*

I.V. INFUSION, ORAL SOLUTION

Adults and children weighing 50 kg (110 lb) or more. 500 mg once daily for 60 days for treatment of inhalation anthrax and 10 to 14 days for treatment of plague.
Infants ages 6 mo and older and children weighing less than 50 kg (110 lb). 8 mg/kg every 12 hr for 60 days for treatment of inhalation anthrax and 10 to 14 days for treatment of plague. *Maximum:* 250 mg/dose.

TABLETS

Adults and children weighing 50 kg (110 lb) or more. 500 mg once daily for 60 days for treatment of inhalation anthrax and 10 to 14 days for treatment of plague.
Children weighing more than 30 kg (66 lb) but less than 50 kg (110 lb). 250 mg every 12 hr for 60 days.

* *To treat acute bacterial sinusitis caused by* Haemophilus influenzae, Moraxella catarrhalis, *or* Streptococcus pneumoniae

I.V. INFUSION, ORAL SOLUTION, TABLETS

Adults. 500 mg daily for 10 to 14 days. Alternatively, 750 mg once daily for 5 days.

* *To treat acute exacerbation of chronic bacterial bronchitis caused by* H. influenzae, H. parainfluenzae, M. catarrhalis, S.pneumoniae, *or* Staphylococcus aureus

I.V. INFUSION, ORAL SOLUTION, TABLETS

Adults. 500 mg once daily for 7 days.

* *To treat community-acquired pneumonia caused by* Chlamydophila pneumoniae, H. influenzae, H. parainfluenzae, Klebsiella pneumoniae, Legionella pneumophila, M. catarrhalis, Mycoplasma pneumoniae, S. aureus, *or* S. pneumoniae

I.V. INFUSION, ORAL SOLUTION, TABLETS

Adults. 500 mg once daily for 7 to 14 days. Alternatively, for infection caused by *C. pneumoniae, H. influenzae, H. parainfluenzae, M. pneumoniae,* or *S. pneumoniae,* 750 mg once daily for 5 days.

∗ *To treat uncomplicated UTI caused by* Escherichia coli, K. pneumoniae, *or* Staphylococcus saprophyticus

I.V. INFUSION, ORAL SOLUTION, TABLETS

Adults. 250 mg once daily for 3 days.

∗ *To treat complicated UTI caused by* Enterococcus faecalis, E. cloacae, E. coli, K. pneumoniae, Proteus mirabilis, *or* Pseudomonas aeruginosa; *acute pyelonephritis caused by* E. coli

I.V. INFUSION, ORAL SOLUTION, TABLETS

Adults. 250 mg once daily for 10 days.

∗ *To treat complicated UTI caused by* E. coli, K. pneumoniae, *or* P. mirabilis, *or acute pyelonephritis caused by* E. coli

I.V. INFUSION, ORAL SOLUTION, TABLETS

Adults. 750 mg once daily for 5 days.

∗ *To treat mild to moderate skin and soft-tissue infections caused by* S. aureus *or* S. pyogenes

I.V. INFUSION, ORAL SOLUTION, TABLETS

Adults. 500 mg once daily for 7 to 10 days.

∗ *To treat complicated skin and soft-tissue infections caused by methicillin-sensitive* E. faecalis, Proteus mirabilis, S. aureus, *or* S. pyogenes; *to treat nosocomial pneumonia caused by* E. coli, H. influenzae, K. pneumoniae, Pseudomonas aeruginosa, S. aureus, Serratia marcescens, *or* S. pneumoniae

I.V. INFUSION, ORAL SOLUTION, TABLETS

Adults. 750 mg once daily for 7 to 14 days.

∗ *To treat chronic bacterial prostatitis caused by* E. coli, E. faecalis, *or* S. epidermidis

I.V. INFUSION, ORAL SOLUTION, TABLETS

Adults. 500 mg once daily for 28 days.

± **DOSAGE ADJUSTMENT** For adult patients with creatinine clearance of 20 to 49 ml/min and dosage is 750 mg daily, dosage interval increased to every 48 hours; for dosage of 500 mg, initial dose of 500 mg given, followed by 250 mg every 24 hours. For adult patients with creatinine clearance of 10 to 19 ml/min or who are receiving dialysis, and dosage is 750 mg, initial dose of 750 mg given, followed by 500 mg every 48 hours; for dosage of 500 mg, initial dose of 500 mg given, followed by 250 mg every 48 hours; and for dosage of 250 mg (no information on dosing adjustment available for adult patient on dialysis at this dosage), dosage interval increased to every 48 hours unless the 250-mg dosage is used to treat uncomplicated UTI, then no dosage adjustment is required. Supplemental doses of levofloxacin are not required following continuous ambulatory peritoneal dialysis or hemodialysis because dialysis is not effective in removing levofloxacin from the body.

Drug Administration

- Administer drug with plenty of fluid to prevent crystalluria.
- Administer dose consistently at the same time(s) daily.

P.O.

- Tablets should be swallowed whole and not chewed, crushed, or split.
- Administer oral solution 1 hr before or 2 hr after eating. Use a calibrated device to measure dosage.
- Administer antacid containing aluminum or magnesium, didanosine, iron, multivitamins with zinc, sucralfate, or zinc at least 2 hr before or after oral solution or tablets of levofloxacin.

I.V.

- Drug is supplied as single-use vials or a premixed solution in single-use flexible container with a concentration of 5 mg/ml.
- To prepare the premixed solution, tear outer wrap at the notch and remove solution container. Check for minute leaks by squeezing the inner bag firmly. Discard if leaks are found or if seal is not intact. Also, discard if solution is cloudy or a precipitate is present. Do not use flexible containers in series connections because an air embolism might result. Do not dilute further. Discard any unused portion.
- To prepare single-use vials, dilute using 0.9% Sodium Chloride Injection, 5% Dextrose in Water, or 5% Dextrose in Water/0.9% Sodium Chloride Injection (see manufacturer's guidelines for other solutions) to a concentration of 5 mg/ml as follows: To achieve a 250 mg desired dosage strength, withdraw 10 ml from a 20 ml vial and add 40 ml of diluent; to achieve a 500 mg desired dosage strength, withdraw 20 ml

from a 20 ml vial and add 80 ml of diluent; and to achieve a 750 mg desired dosage strength, withdraw 30 ml from a 30 ml vial and add 120 ml of diluent. Diluted solution should be clear, slightly yellow, and free of particulate matter. Diluted solution is stable for 72 hr at room temperature, 14 days if refrigerated in plastic containers, and 6 months when frozen. If frozen, thaw only at room temperature or in refrigerator before administering. Do not refreeze after initial thawing.

- Administer a dosage of 250 or 500 mg slowly as an I.V. infusion over 60 min; a dosage of 750 mg slowly over 90 min. Do not administer as a rapid or bolus I.V. injection because hypotension may occur.
- Do not administer by any other route.
- If the same intravenous line is used to administer other drugs, flush line before and after infusion of levofloxacin with a solution compatible with the drug and any other drugs administered via the common I.V. line.
- *Incompatibilities:* Other additives, drugs, or substances; solutions containing multivalent cations

Route	Onset	Peak	Duration
P.O./I.V.	Unknown	1–2 hr	Unknown

Half-life: 6–8 hr

Mechanism of Action

Interferes with bacterial cell replication by inhibiting the bacterial enzyme DNA gyrase, which is essential for repair and replication of bacterial DNA.

Contraindications

Hypersensitivity to levofloxacin, other fluoroquinolones, or their components; myasthenia gravis

Interactions

DRUGS

aluminum-, calcium-, or magnesium-containing antacids; didanosine; iron; sucralfate; zinc: Reduced GI absorption of levofloxacin
cyclosporine: Increased risk of nephrotoxicity
NSAIDs: Possibly increased CNS stimulation and risk of seizures
oral anticoagulants: Increased anticoagulant effect and risk of bleeding
oral antidiabetic drugs: Possibly hyperglycemia or hypoglycemia
theophylline: Increased blood theophylline level and risk of toxicity

Adverse Reactions

CNS: Agitation, anxiety, CNS stimulation, confusion, delirium, depression, disorientation, disturbance in attention, dizziness, electroencephalogram abnormalities, **encephalopathy** (rare), fever, hallucinations, headache, hoarse voice, **increased intracranial pressure**, insomnia, light-headedness, memory impairment, nervousness, nightmares, paranoia, peripheral neuropathy, **pseudotumor cerebri**, psychosis, restlessness, **seizures**, sleep disturbance, **suicidal ideation**, toxic psychoses, tremors
CV: **Aortic dissection**, **arrhythmias**, leukocytoclastic vasculitis, **prolonged QT interval**, **rupture of aortic aneurysm**, tachycardia, **torsades de pointes**, vasculitis, vasodilation
EENT: Blurred vision, decreased visual acuity, diplopia, dysphonia, scotoma, smell or taste perversion, tinnitus, uveitis
ENDO: Hyperglycemia, **hypoglycemia**
GI: Abdominal pain, **acute hepatic failure or necrosis**, anorexia, ***Clostridioides difficile*-associated diarrhea**, constipation, diarrhea, flatulence, **hepatitis**, **hepatotoxicity**, indigestion, jaundice, nausea, **pseudomembranous colitis**, vomiting
GU: **Acute renal failure or insufficiency**, crystalluria, interstitial nephritis, vaginal candidiasis
HEME: **Agranulocytosis**, **aplastic anemia**, eosinophilia, **hemolytic anemia**, **leukopenia**, **pancytopenia**, **prolonged international normalized ratio (INR) and PT**, **thrombocytopenia**
MS: Arthralgia, arthritis, back pain, elevated muscle enzymes, gait abnormality, myalgia, **rhabdomyolysis**, tendon or muscle rupture, tendinopathy
RESP: **Hypersensitivity pneumonitis**
SKIN: **Erythema multiforme**, photosensitivity, pruritus, rash, **Stevens-Johnson syndrome**, **toxic epidermal necrolysis**, urticaria
Other: **Anaphylaxis**, **angioedema**, exacerbation of myasthenia gravis, **multiorgan failure**, serum sickness

Childbearing Considerations

PREGNANCY

- It is not known if drug causes fetal harm.
- Use with caution only if benefit to mother outweighs potential risk to fetus.

LACTATION

- Drug is present in breast milk.
- Breastfeeding is not recommended during drug therapy and for 2 days after last dose; mothers may consider pumping and discarding breast milk during drug therapy and for 2 days after last dose.

Nursing Considerations

! WARNING Know that patients with cardiomyopathy, hypokalemia, or significant bradycardia and those receiving a class IA or III antiarrhythmic shouldn't receive levofloxacin.

- Use levofloxacin cautiously in patients with renal insufficiency. Monitor renal function as appropriate during treatment.
- Use drug cautiously in patients with CNS disorders, such as epilepsy, as well as certain drug therapies, that may lower the seizure threshold. Also, use cautiously in patients taking corticosteroids, especially elderly patients because of increased risk of tendon rupture.
- Expect to obtain culture and sensitivity tests before levofloxacin treatment begins.
- Know that levofloxacin therapy should begin as soon as possible after suspected or confirmed exposure to *Y. pestis*.

! WARNING Monitor patient for a hypersensitivity reaction, which may become life-threatening, such as anaphylaxis or angioedema. A reaction may occur after first dose. If present, notify prescriber, expect drug to be discontinued, and provide supportive care, as needed and ordered.

! WARNING Monitor QT interval if needed. If it lengthens, notify prescriber at once and stop drug.

! WARNING Monitor patient's bowel elimination. If diarrhea develops, obtain stool culture to check for pseudomembranous colitis caused by *Clostridioides difficle*. Diarrhea may be mild or become life-threatening. If confirmed, expect to stop drug and give antibiotics effective against *C. difficile*, as ordered. Also expect to administer electrolytes, fluids, and protein supplementation, as needed and ordered.

! WARNING Monitor blood glucose level, especially in diabetic patient who takes an oral antidiabetic or uses insulin because levofloxacin may alter blood glucose level. If so, notify prescriber, stop drug immediately if patient has hypoglycemia, and provide prescribed treatment because severe cases of hypoglycemia resulting in coma or death have occurred.

! WARNING Be aware that levofloxacin increases risk of aortic aneurysm and dissection within 2 months following drug use, especially in elderly patients.

! WARNING Monitor patient for increased intracranial pressure, seizures, or suicidal behavior or thoughts. Also monitor patient for other persistent, serious, or unusual adverse reactions. Notify prescriber if any such adverse reactions occur and expect to discontinue levofloxacin.

! WARNING Know that fluoroquinolones like levofloxacin have caused disabling and potentially irreversible serious adverse reactions from different body systems that can occur together in the same patient. These reactions can occur within hours to weeks after starting the drug and usually cause central nervous system effects, peripheral neuropathy, tendinitis, and tendon rupture. All ages of patients and patients without any preexisting risk factors have experienced these reactions. Notify prescriber and expect to discontinue levofloxacin immediately at the first signs or symptoms of any serious adverse reactions.

- Watch for evidence of tendon rupture (inflammation, pain, swelling) during and up to several months after therapy, especially in children, elderly patients, patients receiving corticosteroids, and patients with heart, kidney, and lung transplants. Notify prescriber about suspected tendon rupture and have patient rest and refrain from exercise until tendon rupture has been ruled out. If present, expect to provide supportive care, as ordered.

- Be aware that children have a higher incidence of musculoskeletal adverse reactions, especially arthralgia, arthritis, gait abnormality, and tendinopathy. Report any complaint involving the musculoskeletal system promptly to prescriber.

PATIENT TEACHING

- Tell patient how to administer the form of levofloxacin prescribed.
- Advise patient to increase fluid intake during therapy to prevent crystalluria.
- Direct patient to take an antacid containing aluminum or magnesium, didanosine, iron, multivitamins containing sucralfate or zinc at least 2 hours before or after levofloxacin.
- Tell patient to complete the drug as prescribed, even if symptoms subside.

! **WARNING** Alert patient that drug may cause an allergic reaction. If present, tell patient to notify prescriber and, if severe, to seek immediate medical care.

! **WARNING** Urge patient to tell prescriber about severe diarrhea, even if it's more than 2 months after drug therapy ends. Additional treatment may be needed.

! **WARNING** Advise diabetic patient to monitor blood glucose level and report changes. Review how to recognize and treat hypoglycemia. Instruct family or caregiver how to administer glucagon if patient develops severe hypoglycemia and to seek immediate medical care for patient.

- Advise patient to stop taking levofloxacin immediately and notify prescriber if any persistent, serious, or worsening adverse effects occur.
- Tell patient to stop drug and notify prescriber if he develops abnormal changes in motor or sensory function, or if he experiences bruising right after an injury in a tendon area, hearing or feeling a pop or snap in a tendon area or is unable to move the affected area or bear weight. Inform patient tendon problems may be permanent.
- Urge patient to avoid excessive sun exposure and to wear sunscreen because of increased risk of photosensitivity. Tell patient to notify prescriber at first sign of photosensitivity.
- Caution patient to avoid hazardous activities until drug's CNS effects are known and resolved.

levothyroxine sodium

(l-thyroxine sodium, T_4, thyroxine sodium)

Eltroxin (CAN), Ermeza, Euthyrox, Levo-T, Levoxyl, Synthroid, Thyquidity, Tirosint, Tirosint-Sol, Unithroid

Class and Category

Pharmacologic class: Synthetic thyroxine (T_4)
Therapeutic class: Thyroid hormone replacement

Indications and Dosages

∗ *To treat primary, secondary, or tertiary hypothyroidism*

CAPSULES, ORAL SOLUTION, TABLETS

Adults and adolescents in whom growth and puberty are complete. *Initial:* 1.6 mcg/kg once daily. Dosage adjusted by 12.5 to 25 mcg every 4 to 6 wk, as needed. *Usual maintenance dose:* 100 to 125 mcg daily.
Adults with severe long-standing hypothyroidism. *Initial:* 12.5 to 25 mcg daily with dosage adjusted in 12.5- to 25-mcg increments every 2 to 4 wk, as needed.
Elderly patients or patients with cardiac disease. *Initial:* 12.5 to 25 mcg daily, increased gradually every 6 to 8 wk, as needed.
Children ages 12 and older in whom growth and puberty are incomplete. 2 to 3 mcg/kg daily.
Children ages 6 to 12. 4 to 5 mcg/kg daily.

ORAL SOLUTION, TABLETS

Children ages 1 to 5. 5 to 6 mcg/kg daily.
Infants ages 6 mo to 12 mo. 6 to 8 mcg/kg daily.

Infants ages 3 mo to 6 mo. 8 to 10 mcg/kg daily.
Infants and neonates birth to age 3 mo. 10 to 15 mcg/kg daily.
Infants and neonates birth to age 3 mo at risk for cardiac failure. *Initial:* Highly individualized but less than 10 mcg/kg daily with dosage increased every 4 to 6 wk, as needed.

✶ *As adjunct to surgery and radioiodine therapy in the management of thyrotropin-dependent, well-differentiated thyroid cancer*

ORAL SOLUTION, CAPSULES, TABLETS

Adults and children. Highly individualized and based on the target level of thyroid stimulating hormone (TSH) suppression for the stage and clinical status of thyroid cancer.

✶ *To treat myxedema coma*

I.V. INJECTION

Adults. *Initial as loading dose:* 300 to 500 mcg, followed by 50 to 100 mcg once daily until patient able to tolerate drug orally.

±**DOSAGE ADJUSTMENT** For all patients, starting dose and dosage adjustment highly individualized according to patient's age, body weight, cardiovascular status, concomitant medications being taken, co-administered food and the specific nature of the condition being treated. For females of childbearing age who are pregnant, dosage possibly increased during pregnancy. For children at risk for hyperactivity, initial dosage reduced by 75% of normal dosage with dosage increased by 25% of the full recommended replacement dosage weekly until the full replacement dosage is reached.

Drug Administration

P.O.

- Administer once daily, preferably on an empty stomach. Administer tablets one-half to 1 hr before first meal of the day and oral solution 15 min before first meal of the day.
- Administer capsules or tablets with a full glass of water. Have patient swallow drug whole and not chew or divide tablet or open capsule.
- For patient, infants, and children who cannot swallow capsules or tablets, obtain order for oral solution. Alternatively for tablet form, crush tablet, and mix in 5 to 10 ml of breast milk, formula (except soy-based), or water. Administer immediately by dropper or spoon. Do not store mixture. Do not administer in foods that decrease absorption. Do not administer capsule form to children under the age of 6.
- Administer oral solution by squeezing contents of single-dose unit ampule into a cup or glass containing only water. Stir mixture and give to patient to drink immediately. Add more water to cup or glass and have patient drink mixture to obtain the full dose. Alternatively, administer oral solution by squeezing contents into the patient's mouth or onto a spoon before administering without using water.
- Administer at least 4 hr before or after drugs known to interfere with absorption.

I.V.

- Reconstitute drug by adding 5 ml of 0.9% Sodium Chloride Injection to drug vial.
- Shake vial to mix well.
- Administer immediately as an I.V. injection at a rate not to exceed 100 mcg/min.
- Discard any solution left in vial.
- *Incompatibilities:* I.V. solutions except for 0.9% Sodium Chloride Injection; other drugs

Route	Onset	Peak	Duration
P.O.	3–5 days	2–4 hr	Unknown
I.V.	6–8 hr	Unknown	Unknown

Half-life: 3–10 days

Mechanism of Action

Replaces endogenous thyroid hormone, which may exert its physiologic effects by controlling DNA transcription and protein synthesis. Levothyroxine has all the following actions of endogenous thyroid hormone. The drug:

- increases energy expenditure.
- accelerates the rate of cellular oxidation, which stimulates body tissue growth, maturation, and metabolism.
- regulates differentiation and proliferation of stem cells.
- aids in myelination of nerves and development of synaptic processes in the nervous system.
- regulates growth.

- decreases blood and hepatic cholesterol concentrations.
- enhances carbohydrate and protein metabolism, increasing gluconeogenesis and protein synthesis.

Contraindications

Hypersensitivity to levothyroxine or its components; uncorrected adrenal insufficiency

Interactions

DRUGS

5-fluorouracil, clofibrate, estrogens (oral), estrogen-containing oral contraceptives, heroin, methadone, mitotane, tamoxifen: Possibly increased serum thyroxine-binding globulin (TBG) concentration
aluminum- and magnesium-containing antacids, calcium carbonate, cholestyramine, colesevelam, colestipol, ferrous sulfate, kayexalate, lanthanum, orlistat, proton pump inhibitors, sevelamer, simethicone, sucralfate: Possibly decreased absorption and reduced effects of levothyroxine
amiodarone, glucocorticoids: Possibly hyperthyroidism from decreased peripheral conversion of T_4 to T_3, leading to decreased T_3 levels
anabolic steroids, androgens, asparaginase, glucocorticoids, slow-release nicotinic acid: Possibly decreased serum TBG concentration
beta-blockers: Possibly impaired action of beta-blockers and decreased conversion of T_4 to triiodothyronine (T_3)
carbamazepine, fenamates, furosemide (greater than 80 mg I.V.), heparin, hydantoins, NSAIDs, salicylates (greater than 2 g/day): Transient increase in FT4 followed by decreased serum T_4 and normal FT4 and TSH concentrations with continued administration
digoxin: Reduced digoxin effects
insulin, oral antidiabetic drugs: Decreased effectiveness of these drugs
ketamine: Possibly marked hypertension and tachycardia
oral anticoagulants: Altered anticoagulant activity
phenobarbital: Reduces response to thyroxine decreasing effectiveness
rifampin: Accelerates metabolism of levothyroxine
sympathomimetics: Increased risk of coronary insufficiency in patients with coronary artery disease; increased effects of both drugs
tetracyclic and tricyclic antidepressants: Increased therapeutic and toxic effects of both drugs
tyrosine-kinase inhibitors: Possible decreased effectiveness of levothyroxine leading to hypothyroidism

FOODS

cottonseed meal, dietary fiber, soybean flour (infant formula), walnuts: Possibly decreased absorption of levothyroxine from GI tract
grapefruit juice: Possible delayed absorption of levothyroxine and reduced bioavailability

Adverse Reactions

CNS: Anxiety, craniosynostosis (infants with overtreatment), emotional lability, fatigue, fever, headache, heat intolerance, hyperactivity, insomnia, irritability, nervousness, **pseudotumor cerebri** (children), **seizures** (rare), somnolence, tremors
CV: Angina, **arrhythmias**, **cardiac arrest**, **heart failure**, increased blood pressure and pulse, **MI**, palpitations, tachycardia
ENDO: Hyperthyroidism (with over-replacement), **myxedema coma (with undertreatment)**, worsening of diabetic control
GI: Abdominal cramps or pain, diarrhea, dysphagia, elevated liver enzymes, increased appetite, nausea, vomiting
GU: Impaired fertility, menstrual irregularities
MS: Arthralgia, decreased bone mineral density (with over-replacement), muscle spasm or weakness, myalgia, premature closure of the epiphysis (children), slipped capital femoral epiphysis (children)
RESP: Dyspnea, wheezing
SKIN: Alopecia (transient), diaphoresis, flushing, pruritus, rash, urticaria
Other: **Angioedema**, serum sickness, weight gain or loss

Childbearing Considerations

PREGNANCY

- Drug is not known to cause fetal harm and should not be stopped during pregnancy.
- Be aware that pregnancy may increase dosage requirements.

LACTATION

- Drug is present in breast milk.
- Mothers should check with prescriber before breastfeeding.

Nursing Considerations

! **WARNING** Be aware that levothyroxine therapy is not to be used for treatment of obesity or for weight loss. The drug should also not be used to suppress benign thyroid nodules and nontoxic diffuse goiter in iodine-sufficient patients, nor should it be used to treat transient hypothyroidism during the recovery phase of subacute thyroiditis.

! **WARNING** Use levothyroxine cautiously in the elderly and patients with underlying cardiovascular disease. Know that levothyroxine should be started at a lower dose in these patients because overtreatment can increase cardiac contractility, cardiac wall thickness, and heart rate, which can precipitate angina or arrhythmias (atrial fibrillation being the most common arrhythmia in the elderly). Also, use caution in patients with coronary artery disease undergoing surgery while receiving suppressive levothyroxine therapy and in patients receiving sympathomimetic drugs concurrently. Monitor for signs and symptoms of coronary insufficiency.

! **WARNING** Monitor patient for a hypersensitivity reaction, which could become life threatening such as angioedema. If present, notify prescriber immediately and provide supportive care, as needed and ordered.

- Expect to stop biotin and biotin-containing supplements for at least 2 days before thyroid testing because biotin interferes with thyroid hormone immunoassays that are based on a biotin and streptayidin interaction, which may cause an erroneous thyroid hormone test.
- Expect patient to undergo thyroid function tests regularly during levothyroxine therapy. Monitor all patients for signs and symptoms of over- or undertreatment with levothyroxine because drug has a narrow therapeutic index. Overtreatment or undertreatment can negatively affect bone metabolism, cardiovascular function, cognitive function, GI function, glucose and lipid metabolism, growth and development, and reproductive function. In addition, in children with acquired or congenital hypothyroidism, overtreatment may cause craniosynostosis in infants, may adversely affect brain maturation, and may accelerate the bone age and result in premature epiphyseal closure, which will compromise stature for life. Monitor patient's response to titration to detect any of these negative effects and notify prescriber, if present. Especially monitor infants closely during the first 2 weeks of therapy for arrythmias and cardiac overload.
- Know that peak therapeutic effect of levothyroxine may not occur for 4 to 6 weeks.
- Monitor PT of patient who is receiving anticoagulants, as a dosage adjustment may be required.
- Monitor blood glucose level of diabetic patient because drug may worsen glycemic control and result in increased antidiabetic agent or insulin requirement. Carefully monitor patient after starting, changing, or discontinuing levothyroxine.
- Keep in mind when interpreting TBG levels that many disorders and medications can decrease TBG concentration, causing a TBG deficiency.

PATIENT TEACHING

- Inform patient that levothyroxine replaces a hormone that is normally produced by the thyroid gland and that she'll probably need to take drug for life.
- Instruct patient, family, or caregiver how to administer the form of levothyroxine prescribed.
- Emphasize the need to take levothyroxine tablets with a full glass of water to avoid choking, gagging, having tablet stick in throat, and developing heartburn afterward.
- Inform patient that drug may require a few weeks to take effect.
- Advise patient not to stop drug or change dosage unless instructed by prescriber.
- Instruct patient to separate antacids and calcium or iron supplements by at least 4 hours from levothyroxine doses.

! **WARNING** Alert patient that drug may cause an allergic reaction. If present, tell patient to notify prescriber and, if severe, to seek immediate medical care.

! WARNING Instruct patient to report signs of hyperthyroidism, as dosage may need to be decreased. Also, instruct patient to report signs of hypothyroidism as dosage may need to be increased.

- Urge patient to be compliant with laboratory appointments to monitor drug's effectiveness.
- Inform patient that transient hair loss may occur during first few months of levothyroxine therapy.

lidocaine hydrochloride

Lidoderm, Xylocard (CAN)

Class and Category

Pharmacologic class: Amide derivative
Therapeutic class: Class IB antiarrhythmic, local anesthetic

Indications and Dosages

∗ *To treat ventricular arrhythmias occurring during cardiac manipulations, such as cardiac surgery; to treat life-threatening ventricular arrhythmias, such as occurring during acute MI*

I.V. INFUSION AND INJECTION

Adults. *Loading:* 50 to 100 mg (0.70 to 1.4 mg/kg) by I.V. injection given at 25 to 50 mg/min. If desired response isn't achieved after 5 to 10 min, second dose of 25 to 50 mg (or 0.5 to 0.75 mg/kg) given and repeated every 5 min until desired response occurs or maximum dose (300 mg in 1 hr) has been reached. *Maintenance:* 20 to 50 mcg/kg/min (1 to 4 mg/min) by continuous infusion (rarely longer than 24 hr). Smaller bolus dose repeated 15 to 20 min after start of infusion, as needed, to maintain therapeutic blood level. *Maximum:* 300 mg (or 3 mg/kg) over 1 hr.

Children. *Loading:* 1 mg/kg by I.V. injection (not to exceed 100 mg). *Maintenance:* 20 to 50 mcg/kg/min by continuous infusion.

± **DOSAGE ADJUSTMENT** For patients receiving prolonged lidocaine therapy intravenously (greater than 24 hours), dosage reduced. For children, continuous infusion rate should not exceed 20 mcg/kg/min when drug clearance is reduced such as may occur in cardiac arrest, congestive heart failure, and shock. For patients with decreased hepatic function or diminished hepatic blood flow as in heart failure or after cardiac surgery, or elderly patients ages 70 or older, dosage reduced.

∗ *To provide topical anesthesia for mucous membranes or skin*

FILM-FORMING GEL, JELLY, OR OINTMENT

Adults. Thin layer applied to skin or mucous membranes, as needed, before procedure.

∗ *To provide pain relief of postherpetic neuralgia*

TRANSDERMAL PATCH (LIDODERM 5%)

Adults. 1 to 3 patches applied over most painful area for up to 12 hr only once within a 24-hr period.

Drug Administration

I.V.

- Administer I.V. injection as a bolus at a rate of 25 to 50 mg/min.
- Follow manufacturer's guidelines for diluting lidocaine in 1,000 ml of 5% Dextrose in Water.
- Check premixed solutions carefully to ensure correct solution is being used.
- Solution should be clear. If not, discard.
- Use an infusion pump for continuous infusion.
- Administer I.V. infusion at 20 to 50 mcg/kg/ min (1 to 4 mg/min) at the specific rate prescribed. Do not exceed the maximum rate of 4 mg/min, as toxicity risk increases above this rate.
- Reduce continuous infusion dosage, as ordered, if infusion continues beyond 24 hr.
- Cardiac monitoring should be in place when administering lidocaine continuously.
- *Incompatibilities:* None listed by manufacturer

TOPICAL

- Apply lidocaine jelly or ointment to gauze or bandage before applying to skin.

TRANSDERMAL

- Patches may be cut into smaller sizes with scissors prior to removal of the release liner, if needed.
- Apply immediately upon removal from the protective envelope to clean, dry skin. Patch may not stick if it gets wet.

- If patient complains of burning or irritation, remove the patch(es) and do not reapply until irritation is gone.
- Wash hands immediately after applying patch.
- Do not store patch outside of the sealed envelope.
- Fold used patches so that the adhesive side sticks to itself and safely discard.

Route	Onset	Peak	Duration
I.V.	45–90 sec	Unknown	10–20 min
Topical	2–5 min	3–5 min	0.5–1 hr
Transdermal	0.5–3 hr	Unknown	Unknown

Half-life: 1.5–2 hr

Mechanism of Action

Combines with fast sodium channels in myocardial cell membranes, which inhibits sodium influx into cells and decreases ventricular depolarization, as well as automaticity and excitability during diastole. Lidocaine also blocks nerve impulses by decreasing the permeability of neuronal membranes to sodium, which produces local anesthesia.

Contraindications

Adams-Stokes syndrome; hypersensitivity to lidocaine, amide anesthetics, or their components; severe heart block (without artificial pacemaker); Wolff-Parkinson-White syndrome

Interactions

DRUGS

amiodarone, phenytoin, procainamide, propranolol, quinidine: Additive cardiac effects possibly resulting in toxicity; antagonistic cardiac effects
beta-blockers; CYP1A2 inhibitors, such as fluvoxamine; CYP3A4 inhibitors, such as propofol, cimetidine: Increased blood lidocaine level and risk of toxicity
CYP1A2 inducers, CYP3A4 inducers: Decreased blood lidocaine level with decreased effectiveness
digoxin: Increased toxicity

Adverse Reactions

CNS: Agitation; anxiety; apprehension; confusion; difficulty speaking; disorientation; dizziness; drowsiness; euphoria; hallucinations; lethargy; light-headedness; **malignant hyperthermia**; paresthesia; **seizures**; sensation of cold, heat, or numbness; tremors; twitching; unconsciousness
CV: Bradycardia, **cardiac arrest**, **hypotension**, **new or worsening arrhythmias**, tachycardia
EENT: Blurred vision, diplopia, oral hypoesthesia, tinnitus
GI: Nausea, vomiting
HEME: Methemoglobinemia
MS: Dysarthria, muscle weakness, myalgia
RESP: Respiratory arrest or depression
Other: Anaphylaxis; injection-site burning, irritation, petechiae, redness, stinging, swelling, and tenderness; other less severe hypersensitivity reactions; worsened pain

Childbearing Considerations

PREGNANCY

- It is not known if drug causes fetal harm.
- Use with caution only if benefit to mother outweighs potential risk to fetus.

LACTATION

- Drug is present in breast milk.
- Mothers should check with prescriber before breastfeeding.

Nursing Considerations

! **WARNING** Use caution in patients with severe hepatic or renal disease because accumulation of lidocaine may occur and lead to toxicity. Monitor liver and renal function throughout parenteral lidocaine therapy.

! **WARNING** Use caution when administering lidocaine to patients with compromised myocardial function because of risk of electrolyte disturbances or fluid overload. Also, use caution in patients with any form of AV block, including AV block caused by digitalis toxicity, as well as in patients with hypovolemia and shock.

- Monitor patient's ECG continuously when giving lidocaine I.V. to determine effectiveness of drug.

! **WARNING** Observe for respiratory depression after bolus injection and during I.V. infusion of lidocaine.

! **WARNING** Monitor patient for hypersensitivity reactions that can be as severe as anaphylaxis following lidocaine administration. Keep life-support equipment and vasopressors nearby during I.V. use in case of respiratory depression or other reactions. If anaphylaxis occurs, discontinue drug, notify prescriber, and provide supportive care, as needed and ordered.

! **WARNING** Know that if signs of toxicity, such as dizziness occur, notify prescriber and expect to discontinue or slow I.V. infusion. Expect to check blood drug level to determine if a therapeutic level has been exceeded. Therapeutic level is 2 to 5 mcg/ml.

! **WARNING** Monitor for malignant hyperthermia. If present, stop lidocaine administration immediately, notify prescriber, and provide therapeutic countermeasures, as needed and ordered.

- Monitor vital signs as well as electrolyte levels during and after therapy.

PATIENT TEACHING

- Instruct patient how to administer topical form of lidocaine prescribed.
- Inform patient who receives lidocaine as an anesthetic that she'll feel numbness.
- Tell patient to wash hands thoroughly after handling lidocaine topical forms or patch and to avoid getting drug in eyes.

! **WARNING** Tell patient to immediately notify staff if any signs or symptoms of an allergic reaction occurs during I.V. administration. Instruct patient receiving a topical form of lidocaine to notify presriber if an allergic reaction occurs and, if severe, to seek immediate medical care.

- Tell patient prescribed a patch form to remove patch if burning or irritation occurs at the site and not to reapply until irritation is gone.

! **WARNING** Tell patient to report any persistent, serious, or unusual adverse reaction to prescriber.

! **WARNING** Warn patient prescribed a lidocaine patch not to place external heat sources, such as electric blanket or heating pad, on it while wearing it because heat may cause the drug to be absorbed faster, increasing the risk of adverse effects, including toxicity.

! **WARNING** Caution patient to keep lidocaine topical preparations and patches out of reach of children and pets.

linaclotide

Linzess

Class and Category

Pharmacologic class: Guanylate cyclase-C agonist
Therapeutic class: Bowel stimulator

Indications and Dosages

✱ *To treat irritable bowel syndrome with constipation*

CAPSULES

Adults. 290 mcg once daily.

✱ *To treat chronic, idiopathic constipation*

CAPSULES

Adults. 72 or 145 mcg once daily.

✱ *To treat functional constipation in pediatric patients*

CAPSULES

Children ages 6 to 17. 72 mcg once daily.

Drug Administration

P.O.

- Administer on an empty stomach, at least 30 min before the first meal of the day at about the same time each day.
- Capsules should be swallowed whole and not chewed or crushed.
- If patient has difficulty swallowing, capsules can be opened, contents sprinkled on 1 teaspoon of room-temperature applesauce and administered immediately. Ensure that patient does not chew beads. Alternatively, capsule contents may be mixed with 30 ml of room-temperature bottled water, gently swirled for at least 20 sec, and administered immediately. Add another 30 ml of bottled water to beads remaining in cup and repeat process. Do not store mixture for later use. Ensure patient does not eat for 30 min after being given drug mixed in applesauce or water.

- Drug may be administered through a gastrostomy or nasogastric tube by mixing content of capsules with 30 ml of water in a cup; swirl gently for at least 20 sec. Draw mixture up in a catheter-tipped syringe and apply rapid and steady pressure (10 ml/10 sec) to dispense into the tube. Add another 30 ml of water to any beads remaining in cup and repeat process. After administering mixture, flush nasogastric/gastrostomy tube with a minimum of 10 ml of water.

Route	Onset	Peak	Duration
P.O.	1 wk	Unknown	Unknown

Half-life: 11–12 hr

Mechanism of Action

Acts locally on the luminal surface of the intestinal epithelium through activation of guanylate cyclase-C, which increases both extracellular and intracellular concentrations of cyclic guanosine monophosphate (cGMP). Elevation in intracellular cGMP stimulates secretion of bicarbonate and chloride into the intestinal lumen, which increases intestinal fluid and accelerates GI transit to relieve constipation. Increased extracellular cGMP decreases the activity of pain-sensing nerves, resulting in a reduction of intestinal pain present with constipation and irritable bowel syndrome.

Contraindications

Hypersensitivity to linaclotide or its components, known or suspected mechanical GI obstruction, pediatric patients under 2 years of age

Interactions

DRUGS

None reported by manufacturer.

Adverse Reactions

CNS: Fatigue, headache
EENT: Sinusitis
GI: Abdominal distention or pain, defecation urgency, diarrhea (may become severe), dyspepsia, fecal incontinence, flatulence, gastroesophageal reflux, hematochezia, increased risk of viral gastroenteritis, **melena**, nausea, **rectal hemorrhage**, vomiting
RESP: Upper respiratory infection
SKIN: Urticaria
Other: **Dehydration**, **hypersensitivity reactions (anaphylaxis**, **angioedema**, rash, urticaria)

Childbearing Considerations

PREGNANCY

- It is not known if drug can cause fetal harm but is not expected to harm fetus as drug is negligibly absorbed systemically.
- Use with caution only if benefit to mother outweighs potential risk to fetus.

LACTATION

- It is not known if drug is present in breast milk.
- Mothers should check with prescriber before breastfeeding.

Nursing Considerations

! **WARNING** Monitor patient for hypersensitivity reactions, which can become life-threatening, such as anaphylaxis or angioedema. If present, withhold drug, notify prescriber, and provide supportive care, as needed and ordered.

! **WARNING** Monitor patient for diarrhea that may become severe. If severe diarrhea occurs, assess patient for dizziness, electrolyte abnormalities (hypokalemia and hyponatremia), hypotension, and syncope. Notify prescriber if diarrhea occurs. Expect to withhold drug. Also, know that if severe, patient may require hospitalization and intravenous fluid administration.

PATIENT TEACHING

- Instruct patient how to administer linaclotide.

! **WARNING** Alert patient that drug may cause an allergic reaction. If present, tell patient to notify prescriber and, if severe, to seek immediate medical care.

! **WARNING** Advise patient to stop taking linaclotide if severe diarrhea occurs and to contact prescriber immediately.

- Instruct patient to store linaclotide out of the reach of children.

linagliptin

Tradjenta

Class and Category

Pharmacologic class: Dipeptidyl peptidase-4 (DDP-4) enzyme inhibitor
Therapeutic class: Antidiabetic

Indications and Dosages

✱ *As adjunct to improve glycemic control in type 2 diabetes mellitus*

TABLETS

Adults. 5 mg once daily.

±**DOSAGE ADJUSTMENT** For patients taking a supplemental oral hypoglycemic agent or insulin, dosage of those drugs may have to be reduced.

Drug Administration

P.O.

- Administer with or without food but consistently.

Route	Onset	Peak	Duration
P.O.	Unknown	1.5 hr	Unknown

Half-life: 11–12 hr

Mechanism of Action

Inhibits the enzyme, dipeptidyl peptidase-4, that degrades incretin hormones responsible for glucose elevation. This allows levels of incretin hormones to rise, stimulating the release of insulin in a glucose-dependent manner while decreasing the glucagon level in the blood. In addition, glucagon secretion from pancreatic alpha cells is reduced, resulting in a reduction in the amount of glucose released by the liver. These combined actions reduce blood glucose levels, thereby improving glycemic control in type 2 diabetes.

Contraindications

Hypersensitivity to linagliptin or its components

Interactions

DRUGS

CYP3A4 or P-gp inducers (strong), such as rifampin: Decreased linagliptin effectiveness
insulin, sulfonylureas: Increased risk of hypoglycemia

Adverse Reactions

CNS: Headache
CV: Hyperlipidemia, hypertriglyceridemia
EENT: Mouth ulceration, nasopharyngitis, stomatitis
ENDO: **Hypoglycemia**
GI: **Acute pancreatitis**, constipation, diarrhea, elevated lipase level
GU: UTI
MS: Arthralgia (may be disabling and severe); back, extremity, or joint pain; myalgia; **rhabdomyolysis**
RESP: Bronchial hyperreactivity, cough
SKIN: Bullous pemphigoid, exfoliative skin conditions, localized skin exfoliation, rash, urticaria
Other: **Anaphylaxis**, **angioedema**, elevated uric acid, weight gain

Childbearing Considerations

PREGNANCY

- It is not known if drug causes fetal harm.
- Use with caution only if benefit to mother outweighs potential risk to fetus.

LACTATION

- It is not known if drug is present in breast milk.
- Mothers should check with prescriber before breastfeeding.

Nursing Considerations

! **WARNING** Monitor patient for a hypersensitivity reaction, which may become life-threatening such as anaphylaxis or angioedema. If present, notify prescriber, expect drug to be discontinued, and provide supportive care, as needed and ordered.

! **WARNING** Be aware that heart failure has been linked to 2 other drugs in the same class as linagliptin. Use caution when administering linagliptin, especially to patients with a prior history of heart failure or renal impairment. Monitor patient for signs and symptoms of heart failure and report any to prescriber immediately.

! **WARNING** Monitor patient closely for hypoglycemia, especially if another antidiabetic drug, such as insulin or a sulfonylurea, is used concomitantly. If signs and symptoms of hypoglycemia occur, check patient's blood glucose level. If confirmed, treat according to institutional protocol and notify prescriber.

! **WARNING** Monitor patient for signs and symptoms of pancreatitis, such as abdominal pain, fever, nausea, sweating, and vomiting. Notify prescriber if present, and expect drug to be discontinued, as acute pancreatitis may become life-threatening.

- Monitor patient's blood glucose level routinely to determine response to drug. Expect to check patient's glycosylated hemoglobin every 3 to 6 months or as ordered to evaluate long-term blood glucose control.

PATIENT TEACHING

- Instruct patient how to administer linagliptin and what to do if a dose is missed.

! **WARNING** Alert patient that drug may cause an allergic reaction. If present, tell patient to notify prescriber and, if severe, to seek immediate medical care.

! **WARNING** Monitor patient for signs and symptoms of acute pancreatitis, such as persistent severe abdominal pain radiating to the back, which may or may not be accompanied by vomiting, and to seek medical attention immediately.

! **WARNING** Review with patient, family, or caregiver the signs and symptoms of hypoglycemia and how to treat. Urge patient to report hypoglycemia to precriber.

! **WARNING** Review signs and symptoms of heart failure with patient, such as difficulty breathing; swelling or fluid retention, especially in ankles, feet, or legs; unusual tiredness; or fast weight gain. Tell patient to report any such symptoms immediately to prescriber.

- Inform patient that disabling and severe arthralgia may occur with linagliptin therapy beginning within a day of starting therapy or years later. Patient should notify prescriber if severe joint pain occurs.
- Advise patient to report blisters or erosions that occur to prescriber.
- Urge patient to carry identification indicating that patient has diabetes.

linezolid

Zyvox

Class and Category

Pharmacologic class: Oxazolidinone
Therapeutic class: Antibiotic

Indications and Dosages

✶ *To treat vancomycin-resistant* Enterococcus faecium *infections, including concurrent bacteremia*

I.V. INFUSION, ORAL SUSPENSION, TABLETS

Adults and children ages 12 and older. 600 mg every 12 hr for 14 to 28 days.
Neonates ages 7 days and older, infants, and children ages 11 and younger. 10 mg/kg every 8 hr for 14 to 28 days.
Neonates younger than 7 days. 10 mg/kg every 12 hr, increased to every 8 hr when neonate is 7 days old. Given for 14 to 28 days.

✶ *To treat nosocomial pneumonia caused by* Staphylococcus aureus *(methicillin-susceptible and resistant strains) or* Streptococcus pneumoniae *(penicillin-susceptible strains only); to treat community-acquired pneumonia, including accompanying bacteremia, caused by* S. aureus *(methicillin-susceptible strains only) or* S. pneumoniae *(penicillin-susceptible strains only); to treat complicated skin and soft-tissue infections, including diabetic foot infections without concomitant osteomyelitis, caused by* S. aureus *(methicillin-susceptible and resistant strains),* Streptococcus agalactiae, *or* Streptococcus pyogenes

I.V. INFUSION, ORAL SUSPENSION, TABLETS

Adults and children ages 12 and older. 600 mg every 12 hr for 10 to 14 days.
Neonates ages 7 days or older, infants, and children ages 11 and younger. 10 mg/kg every 8 hr for 10 to 14 days.
Neonates younger than 7 days. 10 mg/kg every 12 hr, increased to every 8 hr when neonate is 7 days old. Given for 10 to 14 days.

✶ *To treat uncomplicated skin and soft-tissue infections caused by* S. aureus *(methicillin-susceptible strains only) or* S. pyogenes

ORAL SUSPENSION, TABLETS

Adults. 400 mg every 12 hr for 10 to 14 days.
Children ages 12 and older. 600 mg every 12 hr for 10 to 14 days.
Children ages 5 to 11. 10 mg/kg every 12 hr for 10 to 14 days.
Neonates ages 7 days and older, infants, and children to age 5. 10 mg/kg every 8 hr for 10 to 14 days.
Neonates younger than 7 days. 10 mg/kg every 12 hr, increased to every 8 hr when neonate is 7 days old. Given for 10 to 14 days.

Drug Administration

P.O.

- Administer oral suspension to neonates, infants, and children who cannot swallow tablets.
- Prepare oral suspension by gently tapping bottle to loosen powder. Add about 63 ml distilled water, shake vigorously, then add 60 ml more of distilled water and shake vigorously again. Concentration will be 100 mg/5 ml.
- Before each use, gently invert bottle 3 to 5 times to mix. Do not shake. Use a calibrated device to measure dosage.
- Store oral suspension at room temperature and discard any unused portion after 21 days.
- Tablets should be swallowed whole and not chewed, crushed, or split.

I.V.

- Supplied in single-dose, ready-to-use infusion bags.
- Keep infusion bags in the overwrap until ready to use.
- Check for minute leaks by firmly squeezing the bag. If leaks are detected, discard the solution.
- Solution may exhibit a yellow color that can intensify over time but does not affect potency of drug.
- Do not use with series plastic connections.
- Don't add other drugs to linezolid solution.
- Infuse I.V. solution over 30 to 120 min.
- Flush intravenous line before and after infusion of drug if other drugs will be administered in same line.
- *Incompatibilities:* Amphotericin B, ceftriaxone, chlorpromazine hydrochloride, cotrimoxazole, diazepam, erythromycin lactobionate, pentamidine isethionate, phenytoin sodium, or trimethoprim-sulfamethoxazole; I.V. solutions other than 0.9% Sodium Chloride Injection, 5% Dextrose Injection, or Lactated Ringer's Injection

Route	Onset	Peak	Duration
P.O.	Unknown	1–2 hr	Unknown
I.V.	Unknown	30 min	Unknown

Half-life: 3.4–7 hr

Contraindications

Hypersensitivity to linezolid or its components, use within 14 days of an MAO inhibitor

Interactions

DRUGS

bupropion, buspirone, meperidine, serotonergics, tricyclic antidepressants, triptans: Possibly serotonin syndrome
dopaminergic agents (dobutamine, dopamine), sympathomimetic agents (pseudoephedrine), vasopressive agents (epinephrine, norepinephrine): Increased risk of altered blood pressure
insulin, hypoglycemic drugs: May increase risk for hypoglycemia
MAO inhibitors: Increased risk of life-threatening adverse effects

FOODS

tyramine-containing beverages and foods: Possibly hypertension

Adverse Reactions

CNS: Dizziness, fever, headache, insomnia, peripheral neuropathy, **seizures**, **serotonin syndrome**, vertigo
CV: Hypertension
EENT: Optic neuropathy with possible loss of vision, oral candidiasis, taste alteration, tooth or tongue discoloration
ENDO: Syndrome of inappropriate antidiuretic hormone secretion (SIADH)
GI: Abdominal pain, ***Clostridioides difficile*–associated diarrhea**, constipation, diarrhea, elevated liver enzymes, indigestion, nausea, **pseudomembranous colitis**, vomiting
GU: Vaginal candidiasis
HEME: Anemia, eosinophilia, **leukopenia**, **pancytopenia**, **sideroblastic anemia**, **thrombocytopenia**
MS: **Rhabdomyolysis**

JKL

Mechanism of Action

Inhibits bacterial protein synthesis by interfering with translation of ribonucleic acid (RNA) to protein. In bacteria, protein synthesis begins with binding of a 30S ribosomal subunit and a 50S ribosomal subunit to a messenger RNA (mRNA) molecule to form a 70S initiation complex. The 50S ribosomal subunit consists of 23S ribosomal RNA (rRNA) and other ribosomal subunits. Then, translation begins. Transfer RNA (tRNA) attaches to the 50S subunit and brings specific amino acids into place. As the tRNA and amino acids fall into place, they are joined together by peptide bonds and elongate to form a polypeptide chain, as shown below left. This chain eventually combines with other polypeptide chains to form a complete protein molecule. After translation is complete, the ribosomal subunits fall away and are ready to combine with more mRNA to start the translation process over again.

Binds to a site on the bacterial 23S rRNA of the 50S subunit. This action prevents formation of a functional 70S initiation complex, an essential component of the bacterial translation. Without proper protein production, as shown below right, susceptible bacteria are unable to multiply. Linezolid is bactericidal against most streptococci and bacteriostatic against staphylococci and enterococci.

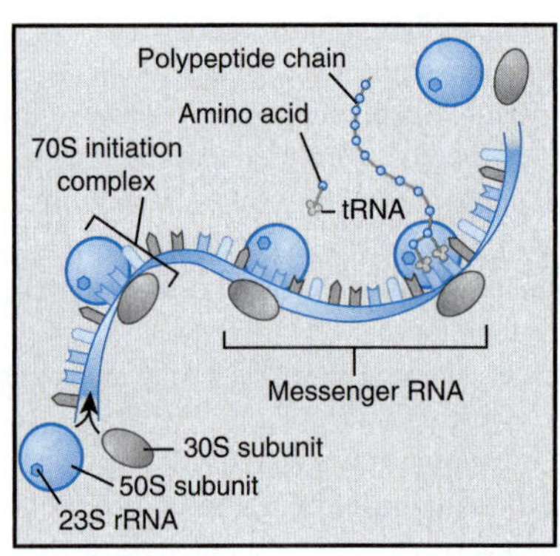

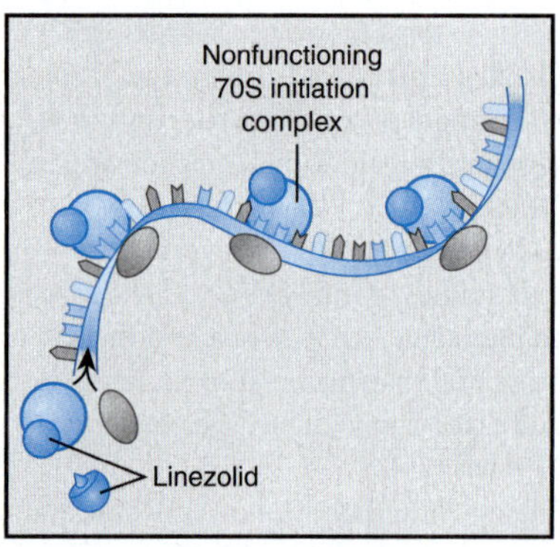

SKIN: Bullous dermatitis, pruritus, rash, **Stevens-Johnson syndrome**, **toxic epidermal necrolysis**
Other: **Anaphylaxis**, **angioedema**, fungal infections, **hyponatremia**, **lactic acidosis**

Childbearing Considerations

PREGNANCY

- It is not known if drug causes fetal harm.
- Use with caution only if benefit to mother outweighs potential risk to fetus.

LACTATION

- Drug is present in breast milk.
- Mothers should check with prescriber before breastfeeding.
- If breastfeeding occurs, mother should monitor infant for diarrhea and vomiting.

REPRODUCTION

- May impair fertility in male patients that may be reversible based on animal studies.

Nursing Considerations

- Obtain body tissue and fluid specimens for culture and sensitivity tests, as ordered, before giving first dose of linezolid. Expect to start drug before test results are known.

! **WARNING** Be aware that linezolid shouldn't be used to treat catheter-related bloodstream infections, catheter-site infections, or infections caused by gram-negative bacteria because the risk of death is higher in these infections.

! **WARNING** Monitor patient for a hypersensitivity reaction that could become life threatening such as anaphylaxis or angioedema. If present, notify prescriber, expect drug to be discontinued, and provide supportive care, as needed and ordered.

! **WARNING** Monitor CBC weekly, as ordered, to detect or track worsening myelosuppression in patients who need more than 2 weeks of therapy, who have preexisting myelosuppression and are receiving drugs that produce bone marrow suppression, who have chronic infection and are receiving or have received antibiotic therapy, who have moderate to severe hepatic impairment, or who have severe renal impairment. Be aware that thrombocytopenia occurs more often in patients with moderate to several hepatic impairment or who have severe renal impairment.

! **WARNING** Monitor patient for signs and symptoms of hyponatremia and SIADH, such as confusion, generalized weakness, and somnolence; if severe, respiratory failure and death may occur. Expect to monitor serum sodium levels regularly in patients at risk, such as the elderly, patients taking diuretics, and patients already at risk for hyponatremia or SIADH. If present, notify prescriber and expect drug to be discontinued.

! **WARNING** Assess patient's bowel pattern daily watching for profuse, watery diarrhea that can occur as long as 2 months after drug has been discontinued. If present, notify prescriber and expect to obtain a stool specimen to determine if cause is *Clostridioides difficile* that may cause mild diarrhea to fatal colitis. If *C. difficile* is confirmed, expect to administer an antibiotic effective against *C. difficile*. Also, expect to administer electrolytes, fluids, and protein supplementation, as needed and ordered.

! **WARNING** Be aware that while linezolid should not be given to patients receiving serotonergic drugs, there are some conditions that may be life-threatening and require the use of linezolid, such as the presence of vancomycin-resistant *Enterococcus faecium* (VRE) or infections, such as nosocomial pneumonia and complicated skin and skin structure infections, including those caused by methicillin-resistant *Staphylococcus aureus* (MRSA). If patient takes buspirone, meperidine, or a serotonergic or tricyclic antidepressant watch closely for signs and symptoms of serotonin syndrome; if monitoring isn't possible, know that linezolid should not be prescribed.

! **WARNING** Monitor patient with a seizure history closely for development of seizure activity.

! **WARNING** Monitor patient for signs and symptoms of rahdomyolysis (dark urine; elevated creatine phosphokinase; muscle pain, tenderness, weakness). If present, notify prescriber, expect drug to be discontinued, and provide supportive care, as needed and ordered.

- Monitor patient with diabetes who is also taking antidiabetic medication because hypoglycemia has been linked to linezolid use in these patients. If hypoglycemia occurs, treat appropriately, and notify prescriber, as dosage of the antidiabetic medication may have to be decreased.
- Notify prescriber if patient develops visual impairment that suggests optic neuropathy, such as blurred vision, changes in color vision or visual acuity, lost vision, or visual field defect. If optic or peripheral neuropathy develops, drug may have to be stopped.
- Know that if patient takes a dopaminergic agent, sympathomimetic agent, or vasopressive agent, monitor blood pressure closely; if monitoring is not possible, know that linezolid should not be prescribed.

PATIENT TEACHING

- Instruct patient how to administer oral form of linezolid prescribed.

! **WARNING** Warn patient with phenylketonuria that oral suspension contains phenylalanine and tablets should be taken instead.

! **WARNING** Instruct patient to avoid beverages and foods that contain large amounts of tyramine, including aged cheese, air-dried or fermented meats, protein-rich foods that have been stored for long periods or poorly refrigerated, red wines, soy sauce, and tap beers.

! **WARNING** Alert patient that drug may cause an allergic reaction. If present, tell patient to notify prescriber and, if severe, to seek immediate medical care.

! **WARNING** Instruct patient to notify prescriber at once about severe diarrhea, even up to 2 months after linezolid therapy has ended, because additional treatment may be needed. Also, advise patient to report repeated episodes of nausea and vomiting as well as any other serious or unusual signs and symptoms that may occur during drug therapy.

! **WARNING** Alert patient that blood tests to check patient's sodium level may be ordered periodically. Review signs and symptoms of hyponatremia and SIADH with patient and family and advise to notify prescriber if present because drug will have to be discontinued if confirmed. Also, tell patient to immediately notify prescriber if other persistent, severe, or unusual signs and symptoms occur.

! **WARNING** Tell patient to notify prescriber immediately if dark urine or muscle pain, tenderness, or weakness occurs.

- Advise diabetic patients prescribed antidiabetic medications to monitor their blood glucose closely and be prepared to treat hypoglycemia if it should occur. If present, tell patient to notify prescriber, as a dosage adjustment may be required in his antidiabetic medication.
- Tell patient to report changes in limb sensation (such as numbness, pins and needles, or tingling) or vision changes because drug may have to be stopped.
- Reassure patient with tooth discoloration that professional dental cleaning can restore tooth color.
- Advise patient not to take over-the-counter cold remedies without consulting prescriber because medications that contain propanolamine or pseudoephedrine may cause or worsen hypertension.
- Alert male patients that drug may impair fertility but that it may be reversible.
- Instruct mothers breastfeeding during drug therapy to monitor their infant for diarrhea and vomiting.

liraglutide

Saxenda, Victoza

Class and Category

Pharmacologic class: Glucagon-like peptide-1 receptor agonist

Therapeutic class: Antidiabetic

Indications and Dosages

* *As adjunct to diet and exercise to improve glycemic control in patients with type 2 diabetes mellitus*

SUBCUTANEOUS INJECTION (VICTOZA)

Adults and children ages 10 and older. *Initial:* 0.6 mg daily for 1 wk, then increased to 1.2 mg daily. Dosage increased to 1.8 mg daily after 1 additional wk, as needed. *Maximum:* 1.8 mg daily.

* *To reduce risk of major adverse cardiovascular events, such as CVA or MI in patients with type 2 diabetes mellitus and established cardiovascular disease*

SUBCUTANEOUS INJECTION (VICTOZA)

Adults. *Initial*: 0.6 mg daily for 1 wk, then increased to 1.2 mg daily.

* *As adjunct for chronic weight management in patients with an initial body mass index of 30 kg/m^2 or greater, or 27 kg/m^2 or greater in the presence of at least one weight-related comorbid condition, such as dyslipidemia, hypertension, or type 2 diabetes mellitus; as adjunct to reduced-calorie diet and increased physical activity for chronic weight management in children 12 years and older with a body weight above 60 kg and an initial BMI corresponding to 30 kg/m^2 for adults (obese) by international cut-offs*

SUBCUTANEOUS INJECTION (SAXENDA)

Adults and children ages 12 and older. *Initial:* 0.6 mg daily for wk 1, increased to 1.2 mg daily for wk 2, increased to 1.8 mg daily for wk 3, increased to 2.4 mg daily for wk 4, and increased to 3 mg daily for wk 5 and onward. *Maximum:* 3 mg daily.

± **DOSAGE ADJUSTMENT** For children who do not tolerate an increased dose during dose escalation, dose reduced to the previous level with dose escalation taking up to 8 weeks.

Also, for children who cannot tolerate a maintenance dose of 3 mg daily, dosage reduced to 2.4 mg daily.

Drug Administration

SUBCUTANEOUS

- Drug is supplied in a multidose prefilled syringe and kept in refrigerator until first use. Discard if pen freezes. Once used, pen may be stored at room temperature for 30 days but should be protected from excessive heat and sunlight.
- May be administered at any time of day but keep administration time consistent.
- Solution should be clear, colorless, and contain no particles.
- Inject drug into abdomen, thigh, or upper arm.
- Rotate sites.
- When patient is also taking insulin, inject at separate injection sites, but can be in same anatomical area. Never mix the 2 drugs.
- If a dose is missed, do not administer an extra dose or increase the dose to make up for the missed dose. Instead, resume the once-daily regimen with the next scheduled dose.
- If more than 3 days have elapsed without liraglutide administration, drug will have to be reinitiated.

Route	Onset	Peak	Duration
SubQ	Unknown	8–12 hr	Unknown

Half-life: 13 hr

Mechanism of Action

Activates the glucagon-like peptide-1 site on pancreatic beta cells, which increases intracellular cyclic AMP, which increases insulin release when blood glucose level is elevated. In addition, because glucagon and insulin levels occur in an inverse relationship to plasma glucose level, increased insulin level will decrease glucagon level, which inhibits glucagon stimulation of the liver that increases plasma glucose level. Although its exact mechanism is unclear, liraglutide also delays gastric emptying, which helps prevent a sudden rise in plasma glucose level after eating. Together these actions work to lower plasma glucose level.

Binds to the glucagon-like peptide-1 receptor and activates it to regulate appetite and calorie intake, resulting in weight loss.

Contraindications

Family or personal history of medullary thyroid cancer, hypersensitivity to liraglutide or its components, pregnancy (Saxenda), presence of multiple endocrine neoplasia syndrome type 2

Interactions

DRUGS

insulin, oral hypoglycemic agents, such as sulfonylureas: Increased risk of hypoglycemia
orally administered drugs: Possibly decreased absorption of these drugs

Adverse Reactions

CNS: Anxiety, asthenia, dizziness, fatigue, fever, headache, insomnia, malaise, **suicidal ideation**
CV: Dyslipidemia, edema, hypertension, **hypotension**, palpitations
EENT: Dry mouth, nasopharyngitis, sinusitis, taste distortion
ENDO: Elevated calcitonin levels, **hypoglycemia**, **medullary thyroid cancer**, **thyroid C-cell hyperplasia**
GI: Abdominal distention or pain, **acute pancreatitis**, anorexia, cholecystitis, cholelithiasis, constipation, diarrhea, dyspepsia, elevated liver or pancreatic enzymes, eructation, flatulence, gastroenteritis, **hemorrhagic and necrotizing pancreatitis**, **hepatitis**, hyperbilirubinemia, ileus, jaundice, nausea, slowed gastric emptying, vomiting
GU: **Acute renal failure**, elevated serum creatinine level, UTI, **worsening of chronic renal failure**
MS: Back pain
RESP: Cough, dyspnea, upper respiratory tract infection
SKIN: Cutaneous amyloidosis, pruritus, rash, urticaria
Other: **Anaphylaxis**; **angioedema**; antiliraglutide antibodies; dehydration; elevated creatine kinase levels; influenza-like symptoms; injection-site reaction, including erythema, pruritus, rash; **malignancies such as breast and papillary thyroid cancer**

Childbearing Considerations

PREGNANCY

- It is not known if Victoza brand of drug causes fetal harm, but animal studies suggest it may.
- Saxenda brand of drug is contraindicated in pregnancy because weight loss offers no benefit to a pregnant person and may result in fetal harm.
- Use Victoza with caution only if benefit to mother outweighs potential risk to fetus.

LACTATION

- It is not known if drug is present in breast milk.
- Mothers should check with prescriber before breastfeeding.

REPRODUCTION

- Females of childbearing age prescribed Saxenda brand of drug need to use effective contraception throughout drug therapy.

Nursing Considerations

! **WARNING** Be aware that liraglutide isn't recommended as first-line therapy for patients with type 2 diabetes mellitus not well controlled with diet and exercise. It also isn't a substitute for insulin therapy. Saxenda brand shouldn't be given with insulin, nor should it be combined with other products intended for weight loss, including herbal preparations, over-the-counter products, or prescription drugs.

! **WARNING** Know that liraglutide shouldn't be given to a patient with a history of thyroid C-cell tumors, including medullary thyroid carcinoma, or to patients with multiple endocrine neoplasia syndrome type 2 because drug may stimulate tumor growth.

- Be aware that dosage of liraglutide given during first week of therapy to lower blood glucose level isn't enough to provide glycemic control but is given to minimize adverse effects when dosage is increased.

! **WARNING** Monitor patient closely for signs and symptoms of a hypersensitivity reaction that may become life-threatening such as anaphylaxis or angioedema, especially in patients with a history of angioedema to other medications. If any hypersensitivity reaction occurs, notify the prescriber, expect drug to be discontinued, and provide supportive care, as needed and ordered.

! **WARNING** Monitor patient for hypoglycemia, especially if he takes another antidiabetic drug, such as a sulfonylurea or insulin. Know that the risk of hypoglycemia is higher in children regardless of concomitant antidiabetic therapies. Report any episode of hypoglycemia because dosage of other antidiabetic may require adjustment. Treat hypoglycemia according to institutional protocol.

! **WARNING** Monitor patients with a history of pancreatitis because drug can cause life threatening pancreatitis in patients with impaired hepatic function. Monitor patient for pancreatitis, especially when therapy starts or dosage increases. Report persistent severe abdominal pain—it may radiate to the back and may be accompanied by vomiting. If pancreatitis is confirmed, expect to stop drug and know that it should not be restarted after episode has been resolved.

! **WARNING** Monitor patients with renal dysfunction because liraglutide may adversely affect renal function causing acute renal failure. Monitor patient's fluid intake, especially if GI dysfunction occurs because dehydration can lead to renal dysfunction that can become severe enough to require dialysis.

! **WARNING** Monitor patient closely for suicidal ideation, such as depression or unusual changes in behavior or mood. If patient becomes suicidal, take safety precautions immediately, discontinue liraglutide therapy, as ordered, and notify prescriber.

! **WARNING** Be aware that because drug delays gastric emptying, pulmonary aspiration may occur when patient undergoes elective surgeries or procedures requiring deep sedation or general anesthesia.

- Monitor patient's blood glucose level and hemoglobin A1C regularly, as ordered, to assess effectiveness of drug when used to treat diabetes mellitus.
- Monitor patient's heart rate regularly. If patient develops a sustained increase in

resting heart rate while taking Saxenda, notify prescriber, as drug will have to be discontinued.

- Monitor patient's serum calcitonin levels, as indicated. Be aware that elevations occur more often when liraglutide dosage is 1.8 mg daily.
- Monitor patient for acute gallbladder disease. Risk is increased in patients who experience a rapid or substantial weight loss, although it may also occur in patients who have lost weight more slowly or less significantly. Notify prescriber if signs and symptoms occur and expect diagnostic testing to be performed.
- Monitor effectiveness of all other oral drugs because liraglutide slows gastric emptying and may impair their absorption. Alert prescriber to any concerns.

PATIENT TEACHING

! WARNING Inform patient of possible risk of medullary thyroid cancer or multiple endocrine neoplasia syndrome type 2 before drug therapy begins. Stress the need to report any symptoms, such as dysphagia, dyspnea, a neck mass, or persistent hoarseness immediately to prescriber.

- Emphasize that liraglutide therapy (Victoza brand) isn't a substitute for diet and exercise when used to treat diabetes mellitus but is used to enhance the effectiveness of these measures.
- Teach patient how to administer liraglutide subcutaneously.

! WARNING Alert patient that drug may cause an allergic reaction. If present, tell patient to notify prescriber and, if severe, to seek immediate medical care.

! WARNING Instruct patient to maintain an adequate fluid intake, as dehydration may cause kidney dysfunction.

! WARNING Alert patient that hypoglycemia can occur with drug use, especially if also taking other antidiabetic drugs and in children regardless of concomitant antidiabetic treatment. Review signs and symptoms of low blood sugar with patient and appropriate treatment.

! WARNING Tell family or caregiver to monitor patient closely for depression or changes in behavior or mood. If suicidal, have them take safety precautions, stop the drug, and seek emergency medical help for patient.

! WARNING Inform patient that drug may increase risk for acute pancreatitis. Tell patient to report persistent severe abdominal pain that may radiate to the back and may be accompanied by vomiting and to stop taking drug.

! WARNING Instruct females of childbearing age prescribed Saxenda to notify prescriber immediately if pregnancy occurs, as drug will have to be discontinued. Also instruct these patients to use an effective contraceptive throughout drug therapy.

! WARNING Alert women that liraglutide does have an effect on preexisting breast neoplasia that may increase risk of breast cancer. In addition, inform all patients that there may be an increase in the development of colorectal neoplasms. Encourage all patients to have cancer screenings done as recommended by their doctor.

! WARNING Tell patient to alert healthcare providers of liraglutide therapy before undergoing elective surgeries or procedures.

- Tell patient to alert prescriber if palpitations or feelings of a racing heartbeat while at rest occur during Saxenda therapy.
- Inform patient that drug may increase risk for gallbladder disease. If abdominal pain, nausea, and vomiting occur, instruct patient to notify prescriber. Also, tell patient to report yellowing of skin or white of the eye along with GI signs and symptoms to prescriber.
- Have patient monitor her weight to assess effectiveness of drug (Saxenda) when prescribed for weight management. Tell patient that Saxenda used for weight loss must be discontinued if she has not achieved a 4% weight loss by 16 weeks.
- Tell patient prescribed Saxenda brand of drug that it should not be given with insulin, nor should it be combined with other products intended for weight loss, including herbal preparations, over-the-counter products, and prescription drugs.

lisdexamfetamine dimesylate

Vyvanse

Class, Category, and Schedule

Pharmacologic class: Amphetamine
Therapeutic class: CNS stimulant
Controlled substance schedule: II

Indications and Dosages

✱ *To treat attention deficit hyperactivity disorder (ADHD)*

CAPSULES, CHEWABLE TABLETS

Adults, adolescents, and children ages 6 and older. *Initial:* 30 mg once daily in the morning, increased, as needed, in increments of 10 or 20 mg daily every wk. *Maximum:* 70 mg daily.

✱ *To treat moderate to severe binge eating disorder*

CAPSULES, CHEWABLE TABLETS

Adults. *Initial:* 30 mg once daily in the morning, increased, as needed, in increments of 20 mg weekly to reach target dosage of 50 to 70 mg/day. *Maximum:* 70 mg daily.

± **DOSAGE ADJUSTMENT** For patients with severe renal impairment (GFR from 15 ml/min to less than 30 ml/min), maximum dose is limited to 50 mg daily. For patients with end-stage renal disease (GFR less than 15 ml/min), maximum dose is limited to 30 mg daily. For patients taking agents that alter urinary pH, dosage adjustments are individualized.

Drug Administration

P.O.

- Administer drug in the morning to avoid insomnia.
- Capsules should be swallowed whole and not chewed or crushed. For patient who cannot swallow the capsule, it may be opened, and contents dissolved in a glass of orange juice or water. Administer immediately. Alternatively, the contents may be mixed with yogurt until completely dispersed and administered immediately.
- Chewable tablets should be chewed thoroughly before swallowing.
- Capsules and chewable tablets are interchangeable on a mg-per-mg basis.

Route	Onset	Peak	Duration
P.O.	2 hr	3.5 hr	10–12 hr

Half-life: < 1 hr

Mechanism of Action

Produces CNS stimulant effects, probably by facilitating release and blocking reuptake of norepinephrine at adrenergic nerve terminals and by stimulating alpha and beta receptors in peripheral nervous system. The drug also releases and blocks reuptake of dopamine in limbic regions of brain. These actions cause decreased motor restlessness and increased alertness. Lisdexamfetamine's action in the treatment of binge eating is unknown.

Contraindications

Hypersensitivity, idiosyncratic reaction to lisdexamfetamine, other sympathomimetic amines, or their components; MAO inhibitor therapy, including intravenous methylene blue and linezolid, within 14 days

Interactions

DRUGS

acidifying agents (urinary), such as ammonium chloride, sodium acid phosphate: Decreased blood level and effects of lisdexamfetamine
alkalinizing agents (urinary), such as acetazolamide, some thiazides: Increased blood level and effects of lisdexamfetamine
buspirone, fentanyl, lithium, MAO inhibitors, selective serotonin reuptake inhibitors, serotonin–norepinephrine reuptake inhibitors, St. John's wort, tricyclic antidepressants, triptans, tryptophan: Increased risk of serotonin syndrome
CYP2 d6 inhibitors, such as fluoxetine, paroxetine, quinidine, ritonavir: Increased exposure to dextroamphetamine; increased risk of serotonin syndrome
MAO inhibitors: Potentiated effects of lisdexamfetamine, possibly hypertensive crisis
tricyclic antidepressants: Possibly increased antidepressant effects and cardiovascular effects can be potentiated

Adverse Reactions

CNS: Affect lability, aggression, agitation, anxiety, depression, dizziness, dyskinesia, dysphoria, energy increase, euphoria, fever,

hallucinations, headache, insomnia, irritability, jittery feeling, mania, mood swings, motor and verbal tics, nightmare, paranoia, paresthesia, psychomotor hyperactivity, psychotic episodes, restlessness, **seizures**, **serotonin syndrome**, somnolence, tremor, worsening of Tourette's syndrome
CV: **Cardiomyopathy**, chest pain, hypertension, increased heart rate, palpitations, peripheral vasculopathy, including Raynaud's phenomenon, tachycardia, ventricular hypertrophy
EENT: Blurred vision, diplopia, dry mouth, mydriasis, oropharyngeal pain, taste alterations, teeth grinding, visual accommodation difficulties
ENDO: Long-term growth suppression
GI: Anorexia, constipation, diarrhea, gastroenteritis, **hepatitis**, intestinal ischemia, nausea, upper abdominal pain, vomiting
GU: Decreased libido, erectile dysfunction, frequent or prolonged erections, priapism, UTI
MS: **Rhabdomyolysis**
RESP: Dyspnea
SKIN: Alopecia, diaphoresis, pruritus, rash, **Stevens-Johnson syndrome**, **toxic epidermal necrolysis**, uncontrolled picking at skin, urticaria
Other: **Anaphylaxis**, **angioedema**, physical or psychological dependence, weight loss

Childbearing Considerations

PREGNANCY

- Pregnancy exposure registry: 1-866-961-2388 or https://womensmentalhealth.org/clinical-and-researchprograms/pregnancyregistry/adhd-medications/.
- Drug may cause fetal harm because as an amphetamine, vasoconstriction occurs, which may decrease placental perfusion. Prenatal or early postnatal exposure can result in long-term neurochemical and behavioral alterations according to animal studies.
- Use with caution only if benefit to mother outweighs potential risk to fetus.

LABOR AND DELIVERY

- Be aware that drug can stimulate uterine contractions, increasing the risk of premature delivery.
- Infants born to mothers taking amphetamines should be monitored for symptoms of withdrawal upon birth, such as agitation, excessive drowsiness, feeding difficulties, and irritability.

LACTATION

- Drug is present in breast milk.
- Breastfeeding is not recommended during drug use.

Nursing Considerations

! WARNING Know that lisdexamfetamine may cause substance use disorder because of its high potential for abuse and misuse, which can lead to addiction. Determine patient's risk and frequently monitor for signs and symptoms of abuse, misuse, and addiction throughout drug therapy because misuse and abuse can lead to an overdose and death. Alert prescriber immediately if abuse and misuse is suspected.

! WARNING Keep in mind lisdexamfetamine shouldn't be given to patients with cardiac abnormalities (structural), cardiomyopathy, or other serious heart problems or rhythm abnormalities because even usual CNS stimulant dosages increase risk of sudden death in patients with these conditions.

- Know that patient should be screened for psychiatric risk factors, such as a family or personal history of aggression or hostility, bipolar disorder, depression, or psychosis before lisdexamfetamine therapy begins because lisdexamfetamine may cause psychiatric adverse reactions. Monitor patients with these disorders throughout drug therapy and alert prescriber if signs and symptoms of psychiatric disorders appear.
- Assess patient for motor and verbal tics and presence of Tourette's syndrome, including a review of family history of these disorders before lisdexamfetamine begins because drug may cause or exacerbate motor and verbal tics and worsen Tourette's syndrome.

! WARNING Monitor patient for a hypersensitivity reaction, which could become life threatening such as anaphylaxis or angioedema. If present, notify prescriber, expect drug to be discontinued, and provide supportive care, as needed and ordered.

! WARNING Monitor patients with heart failure, hypertension, recent MI, or ventricular arrhythmia because drug may increase blood pressure and worsen these conditions. Monitor patient's blood pressure closely throughout drug therapy. Report chest pain or fainting to prescriber immediately.

! WARNING Know that if patient has a history of seizures or EEG abnormality, watch for seizure activity because stimulants may lower seizure threshold. Rarely, lisdexamfetamine may cause seizures in a patient with no history of them. Take seizure precautions for all patients. Notify prescriber if a seizure occurs and expect to discontinue lisdexamfetamine.

! WARNING Monitor patient closely for serotonin syndrome, a rare but serious adverse effect of lisdexamfetamine. Signs and symptoms include agitation, confusion, diaphoresis, diarrhea, fever, hyperactive reflexes, poor coordination, restlessness, shaking, talking or acting with uncontrolled excitement, tremor, and twitching. If symptoms occur, notify prescriber immediately, expect drug to be discontinued, and provide supportive care, as needed and ordered.

- Be aware that therapy may be stopped temporarily to assess continued need for it, as evidenced by a return of attention deficit and hyperactivity.
- Assess growth pattern in pediatric patients because stimulants such as lisdexamfetamine may suppress growth. If so, notify prescriber and expect therapy to be halted.
- Take safety precautions because stimulants may alter accommodation and cause blurred vision.
- Know that lisdexamfetamine can cause a significant elevation in plasma corticosteroid levels, especially in the evening, which may interfere with urinary steroid determinations.

PATIENT TEACHING

- Warn patient, family, or caregiver that drug must be taken exactly as prescribed, and dosage increased only at prescriber's instruction because drug can be abused or lead to dependence.
- Instruct patient, family, or caregiver how to administer form of disdexamfetamine prescribed.

! WARNING Alert patient, family, or caregiver that drug may cause an allergic reaction. If present, tell patient to notify prescriber and stop taking drug. If severe, urge patient to seek immediate medical care.

! WARNING Advise patient, family, or caregiver to immediately report any symptoms that suggest heart disease, such as chest pain or fainting. Also, tell patient, family, or caregiver to report any adverse reactions that are persistent, serious, or unusual.

! WARNING Warn male patients or family or caregiver of male children that painful or prolonged penile erections may occur while taking the drug, especially after a dose increase or during a period of drug withdrawal. In the event this happens, immediate medical attention should be sought.

- Alert patient that drug may cause motor and verbal tics and worsen Tourette's syndrome and to notify prescriber if this occurs.
- Urge patient to avoid hazardous activities until drug effects are known and resolved.
- Instruct patient to tell all prescribers about lisdexamfetamine therapy, as serious drug interactions can occur.
- Instruct patient, family, or caregiver to monitor fingers and toes for soft-tissue breakdown and/or ulceration. If noticed, prescriber should be notified. Reassure patient that signs and symptoms generally improve after the dose is reduced or drug is discontinued.
- Tell females of childbearing age to notify prescriber if pregnancy occurs.
- Inform mothers wanting to breastfeed that breastfeeding is not recommended during lisdexamfetamine therapy.
- Advise patient to keep drug stored in a safe place that can be locked to prevent theft of the drug and out of reach of children. Also stress importance of not giving drug to anyone else.

lisinopril

Qbrelis, Zestril

Class and Category

Pharmacologic class: ACE inhibitor
Therapeutic class: Antihypertensive

Indications and Dosages

✱ *To treat hypertension*

ORAL SOLUTION, TABLETS

Adults. *Initial:* 5 mg (if taking a diuretic) or 10 mg once daily (if no diuretic therapy), adjusted according to blood pressure. *Maintenance:* 20 to 40 mg once daily. Alternatively, 10 to 40 mg once daily. *Maximum:* 80 mg once daily.

Children ages 6 and older with a GFR of at least 30 ml/min. *Initial:* 0.07 mg/kg (maximum 5 mg) once daily, adjusted according to blood pressure. *Maximum:* 0.61 mg/kg (up to 40 mg) daily.

✱ *As adjunct with digitalis and diuretics to treat heart failure*

ORAL SOLUTION, TABLETS

Adults. *Initial:* 5 mg once daily. *Maintenance:* 5 to 20 mg once daily. *Maximum:* 40 mg once daily.

± **DOSAGE ADJUSTMENT** For patients with hyponatremia or creatinine clearance of 30 ml/min or less, initial dosage reduced to 2.5 mg daily with maximum dosage not to exceed 40 mg once daily.

✱ *To improve survival in hemodynamically stable patient within 24 hours of an acute MI*

ORAL SOLUTION, TABLETS

Adults. *Initial:* 5 mg within 24 hr after onset of symptoms, followed by 5 mg after 24 hr and 10 mg after 48 hr and once daily thereafter. *Maintenance:* 10 mg once daily for 6 wk.

± **DOSAGE ADJUSTMENT** For adult patients with baseline systolic blood pressure of 120 mm Hg or less, initial dosage decreased to 2.5 mg daily for first 3 days after MI. If systolic blood pressure falls to 100 mm Hg or less during therapy, maintenance dosage decreased to 2.5 or 5 mg as tolerated; if systolic blood pressure is 90 mm Hg or less for more than 1 hour, drug discontinued. For adult patients, regardless of indication, with impaired renal function (creatinine clearance of 10 to 30 ml/min), initial dosage reduced by half; for patients on hemodialysis or with a creatinine clearance of less than 10 ml/min, initial dose reduced to 2.5 mg once daily. For children with a glomerular filtration rate that falls to less than 30 ml/min, drug discontinued.

Drug Administration

P.O.

- Use a calibrated device when measuring dosage of oral solution.

Route	Onset	Peak	Duration
P.O.	1 hr	6–8 hr	24 hr

Half-life: 12 hr

Mechanism of Action

May reduce blood pressure by inhibiting conversion of angiotensin I to angiotensin II. Angiotensin II is a potent vasoconstrictor that also stimulates adrenal cortex to secrete aldosterone. Lisinopril may also inhibit renal and vascular production of angiotensin II. Decreased release of aldosterone reduces sodium and water reabsorption and increases their excretion, thereby reducing blood pressure.

Contraindications

Concurrent aliskiren use in patients with diabetes; hereditary or idiopathic angioedema or history of angioedema related to previous treatment with an ACE inhibitor; hypersensitivity to lisinopril, other ACE inhibitors, or their components; use of a neprilysin inhibitor such as sacubitril within 36 hours of lisinopril initiation

Interactions

DRUGS

aliskiren (in presence of diabetes or renal impairment), other ACE inhibitors, angiotensin receptor blockers: Increased risk of hypotension, hyperkalemia, and renal impairment

diuretics, other antihypertensives: Increased hypotensive effect

gold (injectable form, such as sodium aurothiomalate): Possibly nitritoid reaction (facial flushing, hypotension, nausea, vomiting)

insulin, oral antidiabetics: Increased risk of hypoglycemia

lithium: Increased blood lithium level and risk of lithium toxicity
mTOR inhibitors, such as everolimus, sirolimus, temsirolimus; neprilysin inhibitors, such as sacubitril: Increased risk for angioedema
NSAIDs: Possibly reduced antihypertensive effect; possibly reduced renal function in patients with preexisting renal dysfunction, the elderly, and patients who are volume-depleted
potassium-sparing diuretics: Increased risk of hyperkalemia
thiazide diuretics: Increased risk of hypokalemia

FOODS

high-potassium diet, potassium-containing salt substitutes: Increased risk of hyperkalemia

Adverse Reactions

CNS: Ataxia, confusion, **CVA**, depression, dizziness, fatigue, hallucinations, headache, insomnia, irritability, memory impairment, mood alterations, nervousness, paresthesia, peripheral neuropathy, somnolence, syncope, transient ischemic attack, tremor, vertigo
CV: **Arrhythmias**, chest pain, fluid overload, **hypotension**, **MI**, orthostatic hypotension, palpitations, peripheral edema, vasculitis
ENDO: Hyperglycemia, syndrome of inappropriate ADH secretion
EENT: Blurred vision, diplopia, dry mouth, olfactory or taste disturbance, photophobia, tinnitus, visual loss
GI: Abdominal pain, anorexia, cholestatic jaundice, constipation, diarrhea, elevated liver enzymes, flatulence, **fulminant hepatic necrosis**, gastritis, **hepatitis**, indigestion, nausea, **pancreatitis**, vomiting
GU: **Acute renal failure**, decreased libido, impotence, **pyelonephritis**
HEME: **Agranulocytosis**, anemia, **hemolytic anemia**, **neutropenia**, **thrombocytopenia**
MS: Arthralgia, arthritis, bone or joint pain, muscle spasms, myalgia
RESP: **Bronchospasm**, cough, dyspnea, paroxysmal nocturnal dyspnea, **pulmonary embolism and infarction**, upper respiratory tract infection
SKIN: Alopecia, cutaneous pseudolymphoma, diaphoresis, erythema, flushing, herpes-zoster, infection, pemphigus, photosensitivity, pruritus, psoriasis, rash, **Stevens-Johnson syndrome**, **toxic epidermal necrolysis**, urticaria
Other: **Anaphylaxis**, **angioedema**, dehydration, gout, **hyperkalemia**, **hyponatremia**, weight gain or loss

Childbearing Considerations

PREGNANCY

- Drug can cause fetal harm. Drug given during the second or third trimester reduces fetal renal function and increases fetal and neonatal morbidity and death. Resulting oligohydramnios can cause fetal lung hypoplasia and skeletal malformations.
- Drug should be discontinued as soon as pregnancy is known.

LACTATION

- It is not known if drug is present in breast milk.
- A decision should be made to discontinue breastfeeding or the drug to avoid potential serious adverse reactions in the breastfed infant.

Nursing Considerations

! WARNING Be aware that lisinopril should not be given to a patient who is hemodynamically unstable after an acute MI.

! WARNING Monitor patient for a hypersensitivity reactions that may become life-threatening, such as anaphylaxis or angioedema. If present, notify prescriber, expect drug to be discontinued, and provide supportive care, as needed and ordered.

! WARNING Monitor patient being dialyzed with high-flux membranes for anaphylaxis. If anaphylaxis occurs, stop dialysis immediately and treat aggressively (antihistamines are ineffective in this situation), as ordered. Anaphylaxis has also occurred with some patients undergoing low-density lipoprotein apheresis with dextran sulfate absorption.

! WARNING Be aware that if patient takes insulin or an oral antidiabetic, monitor blood glucose level closely because risk of hypoglycemia increases, especially during first month of drug therapy.

! **WARNING** Monitor closely patients with fluid volume deficit, heart failure, impaired renal function, or sodium depletion because drug may worsen these conditions.

! **WARNING** Monitor patients with severe aortic senosis or hypertrophic cardiomyopathy because symptomatic hypotension may occur. Monitor blood pressure often, especially during the first 2 weeks of therapy and whenever the dose of lisinopril and/or prescribed diuretic is increased. Also monitor patient for hypotension who is experiencing dehydration, especially if patient experiences diarrhea or vomiting. If excessive hypotension develops, notify prescriber and expect to withhold drug for several days.

! **WARNING** Monitor patient for hepatic dysfunction because lisinopril, an ACE inhibitor, may rarely cause a syndrome that starts with cholestatic jaundice or hepatitis and progresses to fulminant hepatic necrosis. If patient develops jaundice or a marked elevation in liver enzymes, withhold drug and notify prescriber.

! **WARNING** Obtain a CBC and platelet count regularly, as ordered because drug may cause serious adverse hematologic reactions. Monitor patient for signs and symptoms of unexplained bruising or bleeding and infection and notify prescriber, if present.

- Monitor patient's serum creatinine, as ordered because changes in renal function can occur with lisinopril use. If renal function decreases, alert prescriber and expect drug to be withheld or discontinued.
- Monitor patient's serum potassium level, as ordered because drugs that inhibit the renin–angiotensin system such as lisinopril can cause hyperkalemia. Patients at increased risk for developing hyperkalemia include patients with diabetes or renal insufficiency or who are also taking potassium-sparing diuretics, potassium-containing salt substitutes, or potassium supplements.
- Notify prescriber if patient has persistent, nonproductive cough, a common adverse effect of ACE inhibitors, such as lisinopril. Drug will need to be discontinued.

PATIENT TEACHING

- Explain to patient taking lisinopril for hypertension that lisinopril helps to control, but doesn't cure hypertension and that patient may need lifelong therapy.
- Instruct patient how to administer form of lisinopril prescribed.
- Emphasize need to take drug as ordered, even if patient feels well; caution patient not to stop drug without consulting prescriber.
- Instruct patient to report dizziness, especially during first few days of therapy.

! **WARNING** Warn patient that drug may cause an allergic reaction. If present, tell patient to notify prescriber and, if severe, to seek immediate medical care.

! **WARNING** Advise patient to drink adequate fluids and avoid excessive sweating, which can lead to dehydration and hypotension. Make sure she understands that diarrhea, excessive perspiration, and vomiting can also cause hypotension.

! **WARNING** Instruct patient to report signs of unexplained bruising or bleeding or infection, such as fever and sore throat.

! **WARNING** Advise patient who has diabetes and takes insulin or an oral antidiabetic to monitor her blood glucose level closely and watch for symptoms of hypoglycemia.

- Caution her to avoid hazardous activities, such as driving until nervous system symptoms abates.
- Inform patient that persistent, nonproductive cough may develop during lisinopril therapy and prescriber should be notified.
- Caution patient not to use salt substitutes that contain potassium.
- Advise patient to change position slowly to minimize orthostatic hypotension.
- Caution females of childbearing age to notify prescriber immediately if pregnancy occurs because lisinopril must be discontinued.
- Inform mothers that breastfeeding is not recommended during lisinopril therapy.
- Advise patient to inform all prescribers of lisinopril therapy.

lithium carbonate

Carbolith (CAN), Lithane (CAN), Lithobid

lithium citrate

Class and Category

Pharmacologic class: Alkali metal
Therapeutic class: Antimanic

Indications and Dosages

✷ *To treat acute mania and mixed episodes of bipolar disorder; to maintain patients with bipolar disorder*

CAPSULES, TABLETS

Adults and children ages 7 and older weighing more than 30 kg (66 lb). *Initial:* 300 mg 3 times daily, increased every 3 days by 300 mg, as needed. *Acute goal:* 600 mg 2 to 3 times daily. *Maintenance:* 300 to 600 mg 2 to 3 times daily.

Children ages 7 and older weighing 20 (44 lb) to 30 kg (66 lb). *Initial:* 300 mg twice daily, increased 300 mg weekly. *Acute goal:* 600 mg to 1,500 mg in divided doses daily. *Maintenance:* 600 mg to 1,200 mg in divided doses daily.

ORAL SOLUTION

Adults and children ages 7 and older weighing more than 30 kg (66 lb). *Initial:* 8 mEq (5 ml) 3 times daily, increased by 8 mEq (5 ml) every 3 days, as needed. *Acute goal:* 16 mEq (10 ml) 2 to 3 times daily. *Maintenance:* 8 to 16 mEq (5 to 10 ml) 2 to 3 times daily.

Children ages 7 and older weighing 20 kg (44 lb) to 30 kg (66 lb). *Initial:* 8 mEq (5 ml) twice daily, increased by 8 mEq (5 ml) weekly, as needed. *Acute goal:* 16 to 40 mEq (10 to 25 ml) in divided doses daily. *Maintenance:* 16 to 32 mEq (10 to 20 ml) in divided doses daily.

E.R. TABLETS (LITHOBID)

Adults and children ages 12 and older. *Initial:* 900 mg twice daily. *Maintenance:* 600 mg twice daily.

SYRUP (LITHIUM CITRATE)

Adults and children ages 12 and older. Highly individualized. *Usual initial:* 16 mEq (10 ml) 3 times daily. *Usual maintenance:* 8 mEq (5 ml) 3 or 4 times daily.

±**DOSAGE ADJUSTMENT** For elderly patients and patients at risk for lithium toxicity, such as in the presence of severe debilitation or dehydration, or significant cardiovascular or renal disease or who are taking drugs that may affect kidney function, such as ACE inhibitors, angiotensin receptor blockers, diuretics, or NSAIDs, initial dosage may be reduced, and titration done more slowly.

Drug Administration

P.O.

- Do not interchange one form of lithium with another.
- Administer drug in regularly spaced doses consistently.
- Administer drug with water after meals to slow absorption from GI tract and reduce adverse reactions.
- Use a calibrated device when measuring dose of liquid form of drug.
- Capsules and E.R. tablets should be swallowed whole and not chewed, crushed, or opened.

Route	Onset	Peak	Duration
P.O.	5–7 days	1–2 hr	Unknown
P.O./E.R.	5–7 days	4–5 hr	Unknown

Half-life: 18–36 hr

Mechanism of Action

May increase presynaptic degradation of the catecholamine neurotransmitters dopamine, norepinephrine, and serotonin; inhibit their release at neuronal synapses; and decrease postsynaptic receptor sensitivity. These actions may correct overactive catecholamine systems in patients with mania.

Contraindications

Hypersensitivity to lithium or its components

Interactions

DRUGS

ACE inhibitors, angiotensin receptor blockers, diuretics, metronidazole, NSAIDs: Possibly increased blood lithium level and increased risk of toxicity

acetazolamide, sodium bicarbonate, urea, xanthines: Decreased blood lithium level

buspirone, fentanyl, MAO inhibitors, norepinephrine reuptake inhibitors, selective serotonin reuptake inhibitors, St. John's wort, tramadol, tricyclic antidepressants, triptans, tryptophan: Increased risk of serotonin syndrome
calcium channel blockers: Increased risk of neurotoxicity from lithium
calcium iodide, iodinated glycerol, potassium iodide: Possibly increased hypothyroid effects of both drugs
carbamazepine, methyldopa, phenytoin: Possibly increased risk of adverse reactions with these drugs
haloperidol and other antipsychotics: Increased risk of neurotoxicity ranging from extrapyramidal symptoms to neuroleptic malignant syndrome
neuromuscular blockers: Risk of prolonged effects
sodium-glucose cotransporter 2 (SGLT2) inhibitor: Possibly decreased serum lithium concentrations with possible decreased effectiveness of lithium

Adverse Reactions

CNS: Ataxia, **coma**, confusion, depression, disorientation, dizziness, drowsiness, fatigue, headache, lethargy, **seizures**, **serotonin syndrome**, syncope, tremor (in hands), vertigo
CV: **Arrhythmias**, **bradycardia**, **ECG changes**, edema, **hypotension**, palpitations, **peripheral circulatory collapse**, tachycardia, **unmasking of Brugada syndrome**
EENT: Blurred vision, dental caries, dry mouth, exophthalmos
ENDO: Diabetes insipidus, euthyroid goiter, hypothyroidism, **myxedema**, polydipsia
GI: Abdominal distention and pain, anorexia, diarrhea, nausea, vomiting
GU: **Nephrotic syndrome**, polyuria, stress incontinence, urinary frequency
HEME: Leukocytosis
MS: Muscle twitching and weakness
RESP: Dyspnea
SKIN: Abnormally dry skin; acne; alopecia; chronic folliculitis; cutaneous ulcers; dermatitis; dry, thin hair; numbness of skin; pruritus; psoriasis (new onset or exacerbation); rash
Other: **Angioedema**, cold sensitivity, **drug reaction with eosinophilia and systemic symptoms (DRESS)**, weight gain or loss

Childbearing Considerations

PREGNANCY

- Drug may cause fetal harm in first trimester, such as cardiovascular and other anomalies, and especially Ebstein's anomaly.
- Drug may cause fetal harm late in pregnancy with increased risk of neonatal lithium toxicity at birth. Lithium dosage should be decreased or discontinued 2 to 3 days prior to delivery and restarted in the postpartum period at preconception doses.
- Use with caution only if benefit to mother outweighs potential risk to fetus.

LACTATION

- Drug is present in breast milk.
- Breastfeeding is not recommended during drug therapy. However, if a mother chooses to breastfeed, infant should be monitored for signs of lithium toxicity. If present, breastfeeding must be discontinued.

Nursing Considerations

! **WARNING** Be aware that lithium has a narrow therapeutic range. Even a slightly high blood level is dangerous, and some patients show signs of toxicity at normal levels. Be aware that risk of toxicity is increased in patients with electrolyte changes (especially potassium and sodium), recent onset of a concurrent febrile illness, severe debilitation or dehydration, or significant cardiovascular or renal disease, and in patients taking other drugs that affect kidney function, such as ACE inhibitors, angiotensin receptor blockers, diuretics, and NSAIDs. Lithium toxicity signs and symptoms affect many areas of the body and can range from mild to severe and life-threatening symptoms. No antidote for lithium toxicity is available. Notify prescriber immediately if lithium toxicity occurs and expect drug to be discontinued. Provide supportive care, as needed and ordered.

- Expect to monitor blood lithium level 2 or 3 times weekly during first month, and then weekly to monthly during maintenance therapy and when starting or stopping NSAID therapy. In uncomplicated cases, plan to monitor lithium level every 2 to 3 months.

! **WARNING** Monitor patient for a hypersensivity reaction, including skin reaction, which can become life threatening such as angioedema or DRESS. At the first sign of swelling or rash (DRESS may initially only present with a fever or swollen lymph nodes), notify prescriber immediately, expect drug to be discontinued, and provide supportive care, as needed and ordered.

! **WARNING** Be aware that lithium affects extracellular and intracellular potassium ion shift, which can cause ECG changes, such as flattened or inverted T waves; it also can increase the risk of cardiac arrest.

! **WARNING** Monitor patient closely for unexplained palpitations or syncope after starting lithium therapy, as these symptoms may be caused by the unmasking of Brugada syndrome by lithium. Know that Brugada syndrome is a disorder in which electrocardiographic abnormalities occur and can result in sudden death. Patients at risk include those with a family history of Brugada syndrome or a family history of sudden death before the age of 45. Notify prescriber if palpitations or syncope occur and expect to discontinue lithium therapy.

! **WARNING** Monitor patient closely for serotonin syndrome, a rare but serious adverse effect of lithium. Signs and symptoms include agitation, confusion, diaphoresis, diarrhea, fever, hyperactive reflexes, poor coordination, restlessness, shaking, talking or acting with uncontrolled excitement, tremor, and twitching. If symptoms occur, notify prescriber immediately, expect drug to be discontinued, and provide supportive care.

- Ensure that patient's fluid and sodium intake is adequate during treatment.
- Expect prescriber to decrease dosage after acute manic episode is controlled.
- Monitor ECGs, renal and thyroid function test results, and serum electrolyte levels, as appropriate, during lithium treatment. Know that nephrotic syndrome has occurred with lithium use but has resulted in remission after lithium was discontinued.
- Be aware that lithium can cause reversible leukocytosis, which usually peaks within 7 to 10 days of starting therapy; WBC count typically returns to baseline within 10 days after therapy stops.
- Weigh patient daily to detect sudden weight changes.
- Monitor blood glucose level often in diabetic patient because lithium alters glucose tolerance.
- Palpate thyroid gland to detect enlargement because drug may cause goiter.

PATIENT TEACHING

- Instruct patient how to administer form of lithium prescribed.
- Caution patient not to stop taking lithium or adjust dosage without first consulting prescriber.
- Inform patient that frequent urination, nausea, and thirst may occur during the first few days of treatment.

! **WARNING** Alert patient that lithium may cause serious allergic and skin reactions that require immediate reporting to prescriber. If serious, urge patient to seek immediate medical care.

! **WARNING** Instruct patient to seek immediate emergency care if he experiences abnormal heartbeats, fainting, light-headedness, or shortness of breath.

! **WARNING** Instruct patient to report signs of toxicity, such as diarrhea, drowsiness, muscle weakness, tremor, uncoordinated body movements, and vomiting.

- Urge patient to avoid hazardous activities until drug's CNS effects are known and resolved.
- Advise patient to maintain normal fluid and sodium intake.
- Stress importance to females of childbearing age of alerting prescriber of pregnancy.
- Inform mothers that breastfeeding is not recommended during lithium therapy. However, if mother insists on breastfeeding, review signs and symptoms of lithium toxicity and tell her to notify pediatrician immediately if present. Stress that breastfeeding must be discontinued in the presence of lithium toxicity.
- Emphasize importance of complying with scheduled checkups and laboratory tests.

lixisenatide

Adlyxin

Class and Category

Pharmacologic class: Glucagon-like peptide receptor agonist
Therapeutic class: Antidiabetic

Indications and Dosages

* *As adjunct to diet and exercise to improve glycemic control in patients with type 2 diabetes mellitus*

SUBCUTANEOUS INJECTION

Adults. *Initial:* 10 mcg once daily within 1 hr of first meal of the day for 14 days. Increased to 20 mcg once daily on day 15 and thereafter. *Maintenance:* 20 mcg once daily.

Drug Administration

SUBCUTANEOUS

- Inspect solution before administration; it should be clear and colorless.
- Administer drug within 1 hr before patient's first meal of the day.
- Inject drug into patient's abdomen, thighs, or upper arm.
- If a dose is missed, give 1 hr before next meal.
- Rotate sites.
- Protect the pen device containing the drug from light by keeping it in its original packaging until ready for use.
- Do not store pen with needle attached. Unused pens should be stored in refrigerator.
- Prior to first use, store pen in refrigerator. Write date that pen was first used, store pen at room temperature, and discard 14 days later.

Route	Onset	Peak	Duration
SubQ	Unknown	1–3.5 hr	Unknown

Half-life: 3 hr

Mechanism of Action

Decreases glucagon secretion, increases glucose-dependent insulin release, and slows gastric emptying. All of these actions work together to reduce blood glucose levels.

Contraindications

Hypersensitivity to lixisenatide or its components

Interactions

DRUGS

basal insulin, sulfonylureas: Increased risk of hypoglycemia
orally administered drugs: Possibly delayed absorption of orally administered drugs resulting in decreased effectiveness

Adverse Reactions

CNS: Dizziness, headache
EENT: **Altered taste**, **laryngeal edema**
GI: Abdominal distention or pain, **acute pancreatitis**, cholecystitis, cholelithiasis, constipation, diarrhea, dyspepsia, ileus, nausea, vomiting
GU: **Acute kidney injury**, **worsening of chronic renal failure**
RESP: **Bronchospasms**
SKIN: Urticaria
Other: **Anaphylaxis**; **angioedema**; injection-site reactions, such as erythema, pain, and pruritus; lixisenatide-induced antibodies

Childbearing Considerations

PREGNANCY

- Drug may cause fetal harm based on animal studies.
- Use with caution only if benefit to mother outweighs potential risk to fetus.

LACTATION

- It is not known if drug is present in breast milk.
- Mothers should check with prescriber before breastfeeding.

Nursing Considerations

! **WARNING** Monitor patient's renal function before lixisenatide is initiated and during therapy, as ordered. Know that acute kidney injury can occur quickly even in patients who have no history of kidney disease. Patients are at increased risk when they experience dehydration, diarrhea, nausea, or vomiting. Notify prescriber immediately if patient's fluid balance is compromised.

! **WARNING** Monitor patient closely for hypersensitivity reactions that could become life threatening such as anaphylaxis or angioedema. Know that patient with a history of hypersensitivity to other drugs in the same class is at higher risk. If present, notify prescriber, expect drug to be discontinued, and provide supportive care, as needed and ordered.

! **WARNING** Monitor patient for hypoglycemia, especially in patients who also take basal insulin and/or a sulfonylurea. Be prepared to treat hypoglycemia should it occur. Notify prescriber of persistent or severe hypoglycemic episodes, as a dosage reduction in the insulin or sulfonylurea may be needed.

! **WARNING** Monitor patient for signs and symptoms of pancreatitis, including persistent severe abdominal pain, sometimes radiating to the back, that may or may not be accompanied with vomiting. Know that risk increases in patients who have a history of alcohol abuse or cholelithiasis. If pancreatitis is suspected, notify prescriber, expect drug to be discontinued, and provide supportive care, as needed and ordered.

! **WARNING** Know that drug delays gastric emptying, which may cause pulmonary aspiration in patients undergoing elective surgery or procedures requiring deep sedation or general anesthesia.

- Monitor patient for signs and symptoms of acute gallbladder disease. If cholelithiasis is suspected, notify prescriber and expect gallbladder studies to be done. A cholecystectomy may be needed.

PATIENT TEACHING

- Remind patient that lixisenatide does not take the place of dietary measures and exercise also used to control blood sugar.
- Instruct patient, family, or caregiver on how to administer lixisenatide subcutaneously and what to do if a dose is missed.
- Tell patient how to dispose of pen properly and to keep out of reach of children and pets.
- Inform females of childbearing age who are taking oral contraceptives that lixisenatide may interfere with absorption and effectiveness of oral contraceptive. To avoid this, tell patient to take oral contraceptive 1 hour before or 11 hours after administering lixisenatide each day.
- Tell all patients taking oral medications to take them at least 1 hour before administering lixisenatide; if a prescribed drug requires food intake, take it with a meal or snack that does not coincide with lixisenatide administration.

! **WARNING** Alert patient that drug may cause an allergic reaction. If present, tell patient to notify prescriber and, if severe, to seek immediate medical care.

! **WARNING** Encourage patient to be on the alert for hypoglycemia, especially if she is taking basal insulin or sulfonylurea. Review the signs and symptoms of hypoglycemia and how to treat it. If episodes occur frequently or become severe, tell her to notify prescriber, as a dosage reduction may be needed for her basal insulin or sulfonylurea.

! **WARNING** Advise patient to maintain adequate hydration. Emphasize importance of alerting prescriber immediately if she does become dehydrated or develops diarrhea, nausea, or vomiting.

! **WARNING** Review signs and symptoms of pancreatitis with patient and urge her to stop taking drug and notify prescriber, if present.

! **WARNING** Instruct patient to tell all healthcare providers of lixisenatide use, especially if undergoing an elective procedure or surgery.

- Warn patient never to share the pen used to inject lixisenatide even if the needle is changed because of an increased risk for transmission of blood-borne diseases.
- Inform patient that gallbladder problems may occur as a result of lixisenatide therapy. Tell patient to notify prescriber immediately if she develops clay-colored stools, fever, pain in the upper abdomen, and yellowing of eyes or skin.

lofexidine

Lucemyra

Class and Category

Pharmacologic class: Central $alpha_2$-agonist
Therapeutic class: Opioid withdrawal

Indications and Dosages

✱ To mitigate opioid withdrawal symptoms in order to facilitate abrupt opioid discontinuation

TABLETS

Adults. 3 tablets (0.18 mg each) 4 times daily at 5- to 6-hr intervals and continued during the period of peak withdrawal (usually first 5 to 7 days following last use of an opioid, although peak withdrawal may last up to 14 days). Then, dosage gradually reduced over 2 to 4 days by reducing 1 tablet per dose every 1 to 2 days. *Maximum:* 4 tablets (total 0.72 mg) for a single dose, 16 tablets (total 2.88 mg) daily.

± **DOSAGE ADJUSTMENT** For patients experiencing drug-related adverse reactions, dosage reduced, held, or drug discontinued depending on severity of reactions. For patients with moderate hepatic or renal impairment, dosage reduced to 2 tablets 4 times daily; for patients with severe hepatic or renal impairment, including end-stage renal disease or dialysis, dosage reduced to 1 tablet 4 times daily.

Drug Administration

P.O.

- Administer drug with 5 to 6 hr between each dose.
- Give drug with or without food.
- Do not remove desiccant pack from bottle.

Route	Onset	Peak	Duration
P.O.	Unknown	3–5 hr	Unknown

Half-life: 11–13 hr

Mechanism of Action

Binds to receptors on adrenergic neurons to reduce the release of norepinephrine and decrease sympathetic tone, thereby reducing opioid withdrawal symptoms.

Contraindications

Hypersensitivity to lofexidine or its components

Interactions

DRUGS

CNS depressants, such as barbiturates and other sedating drugs: Possibly potentiates effects of CNS depressants

CYP2 d6 inhibitors, such as paroxetine: Increased absorption of lofexidine, increasing risk for bradycardia and orthostatic hypotension

methadone: Increased risk of QT prolongation leading to life-threatening arrythmias

naltrexone (oral): Possibly reduced effectiveness of oral naltrexone if administered within 2 hr of lofexidine

ACTIVITIES

alcohol use: Possibly potentiates CNS depressant effect of alcohol

Adverse Reactions

CNS: Dizziness, insomnia, sedation, somnolence, syncope

CV: Bradycardia, **hypotension**, orthostatic hypotension, **QT prolongation**, **torsades de pointes**

EENT: Dry mouth, tinnitus

Other: Discontinuation effects (anxiety, chills, diarrhea, elevation of blood pressure, extremity pain, hyperhidrosis, insomnia)

Childbearing Considerations

PREGNANCY

- It is not known if drug causes fetal harm.
- Use with caution only if benefit to mother outweighs potential risk to fetus.

LACTATION

- It is not known if drug is present in breast milk.
- Mothers should check with prescriber before breastfeeding.

Nursing Considerations

! WARNING Be aware that lofexidine should not be used in patients with cerebrovascular disease, congenital long QT syndrome, marked bradycardia, recent MI, or severe coronary insufficiency.

- Monitor vital signs before administering each dose of lofexidine because drug may cause a decrease in blood pressure or pulse and may cause syncope.

! WARNING Know that lofexidine prolongs the QT interval. Expect to monitor patient's ECG if he has a history of bradyarrhythmias, congestive heart failure, or hepatic or renal impairment; ECG should also be monitored in patients with electrolyte abnormalities, such as hypokalemia or hypomagnesemia. Know that electrolyte imbalances should be corrected before lofexidine therapy begins.

- Be aware that lofexidine therapy should not be stopped abruptly but gradually withdrawn to reduce the risk of discontinuation symptoms, such as a sudden rise in blood pressure along with anxiety, chills, diarrhea, excessive sweating, extremity pain, and insomnia. If patient stops drug use abruptly, symptoms can be managed by administering the previous lofexidine dose and then subsequently gradually tapering drug dosage downward.

PATIENT TEACHING

- Instruct patient how to administer lofexidine.
- Tell patient that lofexidine therapy will help with opioid withdrawal symptoms but will not completely prevent them.
- Tell patient to take lofexidine exactly as prescribed. Warn patient that stopping drug abruptly can result in a sudden rise in blood pressure along with anxiety, chills, diarrhea, excessive sweating, extremity pain, and insomnia. Caution the patient that drug must be gradually withdrawn.

! **WARNING** Alert patient that lofexidine is not a treatment for opioid use. Tell patient that upon complete opioid discontinuation, he is more likely to have a reduced tolerance to opioids and is at increased risk for a fatal overdose should he resume opioid use. Make sure patient, family, or caregiver are aware of the increased risk of overdose.

! **WARNING** Warn patient to avoid taking any CNS depressant drugs, such as barbiturates, benzodiazepines, or other sedating drugs while taking lofexidine because severe respiratory depression and sedation may occur. Also, warn patient not to drink alcohol while taking drug, for the same reason.

- Tell patient to inform all prescribers of lofexidine therapy and not to take any over-the-counter preparations, including herbal products, without consulting prescriber, as the combination may cause an excessive drop in blood pressure or pulse rate.
- Instruct patient to rise slowly from a lying or sitting position and to maintain adequate hydration, as well as avoid becoming overheated, to help minimize a drop in blood pressure or pulse. Tell patient that if he experiences low blood pressure or decreased pulse rate to withhold drug and notify prescriber for guidance on how to adjust his dose.
- Instruct patient to avoid performing hazardous activities such as driving until the drug's effects on his nervous system are known and resolved.

lorazepam

Ativan, Lorazepam Intensol, Loreer XR

Class, Category, and Schedule

Pharmacologic class: Benzodiazepine
Therapeutic class: Anxiolytic
Controlled substance schedule: IV

Indications and Dosages

✱ *To treat anxiety*

ORAL CONCENTRATE, TABLETS

Adults. *Initial:* 2 to 3 mg 2 or 3 times daily, increased, as needed. *Maximum:* 10 mg daily.

± **DOSAGE ADJUSTMENT** For elderly or debilitated patients, initial dosage may be reduced to 1 to 2 mg daily in divided doses.

E.R. CAPSULES (LOREER XR)

Adults. After stabilization on immediate-release tablet form taken 3 times daily, once daily dosage equal to the total daily dose of tablet form given in the morning.

± **DOSAGE ADJUSTMENT** For patients who will receive a UGT inhibitor during treatment, E.R. capsules will need to be discontinued and replaced with tablet form so dosage can be reduced.

✱ *To treat insomnia caused by anxiety*

ORAL CONCENTRATE, TABLETS

Adults. 2 to 4 mg at bedtime as a single daily dose, as needed.

± **DOSAGE ADJUSTMENT** For elderly or debilitated patients, dosage possibly reduced.

✱ *To provide preoperative sedation*

I.V. INJECTION

Adults. 0.044 mg/kg or 2 mg, whichever is less, 15 to 20 min before procedure. Higher dosage may be required for some patients but not to exceed maximum dose. *Maximum:* 0.05 mg/kg or total of 4 mg.

I.M. INJECTION

Adults. 0.05 mg/kg up to maximum dosage 2 hr before procedure. *Maximum:* 4 mg.

∗ *To treat status epilepticus*

I.M. INJECTION, I.V. INJECTION

Adults. *Initial:* 4 mg I.V. at a rate of 2 mg/min. Repeated in 10 to 15 min if seizures don't subside or recur. I.M. route used only if I.V. route is not accessible. *Maximum:* 8 mg/24 hr.

±**DOSAGE ADJUSTMENT** For patients receiving drug I.M. or I.V. and also taking probenecid or valproate, dosage reduced by 50%. For females of childbearing age, dosage may have to be increased if oral contraceptives are being used.

Drug Administration

- Have emergency resuscitation equipment readily available when administering drug parenterally.

P.O.

- When administering oral concentrate, use calibrated dropper supplied with drug to measure dosage.
- Use only the calibrated dropper provided for oral concentrate. Draw the dose into the dropper and then squeeze the dropper contents into a liquid or onto semi-solid food. Examples of a liquid to use include water, carbonated beverages, or juices or semisolid food such as applesauce or pudding. Gently stir for a few seconds and administer immediately. Do not store mixture for future use.
- Capsules and tablets should be swallowed whole. However, E.R. capsules may be opened and sprinkled over a tablespoon of applesauce, consumed without chewing within 2 hr, and followed by water. Do not store mixture for future use.
- For anxiety, administer in divided doses with the largest dose given before bedtime.
- For insomnia caused by anxiety, administer at bedtime.

I.V.

- Preferred route for treatment of status epilepticus.
- Dilute lorazepam with equal amount of 0.9% Sodium Chloride Injection, 5% Dextrose Injection, or Sterile Water for Injection.
- Gently invert container repeatedly to mix. Do not shake vigorously, as this will result in air entrapment.
- Administer as an I.V. injection slowly, no more than 2 mg/min.
- For preoperative sedation, administer 15 to 20 min before procedure.
- Monitor patient's respirations every 5 to 15 min and keep emergency resuscitation equipment readily available.
- Store unopened multidose vials in refrigerator and protect from light.
- Discard multidose vial after 28 days of initial use.
- *Incompatibilities:* None reported by manufacturer

I.M.

- For status epilepticus, I.M. route used only if I.V. route is not available.
- Inject undiluted deep into large muscle mass, such as gluteus maximus.
- For preoperative sedation, administer 2 hr before procedure.
- Store unopened multidose vials in refrigerator and protect from light.
- Discard multidose vial after 28 days of initial use.

Route	Onset	Peak	Duration
P.O.	1 hr	2 hr	12–24 hr
I.V.	1–3 min	1–1.5 hr	6–8 hr
I.M.	15–30 min	< 3 hr	6–8 hr

Half-life: 10–20 hr

Mechanism of Action

May potentiate the effects of gamma-aminobutyric acid (GABA) and other inhibitory neurotransmitters by binding to specific benzodiazepine receptors in cortical and limbic areas of CNS. GABA inhibits excitatory stimulation, which helps control emotional behavior. Limbic system contains a highly dense area of benzodiazepine receptors, which may explain drug's antianxiety effects. Also, lorazepam hyperpolarizes neuronal cells, thereby interfering with their ability to generate seizures.

Contraindications

For all forms of lorazepam: Acute angle-closure glaucoma; hypersensitivity to

lorazepam, other benzodiazepines, or their components
For parenteral form: Intra-arterial delivery, severe respiratory insufficiency (except in patients requiring anxiety relief and/or diminished recall of events while being mechanically ventilated), sleep apnea syndrome

Interactions

DRUGS

aminophylline, theophylline: Possibly reduced sedative effects of lorazepam
clozapine: Increased risk of ataxia, delirium, excessive salivation, hypotension, marked sedation, and respiratory arrest
CNS depressants: Additive CNS depression, potentially fatal respiratory depression
fentanyl: Possibly decreased therapeutic effects of fentanyl
probenecid, valproate: Possibly increased therapeutic and adverse effects of lorazepam
other benzodiazepines, sedating antihistamines, opioids, tricyclic antidepressants: Increased risk of profound respiratory depression, sedation, and somnolence

ACTIVITIES

alcohol use: Increased CNS depression and severe respiratory depression

Adverse Reactions

CNS: Amnesia, anxiety, ataxia, **coma**, confusion, delusions, depression, dizziness, drowsiness, euphoria, extrapyramidal symptoms, fatigue, headache, hypokinesia, irritability, malaise, nervousness, **seizures**, slurred speech, **suicidal ideation**, tremor, unsteadiness, vertigo
CV: Chest pain, palpitations, tachycardia
EENT: Blurred vision, diplopia, dry mouth, increased salivation, photophobia
ENDO: Syndrome of inappropriate ADH
GI: Abdominal pain, constipation, diarrhea, elevated liver enzymes, jaundice, nausea, thirst, vomiting
GU: Libido changes
HEME: **Agranulocytosis**, **pancytopenia**, **thrombocytopenia**
RESP: **Apnea**, **respiratory depression**, worsening of obstructive pulmonary disease or sleep apnea
SKIN: Diaphoresis
Other: **Anaphylaxis**, injection-site pain (I.M.) or phlebitis (I.V.), physical and psychological dependence, withdrawal symptoms

Childbearing Considerations

PREGNANCY

- Pregnancy exposure registry: 1-866-961-2388 or https://womensmentalhealth.org/pregnancyregistry/.
- Drug may cause fetal harm, such as neurotoxicity. If mother ingests drug for several weeks or more prior to delivery, infant may develop neonatal sedation and withdrawal syndrome.
- Drug should not be used during pregnancy except in life-threatening situations.

LACTATION

- Drug is present in breast milk.
- Mothers should check with prescriber before breastfeeding.
- Infants being breastfed should be observed for inability to suckle, irritability, and sedation.

Nursing Considerations

! **WARNING** Monitor patients closely who have a history of alcohol or drug abuse or a personality disorder because of an increased risk of physical and psychological dependence. Monitor patient closely throughout drug therapy for evidence of abuse or misuse.

! **WARNING** Ensure that a depressed patient is already receiving an antidepressant before starting lorazepam therapy because untreated depression increases risk of suicidal ideation.

! **WARNING** Use extreme caution when giving lorazepam to elderly patients, especially those with compromised respiratory function because drug can cause hypoventilation, respiratory depression, sedation, and unsteadiness. Monitor all patient's respiratory status closely because drug may cause life-threatening respiratory depression.

! **WARNING** Monitor patient for a hypersensitivity reaction, which could become life-threatening, such as anaphylaxis.

If present, notify prescriber, expect drug to be switched to another drug, and provide supportive care, as needed and ordered.

! **WARNING** Monitor patients with encephalopathy or severe hepatic insufficiency because drug may worsen hepatic encephalopathy.

! **WARNING** Be aware that benzodiazepine therapy such as lorazepam should only be used concomitantly with opioids or other CNS depressants in patients for whom other treatment options are inadequate because adverse effects could be profound and possibly result in death. If prescribed together, expect dosing and duration of the opioid or other CNS depressant to be limited. Monitor patient closely for signs and symptoms of profound decrease in consciousness, including coma, sedation, and respiratory depression. Notify prescriber immediately and provide emergency supportive care.

! **WARNING** Monitor CBC and platelet count, as ordered because drug can cause serious hematologic adverse reactions. Monitor patient for bruising, bleeding, and infection.

! **WARNING** Monitor neonate for neonatal sedation and withdrawal syndrome if mother took lorazepam late in pregnancy. Look for hypotonia, lethargy, and respiratory depression in the neonate as well as withdrawal symptoms exhibited by inconsolable crying, feeding difficulties, hyperreflexia, irritability, restlessness, and tremors.

! **WARNING** Know that stopping drug abruptly increases risk of withdrawal symptoms, which may last from weeks to more than 12 months and could be life-threatening. Dosage should be tapered gradually, especially in epileptic patients.

PATIENT TEACHING

- Instruct patient how to administer form of lorazepam prescribed if using drug for anxiety.

! **WARNING** Tell patient to take lorazepam exactly as prescribed and not to increase dosage or frequency because drug can cause addiction and, if misused, could result in overdose or even death. Stress importance of keeping naloxone in the home and instruct family or caregiver how to administer naloxone in the event an overdose occurs. Stress importance of calling 911 if naloxone is administered.

! **WARNING** Urge patient to avoid alcohol while taking lorazepam because it increases drug's CNS depressant effects and can cause severe respiratory depression that may lead to death.

! **WARNING** Alert patient drug can cause an allergic reaction. If present, tell patient to withhold lorazepam until prescriber notified. Urge patient to seek immediate medical care if reaction is severe.

! **WARNING** Warn patient about potentially fatal additive effects of combining lorazepam with an opioid or other CNS depressants. Potentially fatal respiratory depression and sedation may occur. Instruct the patient to inform all prescribers of lorazepam use, especially when pain medication may be prescribed.

! **WARNING** Review signs and symptoms of bleeding and infection control precautions. Tell patient to notify prescriber immediately if signs and symptoms such as bruising, bleeding, or infection occur.

- Advise patient to avoid hazardous activities until drug's CNS effects are known and resolved.
- Instruct patient to report excessive drowsiness and nausea.
- Advise patient to alert prescriber if pregnancy occurs, as drug most likely will need to be discontinued.
- Tell mothers who are breastfeeding during drug therapy to monitor their infant for inability to suckle, irritability, and sedation.

! **WARNING** Advise patient not to stop taking lorazepam without consulting prescriber because of the risk of withdrawal symptoms. Inform patient that withdrawal symptoms could last for weeks to more than 12 months and could be life-threatening.

losartan potassium

Cozaar

Class and Category

Pharmacologic class: Angiotensin II receptor blocker (ARB)
Therapeutic class: Antihypertensive

Indications and Dosages

✷ *To manage hypertension*

ORAL SUSPENSION, TABLETS

Adults. *Initial:* 50 mg once daily. *Maximum:* 100 mg daily.
Children ages 6 and older with an eGFR of 30 ml/min or greater. *Initial:* 0.7 mg/kg (up to 50 mg total) once daily, with dosage adjusted, as needed. *Maximum:* 1.4 mg/kg or 100 mg daily.

✷ *To treat diabetic nephropathy with the presence of an elevated creatinine and proteinuria in patients with type 2 diabetes and hypertension*

ORAL SUSPENSION, TABLETS

Adults. *Initial:* 50 mg once daily, increased to 100 mg once daily, as needed.

✷ *To reduce stroke risk in patients with hypertension and left ventricular hypertrophy*

ORAL SUSPENSION, TABLETS

Adults. *Initial:* 50 mg once daily. Hydrochlorothiazide 12.5 mg daily added and/or dosage increased to 100 mg daily, as needed, followed by hydrochlorothiazide increased to 25 mg, daily, as needed.

± DOSAGE ADJUSTMENT For patients with impaired hepatic function or volume depletion, initial dosage reduced to 25 mg once daily.

Drug Administration

P.O.

- Shake oral suspension before each use.
- Use a calibrated device to measure dosage of oral suspension.
- Store oral suspension in refrigerator for up to 4 wk.

Route	Onset	Peak	Duration
P.O.	6 hr	1–1.5 hr	24 hr

Half-life: 2–6 hr

Mechanism of Action

Blocks binding of angiotensin II to receptor sites in many tissues, including adrenal glands and vascular smooth muscle. Angiotensin II is a potent vasoconstrictor that also stimulates the adrenal cortex to secrete aldosterone. The inhibiting effects of angiotensin II reduce blood pressure.

Decreases left ventricular mass index in patients with left ventricular hypertrophy who also have hypertension. By targeting the renin–angiotensin system, a renoprotective action occurs through the lowering of the albumin excretion rate in patients with type 2 diabetes.

Contraindications

Concurrent aliskiren therapy (in patients with diabetes), hypersensitivity to losartan or its components

Interactions

DRUGS

ACE inhibitors, aliskiren (in patients with diabetes or renal impairment with a glomerular filtration rate less than 60 ml/min), other angiotensin receptor blockers: Increased risk of hyperkalemia, hypotension, and renal dysfunction
lithium: Increased serum lithium levels and risk of lithium toxicity
NSAIDs: Possibly decreased renal function in elderly patients or those with renal dysfunction or volume depletion; possibly decreased effectiveness of losartan
potassium-sparing diuretics, potassium supplements: Increased risk of hyperkalemia

FOODS

high-potassium diet, potassium-containing salt substitutes: Increased risk of hyperkalemia

Adverse Reactions

CNS: Dizziness, fatigue, headache, insomnia, malaise
CV: **Hypotension**
EENT: Nasal congestion
GI: Diarrhea, indigestion, nausea, vomiting
HEME: **Thrombocytopenia**
MS: Back pain, leg pain, muscle spasms
RESP: Cough, upper respiratory tract infection
SKIN: Erythroderma
Other: **Angioedema**, **hyperkalemia**, **hyponatremia**

Childbearing Considerations

PREGNANCY

- Drug can cause fetal harm and should be discontinued as soon as pregnancy is known.
- Drug given during the second or third trimester reduces fetal renal function and increases fetal and neonatal morbidity and death. Resulting oligohydramnios can cause fetal lung hypoplasia and skeletal malformations.

LACTATION

- It is not known if drug is present in breast milk.
- A decision should be made to discontinue breastfeeding or the drug to avoid potential serious adverse reactions in the breastfed infant.

Nursing Considerations

- Know that patients of African descent with hypertension and left ventricular hypertrophy may not benefit from losartan to reduce stroke risk.
- Monitor blood pressure to evaluate drug effectiveness to control hypertension as well as to detect hypotension. Notify prescriber if patient develops dizziness, light-headedness, or syncope.

! **WARNING** Monitor patient for a hypersensitivity reaction, which could become life threatening such as angioedema. If present, notify prescriber, expect drug to be discontinued, and provide supportive care, as needed and ordered.

! **WARNING** Be aware that patients who have renal artery stenosis or severe heart failure may experience acute renal failure from losartan therapy because losartan inhibits the angiotensin–aldosterone system, on which renal function depends. Montior BUN and creatinine levels closely.

! **WARNING** Monitor patient's serum potassium level, as ordered, to detect hyperkalemia and patient for signs and symptoms of hyperkalemia. If present, notify prescriber and expect to implement measures as ordered to decrease the potassium level because hyperkalemia can cause life-threatening adverse effects.

- Monitor patient for muscle pain; rarely, rhabdomyolysis has developed in patients taking other angiotensin II receptor blockers.

PATIENT TEACHING

- Instruct patient how to administer form of lorsartan prescribed.
- Teach patient how to take his blood pressure to monitior effectiveness of drug, if appropriate. Tell patient to notify prescriber immediately if dizziness, fainting, or light-headedness occurs.

! **WARNING** Alert patient that lorsartan may cause an allergic reaction. Tell patient, if present, to notify prescriber and, if severe, to seek immediate medical care.

! **WARNING** Instruct females of childbearing age to notify prescriber immediately if pregnancy occurs as drug may cause fetal harm and will have to be discontinued.

! **WARNING** Review signs and symptoms of hyperkalemia with patient. Instruct patient to avoid potassium-containing salt substitutes because they may increase risk of hyperkalemia. Tell patient to notify prescriber if signs and symptoms of hyperkalemia occur.

- Advise patient to avoid exercising in hot weather and drinking excessive amounts of alcohol; instruct her to notify prescriber if she has prolonged diarrhea, nausea, or vomiting.
- Warn patient to tell all prescribers of losartan therapy.
- Inform mothers breastfeeding should not be undertaken.

lovastatin

(mevinolin)

Altoprev

Class and Category

Pharmacologic class: HMG-CoA reductase inhibitor (statin)
Therapeutic class: Antilipemic

Indications and Dosages

✶ *As adjunct to diet to reduce LDL and total cholesterol levels in patients with primary hypercholesterolemia (Types IIa and IIb); to reduce risk of coronary revascularization procedures, MI, or unstable angina in patients without symptomatic cardiovascular disease and who have average to moderately elevated total-C and LDL-C, and below average HDL-C as primary prevention of coronary heart disease; to slow progression of coronary atherosclerosis in patients with coronary heart disease*

TABLETS

Adults. *Initial:* 20 mg once daily with evening meal for LDL-C reduction of 20% or more, 10 mg daily with evening meal or LDL-C reduction of less than 20%; dosage adjusted after at least 4 wk. *Maximum:* 80 mg daily.

* *As adjunct to diet to reduce apolipoprotein B, LDL-C, and total cholesterol levels in adolescents with heterozygous familial hypercholesterolemia*

TABLETS

Adolescent boys and girls who are at least 1 yr postmenarche and ages 10 to 17. *Initial:* 20 mg daily with the evening meal for LDL-C reduction of 20% or more, 10 mg daily with the evening meal for LDL-C reduction of less than 20%; dosage adjusted after at least 4 wk. *Maintenance:* 10 to 40 mg daily. *Maximum:* 40 mg daily.

* *As adjunct to diet to reduce low-density lipoprotein cholesterol (LDL-C) in patients with primary hyperlipidemia, including heterozygous familial hypercholesterolemia (HeFH); as adjunct to diet to reduce LDL-C and slow the progression of coronary atherosclerosis in patients with coronary heart disease; to reduce risk of MI, unstable angina, and coronary revascularization procedures in patients at high risk for coronary heart disease.*

E.R. TABLETS (ALTOPREV)

Adults. *Initial:* 20 to 60 mg once daily at bedtime. *Maximum:* 60 mg daily.

± **DOSAGE ADJUSTMENT** For patients taking concomitant therapy with amiodarone dosage limited to 40 mg daily; concomitant therapy with danazol, diltiazem, dronedarone, or verapamil, initial dosage reduced to 10 mg (immediate-release) daily and maximum dosage limited to 20 mg daily. For patients who have a creatinine clearance less than 30 ml/min, dosage limited to 20 mg daily and dosage increased, if needed, very carefully.

Drug Administration

P.O.

- Administer immediate-release tablet with evening meal; E.R. tablet at bedtime.
- E.R. tablets and immediate-release tablets should be swallowed whole and not chewed, crushed, or split.
- Give drug 1 hr before or 4 hr after bile acid sequestrant, cholestyramine, or colestipol.

Route	Onset	Peak	Duration
P.O.	Unknown	2–4 hr	Unknown
P.O./E.R.	3 days	14 hr	Unknown

Half-life: 1.1–1.7 hr

Mechanism of Action

Interferes with the hepatic enzyme hydroxymethylglutaryl-coenzyme A reductase. By doing so, lovastatin reduces formation of mevalonic acid (a cholesterol precursor), thus interrupting the pathway by which cholesterol is synthesized. When cholesterol level declines in hepatic cells, LDLs are consumed, which also reduces amount of circulating total cholesterol and serum triglycerides. The decrease in LDLs may result in decreased level of apolipoprotein B, which is found in each LDL particle.

Contraindications

Acute liver failure or decompensated cirrhosis; breastfeeding; concomitant therapy with cobicistat-containing products or strong CYP3A4 inhibitors (such as boceprevir, clarithromycin, erythromycin, HIV protease inhibitors, itraconazole, ketoconazole, nefazodone, posaconazole, telaprevir, telithromycin, voriconazole); hypersensitivity to lovastatin or its components; pregnancy; unexplained elevated liver enzymes

Interactions

DRUGS

amiodarone, boceprevir, cobicistat-containing products, clarithromycin, colchicine, cyclosporine, danazol, diltiazem, dronedarone, erythromycin, fibric acid derivatives, gemfibrozil and other fibrates, HIV protease inhibitors, itraconazole, ketoconazole, nefazodone, niacin (1 g daily or more), posaconazole, ranolazine, telaprevir, telithromycin, verapamil, voriconazole: Increased risk of severe myopathy or rhabdomyolysis

oral anticoagulants: Increased anticoagulant effect and risk of bleeding

ACTIVITIES

alcohol use: Increased lovastatin blood level

FOODS

grapefruit juice (more than 1 qt daily): Increased risk of myopathy or rhabdomyolysis

Adverse Reactions

CNS: Anxiety, asthenia, chills, cognitive impairment, confusion, cranial nerve dysfunction, depression, dizziness, fatigue, fever, headache, insomnia, malaise, memory loss, paresthesia, peripheral nerve palsy, peripheral neuropathy, psychic disturbances, tremor, vertigo

CV: Vasculitis

EENT: Blurred vision, cataracts, ophthalmoplegia, pharyngitis, rhinitis, sinusitis

ENDO: Elevated glycosylated hemoglobin levels, gynecomastia, hyperglycemia, thyroid function abnormalities

GI: Abdominal cramps and pain, anorexia, cholestatic jaundice, **cirrhosis**, constipation, diarrhea, elevated liver enzymes, flatulence, **fulminant hepatic necrosis**, **hepatic failure** (rare), **hepatitis**, hyperbilirubinemia, indigestion, nausea, hepatoma, **pancreatitis**, vomiting

GU: Erectile dysfunction, loss of libido, UTI

HEME: Elevated erythrocyte sedimentation rate (ESR), eosinophilia, **hemolytic anemia**, **leukopenia**, positive antinuclear antibodies (ANA), purpura, **thrombocytopenia**

MS: Arthralgias, arthritis, back pain, immune-mediated necrotizing myopathy, muscle cramps or pain, myalgia, myopathy, myositis, polymyalgia rheumatica, **rhabdomyolysis**

RESP: Cough, dyspnea, **interstitial lung disease**, upper respiratory tract infection

SKIN: Alopecia, changes to hair and nails, dermatomyositis, discolored or dry skin, **erythema multiforme**, flushing, lichen planus, photosensitivity, pruritus, rash, **Stevens-Johnson syndrome**, **toxic epidermal necrolysis**, urticaria

Other: **Anaphylaxis**, **angioedema**, elevated alkaline phosphatase, flu-like syndrome, infections, lupus erythematosus-like syndrome

Childbearing Considerations

PREGNANCY

- Drug may cause fetal harm according to animal studies.
- Drug is contraindicated in pregnancy.

LACTATION

- It is not known if drug is present in breast milk.
- Drug is contraindicated in breastfeeding.

REPRODUCTION

- Females of childbearing age should be advised to use effective contraception during drug treatment.

Nursing Considerations

- Expect patient to be prescribed a standard low-cholesterol diet during therapy.
- Be aware that drug affects mainly total cholesterol and LDL levels; it has only slight effects on HDL and triglyceride levels.
- Monitor patient's lipid panel regularly, as ordered, to determine effectiveness of drug.

! WARNING Montior patient for a hypersensitivity reaction, which could become life threatening such as anaphylaxis or angioedema. If present, notify prescriber, expect drug to be discontinued, and provide supportive care, as needed and ordered.

- Monitor patients closely who have a history of liver disease and patients who consume large amounts of alcohol as drug can adversely affect liver function. Monitor liver enzymes before therapy begins, as ordered. If indicated, expect to measure them during therapy, as ordered. If ALT or AST level reaches or exceeds 3 times upper limit of normal and persists at that level, expect to discontinue lovastatin.

! WARNING Monitor patient closely for muscle pain, tenderness, or weakness suggestive of myopathy. Also, monitor creatine kinase, as ordered. If patient becomes symptomatic or creatine kinase becomes highly elevated, withhold drug, notify prescriber, and expect drug to be discontinued. Be especially alert for myopathy that could become in its more severe form, rhabdomyolysis, in patients with other disorders, such as diabetes complicated with renal dysfunction. Know that risk of myopathy/rhabdomyolysis is dose related and increases with concurrent therapy with many different types of drugs, including other lipid-lowering drugs such as other fibrates or niacin dosage of 1 gram or greater daily.

! **WARNING** Expect to withhold drug temporarily in patients who develop an acute or serious condition predisposing patient to the development of renal failure secondary to rhabdomyolysis. Conditions to be watchful for include hypotension; major surgery or trauma; sepsis; or severe electrolyte, endocrine, or metabolic disorders; or uncontrolled epilepsy. Be mindful that the drug interactions may not be the same for the E.R. formulation of lovastatin as for those encountered with the immediate-release formulation.

! **WARNING** Notify prescriber of any other persistent, serious, or unusual adverse reactions as drug can affect many body systems and cause serious adverse effects.

PATIENT TEACHING

- Inform patient that lovastatin is not a substitute for a low-cholesterol diet and exercise program.
- Instruct patient how to administer form of lovastatin prescribed.
- Tell patient to avoid consuming alcohol or more than 1 quart of grapefruit juice daily while taking drug.

! **WARNING** Stress importance to notify prescriber if females of childbearing age become pregnant as drug is contraindicated in pregnancy. Instruct these patients to use an effective contraceptive throughout drug therapy.

! **WARNING** Alert patient that lovastatin may cause an allergic reaction. If present, tell patient to notify prescriber and, if severe, urge patient to seek immediate medical care.

! **WARNING** Advise patient to report muscle aches, pains, tenderness, or weakness, being especially watchful of these symptoms when dosage is increased. If present, tell the patient to stop taking lovastatin immediately and notify prescriber.

! **WARNING** Instruct patient to report severe GI distress or vision changes, as well as the development of dark urine, fatigue, loss of appetite, right upper abdominal pain, or yellowing of skin.

- Advise patient to avoid performing any hazardous activity, such as driving if cognitive impairment develops until it resolves.
- Tell patient to alert prescriber of any over-the-counter or prescription drugs being taken because serious drug interactions could occur.
- Emphasize the importance of periodic eye examinations during therapy.
- Tell mothers that breastfeeding is contraindicated while taking lovastatin.

lubiprostone

Amitiza

Class and Category

Pharmacologic class: Chloride channel activator
Therapeutic class: GI motility

Indications and Dosages

✷ *To treat chronic idiopathic constipation; to treat opioid-induced constipation in patients with chronic noncancer pain*

CAPSULES

Adults. 24 mcg twice daily.

✷ *To treat irritable bowel syndrome with constipation*

CAPSULES

Women at least 18 yr of age. 8 mcg twice daily.

± **DOSAGE ADJUSTMENT** For patients with chronic idiopathic constipation or opioid-induced constipation who have moderate liver impairment, dosage reduced to 16 mcg twice daily. For patients being treated for any indication who have severe liver impairment, dosage reduced to 8 mcg once daily.

Drug Administration

P.O.

- Administer drug with food and water to reduce nausea.
- Capsules should be swallowed whole and not chewed, crushed, or opened.

Route	Onset	Peak	Duration
P.O.	Unknown	1 hr	Unknown

Half-life: 0.9–1.4 hr

Mechanism of Action

Enhances a chloride-rich intestinal fluid secretion specifically by activating CIC-2, which is a normal constituent of the apical membrane of the human intestine. By increasing intestinal fluid secretion, motility in the intestine is increased, which facilitates the passage of stool to alleviate the symptoms associated with chronic idiopathic constipation. In addition, activation of the apical CIC-2 channels in intestinal epithelial cells bypasses the antisecretory action of opiates through suppression of secretomotor neuron excitability.

Contraindications

Hypersensitivity to lubiprostone or its components, mechanical GI obstruction

Interactions

DRUGS

diphenylheptane opioids, such as methadone: Decreased effectiveness of lubiprostone

Adverse Reactions

CNS: Anxiety, asthenia, depression, dizziness, fatigue, headache, lethargy, malaise, syncope, tremor
CV: Chest discomfort or pain, **hypotension**, palpitations, peripheral edema, tachycardia
EENT: Distortion of sense of smell, dry mouth, pharyngolaryngeal pain, **throat tightness**
GI: Abdominal distention or pain, anorexia, constipation, defecation urgency, diarrhea, dyspepsia, elevated liver enzymes, eructation, fecal incontinence, flatulence, frequent bowel movements, gastritis, gastroesophageal reflux disease, intestinal functional disorder, **ischemic colitis**, nausea, **rectal hemorrhage**, vomiting
GU: Pollakiuria, UTI
MS: Fibromyalgia, joint swelling, muscle cramps or spasms, myalgia
RESP: Cough, dyspnea
SKIN: Cold sweat, erythema, excessive diaphoresis, rash
Other: Flu-like symptoms, generalized pain, **hypokalemia**, swelling, weight gain

Childbearing Considerations

PREGNANCY

- It is not known if drug causes fetal harm.
- Use with caution only if benefit to mother outweighs potential risk to fetus.

LACTATION

- It is not known if drug is present in breast milk.
- Mothers should check with prescriber before breastfeeding.
- If breastfeeding occurs, infant should be monitored for diarrhea.

Nursing Considerations

! **WARNING** Be aware that lubiprostone should not be given to patients with severe diarrhea. Monitor patient for severe diarrhea throughout therapy. If present, expect drug to be discontinued.

! **WARNING** Monitor patient for a hypersensitivity reaction such as throat tightness that could become life-threatening. If present, notify prescriber immediately, withhold drug, and provide supportive care, as needed and ordered.

! **WARNING** Monitor patient's blood pressure for hypotension. Syncope and hypotension have occurred with lubiprostone therapy and sometimes within 1 hour after drug administration, including the first dose. Risk factors include the presence of diarrhea or vomiting or taking drugs known to lower blood pressure.

- Assess patient for dyspnea, which generally has occurred as an acute onset within 30 to 60 minutes after being given the first dose of lubiprostone. Although dyspnea usually resolves within 3 hours after taking drug, it may reoccur with subsequent doses. If it becomes severe or reoccurs, notify prescriber.

PATIENT TEACHING

- Instruct patient how to administer lubiprostone.

- Alert patient that difficulty breathing may occur after the first dose of lubiprostone but generally resolves within 3 hours. Tell patient to notify prescriber if dyspnea occurs and seek immediate medical care.

! **WARNING** Alert patient that an allergic reaction can occur with lubiprostone use. Tell patient to stop taking drug immediately and seek emergency medical care if throat tightness occurs.

! **WARNING** Inform patient of the possibility of diarrhea occurring with lubiprostone therapy. If diarrhea becomes severe, tell patient to stop taking drug and notify prescriber.

- Tell patient that drug may lower his blood pressure to the point of fainting. Caution patient to avoid performing hazardous activities until the effects of drug are known and resolved.
- Instruct patient to inform all prescribers of lubiprostone therapy because drugs known to lower blood pressure increase patient's risk of low blood pressure and possibly fainting.
- Tell mothers who are breastfeeding while taking lubiprostone to monitor the infant for diarrhea.

lumateperone tosylate

Caplyta

Class and Category

Pharmacologic class: Neuroleptic
Therapeutic class: Atypical antipsychotic

Indications and Dosages

∗ *To treat schizophrenia; to treat depressive episodes associated with bipolar I or II disorder as monotherapy or as adjunctive therapy with lithium or valproate*

CAPSULES

Adults. 42 mg once daily.

± **DOSAGE ADJUSTMENT** For patients with moderate or severe hepatic impairment or taking moderate CYP3A4 inhibitors concurrently, dosage reduced to 21 mg once daily. For patients taking strong CYP3A4 inhibitors, dosage reduced to 10.5 mg once daily.

Drug Administration

P.O.

- Administer drug with or without food.

Route	Onset	Peak	Duration
P.O.	Unknown	1–2 hr	Unknown

Half-life: 13–18 hr

Mechanism of Action

May act by being mediated through a combination of antagonist activity of central serotonin 5-HT_{2A} receptors and postsynaptic antagonist activity at central dopamine D_2 receptors.

Contraindications

Hypersensitivity to lumateperone or its components

Interactions

DRUGS

CYP3A4 inducers: Decreased exposure and effectiveness of lumateperone
moderate to strong CYP3A4 inhibitors, UGT inhibitors: Increased exposure and risk of adverse reactions to lumateperone

Adverse Reactions

CNS: Body temperature dysregulation, cognitive and motor impairment, dizziness, dystonia, extrapyramidal symptoms, fatigue, **neuroleptic malignant syndrome**, **seizures**, somnolence, **suicidal ideation**, syncope, tardive dyskinesia
CV: Dyslipidemia, orthostatic hypotension
EENT: Dry mouth
ENDO: Hyperglycemia
GI: Anorexia, dysphagia, nausea, vomiting
HEME: **Agranulocytosis**, **leukopenia**, **neutropenia**
MS: Elevated creatine phosphokinase levels
SKIN: Burning sensation

Childbearing Considerations

PREGNANCY

- Pregnancy exposure registry: 1-866-961-2388 or http://womensmentalhealth.org/clinical-and-research-programs/pregnancyregistry.
- Drug may cause fetal harm if fetus is exposed to drug during the third trimester, as extrapyramidal and/or withdrawal symptoms may occur after delivery.
- Use with caution only if benefit to mother outweighs potential risk to fetus.

LACTATION

- Drug is present in breast milk in low amounts.
- Mothers should check with prescriber before breastfeeding.

REPRODUCTION

- Drug may impair female and male fertility based on animal studies.

Nursing Considerations

! **WARNING** Know that lumateperone shouldn't be used in elderly patients with dementia-related psychosis because drug increases risk of death in these patients. Also, know that lumateperone should not be given to patients with moderate or severe hepatic impairment or to patients taking CYP3A4 inducers or moderate to strong CYP3A4 inhibitors.

- Use lumateperone cautiously in patients at risk for aspiration because drug may cause dysphagia.

! **WARNING** Determine patient's neutrophil count before lumateperone therapy is begun to ensure it is within normal limits. Then, monitor patient's CBC and platelet count regularly, as ordered, because drug can cause serious hematological adverse effects, such as agranulocytosis, leukopenia, and neutropenia. Monitor patient for fever or other signs of infection and report promptly. Know that lumateperone should be discontinued if patient's absolute neutrophil count falls to less than 1,000/mm^3 or patient develops serious hematological adverse reactions.

! **WARNING** Montior patient for seizure activity. Institute seizure precautions, as needed.

! **WARNING** Monitor patient for changes in behavior or thinking suggestive of suicidal ideation. Notify prescriber immediately, if present, and institute suicide precautions.

! **WARNING** Monitor patient for signs and symptoms of neuroleptic malignant syndrome (autonomic instability, delirium, hyperpyrexia, muscle rigidity) and report any such effects to prescriber immediately. Expect lumateperone to be discontinued and appropriate intensive treatment instituted, as prescribed.

- Notify prescriber if patient develops tardive dyskinesia, as it may become irreversible and increases with duration of treatment and cumulative dose. Be aware that tardive dyskinesia can develop after only a relatively brief treatment period, even at low doses, and it may occur after drug has been discontinued.
- Monitor patient's blood glucose and lipid levels as well as weight because drug may cause metabolic changes, such as hyperglycemia, dyslipidemia, and weight gain.
- Assess patient for orthostatic hypotension, especially elderly patients; patients with concomitant treatment with antihypertensive drugs, dehydration, or hypovolemia; patients with known cardiovascular disease; and patients with cerebrovascular disease.
- Institute fall precautions because lumateperone may cause motor and sensory instability, postural hypotension, and somnolence, which may lead to falls.

PATIENT TEACHING

- Instruct patient how to administer lumateperone.

! **WARNING** Review signs and symptoms of infection with patient and stress importance of reporting a suspected infection to prescriber.

! **WARNING** Tell family or caregiver to monitor patient for suicidal thoughts and behaviors, especially during the initial few months of drug therapy and with dosage changes. If present, prescriber should be alerted.

! **WARNING** Alert patient that lumaterperone may cause seizure activity. If a seizure occurs, tell patient to notify prescriber, stop taking drug, and seek immediate medical care.

! **WARNING** Review signs and symptoms of neuroleptic malignant syndrome with patient and family. Urge patient to seek emergency care, if present.

- Encourage patient to inform all prescribers of lumateperone therapy and any other drugs taken, including over-the-counter and herbal products.
- Instruct patient to rise from a lying or sitting position slowly, especially early in drug therapy and when drug is being reinitiated, to avoid a drop in blood pressure. Inform patient that hot tubs, prolonged hot showers, and saunas may worsen this effect.
- Encourage patient to monitor weight and report excessive weight gain. Also, inform patient that drug may increase blood glucose and lipid levels. Review signs and symptoms of hyperglycemia with patient and stress importance of complying with laboratory testing for these metabolic alterations.
- Review signs and symptoms of tardive dyskinesia and tell patient to report these abnormal movements, if present.
- Caution patient to avoid hazardous activities until drug's CNS effects are known and resolved.
- Advise females of childbearing age to notify prescriber if pregnancy occurs. Also, alert mothers that breastfeeding is not recommended during lumateperone therapy.
- Inform patient that drug may impair fertility.

lurasidone hydrochloride

Latuda

Class and Category

Pharmacologic class: Atypical antipsychotic
Therapeutic class: Antipsychotic

Indications and Dosages

✳ *To treat schizophrenia*

TABLETS

Adults. *Initial:* 40 mg once daily, increased, as needed. *Maximum:* 160 mg once daily.
Adolescents ages 13 to 17. *Initial:* 40 mg once daily, increased, as needed. *Maximum:* 80 mg daily.

✳ *To treat depressive episodes associated with bipolar I disorder as monotherapy or adjunctive therapy with either lithium or valproate*

TABLETS

Adults. *Initial:* 20 mg once daily, increased, as needed. *Maximum:* 120 mg once daily.

✳ *To treat depressive episodes associated with bipolar I disorder as monotherapy*

TABLETS

Children ages 10 to 17. *Initial:* 20 mg once daily, increased weekly, as needed. *Usual:* 20 to 40 mg once daily. *Maximum:* 80 mg daily.

Drug Administration

P.O.

- Administer drug with a meal consisting of at least 350 calories.

Route	Onset	Peak	Duration
P.O.	Unknown	1–3 hr	Unknown

Half-life: 18 hr

Mechanism of Action

Mediated possibly through a combination of central dopamine type 2 and serotonin type 2 receptor antagonism to suppress psychotic symptoms and elevate mood.

Contraindications

Concurrent therapy with strong CYP3A4 inducers, such as avasimibe, carbamazepine, phenytoin, rifampin, or St. John's wort; concurrent therapy with strong CYP3A4 inhibitors, such as clarithromycin, ketoconazole, mibefradil, ritonavir, or voriconazole; hypersensitivity to lurasidone or its components

Interactions

DRUGS

CYP3A4 inducers: Possibly decreased effect of lurasidone
CYP3A4 inhibitors: Possibly increased effect of lurasidone

Adverse Reactions

CNS: Agitation, akathisia, anxiety, **CVA**, dizziness, dystonia, extrapyramidal symptoms, fatigue, hypomania or mania activation, impaired cognitive and motor function, insomnia, **neuroleptic malignant syndrome**, parkinsonism, psychomotor hyperactivity, restlessness, **seizures**, somnolence, **suicidal ideation**, syncope, tardive dyskinesia, transient ischemic attacks

CV: Hypertension, orthostatic hypotension, tachycardia
EENT: Blurred vision, dry mouth, increased salivation, oropharyngeal pain, rhinitis, **throat swelling**, **tongue swelling**
ENDO: Hyperglycemia, hyperprolactinemia
GI: Abdominal pain, anorexia, diarrhea, dyspepsia, dysphagia, nausea, vomiting
GU: Elevated creatinine level
HEME: **Agranulocytosis**, **leukopenia**, **neutropenia**
MS: Back pain, **rhabdomyolysis**
RESP: Dyspnea
SKIN: Pruritus, rash, urticaria
Other: Elevated CPK level, **hyponatremia**, weight gain

Childbearing Considerations

PREGNANCY

- Pregnancy exposure registry: 1-866-961-2388 or http://womensmentalhealth.org/clinical-and-research-programs/pregnancyregistry/.
- Drug may cause fetal harm. Neonates exposed to the drug in the third trimester of pregnancy are at risk for extrapyramidal and/or withdrawal symptoms following delivery.
- Use with caution only if benefit to mother outweighs potential risk to fetus.

LACTATION

- It is not known if drug is present in breast milk.
- Mothers should check with prescriber before breastfeeding.

Nursing Considerations

! **WARNING** Be aware that lurasidone should not be used to treat dementia-related psychosis in the elderly because of an increased risk of death, nor in patients at risk for aspiration pneumonia because drug may cause esophageal dysmotility, resulting in dysphagia.

! **WARNING** Use lurasidone cautiously in patients with cardiovascular disease, cerebrovascular disease, or conditions that would predispose them to hypotension. Also, use cautiously in elderly patients because of increased risk of serious cerebrovascular effects, such as stroke or transient ischemic attack.

! **WARNING** Use lurasidone cautiously in patients with a history of seizures or with conditions that lower the seizure threshold, such as Alzheimer's disease.

! **WARNING** Monitor patient for a hypersensitivity reaction, such a pruritus, rash, and urticaria. If present, notify prescriber, expect drug to be discontinued, and provide supportive care, as needed and ordered.

! **WARNING** Monitor patient's CBC, as ordered, because serious adverse hematologic reactions may occur, such as agranulocytosis, leukopenia, and neutropenia. Assess more often during first few months of therapy if patient has a history of drug-induced leukopenia or neutropenia or a significantly low WBC count. If abnormalities occur during therapy, watch for fever or other signs of infection, notify prescriber, and, if severe, expect drug to be discontinued.

! **WARNING** Watch patients closely for suicidal tendencies, especially in children and young adults, and particularly when therapy starts and dosage changes because depression may worsen temporarily during these times.

! **WARNING** Monitor patient closely for neuroleptic malignant syndrome throughout therapy. Notify prescriber immediately of any occurrence.

- Monitor patient's blood glucose level routinely; risk of hyperglycemia may increase.
- Monitor patient for tardive dyskinesia during therapy. Be aware that the occurrence of tardive dyskinesia and the chances of the dyskinesia being irreversible increase the longer therapy continues, as well as with the total cumulative dose. Although less common, tardive dyskinesia may also occur after relatively short periods of therapy at low doses and may even occur after therapy has been discontinued. Monitor patient closely and notify prescriber at once if present.

- Assess patient for fall risk and institute fall precautions.

PATIENT TEACHING

- Instruct patient, family, or caregiver how to administer lurasidone.
- Instruct patient, family, or caregiver that lurasidone must be taken with a meal consisting of at least 350 calories.
- Urge patient to avoid alcohol during lurasidone therapy.

! **WARNING** Alert patient, family, or caregiver that drug may cause seizures. If a seizure occurs, advise to stop drug therapy and seek immediate medical care.

! **WARNING** Alert patient that drug may cause an allergic reaction. If present, tell patient to notify prescriber.

! **WARNING** Alert patient, family, or caregiver that drug may cause suicidal behavior or thoughts. Caution family or caregiver to monitor patient closely and notify prescriber if present. Review suicidal precautions.

! **WARNING** Review infection control measures as well as signs and symptoms of an infection and tell patient to notify prescriber if an infection occurs.

! **WARNING** Stress importance of notifying prescriber if any persistent, serious, or unusual adverse reaction occurs.

- Instruct patient to avoid hazardous activities until drug's effects are known and resolved. Warn patient that falls can also occur due to the effects of drug on the nervous system. Review fall precautions with patient.
- Caution patient to avoid dehydration, exercising strenuously, exposure to extreme heat, or taking medication with anticholinergic activity because lurasidone therapy may interfere with being able to reduce the body's core body temperature.

M

magnesium chloride
Chloromag, Mag-SR

magnesium citrate
(citrate of magnesia)

magnesium gluconate

magnesium hydroxide
(milk of magnesia)
Milk of Magnesia, Pedia-Lax, Phillips' Chewable Tablets, Phillips' Magnesia Tablets (CAN), Phillips' Milk of Magnesia, Phillips' Milk of Magnesia Concentrate

magnesium lactate
Mag-Tab SR Caplets

magnesium oxide
Mag-Ox 400, Maox, Uro-Mag

magnesium sulfate

Class and Category
Pharmacologic class: Mineral
Therapeutic class: Electrolyte replacement

Indications and Dosages
∗ *To correct magnesium deficiency caused by alcoholism, magnesium-depleting drugs, malnutrition, or restricted diet; to prevent magnesium deficiency based on recommended daily allowances according to the National Institutes of Health*

CAPSULES, CHEWABLE TABLETS, CRYSTALS, ENTERIC-COATED TABLETS, E.R. TABLETS, LIQUID, LIQUID CONCENTRATE, ORAL SOLUTION, TABLETS (MAGNESIUM CHLORIDE, CITRATE, GLUCONATE, HYDROXIDE, LACTATE [EXCEPT IN CHILDREN], OXIDE, SULFATE)

Dosage individualized based on severity of deficiency and normal recommended daily allowances listed below.
Adult male ages 31 and older. 420 mg daily.
Adult female ages 31 and older. 320 mg daily (360 mg daily during pregnancy, 320 mg daily during breastfeeding).
Adult male ages 19 to 30. 400 mg daily.
Adult female ages 19 to 30. 310 mg daily (350 mg daily during pregnancy, 310 mg daily during breastfeeding).
Adolescent boys ages 14 to 18. 410 mg daily.
Adolescent girls ages 14 to 18. 360 mg daily (400 mg daily during pregnancy, 360 mg daily during breastfeeding).
Boys and girls ages 9 to 13. 240 mg daily.
Children ages 4 to 8. 130 mg daily.
Children ages 1 to 3. 80 mg daily.
Infants ages 7 to 12 mo. 75 mg daily.
Infants age birth to 6 mo. 30 mg daily.

∗ *To provide magnesium supplementation in total parenteral nutrition (TPN)*

I.V. INFUSION (MAGNESIUM SULFATE)
Adults. *Usual:* 8 to 24 mEq daily added to the TPN solution.

∗ *To treat mild magnesium deficiency*

I.M. INJECTION (MAGNESIUM SULFATE)
Adults. 1 g every 6 hr for 4 doses.

∗ *To treat severe hypomagnesemia*

I.V. INFUSION (MAGNESIUM CHLORIDE)
Adults. 4 g diluted in 250 ml D_5W and infused at no more than 3 ml/min. Then, dosage adjusted according to patient's magnesium level. *Maximum:* 40 g daily.

I.V. INFUSION (MAGNESIUM SULFATE)
Adults. 5 g diluted in 1-liter I.V. solution and infused over 3 hr.

I.M. INJECTION (MAGNESIUM SULFATE)
Adults. 250 mg/kg in divided doses given within a period of 4 hr, as needed.

∗ *To prevent and control seizures in severe preeclampsia or eclampsia*

I.M. INJECTION, I.V. INFUSION OR INJECTION (MAGNESIUM SULFATE)

Adults. *Loading:* 4 g in 5% Dextrose Injection infused generally at a rate not to exceed 150 mg/min or 3.75 ml of a 4% concentration (or its equivalent)/min. Simultaneously, 4 to 5 g I.M. into each buttock using undiluted 50% Magnesium Sulfate Injection, USP followed by 4 to 5 g injected into alternate buttocks every 4 hr, as needed. *Alternatively:* After initial I.V. loading dose, 1 to 2 g/hr administered as a continuous I.V. infusion in place of I.M. dosage. *Maximum:* 40 g/24 hr and for no longer than 5 to 7 days.

∗ *To relieve indigestion with hyperacidity*

CHEWABLE TABLETS, LIQUID, LIQUID CONCENTRATE, ORAL SOLUTION TABLETS (MAGNESIUM HYDROXIDE)

Adults and adolescents. 400 to 1,200 mg (5 to 15 ml liquid or 2.5 to 7.5 ml liquid concentrate) up to 4 times daily with water, or 622 to 1,244 mg (tablets or chewable tablets) up to 4 times daily.

CAPSULES, TABLETS (MAGNESIUM OXIDE)

Adults and adolescents. 140 mg (capsules) 3 times daily or 4 times daily with water or milk, or 400 to 800 mg (tablets) daily.

∗ *To relieve constipation, to evacuate colon for rectal or bowel examination*

LIQUID, LIQUID CONCENTRATE (MAGNESIUM HYDROXIDE)

Adults and children ages 12 and older. 2.4 to 4.8 g (30 to 60 ml) daily as single dose at bedtime or divided doses.

Children ages 6 to 11. 1.2 to 2.4 g (15 to 30 ml)/day as a single dose or in divided doses.

Children ages 2 to 5. 0.4 to 1.2 g (5 to 15 ml) daily as single dose or divided doses.

ORAL SOLUTION (MAGNESIUM CITRATE)

Adults and children ages 12 and older. Up to 10 ounces with 8 ounces of water as a single dose or in divided doses.

Children ages 6 to 11. Up to 5 ounces with 8 ounces of water as a single dose.

CRYSTALS (MAGNESIUM SULFATE)

Adults and children ages 12 and older. 10 to 30 g daily with 8 ounces of water as single dose or divided doses. *Maximum:* 2 times daily.

Children ages 6 to 12. 5 to 10 g with 8 ounces of water as a single dose or divided doses.

±**DOSAGE ADJUSTMENT** For patients with severe renal impairment, dosage including the maximum is reduced to 20 g of magnesium sulfate/48 hr.

Drug Administration

P.O.

- Oral forms are not all interchangeable.
- Chewable tablets should be chewed thoroughly before swallowing, followed by a full glass of water.
- Avoid giving other oral drugs within 2 hr of magnesium-containing antacid.
- Before giving drug as laxative, shake oral solution, liquid, or liquid concentrate well and give with a large amount of water.
- Refrigerate magnesium citrate solution.

I.V.

- Magnesium chloride for injection contains the preservative benzyl alcohol, which may cause fatal toxic syndrome in neonates and premature infants.
- Prepare solution for administration according to manufacturer's guidelines and administer according to condition being treated (see Indication and Dosage section). Use only if solution is clear and container is undamaged.
- For I.V. injection, administer slowly generally at a rate not exceeding 150 mg/min; rapid injection may cause hypotension.
- For I.V. infusion, if drug needs to be diluted (some products such as Magnesium Sulfate in 5% Dextrose injection do not), dilute to a concentration of 20% or less prior to administration using diluents recommended by manufacturer. Infuse at a rate given under indication. Use an infusion pump for administration. Never use series connections.
- Store at room temperature.
- *Incompatibilities:* Alkali carbonates and salicylates (magnesium sulfate); alkali carbonates, arsenates, bicarbonates, phosphates, tartrates (magnesium chloride)

I.M.

- Administer as a deep I.M. injection undiluted (50%) solution in adults but dilute to a 20% or less concentration prior to such injection in children.

Route	Onset	Peak	Duration
P.O.	0.5–6 hr	Unknown	Unknown
I.V.	Immediate	Unknown	30 min
I.M.	1 hr	Unknown	3–4 hr

Half-life: Unknown

Mechanism of Action

Assists all enzymes involved in phosphate transfer reactions that use adenosine triphosphate (ATP) as magnesium is required for normal function of the ATP-dependent sodium-potassium pump in muscle membranes. May effectively treat digitalis glycoside-induced arrhythmias because correction of hypomagnesemia improves the sodium-potassium pump's ability to distribute potassium into intracellular spaces and because magnesium decreases calcium uptake and potassium outflow through myocardial cell membranes. Exerts a hyperosmotic effect in the small intestine causing water retention that distends the bowel and causes the duodenum to secrete cholecystokinin. This substance stimulates fluid secretion and intestinal motility to relieve constipation. Reacts with water to convert magnesium oxide to magnesium hydroxide, which, in turn, rapidly reacts with gastric acid to form water and magnesium chloride, which increases gastric pH to relieve hyperacidity. Depresses the CNS and blocks peripheral neuromuscular impulse transmission by decreasing available acetylcholine to abort seizure activity.

Contraindications

For all forms of magnesium: Hypersensitivity to magnesium salts or any component of magnesium-containing preparations
For magnesium chloride: Coma, marked heart disease, renal impairment
For magnesium sulfate: Heart block, MI, preeclampsia 2 hr or less before delivery (I.V. form)
For use as laxative: Acute abdominal problem (as indicated by abdominal pain, nausea, or vomiting), colostomy or ileostomy, diverticulitis, fecal impaction, intestinal obstruction or perforation, severe renal impairment, ulcerative colitis

Interactions

DRUGS

calcium channel blockers: Possibly enhanced adverse/toxic effects of magnesium salts
calcium salts (I.V.): Possibly neutralization of magnesium sulfate's effects
CNS depressants: Increased CNS depression
digoxin: Possibly heart block and conduction changes
misoprostol: Increased misoprostol-induced diarrhea
neuromuscular blockers: Possibly increased neuromuscular blockade
oral drugs: Possibly decreased absorption of oral drugs when magnesium salts given orally
sodium polystyrene sulfonate resin: Possibly metabolic alkalosis

ACTIVITIES

alcohol use: Increased urinary excretion of magnesium

FOODS

high glucose intake: Increased urinary excretion of magnesium

Adverse Reactions

CNS: Confusion, decreased reflexes, dizziness, syncope
CV: **Arrhythmias**, **hypotension**
GI: Flatulence, vomiting
MS: Muscle cramps
RESP: Dyspnea, **respiratory depression or paralysis**
SKIN: Diaphoresis
Other: **Hypermagnesemia**, **hypersensitivity reactions**, injection-site pain or irritation (I.M. form), laxative dependence, **magnesium toxicity**

M

Childbearing Considerations

PREGNANCY

- It is not known if drug causes fetal harm for some forms of magnesium.
- Magnesium sulfate may cause fetal harm if administered continuously beyond 5 to 7 days to pregnant women, causing hypocalcemia and bone abnormalities in the developing fetus.
- Use with caution only if benefit to mother outweighs potential risk to fetus.

LABOR AND DELIVERY

- Some authorities recommend magnesium chloride and magnesium sulfate not be administered within 2 hr prior to delivery because of the risk of hypermagnesemia-stimulated respiratory depression in the neonate.

- Magnesium sulfate is not approved to treat preterm labor.
- If magnesium sulfate is administered by continuous I.V. infusion, especially for more than 24 hr preceding delivery, to control seizures in a toxemic woman, monitor newborn for signs of magnesium toxicity, including neuromuscular or respiratory depression.

LACTATION

- Drug is present in breast milk.
- Mothers should check with prescriber before breastfeeding.

Nursing Considerations

- Be aware that drug isn't metabolized. Drug remaining in the GI tract produces watery stool within 30 minutes to 3 hours.

! **WARNING** Monitor patient for hypersensitivity reactions. If present, notify prescriber, expect drug to be withheld, and provide supportive care, as needed and ordered.

! **WARNING** Observe for and report early evidence of hypermagnesemia: bradycardia, depressed deep tendon reflexes, diplopia, dyspnea, flushing, hypotension, nausea, slurred speech, vomiting, and weakness.

! **WARNING** Monitor serum electrolyte levels in patients with renal insufficiency because they are at risk for magnesium toxicity.

! **WARNING** Be aware that magnesium may precipitate myasthenic crisis by decreasing patient's sensitivity to acetylcholine.

! **WARNING** Assess frequently the cardiac status of patient taking drugs that lower heart rate, such as beta-blockers because magnesium may aggravate symptoms of heart block.

- Provide adequate diet, exercise, and fluids for patient being treated for constipation.
- Be aware that magnesium salts are not intended for long-term use.

PATIENT TEACHING

- Instruct patient how to administer form of magnesium prescribed.
- Instruct patient to take magnesium-containing antacid between meals and at bedtime. Urge the patient not to take other drugs within 2 hours of the antacid.

! **WARNING** Alert patient that drug may cause an allergic reaction. If present, tell patient to notify prescriber. If severe, urge patient to seek immediate medical care.

! **WARNING** Tell patient to notify prescriber and avoid using magnesium-containing laxative if he has abdominal pain, nausea, or vomiting.

- Caution patient about risk of dependence with long-term laxative use. Teach patient to prevent constipation by increasing dietary fiber and fluid intake and exercising regularly.
- Inform patient that magnesium supplements used to replace electrolytes can cause diarrhea.

mannitol

Aridol, Bronchitol, Osmitrol

Class and Category

Pharmacologic class: Osmotic diuretic
Therapeutic class: Diuretic

Indications and Dosages

✱ *To reduce intracranial pressure and cerebral edema; to reduce intraocular pressure*

I.V. INFUSION (OSMITROL)

Adults and children. *Intracranial pressure:* 0.25 g/kg infused over 30 min and repeated every 6 to 8 hr, as needed. *Intraocular pressure:* 1.5 to 2 g/kg as a single dose of a 15% or 20% solution infused over at least 30 min.

✱ *As adjunct for add-on maintenance therapy to improve pulmonary function in patients with cystic fibrosis*

ORAL INHALATION (BRONCHITOL)

Adults. 400 mg (10 capsules) twice daily with second dose given 2 to 3 hr before bedtime.

✱ *To assess bronchial hyperresponsiveness in patients who do not have clinically apparent asthma*

ORAL INHALATION (ARIDOL)

Adults and children ages 6 and older. Bronchial challenge testing started with 0 mg of mannitol dosage, increased to 5 mg with second dose, 10 mg with third dose, 20 mg with fourth dose, 40 mg with fifth dose, 80 mg with sixth dose, and 160 mg for 3 remaining doses. Doses spaced equally apart. Increased doses given until patient has a positive response or 635 mg of mannitol has been administered.

Drug Administration

I.V.

- Drug is supplied in single-dose containers.
- Crystals may form, especially if solution is chilled. To dissolve, warm the bottle following manufacturer's guidelines and agitate. Cool to body temperature or less before administering. Never administer solution with undissolved crystals.
- Do not place 25% strength in polyvinylchloride bags, as a white flocculent precipitate may form.
- Use an infusion pump and administer with a filter such as a blood filter set to prevent infusion of mannitol crystals.
- To prevent air embolism, use a non-vented infusion set, avoid multiple connections, do not connect flexible containers in series, fully evacuate residual gas in the container prior to administration, do not pressurize the flexible container to increase flow rates, and, if administration is controlled by a pumping device, turn off pump before container runs dry.
- Administer through a large central vein, if possible, because severe infusion-site reactions can occur if administered through a peripheral vein.
- For reduction of intracranial or intraocular pressure, infuse over 30 min.
- If used for eye surgery, infuse 60–90 min before procedure.
- Never administer as an I.V. injection.
- *Incompatibilities:* Blood products, other drugs

ORAL INHALATION

Bronchitol

- Ensure patient has passed the Bronchitol Tolerance Test before first administration.
- Administer a short-acting bronchodilator by oral inhalation, as ordered, 5 to 15 min before each dose.
- Use only with provided inhaler.
- Each capsule contains 40 mg of drug, and each dose will require 10 capsules. Each of the 10 capsules must be inhaled individually once in the morning and once in the evening. Evening dose should be given 2 to 3 hr before bedtime.
- To use inhaler, remove cap and twist open inhaler by turning the mouthpiece.
- Take 1 capsule out of the package and put it in the chamber. (Do not put capsule into the mouthpiece.)
- Hold inhaler upright and turn the mouthpiece until it locks in place.
- Push both buttons at the same time while keeping inhaler upright. Then, release both buttons at the same time. Never keep buttons pressed.
- Hand inhaler to patient; have patient close lips around mouthpiece and take a steady deep breath and then remove inhaler. The patient should then hold breath for 5 sec before exhaling. Do not have patient inhale into inhaler.
- A rattling sound while breathing in should be heard. If it is not heard, have patient tap bottom of inhaler firmly and have patient repeat breathing administration again.
- Afterward, open inhaler, remove empty capsule and throw capsule away. If capsule is not empty, have patient repeat breathing administration again.
- Repeat procedure 9 more times for each dose.
- Inhaler should be discarded and replaced after 7 days of use.
- If inhaler has to be washed, the inhaler should be thoroughly air-dried before the next use.

Aridol

- Use the Aridol Bronchial Challenge Test Kit, when administering test.
- A nose clip may be used, if needed. Once clip is in place, patient should breathe through the mouth.
- To start test, insert 0-mg capsule into inhalation device. Puncture capsule by depressing buttons on side of device slowly, and only once.
- Have patient exhale completely, before inhaling from device in a controlled deep inspiration. At the end of the deep inspiration, start 60-sec timer, have patient hold breath for 5 sec, and exhale through mouth before removal of nose clip.
- After 60 sec, measure the patient's FEV_1 in duplicate (measurement after inhaling the 0 mg capsule is the baseline FEV_1).

- Repeat steps following the mannitol capsule dose instruction schedule that comes with the kit until patient has a positive response (a 15% reduction in FEV_1 from 0-mg baseline or a 10% incremental reduction in FEV_1 between consecutive doses) or 635-mg dose of mannitol has been reached, which indicates a negative test.

Route	Onset	Peak	Duration
I.V.*	1–3 hr	Unknown	Up to 8 hr
I.V.†	30–60 min	Unknown	4–8 hr
I.V.‡	0.5–3 hr	30–60 min	3–8 hr
Inhalation	Unknown	1.5 hr	Unknown

Half-life: 100 min (Osmitrol); 4.7 hr (Aridol, Bronchitol)

*To produce diuresis.
†To decrease intraocular pressure.
‡To decrease intracranial pressure.

Mechanism of Action

For Aridol and Bronchitol: Induces bronchial hyperresponsiveness (Aridol) or improves pulmonary function in cystic fibrosis patients (Bronchitol) in an unknown manner.

For Osmitrol: Elevates plasma osmolality, causing water to flow from tissues, such as brain and eyes, and from CSF, into extracellular fluid, thereby decreasing intracranial and intraocular pressure. Increases the osmolarity of glomerular filtrate, which decreases water reabsorption leading to increased excretion of chloride, sodium, water, and toxic substances Minimizes the hemolytic effects of water used as an irrigant and reduces the movement of hemolyzed blood from the urethra to the systemic circulation, which prevents hemoglobinemia and serious renal complications.

Contraindications

For Aridol: Conditions that may be compromised by induced bronchospasm or repeated spirometry maneuvers such as aortic or cerebral aneurysm, CVA, recent MI, or uncontrolled hypertension; known hypersensitivity to mannitol or to the gelatin used to make capsules

For Bronchitol: Failure to pass the Bronchitol Tolerance Test, hypersensitivity to mannitol or any of the capsule components

For Osmitrol: Active intracranial bleeding (except during craniotomy), anuria, hypersensitivity to mannitol or its components, severe pulmonary vascular congestion or pulmonary edema, severe hypovolemia

Interactions

DRUGS

FOR ARIDOL AND BRONCHITOL

None reported by manufacturer.

FOR OSMITROL

digoxin, drugs that prolong the QT interval, neuromuscular blocking agents: Increased risk of electrolyte imbalances resulting in serious cardiac adverse reactions; increased risk of digitalis toxicity from hypokalemia

diuretics; nephrotoxic drugs, such as aminoglycosides, cyclosporine: Increased risk of renal failure and toxicity

lithium: Initial increased elimination of lithium followed by increased risk of lithium toxicity in patients with hypovolemia or renal impairment

neurotoxic drugs, such as aminoglycosides: Increased risk of CNS toxicity

renally eliminated drugs: Increased elimination and decreased effectiveness of these drugs

Adverse Reactions

FOR ARIDOL

CNS: Dizziness, headache
CV: Chest discomfort
EENT: Gagging, pharyngolaryngeal pain, rhinorrhea, throat irritation
GI: Nausea, vomiting
RESP: **Bronchospasm**, cough, decreased forced expiratory volume, dyspnea, **wheezing**

FOR BRONCHITOL

CNS: Fever
EENT: Oropharyngeal pain
GI: Vomiting
MS: Arthralgia
RESP: **Bronchospasm**, cough, hemoptysis

FOR OSMITROL

CNS: Asthenia, chills, **coma**, confusion, dizziness, fever, headache, lethargy, malaise, **rebound increased intracranial pressure**, **seizures**
CV: Angina-like chest pain, **cardiac arrest**, chest pain, **heart failure**, hypertension, **hypotension**, palpitations, peripheral edema,

tachycardia, thrombophlebitis, **venous thrombosis**
EENT: Blurred vision, dry mouth, rhinitis
GI: Diarrhea, nausea, vomiting
GU: **Acute kidney injury**, **anuria**, **azotemia**, hematuria, oliguria, osmotic nephrosis, polyuria, urine retention
MS: Musculoskeletal stiffness, myalgia
RESP: Cough, dyspnea, **pulmonary edema**
SKIN: Diaphoresis, pruritus, rash, urticaria
Other: **Anaphylaxis**, dehydration, extravasation (with compartment syndrome, swelling, and tissue necrosis), generalized discomfort or pain, **hyperkalemia**, **hypernatremia**, **hyperosmolarity**, hypervolemia, **hypokalemia**, **hyponatremia** (dilutional), hypovolemia, infusion-site reactions (erythema, inflammation, pain, phlebitis, pruritus, or extravasation complications of compartment syndrome, tissue necrosis), **metabolic acidosis**, thirst

Childbearing Considerations

PREGNANCY

- It is not known if drug causes fetal harm. However, use of Bronchitol may increase risk for preterm delivery.
- Use with caution only if benefit to mother outweighs potential risk to fetus.

LACTATION

- It is not known if drug is present in breast milk.
- Mothers should check with prescriber before breastfeeding.

Nursing Considerations

FOR BRONCHITOL

- Know that the Bronchitol Tolerance Test is administered before Bronchitol brand is prescribed to identify patients who are suitable candidates for Bronchitol therapy. The test must be administered by a healthcare practitioner skilled in managing acute bronchospasms. Only patients who experience bronchospasm, a decrease in FEV_1, or a decrease in oxygen saturation with administration of Bronchitol are candidates for drug use.
- Monitor patient's respiratory status to determine effectiveness of Bronchitiol.

! WARNING Monitor patient for bronchospasms during drug therapy that could become severe. If present, notify prescriber and expect to treat bronchospasms, as ordered.

- Monitor patient for hemoptysis. If present, notify prescriber and expect Bronchitol to be discontinued.

FOR ARIDOL

! WARNING Be aware that the bronchial challenge test should not be performed in any patient with clinically apparent asthma or very low baseline pulmonary function tests (less than 70% of the predicted values).

- Know that the bronchial challenge test is for diagnostic purposes only. It should only be conducted by trained professionals.

! WARNING Monitor patients with conditions that may increase sensitivity to bronchoconstriction or other potential effects of the drug.

! WARNING Monitor patient for bronchospasms that could become severe. Have emergency equipment on standby to treat severe bronchospasm that may occur during the test. Expect to administer a short-acting inhaled beta agonist to treat bronchospasm.

FOR OSMITROL

- Know that elderly patients and patients with preexisting renal disease are at greater risk for developing adverse reactions. Expect to administer a test dose of mannitol to evaluate degree of risk, if appropriate. Also, expect to evaluate all patient's cardiac, pulmonary, and renal status and correct any preexisting fluid and electrolyte imbalances before therapy begins, as ordered.

! WARNING Be aware that depending on dosage and duration of mannitol administration, acid–base and electrolyte imbalances may occur, which can be severe and potentially fatal. Monitor central venous pressure, fluid intake and output, and vital signs every hour during I.V. infusion of mannitol. Measure urine output with indwelling urinary catheter, as appropriate. Notify prescriber if renal function worsens and expect mannitol to be discontinued.

! **WARNING** Monitor patient for hypersensitivity reactions, which could become life-threatening, such as anaphylaxis, breathing difficulties, and hypotension; cardiac arrest and death have occurred. If hypersensitivity reactions are present, stop infusion immediately, notify prescriber, and expect to provide supportive emergency care.

! **WARNING** Monitor patient, especially patient with impaired renal function, for CNS toxicity, such as coma, confusion, or lethargy. This may occur as a result of high serum mannitol concentrations or disturbances of electrolyte and acid–base balance caused by mannitol administration. Patients with preexisting compromise of the blood–brain barrier are at increased risk for increasing cerebral edema with mannitol use. Monitor patient closely for a rebound increase in intracranial pressure for at least several hours after mannitol has been discontinued. Know that use of neurotoxic drugs or other diuretics should be avoided, if possible, during mannitol administration.

- Check weight and monitor BUN and serum creatinine electrolyte levels daily, as ordered.
- Expect to monitor patient's cardiac, pulmonary, and renal function as well as signs and symptoms of hyper- or hypovolemia for patient receiving mannitol therapy for reduction in intracranial pressure. Also, expect to monitor this patient's acid–base balance, intracranial pressure, osmol gap, and serum electrolytes and osmolarity.
- Provide frequent mouth care to relieve dry mouth and thirst.
- Know that high concentrations of mannitol may produce false low results for inorganic phosphorus blood concentrations. Mannitol therapy may also produce false positive results in tests for blood ethylene glycol concentrations.

PATIENT TEACHING

FOR BRONCHITOL

- Tell patient that a test must be administered to see if he will benefit from Bronchitol therapy before drug is prescribed.
- Instruct patient how to administer Bronchitol if test indicates drug can be given therapeutically and how to clean inhaler.
- Instruct patient to take each dose, once in the morning and once in the evening. For the evening dose, tell patient to take it at least 2 to 3 hours before bedtime.
- Tell patient to notify prescriber if he sees blood in his sputum, as drug will have to be discontinued.

FOR ARIDOL

- Review how test is to be done with patient beforehand.
- Reassure patient she will not be left alone during the test.
- Inform patient that if test is positive or patient develops significant respiratory symptoms, a short-acting inhaled beta agonist will be given to the patient to relieve symptoms.

FOR OSMITROL

- Inform patient that Osmitrol will be administered by an intravenous infusion.

! **WARNING** Alert patient that Osmitrol may cause an allergic reaction and to notify staff immediately if patient experiences any unusual adverse effects.

! **WARNING** Instruct patient to also report chest pain, difficulty breathing, or pain at I.V. site, along with any other new, persistent, or severe adverse reactions.

- Inform patient that he may experience dry mouth and thirst during mannitol therapy and to request frequent mouth care.

maraviroc

Selzentry

Class and Category

Pharmacologic class: CCR5 co-receptor antagonist

Therapeutic class: Antiretroviral

Indications and Dosages

* *As adjunct to treat CCR5-tropic human immunodeficiency virus type 1 (HIV-1) infection combined with potent CYP3A inhibitors (with or without a potent CYP3A inducer)*

ORAL SOLUTION, TABLETS

Adults and children ages 2 and older weighing 40 kg (88 lb) or more. 150 mg twice daily.

Children ages 2 and older weighing at least 30 kg (66 lb) to less than 40 kg (88 lb). 100 mg twice daily.
Children ages 2 and older weighing at least 20 kg (44 lb) to less than 30 kg (66 lb). 75 mg (tablet) or 80 mg (oral solution) twice daily.
Children ages 2 and older weighing at least 10 kg (22 lb) to less than 20 kg (44 lb). 50 mg (oral solution) twice daily.

* *To treat CCR5-tropic HIV-1 infection combined with potent CYP3A inducers (without a potent CYP3A inhibitor)*

ORAL SOLUTION, TABLETS

Adults. 600 mg twice daily.

* *To treat CCR5-tropic HIV-1 infection in combination with drugs that are not potent CYP3A inducers or inhibitors*

ORAL SOLUTION, TABLETS

Adults and children ages 2 and older weighing at least 30 kg (66 lb). 300 mg twice daily.
Children ages 2 and older weighing 14 kg (30.8 lb) to 30 kg (66 lb). 200 mg twice daily.
Children ages 2 and older weighing 10 kg (22 lb) to 14 kg (30.8 lb). 150 mg twice daily.

ORAL SOLUTION

Infants and children ages 2 and older weighing 6 kg (13.2 lb) to less than 10 kg (22 lb). 100 mg twice daily.
Neonates, infants, and children weighing 4 kg (8.8 lb) to less than 6 kg (13.2 lb). 40 mg twice daily.
Neonates and infants weighing 2 kg (4.4 lb) to less than 4 kg (8.8 lb). 30 mg twice daily.

±**DOSAGE ADJUSTMENT** For adult patients with end stage renal disease on hemodialysis who are receiving noninteracting concomitant drugs and experience postural hypotension, dose reduced to 150 mg twice a day.

Drug Administration

P.O.

- Tablets should be swallowed whole and not crushed.
- Oral solution is available for patient who is unable to swallow tablets or for children weighing at least 2 kg (4.4 lb) but less than 10 kg (22 lb). Measure dosage using dosing syringe that is supplied with drug.
- Open bottle by pushing down firmly on the child-resistant cap and turning counter-clockwise. Do not throw the cap away.
- When using for the first time, remove the press-in bottle adapter and oral syringe from the plastic overwrap. With the bottle on a flat surface, push the ribbed end of the press-in bottle adapter all the way into the neck of the bottle while holding the bottle firmly. Do not remove the press-in bottle adapter from the bottle after it is inserted.
- Choose the oral syringe needed and find the prescribed dose on the oral syringe. Use a 3 ml oral syringe for doses of 2.5 ml or less; a 10 ml oral syringe for doses more than 2.5 ml. Remove air from the oral syringe by pushing plunger to the bottom of the barrel of the syringe to remove excess air.
- Insert oral syringe into the upright bottle through the opening of the press-in bottle adapter until it is firmly in place.
- With oral syringe in place, turn bottle upside down, pull back on the plunger until the top of the plunger is even with the markings on the oral syringe for the prescribed dose. If bubbles are present, fully push the plunger in to empty the oral solution back into the bottle and withdraw dose again. Remove oral syringe by turning bottle upright and place bottle on a flat surface and then remove oral syringe by pulling straight up on the barrel of the oral syringe.
- To administer, place the tip of the oral syringe against the inside of the patient's cheek. Slowly push the plunger all the way down. Make sure patient has time to swallow the drug.
- If prescribed dose is more than 10 ml, the dose will need to be divided.
- Once dose is given close the bottle tightly by turning the child-resistant cap clockwise, leaving the press-in bottle adapter in place.
- Discard oral solution 60 days after first opening the bottle.

Route	Onset	Peak	Duration
P.O.	Unknown	0.5–4 hr	Unknown

Half-life: 14–18 hr

Mechanism of Action

Binds to the human chemokine receptor CCR5 present on the cell membrane selectively, preventing an interaction that would allow CCR5-tropic HIV-1 to enter the cell and replicating.

Contraindications

End-stage renal disease or severe renal impairment in patients receiving potent CYP3A inducers or inhibitors, hypersensitivity to maraviroc or its components

Interactions

DRUGS

CYP3A and P-gp inducers: Decreased effectiveness of maraviroc
CYP3A and P-gp inhibitors: Increased plasma concentration of maraviroc with increased risk of adverse reactions
multidrug resistance-associated protein (MRP)2 and organic anion transporting polypeptide (OATP)1B1 inducers: Possibly decreased effectiveness of maraviroc
multidrug resistance-associated protein (MRP)2 and organic anion transporting polypeptide (OATP)1B1 inhibitors: Possibly increased plasma concentration of maraviroc with increased risk of adverse reactions
St. John's wort: Decreased plasma concentration of maraviroc with substantially decreased effectiveness; increased risk of development of resistance to maraviroc

Adverse Reactions

CNS: Anxiety, changes in levels of consciousness, including loss of consciousness, **CVA**, depression, dizziness, dysesthesias, facial palsy, fever, malaise, memory loss excluding dementia, paresthesia, peripheral neuropathies, **seizures**, sensory abnormalities, sleep disturbances, syncope, tremor
CV: **Acute heart failure**, coronary artery disease, **coronary artery occlusion**, **endocarditis**, hypertension, **MI**, myocardial ischemia, orthostatic hypotension, **unstable angina**
EENT: Conjunctivitis, ear disorders, hemianopia, nasal or ocular infections or inflammations, oral lesions, paranasal sinus disorders, visual field defects
GI: Abdominal distention, appetite disorders, bilirubin increase, bloating, cholestatic jaundice, constipation, elevated pancreatic and liver enzymes, flatulence, gastrointestinal atonic and hypomotility disorders, **hepatic cirrhosis or failure**, **hepatitis**, **hepatotoxicity**, jaundice, **portal vein thrombosis**
GU: Ejaculation and erection disorders, urinary tract signs and symptoms
HEME: Anemias, eosinophilia, **hypoplastic anemia**, **marrow depression**, **neutropenia**
MS: Elevated creatine kinase, joint or muscle aches or pains, myositis, osteonecrosis, **rhabdomyolysis**
RESP: **Breathing difficulties**, cough, respiratory infections
SKIN: Acne, alopecia, apocrine and eccrine gland disorders, benign skin neoplasms, blisters, erythemas, lipodystrophies, nail and nail bed disorders, pruritus, rash (could be severe), **Stevens-Johnson syndrome**, **toxic epidermal necrolysis**
Other: **Angioedema**; **drug reaction with eosinophilia and systemic symptoms (DRESS)**; elevated IgE; generalized discomfort or pain; **immune reconstitution syndrome**; infections such as bacterial, herpes, *Neisseria*, respiratory, tinea, and viral

Childbearing Considerations

- Pregnancy exposure registry: 1-800-258-4263.
- It is not known if drug causes fetal harm.
- Use with caution only if benefit to mother outweighs potential risk to fetus.

LACTATION

- It is not known if drug is present in breast milk.
- The Centers for Disease Control and Prevention recommends that HIV-1 infected mothers not breastfeed to avoid risking postnatal transmission of HIV-1 infection to infants. They also do not recommend breastfeeding because of potential drug-induced adverse reactions in the infant.

Nursing Considerations

- Know that maraviroc is not recommended in patients with dual/mixed- or CXCR4-tropic HIV-1 infections.
- Be sure patient has been checked for CCR5 tropism before treatment with maraviroc is started because it is only effective against this type of infection.

! WARNING Check patient's bilirubin and liver enzyme levels before maraviroc treatment is started and periodically throughout treatment, as ordered, because drug increases risk of hepatotoxicity. Know that patients with a history of liver dysfunction or patients with co-infection with hepatitis B and/or C virus may require additional monitoring. Severe rash or evidence of systemic allergic reactions (including DRESS, eosinophilia, elevated IgE, and other systemic symptoms) has occurred with hepatotoxicity about 1 month after maraviroc therapy was started in some patients. Know that cases of hepatitis have occurred in some patients in the absence of allergic manifestations or who have had no history of hepatic disease.

! **WARNING** Monitor patient closely for a hypersensitivity reaction, including severe skin reactions. Notify prescriber and expect maraviroc to be discontinued immediately if patient develops a hypersensitivity reaction or a rash that is accompanied by blisters, conjunctivitis, eosinophilia, facial edema, fever, joint or muscle aches, lip swelling, malaise, or oral lesions. Know that DRESS may only initially present with a fever or swollen lymph nodes. Be aware that a delay in discontinuing the drug may result in a life-threatening situation. Provide supportive care, as needed and ordered.

! **WARNING** Monitor patient's cardiovascular status throughout maraviroc therapy because, although uncommon, major events such as acute heart failure, endocarditis, hypertension, ischemia, MI, and unstable angina have been reported with maraviroc therapy. Pay close attention to the patient's blood pressure if renal impairment is present because of risk of orthostatic hypotension. Patients with severe renal impairment or end-stage renal disease experiencing orthostatic hypotension should be evaluated for a dosage reduction.

! **WARNING** Be aware that immune reconstitution syndrome has occurred in patients treated with combination antiretroviral therapy, including maraviroc. The inflammatory response predisposes susceptible patients to opportunistic infections such as cytomegalovirus, *Mycobacterium avium* infection, *Pneumocystis jiroveci* pneumonia, or tuberculosis. Autoimmune disorders such as Graves' disease, Guillain-Barré syndrome, or polymyositis have also occurred. Report sudden or unusual adverse reactions to prescriber.

! **WARNING** Know that maraviroc may put patient at increased risk for malignant tumors because of its effect on the immune system.

- Assess patient frequently for signs and symptoms of infection because maraviroc affects some immune cells, placing patient at increased risk.

PATIENT TEACHING

- Instruct patient, family, or caregiver how to administer the form of maraviroc prescribed and what to do if a dose is missed.
- Advise patient to avoid missing doses of maraviroc, as it can result in the development of resistance to drug.

! **WARNING** Inform patient to seek immediate medical attention if signs and symptoms of liver dysfunction or an allergic or skin reaction occurs.

! **WARNING** Advise patients with a history of cardiovascular disease or postural hypotension to notify prescriber if signs and symptoms develop or increase because of an increased risk for cardiovascular events.

- Tell patient to avoid hazardous activities, such as driving, until drug's CNS effects are known and resolved. Urge her to take safety precautions to prevent falling if she has adverse reactions, such as dizziness.
- Instruct patient to alert all prescribers of maraviroc therapy and not to take any over-the-counter medication, including herbal products, without the consent of the prescriber. Inform her that St. John's wort should not be taken while on maraviroc therapy.
- Inform mothers that breastfeeding is not recommended during maraviroc therapy.

memantine hydrochloride

Namenda, Namenda XR

Class and Category

Pharmacologic class: N-methyl-D-aspartate (NMDA) receptor antagonist
Therapeutic class: Antidementia agent

Indications and Dosages

* *To treat moderate to severe dementia of the Alzheimer's type*

ORAL SOLUTION, TABLETS

Adults. *Initial:* 5 mg daily, increased by 5 mg/wk, as needed, to 10 mg daily in 2 divided 5-mg doses; then 15 mg daily with one 5-mg and one 10-mg dose daily; then 20 mg daily in 2 divided 10-mg doses. *Maintenance:* 5 mg once a day up to 10 mg twice a day. *Maximum:* 10 mg twice daily.

E.R. CAPSULES

Adults. *Initial:* 7 mg once daily, increased by 7 mg/wk, as needed, up to 28 mg once daily. *Maximum:* 28 mg once daily.

±**DOSAGE ADJUSTMENT** For patients with severe renal impairment, maintenance dosage reduced to 5 mg twice daily for oral solution and tablet form and 14 mg once daily for E.R. capsules.

Drug Administration

P.O.

- Tablets and capsules should be swallowed whole and not chewed or crushed. However, if patient has difficulty swallowing capsules, open capsule, sprinkle contents on applesauce, and immediately have patient consume entire amount of applesauce.
- For oral solution, use the calibrated device that comes with drug to measure dosage. Once measured, squirt into the corner of patient's mouth. Store at room temperature.
- If a single dose is missed, omit it. If several days of drug therapy are missed, patient will need to begin titration of drug dosage again.

Route	Onset	Peak	Duration
P.O.	Unknown	3–7 hr	Unknown
P.O./E.R.	Unknown	9–12 hr	Unknown

Half-life: 15–24 hr

Contraindications

Hypersensitivity to memantine, amantadine, or their components

Interactions

DRUGS

amantadine, dextromethorphan, ketamine: Possibly additive effects
carbonic anhydrase inhibitors, sodium bicarbonate: Decreased memantine clearance, leading to increased blood drug levels and risk of adverse effects

Adverse Reactions

CNS: Abnormal gait, agitation, akathisia, anxiety, confusion, CVA, delirium, delusions, depression, dizziness, drowsiness, dyskinesia, fatigue, hallucinations, headache, hyperexcitability, insomnia, **neuroleptic malignant syndrome**, psychosis, restlessness, **seizures**, somnolence, **suicidal ideation**, tardive dyskinesia
CV: **AV block**, chest pain, **congestive heart failure**, hypertension, peripheral edema, **prolonged QT interval**, **supraventricular tachycardia**, tachycardia
ENDO: **Hypoglycemia**
GI: **Acute pancreatitis**, anorexia, colitis, constipation, diarrhea, **hepatic failure**, **hepatitis**, ileus, nausea, **pancreatitis**, vomiting
GU: **Acute renal failure**, elevated creatinine levels, impotence, **renal insufficiency**, urinary incontinence, UTI
HEME: **Agranulocytosis**, **leukopenia**, **neutropenia**, **pancytopenia**, **thrombocytopenia**, **thrombotic thrombocytopenic purpura**
MS: Arthralgia, back pain
RESP: Bronchitis, cough, dyspnea, upper respiratory tract infection
SKIN: **Stevens-Johnson syndrome**
Other: Generalized pain, flu-like symptoms

Childbearing Considerations

PREGNANCY

- It is not known if drug causes fetal harm.
- Use with caution only if benefit to mother outweighs potential risk to fetus.

LACTATION

- It is not known if drug is present in breast milk.
- Mothers should check with prescriber before breastfeeding.

Nursing Considerations

- Use memantine cautiously in patients with renal tubular acidosis or severe UTI because these conditions make urine alkaline, reducing memantine excretion and increasing the risk of adverse reactions.

! WARNING Monitor patients with severe hepatic impairment closely because drug undergoes partial hepatic metabolism, which may increase risk of adverse reactions.

! WARNING Monitor patient closely for suicidal behavior or thoughts. If present, notify prescriber and institute suicidal precautions.

! WARNING Monitor patient for seizure activity. Institute seizure precautions, as needed. Notify prescriber if a seizure occurs.

! WARNING Monitor patient for neuroleptic malignant syndrome, which is the most severe form of serotonin syndrome. Be aware that in addition to signs and symptoms of serotonin syndrome (agitation, chills, confusion, diaphoresis, diarrhea, fever, hyperactive reflexes, poor coordination, restlessness, shaking, talking or acting with uncontrolled excitement, tremor, and twitching), neuroleptic malignant syndrome includes autonomic instability with possible changes in vital signs, a high fever, muscle rigidity, and mental status changes.

! WARNING Monitor patient for persistent, serious, or unusual adverse reactions because drug can adversely affect many body systems.

- Monitor patient's response to memantine.

Mechanism of Action

Blocks the excitatory amino acid glutamate on N-methyl-D-aspartate (NMDA) receptor cells in the CNS, which is important in Alzheimer's disease because glutamate levels are abnormally high when brain cells are both active and at rest. Remember that normally, when certain brain cells are resting, magnesium ions block NMDA receptors and prevent influx of calcium and sodium ions and outflow of potassium ions. When learning and memory cells in the brain are active, glutamate engages with NMDA receptors, magnesium ions are removed from NMDA receptors, and cells are depolarized. During depolarization, calcium and sodium ions enter brain cells, and potassium ions leave. Circulating glutamate found in excess in Alzheimer's disease permanently removes magnesium ions and opens ion channels. Increased influx of calcium may damage brain cells and play a major role in Alzheimer's disease with the dying brain cells releasing additional glutamate to worsen the cycle of brain cell destruction. Acting on NMDA receptors of brain cells, drug replaces magnesium, closes ion channels and prevents calcium influx, thereby preventing excessive brain cell death that slows progression of Alzheimer's disease.

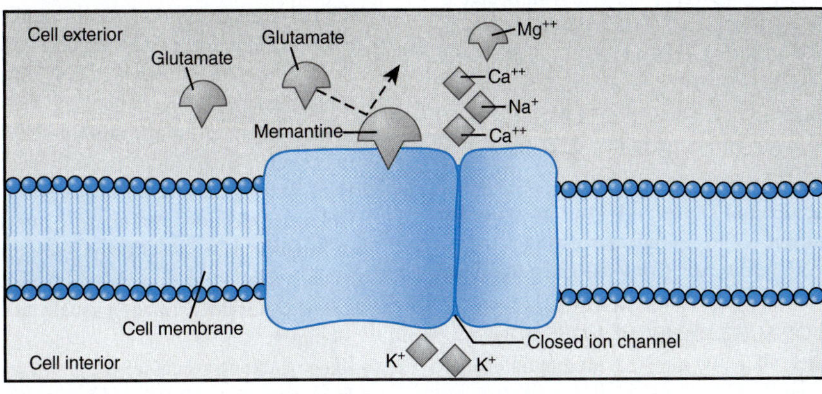

M

PATIENT TEACHING

- Instruct patient how to exactly administer form of memantine prescribed and what to do if a dose is missed. Inform the patient to notify the prescriber if he fails to take drug for several days, as dosage adjustments will be necessary.
- Advise patient to avoid a diet excessively high in fruits and vegetables because these foods contribute to alkaline urine, which can alter memantine clearance and increase adverse reactions.

! **WARNING** Alert family or caregiver that memantine has the potential to cause suicidal thoughts. If present, prescriber should be notified immediately.

! **WARNING** Tell patient to notify prescriber if persistent, serious, or unusual adverse reactions occurs, including seizures.

- Caution patient to avoid hazardous activities until drug's CNS effects are known and resolved.

meperidine hydrochloride (pethidine hydrochloride)

Demerol

Class, Category, and Schedule

Pharmacologic class: Opioid
Therapeutic class: Opioid analgesic
Controlled substance schedule: II

Indications and Dosages

✱ *To relieve pain severe enough to require opioid treatment and for which alternative treatment options such as nonopioid analgesics or opioid combination products are inadequate or not tolerated*

ORAL SOLUTION, TABLETS, I.M. OR SUBCUTANEOUS INJECTION

Adults. 50 to 150 mg every 3 to 4 hr, as needed.
Children. 1.1 to 1.8 mg/kg every 3 to 4 hr, as needed. *Maximum:* Not to exceed adult dose.

✱ *To provide preoperative sedation*

I.M. OR SUBCUTANEOUS INJECTION

Adults. 50 to 100 mg 30 to 90 min before surgery.
Children. 1.1 to 2.2 mg/kg 30 to 90 min before surgery. *Maximum:* Not to exceed adult dose.

✱ *As adjunct to anesthesia*

I.V. INFUSION OR INJECTION

Adults. Individualized. Repeated slow injections of fractional doses such as 10-mg/ml solution or continuous infusion of dilute solution (1 mg/ml) titrated, as needed.

✱ *To provide obstetric analgesia*

I.M. OR SUBCUTANEOUS INJECTION

Adults. 50 to 100 mg given with regular, painful contractions; repeated every 1 to 3 hr.

± **DOSAGE ADJUSTMENT** For elderly patients, total daily dosage decreased. For patients receiving phenothiazines, or tranquilizers concurrently, dosage proportionately reduced by 25% to 50%. For patients with hepatic or renal impairment and receiving drug intravenously, dosage titrated slowly.

Drug Administration

P.O.

- Dosing errors related to confusion between milligrams (mg) and milliliters (ml), and different concentrations of oral solutions can result in accidental overdose and death. Check dosage and concentration of oral solution carefully before administering.
- Dilute oral solution in half a glass of water because undiluted solution may exert a slight topical anesthetic effect on mucous membranes.
- Use calibrated device when measuring dosage of oral solution.

I.V.

- Patient should be lying down during I.V. administration.
- Inspect for particulate matter and discoloration prior to administration. Do not use if color is darker than pale yellow or discolored in any other way, or contains preciptiate.
- For I.V. injection, administer diluted and inject very slowly.
- For I.V. infusion, mix with 0.9% Sodium Chloride Injection, 5% Dextrose Injection, or Ringer's or Lactated Ringer's solution to a concentration of 1 mg/ml. Administer as a slow continuous infusion usually at 15 to 35 mg/hr.
- Keep naloxone available.
- *Incompatibilities:* None listed by manufacturer

I.M.

- Inject into a large muscle mass.

SUBCUTANEOUS

- Subcutaneous injection is painful and isn't recommended unless no other route can be used.

Route	Onset	Peak	Duration
P.O.	15 min	1–1.5 hr	2–4 hr
I.V.	1 min	5–7 min	2–4 hr
I.M., SubQ	10–15 min	30–50 min	2–4 hr

Half-life: 2.5–4 hr

Mechanism of Action

Binds with opiate receptors in the spinal cord and higher levels of the CNS thereby stimulating kappa and mu receptors, which alters the perception of and emotional response to pain.

Contraindications

Acute or severe bronchial asthma in an unmonitored setting or in the absence of resuscitative equipment; hypersensitivity to meperidine or its components; known or suspected GI obstruction, including paralytic ileus; significant respiratory depression; use within 14 days of MAO inhibitor therapy

Interactions

DRUGS

5-HT$_3$ receptor antagonists, drugs that affect the serotonin neurotransmitter system (mirtazapine, tramadol, trazodone), MAO inhibitors including I.V. methylene blue and linezolid, selected muscle relaxants (cyclobenzaprine, metaxalone), selective serotonin reuptake inhibitors (SSRIs), serotonin and norepinephrine reuptake inhibitors (SNRIs), tricyclic antidepressants, triptans: Increased risk of serotonin syndrome

acyclovir: Possibly increased blood meperidine level

anticholinergics: Increased risk of severe constipation, which may lead to paralytic ileus; increased risk of urinary retention

benzodiazepines, CNS depressants, muscle relaxants, other opioids, sedating antihistamines, tricyclic antidepressants: Increased risk of significant respiratory depression and other life-threatening adverse effects

cimetidine: Reduced clearance and volume of distribution of meperidine

CYP3A4 inducers, such as carbamazepine, phenytoin, rifampin: Increased clearance of meperidine with decreased effectiveness

CYP3A4 inhibitors, such as azole-antifungals, macrolide antibiotics, protease inhibitors: Decreased clearance of meperidine resulting in increased or prolonged opioid effects

diuretics: Reduced effectiveness of diuretics

mixed agonist/antagonist and partial agonist opioid analgesics, such as buprenorphine, butorphanol, nalbuphine, pentazocine: Decreased analgesic effect of meperidine; possibly precipitation of withdrawal symptoms

MAO inhibitors: Increased risk of coma, hypotension, or severe respiratory depression

muscle relaxants: Possibly enhanced neuromuscular blocking action of skeletal muscle relaxants; increased degree of respiratory depression

ACTIVITIES

alcohol use: Possibly increased CNS and respiratory depression and hypotension

Adverse Reactions

CNS: Agitation, confusion, delirium, depression, dizziness, drowsiness, headache, **increased intracranial pressure**, lack of coordination, malaise, mood changes, nervousness, nightmares, restlessness, **seizures**, syncope, transient hallucinations or disorientation, tremor, weakness

CV: **Hypotension**, orthostatic hypotension, tachycardia

EENT: Blurred vision, diplopia, dry mouth

ENDO: **Adrenal insufficiency**, **hypoglycemia**

GI: Abdominal cramps or pain, anorexia, constipation, ileus, nausea, vomiting

GU: Decreased libido, dysuria, erectile dysfunction, impotence, infertility, lack of menstruation, urinary frequency, urine retention

MS: Involuntary muscle movements

RESP: Dyspnea, **respiratory arrest or depression**, wheezing

SKIN: Diaphoresis, flushing, pruritus, rash, urticaria

Other: **Anaphylaxis**; injection-site pain, redness, or swelling; physical and psychological dependence; opioid-induced allodynia and hyperalgesia

Childbearing Considerations

PREGNANCY

- Drug may cause fetal harm.
- Prolonged use of drug during pregnancy can result in neonatal opioid withdrawal syndrome (NOWS), which may be life-threatening if not recognized and treated.
- Avoid prolonged use during pregnancy. Use with caution only if benefit to mother outweighs potential risk to fetus.

LABOR AND DELIVERY

- Drug is not recommended for use in pregnant women immediately before or during labor. Opioids may alter length of time of labor.
- Opioids cross the placental barrier and may produce respiratory depression and psycho-physiologic effects in the newborn. Monitor newborn closely for signs of excess sedation and respiratory depression.
- An opioid antagonist, such as naloxone, must be available at the time of delivery in the event it is needed to reverse opioid-induced respiratory depression in the neonate.

LACTATION

- Drug is present in breast milk.
- Mothers should check with prescriber before breastfeeding.
- If breastfeeding occurs, monitor infant for excess sedation and respiratory depression and for withdrawal symptoms when breastfeeding is stopped.

REPRODUCTION

- Chronic use of opioids may reduce fertility.

Nursing Considerations

! **WARNING** Be aware that use of opioids, such as meperidine, may lead to abuse, addiction, misuse, overdose, and possibly death. Because of this, a Risk Evaluation and Mitigation Strategy (REMS) is required. Monitor patient for evidence of physical dependence or abuse throughout meperidine therapy. Know that addiction can occur not only in those who abuse or misuse drug but also in patients who are appropriately prescribed the drug at recommended doses. Be aware that excessive use of meperidine may not only lead to abuse, addiction, and misuse, it can lead to overdose, and possibly death. Monitor patient's intake of drug closely.

! **WARNING** Monitor patient for a hypersensitivity reaction, which could become life-threatening, such as anaphylaxis. If present, notify prescriber, expect drug to be switched to another analgesic, and provide supportive care, as needed and ordered.

! **WARNING** Monitor patient's respiratory and cardiovascular status during treatment. Notify prescriber immediately and expect to discontinue drug if respiratory rate falls to less than 12 breaths/minute or if respiratory depth decreases because serious, life-threatening, or fatal respiratory depression may occur. Monitor patient especially during initiation or following a dose increase.

! **WARNING** Monitor patient's vital signs closely, especially after initiating or titrating dose of meperidine. Know that in addition to respiratory depression, meperidine may cause severe hypotension, especially in patients whose blood pressure is already compromised by a depleted blood volume or after concurrent administration of drugs that decrease blood pressure.

! **WARNING** Monitor cachectic, debilitated or elderly patients, especially when initiating and titrating therapy, as they are at increased risk for adverse effects, especially respiratory depression.

! **WARNING** Be aware that meperidine should only be used concomitantly with benzodiazepine and other CNS depressants therapy in patients for whom other treatment options are inadequate. If prescribed together, expect dosing and duration of meperidine to be limited. Monitor patient closely for signs and symptoms of a decrease in consciousness, including coma, profound sedation, and significant respiratory depression. Notify prescriber immediately and provide emergency supportive care, as death may occur.

! **WARNING** Monitor patient's blood glucose level, especially if diabetic, because opioids may cause hypoglycemia.

! **WARNING** Monitor patients with hepatic or renal dysfunction for signs and symptoms of CNS and respiratory depression because meperidine and/or its active metabolite may accumulate in these patients.

! **WARNING** Monitor patients closely who may be susceptible to the intracranial effects of carbon dioxide retention from respiratory depression caused by meperidine therapy, such as patients with head injuries or those who have a preexisting elevation in intracranial pressure.

! **WARNING** Be aware that concomitant use with CYP3A4 inhibitors or discontinuation of CYP3A4 inducers can result in fatal overdose of meperidine.

! **WARNING** Monitor patient for adrenal insufficiency. Although rare, it can be life-threatening. Monitor patient for anorexia, dizziness, fatigue, hypotension, nausea, vomiting, or weakness. Notify prescriber if adrenal insufficiency is suspected and expect diagnostic testing to be done. If confirmed, expect to administer corticosteroids and wean patient off meperidine, if possible.

! **WARNING** Know that many drugs may interact with opioids, such as meperidine, to cause serotonin syndrome. Monitor patient closely for signs and symptoms such as agitation, diaphoresis, diarrhea, fever, hallucinations, labile blood pressure, muscle twitching or stiffness, nausea, shakiness, shivering, tachycardia, trouble with coordination, or vomiting. Notify prescriber at once because serotonin syndrome may be life-threatening. Be prepared to discontinue drug, if possible and ordered, and provide supportive care.

! **WARNING** Know that prolonged use may increase risk of toxicity exhibited by seizures from the accumulation of the meperidine metabolite, normeperidine. Also, monitor patients with a seizure history or disorder because meperidine may cause or worsen seizures.

! **WARNING** Know that chronic maternal use of meperidine during pregnancy can result in neonatal opioid withdrawal syndrome (NOWS), which may be life-threatening if not recognized and treated appropriately. NOWS occurs when a newborn has been exposed to opioid drugs like meperidine for a prolonged period while in utero.

- Know that meperidine may cause spasm of the sphincter of Oddi and elevate serum amylase level. Monitor patients with biliary tract disease, including acute pancreatitis, for worsening symptoms.
- Monitor patient for a paradoxic increase in pain known as opioid-induced hyperalgesia or an increase in sensitivity to pain known as opioid-induced allodynia, especially when meperidine dosage increases. Do not confuse this with tolerance, which is the need for increasing doses of opioids to maintain an effect. If opioid-induced allodynia and hyperalgesia is suspected, notify prescriber and expect dosage to be decreased or opioid rotation to be prescribed.
- Monitor patient's bowel function to detect constipation and assess the need for stool softeners.
- Expect withdrawal symptoms to occur if drug is abruptly withdrawn after long-term use.

PATIENT TEACHING

- Inform patient that meperidine is a controlled substance.
- Instruct patient how to administer form of meperidine prescribed.
- Advise patient to take drug exactly, as prescribed. Advise patient not to increase dosage but to notify prescriber if meperidine becomes ineffective or pain increases when dosage increases.

! **WARNING** Warn patient that meperidine use can lead to abuse, addiction, misuse, overdose, and possibly death, even with normal dosing. Stress importance of patient not increasing dosage or frequency of administration without consulting prescriber. Encourage family or caregiver to obtain naloxone for home use; if and when it's needed, it will be readily available. Review signs and symptoms of an opioid overdose and how to administer naloxone. Stress importance of the need to call 911 if naloxone is administered.

! **WARNING** Warn patient not to consume alcohol or take sedatives or tranquilizers without prescriber knowledge, as severe respiratory depression can occur and may lead to death. Tell patient to notify all prescribers of meperidine use.

! **WARNING** Alert patient that meperidine may cause an allergic reaction. Tell patient to notify prescriber if present and to seek immediate medical care, if severe.

! **WARNING** Review signs and symptoms of hypoglycemia with all patients, including diabetics and how to treat it if it should occur. Urge patient to seek immediate medical care if hypoglycemia becomes severe.

! **WARNING** Alert patient that meperidine therapy may cause his blood pressure or respiratory rate to drop. If patient feels lightheaded, faints, or has difficulty breathing, urge patient to seek immediate medical care.

! **WARNING** Stress importance of notifying prescriber if other persistent, serious, or unusual adverse reactions occur while taking meperidine.

! **WARNING** Caution pregnant patient not to increase dosage or take drug for a prolonged period, as adverse effects can cause infant to experience life-threatening withdrawal when born.

! **WARNING** Stress importance of keeping meperidine out of the reach of children, as ingestion may lead to a fatal overdose.

! **WARNING** Tell breastfeeding mothers to monitor infant for excess sedation and respiratory depression and for withdrawal symptoms when breastfeeding is stopped.

- Instruct patient to report constipation, severe nausea, and shortness of breath.
- Advise patient to avoid hazardous activities until drug's CNS effects are known and resolved.
- Inform patient that long-term use of opioids, such as meperidine, may decrease sex hormone levels, causing decreased libido, erectile dysfunction, impotence, infertility, or lack of menstruation. Encourage patient to report any symptoms to prescriber.
- Instruct patient to notify all prescribers of opioid use.
- Inform patient who has been receiving meperidine for more than a few weeks and the drug is to be discontinued, to taper dosage off, as abrupt discontinuation could precipitate withdrawal symptoms.

meropenem

Class and Category

Pharmacologic class: Carbapenem
Therapeutic class: Antibiotic

Indications and Dosages

* *To treat complicated intra-abdominal infections caused by susceptible strains of viridans group streptococci,* Bacteroides fragilis, B. thetaiotaomicron, Escherichia coli, Klebsiella pneumoniae, Peptostreptococcus *species, or* Pseudomonas aeruginosa

I.V. INFUSION OR INJECTION

Adults and children weighing more than 50 kg (110 lb). 1 g every 8 hr.
Children ages 3 mo and older weighing less than 50 kg (110 lb). 20 mg/kg every 8 hr. *Maximum:* 1 g every 8 hr.

I.V. INFUSION

Infants with gestational ages 32 wk and older and postnatal ages 2 wk and older. 30 mg/kg every 8 hr.
Infants with gestational ages 32 wk and older but postnatal age less than 2 wk or infants with gestational age less than 32 wk but postnatal ages 2 wk or older. 20 mg/kg every 8 hr.
Infants with gestational age less than 32 wk and postnatal age less than 2 wk. 20 mg/kg every 12 hr.

* *To treat complicated skin and skin structure infections caused by* B. fragilis, Enterococcus faecalis *(excluding vancomycin-resistant isolates),* E. coli, Peptostreptococcus *species,* Proteus mirabilis, P. aeruginosa, Staphylococcus aureus, Streptococcus agalactiae, S. pyogenes, *or viridans group* streptococci

I.V. INFUSION OR INJECTION

Adults and children weighing more than 50 kg (110 lb). 500 mg (1 g if caused by *Pseudomonas aeruginosa*) every 8 hr.

Children ages 3 mo and older weighing 50 kg (110 lb) or less. 10 mg/kg (20 mg/kg if caused by *Pseudomonas aeruginosa*) every 8 hr. *Maximum:* 500 mg every 8 hr.

* *To treat bacterial meningitis caused by* Haemophilus influenzae, Neisseria meningitidis, *or* Streptococcus pneumoniae *(penicillin-susceptible isolates)*

I.V. INFUSION OR INJECTION

Children weighing more than 50 kg (110 lb). 2 g every 8 hr.

Children ages 3 mo and older weighing 50 kg (110 lb) or less. 40 mg/kg every 8 hr. *Maximum:* 2 g every 8 hr.

±**DOSAGE ADJUSTMENT** For adult patients with a creatinine clearance of 26 to 50 ml/min, dosage interval increased to every 12 hours. For adult patients with a creatinine clearance of 10 to 25 ml/min, dosage reduced by half and given every 12 hours. For adult patients with creatinine clearance less than 10 ml/min, dosage reduced by half and given every 24 hours. There are no guidelines for children with renal impairment.

Drug Administration

I.V.

- For I.V. injection, add 10 ml Sterile Water for Injection to 500-mg vial, or 20 ml to 1-g vial of drug. Shake to dissolve and let stand until clear. Administer over 3 to 5 min. Once reconstituted, drug may be stored for up to 3 hr at room temperature or for 13 hr if refrigerated.
- For I.V. infusion, drug vials may be directly reconstituted with 0.9% Sodium Chloride Injection or 5% Dextrose Injection. Alternatively, a drug vial may be reconstituted, then the resulting solution added to 0.9% Sodium Chloride Injection or 5% Dextrose Injection container and further diluted. Solutions for infusion should have a concentration ranging from 1 mg/ml to 20 mg/ml. Infuse over 15 to 30 min. If mixed with 0.9% Sodium Chloride Injection, solution may be stored for 1 hr at room temperature and up to 15 hr if refrigerated. If mixed with 5% Dextrose Injection, solution must be used immediately.
- Follow manufacturer's guidelines for preparing ADD-Vantage vials for administration.
- Do not use flexible container in series plastic connections.
- *Incompatibilities:* Other drugs, including solutions containing other drugs

Route	Onset	Peak	Duration
I.V.	Unknown	1 hr	Unknown

Half-life: 1–1.5 hr

Mechanism of Action

Penetrates cell walls of most gram-negative and gram-positive bacteria, inactivating penicillin-binding proteins thereby inhibiting bacterial cell wall synthesis, which causes cell death.

Contraindications

Hypersensitivity to meropenem, other carbapenem drugs, beta-lactams, or their components

Interactions

DRUGS

probenecid: Inhibited renal excretion of meropenem increasing meropenem plasma concentrations

valproic acid: Possibly reduced blood level of valproic acid to subtherapeutic level

Adverse Reactions

CNS: Headache, paresthesia, **seizures**

CV: **Shock**

EENT: Epistaxis, glossitis, oral candidiasis

GI: Anorexia, constipation, ***Clostridioides difficile*-associated diarrhea**, diarrhea, elevated liver enzymes, nausea, **pseudomembranous colitis**, vomiting

GU: Elevated BUN and serum creatinine levels, hematuria, **renal failure**

HEME: **Agranulocytosis**, **hemolytic anemia**, **leukopenia**, **neutropenia**, positive Coombs' test

MS: **Rhabdomyolysis**

RESP: **Apnea**, dyspnea

SKIN: Acute generalized exanthematous pustulosis, diaper rash from candidiasis (children), **erythema multiforme**, pruritus, rash, **Stevens-Johnson syndrome**, **toxic epidermal necrolysis**

Other: **Anaphylaxis**; **angioedema**; **drug reaction with eosinophilia and systemic symptoms (DRESS)**; injection-site inflammation, pain, phlebitis, or thrombophlebitis; **sepsis**

Childbearing Considerations

PREGNANCY

- It is not known if drug causes fetal harm.
- Use with caution only if benefit to mother outweighs potential risk to fetus.

LACTATION

- Drug is present in breast milk.
- Mothers should check with prescriber before breastfeeding.

Nursing Considerations

- Obtain body fluid and tissue samples, as ordered, for culture and sensitivity testing. Expect to review test results, if possible, before giving first dose of meropenem.

! **WARNING** Be aware that fatal hypersensitivity reactions have occurred with meropenem use. Determine whether patient has had previous reactions to antibiotics or other allergens. Monitor patient closely and stop drug immediately if signs and symptoms of anaphylaxis occur. Notify prescriber and expect to provide supportive emergency care, as needed and ordered.

! **WARNING** Monitor patient for blister formation, rash, and other cutaneous abnormalities because drug may cause severe cutaneous adverse reactions that may become life-threatening. Know that DRESS may only initially present with a fever or swollen lymph glands. At first sign of skin abnormality, stop drug therapy immediately and notify prescriber.

! **WARNING** Monitor patient closely for diarrhea, which may indicate pseudomembranous colitis caused by *Clostridioides difficile*, which may be mild or become life-threatening. If diarrhea occurs, notify prescriber, and expect to obtain a stool specimen. If confirmed, expect meropenem to be discontinued and be prepared to treat with an antibiotic effective against *C. difficile*, as ordered. Also, expect to give electrolytes, fluids, and protein supplementation, as needed and ordered.

! **WARNING** Take seizure precautions according to facility policy, especially for patients with bacterial meningitis, CNS, or renal disorders because of an increased risk of seizures with meropenem.

! **WARNING** Monitor patient with creatinine clearance of 10 to 26 ml/min for signs and symptoms of renal failure as well as for heart failure, seizures, or shock.

! **WARNING** Expect to monitor patient's CBC regularly, as ordered, because drug can cause serious hematologic adverse reactions, which could become life-threatening.

PATIENT TEACHING

- Inform patient that meropenem will be administered intravenously.

! **WARNING** Tell patient to immediately report difficulty breathing, injection-site pain, skin changes (blister formation, rash), and sore mouth.

! **WARNING** Alert patient to notify staff immediately if an allergic reaction occurs with meropenem administration.

! **WARNING** Urge patient to tell prescriber about diarrhea that is severe or lasts longer than 3 days. Remind patient that bloody or watery stools can occur 2 or more months after antibiotic therapy and can be serious, requiring prompt treatment.

- Instruct patient to avoid hazardous activities until drug's CNS effects are known and resolved.

mesalamine

Apriso, Canasa, Delzicol, Lialda, Pentasa, Rowasa, Salofalk (CAN), sfROWASA

Class and Category

Pharmacologic class: Aminosalicylate
Therapeutic class: Anti-inflammatory

Indications and Dosages

∗ *To treat actively mild to moderate ulcerative colitis*

D.R. CAPSULES (DELZICOL)

Adults. *Initial:* 800 mg 3 times daily for 6 wk. **Children ages 5 and older weighing 54 kg (118.8 lb) to 90 kg (198 lb).** 27 to 44 mg/kg/day in 2 divided doses given in morning and afternoon for 6 wk. *Maximum:* 2.4 g daily.

Children ages 5 and older weighing 33 kg (72.6 lb) to less than 54 kg (118.8 lb). 37 to 61 mg/kg/day in 2 divided doses given in morning and afternoon for 6 wk. *Maximum:* 2 g daily.
Children ages 5 and older weighing 17 kg (37.4 lb) to less than 33 kg (72.6 lb). 36 to 71 mg/kg/day in 2 divided doses given in morning and afternoon for 6 wk. *Maximum:* 1.2 g daily.

D.R. TABLETS (LIALDA)

Children weighing more than 50 kg (110 lb). 4.8 g once daily with a meal for 8 wk, then reduced to 2.4 g once daily with a meal.
Children weighing more than 35 kg (77 lb) to and including 50 kg (110 lb). 3.6 g once daily with a meal for 8 wk, then reduced to 2.4 g once daily after wk 8 with a meal.
Children weighing 24 kg (52.8 lb) to 35 kg (77 lb). 2.4 g once daily with a meal for 8 wk then reduced to 1.2 g once daily after wk 8 with a meal.

* *To induce remission in patients with actively mild to moderate ulcerative colitis.*

D.R. TABLETS (LIALDA)

Adults. *Initial:* 2.4 or 4.8 g once daily with a meal.

E.R. CAPSULES (PENTASA)

Adults. 1 g four times daily.

* *To maintain remission in patients with mild to moderate ulcerative colitis*

D.R. CAPSULES (DELZICOL)

Adults. 1.6 g daily in 2 to 4 divided doses.

D.R. TABLETS (LIALDA)

Adults. 2.4 g once daily with a meal.

E.R. CAPSULES (APRISO)

Adults. 1.5 g once daily in the morning.

E.R. CAPSULES (PENTASA)

Adults. 1 g four times daily.

* *To treat mild to moderate distal ulcerative colitis, proctitis, and proctosigmoiditis*

RECTAL SUSPENSION (ROWASA, SFROWASA)

Adults. 4 g (60 ml) daily at bedtime for 3 to 6 wk.

* *To treat actively mild to moderate ulcerative proctitis*

SUPPOSITORIES (CANASA)

Adults. 1 g once daily at bedtime for 3 to 6 wk.

Drug Administration

P.O.

- Do not interchange or substitute one brand for another or the strength of the same brand for another.
- Capsules and tablets should be swallowed whole and not chewed, crushed, or split/opened. An exception is Delzicol capsules, which can be opened, and the inner tablets swallowed and Pentasa capsules, which can be opened and contents sprinkled onto applesauce or yogurt and mixture consumed immediately.
- Do not coadminister drug with antacids.
- Ensure that patient is well hydrated.
- Administer Lialda brand with food.

P.R.

- Administer suppository at bedtime. Do not cut or break suppository. Ensure that suppository is firm before inserting it. If it's too soft, chill in refrigerator for 30 min or run under cold water before removing wrapper. Moisten with water-soluble lubricant or tap water before insertion. Have patient retain suppository for 1 to 3 hr. Avoid suppository touching surfaces to prevent staining.
- To administer rectal suspension, shake suspension bottle before each dose, then remove protective covering from applicator tip. Place patient on left side or in a knee-chest position. Insert applicator tip gently into the rectum pointing toward the umbilicus. Squeeze bottle in a steady manner. Have patient remain in the position for at least 30 min. Give suspension at bedtime so patient can retain for prescribed time of about 8 hr, if possible. Retention time ranges from 3.5 to 12 hr.
- Have patient drink an adequate amount of fluids during treatment.
- Suspension may darken slightly over time, but this change doesn't affect potency. Discard rectal suspension that turns dark brown.

Route	Onset	Peak	Duration
P.O.	1 wk–3 mo	3–12 hr	Unknown
P.R.	Unknown	4–7 hr	Unknown

Half-life: 7–12 hr

Mechanism of Action

May reduce inflammation by inhibiting the enzyme cyclooxygenase and decreasing production of arachidonic acid metabolites, which may be increased in patients with inflammatory bowel disease. May also reduce inflammation by interfering with leukotriene synthesis and inhibiting the enzyme lipoxygenase, both of which take part in inflammatory response.

Contraindications

Hypersensitivity to mesalamine, other salicylates, including aminosalicylates, or their components

Interactions

DRUGS

azathioprine, 6-mercaptopurine: Possibly increased risk for blood disorders
nephrotoxic agents, including NSAIDs: Possibly increased risk of nephrotoxicity

Adverse Reactions

CNS: Chills, confusion, depression, dizziness, drug fever, emotional lability, fatigue, fever, **Guillain-Barré syndrome**, headache (severe), **intracranial hypertension**, peripheral neuropathy, somnolence, transverse myelitis, tremor, vertigo, weakness
CV: Chest pain, **myocarditis**, **pericardial effusion**, **pericarditis**, T wave abnormalities
EENT: Blurred vision, dry mouth, pharyngitis, rhinitis, sinusitis, swelling of eye, taste perversion, tinnitus
GI: Abdominal cramps or pain (severe), anal pruritus, anorexia, bloody diarrhea, cholecystitis, **cirrhosis**, colitis, constipation, diarrhea, discoloration of feces, distention (abdomen), elevated liver enzymes, feeling of incomplete defecation, flatulence, gastritis, **GI bleeding**, **hepatitis**, **hepatotoxicity**, indigestion, jaundice, Kawasaki-like syndrome, **liver failure or necrosis**, mucous stools, nausea, **pancreatitis**, **perforated peptic ulcer**, rectal discharge or pain, vomiting
GU: **Acute or chronic renal failure**, decreased libido, dysmenorrhea, dysuria, epididymitis, hematuria, interstitial nephritis, menorrhagia, minimal change disease, nephrogenic diabetes insipidus, nephrolithiasis, nephrotic syndrome, **nephrotoxicity**, reversible oligospermia, urinary frequency and urgency
HEME: **Agranulocytosis**, anemia, **aplastic anemia**, eosinophilia, **granulocytopenia**, **leukopenia**, lymphadenopathy, **neutropenia**, **pancytopenia**, **thrombocytopenia**
MS: Back pain, dysarthria, myalgia
RESP: **Allergic alveolitis**, **asthma exacerbation**, bronchitis, **eosinophilic or interstitial pneumonitis**, **fibrosing alveolitis**, **interstitial lung disease**, pleurisy/pleuritis, **pneumonitis**
SKIN: Acne, acute generalized exanthematous pustulosis (AGEP), alopecia, diaphoresis, dryness, erythema, including erythema nodosum, photosensitivity, psoriasis, pruritus, pyoderma gangrenosum, rash, **Stevens-Johnson syndrome**, **toxic epidermal necrolysis (TEN)**, urticaria
Other: **Acute intolerance syndrome**, **anaphylaxis**, **angioedema**, **drug reaction with eosinophilia and systemic symptoms (DRESS)**, gout, systemic lupus erythematosus or lupus-like syndrome

Childbearing Considerations

PREGNANCY

- It is not known if drug causes fetal harm although it does cross the placental barrier.
- Use with caution only if benefit to mother outweighs potential risk to fetus.

LACTATION

- Drug is present in breast milk.
- Mothers should check with prescriber before breastfeeding.
- If breastfeeding occurs, infant should be monitored for diarrhea.

Nursing Considerations

! WARNING Monitor patients for a hypersensitivity reaction, especially patients with sulfite sensitivity. Some drug formulations contain sulfites, which may cause hypersensitivity reactions in these patients. Know that hypersensitivity reactions may affect internal organs, such as the heart (myocarditis, pericarditis), kidneys (nephritis), liver (hepatitis), and lungs (pneumonitis), as well as cause hematologic adverse effects. If hypersensitivity is suspected, notify prescriber immediately, expect mesalamine to be discontinued, and provide supportive care, as ordered.

! WARNING Monitor patient for serious skin reactions. Expect drug to be discontinued at the first sign or symptom of a rash or severe cutaneous adverse reactions. Be aware that DRESS may only initially present with a fever or swollen lymph nodes.

! WARNING Monitor patient's CBC with differential for eosinophilia, which may indicate an hypersensitivity reaction, and other hematological adverse reactions. Know that patients ages 65 and older are at increased risk for blood dyscrasias, such as agranulocytosis, neutropenia, and pancytopenia.

! WARNING Expect to assess patient's hepatic function before mesalamine begins and then periodically throughout therapy, as ordered. Monitor patient closely for hepatic dysfunction, especially patients with liver disease because hepatic dysfunction may become severe causing hepatotoxicity or hepatic failure. Notify prescriber if liver enzymes become elevated.

! WARNING Expect to assess patient's renal function prior to the initiation of mesalamine therapy and then periodically throughout therapy, as ordered, because drug may cause renal impairment, which could lead to nephrotoxicity or renal failure. Patients at risk include patients taking concomitant nephrotoxic drugs or who have a history of renal disease or known renal impairment. If renal function decreases during therapy, notify prescriber and expect drug to be discontinued.

! WARNING Monitor patient for signs and symptoms of acute intolerance syndrome, such as acute abdominal pain, bloody diarrhea, fever, headache, and rash. If suspected, expect to discontinue mesalamine therapy and provide supportive care, as needed and ordered.

- Be aware that mesalamine may interfere with the measurement of urinary normetanephrine, producing falsely elevated test results if the test is done by liquid chromatography with electrochemical detection.
- Know that patients with preexisting skin conditions, such as atopic dermatitis and atopic eczema are at higher risk for more severe photosensitivity reactions.

PATIENT TEACHING

- Instruct patient how to administer brand of mesalamine prescribed.
- Tell patient to avoid taking mesalamine with antacids.
- Encourage patient to drink an adequate amount of fluids.

! WARNING Alert patient that drug may cause an allergic reaction. Tell patient to notify prescriber if an allergic reaction occurs. If severe, urge patient to seek immediate medical care.

! WARNING Advise patient to stop taking drug and to notify prescriber immediately if serious skin adverse reactions occurs.

! WARNING Advise patient to notify prescriber immediately about abdominal cramps or pain, bloody diarrhea, fever, headache, or any other adverse effects that are persistent, severe, or worsen during mesalamine therapy.

! WARNING Advise patient to take sun precautions such as using sunscreen and protective clothing while outdoors, as drug may cause photosensitivity reactions that could be severe, especially in patient with preexisting skin conditions.

- Tell patient to alert all prescribers of mesalamine therapy because of potential drug interactions, especially those drugs that increase sensitivity to sun and UV light.
- Alert patient that urine may be come discolored if it comes into contact with any surface treated with bleach. However, tell patient if urine is discolored before contact with any surface or water, prescriber should be notified.
- Tell mothers who are breastfeeding to monitor their infant for diarrhea.

metformin hydrochloride

Glumetza

Class and Category

Pharmacologic class: Biguanide
Therapeutic class: Antidiabetic

Indications and Dosages

✱ *As adjunct to reduce blood glucose level in type 2 diabetes mellitus*

ORAL SOLUTION

Adults. *Initial:* 500 mg twice daily or 850 mg once daily with meals, increased by 500 mg/wk or by 850 mg every 2 wk until desired response occurs. *Maximum:* 2,550 mg daily given in divided doses.

Children ages 10 and older. 500 mg twice daily with meals, increased as prescribed by 500 mg/wk until desired response occurs. *Maximum:* 2,000 mg daily in divided doses.

±**DOSAGE ADJUSTMENT** For patients not tolerating maximum dosage, total daily dose may be divided into 3 doses and given with meals.

E.R. TABLETS (GLUMETZA)

Adults. *Initial:* 500 mg once daily with evening meal. Increased by 500 mg every 1 to 2 wk, as needed. *Maximum:* 2,000 mg daily.

Drug Administration

P.O.

- Administer twice-daily dosages with meals, once in the morning and once in the evening.
- Administer once-daily dosages of immediate-release tablets with morning meal.
- Administer extended-release tablets with evening meal.
- Extended-release tablets should be swallowed whole and not chewed, crushed, or split.
- Measure oral solution using the provided dosing cup.

Route	Onset	Peak	Duration
P.O.	3 hr	2–3 hr	Unknown
P.O./Solution	Unknown	3.5–6.5 hr	Unknown
P.O./E.R.	Unknown	4–8 hr	Unknown

Half-life: 4–9 hr

Mechanism of Action

May promote storage of excess glucose as glycogen in the liver, which reduces glucose production. Improves glucose use possibly by adipose tissue and skeletal muscle increasing glucose transport across cell membranes. May also increase the number of insulin receptors on cell membranes and make them more sensitive to insulin. Decreases blood total cholesterol and triglyceride levels modestly.

Contraindications

Acute or chronic metabolic acidosis, including diabetic ketoacidosis with or without coma; hypersensitivity to metformin or its components; severe renal disease (estimated glomerular filtration rate below 30 ml/min)

Interactions

DRUGS

calcium channel blockers, corticosteroids, estrogens, isoniazid, nicotinic acid, oral contraceptives, phenothiazines, phenytoin, sympathomimetics, thiazide and other diuretics, thyroid drugs: Possibly reduced effectiveness of metformin resulting in hyperglycemia

carbonic anhydrase inhibitors, such as acetazolamide, dichlorphenamide, topiramate, zonisamide: Possibly increased risk of lactic acidosis

cimetidine, dolutegravir, ranolazine, vandetanib: Increased blood metformin level and possibly increased risk of lactic acidosis

insulin, sulfonylureas: Increased risk of hypoglycemia

ACTIVITIES

alcohol use: Increased risk of hypoglycemia and lactate formation

Adverse Reactions

CNS: Headache

EENT: Metallic taste

ENDO: **Hypoglycemia**

GI: Abdominal distention, anorexia, constipation, diarrhea, flatulence, **hepatic injury**, indigestion, nausea, vomiting

HEME: **Aplastic anemia**, megaloblastic anemia, **thrombocytopenia**

SKIN: Photosensitivity, rash

Other: **Lactic acidosis**, vitamin B_{12} deficiency (with immediate-release formulation), weight loss

Childbearing Considerations

PREGNANCY

- It is not known if drug causes fetal harm although it does cross the placental barrier.
- Use with caution only if benefit to mother outweighs potential risk to fetus.

LACTATION

- Drug is present in breast milk.
- Mothers should check with prescriber before breastfeeding.

REPRODUCTION

- Caution females of childbearing age of the potential for unintended pregnancy as drug may cause ovulation in some anovulatory women.

Nursing Considerations

! WARNING Know that metformin should never be given to a patient with severe renal impairment (eGFR below 30 ml/min). Be aware that initiation of metformin is not recommended in patients who have an eGFR between 45 and 60 ml/min. Also, be aware that metformin is not recommended for use in patients with hepatic impairment because of risk of lactic acidosis. Expect to assess patient's eGFR at least annually. Anticipate that the elderly and those at increased risk for renal impairment may be tested more frequently.

- Expect prescriber to alter dosage if patient has a condition that decreases or delays gastric emptying, such as diarrhea, gastroparesis, GI obstruction, ileus, or vomiting.

! WARNING Monitor patient closely for signs and symptoms of lactic acidosis that often are subtle and nonspecific, such as abdominal pain, increased somnolence, malaise, myalgias, and respiratory distress. Know that hypotension and resistant bradyarrhythmias have occurred with severe acidosis. Be aware that most cases of lactic acidosis have occurred in patients with significant renal impairment because metformin is substantially excreted by the kidneys. Other risk factors include being age 65 or older; certain drug interactions, such as carbonic anhydrase inhibitors; excessive alcohol intake; hepatic impairment; hypoxic states; radiologic studies with contrast; sepsis, and withholding of fluids and food, which increases risk of volume depletion. Expect drug to be withheld if patient becomes dehydrated. If lactic acidosis is suspected, notify prescriber, expect metformin to be immediately discontinued, and provide appropriate supportive care. Know that prompt hemodialysis may be needed to correct the acidosis and remove the accumulated metformin.

! WARNING Know that iodinated contrast media used in radiographic studies increase risk of renal failure and lactic acidosis during metformin therapy. Expect to withhold drug for 48 hours before and after testing.

- Monitor patient's blood glucose level to evaluate drug effectiveness. Assess for hyperglycemia and the need for insulin during times of increased stress, such as infection and surgery.
- Expect yearly measurements of patient's hematologic status as well as vitamin B_{12} level. Be aware that vitamin B_{12} deficiency has occurred with use of the immediate-release formulation of metformin.

PATIENT TEACHING

- Instruct patient how to administer form of metformin prescribed.
- Direct patient to take drug exactly as prescribed and not to change the dosage or frequency unless instructed.
- Caution patient to avoid alcohol, which can increase the risk of hypoglycemia and lactic acidosis.
- Emphasize importance of checking blood glucose level regularly, controlling weight, exercising regularly, and following prescribed diet.
- Teach patient how to recognize hyperglycemia and hypoglycemia. Urge the patient to notify prescriber of abnormal blood glucose level. Advise patient to expect glycosylated hemoglobin every 3 months until blood glucose is controlled.

! WARNING Instruct patient to report early signs of lactic acidosis, including drowsiness, hyperventilation, malaise, and muscle pain.

- Alert females of childbearing age that metformin may cause ovulation in some premenopausal anovulatory women, which may lead to unintended pregnancy.

methadone hydrochloride

Metadol (CAN), Methadose

Class, Category, and Schedule

Pharmacologic class: Opioid
Therapeutic class: Opioid agonist
Controlled substance schedule: II

Indications and Dosages

✱ *To manage opioid detoxification and then maintenance of opioid abstinence*

DISPERSIBLE TABLETS, ORAL CONCENTRATE, ORAL SOLUTION, TABLETS

Adults. *Initial on day 1:* 20 to 30 mg as a single dose, followed by 5 to 10 mg 2 to 4 hr later, as needed. *Maximum for day 1:* 40 mg. *Maintenance:* Highly individualized with dosage adjustments made until opioid withdrawal symptoms have ceased for 24 hr, which usually requires doses between 80 to 120 mg/day. *Maximum:* 120 mg daily.

I.M., I.V., OR SUBCUTANEOUS INJECTION

Hospitalized adults unable to take drug orally. Highly individualized.

± **DOSAGE ADJUSTMENT** For patients who had used oral methadone prior to hospitalization, dosage initially decreased by 50%.

✱ *To manage moderate to severe pain when a continuous, around-the-clock opioid analgesic is needed for an extended period of time and for which alternative treatment options are inadequate*

TABLETS

Adults. *Initial:* 2.5 mg every 8 to 12 hr increased slowly, as needed, every 3 to 5 days.

I.M., I.V., OR SUBCUTANEOUS INJECTION

Adults unable to take drug orally. *Initial:* 2.5 to 10 mg every 8 to 12 hr increased slowly, as needed, every 3 to 5 days.

± **DOSAGE ADJUSTMENT** For elderly patients and patients with hepatic or renal dysfunction, initial dose reduced. For patients converting from one form of methadone to another, follow manufacturer's guidelines.

Drug Administration

- Store all forms of drug at room temperature. Protect from light.
- Make sure opioid antagonist (naloxone) and equipment for administering oxygen and controlling respiration are nearby before giving methadone.

P.O.

- For liquid forms not in a ready-to-drink solution, dilute with at least 120-ml water or an acidic beverage such as orange juice and use a calibrated device to measure dosage.
- Dissolve dispersible tablets in 120 ml of water, orange juice, or citrus-flavored non-alcoholic beverage before giving. Administer immediately. Dispersible tablet may not completely dissolve in water. If a residue remains in the cup after initial administration with water, add a small amount of liquid to the cup and give to patient to drink to ensure that all of the drug has been ingested. Do not store mixture.

I.V.

- Follow manufacturer's guidelines for preparation and administration of drug, as it is highly individualized.
- *Incompatibilities:* None reported by manufacturer.

I.M.

- Preferred parenteral route.
- Inject into a large muscle mass.
- Rotate sites.

SUBCUTANEOUS

- Rotate sites.

Route	Onset	Peak	Duration
P.O.	30–60 min	1–7 hr	4–8 hr
I.V.	Unknown	Unknown	4–8 hr
I.M./SubQ	10–20 min	Unknown	4–8 hr

Half-life: 8–59 hr.

Mechanism of Action

Binds with and activates opioid receptors (primarily mu receptors) in spinal cord and higher levels of CNS to produce analgesia and euphoric effects.

Contraindications

Acute or severe bronchial asthma in unmonitored setting or in absence of resuscitative equipment, hypersensitivity to methadone or its components, paralytic ileus, significant respiratory depression

Interactions

DRUGS

5-HT$_3$ receptor antagonists, certain muscle relaxants (cyclobenzaprine, metaxalone), drugs that affect the serotonin neurotransmitter system (mirtazapine, tramadol, trazodone), I.V. methylene blue, linezolid, MAO inhibitors, selective serotonin reuptake inhibitors (SSRIs), serotonin and norepinephrine reuptake inhibitors (SNRIs),

tricyclic antidepressants, triptans: Increased risk of serotonin syndrome
anticholinergics: Possibly severe constipation leading to ileus; urine retention
benzodiazepines, CNS depressants, other opioids, sedating antihistamines, tricyclic antidepressants: Increased risk of significant respiratory depression and other life-threatening adverse effects
CYP3A4, CYP2B6, CYP2C19, CYP2C9 inducers, such as carbamazepine, phenobarbital, phenytoin, rifampin, St. John's wort: Decreased methadone concentration, resulting in decreased efficacy or onset of withdrawal symptoms in patients dependent on methadone
CYP3A4, CYP2B6, CYP2C19, CYP2C9, CYP2D6 inhibitors, such as azole-antifungal agents, macrolide antibiotics, protease inhibitors, some selective serotonin reuptake inhibitors (fluvoxamine, sertraline): Increased methadone concentration, resulting in increased or prolonged opioid effects that may result in a fatal overdose
desipramine: Increased plasma desipramine levels
didanosine, stavudine: Decreased area under the concentration-time curve and peak levels of these drugs
diuretics: Decreased diuresis
diuretics, laxatives, mineralocorticoid hormones: Increased risk of electrolyte disturbances and prolonged QT interval
MAO inhibitors: Possibly increased risk of opioid toxicity or serotonin syndrome
mixed agonist-antagonist analgesics and partial agonist opioid analgesics, such as buprenorphine, butorphanol, nalbuphine, pentazocine: Possibly reduced analgesic effect of methadone; possibly precipitation of withdrawal symptoms
muscle relaxants: Possibly enhanced neuromuscular blocking action of skeletal muscle relaxants; increased degree of respiratory depression
zidovudine: Increased zidovudine levels possibly resulting in toxic effects

ACTIVITIES

alcohol use: Increased CNS and respiratory depression, possibly hypotension

Adverse Reactions

CNS: Agitation, amnesia, anxiety, asthenia, **coma**, confusion, decreased concentration, delirium, delusions, depression, dizziness, drowsiness, dysphoria, euphoria, fever, hallucinations, headache, insomnia, lethargy, light-headedness, malaise, psychosis, restlessness, sedation, **seizures**, syncope, tremor
CV: **Bradycardia**, **cardiac arrest**, **cardiomyopathy**, edema, **heart failure**, **hypotension**, orthostatic hypotension, palpitations, phlebitis, **prolonged QT interval**, **shock**, tachycardia, **torsades de pointes**, T-wave inversion on ECG, **ventricular fibrillation or tachycardia**
EENT: Blurred vision, diplopia, dry mouth, glossitis, **laryngeal edema or laryngospasm**, miosis, nystagmus, rhinitis, strabismus
ENDO: **Adrenal insufficiency**, **hypoglycemia**
GI: Abdominal cramps or pain, anorexia, biliary tract spasm, constipation, diarrhea, dysphagia, elevated liver enzymes, gastroesophageal reflux, hiccups, ileus and **toxic megacolon** (in patients with inflammatory bowel disease), indigestion, nausea, vomiting
GU: Amenorrhea, decreased ejaculate potency, decreased libido, difficult ejaculation, impotence, infertility, lack of menstruation, urinary hesitancy, urine retention
HEME: Anemia, **leukopenia**, **thrombocytopenia**
MS: Arthralgia
RESP: **Apnea**, **asthma exacerbation**, **atelectasis**, **bronchospasm**, depressed cough reflex, **hypoventilation**, **pulmonary edema**, **respiratory arrest or depression**, wheezing
SKIN: Diaphoresis, flushing
Other: **Angioedema and other hypersensitivity reactions**; **hypokalemia**; **hypomagnesemia**; injection-site edema, pain, rash, or redness; physical and psychological dependence; weight gain; withdrawal symptoms

Childbearing Considerations

PREGNANCY

- Drug may cause fetal harm.
- Prolonged use of drug during pregnancy can result in neonatal opioid withdrawal syndrome (NOWS), which may be life-threatening if not recognized and treated.
- Use with extreme caution only if benefit to mother outweighs potential risk to fetus.

- Pregnancy can decrease the terminal half-life of drug during the second and third trimesters resulting in possible withdrawal symptoms in some pregnant women. To avoid this, dosage may have to be increased or the dosing interval decreased to achieve therapeutic effect.

LABOR AND DELIVERY

- Opioid-dependent women on methadone maintenance therapy may need additional analgesia during labor.
- Opioids cross the placental barrier and may produce respiratory depression and psycho-physiologic effects in the newborn. Monitor newborn closely for signs of excess sedation and respiratory depression.
- An opioid antagonist, such as naloxone, must be available at the time of delivery in the event it is needed to reverse opioid-induced respiratory depression in the neonate.

LACTATION

- Drug is present in breast milk.
- Mothers should check with prescriber before breastfeeding.
- If breastfeeding occurs, monitor infant for excess sedation and respiratory depression.

REPRODUCTION

- Chronic use of opioids may reduce fertility.

Nursing Considerations

- Be aware that use of methadone requires a Risk Evaluation and Mitigation Strategy (REMS) before drug can be dispensed, to ensure that the benefits outweigh the risks of abuse, addiction, and misuse.

! **WARNING** Assess patient's current drug use, including all prescription and over-the-counter drugs before therapy begins. Be aware that excessive use of methadone may lead to abuse, addiction, misuse, overdose, and possibly death. Monitor patient's intake of drug closely.

! **WARNING** Give drug cautiously to patients at risk for a prolonged QT interval, such as those with cardiac hypertrophy, hypokalemia, or hypomagnesemia; those with a history of cardiac conduction abnormalities; and those taking diuretics or medications that affect cardiac conduction.

! **WARNING** Be aware that patients tolerant to other opioids may be incompletely tolerant to methadone. A high degree of "opioid tolerance" does not eliminate the possibility of methadone toxicity. Some patients have died during conversion from chronic high-dose therapy with other opioid agonists. Monitor patient closely during the conversion process.

! **WARNING** Monitor patient for a hypersensitivity reaction, which could become life-threatening such as angioedema. If present, notify prescriber, expect drug to be discontinued and another drug substituted, and provide supportive care, as needed and ordered.

- Monitor patient for expected excessive confusion, drowsiness, or unsteadiness during first 3 to 5 days of therapy, and notify prescriber if effects continue to worsen or persist beyond this time.

! **WARNING** Monitor circulatory and respiratory status carefully and often during methadone therapy, especially when drug therapy is initiated and when patient is being converted to methadone, because cardiac arrest, circulatory or respiratory depression, hypotension, respiratory arrest, and shock can develop. Life-threatening respiratory depression can occur even when drug is being used as prescribed and is not abused or misused. Be especially vigilant with cachectic, debilitated, and elderly patients, who are at higher risk for developing respiratory depression. Assess patient for excessive or persistent sedation; dosage may have to be adjusted.

! **WARNING** Monitor patients closely with conditions accompanied by hypercapnia or hypoxia or decreased respiratory reserve, such as asthma, chronic obstructive pulmonary disease or cor pulmonale, CNS depression or coma, kyphoscoliosis, myxedema, severe obesity, or sleep apnea syndrome. This is because methadone, even with usual therapeutic doses, may decrease respiratory drive while simultaneously increasing airway resistance to the point of apnea. Know that the peak respiratory depressant effect of methadone occurs later and persists longer than the peak analgesic effect. Monitor patient's respiratory status closely, especially when initiating drug or following a dosage increase.

! **WARNING** Monitor patients, especially the elderly, for cardiac arrhythmias, hypotension, hypovolemia, orthostatic hypotension, and vasovagal syncope because methadone may produce cholinergic effects in patients with cardiac disease, resulting in bradycardia and peripheral vasodilation; dosage decrease may be indicated.

! **WARNING** Monitor patients with seizure disorders because methadone may induce or aggravate seizure activity.

! **WARNING** Monitor patients who have head injuries or other conditions that may increase intracranial pressure (ICP) because methadone may further increase ICP.

! **WARNING** Monitor patient for adrenal insufficiency. Although rare, it can be life-threatening. Monitor patient for anorexia, dizziness, fatigue, hypotension, nausea, vomiting, or weakness. Notify prescriber if adrenal insufficiency is suspected and expect diagnostic testing to be done. If confirmed, expect to administer corticosteroids and wean patient off methadone, if possible.

! **WARNING** Know that benzodiazepine and other CNS depressant therapy should only be used concomitantly in patients for whom other treatment options are inadequate. If prescribed together, expect dosing and duration of methadone to be limited. Monitor patient closely for signs and symptoms of a decrease in consciousness, including coma, profound sedation, and significant respiratory depression. Notify prescriber immediately and provide emergency supportive care, as death may occur.

! **WARNING** Know that many drugs may interact with opioids, such as methadone, to cause serotonin syndrome. Monitor patient closely for signs and symptoms such as agitation, diaphoresis, diarrhea, fever, hallucinations, labile blood pressure, muscle twitching or stiffness, nausea, shakiness, shivering, tachycardia, trouble with coordination, or vomiting. Notify prescriber at once because serotonin syndrome may be life-threatening. Be prepared to discontinue drug, if possible and ordered. Expect to provide supportive care, as needed and ordered. Also, be aware that concomitant use of methadone with CYP3A4, CYP2B6, CYP2C19, or CYP2D6 inhibitors or discontinuation of concomitantly used CYP3A4, CYP2B6, CYP2C19, or CYP2C9 inducers can result in a fatal overdose.

! **WARNING** Know that chronic maternal use of methadone during pregnancy can result in NOWS, which may be life-threatening if not recognized and treated appropriately.

! **WARNING** Know that breastfeeding mothers on maintenance therapy put their infants at risk of withdrawal symptoms if they abruptly stop breastfeeding or discontinue methadone therapy. Methadone also accumulates in CNS tissue, increasing the risk of seizures in infants.

- Monitor patient for pain because maintenance dosage doesn't provide pain relief; patients with tolerance to opiate agonists, including those with chronic cancer pain, may require a higher dosage.
- Monitor patients who are pregnant or who have liver or renal impairment for increased adverse effects from methadone because drug may have a prolonged duration and cumulative effect in these patients. Methadone may prolong labor by reducing duration, frequency, or strength of uterine contractions, so expect dosage to be tapered before third trimester of pregnancy.
- Check plasma amylase and lipase levels in patients who develop biliary tract spasms because levels may increase up to 15 times normal. Notify prescriber immediately of any significant or sustained increase.
- Monitor patients with prostatic hypertrophy, renal disease, or urethral stricture for urine retention and oliguria because methadone can increase tension of detrusor muscle.
- Anticipate need to treat patient's symptoms of anxiety because methadone doesn't have antianxiety effects. Be aware that anxiety

may be confused with symptoms of opioid abstinence.

- Assess patient for withdrawal symptoms with long-term methadone use. Avoid abrupt discontinuation because withdrawal symptoms will occur within 3 to 4 days after last dose.

PATIENT TEACHING

- Instruct patient how to administer form of methadone prescribed.

! **WARNING** Inform patient that misuse of drug either by taking excessive amounts or by taking drug for prolonged periods of time can lead to addiction, overdose, or even death. Therefore, tell patient to take drug exactly as prescribed and for the shortest time possible.

! **WARNING** Warn patient and family that an opioid overdose can result in death. Instruct family or caregiver on the signs and symptoms of an overdose, including respiratory depression. Stress importance of having naloxone available for emergency use in the event patient experiences an opioid overdose. Instruct family or caregiver how to administer naloxone and stress the need to call 911 right away because naloxone effects are only temporary.

! **WARNING** Alert patient that drug may cause an allergic reaction. If present, tell patient to notify prescriber and, if severe, to seek immediate medical care.

! **WARNING** Review signs and symptoms of hypoglycemia with all patients, including diabetics and how to treat it if it should occur. Urge patient to seek immediate medical care if hypoglycemia becomes severe.

- Instruct patient to notify prescriber of worsening or breakthrough pain because dosage may have to be adjusted.

! **WARNING** Urge patient to notify prescriber if he experiences dizziness, light-headedness, palpitations, or syncope, which may be caused by methadone-induced arrhythmias. Also, tell patient to notify prescriber immediately of any other persistent, serious, or unusual adverse reactions, especially if respirations slow or breathing becomes difficult.

! **WARNING** Advise patient to notify prescriber of all other drugs he's currently taking, including benzodiazepines, and to avoid alcohol and other depressants, such as sleeping pills and tranquilizers, because they may increase drug's CNS depressant effects and cause severe respiratory depression that could result in death.

! **WARNING** Instruct patient, family, or caregiver to keep methadone out of the reach of children because accidental ingestion can be fatal.

- Instruct patient to avoid potentially hazardous activities or those that require mental alertness because methadone therapy may cause drowsiness or sleepiness.
- Teach patient to change positions slowly to minimize the effects of orthostatic hypotension.
- Instruct females of childbearing age to notify prescriber if she becomes pregnant.
- Advise patient that drug may cause severe constipation and to take measures to avoid constipation. If unresolved or severe, tell patient to seek medical attention.
- Inform patient that long-term use of opioids like methadone may decrease sex hormone levels, causing decreased libido, erectile dysfunction, impotence, infertility, or lack of menstruation. Encourage patient to report any symptoms.
- Inform patient that abrupt cessation of methadone therapy can precipitate withdrawal symptoms. Urge the patient to notify prescriber if he develops any concerns over therapy.
- Tell breastfeeding mothers to monitor infant for excess sedation and respiratory depression.

methimazole

Tapazole

Class and Category

Pharmacologic class: Thyroid hormone antagonist

Therapeutic class: Antithyroid

Indications and Dosages

∗ *To treat hyperthyroidism in preparation for radioactive iodine therapy or thyroidectomy; to treat Graves' disease with hyperthyroidism or toxic multinodular goiter for whom radioactive iodine therapy or surgery is not an appropriate treatment option*

TABLETS

Adults. *Initial:* 15 mg daily for mild hyperthyroidism, 30 to 40 mg daily for moderate hyperthyroidism, and 60 mg daily for severe hyperthyroidism given in divided doses 3 times daily 8 hr apart for 6 to 8 wk or until euthyroid level is reached. *Maintenance:* 5 to 15 mg daily.
Children. *Initial:* 0.4 mg/kg daily in divided doses 3 times daily 8 hr apart. *Maintenance:* 0.2 mg/kg daily.

Drug Administration

P.O.

- Ensure drug is given at consistently 8 hr apart.
- May give with or without food.

Route	Onset	Peak	Duration
P.O.	12–18 hr	1–2 hr	36–72 hr

Half-life: 4–6 hr

Mechanism of Action

Interferes directly with thyroid hormone synthesis in the thyroid gland by inhibiting iodide incorporation into thyroglobulin thereby depleting thyroglobulin stores and the circulating thyroid hormone level to drop.

Contraindications

Breastfeeding, hypersensitivity to methimazole or its components

Interactions

DRUGS

beta-blockers: Possibly increased blood levels of these drugs when patient becomes euthyroid
digoxin: Possibly increased blood digoxin level when patient becomes euthyroid
oral anticoagulants: Possibly action of oral anticoagulants may be potentiated
theophylline: Increased blood theophylline level when patient becomes euthyroid

Adverse Reactions

CNS: Drowsiness, headache, paresthesia, vertigo
CV: Edema
EENT: Loss of taste
ENDO: Hypothyroidism
GI: Diarrhea, indigestion, jaundice, nausea, vomiting
HEME: **Agranulocytosis, aplastic anemia, leukopenia, thrombocytopenia**
MS: Arthralgia, myalgia
SKIN: Alopecia, pruritus, rash, skin discoloration, urticaria
Other: Lupus-like symptoms, lymphadenopathy

Childbearing Considerations

PREGNANCY

- Drug may cause fetal harm as it crosses the placental barrier and can induce goiter and even cretinism in the developing fetus. In addition, rare cases of congenital defects have occurred in infants born to mothers who received the drug during pregnancy.
- If pregnancy occurs, it is recommended that drug be discontinued, and an alternative drug substituted during the pregnancy.

LACTATION

- Drug is present in breast milk.
- Mothers should check with prescriber before breastfeeding.

Nursing Considerations

- Closely monitor thyroid function test results during methimazole therapy.

! **WARNING** Monitor patient's CBC results to detect abnormalities caused by inhibition of myelopoiesis, which could become quite serious even life-threatening. Assess patient for bruising, unexplained bleeding, and infection. Institute bleeding and infection control measures, if needed.

- Watch for signs and symptoms of hypothyroidism, such as cold intolerance, depression, and edema as dosage will need to be decreased.
- Be aware that hyperthyroidism may increase metabolic clearance of beta-blockers and theophylline and that dosages of these drugs may have to be reduced as the patient's thyroid condition becomes corrected.

PATIENT TEACHING

- Instruct patient how to administer methimazole therapy.

! **WARNING** Instruct patient to notify prescriber immediately about cold intolerance, fever, sore throat, tiredness, and unusual bleeding or bruising.

M

! **WARNING** Tell females of childbearing age to notify prescriber if pregnancy occurs as drug is not recommended during pregnancy.

- Explain about possible hair loss or thinning during and for months after therapy.

methocarbamol

Class and Category

Pharmacologic class: Carbamate derivative
Therapeutic class: Skeletal muscle relaxant

Indications and Dosages

* *As adjunct to rest, physical therapy, and other measures to relieve discomfort caused by acute, painful musculoskeletal conditions*

TABLETS

Adults. *Initial:* 1,500 mg 4 times daily for 2 to 3 days. *For severe discomfort:* 8,000 mg daily in divided doses for 2 to 3 days, followed by maintenance dosage. *Maintenance:* 1,000 mg 4 times daily. Alternatively for maintenance, 750 mg every 4 hr, or 1,500 mg 3 times daily.

I.M. INJECTION, I.V. INJECTION

Adults. *Initial:* 1 g followed by 1 g every 8 hr, as needed, for a total of 3 g in 24 hr. Then, 1 g every 8 hr for no longer than 2 more days, as needed. *Maximum:* 3 g daily for no longer than 3 days.

* *To provide supportive therapy for tetanus*

TABLETS

Adults and adolescents. Up to 24 g daily in divided doses given by nasogastric tube.

I.V. INFUSION OR INJECTION

Adults. *Initial:* 1 or 2 g injected at 300 mg/min (3 ml/min) followed by an additional 1 or 2 g infused at a rate not to exceed 3 ml/min for a total dose of up to 3 g. Dosing procedure repeated every 6 hr, as needed, until nasogastric tube can be inserted, and oral therapy begun.
Children. *Initial:* 500 mg/m^2/dose or 15 mg/kg and repeated every 6 hr, as needed. *Maximum:* 1.8 g/m^2/day for 3 consecutive days only.

Drug Administration

P.O.

- Administer tablets with food or milk to minimize nausea.
- Crush tablets and mix with water or saline solution for administration by NG tube.

I.V.

- For I.V. injection, administer undiluted into the vein or give through infusion line at a maximum rate of 300 mg/min (3 ml/min).
- For I.V. infusion, add 1 g (1 vial) of drug to no more than 250 ml 0.9% Sodium Chloride Injection or 5% Dextrose in Water. Once prepared administer immediately. Do not refrigerate. Infusion rate should not exceed 300 mg (3 ml)/min to avoid hypotension and seizures.
- Care should be taken to avoid extravasation because thrombophlebitis may occur.
- Keep patient recumbent during I.V. administration and for at least 15 min afterward. Then, have the patient rise slowly.
- *Incompatibilities:* None reported by manufacturer

I.M.

- Inject deep into large muscle, such as the gluteus.
- Give no more than 500 mg (5 ml) into each gluteal region.
- Don't give methocarbamol by subcutaneous route.

Route	Onset	Peak	Duration
P.O.	30 min	2 hr	Unknown
I.V.	Immediate	Unknown	Unknown
I.M.	Unknown	Unknown	Unknown

Half-life: 1–2 hr

Mechanism of Action

May depress CNS, which leads to sedation and reduced skeletal muscle spasms. Alters perception of pain also.

Contraindications

Hypersensitivity to methocarbamol or its components

Interactions

DRUGS

anticholinesterase drugs: Possibly inhibit the effect of these drugs such as pyridostigmine bromide.
CNS depressants: Increased CNS depression

ACTIVITIES

alcohol use: Increased CNS depression

Adverse Reactions

CNS: Dizziness, drowsiness, fever, headache, light-headedness, **seizures (I.V.)**, syncope, vertigo, weakness
CV: **Bradycardia**, **hypotension**, and thrombophlebitis (parenteral)
EENT: Blurred vision, conjunctivitis, diplopia, metallic taste, nasal congestion, nystagmus
GI: Nausea
GU: Black, brown, or green urine
SKIN: Flushing, pruritus, rash, urticaria
Other: **Anaphylaxis (parenteral)**, **angioedema**, injection-site irritation or pain (I.M.), injection-site sloughing (I.V.)

Childbearing Considerations

PREGNANCY

- Drug may cause fetal harm. Reports of congenital abnormalities following in utero exposure to drug have occurred.
- Drug should not be given to females of childbearing age who are or may become pregnant, especially early in pregnancy unless the benefit to mother outweighs potential risk to fetus.

LACTATION

- It is not known if drug is present in breast milk.
- Mothers should check with prescriber before breastfeeding.

REPRODUCTION

- Females of childbearing age should use effective contraception during drug therapy.

Nursing Considerations

! **WARNING** Be aware that the parenteral dosage form shouldn't be used in patients with renal dysfunction because the polyethylene glycol 300 vehicle is nephrotoxic.

! **WARNING** Monitor patient for hypersensitivity reactions, which could become life-threatening such as anaphylaxis or angioedema, especially with parenteral administration. If present, notify prescriber, expect drug to be discontinued, and provide supportive care, as needed and ordered.

! **WARNING** Monitor patient's vital signs closely as drug may cause bradycardia and hypotension.

PATIENT TEACHING

- Tell patient to take oral drug exactly as prescribed.
- Instruct patient to avoid alcohol and other CNS depressants during therapy.

! **WARNING** Instruct patient to report signs and symptoms of an allergic reaction and to stop taking drug. If severe, urge patient to seek immediate emergency care.

! **WARNING** Tell patient to notify prescriber if patient faints, feels lightheaded or dizzy, or notices his pulse is significantly slower than normal.

! **WARNING** Urge females of childbearing age to use effective contraception during drug therapy and to notify prescriber if pregnancy occurs as drug may need to be discontinued.

- Inform patient that urine may turn black, brown, or green until methocarbamol is discontinued.
- Advise patient to avoid hazardous activities until drug's CNS effects are known and resolved.

methotrexate (amethopterin)

Jylamvo, Otrexup, Rasuvo, Reditrex, Xatmep

methotrexate sodium

Trexall

Class and Category

Pharmacologic class: Folate antagonist (antimetabolite)
Therapeutic class: Antineoplastic

Indications and Dosages

✱ *To treat severe psoriasis unresponsive to other therapy*

ORAL SOLUTION (JYLAMVO), TABLETS (TREXALL)

Adults. 10 to 25 mg once weekly. *Maximum:* 30 mg/wk.

I.M. OR I.V. INJECTION (METHOTREXATE SODIUM), SUBCUTANEOUS INJECTION (OTREXUP, RASUVO, REDITREX)

Adults. 10 to 25 mg as a single dose weekly. *Maximum:* 25 to 30 mg weekly depending on product being used.

✶ *To treat severe rheumatoid arthritis unresponsive to other therapy*

ORAL SOLUTION (JYLAMVO) TABLETS (TREXALL)

Adults. 7.5 mg once weekly. *Maximum:* 20 mg/wk.

I.M. INJECTION (METHOTREXATE SODIUM), SUBCUTANEOUS INJECTION (OTREXUP, RASUVO, REDITREX, TREXALL)

Adults. 7.5 mg once weekly, then gradually increased to achieve an optimal response. *Maximum:* 20 mg/wk.

✶ *To treat active polyarticular juvenile idiopathic arthritis unresponsive to other therapy*

ORAL SOLUTION (JYLAMVO, XATMEP), I.M. INJECTION (METHOTREXATE SODIUM), SUBCUTANEOUS INJECTION (OTREXUP, RASUVO, REDITREX), TABLETS (TREXALL)

Children ages 2 to 16. *Initial:* 10 mg/m^2 once weekly, increased gradually, as needed. *Maximum:* 30 mg/m^2/wk although even doses higher than 20 mg/m^2/wk significantly increases risk of adverse reactions.

✶ *To treat neoplastic disease (acute lymphoblastic leukemia, breast cancer, gestational trophoblastic neoplasia, meningeal leukemia, non-Hodgkin's lymphoma, osteosarcoma, squamous cell carcinoma of the head and neck)*

I.M. OR I.V. INJECTION (METHOTREXATE SODIUM), INTRATHECAL (METHOTREXATE), TABLETS (TREXALL)

Adults and children. Highly individualized depending on type of neoplasm present and product being used. I.M. injection administered only in certain types of neoplastic diseases.

✶ *To treat acute lymphoblastic leukemia as part of a combination chemotherapy maintenance regimen*

ORAL SOLUTION (JYLAMVO, XATMEP), TABLETS (TREXALL)

Adults and children. *Initial:* 20 mg/m^2 once weekly, followed by dosage adjustments based on patient's absolute neutrophil count and platelet count, as needed.

✶ *To treat mycosis fungoides (cutaneous T-cell lymphoma) as monotherapy or part of combination chemotherapy regimen*

ORAL SOLUTION (JYLAMVO), TABLETS (TREXALL)

Adults. 25 to 75 mg once weekly as monotherapy or 10 mg/m^2 twice weekly as part of a combination chemotherapy regimen.

✶ *To treat relapsed or refractory non-Hodgkin lymphomas as part of a combination chemotherapy regimen*

ORAL SOLUTION (JYLAMVO), TABLETS (TREXALL)

Adults. 2.5 mg 2 to 4 times per wk. *Maximum:* 10 mg per wk.

± **DOSAGE ADJUSTMENT** For patients with hepatic or renal failure, a reduced dose may be required. For patients being treated for neoplastic disease, dose may need to be withheld or drug discontinued for serious adverse reactions.

Drug Administration

- Verify pregnancy status before initiating drug therapy in females of childbearing age.

P.O.

- Follow facility policy for handling and disposing drug because it is cytotoxic.
- Tablets should be swallowed whole and not chewed, crushed, or split.
- Administer at least 1 hr before or 2 hr after food or drink except for water.
- Use a calibrated device when measuring oral solution dosage. Store solution in refrigerator or at room temperature. If stored at room temperature, discard after 60 days (Xatmep) or 90 days (Jylamvo).

I.V.

- Follow facility policy for preparing and handling drug; parenteral form poses a risk of carcinogenicity, mutagenicity, and teratogenicity. Avoid skin contact.
- Use only preservative-free formulation of methotrexate when administering high-dose therapy or when drug is administered intrathecally to neonates or low-birth-weight infants.
- Follow manufacturer's guidelines for preparation and administration, as guidelines vary between products and dosages.

- Drug can be diluted with 0.9% Sodium Chloride Injection immediately before administration. Once diluted, drug should be used within 4 hr if stored at room temperature or 24 hr if stored in refrigerator.
- Monitor injection site for evidence of necrosis or other local reactions. If present, notify prescriber immediately.
- Expect to administer leucovorin rescue in patients receiving intermediate- or high-dose regimens for neoplastic disorders. Expect to administer folic acid or folinic acid to patients being treated for polyarticular juvenile idiopathic arthritis, psoriasis, or rheumatoid arthritis to reduce the risk of adverse reactions to the drug.
- *Incompatibilities:* None reported by manufacturer.

I.M.

- Follow facility policy for preparing and handling drug; parenteral form poses a risk of carcinogenicity, mutagenicity, and teratogenicity. Avoid skin contact.
- Monitor injection site for evidence of necrosis or other local reactions. If present, notify prescriber immediately.
- Rotate sites.

SUBCUTANEOUS

- Follow facility policy for preparing and handling drug; subcutaneous form poses a risk of carcinogenicity, mutagenicity, and teratogenicity. Avoid skin contact.
- Administer Otrexup and Rasuvo injection using the single-dose auto-injector. If dosage not available with auto-injector, use a different formulation.
- Administer injection into patient's abdomen or thigh only.
- Monitor injection site for evidence of necrosis or other local reactions. If present, notify prescriber immediately.

INTRATHECAL

- Follow facility policy for preparing and handling drug; intrathecal form poses a risk of carcinogenicity, mutagenicity, and teratogenicity. Avoid skin contact.
- Use only preservative-free form.
- Administered only by person skilled in intrathecal injections.
- Monitor injection site for evidence of necrosis or other local reactions. If present, notify prescriber immediately.

Route	Onset	Peak	Duration
P.O.	Unknown	1–2 hr	Unknown
I.V.	Unknown	Unknown	Unknown
I.M.	Unknown	30–60 min	Unknown
SubQ	Unknown	1–2 hr	Unknown
Intrathecal	Unknown	Unknown	Unknown

Half-life: 3–15 hr

Mechanism of Action

May exert immunosuppressive effects by inhibiting replication and function of T and possibly B lymphocytes. Slows rapidly growing cells, such as epithelial skin cells in psoriasis by possibly inhibiting dihydrofolate reductase, the enzyme that reduces folic acid to tetrahydrofolic acid. Interferes with DNA synthesis and cell reproduction in rapidly proliferating cells through inhibition of tetrahydrofolic acid. Interrupts the process that causes inflammation to prevent damage to joints.

Contraindications

For all conditions: Breastfeeding, hypersensitivity to methotrexate or its components

For treatment of psoriasis or rheumatoid arthritis: Alcoholism; alcoholic liver disease; chronic liver disease; laboratory evidence or overt immunodeficiency syndromes; pregnancy; preexisting blood dyscrasias, such as bone marrow hypoplasia, leukopenia, significant anemia, or thrombocytopenia

Interactions

DRUGS

bone marrow depressants: Possibly increased bone marrow depression

chloramphenicol, nonabsorbable broad-spectrum antibiotics, tetracycline: Possibly decreased methotrexate absorption

co-trimoxazole: Possibly increased bone marrow suppression

folic acid: Possibly decreased effectiveness of methotrexate

hepatotoxic drugs: Increased risk of hepatotoxicity

NSAIDs, penicillins, phenylbutazone, phenytoin, probenecid, salicylates, sulfonamides: Increased risk of methotrexate toxicity

theophylline: Possibly increased risk of theophylline toxicity
vaccines: Risk of disseminated infection with live-virus vaccines, risk of suppressed response to killed-virus vaccines

ACTIVITIES

alcohol use: Increased risk of hepatotoxicity

Adverse Reactions

CNS: Aphasia, **cerebral thrombosis**, chills, dizziness, drowsiness, fatigue, fever, headache, hemiparesis, **leukoencephalopathy**, malaise, paresis, **seizures**
CV: Chest pain, **deep vein thrombosis**, **hypotension**, **pericardial effusion**, **pericarditis**, **thromboembolism**
ENDO: Gynecomastia
EENT: Blurred vision, conjunctivitis, gingivitis, glossitis, pharyngitis, stomatitis, transient blindness, tinnitus
GI: Abdominal pain, anorexia, **cirrhosis**, diarrhea, elevated liver enzymes, enteritis, **GI bleeding** and ulceration, **hepatitis**, **hepatotoxicity**, nausea, **pancreatitis**, vomiting
GU: Cystitis, hematuria, infertility, menstrual dysfunction, nephropathy, **renal failure**, **tubular necrosis**, vaginal discharge
HEME: Anemia, **aplastic anemia**, **leukopenia**, **neutropenia**, **pancytopenia**, **thrombocytopenia**
MS: Arthralgia, dysarthria, myalgia, stress fracture
RESP: Dry nonproductive cough, dyspnea, **interstitial pneumonitis**, pneumonia, **pulmonary fibrosis or failure**, **pulmonary infiltrates**
SKIN: Acne, alopecia, altered skin pigmentation, ecchymosis, **erythema multiforme**, **exfoliative dermatitis**, furunculosis, necrosis, photosensitivity, pruritus, psoriatic lesions, rash, **Stevens-Johnson syndrome**, telangiectasia, **toxic epidermal necrolysis**, ulceration, urticaria
Other: **Anaphylaxis**, increased risk of infection, injection site necrosis or reaction, lymphadenopathy, **lymphoproliferative disease**

Childbearing Considerations

PREGNANCY

- Drug can cause fetal harm, such as embryotoxicity and fetal defects or death.
- Drug is contraindicated in pregnant women with psoriasis or rheumatoid arthritis and should be used in the treatment of neoplastic disease only if benefit to the mother outweighs the risk to the fetus.
- A negative pregnancy test should be obtained before drug therapy is started.

LACTATION

- Drug may be present in breast milk.
- Breastfeeding should not be undertaken during drug therapy and for 1 wk after final dose because it may cause myelosuppression in the breastfed infant.

REPRODUCTION

- Because of fetal harm, both partners should avoid conception during and after drug is discontinued for 3 mo for male patients and 6 mo for female patients.
- Drug may cause fertility impairment, menstrual dysfunction, and oligospermia during drug therapy. It is not known if infertility is reversible.

Nursing Considerations

! **WARNING** Ensure that females of childbearing age have a negative pregnancy test before starting methotrexate therapy.

- Ensure patient is current on immunizations prior to starting methotrexate. Immunization with live vaccines is not recommended during treatment.

! **WARNING** Monitor results of CBC, chest x-ray, liver and renal function tests, and urinalysis before and during treatment because drug can cause serious adverse reactions to many systems, some of which could be life-threatening. Follow standard precautions such as infection control measures because drug can cause immunosuppression. Also, monitor patient for bruising or unexplained bleeding. Notify prescriber of any other persistent, serious, or unusual signs and symptoms.

! **WARNING** Monitor patient for hypersensitivity reactions to drug because severe reactions such as anaphylaxis have occurred with drug use. Report any such reactions immediately, expect drug to be discontinued and provide supportive care, as needed and ordered.

- Increase patient's fluid intake to 2 to 3 L daily, unless contraindicated, to reduce the risk of adverse genitourinary tract reactions.
- Be aware that high doses of methotrexate can impair renal elimination by forming crystals that obstruct urine flow. To prevent drug precipitation, alkalinize patient's urine with sodium bicarbonate tablets, as ordered.
- Be aware that if patient becomes dehydrated from vomiting, prescriber should be notified, and expect to withhold drug until patient recovers.
- Be aware that methotrexate resistance may develop with prolonged use.

PATIENT TEACHING

- Prepare a calendar of treatment days for patient and emphasize importance of following instructions exactly.
- Instruct patient, family, or caregiver how to administer the oral form of methotrexate prescribed.
- Instruct patient to avoid alcohol during methotrexate therapy. Tell patients being treated for cancer to also avoid folic acid or folinic acid unless they are directed to do so by the prescriber. However, tell patients being treated for polyarticular juvenile idiopathic arthritis, psoriasis, or rheumatoid arthritis that folic acid or folinic acid therapy may be needed to reduce the risk of adverse reactions to the drug.

! **WARNING** Alert patient to notify prescriber if an allergic reaction occurs; if severe, advise patient to seek immediate medical care.

! **WARNING** Urge patient to notify prescriber if persistent, serious, or unusual adverse reactions occur. Instruct patient on infection control measures and bleeding precautions to take while receiving methotrexate.

! **WARNING** Urge females of childbearing age to use reliable contraception during methotrexate therapy and for 6 months after last dose. Urge male patient or female partner of childbearing age to use reliable contraception during methotrexate therapy and for 3 months after last dose. Tell these patients to notify prescriber immediately if pregnancy occurs.

- Tell patient to inform all prescribers of methotrexate therapy as well as any concomitant drugs they may be taking, including over-the-counter drugs, herbal products, and vitamins.
- Advise patient not to receive live vaccines during methotrexate therapy.
- Encourage frequent mouth care to reduce the risk of mouth sores.
- Instruct patient to use sunblock when exposed to sunlight.
- Tell mothers not to breastfeed during drug therapy and for 1 week following final dose.

methoxypolyethylene glycol-epoetin beta

Mircera

Class and Category

Pharmacological class: Erythropoietin stimulating protein
Therapeutic class: Antianemic

Indications and Dosages

∗ *To treat anemia associated with chronic renal failure*

I.V. INJECTION, SUBCUTANEOUS INJECTION

Adults on dialysis and not currently being treated with an erythropoiesis-stimulating agent (ESA). *Initial:* 0.6 mcg/kg every 2 wk, increased or decreased by 25% monthly, as needed. *Maintenance:* Twice that of every 2-wk dose given every 4 wk and subsequently titrated, as needed.
Adults not on dailysis and not currently being treated with an ESA. 1.2 mcg/kg once a mo subcutaneously. Alternatively, 0.6 mcg/kg every 2 wk I.V. *Maintenance:* Twice that of every 2-wk dose given every 4 wk and subsequently titrated, as needed.
Adults stabilized on less than 8,000 units/wk of epoetin alfa or 40 mcg/wk of darbepoetin alfa. 60 mcg every 2 wk or 120 mcg every 4 wk.
Adults stabilized on 8,000 to 16,000 units/wk of epoetin alfa or 40 to 80 mcg/wk of darbepoetin alfa. 100 mcg every 2 wk or 200 mcg every 4 wk.

M

Adults stabilized on more than 16,000 units/wk of epoetin alfa or more than 80 mcg/wk of darbepoetin alfa. 180 mcg every 2 wk or 360 mcg every 4 wk.

I.V. INJECTION

Children ages 3 mo to 17 yr on or not on diaylsis who are converting from another erythropoiesis-stimulating agent (ESA) after hemoglobin level stabilized with an ESA. Initial dose calculated based on the total weekly erythropoiesis-stimulating agent (ESA) dose at the time of conversion and given once every 4 wk.

±**DOSAGE ADJUSTMENT** For all patients with chronic kidney disease who experience a rapid hemoglobulin increase of more than 1 g/dl in any 2-week period, dosage reduced by 25% or more, as needed. For adult patients on dialysis, if hemoglobin is approaching or exceeding 11 g/dl, dosage reduced or interrupted. If drug withheld until hemoglobin begins to decrease; then drug restarted at a dose 25% less than previously given. For all patients when hemoglobin doesn't increase by 1 g/dl after 4 weeks of therapy, dosage increased by 25%. For all patients with hypertension that is difficult to control, dose reduced, or drug withheld.

Drug Administration

I.V.

- Drug packaged as single-dose prefilled syringes.
- Drug contains no preservatives, so discard any unused portion.
- Do not pool unused portions from the prefilled syringes.
- Do not use the prefilled syringe more than once. Prefilled syringes are not to be used to administer partial doses.
- For patients who are less than 6 years of age, use the same route of administration as the previous ESA when switching from another ESA.
- Inspect solution in syringe. Do not use if not colorless to slightly yellow or if particulate matter is visible.
- Fully depress the plunger during injection for the needle guard to activate.
- Store in original cartons.
- Avoid vigorous shaking or prolonged exposure to light.
- Store in refrigerator. Store also at room temperature (for no more than 30 days).
- *Incompatibilities:* Parenteral solutions, other drugs mixed in prefilled syringes

SUBCUTANEOUS

- Follow guidelines for I.V. administration.
- Administer in the abdomen, arm, or thigh.
- Rotate sites.

Route	Onset	Peak	Duration
I.V., SubQ	7–15 days	72 hr	Unknown

Half-life: 134 hr

Mechanism of Action

Stimulates release of reticulocytes from bone marrow into the bloodstream, where they develop into mature RBCs.

Contraindications

Hypersensitivity to methoxypolyethylene glycol-epoetin beta or its components, pure red cell aplasia, uncontrolled hypertension

Interactions

DRUGS

None reported by manufacturer.

Adverse Reactions

CNS: **CVA**, headache, **seizures**
CV: Chest pain, **congestive heart failure**, **deep vein thrombosis**, hypertension, **hypotension**, **MI**, tachycardia, vascular access thrombosis
EENT: Nasopharyngitis
GI: Constipation, diarrhea, **GI bleeding**, vomiting
GU: UTI
HEME: **Severe anemia**, **including pure red cell aplasia**
MS: Back or limb pain, muscle spasms
RESP: **Bronchospasms**, cough, upper respiratory tract infection
SKIN: Erythema, pruritus, rash, **Stevens-Johnson syndrome**, **toxic epidermal necrolysis**, urticaria
Other: **Anaphylaxis**, **angioedema**, antibody formation to drug

Childbearing Considerations

PREGNANCY

- It is not known if drug causes fetal harm.
- Use with caution only if benefit to mother outweighs potential risk to fetus.

LACTATION

- It is not known if drug is present in breast milk.
- Mothers should check with prescriber before breastfeeding.

Nursing Considerations

- Use caution when administering drug to patients who have conditions that could decrease or delay response to drug, such as aluminum intoxication, folic acid deficiency, hemolysis, infection, inflammation, iron deficiency, osteitis (fibrosa cystica), or vitamin B_{12} deficiency.
- Monitor drug effectiveness by checking hemoglobin every 2 weeks until stabilized and maintenance dose has been established. Then, expect hemoglobin to be monitored at least monthly unless dosage adjustment is needed.

! WARNING Know that target hemoglobin shouldn't exceed 11 g/dl because it increases risk of life-threatening adverse cardiovascular effects. Keep in mind the risk of hypertensive or thrombotic complications increases if hemoglobin rises more than 1 g/dl over 2 weeks.

- Expect to give an iron supplement because iron requirements rise when erythropoiesis consumes existing iron stores.

! WARNING Monitor patient for hypersensitivity reactions, which could become life-threatening, such as anaphylaxis and angioedema. If present, stop drug immediately, notify prescriber, and expect to provide supportive care, as needed and ordered.

! WARNING Monitor patient for seizures, especially during the first couple months of therapy.

! WARNING Monitor patients closely with a cardiovascular disorder caused by a history of hypertension or vascular disease. Monitor patient's blood pressure. Be aware that if patient's blood pressure is difficult to control even with dietary measures or drug therapy, dose of methoxypolyethylene glycol-epoetin beta should be reduced or drug withheld until blood pressure is controlled.

! WARNING Monitor patients with a serious hematologic disorder, such as hypercoagulation, myelodysplastic syndrome, or sickle cell disease.

! WARNING Notify prescriber if patient has sudden loss of response to drug, evidenced by low reticulocyte count or severe anemia. Anti-erythropoietin antibody-related anemia may be present, which requires stopping drug and any other erythropoietic proteins.

PATIENT TEACHING

- Instruct patient how to self-administer drug subcutaneously, if prescribed. Explain to family or caregiver, if patient is a child, that children under age 17 should not inject drug.
- Stress importance of complying with dosage regimen.
- Encourage patient to eat iron-rich foods.

! WARNING Warn patient to stop taking drug immediately if an allergic reaction occurs and notify prescriber. If serious, tell patient to seek immediate medical care.

! WARNING Advise patient that the risk of seizures is highest during the first couple of months of methoxypolyethylene glycol-epoetin beta therapy. Urge the patient to avoid hazardous activities during this time and institute seizure precautions.

! WARNING Review possible adverse reactions, and urge patient to notify prescriber about any persistent, serious, or unusual adverse reactions, especially anemia manifestations as this may indicate drug has lost its effectiveness.

- Stress importance of keeping follow-up laboratory and medical appointments.

methyldopa

Class and Category

Pharmacologic class: Central alpha agonist
Therapeutic class: Antihypertensive

Indications and Dosages

✶ *To manage hypertension*

TABLETS

Adults. *Initial:* 250 mg 2 or 3 times daily for first 48 hr, decreased or increased, as needed, after 2 days with adjustments made no less than every 2 days. *Maintenance:* 500 to 2,000 mg daily in divided doses twice daily to 4 times daily. *Maximum:* 3,000 mg daily.
Children. *Initial:* 10 mg/kg daily in divided doses twice daily to 4 times daily for first 48 hr, decreased or increased, as needed, after 2 days with adjustments made no less than every 2 days. *Maximum:* 65 mg/kg or 3,000 mg daily, whichever is less.

±**DOSAGE ADJUSTMENT** For patients receiving other antihypertensives other than thiazides, initial dosage limited to 500 mg daily in divided doses.

Drug Administration

P.O.

- Drug should be administered consistently at same time each day.
- To minimize sedation, administer dosage increases in the evening.
- Store at room temperature.

Route	Onset	Peak	Duration
P.O.	3–6 hr	2–4 hr	12–48 hr

Half-life: 1.5–2 hr

Mechanism of Action

Decarboxylated in the body to produce alpha-methylnorepinephrine, a metabolite that stimulates central inhibitory alpha-adrenergic receptors thereby possibly reducing blood pressure by decreasing sympathetic stimulation of heart and peripheral vascular system.

Contraindications

Active hepatic disease, hypersensitivity to methyldopa or its components, impaired hepatic function from previous methyldopa therapy, use within 14 days of MAO inhibitor

Interactions

DRUGS

anesthetics: Possibly enhanced effect requiring reduced dosage of anesthetics
antihypertensives: Increased hypotension
CNS depressants: Possibly increased CNS depression
ferrous gluconate, ferrous sulfate: Decreased bioavailability of methyldopa
lithium: Increased risk of lithium toxicity
MAO inhibitors: Possibly hallucinations, headaches, hyperexcitability, and severe hypertension

ACTIVITIES

alcohol use: Possibly increased CNS depression

Adverse Reactions

CNS: Decreased concentration, depression, dizziness, drowsiness, fever, headache, involuntary motor activity, memory loss (transient), nightmares, paresthesia, parkinsonism, sedation, vertigo, weakness
CV: Angina, **bradycardia**, edema, **heart failure**, **myocarditis**, orthostatic hypotension
EENT: Black or sore tongue, dry mouth, nasal congestion
ENDO: Gynecomastia
GI: Constipation, diarrhea, flatulence, **hepatic necrosis**, **hepatitis**, jaundice, nausea, **pancreatitis**, vomiting
GU: Decreased libido, impotence
HEME: **Agranulocytosis**, **hemolytic anemia**, **leukopenia**, positive Coombs' test, positive tests for ANA and rheumatoid factor, **thrombocytopenia**
SKIN: Eczema, rash, urticaria
Other: Weight gain

Childbearing Considerations

PREGNANCY

- It is not known if drug causes fetal harm.
- Use with caution only if benefit to mother outweighs potential risk to fetus.

LACTATION

- Drug is present in breast milk.
- Mothers should check with prescriber before breastfeeding.

Nursing Considerations

! **WARNING** Obtain CBC and differential results before and periodically during methyldopa therapy, as ordered because drug can cause serious adverse to life-threatening hematologic reactions.

- Monitor blood pressure regularly during therapy to determine effectiveness of drug.

! **WARNING** Notify prescriber if patient has signs of heart failure such as dyspnea, edema, hypertension, or weight gain. Expect drug to be discontinued.

! **WARNING** Monitor results of Coombs' test; a positive result after several months of treatment indicates that patient has hemolytic anemia. Expect to discontinue drug.

- Monitor patient for involuntary, rapid, jerky movements in patients with severe bilateral cerebrovascular disease. Know that drug will need to be discontinued, if present.
- Be aware that hypertension may return within 48 hours after stopping drug.

PATIENT TEACHING

- Instruct patient how to administer methyldopa.
- Tell patient to take methyldopa exactly as prescribed and not to skip a dose. Explain that hypertension can return within 48 hours after stopping drug.
- Caution patient not to stop drug abruptly; doing so may cause withdrawal symptoms, such as headache, hypertension, increased sweating, nausea, and tremor.

! **WARNING** Direct patient to notify prescriber about bruising, chest pain, fever, involuntary jerky movements, prolonged dizziness, rash, and yellow eyes or skin.

- Instruct patient to weigh daily and to report a gain of more than 5 lb (2.3 kg) in 2 days.
- Advise patient to change position slowly to minimize orthostatic hypotension.

methylnaltrexone bromide

Relistor

Class and Category

Pharmacologic class: Peripheral mu-opioid receptor antagonist
Therapeutic class: GI effector

Indications and Dosages

✷ *To treat opioid-induced constipation in patients with advanced illness and not responsive to laxative therapy.*

SUBCUTANEOUS INJECTION

Adults weighing more than 114 kg (251 lb). 0.15 mg/kg every other day, as needed.
Adults weighing 62 to 114 kg (136 to 251 lb). 12 mg every other day, as needed.
Adults weighing 38 to less than 62 kg (84 to less than 136 lb). 8 mg every other day, as needed.
Adults weighing less than 38 kg (84 lb). 0.15 mg/kg every other day, as needed.

±**DOSAGE ADJUSTMENT** For patients with moderate to severe renal impairment, dosage reduced by half.

✷ *To treat opioid-induced constipation in patients with chronic noncancer pain*

SUBCUTANEOUS INJECTION

Adults. 12 mg once daily.

TABLETS

Adults. 450 mg once daily in the morning at least 30 min before first meal.

±**DOSAGE ADJUSTMENT** For patients with chronic noncancer pain with moderate to severe renal impairment (creatinine clearance less than 60 ml/min) taking tablet form, daily dosage reduced to 150 mg once daily and subcutaneous injection dosage reduced to 6 mg once daily. For patients with chronic noncancer pain with moderate to severe hepatic impairment, dosage reduced to 150 mg once daily for tablet form. For patients with severe hepatic impairment taking injection form, dosage reduced by half.

Drug Administration

P.O.

- Administer with water on an empty stomach at least 30 min before first meal of the day.

SUBCUTANEOUS

- Use the prefilled syringe only for patients who require a dose of 8 or 12 mg. Use the drug vial for administration for patients who require other doses.
- To determine volume of drug to give to patients weighing more than 114 kg (251 lb) or less than 38 kg (84 lb), multiply patient's weight in kilograms by 0.00375 and round up to the nearest 0.1 ml. For patients weighing 62 to 114 kg (136 to 251 lb), injection volume administered should be 0.3 ml. For patients weighing 38 to less than 62 kg (84 to less than 136 lb), injection volume administered should be 0.2 ml.
- Solution should be clear and colorless to pale yellow.

M

- Once drug is drawn from vial into syringe, drug is stable for 24 hr at room temperature.
- Inject into abdomen, thigh, or upper arm.
- Rotate injection sites.

Route	Onset	Peak	Duration
P.O.	30–60 min	30 min	Unknown
SubQ	Unknown	0.5 hr	Unknown

Half-life: 8 hr

Mechanism of Action

Binds to peripherally acting mu-opioid receptors in the GI tract, preventing opioid-induced slowing of GI motility and transit time, which then relieves constipation.

Contraindications

Hypersensitivity to methylnaltrexone bromide or its components, GI obstruction

Interactions

DRUGS

other opioid antagonists: Possible additive effects and increased risk of opioid withdrawal

Adverse Reactions

CNS: Anxiety, chills, dizziness, headache, malaise, tremor
EENT: Rhinorrhea
ENDO: Hot flashes
GI: Abdominal distention, pain, or tenderness; diarrhea; flatulence; GI cramping, **GI perforation**; nausea; vomiting
MS: Muscle spasms
SKIN: Excessive diaphoresis, piloerection

Childbearing Considerations

PREGNANCY

- Drug may cause fetal harm as drug may precipitate opioid withdrawal in a fetus.
- Use with caution only if benefit to mother outweighs potential risk to fetus.

LACTATION

- It is not known if drug is present in breast milk.
- Breastfeeding should not be undertaken during drug therapy.

Nursing Considerations

! **WARNING** Use methylnaltrexone cautiously in patients with known or suspected lesions of the GI tract as well as conditions that may affect the structural integrity of the GI tract wall, such as diverticular disease, infiltrative GI tract malignancies, Ogilvie's syndrome, peptic ulcer disease, and peritoneal metastases, because of increased risk of GI perforation.

! **WARNING** Monitor patient for development of persistent, severe, or worsening abdominal pain because GI perforation may occur with severe constipation that has not responded to methylnaltrexone therapy. Notify prescriber immediately and expect drug to be discontinued.

! **WARNING** Notify prescriber about persistent or severe diarrhea that may lead to severe dehydration and expect drug to be discontinued. Be aware that elderly patients experience a higher incidence of diarrhea.

- Monitor patient for symptoms of opioid withdrawal, such as abdominal pain, anxiety, chills, diaphoresis, diarrhea, or yawning that has occurred with methylnaltrexone therapy. Patients at greatest risk for opioid withdrawal are those who have disruptions to the blood–brain barrier with opioid administration.

PATIENT TEACHING

- Instruct patient how to administer oral form of methylnaltrexone or instruct patient, family, or caregiver how to prepare and administer the drug subcutaneously, if prescribed.
- Inform patient that a bowel movement may occur within 30 minutes after drug has been administered so patient should be near a toilet after administration.

! **WARNING** Advise patient that if abdominal pain, nausea, persistent or severe diarrhea, or vomiting that is new or worsens occurs, prescriber should be notified, and drug discontinued.

- Reassure patient that drug is not a controlled substance.
- Tell patient to stop taking methylnaltrexone if she stops taking opioid pain medication.
- Inform mothers breastfeeding should not be undertaken during drug therapy.

methylphenidate hydrochloride

Aptensio XR, Concerta, Cotempla XR-ODT, Daytrana, Jornay PM, Methylin, QuilliChew ER, Quillivant XR, Relexxii, Ritalin, Ritalin LA, Ritalin SR

Class, Category, and Schedule

Pharmacologic class: Piperidine
Therapeutic class: CNS stimulant
Controlled substance schedule: II

Indications and Dosages

* *To treat attention-deficit hyperactivity disorder (ADHD)*

CHEWABLE TABLETS (METHYLIN), ORAL SOLUTION, (METHYLIN), TABLETS (METHYLIN, RITALIN)

Adults. *Initial:* 20 to 30 mg in divided doses 2 or 3 times daily 30 to 45 min before breakfast and lunch, and a third dose between 2 and 4 pm, as needed. *Maximum:* 60 mg daily in 2 or 3 divided doses.
Children ages 6 and older. *Initial:* 5 mg twice daily 30 to 45 min before breakfast and lunch; increased by 5 to 10 mg daily at 1-wk intervals. *Maximum:* 60 mg daily in 2 to 3 divided doses.

S.R. TABLETS (RITALIN SR)

Adults and children ages 6 and older who are switching from immediate-release to sustained-release form. *Initial:* If dosage same as immediate release and not taken more frequently than every 8 hr, sustained-release dosage taken once daily before breakfast. *Maximum:* 60 mg once daily before breakfast.

E.R. CAPSULES (RITALIN LA)

Adults and children ages 6 to 12. *Initial:* 10 or 20 mg once daily, increased weekly in increments of 10 mg, as needed. *Maximum:* 60 mg daily.

± **DOSAGE ADJUSTMENT** For patients switching from Ritalin twice daily, if previous dose was 10 mg twice daily, dosage changed to 20 mg once daily; if previous dose was 15 mg twice daily, dosage changed to 30 mg once daily; if previous dose was 20 mg twice daily, dosage changed to 40 mg once daily; and if previous dose was 30 mg twice daily, dosage changed to 60 mg once daily.

E.R. ORAL SUSPENSION (QUILLIVANT XR)

Adults and children ages 6 and older. *Initially:* 20 mg once daily in morning; increased weekly in increments of 10 to 20 mg, as needed. *Maximum:* 60 mg daily.

E.R. TABLETS (CONCERTA, RELEXXII)

Adults ages 18 to 65 and children ages 6 and older who are methylphenidate naive. 18 mg daily before breakfast for children and adolescents and 18 mg to 36 mg once daily before breakfast for adults; increased in 18-mg increments at 1-wk intervals. *Maximum:* 72 mg daily (adults and children over age 12), 54 mg/day (children ages 6 to 12).
Adults and children ages 6 and older who are currently taking immediate-release methylphenidate tablets. If previous dosage was 5 mg twice daily or 3 times daily, dosage switched to 18 mg once daily in morning; if previous dosage was 10 mg twice daily or 3 times daily, dosage switched to 36 mg once daily in morning; if previous dosage was 15 mg twice daily or 3 times daily, dosage switched to 54 mg in the morning; and for adults only if dosage was 20 mg twice daily or 3 times daily, dosage switched to 72 mg in the morning.

E.R. CAPSULES (APTENSIO XR)

Adults and children ages 6 and older. *Initial:* 10 mg once daily in morning, increased by 10 mg once daily weekly, as needed. *Maximum:* 60 mg once a day in the morning.

ORALLY DISINTEGRATING TABLET (COTEMPLA XR-ODT)

Children ages 6 to 17. *Initial:* 17.3 mg once daily in the morning, then titrated weekly in increments of 8.6 mg to 17.3 mg. *Maximum:* 51.8 mg daily.

E.R. CHEWABLE TABLETS (QUILLICHEWER)

Adults and children ages 6 and older. *Initial:* 20 mg once daily in the morning, increased weekly in increments of 10 mg, 15 mg, or 20 mg daily, as needed. *Maximum:* 60 mg once daily in the morning.

E.R. CAPSULES (JORNAY PM)

Adults and children ages 6 and older. 20 mg once daily in evening, increased weekly in increments of 20 mg, as needed. *Maximum:* 100 mg once daily.

TRANSDERMAL PATCH (DAYTRANA)

Adults and children ages 6 and older. *Initial:* 10-mg (12.5-cm^2) patch worn 9 hr daily for wk 1; 15-mg (18.75-cm^2) patch worn 9 hr daily for wk 2; 20-mg (25-cm^2) patch worn 9 hr daily for wk 3; 30-mg (37.5-cm^2) patch worn 9 hr daily for wk 4 and thereafter. *Maximum:* 30-mg (37.5-cm^2) patch worn 9 hr daily.

* *To treat narcolepsy*

CHEWABLE TABLETS (METHYLIN), ORAL SOLUTION, TABLETS (METHYLIN, RITALIN)

Adults. *Initial:* 20 to 30 mg in divided doses daily 30 to 45 min before meals. *Maximum:* 60 mg daily in 2 or 3 divided doses.

Children ages 6 and older. *Initial:* 5 mg twice daily before breakfast and lunch, increased weekly in increments of 5 to 10 mg weekly, as needed. *Maximum:* 60 mg daily in divided doses.

S.R. TABLETS (RITALIN SR)

Adults who are switching from immediate-release to sustained-release form. *Initial:* If dosage same as immediate release and not taken more frequently than every 8 hr, dosage same for sustained release taken once daily before breakfast, increased by 10 mg weekly, as needed. *Maximum:* 60 mg once daily before breakfast.

Drug Administration

P.O.

- Administer in relationship to meals or time of day according to product being administered. See Indications and Dosages section.
- Administer last dose of the day by 6 p.m., except for Jornay PM, which is administered in the evening.
- Chewable tablets should be thoroughly chewed before swallowing and administered with a full glass of water or another type of beverage.
- Tablets and capsules should be swallowed whole and not chewed, crushed, or split/opened, except for Aptensio XR, Jornay PM, or Ritalin LA, which may be opened, and contents sprinkled onto a small amount of cool applesauce and ingested immediately. Follow with water.
- Vigorously shake oral suspension bottle made by pharmacist for at least 10 sec before each dose. If using the oral dosing dispenser, remove the bottle cap and confirm that the bottle adapter has been inserted into the top of the bottle. Insert the tip of the oral dosing dispenser provided into the bottle adapter, turn bottle upside down, and withdraw prescribed amount of liquid into the oral dosing dispenser. Then, remove the filled oral dosing dispenser from bottle and dispense drug directly into patient's mouth. Replace the bottle cap and wash the oral dosing dispenser after each use. Store at room temperature. Discard after 4 mo.
- Use calibrated device to measure dosage of oral solution.
- Administer orally disintegrating tablets with dry, gloved hands by first peeling back the foil on the blister pack. Do not push tablet through the foil. Carefully remove tablet from blister pack and place on patient's tongue. There is no need for patient to take a drink following administration.

TRANSDERMAL

- After opening pouch and removing protective liner, apply patch to a clean, dry area on patient's hip. Press patch firmly in place for about 30 sec.
- Avoid applying patch to skin that's damaged, irritated, or oily and avoid the waistline, where clothing may dislodge the patch.
- Have patient avoid bathing, showering, or swimming while patch is on because water can interfere with patch adherence.
- Do not apply or re-apply patch with common adhesives, dressings, or tape. Instead if a patch does fall off, a new patch may be applied, but the total exposure time for the day shouldn't exceed 9 hr.
- Rotate application site by applying on other hip.

Route	Onset	Peak	Duration
P.O. (tablets)	20–60 min	2–4 hr	3–6 hr
P.O./E.R.	20–60 min	8–12 hr	Unknown
P.O./S.R.	20–60 min	3–8 hr	Unknown
P.O. (E.R. once daily)	Unknown	Unknown	About 12 hr
Transdermal	2 hr	8–10 hr	10 hr

Half-life: 3–8 hr

Mechanism of Action

Blocks the reuptake mechanism of dopaminergic neurons in the cerebral cortex and subcortical structures of the brain, including the thalamus, decreasing motor restlessness, and improving concentration. May trigger sympathomimetic activity to produce decreased fatigue and increase alertness and motor activity in patients with narcolepsy.

Contraindications

Agitation, marked anxiety, tension; glaucoma; hypersensitivity to methylphenidate or its components; tics or diagnosis or history of Tourette's syndrome; use within 14 days of an MAO inhibitor

Interactions

DRUGS

anticonvulsants, oral anticoagulants, phenylbutazone, tricyclic antidepressants: Inhibited metabolism and increased blood levels of these drugs
antihypertensives: Decreased effectiveness of antihypertensives
buspirone, fentanyl, lithium, MAO inhibitors, selective serotonin reuptake inhibitors, serotonin–norepinephrine reuptake inhibitors, St. John's wort, tricyclic antidepressants, triptans, tryptophan: Increased risk of serotonin syndrome
gastric pH modulators: May interfere with the pharmacodynamics of orally disintegrating tablet form
halogenated anesthetics: May increase risk of sudden blood pressure and heart rate elevation during surgery
MAO inhibitors: Possibly increased adverse effects of methylphenidate, possibly severe hypertension
risperidone: Increased risk of extrapyramidal symptoms

ACTIVITIES

alcohol use: Possibly increased CNS effects; with long-acting forms, possible increased adverse effects

FOODS

caffeine: Increased methylphenidate effects

Adverse Reactions

CNS: Aggressiveness, agitation, anger, anxiety, cerebral arteritis, **cerebral occlusion**, confusion, **CVA**, depression, disorientation, dizziness, drowsiness, dyskinesia, emotional lability, excessive talkativeness, extrapyramidal disorder, fatigue, fever, hallucinations, headache, hyperactivity, hypomania, insomnia, irritability, ischemic neurologic defects (reversible), lability of affect, lethargy, mania, migraine, motor and verbal tics, nervousness, **neuroleptic malignant syndrome**, obsessive–compulsive disorder (rare), paresthesia, psychosis, restlessness, sedation, **seizures**, somnolence, **suicidal ideation**, transient mood depression, tension, tremor, Tourette's syndrome (rare), toxic psychosis, vertigo
CV: Angina, **arrhythmias**, **bradycardia**, **cardiac arrest**, chest discomfort or pain, **extrasystoles**, hypertension, **hypotension**, **MI**, necrotizing vasculitis, palpitations, peripheral vasculopathy, including Raynaud's phenomenon, **sudden death**, **supraventricular tachycardia**, tachycardia, vasculitis
EENT: Accommodation abnormality, acute angle closure glaucoma, blurred vision, diplopia, dry mouth or throat, increased intraocular pressure, mydriasis, nasopharyngitis, pharyngitis, rhinitis, sinusitis, trismus (restricted opening of mouth), vision changes
ENDO: Dysmenorrhea, growth suppression in children with long-term use, gynecomastia
GI: Abdominal pain, anorexia, constipation, diarrhea, dyspepsia, elevated bilirubin and liver enzymes, **hepatotoxicity**, nausea, **severe hepatic failure or injury**, vomiting
GU: Decreased libido, hematuria, priapism
HEME: Anemia, **decreased platelet count**, **leukopenia**, **pancytopenia**, **thrombocytopenia**, **thrombocytopenic purpura**
MS: Arthralgia, myalgia, muscle tightness or twitching, **rhabdomyolysis**
RESP: Cough, dyspnea, upper respiratory tract infection
SKIN: Allergic contact dermatitis, alopecia, application-site reactions (transdermal patch), bullous skin conditions, chemical leukoderma (persistent loss of skin pigmentation with transdermal patch), erythema, **erythema multiforme**, exanthemas, excessive diaphoresis, **exfoliative dermatitis**, fixed drug eruption, pruritus, rash, urticaria

Other: **Anaphylaxis**, **angioedema**, elevated alkaline phosphatase, physical and psychological dependence, weight loss (prolonged use)

Childbearing Considerations

PREGNANCY

- Pregnancy exposure registry: 1-866-961-2388 or https://womensmentalhealth.org/adhd-medications/.
- It is not known if drug causes fetal harm.
- Use with caution only if benefit to mother outweighs potential risk to fetus.

LACTATION

- Drug is present in breast milk.
- Mothers should check with prescriber before breastfeeding.
- If breastfeeding occurs, infant should be monitored for agitation, anorexia, insomnia, and reduced weight gain.

Nursing Considerations

! WARNING Know that drug should not be administered to patients with cardiomyopathy, coronary artery disease, known structural cardiac abnormalities, serious cardiac arrhythmia, or other serious cardiac disease because sudden death has occurred during methylphenidate therapy.

! WARNING Keep in mind that, when signs and symptoms of ADHD occur with acute stress reactions or with preexisting structural cardiac abnormalities or other serious heart problems, methylphenidate usually isn't indicated because of possible worsened reaction or sudden death.

- Expect patient with significant hyperopia or abnormally increased intraocular pressure to be evaluated by an ophthalmologist before drug therapy begins because drug may cause angle closure glaucoma and increased intraocular pressure.
- Assess patient and family history of tics and Tourette's syndrome before drug therapy begins because drug can cause or exacerbate motor and verbal tics and Tourette's syndrome. Monitor patient closely throughout drug therapy.

! WARNING Be aware that methylphenidate has a high potential for abuse, addiction, and misuse with possibility of overdose, and possibly death, especially with excessive dosage. Monitor patient for evidence of physical dependence or abuse throughout methylphenidate therapy. Monitor patient's intake of drug closely.

! WARNING Know that the E.R. tablet form (Concerta) shouldn't be given to patients with esophageal motility disorders; drug may cause GI obstruction because tablet doesn't change shape in GI tract.

! WARNING Monitor patient for suicidal behavior or thinking. Watch patient closely (especially children, adolescents, and young adults), for suicidal tendencies, particularly when therapy starts and dosage changes, because depression may worsen temporarily during these times, possibly leading to suicidal ideation.

! WARNING Monitor patient for a hypersensitivity reaction, which could become life-threatening, such as anaphylaxis or angioedema. If present, notify prescriber, expect drug to be discontinued, and provide supportive care, as needed and ordered.

- Monitor transdermal patch application site for erythema. If more intense reactions occur with erythema, such as local edema or papule or vesicle formation that doesn't improve within 48 hours after patch is removed from irritated site or that spreads beyond the patch site, further diagnostic testing is required to determine presence of allergic contact dermatitis.

! WARNING Know that patients with allergic contact dermatitis from transdermal patch may develop systemic allergy reaction if methylphenidate is taken by another route, such as by mouth. Monitor patient closely if route of administration changes and report any evidence of flare-up of previous dermatitis or positive patch-test sites, generalized skin eruptions in previously unaffected skin, or other symptoms, such as arthralgia, diarrhea, fever, headache, malaise, or vomiting because drug may have to be discontinued.

! WARNING Be alert for seizure activity in patients receiving methylphenidate as drug-induced seizures may occur.

! **WARNING** Be aware that methylphenidate may induce CNS stimulation and psychosis and may worsen behavior disturbances and thought disorders in patients who already have psychosis. Use drug cautiously in patients with psychosis. Monitor children and adolescents for first-time psychotic or manic symptoms. If present, notify prescriber and expect drug to be discontinued.

! **WARNING** Monitor patient for other persistent, serious, or unusual adverse reactions because drug can cause multiple adverse reactions from many body systems.

! **WARNING** Monitor patient closely for serotonin syndrome, a rare but serious adverse effect of methylphenidate when taken in combination with serotonergic drugs. Signs and symptoms include agitation, confusion, diaphoresis, diarrhea, fever, hyperactive reflexes, poor coordination, restlessness, shaking, talking or acting with uncontrolled excitement, tremor, and twitching. If symptoms occur, notify prescriber immediately, expect drug to be discontinued, and provide supportive care.

- Monitor patient's blood pressure and heart rate during drug therapy because drug may cause hypertension and tachycardia. Expect methylphenidate to be withheld on the day of surgery if patient will be receiving anesthetics because concurrent use with halogenated anesthetics may increase the risk of sudden blood pressure and heart rate elevation during surgery.
- Inspect patient's fingers and toes for signs of peripheral vasculopathy, such as digital ulceration and/or soft-tissue breakdown. Although usually mild and intermittent, more severe manifestation may occur. Notify prescriber, if present, and expect dose to be reduced or drug discontinued.
- Monitor growth in children. Report failure to grow or gain weight and expect to stop drug.

! **WARNING** Avoid stopping drug abruptly after long-term use because doing so may unmask dysphoria, paranoia, severe depression, or suicidal thoughts.

PATIENT TEACHING

- Instruct patient, family, or caregiver how to administer form of methylphenidate prescribed.

! **WARNING** Warn patient that methylphenidate is a controlled substance and can be abused and lead to dependence. Dosage should not be increased, or dosage interval shortened without prescriber knowledge. Encourage family or caregiver to obtain naloxone for home use; if and when it's needed, it will be readily available. Review signs and symptoms of an overdose and how to administer naloxone. Stress importance of the need to call 911 if naloxone is administered.

- Alert patient taking drug long term that prescriber may take patient off drug periodically to determine continued need.
- Advise patient to avoid alcohol while taking methylphenidate.

! **WARNING** Urge family or caregiver to watch patient closely for suicidal tendencies, especially when therapy starts or dosage changes and particularly if patient is a child, teenager, or young adult.

! **WARNING** Alert patient, family, or caregiver that drug may cause an allergic reaction. If present, tell them to notify prescriber and stop drug therapy. If reaction is severe, patient should seek immediate medical care.

! **WARNING** Warn patient, family, or caregiver drug may cause seizures. If a seizure occurs, tell patient to notify prescriber and seek immediate medical care.

! **WARNING** Alert patient, family, or caregiver that psychotic or manic symptoms, even without a prior history, may occur and should be reported to prescriber.

! **WARNING** Warn male patients and family, or caregiver of male children that painful or prolonged penile erections may occur while taking the drug, especially after a dosage increase or during period of drug withdrawal. In the event that this happens, immediate medical attention should be sought.

! **WARNING** Instruct patient, family, or caregiver to report other adverse reactions that may be persistent, serious, or unusual because drug can adversely affect many body systems such as causing symptoms of a heart attack or stroke.

- Advise patient, family, or caregiver if new tics or worsening of tics or Tourette's occurs to notify prescriber.
- Instruct patient to tell all prescribers about methylphenidate therapy, as serious drug interactions can occur.
- Inform family or caregiver of children on long-term therapy that drug may delay growth.
- Instruct patient, family, or caregiver to monitor fingers and toes for ulceration and/or soft-tissue breakdown. If noticed, prescriber should be called. Reassure patient that signs and symptoms generally improve after the dose is reduced or drug is discontinued.
- Inform mothers who are breastfeeding to monitor their infant for agitation, anorexia, insomnia, and reduced weight gain.
- Instruct patient, family, or caregiver to keep drug in a safe place, preferably locked, to prevent theft and not to share drug with anyone. Also instruct patient how to safely dispose of unused or expired drug.

! **WARNING** Urge patient to avoid stopping drug abruptly after long-term use because doing so may unmask dysphoria, paranoia, severe depression, or suicidal thoughts.

methylprednisolone

Medrol

methylprednisolone acetate

Depo-Medrol

methylprednisolone sodium succinate

Solu-Medrol

Class and Category

Pharmacologic class: Glucocorticoid
Therapeutic class: Corticosteroid

Indications and Dosages

✱ To treat immune and inflammatory disorders

TABLETS (METHYLPREDNISOLONE)

Adults. 4 to 48 mg daily as a single dose or in divided doses. Alternatively, twice the daily dose every other day.
Children. 0.11 to 1.66 mg/kg daily in divided doses 3 times daily or 4 times daily.

I.M. INJECTION, I.V. INFUSION, I.V. INJECTION (METHYLPREDNISOLONE SODIUM SUCCINATE)

Adults. *Initial:* 10 to 40 mg with subsequent doses dictated by patient's response and condition being treated.
Children. 0.11 to 1.66 mg/kg daily in divided doses 3 times daily or 4 times daily.

I.M. INJECTION (METHYLPREDNISOLONE ACETATE)

Adults. *Initial:* 4 to 120 mg daily according to clinical response.

INTRA-ARTICULAR, INTRALESIONAL, OR SOFT-TISSUE INJECTION (METHYLPREDNISOLONE ACETATE)

Adults. 4 to 10 mg for small joints; 10 to 40 mg for medium joints; and 20 to 80 mg for large joints every 1 to 5 wk, according to clinical response.

Drug Administration

P.O.

- Give drug with food to minimize GI irritation and indigestion.
- For once-daily dosing, give in the morning to coincide with normal cortisol secretion.

I.V.

- Store drug at room temperature. Protect from light.
- Never administer methylprednisolone acetate intravenously.
- Use only the accompanying diluent or Bacteriostatic Water for Injection with Benzyl Alcohol for reconstitution.
- Do not use formulations containing benzyl alcohol in neonates. Instead, use preservative-free formulations.
- Compatible diluents include 0.9% Sodium Chloride Injection, 5% Dextrose in Water, and 5% Dextrose in Water/0.9% Sodium Chloride Injection.
- Reconstitute and further dilute drug following manufacturer's guidelines.

- When using the ACT-O-VIAL system, press down on plastic activator to force diluent into the lower compartment. Gently agitate to mix solution. After removing plastic tab covering center of stopper and sterilizing stopper, insert needle squarely through center of stopper until tip is just visible. Invert vial and withdraw dose. Then, continue to follow manufacturer's guidelines.
- For I.V. injection, administer diluted drug directly into a vein or through a free-flowing compatible I.V. solution over at least 5 min.
- For I.V. infusion, administer diluted drug over 30 min for doses less than 0.5 g and over at least 30 to 60 min for doses greater than 0.5 g or 30 mg/kg.
- Discard mixed solution after 48 hr.
- *Incompatibilities:* None reported by manufacturer.

I.M.

- Inject slowly and deeply into gluteal muscle.
- Do not inject into deltoid muscle because of risk of subcutaneous atrophy.
- If a large dose is prescribed, divide dose into several small injections rather than administering as a single large dose.
- Rotate sites.

INTRA-ARTICULAR/INTRALESIONAL/ SOFT-TISSUE INJECTIONS

- Administered by healthcare professional trained in these types of injections.

Route	Onset	Peak	Duration
P.O.	Rapid	1–2 hr	30–36 hr
I.V.	< 1 hr	0.8 hr	12 hr
I.M.	6–48 hr	4–8 days	1–4 wk
Intra-articular/ intralesional/ soft tissue	Rapid	7 days	1–5 wk

Half-life: 12–36 hr

Mechanism of Action

Binds to intracellular glucocorticoid receptors and suppresses inflammatory and immune responses by inhibiting accumulation of monocytes and neutrophils at inflammation sites, stabilizing lysosomal membranes, suppressing the antigen response of macrophages and helper T cells, and inhibiting the synthesis of inflammatory response mediators, such as cytokines, interleukins, and prostaglandins.

Contraindications

Hypersensitivity to methylprednisolone or its components, idiopathic thrombocytopenic purpura (I.M.), intrathecal administration, premature infants (preparations containing benzyl alcohol), systemic fungal infections

Interactions

DRUGS

aminoglutethimide: Possibly loss of methylprednisolone-induced adrenal suppression
amphotericin B, potassium-depleting diuretics: Possibly severe hypokalemia
anticholinesterases: Possibly severe weakness in patients with myasthenia gravis
aspirin, NSAIDs: Increased risk of adverse GI effects and bleeding
barbiturates, carbamazepine, phenytoin, rifampin: Decreased blood methylprednisolone level
cholestyramine: Possibly increased methylprednisolone clearance
cyclosporine: Increased activity of both drugs
digoxin: Possibly hypokalemia-induced arrhythmias and digitalis toxicity
estrogens, oral contraceptives: Possibly increased therapeutic and toxic effects of methylprednisolone
insulin, oral antidiabetic drugs: Possibly increased blood glucose level
isoniazid: Possibly decreased therapeutic effects of isoniazid
ketoconazole, macrolide antibiotics, such as erythromycin and troleandomycin: Decreased methylprednisolone clearance and increased risk of adverse effects
oral anticoagulants, thrombolytics: Increased risk of decreased therapeutic effects of these drugs
vaccines: Decreased antibody response and increased risk of neurologic complications

ACTIVITIES

alcohol use: Increased risk of adverse GI effects, including bleeding

Adverse Reactions

CNS: Ataxia, behavioral changes, depression, dizziness, euphoria, fatigue,

headache, **increased intracranial pressure with papilledema**, insomnia, malaise, mood changes, neuropathy, paresthesia, restlessness, **seizures**, steroid psychosis, syncope, vertigo
CV: **Arrhythmias**, **cardiac arrest**, edema, **fat embolism**, **heart failure**, hypertension, **hypertrophic cardiomyopathy** (premature infants), **hypotension**, **myocardial rupture following recent MI**, tachycardia, **thromboembolism**, thrombophlebitis
EENT: Exophthalmos, glaucoma, increased intraocular pressure, nystagmus, posterior subcapsular cataracts
ENDO: **Adrenal insufficiency**, cushingoid symptoms (buffalo hump, central obesity, moon face, supraclavicular fat pad enlargement), diabetes mellitus, growth suppression in children, hyperglycemia
GI: Abdominal distention, **acute hepatitis**, elevated liver enzymes, hepatomegaly, hiccups, increased appetite, **melena**, nausea, **pancreatitis**, peptic ulcer, ulcerative esophagitis, vomiting
GU: Amenorrhea, glycosuria, menstrual irregularities, perineal burning or tingling
HEME: Easy bruising, leukocytosis
MS: Arthralgia; aseptic necrosis of femoral and humeral heads; Charcot-like arthropathy; compression fractures; muscle atrophy, twitching, or weakness; myalgia; osteoporosis; spontaneous fractures; steroid myopathy; tendon rupture
RESP: **Pulmonary edema**
SKIN: Acne; allergic dermatitis; altered skin pigmentation; diaphoresis; dry, scaly skin; erythema; hirsutism; necrotizing vasculitis; petechiae; purpura; rash; scarring; sterile abscess; striae; subcutaneous fat atrophy; thin, fragile skin; urticaria
Other: Activation of latent infections, **anaphylaxis**, **angioedema**, exacerbation of systemic fungal infections, **hypernatremia**, **hypocalcemia**, **hypokalemia**, **hypokalemic alkalosis**, impaired wound healing, masking of signs of infection, **metabolic alkalosis**, negative nitrogen balance from protein catabolism, suppressed skin test reaction, **tumor lysis syndrome (in presence of malignancies)**, weight gain

Childbearing Considerations

PREGNANCY

- Drug may cause fetal harm. Some formulations contain benzyl alcohol, which can cross the placental barrier and cause "gasping syndrome" in premature infants when born.
- Use with caution only if benefit to mother outweighs potential risk to fetus.
- Infants born to mothers who have received corticosteroids during pregnancy should be observed for hypoadrenalism.

LACTATION

- Drug appears in breast milk and could suppress growth, interfere with endogenous corticosteroid production, or cause other adverse effects if infant is breastfed.
- A decision should be made to discontinue breastfeeding or the drug to avoid potential serious adverse reactions in the breastfed infant.

Nursing Considerations

! **WARNING** Know that high doses of methylprednisolone should not be used for the treatment of traumatic brain injury because of increased risk of death. Preparations containing benzyl alcohol should not be used to treat pediatric patients because of risk of "gasping syndrome."

- Know that high doses of methylprednisolone should not be used in patients with active ocular herpes simplex because of risk of corneal perforation.

! **WARNING** Administer methylprednisolone with extreme caution in patients with a recent MI because corticosteroid use may increase risk of left ventricular free wall rupture.

! **WARNING** Use cautiously in patients with congestive heart failure or renal insufficiency because sodium retention and edema can occur in patients taking a corticosteroid. Also, use cautiously in patients with diverticulitis, fresh intestinal anastomoses, nonspecific ulcerative colitis, or peptic ulcer; these conditions increase risk of perforation during corticosteroid therapy. In addition, use caution in patients with systemic sclerosis, because drug may increase risk of scleroderma renal crisis.

! **WARNING** Monitor patient for a hypersensitivity reaction, which could become life-threatening, such as anaphylaxis or angioedema. If present, notify prescriber, expect drug to be switched to a different steroid, and provide supportive care, as needed and ordered.

! **WARNING** Closely monitor patient for signs of infection because drug may mask them or may worsen systemic fungal infections or active latent disease. Be aware that chickenpox and measles can become life-threatening in patients taking a corticosteroid.

! **WARNING** Expect to taper long-term therapy when discontinuing drug to avoid possibly fatal acute adrenocortical insufficiency and expect dosage to be increased during times of stress.

! **WARNING** Monitor patient's liver enzymes, as ordered, especially in patients receiving high doses. This is important because, although rare, this can develop into a toxic form of acute hepatitis. The onset of liver dysfunction can occur several weeks or even longer after administration of methylprednisolone. Notify prescriber if liver dysfunction is suspected and expect drug to be discontinued, as condition can develop into acute liver failure and death.

! **WARNING** Monitor patients with malignancies, including hematological malignancies and solid tumors for tumor lysis syndrome. Patients at higher risk include patients with high sensitivity to cytotoxic agents, high tumor burden, or have a high proliferative rate.

- Assess for possible depression or psychotic episodes during therapy.
- Protect patient from falling, especially elderly patient at risk for fractures from osteoporosis.
- Monitor blood glucose level; dosage of insulin or oral antidiabetic drug may have to be adjusted in diabetic patient.
- Be aware that changes in thyroid function, such as development of hyperthyroidism or hypothyroidism, may require dosage adjustment in chronic therapy because metabolic clearance of methylprednisolone is affected by thyroid activity.
- Know that skin testing should be avoided during methylprednisolone therapy because drug may suppress reaction.

PATIENT TEACHING

- Instruct patient how to administer oral form of methylprednisolone and what to do if a dose is missed.
- Urge patient to take calcium supplements, vitamin D, or both if recommended by prescriber.
- Inform patient that insomnia and restlessness usually resolve after 1 to 3 weeks.

! **WARNING** Caution patient not to stop taking methylprednisolone abruptly, especially if taking drug long-term or to change dosage without consulting prescriber.

! **WARNING** Alert patient that drug may cause an allergic reaction. Tell patient to notify prescriber if an allergic reaction occurs and to seek immediate medical care, if severe.

! **WARNING** Review signs and symptoms of infection and infection control measures to implement such as avoiding people with contagious diseases. Warn patient to immediate notify prescriber if chickenpox or measles exposure occurs, especially if patient has never experienced these infections or if other signs and symptoms of infection occur.

! **WARNING** Review signs and symptoms of tumor lysis syndrome (GI and urinary symptoms, hyperkalemia, and hypocalcemia) with patients with a malignancy and stress importance of alerting prescriber immediately, if present.

! **WARNING** Urge patient to notify prescriber immediately of signs of impending adrenocortical insufficiency, such as anorexia, dizziness, fainting, fatigue, fever, joint pain, muscle weakness, or nausea; and swelling or sudden weight gain. Also, tell patient to notify prescriber immediately of black or tarry stools or any other persistent, serious, or unusual adverse reactions.

- Instruct patients with diabetes to monitor his blood glucose level closely as drug can affect blood glucose control.

- Instruct patient not to obtain vaccinations unless approved by prescriber.
- Explain the need for regular exercise or physical therapy to maintain muscle mass.
- Inform mothers wishing to breastfeed that breastfeeding needs to be discontinued during drug therapy or drug will have to be discontinued.
- Advise patient to carry medical identification that documents his need for long-term corticosteroid therapy.

metoclopramide

Gimoti

metoclopramide hydrochloride

Reglan

Class and Category

Pharmacologic class: Dopamine-2 receptor antagonist
Therapeutic class: Antiemetic, upper GI stimulant

Indications and Dosages

✶ *To treat acute and recurrent diabetic gastroparesis*

ORALLY DISINTEGRATING TABLETS, ORAL SOLUTION, TABLETS

Adults experiencing mild symptoms. 10 mg 4 times daily before each meal and at bedtime for 2 to 8 wk. *Maximum:* 40 mg daily in divided doses; no longer than 12 wk.

I.M. OR I.V. INJECTION

Adults experiencing severe symptoms. 10 mg 4 times daily for up to 10 days followed by oral dosing for 2 to 8 wk. I.V. injection given undiluted slowly over 1 to 2 min.

NASAL SPRAY (GIMOTI)

Adults less than 65 yr of age. 15 mg (1 spray) in one nostril 4 times daily 30 min before meals and at bedtime for 2 to 8 wk. *Maximum:* 60 mg (4 sprays) daily; no longer than 12 wk.

±**DOSAGE ADJUSTMENT** For patients ages 65 and older, nasal spray not used for initial therapy. For elderly patient already stabilized on a dosage of 10 mg 4 times daily with another form of drug, patient may be switched to nasal spray with a dosage of 15 mg (1 spray) in one nostril 4 times daily for 2 to 8 weeks.

✶ *To treat gastroesophageal reflux disease (GERD)*

ORALLY DISINTEGRATING TABLETS, ORAL SOLUTION, TABLETS

Adults. *Continuous dosing:* 10 to 15 mg 4 times daily 30 min before meals and at bedtime for 4 to 12 wk. *Intermittent dosing:* Up to 20 mg as a single dose prior to provoking situation. *Maximum:* 60 mg daily in divided doses; no longer than 12 wk.

±**DOSAGE ADJUSTMENT** For patients with diabetic gastroparesis or GERD who are taking tablet form (not orally disintegrating tablet) and are elderly, dosage reduced to 5 mg 4 times daily. For patients who are CYP2D6 poor metabolizers or have moderate to severe hepatic or renal impairment or are taking strong CYP2D6 inhibitors, such as bupropion, fluoxetine, paroxetine, or quinidine, dosage reduced to 5 mg 4 times daily or 10 mg 3 times daily with maximum dosage reduced to 30 mg daily. For patients with end-stage renal disease, including those treated with continuous ambulatory peritoneal dialysis or hemodialysis, dosage reduced to 5 mg 4 times daily or 10 mg twice daily with maximum dosage reduced to 20 mg daily. For patients who are taking orally disintegrating tablets or oral solution and have a creatinine clearance of less than 40 ml/min, dosage reduced by 50%.

✶ *To prevent or reduce nausea and vomiting from emetogenic cancer chemotherapy*

I.V. INFUSION

Adults receiving less emetogenic regimens. 1 mg/kg infused over at least 15 min 30 min before chemotherapy and repeated every 2 hr for 2 additional doses, then every 3 hr for 3 doses.

Adults receiving highly emetogenic regimens with drugs, such as cisplatin or dacarbazine. 2 mg/kg infused over at least 15 min 30 min before chemotherapy and repeated every 2 hr for 2 additional doses, then every 3 hr for 3 doses.

✶ *To prevent postoperative nausea and vomiting*

I.M. INJECTION

Adults. 10 to 20 mg given at or near end of surgery.

✱ *To facilitate small bowel intubation; to aid in radiological examinations*

I.V. INJECTION

Adults and adolescents over age 14. 10 mg as a single undiluted dose given over 1 to 2 min.

Children ages 6 to 14. 2.5 to 5 mg as a single undiluted dose given over 1 to 2 min.

Children under the age of 6. 0.1 mg/kg as a single undiluted dose given over 1 to 2 min.

±**DOSAGE ADJUSTMENT** For patients with a creatinine clearance less than 40 ml/min, parenteral dosages reduced by half.

Drug Administration

P.O.

- Give oral solution and tablets 30 min before meals and at bedtime when used to treat gastroparesis and GERD. A single dose may be given prior to provoking situation for GERD.
- Use a calibrated device to measure dosage of oral solution.
- Give orally disintegrating tablets 30 min before each meal and at bedtime. A single dose may be given prior to provoking situation for GERD. Remove orally disintegrating tablet from sealed blister (do not push tablet through covering) with dry, gloved hand and give to patient to place on her tongue. If the orally disintegrating tablet breaks or crumbles, discard and obtain a new one.

I.V.

- I.V. injection is given for doses of 10 mg or less. Inject undiluted over 1 to 2 min.
- I.V. infusion is used for doses greater than 10 mg. Dilute in 50 ml 0.9% Sodium Chloride Injection (preferred solution), 5% Dextrose in Water, 5% Dextrose in Water/0.45% Sodium Chloride Injection, Lactated Ringer's, or Ringer's solution. Infuse over at least 15 min. Diluted drug can be stored for 48 hr if refrigerated or if diluted with 0.9% Sodium Chloride it may be frozen for up to 4 weeks. It does not need to be protected from light if diluted solution is administered within 24 hours. If protected from light and refrigerated, it may be administered up to 48 hours.
- Avoid rapid I.V. delivery because it may cause anxiety, restlessness, and drowsiness.
- *Incompatibilities:* Cephalothin sodium, chloramphenicol, sodium bicarbonate

I.M.

- Inject into a large muscle mass.
- Rotate sites.

INTRANASAL

- Administer 30 min before each meal and at bedtime.
- Prime spray bottle before first use by pressing down firmly and releasing 10 times on the finger flange (a spray should appear after the first few times of pressing down).
- Have the patient place the tip of the spray nozzle under 1 nostril and lean head slightly forward so the tip is aimed away from the septum and toward the back of the nose. Then have patient close the other nostril with the other index finger and move spray pump upwards so tip of nozzle is in the nostril. To ensure a full dose, have patient hold the bottle upright while pressing down firmly and completely on finger flange and release while inhaling slowly through the open nostril. Have patient remove the nozzle tip from nostril and exhale slowly through mouth.
- If uncertain that the spray has entered the nose, do not repeat the dose but administer dose at the next scheduled time. Likewise, if a dose is missed, do not make up for the missed dose or double the next dose.
- Wipe the spray nozzle with a clean tissue.
- Clear a nozzle that has become clogged by removing the spray nozzle and soaking it in warm water and then rinse. Do not insert a pin or other sharp object into nozzle to clear clog. Dry spray nozzle at room temperature and when dry place back on the spray bottle.
- Discard nasal spray 4 wk after opening even if bottle contains unused drug.

Route	Onset	Peak	Duration
P.O.	30–60 min	1–2 hr	1–2 hr
I.V.	1–3 min	15 min	1–2 hr
I.M.	10–15 min	Unknown	1–2 hr
Intranasal	30–60 min	Unknown	Unknown

Half-life: 5–6 hr; 8 hr (nasal spray)

Mechanism of Action

Antagonizes the inhibitory effect of dopamine on GI smooth muscle. This causes gastric contraction, which promotes gastric emptying and peristalsis, and also reduces gastroesophageal reflux. Blocks dopaminergic receptors in the chemoreceptor trigger zone, preventing nausea and vomiting.

Contraindications

Catecholamine-releasing paragangliomas; epilepsy; history of dystonic reaction or tardive dyskinesia to metoclopramide; hypersensitivity to metoclopramide or its components; pheochromocytoma; when stimulation of GI motility might be dangerous, such as in the presence of GI hemorrhage, mechanical obstruction, or perforation

Interactions

DRUGS

anticholinergics, antidiarrheals, antiperistaltics, antipsychotic drugs: Potential for additive effects, including increased frequency and severity of neuroleptic malignant syndrome, other extrapyramidal symptoms, and tardive dyskinesia
CNS depressants, such as anxiolytics, hypnotics, opiates, sedatives: Increased risk of CNS depression
atovaquone, cimetidine, digoxin, posaconazole (oral suspension): Decreased absorption and reduced effectiveness of these drugs
CNS depressants: Possibly increased CNS depression
cyclosporine, sirolimus, tacrolimus: Increased absorption and risk of adverse effects
CYP2D6 inhibitors (strong), such as bupropion, fluoxetine, paroxetine, quinidine: Increased plasma concentrations of metoclopramide; risk of exacerbation of extrapyramidal symptoms
dopaminergic agonists and other drugs that increase dopamine concentrations, such as apomorphine, bromocriptine, cabergoline, levodopa, pramipexole, ropinirole, rotigotine: Decreased effectiveness of metoclopramide; potential for exacerbation of symptoms, such as parkinsonism
MAO inhibitors: Increased risk of severe hypertension
mivacurium, succinylcholine: Enhanced neuromuscular blockade
serotonergic drugs: Possible development of serotonin syndrome

ACTIVITIES

alcohol use: Risk of increased CNS depression

Adverse Reactions

CNS: Agitation, anxiety, confusion, depression, dizziness, drowsiness, extrapyramidal reactions (motor restlessness, parkinsonism, tardive dyskinesia), fatigue, hallucinations, headache, insomnia, irritability, lassitude, nervousness, **neuroleptic malignant syndrome**, panic reaction, restlessness, **seizures**, **suicidal ideation**
CV: **AV block**, **bradycardia**, fluid retention, **heart failure**, hypertension, **hypotension**, **supraventricular tachycardia**
EENT: Dry mouth, glossal edema, **laryngeal edema**, visual disturbances
ENDO: Galactorrhea, gynecomastia, hyperprolactinemia
GI: Constipation, diarrhea, nausea
GU: Impotence, menstrual irregularities, urinary frequency or incontinence
HEME: **Agranulocytosis**, **leukopenia**, **methemoglobinemia**, **neutropenia**, **sulfhemoglobinemia**
RESP: **Bronchospasm**
SKIN: Rash, urticaria
Other: **Angioedema**, porphyria, restless leg syndrome

Childbearing Considerations

PREGNANCY

- It is not known if drug causes fetal harm.
- Use with caution only if benefit to mother outweighs potential risk to fetus.

LABOR AND DELIVERY

- Drug crosses the placental barrier and may cause extrapyramidal signs and methemoglobinemia in the neonate if given to mother during delivery.
- Use with caution only if benefit to mother outweighs potential risk to fetus.

LACTATION

- Drug is present in breast milk and may cause GI adverse effects in the breastfed infant such as intestinal discomfort and increased intestinal gas formation as well as extrapyramidal signs (dystonias) and methemoglobinemia.
- Mothers should check with prescriber before breastfeeding.

Nursing Considerations

- Know that orally disintegrating tablets are not recommended for use in children because of increased risk of tardive dyskinesia and other extrapyramidal symptoms.

! WARNING Be aware that metoclopramide therapy should not be used in patients with depression because of increased risk of suicidal ideation. Monitor patient for suicidal ideation throughout drug therapy because it can occur even in patients without depression.

! WARNING Know that drug should not be given to patients with a history of hypertension or patients taking monoamine oxidase inhibitors because of increased risk of hypertension that could lead to a hypertensive crisis. Monitor blood pressure throughout therapy. Expect drug to be discontinued in any patient with a rapid rise in blood pressure.

- Assess patient for signs of intestinal obstruction, such as abnormal bowel sounds, diarrhea, nausea, and vomiting, before administering metoclopramide. Notify prescriber if detected.

! WARNING Monitor patient for a hypersensitivity reaction, which may become life-threatening, such as angioedema. If present, notify prescriber, expect drug to be discontinued, and provide supportive care, as needed and ordered.

! WARNING Notify prescriber if patient shows signs of toxicity, such as disorientation, drowsiness, and extrapyramidal reactions.

! WARNING Monitor patient's CBC periodically, as ordered, for abnormalities because drug can cause serious to life-threatening adverse hematologic reactions. Observe patient for signs of bruising, unexplained bleeding, or infection and report to prescriber, if present.

! WARNING Watch closely for tardive dyskinesia, especially in the elderly, women, and patients with diabetes because this serious adverse effect is often irreversible even after therapy stops. Therapy lasting longer than 12 weeks isn't recommended because risk of tardive dyskinesia increases the longer the patient takes metoclopramide. Risk also has been linked to total cumulative dose so prescriber must take this into account when setting dosage. Also, be aware that drug can cause other extrapyramidal symptoms besides tardive dyskinesia. For example, though rare, drug may cause dystonic reactions such as dyspnea and stridor, possibly caused by laryngospasm. At first sign of involuntary movements of face, tongue, or limbs, or any other abnormal sign or symptom, notify prescriber and expect to discontinue drug.

! WARNING Monitor patient with NADH-cytochrome b5 reductase deficiency because metoclopramide increases risk of methemoglobinemia and sulfhemoglobinemia. For patients with glucose-6-phosphate dehydrogenase (G6PD) deficiency, methylene blue treatment is not recommended if metoclopramide-induced methemoglobinemia occurs because the treatment may cause hemolytic anemia in these patients, which may be fatal.

! WARNING Monitor patient closely for neuroleptic malignant syndrome, a rare but potentially fatal disorder characterized by altered level of consciousness, arrhythmias, diaphoresis, hyperthermia, irregular pulse or blood pressure, muscle rigidity, and tachycardia. Know that risk increases in patients experiencing a toxic reaction to metoclopramide as a result of overdosage or receiving concomitant treatment with another drug associated with neuroleptic malignant syndrome. Expect metoclopramide to be discontinued immediately, if present.

- Monitor patient, especially a patient with heart failure or cirrhosis, for possible fluid retention or volume overload due to transient increase in plasma aldosterone level. Expect metoclopramide to be discontinued if fluid retention occurs.

PATIENT TEACHING

- Instruct patient on how to take the form of metoclopramide prescribed.
- Urge patient to avoid alcohol and CNS depressants while taking metoclopramide.

! **WARNING** Alert patient that drug may cause an allergic reaction. Tell patient to notify prescriber if an allergic reaction occurs and to seek immediate medical care, if severe.

! **WARNING** Warn family or caregiver to monitor patient for abnormal behavior or thoughts that may be suggestive of suicidal ideation. If concerns are raised, urge them to contact prescriber.

! **WARNING** Stress importance to mothers who are breastfeeding while taking metoclopramide to notify pediatrician of any adverse effects noticed in infant and to stop breastfeeding or consult prescriber about stopping drug therapy.

! **WARNING** Tell patient to immediately report involuntary movements of face, eyes, tongue, or hands, including lip smacking, chewing, puckering of mouth, frowning, scowling, sticking out tongue, blinking, moving eyes, or shaking arms and legs.

! **WARNING** Stress importance of reporting other signs and symptoms that are persistent, severe, or unusual.

- Advise against activities that require alertness.
- Urge patient to tell all prescribers about metoclopramide therapy.

metolazone

Class and Category

Pharmacologic class: Thiazide-like diuretic
Therapeutic class: Diuretic

Indications and Dosages

* *To manage mild to moderate hypertension*

TABLETS

Adults. 2.5 to 5 mg once daily.

* *To manage edema from heart failure or renal disease*

TABLETS

Adults. 5 to 10 mg once daily for edema of heart failure; 5 to 20 mg once daily for edema of renal disease.

Drug Administration

P.O.

- Administer at same time every day in the morning.

Route	Onset	Peak	Duration
P.O.	1 hr	8 hr	24 hr

Half-life: 6–14 hr

Mechanism of Action

Promotes renal excretion of sodium and water by inhibiting their reabsorption in distal convoluted tubules causing extracellular fluid volume and plasma to be reduced, which reduces blood pressure. Helps to reduce blood pressure also by decreasing peripheral vascular resistance.

Contraindications

Anuria, hepatic coma or precoma, hypersensitivity to metolazone or its components

Interactions

DRUGS

ACTH or corticosteroids: Possible increased risk of hypokalemia and salt and water retention
antigout drugs: Increased blood uric acid level and risk of gout attack
barbiturates, narcotics, other antihypertensives: Increased risk of orthostatic hypotension
digoxin: Increased risk of electrolyte imbalances and digoxin-induced arrhythmias
diuretics: Additive effects of both drugs, possibly leading to electrolyte imbalances and severe hypovolemia
hydralazine: Possibly interference with the natriuretic action of metolazone
insulin, oral antidiabetic drugs: Decreased effectiveness of these drugs, increased risk of hyperglycemia
lithium: Increased risk of lithium toxicity
neuromuscular blockers: Increased risk of hypokalemia and neuromuscular blockade, increased risk of respiratory depression
NSAIDs, sympathomimetics: Possibly decreased metolazone effectiveness

ACTIVITIES

alcohol use: Increased risk of orthostatic hypotension

Adverse Reactions

CNS: Anxiety, chills, depression, dizziness, drowsiness, headache, insomnia, neuropathy, paresthesia, restlessness, syncope, weakness

CV: Chest pain, cold extremities, orthostatic hypotension, palpitations, peripheral edema, vasculitis, **venous thrombosis**
EENT: Bitter taste, blurred vision, dry mouth, epistaxis, pharyngitis, sinus congestion, tinnitus
ENDO: Hyperglycemia
GI: Abdominal pain, anorexia, cholecystitis, constipation, diarrhea, **hepatic dysfunction**, **hepatitis**, indigestion, nausea, **pancreatitis**, vomiting
GU: Decreased libido, glycosuria, impotence
HEME: **Agranulocytosis**, **aplastic anemia**, **leukopenia**, **thrombocytopenia**
MS: Arthralgia, myalgia
RESP: Cough
SKIN: Dry skin, necrosis, petechiae, photosensitivity, pruritus, rash, urticaria
Other: Gout, hypochloremia, **hypokalemia**, **hyponatremia**, hypovolemia, **metabolic alkalosis**

Childbearing Considerations

PREGNANCY

- Drug may cause fetal harm such as fetal or neonatal jaundice, thrombocytopenia, and possibly other adverse reactions that have occurred in adults.
- Use with caution only if benefit to mother outweighs potential risk to fetus.

LACTATION

- Drug is present in breast milk.
- Breastfeeding is not recommended during drug therapy.

Nursing Considerations

- Anticipate giving metolazone with a loop diuretic if patient responds poorly to loop diuretic therapy alone.
- Measure patient's fluid intake and output and daily weight to monitor drug's diuretic effect.

! WARNING Monitor blood chemistry test results and assess for evidence of hypochloremia, hypokalemia, and, possibly, mild metabolic alkalosis. Also monitor patient's CBC, as ordered, because drug can cause serious adverse hematological reactions.

- Monitor serum calcium and uric acid levels, especially if patient has a history of gout or renal calculi. Metolazone may slightly increase calcium reabsorption and decrease uric acid excretion.

PATIENT TEACHING

- Inform patient that metolazone controls but doesn't cure hypertension. Discuss possible need for lifelong therapy and consequences of uncontrolled hypertension.
- Instruct patient how to administer metolazone.
- Emphasize the importance of diet control, especially limiting sodium intake, and maintaining a normal weight.

! WARNING Urge patient to notify prescriber about persistent, severe diarrhea, nausea, or vomiting, which can cause dehydration and orthostatic hypotension. Also, tell patient to notify prescriber if persistent, serious, or unusual adverse reactions occur.

- Advise patient to change position slowly to minimize orthostatic hypotension.
- Inform diabetic patient that metolazone may increase blood glucose level and that he should check his level often.
- Inform mothers that breastfeeding is not recommended during metolazone therapy.

metoprolol succinate

Kapspargo Sprinkle, Toprol-XL

metoprolol tartrate

Lopresor (CAN), Lopresor SR (CAN), Lopressor

M

Class and Category

Pharmacologic class: Beta$_1$-adrenergic blocker
Therapeutic class: Antianginal, antihypertensive

Indications and Dosages

* *To manage hypertension, alone or with other antihypertensives*

E.R. CAPSULES (KAPSPARGO SPRINKLE), E.R. TABLETS (TOPROL-XL)

Adults. *Initial:* 25 to 100 mg once daily, adjusted weekly or longer, as needed. *Maximum:* 400 mg daily.
Children ages 6 and older. *Initial:* 1 mg/kg (maximum 50 mg) once daily, adjusted weekly, as needed. *Maximum:* 2 mg/kg (maximum 200 mg) once daily.

TABLETS (LOPRESSOR)

Adults. *Initial:* 100 mg once daily or 50 mg twice daily increased weekly, as needed, to achieve optimum blood pressure control. *Usual effective dose:* 100 to 450 mg daily. *Maximum:* 450 mg daily as a single dose or in divided doses.

✱ *To treat hemodynamically stable patients with definite or suspected acute MI to reduce cardiovascular mortality*

TABLETS (LOPRESSOR), I.V. INJECTION (LOPRESSOR)

Adults. *Initial:* 5 mg by I.V. bolus every 2 min for 3 doses followed by 25 to 50 mg P.O. every 6 hr for 48 hr, starting 15 min after final I.V. dose. *Maintenance:* 100 mg P.O. twice daily for at least 3 mo.

±**DOSAGE ADJUSTMENT** For patients who develop an intolerance to oral dose, dosage reduced to 25 mg.

✱ *To treat angina pectoris long-term; to reduce angina attacks; to improve exercise tolerance*

E.R. CAPSULES (KAPSPARGO SPRINKLE), E.R. TABLETS (TOPROL-XL)

Adults. 100 mg once daily, increased weekly, as needed. *Maximum:* 400 mg daily.

TABLETS (LOPRESSOR)

Adults. *Initial:* 50 mg twice daily, adjusted weekly in increments of 50 mg twice daily, as needed. *Maximum:* 400 mg daily.

✱ *To reduce risk of cardiovascular mortality and heart-failure hospitalization in patients with heart failure*

E.R. TABLETS (TOPROL-XL)

Adults. *Initial:* 25 mg once daily for class II heart failure or 12.5 mg once daily for more severe heart failure for 2 wk. Then, dosage doubled every 2 wk, as tolerated. *Maximum:* 200 mg daily.

E.R. CAPSULES (KAPSPARGO SPRINKLE)

Adults. *Initial:* 25 mg once daily for 2 wk. Then, dosage doubled every 2 wk, as tolerated. *Maximum:* 200 mg daily.

±**DOSAGE ADJUSTMENT** For elderly patients or patients with hepatic impairment, initial dosage reduced with gradual dose titration. For patients who experience symptomatic bradycardia, dosage reduced.

Drug Administration

P.O.

- Administer with or immediately after a meal.
- Tablets may be cut in half, but not chewed or crushed and should be swallowed as a whole or half of tablet, if split.
- For patient unable to swallow E.R. capsules, open capsule and sprinkle over soft food, such as applesauce, pudding, or yogurt. Mixture must be swallowed within 60 min and never stored for later use.
- E.R. capsule form can be administered via a nasogastric tube by mixing contents of opened capsule with 15 ml of water and drawing mixture up into a syringe. Gently shake mixture for about 10 sec, then flush it through a 12 French or larger nasogastric tube. Ensure no pellets are left in the syringe. Rinse the tube with water until all of drug is washed out.

I.V.

- Administer drug undiluted as an I.V. injection over 2 min.
- Drug should only be administered in a coronary care or intensive care setting.
- *Incompatibilities:* None reported by manufacturer

Route	Onset	Peak	Duration
P.O.	15 min	1 hr	3–6.5 hr
P.O. (E.R.)	15 min	6–12 hr	24 hr
I.V.	5 min	20 min	5–8 hr

Half-life: 3–7 hr

Mechanism of Action

Inhibits stimulation of beta$_1$-receptor sites, located mainly in the heart, resulting in decreased cardiac excitability, cardiac output, and myocardial oxygen demand to help relieve angina, minimize cardiac tissue damage from a myocardial infarction, and help relieve symptoms of heart failure. Helps reduce blood pressure also by decreasing renal release of renin.

Contraindications

For all indications: Hypersensitivity to metoprolol, other beta-blockers, or their components

For angina and hypertension: Cardiogenic shock, heart block greater than first degree, overt cardiac failure, sinus bradycardia

For MI: Heart rate less than 45 beats/min, moderate to severe cardiac failure, second- and third-degree heart block, significant first-degree heart block (P-R interval 0.24 sec or greater), systolic blood pressure less than 100 mm Hg

Interactions

DRUGS

alpha-adrenergic agents, such as alpha-methyldopa, betanidine, guanethidine, reserpine: Possibly increased antihypertensive effects
calcium channel blockers: Increased risk of additive reduction in myocardial contractility
catecholamine-depleting drugs, such as reserpine: Possibly additive effect resulting in hypotension or marked bradycardia
CYP2D6 inhibitors, such as antiarrhythmics (propafenone, quinidine), antidepressants (bupropion, clomipramine, desipramine, fluoxetine, fluvoxamine, paroxetine, sertraline), antifungals (terbinafine), antihistamines (diphenhydramine), antimalarials (hydroxychloroquine, quinidine), antipsychotics (chlorpromazine, fluphenazine, haloperidol, thioridazine), antiretrovirals (ritonavir): Increased plasma metoprolol level causing decrease in the cardioselectivity of metoprolol
clonidine: Increased risk of bradycardia and hypotension; increased risk of rebound hypertension when clonidine is discontinued
digoxin, other beta-blockers: Decreased heart rate and slowed atrioventricular conduction
dipyridamole: Possibly altered heart rate
ergot alkaloids: Possibly enhanced vasoconstrictive action of ergot alkaloids
hydralazine: Increased metoprolol concentration
MAO inhibitors: Possibly significant hypertension
other antihypertensives: Additive hypotensive effect
prazosin: Possibly increased postural hypotensive effect of first dose of prazosin

FOODS

all foods: Increased bioavailability of metoprolol

Adverse Reactions

CNS: Anxiety, confusion, **CVA**, depression, dizziness, drowsiness, fatigue, hallucinations, headache, insomnia, nightmares, paresthesia, short-term memory loss, somnolence, syncope, tiredness, vertigo, weakness
CV: Angina, **arrhythmias (including AV block and bradycardia)**, **arterial insufficiency**, **cardiac arrest**, **cardiogenic shock**, chest pain, decreased HDL level, increased triglyceride levels, gangrene of extremity, **heart failure**, hypertension, orthostatic hypotension, palpitations, peripheral edema
EENT: Blurred vision, dry eyes or mouth, nasal congestion, rhinitis, taste disturbance, tinnitus
ENDO: **Hypoglycemia**
GI: Constipation, diarrhea, flatulence, heartburn, **hepatitis**, nausea, vomiting
GU: Decreased libido, impotence
HEME: **Agranulocytosis**, **leukopenia**, **thrombocytopenia**
MS: Arthralgia, back pain, myalgia
RESP: **Bronchospasm**, dyspnea, shortness of breath
SKIN: Alopecia, diaphoresis, photosensitivity, pruritus, rash, urticaria, worsening of psoriasis

Childbearing Considerations

PREGNANCY

- It is not known if drug causes fetal harm. However, drug crosses the placenta, placing the fetus at risk for bradycardia, hypoglycemia, hypotension, and respiratory depression at birth.
- Use with caution only if benefit to mother outweighs potential risk to fetus.
- Mothers with hypertension have an increased risk for pre-eclampsia, gestational diabetes, premature delivery, and delivery complications.

LACTATION

- Drug is present in breast milk.
- Mothers should check with prescriber before breastfeeding.
- If breastfeeding occurs with a mother who is a slow metabolizer of drug, breastfed infant should be monitored for bradycardia and other symptoms of beta-blockade such as constipation, diarrhea, or dry eyes, mouth, or skin.

REPRODUCTION

- Drug may cause erectile dysfunction and inhibit sperm motility.

Nursing Considerations

! WARNING Know that beta-blockers such as metoprolol should not be given to patients with bronchospastic disease because drug can exacerbate bronchospasm. However, metoprolol may be given to these patients for initial treatment of an MI but bronchodilators should be readily available for use or administered concomitantly.

! **WARNING** Know that patients undergoing noncardiac major surgery should not begin a high-dose regimen using E.R. metoprolol because such use in patients with cardiovascular risk factors has been associated with bradycardia, hypotension, stroke, and death. However, also be aware that beta-blocker therapy such as metoprolol that is already in place should not be routinely discontinued prior to major surgery.

! **WARNING** Be aware that if patient has pheochromocytoma, alpha-blocker therapy should start first, followed by metoprolol to prevent paradoxical increase in blood pressure from attenuation of beta-mediated vasodilation in skeletal muscle.

! **WARNING** Substituting metoprolol for clonidine requires gradually reducing clonidine and increasing metoprolol dosage over several days. This is because given together, these drugs have additive hypotensive effects.

- Use cautiously in patients with angina or hypertension who have congestive heart failure because beta-blockers such as metoprolol can further depress myocardial contractility, worsening heart failure. If worsening heart failure occurs, expect diuretic therapy to be increased and measures to stabilize patient utilized before administering the next dose. Expect to decrease the metoprolol dosage if patient with heart failure develops symptomatic bradycardia.

! **WARNING** Assess patient's ECG before metoprolol therapy is begun and then throughout drug therapy, as ordered, because patients taking metoprolol may be at risk for bradycardia including cardiac arrest, heart block, and sinus pause. Patients at risk include patients with conduction disorders (including Wolff-Parkinson-White), first-degree AV block, sinus node dysfunction or use of drugs concomitantly that cause bradycardia. Monitor patient closely for bradycardia. If severe, notify prescriber, expect dosage to be reduced or drug discontinued. Prepare for the possibility of assisting with insertion of temporary pacemaker.

! **WARNING** Be aware that patients with a history of severe anaphylactic reactions may be more reactive to repeated challenges of the allergen while taking beta-blocker therapy, such as metoprolol, and may be unresponsive to the usual doses of epinephrine used to treat an allergic reaction.

! **WARNING** Monitor patient for hypoglycemia, especially in patients with diabetes or when patient is in a fasting state or is vomiting. Also, know that beta-blockers like metoprolol may prevent early warning signs of hypoglycemia, such as tachycardia. Be aware that this may increase the risk for severe or prolonged hypoglycemia at any time during drug therapy. Treat hypoglycemia according to institutional protocol and alert prescriber if hypoglycemia occurs frequently or becomes severe.

- Monitor patient with hyperthyroidism closely because beta-adrenergic blockers, such as metoprolol, may mask signs of hyperthyroidism, such as tachycardia. Also, know that abrupt discontinuation of metoprolol should be avoided because thyroid storm could be precipitated.
- Monitor patient with peripheral vascular disease for evidence of arterial insufficiency (coldness, pain, and pallor in affected extremity). Metoprolol can precipitate or aggravate peripheral vascular disease.

! **WARNING** Expect to taper dosage over 1 to 2 weeks when drug is discontinued; stopping abruptly can cause MI, myocardial ischemia, severe hypertension, or ventricular arrhythmias, especially in patients with cardiac disease.

PATIENT TEACHING

- Instruct patient how to administer form of metoprolol prescribed.

! **WARNING** Caution patient not to stop drug abruptly as serious to life-threatening reactions can occur. For example, if a patient with hyperthyroidism abruptly stops drug, it can precipitate a medical emergency called thyroid storm.

! **WARNING** Warn patient with a history of severe anaphylactic reactions that he may be more reactive to repeated challenges of the allergen while taking beta-blocker therapy, such as metoprolol, Stress importance of seeking immediate medical care at the first sign of an allergic reaction to anything.

! **WARNING** Teach patient how to take a radial pulse. Advise patient to notify prescriber if pulse rate falls below 60 beats/min or is significantly lower than usual.

! **WARNING** Tell patient to contact prescriber if breathing difficulties occur, edema or other signs of heart failure worsen, or if other persistent, serious, or unusual adverse reactions occur.

! **WARNING** Review signs and symptoms of hypoglycemia with patient and family or caregiver. Warn patient, family, or caregiver severe hypoglycemia may occur if patient is unable to eat regularly or vomiting occurs. Instruct patient, family, or caregiver on how to manage hypoglycemia. Tell patient to alert prescriber if hypoglycemia occurs frequently. If hypoglycemia is severe, urge patient to seek immediate emergency care.

! **WARNING** Warn breastfeeding mother who is a slow metabolizer of drug, to monitor her breastfed infant for a slow heart rate and other symptoms of beta-blockade such as constipation, diarrhea, or dry eyes, mouth, or skin. If present, she should notify pediatrician immediately.

- Advise patient to avoid performing hazardous activities such as driving until effects of drug are known and resolved.
- Advise patient with peripheral vascular disease to watch for coldness, pain, and pallor in affected extremity as drug can precipitate or aggravate peripheral vascular disease.

metronidazole

Flagyl, Flagyl I.V. RTU, Likmez, Metro I.V.

Class and Category

Pharmacologic class: Nitroimidazole
Therapeutic class: Antiprotozoal

Indications and Dosages

* *To treat systemic anaerobic infections caused by susceptible anaerobic bacteria*

CAPSULES, ORAL SUSPENSION (LIKMEZ), TABLETS

Adults. 7.5 mg/kg every 6 hr for 7 to 10 days. Infections of bone and joint, endocardium, or lower respiratory tract infections may require longer treatment. *Maximum:* 4,000 mg daily.

I.V. INFUSION

Adults. *Initial:* 15 mg/kg infused over 1 hr as a single dose and then 7.5 mg/kg infused over 1 hr every 6 hr for 7 to 10 days. Infections of bone and joint, endocardium, or lower respiratory tract infections may require longer treatment. *Maximum:* 4,000 mg daily.

* *To treat amebiasis*

CAPSULES, ORAL SUSPENSION (LIKMEZ), TABLETS

Adults. *For acute amebic dysentery:* 750 mg 3 times daily for 5 to 10 days. *For amebic liver abscess:* 500 (oral suspension, tablets) or 750 mg (tablets, capsules, or oral suspension) 3 times daily for 5 to 10 days.
Children. 35 to 50 mg/kg/24 hr in 3 divided doses daily for 10 days. *Maximum:* 2,250 mg/24 hr (750 mg/dose or 7.5 ml/dose) for 10 days.

* *To treat trichomoniasis* (Trichomonas vaginalis)

TABLETS

Adults. 2,000 mg as a single dose, 1,000 mg twice daily for 1 day, or 250 mg 3 times daily for 7 days.

CAPSULES

Adults. 375 mg 2 times daily for 7 days.

ORAL SUSPENSION (LIKMEZ)

Adults. 2 g (20 ml) given as a single dose, or 2 divided doses of 1 g (10 ml) given on the same day. Alternatively, 250 mg (2.5 ml) 3 times daily for 7 consecutive days.

* *To treat bacterial vaginosis*

✱ *To prevent postoperative bowel infection in elective colorectal surgery, which is contaminated or potentially contaminated*

I.V. INFUSION

Adults. 15 mg/kg infused over 30 to 60 min and completed 1 hr before surgery and then 7.5 mg/kg infused over 30 to 60 min 6 and 12 hr after initial dose.

E.R. TABLETS

Adult nonpregnant women and postmenarchal adolescents. 750 mg once daily for 7 days.

±**DOSAGE ADJUSTMENT** For patients with severe hepatic impairment, dosage reduced by 50%. For patients with end-stage renal failure receiving hemodialysis and the administration of drug cannot be separated from the dialysis session, a supplemental dose of the drug is recommended to be given following hemodialysis.

✱ *Topical and vaginal forms presented in appendix*

Drug Administration

P.O.

- Administer immediate-release drug with food to minimize adverse GI reactions.
- Administer E.R. tablets 1 hr before or 2 hr after a meal.
- Capsules and tablets should be swallowed whole and not chewed, crushed, or split/opened.
- Shake oral suspension bottle well and use a calibrated oral dosing device to correctly measure dosage.

I.V.

- Do not use aluminum equipment such as needles or cannulae that would come in contact with drug solution, as precipitates may form.
- Don't give drug by I.V. injection; administer only as a slow I.V. infusion.
- Do not use if solution is cloudy or precipitated or if the seal is not intact.
- For use of Viaflex plus plastic container, do not connect flexible plastic containers in series or pressurize intravenous solutions contained in flexible plastic containers to increase flow rate because an air embolism could result when administering drug. In addition, vented intravenous administration sets with the vent in the open position should not be used with flexible plastic containers.
- Discontinue primary I.V. infusion during metronidazole infusion.
- Using ready-to-use solutions (no buffering or dilution required), infuse over 30 to 60 min for prophylactic use; 60 min for treatment of systemic anaerobic infections.
- Change intravenous administration equipment at least once every 24 hr.
- Store at room temperature. Refrigeration may cause precipitation to occur.
- *Incompatibilities:* Aztreonam, cefamandole nafate, cefoxitin, penicillin G, and other additives, drugs, or solutions; I.V. equipment made of aluminum

Route	Onset	Peak	Duration
P.O.	Unknown	1–2 hr	Unknown
P.O./E.R.	15 min	4.6–6.8 hr	Unknown
I.V.	Immediate	1 hr	Unknown

Half-life: 8 hr

Mechanism of Action

Undergoes intracellular chemical reduction during anaerobic metabolism, which damages DNA's helical structure and breaks its strands thereby inhibiting bacterial nucleic acid synthesis and causing cell death.

Contraindications

Alcohol use, including products containing propylene glycol during and for at least 3 days after metronidazole therapy; Cockayne syndrome; hypersensitivity to metronidazole, other nitroimidazole derivatives, or their components; use of disulfiram within past 2 wk

Interactions

DRUGS

5-fluorouracil: Decreased clearance of 5-fluorouracil and potential for 5-fluorouracil toxicity

amiodarone, carbamazepine, cyclosporine, phenytoin, quinidine, tacrolimus: Increased plasma levels of these drugs

busulfan: Increased risk of serious busulfan toxicity

cimetidine and other drugs that inhibit CYP450 enzymes: Possibly delayed elimination and increased blood level of metronidazole

disulfiram: Possibly combined toxicity, with confusion and psychotic reactions

drugs known to prolong QT interval: Increased risk of QT prolongation
lithium: Possible development of elevated lithium levels with potential for toxicity in patients on high doses
oral anticoagulants: Possibly increased anticoagulant effect
phenobarbital, phenytoin, and other drugs that induce microsomal liver enzyme activity: Possibly accelerated elimination of metronidazole and decreased effectiveness

ACTIVITIES

alcohol use: Possibly disulfiram-like effects

Adverse Reactions

CNS: Aseptic meningitis (parenteral form), asthenia, ataxia, chills, confusion, depression, dizziness, dysarthria, **encephalopathy**, fever, headache, hypoesthesia, incoordination, insomnia, irritability, jumpy eye movements, light-headedness, malaise, numbness, paresthesia, peripheral neuropathy, psychosis, **seizures** (high doses), somnolence, syncope, vertigo, weakness
CV: Chest pain, **hypotension,** palpitations, peripheral edema, **prolonged QT interval**, tachycardia
EENT: Dry mouth, furry tongue, glossitis, hearing impairment or loss, metallic taste, nasal congestion, nystagmus, optic neuropathy, pharyngitis, rhinitis, sinusitis, stomatitis, tinnitus
GI: Abdominal cramps or pain, anorexia, constipation, diarrhea, elevated liver enzymes, epigastric distress, **hepatic failure or hepatotoxicity** (patients with Cockayne syndrome), nausea, **pancreatitis**, vomiting
GU: Burning or irritation of sexual partner's penis, candidal cervicitis or vaginitis, chromaturia, dark urine, decreased libido, dryness of vagina or vulva, dysmenorrhea, dyspareunia, dysuria, genital pruritus, moniliasis, proctitis, urinary frequency, UTI
HEME: Agranulocytosis, eosinophilia, **leukopenia**, **neutropenia**, **thrombocytopenia**
MS: Arthralgia, back pain, dysarthria, muscle spasms, myalgia
RESP: Dyspnea, risk of upper respiratory infection
SKIN: Acute generalized exanthematous pustulosis (AGEP), burning or stinging sensation, dermatitis bullous, erythema, erythematous rash, fixed drug eruption, flushing, hyperhidrosis, pruritus, rash, **Stevens-Johnson syndrome**, **toxic epidermal necrolysis**, urticaria
Other: Anaphylaxis angioedema; bacterial infection; **drug reaction with eosinophilia and systemic symptoms (DRESS)**; flu-like symptoms; infusion-site edema, pain, or tenderness

Childbearing Considerations

PREGNANCY

- It is not known if drug causes fetal harm although drug does cross the placental barrier.
- Use with caution only if benefit to mother outweighs potential risk to fetus.

LACTATION

- Drug is present in breast milk.
- A decision should be made to discontinue breastfeeding or the drug to avoid potential serious adverse reactions in the breastfed infant. Alternatively, mothers may choose to pump and discard breast milk for the duration of drug therapy and for 48 hr after therapy ends.

Nursing Considerations

! **WARNING** Monitor patient for a hypersensitivity reaction, which could become life-threatening, such as anaphylaxis or angioedema as well as severe skin reactions such as DRESS. If signs and symptoms of a hypersensitivity or skin reaction occurs (DRESS may only initially present with a fever or swollen lymph nodes), notify prescriber immediately, expect drug to be discontinued (and infusion stopped if IV route used), and provide supportive care, as needed and ordered.

! **WARNING** Use parenteral metronidazole with extreme caution in patients with Cockayne syndrome because acute hepatic failure and severe hepatotoxicity have occurred as rapidly as within 2 days, with some fatalities. If no other treatment is available, expect to obtain liver function studies before metronidazole is given parenterally, again within the first 2 to 3 days after treatment is initiated, frequently during therapy, and at the end of therapy. Also, monitor patient with severe liver disease receiving any form of the drug because

M

slowed metronidazole metabolism may cause drug to accumulate in body and increase the risk of serious to life-threatening adverse effects, If liver enzymes become elevated, expect metronidazole to be discontinued and liver enzymes monitored until they have returned to baseline values.

- Be aware that parenteral form of metronidazole contains 790 mg of sodium per 100 ml. Monitor patients predisposed to edema or who are receiving corticosteroids or a reduced-sodium diet.

! **WARNING** Monitor patient's neurologic status, especially in patients with CNS diseases throughout metronidazole therapy because drug may cause serious to life-threatening neurological effects such as encephalopathy, meningitis (with I.V. administration), or seizures. If abnormal neurologic signs and symptoms occur, notify prescriber and expect to discontinue drug. Be aware that prolonged oral administration of the drug may cause persistent peripheral neuropathy.

! **WARNING** Monitor patients with blood dyscrasias or a history of such because metronidazole therapy has caused agranulocytosis, leukopenia, and neutropenia in some patients. Monitor CBC if therapy lasts longer than 10 days or if second course of treatment is needed.

! **WARNING** Monitor patient with Crohn's disease closely who is exposed to metronidazole at high doses for extended periods of time because these patients have an increased risk of cancers, such as breast and colon cancers.

- Monitor patients with end-stage renal disease who are not on hemodialysis or patients with severe renal impairment for adverse reactions because reduced urinary excretion may cause metronidazole and its metabolites to accumulate in the body.
- Assess patient for fungal superinfections. Candidiasis may occur and present with more serious symptoms during therapy with metronidazole and require treatment with a candidacidal agent.
- Be aware that metronidazole may interfere with certain chemistry values, such as alanine aminotransferase (ALT), aspartate aminotransferase (AST), glucose hexokinase, lactate dehydrogenase (LDH), and triglycerides.

PATIENT TEACHING

- Instruct patient how to administer oral form of metronidazole prescribed.
- Urge patient to complete the entire course of therapy. However, instruct patient to notify prescriber if no improvement occurs within a few days of taking oral form of drug.
- Caution patient to avoid alcohol during therapy and for at least 3 days afterward.

! **WARNING** Alert patient that drug may cause an allergic or skin allergic reaction that could be quite serious. Stress importance of stopping drug, notifying prescriber immediately if an allergic or skin reaction occurs, and seeking immediate medical care, if severe.

! **WARNING** Tell patient with Cockayne syndrome or patients with liver disease to stop drug immediately if signs and symptoms of liver dysfunction occur, such as abdominal pain, change in skin or stool color, or nausea, and to notify prescriber.

! **WARNING** Advise patient to notify prescriber of any persistent, serious, or unusual adverse effects because drug can cause many different types of adverse effects, some of which can be life-threatening.

- Advise patient to avoid hazardous activities until drug's CNS effects are known and resolved.
- Suggest ice chips or sugarless hard candy or gum if patient reports dry mouth; suggest a dental visit if dryness lasts longer than 2 weeks.
- Inform mothers who are breastfeeding that breastfeeding should be discontinued during drug therapy. Alternatively, tell mothers they may choose to pump and discard breast milk for the duration of drug therapy and for 48 hours after therapy ends.
- Inform patient with trichomoniasis that her male sexual partners should wear condoms during her treatment and that they may need treatment themselves to prevent reinfection.
- Urge patient to follow up with prescriber to make sure infection is gone.

micafungin sodium

Mycamine

Class and Category

Pharmacologic class: Echinocandin
Therapeutic class: Antifungal

Indications and Dosages

∗ *To treat esophageal candidiasis*

I.V. INFUSION

Adults. 150 mg once daily for 10 to 30 days (mean duration: 15 days).
Children ages 4 mo and older weighing more than 30 kg (66 lb). 2.5 mg/kg once daily. *Maximum:* 150 mg once daily.
Children ages 4 mo and older weighing 30 kg (66 lb) or less. 3 mg/kg once daily.

∗ *To prevent* Candida *infection in patients undergoing hematopoietic stem cell transplantation*

I.V. INFUSION

Adults. 50 mg once daily for 6 to 51 days (mean duration: 19 days).
Children ages 4 mo and older. 1 mg/kg once daily. *Maximum:* 50 mg once daily.

∗ *To treat candidemia, acute disseminated candidiasis, and* Candida *peritonitis and abscesses*

I.V. INFUSION

Adults. 100 mg once daily for 10 to 47 days (mean duration: 15 days).
Children ages 4 mo and older. 2 mg/kg once daily. *Maximum:* 100 mg once daily.

∗ *To treat candidemia, acute disseminated candidiasis, and* Candida *peritonitis and abscesses without meningoencephalitis and/or ocular dissemination*

I.V. INFUSION

Children younger than 4 mo of age. 4 mg/kg once daily.

Drug Administration

I.V.

- Reconstitute by adding 5 ml of 0.9% Sodium Chloride Injection (without a bacteriostatic agent) or 5% Dextrose Injection to each 50-mg vial to yield 10 mg/ml and to each 100-mg vial to yield 20 mg/ml.
- Swirl vial gently to minimize excessive foaming.
- Reconstituted solution may be stored for up to 24 hr at room temperature. Protect from light.
- For adult patients, add reconstituted solution to 100 ml 0.9% Sodium Chloride Injection or 5% Dextrose Injection.
- For pediatric patients, follow manufacturer's guidelines for calculating volume to use for dilution.
- Infuse over 1 hr for both adults and children after flushing an existing I.V. line with 0.9% Sodium Chloride Injection. Protect diluted solution from light, although the infusion drip chamber or tubing need not be covered.
- Administer pediatric concentrations greater than 1.5 mg/ml through a central catheter to minimize risk of infusion reactions.
- Monitor infusion rate carefully because infusions that took less than 1 hr to infuse have been associated with more frequent hypersensitivity reactions.
- *Incompatibilities:* Other drugs

Route	Onset	Peak	Duration
I.V.	Unknown	Unknown	Unknown

Half-life: 11–21 hr

Mechanism of Action

Inhibits synthesis of 1,3-beta-D-glucan, which is an essential component of the *Candida* fungal cell wall. Without 1,3-beta-D-glucan, the fungal cell dies.

Contraindications

Hypersensitivity to micafungin, other echinocandins, or their components

Interactions

DRUGS

itraconazole, nifedipine, sirolimus: Increased plasma levels of these drugs

Adverse Reactions

CNS: Anxiety, delirium, dizziness, dysgeusia, fatigue, fever, headache, insomnia, **intracranial hemorrhage**, rigors, **seizures**, somnolence
CV: Arrhythmia, **atrial fibrillation**, **bradycardia**, **cardiac arrest**, **deep vein thrombosis**, hypertension, **hypotension**, **MI**, peripheral edema, phlebitis, tachycardia, **shock**, vasodilation
EENT: Epistaxis, mucosal inflammation

ENDO: Hyperglycemia, **hypoglycemia**
GI: Abdominal pain, anorexia, constipation, diarrhea, dyspepsia, elevated liver enzymes, **hepatic dysfunction**, **hepatitis**, hiccups, hyperbilirubinemia, jaundice, nausea, vomiting, **worsening hepatic failure**
GU: **Acute renal failure**, **anuria**, elevated blood urea and serum creatinine levels, oliguria, **renal tubular necrosis**
HEME: Anemia, **coagulopathy**, **disseminated intravascular coagulation (DIC)**, eosinophilia, **hemolytic anemia**, **leukopenia**, **lymphopenia**, **neutropenia**, **pancytopenia**, **thrombocytopenia**
RESP: **Apnea**, cough, **cyanosis**, dyspnea, **hypoxia**, pneumonia, **pulmonary embolism**
SKIN: Erythema, **erythema multiforme**, flushing, necrosis, pruritus, rash, **Stevens-Johnson syndrome**, **toxic epidermal necrolysis**, urticaria
Other: **Acidosis**, **anaphylaxis**, **angioedema**, bacteremia, **hyperkalemia**, **hypernatremia**, **hypocalcemia**, **hypokalemia**, **hypomagnesemia**, **hyponatremia**, **hypophosphatemia**, injection-site reactions, including phlebitis and thrombophlebitis, **sepsis**

Childbearing Considerations

PREGNANCY

- Drug may cause fetal harm based on animal studies.
- Use with caution only if benefit to mother outweighs potential risk to fetus.

LACTATION

- It is not known if drug is present in breast milk.
- Mothers should check with prescriber before breastfeeding.

Nursing Considerations

! **WARNING** Monitor patient closely for hypersensitivity reactions, which could become life-threatening, such as anaphylaxis and angioedema. Stop infusion immediately, if present, notify prescriber, and provide supportive care, as needed and ordered.

! **WARNING** Monitor patient's vital signs closely as life-threatening cardiovascular or respiratory adverse reactions may occur with drug use.

! **WARNING** Monitor patient's liver and renal function closely throughout therapy because liver and renal abnormalities may occur in patients receiving micafungin, some of which could become life-threatening, such as acute renal failure or worsening hepatic failure.

! **WARNING** Monitor hematologic status closely because hematologic abnormalities may occur, which could become life-threatening. Monitor patient for bruising, unexplained bleeding, or infections. If patient's condition worsens, expect micafungin to be discontinued.

- Expect to monitor patient's blood glucose level and electrolytes, as ordered, as drug may cause alterations.

PATIENT TEACHING

- Inform patient that micafungin will be administered intravenously.

! **WARNING** Stress importance of notifying staff immediately if difficulty breathing or swallowing occurs, or other signs of an allergic reaction occurs. Also instruct patient to report any infusion-site discomfort immediately.

! **WARNING** Tell patient to report any persistent, serious, or unusual signs and symptoms to prescriber.

midazolam

Nayzilam

midazolam hydrochloride

Seizalam

Class, Category, and Schedule

Pharmacologic class: Benzodiazepine
Therapeutic class: Sedative-hypnotic
Controlled substance schedule: IV

Indications and Dosages

✱ *To induce amnesia and sedation and relieve anxiety prior to diagnostic, endocscopic, or therapeutic procedures*

SYRUP

Children ages 6 to 16 and cooperative children. 0.25 to 0.5 mg/kg as a single dose 30 to 45 min before surgery. *Usual:* 0.5 mg/kg. *Maximum:* 20 mg.

Children ages 6 mo to 6 yr and less cooperative children. 0.25 to 1 mg/kg as a single dose 30 to 45 min before surgery. *Maximum:* 20 mg.

±DOSAGE ADJUSTMENT For children with cardiac or respiratory compromise, high-risk children, and children who have received concomitant narcotics or other CNS depressants, dosage kept at 0.25 mg/kg. For obese children, dose should be calculated based on ideal body weight.

I.V. INJECTION

Adults ages 60 and older and adults who are debilitated or chronically ill. *Initial:* 1 to 1.5 mg over 2 min immediately before procedure. After 2-min waiting period, an additional 1-mg dose given, as needed. *Maintenance:* After another 2-min waiting period, dosage adjusted to desired level in 25% increments every 2 min, as needed. *Maximum:* 3.5 mg total initial dosage.

Adults under age 60 and adolescents. *Initial:* Up to 2.5 mg over 2 min immediately before procedure. After 2-min waiting period, dosage adjusted to desired level in 25% increments, as needed, with smaller doses and 2 min between each dose. *Maximum:* 5 mg.

Children ages 6 to 12. *Initial:* 0.025 to 0.05 mg/kg, over 2 min up to 0.4 mg/kg, as needed, immediately before procedure. *Maintenance:* After a 2- to 3-min waiting period, dosage adjusted, as needed. *Maximum:* 10 mg.

Children ages 6 mo to 5 yr. *Initial:* 0.05 to 0.1 mg/kg, over 2 min up to 0.6 mg/kg, as needed, immediately before procedure. *Maintenance:* After waiting 2 to 3 min, dosage adjusted, as needed. *Maximum:* 6 mg.

I.M. INJECTION

Adults ages 60 and older. 0.02 to 0.05 mg/kg as a single dose 30 to 60 min before surgery.

Adults under ages 60 and adolescents. 0.07 to 0.08 mg/kg as a single dose 30 to 60 min before surgery.

Children ages 6 mo to 12 yr. 0.1 to 0.15 mg/kg, up to 0.5 mg/kg for more anxious patients as a single dose 30 to 60 min before surgery. *Maximum:* 10 mg.

±DOSAGE ADJUSTMENT For elderly patients and patients who are chronically ill, maintenance dosage reduced by 50%. For adults who have been premedicated with an opiate, maintenance dosage reduced by 25%.

* *To induce general anesthesia*

I.V. INJECTION

Adults older than 55. 0.3 mg/kg over 20 to 30 sec (if not premedicated) or 0.2 mg/kg over 20 to 30 sec (if premedicated). After 2-min waiting period, additional doses given, as needed, in increments of 25% of initial dose.

Adults under the age of 55. 0.3 to 0.35 mg/kg over 20 to 30 sec (if not premedicated) or 0.25 mg/kg over 20 to 30 sec (if premedicated). After 2-min waiting period, additional doses given, as needed, in increments of 25% of initial dose.

* *To provide sedation for intubated and mechanically ventilated patients as a component of anesthesia or during treatment in a critical care setting*

I.V. INFUSION

Adults. *Initial:* 0.01 to 0.05 mg/kg infused over several min, repeated at 10- to 15-min intervals until adequate sedation occurs. *Maintenance:* 0.02 to 0.10 mg/kg/hr initially and adjusted, as needed. After achieving desired level of sedation, infusion rate decreased every few hr, as needed, until minimum effective infusion rate is determined.

Children. *Initial bolus:* 0.05 to 0.2 mg/kg infused over several min. *Maintenance:* 0.06 to 0.12 mg/kg/hr by continuous infusion with dosage adjusted, as needed, to maintain effect.

Infants over age 32 wk. 0.06 mg/kg/hr by continuous infusion with rate adjusted, as needed.

Infants under age 32 wk. *Initial:* 0.03 mg/kg/hr by continuous infusion with rate adjusted, as needed.

±DOSAGE ADJUSTMENT For children who are hemodynamically compromised, the usual loading dose is titrated in small increments, separated by 2 to 3 min.

* *To treat acute, intermittent, stereotypic episodes of frequent seizure activity (i.e., seizure clusters, acute repetitive seizures) that are distinct from a patient's usual seizure pattern in patients with epilepsy*

NASAL SPRAY (NAYZILAM)

Adults and children ages 12 and older. 5 mg (1 spray) into one nostril. After 10 min, an additional 5 mg (1 spray) into the opposite nostril, as needed. *Maximum:* 10 mg (2 sprays) to treat a single episode and used no more than one episode every 3 days and no more than 5 episodes a mo.

∗ *To treat status epilepticus*

I.M. INJECTION (SEIZALAM)

Adults. 10 mg as a single dose.

Drug Administration

- Dosage must be individualized.
- Drug may cause respiratory depression and arrest. For all forms, have appropriate resuscitative drugs and equipment readily available during drug therapy, as well as staff knowledgeable and skilled in airway management.
- Drug forms other than nasal spray should only be administered in settings in which patient's cardiac and respiratory functions can be continuously monitored.

P.O.

- Syrup form can cause same severe respiratory symptoms as parenteral form.
- To use oral dispenser that comes with bottle, push plunger completely down toward the tip of the oral dispenser and insert tip firmly into opening of the bottle adapter.
- Turn entire bottle and oral dispenser upside down. Pull plunger out slowly until the desired dosage is withdrawn into the oral dispenser. Turn entire unit right side up and remove the oral dispenser slowly from the bottle. Cover tip with cap until ready to administer.
- Administer directly into patient's mouth. Do not dilute with any liquid.

I.V.

- Never administer excessive single doses or by rapid administration because airway obstruction or respiratory arrest or depression may occur.
- Avoid administering by any other parenteral route, especially intra-arterially.
- Drug may be mixed in same syringe with atropine sulfate, meperidine hydrochloride, morphine sulfate, or scopolamine hydrobromide, as needed. The resulting solution is stable for 30 min.
- Follow manufacturer's guidelines if using the Carpuject Syringe with the reusable Carpuject Holder.
- Administration rates determined by purpose of drug therapy. See Indications and Dosages section.
- Midazolam at a concentration of 0.5 mg/ml is compatible with 0.9% Sodium Chloride, or 5% Dextrose in Water for up to 24 hr and with Lactated Ringer's solution for up to 4 hr; 1-mg/ml or 5-mg/ml formulations are compatible with 0.9% Sodium Chloride Injection or 5% Dextrose in Water.
- For I.V. injection, administer slowly over at least 2 min and wait at least 2 min to evaluate therapeutic effects when initiating or titrating doses. For I.V. infusion, infuse at the rate specified (see Indications and Dosages section). Rate adjusted as needed.
- *Incompatibilities:* None reported by manufacturer.

I.M.

- Administer deeply into a large muscle mass except for Seizalam, which should be injected only into the mid-outer thigh.
- Rotate sites for additional dosages.

INTRANASAL

- Drug available as a single-dose nasal spray unit. Do not open blister packaging until ready to use.
- Do not test or prime unit before use and discard if the nasal spray unit appears damaged.
- When ready to administer drug, remove nasal spray unit from blister package carefully. Hand nasal spray unit to patient and tell patient to hold the nasal spray unit with thumb on the plunger and middle and index fingers on each side of the nozzle. Have patient place the tip of the nozzle into one nostril until fingers on either side of the nozzle touch the bottom of the nose. Then have patient press the plunger firmly to deliver the dose using only one motion. It is not necessary to have the patient breathe deeply when drug is administered. Discard the nasal spray unit and packaging.
- Do not administer a second dose if patient's breathing is compromised.
- Store at room temperature.

Route	Onset	Peak	Duration
P.O.	10–20 min	45–60 min	2–6 hr
I.V.	3–5 min	3–5 min	2–6 hr
I.M.	15 min	0.5–1 hr	2–6 hr
Intranasal	10 min	0.5–2 hr	4 hr

Half-life: 1.5–2.5 hr

Mechanism of Action

May exert sedating effect by increasing activity of gamma-aminobutyric acid, a major inhibitory neurotransmitter in the brain thereby producing a calming effect, which relaxes skeletal muscles, and—at high doses—induces sleep.

Contraindications

Acute angle closure glaucoma; acute pulmonary insufficiency; hypersensitivity to midazolam, other benzodiazepines, or their components; severe chronic obstructive pulmonary disease

Interactions

DRUGS

cimetidine, diltiazem, erythromycin, fluconazole, itraconazole, ketoconazole, ritonavir, saquinavir, verapamil: Intense and prolonged sedation caused by reduced midazolam metabolism
CNS depressants (secobarbital), droperidol-fentanyl combination, opioids (fentanyl, meperidine, morphine): Possibly increased CNS and respiratory depression and hypotension
halothane: Reduced minimum alveolar concentration of halothane required during maintenance of anesthesia
pancuronium: Potentiated effect of pancuronium
sodium valproate: Increased effect of midazolam
thiopental: Slight reduction in dosage requirement of thiopental following I.M. midazolam

Adverse Reactions

CNS: Agitation, delirium, or dreaming during emergence from anesthesia; anxiety; ataxia; chills; combativeness; confusion; dizziness; drowsiness; euphoria; excessive sedation; headache; impaired cognitive function; insomnia; lethargy; nervousness; nightmares; paresthesia; prolonged emergence from anesthesia; restlessness; retrograde amnesia; sleep disturbance; slurred speech; **suicidal ideation** (nasal spray form); weakness; yawning
CV: **Cardiac arrest**, **hypotension**, **nodal rhythm**, **PVCs**, tachycardia, **vasovagal episodes**
EENT: Blurred vision, diplopia, or other vision changes; increased salivation; **laryngospasm**; miosis; nystagmus; toothache
GI: Hiccups, nausea, retching, vomiting
RESP: **Airway obstruction**, **bradypnea**, **bronchospasm**, coughing, decreased tidal volume, dyspnea, hyperventilation, **respiratory arrest**, **shallow breathing**, tachypnea, wheezing
SKIN: Pruritus, rash, urticaria
Other: Injection-site burning, edema, induration, pain, redness, and tenderness; physical or psychological dependence, withdrawal reactions

Childbearing Considerations

PREGNANCY

- Pregnancy exposure registry for Nayzilam and Seizalam brands: 1-888-233-2334 or http://www.aedpregnancyregistry.org/.
- Drug may cause fetal harm based on benzodiazepines as a class such as an increased risk of congenital malformations if given in the first trimester.
- Drug is not recommended in pregnancy because other benzodiazepines given in the last wk of pregnancy have resulted in neonatal CNS depression. Withdrawal can occur in neonates when mother has used the nasal spray form during the later stages of pregnancy.

LABOR AND DELIVERY

- Drug is not recommended for use during labor and delivery as administration may result in a floppy infant syndrome, which occurs mainly within the first hours after birth and may last up to 14 days.

LACTATION

- Drug is excreted in breast milk.
- Mothers should check with prescriber before breastfeeding.
- If mother has received drug for anesthesia or sedation, breastmilk should be discarded for at least 4 to 8 hr after drug was administered.

- If nasal spray formulation is used with breastfeeding, infant should be monitored for lethargy, poor sucking, and somnolence.

Nursing Considerations

! **WARNING** Know that repeated or lengthy use of sedation drugs such as midazolam and general anesthetics during procedures or surgeries should be avoided in children younger than 3 years of age or in pregnant women during their third trimester because the combined use may affect the development of children's brains.

! **WARNING** Determine before administering midazolam whether patient consumes alcohol or takes antibiotics, antihypertensives, or protease inhibitors because these substances can produce an intense and prolonged sedative effect when taken with midazolam.

! **WARNING** Assess patient's current drug use, including all prescription and over-the-counter drugs before nasal spray therapy begins. Be aware that excessive use of nasal spray may lead to abuse, addiction, misuse, overdose, and possibly death. Monitor patient's intake of drug closely and patient's behavior.

! **WARNING** Know that even though nasal spray form is indicated only for intermittent use by the patient, if it is used more often than recommended, is stopped abruptly, or a rapid dosage reduction occurs, an acute withdrawal reaction may occur that could be life-threatening. In addition, a protracted withdrawal syndrome may occur that could last weeks to more than 12 months. Expect dosage to be tapered before being totally discontinued if patient has abused the use of the drug.

! **WARNING** Monitor patient's vital signs closely as midazolam can cause life-threatening cardiovascular and respiratory adverse reactions.

! **WARNING** Be aware that concomitant use of benzodiazepines such as midazolam with opioids may result in coma, profound sedation, respiratory depression, and death. Monitor patient closely.

- Assess level of consciousness frequently because the range between sedation and unconsciousness or disorientation is narrow with midazolam.
- Be aware that recovery time for drug administered for surgery or procedures is usually 2 hours but may be up to 6 hours.

PATIENT TEACHING

! **WARNING** Instruct patient how to administer nasal spray form, if prescribed for seizure activity. Stress importance of avoiding opioid use unless under supervision of a prescriber because of risk of severe respiratory depression and sedation.

! **WARNING** Stress importance of not taking a second dose of nasal spray if breathing difficulties occur and to seek immediate emergency attention.

! **WARNING** Inform patient that misuse of nasal spray, either by taking excessive amounts or by taking drug for prolonged periods of time, can lead to addiction, overdose, or even death. Stress importance of taking drug exactly as prescribed. Encourage family or caregiver to have naloxone in the home and instruct how to use it. Stress importance of calling 911 if naloxone is administered.

! **WARNING** Instruct patient prescribed nasal spray form to avoid alcohol or other CNS depressants during midazolam nasal spray therapy to avoid risk of airway obstruction, apnea, or profound hypoventilation. Also, instruct patient to avoid alcohol and other CNS depressants for 24 hours after receiving drug for surgery or a procedure, as directed by prescriber.

! **WARNING** Urge family or caregiver to watch patient taking nasal spray closely for suicidal tendencies, especially when therapy starts or dosage changes.

! **WARNING** Warn patient that if nasal spray is abused and abrupt cessation of drug therapy occurs, it can precipitate acute withdrawal symptoms, which could be life-threatening or last from a few weeks to over 12 months.

- Inform patient that he may not remember procedure because midazolam produces amnesia.

- Advise patient to avoid hazardous activities until drug's adverse CNS effects, such as dizziness and drowsiness, have worn off.
- Inform breastfeeding mothers who have received drug for anesthesia or sedation, that breastmilk should be discarded for at least 4 to 8 hours after drug was administered. If a breastfeeding mother is using the nasal form of the drug, tell her to monitor her infant for lethargy, poor sucking, and somnolence.

miglitol

Glyset

Class and Category

Pharmacologic class: Alpha glucosidase inhibitor
Therapeutic class: Antidiabetic

Indications and Dosages

As adjunct to manage type 2 diabetes mellitus

TABLETS

Adults. *Initial:* 25 mg 3 times daily. After 4 to 8 wk, dosage increased to 50 mg 3 times daily for 3 mo, as needed, with a further increase to 100 mg 3 times daily, as needed. Alternatively, 25 mg once daily and gradually increased to 25 mg 3 times daily before further dosage increased 4 to 8 wk later. *Maximum:* 100 mg 3 times daily.

±**DOSAGE ADJUSTMENT** For patients experiencing persistent GI symptoms, dosage reduced or drug discontinued.

Drug Administration

P.O.

- Administer drug when patient takes first bite of each main meal.

Route	Onset	Peak	Duration
P.O.	Rapid	2–3 hr	Unknown

Half-life: 2 hr

Mechanism of Action

Inhibits intestinal glucoside hydrolase enzymes (normally hydrolyze disaccharides and oligosaccharides to glucose and other monosaccharides), causing a delay carbohydrate absorption and digestion and reducing postprandial blood glucose level.

Contraindications

Chronic intestinal diseases associated with marked disorders of absorption or digestion, colonic ulceration, conditions that may deteriorate as a result of increased gas formation in the intestine, diabetic ketoacidosis, hypersensitivity to miglitol or its components, inflammatory bowel disease, partial intestinal obstruction, predisposition to intestinal obstruction

Interactions

DRUGS

digestive enzyme preparations, intestinal adsorbents (activated charcoal): Decreased miglitol effects
digoxin: Possibly decreased blood digoxin level
insulin, sulfonylureas: Increased risk and severity of hypoglycemia
propranolol: Decreased bioavailability of these drugs

Adverse Reactions

GI: Abdominal distention or pain; diarrhea; flatulence; **hepatotoxicity**; ileus, including paralytic ileus, nausea, pneumatosis cystoides intestinalis (rare), subileus
HEME: Low serum iron level
SKIN: Rash (transient)

Childbearing Considerations

PREGNANCY

- It is not known if drug causes fetal harm.
- Use with caution only if benefit to mother outweighs potential risk to fetus.

LACTATION

- Drug is present in breast milk.
- Breastfeeding is not recommended during drug therapy.

Nursing Considerations

- Use miglitol cautiously in patient with serum creatinine level above 2 mg/dl or creatinine clearance above 25 ml/min.
- Review patient's HbA1C level, as ordered, to monitor long-term glucose control.
- Monitor patient for evidence of overdose, such as transient increases in abdominal discomfort, diarrhea, and flatulence (but not hypoglycemia).

! **WARNING** Monitor patient's liver enzymes, as ordered and patient for signs and symptoms of liver dysfunction because miglitol may cause liver dysfunction that could progress to hepatotoxicity.

! **WARNING** Be aware that some patients with type 2 diabetes also may receive insulin or a sulfonylurea as adjunct to miglitol therapy. Monitor these patients closely for hypoglycemia because insulin and sulfonylureas may cause hypoglycemia, and miglitol therapy may make it more severe. If hypoglycemia occurs, use an oral glucose product such as dextrose to treat mild to moderate hypoglycemia rather than sucrose, whose hydrolysis to fructose and glucose is inhibited by miglitol.

! **WARNING** Monitor patient for constipation, diarrhea, mucus discharge, or rectal bleeding suggestive of pneumatosis cystoides intestinalis. If suspected, notify prescriber and prepare patient for diagnostic imaging, as ordered. If confirmed, expect drug to be discontinued.

PATIENT TEACHING

- Explain that miglitol is an adjunct to diet, which is the primary treatment for type 2 diabetes mellitus.
- Instruct patient how to administer miglitol.
- Explain importance of monitoring blood glucose levels.

! **WARNING** Review signs and symptoms of liver dysfunction with patient and stress importance of notifying prescriber if present.

! **WARNING** Instruct patient, family, or caregiver on the signs and symptoms of hypoglycemia if patient takes other drugs for blood glucose control and how to treat hypoglycemia. Tell patient to notify prescriber if hypoglycemia occurs frequently or is severe. Inform patient that if miglitol is the only drug patient takes to control blood glucose level, it won't cause hypoglycemia.

! **WARNING** Explain that adverse GI reactions usually decrease in frequency and intensity over time. However, instruct patient to report to prescriber immediately if signs and symptoms such as diarrhea, mucus discharge, persistent or severe constipation, or rectal bleeding occurs.

- Inform mothers breastfeeding is not recommended during drug therapy.

milnacipran hydrochloride

Savella

Class and Category

Pharmacologic class: Selective norepinephrine and serotonin reuptake inhibitor SNRI
Therapeutic class: Antifibromyalgia

Indications and Dosages

* *To manage fibromyalgia*

TABLETS

Adults. *Initial:* 12.5 mg on day 1; 12.5 mg twice daily on days 2 and 3; 25 mg twice daily on days 4 through 7; and then 50 mg twice daily. May be further increased, as needed, to 100 mg twice daily. *Usual:* 50 mg twice daily. *Maximum:* 100 mg twice daily.

± **DOSAGE ADJUSTMENT** For patients with severe renal impairment (creatinine clearance of 5 to 29 ml/min), maintenance dosage decreased by 50%. If tolerated, dosage may then be increased to 100 mg in two divided doses.

Drug Administration

P.O.

- Administer with or without food but giving with food improves tolerability.

Route	Onset	Peak	Duration
P.O.	Unknown	2–4 hr	Unknown

Half-life: 6–8 hr

Mechanism of Action

Inhibits reuptake of norepinephrine and serotonin by CNS neurons without affecting uptake of dopamine or other neurotransmitters, thereby increasing amount of norepinephrine and serotonin available in nerve synapses to improve symptoms of fibromyalgia, including central analgesic effect.

Contraindications

Hypersensitivity to milnacipran or its components, use within 14 days of MAO inhibitor, including I.V. methylene blue and linezolid

Interactions

DRUGS

amphetamines, buspirone, fentanyl, I.V. methylene blue, linezolid, lithium, MAO inhibitors, selective serotonin reuptake inhibitors, serotonin–norepinephrine reuptake inhibitors, St. John's wort, tramadol, tricyclic antidepressants, triptans: Increased risk of serotonin syndrome
clomipramine: Increased risk of euphoria and postural hypotension
anticoagulants (aspirin, NSAIDs, warfarin), antiplatelets: Increased risk of bleeding
clonidine: Possibly inhibited antihypertensive effect
CNS-active drugs: Possibly increased CNS effects
digoxin: Possibly increased risk of postural hypotension and tachycardia
epinephrine, norepinephrine: Increased risk of arrhythmias and paroxysmal hypertension
MAO inhibitors: Possibly hyperpyretic episodes, hypertensive crisis, serotonin syndrome, and severe seizures

ACTIVITIES

alcohol use: Increased risk of liver impairment

Adverse Reactions

CNS: Aggression, anger, anxiety, chills, delirium, depression, dizziness, fatigue, fever, hallucinations, headache, **homicidal ideation**, hypoesthesia, insomnia, irritability, loss of consciousness, migraine, **neuroleptic malignant syndrome**, paresthesia, parkinsonism, **seizures**, **serotonin syndrome**, **suicidal ideation**, tremor
CV: Chest pain, hypercholesterolemia, hypertension, **hypertensive crisis**, increased heart rate, palpitations, peripheral edema, **supraventricular tachycardia**, tachycardia, **Takotsubo cardiomyopathy**
EENT: Accommodation abnormality, angle closure glaucoma, blurred vision, dry mouth, mydriasis
ENDO: Galactorrhea, hot flashes, hyperprolactinemia
GI: Abdominal distention or pain, **acute pancreatitis**, anorexia, constipation, diarrhea, dyspepsia, elevated liver enzymes, gastroesophageal reflux, flatulence, **hepatitis**, jaundice, liver dysfunction, nausea, vomiting
GU: **Acute renal failure**, cystitis, decreased libido, delayed or absent orgasm (females), dysuria, ejaculation disorder, erectile dysfunction, prostatitis, scrotal or testicular pain, testicular swelling, urethral pain, urinary hesitation, urine retention, UTI
HEME: **Leukopenia**, **neutropenia**, **thrombocytopenia**
MS: **Rhabdomyolysis**
RESP: Dyspnea, upper respiratory infection
SKIN: **Erythema multiforme**, flushing, hyperhidrosis, night sweats, pruritus, rash, **Stevens-Johnson syndrome**
Other: **Hyponatremia**, weight gain or loss

Childbearing Considerations

PREGNANCY

- Pregnancy exposure registry: 1-877-643-3010, email: pregnancyregistries@incresearch.com, or www.savellapregnancyregistry.com.
- Drug may cause fetal harm, especially if given during the third trimester. Neonate may require prolonged hospitalization, respiratory support, and tube feeding immediately upon birth.
- Use with caution only if benefit to mother outweighs potential risk to fetus.

LACTATION

- Drug is present in breast milk.
- Mothers should check with prescriber before breastfeeding.

M

Nursing Considerations

! **WARNING** Know that at least 14 days should elapse between stopping an MAO inhibitor and starting milnacipran. At least 5 days should elapse between stopping milnacipran and starting an MAO inhibitor.

! **WARNING** Keep in mind that because milnacipran may aggravate liver disease, it shouldn't be given to patients with alcohol addiction or chronic liver disease. Monitor patient's liver function. If jaundice or signs and symptoms of liver dysfunction occur, notify prescriber and expect drug to be discontinued.

- Ensure patient has had an ophthalmic examination before milnacipran therapy is begun because pupillary dilation that occurs with drug use may trigger an angle closure glaucoma attack in a patient with anatomically narrow angle who does not have a patent iridectomy.

! **WARNING** Measure patient's blood pressure and heart rate before starting and periodically during milnacipran therapy because drug can raise blood pressure and heart rate. Monitor patient with cardiac disease or hypertension closely. If hypertension or tachycardia occurs and persists, notify prescriber and expect to reduce dosage or discontinue drug because life-threatening hypertensive crisis or supraventricular tachycardia may occur.

! **WARNING** Watch for hypersensitivity reactions, especially in patients with aspirin sensitivity, because drug contains the yellow dye tartrazine.

! **WARNING** Watch closely for suicidal tendencies, especially when therapy starts and dosage changes.

! **WARNING** Monitor patient for seizure activity. If present, notify prescriber and institute seizure precautions.

! **WARNING** Check patient's serum sodium level, as ordered, because drug may cause hyponatremia, especially in elderly patients, patients taking diuretics, and patients who are volume depleted.

! **WARNING** Monitor patient closely for serotonin syndrome, a rare but serious adverse effect of selective serotonin reuptake inhibitors, such as milnacipran. Signs and symptoms include agitation, confusion, diaphoresis, diarrhea, fever, hyperactive reflexes, poor coordination, restlessness, shaking, talking or acting with uncontrolled excitement, tremor, and twitching. In its most severe form, it can resemble neuroleptic malignant syndrome with autonomic instability with possible rapid fluctuation of vital signs, mental status changes, and muscle rigidity. If symptoms occur, notify prescriber immediately, expect to discontinue drug, and provide supportive care.

- Monitor patient with mild to moderate renal impairment or patients who have a history of dysuria, especially men with prostatic hypertrophy, prostatitis, and other lower urinary tract obstructive disorders for renal dysfunction.

! **WARNING** Monitor patient for any other persistent, severe, or unusual adverse reactions because drug can adversely affect multiple body systems.

- Expect to taper drug when no longer needed, as ordered, to minimize adverse reactions.

PATIENT TEACHING

- Instruct patient how to administer milnacipran.
- Caution patient to avoid aspirin and NSAIDs, if possible, while taking milnacipran.

! **WARNING** Caution patient against stopping drug abruptly because serious adverse effects may result.

! **WARNING** Tell patient to have his blood pressure and pulse monitored regularly throughout milnacipran therapy and to notify prescriber if a persistent elevation occurs because it may become serious if not treated.

! **WARNING** Urge family or caregiver to watch patient closely for suicidal tendencies, especially when therapy starts or dosage changes.

! **WARNING** Alert patient, family, or caregiver that drug may cause seizures. If a seizure occurs, patient should seek immediate medical care.

! **WARNING** Instruct patient to notify prescriber if dysuria occurs or any other persistent, severe, or unusual adverse reactions as some may become quite serious.

! **WARNING** Alert pregnant patients to notify prescriber when pregnancy is advancing to the third trimester as drug may need to be discontinued.

- Instruct patient to alert all prescribers about milnacipran therapy.
- Advise patient to avoid activities, such as driving, that require alertness until the CNS effects of milnacipran are known and resolved.
- Have patient speak with prescriber about sexual dysfunction concerns, if present.

milrinone lactate

Class and Category

Pharmacologic class: Phosphodiesterase 3 inhibitor
Therapeutic class: Inotropic

Indications and Dosages

✱ *To provide short-term treatment of acute decompensated heart failure*

I.V. INFUSION

Adults. *Loading:* 50 mcg/kg slowly over 10 min followed by 0.375 to 0.75 mcg/kg/min as a continuous infusion with infusion rate adjusted, as needed. *Maximum:* 1.13 mg/kg daily.

±**DOSAGE ADJUSTMENT** For all patients, dosage adjusted according to cardiac output, pulmonary artery wedge pressure (PAWP), and clinical response. For patients with a creatinine clearance of 50 ml/min, infusion rate reduced to 0.43 mcg/kg/min; if 40 ml/min, infusion rate reduced to 0.38 mcg/kg/min; if 30 ml/min, infusion rate reduced to 0.33 mcg/kg/min; if 20 ml/min, infusion rate reduced to 0.28 mcg/kg/min; if 10 ml/min, infusion rate reduced to 0.23 mcg/kg/min; and if 5 ml/min, infusion rate reduced to 0.2 mcg/kg/min.

Drug Administration

I.V.

- For I.V. infusion used for loading dose, infuse drug directly into I.V. line with compatible solution slowly over 10 min. Drug may be given undiluted but diluting to a rounded total volume of 10 or 20 ml may simplify controlling the rate of delivery. Use a controlled-rate infusion device for administration.
- For continuous I.V. infusion, dilute drug with 0.45% or 0.9% Sodium Chloride Injection or 5% Dextrose Injection to achieve a 200-mcg/ml concentration using 1-mg/ml vial as follows: Add 40 ml of above solution to 10 ml of drug to achieve a total volume of 50 ml or add 80 ml of above solution to 20 ml of drug to achieve a total volume of 100 ml. Using a calibrated electronic infusion device, infuse continuously at a rate between 0.375 mcg/kg/min up to 0.75 mcg/kg/min depending on patient's needs and response to drug but not exceeding 1.13 mg/kg/day. Discard unused portion in vial.
- Be aware drug also comes premixed and does not require further dilution.
- Store unused vials at room temperature, avoiding excessive heat or cold.
- *Incompatibilities:* None reported by manufacturer.

Route	Onset	Peak	Duration
I.V.	5–15 min	1–2 hr	3–6 hr

Half-life: 2.5 hr

Contraindications

Hypersensitivity to milrinone or its components

Interactions

DRUGS

None reported by manufacturer.

Adverse Reactions

CNS: Headache, tremor
CV: Angina, **hypotension**, **supraventricular arrhythmias**, **ventricular ectopic activity**, **torsades de pointes**, **ventricular fibrillation** and **tachycardia**
GI: Liver function test abnormalities
HEME: **Thrombocytopenia**
RESP: **Bronchospasm**
SKIN: Rash
Other: **Anaphylactic shock**, **hypokalemia**, infusion-site reactions (pain, redness, swelling)

Childbearing Considerations

PREGNANCY

- It is not known if drug causes fetal harm.
- Use with caution only if benefit to mother outweighs potential risk to fetus.

LACTATION

- It is not known if drug is present in breast milk.
- Mothers should check with prescriber before breastfeeding.

Nursing Considerations

- Expect patient to receive digoxin before starting milrinone, if needed, which can increase ventricular response rate.

Mechanism of Action

Increases the force of myocardial contraction—and cardiac output—by blocking the enzyme phosphodiesterase. Normally, this enzyme is activated by hormones binding to cell membrane receptors. As shown below left, phosphodiesterase normally degrades intracellular cAMP, which restricts calcium movement into myocardial cells. By inhibiting phosphodiesterase, as shown below right, milrinone slows the rate of cAMP degradation, increasing the intracellular cAMP level and the amount of calcium that enters myocardial cells. In blood vessels, increased cAMP causes smooth-muscle relaxation, which improves cardiac output by reducing preload and afterload.

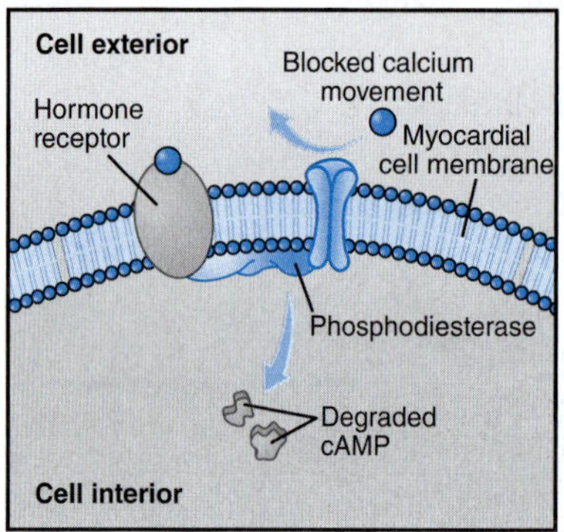

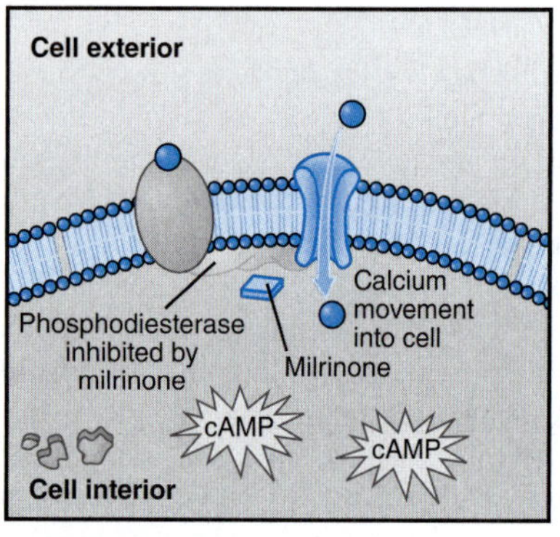

! WARNING Ensure continuous ECG monitoring is present during milrinone therapy because drug can cause life-threatening arrhythmias such as torsades de pointes and ventricular fibrillation and tachycardia.

- Monitor blood pressure, cardiac output, fluid status, heart rate, pulmonary artery wedge pressure, and weight during therapy to determine drug effectiveness. Notify prescriber at once and expect to stop drug if severe hypotension develops or significant changes occurs in other monitoring parameters.

! WARNING Monitor patient for a hypersensitivity reaction, which could become life-threatening, such as anaphylaxis. If present, notify prescriber immediately, expect drug to be discontinued, and provide supportive care, as needed and ordered.

! WARNING Check platelet count before and periodically during infusion, as ordered. Monitor patient for bruising and unexpected bleeding. Expect to discontinue drug if platelet count falls below 150,000/mm^3 or patient develops major bleeding.

- Monitor liver and renal function test results and serum electrolyte levels. Notify prescriber of abnormalities.

PATIENT TEACHING

- Inform patient that drug is administered intravenously.
- Reassure patient that he will be monitored constantly during therapy.

! WARNING Tell patient to alert staff immediately if feeling ill or unusual.

minocycline hydrochloride

Dynacin, Emrosi, Minocin, Minolira, Ximino

Class and Category

Pharmacologic class: Tetracycline
Therapeutic class: Antibiotic

Indications and Dosages

* *To treat infections as follows: bartonellosis due to* Bartonella bacilliformis; *brucellosis due to* Brucella *species;* Campylobacter fetus *infections caused by* Campylobacter fetus; *chancroid caused* by Haemophilus ducreyi; *cholera caused by* Vibrio cholerae; *granuloma inguinale caused by* Klebsiella granulomatis; *inclusion conjunctivitis caused by* Chlamydia trachomatis; *lymphogranuloma venereum caused by* Chlamydia trachomatis; *plague caused by* Yersinia pestis; *psittacosis due to* Chlamydophila psittaci; *relapsing fever due to* Borrelia recurrentis; *respiratory tract infections caused by* Mycoplasma pneumoniae; *Rocky Mountain spotted fever, typhus fever and the typhus group, Q fever, rickettsialpox, and tick fevers caused* by rickettsiae; *trachoma caused by* Chlamydia trachomatis; *or tularemia due to* Francisella tularensis; *other gram-negative infections caused by* Acinetobacter *species,* Escherichia coli, Klebsiella aerogenes, *or* Shigella species; *respiratory tract infections caused by* Haemophilus influenza *or respiratory tract and urinary tract infections caused by* Klebsiella *species; other gram-positive infections, such as skin and skin structure infections caused by* Staphylococcus aureus *or upper respiratory tract infections caused by* Streptococcus pneumoniae; *and infections when penicillin is contraindicated such as actinomycosis caused by* Actinomyces israelii, *anthrax due to* Bacillus anthracis, *infections caused by* Clostridioides *species, listeriosis due to* Listeria *monocytogenes, syphilis caused by* Treponema pallidum *subspecies* pallidum, *Vincent's infection caused by* Fusobacterium fusiforme, *uncomplicated urethritis in men or infections in women caused by* Neisseria gonorrhoeae, *or yaws caused by* Treponema pallidum *subspecies* pertenue

CAPSULES, TABLETS

Adults and adolescents. *Initial:* 200 mg followed by 100 mg every 12 hr. Alternatively, 100 to 200 mg initially, followed by 50 mg every 6 hr.

Children ages 8 and older. *Initial:* 4 mg/kg followed by 2 mg/kg every 12 hr. *Maximum:* 200 mg as initial dose; 100 mg/dose for remainder doses.

I.V. INFUSION

Adults and adolescents. *Initial:* 200 mg followed by 100 mg every 12 hr. *Maximum:* 200 mg daily. Infused over 1 hr.

Children ages 8 and older. *Initial:* 4 mg/kg followed by 2 mg/kg every 12 hr. *Maximum:* Not to exceed adult dose. Infused over 1 hr.

± **DOSAGE ADJUSTMENT** For patients with renal impairment, dosage decreased or dosage interval increased; dosage not to exceed 200 mg daily. Duration of therapy varies depending on severity and type of infection.

* *To treat uncomplicated gonorrhea from* Neisseria gonorrhoeae *in nonpregnant patients allergic to penicillin*

CAPSULES, TABLETS

Adults and adolescents. *Initial:* 200 mg followed by 100 mg every 12 hr for at least 4 days.

* *To treat uncomplicated gonococcal urethritis in men allergic to penicillin*

CAPSULES, TABLETS

Adult male. 100 mg every 12 hr for 5 days.

* *To treat asymptomatic meningococcal carriers with* Neisseria meningitidis *in nasopharynx*

CAPSULES, TABLETS

Adults and adolescents. 100 mg every 12 hr for 5 days.

* *To treat infections caused by* Mycobacterium marinum

CAPSULES, TABLETS

Adults. 100 mg every 12 hr for 6 to 8 wk.

* *To treat uncomplicated nongonococcal endocervical, rectal, or urethral infection caused by* Chlamydia trachomatis *or* Ureaplasma urealyticum

CAPSULES, TABLETS

Adults. 100 mg every 12 hr for at least 7 days.

* *To treat syphilis caused by* Treponema pallidum *in patients allergic to penicillin*

CAPSULES, TABLETS

Adults. *Initial:* 200 mg, followed by 100 mg every 12 hr for 10 to 15 days.

* *To treat acne, including inflammatory, nonnodular, moderate to severe*

CAPSULES, TABLETS

Adults and children ages 8 and older. 50 to 100 mg twice daily for up to 12 wks.

E.R. CAPSULES (XIMINO)

Adults and children ages 12 and older. 1 mg/kg/dose once daily for 12 wk.

E.R. TABLETS (MINOLIRA)

Adults weighing 126 to 136 kg (277 to 299 lb). 135 mg once daily.
Adults weighing 90 to 125 kg (198 to 275 lb). 105 mg once daily.
Adults weighing 60 to 89 kg (132 to 196 lb). 67.5 mg (one-half of the 135 mg-tablet) once daily.
Adults weighing 45 to 59 kg (99 to 130 lb). 52.5 mg (one-half of the 105-mg tablet) once daily.

E.R. CAPSULES (EMROSI)

Adults. 40 mg once daily.

Drug Administration

P.O.

- Administer drug with a full glass of water or milk, or with food.
- Capsules, E.R. tablets, and immediate-release tablets should be swallowed whole and not chewed, crushed, or split with the exception of Minolira, which is scored for splitting, if needed.
- Ensure that patient does not lie down immediately after administration and do not administer drug 1 hr before bedtime, to minimize esophageal and GI irritation.
- Do not administer drug within 2 hr of an antacid or 3 hr of an iron preparation.

I.V.

- I.V. route used only when oral administration is not possible.
- Reconstitute each 100-mg vial with 5 ml Sterile Water for Injection.
- Immediately further dilute in 100 to 1,000 ml 0.9% Sodium Chloride Injection, 5% Dextrose in Water, 5% Dextrose Injection with 0.9% Sodium Chloride Injection, or further dilute in 250 to 1,000 ml with Lactated Ringer's Injection.
- Flush I.V. line with any of the above diluents before and after administration if I.V. line is used for administration of other drugs.
- Infuse over 60 min.
- Store reconstituted drug at room temperature for up to 4 hr or refrigerated for up to 24 hr.
- *Incompatibilities:* Calcium-containing solutions (except for Lactated Ringer's Injection), other drugs

Route	Onset	Peak	Duration
P.O.	Unknown	1–4 hr	Unknown
P.O./E.R.	Unknown	3.5–4 hr	Unknown
I.V.	Unknown	Unknown	Unknown

Half-life: 2.7–5.5 hr

Mechanism of Action

Inhibits bacterial protein synthesis by competitively binding to the 30S ribosomal subunit of the mRNA–ribosome complex of certain organisms.

Contraindications

Hypersensitivity to minocycline, other tetracyclines, or their components

Interactions

DRUGS

aluminum-, calcium-, or magnesium-containing antacids; calcium supplements; choline and magnesium salicylates; iron-containing preparations; magnesium-containing laxatives; sodium bicarbonate: Possibly formation of nonabsorbable complex, impaired minocycline absorption
atazanavir: Possibly decreased serum concentration of atazanavir
BCG (immunization or intravesical): Possibly decreased effectiveness of BCG
bile acid sequestrants, calcium salts: Decreased minocycline absorption
bismuth subsalicylate: Possibly decreased serum concentration of minocycline
cholera or typhoid vaccines: Possibly diminished effectiveness of vaccines
CNS depressants: Possibly enhanced CNS depressant effect
lactobacillus and estriol: Possibly diminished effectiveness of these products
lanthanum: Possible decreased effectiveness of minocycline
mecamylamine: Possibly enhanced neuromuscular blocking effect of mecamylamine
methoxyflurane: Increased risk of nephrotoxicity
mipomersen: Possibly enhanced hepatotoxicity of mipomersen
multivitamins/minerals: Possibly decreased concentration of minocycline
neuromuscular blocking agents: Enhanced neuromuscular blocking effect of these agents

penicillin: Interference with bactericidal action of penicillin
quinapril: Possibly decreased effectiveness of minocycline
retinoic acid derivatives: Possibly enhanced adverse effects of these drugs
sucralfate, zinc salts: Possibly decreased absorption of minocycline
sucroferric oxyhydroxide: Possibly decreased serum concentration of minocycline
vitamin K antagonists: Possibly enhanced anticoagulant effect of vitamin K antagonists

Adverse Reactions

CNS: Dizziness, fever, headache, **intracranial hypertension**, light-headedness, unsteadiness, vertigo
CV: **Myocarditis**, **pericarditis**
EENT: Blurred vision, darkened or discolored tongue, glossitis, papilledema, tooth discoloration, vision changes
ENDO: **Thyroid cancer**, thyroid function abnormality
GI: Abdominal cramps or pain, anorexia, ***Clostridioides difficile*-associated diarrhea**, diarrhea, dysphagia, enterocolitis, esophageal irritation and ulceration, **hepatitis**, **hepatotoxicity**, indigestion, **jaundice**, nausea, **pancreatitis**, **pseudomembranous colitis**, vomiting
GU: Genital candidiasis, **nephritis**, **nephrotoxicity**
HEME: Eosinophilia, **hemolytic anemia**, **neutropenia**, **thrombocytopenia**, **thrombocytopenic purpura**
MS: Arthralgia, myopathy (transient)
RESP: **Pneumonitis**, **pulmonary infiltrates**
SKIN: **Erythema multiforme**, **exfoliative dermatitis**, brown pigmentation of skin and mucous membranes, **erythema multiforme**, erythematous and maculopapular rash, **exfoliative dermatitis**, onycholysis, photosensitivity, pruritus, purpura (anaphylactoid), rash, **Stevens-Johnson syndrome**, urticaria
Other: **Anaphylaxis**, **angioedema**, serum sickness-like reaction, systemic lupus erythematosus exacerbation

Childbearing Considerations

PREGNANCY

- Drug may cause fetal harm as it crosses the placental barrier and may discolor teeth.
- Like other tetracyclines, rare reports of congenital anomalies, including limb reduction have been reported.
- Drug is not recommended for use during pregnancy.

LACTATION

- Drug is present in breast milk.
- A decision should be made to discontinue breastfeeding or the drug to avoid potential serious adverse reactions in the breastfed infant.

Nursing Considerations

! WARNING Obtain blood, hepatic, and renal test results before and during long-term therapy, as ordered. Monitor patients with hepatic or renal dysfunction and in those taking other hepatotoxic drugs during drug therapy because drugs may cause nephrotoxicity or hepatotoxicity.

! WARNING Monitor patient for hypersensitivity reactions, which could become life-threatening, such as anaphylaxis or angioedema. If present, notify prescriber, withhold drug, and expect to provide supportive care, as needed and ordered.

! WARNING Monitor patient for development of foul-smelling diarrhea, which suggests *Clostridioides difficile* that may range from mild diarrhea to fatal colitis. If present, notify prescriber, obtain stool culture, and expect minocycline to be discontinued, if confirmed. In addition, expect an antibiotic treatment for *C. difficile* to be administered as well as electrolyte, fluid, and protein supplementation administered, as needed and ordered.

! WARNING Monitor patient for signs and symptoms of thyroid cancer such as alteration in thyroid function or presence of nodule in patients receiving minocycline therapy over prolonged periods.

! WARNING Monitor patient's CBC and platelet count throughout drug therapy, as ordered, because drug can cause serious adverse hematologic reactions. Also, monitor patient for bruising, unexplained bleeding, and infection. Monitor PT in patient who also takes an anticoagulant during minocycline therapy.

! **WARNING** Monitor patient for blurred vision or headache because benign intracranial hypertension has occurred with the use of minocycline. If present, notify prescriber and expect drug to be discontinued. Know that although intracranial hypertension usually resolves after drug is discontinued, permanent visual loss can occur. Expect patient with suspected intracranial hypertension to undergo a prompt ophthalmologic evaluation and be monitored until vision is stabilized, as intracranial pressure can remain elevated for weeks after drug is discontinued.

- Assess patient for signs of superinfection; if signs appear, notify prescriber, discontinue minocycline, and start appropriate therapy, as ordered.

PATIENT TEACHING

- Instruct patient how to administer the oral form of minocycline prescribed.
- Instruct patient not to take minocycline within 2 hours of an antacid or 3 hours of an iron preparation.
- Urge patient to complete full course of treatment even if he feels better before finishing. However, instruct patient to notify prescriber if no improvement occurs in a few days.

! **WARNING** Alert patient that drug may cause an allergic reaction. Tell patient to withhold drug and notify prescriber if an allergic reaction occurs. Urge patient to seek immediate emergency care if reaction is severe.

! **WARNING** Explain that diarrhea may occur up to 2 months after completing therapy; urge patient to notify prescriber if it occurs because it could be severe.

! **WARNING** Urge patient to notify prescriber immediately if bruising, unexplained bleeding, or an infection occurs.

! **WARNING** Instruct patient to notify prescriber immediately about blurred vision, dizziness, headache, and unsteadiness as well as any other persistent, serious, or unusual adverse reactions.

- Advise patient to avoid prolonged exposure to sun or sunlamps during therapy.
- Inform females of childbearing age to notify prescriber if pregnancy occurs.
- Tell breastfeeding mothers that breastfeeding must be discontinued during drug therapy or drug will need to be discontinued.

mirabegron

Myrbetriq, Myrbetriq Granules

Class and Category

Pharmacologic class: Beta-3 adrenergic agonist
Therapeutic class: Bladder antispasmodic

Indications and Dosages

* *To treat overactive bladder with symptoms of urge urinary incontinence, urgency, and urinary frequency as monotherapy or in combination with solifenacin succinate*

E.R. TABLETS

Adults. *Initial*: 25 mg once daily, increased, as needed, to 50 mg once daily after 4 to 8 wk.

± **DOSAGE ADJUSTMENT** For patients with moderate hepatic impairment or severe renal impairment, dosage should not exceed 25 mg once daily.

* *To treat pediatric neurogenic detrusor overactivity (NDO)*

E.R. TABLETS

Children ages 3 and older weighing 35 kg (77 lb) or more. 25 mg once daily, increased to 50 mg once daily after 4 to 8 wk, as needed.

± **DOSAGE ADJUSTMENT** For children with severe hepatic or renal impairment and weighing 35 kg (77 lb) or more, dosage should not exceed 25 mg once daily.

E.R. ORAL SUSPENSION

Children ages 3 and older weighing 35 kg (77 lb) or more. 48 mg (6 ml) once daily, increased to 80 mg (10 ml) once daily after 4 to 8 wk, as needed. *Maximum:* 80 mg (10 ml) once daily.

Children ages 3 and older weighing 22 kg (48.4 lb) to less than 35 kg (77 lb). 32 mg (4 ml) once daily, increased to 64 mg (8 ml) once daily after 4 to 8 wk, as needed.

Children ages 3 and older weighing 11 kg (24.2 lb) to less than 22 kg (48.4 lb). 24 mg (3 ml) once daily, increased to 48 mg (6 ml) once daily after 4 to 8 wk, as needed.

±**DOSAGE ADJUSTMENT** For children with severe renal dysfunction (eGFR of 15 to 29 ml/min) and weighing 35 kg (77 lb) or more, dosage should not exceed 48 mg (6 ml); for children with renal dysfunction (eGFR of 15 to 29 ml/min) and weighing 22 kg (48.4 lb) to less than 35 kg (77 lb), dosage should not exceed 32 mg (4 ml); and for children with renal dysfunction (eGFR of 15 to 29 ml/min) and weighing 11 kg (24.2 lb) to less than 22 kg (48.4 lb), dosage should not exceed 24 mg (3 ml). For children with mild hepatic impairment and weighing 35 kg (77 lb) or more, dosage should not exceed 48 mg (6 ml) and maximum dose of 80 mg (10 ml); for children with moderate hepatic impairment and weighing 35 kg (77 lb) or more, dosage should not exceed 48 mg (6 ml and maximum dose of 48 mg (6 ml); for children with mild to moderate hepatic impairment and weighing 22 kg (48.4 lb) to less than 35 kg (77 lb), dosage should not exceed 32 mg (4 ml) and maximum dose of 64 mg (8 ml) for mild impairment and 32 mg (4 ml) for moderate impairment; and for children with mild to moderate hepatic impairment and weighing 11 kg (24.2 lb) to less than 22 kg (48.4 lb), dosage should not exceed 24 mg (3 ml) with maximum dose of 48 mg (6 ml for mild impairment and 24 mg (3 ml) for moderate impairment.

Drug Administration

P.O.

- Do not interchange E.R. tablets with E.R. oral suspension.
- A recommended adult dosage for E.R. oral suspension has not been determined.
- Do not combine E.R. tablets and E.R. oral suspension to achieve a total dose.
- Administer E.R. tablets with water. E.R. tablets should not be chewed, crushed, or divided. Adults may take tablets with or without food; children should take tablets with food.
- To make E.R. suspension, tap closed bottle several times to loosen granules, then add 100 ml of water to bottle and shake vigorously for 1 min. Then, let stand for 10 to 30 min followed by shaking bottle vigorously again for 1 min (suspension will contain 8 mg/ml of drug). If granules have not dispersed, shake vigorously for another 1 min. Measure dosage using a calibrated device. Administer with food. Store suspension at room temperature for up to 28 days and then discard.
- If a dose is missed and less than 12 hr has passed since missed dose, administer drug; if more than 12 hr has passed, skip missed dose.

Route	Onset	Peak	Duration
P.O.	Unknown	3.5 hr	Unknown

Half-life: 50 hr

Mechanism of Action

Relaxes the detrusor smooth muscle during the storage phase of the urinary bladder fill-void cycle by activating the beta-3 adrenergic receptor, which increases bladder capacity. Increased bladder capacity causes urge sensation to decrease, which in turn decreases urinary frequency.

Contraindications

Hypersensitivity to mirabegron or its components

Interactions

DRUGS

CYP2D6 substrates, such as desipramine, flecainide, metoprolol, propafenone, thioridazine: Increased blood levels of these drugs
digoxin: Increased risk of digoxin toxicity
warfarin: Possibly changes in INR and prothrombin time with multiple doses of warfarin

Adverse Reactions

CNS: Anxiety, confusion, dizziness, fatigue, hallucinations, headache, insomnia
CV: **Atrial fibrillation**, elevated LDH levels, hypertension, palpitations, tachycardia
EENT: Dry mouth, glaucoma, nasopharyngitis, rhinitis, sinusitis
GI: Abdominal distention or pain, constipation, diarrhea, dyspepsia, elevated liver enzymes, gastritis, nausea
GU: Bladder pain, cystitis, nephrolithiasis, **prostate cancer**, urinary retention, UTI, vaginal infections, vulvovaginal pruritus
MS: Arthralgia, back pain
RESP: Cough (children)
SKIN: Acute febrile neutrophilic dermatosis (Sweet's syndrome), pruritus, rash, **Stevens-Johnson syndrome**

M

Other: Angioedema, flu-like symptoms

Childbearing Considerations

PREGNANCY

- It is not known if drug causes fetal harm.
- Use with caution only if benefit to mother outweighs potential risk to fetus.

LACTATION

- It is not known if drug is present in breast milk.
- Mothers should check with prescriber before breastfeeding.

Nursing Considerations

! **WARNING** Know that mirabegron should not be given to patients with severe uncontrolled hypertension (defined as systolic blood pressure 180 mm Hg or higher and/or diastolic blood pressure 110 mm Hg or higher) because drug can increase blood pressure. Monitor patient's blood pressure regularly and report persistent or significant increases to prescriber.

! **WARNING** Be aware that mirabegron should not be given to patients with end-stage renal disease or to patients with severe hepatic impairment because drug has not been studied in these conditions, and adverse effects are unknown.

! **WARNING** Monitor patient closely for a hypersensitivity reaction such as angioedema of the face, larynx, lips, and tongue, which may occur as soon as the first dose or hours after the first dose or after multiple doses. Be prepared to administer emergency treatment for life-threatening upper airway swelling, as ordered, and maintain a patent airway. Notify prescriber and expect drug to be discontinued. Provide additional supportive care, as needed and ordered.

- Monitor patients with bladder outlet obstruction and in patients taking antimuscarinic drugs for the treatment of this condition because drug may cause urinary retention.

PATIENT TEACHING

- Instruct patient, family, or caregiver how to administer oral form of drug prescribed and what to do if a dose is missed.

! **WARNING** Alert patient that serious allergic reactions can occur. If present, tell patient to notify prescriber and, if severe (swelling around face, neck, or tongue) to seek immediate medical care.

- Warn patient that drug may increase blood pressure. Encourage patient to have his blood pressure checked regularly, especially if he has hypertension.
- Review common adverse effects of drug with patient. Tell patient to notify prescriber if he experiences a decrease in urinary output despite a normal intake. Also, remind patient that drug may cause itching, rapid heartbeat, rash, or urinary tract infections and to alert prescriber, if present.

mirikizumab-mrkz

Omvoh

Class and Category

Pharmacologic class: Intereleukin-23 antagonist monoclonal antibody
Therapeutic class: Anti-inflammatory

Indications and Dosages

∗ *To treat moderate to severe active ulcerative colitis*

I.V. INFUSION, SUBCUTANEOUS INJECTION

Adults. *Induction:* 300 mg I.V. infused over at least 30 min and repeated at wk 4 and again at wk 8. *Maintenance:* 200 mg (given as 2 consecutive injections of 100 mg each) subcutaneously at wk 12 and every 4 wk thereafter.

∗ *To treat moderate to severe active Crohn's disease*

I.V. INFUSION, SUBCUTANEOUS INJECTION

Adults. *Induction:* 900 mg I.V. infused over at least 90 min and repeated at wk 4 and again at wk 8 *Maintenance:* 300 mg (given as 2 consecutive injections of 100 mg and 200 mg in any order) subcutaneously at wk 12 and every 4 wk thereafter.

Drug Administration

I.V.

- Each vial is for single use.

- Solution should be clear to opalescent, colorless to slightly yellow to slightly brown and free of visible particles.
- Know that for Crohn's disease, 45 ml of the infusion bag solution should be discarded prior to adding drug vial contents.
- Use an 18 G to 21 G needle to withdraw 15 ml for 300 mg dose and 45 ml for 900 mg dose of drug from vial and transfer to an infusion bag ranging in size from 50 ml to 250 ml for 300 mg dose and 100 ml or 250 ml for 900 mg dose of 0.9% Sodium Chloride Injection or 5% Dextrose Injection.
- Gently invert infusion bag. Do not shake.
- Connect infusion set to infusion bag and prime the line.
- Start infusion immediately after preparation or if diluted solution was stored in the refrigeration, allow solution to warm to room temperature prior to the start of the IV infusion. Infuse over at least 30 min for 300 mg dose and at least 90 min for 900 mg dose.
- When infusion is finished, flush the line with 0.9% Sodium Chloride Injection or 5% Dextrose Injection solution and flush at the same infusion rate as when the drug was administered. The time required to flush the drug solution from the infusion line is in addition to the minimum 30-minute or 90-min infusion time.
- If diluted infusion solution is not used immediately, store in refrigerator and use within 48 hr. Diluted infusion solution should not be stored at room temperature no more than 5 hr, starting from the time of vial puncture. Keep drug away from direct heat or light and do not freeze the diluted infusion solution.
- *Incompatibilities:* Other drugs, other solutions other than 0.9% Sodium Chloride Injection or 5% Dextrose Injection

SUBCUTANEOUS

- The 200 mg/2ml prefilled pen and prefilled syringe are to be used only for maintenance treatment of Crohn's disease.
- Use 2 prefilled pens or syringes to achieve a full maintenance dose.
- Remove prefilled pens or syringes from refrigerator and leave at room temperature for 30 min. Do not shake the pens or syringes.
- Solution should be clear to opalescent, colorless to slightly yellow to slightly brown and free of visible particles.
- Inject subcutaneously into the abdomen, back of upper arm, or thigh. Do not inject into areas where skin is bruised, erythematous, indurated, or tender.
- Rotate sites.
- Discard any unused product as drug does not contain preservations.
- Administer a missed dose as soon as possible, then resume dosing every 4 wk.

Route	Onset	Peak	Duration
I.V., SubQ.	Unknown.	5 days.	Unknown

Half-life: 9.3 days

Mechanism of Action

Binds selectively to the p 19 subunit of human IL-23 cytokine to inhibit the release of pro-inflammatory cytokines and chemokines. This action decreases intestinal inflammation.

Contraindications

Hypersensitivity to mirikizumab-mrkz or any of its components

Interactions

CYP450 substrates: Possibly decreased CYP450 substrate exposure

live vaccines: May increase risk of infection from vaccine

Adverse Reactions

GI: Elevated liver enzymes, **hepatotoxicity**

MS: Arthralgia

RESP: Upper respiratory infections

SKIN: Rash

Other: **Anaphylaxis**, infections including herpes viral infections, injection site reactions (mucocutaneous erythema, pain, pruritis, urticaria), tuberculosis (TB) reactivation

Childbearing Considerations

PREGNANCY

- Pregnancy exposure registry: 1-800-545-5979.
- It is not known if drug can cause fetal harm. However, as a monoclonal antibody, it does cross the placenta peaking in the third trimester and may cause immunosuppression in the utero-exposed infant.

- Use with caution only if benefit to mother outweighs potential risk to fetus.

LACTATION

- It is not known if drug is present in breast milk.
- Mother should check with prescriber before breastfeeding.

Nursing Considerations

! **WARNING** Know that mirikizumab-mrkz therapy should not be initiated in patients with a significant active infection until the infection is resolved or adequately treated. Monitor the patient closely during mirikizumab-mrkz therapy, especially if patient has a chronic infection or a history of recurrent infections. If an infection occurs or becomes acute or if an infection is not responding to therapy, continue to monitor the patient closely and expect drug to be withheld until the infection is resolved.

- Be aware that patients should be evaluated for TB before mirikizumab-mrkz is begun. Know that mirikizumab-mrkz therapy should not be used in patients with active TB. Expect to administer anti-TB therapy for patients with latent TB, or in patients with a past history of active or latent TB in whom an appropriate course of therapy cannot be confirmed.

! **WARNING** Know that patients with liver cirrhosis should not receive mirikizumab-mrkz therapy. Determine a baseline for liver enzymes at start of therapy for other patients and continue to monitor liver function for at least 24 weeks of therapy and periodically thereafter, as ordered. Expect drug to be withheld if patient develops liver dysfunction until drug-induced liver dysfunction is ruled out.

- Ensure that patient is up to date on immunizations before therapy with mirikizumab-mrkz is begun. Know that patient should not receive any live vaccines while taking drug.

! **WARNING** Monitor patient for a hypersensitivity reaction, which could become life-threatening, such as anaphylaxis during I.V. infusion. Other infusion-related hypersensitivity reactions include mucocutaneous erythema and pruritis, especially during induction. If a severe reaction occurs, discontinue I.V. infusion immediately, notify prescriber, and provide supportive care, as needed and ordered.

PATIENT TEACHING

- Instruct patient or family on how to administer a mirikizumab-mrkz subcutaneous injection and what to do if a dose is missed.

! **WARNING** Instruct patient on infection control precautions. Stress importance of alerting prescriber if signs and symptoms of an infection occur.

! **WARNING** Stress importance of reporting any allergic reactions, especially during the I.V. infusion.

! **WARNING** Review signs and symptoms of liver dysfunction with patient (abdominal pain, dark urine, fatigue, jaundice, nausea, and vomiting) and encourage patient to notify prescriber if present.

- Warn patient to avoid immunizations with live vaccines.
- Educate patient on the symptoms of TB (cough, difficulty breathing, unexplained fever) and to notify prescriber, if present.
- Inform mothers who had received drug during pregnancy to alert pediatrician because live virus immunizations should be delayed for a minimum of 2 months after infant is born.

mirtazapine

Remeron, Remeron SolTab

Class and Category

Pharmacologic class: Tetracyclic antidepressant
Therapeutic class: Antidepressant

Indications and Dosages

∗ *To treat major depression*

ORAL DISINTEGRATING TABLETS, TABLETS

Adults. *Initial:* 15 mg daily at bedtime. Increased, as needed and tolerated, at 1- to 2-wk intervals. *Maximum:* 45 mg daily.

±**DOSAGE ADJUSTMENT** For patients taking strong CYP3A inducers (carbamazepine, phenytoin, rifampin) concomitantly, dosage increased. For patients taking cimetidine or strong CYP3A inhibitors (clarithromycin, ketoconazole) concomitantly, dosage decreased.

Drug Administration

P.O.

- Administer dose preferably at bedtime with water.
- Tablets should be swallowed whole and not chewed, crushed, or split.
- Remove oral disintegrating tablets gently from blister pack with dry, gloved hands. Patient should place tablet on tongue and let it dissolve, which will occur within 30 sec. Orally disintegrating tablets should not be swallowed whole and should not be chewed or crushed. Water may be taken once tablet has dissolved.

Route	Onset	Peak	Duration
P.O.	Unknown	2 hr	Unknown

Half-life: 20–40 hr

Mechanism of Action

May inhibit neuronal reuptake of norepinephrine and serotonin to increase the action of these neurotransmitters in nerve cells. Increased neuronal serotonin and norepinephrine levels may elevate mood.

Contraindications

Hypersensitivity to mirtazapine or its components; use within 14 days of an MAO inhibitor, including I.V. methylene blue and linezolid

Interactions

DRUGS

anxiolytics, hypnotics, other CNS depressants (including sedatives): Increased CNS depression
CYP3A4 inducers, such as carbamazepine, phenytoin, rifampicin: Decreased mirtazapine effects and effectiveness
CYP3A4 inhibitors, such as azole-antifungals, cimetidine, CYP3A4 inhibitors, erythromycin, HIV protease inhibitors, ketoconazole, nefazodone: Increased serum mirtazapine effects and risk of adverse reactions
MAO inhibitors, including I.V. methylene blue and linezolid; other serotonergic drugs: Possibly hyperpyrexia, hypertension, seizures, and serotonin syndrome
QTc-prolonging drugs: Increased risk of QT prolongation and/or ventricular arrhythmias, such as torsades de pointes
warfarin: Possible increase in INR

ACTIVITIES

alcohol use: Increased CNS depression

Adverse Reactions

CNS: Agitation, akathisia, amnesia, anxiety, apathy, asthenia, ataxia, **cerebral ischemia**, chills, confusion, delirium, delusions, depersonalization, depression, dizziness, dream disturbances, drowsiness, dyskinesia, dystonia, emotional lability, euphoria, extrapyramidal reactions, fever, hallucinations, hostility, hyperkinesia, hyperreflexia, hypoesthesia, hypokinesia, lack of coordination, malaise, mania, migraine headache, **neuroleptic malignant syndrome-like reactions**, neurosis, paranoia, paresthesia, psychomotor restlessness, **seizures**, **serotonin syndrome**, somnambulism (ambulation and other complex behaviors out of bed), somnolence, syncope, tremor, vertigo
CV: Angina, **bradycardia**, edema, hypercholesterolemia, hypertension, hypertriglyceridemia, **hypotension**, **MI**, orthostatic hypotension, peripheral edema, **PVCs**, **torsades de pointes**, vasodilation, **ventricular arrhythmia**
EENT: Accommodation disturbances, conjunctivitis, dry mouth, earache, epistaxis, eye pain, gingival bleeding, glaucoma, glossitis, hearing loss, hyperacusis, keratoconjunctivitis, lacrimation, pharyngitis, sinusitis, stomatitis
ENDO: Breast pain, galactorrhea, gynecomastia, hyperprolactinemia
GI: Abdominal distention and pain, anorexia, cholecystitis, colitis, constipation, elevated ALT level, eructation, increased appetite, nausea, thirst, vomiting
GU: Amenorrhea, cystitis, dysmenorrhea, dysuria, hematuria, impotence, increased libido, leukorrhea, renal calculi, urinary frequency and incontinence, urine retention, UTI, vaginitis
HEME: **Agranulocytosis**, **neutropenia**

MS: Arthralgia, back pain, dysarthria, elevated creatine kinase blood level, muscle twitching, myalgia, myasthenia, neck pain and rigidity, **rhabdomyolysis**
RESP: **Asthma**, bronchitis, cough, dyspnea, pneumonia
SKIN: Acne, alopecia, bullous dermatitis, dry skin, **erythema multiforme**, **exfoliative dermatitis**, photosensitivity, pruritus, rash, **Stevens-Johnson syndrome**, **toxic epidermal necrolysis**
Other: **Angioedema**, dehydration, flu-like symptoms, herpes simplex, **hyponatremia**, weight change

Childbearing Considerations

PREGNANCY

- Pregnancy exposure registry: 1-844-405-6185 or https://womensmentalhealth.org/clinical-and-research-programs/pregnancyregistry/antidepressants/.
- It is not known if drug causes fetal harm.
- Use with caution only if benefit to mother outweighs potential risk to fetus.

LACTATION

- Drug may be present in breast milk.
- Mothers should check with prescriber before breastfeeding.

Nursing Considerations

! **WARNING** Don't give drug within 14 days of an MAO inhibitor or concurrent therapy with serotonin-precursors, such as L-tryptophan and oxitriptan, to avoid serious, possibly fatal, serotonin syndrome reaction.

- Expect mirtazapine therapy to last 6 months or longer for acute depression.
- Monitor patient closely, especially during the first few weeks of therapy, for the development of akathisia, an unpleasant or distressing restlessness and need to move, often accompanied by an inability to sit or stand still. Notify prescriber, if present, and know that increasing the dose may worsen patient's condition.

! **WARNING** Monitor patient for hypersensitivity, which could become life-threatening, such as angioedema. If present, stop drug, notify prescriber, and provide supportive care, as needed and ordered.

! **WARNING** Watch closely for suicidal tendencies, especially when therapy starts or dosage changes, because depression may briefly worsen.

! **WARNING** Monitor patient, especially elderly patients and in those receiving concurrent medication known to cause hyponatremia because drug may lower the serum sodium level in these patients. Monitor serum sodium regularly throughout drug therapy, as ordered and patients for symptoms of hyponatremia.

! **WARNING** Monitor patients receiving other serotonergic drugs, such as lithium, St. John's wort, tramadol, triptans, and most tricyclic antidepressants, because of increased risk for serotonin syndrome. Know that serotonin syndrome can occur as an adverse drug reaction to mirtazapine therapy without the concomitant use of other drugs. Monitor patient closely for signs and symptoms of serotonin syndrome, such as alteration in vital signs, GI symptoms, mental status changes, or neuromuscular abnormalities. Its most severe form resembles neuroleptic malignant syndrome and presents with autonomic instability with possible rapid changes in vital signs, hyperthermia, mental status changes, and muscle rigidity. If any of these symptoms occur, notify prescriber immediately, provide supportive care, as needed and ordered, and expect mirtazapine to be discontinued.

! **WARNING** Monitor patient closely for infection (fever, pharyngitis, stomatitis), which may be linked to a low WBC count. If these signs occur, notify prescriber and expect to stop drug.

! **WARNING** Monitor patient for any other persistent, serious, or unusual adverse reaction because drug can adversely affect many body systems with the potential to cause serious effects.

- Be aware that mirtazapine therapy should not be discontinued abruptly because adverse reactions may occur.

PATIENT TEACHING

- Advise patient that drug may cause mild pupillary dilation, which may lead to an episode of acute closure glaucoma. Encourage patient to have an eye exam before starting therapy to see if he is at risk.

! WARNING Inform phenylketonuric patient that mirtazapine disintegrating tablets contain phenylalanine 2.6 mg per 15-mg tablet, 5.2 mg per 30-mg tablet, and 7.8 mg per 45-mg tablet.

- Instruct patient how to administer form of mirtazapine prescribed.
- Instruct patient to avoid alcohol and other CNS depressants during therapy and for up to 7 days after drug is discontinued.
- Caution patient not to discontinue mirtazapine therapy abruptly.

! WARNING Alert patient that drug may cause an allergic reaction. If present, tell patient to notify prescriber and, if severe to seek immediate medical attention.

! WARNING Instruct patient to notify prescriber at once about chills, fever, mouth irritation, sore throat, and other signs of infection. Tell patient to notify prescriber immediately of any other persistent, serious, or unusual adverse reactions.

- Advise patient to avoid hazardous activities until drug's CNS effects are known and resolved.
- Direct patient to change position slowly to minimize the effects of orthostatic hypotension.
- Encourage patient to visit prescriber regularly during therapy to monitor progress.

mitoxantrone hydrochloride

Class and Category

Pharmacologic class: Anthracenedione
Therapeutic class: Antineoplastic

Indications and Dosages

✱ *To reduce neurologic disability and frequency of relapses in patients with secondary (chronic) progressive, progressive relapsing, or worsening relapsing-remitting multiple sclerosis (patients whose neurologic status is significantly abnormal between relapses)*

I.V. INFUSION

Adults. 12 mg/m^2 infused over 5 to 15 min every 3 mo and dosage adjusted, as needed. *Maximum:* Cumulative lifetime dose of 140 mg/m^2.

✱ *As adjunct to treat pain related to advanced hormone-refractory prostate cancer*

I.V. INFUSION

Adults. 12 to 14 mg/m^2 infused over 5 to 15 min every 21 days.

✱ *As adjunct to treat acute nonlymphocytic leukemia (ANLL)*

I.V. INFUSION

Adults. *Induction:* 12 mg/m^2 infused over no less than 3 min on days 1 to 3 with 100 mg/m^2 of cytarabine as a continuous 24-hr infusion on days 1 to 7. If patient's antileukemic response is inadequate or incomplete, second induction course is given at same dosage but only for 2 days with mitoxantrone and 5 days for cytarabine.

Drug Administration

I.V.

- Follow facility policy for handling antineoplastics. Be aware that manufacturer recommends goggles, gloves, and a gown during drug preparation and delivery.
- After penetration of multidose stopper, store undiluted drug concentrate for up to 7 days at room temperature or 14 days refrigerated. Avoid freezing drug.
- Before administering drug, dilute it in at least 50 ml of 0.9% Sodium Chloride Injection or 5% Dextrose in Water. Drug may be further diluted with 0.9% Sodium Chloride Injection, 5% Dextrose in Water, or 5% Dextrose in Water with 0.9% Sodium Chloride Injection. Use immediately.
- Administer diluted solution slowly into the tubing as a freely running intravenous infusion of 0.9% Sodium Chloride Injection or 5% Dextrose in Water over no less than 3 min. A short infusion should be administered over 5 to 15 min.
- Drug shouldn't be given intra-arterially, intramuscularly, intrathecally, or subcutaneously because of possible severe adverse reactions.
- If mitoxantrone solution contacts skin or mucosa, the area should be washed

thoroughly with warm water. If it contacts eyes, irrigate them thoroughly with water or Normal Saline solution.

- Discard unused diluted solution immediately because it contains no preservatives.
- If any signs of extravasation occur (bluish discoloration, burning, erythema, pain, swelling, or ulceration), stop infusion immediately and notify prescriber. Reinsert I.V. line in another large vein and resume administration slowly. Apply ice bags intermittently to affected site and elevate affected extremity. Extravasation reactions may progress so site should be assessed frequently. Be aware a surgical consult may be needed if there is any sign of a local reaction.
- *Incompatibilities:* Other drugs

Route	Onset	Peak	Duration
I.V.	Unknown	Unknown	Unknown

Half-life: 23–215 hr

Mechanism of Action

Binds to DNA, causing cross-linkage and strand breakage, interfering with RNA synthesis, and inhibiting topoisomerase II, an enzyme that uncoils and repairs damaged DNA. Produces a cytocidal effect on proliferating and nonproliferating cells that doesn't appear to be cell-cycle specific. Inhibits B-cell, T-cell, and macrophage proliferation and impairs antigen function.

Contraindications

Hypersensitivity to mitoxantrone or its components

Interactions

DRUGS

vaccines, killed virus: Decreased antibody response to vaccine

vaccines, live virus: Increased risk of replication of and adverse effects of vaccine virus, decreased antibody response to vaccine

Adverse Reactions

CNS: Headache, **seizures**

CV: **Arrhythmias**, **cardiotoxicity**, chest pain, **congestive heart failure**, decreased left ventricular ejection fraction, **ECG changes**

EENT: Blue-colored cornea, conjunctivitis, mucositis, stomatitis

GI: Abdominal pain, diarrhea, elevated liver enzymes, **GI bleeding**, jaundice, nausea, vomiting

GU: Blue-green urine, **renal failure**

HEME: **Acute myelogenous leukemia**, **leukopenia**, **other leukemias**, **thrombocytopenia**

MS: Myelodysplasia

RESP: Cough, dyspnea

SKIN: Alopecia, extravasation

Other: **Anaphylaxis and other hypersensitivity reactions**, hyperuricemia, infection, infusion-site pain or redness

Childbearing Considerations

PREGNANCY

- Drug may cause fetal harm.
- A negative pregnancy test must be obtained prior to each dose.
- Drug should not be given to pregnant women.

LACTATION

- Drug is present in breast milk.
- Breastfeeding should be discontinued prior to drug therapy.

REPRODUCTION

- Females of childbearing age should use an effective form of contraception during drug therapy.

Nursing Considerations

! **WARNING** Be aware that drug shouldn't be given to patient with multiple sclerosis whose neutrophil count is less than 1,500/mm^3.

! **WARNING** Ensure females of childbearing age have a negative pregnancy test before drug is administered and before each course of therapy as drug may cause fetal harm.

- Know that before mitoxantrone therapy and before each dose, expect patient to have an ECG and evaluation of left ventricular ejection fraction. If patient's left ventricular ejection fraction drops below normal, expect drug to be discontinued.
- Check liver enzymes, as ordered, before each course of therapy. Also, expect to obtain CBC with platelet count, and hematocrit and hemoglobin levels before therapy begins and before each course of therapy.

! **WARNING** Monitor I.V. site closely for extravasation, which may cause a severe reaction.

! WARNING Monitor patient for a hypersensitivity reaction, which may become life-threatening, such as anaphylaxis. If present, notify prescriber, expect drug to be discontinued and provide supportive care, as needed and ordered.

! WARNING Be aware that if severe or life-threatening nonhematologic or hematologic toxicity occurs during first induction course, the second course will probably be withheld until it resolves. Know that if patient develops thrombocytopenia, precautions should be taken per facility policy. Assess patient for evidence of infection, such as fever, if leukopenia occurs. Expect to obtain appropriate specimens for culture and sensitivity testing. Monitor patients with chickenpox or recent exposure and patients with herpes zoster for severe, generalized disease.

! WARNING Assess patient for cardiac dysfunction throughout therapy. Watch for evidence of cardiotoxicity, such as arrhythmias and chest pain, in patient with heart disease. Risk increases when cumulative dose reaches 140 mg/m^2 in cancer or 100 mg/m^2 in multiple sclerosis. Notify prescriber of any significant changes and expect drug to be discontinued. Be aware that congestive heart failure may occur months or years after drug has been discontinued.

! WARNING Be aware that patients receiving mitoxantrone in combination with other antineoplastics or radiation therapy or who have multiple sclerosis are at risk for developing secondary leukemia, including acute myelogenous leukemia.

- Monitor blood uric acid level for hyperuricemia in patients with a history of gout or renal calculi and will be receiving drug for leukemia. Expect to give allopurinol, as prescribed, to prevent uric acid nephropathy.

PATIENT TEACHING

- Advise patient to complete dental work, if possible, before treatment begins or defer it until blood counts return to normal; drug may delay healing and cause gingival bleeding. Teach patient proper oral hygiene and advise use of a toothbrush with soft bristles.
- Alert females of childbearing age a negative pregnancy test must be obtained before drug therapy begins and before each course of therapy is given. Instruct females of childbearing age to use an effective contraceptive throughout drug therapy to avoid pregnancy but if pregnancy occurs to notify prescriber immediately.
- Inform patient that drug will be given intravenously.

! WARNING Instruct patient to notify medical personnel immediately if a bluish discoloration, burning, pain, redness, swelling, or ulceration occurs at intravenous site used to administer drug.

- Urge patient to drink plenty of fluid to increase urine output and uric acid excretion.
- Explain that urine may appear blue-green for 24 hours after treatment and that the whites of the eyes may appear blue. Emphasize that these effects are temporary and harmless. Explain that hair loss is possible, but that hair should return after therapy ends.

! WARNING Caution patient not to receive immunizations unless approved by prescriber. Also, advise persons who live in same household as patient to avoid receiving immunization with oral polio vaccine. Tell patient to avoid persons who recently received the oral polio vaccine or to wear a mask over his nose and mouth.

! WARNING Instruct patient to avoid persons with infections if bone marrow depression occurs. Advise patient to contact prescriber if chills, cough, fever, hoarseness, lower back or side pain, or difficult or painful urination occurs; these changes may signal an infection.

! WARNING Tell patient to contact prescriber immediately if he has black or tarry stools, unusual bleeding or bruising, blood in urine or stool, or pinpoint red spots on his skin. Emphasize the need to avoid accidental cuts, as from fingernail clippers or a razor, because of possible excessive bleeding or infection.

- Caution patient to avoid contact sports or activities that may cause bruising or injury.
- Tell mothers breastfeeding should be avoided during drug therapy.
- Emphasize the importance of complying with the dosage regimen and keeping follow-up medical and laboratory appointments.

! **WARNING** Urge patient to comply with yearly examinations after therapy ends to check for late-occurring drug-induced heart problems. Tell patient to report a fast or uneven heartbeat, swelling in ankles or legs, or trouble breathing even after drug has been discontinued.

modafinil

Provigil

Class, Category, and Schedule

Pharmacologic class: Analeptic
Therapeutic class: CNS stimulant
Controlled substance schedule: IV

Indications and Dosages

∗ *To improve daytime wakefulness in patients with narcolepsy, obstructive sleep apnea-hypopnea syndrome, and shift work sleep disorder*

TABLETS

Adults. 200 mg daily in morning or 1 hr before starting work shift. *Maximum:* 400 mg daily.

± **DOSAGE ADJUSTMENT** For patients with severe hepatic impairment, dosage should be reduced by 50%.

Drug Administration

P.O.

- Administer daily dose in morning or 1 hr before starting work shift.
- Administer drug on an empty stomach, if possible, because food may delay drug's absorption and onset of action.

Route	Onset	Peak	Duration
P.O.	Unknown	2–4 hr	Unknown

Half-life: 15 hr

Mechanism of Action

May inhibit the release of gamma-aminobutyric acid (GABA), the most common inhibitory neurotransmitter, or CNS depressant, in the brain. Increases also the release of glutamate, an excitatory neurotransmitter, or CNS stimulant, in the hippocampus and thalamus. These 2 actions may improve wakefulness.

Contraindications

Hypersensitivity to modafinil, armodafinil, or their components

Interactions

DRUGS

CYP2C19 substrates, such as clomipramine, diazepam, omeprazole, phenytoin, propranolol: Increased systemic exposure of these drugs
CYP3A4/5 substrates, such as cyclosporine, midazolam, steroidal contraceptives, triazolam: Decreased systemic exposure of these drugs, with steroidal contraceptives continuing to have decreased effectiveness for 1 mo after modafinil is discontinued
MAO inhibitors: Increased risk of adverse effects
warfarin: Possibly decreased warfarin metabolism and increased risk of bleeding

Adverse Reactions

CNS: Aggressiveness, agitation, anxiety, confusion, delusions, depression, hallucinations, headache, insomnia, mania, nervousness, psychomotor hyperactivity, psychosis, **suicidal ideation**
GI: Nausea
HEME: **Agranulocytosis**
SKIN: Rash, **Stevens-Johnson syndrome**, **toxic epidermal necrolysis**
Other: **Anaphylaxis**, **angioedema**, **drug reaction with eosinophilia and systemic symptoms (DRESS)**, infection, **multiorgan hypersensitivity**, physical and psychological dependency

Childbearing Considerations

PREGNANCY

- Pregnancy exposure registry: 1-866-404-4106.
- Drug may cause fetal harm such as intrauterine growth restriction and spontaneous abortion based on animal studies.

- Use with caution only if benefit to mother outweighs potential risk to fetus.

LACTATION

- It is not known if drug is present in breast milk.
- Mothers should check with prescriber before breastfeeding.

REPRODUCTION

- Females of childbearing age using steroidal contraceptives (including depot or implantable contraceptives) should be advised to use an alternative contraceptive method during drug therapy and for 1 mo after drug is discontinued.

Nursing Considerations

! **WARNING** Keep in mind that modafinil shouldn't be given to patients with mitral valve prolapse syndrome or a history of left ventricular hypertrophy because drug may cause ischemic changes.

- Use cautiously in patients with recent MI or unstable angina because effect of drug is unknown in these disorders.
- Use cautiously in patients with a history of depression, mania, or psychosis because these conditions may worsen during therapy and may require modafinil to be stopped. Know that giving drug to patient with emotional instability, a history of psychosis, or psychological illness with psychotic features, will require baseline behavioral assessment and frequent clinical observation.

! **WARNING** Monitor patient with a history of alcoholism, stimulant abuse, or other substance abuse for compliance with modafinil therapy. Observe for signs of abuse or misuse, including drug-seeking behavior, frequent prescription refill requests, or increased frequency of dosing. Also, watch for evidence of excessive modafinil dosage, including aggressiveness, anxiety, confusion, decreased prothrombin time, diarrhea, irritability, nausea, nervousness, palpitations, sleep disturbances, and tremor. Report findings or suspicions to prescriber.

- Be aware that modafinil, like other CNS stimulants, may alter feelings, judgment, mood, motor skills, perception, thinking, and signs that patient needs sleep.

! **WARNING** Monitor patient for signs and symptoms of hypersensitivity, including severe cutaneous reactions such as DRESS. If hypersenstivity occurs or a severe skin reaction is present such as a rash (DRESS may only initially present with a fever or swollen lymph nodes), notify prescriber, expect to discontinue drug, and provide supportive care, as needed and ordered.

! **WARNING** Watch closely for suicidal tendencies, especially in patients with a psychiatric history.

PATIENT TEACHING

- Inform patient that modafinil can help but not cure narcolepsy and that drug's full effects may not be seen right away.
- Instruct patient how to administer modafinil.

! **WARNING** Warn patient that modafinil is a controlled substance and can cause dependency. Stress importance of not increasing dosage or frequency of taking drug without consulting prescriber. Tell patient to keep drug stored in a safe place to avoid theft and away from children.

- Advise patient to avoid alcohol while taking modafinil.
- Caution patient to avoid excessive intake of beverages, foods, and over-the-counter drugs that contain caffeine because caffeine may lead to increased CNS stimulation. If he drinks grapefruit juice, encourage the patient to drink a consistent amount daily.
- Encourage a regular sleeping pattern.

! **WARNING** Alert patient that drug may cause an allergic reaction. If present, tell patient to notify prescriber and, if serious, stress importance of stopping drug, seeking immediate medical care, and contacting prescriber if serious or unusual adverse reactions occur, including the appearance of blisters, difficulty breathing or swallowing, hives, mouth sores, peeling skin, or a rash.

! WARNING Urge family or caregiver to watch patient closely for abnormal behaviors, including suicidal tendencies, especially if patient has a psychiatric history. Urge patient or family or caregiver to report anxiety, chest pain, depression, or evidence of mania or psychosis to prescriber.

- Inform patient that drug can affect concentration and function and can hide signs of fatigue. Urge the patient not to drive or perform activities that require mental alertness until full CNS effects are known and resolved.
- Inform females of childbearing age that modafinil can decrease the effectiveness of certain contraceptives, including birth control pills and implantable hormonal contraceptives. If she uses such contraceptives, urge her to use an alternate birth control method during modafinil therapy and for up to 1 month after she stops taking the drug. If pregnancy occurs or is suspected, tell her to notify prescriber.
- Advise patient to keep follow-up appointments with prescriber so that her progress can be monitored.

mometasone furoate

Asmanex HFA, Asmanex Twisthaler

mometasone furoate monohydrate

Nasonex, Nasonex 24 hr Allergy

Class and Category

Pharmacologic class: Glucocorticoid
Therapeutic class: Anti-inflammatory

Indications and Dosages

∗ *To prevent seasonal allergic rhinitis*

NASAL SPRAY (NASONEX)

Adults and adolescents ages 12 and older. 100 mcg (2 sprays) in each nostril once daily, started 2 to 4 wk prior to anticipated start of pollen season, if known.

∗ *To treat chronic rhinosinusitis with nasal polyps*

NASAL SPRAY (NASONEX)

Adults. 100 mcg (2 sprays) in each nostril once or twice daily.

∗ *To treat patients with nasal polyps who have had ethmoid sinus surgery*

SINUS IMPLANT (SINUVA)

Adults. Implant placed under endoscopic visualization. Removed in 90 days or earlier, if needed, using standard surgical instruments.

∗ *To maintain asthma control*

ORAL INHALATION (ASMANEX TWISTHALER)

Adults and children ages 12 and older who have been taking bronchodilators alone or inhaled corticosteroids. *Initial:* 220 mcg (1 inhalation) once daily in the evening, and increased, as needed. *Maximum:* 440 mcg once daily in the evening or in divided doses of 220 mcg and given twice daily in morning and evening.
Adults and children ages 12 and older who have taken oral corticosteroids. 440 mcg (2 inhalations) twice daily in morning and evening. *Maximum:* 880 mcg daily.
Children ages 4 to 11 regardless of prior therapy. 110 mcg (1 inhalation) once daily in the evening. *Maximum:* 110 mcg daily.

ORAL INHALATION (ASMANEX HFA)

Adults and children ages 12 and older not taking an inhaled corticosteroid. *Initial:* Using a 100-mcg inhaler, 2 inhalations twice daily, increased, as needed, after 2 wk. *Maximum:* Using a 200-mcg inhaler, 2 inhalations twice daily for maximum dosage of 800 mcg/day.
Adults and children ages 12 and older taking oral corticosteroid therapy. *Initial:* Using a 200-mcg inhaler, 2 inhalations twice daily, increased, as needed, after 2 wk. *Maximum:* Using a 200-mcg inhaler, 2 inhalations twice daily for maximum dosage of 800 mcg/day.
Children ages 5 to less than 12. Using a 50-mcg inhaler, 2 inhalations twice daily. *Maximum:* 200 mcg daily.

Drug Administration

ORAL INHALATION

Asmanex Twisthaler

- Asmanex Twisthaler contains small amounts of lactose, which contains trace levels of milk proteins. Do not administer to patients with a milk protein allergy because anaphylactic reactions have occurred.

- Administer once-daily dose for asthma control in the evening; twice daily in the morning and evening.
- Place inhaler in an upright position. Twist cap counterclockwise while holding colored base, making sure indented arrow (on white portion of the inhaler directly above the colored base) is pointing to the dose counter. Removing the cap loads inhaler with drug, and the dose counter on the base will count down by 1.
- Have patient take a full breath in and out, and then place mouthpiece in patient's mouth. Have patient firmly close lips around mouthpiece, taking care not to cover ventilation holes on the inhaler. Then, have patient take a fast, deep breath. Patient may not feel, smell, or taste anything with the inhalation. After taking the breath, patient should remove inhaler from mouth and hold breath for about 10 sec. Patient should not exhale into the inhaler.
- Have patient rinse mouth with water and spit out contents afterward without swallowing the water.
- Wipe the mouthpiece dry, if needed, and replace the cap right away, turning it clockwise while pressing down. A click should be heard when the cap is fully closed.
- Write down the date inhaler is opened and discard it 45 days from that date or when dose counter reads 00, whichever comes first.

Asmanex HFA

- Remove cap from the mouthpiece of the actuator. If using the inhaler for the first time, prime it by releasing 4 test sprays into the air, away from face, shaking well before each spray. If inhaler has not been used for more than 5 days, inhaler requires priming again.
- Use only the Asmanex HFA canister with the Asmanex HFA actuator.
- Shake inhaler before each use.
- Have patient breathe out as fully as possible through mouth.
- Holding the inhaler in an upright position, have patient insert the mouthpiece into mouth, and close lips around it.
- Patient should take a deep breath in slowly through mouth and while doing this press down firmly and fully on the top of the canister until it stops moving in the actuator. Then, patient should take finger off the canister.
- When patient is finished breathing in, have patient hold breath as long as possible (10 sec, if possible). Then, inhaler is removed from mouth and patient should breathe out through nose, while keeping lips closed.
- Wait at least 30 sec before administering second inhalation and then shake inhaler well again and repeat earlier steps.
- Replace cap over the mouthpiece right away after use.
- Do not wash inhaler in water but wipe the mouthpiece clean using a dry wipe after every 7 days of use.
- Have patient rinse mouth after each use of oral inhaler to help prevent mouth and throat dryness, relieve throat irritation, and prevent oropharyngeal infection.

INTRANASAL

Nasonex

- Prime nasal spray bottle before using for the first time by pressing down and releasing pump 10 times or until a fine spray appears. If drug is not used for more than 1 wk, container will have to be reprimed by spraying 2 times or until a fine spray appears.
- Shake container before each use.
- Have patient blow nose, tilt head slightly forward, and insert tube into a nostril, pointing toward inner corner of eye, away from nasal septum.
- Have patient hold the other nostril closed and spray while inhaling gently.
- Repeat the procedure in the other nostril.

Sinuva

- Implant inserted by physicians trained in otolaryngology.
- To prepare for insert, open package. Do not use if package is already opened, the package or product is damaged, or has evidence of gross contamination.
- Avoid bending, damaging, or twisting implant.
- Implant should not be compressed and loaded into the delivery system more than 2 times.

- Follow manufacturer's guidelines when assisting physician in removal of the implant.

Route	Onset	Peak	Duration
Inhalation	Unknown	1–2.5 hr	Unknown
Intranasal, including implant	Unknown	Unknown	Unknown

Half-life: 5–6 hr

Mechanism of Action

Inhibits the activity of cells and mediators active in the inflammatory response, possibly by decreasing influx of inflammatory cells into nasal passages and thereby decreasing nasal inflammation. Decreasing the inflammatory response in lung tissue helps to relieve asthma symptoms.

Contraindications

For all forms: Hypersensitivity to mometasone or its components
For Asmanex HFA: Status asthmaticus or other asthma episodes that require emergency care
For Asmanex Twisthaler: Hypersensitivity to milk proteins, status asthmaticus, or other asthma episodes that require emergency care
For Sinuva Sinus Implant: Hypersensitivity to mometasone, any of the copolymers of the implant, or their components

Interactions

DRUGS

strong CYP4503A4 inhibitors, such as atazanavir, clarithromycin, cobicistat-containing products, indinavir, itraconazole, ketoconazole, nefazodone, nelfinavir, ritonavir, saquinavir, telithromycin: Increased plasma mometasone levels leading to possible increased adverse reactions

Adverse Reactions

CNS: Headache, presyncope (implant)
CV: Chest pain
EENT: Blurred vision, cataracts, conjunctivitis, dry mouth, earache, epistaxis (nasal spray), glaucoma, nasal irritation, nasal perforation (nasal spray), nasopharyngitis, oral and pharyngeal candidiasis (nasal spray), otitis media, pharyngitis, rhinitis, sinusitis, **throat tightness**, unpleasant taste. *For implant:* Epistaxis; implant migration; nasal infection, irritation, pain, perforation
ENDO: **Adrenal insufficiency**, growth suppression (children), hypercorticism (with higher-than-recommended doses)
GI: Diarrhea, dyspepsia, nausea, vomiting
GU: Dysmenorrhea
MS: Arthralgia, decreased bone mineral density, myalgia, pain
RESP: **Asthma aggravation**, bronchitis, **bronchospasm**, increased cough, upper respiratory tract infection, wheezing
SKIN: Pruritus, rash, urticaria
Other: **Anaphylaxis**, **angioedema**, flu-like symptoms, immunosuppression, impaired wound healing, viral infection

Childbearing Considerations

PREGNANCY

- It is not known if drug causes fetal harm.
- Use with caution only if benefit to mother outweighs potential risk to fetus.

LACTATION

- It is not known if drug is present in breast milk, although other corticosteroids are.
- Mothers should check with prescriber before breastfeeding.

Nursing Considerations

! **WARNING** Be aware that oral inhalation should not be used to treat bronchospasm or other acute episodes of asthma. Ensure that a short-acting $beta_2$ agonist, such as albuterol, is available, if needed, to treat acute asthma symptoms.

! **WARNING** Be aware that a sinus implant is now available as a nonsurgical treatment for nasal polyps but it should not be used in patients with nasal ulcers or trauma.

! **WARNING** Know that mometasone is not recommended to be given to patients with ocular herpes simplex; tubercular infection; or untreated bacterial, fungal, or systemic viral infection because drug may worsen infection causing it to become quite serious as drug causes immunosuppression.

- Expect to taper prescribed oral corticosteroid therapy slowly 1 week after patient changes to mometasone. Expect to reduce dosage by no more than 2.5 mg daily at weekly intervals, if patient takes prednisone. Monitor patient for symptoms of systemically active corticosteroid withdrawal, such as depression, joint and muscle pain, and lassitude, despite maintenance or even improvement of respiratory symptoms.

! **WARNING** Notify prescriber immediately if patient has bronchospasm after mometasone oral inhalation and expect to give a fast-acting inhaled bronchodilator, discontinue mometasone, and use an alternate drug, as ordered.

! **WARNING** Monitor patient for a hypersensitivity reaction, which could become life-threatening, such as anaphylaxis or angioedema. Be aware that allergic conditions that may have been masked by corticosteroid therapy when switching patient from systemic corticosteroid to mometasone may become evident. If a hypersensitivity reaction occurs, notify prescriber, expect drug to be switched to another drug, and provide supportive care, as needed and ordered.

! **WARNING** Assess patient switched from systemic corticosteroid to mometasone for adrenal insufficiency (fatigue, hypotension, lassitude, nausea, vomiting, weakness) during initial treatment and during infection, stress, surgery, trauma, or an electrolyte-depleting condition. Notify prescriber immediately if signs or symptoms arise because adrenal insufficiency may be life-threatening. Hypothalamic-pituitary-adrenal axis function may take several months to recover after systemic corticosteroids are discontinued. Abrupt withdrawal of mometasone also may precipitate adrenal insufficiency. Know that drug may cause hypercortisolism in patients who exceed the recommended dosages.

! **WARNING** Notify prescriber if an infection is suspected because it can become severe or even life-threatening as mometasone causes immunosuppression. Be aware that if patient is exposed to chickenpox, prescriber may order varicella-zoster immune globulin to be given or, if chickenpox develops, treatment with antiviral agents may be prescribed. In addition, if patient is exposed to measles, prophylaxis with pooled I.M. immunoglobulin may be prescribed.

- Monitor patient using nasal spray for local nasal adverse reactions such as *Candida* infection, epistaxis, and nasal septum perforation. Assess nasal mucosa regularly for changes if nasal spray is used over several months or longer. Report oropharyngeal candidiasis and expect patient to receive appropriate antifungal therapy while remaining on mometasone therapy. If candidiasis is severe, however, mometasone therapy may have to be temporarily halted.
- Closely monitor a child's growth pattern; drug may stunt growth.

PATIENT TEACHING

- Instruct patient how to administer form of mometasone prescribed.
- Tell patient to take drug exactly as prescribed and not to change dosage without consulting with prescriber first.

! **WARNING** Review procedure for inserting implant. Tell patient it will stay in place for up to 90 days. Tell patient to report any adverse reactions, especially nasal bleeding or infection and signs of migration, such as choking, throat irritation, or swallowing of the implant.

! **WARNING** Stress importance of seeking immediate medical care if bronchospasms occur after administration of mometasone. Also, caution patient not to use mometasone oral inhalation, if prescribed, to relieve acute bronchospasm and to notify prescriber if rescue inhaler is required more often or doesn't seem to be as effective.

- Instruct patient to contact prescriber if symptoms persist or worsen after 3 weeks.

! **WARNING** Urge patient to seek emergency care if allergic reactions occur and to stop taking drug.

! **WARNING** Tell patient to report symptoms of adrenal insufficiency such as fatigue, hypotension, lassitude, nausea, vomiting, or weakness during initial treatment and during infection, stress, surgery, trauma, or an electrolyte-depleting condition. Notify prescriber immediately if signs or symptoms arise. Keep in mind that if patient switches from an oral corticosteroid to mometasone, she should be advised to carry or wear medical identification indicating the need for supplemental systemic corticosteroids if situations mentioned above occur.

! **WARNING** Caution patient about risk for infection. Review infection control measures patient should use such as avoiding exposure to chickenpox and measles. If exposed, patient should contact prescriber immediately. Also, alert patient of potential worsening of existing infections.

- Review adverse reactions with patient and family or caregiver and to contact prescriber if bothersome, persistent, severe, or unusual adverse reactions occur.

monomethyl fumarate

Bafiertam

Class and Category

Pharmacologic class: Nuclear factor erythroid-2 related factor 2 (Nrf2) activator
Therapeutic class: Immunomodulator

Indications and Dosages

∗ *To treat relapsing forms of multiple sclerosis, including active secondary progressive disease, clinically isolated syndrome, or relapsing-remitting disease*

D.R. CAPSULES

Adults. 95 mg twice daily for 7 days, then increased to 190 mg twice daily. *Maintenance:* 190 mg twice daily.

± **DOSAGE ADJUSTMENT** For patients unable to tolerate maintenance dose, dosage decreased to 95 mg twice daily for up to 4 weeks before resuming maintenance dosage of 190 mg twice daily.

Drug Administration

P.O.

- Expect to administer nonenteric-coated aspirin up to a dose of 325 mg 30 min before monomethyl fumarate administration to reduce severity of flushing.
- May be taken with or without food.
- Capsules should be swallowed whole without chewing, crushing, or opening capsule.

Route	Onset	Peak	Duration
P.O.	Unknown	4.03 hr	Unknown

Half-life: 0.5 hr

Mechanism of Action

May act by decreasing inflammation and preventing nerve damage associated with multiple sclerosis.

Contraindications

Concurrent therapy with dimethyl fumarate or diroximel fumarate; hypersensitivity to dimethyl fumarate, diroximel fumarate, monomethyl fumarate, or their components

Interactions

DRUGS

dimethyl fumarate, diroximel fumarate: Increased serum monomethyl fumarate levels, increasing risk of adverse reactions

Adverse Reactions

CNS: **Progressive multifocal leukoencephalopathy**
EENT: Rhinorrhea
GI: Abdominal pain; **acute pancreatitis**; diarrhea; dyspepsia; elevated bilirubin and liver enzymes; **GI hemorrhage**, **obstruction**, **perforation**, **and ulceration**; **liver injury**; nausea; vomiting
GU: Albumin in urine
HEME: Eosinophilia (transient), lymphopenia
SKIN: Alopecia, erythema, flushing, pruritus, rash
Other: **Anaphylaxis**, **angioedema**, herpes zoster and other serious opportunistic infections

Childbearing Considerations

PREGNANCY

- Pregnancy exposure registry: 1-866-663-9564.
- It is not known if drug can cause fetal harm, although animal studies suggest fetal harm may occur.
- Use with caution only if benefit to mother outweighs potential risk to fetus.

LACTATION

- It is not known if drug is present in breast milk.

- Mothers should check with prescriber before breastfeeding.

Nursing Considerations

- Ensure that the following tests have been done prior to beginning monomethyl fumarate therapy: alkaline phosphatase, complete blood cell count (including lymphocyte count), serum aminotransferase, and total bilirubin levels. A baseline is needed because of drug's ability to cause liver damage and lymphopenia once therapy starts.
- Monitor patient's complete blood cell count, including lymphocyte count, for 6 months after drug therapy starts and then every 6 to 12 months, as indicated, because monomethyl fumarate can decrease lymphocyte counts. Be aware that interruption of drug therapy may be needed if lymphocyte counts decrease to less than 0.5 3 10^9/L and persisting more than 6 months.

! **WARNING** Monitor patient for a hypersensitivity reaction, which could become life-threatening, such as anaphylaxis and angioedema. Know reaction can occur after the first dose as well as any time during treatment. If present, discontinue monomethyl fumarate, notify prescriber and provide supportive therapy, as needed and ordered.

! **WARNING** Monitor patient's liver alkaline phosphatase, serum aminotransferase, and total bilirubin levels during treatment because monomethyl fumarate can cause liver injury. Expect drug to be discontinued if liver injury is suspected.

! **WARNING** Monitor patient for signs and symptoms of herpes zoster and other serious opportunistic infections that can affect the patient's brain, ears, eyes, GI tract, lungs, meninges, skin, or spinal cord. These infections can become serious. If present, notify prescriber and provide appropriate treatment, as ordered. If patient develops herpes zoster or other infections become serious, monomethyl fumarate may have to be discontinued.

! **WARNING** Monitor patient for serious GI adverse reactions that may become life-threatening, such as hemorrhage, obstruction, perforation, and ulceration. Notify prescriber immediately, if present. Be aware that less serious GI adverse reactions such as abdominal pain, diarrhea, dyspepsia, nausea, and vomiting may also occur, especially early in monomethyl fumarate therapy but usually decrease over time.

! **WARNING** Be aware that progressive multifocal leukoencephalopathy (PML) has occurred with the prodrug of monomethyl fumarate, especially in patients who develop lymphopenia. The majority of cases occurred in patients with lymphocyte counts less than 0.5×10^9/L. Notify prescriber at first sign of PML, withhold drug, and expect patient to undergo a diagnostic workup to confirm diagnosis. Signs and symptoms to be alert for include changes in thinking, memory, and orientation that lead to confusion; disturbances of vision; personality changes; and progressive clumsiness or weakness on one side of the body. Be aware that these changes can gradually occur over days to weeks.

PATIENT TEACHING

- Instruct patient how to administer monomethyl fumarate.
- Tell patient to keep unopened bottles of drug in refrigerator and opened bottle at room temperature.
- Encourage patient to comply with blood tests that will be required before and during monomethyl fumarate therapy.

! **WARNING** Alert patient that drug may cause an allergic reaction. If present, tell patient to notify prescriber and, if severe, to seek immediate medical care.

! **WARNING** Alert patient that flushing and GI adverse reactions (abdominal pain, diarrhea, and nausea) are the most common reactions to monomethyl fumarate therapy and may diminish over time. Let patient know that taking a nonenteric-coated aspirin, if not contraindicated, prior to taking drug may help reduce flushing. Warn patient that more serious GI adverse reactions may occur and to notify prescriber if bloody diarrhea or vomiting occurs or severe abdominal pain or other severe GI reactions, if present.

! **WARNING** Review infection control measures and tell patient to alert prescriber if signs and symptoms of herpes zoster or other infections develop.

! **WARNING** Instruct patient to notify prescriber if other persistent, serious, or unusual adverse reactions occur.

montelukast sodium

Singulair

Class and Category

Pharmacologic class: Leukotriene receptor antagonist
Therapeutic class: Antiallergen, antiasthmatic

Indications and Dosages

✶ *To prevent or treat asthma*

TABLETS

Adults and adolescents ages 15 and older. 10 mg once daily in evening. *Maximum:* 10 mg daily.

CHEWABLE TABLETS

Children ages 6 to 14. 5 mg once daily in evening. *Maximum:* 5 mg daily.
Children ages 2 to 5. 4 mg once daily in evening. *Maximum:* 4 mg daily.

ORAL GRANULES

Children ages 12 mo to 23 mo. 4 mg once daily in evening. *Maximum:* 4 mg daily.

✶ *To treat seasonal allergic rhinitis*

TABLETS

Adults and adolescents ages 15 and older. 10 mg once daily.

CHEWABLE TABLETS

Children ages 6 to 14. 5 mg once daily.
Children ages 2 to 5. 4 mg once daily.

ORAL GRANULES

Children ages 2 to 5. 4 mg once daily.

✶ *To treat perennial allergic rhinitis*

TABLETS

Adults and adolescents ages 15 and older. 10 mg once daily.

CHEWABLE TABLETS

Children ages 6 to 14. 5 mg once daily.
Children ages 2 to 5. 4 mg once daily.

ORAL GRANULES

Children ages 6 mo to 23 mo. 4 mg once daily.

✶ *To prevent exercise-induced bronchoconstriction*

TABLETS

Adults and adolescents ages 15 and older. 10 mg at least 2 hr before exercise. *Maximum:* 10 mg in 24 hr.

CHEWABLE TABLETS

Children ages 6 to 14. 5 mg at least 2 hr before exercise. *Maximum:* 5 mg in 24 hr.

Drug Administration

P.O.

- Administer drug used to prevent or treat asthma in the evening.
- Administer drug to prevent exercise-induced bronchoconstriction at least 2 hr before exercise.
- Administer all forms of drug used to treat rhinitis at any time of day but be consistent.
- Tablets should be swallowed whole and not chewed, crushed, or split.
- Chewable tablets should be thoroughly chewed before swallowing.
- To administer oral granules, pour contents directly into child's mouth or mix with 1 teaspoon of ice cream or cold or room-temperature applesauce, carrots, or rice—but not liquids (except for breast milk or baby formula) or other foods—just before administration. Liquids may be given after drug has been administered. Once packet is opened, the full dose must be administered within 15 min. Drug must not be stored for future use if mixed with food.

Route	Onset	Peak	Duration
P.O.	Unknown	3–4 hr	Unknown
P.O./Chewable	Unknown	1–2.5 hr	Unknown
P.O./Granules	Unknown	1–3 hr	Unknown

Half-life: 2.7–5.5 hr

Mechanism of Action

Antagonizes receptors for cysteinyl leukotrienes, produced by arachidonic acid metabolism and released from eosinophils, mast cells, and other cells. Remember when cysteinyl leukotrienes bind to receptors in bronchial airways, they increase endothelial membrane permeability, which leads to airway edema, smooth-muscle contraction, and altered activity of cells in asthma's inflammatory process. Blocking these effects improves both nasal and respiratory symptoms.

Contraindications

Hypersensitivity to montelukast or its components

Interactions

DRUGS

phenobarbital: Decreased amount of circulating montelukast

Adverse Reactions

CNS: Aggression, agitation, anxiousness, asthenia, attention disturbance, depression, disorientation, dizziness, dream abnormalities, drowsiness, fatigue, fever, hallucinations, headache, hostility, hypoesthesia, insomnia, irritability, memory impairment, obsessive–compulsive symptoms, paresthesia, restlessness, **seizures**, sleep walking, somnambulism, somnolence, stuttering, **suicidal ideation**, tic, tremor
CV: Edema, palpitations
EENT: Conjunctivitis, dental pain or tooth infection, epistaxis, laryngitis, myopia (children), nasal congestion, otitis media, pharyngitis, rhinitis (children), rhinorrhea, sinusitis, tonsillitis
GI: Abdominal pain, **cholestatic hepatitis**, diarrhea, dyspepsia, elevated liver enzymes, **hepatic eosinophilic infiltration**, **hepatotoxicity**, indigestion, infectious gastroenteritis, nausea, **pancreatitis**, vomiting
GU: Enuresis (children), pyuria
HEME: **Increased bleeding tendency**, systemic eosinophilia, **thrombocytopenia**
MS: Arthralgia, muscle cramps, myalgia
RESP: Acute bronchitis (children), cough, pneumonia (children), **pulmonary eosinophilia**, upper respiratory tract infection, wheezing (children)
SKIN: **Atopic dermatitis (children)**, **bruising**, **eczema (children)**, **erythema multiforme**, erythema nodosum, pruritus, rash, skin infection (children), **Stevens-Johnson syndrome**, **toxic epidermal necrolysis**, urticaria
Other: **Anaphylaxis**, **angioedema**; flu-like syndrome, varicella (children), viral-like infection (in children)

Childbearing Considerations

PREGNANCY

- It is not known if drug causes fetal harm.
- Use with caution only if benefit to mother outweighs potential risk to fetus.

LACTATION

- Drug is present in breast milk.
- Mothers should check with prescriber before breastfeeding.

Nursing Considerations

! WARNING Know that montelukast shouldn't be used to treat acute asthma attack or status asthmaticus.

! WARNING Keep in mind that montelukast shouldn't be abruptly substituted for inhaled or oral corticosteroids; expect to taper corticosteroid dosage gradually, as directed.

! WARNING Monitor patient for a hypersensitivity reaction, which could become life-threatening, such as anaphylaxis or angioedema. If present, notify prescriber, expect drug to be discontinued, and provide supportive care, as needed and ordered.

! WARNING Watch patient closely for suicidal tendencies during montelukast therapy, especially when therapy starts or dosage changes.

- Monitor patient for adverse reactions, such as eosinophilia, cardiac and pulmonary symptoms, and vasculitis in patient undergoing corticosteroid withdrawal. Notify prescriber if such reactions occur.
- Monitor patient for adverse neuropsychiatric effects that may become serious and may occur even after drug is discontinued. Notify prescriber if present. Drug may have to be discontinued if still being taken by patient.

PATIENT TEACHING

! WARNING Inform patient, family or caregiver that chewable tablet contains phenylalanine and should not be taken by a patient who has phenylketonuria.

- Advise patient how to administer form of montelukast prescribed and to take drug even when feeling well.
- Urge the patient not to decrease dosage or stop taking other prescribed allergy or asthma drugs unless instructed by prescriber.

M

! **WARNING** Caution patient prescribed drug for asthma not to use drug for acute asthma attack or status asthmaticus; make sure he has appropriate short-acting rescue drug available. Instruct patient prescribed drug for asthma to notify prescriber if he needs a short-acting inhaled bronchodilator more often than usual, or more often than prescribed, to control symptoms.

! **WARNING** Caution patient with aspirin sensitivity to avoid aspirin and NSAIDs during montelukast therapy. Montelukast may not effectively reduce bronchospasm in such a patient.

! **WARNING** Alert patient that drug may cause an allergic reaction. If present, tell patient to notify prescriber and, if severe, to seek immediate medical care.

! **WARNING** Instruct patient to report increased bleeding tendency or severe skin reaction that occurs without warning immediately to prescriber.

! **WARNING** Urge family or caregiver to watch patient closely for abnormal behaviors, including depression, stuttering, or suicidal tendencies, during therapy, and urge them to notify prescriber if present and to stop taking drug.

morphine sulfate

Duramorph PF, Infumorph, M-Eslon (CAN), Mitigo, MS Contin, Statex (CAN)

Class, Category, and Schedule

Pharmacologic class: Opioid
Therapeutic class: Opioid analgesic
Controlled substance schedule: II

Indications and Dosages

∗ *To relieve pain severe enough to require opioid treatment and for which alternative treatment options such as nonopioid analgesics or opioid combination products are inadequate or not tolerated*

TABLETS

Adults. 15 to 30 mg every 4 hr, as needed.
Children weighing at least 50 kg (110 lb). *Initial:* 15 mg every 4 hr, as needed. *Maximum:* 30 mg for initial dose.

ORAL SOLUTION

Adults. 10 to 20 mg every 4 hr, as needed.
Children ages 2 to 17. 0.15 to 0.3 mg/kg (acute pain only and only certain brands), as needed.

I.M. INJECTION

Adults. 10 mg every 4 hr, as needed.

I.V. INFUSION

Adults. Highly individualized and dependent on product being used and patient's response.

I.V. INJECTION

Adults. 0.1 to 0.2 mg/kg every 4 hr, as needed.

EPIDURAL INJECTION (MORPHINE SULFATE PRESERVATIVE FREE)

Adults. *Initial:* 5 mg as a single dose. If pain isn't relieved after 1 hr, 1-mg to 2-mg doses given at appropriate intervals to relieve pain. *Maximum:* 10 mg/24 hr.

EPIDURAL INJECTION (INFUMORPH)

Adults with no tolerance to opioids. *Initial:* 3.5 to 7.5 mg/day.
Adults with some tolerance to opioids. *Initial:* 4.5 to 10 mg/day.

INTRATHECAL INJECTION (MORPHINE SULFATE PRESERVATIVE FREE)

Adults. 0.2 to 1 mg as a single dose.

INTRATHECAL INJECTION (INFUMORPH)

Adults with no tolerance to opioids. *Initial:* 0.2 to 1 mg/day.
Adults with some tolerance to opioids. *Initial:* 1 to 10 mg/day.

SUPPOSITORIES

Adults. 10 to 20 mg every 4 hr, as needed.
Children. Individualized dosage based on patient's age, size, and need.

∗ *To manage moderate to severe pain when a continuous, around-the-clock opioid analgesic is needed for an extended period of time*

E.R. CAPSULES

Adults who are not opioid tolerant. *Initial:* 30 mg every 24 hr, as needed.
Adults converting from other oral morphine formulations: Total previous daily dose every 24 hr. Alternatively, one-half total previous daily dose every 12 hr.
Adults converting from parenteral morphine. Highly individualized. *Usual:*

3 times the previous daily parenteral morphine dosage.
Adults converting from other nonmorphine opioids (oral or parenteral). Highly individualized. *Usual:* Half of the estimated daily morphine requirements every 24 hr, and then increased, as needed.

E.R. TABLETS (MS CONTIN)

Adults who are opioid-naive. 15 mg every 8 or 12 hr.
Adults who are not opioid tolerant. 15 mg every 12 hr as needed.
Adults converting from other oral morphine formulations. One-half of patient's previous 24-hr requirements every 12 hr. Alternatively, one-third of patient's previous 24-hr requirements every 8 hr.
Adults converting from parenteral morphine. Highly individualized. *Usual:* 3 times the previous daily parenteral morphine dosage.
Adults converting from other parenteral or oral nonmorphine opioids. Highly individualized. *Usual:* Half of the estimated daily morphine requirements, and then increased, as needed.

Drug Administration

- Ensure that before giving morphine, opioid antagonist and equipment for oxygen delivery and respiration are available.
- Store morphine at room temperature.
- Avoid medication errors by checking dosage (mg vs. ml), concentration, and product being used.
- Have naloxone readily available.

P.O.

- Give oral form with food or milk to minimize adverse GI reactions, as needed.
- Use dosing syringe or dosing cup that comes with product to measure dosage of oral solution. Use only 2 mg/ml or 4 mg/ml strengths for children. Never use the 20 mg/ml strength for children.
- Tablets should not be chewed, crushed, or dissolved (pellets) in mouth.
- ER capsules should be swallowed whole, or capsules can be opened, and contents sprinkled on applesauce (at room temperature or cooler). It can also be given through a gastrostomy tube (but not a nasogastric tube) by first flushing the tube with water; then sprinkle pellets into 10 ml of water. Using a funnel, swirl the pellets and water into the tube. Rinse container with another 10 ml and pour this into the funnel. Repeat rinsing until no pellets remain in the container.
- E.R. forms of morphine aren't interchangeable.

I.V.

- Have an opioid antagonist (naloxone) immediately available before administering morphine I.V.
- Discard injection solution that is discolored or darker than pale yellow or that contains precipitates that don't dissolve with shaking.
- Don't use highly concentrated solutions (such as 10 to 25 mg/ml) for single-dose administration. These solutions are intended for use in continuous, controlled microinfusion devices.
- For direct I.V. injection, inject directly into tubing of free-flowing I.V. solution slowly over 4 to 5 min. Rapid I.V. injection may increase adverse reactions.
- For continuous I.V. infusion, dilute drug in 0.9% Sodium Chloride or 5% Dextrose in Water. Follow manufacturer's instructions for amount of diluent to use. Administer with infusion-control device. Adjust dose and rate based on patient response, as prescribed.
- *Incompatibilities:* None reported by manufacturer.

I.M.

- Avoid I.M. route for long-term therapy because of injection-site irritation.
- Inject into a large muscle mass.
- Rotate sites.

INTRATHECAL

- Drug administered intrathecally only by healthcare professional skilled in this type of injection.

EPIDURAL

- Drug administered epidurally only by healthcare professional skilled in this type of injection.
- Dosage must be individualized according to patient's age, body mass, physical status, previous experience with opioids, risk factors for respiratory depression, and drugs to be coadministered before or during surgery.

P.R.

- If rectal suppository is too soft to insert, refrigerate for 30 min or run wrapped suppository under cold tap water.
- Moisten suppository before inserting.

Route	Onset	Peak	Duration
P.O.	15–30 min	> 1 hr	3–5 hr
P.O. (E.R.)	1–2 hr	3–4 hr	8–24 hr
I.V.	> 5 min	20 min	4–5 hr
I.M.	10–30 min	30–60 min	4–5 hr
Epidural	15–60 min	15–60 min	24 hr
Intrathecal	15–60 min	30–60 min	24 hr
P.R.	20–60 min	20–60 min	3–7 hr

Half-life: 1.5–4.5 hr

Mechanism of Action

Binds with and activates opioid receptors (mainly mu receptors) in brain and spinal cord to produce analgesia and euphoria.

Contraindications

For all forms: Acute or severe bronchial asthma in an unmonitored setting or in the absence of resuscitative equipment; GI obstruction, including paralytic ileus; hypersensitivity to morphine sulfate or its components; significant respiratory depression; use of MAO inhibitors within past 14 days

For neuraxial administration: Concomitant anticoagulant therapy, infection at the injection microinfusion site, presence of any other concomitant therapy or medical condition that would render epidural or intrathecal administration of morphine especially hazardous

Interactions

DRUGS

5-HT$_3$ receptor antagonists; cyclobenzaprine; linezolid; methylene blue; selected psychiatric drugs, such as amoxapine, buspirone, lithium, mirtazapine, nefazodone, trazodone, vilazodone; selective serotonin reuptake inhibitors; serotonin–norepinephrine reuptake inhibitors; St. John's wort; tricyclic antidepressants; tramadol; triptans; tryptophan: Increased risk of serotonin syndrome

anticholinergics: Possibly severe constipation leading to ileus, urine retention

antipsychotics, anxiolytics, benzodiazepines, cimetidine, CNS depressants, general anesthetics, muscle relaxants, other opioids, neuroleptics, P-glycoprotein inhibitors, psychotropic drugs, sedating antihistamines, sedative/hypnotics, tranquilizers, tricyclic antidepressants: Increased additive effects increasing risk of coma, hypotension, profound sedation, respiratory depression, death

diuretics: Decreased diuretic efficacy

MAO inhibitors: Increased risk of opioid toxicity (coma, respiratory depression) or serotonin syndrome

mixed agonist-antagonist and partial agonist analgesics, such as butorphanol, buprenorphine, nalbuphine, pentazocine: Possibly withdrawal symptoms or reduced analgesic effect

oral P2Y12 inhibitors: Decreased absorption and peak concentration of oral P2Y12 inhibitors and delayed onset of antiplatelet effect when given with intravenous morphine sulfate

skeletal muscle relaxants: Enhanced neuromuscular blocking action of skeletal muscle relaxants; increased degree of respiratory depression

ACTIVITIES

alcohol use: Increased morphine plasma levels and potentially fatal overdose of morphine from increased CNS and respiratory depression and hypotension

Adverse Reactions

CNS: Agitation, amnesia, anxiety, ataxia, chills, **coma**, confusion, decreased concentration, delirium, delusions, depression, dizziness, dream abnormalities, drowsiness, edema, euphoria, fever, gait disturbance, hallucinations, headache, **increased intracranial pressure**, insomnia, lethargy, light-headedness, malaise, mood alterations, psychosis, restlessness, rigidity, sedation, **seizures**, syncope, thinking disturbances, tremor, uncoordinated muscle movements, unresponsiveness, vertigo, weakness

CV: **Bradycardia**, **cardiac arrest**, edema, hypertension, **hypotension**, orthostatic hypotension, palpitations, **shock**, tachycardia, vasodilation

EENT: Amblyopia, blurred vision, diplopia, dry mouth, eye pain, hiccup, **laryngeal**

edema or laryngospasm (allergic), miosis, nystagmus, rhinitis, taste or voice alteration
ENDO: **Adrenal insufficiency** (rare), hypogonadism
GI: Abdominal cramps or pain, anorexia, biliary tract spasm, constipation, diarrhea, dysphagia, elevated liver enzymes, flatulence, gastroenteritis, gastroesophageal reflux, hiccups, ileus (in patients with inflammatory bowel disease) indigestion, **intestinal obstruction**, nausea, **toxic megacolon** (in patients with inflammatory bowel disease), vomiting
GU: Decreased ejaculate potency, decreased libido, difficult ejaculation, dysuria, impotence, infertility, menstrual irregularities, oliguria, prolonged labor, urinary hesitancy, urine retention
HEME: Anemia, **leukopenia**, **thrombocytopenia**
MS: Arthralgia, decreased bone mineral density, skeletal muscle rigidity
RESP: **Apnea**, **asthma exacerbation**, **atelectasis**, **bronchospasm**, decreased oxygen saturation, depressed cough reflex, **hypoventilation**, **pulmonary edema**, **respiratory arrest and depression**, wheezing
SKIN: Diaphoresis, dryness, flushing, pallor, pruritus, rash, urticaria
Other: **Anaphylaxis**, **angioedema**, **or other hypersenstivity reactions**; injection-site edema, pain, rash, or redness; opioid-induced allodynia and hyperalgesia; physical and psychological dependence; weight loss; withdrawal symptoms

Childbearing Considerations

PREGNANCY

- Drug may cause fetal harm.
- Prolonged use of drug during pregnancy can result in neonatal opioid withdrawal syndrome (NOWS), which may be life-threatening if not recognized and treated.
- Avoid prolonged use during pregnancy. Use with caution only if benefit to mother outweighs potential risk to fetus.

LABOR AND DELIVERY

- Drug is not recommended for use in pregnant women immediately before or during labor. Opioids may alter length of time of labor.
- Opioids cross the placental barrier and may produce respiratory depression and psycho-physiologic effects in the neonate. Monitor neonate closely for signs of excess sedation and respiratory depression.
- An opioid antagonist, such as naloxone, must be available at the time of delivery in the event it is needed to reverse opioid-induced respiratory depression in the neonate.

LACTATION

- Drug is present in breast milk.
- Patient should check with prescriber before breastfeeding.
- Beastfed infant may develop respiratory depression and excess sedation as well as withdrawal symptoms when mother stops taking morphine or breastfeeding stops.

REPRODUCTION

- Chronic use of opioids may reduce fertility.

Nursing Considerations

! WARNING Know that mixed agonist/antagonist (butorphanol, nalbuphine, or pentazocine) or partial agonist (buprenorphine) analgesics should not be administered to patients taking a full opioid agonist such as morphine because doing so may decrease analgesic effect and/or precipitate withdrawal symptoms.

! WARNING Be aware that morphine can lead to abuse, addiction, and misuse. To ensure that benefits of morphine therapy outweigh risks, a Risk Evaluation and Mitigation Strategy (REMS) is required. Monitor patient for evidence of physical dependence or abuse. Know that addiction can occur not only in those who obtain the drug illicitly but also in patients who are appropriately prescribed the drug at recommended doses. Be aware that excessive use of morphine may not only lead to abuse, addiction, and misuse, it can lead to overdose, and possibly death. Monitor patient's intake of drug closely.

- Monitor effectiveness of morphine to relieve pain; consult prescriber, as needed.
- Monitor patient for excessive or persistent sedation; dosage may have to be adjusted.

! WARNING Monitor patient for hypersenstivity reactions, which could become life-threatening such as anaphylaxis or angioedema. If present, notify prescriber, expect drug to be discontinued, and provide supportive care, as needed and ordered.

! WARNING Use extreme caution when administering morphine to patients with conditions accompanied by hypercapnia, hypoxia, or decreased respiratory reserve, such as asthma, chronic obstructive pulmonary disease (COPD), or cor pulmonale. This is because even with usual therapeutic doses, morphine may decrease respiratory drive while simultaneously increasing airway resistance to the point of apnea. Monitor patient's respiratory status closely, especially during the initiation of therapy or following a dose increase.

! WARNING Know that if patient is receiving a continuous morphine infusion, watch for and notify prescriber about new neurologic signs or symptoms. Inflammatory masses (such as granulomas) have caused serious neurologic reactions, including paralysis.

! WARNING Monitor respiratory status carefully and frequently during morphine therapy, especially when drug therapy is initiated and when patient is being converted to morphine because respiratory depression can develop. Be especially vigilant with cachectic, debilitated, and elderly patients who are at higher risk.

! WARNING Expect to administer morphine carefully to patients who may be at risk for carbon dioxide retention (e.g., those with brain tumors or increased intracranial pressure). Monitor for signs of sedation and respiratory depression, especially when initiating therapy. Morphine may reduce respiratory drive, and the resultant carbon dioxide retention can further increase intracranial pressure. Also, know that opioids like morphine may obscure signs and symptoms in a patient with a head injury.

! WARNING Monitor patients closely whose ability to maintain a normal blood pressure is already compromised by a reduced blood volume or concurrent administration of certain CNS depressant drugs; the drug may cause severe hypotension in these patients, especially when initiating or titrating the dose of morphine. Assess blood pressure frequently.

! WARNING Know that morphine may have a prolonged duration and cumulative effect in patients with impaired hepatic or renal function.

! WARNING Be aware that elderly patients may have increased sensitivity to morphine with drug decreasing cardiac, hepatic, or renal function more often. Expect dosage to be started at the low end of the dosing range and titrated slowly. Also monitor the elderly for more frequent signs of CNS and respiratory depression.

! WARNING Know that morphine should only be used concomitantly with benzodiazepine and other CNS depressant therapy in patients for whom other treatment options are inadequate. If prescribed together, expect dosing and duration of morphine to be limited. Monitor patient closely for signs and symptoms of a decrease in consciousness, including coma, profound sedation, and significant respiratory depression. Ensure that naloxone is readily available to treat significant respiratory depression and profound sedation. Notify prescriber immediately and provide additional emergency supportive care, as death may occur.

! WARNING Monitor patients with sleep-related breathing disorders because morphine increases the risk of central sleep apnea in a dose-dependent fashion. If patient has central sleep apnea, know that morphine dosage may have to be reduced.

! WARNING Monitor patient with a seizure disorder for increased seizure activity because morphine may worsen the disorder.

! WARNING Monitor patient's blood glucose level, especially if patient is a diabetic because opioids like morphine may cause hypoglycemia.

! WARNING Know that chronic maternal use of morphine during pregnancy can result in NOWS, which may be life-threatening if not recognized and treated appropriately. NOWS occurs when a newborn has been exposed to opioid drugs, such as morphine for a prolonged period while in utero.

! WARNING Know that many drugs may interact with opioids like morphine to cause serotonin syndrome. Monitor patient closely for signs and symptoms, such as agitation, diaphoresis, diarrhea, fever, hallucinations, labile blood pressure, muscle twitching or stiffness, nausea, shakiness, shivering, tachycardia, trouble with coordination, or vomiting. Notify prescriber at once because serotonin syndrome may be life-threatening. Be prepared to discontinue drug, if possible and ordered, and provide supportive care.

! WARNING Monitor patient for adrenal insufficiency. Although rare, it can be life-threatening. Monitor patient for anorexia, dizziness, fatigue, hypotension, nausea, vomiting, and weakness. Notify prescriber if adrenal insufficiency is suspected and expect diagnostic testing to be done. If confirmed, expect to administer corticosteroids and wean patient off morphine, if possible.

- Monitor patient for paradoxic increase in pain known as opioid-induced hyperalgesia or an increase in sensitivity to pain known as allodynia, especially when morphine dosage increases. Do not confuse this with tolerance, which is the need for increasing doses of opioids to maintain an effect. If opioid-induced allodynia or hyperalgesia is suspected, notify prescriber and expect dosage to be decreased or opioid rotation to be prescribed.
- Know that morphine may cause spasm of the sphincter of Oddi and elevate serum amylase levels. Monitor patients with biliary tract disease, including acute pancreatitis for worsening symptoms.
- Keep in mind when discontinuing morphine in patients receiving more than 30 mg daily, expect prescriber to reduce daily dose by about one-half for 2 days and then by 25% every 2 days thereafter until total dose reaches initial amount recommended for patients who haven't received opioids (15 to 30 mg daily). This regimen minimizes the risk of withdrawal symptoms such as body aches, diaphoresis, diarrhea, fever, piloerection, rhinorrhea, sneezing, and yawning.

PATIENT TEACHING

- Instruct patient how to take form of morphine prescribed.

! WARNING Stress importance of taking drug exactly as prescribed and before pain is severe. Also, instruct not to take more drug than prescribed and not to take it longer than absolutely needed because excessive or prolonged use can lead to abuse, addiction, misuse, overdose, and possibly death.

- Advise patient to notify prescriber for worsening or breakthrough pain or pain increases when dose is increased.

! WARNING Encourage family or caregiver to have naloxone in household to treat an emergency opioid overdose. Instruct on how to recognize respiratory depression and how to give naloxone. Emphasize that even if naloxone is given, 911 should be called immediately with naloxone administration.

! WARNING Urge patient to avoid alcohol and other CNS depressants, including benzodiazepines, during therapy without prescriber knowledge, as severe respiratory depression can occur and may lead to death.

! WARNING Warn patient to keep drug out of reach of children, as accidental ingestion may cause death. Also, remind patient that drug is a controlled substance. Patient should take steps to protect drug from theft.

! WARNING Alert patient that morphine may cause an allergic reaction. If present, tell patient to notify prescriber and, if severe, to seek immediate medical care.

! WARNING Stress importance of notifying prescriber of persistent, serious, or unusual adverse reactions, especially breathing problems.

! WARNING Inform breastfeeding mothers to monitor their infant for respiratory depression and excess sedation. Warn mother infant may experience withdrawal symptoms when mother either stops taking morphine or stops breastfeeding. Encourage her to consult pediatrician before morphine therapy or breastfeeding will stop.

! WARNING Advise females of childbearing age to notify prescriber if she becomes pregnant. Chronic morphine use during pregnancy may cause physical dependence in fetus and withdrawal in neonate.

! **WARNING** Tell patient to alert all prescribers of morphine use. This is important because a potentially fatal effect can occur when an opioid such as morphine is combined with a benzodiazepine.

- Warn patient not to discontinue morphine use abruptly if more than a few weeks of use has occurred, as withdrawal symptoms may develop such as anxiety, decreased appetite, excessive tearing, irritability, muscle aches or twitching, rapid heart rate, or yawning.
- Advise patient to avoid potentially hazardous activities during morphine therapy.
- Tell patient to change positions slowly to minimize orthostatic hypotension.
- Inform patient that long-term use of opioids such as morphine may decrease sex hormone levels, causing decreased libido, erectile dysfunction, impotence, infertility, or lack of menstruation. Encourage patient to report any symptoms.
- Instruct patient that when morphine is no longer needed, patient should dispose of drug promptly. Expired, unused, or unwanted drug can be disposed of by flushing the drug down the toilet if a drug take-back option is not available.

moxifloxacin hydrochloride

Class and Category

Pharmacologic class: Fluoroquinolone
Therapeutic class: Antibiotic

Indications and Dosages

* *To treat acute sinusitis caused by* Haemophilus influenzae, Moraxella catarrhalis, *or* Streptococcus pneumoniae; *to treat mild to moderate community-acquired pneumonia caused by* Chlamydia pneumoniae, H. influenzae, Klebsiella pneumoniae, M. catarrhalis, Mycoplasma pneumoniae, Staphylococcus aureus, *or* S.pneumoniae *(including penicillin-resistant or multi-drug-resistant strains)*

I.V. INFUSION, TABLETS

Adults. 400 mg every 24 hr for 10 days for acute sinusitis and 7 to 14 days for community-acquired pneumonia.

* *To treat acute exacerbation of chronic bronchitis caused by* H. influenzae, H. parainfluenzae, Klebsiella pneumoniae, M. catarrhalis, S. pneumoniae, *or* Staphylococcus aureus

I.V. INFUSION, TABLETS

Adults. 400 mg every 24 hr for 5 days.

* *To treat uncomplicated skin and soft-tissue infections caused by* S. aureus *or* Streptococcus pyogenes

I.V. INFUSION, TABLETS

Adults. 400 mg every 24 hr for 7 days.

* *To treat complicated skin and skin structure infections caused* by Enterobacter cloacae, E. coli, K. pneumoniae, *or* S. aureus

I.V. INFUSION, TABLETS

Adults. 400 mg every 24 hr for 7 to 21 days.

* *To treat complicated intra-abdominal infections, including polymicrobial infections such as abscesses caused by* Bacteroides fragilis, B. thetaiotaomicron, Clostridium perfringens, Enterococcus faecalis, E. coli, Peptostreptococcus *species,* Proteus mirabilis, Streptococcus anginosus, *or* S. constellatus

I.V. INFUSION, TABLETS

Adults. 400 mg every 24 hr for 5 to 14 days with initial dosage given as I.V. infusion.

* *To prevent or treat plague, including pneumonic and septicemic plague, caused by* Yersinia pestis

I.V. INFUSION, TABLETS

Adults. 400 mg every 24 hr for 10 to 14 days after exposure confirmed or suspected.

Drug Administration

P.O.

- Administer drug with or without food and administer consistently at about the same time of day.
- Administer drug at least 4 hr before and 8 hr after aluminum- or magnesium-containing antacids, didanosine chewable buffered tablets or powder for oral solution prepared, multivitamins containing iron or zinc, or sucralfate.

I.V.

- Flush I.V. line before and after infusion with a compatible solution, such as 0.9% Sodium Chloride Injection, 5% Dextrose Injection, or Lactated Ringer's solution.

- Stop other solutions during moxifloxacin infusion.
- Infuse drug over 60 min using ready-to-use flexible bags with 400 mg of moxifloxacin in 250 ml of 0.9% Sodium Chloride Injection. Don't dilute further.
- Do not give by rapid or bolus I.V. injection.
- Don't refrigerate drug because precipitation will occur.
- Discard any unused portion; premixed bags are for single use only.
- *Incompatibilities:* Other I.V. additives or drugs

Route	Onset	Peak	Duration
P.O./I.V.	Unknown	Unknown	Unknown

Half-life: 12 hr

Mechanism of Action

Inhibits synthesis of bacterial enzyme DNA gyrase by counteracting excessive supercoiling of DNA during replication or transcription. Inhibiting DNA gyrase causes rapid- and slow-growing bacterial cells to die.

Contraindications

Hypersensitivity to moxifloxacin, other fluoroquinolones, or their components; myasthenia gravis

Interactions

DRUGS

aluminum- or magnesium-containing antacids; drug formulations with divalent or trivalent cations, such as didanosine chewable buffered tablets or powder for oral solution; metal cations, such as iron; multivitamins containing iron or zinc; sucralfate: Possibly substantial interference with moxifloxacin absorption, causing low blood moxifloxacin level
antidiabetic agents: Increased risk of either hyperglycemia or hypoglycemia
class IA antiarrhythmics, such as quinidine; class III antiarrhythmics, such as sotalol; other drugs known to prolong QTc interval, such as antipsychotics, cisapride, disopyramide erythromycin, pentamidine and tricyclic antidepressants: Possibly prolonged QTc interval
corticosteroids: Increased risk of Achilles and other tendon ruptures
NSAIDs: Increased risk of CNS stimulation and seizures
warfarin: Possibly increased anticoagulation

Adverse Reactions

CNS: Abnormal gait, agitation, altered coordination, anxiety, confusion, delirium, depression, disorientation, disturbance in attention, dizziness, fever, hallucinations, headache, **increased intracranial pressure (including pseudotumor cerebri)**, insomnia, memory impairment, nervousness, paranoia, peripheral neuropathy, psychosis, psychotic reaction, **seizures**, **suicidal ideation**, syncope, **toxic psychosis**, tremors
CV: **Aortic dissection**, hypertension, **hypotension**, palpitations, peripheral edema, **prolonged QT interval**, **rupture of aortic aneurysm**, tachycardia, vasculitis, vasodilation, **ventricular tachyarrhythmias**
EENT: Altered taste, deafness or other hearing impairments, **laryngeal edema**, vision loss
ENDO: Hyperglycemia, **hypoglycemia**
GI: Abdominal pain, abnormal liver enzymes, **acute hepatic necrosis**, **cholestatic hepatitis**, ***Clostridioides difficile*–associated diarrhea**, diarrhea, dyspepsia, **hepatic failure**, **hepatitis**, jaundice, nausea, **pseudomembranous colitis**, vomiting
GU: **Acute renal insufficiency or failure**, interstitial nephritis
HEME: **Agranulocytosis**, **aplastic anemia**, eosinophilia, **hemolytic anemia**, **leukopenia**, **pancytopenia**, **prolonged prothrombin time**, **thrombocytopenia**
MS: Arthralgia; muscle weakness; myalgia; tendon inflammation, pain, or rupture
RESP: **Allergic pneumonitis**
SKIN: Photosensitivity, rash, **Stevens-Johnson syndrome**, **toxic epidermalnecrolysis**
Other: **Anaphylaxis**, **anaphylactic shock**, **angioedema**, serum sickness, worsening of myasthenia gravis

Childbearing Considerations

PREGNANCY

- It is not known if drug causes fetal harm.
- Use with caution only if benefit to mother outweighs potential risk to fetus.

LACTATION

- Drug may be present in breast milk.
- Breastfeeding is not recommended during drug therapy.

M

Nursing Considerations

! WARNING Be aware that if patient has hypokalemia, expect to correct it before beginning moxifloxacin therapy to prevent arrhythmias. Monitor serum potassium level, as ordered, during therapy to assess for hypokalemia.

! WARNING Determine if patient has a history of CNS disorders, such as cerebral arteriosclerosis or epilepsy because drug may lower seizure threshold. Notify prescriber before starting drug and take seizure precautions.

! WARNING Be aware that there is an increased risk of aortic aneurysm and dissection within 2 months following use of moxifloxacin as a fluroquinolone, especially in elderly patients. Moxifloxacin should be reserved for patients with a known aortic aneurysm or patients who are at greater risk for aortic aneurysms only when there are no alternative antibacterial therapies available.

! WARNING Keep in mind before starting moxifloxacin therapy, determine if patient takes a class IA antiarrhythmic, such as quinidine; a class III antiarrhythmic, such as sotalol; or other drugs that prolong the QTc interval, such as antipsychotics, cisapride, erythromycin, or tricyclic antidepressants. These drugs should be avoided in patients taking moxifloxacin because they may prolong the QTc interval and lead to life-threatening ventricular tachycardia or torsades de pointes. Monitor patient closely throughout therapy, especially if he has significant acute myocardial ischemia or bradycardia, because these conditions increase risk of prolonging the QTc interval.

- Expect to obtain a 12-lead ECG before therapy begins to assess patient for a prolonged QTc interval. Ask patient if he or a blood relative has a history of prolonged QTc interval. Monitor elderly patients closely; they may have increased risk of prolonged QTc interval.
- Obtain a fluid or tissue specimen for culture and sensitivity, as ordered. Expect to begin therapy before results are available.

! WARNING Monitor patient for hypersensitivity reactions, which could become life-threatening such as anaphylaxis or angioedema. If present, notify prescriber, expect drug to be discontinued, and provide supportive care, as needed and ordered.

! WARNING Monitor patient for diarrhea. If profuse, watery diarrhea develops, contact prescriber and expect to obtain a stool specimen to rule out pseudomembranous colitis caused by *Clostridioides difficile*. It may be mild or become life-threatening. If confirmed, expect to withhold moxifloxacin and treat with an antibiotic effective against *C. difficile*, as ordered. Also, expect electrolytes, fluids, and protein supplementation to be administered, as needed and ordered.

! WARNING Monitor patient for CNS (including psychiatric) adverse reactions, such as confusion, depression, dizziness, hallucinations, peripheral neuropathy, psychosis, suicidal ideation, and tremors. If any occurs, notify prescriber and expect moxifloxacin to be discontinued.

- Monitor patients with liver dysfunction, including cirrhosis, because drug may adversely affect liver function.

! WARNING Know that fluoroquinolones, such as moxifloxacin, have caused disabling and potentially irreversible serious adverse reactions from different body systems that can occur together in the same patient. These reactions can occur within hours to weeks after starting the drug. All ages of patients and patients without any preexisting risk factors have experienced these reactions. Notify prescriber and expect to discontinue moxifloxacin immediately at the first signs or symptoms of any serious adverse reactions

! WARNING Monitor patient's blood glucose, especially in diabetic patients receiving concomitant treatment with insulin or an oral hypoglycemic agent, for changes in blood glucose levels. If dysglycemia occurs, treat according to standard of care and expect that drug may have to be discontinued.

- Monitor patients who are prone to tendinitis, such as athletes, the elderly, and those taking corticosteroids, for complaints of tendon inflammation, pain, or rupture. If present, notify prescriber and expect to discontinue moxifloxacin, place patient on bedrest with no exercise of affected limb, and obtain diagnostic tests to confirm rupture.

PATIENT TEACHING

- Instruct patient how to administer oral form of moxifloxacin.
- Caution patient to complete the prescribed course of therapy even if feeling better.
- Teach patient to take drug at least 4 hours before and 8 hours after aluminum- or magnesium-containing antacids, didanosine chewable buffered tablets or oral solution prepared from powder, multivitamins containing iron or zinc, or sucralfate.
- Urge patient to drink plenty of fluids while taking moxifloxacin.

! **WARNING** Alert patient that drug may cause an allergic reaction. If present, tell patient to notify prescriber and, if severe, to seek immediate medical care. Caution patient to stop drug and notify prescriber if he has a rash, trouble breathing, or other signs of an allergic reaction. Also, advise patient to stop taking moxifloxacin immediately and notify prescriber if any other persistent, serious, or worsening adverse effects occur.

! **WARNING** Urge patient to tell prescriber if diarrhea develops, even more than 2 months after moxifloxacin therapy ends.

! **WARNING** Urge patient to notify prescriber at once about fainting or palpitations because they may indicate a serious arrhythmia. Also, tell patient to seek emergency help immediately if patient develops sudden back, chest, or stomach pain.

! **WARNING** Warn patient, especially diabetics, that moxifloxacin may alter blood glucose levels. Review signs and symptoms of hyperglycemia and hypoglycemia. Tell patient to report symptomatic changes in blood glucose levels to prescriber and review how to treat hypoglycemia.

! **WARNING** Tell patient to notify prescriber if motor or sensory changes occur. Also, alert patient, family, or caregiver that drug may cause suicidal behavior or thoughts. Tell them to monitor patient closely and to notify prescriber of any concerns.

- Urge patient to stop any exercise and contact prescriber immediately if he develops tendon inflammation, pain, or rupture.
- Caution patient to avoid hazardous activities until adverse CNS effects are known and resolved.
- Tell patient to avoid excessive exposure to sunlight or artificial ultraviolet light because severe sunburn may result. Instruct patient to notify prescriber if sunburn develops because moxifloxacin may have to be discontinued.
- Inform mothers breastfeeding is not recommended during drug therapy.

mycophenolate mofetil

CellCept, Myhibbin

mycophenolate mofetil hydrochloride

CellCept Intravenous

mycophenolic acid

Myfortic

M

Class and Category

Pharmacologic class: Mycophenolic acid
Therapeutic class: Immunosuppressant

Indications and Dosages

* *To prevent organ rejection in patients receiving allogenic kidney transplants*

CAPSULES, I.V. INFUSION, ORAL SUSPENSION, TABLETS

Adults. 1 g twice daily. I.V. infused over no less than 2 hr.

D.R. TABLETS

Adults. 720 mg twice daily.

Children ages 5 and older who are at least 6 mo post kidney transplant. 400 mg/m^2 twice daily.

Children ages 5 and older who are at least 6 mo post kidney transplant with a body surface area between 1.19 to 1.58 m^2. 540 mg twice daily.

Children ages 5 and older who are at least 6 mo post kidney transplant with a body surface area greater than 1.58 m^2. 720 mg twice daily.

ORAL SUSPENSION

Children ages 3 mo and older. 600 mg/m^2 twice daily. *Maximum:* 2 g (10 ml) daily in 2 divided doses.

CAPSULES

Children with body surface area of 1.25 m^2 to less than 1.5 m^2. 750 mg twice daily.

CAPSULES, TABLETS

Children with body surface area of 1.5 m^2 or greater. 1 g twice daily.

✱ *To prevent organ rejection in patients receiving allogenic heart transplants*

CAPSULES, I.V. INFUSION, ORAL SUSPENSION, TABLETS

Adults. 1.5 g twice daily. I.V. infused over no less than 2 hr.

ORAL SUSPENSION

Children ages 3 mo and older. 600 mg/m^2 twice daily and, if tolerated, increased to 900 mg/m^2 twice daily. *Maximum:* 3 g (15 ml) daily in 2 divided doses.

CAPSULES

Children with body surface area of 1.25 m^2 to less than 1.5 m^2. 750 mg twice daily.

CAPSULES, TABLETS

Children with body surface area of 1.5 m^2 or greater. 1 g twice daily.

✱ *To prevent organ rejection in patients receiving allogenic liver transplants*

I.V. INFUSION

Adults. 1 g twice daily. I.V. infused over no less than 2 hr.

CAPSULES, ORAL SUSPENSION, TABLETS

Adults. 1.5 g twice daily.

ORAL SUSPENSION

Children ages 3 mo and older. 600 mg/m^2 twice daily and, if tolerated, increased to 900 mg/m^2 twice daily. *Maximum:* 3 g (15 ml) daily in 2 divided doses.

CAPSULES

Children with body surface area of 1.25 m^2 to less than 1.5 m^2. 750 mg twice daily.

CAPSULES, TABLETS

Children with body surface area of 1.5 m^2 or greater. 1 g twice daily.

± **DOSAGE ADJUSTMENT** For patients who develop an absolute neutrophil count of less than $1.3 \times 10^3/\mu L$, dosage reduced or therapy interrupted.

Drug Administration

- Handle drug similarly to a chemotherapeutic drug because mycophenolate mofetil is embryotoxic and genotoxic and may have mutagenic properties.
- Avoid inhalation or contact of skin or mucous membranes with the powder found in capsules or oral suspension. If contact occurs, wash area thoroughly with soap and water; rinse eyes with plain water.

P.O.

- Capsules, oral suspension, or tablets should not be used interchangeably with D.R. tablets.
- Capsules and tablets should be swallowed whole and not chewed, crushed, or split/opened.
- Administer on an empty stomach 1 hr before or 2 hr after a meal. However, in stable transplant patients, drug may be taken with food, if needed.
- Know that a pharmacist will reconstitute oral suspension.
- When giving oral suspension, don't mix with any other drugs.
- Ask patient about history of phenylketonuria before initial administration because oral suspension contains aspartame.
- Oral suspension can be administered through an 8 F or larger nasogastric tube.
- Store drug at room temperature. Oral suspension also may be stored in refrigerator. Discard oral suspension once mixed after 60 days.

I.V.

- Expect to switch patient receiving drug I.V. to oral form as soon as possible, as ordered.
- Reconstitute with 14 ml of 5% Dextrose in Water for each vial (2 vials will be needed for 1-g dose; 3 vials for 1.5-g dose), then shake gently.
- Further dilute 1-g dose with 140 ml of 5% Dextrose in Water and 210 ml for 1.5-g dose.
- Administer within 4 hr once reconstituted and diluted.
- Administer infusion over no less than 2 hr. Never administer by rapid or bolus I.V. injection.
- *Incompatibilities:* Other I.V. drugs and solutions

Route	Onset	Peak	Duration
P.O.	Unknown	0.5–2 hr	Unknown
P.O./D.R.	Unknown	1.5–2.7 hr	Unknown
I.V.	Unknown	Unknown	Unknown

Half-life: 8–18 hr

Mechanism of Action

Hydrolyzes to form mycophenolic acid (MPA), inhibits guanosine nucleotide synthesis, and proliferation of T and B lymphocytes. Suppresses antibody formation also by B lymphocytes and prevents glycosylation of lymphocyte and monocyte glycoproteins involved in adhesion to endothelial cells. May inhibit also leukocytes from sites of inflammation and graft rejection, which may explain how mycophenolate mofetil prolongs allogeneic transplant survival.

Contraindications

Hypersensitivity to mycophenolate mofetil, mycophenolic acid, mycophenolate sodium, or any of their components; hypersensitivity to polysorbate 80 (I.V. form)

Interactions

DRUGS

acyclovir, ganciclovir, probenecid, valacyclovir, valganciclovir: Increased plasma concentrations and/or adverse reactions of these drugs
aminoglycosides, bile acid sequestrants, cephalosporins, cyclosporine A, fluoroquinolones, penicillins, rifampin, sulfamethoxazole/trimethoprim: Decreased effectiveness of mycophenolate mofetil
antacids with aluminum and magnesium hydroxides, sevelamer: Decreased absorption of oral mycophenolate mofetil
isavuconazole: Increased risk of adverse reactions caused by mycophenolate mofetil
live vaccines: Decreased effectiveness of live vaccines
oral contraceptives (combination): Possibly decreased effectiveness of oral contraceptives
proton pump inhibitors, such as lansoprazole, pantoprazole: Possibly decreased effectiveness of mycophenolate mofetil
telmisartan: Decreased mycophenolate mofetil system exposure reducing effectiveness

Adverse Reactions

CNS: Agitation, anxiety, asthenia, chills, confusion, delirium, depression, dizziness, emotional lability, fever, hallucinations, headache, hypertonia, hypesthesia, insomnia, malaise, meningitis, nervousness, neuropathy, paresthesia, **progressive multifocal leukoencephalopathy**, psychosis, **seizures**, somnolence, syncope, thinking abnormality, tremor, vertigo
CV: Angina pectoris, **arrhythmias**, **arterial thrombosis**, **atrial fibrillation or flutter**, **bradycardia**, **cardiac arrest**, CV disorder, **congestive heart failure**, **extrasystoles**, generalized edema, **hemorrhage**, hypercholesterolemia, hyperlipemia, hypertension, **hypotension**, increased lactic dehydrogenase, increased SGOT and SGPT, increased venous pressure, **infectious endocarditis**, orthostatic hypotension, palpitations, **pericardial effusion**, peripheral edema, peripheral vascular disorder, **supraventricular tachycardia**, **thrombosis**, vasodilation, vasospasm, **ventricular extrasystole**, **ventricular tachycardia**
EENT: Amblyopia, cataract, conjunctivitis, deafness, dry mouth, ear disorder or pain, epistaxis, eye hemorrhage, gingivitis, gum hyperplasia, lacrimation disorder, mouth ulceration, oral candidiasis, pharyngitis, rhinitis, sinusitis, stomatitis, tinnitus, vision abnormality, voice alteration

ENDO: Cushing's syndrome, diabetes mellitus, hypercalcemia, **hypoglycemia**, hypothyroidism, parathyroid disorder
GI: Abdomen enlargement or pain, anorexia, ascites, cholangitis, cholestatic jaundice, colitis, constipation, diarrhea, dyspepsia, dysphagia, elevated liver enzymes, esophagitis, flatulence, gastritis, gastroenteritis, GI candidiasis, **GI hemorrhage or perforation**, GI infection, **hepatitis**, hernia, ileus, intestinal villous atrophy, jaundice, **liver damage**, **melena**, nausea, **pancreatitis**, **peritonitis**, **reactivation of hepatitis B or hepatitis C**, rectal disorder, stomach ulcer, **ulceration of GI tract**, vomiting
GU: Albuminuria; bilirubinemia; BK virus-related nephropathy; dysuria; hematuria; hydronephrosis; impotence; increased BUN or creatinine levels; **kidney tubular necrosis**; nocturia; oliguria; pain; polyomavirus-associated nephropathy; prostatic disorder; **pyelonephritis**; **renal failure**; scrotal edema; urinary tract disorder or infection; urine abnormality, frequency, incontinence, or retention
HEME: Anemia, **agranulocytosis**, **bone marrow failure**, **coagulation disorder**, hypochromic anemia, hypogammaglobulinemia, **increased prothrombin time or thromboplastin time**, leukocytosis, **leukopenia**, lymphopenia, **neutropenia**, **pancytopenia**, polycythemia, pure red cell aplasia, **thrombocytopenia**
MS: Arthralgia; back, neck or pelvic pain; joint disorder; leg cramps; myalgia; myasthenia; osteomyelitis; osteoporosis
RESP: **Apnea**; **asthma**; **atelectasis**; bronchiectasis; bronchitis; candidiasis; cough; dyspnea; **hemoptysis**; hyperventilation; **hypoxia**; interstitial lung disease; **neoplasm**; pleural effusion; pneumonia; **pneumothorax**; **pulmonary edema**, **fibrosis**, **or hypertension**; **respiratory acidosis** or infection; sputum increase; **wheezing**
SKIN: Abscess; acne; alopecia; benign neoplasm, **carcinoma**, hypertrophy, or ulcer; cellulite; ecchymosis; fungal dermatitis; hirsutism; pallor; petechiae; pruritus; rash; sweating; vesiculobullous rash
Other: Abnormal healing; **acidosis**; activation of latent infections (such as tuberculosis); acute inflammatory syndrome; **alkalosis**; **angioedema**; bacterial, fungal, protozoal, and viral infections, including opportunistic infections; congenital defects; cyst; de novo purine synthesis inhibitors-associated acute inflammatory syndrome; dehydration; flu-like syndrome; gout; hiccup; **hyperkalemia**; **hypersensitivity reactions**; hyperuricemia; hypervolemia; **hypocalcemia**; hypochloremia; **hypokalemia**; **hypomagnesemia**; **hyponatremia**; **hypophosphatemia**; hypoproteinemia; immunosuppression; increased alkaline phosphatase; increased gamma glutamyl transpeptidase; **Kaposi's sarcoma**; lymphocele; lympnadenopathy, **lymphoma**; **malignancies**; **sepsis**; thirst; weight gain or loss

Childbearing Considerations

PREGNANCY

- Pregnancy exposure registry: 1-800-617-8191 or www.mycophenolateREMS.com.
- Drug causes fetal harm, such as an increased risk of first-trimester pregnancy loss, and an increased risk of multiple congenital malformations in multiple organ systems.
- A negative pregnancy test should be performed and a second one done 8 to 10 days later before drug therapy is begun.
- Drug is not recommended for use during pregnancy.

LACTATION

- It is not known if drug is present in breast milk.
- Mothers should check with prescriber before breastfeeding.

REPRODUCTION

- Know that females of childbearing age must receive contraceptive counseling and use at least 2 contraceptives simultaneously throughout drug therapy and for 6 wk following drug discontinuation unless abstinence is practiced, an intrauterine device is in place, or tubal ligation or vasectomy in male partner has occurred.
- Know that male patients and their female partner of childbearing age must also receive contraceptive counseling and use an effective contraceptive throughout drug therapy and for 90 days following drug discontinuation unless abstinence is practiced.

- Inform females of childbearing age that drug may make combination oral hormonal contraceptives ineffective.
- Females of childbearing age or female partner of childbearing age should be made aware that follow-up pregnancy testing will be done during drug use.
- Instruct male patients not to donate sperm during drug therapy and for at least 90 days following drug discontinuation.

Nursing Considerations

! **WARNING** Keep in mind, before starting mycophenolate therapy in females of childbearing age, to make sure a negative pregnancy test within 1 week of starting therapy is done, using a test with a sensitivity of at least 25 mIU/ml. Therapy shouldn't start until results are confirmed.

! **WARNING** Know that mycophenolate mofetil therapy should be avoided in patients with hypoxanthine-guanine phosphoribosyl-transferase deficiency because drug may exacerbate disease symptoms.

- Know that corticosteroids and cyclosporine should be used with mycophenolate mofetil therapy.
- Obtain CBC weekly during first month of therapy, twice monthly for the second and third months of therapy, and then monthly through the first year, as ordered. Notify prescriber of any abnormalities. If significant, anticipate dosage reduction if absolutely necessary because reduced immunosuppression increases the risk of organ rejection. Also, provide supportive care, as ordered.

! **WARNING** Monitor patient for a hypersensitivity reaction, which may become life-thretening such as angioedema. If present, notify prescriber, expect drug to be switched to a different drug, and provide supportive care, as needed and ordered.

! **WARNING** Know that patient may be at increased risk for bacterial, fungal, protozoal, and viral infections, including opportunistic infections and viral reactivation of hepatitis B and C, which may lead to hospitalization and possibly fatal outcome. Monitor patient for signs and symptoms of infection and institute infection control measures. Expect to stop drug or reduce the dose and provide supportive care, as ordered, if neutropenia develops.

! **WARNING** Monitor patient for acute inflammatory syndrome characterized by arthralgias, arthritis, elevated inflammatory markers, fever, and muscle pain. Symptoms may occur weeks to months after drug is initiated or after a dosage increase. If present, expect drug to be discontinued and patient to improve within 24 to 48 hours.

! **WARNING** Know that mycophenolate mofetil therapy has been associated with JC-virus-associated progressive multifocal leukoencephalopathy that can be life-threatening. Monitor patient for apathy, ataxia, cognitive deficiencies, and confusion. Report suspicions of disorder immediately to prescriber. Also, know that patient is at increased risk for other viral infections, such as cytomegalovirus infections, COVID-19 infections, and polyomavirus-associated nephropathy. Expect dosage to be reduced or drug possibly discontinued in patients who develop new infections or reactivated viral infections.

! **WARNING** Monitor patient for other persistent, serious, or unusual adverse effects because drug can affect many systems with the potential for adverse reactions.

- Monitor patient's serum creatinine levels, as ordered, to detect changes in kidney function because drug may cause polyomavirus-associated nephropathy. Notify prescriber if changes occur and expect dosage to be reduced, if needed.

PATIENT TEACHING

! **WARNING** Advise females of childbearing age that 2 forms of contraceptives should be used simultaneously before beginning mycophenolate mofetil therapy, during therapy, and for 6 weeks following discontinuation of therapy because of potential for fetal harm. Tell male patients that they and their female partner of childbearing age should use effective contraception during therapy and for

90 days following discontinuation of therapy. Inform females of childbearing age who use combination oral contraceptives that drug may decrease effectiveness of oral contraceptives. Urge patient to notify prescriber immediately if pregnancy occurs because drug increases risk of first-trimester pregnancy loss and congenital malformations.

! **WARNING** Tell patient about increased risk of lymphomas or other malignancies, especially of the skin, before therapy starts. Tell patient to report any unusual signs or symptoms to prescriber.

- Instruct patient how to take form of mycophenolate mofetil prescribed.
- Advise patient not to take antacids at the same time as oral mycophenolate mofetil because some antacids can decrease drug's absorption.
- Tell patient that frequent laboratory tests may be needed during therapy. Emphasize that having these tests done is essential to continuing therapy.

! **WARNING** Alert patient that drug may cause an allergic reaction. If present, tell patient to notify prescriber and, if severe, to seek immediate medical care.

! **WARNING** Caution patient to avoid contact with people who have infections because drug causes immunosuppression, placing patient at increased risk for developing an infection. Urge patient to report any signs of infection to prescriber immediately. Stress importance of not receiving live vaccines during therapy and to avoid people who have received such vaccines or to wear a protective mask when patient is around them.

! **WARNING** Urge patient to report any signs of unexpected bleeding or bruising, or any other sign of bone marrow depression immediately. Also, instruct patient to report any persistent, serious, or unusual adverse reactions to prescriber as drug dosage may need to be reduced or drug discontinued.

! **WARNING** Urge patient to notify prescriber if persistent, serious, or unusual adverse reactions occur.

! **WARNING** Advise patient to avoid exposure to direct sunlight an UV light and to wear sunscreen when outdoors because of increased risk for skin cancer.

- Caution patient not to engage in hazardous activities such as driving a car or using machines until the effects of the drug are known and patient is not experiencing confusion, dizziness, low blood pressure, somnolence, or tremors.
- Emphasize importance of follow-up care to monitor the drug's effectiveness and possible adverse effects because of the increased risk for cancer and infections as a result of immunosuppression.

! **WARNING** Caution patient not to donate blood during therapy and for at least 6 weeks following discontinuation of drug. Tell male patients not to donate semen during therapy and for 90 days following discontinuation of drug.

N O

nadolol
Corgard

Class and Category
Pharmacologic class: Nonselective beta-blocker
Therapeutic class: Antianginal, antihypertensive

Indications and Dosages
✱ To manage hypertension, alone or with other antihypertensives

TABLETS

Adults. *Initial:* 40 mg once daily, increased by 40 to 80 mg, as needed. *Maintenance:* 40 to 80 once mg daily. *Maximum:* 320 mg daily.

✱ To manage angina pectoris as long-term therapy

TABLETS

Adults. *Initial:* 40 mg once daily, increased by 40 to 80 mg once daily every 3 to 7 days, as needed. *Maintenance:* 40 to 80 mg daily. *Maximum:* 240 mg daily.

±**DOSAGE ADJUSTMENT** For patients with renal impairment, interval possibly increased to every 24 to 36 hours if creatinine clearance is 31 to 50 ml/min; to every 24 to 48 hours if it's 10 to 30 ml/min; or to every 40 to 60 hours if it's less than 10 ml/min.

Drug Administration
P.O.

- Check apical pulse before administering drug. If slower than 60 beats/min, notify prescriber and withhold drug.
- Administer drug once daily at about the same time of day without regard to meals.
- Store at room temperature, avoiding excessive heat. Protect from light.
- If dose is missed, administer it as soon as possible unless it is less than 8 hr away from next dose.

Route	Onset	Peak	Duration
P.O.	1 hr	3–4 hr	24 hr

Half-life: 10–24 hr

Mechanism of Action
Blocks $alpha_1$ and $beta_2$ receptors selectively in vascular smooth muscle and $beta_1$ receptors in the heart, thereby reducing peripheral vascular resistance and blood pressure. Decreases cardiac excitability, cardiac output, and myocardial oxygen demand because of its potent beta-blocker action, thus reducing angina. Prevents reflex tachycardia also, which typically occurs with most alpha-blockers.

Contraindications
Bronchial asthma; cardiogenic shock; heart failure; hypersensitivity to nadolol, other beta-blockers, or their components; second- or third-degree AV block; sinus bradycardia

Interactions
DRUGS

digoxin: Increased risk of bradycardia
epinephrine: Possibly unresponsive to usual doses of epinephrine used to treat allergic reaction
general anesthetics: Increased risk of hypotension and myocardial depression
insulin, oral antidiabetic drugs: Possibly increased risk of hyperglycemia and hypoglycemia
reserpine and other catecholamine-depleting drugs: Increased risk of bradycardia and hypotension

Adverse Reactions
CNS: Anxiety, depression, dizziness, drowsiness, fatigue, headache, paresthesia, syncope, vertigo, weakness, yawning
CV: **Bradycardia**, chest pain, edema, **heart block**, **heart failure**, **hypotension**, orthostatic hypotension, **ventricular arrhythmias**
EENT: Nasal congestion, taste perversion
ENDO: **Hypoglycemia**
GI: Dyspepsia, elevated liver enzymes, **hepatic necrosis**, **hepatitis**, jaundice, nausea, vomiting
GU: Ejaculation failure, impotence
RESP: Cough, dyspnea, wheezing
SKIN: Pruritus, scalp tingling

Childbearing Considerations
PREGNANCY

- It is not known if drug causes fetal harm.
- Use with caution only if benefit to mother outweighs potential risk to fetus.

LABOR AND DELIVERY

- Monitor neonate whose mothers are receiving nadolol at parturition for bradycardia, hypoglycemia, or other associated symptoms.

LACTATION

- Drug is present in breast milk.
- A decision should be made to discontinue breastfeeding or the drug to avoid potential serious adverse reactions in the breastfed infant.

Nursing Considerations

- Anticipate that drug may worsen psoriasis; in patients with myasthenia gravis, it may worsen muscle weakness and diplopia.
- Be aware that chronic beta-blocker therapy, such as nadolol, is not routinely withheld prior to major surgery because the benefits outweigh the risks associated with its use with general anesthesia and surgical procedures.

! **WARNING** Monitor patient for signs and symptoms of hypoglycemia, especially if patient has diabetes mellitus or patients are fasting because of not eating regularly, surgery, or are vomiting. Know that beta-blockers like nadolol may prevent early warning signs of hypoglycemia, such as tachycardia and may increase the risk for severe or prolonged hypoglycemia at any time during treatment. Be prepared to treat hypoglycemia according to institutional guidelines and notify prescriber.

! **WARNING** Monitor patient's vital signs to detect bradycardia, irregular heart beat, or hypotension. Also, monitor patient for signs and symptoms of heart failure or any other persistent, serious, or unusual adverse reactions.

! **WARNING** Withdraw drug gradually over 2 weeks, or as ordered, to avoid MI caused by unopposed beta stimulation or thyroid storm caused by underlying hyperthyroidism. Expect drug to mask tachycardia caused by hyperthyroidism.

PATIENT TEACHING

- Instruct patient how to to administer nadolol and what to do if a dose is missed.
- Teach patient how to take a radial pulse and direct patient to do so before each dose of nadolol. Instruct patient to notify prescriber if pulse rate falls below 60 beats/minute.

! **WARNING** Caution patient not to stop taking nadolol abruptly or change dosage.

! **WARNING** Instruct patient on the signs and symptoms of low blood glucose and inform patient that nadolol therapy may mask early signs such as a rapid heart rate and may increase risk of severe or prolonged hypoglycemia, especially if patient has diabetes or patient is not eating regularly, fasting because of surgery, or is vomiting. Instruct patient how to treat low blood glucose and to notify prescriber if present and to seek immediate medical care, if severe.

! **WARNING** Review signs of impending heart failure and urge patient to notify prescriber immediately if they occur.

- Tell mothers breastfeeding should not be undertaken during drug therapy or drug will need to be discontinued.

nafcillin sodium

Class and Category

Pharmacologic class: Penicillin
Therapeutic class: Antibiotic

Indications and Dosages

∗ *To treat infections caused by penicillinase-producing* Staphylococcus aureus

I.V. INFUSION, I.V. INJECTION

Adults. *For mild to moderate infections:* 500 mg every 4 hr. *For severe infections:* 1,000 mg every 4 hr. I.V. injection given over 5 to 10 min; I.V. infusion given over 30 to 60 min.

I.M. INJECTION

Adults. *For mild to moderate infections:* 500 mg every 4 to 6 hr. *For severe infections:* 1,000 mg every 4 hr.
Infants and children weighing less than 40 kg (88 lb). 25 mg/kg twice daily
Neonates. 10 mg/kg twice daily.

± **DOSAGE ADJUSTMENT** For patients of all ages, duration of therapy continued for at least 48 hours after patient is afebrile, asymptomatic, and cultures are negative. Severe infections require at least 14 days of therapy, although endocarditis and osteomyelitis may require a longer duration of therapy.

Drug Administration

I.V.

- For I.V. injection, reconstitute with 15 to 30 ml of Sterile Water for Injection or 0.9% Sodium Chloride Injection. Inject directly into a vein or through the tubing of an intravenous infusion. Administer over 5 to 10 min.
- For I.V. infusion, drug is available as a premixed solution or powder for injection. Reconstitute powder with 15 to 30 ml of Sterile Water for Injection or 0.9% Sodium Chloride Injection. Further dilute following manufacturer's guidelines prior to administration. Infuse over 30 to 60 min.
- *Incompatibilities:* Other drugs

I.M.

- Reconstitute with Sterile Water for Injection, 0.9% Sodium Chloride Injection, or Bacteriostatic Water for Injection by adding 3.4 ml to a 1-g bottle and 6.6 ml to a 2-g bottle to provide a concentration of 250 mg/ml. Do not use Bacteriostatic Water for Injection when reconstituting drug to be administered to neonates.
- Inject the clear solution immediately deep into the gluteal muscle.
- Rotate sites.
- Reconstituted solution is stable for 3 days at room temperature and 7 days refrigerated.

Route	Onset	Peak	Duration
I.V.	Immediate	Immediate	Unknown
I.M.	Unknown	30–60 min	Unknown

Half-life: 33–61 min

Mechanism of Action

Binds to certain penicillin-binding proteins in bacterial cell walls, thereby inhibiting the final stage of bacterial cell wall synthesis to cause cell lysis. Bolstered by its chemical composition; its unique side chain resists destruction by beta-lactamases.

Contraindications

Hypersensitivity to nafcillin, other penicillins, or their components

Interactions

DRUGS

cyclosporine: Increased risk of subtherapeutic cyclosporine levels
tetracycline: Possible antagonized bactericidal effect of nafcillin
warfarin: Decreased effectiveness of warfarin

Adverse Reactions

CNS: Depression, fever, headache, **seizures**
CV: **Hypotension**, **vascular collapse**
EENT: Black or hairy tongue, **laryngospasm**, oral candidiasis, stomatitis
GI: Abdominal pain, cholestasis, ***Clostridioides difficile*-associated diarrhea**, diarrhea, elevated liver enzymes, nausea, **pseudomembranous colitis**, vomiting
GU: **Acute kidney injury**, hematuria, interstitial nephritis, proteinuria, **renal tubular damage**, vaginitis
HEME: **Agranulocytosis**, **bone marrow depression**, **leukopenia**, **neutropenia**
RESP: **Bronchospasm**
SKIN: **Exfoliative dermatitis**, pruritus, rash, urticaria
Other: **Anaphylaxis**; **angioedema**; **hypokalemia**; injection-site pain, redness, and swelling; phlebitis; serum sickness-like reaction; skin sloughing; thrombophlebitis; tissue necrosis (severe)

Childbearing Considerations

PREGNANCY

- It is not known if drug causes fetal harm.
- Use with caution only if benefit to mother outweighs potential risk to fetus.

LACTATION

- Drug is present in breast milk.
- Mothers should check with prescriber before breastfeeding.

Nursing Considerations

- Obtain body fluid or tissue samples for culture and sensitivity testing, as ordered, and obtain test results, if possible, before giving nafcillin.
- Expect to have the following laboratory tests ordered before and then periodically during nafcillin therapy: alkaline phosphatase, bilirubin, blood urea nitrogen, creatinine, liver enzymes, and urinalysis; this provides a baseline and then allows monitoring for adverse effects stemming from nafcillin therapy.

- Know that when giving nafcillin to patient at risk for fluid overload or hypertension, each gram contains 2.5 mEq sodium.

! **WARNING** Monitor patient for hypersensitivity reactions, which could become life-threatening, such as anaphylaxis or angioedema. If present, stop drug, notify prescriber, and provide supportive care, as needed and ordered.

! **WARNING** Watch for evidence of pseudomembranous colitis, especially in elderly, immunocompromised, or debilitated patients who receive large doses of nafcillin. If profuse, watery diarrhea develops, contact prescriber and expect to obtain a stool specimen to rule out pseudomembranous colitis caused by *Clostridioides difficile*. It may be mild or become life-threatening. If confirmed, notify prescriber and expect to withhold nafcillin and treat with an antibiotic effective against *C. difficile*, as ordered. Also, expect to administer electrolytes, fluids, and protein supplementation, as needed and ordered.

! **WARNING** Montior patient for adverse hematological reactions that could become life-threatening. Monitor patient for signs and symptoms of an infection or infection being treated by nafcillin becoming worse. If present, expect to obtain a CBC and if confirmed, notify prescriber, expect drug to be discontinued, and a different antibiotic prescribed

PATIENT TEACHING

- Inform patient that drug is given either intravenously or as an intramuscular injection.

! **WARNING** Advise patient that drug can cause an allergic reaction. Tell patient to notify staff if chills, fever, GI distress, rash or any other serious or unusual reactions are experienced.

! **WARNING** Urge patient to tell prescriber if diarrhea develops, even 2 or more months after nafcillin therapy ends.

nalbuphine hydrochloride

Class and Category

Pharmacologic class: Opioid
Therapeutic class: Opioid analgesic

Indications and Dosages

✶ To relieve pain severe enough to require an opioid analgesic and for which alternative treatment options such as nonopioid analgesics or opioid combination products are inadequate or not tolerated

I.M., I.V., OR SUBCUTANEOUS INJECTION

Adults weighing 70 kg (154 lb). 10 mg every 3 to 6 hr and adjusted, as needed. I.V. injection given over 2 to 3 min.

±**DOSAGE ADJUSTMENT** For patients who weigh more or less than 70 kg, take other medications concurrently, have a different level of severity of pain, or have a different physical status, dosage may need to be adjusted. For nontolerant patients, single maximum dose should not exceed 20 mg and maximum total daily dose should not exceed 160 mg.

✶ As adjunct to balanced anesthesia, for obstetrical analgesia during labor and delivery, and for preoperative and postoperative analgesia

I.V. INJECTION

Adults. 0.3 to 3 mg/kg given over 10 to 15 min followed by 0.25 to 0.5 mg/kg, as needed.

Drug Administration

- Keep resuscitation equipment and naloxone readily available to reverse nalbuphine's effects, as needed.
- Store ampuls in carton until ready to use and protect from light.

I.V.

- For direct I.V. injection used as an analgesic, inject slowly through an I.V. line with a compatible infusing solution such as 0.9% Sodium Chloride Injection, 5% Dextrose in Water, and Lactated Ringer's solution.
- For direct I.V. injection used as adjunct to balance anesthesia, inject drug over 10 to 15 min.
- *Incompatibilities:* None reported by manufacturer.

I.M.

- Rotate sites.

SUBCUTANEOUS

- Rotate sites.

Route	Onset	Peak	Duration
I.V.	2–3 min	2–3 min	3–6 hr
I.M.	15 min	30 min	3–6 hr
SubQ	15 min	Unknown	3–6 hr

Half-life: 5 hr

Mechanism of Action

Binds with and stimulates kappa and mu opiate receptors in the spinal cord and higher levels in the CNS to alter the perception of and emotional response to pain.

Contraindications

Acute or severe bronchial asthma in an unmonitored setting or in the absence of resuscitative equipment; GI obstruction, including paralytic ileus; hypersensitivity to nalbuphine or any of its components; significant respiratory depression

Interactions

DRUGS

5-HT$_3$ receptor antagonists, cyclobenzaprine; metaxalone; methylene blue (I.V.); selected psychiatric drugs, such as buspirone, lithium, mirtazapine, nefazodone, trazodone, vilazodone; selective serotonin reuptake inhibitors; serotonin–norepinephrine reuptake inhibitors; St. John's wort; tramadol; tricyclic antidepressants; triptans; tryptophan: Increased risk of serotonin syndrome

anticholinergics: Increased risk of severe constipation and urine retention

antipsychotics, anxiolytics, benzodiazepines, CNS depressants, general anesthetics, muscle relaxants, other opioids, other sedative/hypnotics, sedating antihistamines, tranquilizers, tricyclic antidepressants: Increased risk of coma, severe respiratory depression, profound sedation, and death

diuretics: Reduced effectiveness of diuretics

MAO inhibitors: Risk of opioid toxicity or serotonin syndrome

neuromuscular blockers: Increased risk of respiratory depression severity

ACTIVITIES

alcohol use: Increased risk of coma, hypotension, profound sedation, and respiratory depression

Adverse Reactions

CNS: Agitation, anxiety, confusion, decreased level of consciousness, depression, dizziness, euphoria, fatigue, fever, hallucinations, headache, nervousness, restlessness, **seizures**, somnolence, syncope, tiredness, tremor, weakness

CV: Hypertension, **hypotension**, tachycardia

EENT: Blurred vision, diplopia, dry mouth

ENDO: **Adrenal insufficiency**, **hypoglycemia**

GI: Abdominal cramps or pain, anorexia, constipation, nausea, vomiting

GU: Decreased libido, decreased urine output, impotency, infertility, lack of menstruation, ureteral spasm

RESP: Dyspnea, **pulmonary edema**, **respiratory depression**, wheezing

SKIN: Diaphoresis, flushing, pruritus, rash, sensation of warmth, urticaria

Other: **Hypersensitivity reactions**, injection-site burning, pain, redness, swelling, and warmth; opioid induced allodynia and hyperalgesia; physical and psychological dependency

Childbearing Considerations

PREGNANCY

- Drug may cause fetal harm.
- Prolonged use of drug during pregnancy can result in neonatal opioid withdrawal syndrome (NOWS), which may be life-threatening if not recognized and treated.
- Avoid prolonged use during pregnancy. Use with caution only if benefit to mother outweighs potential risk to fetus.

LABOR AND DELIVERY

- Drug is not recommended for use in pregnant women immediately before or during labor as drug can cause severe fetal bradycardia. Opioids may alter length of time of labor.
- Opioids cross the placental barrier and may produce respiratory depression and psycho-physiologic effects in the newborn. Monitor neonate closely for signs of excess sedation and respiratory depression.
- An opioid antagonist, such as naloxone, must be available at the time of delivery in the event it is needed to reverse opioid-induced respiratory depression in the neonate.

LACTATION

- Drug is present in breast milk.

- Mothers should check with prescriber before breastfeeding.
- If breastfeeding occurs, monitor infant for excess sedation and respiratory depression.

REPRODUCTION

- Chronic use of opioids may reduce fertility.

Nursing Considerations

! WARNING Be aware that nalbuphine can lead to abuse, addiction, and misuse. Monitor patient for evidence of physical/psychological dependence or abuse. Be aware that excessive use of nalbuphine may not only lead to abuse, addiction, and misuse, it can lead to overdose, and possibly death. Also, know that overestimating the nalbuphine dosage when comverting patients from another opioid product can result in a fatal overdose with the first dose. Monitor patient and intake of drug closely.

! WARNING Know that full opioid agonist analgesics should not be administered to patients receiving a mixed agonist/antagonist like nalbuphine because doing so may decrease analgesic effect and/or precipitate withdrawal symptoms.

- Monitor effectiveness of nalbuphine to relieve pain; consult prescriber, as needed. Monitor patient for paradoxic increase in pain known as opioid-induced hyperalgesia or an increase in sensitivity to pain known as opioid-induced allodynia, especially when dosage increases. Do not confuse this with tolerance, which is the need for increasing doses of opioids to maintain an effect. If opioid-induced allodynia or hyperalgesia is suspected, notify prescriber and expect dosage to be decreased or opioid rotation to be prescribed.

! WARNING Monitor patient for a hypersensitivity reaction, which may become life-threatening, including death. If present, notify prescriber, expect drug to be discontinued, and provide supportive care, as needed and ordered.

! WARNING Monitor respiratory status carefully and frequently during nalbuphine therapy, especially when drug therapy is initiated because respiratory depression can develop and can become life-threatening or fatal. Be especially vigilant with cachectic, debilitated, and elderly patients who are at higher risk as well as patients with chronic pulmonary disease or cor pulmonale and those with a significant decreased respiratory reserve, hypercapnia, hypoxia, or preexisting respiratory depression. Know that carbon dioxide retention from respiratory depression may increase the sedating effects of nalbuphine. Know that lowest dosage should be used when initiating drug therapy in these patients and dosage titrated slowly.

! WARNING Monitor patients closely whose ability to maintain a normal blood pressure is already compromised by a reduced blood volume or concurrent administration of certain CNS depressant drugs; the drug may cause severe hypotension in these patients, especially when initiating or titrating the dose of nalbuphine. Assess blood pressure frequently.

! WARNING Montior patient's blood glucose level because hypoglycemia can occur in patients taking opioids such as nalbuphine. If present, treat according to institutional protocol and notify prescriber.

! WARNING Be aware that nalbuphine should only be used concomitantly with benzodiazepine therapy in patients for whom other treatment options are inadequate. If prescribed together, expect dosing and duration of nalbuphine to be limited. Monitor patient closely for signs and symptoms of a decrease in consciousness, including coma, profound sedation, and significant respiratory depression. Notify prescriber immediately and provide emergency supportive care, as death may occur.

! WARNING Know that opioids like nalbuphine can cause sleep-related breathing disorders, including central sleep apnea and sleep-related hypoxemia in a dose-dependent fashion. Expect dosage to be decreased if patient has or develops these disorders.

! WARNING Know that drug may cause seizures. Monitor patient closely.

! **WARNING** Monitor patient for adrenal insufficiency. Although rare, it can be life-threatening. Monitor patient for anorexia, dizziness, fatigue, hypotension, nausea, vomiting, and weakness. Notify prescriber if adrenal insufficiency is suspected and expect diagnostic testing to be done. If confirmed, expect to administer corticosteroids and wean patient off nalbuphine if possible.

! **WARNING** Be aware that chronic maternal use of nalbuphine during pregnancy can result in NOWS, which may be life-threatening if not recognized and treated appropriately. NOWS occurs when a newborn has been exposed to opioid drugs like nalbuphine for a prolonged period while in utero.

! **WARNING** Know that many drugs may interact with opioids like nalbuphine to cause serotonin syndrome. Monitor patient closely for signs and symptoms, such as agitation, diaphoresis, diarrhea, fever, hallucinations, labile blood pressure, muscle twitching or stiffness, nausea, shakiness, shivering, tachycardia, trouble with coordination, or vomiting. Notify prescriber at once because serotonin syndrome may be life-threatening. Be prepared to discontinue drug, if possible and ordered, and provide supportive care.

- Anticipate that nalbuphine may cause spasm of the sphincter of Oddi and elevate serum amylase levels. Monitor patients with biliary tract disease, including acute pancreatitis for worsening symptoms.
- Be aware that during prolonged use, a stool softener may be needed to minimize constipation.

! **WARNING** Know that if patient is opioid-dependent, drug should not be discontinued abruptly. Expect drug to be gradually tapered by 25% to 50% every 2 to 4 days. During this time, monitor patient for withdrawal symptoms, such as abdominal cramps, anorexia, anxiety, backache, bone or joint pain, confusion, depression, diaphoresis, dysphoria, erythema, fear, fever, irritability, labile blood pressure and pulse, lacrimation, muscle spasms, myalgia, mydriasis, nasal congestion, nausea, opioid craving, piloerection, restlessness, rhinorrhea, sensation of crawling skin, sleep disturbances, tremor, uneasiness, vomiting, and yawning.

PATIENT TEACHING

- Inform patient that drug is only available in the form of an injection. Instruct patient how to administer nalbuphine as a subcutaneous injection, if prescribed.

! **WARNING** Warn patient excessive or prolonged use can lead to abuse, addiction, misuse, overdose, and possibly death. Encourage family or caregiver to have naloxone in the home and instruct how to use it. Stress importance of calling 911 if naloxone is administered.

- Tell patient to avoid increasing dosage or the frequency taken without consulting prescriber if pain relief is not adequate. Also notify prescriber if pain actually increases when dosage increases or increased sensitivity to pain or new pain develops while taking nalbuphine.

! **WARNING** Warn patient not to consume alcohol or take a benzodiazepine without prescriber knowledge while taking nalbuphine, as severe respiratory depression can occur and may lead to death. Inform patient about potentially fatal additive effects of combining a benzodiazepine with an opioid. Instruct patient to inform all prescribers of nalbuphine use.

! **WARNING** Alert patient that drug may cause an allergic reaction that could be severe. If present, tell patient to notify prescriber and, if severe, to seek immediate medical care.

! **WARNING** Instruct patient to notify prescriber if any persistent, severe, or unusual adverse reactions occur.

! **WARNING** Instruct patient to notify all prescribers of opioid use because serious drug interactions can occur.

! **WARNING** Stress importance of patient not sharing drug with others and to take steps to prevent theft of drug.

- Advise patient to avoid hazardous activities until nalbuphine's CNS effects are known and resolved.
- Counsel patient against making important decisions while receiving drug because it may cloud judgment.
- Inform patient that long-term use of opioids like nalbuphine may decrease sex hormone levels, causing decreased libido, erectile dysfunction, impotence, infertility, or lack of menstruation. Encourage patient to report any symptoms to prescriber.
- Instruct females of childbearing age to notify prescriber if pregnancy occurs as chronic use during pregnancy may cause fetal harm.
- Advise breastfeeding mothers to monitor their infant for excess sedation and respiratory depression.

! **WARNING** Advise patient who has taken nalbuphine long term to not discontinue drug abruptly as withdrawal symptoms can occur.

naldemedine

Symproic

Class and Category

Pharmacologic class: Opioid receptor antagonist
Therapeutic class: Opioid antagonist of GI tract

Indications and Dosages

✶ *To treat opioid-induced constipation in patients with chronic noncancer pain*

TABLETS

Adults. 0.2 mg once daily.

Drug Administration

P.O.

- May be administered with or without food.
- Keep in light-resistant container until ready to administer.

Route	Onset	Peak	Duration
P.O.	Unknown	45 min	Unknown

Half-life: 11 hr

Mechanism of Action

Functions as a peripherally acting mu-opioid receptor antagonist in the GI tract to decrease the constipating effects of opioids.

Contraindications

GI obstruction or increased risk of recurrent obstruction due to the potential for GI perforation, hypersensitivity to naldemedine or its components

Interactions

DRUGS

moderate CYP3A inhibitors, such as aprepitant, atazanavir, diltiazem, erythromycin, fluconazole; P-glycoprotein inhibitors, such as amiodarone, captopril, cyclosporine, quercetin, quinidine, verapamil; strong CYP3A inhibitors, such as itraconazole: Increased plasma naldemedine concentrations increasing risk of adverse reactions
other opioid antagonists: Possible additive effect of opioid receptor antagonism and increased risk of opioid withdrawal
strong CYP3A inducers, such as carbamazepine, phenytoin, rifampin, St. John's wort: Significant decrease in plasma naldemedine concentrations, which may decrease effectiveness

Adverse Reactions

GI: Abdominal pain, diarrhea, gastroenteritis, **GI perforation**, nausea, vomiting
RESP: **Bronchospasm**
SKIN: Rash
Other: Opioid withdrawal

Childbearing Considerations

PREGNANCY

- Drug may cause fetal harm.
- Crosses the placental barrier and may precipitate neonatal opioid withdrawal syndrome (NOWS), which may be life-threatening if not recognized and treated.
- Use with caution only if benefit to mother outweighs potential risk to fetus.

LACTATION

- It is not known if drug is present in breast milk.
- A decision should be made to discontinue breastfeeding or the drug to avoid potential serious adverse reactions in the breastfed infant.

Nursing Considerations

- Know that patients receiving opioids for less than a month may be less responsive to naldemedine therapy.
- Expect naldemedine to be discontinued if treatment with an opioid pain medication is discontinued.

! **WARNING** Know that drug may cause bronchospasms. If present, notify prescriber, stop drug, and provide measures to relieve bronchospasms, as ordered.

! **WARNING** Monitor patient closely for abdominal pain. Know that GI perforation has occurred with use of another peripherally acting opioid antagonist in patients with conditions that affect the GI tract wall integrity, such as diverticular disease, infiltrative GI tract malignancies, Ogilvie syndrome, peptic ulcer disease, or peritoneal metastases. Patients with Crohn's disease may be at increased risk for GI perforation. Notify prescriber immediately if abdominal pain becomes persistent, severe, or worsens. Expect drug to be discontinued.

- Monitor patient for signs and symptoms of opioid withdrawal, such as abdominal pain, chills, diarrhea, feeling cold, fever, flushing, hyperhidrosis, increased lacrimation, nausea, and vomiting. Patients who develop disruptions to the blood–brain barrier may be at increased risk for opioid withdrawal or reduced analgesia.

PATIENT TEACHING

- Instruct patient how to administer naldemedine.
- Inform patient that naldemedine should be discontinued if treatment with the opioid pain medication is discontinued.
- Tell patient that the most common side effects of naldemedine include abdominal pain, diarrhea, nausea, and vomiting.

! **WARNING** Alert patient that bronchospasms may occur with drug administration. If present, tell patient to stop taking drug and seek immediate medical care.

! **WARNING** Advise patient to seek immediate emergency care if persistent, severe, or worsening abdominal pain occurs.

- Review the signs and symptoms of withdrawal with patient and tell her to notify prescriber if these symptoms occur.
- Inform females of childbearing age to notify prescriber if pregnancy occurs.
- Inform mothers that breastfeeding is not recommended. However, if mother insists tell her the drug will have to be discontinued.

NEW!

nalmefene hydrochloride

Zurnai

Class and Category

Pharmacologic class: Opioid antagonist
Therapeutic class: Antidote

Indications and Dosages

∗ *To provide emergency treatment of known or suspected opioid overdose caused by natural or synthetic opioids as manifested by respiratory and/or CNS depression*

I.M. INJECTION, SUBCUTANEOUS INJECTION

Adults and children ages 12 and older. *Initial:* 1.5 mg with dose repeated after 2 to 5 min if desired response is not obtained. Additional doses of 1.5 mg given every 2 to 5 min, as needed, until emergency medical assistance arrives.

± **DOSAGE ADJUSTMENT** For patients receiving partial agonists or mixed agonist/antagonists, such as buprenorphine and pentazocine, repeated dosing of nalmefene may be required.

Drug Administration

I.M., SUBCUTANEOUS INJECTION

- Keep resuscitation equipment readily available during drug administration.
- Do not prime or test drug prior to administration. Each auto-injector can only be used one time.
- Solution should be clear, free of particulates, and the glass container undamaged before administration.
- Inject drug intramuscularly or subcutaneously as soon as possible into the anterolateral aspect of the thigh, through clothing, if necessary, because prolonged respiratory depression may cause CNS damage or even death.

- To administer drug, place needle guard against outer thigh. Press the needle end firmly into the injection site until you hear a click and then hold for 3 sec. After 3 sec, the viewing window should turn completely orange indicating the dose has been given. Remove device from injection site.
- Move patient onto their side.
- Know that additional doses may be needed. Re-administer using a new auto-injector, every 2 to 5 min, if patient does not respond or responds and then relapses into respiratory depression.
- Institute immediate emergency medical assistance after administering first dose. Remain with patient and observe patient closely until emergency personnel arrive, even if patient wakes up.

Route	Onset	Peak	Duration
I.M., SubQ	2.5-5 min	5-15 min	Unknown

Half-life: 9.07 hr

Mechanism of Action

Antagonizes (briefly and competitively) mu, kappa, and sigma receptors in the CNS, thus reversing analgesia, hypotension, respiratory depression, and sedation caused by most opioids. Mu receptors are responsible for analgesia, euphoria, miosis, and respiratory depression. Kappa receptors are responsible for analgesia and sedation. Sigma receptors control dysphoria and other delusional states.

Contraindications

Hypersensitivity to nalmefene hydrochloride or its components

Interactions

DRUGS

opioids: Possible precipitation of opioid withdrawal in opioid dependent patients

Adverse Reactions

CNS: Agitation, allodynia (feeling pain at a site where normally pain is not felt), burning sensation, chills, confusion, depression, dizziness, feeling abnormal or hot, fever, headache, irritability, myoclonus, nervousness, **recurrent CNS depression**, somnolence, tremor
CV: **Arrhythmia**, **bradycardia**, hypertension, **hypotension**, palpitations, tachycardia, vasodilatation
EENT: Dry mouth, ear discomfort, pharyngitis, tinnitus
ENDO: Hot flashes
GI: Diarrhea, nausea, vomiting
GU: Urinary retention
RESP: **Recurrent respiratory depression**
SKIN: Flushing, pruritus
Other: **Precipitation of acute**, **severe opioid withdrawal** (in opioid dependent patients)

Childbearing Considerations

PREGNANCY

- It is not known if drug can cause fetal harm.
- Use with caution only if benefit to mother outweighs potential risk to fetus.

LABOR AND DELIVERY

- If drug is given to an opioid dependent pregnant woman giving birth, monitor neonate for opioid withdrawal symptoms such as excessive crying, hyperactive reflexes, and seizures.

LACTATION

- It is not known if drug is present in breast milk.
- Mothers should check with prescriber before breastfeeding.

Nursing Considerations

! WARNING Be aware that an opioid overdose is a medical emergency and treatment should not be withheld even if patient is pregnant as lack of treatment may cause death of patient including a pregnant patient and her fetus.

! WARNING Monitor patient after administration of nalmefene for recurrent CNS and respiratory depression and be prepared to administer additional doses 2 to 5 minutes apart, as needed. Also, be prepared to administer additional resuscitative and supportive measures, as needed, after calling for emergency medical assistance.

! WARNING Monitor patients who are opioid dependent for an acute withdrawal syndrome exhibited by abdominal cramps, body aches, diarrhea, fever, increased blood pressure, irritability, nausea, nervousness, piloerection, restlessness, runny nose, shivering or trembling, sneezing, sweating, tachycardia, vomiting, yawning, weakness. Aggressive behavior may also occur.

! WARNING Monitor patient closely for abrupt reversal of opioid depression in patients in both emergency department and postoperative settings. Monitor patient for sudden onset of cardiovascular instability (cardiac arrest, hypotension, hypertension, pulmonary edema, tachycardia, ventricular tachycardia and fibrillation) or other signs and symptoms such as nausea, seizures, sweating, and tremulousness. Know that patients at greatest risk are patients with pre-existing cardiovascular disorders or patients who have received other drugs that may have similar adverse cardiovascular effects.

- Be aware that reversal of respiratory depression by mixed agonist/antagonists or partial agonists such as buprenorphine and pentazocine may not be complete. For example, buprenorphine has a long duration of action causing antagonism to cause a gradual onset of reversal effects and a decreased duration of action of the normally prolonged respiratory depression.

PATIENT TEACHING

- Instruct family or caregiver how to recognize an opioid overdose. Teach them how to administer nalmefene including the need to position patient in a side lying position.
- Stress importance of calling 911 after administering drug and that additional doses may be needed while waiting for emergency medical assistance to arrive.

! WARNING Warn opioid dependent patient, family, or caregiver that drug may precipitate opioid withdrawal. Stress importance to patient of not attempting to overcome the opioid blockade with high or repeated doses of exogenous opioids because this could cause opioid intoxication and even death.

naloxegol oxalate

Movantik

Class and Category

Pharmacologic class: Opioid receptor antagonist

Therapeutic class: Opioid antagonist of gastrointestinal tract

Indications and Dosages

** To treat opioid-induced constipation in patients with chronic noncancer pain*

TABLETS

Adults. 25 mg once daily.

± **DOSAGE ADJUSTMENT** For patients unable to tolerate naloxegol at the normal dose, dosage reduced to 12.5 mg once daily. For patients with renal impairment (creatinine clearance less than 60 ml/min), and patients taking moderate CYP3A4 inhibitor drugs, such as diltiazem, erythromycin, or verapamil, initial dosage reduced to 12.5 mg once daily. For patients with renal impairment who are tolerating the lower dose well, dosage increased to 25 mg once daily.

Drug Administration

P.O.

- Administer drug on an empty stomach at least 1 hr prior to the first meal of the day or 2 hr after the meal.
- Do not administer with grapefruit juice.
- Tablet can be crushed to a powder and mixed with 4 ounces of water for patient who is unable to swallow tablet whole. Once mixed, patient must drink mixture immediately. Refill same glass with 4 ounces of water, stir, and have patient drink contents again.
- Drug may be administered through a nasogastric tube. Flush tube with 30 ml of water using a 60-ml syringe. Crush tablet to a powder in a container and mix with 60 ml of water. Draw up mixture using the 60-ml syringe and administer contents through the nasogastric tube. Add about 60 ml of water to same container used to prepare the dose. Draw up the water using the same 60-ml syringe and use all the water to flush the nasogastric tube and any remaining drug from the nasogastric tube into the stomach.

Route	Onset	Peak	Duration
P.O.	6–12 hr	2–3 hr	Unknown

Half-life: 6–11 hr

Mechanism of Action

Functions as a peripherally acting mu-opioid receptor antagonist in tissues such as the gastrointestinal tract, thereby decreasing the constipating effects of opioids.

Contraindications

Concomitant therapy with strong CYP3A4 inhibitors, such as clarithromycin and ketoconazole; GI obstruction or risk of recurrent obstruction due to potential for GI perforation; hypersensitivity to naloxegol or its components

Interactions

DRUGS

CYP3A4 inducers, such as carbamazepine, rifampin, St. John's wort: Decreased plasma naloxegol levels and effectiveness
CYP3A4 inhibitors, such as clarithromycin, diltiazem, erythromycin, itraconazole, ketoconazole, verapamil: Increased plasma naloxegol levels, possibly increasing risk of adverse reactions, including opioid withdrawal
other opioid antagonists: Potential for additive effects and increased risk of opioid withdrawal

FOOD

grapefruit, grapefruit juice: Increased plasma naloxegol levels

Adverse Reactions

CNS: Headache
GI: Abdominal pain (may become severe), diarrhea, flatulence, **GI perforation**, nausea, vomiting
SKIN: Diaphoresis, rash, urticaria
Other: **Angioedema**, opioid withdrawal

Childbearing Considerations

PREGNANCY

- Drug may cause fetal harm.
- Use of drug during pregnancy may precipitate neonatal opioid withdrawal syndrome (NOWS), which may be life-threatening if not recognized and treated.
- Use with caution only if benefit to mother outweighs potential risk to fetus.

LACTATION

- It is not known if drug is present in breast milk.
- Drug is not recommended for use in a mother who is breastfeeding.

Nursing Considerations

- Expect all maintenance laxative therapy to be discontinued prior to patient starting naloxegol therapy but know that laxatives may be given, as ordered and if needed, after 3 days of naloxegol therapy.
- Know that patients receiving opioids for less than a month may be less responsive to naloxegol therapy while patients who have taken opioids for at least 4 weeks prior to starting naloxegol may have an increased response to naloxegol because of sustained exposure to opioids.

! WARNING Monitor patient for a hypersensitivity reaction, which could become life-threatening, such as angioedema. If present, notify prescriber, expect drug to be discontinued, and provide supportive care, as needed and ordered.

! WARNING Monitor patient for the development of persistent, severe, or worsening abdominal pain and/or diarrhea because GI perforation has occurred with use of naloxegol. Symptoms generally occur within a few days of starting naloxegol therapy. If this type of abdominal pain occurs, withhold drug and notify prescriber. Know that drug may be restarted at a lower dose (12.5 mg daily) once symptoms have resolved and if drug is still needed.

- Monitor patient for opioid withdrawal symptoms, such as abdominal pain, anxiety, chills, diaphoresis, diarrhea, irritability, and yawning. Clusters of these symptoms may occur with naloxegol therapy, especially if patient is receiving methadone or has a disruption in opioid therapy.
- Know that if opioid therapy is discontinued, naloxegol therapy should be discontinued.

PATIENT TEACHING

- Tell patient to stop all maintenance laxative therapy prior to starting naloxegol therapy. Reassure the patient that laxatives may be used, if needed, after the first 3 days of therapy.
- Instruct patient how to administer form of naloxegol prescribed.
- Remind patient not to consume grapefruit or grapefruit juice while taking naloxegol.
- Tell patient to notify prescriber if opioid therapy is discontinued because drug also will need to be discontinued.
- Advise patient to inform prescriber of all medications being taken, including over-the-counter drugs and any new drug therapy begun once naloxegol therapy begins.

! **WARNING** Alert patient that drug may cause an allergic reaction. If present, tell patient to notify prescriber, and, if severe, to seek immediate medical care.

! **WARNING** Instruct patient to stop drug and seek medical attention promptly if persistent, severe, or worsening abdominal pain and/or diarrhea develops. Tell patient symptoms may occur a few days after starting treatment.

! **WARNING** Warn patient that opioid withdrawal symptoms may occur while taking naloxegol and to notify prescriber.

- Caution females of childbearing age to notify prescriber if pregnancy occurs.
- Advise mothers breastfeeding should not be undertaken.

naloxone hydrochloride

Kloxxado, Narcan, Rezenopy, Rivive, Zimhi

Class and Category

Pharmacologic class: Opioid antagonist
Therapeutic class: Antidote

Indications and Dosages

✱ *To treat known or suspected opioid overdose as manifested by CNS or respiratory depression*

I.M., I.V., OR SUBCUTANEOUS INJECTION (NARCAN)

Adults. 0.4 to 2 mg repeated every 2 to 3 min, as needed. If no response after 10 mg, patient may not have opioid-induced respiratory depression.
Children. 0.01 mg/kg as a single dose I.V.; if no improvement, 0.1 mg/kg given I.V. as a second dose. If I.V. route is not available, drug may be given as an I.M. or subcutaneous injection in divided doses.

NASAL SPRAY (NARCAN)

Adults and children. 4 mg (1 spray) into 1 nostril and repeated every 2 to 3 min, as needed, alternating nostrils with each dose.

NASAL SPRAY (KLOXXADO)

Adults and children. 8 mg (1 spray) repeated every 2 to 3 min, as needed, alternating nostrils with each dose.

NASAL SPRAY (RIVIVE)

Adults and children. 3 mg (1 spray) into 1 nostril and repeated every 2 to 3 min, as needed, alternating nostrils with each dose.

NASAL SPRAY (REZENOPY)

Adults and children. 10 mg (1 spray into 1 nostril) and repeated every 2 to 3 min, as needed, alternating nostrils with each dose.

± **DOSAGE ADJUSTMENT** For patients who receive reversal of respiratory depression through partial agonists or mixed agonist/antagonists, such as buprenorphine and pentazocine, effect may be incomplete requiring higher doses or repeat administration of nasal spray.

I.M. OR SUBCUTANEOUS INJECTION (ZIMHI)

Adults and children. 5 mg/0.5 ml repeated every 2 to 3 min.

✱ *To treat postoperative opioid-induced respiratory depression*

I.V. INJECTION (NARCAN)

Adults. *Initial:* 0.1 to 0.2 mg every 2 to 3 min until desired response occurs. Additional doses given every 1 to 2 hr, as needed, based on patient response.
Children. *Initial:* 0.005 to 0.01 mg every 2 to 3 min until desired response occurs. Additional doses given every 1 to 2 hr, as needed, based on patient response.

✱ *To reverse opioid-induced depression*

I.M., I.V., OR SUBCUTANEOUS INJECTION (NARCAN)

Adults. *Initial:* 0.1 mg to 0.2 mg every 2 to 3 min until desired response occurs. Additional doses given every 1 to 2 hr, as needed, based on patient response.
Children. *Initial:* 0.005 mg to 0.01 mg, repeated every 2 to 3 min, as needed.
Neonates. *Initial:* 0.01 mg/kg repeated every 2 to 3 min, as needed.

✱ *As adjunct to treat hypotension caused by septic shock*

I.V. INFUSION OR INJECTION (NARCAN)

Adults. Highly individualized.

Drug Administration

- Keep resuscitation equipment readily available during drug administration.
- Administer parenteral drug by I.V. route whenever possible.

- Place patient in the supine position before administering drug and then reposition to the lateral recumbent position after administering drug. Reposition patient with each dose administered.

I.V.

Narcan

- For I.V. injection, give undiluted as a bolus using the single-dose prefilled syringe.
- For I.V. infusion, dilute 2 mg of drug in 500 ml of 0.9% Sodium Chloride Injection or 5% Dextrose solution to provide a concentration of 0.004 mg/ml. Infuse at a rate titrated to patient's response.
- Discard any unused diluted solution after 24 hr.
- *Incompatibilities:* Preparations containing bisulfite, metabisulfite, long-chain or high-molecular-weight anions; solutions with an alkaline pH; other drugs

I.M.

- Inject Narcan into large muscle of arm, buttocks, or thigh using the single-dose prefilled syringe.
- Inject Zimhi into the anterolateral aspect of the thigh following manufacturer's instructions for use of the device. Administer through clothing if necessary. In children under the age of 1, pinch up the thigh muscle while administering the dose.
- If more than 1 dose is needed, rotate sites.

SUBCUTANEOUS

- Inject Narcan into subcutaneous tissue using the single-dose prefilled syringe.
- Inject Zimhi into the anterolateral aspect of the thigh following manufacturer's instructions for use of the device. Administer through clothing if necessary. In children under the age of 1, pinch up the thigh muscle while administering the dose.
- If more than 1 dose is needed, rotate sites.

NASAL SPRAY

Kloxxado, Narcan, Rezenopy, Rivive

- Each nasal spray contains a single dose and cannot be reused.
- Make sure device nozzle is inserted in either one of patient's nostrils. Provide support to the back of patient's neck to allow the head to tilt back.
- Do not prime or test the device prior to administration. Press firmly on the device plunger to administer the dose. Remove the device nozzle from patient's nostril after use.
- If repeat doses are needed, alternate nostrils, using a new container each time.

Route	Onset	Peak	Duration
I.V.	1–2 min	5–15 min	45–60 min
I.M., SubQ	2–5 min	5–15 min	1–2 hr
Intranasal	8–13 min	20–30 min	30–120 min

Half-life: 30–90 min; 2 hr (intranasal)

Mechanism of Action

Antagonizes (briefly and competitively) mu, kappa, and sigma receptors in the CNS, thus reversing analgesia, hypotension, respiratory depression, and sedation caused by most opioids. Mu receptors are responsible for analgesia, euphoria, miosis, and respiratory depression. Kappa receptors are responsible for analgesia and sedation. Sigma receptors control dysphoria and other delusional states.

Contraindications

Hypersensitivity to naloxone or its components

Interactions

DRUGS

naloxegol: Possibly increased risk of opioid withdrawal

Adverse Reactions

CNS: Excitement, headache, irritability, nervousness, restlessness, **seizures**, tremor, violent behavior

CV: **Cardiac arrest**, **hypotension**, **severe hypertension**, **ventricular fibrillation**, **ventricular tachycardia**

EENT: Nasal congestion, dryness, edema, inflammation, or pain (spray form); toothache

GI: Constipation, nausea, vomiting

MS: Muscle spasms, musculoskeletal pain

RESP: Dyspnea, **pulmonary edema**

SKIN: Diaphoresis, xeroderma

Other: Withdrawal symptoms

Childbearing Considerations

PREGNANCY

- Drug may cause fetal harm.
- Drug crosses the placental barrier and may precipitate withdrawal (maybe severe) in

the fetus, as well as in the opioid-dependent mother.

- Monitor fetus for signs of distress after drug is given and until fetus and mother are stable.

LACTATION

- It is not known if drug is present in breast milk.
- Mothers should check with prescriber before breastfeeding following drug administration.

Nursing Considerations

! **WARNING** Anticipate that rapid reversal of opioid effects can cause diaphoresis, nausea, and vomiting, in addition to serious adverse effects, such as hypotension, pulmonary edema, seizures, and ventricular arrhythmias. Monitor patient closely, especially patients at risk because of the presence of preexisting cardiovascular disorders or who are receiving drugs that cause similar adverse cardiovascular effects.

! **WARNING** Watch for opioid withdrawal symptoms, especially when giving naloxone to opioid-dependent patient. Symptoms may include abdominal cramps, anorexia, anxiety, backache, bone or joint pain, confusion, depression, diaphoresis, dysphoria, erythema, fear, fever, irritability, labile blood pressure and pulse, lacrimation, muscle spasms, myalgia, mydriasis, nasal congestion, nausea, opioid craving, piloerection, restlessness, rhinorrhea, sensation of crawling skin, sleep disturbances, tremor, uneasiness, vomiting, and yawning.

! **WARNING** Be aware that naloxone may precipitate withdrawal (may be severe) in the fetus, as well as in the opioid-dependent mother. Monitor mother and fetus for signs of distress after drug is given.

! **WARNING** Monitor patient in postoperative setting who has received naloxone because abrupt postoperative reversal of opioid depression after using naloxone may cause serious adverse effects. Excessive doses of naloxone in the postoperative setting have also caused significant reversal of analgesia and have caused patient to become agitated.

- Expect patient with hepatic or renal dysfunction to have increased circulating blood naloxone level.

PATIENT TEACHING

- Inform family or caregiver that naloxone will reverse opioid-induced adverse reactions. Instruct them on the signs and symptoms of an opioid overdose, such as inability of patient to wake up and patient developing severe breathing problems.
- Instruct family or caregiver on how to administer naloxone by nasal spray (Kloxxado, Narcan, Rezenopy, Rivive) or via an injection. Alert family or caregiver using Zimhi injectable form that drug should only be administered by individuals who are 12 years and older. Inform family or caregiver that Narcan or Revive nasal spray can be purchased as an over-the-counter drug.

! **WARNING** Stress importance of calling 911 immediately after administration. Instruct family or caregiver to repeat dosage every 2 to 3 minutes if patient does not respond until emergency medical personnel arrive. Remind family or caregiver that each dose requires the use of a new device.

naltrexone

Vivitrol

naltrexone hydrochloride

Revia (CAN)

Class and Category

Pharmacologic class: Opioid antagonist
Therapeutic class: Opioid and alcohol blocker

Indications and Dosages

∗ *To provide blockade of the effects of exogenously administered opioids*

TABLETS

Adults. *Initial:* 25 mg, and if no withdrawal symptoms occur, dosage increased the following day to 50 mg and then 50 mg given once daily thereafter. Alternatively, 50 mg every weekday with 100-mg dose on

Saturday, 100 mg every other day, or 150 mg every third day.

∗ *To prevent relapse to opioid dependence following opioid detoxification*

I.M. INJECTION (VIVITROL)

Adults. 380 mg every 4 wk or once monthly.

∗ *As adjunct to treat alcoholism*

TABLETS

Adults. 50 mg daily for up to 12 wk.

I.M. INJECTION (VIVITROL)

Adults. 380 mg every 4 wk or once monthly.

Drug Administration

- Don't administer drug to patients who have not been free of short-acting opioids for at least 7 to 10 days.
- A naloxone challenge test may have to be done before drug therapy begins.

P.O.

- Give drug with antacids or food if GI upset occurs.

I.M.

- If drug is stored in refrigerator, allow it to warm up to room temperature before administering. The suspension should be milky white and not contain clumps.
- Dilute using only diluent supplied in carton. Don't substitute any components for components in carton.
- Inject deep into the gluteal muscle using only the needles supplied in the carton (1½-inch and 2-inch needles). Do not use any other needle. Choose the 1½-needle for very lean patients and the 2-inch needle for patients with a larger amount of subcutaneous tissue overlying the gluteal muscle. Either needle size may be used for patients with average body size.
- Rotate sites using other gluteal muscle for next injection.
- Store entire dose pack in refrigerator; unrefrigerated drug can be stored at room temperature for no more than 7 days.
- Avoid administering as a subcutaneous injection because of increased risk of severe injection-site reactions.
- Never give drug intravenously.
- Inspect injection site for reactions. Report any such findings to prescriber because abscesses and site necrosis may occur and may require surgical intervention.

Route	Onset	Peak	Duration
P.O.	15–30 min	1 hr	24–72 hr
I.M.	Unknown	2 hr	Unknown

Half-life: 12–17 hr

Mechanism of Action

Displaces opioid agonists from—or blocks them from binding with—delta, kappa, and mu receptors with the blockade reversing the euphoric effect of opioids. The action in treating alcoholism is unknown but is thought to be related to the endogenous opioid system.

Contraindications

Acute opioid withdrawal; concurrent therapy with opioid analgesics; dependency on opioids, including those currently maintained on opiate agonists (methadone) or partial agonists (buprenorphine); failure of the naloxone challenge test or patient has a positive urine screen for opioids; hypersensitivity to naltrexone or its components

Interactions

DRUGS

disulfiram: Increased risk of hepatoxicity
opioid analgesics: Reversal of analgesic and adverse effects of these drugs, possibly withdrawal symptoms in opioid-dependent patients
thioridazine: Increased lethargy and somnolence

Adverse Reactions

CNS: Abnormal thinking, agitation, anxiety, asthenia, chills, confusion, depression, dizziness, euphoria, fatigue, fever, hallucinations, headache, hyperkinesia, insomnia, irritability, malaise, nervousness, restlessness, somnolence, **suicidal ideation**, syncope, tremor
CV: Chest pain, edema, hypertension, palpitations, tachycardia
EENT: Blurred vision, burning eyes, conjunctivitis, dry mouth, eyelid swelling, hoarseness, pharyngitis, rhinitis, sneezing, tinnitus, vision abnormalities
ENDO: Hot flashes
GI: Abdominal cramps, anorexia, constipation, diarrhea, elevated liver

enzymes, GI ulceration, **hepatotoxicity** (excessive doses), nausea, vomiting
GU: Difficult ejaculation, urinary frequency
HEME: **Idiopathic thrombocytopenic purpura**
MS: Arthralgia, back pain or stiffness, joint stiffness, muscle cramps, myalgia
RESP: Cough, dyspnea, **eosinophilic pneumonia**, upper respiratory tract infection
SKIN: Increased sweating, pruritus, rash
Other: **Anaphylaxis**; injection-site reactions, such as bruising, erythema, induration, pain, tenderness; thirst

Childbearing Considerations

PREGNANCY

- It is not known if drug causes fetal harm.
- Use with caution only if benefit to mother outweighs potential risk to fetus.

LACTATION

- Drug may be present in breast milk.
- Mothers should check with prescriber before breastfeeding.

Nursing Considerations

! **WARNING** Use naltrexone cautiously in patients with hemophilia, severe hepatic failure, severe renal impairment, or thrombocytopenia.

- Prepare patient for naloxone challenge test if there are any doubts about patient's abstinence of 7 to 10 days.
- Anticipate that some patients may need treatment for up to 1 year. Be aware that drug can be given as an I.M. injection every 4 weeks if compliance with oral dosage is problematic.

! **WARNING** Monitor patient for hypersensitivity, which could become life-threatening, such as anaphylaxis. If present, notify prescriber, expect drug to be discontinued, and provide supportive care, as needed and ordered.

! **WARNING** Watch patient closely for suicidal tendencies throughout naltrexone therapy.

! **WARNING** Monitor patient's liver enzymes, as ordered, and patient for signs and symptoms of liver dysfunction because naltrexone may possibly cause hepatotoxicity. Notify prescriber of any abnormalities.

! **WARNING** Be aware that patients who receive naltrexone and need pain management are more likely to have longer, deeper respiratory depression and histamine-release reactions (such as bronchoconstriction, facial swelling, generalized erythema, and itching) if given an opioid analgesic. Expect alternative analgesics to be used, such as conscious sedation with a benzodiazepine, general anesthesia, nonopioid analgesics, or regional anesthesia. If an opioid analgesic must be used, monitor patient closely.

! **WARNING** Be aware that after opioid detoxification, patients may have lowered tolerance to opioids that could result in life-threatening circulatory collapse or respiratory compromise if patient uses previously tolerated doses of opioids.

PATIENT TEACHING

- Instruct patient how to administer oral naltrexone.
- Instruct patient to take oral drug with an antacid or food if stomach upset occurs.
- Tell patient struggling with compliance of taking oral naltrexone that drug can be administered as an injection once a month by a healthcare provider.
- Explain that patient may have nausea after first injection but that it is usually mild and subsides within a few days. Most patients don't have nausea with repeat doses.
- Inform patient that naltrexone doesn't eliminate or diminish alcohol withdrawal symptoms.

! **WARNING** Alert patient that drug may cause an allergic reaction. If present, tell patient to notify prescriber and, if severe, to seek immediate medical care.

! **WARNING** Urge family or caregiver to watch patient closely for abnormal behaviors, including suicidal tendencies, even after patient stops taking naltrexone.

! **WARNING** Warn patient that drug may cause liver damage. Tell her to report any signs of liver dysfunction, such as anorexia, digestive problems, or yellowing of skin or whites of her eyes.

! **WARNING** Caution patient against taking opioids during naltrexone therapy or in the future because she'll be more sensitive to them. In fact, strongly warn patient that taking large doses of heroin or any other opioid (including levo-alpha-acetyl-methadol [LAAM] or methadone) while taking naltrexone could lead to coma, serious injury, or death. Emphasize importance of having access to naloxone for emergency treatment of opioid overdose. Instruct family or caregiver when and how to administer naloxone, if needed.

- Tell patient to report adverse reactions promptly, especially abdominal pain, coughing, dyspnea, jaundice, and wheezing. Also, tell patient to report any injection-site reactions to prescriber, especially if reaction does not improve in 1 month following the injection or worsens, as further treatment may be necessary.
- Caution patient to avoid performing hazardous activities, such as driving, until CNS effects of drug are known and resolved.
- Inform patient about nonopioid treatments for cough, diarrhea, and pain.
- Tell patient while taking drug she may not experience the expected effects from opioid-containing analgesic, antidiarrheal, or antitussive drugs.
- Instruct patient to carry medical identification that lists naltrexone therapy.

naproxen

EC-Naprosyn, Naprosyn

naproxen sodium

Aleve, Anaprox DS, Flanax, Mediproxen, Naprelan

Class and Category

Pharmacologic class: NSAID
Therapeutic class: Analgesic

Indications and Dosages

∗ *To relieve mild to moderate musculoskeletal inflammation, including ankylosing spondylitis, osteoarthritis, and rheumatoid arthritis*

ORAL SUSPENSION, TABLETS (NAPROXEN)

Adults. 250 to 500 mg twice daily. *Maximum:* 1,500 mg daily for limited periods.

D.R. TABLETS (EC-NAPROSYN)

Adults. 375 or 500 mg twice daily. *Maximum:* 1,500 mg daily.

E.R. TABLETS (NAPROXEN SODIUM)

Adults. 750 to 1,000 mg daily. *Maximum:* 1,500 mg daily.

TABLETS (ANAPROX DS)

Adults. 275 to 550 mg twice daily. *Maximum:* 1,500 mg daily for limited periods.

∗ *To relieve symptoms of juvenile rheumatoid arthritis and other inflammatory conditions in children*

ORAL SUSPENSION (NAPROXEN)

Children ages 2 and older. 10 mg/kg daily in divided doses twice daily.

∗ *To relieve symptoms of acute gout*

ORAL SUSPENSION, TABLETS (NAPROXEN)

Adults. *Initial:* 750 mg, then 250 mg every 8 hr until symptoms subside.

TABLETS (NAPROXEN SODIUM)

Adults. *Initial:* 825 mg, then 275 mg every 8 hr until symptoms subside.

∗ *To relieve mild to moderate pain, including acute tendinitis and bursitis, arthralgia, dysmenorrhea, and myalgia*

ORAL SUSPENSION, TABLETS (NAPROXEN)

Adults. *Initial:* 500 mg, then 500 mg every 12 hr or 250 mg every 6 to 8 hr, as needed. *Maximum:* 1,250 mg on day 1; 1000 mg daily thereafter.

TABLETS (NAPROXEN SODIUM)

Adults. *Initial:* 550 mg followed by 550 mg every 12 hr. Alternatively, 275 mg every 6 to 8 hr, as needed. *Maximum:* 1,375 mg for initial total daily dose; subsequent days total daily dose should not exceed 1,100 mg.

∗ *To relieve fever and mild to moderate musculoskeletal inflammation or pain*

CAPLET, CAPSULES, TABLETS (OTC NAPROXEN SODIUM)

Adults and adolescents. 220 mg every 8 to 12 hr, as needed. Alternatively, 440 mg and then 220 mg 12 hr later daily, as needed. *Maximum:* 660 mg daily for 10 days unless directed otherwise.

±**DOSAGE ADJUSTMENT** For patients over age 65, dosage reduced.

Drug Administration

P.O.

- Different dose strengths and formulations such as oral suspension or tablets are not always bioequivalent and should not be interchanged when changing formulation.
- D.R., E.R., and film-coated tablets should be swallowed whole and not broken, chewed, or crushed.
- Administer drug with food and a full glass of water to reduce GI distress.
- Have patient remain upright for 15 to 30 min after administration of tablet to prevent drug from lodging in esophagus and causing irritation.
- Shake suspension well before administering. Use a calibrated device to measure dosage.

Route	Onset	Peak	Duration
P.O.	30–60 min	2–4 hr	< 12 hr
P.O./D.R./E.R.	30–60 min	2–12 hr	< 12 hr

Half-life: 12–17 hr

Mechanism of Action

Reduces symptoms of inflammation and relieves pain by blocking cyclooxygenase, the enzyme needed to synthesize prostaglandins, which mediate the inflammatory response and cause local pain, swelling, and vasodilation. Reduction of fever probably stems from effects on the hypothalamus, which increases peripheral blood flow, causing vasodilation and heat dissipation.

Contraindications

History of asthma, urticaria, or other allergic-type reactions induced by aspirin or other NSAIDs; hypersensitivity to naproxen or its components; postoperatively for pain management after coronary artery bypass graft (CABG) surgery

Interactions

DRUGS

ACE inhibitors, angiotensin receptor blockers (ARBs): Decreased antihypertensive effects; increased risk of renal dysfunction, especially in the elderly and those with impaired renal function or volume depletion

aluminum hydroxide or magnesium oxide antacids, cholestyramine, sucralfate: Possibly delayed absorption of naproxen

anticoagulants, antiplatelets, selective serotonin reuptake inhibitors, serotonin–norepinephrine reuptake inhibitors: Prolonged PT, increased risk of bleeding

aspirin: Decreased aspirin effectiveness with its antiplatelet effect taken to protect against CVA or MI; increased risk of GI adverse reactions compared to use of NSAID alone

beta-blockers: Decreased antihypertensive effects of these drugs

cyclosporine: Increased risk of nephrotoxicity

digoxin: Increased blood digoxin level and risk of digitalis toxicity

diuretics: Decreased diuretic effectiveness

lithium: Increased risk of lithium toxicity

methotrexate: Increased risk of methotrexate toxicity

other albumin-bound drugs: Increased risk of interference with binding requiring dosage changes of these drugs

other NSAIDs, salicylates: Increased risk of GI toxicity

pemetrexed: Increased risk of pemetrexed-associated GI and renal toxicity, myelosuppression

probenecid: Increased risk of naproxen toxicity

ACTIVITIES

alcohol use, smoking: Increased risk of naproxen-induced GI ulceration

Adverse Reactions

CNS: **Aseptic meningitis**, chills, cognitive impairment, **CVA**, decreased concentration, depression, dizziness, dream disturbances, drowsiness, fever, headache, insomnia, light-headedness, malaise, **seizures**, vertigo

CV: Edema, **heart failure**, hypertension, **MI**, palpitations, tachycardia, vasculitis

EENT: **Papilledema**, papillitis, retrobulbar optic neuritis, stomatitis, tinnitus, vision or hearing changes

ENDO: Hyperglycemia, **hypoglycemia**

GI: Abdominal pain, anorexia, colitis, constipation, diarrhea, diverticulitis, dyspepsia, dysphagia, elevated liver enzymes, esophagitis, flatulence, gastritis, gastroenteritis, gastroesophageal reflux disease, **GI bleeding** and ulceration, heartburn, hematemesis, **hepatitis**, indigestion, **melena**, nausea, **pancreatitis**, **perforation of intestines or stomach**, vomiting
GU: Elevated serum creatinine level, **glomerulonephritis**, hematuria, infertility (in women), interstitial nephritis, menstrual irregularities, **nephrotic syndrome**, **renal failure**, **renal papillary necrosis**
HEME: **Agranulocytosis**, anemia, **aplastic anemia**, eosinophilia, **granulocytopenia**, **hemolytic anemia**, **leukopenia**, **neutropenia**, **pancytopenia**, **thrombocytopenia**
MS: Muscle weakness, myalgia
RESP: **Asthma**, dyspnea, **eosinophilic pneumonitis**, **respiratory depression**
SKIN: Acute generalized exanthematous pustulosis, alopecia, diaphoresis, ecchymosis, **erythema multiforme**, **exfoliative dermatitis**, fixed drug eruptions, photosensitivity, pruritus, pseudoporphyria, purpura, rash, **Stevens-Johnson syndrome**, **toxic epidermal necrolysis**, urticaria
Other: **Anaphylaxis**, **angioedema**, **drug reaction with eosinophilia and systemic symptoms (DRESS)**, **hyperkalemia**, systemic lupus erythematosus

Childbearing Considerations

PREGNANCY

- Drug increases risk of premature closure of the fetal ductus arteriosus if given during the third trimester of pregnancy.
- Drug can cause fetal renal dysfunction leading to oligohydramnios and possibly neonatal renal impairment if given at or after 20 wk of gestation.
- Drug should be avoided in pregnant women starting at 30 wk of gestation and onward.
- Drug should only be given, if absolutely needed, using lowest dose and shortest duration possible between 20 and 30 wk of gestation.

LACTATION

- Drug is present in breast milk.
- Mothers should check with prescriber before breastfeeding.

REPRODUCTION

- Drug may delay or prevent rupture of ovarian follicles, which may cause reversible infertility in some women.
- Drug should not be used in females of childbearing age who have difficulty conceiving or who are undergoing investigation of infertility.

Nursing Considerations

! **WARNING** Be aware that NSAIDs like naproxen should be avoided in patients with a recent MI because risk of reinfarction increases with NSAID therapy. If therapy is unavoidable, monitor patient closely for signs of cardiac ischemia.

! **WARNING** Know that the risk of heart failure increases with use of NSAIDs, such as naproxen. NSAIDs should not be used in patients with severe heart failure but, if unavoidable, monitor patient for worsening of heart failure.

! **WARNING** Be aware that naproxen may decrease benefit of aspirin when taken for a heart attack or stroke.

- Monitor patient for effectiveness of naproxen therapy.

! **WARNING** Assess patient for a hypersensitivity or skin reaction that may occur without warning even in patients without a history of hypersensitivity to NSAIDs. Reaction could become life-threatening, such as anaphylaxis or DRESS. At first sign of a hypersensitivity or skin reaction (DRESS may only initially present with a fever or swollen lymph nodes), stop drug and notify prescriber. Be prepared to give supportive care, as needed and ordered.

! **WARNING** Monitor patients, especially patients with a history of GI bleeding or ulcer disease for serious GI tract bleeding, perforation, and ulceration, which may occur without warning. Elderly patients are at greater risk. To minimize risk, give drug with food and expect use to be for the shortest time possible in these patients. If GI distress occurs, withhold drug and notify prescriber immediately.

- Monitor patient—especially if elderly or receiving long-term naproxen therapy—for less common but serious adverse GI reactions, including anorexia, constipation, diverticulitis, dysphagia, esophagitis, gastritis, gastroenteritis, gastroesophageal reflux disease, hemorrhoids, hiatal hernia, melena, stomatitis, and vomiting.

! **WARNING** Monitor patient closely for thrombotic events, including MI and stroke because NSAIDs increase the risk, especially if used in higher doses than recommended or for extended periods of time. These events have occurred even in patients who do not have a history or risk factors for cardiovascular disease. Monitor patient for warning signs, such as chest pain, slurring of speech, shortness of breath, or weakness. If present, withhold naproxen, alert prescriber immediately, and provide supportive care as prescribed.

! **WARNING** Monitor liver enzymes because, in rare cases, elevations may progress to severe hepatic reactions, including fatal hepatitis, hepatic failure, or liver necrosis.

! **WARNING** Monitor BUN and serum creatinine levels, especially in elderly patients; patients taking diuretics, ACE inhibitors, or ARBs; and patients with heart failure; hepatic dysfunction; hypovolemia; or impaired renal function as naproxen may cause renal failure. Be aware that naproxen is not recommended for patients with advanced renal disease. Rehydrate a dehydrated patient before giving drug.

- Monitor CBC for decreased hemoglobin and hematocrit because drug may worsen anemia. Be aware that if patient has bone marrow suppression or is receiving treatment with an antineoplastic drug, laboratory results (including WBC count) must be monitored; watch for evidence of infection because anti-inflammatory and antipyretic actions of naproxen may mask signs and symptoms, such as fever and pain.
- Monitor patients for hypertension as well as patients who already have hypertension because drug may cause hypertension or worsen it. Monitor blood pressure closely. Also, watch for fluid retention because of naproxen's sodium content.
- Assess drug effectiveness in ankylosing spondylitis, as evidenced by decreased morning stiffness, night pain, and pain at rest; in osteoarthritis: decreased joint pain or tenderness and increased ability to perform daily activities, mobility, and range of motion; in rheumatoid arthritis: decreased joint swelling and morning stiffness and increased mobility; in acute gouty arthritis: decreased heat, pain, swelling, and tenderness in affected joints.
- Tell prescriber if patient complains of vision changes; patient may need ophthalmic exam.

PATIENT TEACHING

! **WARNING** Advise patient to consult prescriber before taking naproxen-containing over-the-counter products if asthma, bleeding problems, heart or kidney disease, high blood pressure, or ulcers are present; a need for diuretic therapy; persistent stomach problems, such as heartburn, stomach pain, or upset stomach; or serious adverse effects from previous use of fever reducers or pain relievers.

! **WARNING** Tell pregnant patient to avoid taking naproxen-containing products 30 weeks or later in pregnancy and females of childbearing age trying to conceive. Also tell pregnant patient not to take naproxen-containing products between 20 and 30 weeks of pregnancy, unless directed to do so by prescriber.

- Instruct patient how to administer form of naproxen prescribed.

! **WARNING** Caution patient not to exceed recommended dosage, take for longer than directed, or take for more than 10 days without consulting prescriber because serious adverse reactions, such as a heart attack, heart failure, or stroke, may occur.

! **WARNING** Alert patient to allergic reactions and rare but serious skin reactions. If present, tell patient to notify prescriber and, if severe, to seek immediate medical care.

! **WARNING** Inform patient that naproxen may increase risk of serious adverse GI reactions; stress the importance of seeking immediate medical attention for such signs and symptoms as abdominal or epigastric pain, black or tarry stools, indigestion, or vomiting blood or material that looks like coffee grounds.

! **WARNING** Explain that naproxen may increase risk of serious adverse cardiovascular reactions; urge patient to seek immediate medical attention if signs or symptoms arise, such as chest pain, edema, shortness of breath, slurring of speech, unexplained weight gain, and weakness.

! **WARNING** Tell patient to notify prescriber immediately if other persistent, serious, or unusual adverse reactions occur.

- Caution patient to avoid hazardous activities until drug's CNS effects are known and resolved.
- Urge patient to keep scheduled appointments with prescriber to monitor progress.

naratriptan hydrochloride

Class and Category

Pharmacologic class: Selective serotonin 5-HT receptor agonist
Therapeutic class: Antimigraine

Indications and Dosages

∗ *To relieve acute migraine with or without aura*

TABLETS

Adults. 1 or 2.5 mg as a single dose, repeated once in 4 hr, as needed, if headache returns or only partial relief obtained. *Maximum:* 5 mg daily; 4 migraine attacks/30 days.

±**DOSAGE ADJUSTMENT** For patients with mild to moderate hepatic or renal impairment, initial dose not to exceed 1 mg and maximum dosage reduced to 2.5 mg daily.

Drug Administration

P.O.

- Administer drug as soon as symptoms of a migraine appear.
- Tablet should be swallowed whole with water.
- Store away from heat and light.

Route	Onset	Peak	Duration
P.O.	1–2 hr	2–3 hr	Unknown

Half-life: 6 hr

Mechanism of Action

Binds to receptors on intracranial blood vessels and sensory nerves in trigeminal-vascular system to stimulate negative feedback, which halts serotonin release. Constricts dilated and inflamed cranial vessels in the carotid circulation and inhibits production of proinflammatory neuropeptides selectively to relieve migraine pain.

Contraindications

History of basilar or hemiplegic migraine, coronary artery disease, coronary artery vasospasm, stroke, or transient ischemic attack; hypersensitivity to naratriptan or its components; ischemic bowel disease; peripheral vascular disease; recent (within 24 hr) use of another 5-HT_1 agonist or an ergotamine-containing drug; severe hepatic or renal impairment; uncontrolled hypertension; Wolff-Parkinson-White syndrome or other cardiac accessory conduction pathway disorders

Interactions

DRUGS

ergot-containing drugs: Possibly additive or prolonged vasospastic reactions
MAO inhibitors, selective serotonin reuptake inhibitors, serotonin–norepinephrine reuptake inhibitors, tricyclic antidepressants, triptans: Increased risk of serotonin syndrome
other selective serotonin 5-HT receptor agonists (including triptans): Possibly additive risk of vasospastic reactions

Adverse Reactions

CNS: Dizziness, drowsiness, fatigue, malaise, paresthesia
CV: **Chest heaviness**, **pain**, **or pressure**; hypertension; **hypertensive crisis**
EENT: Decreased salivation, otitis media, pharyngitis, photophobia, rhinitis, **throat tightness**
GI: Nausea, vomiting
Other: **Anaphylaxis**, **angioedema**

Childbearing Considerations

PREGNANCY

- It is not known if drug causes fetal harm.

- Use with caution only if benefit to mother outweighs potential risk to fetus.
- Females of childbearing age with migraine may be at increased risk of preeclampsia during pregnancy.

LACTATION

- It is not known if drug is present in breast milk.
- Mothers should check with prescriber before breastfeeding.

Nursing Considerations

! **WARNING** Monitor patient for a hypersensitivity reaction, which could become life-threatening, such as anaphylaxis or angioedema. If present, notify prescriber, expect drug to be discontinued, and provide supportive care, as needed and ordered.

! **WARNING** Know that because naratriptan therapy can cause coronary artery vasospasm, monitor patient with coronary artery disease for signs or symptoms of angina while taking drug. Because naratriptan may also cause peripheral vasospastic reactions, such as ischemic bowel disease, monitor patient for abdominal pain and bloody diarrhea.

! **WARNING** Monitor patient closely for serotonin syndrome if she is taking naratriptan along with a selective serotonin reuptake inhibitor or serotonin–norepinephrine reuptake inhibitor. Notify prescriber immediately if the patient exhibits agitation, coma, diarrhea, hallucinations, hyperreflexia, hyperthermia, incoordination, labile blood pressure, nausea, tachycardia, or vomiting because serotonin syndrome can be life-threatening. Provide supportive care, as needed and ordered.

- Monitor patient for hypertension during naratriptan therapy even in patients with no history of hypertension because drug can cause significant elevation in blood pressure.
- Be prepared to perform a complete neurovascular assessment in any patient who reports an unusual headache or who fails to respond to first dose of naratriptan.

PATIENT TEACHING

- Inform patient that naratriptan used to treat acute migraine attacks won't prevent or reduce the number of migraines.
- Instruct patient how to administer naratriptan.

! **WARNING** Alert patient drug may cause an allergic reaction. If present, tell patient to notify prescriber and, if severe, to seek immediate medical care.

- Advise patient not to take more than maximum prescribed amount of naratriptan during any 24-hour period or to exceed treating headache more than 4 times each month. Overuse can cause headaches to become worse or increase frequency of migraine attacks. Advise patient to seek reevaluation by prescriber if she has more than 4 headaches during any 30-day period while taking naratriptan.
- Urge patient to inform all prescribers that she is receiving naratriptan therapy because serious drug interactions may occur.

natalizumab

Tysabri

Class and Category

Pharmacologic class: Monoclonal antibody
Therapeutic class: Immunomodulator

Indications and Dosages

∗ *To treat relapsing forms of multiple sclerosis, including active secondary progressive disease, clinically isolated syndrome, and relapsing-remitting disease; to induce and maintain remission in moderately to severely active Crohn's disease with evidence of inflammation in patients who had inadequate response to or are unable to tolerate conventional therapy and inhibitors of tumor necrosis factor alpha*

I.V. INFUSION

Adults. 300 mg every 4 wk.

Drug Administration

I.V.

- Inspect drug solution before preparing for administration. Solution should be colorless, clear to slightly opalescent.
- Withdraw 15 ml of drug from drug vial and inject into 100 ml of 0.9% Sodium Chloride Injection. Do not use any other diluents.
- Gently invert solution to mix completely. Do not shake.

- Infuse drug over 1 hr. Do not give by I.V. push or bolus.
- After infusion, flush line with 0.9% Sodium Chloride Injection.
- Refrigerate drug and use within 48 hr if not used immediately. If refrigerated, allow to warm to room temperature before using.
- Observe patient during infusion and for 1 hr after infusion is complete for the first 12 infusions. At first sign of a hypersensitivity reaction evidenced by chest pain, dizziness, dyspnea, fever, flushing, hypotension, nausea, pruritis, rash, rigors, or urticaria, discontinue drug and notify prescriber. Risk for an infusion reaction increases if natalizumab therapy was interrupted for a period of time. Continue to observe patient for infusion reactions for the 13th and subsequent infusions, as needed.
- *Incompatibilities:* Other drugs, solutions other than 0.9% Sodium Chloride Injection

Route	Onset	Peak	Duration
I.V.	Unknown	Unknown	Unknown

Half-life: 12–20 days

Mechanism of Action

Inhibits migration of leukocytes from vascular space, increasing the number of circulating leukocytes by binding to integrins on the surface of leukocytes (except neutrophils) and inhibiting adhesion of leukocytes to their counter receptors to help relieve symptoms of Crohn's disease. Be aware that in multiple sclerosis, lesions probably occur when activated inflammatory cells, including T-lymphocytes, cross the blood–brain barrier.

Contraindications

History of or presence of progressive multifocal leukoencephalopathy, hypersensitivity to natalizumab or its components

Interactions

DRUGS

antineoplastics, immunomodulating agents, immunosuppressants, inhibitors of TNF-α: Increased risk of life-threatening infection

Adverse Reactions

CNS: Depression, dizziness, **encephalitis**, fatigue, headache, **herpes encephalitis**, **meningitis**, **progressive multifocal leukoencephalopathy (PML)**, rigors, somnolence, **suicidal ideation**, vertigo

CV: Chest discomfort, peripheral edema

EENT: Acute retinal necrosis, sinusitis, tonsillitis, tooth infection

GI: Abdominal discomfort, cholelithiasis, diarrhea, elevated liver enzymes, gastroenteritis, **hepatotoxicity**, jaundice, nausea

GU: Amenorrhea; dysmenorrhea; irregular menstruation; ovarian cysts; UTI; urinary frequency, incontinence, or urgency; vaginitis

HEME: **Hemolytic anemia**, **immune thrombocytopenic purpura**, **thrombocytopenia**

MS: Arthralgia, back or limb pain, joint swelling, muscle cramp

RESP: Cough, pneumonia or other respiratory tract infection

SKIN: Dermatitis, night sweats, pruritus, rash, urticaria

Other: **Acute hypersensitivity reaction such as anaphylaxis**, antibody formation, flu-like illness, herpes, **immune reconstitution inflammatory syndrome**, opportunistic infections, weight gain or loss

Childbearing Considerations

PREGNANCY

- Drug may cause fetal harm as neonatal thrombocytopenia, with possible anemia, may occur.
- Expect to obtain a CBC in neonates exposed to drug in utero.
- Use with caution only if benefit to mother outweighs potential risk to fetus.

LACTATION

- Drug is present in breast milk.
- Mothers should check with prescriber before breastfeeding.

Nursing Considerations

- Make sure patient has enrolled in the TOUCH prescribing program before giving natalizumab. Once patient has signed and initialed the TOUCH program enrollment form, place original signed form in the patient's medical record, send a copy to Biogen Idec, and give a copy to patient. Be aware that patient needs to be evaluated 3 months after the first infusion, 6 months after the first infusion, every 6 months thereafter, and for at least 6 months after drug is discontinued. Know that a patient status report and reauthorization questionnaire must also be submitted 6 months after drug is initiated and every 6 months thereafter.

- Be aware that all atypical and serious opportunistic infections must be reported to Biogen Idec at 1-800-456-2255 and the FDA's MedWatch Program at 1-800-FDA-1088.
- Make sure patient with multiple sclerosis has had an MRI of the brain before starting natalizumab therapy. It will help distinguish evidence of multiple sclerosis from PML symptoms if they occur after therapy starts. Also, know that the following 3 factors increase the risk of PML in patients treated with natalizumab: longer treatment duration, especially beyond 2 years; prior treatment with an immunosuppressant; and the presence of anti-JCV antibodies.

! **WARNING** Monitor patient for a hypersensitivity reaction that usually occurs within the first 2 hours of the start of the drug infusion and could become life-threatening, such as anaphylaxis. If present, stop infusion, notify prescriber, and provide supportive care, as needed and ordered. A reaction most commonly occurs in patients with antibodies to the drug. Know that antibodies detected within first 6 months may be transient and may disappear with continued dosing. Antibody testing may be necessary and usually is done 3 months after an initial positive result to determine if antibodies are persistent. If antibodies are present, patient should not be retreated with drug.

! **WARNING** Monitor patient closely for evidence of PML, a viral brain infection that may be disabling or fatal because natalizumab increases the risk. Patients at increased risk include those who have received natalizumab for longer than 2 years, have had prior treatment with an immunosuppressant, and who have anti-JCV antibodies. If patient has unexplained neurologic changes, notify prescriber, withhold natalizumab, and prepare patient for a gadolinium-enhanced brain MRI and possible cerebrospinal fluid analysis, as ordered. Be aware that immune reconstitution inflammatory syndrome may occur in patients who develop PML, even when drug has been discontinued. Monitor patients for evidence of an overwhelming inflammatory response either to an opportunistic infection or the paradoxical symptomatic relapse of a prior infection despite it having been treated successfully in the past.

! **WARNING** Assess patient for evidence of other infections besides PML because natalizumab may adversely affect immune system, increasing risk of infection. For example, drug increases the risk for encephalitis and meningitis as well as acute retinal necrosis caused by herpes simplex and varicella-zoster viruses that could become life-threatening or result in blindness. Other infections that may occur but are uncommon may include aspergilloma, *Candida* pneumonia, cryptococcal fungemia, or pulmonary mycobacterium avium intracellulare. If infection occurs, expect to obtain appropriate specimens for culture and sensitivity and to treat accordingly, as ordered. If infection is serious, expect drug to be discontinued.

! **WARNING** Assess patient's liver function regularly, as ordered, because natalizumab may cause significant liver damage. Expect drug to be discontinued if patient becomes jaundiced or liver enzymes become elevated.

! **WARNING** Monitor patient's platelet counts for thrombocytopenia, as ordered. If suspected, notify prescriber and expect drug to be discontinued.

- Be aware that if patient with Crohn's disease has no therapeutic response after 12 weeks, natalizumab should be discontinued. If patient is on chronic oral corticosteroid therapy, expect tapering of oral corticosteroid dose to begin. If patient can't be tapered off oral corticosteroids within 6 months of starting natalizumab therapy, expect natalizumab to be discontinued. Likewise, if patient needs additional steroid use that extends beyond 3 months in a calendar year to control signs and symptoms of Crohn's disease, expect natalizumab to be discontinued.
- Ensure that when natalizumab is discontinued, patient completes the "Initial Discontinuation Questionnaire," and then has an appointment in 6 months to complete the "6-Month Discontinuation Questionnaire."

PATIENT TEACHING

- Instruct patient on benefits and risks of natalizumab therapy and provide medication guide for patient to read before therapy begins.
- Encourage patient to ask questions before signing the enrollment form.
- Inform patient that natalizumab is given intravenously every 4 weeks and that each infusion lasts about 1 hour.

! **WARNING** Alert patient that drug may cause an allergic or infusion reaction. Tell patient to alert staff if any symptoms occur during infusion. After infusion, tell patient to alert prescriber if present and, if severe, to seek immediate medical care.

- Emphasize need to report any worsening symptoms that persist over several days.

! **WARNING** Review signs and symptoms of PML with patient, family, or caregiver. Tell them that signs and symptoms suggestive of PML can occur up to 6 months after drug is discontinued and should be reported immediately.

! **WARNING** Review infection control measures with patient. Instruct patient to avoid people who have infections. Advise patient, family, or caregiver to report confusion, cough, fever, headache, lower-back or side pain, or other unexplained signs and symptoms because they may indicate infection.

! **WARNING** Review bleeding precautions with patient. Advise patient to notify prescriber if bleeding is difficult to stop, including from gums, nose, or a cut; easy bruising; heavier menstrual periods than normal; and small, scattered, spots on skin that appear pink, purple, or red.

! **WARNING** Review signs and symptoms of liver dysfunction and urge patient to report abdominal pain, fatigue, and jaundice immediately to prescriber.

! **WARNING** Tell patient to report decreased visual acuity or eye pain or redness, as these may be early signs of acute retinal necrosis caused by a herpes virus.

- Tell patient to inform all healthcare providers that he is receiving natalizumab therapy.
- Stress the need to have follow-up visits 3 months after first infusion, 6 months after first infusion, and at least every 6 months thereafter.

nateglinide

Class and Category

Pharmacologic class: Meglitinide
Therapeutic class: Antidiabetic

Indications and Dosages

∗ *As adjunct to diet and exercise to control blood glucose level in type 2 diabetes mellitus*

TABLETS

Adults. 120 mg 3 times daily 30 min before meals.

± **DOSAGE ADJUSTMENT** For patients with near goal glycemic control, dosage reduced to 60 mg 3 times daily.

Drug Administration

P.O.

- Administer within 30 min before meals to reduce risk of hypoglycemia.
- Do not administer if a meal is skipped.

Route	Onset	Peak	Duration
P.O.	20 min	1 hr	4 hr

Half-life: 1.5 hr

Contraindications

Hypersensitivity to nateglinide or its components

Interactions

DRUGS

beta-blockers, clonidine, guanethidine, reserpine: Possibly blunted signs and symptoms of hypoglycemia
corticosteroids, phenytoin, rifampin, somatostatin analogues (lanreotide, octreotide), somatropin, St. John's wort, sympathomimetics, thiazide diuretics, thyroid products: Possibly reduced hypoglycemic effects of nateglinide
CYP2C9 substrate poor metabolizers, CYP2C9 inhibitors (amiodarone, fluconazole, sulfinpyrazone), glucomannan, guanethidine, gymnema sylvestre, MAO inhibitors, methandrostenolone and other anabolic

Mechanism of Action

Stimulates the release of insulin from functioning beta cells of the pancreas. Interacting with the adenosine triphosphatase (ATP)-potassium channel on the beta cell membrane, nateglinide prevents potassium (K+) from leaving the cell causing the beta cell to depolarize and the cell membrane's calcium channel to open. Consequently, calcium (Ca++) moves into the cell and insulin moves out of it. Remember that the extent of insulin release is glucose dependent; the lower the glucose level, the less insulin is secreted from the cell. Promoting insulin secretion improves glucose tolerance.

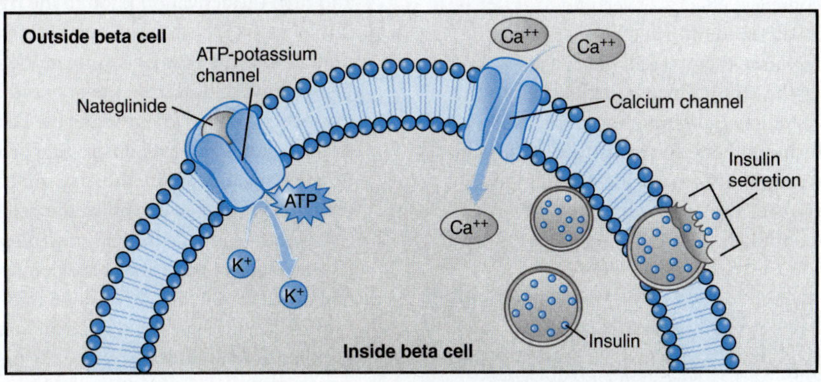

hormones nonselective beta-adrenergic blockers, NSAIDs, salicylates, somatostatin analogues: Possibly additive hypoglycemic effects of nateglinide

ACTIVITIES

alcohol use: Increased risk of hypoglycemia

Adverse Reactions

CNS: Dizziness
ENDO: **Hypoglycemia**
GI: **Cholestatic hepatitis**, diarrhea, elevated liver enzymes, jaundice
MS: Arthropathy, back pain
RESP: Bronchitis, cough, upper respiratory tract infection
SKIN: Pruritus, rash, urticaria
Other: Flu-like symptoms

Childbearing Considerations

PREGNANCY

- It is not known if drug causes fetal harm.
- Use with caution only if benefit to mother outweighs potential risk to fetus.

LACTATION

- It is not known if drug is present in breast milk.
- A decision should be made to discontinue breastfeeding or the drug to avoid potential serious adverse reactions in the breastfed infant, such as hypoglycemia.

Nursing Considerations

- Monitor fasting glucose and HbA1C levels periodically, as ordered, to evaluate drug effectiveness.
- Monitor patient often in event of fever, infection, surgery, or trauma because transient loss of glucose control may occur, requiring an alteration in therapy.

! WARNING Know that patients who are poor metabolizers of CYP2CP substrates are at increased risk of developing hypoglycemia because they may experience an additive hypoglycemic effect from nateglinide therapy.

PATIENT TEACHING

- Instruct patient how to administer nateglinide.
- Advise patient to skip scheduled dose if a meal is skipped, to reduce the risk of hypoglycemia.

! WARNING Tell patient how to recognize hyperglycemia and hypoglycemia. Advise patient to notify prescriber if blood glucose level is persistently abnormal. Review how to treat hypoglycemia. Inform patient that insufficient calorie intake, persistent consumption of alcohol, and strenuous exercise increase risk of hypoglycemia. Alert patients who are poor metabolizers of CYP2CP substrates that they may experience an additive hypoglycemic effect during nateglinide therapy.

- Advise patient to monitor blood glucose level and to keep follow-up appointments to monitor HbA1C level because drug may become less effective overtime.
- Tell patient to inform all prescribers of nateglinide therapy and not to take any over-the-counter drugs, including herbal preparations, without prescriber's knowledge.
- Inform mothers that breastfeeding should not be undertaken during nateglinide therapy or the drug will need to be discontinued.

NEW!

nemolizumab-ilto

Nemluvio

Class and Category

Pharmacologic class: Interluekin-31 receptor antagonist

Therapeutic class: Anti-inflammatory

Indications and Dosages

✶ *As adjunct to treat moderate-to-severe atopic dermatitis in combination with topical corticosteroids and/or calcineurin inhibitors when disease is not adequately controlled with topical prescription therapies*

SUBCUTANEOUS INJECTION

Adults and children 12 yrs and older. *Initial:* 60 mg (two 30 mg injections), followed by 30 mg every 4 wk. After 16 wk, if skin is clear or almost clear, frequency of injection is increased to every 8 wk.

✶ *To treat prurigo nodularis*

SUBCUTANEOUS INJECTION

Adults weighing 90 kg (198 lb) or more. *Initial:* 60 mg (two 30 mg injections), followed by 60 mg every 4 wk.

Adults weighing less than 90 kg (198 lb). Initial: 60 mg (two 30 mg injections), followed by 30 mg every 4 wk.

Drug Administration

SUBCUTANEOUS

- Remove drug pen from refrigerator and allow to reach room temperature, which may take 30 to 45 min. Injecting the drug cold might cause pain at injection site.
- Powder should be white in one chamber and a clear diluent in the other chamber. Do not use if powder is discolored or diluent is cloudy or contains visible particles. Also, do not use if pen is dropped or appears cracked or damaged.
- Reconstitute by holding the pen upright and turn the activation knob to the right until it stops. This begins transferring the diluent into the powder chamber. Watch the inspection window until the gray rod has stopped moving. Do not shake the pen at any time during the reconstituting process because shaking before the gray rod has completely stopped can affect the drug dose.
- Once drug is reconstituted (gray rod has completely stopped), shake the pen up and down for 30 sec. Then wait 5 min for bubbles to decrease. If the drug has not dissolved completely, shake the pen up and down again for 30 sec and wait an additional 5 min. A small foam layer or a few small air bubbles may remain in dissolved drug and is normal. Do not use the pen if the dissolved drug is cloudy or contains any particles.
- Holding the pen upright, twist the gray cap until the orange needle guard pops up. Gently pull the cap off the orange needle. If cap cannot be removed, make sure the activation knob is turned completely to the right until it stops.
- Administer in abdomen (2 inches away from navel), upper outer arm, or in the upper thigh. Do not inject into an area that is bruised, red, tender, or in areas containing scars or stretch marks. If a second injection is needed, inject in a different site, which is at least 1 inch away from first injection.
- Place the pen vertically on the injection site so that the orange needle guard is flat against the skin, and you can easily see the inspection window during injection. Gently push the pen down until the orange needle guard is completely pushed in. The injection will start right away with a click and the orange rod will begin to move down the inspection window. Do not lift the pen yet and keep pushing down. Hold slowly and count to 15. Check the inspection window

to make sure the orange rod and gray rod have stopped, indicating the injection is completed. It is normal that the orange rod does not cover the whole inspection window at the end of the injection. Lift the pen straight up from the skin. The orange needle guard will lock in place to cover the needle. Do not rub injection site but instead press a cotton ball or gauze over the injection site, if bleeding occurs.

- Administer drug within 4 hr once it has been reconstituted. Know that drug can be kept at room temperature during this time. If not used within 4 hr, discard pen and start again.

Route	Onset	Peak	Duration
SubQ	Unknown	6 days	Unknown

Half-life: 18.9 days

Mechanism of Action

Binds to human interleukin-31 (IL-31) to inhibit its interaction with selected IL-31 receptors. This action inhibits the release of proinflammatory cytokines and chemokines to reduce epidermal dysregulation, fibrosis, inflammation, and pruritus present in atopic dermatitis and prurigo nodularis.

Contraindications

Hypersensitivity to nemolizumab-ilto or its components

Interactions

DRUGS

live vaccines: Possibly increased risk of infection

Adverse Reactions

CNS: Headache (including migraine)
MS: Arthralgia, myalgia
SKIN: Urticaria
Other: **Angioedema**, herpes zoster, injection site reactions

Childbearing Considerations

PREGNANCY

- It is not known if drug can cause fetal harm. However, because endogenous IgG antibodies cross the placenta, which increases as pregnancy progresses and peaks during the third trimester, neonate should be monitored for serious infections during the first 3 months of life.
- Use with caution only if benefit to mother outweighs potential risk to fetus.

LACTATION

- It is not known if drug is present in breast milk.
- Mothers should check with prescriber before breastfeeding

Nursing Considerations

- Ensure that all appropriate vaccinations have been completed before nemolizumab-ilto therapy begins because drug may alter patient's immune response. Know that live vaccines should be avoid during drug treatment.

! WARNING Monitor patient closely for a hypersensitivity reaction such as angioedema. If present, notify prescriber immediately, expect drug to be discontinued, and provide supportive care, as needed and ordered.

- Know that when treatment for atopic dermatitis has shown that the disease has sufficiently improved, expect topical therapies to be discontinued.

PATIENT TEACHING

- Train patient, family, or caregiver how to administer drug by a subcutaneous injection and what injection sites to use. Tell parents of children who are 12 and older that the child may administer the injection but only under supervision.
- Stress importance of complying with the dosing schedule and what to do if a dose is missed.

! WARNING Alert patient that drug may cause an allergic reaction. If an allergic reaction is present, tell patient to notify prescriber and, if severe, to seek immediate medical care.

! WARNING Tell patient to inform all prescribers of nemolizumab-ilto therapy before any potential vaccination. Warn patient not to receive live vaccines.

nicardipine hydrochloride

Class and Category

Pharmacologic class: Calcium channel blocker
Therapeutic class: Antianginal, antihypertensive

Indications and Dosages

∗ To manage chronic stable angina pectoris as monotherapy or adjunct with beta-blockers

CAPSULES

Adults. 20 mg 3 times daily, increased every 3 days, as needed. *Maintenance:* 20 to 40 mg 3 times daily.

±**DOSAGE ADJUSTMENT** For patients with impaired liver function, initial dose reduced to 20 mg twice daily with a slow titration. For patients with impaired renal function, initial dosage of 20 mg 3 times daily kept but titration done slower.

∗ To manage hypertension as monotherapy or as adjunct with other antihypertensives

CAPSULES

Adults. 20 mg 3 times daily, increased every 3 days, as needed. *Maintenance:* 20 to 40 mg 3 times daily.

±**DOSAGE ADJUSTMENT** For patients with impaired liver function, initial dose reduced to 20 mg twice daily with slow titration. For patients with impaired renal function, initial dosage of 20 mg 3 times daily kept but titration done slower.

∗ To control hypertension when oral therapy is not desirable or feasible

I.V. INFUSION

Adults just starting nicardipine. *Initial:* 5 mg/hr; increased by 2.5 mg/hr every 5 to 15 min, as needed. *Maximum:* 15 mg/hr. *For patients achieving blood pressure goal:* Dosage reduced to 3 mg/hr.

Adults substituting parenteral form for oral form of nicardipine. *Initial:* 0.5 mg/hr substituted for 20 mg 3 times daily; 1.2 mg/hr substituted for 30 mg 3 times daily; and 2.2 mg/hr substituted for 40 mg 3 times daily.

±**DOSAGE ADJUSTMENT** For patients with heart failure or impaired hepatic or renal function, dosage titrated slowly to achieve blood pressure goal.

Drug Administration

P.O.

- Capsules should be swallowed whole and not chewed, crushed, or opened.
- May be administered with food but avoid giving with a high-fat meal or grapefruit juice.

I.V.

- Inspect solution in vial. It should appear clear and yellow in color.
- Dilute each 25-mg vial of nicardipine with 240 ml of a suitable diluent to yield 0.1 mg/ml. Solutions that can be used include 0.45% or 0.9% Sodium Chloride Injection, 5% Dextrose in Water, 5% Dextrose Injection and either 0.45% or 0.9% Sodium Chloride Injection combined or 5% Dextrose Injection with 40 mEq of potassium.
- If using premixed nicardipine (no dilution required), strength must be checked carefully because drug comes as single strength (20 mg nicardipine in 200 ml of solution, providing 0.1 mg/ml) or double strength (40 mg nicardipine in 200 ml of solution, providing 0.2 mg/ml). Also check for minute leaks prior to use by squeezing bag firmly.
- Administer drug through large peripheral veins or central veins.
- Administer continuous infusion with I.V. pump or controller, and adjust according to patient's blood pressure, as prescribed.
- Titrate infusion dosage slowly in patients receiving a beta-blocker and in patients with heart failure or significant left ventricular dysfunction because of possible negative inotropic effects. Also, patients with renal impairment require a more gradual titration.
- Stop infusion if hypotension or tachycardia occurs and notify prescriber. Expect to restart infusion at a lower dose once patient's blood pressure and heart rate have stabliized.
- Change peripheral I.V. site every 12 hr, if feasible.
- Give first dose of oral nicardipine 1 hr before stopping I.V. infusion, as ordered.
- Use solution within 24 hr if stored at room temperature.
- *Incompatibilities:* Lactated Ringer's or Sodium Bicarbonate solution through same I.V. line, other drugs

Route	Onset	Peak	Duration
P.O.	0.5–2 hr	0.5–2 hr	< 8 hr
I.V.	10–20 min	45 min	3 hr

Half-life: 8.5 hr

Mechanism of Action

May slow extracellular calcium movement into myocardial and vascular smooth-muscle cells by deforming calcium channels in cell membranes, inhibiting ion-controlled gating mechanisms, and interfering with calcium release from the sarcoplasmic reticulum. Decreasing the intracellular calcium level inhibits smooth-muscle cell contraction and dilates coronary and systemic arteries leading to decreased myocardial oxygen requirements and reduced afterload, blood pressure, and peripheral resistance.

Contraindications

Advanced aortic stenosis, hypersensitivity to nicardipine and its components

Interactions

DRUGS

cimetidine: Increased nicardipine bioavailability
cyclosporine: Increased plasma cyclosporine levels
digoxin: Transiently increased blood digoxin level, increased risk of digitalis toxicity
fentanyl: Possibly severe hypotension
tacrolimus: Increased plasma tacrolimus levels

FOODS

grapefruit, grapefruit juice: Possibly increased bioavailability of nicardipine
high-fat meals: Decreased blood nicardipine level

Adverse Reactions

CNS: Anxiety, asthenia, ataxia, confusion, dizziness, drowsiness, headache, nervousness, paresthesia, psychiatric disturbance, syncope, tremor, weakness
CV: **Bradycardia**, chest pain, exacerbation of angina (chronic therapy), **heart failure**, **hypotension**, orthostatic hypotension, palpitations, peripheral edema, tachycardia
EENT: Altered taste, blurred vision, dry mouth, epistaxis, gingival hyperplasia, pharyngitis, rhinitis, tinnitus
ENDO: Gynecomastia, hyperglycemia
GI: Anorexia, constipation, diarrhea, elevated liver enzymes, indigestion, nausea, thirst, vomiting
GU: Dysuria, nocturia, polyuria, sexual dysfunction, urinary frequency
HEME: Anemia, **leukopenia**, **thrombocytopenia**
MS: Joint stiffness, muscle spasms
RESP: Bronchitis, cough, **decreased oxygen saturation**, upper respiratory tract infection
SKIN: Dermatitis, diaphoresis, **erythema multiforme**, flushing, photosensitivity, pruritus, rash, **Stevens-Johnson syndrome**, urticaria
Other: **Hypokalemia**, injection-site irritation, weight gain

Childbearing Considerations

PREGNANCY

- Drug may cause fetal harm, such as transient fetal heart rate decelerations and neonatal hypotension when drug is given intravenously.
- Drug may also cause maternal harm causing such adverse reactions as dizziness, flushing, headache, hypotension, nausea, and reflex tachycardia when administered intravenously.
- Use with caution only if benefit to mother outweighs potential risk to fetus.

LACTATION

- Drug is present in breast milk.
- Breastfeeding is not recommended by some manufacturers.

Nursing Considerations

- Check blood pressure and pulse rate before nicardipine therapy begins, during dosage changes, and periodically throughout therapy. During prolonged therapy, periodically assess ECG tracings for arrhythmias and other changes.

! **WARNING** Monitor fluid intake and output and daily weight for signs of fluid retention, which may precipitate heart failure. Also, assess for signs of heart failure, such as crackles, dyspnea, jugular vein distention, peripheral edema, and weight gain.

! **WARNING** Monitor patient with angina for increases in duration, frequency, or severity of symptoms because with chronic use of oral nicardipine (rarely with I.V. administration), exacerbation of angina may occur.

! **WARNING** Monitor serum potassium level during prolonged therapy. Hypokalemia increases the risk of arrhythmias.

! **WARNING** Monitor patients who take a beta-blocker or have heart failure or significant left ventricular dysfunction because of drug's negative inotropic effect on some patients.

! **WARNING** Monitor pregnant patient receiving drug intravenously for adverse reactions such as dizziness, flushing, headache, hypotension, nausea, and reflex tachycardia. Also monitor fetal heart rate and once baby is born monitor for hypotension.

- Expect to periodically monitor hepatic and renal function test results during prolonged therapy. Anticipate drug dosage to be titrated slowly in these patients. Expect elevated liver enzymes to return to normal after drug is discontinued.

! **WARNING** Expect to taper dosage gradually before discontinuing drug. Otherwise, angina or dangerously high blood pressure could result.

PATIENT TEACHING

- Instruct patient how to administer oral nicardipine. Urge patient to take nicardipine even if she feels well.
- Teach patient how to take her pulse daily and urge her to notify prescriber immediately if it falls below 50 beats/minute.
- Teach patient how to measure blood pressure and urge her to do so weekly if drug was prescribed for hypertension. Suggest that she keep a log of blood pressure readings and take it to follow-up visits.

! **WARNING** Caution patient against stopping nicardipine abruptly because angina or dangerously high blood pressure could result.

! **WARNING** Advise patient to notify prescriber immediately about chest pain that's not relieved by rest or nitroglycerin, constipation, irregular heartbeats, nausea, pronounced dizziness, severe or persistent headache, and swelling of hands or feet.

! **WARNING** Instruct patient to notify prescriber if persistent, serious, or unusual adverse reactions occur.

- Advise patient to change position slowly to minimize orthostatic hypotension.
- Urge patient to avoid potentially hazardous activities until drug's CNS effects are known and resolved.
- Encourage patient to comply with suggested lifestyle changes, such as alcohol moderation, low-fat and low-sodium diet, regular exercise, smoking cessation, stress management, and weight reduction.
- Inform patient that hot tubs, prolonged hot showers, or saunas may cause dizziness or fainting.
- Instruct patient to avoid prolonged sun exposure and to use sunscreen when going outdoors.
- Inform mothers that breastfeeding may not be recommended during drug therapy.

nicotine nasal solution

Nicotrol NS

nicotine polacrilex

Nicorette, Nicorette Plus (CAN)

nicotine transdermal system

Habitrol, NicoDerm CQ, Nicotine Transdermal System Patch Kit, Nicotrol

Class and Category

Pharmacologic class: Nicotinic agonist
Therapeutic class: Smoking cessation adjunct

Indications and Dosages

∗ *As adjunct to smoking cessation for the relief of nicotine withdrawal symptoms, including craving*

CHEWING GUM (NICORETTE, NICORETTE PLUS)

Adults. *Initial for patient who smokes first cigarette later than 30 min after waking up:* 2 mg (1 piece). *Initial for patient who smokes first cigarette within 30 min of waking up:* 4 mg (1 piece). Subsequently, 2 mg or 4 mg every 1 to 2 hr, for 1 to 6 wk (with at least 9 pieces daily for the first 6 wk); then 2 or 4 mg every 2 to 4 hr for 7 to 9 wk; and then 2 or 4 mg every 4 to 8 hr for 10 to 12 wk. *Maximum:* 24 pieces daily for no longer than 12 wk.

NASAL SPRAY (NICOTROL NS)

Adults. 1 mg (2 sprays, 1 spray in each nostril) or 2 mg (4 sprays, 2 sprays in each nostril) hourly and then increased, as needed. *Maximum:* 5 mg/hr or 40 mg (80 sprays) daily for up to 3 mo.

LOZENGES (NICORETTE)

Adults who smoke first cigarette more than 30 min after waking up. 2 mg (1 lozenge)

every 1 to 2 hr for wk 1–6 (with at least 9 lozenges used per day during the first 6 wk): 1 lozenge every 2 to 4 hr for wk 7–9; 1 lozenge every 4 to 8 hr for wk 10–12. *Maximum:* No more than 1 lozenge at a time, no use of lozenges continuously 1 after another, no more than 5 lozenges in 6 hr; no more than 20 lozenges daily. Not to be used longer than 12 wk.

Adults who smoke first cigarette within 30 min after waking up. 4 mg (1 lozenge) every 1 to 2 hr for wk 1–6 (with at least 9 lozenges used per day during the first 6 wk); 1 lozenge every 2 to 4 hr for wk 7–9; 1 lozenge every 4 to 8 hr for wk 10–12. *Maximum:* No more than 1 lozenge at a time, no use of lozenges continuously 1 after another, no more than 5 lozenges in 6 hr; no more than 20 lozenges daily. Not to be used longer than 12 wk.

TRANSDERMAL PATCH (NICOTROL)

Adults who smoke more than 10 cigarettes a day. 15-mg patch 1 time daily for 6 wk, then 10-mg patch once daily for 2 wk, then 5-mg patch 1 time daily for 2 wk.

Adults who smoke 10 or less cigarettes a day. 10-mg patch once daily for 6 wk, then 5-mg patch 1 time daily for 2 wk.

TRANSDERMAL SYSTEM (HABITROL, NICODERM CQ, NICOTINE TRANSDERMAL SYSTEM PATCH KIT)

Adults who smoke more than 10 cigarettes a day. 21-mg patch daily for wk 1 through 4; 14-mg patch daily for wk 5 and 6; 7-mg patch daily for wk 7 and 8.

Adults who smoke 10 cigarettes or less a day. 14-mg patch daily for 6 wk followed by 7-mg patch daily for 2 additional wk.

±**DOSAGE ADJUSTMENT** For patients with moderate to severe hepatic or renal impairment, dosage may have to be reduced.

Drug Administration

P.O.

- For chewing gum or lozenges, patient must wait at least 15 min after drinking coffee, juice, soft drink, tea, or wine before using these forms of drug.
- Gum should be chewed until a tingling sensation or peppery taste occurs and then gum placed in cheek until sensation or taste subsides. Gum then should be moved to a different site until tingling or taste returns and then subsides, repeating until there is no longer a sensation—usually about 30 min. Caution against swallowing the gum.
- For lozenges, tell patient to allow lozenge to slowly dissolve and minimize swallowing. The lozenge should not be chewed or swallowed but moved from one side of mouth to the other until it is completely dissolved. It will take about 20 to 30 min.

INTRANASAL

- Have patient tilt head back and spray into a nostril. Caution against inhaling, sniffing, or swallowing spray during administration because nicotine is absorbed through nasal and oral mucosa.
- Warn patient a hot, peppery feeling in back of throat or nose, coughing, running nose, sneezing, or watery eyes may occur during first week of use but these symptoms will subside in a few days.
- Prime pump before first use and when not used for 24 hr by pressing up on bottom with thumb; pump into a tissue until a fine spray is seen (6 to 8 times).
- Have patient blow nose, tilt head back slightly and insert tip of bottle into nostril. While patient breaths through mouth, spray once in each nostril having patient avoid sniffing or inhaling while spraying. If nose runs, have patient gently sniff to keep drug in nose. Have patient wait 2 to 3 minutes before blowing nose.
- Prolonged use of nasal form may cause dependence.

TRANSDERMAL

- Open package immediately before use. Do not cut patch or use a patch that's damaged upon opening protective pouch.
- Apply system to a clean, dry, hairless site on outer arm or upper body. Do not apply to skin that has had creams, lotions, or oils applied to the skin. Also, do not apply to damaged skin. Save pouch for disposal of patch after use.
- After removing backing, press on skin for 10 sec.
- Apply patch consistently at about the same time of day. Change systems and rotate sites every 24 hr.
- Do not use same site for 7 days. Do not apply more than 1 patch at a time.
- After removing patch, fold sticky ends together, put in pouch, and discard.
- Wash hands.

Route	Onset	Peak	Duration
P.O.	Unknown	30 min	Unknown
Intranasal	Rapid	10–20 min	Unknown
Transdermal	Unknown	2–8 hr	24 hr

Half-life: 1–4 hr

Mechanism of Action

Binds selectively to nicotinic-cholinergic receptors at autonomic ganglia, in the adrenal medulla, at neuromuscular junctions, and in the brain. Reduces nicotine craving and withdrawal symptoms by providing a lower dose of nicotine than cigarettes.

Contraindications

Hypersensitivity to nicotine or its components, including menthol or soy

Interactions

DRUGS

acetaminophen, adrenergic antagonists (labetalol, prazosin), beta-blockers, imipramine, insulin, oxazepam, pentazocine, theophylline: Possibly increased therapeutic effects of these drugs (chewing gum, nasal spray, transdermal system)

adrenergic agonists (isoproterenol): Decreased effectiveness of these drugs

FOODS

acidic beverages (citrus juices, coffee, soft drinks, tea, wine): Decreased nicotine absorption from gum if beverages consumed within 15 min before or while chewing gum

caffeine: Increased effects of caffeine (chewing gum, nasal spray, transdermal system)

Adverse Reactions

CNS: Dizziness, dream disturbances, drowsiness, headache, irritability, light-headedness, nervousness (chewing gum, transdermal system); amnesia, confusion, difficulty speaking, headache, migraine headache, paresthesia, **seizures** (nasal spray)

CV: **Arrhythmias** (all forms); chest pain (nasal spray); hypertension (chewing gum, transdermal system); peripheral edema (nasal spray)

EENT: Increased salivation, injury to teeth or dental work, mouth injury, oral blistering, pharyngitis, stomatitis (chewing gum); altered taste, dry mouth (chewing gum, transdermal system); altered smell and taste, burning eyes, dry mouth, earache, epistaxis, gum disorders, hoarseness, lacrimation, mouth and tongue swelling, nasal blisters, nasal irritation or ulceration, pharyngitis, rhinitis, sinus problems, sneezing, vision changes (nasal spray); altered taste, lacrimation, pharyngitis, rhinitis, sinusitis

GI: Eructation (chewing gum); abdominal pain, constipation, diarrhea, flatulence, increased appetite, indigestion, nausea, vomiting (chewing gum, transdermal system); abdominal pain, constipation, diarrhea, dysphagia, flatulence, hiccups, indigestion, nausea (nasal spray)

GU: Dysmenorrhea (chewing gum, transdermal system); menstrual irregularities (nasal spray)

MS: Jaw and neck pain (chewing gum); arthralgia, myalgia (chewing gum, transdermal system); arthralgia, back pain, myalgia (nasal spray)

RESP: Cough (chewing gum, transdermal system); bronchitis, **bronchospasm**, chest tightness, cough, dyspnea, increased sputum production (nasal spray)

SKIN: Diaphoresis, erythema, pruritus, rash, urticaria (chewing gum, transdermal system); acne, flushing of face, pruritus, purpura, rash (nasal spray)

Other: **Anaphylaxis and other hypersensitivity reactions**, delayed wound healing, flu-like symptoms, generalized pain, physical dependence, withdrawal symptoms

Childbearing Considerations

PREGNANCY

- Drug may cause fetal harm.
- Drug use is not recommended during pregnancy.

LACTATION

- Drug is present in breast milk.
- Mothers should check with prescriber before breastfeeding.

Nursing Considerations

- Know that drug should be used with caution in patients with hyperthyroidism, insulin-dependent diabetes, or pheochromocytoma because nicotine releases catecholamines from the adrenal medulla, which affects the drug dosing treatment of these disorders.
- Use caution when nicotine is given with patients with active gastric or peptic ulcers or who have esophagitis because nicotine delays healing in ulcer disease.

! **WARNING** Monitor patient for hypersensitivity reaction. Notify prescriber, if present, and expect nicotine product to be discontinued. If reaction is serious, expect to provide supportive care, as needed and ordered.

! **WARNING** Monitor patient, especially if patient has asthma or COPD, for bronchospasms after drug administration. If present, notify prescriber immediately.

! **WARNING** Remove patch before patient has an MRI to prevent burns.

PATIENT TEACHING

- Advise patient to notify prescriber about other conditions or drugs patient may have or takes before starting nicotine therapy.
- Instruct patient on how to use nicotine product prescribed and encourage patient to read and follow package instructions to obtain best results.

! **WARNING** Emphasize that patient must stop smoking as soon as nicotine treatment starts to avoid toxicity.

! **WARNING** Alert patient that drug may cause an allergic reaction. If present, tell patient to notify prescriber and, if severe, to seek immediate medical care.

! **WARNING** Review signs and symptoms of a nicotine overdose. If present, tell patient to notify prescriber and, if severe, to seek immediate medical care.

! **WARNING** Inform patient, especially if patient has asthma or COPD, that nicotine may cause bronchospasms. If patient develops difficulty breathing after taking a nicotine product, tell patient to notify prescriber and seek immediate medical care.

! **WARNING** Urge patient to keep all unused nicotine forms safely away from children and pets and to discard used forms carefully. (Enough nicotine may remain in used systems to poison children and pets.) Instruct patient to contact a poison control center immediately if a child may have ingested nicotine.

- Inform patient that it may take several attempts to stop smoking. Urge patient to join a smoking cessation program.
- Tell females of childbearing age to notify prescriber if pregnancy occurs as drug is not recommended during pregnancy.

nifedipine

Adalat XL (CAN), Afeditab CR, Procardia, Procardia XL

Class and Category

Pharmacologic class: Calcium channel blocker
Therapeutic class: Antianginal, antihypertensive

Indications and Dosages

∗ *To manage chronic stable angina, vasospastic angina*

CAPSULES (PROCARDIA)

Adults. *Initial:* 10 mg 3 times daily, increased over 1 to 2 wk, as needed. *Maintenance:* 10 to 20 mg 3 times daily. *Maximum:* 180 mg daily, 30 mg/dose.

E.R. TABLETS (PROCARDIA XL)

Adults. *Initial:* 30 or 60 mg once daily, increased over 7 to 14 days, as needed. *Maximum:* 120 mg daily.

E.R. TABLETS (ADALAT XL)

Adults. *Initial:* 30 mg once daily, increased, as needed, over 7 to 14 days. *Maximum:* 90 mg daily.

∗ *To manage hypertension*

E.R. TABLETS (AFEDITAB CR)

Adults. *Initial:* 30 mg once daily, increased, as needed, over 7 to 14 days. *Maintenance:* 30 to 60 mg daily. *Maximum:* 90 mg daily.

E.R. TABLETS (ADALAT XL)

Adults. *Initial:* 20 or 30 mg daily, increased over 7 to 14 days, as needed. *Maintenance:* 30 to 60 mg daily. *Maximum:* 90 mg daily.

E.R. TABLETS (PROCARDIA XL)

Adults. 30 or 60 mg daily, increased over 7 to 14 days, as needed. *Maximum:* 120 mg daily.

± **DOSAGE ADJUSTMENT** For elderly patients and those with heart failure or impaired hepatic or renal function, dosage initiated at lower end of dosage range.

Drug Administration

P.O.

- Capsules and E.R. tablets should be swallowed whole and not chewed, crushed, or opened. E.R. tablets should be administered on an empty stomach;

N O

immediate-release capsules can be administered with or without food.

- Do not administer with grapefruit juice.

Route	Onset	Peak	Duration
P.O.	30–60 min	30–120 min	8 hr
P.O./E.R.	20 min	6 hr	24 hr

Half-life: 2–7 hr

Mechanism of Action

May slow movement of calcium into myocardial and vascular smooth-muscle cells by deforming calcium channels in cell membranes, inhibiting ion-controlled gating mechanisms, and disrupting calcium release from sarcoplasmic reticulum. Decreasing intracellular calcium level inhibits smooth-muscle cell contraction and dilates arteries, which decreases myocardial oxygen demand, peripheral resistance, blood pressure, and afterload.

Contraindications

Hypersensitivity to nifedipine or its components

Interactions

DRUGS

cimetidine, clarithromycin, erythromycin, fentanyl, fluconazole, fluoxetine, indinavir, itraconazole, nefazodone, nelfinavir, saquinavir: Increased risk of hypotension
beta-blockers: Increased risk of profound hypotension, heart failure, and worsening of angina
digoxin: Transiently increased blood digoxin level, increased risk of digitalis toxicity
oral anticoagulants: Possibly increased prothrombin time
phenytoin: Decreased systemic exposure of nifedipine
quinidine: Possibly decreased plasma quinidine level

FOODS

grapefruit, grapefruit juice: Possibly increased bioavailability of nifedipine

Adverse Reactions

CNS: Anxiety, ataxia, confusion, dizziness, drowsiness, headache, nervousness (possibly extreme), nightmares, paresthesia, psychiatric disturbance, syncope, tremor, weakness
CV: **Bradycardia**, chest pain, **heart failure**, **hypotension**, palpitations, peripheral edema, tachycardia
EENT: Altered taste, blurred vision, dry mouth, epistaxis, gingival hyperplasia, nasal congestion, pharyngitis, sinusitis, tinnitus
ENDO: Gynecomastia, hyperglycemia
GI: Anorexia; constipation; diarrhea; dyspepsia; elevated liver enzymes; **GI bleeding**, irritation, or **obstruction**; **hepatitis**; nausea; vomiting
GU: Dysuria, nocturia, polyuria, sexual dysfunction, urinary frequency
HEME: Anemia, **leukopenia**, positive Coombs' test, **thrombocytopenia**
MS: Joint stiffness, muscle cramps
RESP: Chest congestion, cough, dyspnea, respiratory tract infection, wheezing
SKIN: Acute generalized exanthematous pustulosis, diaphoresis, **erythema multiforme**, **exfoliative dermatitis**, flushing, photosensitivity, pruritus, rash, **Stevens-Johnson syndrome**, **toxic epidermal necrolysis**, urticaria

Childbearing Considerations

PREGNANCY

- Drug may cause fetal harm, according to animal studies.
- Use with caution only if benefit to mother outweighs potential risk to fetus.

LACTATION

- Drug is present in breast milk.
- Mothers should check with prescriber before breastfeeding.

Nursing Considerations

! WARNING Be aware that patients with galactose intolerance should not take nifedipine because drug contains lactose. The capsule form of nifedipine should not be used to treat hypertension because its effects on blood pressure are not known.

- Use cautiously in patients with cirrhosis because it is unknown how nifedipine exposure may be altered in these patients.

! WARNING Keep in mind that because of the drug's negative inotropic effect on some patients, frequently monitor heart rate and rhythm, as well as blood pressure, especially in patients who take a beta-blocker or have heart failure, significant left ventricular dysfunction, or tight aortic stenosis.

! **WARNING** Monitor fluid intake/output and daily weight; fluid retention may lead to heart failure. Also, assess for signs of heart failure, such as crackles, dyspnea, jugular vein distention, peripheral edema, and weight gain.

! **WARNING** Avoid abruptly stopping nifedipine therapy and instead taper it, as prescribed, over 7 to 14 days to avoid precipitating angina.

PATIENT TEACHING

- Instruct patient how to administer form of nifedipine prescribed. Urge patient to take nifedipine exactly as prescribed, even when she's feeling well.
- Advise patient to notify prescriber if she misses 2 or more doses.
- Urge patient not to take drug with grapefruit juice. Urge patient to avoid alcoholic beverages because they may worsen dizziness, drowsiness, and hypotension.
- Inform patient taking E.R. tablets that their empty shells may appear in stool but this is a harmless effect.
- Teach patient to measure blood pressure and pulse rate and advise patient to call prescriber if they drop below accepted levels. Suggest keeping a log of weekly measurements and taking it to follow-up visits.

! **WARNING** Caution patient against stopping nifedipine abruptly because angina or dangerously high blood pressure could result.

! **WARNING** Instruct patient to notify prescriber immediately about chest pain, difficulty breathing, ringing in ears, and swollen gums.

- Advise patient to avoid hazardous activities until drug's CNS effects are known and resolved.
- Teach patient to minimize constipation by increasing her intake of fluids, if allowed, and dietary fiber.
- Emphasize the need to comply with prescribed lifestyle changes, such as low-fat or low-sodium diet, regular exercise, smoking cessation, stress reduction, and weight reduction.
- Emphasize the need for good oral hygiene and regular dental visits.
- Caution patient that hot tubs, prolonged hot showers, and saunas may cause dizziness and fainting.
- Advise patient to avoid prolonged sun exposure and to wear sunscreen outdoors.
- Tell females of childbearing age to notify prescriber if pregnancy occurs.

nirmatrelvir

Class and Category

Pharmacologic class: Protease inhibitor
Therapeutic class: Antiviral

Indications and Dosages

✱ *As adjunct to treat mild to moderate coronavirus disease 2019 (COVID-19) in patients at high risk for progression to severe COVID-19, including hospitalization or death with positive results of direct severe acute respiratory syndrome coronavirus 2 (SARS-CoV-2) viral testing and who are at high risk for progression to severe COVID-19, including hospitalization or death.*

P.O.

Adults. 300 mg with 100 mg ritonavir twice daily for 5 days.

± **DOSAGE ADJUSTMENT** For patients with moderate impaired renal function (eGFR of 30 to less than 60 ml/min), dosage reduced to 150 mg (no dosage change for ritonavir). For patients with severe renal impairment (eGFR less than 30 ml/min), including patients on hemodialysis, dosage interval decreased on day 1 to once daily for both nirmatrelvir and ritonavir and dosage decreased to 150 mg and dosage interval decreased to once daily for both drugs for days 2 to 5.

Drug Administration

TABLET

- Know that nirmatrelvir and ritonavir are copackaged for oral use and supplied under the trade name of Paxlovid even though the 2 drugs are not combined into 1 tablet but are administered as 2 different drugs.
- Administer both nirmatrelvir and ritonavir tablets together at the same time with

or without food because failure to do so may result in insufficient plasma levels of nirmatrelvir to achieve desired results.

- For patients receiving hemodialysis, drug should be administered after hemodialysis.
- Have patient swallow the tablet whole and not break, chew, or crush the tablet.
- If a dose is missed and it is within 8 hr of the scheduled administration time of the missed dose, administer and resume the normal dosing schedule. If it is more than 8 hr since the missed dose, skip the missed dose and resume the normal dosing schedule.

Route	Onset	Peak	Duration
P.O.	Unknown	Unknown	Unknown

Half-life: 6.05 hr

Mechanism of Action

Inhibits the activity of SARS-CoV-2 main protease (Mpro), rendering it incapable of processing polyprotein precursors, which prevents viral replication.

Contraindications

Concurrent therapy with drugs that are highly dependent on CYP3A for clearance and for which elevated concentrations are associated with serious and/or life-threatening reactions, such as alpha$_1$-adrenoreceptor antagonist (alfuzosin), analgesics (pethidine, piroxicam, propoxyphene), antianginal (ranolazine), antiarrhythmics (amiodarone, dronedarone, flecainide, propafenone, quinidine), anti-gout (colchicine), antipsychotics (clozapine, lurasidone, pimozide), ergot derivatives (dihydroergotamine, ergotamine, methylergonovine), HMG-CoA reductase inhibitors (lovastatin, simvastatin), PDE-5 inhibitor when used for pulmonary arterial hypertension (sildenafil [Revatio]), and sedative/hypnotics (oral midazolam, triazolam); hypersensitivity to nirmatrelvir or ritonavir or any of their components; within recent discontinuation of potent CYP3A inducers where significantly reduced nirmatrelvir or ritonavir plasma concentrations may be associated with the potential for loss of virologic response and possible resistance such as anticancer drugs (apalutamide), anticonvulsants (carbamazepine, phenobarbital, phenytoin), antimycobacterials (rifampin), and herbal products (St. John's wort)

Interactions

DRUGS

antiarrhythmics (bepridil, systemic lidocaine): Increased risk of change in therapeutic concentration for antiarrhythmics

anticancer drugs (abemaciclib, ceritinib, dasatinib, encorafenib, ibrutinib, ivosidenib, neratinib, nilotinib, venetoclax, vinblastine, vincristine): Potential for significant adverse reactions

anticoagulants (rivaroxaban, warfarin): Increased risk of INR change (warfarin) or bleeding (rivaroxaban)

antidepressants (bupropion, trazodone): Change in therapeutic response (bupropion) or increased risk of adverse reactions of dizziness, hypotension, nausea, and syncope (trazodone)

antifungals (ketoconazole, isavuconazonium sulfate, itraconazole): Plasma concentration increased with increased risk of adverse reactions

anti-HIV drugs (bictegravir/emtricitabine/tenofovir, didanosine, delavirdine, efavirenz, maraviroc, nevirapine, raltegravir, zidovudine): Change in plasma concentration either affecting effectiveness of the anti-HIV drug or increasing risk of adverse reactions

anti-infective (clarithromycin, erythromycin), anti-HIV protease inhibitors (amprenavir, atazanavir, darunavir, fosamprenavir, indinavir, nelfinavir, saquinavir, tipranavir), antimycobacterial (bedaquiline, rifabutin), bosentan, calcium channel blockers (amlodipine, diltiazem, felodipine, nicardipine, nifedipine), digoxin, fentanyl, hepatitis C direct-acting antivirals (elbasvir/grazoprevir, glecaprevir/pibrentasvir, ombitasvir, paritaprevir, ritonavir and dasabuvir, sofosbuvir/velpatasvir/voxilaprevir), HMG-CoA reductase inhibitors (atorvastatin, rosuvastatin), immunosuppressants (cyclosporine, sirolimus, tacrolimus), parenteral midazolam, quetiapine, salmeterol, systemic corticosteroids (betamethasone, budesonide, ciclesonide, dexamethasone, fluticasone, methylprednisolone, mometasone, prednisone, triamcinolone): Increased plasma concentrations of these drugs increasing risk of adverse reactions

hormonal contraceptive (ethinyl estradiol): Decreased effectiveness of ethinyl estradiol

methadone, voriconazole: Decreased plasma concentration of these drugs

∗ *Refer to manufacturer's guidelines for ritonavir drug interactions.*

Adverse Reactions

CV: Hypertension
EENT: Alteration in taste
GI: Diarrhea
MS: Myalgia
SKIN: **Stevens-Johnson syndrome** (with Paxlovid combination), **toxic epidermal necrolysis** (with Paxlovid combination)
Other: **Anaphylaxis and other hypersensitivity reactions** (with Paxlovid combination)

∗ *Refer to manufacturer's's guidelines for ritonavir adverse drug reactions.*

Childbearing Considerations

PREGNANCY

- It is not known if drug can cause fetal harm.
- Use with caution only if benefit to mother outweighs potential risk to fetus.

LACTATION

- Drug is present in breast milk in small amounts.
- Mothers should check with prescriber before breastfeeding.

REPRODUCTION

- Females of childbearing age using a combined hormonal contraceptive should use an effective alternative contraceptive method or an additional barrier method of contraception during drug therapy.

Nursing Considerations

- Know that nirmatrelvir in combination with ritonavir under the trade name of Paxlovid has now received full FDA approval to treat COVID-19. However, be aware that drug is not authorized for use to treat patients hospitalized due to COVID-19. It is also not authorized for use for longer than 5 consecutive days and it is not authorized for preexposure or postexposure to prevent COVID-19. Drug is also not recommended for patients with severe hepatic impairment.

! WARNING Be aware that because nirmatrelvir is given with ritonavir, a risk of HIV-1 resistance to HIV protease inhibitors may develop in patients with uncontrolled or undiagnosed HIV-1 infection.

- Expect patient who is started on nirmatrelvir therapy and then requires hospitalization to continue on to complete the full 5-day treatment course at the prescriber's discretion.
- Continue isolation protocols according to public health recommendations during drug therapy to minimize the transmission of SARS-CoV-2 virus.

! WARNING Monitor patient for hypersensitivity reaction because the combined use of nirmatrelvir and ritonavir under the name of Paxlovid have caused anaphylaxis and other hypersensitivity reactions including serious skin reaction such as Stevens-Johnson syndrome and toxic epidermal necrolysis. If present, notify prescriber and expect drug to be discontinued. Provide supportive care, as needed and ordered.

! WARNING Monitor patient closely with preexisting liver disease, liver enzyme abnormalities, or hepatitis, as clinical hepatitis, jaundice, and transaminase elevations have occurred in patients receiving ritonavir.

PATIENT TEACHING

- Ensure that patient has received the "Fact Sheet for Patients, Parents, and Caregivers."

! WARNING Tell patient to alert prescriber of all drug therapies taken before drug is administered, as nirmatrelvir/ritonavir combination can cause many drug interactions, resulting in adverse reactions that could be severe.

- Instruct patient how to administer nirmatrelvir and what to do if a dose is missed.
- Stress importance of completing the full 5-day treatment with nirmatrelvir in combination with ritonavir.
- Stress need for patient to continue isolation per public health recommendations.

! WARNING Inform patient that an allergic reaction may occur with nirmatrelvir. If present, advise patient or caregiver to notify prescriber and, if serious, patient should seek immediate medical care.

> ! **WARNING** Tell patient to notify prescriber if persistent, serious, or unusual adverse reactions occur.

- Inform females of childbearing age using a combined hormonal contraceptive that she should use an effective alternative contraceptive method or an additional barrier method of contraception during drug therapy.
- Encourage mothers who are breastfeeding to discuss continued breastfeeding during COVID-19 infection treatment with prescriber before doing so.

nitrofurantoin

Furadantin, Macrobid, Macrodantin

Class and Category

Pharmacologic class: Nitrofuran
Therapeutic class: Antibiotic

Indications and Dosages

∗ *To treat acute cystitis due to* Enterococci, Escherichia coli, *or* Staphylococcus aureus; *certain strains of* Enterobacter *or* Klebsiella *species*

CAPSULES, ORAL SUSPENSION

Adults and adolescents. 50 to 100 mg 4 times daily with meals and at bedtime and continued for 1 wk or at least 3 days after urine is negative for bacteria. Alternatively using Macrobid, 100 mg every 12 hr for 7 days.
Children ages 1 mo and older. 5 to 7 mg/kg/day in 4 divided doses, continued for 1 wk or at least 3 days after urine is negative for bacteria.

∗ *To suppress chronic cystitis*

CAPSULES, ORAL SUSPENSION

Adults. 50 to 100 mg daily at bedtime.
Children ages 1 mo and older. 1 to 2 mg/kg daily at bedtime or 2 divided doses and given every 12 hr.

Drug Administration

P.O.

- Give drug with food or milk to minimize GI upset.
- Capsules should be swallowed whole and not chewed, crushed, or opened.
- Shake suspension before pouring dose and use a calibrated device to measure dose. Mix with food or milk, as needed.
- Administer drug used to suppress chronic cystitis once daily at bedtime.

Route	Onset	Peak	Duration
P.O.	Unknown	30 min	Unknown

Half-life: 20–60 min

Mechanism of Action

Alters or inactivates bacterial ribosomal proteins and other macromolecules thereby inhibiting aerobic energy metabolism, bacterial protein synthesis, cell wall synthesis, DNA synthesis, and RNA synthesis. Remember that nitrofurantoin is bacteriostatic at low doses and bactericidal at higher doses.

Contraindications

Acute porphyria (Macrobid, Macrodantin); age under 1 mo (Furadantin), under 3 mo (Macrodantin), or ages 12 and under (Macrobid); anuria; creatinine clearance less than 60 ml/min; G6PD (Macrobid, Macrodantin); history of cholestatic jaundice or hepatic dysfunction with previous nitrofurantoin therapy; hypersensitivity to nitrofurantoin, other nitrofurans, or their components; oliguria; pregnancy near term (38 to 42 wk)

Interactions

DRUGS

antacids containing magnesium trisilicate: Decreased nitrofurantoin absorption
live vaccines: Possibly diminished therapeutic effect of the vaccines
uricosuric, such as probenecid, sulfinpyrazone: Increased nitrofurantoin serum levels with increased risk of toxicity; decreased urinary levels with decreased effectiveness

FOODS

all foods: Delays gastric emptying, thus increasing absorption

Adverse Reactions

CNS: Chills, confusion, depression, headache, **neurotoxicity**, peripheral neuropathy
CV: Vasculitis
EENT: Optic neuritis, parotitis, tooth discoloration

GI: Abdominal pain, anorexia, cholestatic jaundice, **Clostridioides difficile–associated diarrhea (CDAD)**, diarrhea, **hepatic necrosis**, **hepatitis**, jaundice, nausea, **pancreatitis**, **pseudomembranous colitis**, vomiting
GU: Rust-colored to brown urine
HEME: **Aplastic anemia**, **granulocytopenia**, **hemolytic anemia**, **leukopenia**, megaloblastic anemia, **methemoglobinemia**, **thrombocytopenia**
MS: Arthralgia, myalgia
RESP: **Asthma** (in asthmatic patients), **cyanosis**, **interstitial pneumonitis**, **pulmonary fibrosis**
SKIN: Alopecia; eczematous, erythematous, or maculopapular eruptions; **erythema multiforme**; **exfoliative dermatitis**; pruritus; rash; **Stevens-Johnson syndrome**
Other: **Anaphylaxis**, **angioedema**, drug-induced fever, lupus-like syndrome

Childbearing Considerations

PREGNANCY

- Drug can cause fetal harm if administered between 38 and 42 wk gestation due to possible hemolytic anemia occurring in the neonate.
- Use with caution only if benefit to mother outweighs potential risk to fetus before week 38 gestation; contraindicated from 38 gestation on.

LABOR AND DELIVERY

- Drug is contraindicated when labor is imminent, during labor and delivery, and in the neonate under 1 mo of age because drug may cause hemolytic anemia in the fetus and neonate.

LACTATION

- Drug is present in breast milk.
- A decision should be made to discontinue breastfeeding or the drug to avoid potential serious adverse reactions in the breastfed infant.

Nursing Considerations

! WARNING Know that nitrofurantoin is contraindicated in a pregnant patient from 38 weeks gestation on because of possible hemolytic anemia developing in the neonate.

- Obtain a specimen of patient's urine for culture and sensitivity tests, as ordered; review test results if possible before giving nitrofurantoin.

! WARNING Monitor patient for a hypersensitivity reaction, which could become life-threatening, such as anaphylaxis and angioedema. If present, notify prescriber, expect drug to be discontinued, and provide supportive care, as needed and ordered.

! WARNING Monitor patient for evidence of superinfection, such as abdominal pain, diarrhea, and fever. If patient develops diarrhea, it may indicate pseudomembranous colitis caused by *Clostridioides difficile,* which can range from being mild to fatal colitis. Notify prescriber and expect to obtain a stool specimen to confirm presence of *C. difficile.* If confirmed, expect to withhold nitrofurantoin and treat with an antibiotic effective against *C. difficile.* Also, expect to administer electrolytes, fluids, and protein supplementation, as needed and ordered.

! WARNING Monitor patient for hepatic and pulmonary abnormalities because rare but severe reactions have occurred with nitrofurantoin use, especially in the elderly.

! WARNING Monitor patient's CBC and platelet count, and patient for bruising, unexplained bleeding, and infection because drug may cause severe adverse hematological reactions.

- Observe patient for changes in nervous function because peripheral neuropathy, although uncommon, may become severe or irreversible. Patients with anemia, debilitating disease, diabetes mellitus, electrolyte imbalance, renal impairment, or vitamin B deficiency are at higher risk for peripheral neuropathy.

PATIENT TEACHING

! WARNING Alert pregnant patient that nitrofurantoin should not be administered from 38 weeks gestation onward because drug can cause serious harm in the neonate.

- Instruct patient how to administer form of nitrofurantoin prescribed.
- Tell patient to complete prescribed course of therapy even if symptoms subside before course is completed.

- Caution patient against taking any antacid preparations that contain magnesium trisilicate during therapy.
- Explain that urine may turn brown, orange, or rust-colored during therapy.

! **WARNING** Alert patient that drug may cause an allergic reaction. If present, tell patient to notify prescriber and, if severe, to seek immediate medical care.

! **WARNING** Urge patient to tell prescriber about diarrhea that's severe or lasts longer than 3 days. Explain that bloody or watery stools can occur 2 or more months after nitrofurantoin therapy and can be serious, requiring prompt treatment.

! **WARNING** Review bleeding and infection control measures to take. Urge patient to notify prescriber immediately if bruising, unexplained bleeding, or a different infection occurs.

! **WARNING** Urge patient to report any other persistent, serious, and unusual adverse reactions.

- Inform patient that drug may cause peripheral neuropathy, which could become severe. Tell patient to notify prescriber if sensation changes occur in extremities.
- Inform breastfeeding mothers that breastfeeding or the drug needs to be discontinued.

nitroglycerin

(glyceryl trinitrate)

Nitro-Bid Ointment 2%, Nitro-Dur Patch, Nitrolingual Pumpspray, NitroMist, Nitrostat, Rectiv, Trinipatch (CAN)

Class and Category

Pharmacologic class: Nitrate
Therapeutic class: Antianginal, vasodilator

Indications and Dosages

∗ *To prevent anginal attacks due to coronary artery disease*

TOPICAL OINTMENT (NITRO-BID)

Adults. *Initial:* 1/2 inch of 2% ointment twice daily with first dose applied upon awakening and second dose 6 hr later. Dosage increased, in ½-inch increments as needed. Ointment removed daily to provide a 10- to 12-hr nitrate free interval.

TRANSDERMAL PATCH (NITRO-DUR PATCH, TRINIPATCH)

Adults. *Initial:* 0.2 to 0.4 mg/hr worn 12 to 14 hr, with dosage increased or decreased, as needed.

∗ *To treat acute angina pectoris; to reduce or limit anginal attacks before events that might precipitate an acute attack*

S.L. TABLETS (NITROSTAT)

Adults. *For acute attack:* 0.3 to 0.6 mg (1 tablet) every 5 min up to 3 tablets, as needed. *For use before a precipitating event:* 0.3 to 0.6 mg (1 tablet) taken 5 to 10 min before a precipitating event. *Maximum:* 3 tablets in 15 min.

TRANSLINGUAL SPRAY (NITROLINGUAL, NITROMIST)

Adults. *For acute attack:* 1 or 2 metered doses (400 or 800 mcg) onto or under tongue then 1 metered dose of 400 mcg repeated every 5 min, as needed, for no more than 3 metered doses total including initial dose. *For before a precipitating event:* 1 or 2 metered doses (400 or 800 mcg) onto or under tongue and taken 5 to 10 min before an event that might precipitate an acute attack. *Maximum:* 3 metered doses within 15 min.

∗ *To treat perioperative hypertension; to control congestive heart failure in the setting of acute MI; to treat angina pectoris in patients who have not responded to sublingual nitroglycerin and beta blockers; to induce intraoperative hypotension*

I.V. INFUSION (NITROGLYCERIN)

Adults. Highly individualized. *Suggested initial:* 5 mcg/min, increased by 5 mcg/min every 3 to 5 min to 20 mcg/min, as needed, and then by 10 to 20 mcg/min every 3 to 5 min if higher dosage is needed.

∗ *To treat moderate to severe pain associated with chronic anal fissure*

RECTAL OINTMENT (RECTIV)

Adults. 1 inch (375 mg) of ointment equivalent to 1.5 mg of nitroglycerin to intra-anal area every 12 hr for up to 3 wk.

Drug Administration

- Time administration according to route of administration and condition being treated. See Indications and Dosages section.

SUBLINGUAL

- Place S.L. tablet under patient's tongue and make sure it dissolves completely. Tablet should not be chewed, crushed, or swallowed.

TRANSLINGUAL

- Prime container when using for first time by spraying into the air 10 times if using Nitromist or 5 times if using Nitrolingual. If container is not used for 6 wk, it will have to be reprimed by spraying it twice if using Nitromist or once if using Nitrolingual. If Nitrolingual has not been used for 3 mo or longer, reprime with up to 5 sprays.
- Don't shake container before administering.
- Have patient assume a sitting position. Then, have patient spray drug under or on the tongue and close mouth immediately after administration. Ensure patient does not inhale the spray. Patient should wait at least 10 sec, if possible, before swallowing.
- Do not allow patient to rinse mouth or spit for 5 to 10 min after administration.

I.V.

- Dilute only in 0.9% Sodium Chloride Injection or 5% Dextrose in Water. Do not mix with other infusions. For example, add 50 mg of nitroglycerin into a 500 ml glass bottle to yield a final concentration of 100 mcg/ml; dilute 5 mg into 100 ml will yield a final concentration of 50 mcg/ml. Concentration may be increased after initial dosage titration to limit fluids being given to the patient but concentration should never exceed 400 mcg/ml. If concentration is adjusted, flush or replace the infusion set before a new concentration is given.
- Always mix in a glass bottle, not a container made of polyvinyl chloride. Invert bottle several times to assure uniform dilution. Use with a nonabsorbent tubing infusion set.
- Don't use a filter because plastic absorbs drug.
- Administer with infusion pump.
- *Incompatibilities:* Other drugs

TOPICAL

- For ointment, measure dosage by means of the dose measuring applicator supplied by manufacturer. Place the applicator on a flat surface printed side down. Squeeze the prescribed amount from tube onto the applicator. Then, place applicator paper on hairless area of body and spread in a thin, even layer over an area at least 2 inches by 3 inches. Do not rub in. Don't place on cuts or irritated areas.
- Cover with plastic film and tape in place. Wash hands after application. Rotate sites.
- Remove any excess ointment from previous site before applying next dose. Store at room temperature.

TRANSDERMAL

- Open transdermal patch package immediately before use. Apply patch to hairless area, and press edges to seal. Rotate sites. Store at room temperature.
- Remove patch after 12 to 14 hr daily, wash area with soap and water.
- If patient needs cardioversion or defibrillation, remove transdermal patch before procedure.

P.R.

- Cover finger with a finger cot or hand with a disposable surgical glove. Apply 1 inch of ointment onto a covered finger. Insert gently into the anal canal no further than the first finger joint. Remove finger. If this cannot be done because of pain, apply directly to the outside of the anus. Remove finger cot or glove, and wash hands.

Route	Onset	Peak	Duration
I.V.	Immediate	1–2 min	3–5 min
S.L.	1–3 min	5–7 min	25 min
Translingual	1–3 min	4–15 min	25 min
Topical	15–30 min	1 hr	7 hr
Transdermal	In 30 min	2 hr	10–12 hr
P.R.	Unknown	Unknown	Unknown

Half-life: 1–4 min

Mechanism of Action

May interact with nitrate receptors in vascular smooth-muscle cell membranes to reduce nitroglycerin to nitric oxide, which activates the enzyme guanylate cyclase, increasing intracellular formation of cGMP. Increased cGMP level may relax vascular smooth muscle by forcing calcium out of muscle cells, causing vasodilation. Venous dilation decreases venous return to the heart, reducing left ventricular end-diastolic pressure and pulmonary artery wedge pressure. Arterial dilation decreases systemic arterial pressure, systemic vascular resistance, and mean arterial pressure. Thus, nitroglycerin reduces preload and afterload, decreasing myocardial workload and oxygen demand. Dilates coronary arteries also, increasing blood flow to ischemic myocardial tissue and provides analgesic effects in anal tissue.

Contraindications

Acute MI (S.L.), angle-closure glaucoma, cerebral hemorrhage, circulatory failure and shock, concurrent use of phosphodiesterase inhibitors (avanafil, sildenafil, tadalafil, vardenafil) or riociguat, constrictive pericarditis (I.V.), head trauma, hypersensitivity to adhesive in transdermal form, hypersensitivity to nitrates, or their components, hypotension (I.V.), hypovolemia (I.V.), inadequate cerebral circulation (I.V.), increased intracranial pressure, orthostatic hypotension, pericardial tamponade (I.V.), restrictive cardiomyopathy (I.V.), severe anemia

Interactions

DRUGS

antihypertensives, beta-adrenergic blockers, calcium channel blockers: Increased risk of additive hypotensive effects
aspirin: Increased nitroglycerin concentrations enhancing vasodilatory and hemodynamic effects of nitroglycerin
ergotamine and related drugs: Possibly precipitate angina (oral nitroglycerin)
heparin: Possibly decreased anticoagulant effect of heparin
phosphodiesterase inhibitors (such as avanafil, sildenafil, tadalafil, vardenafil), riociguat: Possibly severe hypotensive effect of nitroglycerin
tissue-type plasminogen activator (t-PA): Decreases thrombolytic effect of t-PA.

ACTIVITIES

alcohol use: Possibly increased orthostatic hypotension

Adverse Reactions

CNS: Agitation, anxiety, dizziness, drowsiness, headache, insomnia, restlessness, syncope, weakness
CV: **Arrhythmias**, edema, **hypotension**, orthostatic hypotension, palpitations, tachycardia
EENT: Blurred vision, burning or tingling in mouth (S.L. forms), dry mouth
GI: Abdominal pain, diarrhea, indigestion, nausea, vomiting
GU: Dysuria, impotence, urinary frequency
HEME: **Methemoglobinemia**
MS: Arthralgia
RESP: Bronchitis, pneumonia, transient hypoxemia
SKIN: Contact dermatitis (transdermal forms), **exfoliative dermatitis**, flushing of face and neck, rash
Other: **Hypersensitivity reactions**

Childbearing Considerations

PREGNANCY

- It is not known if drug causes fetal harm.
- Use with caution only if benefit to mother outweighs potential risk to fetus.

LACTATION

- It is not known if drug is present in breast milk.
- Mothers should check with prescriber before breastfeeding.

Nursing Considerations

! **WARNING** Use nitroglycerin cautiously in elderly patients, especially those who are volume-depleted or taking several medications because of the increased risk of falls and hypotension. Hypotension may be accompanied by angina and paradoxical slowing of the heart rate. Hypotension may become severe, especially in patients in an upright position, even with small doses, particularly in patients with aortic or mitral stenosis, constrictive pericarditis, or who are already experiencing hypotension. Symptoms of severe hypotension include collapse, nausea, pallor, perspiration, syncope, vomiting, and weakness. Notify prescriber immediately if these occur, and provide appropriate treatment, as ordered.

! **WARNING** Use nitroglycerin cautiously in patients with hypertrophic obstructive cardiomyopathy because nitrate therapy may aggravate angina in this condition.

- Monitor patient for headache, especially at the beginning of therapy. If headache is severe, notify prescriber as dosage may need to be reduced. Treat headache with acetaminophen or a NSAID, as ordered. Know that tolerance usually develops if therapy continued.

- Check vital signs before every dosage adjustment and often during therapy.
- Monitor heart and breath sounds frequently, level of consciousness, fluid intake and output, and pulmonary artery wedge pressure, if possible.

! **WARNING** Monitor patient for a hypersensitivity reaction. If present, notify prescriber, expect drug to be switched to another drug, and provide supportive care, as needed and ordered.

! **WARNING** Assess patient for evidence of overdose, such as confusion, diaphoresis, dyspnea, flushing, headache, hypotension, nausea, palpitations, tachycardia, vertigo, vision changes, and vomiting. Treat as prescribed by removing nitroglycerin source, if possible; elevating legs above heart level; and providing supportive care, as needed and ordered to treat severe hypotension.

- Plan a nitroglycerin-free period of about 10 to 12 hours each day, if ordered, to maintain therapeutic effects and avoid tolerance.

PATIENT TEACHING

- Instruct patient on how to take type of nitroglycerin product prescribed and encourage patient to read and follow package instructions to obtain full benefits of drug.
- Teach patient to recognize signs and symptoms of angina pectoris, including chest fullness, pain, and pressure, possibly with sweating and nausea. Pain may radiate down left arm or into neck or jaw. Inform women and those with diabetes mellitus or hypertension that they may feel only fatigue and shortness of breath.

! **WARNING** Tell patient taking nitroglycerin for an acute angina attack that if relief is not obtained after taking 3 doses 5 minutes apart, to call 911 or have family or caretaker make the call.

- Inform patient that nitroglycerin commonly causes headache, which typically resolves after a few days of continuous therapy. Suggest taking acetaminophen, as needed, and not contraindicated.
- Urge patient to avoid alcohol and erectile dysfunction drugs during therapy.
- Inform patient that prescriber may order a 10- to 12-hour drug-free period at night (or at another time if she has chest pain at night or in the morning) to prevent drug tolerance. Also, inform patient that drug should be taken as prescribed, as excessive use may lead to tolerance as well.

! **WARNING** Alert patient nitroglycerin may cause an allergic reaction. Tell patient to notify prescriber if an allergic reaction occurs and, if severe, to seek immediate medical care.

! **WARNING** Advise patient to notify prescriber of any persistent, serious, or unusual adverse reactions.

- Inform patient that swimming or bathing doesn't affect topical or transdermal form but that electric blankets, hot tubs, magnetic therapy over the site, and prolonged hot showers and saunas should not be used because this may increase drug absorption and cause dizziness and hypotension.
- Advise patient to notify prescriber immediately about blurred vision, dizziness, and severe headache.
- Suggest that patient change positions slowly to minimize orthostatic hypotension.
- Advise patient to avoid hazardous activities until drug's CNS effects are known and resolved.
- Advise patient to alert all prescribers of nitroglycerin use because of potential drug interactions.

nitroprusside sodium

Nipride (CAN), Nitropress, Nipride RTU

Class and Category

Pharmacologic class: Vasodilator
Therapeutic class: Antihypertensive, vasodilator

Indications and Dosages

* *To treat hypertensive crisis and acute heart failure; to produce controlled hypotension in order to reduce bleeding during surgery*

I.V. INFUSION

Adults and children. *Initial:* 0.3 mcg/kg/min, increased gradually, waiting at least 5 min between titrations, as needed, until desired level is reached. *Maximum:* 10 mcg/kg/min.

±**DOSAGE ADJUSTMENT** For patients with renal impairment (eGFR less than 30 ml/min) mean infusion rate should not exceed 3 mcg/kg/min. For patients with anuria, mean infusion rate should not exceed 1 mcg/kg/min.

Drug Administration

I.V.

- Obtain baseline vital signs before administering nitroprusside.
- Dilute concentrated drug solution with 250 to 1,000 ml 5% Dextrose in Water to produce concentrations of 50 to 200 mcg/ml.
- Don't use solution if it contains particles or is blue, green, red, or darker than faint brown.
- Diluted solution is stable at room temperature for 24 hr when protected from light.
- Use an infusion pump for administration. Never administer undiluted or as an I.V. injection.
- Place opaque cover over infusion container because drug is metabolized by light. I.V. tubing need not be covered.
- Keep patient supine when starting drug or titrating dose up or down.
- Infuse piggybacked into a peripheral vein through a main I.V. line with no other drug being infused at the same time. Do not change rate of main I.V. solution while nitroprusside is being infused.
- Monitor blood pressure continuously with intra-arterial pressure monitor. Record blood pressure every 5 min at start of infusion and every 15 min thereafter.
- If severe hypotension occurs, stop infusion immediately and notify prescriber. Because of drug's short half-life, drug effects on blood pressure are quickly reversed.
- *Incompatibilities:* Other drugs

Route	Onset	Peak	Duration
I.V.	Immediate	1–2 min	1–10 min

Half-life: 2 min

Mechanism of Action

May interact with nitrate receptors in vascular smooth-muscle cell membranes to reduce nitroprusside to nitric oxide and then activates intracellular guanylate cyclase, which increases the cGMP level. Increased cGMP level may relax vascular smooth muscle by forcing calcium out of muscle cells. Relaxing smooth muscles cause arteries and veins to dilate, which reduces peripheral vascular resistance and blood pressure.

Contraindications

Acute heart failure associated with decreased peripheral vascular resistance, concomitant use of riociguat, compensatory hypertension when primary hemodynamic lesion is aortic coarctation or arteriovenous shunting, congenital optic atrophy, decreased cerebral perfusion, hypersensitivity to nitroprusside or its components, tobacco-induced amblyopia, use of PDE-5 inhibitors, used to produce hypotension during surgery in patients with inadequate circulation or in moribund patients (A.S.A. class 5E) requiring emergency surgery

Interactions

DRUGS

ganglionic blockers, inhaled anesthetics, negative inotropic agents: Increased hypotensive effect

PDE-5 inhibitors, riociguat: Increased risk of hypotension

Adverse Reactions

CNS: Anxiety, dizziness, headache, **increased intracranial pressure**, nervousness, restlessness

CV: **Hypotension**, tachycardia

ENDO: Hypothyroidism

GI: Abdominal pain, ileus, nausea, vomiting

HEME: **Methemoglobinemia**

MS: Muscle twitching

SKIN: Diaphoresis, flushing, rash

Other: **Cyanide toxicity**, infusion-site phlebitis, **thiocyanate toxicity**

Childbearing Considerations

PREGNANCY

- It is not known if drug causes fetal harm.
- Use with caution only if benefit to mother outweighs potential risk to fetus.

LACTATION

- It is not known if drug is present in breast milk.
- Once patient's condition has stabilized, prescriber should be consulted as to when breastfeeding may resume, if at all.

Nursing Considerations

- Obtain baseline vital signs before administering nitroprusside.
- Monitor blood pressure continuously with intra-arterial pressure monitor. Record blood pressure every 5 minutes at start of infusion and every 15 minutes thereafter.

! **WARNING** Be aware that if patient has severe heart failure, expect to administer an inotropic drug, such as dopamine or dobutamine, as prescribed.

! **WARNING** Be aware cyanide toxicity can occur when nitroprusside is administered faster than 2 mcg/min because cyanide is generated faster than the patient can eliminate it in the form of thiocyanate. Monitor serum thiocyanate level at least every 72 hours for patients at risk, as ordered; levels above 100 mcg/ml are associated with toxicity. Monitor patient for evidence of cyanide toxicity (absence of reflexes, coma, distant heart sounds, hypotension, metabolic acidosis, mydriasis, pink skin, shallow respirations, and weak pulse). If present, stop nitroprusside immediately, notify prescriber, and provide supportive care, as needed and ordered.

PATIENT TEACHING

- Inform patient drug will be admininstered intravenously and that he will be monitored very closely throughout nitroprusside therapy.

! **WARNING** Instruct patient to notify nurse immediately if serious or unusual symptoms are experienced such as dizziness caused by a sudden, severe drop in blood pressure.

- Advise patient to change position slowly to minimize dizziness.

norepinephrine bitartrate

(levarterenol bitartrate)

Levophed

Class and Category

Pharmacologic class: Sympathomimetic
Therapeutic class: Vasopressor

Indications and Dosages

✱ *To manage blood pressure in acute hypotensive states such as blood transfusion, drug adverse effect, MI, during or post pheochromocytomectomy, poliomyelitis, spinal anesthesia, and sympathectomy reactions; as adjunct to treat cardiac arrest and profound hypotension*

I.V. INFUSION

Adults. *Initial average dose:* 8 to 12 mcg/min. Then, titrated to maintain systolic blood pressure between 80 to 100 mm Hg in patients previously not hypertensive and 40 mm Hg below preexisting systolic blood pressure in patients previously hypertensive. *Maintenance:* 2 to 4 mcg/min.

Drug Administration

I.V.

- Dilute by adding 4 mg of drug to 1,000 ml of 5% Dextrose Injection or 5% Dextrose Injection with 0.9% Sodium Chloride solution to yield a concentration of 4 mcg/ml. Do not use 0.9% Sodium Chloride Injection alone. Never administer undiluted.
- Solution should be colorless. Do not use if it contains particles or is discolored such as a pinkish or darker than a slightly yellow color.
- Give drug using a flow-control device.
- Infuse through a central line or large peripheral vein to avoid extravasation. Do not infuse into leg veins in the elderly or in patients with occlusive vascular disease of the legs.
- Avoid using a catheter tie-in technique, if possible.
- Check blood pressure every 2 to 3 min, preferably by direct intra-arterial monitoring, until stabilized and then every 5 min.
- If extravasation occurs, it can cause severe tissue damage and necrosis. Notify prescriber and expect prescriber to give multiple subcutaneous injections of phentolamine (5 to 10 mg diluted in 10 to 15 ml of 0.9% Sodium Chloride Injection) around extravasated peripheral infusion site.
- If blanching occurs along vein, change infusion site and notify prescriber at once.

- When discontinuing infusion, reduce the flow rate gradually. Avoid abrupt withdrawal.
- *Incompatibilities:* Alkalis, iron salts, or oxidizing agents; whole blood or plasma

Route	Onset	Peak	Duration
I.V.	Immediate	1–2 min	1–10 min

Half-life: 1–2.5 min

Mechanism of Action

Inhibits adenyl cyclase and directly stimulates alpha-adrenergic receptors, which inhibits cAMP production. Inhibition of cAMP constricts arteries and veins and increases peripheral vascular resistance and systolic blood pressure.

Contraindications

Concurrent use of cyclopropane and hydrocarbon inhalation anesthetics, hypersensitivity to norepinephrine or its components, hypovolemia (except as an emergency measure), mesenteric or peripheral vascular thrombosis (except as an emergency measure), profound hypercarbia or hypoxia

Interactions

DRUGS

cyclopropane and halothane anesthetics: Increased cardiac autonomic irritability, sensitizing the myocardium to the action of norepinephrine

MAO inhibitors of the imipramine or triptyline types: May cause prolonged, severe hypertension

Adverse Reactions

CNS: Anxiety, dizziness, headache, insomnia, nervousness, tremor, weakness

CV: Angina, **bradycardia**, **ECG changes**, edema, hypertension, **hypotension**, palpitations, peripheral vascular insufficiency (including gangrene), **PVCs**, sinus tachycardia

GI: Nausea, vomiting

GU: Decreased renal perfusion

RESP: Apnea, dyspnea

SKIN: Pallor

Other: **Hypersensitivity reactions**, infusion-site sloughing and tissue necrosis, **metabolic acidosis**

Childbearing Considerations

PREGNANCY

- It is not known if drug causes fetal harm.
- Use with caution only if benefit to mother outweighs potential risk to fetus.

LACTATION

- It is not known if drug is present in breast milk.
- Mothers should check with prescriber before breastfeeding.

Nursing Considerations

- Expect to correct hypovolemia before administering norepinephrine.

> **! WARNING** Use extreme caution when administering norepinephrine in patients also receiving antidepressants of the impramine or triptyline types or MAO inhibitors because severe, prolonged hypertension may occur.

- Check blood pressure every 2 to 3 minutes, preferably by direct intra-arterial monitoring, until stabilized and then every 5 minutes.
- Monitor continuous ECG during therapy.

> **! WARNING** Monitor patient for hypersensitivity reaction that could become life-threatening, especially for patients with asthma. This is because norepinephrine contains sodium metabisulfite, which can trigger an allergic reaction for patients with a sulfite allergy. If a hypersensitivity reaction occurs during norepinephrine therapy, notify prescriber immediately.

PATIENT TEACHING

- Urge patient to immediately report burning, leaking, or tingling around I.V. site.

> **! WARNING** Alert patient who is conscious to notify staff immediately if he experiences a sudden different feeling of not feeling well that could be suggestive of an allergic reaction.

nortriptyline hydrochloride

Aventyl (CAN), Pamelor

Class and Category

Pharmacologic class: Tricyclic antidepressant (TCA)

Therapeutic class: Antidepressant

Indications and Dosages

* *To treat depression*

CAPSULES, ORAL SOLUTION

Adults. *Initial:* 25 mg 3 times daily or 4 times daily, increased, as needed. Alternatively, total daily dose 1 time daily. *Maximum:* 150 mg daily.

Adolescents and the elderly. 30 to 50 mg daily in divided doses. Alternatively, total daily dose 1 time daily.

Drug Administration

P.O.

- Capsules should be swallowed whole and not chewed, crushed, or opened.
- Use a calibrated device when measuring dosage for oral solution.

Route	Onset	Peak	Duration
P.O.	Unknown	7–8.5 hr	Unknown

Half-life: 16–38 hr

Mechanism of Action

May interfere with reuptake of serotonin (and possibly other neurotransmitters) at presynaptic neurons, thus enhancing serotonin's effects at postsynaptic receptors. Restoring normal neurotransmitter levels at nerve synapses may elevate mood.

Contraindications

Acute recovery phase of MI; hypersensitivity to nortriptyline, other dibenzazepines, tricyclic antidepressants, or their components; use within 14 days of MAO inhibitor therapy, including intravenous methylene blue or linezolid

Interactions

DRUGS

barbiturates, CNS depressants: Possibly increased CNS depression

chlorpropamide: Possibly significant hypoglycemia

cimetidine: Increased plasma concentrations of nortriptyline

MAO inhibitors (including I.V. methylene blue, linezolid), serotonergic drugs (buspirone, fentanyl, lithium, St. John's wort, tramadol, tricyclic antidepressants, triptans, tryptophan): Increased risk of serotonin syndrome

P4502D6 inhibitors, such as cimetidine, fluoxetine and other antidepressants, phenothiazines, quinidine, selective serotonin reuptake inhibitors, type IC antiarrhythmics (flecainide, propafenone): Possibly increased plasma concentration of these drugs with possible increase in adverse reactions

other anticholinergics, sympathomimetic drugs: Increased risk of profound hypertension

reserpine: Possibly produce a stimulating effect

ACTIVITIES

alcohol use: Increased alcohol effects, CNS and respiratory depression, hypertension

Adverse Reactions

CNS: Ataxia, confusion, **CVA**, delirium, dizziness, drowsiness, excitation, hallucinations, headache, insomnia, nervousness, nightmares, parkinsonism, **serotonin syndrome**, **suicidal ideation**, tremor

CV: **Arrhythmias**, orthostatic hypotension, **unmasking of Brugada syndrome**

EENT: Angle-closure glaucoma, blurred vision, dry mouth, increased intraocular pressure, taste perversion

GI: Constipation, diarrhea, heartburn, ileus, increased appetite, nausea, vomiting

GU: Sexual dysfunction, urine retention

HEME: **Bone marrow depression**

RESP: Wheezing

SKIN: Diaphoresis, urticaria

Other: Weight gain

Childbearing Considerations

PREGNANCY

- It is not known if drug causes fetal harm.
- Use with caution only if benefit to mother outweighs potential risk to fetus.

LACTATION

- Drug is present in breast milk.
- Mothers should check with prescriber before breastfeeding.

Nursing Considerations

- Expect to stop MAO inhibitor therapy, including intravenous methylene blue and linezolid, if prescribed, 10 to 14 days before starting nortriptyline.

! **WARNING** Know that nortriptyline should be avoided in patients with Brugada syndrome or those suspected of having the disorder because Brugada syndrome can cause abnormal ECG findings and syncope as well as increasing the risk of sudden death.

- Be aware that oral solution (10 mg/5 ml) is 4% alcohol.
- Monitor blood nortriptyline level; therapeutic range is 50 to 150 ng/ml.

! **WARNING** Watch patient closely (especially adolescents and young adults), for suicidal tendencies, particularly when therapy starts and dosage changes because depression may worsen temporarily during these times.

! **WARNING** Monitor patient for possible serotonin syndrome, characterized by agitation, chills, confusion, diaphoresis, diarrhea, fever, hyperactive reflexes, poor coordination, restlessness, shaking, talking or acting with uncontrolled excitement, tremor, and twitching. Notify prescriber immediately if serotonin syndrome is suspected because it can become life-threatening and expect to discontinue nortriptyline therapy.

- Monitor ECG tracing to detect arrhythmias.

PATIENT TEACHING

! **WARNING** Tell patient to inform prescriber if there is a family history of sudden unexplained death before the age of 45 before nortriptyline therapy is begun or if abnormal heartbeat or unexplained fainting occurs during nortriptyline therapy.

- Advise patient that drug may cause mild pupillary dilation, which may lead to an episode of acute angle-closure glaucoma. Encourage patient to have an eye exam before starting therapy to see if he is at risk.
- Instruct patient how to administer form of nortriptyline prescribed.
- Tell patient that oral solution contains alcohol and to alert prescriber if alcohol consumption is an issue for the patient.
- Discourage drinking alcoholic beverages during therapy because of increased CNS effects.
- Explain that improvement may take weeks.

! **WARNING** Urge family or caregiver to watch patient closely for suicidal tendencies, especially when therapy starts or dosage changes and particularly if patient is a teenager or young adult.

! **WARNING** Tell patient to notify prescriber of any persistent, serious, or unusual adverse reaction.

- Advise patient to avoid hazardous activities until drug's CNS effects are known and resolved.
- Instruct patient to change position slowly to minimize orthostatic hypotension.
- Suggest that patient minimize constipation by drinking plenty of fluids (if allowed), exercising regularly, and eating high-fiber foods.

nystatin

Class and Category

Pharmacologic class: Polyene macrolide
Therapeutic class: Antifungal

Indications and Dosages

∗ *To treat oral candidiasis (thrush)*

ORAL SUSPENSION

Adults and children. 400,000 to 600,000 units (4 to 6 ml) swished and swallowed 4 times daily until at least 48 hr after symptoms subside.
Infants. 200,000 units (2 ml) with dosage divided in half and applied to each side of mouth 4 times daily until at least 48 hr after symptoms subside.

∗ *To treat non-esophageal mucus membrane intestinal candidiasis*

TABLETS

Adults. 500,000 to 1,000,000 units (1 to 2 tablets) every 8 hr until at least 48 hr after symptoms subside.

∗ *Topical use found in Appendix*

Drug Administration

P.O.

- Shake oral suspension well before measuring dose.
- Use supplied dropper or a calibrated syringe to measure dosage.
- Oral suspension should be swished and retained in mouth for several minutes before patient swallows it.
- When using powder form, prepare only a single dose at a time because it does not

contain preservatives. Add prescribed dosage to about 4 ounces of water. Stir well and divide into smaller portions. Administer immediately using 1 portion at a time until entire volume is used.

- Administer to infants by swabbing oral suspension on both sides of mouth or drop one-half the dose on each side of tongue. Avoid feeding for 5 to 10 min.

Route	Onset	Peak	Duration
P.O.	24–72 hr	Unknown	Unknown

Half-life: 16–38 hr

Mechanism of Action

Binds to sterols in fungal cell membranes, impairing membrane integrity and causing cells to lose intracellular potassium and other cellular contents and, eventually, die.

Contraindications

Hypersensitivity to nystatin or its components

Interactions

DRUGS

None reported by manufacturer.

Adverse Reactions

ENDO: Hyperglycemia (oral suspension)
GI: Abdominal pain, diarrhea, nausea, vomiting (oral forms)

Childbearing Considerations

PREGNANCY

- It is not known if drug causes fetal harm.
- Use with caution only if benefit to mother outweighs potential risk to fetus.

LACTATION

- It is not known if drug is present in breast milk.
- Mothers should check with prescriber before breastfeeding.

Nursing Considerations

- Monitor patient for adverse reactions.

PATIENT TEACHING

- Instruct patient how to administer form of nystatin prescribed.
- Review adverse reactions with patient and to report them to prescriber if prolonged or severe.

ocrelizumab

Ocrevus

Class and Category

Pharmacologic class: Monoclonal antibody
Therapeutic class: Anti-multiple sclerotic

Indications and Dosages

✱ *To treat primary progressive multiple sclerosis; to treat relapsing forms of multiple sclerosis, including active secondary progressive disease, clinically isolated syndrome, or relapsing-remitting disease*

I.V. INFUSION

Adults. *Initial:* 300 mg, followed 2 wk later by a second 300-mg infusion. *Maintenance:* Single infusion of 600 mg every 6 mo beginning 6 mo after first 300-mg dose. See Drug Administration for infusion rate for initial and maintenance dosages.

Drug Administration

- Expect to premedicate patient with 100 mg of methylprednisolone (or an equivalent corticosteroid) intravenously, as ordered, about 30 min before each ocrelizumab infusion, to reduce the frequency and severity of infusion reactions. Also, expect to premedicate patient with an antihistamine such as diphenhydramine about 30 to 60 min prior to each ocrelizumab infusion to further reduce infusion reactions. Know that the administration of an antipyretic such as acetaminophen may also be ordered.

I.V.

- Do not shake drug vial.
- Withdraw prescribed dose and dilute in an infusion bag containing 0.9% Sodium Chloride Injection to a final drug concentration of approximately 1.2 mg/ml. For example, withdraw 10 ml (300 mg) from vial and inject into a 250-ml infusion bag or withdraw 20 ml (600 mg) from vial and inject into a 500-ml infusion bag. Do not use any other diluents to dilute ocrelizumab.
- Prepared solution can be stored for up to 24 hr in the refrigerator or 8 hr at room temperature, which must include the infusion time.

- If prepared solution was refrigerated, allow solution to warm to room temperature before administering.
- Administer the diluted solution through a dedicated line using an infusion set with a 0.2- or 0.22-micron in-line filter.
- Infuse initial 2 doses starting at 30 ml per hr, then increased by 30 ml per hr every 30 min to maximum infusion rate of 180 ml per hr with an infusion duration of 2.5 hr or longer.
- Infuse maintenance dose starting at 40 ml per hr, increased by 40 ml per hr every 30 min with maximum infusion of 200 ml per hr and duration of infusion 3.5 hr or longer. Alternatively, if patient has had no prior serious infusion reaction with any previous infusion, begin infusing drug at 100 ml per hr for the first 15 min, increase to 200 ml per hr for the next 15 min, then increase to 250 ml per hr for the next 30 min followed by an increase to 300 ml per hr for the remaining 60 min with an infusion duration of 2 hr or longer.
- Monitor patient for life-threatening infusion reactions. If present, stop infusion immediately, provide supportive care, as ordered, and know that drug will be permanently discontinued. If infusion reaction is not life-threatening but severe, expect to immediately interrupt the infusion and provide supportive treatment, as ordered and needed. Expect to restart the infusion only after all symptoms have resolved. When restarting, expect to restart at half the infusion rate at the time of onset of the infusion reaction. If this rate is tolerated, increase the rate per the standard protocol. If patient is experiencing a mild to moderate infusion reaction, expect to reduce the infusion rate to half the rate at the onset of the infusion reaction and maintain the reduced rate for at least 30 minutes. If this rate is tolerated, expect to increase the rate per the standard protocol. Monitor patient for infusion reactions for at least 1 hr after completion of the infusion.
- Expect to administer a planned infusion that is missed as soon as possible. It should not be withheld until the next scheduled dose. Reset the dose schedule to administer the next sequential dose 6 mo after the missed dose is administered because doses must be separated by at least 5 mo.
- *Incompatibilities:* Solutions other than 0.9% Sodium Chloride Injection

Route	Onset	Peak	Duration
I.V.	14 days	Unknown	72 wk

Half-life: 26 days

Mechanism of Action

Thought to involve binding to CD20, a cell surface antigen on pre-B and mature B lymphocytes, which results in antibody-dependent cellular cytolysis and complement-mediated lysis to possibly relieve symptoms of multiple sclerosis.

Contraindications

Active hepatitis B virus infection, hypersensitivity to ocrelizumab or its components

Interactions

DRUGS

other immune-modulating or immunosuppressants: Increased risk of immunosuppression

vaccines (live or live-attenuated): Possibly decreased effectiveness or increased risk of infection

Adverse Reactions

CNS: Depression, dizziness, fatigue, fever, headache, **progressive multifocal leukoencephalopathy (PML)**

CV: **Hypotension**, peripheral edema, tachycardia

EENT: **Laryngeal or pharyngeal edema**, oropharyngeal pain, throat irritation

GI: Diarrhea, **immune-mediated colitis**, nausea

HEME: **Neutropenia**

MS: Back or extremity pain

RESP: **Bronchospasms**, cough, dyspnea, respiratory infections

SKIN: Erythema, flushing, pruritus, pyoderma gangrenosum (large painful sores), rash, skin infections, urticaria

Other: **Anaphylaxis**; anti-ocrelizumab antibody formation; bacterial, fungal, parasitic, and new or reactivated viral infections (may become severe); decreased immunoglobulins; infusion reactions (may become severe)

Childbearing Considerations

PREGNANCY

- Pregnancy exposure registry: 1-833-872-4370 or www.ocrevuspregnancyregistry.com.
- It is not known if drug causes fetal harm. However, as a humanized monoclonal antibody, it may cross the placental barrier. This may increase the potential for transient peripheral B-cell depletion and lymphocytopenia in the neonate.
- The safety and effectiveness of vaccine administration in these infants are unknown. Live or live-attenuated vaccines should not be administered to infant exposed to the drug in utero before confirming the recovery of B-cell counts.
- Use with caution only if benefit to mother outweighs potential risk to fetus.

LACTATION

- It is not known if drug is present in breast milk.
- Mothers should check with prescriber before breastfeeding.

REPRODUCTION

- Females of childbearing age need to use effective contraception during drug therapy and for 6 mo after the last drug dose.

Nursing Considerations

- Expect to perform hepatitis B virus (HBV) screening, as ordered, prior to initiating ocrelizumab therapy because drug is contraindicated in patients with active HBV that has been confirmed by positive test results.
- Administer all necessary immunizations, as ordered, according to guidelines at least 4 weeks prior to initiation of ocrelizumab therapy for live or live-attenuated vaccines and, whenever possible, at least 2 weeks before initiation of ocrelizumab therapy for nonlive vaccines. This is because drug may interfere with effectiveness of nonlive vaccines, and safety of immunization with live or live-attenuated vaccines following ocrelizumab therapy is unknown.

! **WARNING** Assess patient for evidence of an active infection prior to every infusion of ocrelizumab. Serious, including life-threatening or fatal, bacterial, fungal, parasitic, and new or reactivated viral infections have occurred with ocrelizumab therapy by herpes simplex virus and varicella zoster virus may occur at any time during drug therapy with ocrelizumab and may become life-threatening. Infections may include central nervous system infections such as encephalitis or meningitis, disseminated skin and soft-tissue infections, and intraocular infections. Monitor patient closely during therapy and institute infection control measures, as needed. If present, know that the infusion must be delayed until the infection is resolved.

! **WARNING** Monitor patient for a hypersensitivity reaction which could become life-threatening, such as anaphylaxis. If present, notify prescriber, expect drug to be discontinued, and provide supportive care, as needed and ordered.

! **WARNING** Notify prescriber immediately if patient experiences bronchospasms with administration of the drug. Provide supportive care, as needed and ordered until bronchospasms cease.

! **WARNING** Know that PML has occurred in patients treated with ocrelizumab. Patients at risk include patients who are immunocompromised or receive polytherapy with immunosuppressants. Monitor patient for PML, which may include changes in memory, orientation, or thinking that could lead to confusion and personality changes. Other symptoms include clumsiness of limbs, disturbance of vision, and progressive weakness on 1 side of the body. If present, notify prescriber immediately because PML usually leads to death or severe disability.

! **WARNING** Monitor patient for immune-mediated colitis, which can present as an acute onset and be severe. Know that onset may range from weeks to years. If new or persistent diarrhea or other GI signs and symptoms occur, notify prescriber, expect drug to be discontinued, and systemic corticosteroids ordered. Be aware that in some cases, hospitalization may be required, including surgical intervention.

PATIENT TEACHING

- Explain the importance of as well as the risks associated with ocrelizumab therapy before drug is administered.

! **WARNING** Tell patient medication will be given before the infusion to lessen or prevent infusion reactions. However, inform patient that infusion reactions may occur up to 24 hours after the infusion and include allergic types of signs and symptoms. If adverse reactions occur in this time frame, patient should notify prescriber and if reactions are severe, seek immediate emergency medical care.

! **WARNING** Alert patient that drug may cause bronchospasms with administration. Tell patient to inform staff if difficulty breathing occurs or seek immediate medical care if difficulty breathing occurs at home.

! **WARNING** Tell patient to notify prescriber if a sudden onset of diarrhea or persistent diarrhea occurs that may include black, tarry stools or stools that have blood or mucus in them along with severe stomach pain or tenderness.

! **WARNING** Instruct family or caregiver to report changes in memory, orientation, or thinking by patient that could lead to confusion and personality changes. Other symptoms to report include clumsiness of limbs, disturbance of vision, and progressive weakness on 1 side of the body. If present, urge family or caregiver to notify prescriber immediately.

! **WARNING** Review signs and symptoms of infection with patient. Encourage patient to use infection control measures in daily life. If present (chills, fever, painful urination, or persistent cough), tell patient to immediately notify prescriber.

! **WARNING** Stress importance of reporting to prescriber any other persistent, severe, or unusual signs and symptoms.

! **WARNING** Inform patient that ocrelizumab may increase risk of breast cancer. Stress importance of following standard breast cancer screening guidelines.

- Inform patient that live or live-attenuated vaccines should not be given within 4 weeks of starting drug therapy and for 2 weeks prior to starting drug therapy for nonlive vaccines. Also, tell mothers of infants exposed to drug during pregnancy to inform pediatrician of exposure before any live or live-attenuated vaccines are administered to the infant.
- Instruct females of childbearing age to use effective contraception during drug therapy and for 6 months after the last drug dose. Also tell them to alert prescriber if pregnancy should occur.

ofatumumab

Kesimpta

Class and Category

Pharmacologic class: CD20-directed cytolytic antibody
Therapeutic class: Anti-multiple sclerotic

Indications and Dosages

∗ *To treat relapsing forms of multiple sclerosis, including active secondary progressive disease, clinically isolated syndrome, and relapsing-remitting disease*

SUBCUTANEOUS INJECTION

Adults. *Initial:* 20 mg, repeated at wk 1 and 2. *Maintenance:* 20 mg monthly starting at wk 4.

Drug Administration

SUBCUTANEOUS

- Remove prefilled pen or syringe from refrigerator and allow drug to reach room temperature (15–30 min).
- Inspect drug solution. Discard if particles are visible or solution appears cloudy.
- Do not shake prefilled pens or syringes.
- To administer drug using the prefilled Sensoready pen, remember that if pen is dropped, it must be discarded. Use the pen within 5 min of removing the cap. Inject subcutaneously at a 90 degree angle into the abdomen, thigh, or outer upper arm. Two loud clicks will be heard: First click indicates injection has started, second click indicates the injection is almost complete. Keep holding the pen firmly against the skin until the green indicator fills the window and stops moving. Remove pen from skin. Do not rub injection site.

- To administer drug using the prefilled syringe, do not remove needle cap until just before giving injection. Avoid touching the syringe guard wings before use because this may cause the needle guard to be activated too early. Insert needle at a 45 degree angle into the abdomen, thigh, or outer upper arm. At the end of the injection but before removing needle from skin, place fingers on syringe finger grips. Slowly press down on the plunger head as far as it will go, so the plunger head is completely between the syringe guard wings. Continue to press fully on the plunger head for an additional 5 sec. Hold the syringe in place for the full 5 sec. Then slowly release the plunger head until the needle is covered and remove syringe from injection site. Do not rub injection site.
- Do not inject into abnormal areas or where skin is bruised, hard, red, scaly, or tender.
- Monitor patient for life-threatening infusion reactions. If present, stop infusion immediately, provide supportive care, as ordered, and know that drug will be permanently discontinued. If infusion reaction is not life-threatening but severe, expect to immediately interrupt the infusion and provide supportive treatment, as ordered and needed. Expect to restart the infusion only after all symptoms have resolved. When restarting, expect to restart under close supervision. If only a mild to moderate injection-related reaction occurs, expect infusion to continue.
- Prefilled pens and syringes are for 1-time use.
- Store in refrigerator until ready to use. If needed, drug may be stored up to 7 days at room temperature, then it must be discarded.

Route	Onset	Peak	Duration
SubQ	Unknown	Unknown	Unknown

Half-life: 16 days

Mechanism of Action

Thought to involve binding to CD20, a cell surface antigen present on pre-B and mature B lymphocytes, which results in antibody-dependent cellular cytolysis and complement-mediated lysis to possibly relieve symptoms of multiple sclerosis.

Contraindications

Active hepatitis B viral (HBV) infection, hypersensitivity to ofatumumab or its components

Interactions

DRUGS

immunosuppressive drugs, such as systemic corticosteroids: Increased risk of infection
live-attenuated or live vaccines: Increased risk of adverse effects

Adverse Reactions

CNS: Dizziness, headache, **progressive multifocal leukoencephalopathy (PML)**
EENT: **Laryngeal or pharyngeal edema**, oropharyngeal pain, throat irritation
CV: **Hypotension**, tachycardia
GI: Nausea
GU: UTI
MS: Back pain
RESP: **Bronchospasms**, dyspnea, upper respiratory infections
SKIN: Erythema, flushing, pruritus, rash, urticaria
Other: **Anaphylaxis**, **angioedema**, anti-ofatumumab antibody formation, decreased blood immunoglobulin levels (especially immunoglobulin M), infections (bacterial, fungal, and new or reactivated viral infections), injection-related systemic reactions (chills, fatigue, fever, headache, myalgia), injection-site local reactions (erythema, pain, pruritus, swelling)

Childbearing Considerations

PREGNANCY

- Pregnancy exposure registry: 1-877-311-8972 or www.mothertobaby.org/join-study or email: MotherToBaby@health.ucsd.edu.
- It is not known if drug causes fetal harm, but animal studies suggest that fetal harm can occur due to fetal B-cell lymphopenia and reduced antibody response.
- Use with caution only if benefit to mother outweighs potential risk to fetus.
- If infant was exposed to drug in utero, live or live-attenuated vaccines should be withheld until B-cell counts have recovered.

LACTATION

- It is not known if drug is present in breast milk.
- Mothers should check with prescriber before breastfeeding.

REPRODUCTION

- Females of childbearing age should use effective contraception during drug therapy and for 6 mo after drug is discontinued.

Nursing Considerations

! **WARNING** Determine that screenings for HBV and quantitative serum immunoglobulins have been done before first dose is given. Therapy with ofatumumab is contraindicated in the presence of HBV. Therapy may have to be withheld in patients with low serum immunoglobulins until levels are higher.

- Ensure that all immunizations according to immunization guidelines have been administered to patient at least 4 weeks prior to starting of ofatumumab for live or live-attenuated vaccines, and whenever possible, at least 2 weeks before for inactivated vaccines.

! **WARNING** Expect initiation of therapy to be delayed if patient has an active infection until infection is resolved. Be aware patient is at risk for infections, including serious bacterial, fungal, and new or reactivated viral infections during therapy. Some infections may become life-threatening. Monitor patient for infections throughout drug therapy and institute infection control measures. Notify prescriber if an infection is suspected.

! **WARNING** Monitor patient for a hypersensitivity reaction, which may become life-threatening such as anaphylaxis or angioedema. If present, notify prescriber, stop infusion immediately, expect drug to be discontinued, and provide supportive care, as needed and ordered.

- Monitor patient for injection type adverse reactions such as chills, fatigue, fever, headache, and myalgia as well as local reactions at injection site such as erythema, itching, pain, or swelling.

! **WARNING** Be aware that progressive multifocal leukoencephalopathy (PML) has the potential to occur with ofatumumab therapy. Notify prescriber at the first sign of PML, withhold drug, and expect patient to undergo a diagnostic workup to confirm diagnosis. Signs and symptoms to be alert for include changes in thinking, memory, and orientation that lead to confusion; disturbances of vision; personality changes; and progressive clumsiness or weakness on 1side of the body. Be aware that these changes can gradually occur over days to weeks. Expect drug to be discontinued if PML is confirmed.

PATIENT TEACHING

- Teach patient and family or caregiver how to administer drug as a subcutaneous injection and what to do if a dose is missed.
- Tell patient that injection-site reactions may occur, usually within 24 hours and predominantly after the first injection. If present, tell patient to notify prescriber.

! **WARNING** Alert patient that drug may cause an allergic reaction. Tell patient to alert staff immediately if suddenly not feeling well or experiencing signs and symptoms of an allergic reaction.

! **WARNING** Review signs and symptoms of infection and infection control measures. Stress importance of notifying prescriber if an infection occurs, as it can become quite serious.

! **WARNING** Instruct patient to notify prescriber if other persistent, severe, or unusual signs and symptoms occur after drug therapy is initiated.

- Inform patient that vaccines should not be received during ofatumumab therapy. Inform mothers who were treated with drug during pregnancy not to have their infants receive live or live-attenuated vaccines until pediatrician indicates it is safe to do so.
- Advise females of childbearing age to use effective contraception during drug therapy and for 6 months after drug has been discontinued. Also, instruct these patients to alert prescriber if pregnancy occurs.

ofloxacin

Class and Category

Pharmacologic class: Fluoroquinolone
Therapeutic class: Antibiotic

Indications and Dosages

∗ *To treat acute, uncomplicated cystitis caused by* Escherichia coli *or* Klebsiella pneumoniae

TABLETS

Adults. 200 mg every 12 hr for 3 days.

∗ *To treat uncomplicated cystitis caused by* Citrobacter diversus, Enterobacter aerogenes, Proteus mirabilis, *or* Pseudomonas aeruginosa

TABLETS

Adults. 200 mg every 12 hr for 7 days.

∗ *To treat complicated UTI caused by* C. diversus, E. coli, K. pneumoniae, P. mirabilis, *or* P. aeruginosa

Adults. 200 mg every 12 hr for 10 days.

∗ *To treat pelvic inflammatory disease caused by susceptible organisms*

TABLETS

Adults. 400 mg every 12 hr with metronidazole P.O. for 10 to 14 days.

∗ *To treat prostatitis caused by* E. coli

TABLETS

Adults. 300 mg every 12 hr for 6 wk.

∗ *To treat acute, uncomplicated urethral and cervical gonorrhea caused by* Neisseria gonorrhoeae

TABLETS

Adults. 400 mg as a single dose.

∗ *To treat nongonococcal cervicitis/urethritis caused by* Chlamydia trachomatis; *to treat mixed infection of the cervix and urethra caused by* C. trachomatis *and* N. gonorrhaeae

TABLETS

Adults. 300 mg every 12 hr for 7 days.

∗ *To treat acute exacerbation of chronic bronchitis or community-acquired pneumonia caused by* Haemophilus influenzae *or* Streptococcus pneumoniae; *to treat uncomplicated skin and soft-tissue infections caused by* Proteus mirabilis, Staphylococcus aureus, *or* Streptococcus pyogenes

TABLETS

Adults. 400 mg every 12 hr for 10 to 14 days.

±**DOSAGE ADJUSTMENT** For patients with creatinine clearance of 20 to 50 ml/min, after initial dose, dosing interval increased to every 24 hours; if creatinine clearance is less than 20 ml/min after initial dose, dosage reduced by 50% and given every 24 hours. For patients with severe liver dysfunction, maximum dose limited to 400 mg daily.

Drug Administration

P.O.

- Administer each dose with a full glass of water.
- Do not administer antacids, iron or zinc preparations, or other drugs (such as didanosine and sucralfate) within 2 hr of drug, to prevent decreased or delayed drug absorption.

Route	Onset	Peak	Duration
P.O.	Unknown	0.5–2 hr	Unknown

Half-life: 4–8 hr

Mechanism of Action

Inhibits synthesis of the bacterial enzyme DNA gyrase by counteracting excessive supercoiling of DNA during replication or transcription. Inhibition of DNA gyrase causes rapid- and slow-growing bacterial cells to die.

Contraindications

Hypersensitivity to ofloxacin, other fluoroquinolones, or their components

Interactions

DRUGS

aluminum-, calcium-, or magnesium-containing antacids; didanosine; ferrous sulfate; magnesium-containing laxatives; multivitamins; sevelamer; sucralfate; zinc: Decreased absorption of ofloxacin

insulin, oral antidiabetic drugs: Possibly disturbance in blood glucose control with these agents

NSAIDs: Possibly increased risk of CNS stimulation and seizures

theophylline: Increased risk of theophylline-related adverse reactions

procainamide: Decreased renal clearance of procainamide

warfarin: Possibly increased anticoagulant activity and risk of bleeding

Adverse Reactions

CNS: Aggressiveness, agitation, ataxia, **CVA**, delirium, disorientation, disturbance in attention, dizziness, drowsiness, emotional lability, exacerbation of extrapyramidal disorders and myasthenia gravis, fever, headache, incoordination, insomnia, lightheadedness, mania, memory impairment, nervousness, peripheral neuropathy, psychotic reactions, restlessness, **suicidal ideation**, syncope
CV: **Arrhythmias**, **prolonged QT interval**, **severe hypotension**, **torsades de pointes**, vasculitis
EENT: Blurred vision; conjunctivitis; diplopia; disturbances in equilibrium, hearing, smell, and taste
ENDO: Hyperglycemia, **hypoglycemia**
GI: Abdominal cramps or pain, **acute hepatic necrosis or failure**, ***Clostridioides difficile*-associated diarrhea**, diarrhea, **hepatitis**, jaundice, nausea, **pseudomembranous colitis**, vomiting
GU: **Acute renal insufficiency or failure**, interstitial nephritis, renal calculi, vaginal candidiasis
HEME: **Agranulocytosis**, **aplastic or hemolytic anemia**, **leukopenia**, **pancytopenia**, **thrombocytopenia**
MS: Arthralgia; myalgia; **rhabdomyolysis**; tendinitis; tendon inflammation, pain, or rupture
RESP: **Hypersensitivity pneumonitis**, **pulmonary edema**
SKIN: Blisters, diaphoresis, erythema, **erythema multiforme**, **exfoliative dermatitis**, hyperpigmentation, photosensitivity, pruritus, rash, **Stevens-Johnson syndrome**, **toxic epidermal necrolysis**, urticaria, vesiculobullous eruption
Other: **Acidosis**, **anaphylaxis**, serum sickness

Childbearing Considerations

PREGNANCY

- It is not known if drug causes fetal harm.
- Use with caution only if benefit to mother outweighs potential risk to fetus.

LACTATION

- Drug is present in breast milk.
- A decision should be made to discontinue breastfeeding or the drug to avoid potential serious adverse reactions in the breastfed infant.

Nursing Considerations

! **WARNING** Know that because of increased risk of prolonged QT interval, ofloxacin shouldn't be used if patient has had a prolonged QT interval, has an uncorrected electrolyte disorder, or takes a class IA or class III antiarrhythmic. Monitor elderly patients closely because risk of prolonged QT interval may be increased in this group.

- Avoid use of ofloxacin in patients with myasthenia gravis because drug can cause exacerbation of muscle weakness that may become severe enough to require ventilatory support or even result in death.
- Maintain adequate hydration to prevent development of highly concentrated urine and crystalluria.

! **WARNING** Monitor patient closely for hypersensitivity, which may become life-threatening such as anaphylaxis and may occur as early as first dose. If present, notify prescriber immediately, expect to discontinue drug, and provide supportive care, as needed and ordered.

! **WARNING** Monitor patient for a change in behavior or thinking because drug may cause suicidal ideation.

! **WARNING** Monitor patient for skin reactions because ofloxacin can cause multiple skin reactions, some of which could be quite severe. At the first sign of a rash or other skin abnormality, notify prescriber and expect drug to be discontinued. Provide supportive care, as needed and ordered.

! **WARNING** Notify prescriber if diarrhea develops because it may indicate pseudomembranous colitis caused by *Clostridioides difficile*, which can range from being mild to fatal colitis. If diarrhea occurs, notify prescriber and expect a stool specimen to be obtained to confirm diagnosis. If confirmed, expect prescriber to discontinue ofloxacin and order an antibacterial agent effective against *C. difficile*. Also expect to administer electrolytes, fluids, and protein supplementation, as needed and ordered.

! **WARNING** Be aware that an increased risk of aortic aneurysm and dissection within 2 months of fluoroquinolone therapy has occurred in patients, especially elderly patients. Know that ofloxacin should only be used in patients with a known aortic aneurysm or patients at greater risk for aortic aneurysms when there are no alternative antibacterial treatments available.

! **WARNING** Expect an increased risk of toxicity may occur in patients with severe hepatic disease, including cirrhosis.

! **WARNING** Be aware that ofloxacin may stimulate the CNS and aggravate seizure disorders. Also, know that the drug may cause many psychiatric adverse reactions. Monitor patient closely.

! **WARNING** Monitor patient closely for hypoglycemia, especially if patient is elderly, has diabetes or renal insufficiency, or is taking hypoglycemic drugs such as sulfonylureas. Hypoglycemia can become severe and result in coma. Treat hypoglycemia quickly and effectively. Notify prescriber of incident and expect that drug may be replaced with a different antibiotic for this patient.

- Know that fluoroquinolones like ofloxacin have caused disabling and potentially irreversible serious adverse reactions from different body systems that can occur together in the same patient. These reactions can occur within hours to weeks after starting the drug and usually cause CNS effects; peripheral neuropathy (altered sense of light touch, pain, position sense, temperature, or vibration along with burning, numbness, pain, tingling, weakness), which could be permanent; a severe photosensitivity reaction; and tendinitis, and tendon rupture, which occurs more often in the elderly or patients taking corticosteroids. All ages of patients and patients without any preexisting risk factors have experienced these reactions. Notify prescriber and expect to discontinue ofloxacin immediately at the first signs or symptoms of any serious adverse reactions. If patient experiences tendon rupture expect patient to be put on immediate bed rest.
- Be alert for secondary fungal infection.

PATIENT TEACHING

- Instruct patient how to administer ofloxacin.
- Tell patient to complete full course of ofloxacin therapy exactly as prescribed, even if he feels better before it's complete.
- Tell patient to maintain adequate hydration throughout drug therapy.
- Urge patient not to take antacids, iron or zinc preparations, or other drugs (such as didanosine and sucralfate), within 2 hours of ofloxacin to prevent decreased or delayed drug absorption.

! **WARNING** Alert patient that drug may cause an allergic reaction. If present, tell patient to notify prescriber and, if severe, to seek immediate medical care.

! **WARNING** Instruct patient on the signs and symptoms of hypoglycemia even if patient does not have diabetes. Tell patient to notify prescriber immediately if he develops a hypoglycemic reaction and instruct patient how to treat the reaction.

! **WARNING** Alert patient and family or caregiver that drug may cause suicidal thoughts. Tell family or caregiver to alert prescriber immediately if patient exhibits suicidal behavior or thinking.

! **WARNING** Tell patient to notify prescriber immediately at the first sign of a rash or other skin abnormality.

! **WARNING** Advise patient to notify prescriber if diarrhea develops, even up to 2 months after ofloxacin therapy ends. Additional therapy may be needed.

! **WARNING** Advise patient to notify prescriber immediately about abnormal motor or sensory function, burning skin, hives, itching, rapid heart rate, rash, and tendon pain. Also, advise patient to stop taking ofloxacin immediately and notify prescriber if any other persistent, serious, or worsening adverse effects occur.

- Advise patient to avoid hazardous activities until CNS effects of drug are known and resolved.
- Tell patient to limit exposure to sun and ultraviolet light to prevent phototoxicity

olanzapine

Zyprexa, Zyprexa IntraMuscular, Zyprexa Zydis

olanzapine pamoate monohydrate

Zyprexa Relprevv

Class and Category

Pharmacologic class: Thienobenzodiazepine derivative
Therapeutic class: Antipsychotic

Indications and Dosages

✱ *To treat schizophrenia*

ORALLY DISINTEGRATING TABLETS, TABLETS

Adults. *Initial:* 5 to 10 mg once daily. *Target:* 10 mg once daily. Once 10 mg daily dosage reached, additional dosage adjustment made in 5-mg increments every wk, as needed. *Maintenance:* 10 mg once daily. *Maximum:* 20 mg daily.
Adolescents ages 13 and older. *Initial:* 2.5 to 5 mg once daily. Target: 10 mg once daily. Once 10 mg daily dosage reached, increased in increments of 2.5 mg or 5 mg, as needed. *Maintenance:* 10 mg once daily. *Maximum:* 20 mg daily.

I.M. INJECTION-ER (ZYPREXA RELPREVV)

Adults who have been taking 10 mg daily orally. *Initial:* 210 mg every 2 wk for first 8 wk, then decreased to 150 mg every 2 wk. Alternatively, 405 mg every 4 wk for first 8 wk, then decreased to 300 mg every 4 wk.
Adults who have been taking 15 mg daily orally. *Initial:* 300 mg every 2 wk for 8 wk, then decreased to 210 mg every 2 wk or 405 mg every 4 wk.
Adults who have been taking 20 mg daily orally. 300 mg every 2 wk.

✱ *To treat manic phase of bipolar I disorder (manic or mixed episodes)*

ORALLY DISINTEGRATING TABLETS, TABLETS

Adults. *Initial:* 10 to 15 mg once daily decreased or increased in 5-mg increments no less than every 24 hr, as needed. *Maintenance:* 5 to 20 mg daily. *Maximum:* 20 mg daily.
Adolescents ages 13 and older. *Initial:* 2.5 to 5 mg once daily, increased, as needed, in 2.5- or 5-mg increments. *Maintenance:* Lowest dose needed to maintain remission. *Maximum:* 20 mg daily.

✱ *As adjunct to lithium or valproate therapy to treat bipolar I disorder*

ORALLY DISINTEGRATING TABLETS, TABLETS

Adults. *Initial:* 10 mg once daily with lithium or valproate sodium, increased or decreased by 5 mg no less than every 24 hr, as needed. *Maintenance:* 5 to 20 mg/day. *Maximum:* 20 mg daily.

✱ *To treat agitation associated with schizophrenia and bipolar I mania*

I.M. INJECTION (ZYPREXA INTRAMUSCULAR)

Adults. 2.5 to 10 mg, as needed. Repeat, as needed, every 2 to 4 hr for total of 3 doses. *Maximum:* 3 doses of 10 mg administered with second dose given after 2 hr and third dose given 4 hr after second dose providing patient is not exhibiting orthostatic hypotension.

± **DOSAGE ADJUSTMENT** For debilitated patients, those prone to hypotension, and female nonsmokers age 65 and older receiving a short-acting oral form, initial dosage possibly reduced to 5 mg. For elderly patients, receiving the short-acting I.M. form, dosage should not exceed 5 mg. For debilitated patients, female nonsmokers age 65 and older, and those prone to hypotension receiving the short-acting I.M. form, initial dosage decreased to 2.5 mg. For patients who are debilitated, female nonsmokers age 65 and older, or those prone to hypotension receiving the extended-release I.M. form, dosage decreased to 150 mg every 4 weeks.

Drug Administration

P.O.

- For oral disintegrating tablets, open sachet and peel back foil on blister. Do not push tablet through foil. Immediately upon opening the blister, remove tablet with dry, gloved hands. Place tablet on patient's tongue. It can be swallowed after it dissolves with or without liquid.

I.M.

- Keep patient recumbent after I.M. injection of olanzapine if bradycardia, dizziness, drowsiness, or hypoventilation occurs. Don't let patient sit or stand up until blood pressure and heart rate have returned to baseline.
- There are 2 formulations for I.M. injection. One is an immediate-release formulation and one is an extended release. They are not interchangeable. When administering drug intramuscularly, make sure the right formulation is being administered.

Immediate-release formulation

- Reconstitute by dissolving contents of vial in 2.1 ml using only Sterile Water for Injection to yield 5 mg/ml.
- Solution should be clear yellow.
- Administer within 1 hr after reconstitution.
- Inject I.M. slowly, deep into muscle mass.

Extended-release formulation

- Reconstitute using only the diluent provided as follows: for 150- or 210-mg dose, use 1.3 ml of diluent; for 300-mg dose, use 1.8 ml of diluent; and for 405-mg dose, use 2.3 ml of diluent.
- Loosen the powder in the vial by lightly tapping the vial.
- Withdraw predetermined diluent into syringe. Inject into powder vial and withdraw air to equalize pressure. Remove needle and hold vial upright.
- Pad a hard surface, then tap vial firmly and repeatedly on the surface until no powder is visible. Shake vial vigorously until suspension appears smooth and consistent in color and texture (yellow and opaque). If foam has formed, let vial stand until it has dissipated.
- Administer immediately or, if stored at room temperature for up to 24 hr, remember that drug vial must be vigorously shaken to resuspend solution prior to administration.
- Attach new needle to syringe and slowly withdraw desired amount into the syringe. Remove needle from syringe.
- Administer by first attaching a 19 G (1.5-inch) needle or larger to syringe to prevent clogging. Obese patients may need a 2-inch needle. Inject deeply into the gluteal muscle. Aspirate for several sec to ensure that no blood appears and then inject with steady, continuous pressure. Withdraw needle. Do not massage injection site.
- Following the injection of extended-release olanzapine, patient may experience a syndrome similar to an olanzapine overdose, with delirium and sedation being the primary symptoms. Patient must be observed for at least 3 hr following each injection for this syndrome. Notify prescriber immediately if it should occur.

Route	Onset	Peak	Duration
P.O.	Unknown	6 hr	Unknown
I.M.	Unknown	15–45 min	Unknown
I.M./E.R.	Unknown	7 days	Unknown

Half-life: 21–54 hr (P.O.); 30 days (I.M.)

Mechanism of Action

May achieve antipsychotic effects by antagonizing dopamine and serotonin receptors. Binding competitively to and antagonism of the muscarinic receptors M_1 through M_5 accounts for the drug's antichoinergic effects.

Contraindications

Hypersensitivity to olanzapine or its components

Interactions

DRUGS

anticholinergic drugs: May increase risk for severe GI adverse reactions related to hypomotility
antihypertensives: Increased effects of antihypertensives, increased risk of hypotension
carbamazepine, rifampin: Increased olanzapine clearance
charcoal: Reduced olanzapine level by about 60%; interferes with olanzapine effectiveness
CNS depressants: Additive CNS depression, potentiated orthostatic hypotension
diazepam: Potentiated orthostatic hypotension
dopamine agonists, levodopa: Antagonized effects of these drugs
fluoxetine, fluvoxamine: Decreased olanzapine clearance
lorazepam (parenteral): Possibly increased somnolence with I.M. olanzapine injection

ACTIVITIES

alcohol use: Potentiated orthostatic hypotension

smoking: Decreased blood olanzapine level

Adverse Reactions

CNS: Abnormal gait, agitation, akathisia, altered thermoregulation, amnesia, anxiety, asthenia, dizziness, euphoria, fatigue, fever, headache, hypertonia, insomnia, motor and sensory instability, nervousness, **neuroleptic malignant syndrome**, restless leg syndrome, restlessness, somnolence, stuttering, **suicidal ideation**, syncope, tardive dyskinesia, thirst, tremor

CV: **Bradycardia**, chest pain, elevated triglyceride levels, hyperlipidemia, hypertension, **hypotension**, orthostatic hypotension, peripheral edema, tachycardia, **venous thromboembolic events**

EENT: Amblyopia, dry mouth, increased salivation, pharyngitis, rhinitis

ENDO: **Diabetic coma**, **diabetic ketoacidosis**, hyperglycemia, **hyperprolactinemia**

GI: Abdominal pain, **cholestatic** or **mixed liver injury**, constipation, dysphagia, elevated liver enzymes, **hepatitis**, increased appetite, jaundice, nausea, **pancreatitis**, vomiting

GU: Priapism, urinary incontinence, UTI

HEME: **Agranulocytosis**, **leukopenia**, **neutropenia**

MS: Arthralgia; back, joint, or limb pain; muscle spasms and twitching; **rhabdomyolysis**

RESP: Cough, **pulmonary embolism**

SKIN: **Ecchymosis**, photosensitivity, pruritus, rash, urticaria

Other: **Anaphylaxis**, **angioedema**, discontinuation reaction, **drug reaction with eosinophilia and systemic symptoms (DRESS)**, flu-like symptoms, injection-site abscess, weight gain

Childbearing Considerations

PREGNANCY

- Pregnancy exposure registry: 1-866-961-2388 or http://womensmentalhealth.org/clinical-and-research-programs/pregnancyregistry/.
- Drug may cause fetal harm, as exposure to drug during the third trimester of pregnancy increases the risk for extrapyramidal and/or withdrawal symptoms following delivery.
- Use with caution only if benefit to mother outweighs potential risk to fetus.

LACTATION

- Drug is present in breast milk.
- Mothers should check with prescriber before breastfeeding. However, if breastfeeding occurs, infant should be monitored for excess sedation, extrapyramidal symptoms, poor feeding, and irritability.

REPRODUCTION

- Drug may cause an increase in serum prolactin levels, which may lead to a reversible reduction in fertility in females of childbearing age.

Nursing Considerations

! **WARNING** Be aware that olanzapine shouldn't be used for elderly patients with dementia-related psychosis because drug increases risk of death in these patients.

! **WARNING** Monitor patient for a hypersensitivity reaction, which could become life-threatening, such as anaphylaxis and angioedema. If present, notify prescriber, expect drug to be discontinued, and provide supportive care, as needed and ordered.

! **WARNING** Know that olanzapine may cause a drug reaction with eosinophilia and systemic symptoms called DRESS. Although uncommon, it can become fatal. Assess patient regularly for a cutaneous reaction exhibited by eosinophilia, exfoliative dermatitis, fever, lymphadenopathy, or rash. Know that systemic complications such as hepatitis, myocarditis and/or pericarditis, nephritis, or pneumonitis also may occur. If suspected, stop olanzapine and notify prescriber immediately. Expect to provide supportive care, as ordered.

! **WARNING** Monitor CBC often during first few months of therapy, especially if patient has low WBC count or history of drug-induced leukopenia or neutropenia. If WBC count declines, and especially if neutrophil count drops below 1,000/mm^3, expect olanzapine to be discontinued. If neutropenia is significant, also monitor patient for fever or other evidence of infection and provide appropriate treatment, as prescribed.

! **WARNING** Monitor patients with a current diagnosis or prior history of angle-closure glaucoma, constipation, paralytic ileus or related conditions, significant prostatic hypertrophy, or urinary retention because of drug's cholinergic antagonism.

! **WARNING** Monitor patients with hepatic impairment or conditions associated with limited hepatic functional reserve and in patients who are being treated with potentially hepatotoxic drugs. Also, monitor patients with known cardiovascular or cerebrovascular disease and conditions that would predispose patient to hypotension, such as presence of dehydration, hypovolemia, or treatment with antihypertensive medications because of the increased risk for bradycardia, hypotension, and syncope.

! **WARNING** Watch patient closely (especially adolescent and young adults), for suicidal tendencies, particularly when therapy starts and dosage changes because depression may worsen temporarily during these times, possibly leading to suicidal ideation.

! **WARNING** Monitor patient for seizures, especially patients with a history of seizures because drug may cause seizures. Institute seizure precautions, as appropriate.

! **WARNING** Monitor patient's blood glucose level routinely because olanzapine may increase risk of hyperglycemia.

! **WARNING** Be alert for and immediately report signs of neuroleptic malignant syndrome.

- Monitor patient's blood pressure routinely during therapy because olanzapine may cause orthostatic hypotension.
- Assess daily weight to detect fluid retention or metabolic changes.
- Notify prescriber if patient develops tardive dyskinesia or urinary incontinence.
- Monitor patient's lipid levels throughout therapy, as ordered, because olanzapine may cause significant elevations.
- Be aware that drug may cause hyperprolactinemia, which, in turn, may reduce pituitary gonadotropin secretion. This then inhibits reproductive function by impairing gonadal steroidogenesis in both female and male patients. In addition, long-standing hyperprolactinemia may decrease bone density in patient when it is associated with hypogonadism.
- Institute fall precautions, especially in patients with conditions, diseases, or concurrent drug therapy that could exacerbate effects of motor and sensory instability, postural hypotension, and somnolence.

PATIENT TEACHING

! **WARNING** Warn patient with phenylketonuria that disintegrating olanzapine tablets contain phenylalanine.

- Instruct patient how to administer oral form of olanzapine prescribed.
- Tell patient receiving the extended-release parenteral form of olanzapine that she will need to be monitored for at least 3 hours following the injection. Stress importance of reporting any unusual symptoms, including altered thoughts and lethargy, immediately to healthcare professional.
- Advise patient to avoid alcohol and smoking during olanzapine therapy.

! **WARNING** Alert patient that drug may cause an allergic or severe skin reaction. If present, tell patient to notify prescriber immediately at the first sign of an allergic or skin reaction, such as a rash and seek immediate medical care.

! **WARNING** Urge family or caregiver to watch patient closely for suicidal tendencies, especially when therapy starts or dosage changes and particularly if patient is a teenager or young adult.

! **WARNING** Advise patient to notify prescriber immediately if persistent, serious, or unusual adverse reactions occur.

- Urge patient to avoid hazardous activities until drug's CNS effects are known and resolved. Also, inform patient of increased risk for falls because of potential CNS effects. Review fall precautions with patient.
- Instruct patient to change position slowly to minimize effects of orthostatic hypotension.
- Encourage patient to weigh self frequently to detect weight gain. If diabetes is present,

also instruct patient to monitor blood glucose level closely.

- Warn females of childbearing age that chronic olanzapine therapy may alter reproductive function through olanzapine-induced hyperprolactinemia causing amenorrhea. If reproductive adverse effects occur, patient should notify prescriber. Also, tell pregnant patient to alert prescriber when she enters the third trimester of her pregnancy as drug may need to be discontinued.
- Advise mothers breastfeeding during drug therapy to monitor their infant for excess sedation, extrapyramidal symptoms, poor feeding, and irritability.

oliceridine

Olinvyk

Class, Category, and Schedule

Pharmacologic class: Opioid agonist
Therapeutic class: Analgesic
Controlled substance schedule: II

Indications and Dosages

* *To manage acute pain severe enough to require an intravenous opioid analgesic for patient for whom alternative treatments are inadequate*

I.V. INJECTION

Adults. *Initial:* 1.5 mg followed by 0.35-mg to 0.5-mg demand dose with a 6-min lockout. Supplemental doses of 0.75 mg may be given by healthcare provider beginning 1 hr after initial dose and hourly thereafter, as needed. *Maximum:* 3 mg as a single dose; 27 mg daily for no longer than 48 hr.

±**DOSAGE ADJUSTMENT** For patients experiencing unacceptable opioid-related adverse reaction, dosage may be reduced with dosage adjustment made to obtain an appropriate balance between management of pain and opioid-related adverse reactions.

Drug Administration

I.V.

- Initiation of oliceridine dosing regimen should take into account patient's severity of pain, patient response, prior analgesic treatment experience, and risk factors for addiction, abuse, and misuse.
- Use of oliceridine (30 mg/30 ml) vial is intended for patient-controlled analgesia (PCA) only. Set demand dose with a 6-min lockout.
- Draw oliceridine directly from vial into PCA syringe or I.V. bag without diluting.
- Know that drug solution should be clear and colorless.
- Know that if analgesia is still required with a 27-mg cumulative daily dose before 24 hr are up, an alternative analgesic regimen should be administered, as prescribed, until oliceridine can be resumed the next day. Alternative analgesia may include multimodal therapies.
- Have naloxone readily available.
- *Incompatibilities:* None reported by manufacturer

Route	Onset	Peak	Duration
I.V.	2–5 min	Unknown	Unknown

Half-life: 1.3–3 hr

Mechanism of Action

Action of analgesic action unknown but specific CNS opioid receptors with opioid-like activity have been identified throughout the brain and spinal cord and are thought to play a role in the analgesic effects of oliceridine.

Contraindications

Acute or severe bronchial asthma in an unmonitored setting or in the absence of resuscitative equipment; GI obstruction, including paralytic ileus; hypersensitivity to oliceridine or its components; significant respiratory depression

Interactions

DRUGS

anticholinergic drugs: Possibly increased risk of urinary retention and/or severe constipation, which may lead to paralytic ileus

benzodiazepines and other CNS depressants (antipsychotics, anxiolytics, general anesthetics, muscle relaxants, other opioids, tranquilizers): Increased risk of coma, hypotension, profound sedation, respiratory depression, death

CYP2D6 moderate to strong inhibitors (bupropion, fluoxetine, paroxetine, quinidine), CYP3A4 moderate to strong inhibitors

(antiretroviral agents, azole antifungal agents such as ketoconazole, macrolide antibiotics such as erythromycin, NS3/4A inhibitors, protease inhibitors such as ritonavir, selective serotonin reuptake inhibitors): Possibly increased plasma concentration of oliceridine, causing increased or prolonged opioid effects
CYP3A4 inducers (carbamazepine, phenytoin, rifampin): Possibly reduced plasma concentration of oliceridine, causing decreased effectiveness
diuretics: Possibly reduced effectiveness of diuretics
mixed agonist/antagonist, partial agonist opioid analgesics such as buprenorphine, butorphanol, nalbuphine, pentazocine: Possibly reduced analgesic effect of oliceridine and/or precipitation of withdrawal symptoms
muscle relaxants: Possibly enhanced neuromuscular blocking action of skeletal muscle relaxants and increased degree of respiratory depression
serotonergic drugs (5-HT_3 receptor antagonists; certain muscle relaxants such as cyclobenzaprine and metaxalone; drugs that affect the serotonin neurotransmitter system, such as mirtazapine, tramadol, trazodone; MAO inhibitors such as drugs used to treat psychiatric disorders and I.V. methylene blue, linezolid; norepinephrine reuptake inhibitors; selective serotonin reuptake inhibitors): Possibly development of serotonin syndrome

ACTIVITIES

alcohol: Increased risk of coma, hypotension, profound sedation, respiratory depression, and death

Adverse Reactions

CNS: Anxiety, dizziness, fever, headache, insomnia, restlessness, sedation, **seizures**, somnolence
CV: Increased blood pressure, **QT prolongation**, **severe hypotension**, tachycardia
EENT: Dry mouth
ENDO: **Adrenal insufficiency**, androgen deficiency, hypoglycemia
GI: Constipation, diarrhea, dyspepsia, elevated amylase or liver enzymes, flatulence, nausea, spasm of sphincter of Oddi, vomiting
HEME: Anemia
MS: Back pain, muscle spasms
RESP: Cough, decreased oxygen saturation, dyspnea, **hypoxia**, **respiratory depression**
SKIN: Excessive diaphoresis, flushing, hot flush, pruritus, rash, urticaria
Other: **Anaphylaxis**, **hypocalcemia**, **hypokalemia**, **hypomagnesemia**, **hypophosphatemia**, infusion site extravasation, opioid-induced allodynia and hyperalgesia, physical and psychological dependence, withdrawal

Childbearing Considerations

PREGNANCY

- Drug may cause fetal harm.
- Prolonged use of drug during pregnancy can result in neonatal opioid withdrawal syndrome (NOWS), which may be life-threatening if not recognized and treated.
- Avoid prolonged use during pregnancy. Use with caution only if benefit to mother outweighs potential risk to fetus.

LABOR AND DELIVERY

- Drug is not recommended for use in pregnant women immediately before or during labor. Opioids may alter length of time of labor.
- Opioids cross the placental barrier and may produce respiratory depression and psychological effects in the neonate. Monitor neonate closely for signs of excess sedation and respiratory depression.
- An opioid antagonist, such as naloxone, must be available at the time of delivery in case it is needed to reverse opioid-induced respiratory depression in the neonate.

LACTATION

- It is not known if drug is present in breast milk.
- Mothers should check with prescriber before breastfeeding once patient has been discharged from hospital.
- If breastfeeding occurs shortly after drug has been discontinued, monitor infant for excess sedation and respiratory depression.

REPRODUCTION

- Chronic use of opioids may reduce fertility.

Nursing Considerations

! WARNING Know that oliceridine should be avoided in patients who are in a coma or have impaired consciousness because drug can obscure their clinical course. Also, know that patients susceptible to the intracranial effects of carbon dioxide retention, such as patients with brain tumors or head injury, may develop further increased intracranial pressure because of oliceridine's ability to reduce respiratory drive, which causes carbon dioxide retention.

! **WARNING** Be aware that use of opioids like oliceridine may lead to abuse, addiction, misuse, overdose, and possibly death. Addiction can occur even with appropriately prescribed dosages. Know that drug should only be used in patients when alternative treatment options have not been tolerated or not expected to be tolerated or alternative treatment has not provided adquate analgesia or are not expected to provide adequate analgesia. Monitor patient's intake of drug closely and for evidence of physical and psychological dependence.

! **WARNING** Know that cumulative total daily dose of oliceridine should not exceed 27 mg daily because of risk of QT prolongation. Also, monitor patient using PCA for signs of excessive sedation, respiratory depression, or other adverse effects because PCA administration has resulted in adverse outcomes and episodes of respiratory depression.

! **WARNING** Be aware that overestimating the oliceridine dosage when converting patients from another opioid product can result in a fatal overdose with the first dose. Double check dosage before administering. Know that an initial 1-mg dose of oliceridine is approximately equipotent to 5 mg of morphine.

- Monitor effectiveness of oliceridine to relieve pain. Attempt to identify source of increased pain, especially if level of pain increases after dosage stabilization. Consult prescriber about dosage adjustment because patient may have developed a paradoxic increase in pain known as opioid-induced hyperalgesia or an increase in sensitivity to pain known as opioid-induced allodynia, especially when dosage increases. Do not confuse this with tolerance, which is the need for increasing doses of opioids to maintain an effect. If opioid-induced allodynia or hyperalgesia is suspected, expect dosage to be decreased or opioid rotation to be prescribed.

! **WARNING** Monitor patient's blood pressure closely, especially when initiating oliceridine therapy and when titrating dose because drug may cause severe hypotension and syncope in ambulatory patients due to its vasodilatory effects. Be aware that risk of hypotension is greater in patients who have already been compromised by a reduced blood volume or are receiving concurrent therapy with certain CNS depressant drugs, such as general anesthetics and phenothiazines.

! **WARNING** Monitor patient for a hypersensitivity reaction such as anaphylaxis. If present, notify prescriber, expect drug to be switched to a different analagesic, and provide supportive care, as needed and ordered.

! **WARNING** Monitor patients closely with conditions accompanied by hypoxia or decreased respiratory reserve, such as asthma, COPD, or cor pulmonale. This is because even with usual therapeutic dosages, oliceridine may decrease respiratory drive while simultaneously increasing airway resistance to the point of apnea. Monitor patient's respiratory status closely, especially in cachectic, debilitated, and elderly patients and in patients with chronic pulmonary disease. Respiratory depression may occur at any time but is most likely to occur during initiation of therapy or following a dosage increase. Have resuscitative equipment nearby and be prepared to administer supportive measures and use of opioid antagonists, as ordered.

! **WARNING** Know that opioids such as oliceridine can cause sleep-related breathing disorders, such as central sleep apnea and sleep-related hypoxemia. Risk for central sleep apnea increases in a dose-dependent fashion. If central sleep apnea occurs, notify prescriber, as dosage may have to be reduced.

! **WARNING** Moniator patient's blood glucose level because opioids like oliceridine may cause hypoglycemia. Be prepared to treat if hypoglycemia occurs and notify prescriber.

! **WARNING** Know that chronic use of oliceridine continued to end of pregnancy may result in neonatal opioid withdrawal syndrome (NOWS), which may be life-threatening if not recognized and treated appropriately. NOWS occurs when a newborn has been exposed to opioid drugs for a prolonged period while in utero.

! **WARNING** Monitor patient for adrenal insufficiency. Although rare, it can be life-threatening. Monitor patient for anorexia, dizziness, fatigue, hypotension, nausea, vomiting, or weakness. Notify prescriber if adrenal insufficiency is suspected and expect diagnostic testing to be done. If confirmed, expect to administer corticosteroids and wean patient off oliceridine, if possible.

! **WARNING** Monitor patients with seizure disorders closely because oliceridine may induce or aggravate seizures. Institute seizure precautions, as appropriate.

! **WARNING** Be aware that oliceridine should only be used concomitantly with benzodiazepine or other CNS depressant therapy in patients for whom other treatment options are inadequate. If prescribed together, expect dosing and duration of oliceridine and/or benzodiazepine or other CNS depressant to be limited. Monitor patient closely for signs and symptoms of a decrease in consciousness, including coma, profound sedation, and significant respiratory depression. Notify prescriber immediately and provide emergency supportive care, as death may occur.

! **WARNING** Monitor patients with decreased CYP2D6 function (poor metabolizers of CYP2D6 or normal metabolizers taking moderate or strong CYP2D6 inhibitors) or patients who are receiving concomitant therapy with CYP3A4 inhibitors and inducers, including when discontinuation occurs because of increased risk of prolonged opioid adverse reactions and exacerbated respiratory depression.

! **WARNING** Know that many drugs may interact with opioids like oliceridine to cause serotonin syndrome. Monitor patient closely for signs and symptoms, such as agitation, diaphoresis, diarrhea, fever, hallucinations, labile blood pressure, muscle twitching or stiffness, nausea, shakiness, shivering, tachycardia, trouble with coordination, or vomiting. Notify prescriber at once because serotonin syndrome may be life-threatening. Be prepared to discontinue drug, if possible and ordered, and provide supportive care.

- Monitor patients with biliary tract disease for worsening symptoms because oliceridine may cause spasm of the sphincter of Oddi.
- Know that oliceridine therapy should not be abruptly discontinued in a physically dependent patient. Instead, taper dose gradually while monitoring for withdrawal. If patient exhibits withdrawal signs and symptoms, be aware that dose should be raised to the previous level and then tapered more slowly, either by increasing the interval between decreases, decreasing the amount of dosage change, or both, as prescribed.

PATIENT TEACHING

- Explain to patient how PCA works, including the use of a 6-minute lockout for oliceridine.

! **WARNING** Alert patient to the possibility of addiction even with prescribed dosages and to use demand doses only as truly needed.

- Inform patient to keep staff informed about the degree of pain relief achieved with oliceridine administration. Also alert patient to notify staff if pain increases when dosage increases or patient experiences increased sensitivity to pain because a dosage adjustment may be needed.

! **WARNING** Alert patient that drug may cause an allergic reaction. Urge patient to promptly notify staff if an allergic reaction develops while receiving oliceridine.

! **WARNING** Inform patient that drug can cause severe constipation and to notify prescriber, if present.

! **WARNING** Instruct patient to alert staff of any other persistent, serious, or unusual adverse effects.

! **WARNING** Tell mothers that if breastfeeding occurs shortly after drug has been discontinued, mother should monitor infant for excess sedation and respiratory depression.

olmesartan medoxomil

Benicar

Class and Category

Pharmacologic class: Angiotensin II receptor blocker (ARB)
Therapeutic class: Antihypertensive

Indications and Dosages

* *To manage or as adjunct to manage hypertension*

ORAL SUSPENSION, TABLETS

Adults, adolescents, and children ages 6 and older weighing 35 kg (77 lb) or more. *Initial:* 20 mg daily, increased in 2 wk to 40 mg daily, as needed. *Maximum:* 40 mg daily.

Adolescents and children age 6 and older weighing 20 kg (44 lb) to less than 35 kg (77 lb). *Initial:* 10 mg daily, increased in 2 wk to 20 mg daily, as needed. *Maximum:* 20 mg daily.

± **DOSAGE ADJUSTMENT** For patients with possible depletion of intravascular volume, such as those treated with diuretics, especially if impaired renal function is present, lower starting dosage is recommended.

Drug Administration

P.O.

- For patient who cannot swallow tablets, have pharmacist make a suspension form.
- Shake the oral suspension well before each use. Use a calibrated device to measure dosage of oral suspension. Refrigerate the oral suspension for up to 4 wk. Return promptly to the refrigerator after each use.

Route	Onset	Peak	Duration
P.O.	< 2 wk	1–2 hr	24 hr

Half-life: 13 hr

Contraindications

Aliskiren therapy in patients with diabetes or renal impairment (GFR less than 60 ml/min), hypersensitivity to olmesartan medoxomil or its components

Interactions

DRUGS

ACE inhibitors, aliskiren (in patients with diabetes or renal impairment), other angiotensin receptor blockers: Increased risk of hyperkalemia, hypotension, and renal dysfunction
colesevelam: Reduced effectiveness of olmesartan
drugs that may increase potassium levels, such as heparin, potassium-sparing diuretics, potassium supplements: Increased risk of hyperkalemia
lithium: Increased serum lithium level with possible toxicity
NSAIDs: Increased risk of renal dysfunction in elderly patients and patients who are volume-depleted or have preexisting renal dysfunction; increased antihypertensive effect of olmesartan

FOOD

salt substitutes containing potassium: Increased risk of hyperkalemia

Adverse Reactions

CNS: Asthenia, dizziness, fatigue, headache, insomnia, vertigo
CV: Chest pain, hypercholesterolemia, hyperlipidemia, hypertriglyceridemia, peripheral edema, tachycardia
EENT: Pharyngitis, rhinitis, sinusitis
ENDO: Hyperglycemia
GI: Abdominal pain, diarrhea, gastroenteritis, indigestion, nausea, sprue-like enteropathy, vomiting
GU: **Acute renal failure**, elevated BUN and serum creatinine levels, hematuria, UTI
MS: Arthralgia, arthritis, back pain, myalgia, **rhabdomyolysis**, skeletal pain
RESP: Bronchitis, cough, upper respiratory tract infection
SKIN: Alopecia, pruritus, rash, urticaria
Other: **Anaphylaxis**, **angioedema**, **hyperkalemia**, hyperuricemia, increased CK level, flu-like symptoms, pain

Childbearing Considerations

PREGNANCY

- Drug causes fetal harm.
- Drug given during the second or third trimester reduces fetal renal function and

Mechanism of Action

Blocks angiotensin II from binding to receptor sites in many tissues, including adrenal glands and vascular smooth muscle to reduce blood pressure by allowing angiotensin II, a potent vasoconstrictor, to stimulate the adrenal cortex to secrete aldosterone and inhibit the effects of angiotensin II.

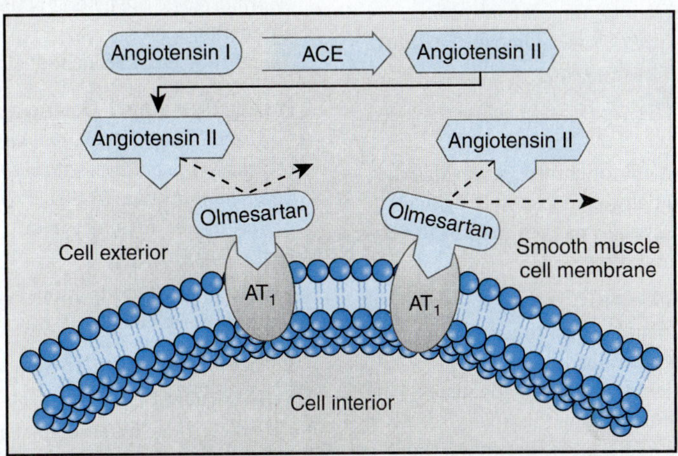

increases fetal and neonatal morbidity and death. Resulting oligohydramnios can cause fetal lung hypoplasia and skeletal malformations.

- Drug should be discontinued as soon as pregnancy is known.

LACTATION

- It is not known if drug is present in breast milk.
- A decision should be made to discontinue breastfeeding or the drug to avoid potential adverse reactions in the breastfed infant.

Nursing Considerations

- Expect to correct known or suspected hypovolemia, before beginning olmesartan therapy.
- Monitor blood pressure frequently to assess effectiveness of therapy. If blood pressure isn't controlled with olmesartan alone, expect to administer a diuretic, such as hydrochlorothiazide, as prescribed, but know that use of diuretics or other antihypertensive drugs during olmesartan therapy increases the risk of hypotension.
- Know that if patient also receives a diuretic, adequate hydration should be provided, as appropriate, to help prevent hypovolemia. Watch for evidence of hypovolemia, such as hypotension with dizziness and fainting.

! **WARNING** Expect to discontinue drug temporarily if patient experiences hypotension. Place patient in supine position immediately and prepare to administer normal saline solution I.V., as prescribed. Expect to resume drug therapy after blood pressure stabilizes.

! **WARNING** Monitor patient for a hypersensivity reaction, which could become life-threatening, such as anaphylaxis. If present, notify prescriber, expect drug to be discontinued, and provide supportive care, as needed and ordered.

! **WARNING** Monitor patient for increased BUN and serum creatinine levels, especially in a patient with impaired renal function because drug may cause acute renal failure. If increased levels are significant or persist, notify prescriber immediately.

! **WARNING** Monitor patient's electrolytes regularly, as ordered, and observe patient for signs and symptoms of electrolyte imbalances, especially hyperkalemia, because drug inhibits the renin–angiotensin system and may cause hyperkalemia. Be aware risks for hyperkalemia include concomitant use of potassium-sparing diuretics and potassium supplements and/or potassium containing salt substitutes. In addition, patients with diabetes mellitus or renal insufficiency are also at risk for hyperkalemia.

- Monitor patient for chronic severe diarrhea and substantial weight loss, as drug may cause these symptoms even months to years after drug initiation.

PATIENT TEACHING

- Instruct patient how to administer form of olmesartan prescribed.
- Advise patient to maintain adequate hydration during drug therapy. Also, tell patient to avoid exercise in hot weather and excessive alcohol use to reduce the risk of dehydration and hypotension. Also, instruct the patient to notify prescriber if he has prolonged diarrhea, nausea, or vomiting.

! WARNING Alert patient that drug may cause an allergic reaction. If present, tell patient to notify prescriber and, if severe, to seek immediate medical care.

! WARNING Review signs and symptoms of electrolyte imbalances and urge patient to contact prescriber immediately if present. Encourage patient to comply with routine laboratory appointments to monitor electrolyte levels.

- Caution patient to avoid hazardous activities until drug's CNS effects are known and resolved.
- Advise females of childbearing age to notify prescriber immediately if pregnancy occurs.
- Inform mothers breastfeeding should not be undertaken during olmesartan therapy; otherwise the drug will need to be discontinued.

olodaterol

Striverdi Respimat

Class and Category

Pharmacologic class: Long-acting beta$_2$-adrenergic agonist
Therapeutic class: Bronchodilator

Indications and Dosages

✶ *To provide long-term maintenance for airflow obstruction in patients with chronic obstructive pulmonary disease (COPD), including chronic bronchitis and/or emphysema*

ORAL INHALATION

Adults. 5 mcg (2 inhalations) once daily at same time each day.

Drug Administration

INHALATION

- Load cartridge into the inhaler. Prime before first use by actuating inhaler toward the ground until an aerosol cloud is visible, and then repeat the process 3 more times. If not used for more than 3 days, actuate inhaler once before use; if not used for more than 21 days, reprime the same way as if using inhaler for the first time.
- Use inhalation spray only with the Striverdi Respimat inhaler. Do not use to administer other drugs.
- Administer by first pressing the safety catch while firmly pulling off the clear base with other hand. Do not touch the piercing element. Insert the narrow end of the cartridge into the inhaler. Place inhaler on a firm surface and push down firmly until it clicks. Replace the clear base. Then, turn the clear base in the direction of the arrows on the label until it clicks. Open the cap until it snaps fully open. Prime the inhaler, if needed, as explained above. Device is ready for use.
- Have patient breathe out slowly and fully, then have patient close lips around the mouthpiece without covering the air vents. Have patient breathe in slowly through the mouth while pressing the dose release button. Patient should continue to finish the slow breath and then hold breath for 10 sec, if able.

- Repeat for second inhalation. Close cap when finished.
- Inhaler will lock after 60 actuations (30-day supply), signifying it is empty.
- Discard after 3 mo or when locking mechanism is engaged, whichever comes first.

Route	Onset	Peak	Duration
Inhalation	5 min	10–20 min	24 hr

Half-life: 7.5 hr

Mechanism of Action

Binding and activating beta$_2$-adrenoceptors in the airways stimulates intracellular adenyl cyclase (an enzyme that mediates the synthesis of cyclic-3′ 5′-adenosine monophosphate [cAMP]), which elevates levels of cAMP to cause bronchodilation by relaxing airway smooth-muscle cells.

Contraindications

Asthma without use of a long-term asthma control drug, hypersensitivity to olodaterol or its components

Interactions

DRUGS

adrenergic agents: Potentiated sympathetic effects
beta-blockers: Decreased effectiveness of olodaterol and beta-blockers; possibly severe bronchospasm
diuretics, steroids, xanthine derivatives: Increased risk of hypokalemia
drugs known to prolong QT interval, MAO inhibitors, tricyclic antidepressants: Possibly adverse cardiovascular effects
ketoconazole: Possibly increased serum olodaterol level
non-potassium-sparing diuretics: Possibly increased risk of ECG changes and hypokalemia

Adverse Reactions

CNS: Dizziness, fever
CV: **Atrial fibrillation**, chest pain, **ECG changes**, palpitations, tachycardia
EENT: Nasopharyngitis
ENDO: Hyperglycemia
GI: Constipation, diarrhea
GU: UTI
MS: Arthralgia, back pain
RESP: Bronchitis, COPD exacerbation, cough, **paradoxical bronchospasms**, pneumonia, upper respiratory infection
SKIN: Rash
Other: **Anaphylaxis, angioedema, and other immediate hypersensitivity reactions**; **hypokalemia**

Childbearing Considerations

PREGNANCY

- It is not known if drug causes fetal harm.
- Use with caution only if benefit to mother outweighs potential risk to fetus.

LABOR AND DELIVERY

- Drug may inhibit labor due to a relaxant effect on uterine smooth muscle.

LACTATION

- It is not known if drug is present in breast milk.
- Mothers should check with prescriber before breastfeeding.

Nursing Considerations

! WARNING Know that olodaterol therapy should not be used in patients with acutely deteriorating COPD, which may be a life-threatening condition. It should also not be used for relief of acute episodes of bronchospasm.

! WARNING Watch patient closely for paradoxical bronchospasm. If present, discontinue olodaterol therapy immediately, notify prescriber, and implement treatment according to standard of care.

! WARNING Monitor patient for worsening or deteriorating asthma because asthma-related deaths have increased in patients receiving salmeterol, a drug in the same class as olodaterol. Be aware that use of long-acting beta$_2$-adrenergic agonists, such as olodaterol, is contraindicated in patients with asthma without the use of a long-term asthma control medication, such as an inhaled corticosteroid. Monitor patient closely and notify prescriber immediately of any changes in patient's respiratory status.

! WARNING Watch patient closely for hypersensitivity reactions, which could become life-threatening, such as anaphylaxis or angioedema. Some hypersensitivity reactions may be immediate. If present, stop olodaterol therapy immediately, notify prescriber, and provide supportive care, as needed and ordered.

! **WARNING** Monitor patients with seizure disorders or thyrotoxicosis; and patients who are unusually responsive to sympathomimetic amines or are at risk for developing prolonged QT interval as serious adverse effects can occur.

! **WARNING** Monitor patients with a history of cardiovascular disorders such as arrhythmias, coronary insufficiency, hypertension, or hypertrophic obstructive cardiomyopathy. Notify prescriber of any significant increases in blood pressure or pulse rate or worsening of chronic conditions. Olodaterol may also cause ECG changes, such as flattening of the T wave, prolonged QT interval, and ST-segment depression. Drug may have to be discontinued if such reactions occur.

! **WARNING** Monitor patient's serum potassium level and assess for signs and symptoms of hypokalemia, especially if patient has severe COPD because hypokalemia may be made worse by hypoxia and concomitant treatment.

PATIENT TEACHING

- Advise patient, especially if she has a significant cardiac history, to inform prescriber of any other drugs she is taking before beginning olodaterol therapy and to keep prescriber informed of any new drug therapies while taking olodaterol.
- Instruct patient how to administer olodaterol.
- Caution patient not to increase olodaterol dosage or frequency without consulting prescriber because serious adverse reactions may occur.
- Urge patient to notify prescriber if her symptoms worsen, if olodaterol becomes less effective, or if she needs more inhalations of her prescribed short-acting beta$_2$-agonist than usual. This may indicate that her condition is worsening.

! **WARNING** Tell patient that olodaterol may cause paradoxical bronchospasms. If present, tell patient to discontinue drug and notify prescriber. If severe or unrelieved, stress importance of seeking emergency treatment to relieve bronchospasms.

! **WARNING** Alert patient that drug may cause an allergic reaction. If present, tell patient to notify prescriber and, if severe to seek immediate medical care.

! **WARNING** Instruct patient to notify prescriber immediately if chest pain, palpitations, rapid heart rate, or other troublesome effects are experienced while taking olodaterol because dosage may have to be adjusted.

omadacycline

Nuzyra

Class and Category

Pharmacologic class: Aminomethylcycline of the tetracycline class
Therapeutic class: Antibacterial

Indications and Dosages

∗ *To treat community-acquired bacterial pneumonia caused by* Chlamydophila pneumoniae, Haemophilus influenzae, H. parainfluenzae, Klebsiella pneumoniae, Legionella pneumophilia, Mycoplasma pneumoniae, Staphylococcus aureus *(methicillin-susceptible isolates),* or Streptococcus pneumoniae

I.V. INFUSION, TABLETS

Adults. *Loading:* 200-mg I.V. infused over 60 min once on day 1. Alternatively, 100-mg I.V. infused over 30 min twice on day 1 or 300 mg P.O. twice daily on day 1. *Maintenance:* 100 mg once daily I.V. infused over 30 min once daily for total of 7 to 14 days. Alternatively, 300 mg P.O. once daily for total of 7 to 14 days.

∗ *To treat acute bacterial skin structure and skin infections caused by* Enterobacter cloacae, Enterococcus faecalis, K. pneumoniae, S.anginosus *group,* S. aureus *(methicillin-susceptible and-resistant isolates),* S. lugdunensis, *or* S. pyogenes

I.V. INFUSION, TABLETS

Adults. *Loading:* 200-mg I.V. infused over 60 min once on day 1. Alternatively, 100-mg I.V. infused over 30 min twice on day 1 or 450 mg P.O. once daily on day 1 and day 2. *Maintenance:* 100-mg I.V. infused over 30 min once daily for total of 7 to 14 days. Alternatively, 300 mg P.O. once daily for total of 7 to 14 days.

Drug Administration

P.O.

- Administer oral tablets with water after patient has fasted for at least 4 hr.
- After administration, patient should not drink (except water) or eat for 2 hr and not ingest any antacids, dairy products, iron preparations, or multivitamins for 4 hr after administration.

I.V.

- Reconstitute each 100-mg vial with 5 ml of 0.9% Sodium Chloride Injection, 5% Dextrose Injection, or Sterile Water for Injection.
- Gently swirl contents and let vial stand until the cake has completely dissolved and any foam disperses. Do not shake vial. If needed, invert vial to dissolve any remaining powder and swirl gently, to prevent foaming. Reconstituted solution should be yellow to dark orange in color; if not, discard solution.
- Dilute further within 1 hr by withdrawing reconstituted solution from vial and adding it to 100 ml of 0.9% Sodium Chloride Injection or 5% Dextrose Injection in an intravenous bag. Concentration of the final diluted infusion solution will be either 1 mg/ml or 2 mg/ml depending on number of vials reconstituted.
- Use within 24 hr if diluted drug is left at room temperature or within 7 days, if refrigerated.
- If refrigerated, remove infusion bag from refrigerator and allow infusion bag to reach room temperature prior to use.
- Administer total infusion over 60 min for a 200-mg dose or a total infusion time of 30 min for a 100-mg dose.
- Infuse through a dedicated line or through a Y-site.
- If the same intravenous line is used for sequential infusion of several drugs, flush with 0.9% Sodium Chloride Injection or 5% Dextrose Injection before and after infusion.
- *Incompatibilities:* Other drugs, solutions other than 0.9% Sodium Chloride Injection, 5% Dextrose Injection, or Sterile Water

Route	Onset	Peak	Duration
P.O.	Unknown	2.5 hr	Unknown
I.V.	Unknown	0.5 hr	Unknown

Half-life: 15.5–16.8 hr

Mechanism of Action

Binds to the 30S ribosomal subunit and blocks protein synthesis, exerting a bacteriostatic effect as well as a bactericidal effect against some isolates of *S. pneumoniae* and *H. influenzae*.

Contraindications

Hypersensitivity to omadacycline, other tetracycline-class antibacterial drugs, or their components

Interactions

DRUGS

antacids containing aluminum, calcium, or magnesium; bismuth subsalicylate; iron preparations: Decreased absorption of oral omadacycline

anticoagulant drugs: Depressed plasma prothrombin activity

FOODS

all foods, especially dairy products: Decreased absorption of oral omadacycline

Adverse Reactions

CNS: Fatigue, headache, insomnia, lethargy, vertigo

CV: **Atrial fibrillation**, hypertension, tachycardia

EENT: Oral candidiasis, oropharyngeal pain, taste distortion

GI: Abdominal pain, ***Clostridioides difficile*–associated diarrhea**, constipation, diarrhea, dyspepsia, elevated bilirubin and liver enzymes, elevated lipase levels, nausea, vomiting

GU: Vulvovaginal mycotic infection

HEME: Anemia, thrombocytosis

SKIN: Excessive diaphoresis, erythema, pruritus, urticaria

Other: Elevated alkaline phosphatase or creatinine phosphokinase, **hypersensitivity reactions**, infusion-site reactions (erythema, induration, inflammation, irritation, pain, swelling)

Childbearing Considerations

PREGNANCY

- Drug causes fetal harm such as adverse effects on skeleton growth and tooth development when given during the second and third trimester.
- The use of drug during last half of pregnancy may cause permanent discoloration of the child's teeth.
- Drug should not be used during pregnancy unless there is no alternative and benefit to mother outweighs potential risk to fetus.

LACTATION

- It is not known if drug is present in breast milk.
- Breastfeeding is not recommended during drug therapy and for 4 days following the last dose.

REPRODUCTION

- Females of childbearing age should use effective contraception during drug therapy.
- Drug may reduce ovulation and increase embryonic loss in females of childbearing age, according to animal studies.
- Drug may cause injury to the testis and reduced motility and reduced sperm counts in male patients, according to animal studies.

Nursing Considerations

! **WARNING** Be aware that patients treated for community-acquired bacterial pneumonia with omadacycline may have a higher risk of death, especially patients over the age of 65 and patients with multiple disorders. Monitor patients with pneumonia closely for worsening and/or complications of infection and underlying conditions.

! **WARNING** Monitor patient for hypersensitivity reactions. Know that other tetracyclines have caused reactions, including anaphylaxis. If patient develops a reaction, notify prescriber and expect drug to be discontinued. Provide supportive care, as ordered and required.

! **WARNING** Assess patient for signs of secondary infection, such as profuse, watery diarrhea. If such diarrhea develops, contact prescriber and expect to obtain a stool specimen to rule out pseudomembranous colitis caused by *Clostridioides difficile*. Know that CDAD can range from being mild to causing fatal colitis. If *C. difficile* is confirmed, expect drug to be discontinued and an antibiotic effective against *C. difficile* ordered. Also, expect to administer electrolytes, fluids, and protein supplementation, as needed and ordered.

! **WARNING** Monitor patient for tetracycline-class effects, such as abnormal liver function tests, acidosis, azotemia, hyperphosphatemia, increased BUN, pancreatitis, photosensitivity, and pseudotumor cerebri. Expect omadacycline to be discontinued if any of these adverse reactions occurs.

PATIENT TEACHING

- Instruct patient how to administer oral omadacycline.
- Inform patient that nausea and vomiting may occur with omadacycline use, especially if patient received the oral loading dose for treatment of acute bacterial skin and skin structure infections.

! **WARNING** Alert patient that drug may cause an allergic reaction. If present, tell patient to notify staff if receiving drug intravenously. If receiving oral form of drug tell patient to stop drug and notify prescriber. If serious, tell patient to seek immediate medical care.

! **WARNING** Alert patient that diarrhea is a common problem with antibacterial drugs. However, urge patient to notify prescriber if diarrhea becomes severe. Inform patient that bloody or watery stools can occur even after omadacycline therapy has been discontinued.

! **WARNING** Tell patient to notify prescriber if any other persistent, serious, or unusual adverse reactions occur.

- Instruct females of childbearing age to use effective contraception during drug therapy and to notify prescriber if pregnancy occurs as drug will have to be discontinued. Alert male patients to possible adverse effects on reproduction.

- Advise mothers not to breastfeed their infant during omadacycline therapy and for 4 days after the last dose of drug.

omalizumab

Xolair

Class and Category

Pharmacologic class: Monoclonal antibody
Therapeutic class: Antiallergenic, antiasthmatic

Indications and Dosages

* *To treat moderate to severe persistent asthma in patients with positive skin test or in vitro reactivity to a perennial aeroallergen and symptoms have been inadequately controlled with inhaled corticosteroids*

SUBCUTANEOUS INJECTION

Adults and children ages 6 and older. 75 to 375 mg every 2 or 4 wk. Dose and frequency determined by body weight and blood IgE levels.

± **DOSAGE ADJUSTMENT** For patients with significant changes in body weight, dosage will need to be adjusted.

* *As add-on maintenance treatment for chronic rhinosinusitis with nasal polyps (CRSwNP) for patients with inadequate response to nasal corticosteroids*

SUBCUTANEOUS INJECTION

Adults. 75 mg to 600 mg every 2 to 4 wk. Dose and frequency determined by body weight and blood IgE levels.

± **DOSAGE ADJUSTMENT** For patients with significant changes in body weight, dosage will need to be adjusted.

* *To treat chronic idiopathic urticaria in patients who remain symptomatic despite H_1 antihistamine treatment*

SUBCUTANEOUS INJECTION

Adults and adolescents ages 12 and older. 150 or 300 mg every 4 wk.

* *To reduce allergic reactions (Type 1), including anaphylaxis that may occur with accidental exposure to one or more foods in patients with IgE-mediated food allergy*

SUBCUTANEOUS INJECTION

Adults and children ages 1 and older. 75 mg to 600 mg every 2 to 4 wk. Dose and frequency determined by body weight and blood IgE levels.

± **DOSAGE ADJUSTMENT** For patients with significant changes in body weight, dosage will need to be adjusted.

Drug Administration

SUBCUTANEOUS

Autoinjector

- Use only in patients ages 12 and older.
- Determine number of autoinjectors needed for dosage based on manufacturer's guidelines. Autoinjector is available in 3 strengths; ensure right combination of autoinjectors are used to administer dose if more than 1 autoinjector is required.
- Take autoinjector(s) out of refrigerator and set on a clean, flat surface for at least 30 to 45 min to allow drug to reach room temperature. Do not use heat sources to speed up warming process.
- When removing autoinjector from carton, do not turn carton upside down, do not remove cap until ready to inject, and do not hold autoinjector by the cap but instead hold the middle of the autoinjector.
- Solution should appear clear and colorless to pale brownish-yellow. Some air bubbles may be present.
- Sites to inject drug are the abdomen or anterior thigh surface.
- To inject, remove cap by pulling straight off. Do not twist the cap. Hold the autoinjector with needle guard directly against the skin at a 90-degree angle. Press straight down and hold autoinjector firmly against the skin. The first click heard indicates the injection has started. Green indicator will move within viewing window. Listen for the second click. This indicates injection is almost done. Keep holding autoinjector until green indicator has stopped moving and completely fills the viewing window. Remove autoinjector from skin. Do not rub the injection site.
- If more than 1 injection is needed, use a new autoinjector for each injection and inject at least 1 in apart form each other.

Prefilled syringes

- Used in patients of all ages.

- Determine the number of prefilled syringes needed for dosage based on manufacturer's guidelines taking into account body weight for patients younger than 12. Prefilled syringes are available in 3 dosage strengths; ensure right combination of syringes are used to administer dose if more than 1 syringe is required.
- Needle cap on syringes contain natural rubber latex, which may cause allergic reactions in latex sensitive individuals.
- Remove syringe(s) from refrigerator and place on a clean, flat surface for at least 30 to 45 min to allow drug to warm to room temperature. Do not use heat sources to speed up warming process.
- Take syringe out of blister package being careful not to flip the blister pack upside down and when removing syringe from blister pack hold the middle part of the syringe.
- Solution in syringe should be clear and colorless to pale brownish yellow. Some air bubbles may be present.
- Do not inject more than 150 mg per injection site.
- Inject into the abdomen or anterior aspect of thigh. Remove cap by pulling straight off. Do not twist the cap. Pinch skin. Inject needle all the way into the pinched skin at a 45-degree angle. Slowly push plunger all the way down until the plunger head is between the safety guard wings. Release the plunger and allow needle to be covered by needle-shield. Do not rub injection site.
- If dosage requires more than 1 injection, inject each one at least 1 in apart form each other.

Lyophilized powder

- Determine number of vials needed to be reconstituted (each vial delivers 150 mg/1.2 ml).
- Reconstitute each vial by adding 1.4 ml Sterile Water for Injection into a 3-ml syringe with a 1-inch 18 G needle. Place drug vial upright and inject Sterile Water for Injection into vial.
- Gently swirl upright vial for about 1 min to evenly wet powder. Don't shake. Every 5 min, gently swirl for 5 to 10 sec until solution contains no gel-like particles, which usually takes 15 to 20 min. Discard if powder takes longer than 40 min to dissolve and start with a new vial. Solution should be clear or slightly opalescent and may have a few small bubbles or foam around edge of vial.
- Use reconstituted omalizumab solution within 8 hr if refrigerated or 4 hr if stored at room temperature. Protect from sunlight.
- Remove reconstituted omalizumab from vial by inverting vial for 15 sec to let solution drain toward stopper. Using a new 3-ml syringe with a 1-in, 18 G needle, insert needle into inverted vial and position needle tip at the very bottom of solution in the vial stopper. Then, pull plunger all the way back to end of syringe barrel to remove all solution from inverted vial. To obtain full 150-mg dose (1 vial containing 1.2 ml of reconstituted omalizumab), all of the product must be withdrawn from vial before expelling any air or excess solution from syringe (0.6 ml will need to be expelled to obtain a dose of 75 mg). Replace needle with a 25 G needle for administration.
- Inject as a subcutaneous injection into the abdomen or anterior aspect of thigh. Injection may take up to 15 sec to administer.
- If more than 1 injection is required, administer each injection at least 1 in apart.
- If skin contact occurred while preparing or administering drug, wash area with water.
- Autoinjectors, prefilled syringes, and vials should be stored in refrigerator until ready for use. If autoinjector or prefilled syringe is removed from refrigerator and then placed back in the refrigerator without being used, total combined time out of the refrigerator should not exceed 2 days.

Route	Onset	Peak	Duration
SubQ	Unknown	7–8 days	Unknown

Half-life: 24–26 days

Mechanism of Action

Helps reduce inflammation by binding to circulating IgE and keeping it from binding to mast cells to inhibit degranulation and block release of histamine and other chemical mediators. Remember that in asthma, inflammation results when antigen reexposure causes mast cells to degranulate and release histamine and chemical mediators. Blocking these responses helps asthma and chronic rhinosinusitis with nasal polyp symptoms and urticaria to be less likely to develop.

Contraindications

Hypersensitivity to omalizumab or its components

Interactions

DRUGS

None reported by manufacturer.

Adverse Reactions

CNS: Anxiety, dizziness, fatigue, fever, headache, vertigo
CV: Peripheral edema
EENT: Earache, epistaxis, nasopharyngitis, oropharyngeal pain, otitis media, pharyngitis, sinusitis
GI: Gastroenteritis, nausea, upper abdominal pain
HEME: Eosinophilic conditions, **thrombocytopenia (severe)**
MS: Arm or leg pain, arthralgia, fractures, myalgia,
RESP: **Asthma**, bronchitis, cough, upper respiratory tract infection
SKIN: Alopecia, dermatitis, pruritus, rash, urticaria
Other: **Anaphylaxis**; antibodies to omalizumab; eosinophilic conditions; fungal infections; generalized pain; injection-site bruising, burning, hive or mass formation, induration, inflammation, itching, pain, redness, stinging, and warmth; lymphadenopathy; **malignancies**

Childbearing Considerations

PREGNANCY

- It is not known if drug causes fetal harm, but drug crosses the placental barrier.
- Drug is not recommended for use in pregnant patients.

LACTATION

- It is not known if drug is present in breast milk.
- Mothers should check with prescriber before breastfeeding.

Nursing Considerations

- Record patient's weight, and obtain blood IgE levels, as ordered, before starting omalizumab prescribed to treat asthma or chronic rhinosinusitis with nasal polps; dosage and dosing frequency are based on these factors.
- Be aware that inhaled or systemic corticosteroids should not be discontinued abruptly upon initiation of omalizumab therapy for asthma or chronic rhinosinusitis with nasal polyps. Instead, dosage should be discontinued gradually.

! **WARNING** Do not administer omalizumab for emergency treatment of allergic reactions, including anaphylaxis.

! **WARNING** Monitor patient closely for hypersensitivity reactions, particularly for first 2 hours after administration. Although rare, anaphylaxis has occurred as early as first dose and as late as more than 1 year after starting regular treatment. Be aware that patients with a history of anaphylaxis to drugs, foods, or other causes are at increased risk of omalizumab induced anaphylaxis. Monitor patient closely and keep emergency medication and equipment readily available. If present, notify prescriber immediately, expect drug to be discontinued and provide supportive care, as needed and ordered.

! **WARNING** Monitor patient's platelet count and patient for bleeding which could become severe. Institute bleeding precautions. Notify prescriber of any abnormalities.

! **WARNING** Monitor patient closely for signs of cancer because drug increases risk. Report any abnormal findings to prescriber.

- Monitor patient for persistent, serious, or unusual adverse reactions.
- Know that serum total IgE levels obtained less than 1 year following omalizumab discontinuation should not be used to reassess dosing regimen because these levels may not reflect steady-state free IgE levels. Elevated IgE levels may persist for up to 1 year following discontinuation of drug.

PATIENT TEACHING

! **WARNING** Explain that omalizumab prescribed for the treatment of asthma isn't used to treat acute bronchospasm or status asthmaticus. Tell patient to notify prescriber if asthma remains uncontrolled or worsens after initiation of omalizumab therapy.

! **WARNING** Tell patient omalizumab can not be used to treat emergency allergic reactions, including severe reactions.

- Tell patient not to abruptly stop any prescribed systemic or inhaled corticosteroid when starting omalizumab therapy because steroid dosage must be tapered gradually under prescriber's supervision. Also tell patient not to decrease dose or stop taking any other drugs or allergen immunotherapy unless directed to do so by prescriber because it takes time for improvement to occur in condition being treated.
- Alert patient that prefilled syringe needle cover contains latex and should not be used if allergic to latex. Have patient notify prescriber of latex allergy.
- Instruct patient or caregiver how to administer drug as a subcutaneous injection. Tell family or caregiver that if patient is under the age of 12 years, injection should be administered by an adult. If more than 1 injection (more than a 150 mg dose) is required, dosage should be split and injected in more than 1 injection site. Tell patient all injections should be administered consecutively and at 1 sitting.
- Caution patient that any improvement in his condition may take time.

! WARNING Alert patient that drug may cause an allergic reaction. If present, tell patient to notify prescriber and, if severe, to seek immediate medical care.

! WARNING Inform patient of risk of malignancy and suggest routine cancer screening. Instruct patient to notify prescriber of any unsual adverse reactions.

- Urge females of childbearing age, if she becomes pregnant, to notify prescriber as drug is not recommended for use during pregnancy.
- Encourage patient to comply with regularly scheduled prescriber visits.

omega-3-acid ethyl esters

Lovaza, Vascepa

Class and Category

Pharmacologic class: Ethyl esters
Therapeutic class: Antilipemic

Indications and Dosages

✱ As adjunct to diet to reduce severe triglyceride level that is equal to or exceeds 500 mg/dl

CAPSULES

Adults. 4 g once daily (Lovaza only) or 2 g twice daily (Vascepa with food).

✱ As adjunct to maximally tolerated statin therapy to reduce the risk of coronary revascularization, MI, stroke, and unstable angina in patients requiring hospitalization and who have elevated triglyceride levels of 150 mg/dl or greater with established cardiovascular disease or diabetes mellitus and 2 or more additional risk factors for cardiovascular disease

CAPSULES (VASCEPA)

Adults. 2 g twice daily with food.

Drug Administration

P.O.

- Capsules should be swallowed whole and not chewed, crushed, or opened.
- Administer Vascepa brand with food.

Route	Onset	Peak	Duration
P.O.	Unknown	5 hr	Unknown

Half-life: 89 hr

Mechanism of Action

May inhibit very-low-density lipoprotein and triglyceride synthesis in the liver to reduce triglyceride synthesis, which causes plasma triglyceride levels to decrease.

Contraindications

Hypersensitivity to omega-3-acid ethyl esters or their components

Interactions

DRUGS

anticoagulants, antiplatelets: Possibly increased bleeding time

Adverse Reactions

CV: Angina pectoris
EENT: Halitosis, nosebleeds, taste perversion
GI: Diarrhea, dyspepsia, eructation, nausea, vomiting
HEME: **Prolonged bleeding time, hemorrhagic diathesis**
MS: Back pain
SKIN: Bruising, rash, urticaria
Other: **Anaphylaxis**, flu-like symptoms

Childbearing Considerations

PREGNANCY

- It is not known if drug causes fetal harm.
- Use with caution only if benefit to mother outweighs potential risk to fetus.

LACTATION

- Drug is present in breast milk.
- Mothers should check with prescriber before breastfeeding.

Nursing Considerations

- Be aware that drugs known to increase triglyceride levels, such as beta-blockers, thiazide diuretics, and estrogens, should be discontinued or changed, if possible, before omega-3 ethyl ester therapy starts.
- Expect to check patient's triglyceride level before starting drug therapy and periodically throughout omega-3-acid ethyl ester therapy to determine effectiveness.
- Expect to stop omega-3-acid ethyl ester therapy after 2 months if patient's triglyceride level doesn't decrease as expected.

! **WARNING** Monitor patient for hypersensitivity reactions to drug that could become life-threatening, such as anaphylaxis. If present, notify prescriber, expect drug to be discontinued, and provide supportive care, as needed and ordered.

! **WARNING** Monitor patient with history of paroxysmal or persistent atrial fibrillation for recurrences of symptomatic atrial fibrillation or flutter, especially within the first 2 to 3 months of initiating omega-3 ethyl ester therapy.

PATIENT TEACHING

- Instruct patient how to take brand of omega-3-ethyl ester prescribed.

! **WARNING** Alert patient that drug may cause an allergic reaction. If present, tell patient to notify prescriber and, if severe, to seek immediate medical care. Also stress importance of patient alerting prescriber if chest pain occurs. If chest pain is not relieved quickly, urge patient to seek immediate medical care.

! **WARNING** Warn patient with a history of atrial fibrillation to notify prescriber if pulse becomes irregular.

- Explain that patient will need periodic laboratory tests to evaluate therapy.

omega 3-carboxylic acids

Epanova

Class and Category

Pharmacologic class: Fish oil derivative
Therapeutic class: Antilipemic

Indications and Dosages

✱ *As adjunct to diet to reduce triglyceride levels in patients with severe (equal to or greater than 500 mg/dl) hypertriglyceridemia*

CAPSULES

Adults. 2 or 4 g once daily.

Drug Administration

P.O.

- Capsules should be swallowed whole and not chewed, crushed, or opened.
- If a dose is missed, administer it as soon as possible but do not double the dose to make up for a missed dose.

Route	Onset	Peak	Duration
P.O.	Unknown	5–9 hr	Unknown

Half-life: 37–46 hr

Mechanism of Action

May reduce synthesis of triglycerides in the liver by inhibiting acyl-CoA-1,2 diacylglycerol acyltransferase, increasing mitochondrial and peroxisomal beta oxidation in the liver, decreasing lipogenesis in the liver, and increasing plasma lipoprotein lipase activity.

Contraindications

Hypersensitivity to omega 3-carboxylic acids or its components

Interactions

DRUGS

anticoagulants, antiplatelet agents: Possibly increased risk of bleeding

Adverse Reactions

CNS: Fatigue
CV: Elevated LDL-C levels
EENT: Difficulty swallowing, nasopharyngitis
GI: Abdominal discomfort, distention, or pain; constipation; diarrhea; eructation; flatulence; nausea; vomiting
MS: Arthralgia

Childbearing Considerations

PREGNANCY

- It is not known if drug causes fetal harm.
- Use with caution only if benefit to mother outweighs potential risk to fetus.

LACTATION

- It is not known if drug is present in breast milk.
- Mothers should check with prescriber before breastfeeding.

Nursing Considerations

! **WARNING** Monitor patient for signs and symptoms of a hypersensitivity reaction because omega 3-carboxylic acids contain polyunsaturated free fatty acids derived from fish oils and it is not known if cross-sensitivity exists. If present, notify prescriber, expect drug to be discontinued, and provide supportive care, as needed and ordered.

- Monitor LDL-C levels, as ordered, periodically during therapy with omega 3-carboxylic acids because drug may increase these levels in some patients.

PATIENT TEACHING

- Instruct patient how to administer omega 3-carboxylic acids and what to do if a dose is missed.
- Inform patient that drug therapy is not a substitution for dietary measures. Adherence to dietary restrictions must be continued.

! **WARNING** Tell patient to notify prescriber if any signs or symptoms of an allergic reaction occur and to seek immediate medical care, if severe.

omeprazole

Losec (CAN), Prilosec

omeprazole magnesium

Prilosec, Prilosec OTC

Class and Category

Pharmacologic class: Proton pump inhibitor
Therapeutic class: Antiulcer

Indications and Dosages

∗ *To treat frequent heartburn that occurs 2 or more days a week*

D.R. TABLETS, D.R. TABLETS ODT

Adults. 20 mg once daily before eating in the morning for 14 days. *Maximum:* No more than a 14 day course every 4 mo.

∗ *To treat symptomatic gastroesophageal reflux disease (GERD)*

D.R CAPSULES, D.R. ORAL SUSPENSION

Adults and adolescents ages 16 and older. 20 mg once daily for 4 wk.
Children ages 1 to 16 weighing 20 kg (44 lb) or more. 20 mg once daily for up to 4 wk.
Children ages 1 to 16 weighing 10 kg (22 lb) to less than 20 kg (44 lb). 10 mg once daily for up to 4 wk.
Children ages 1 to 16 weighing 5 kg (11 lb) to less than 10 kg (22 lb). 5 mg once daily for up to 4 wk.

∗ *To treat erosive esophagitis due to acid mediated GERD*

D.R. CAPSULES, D.R. ORAL SUSPENSION

Adults and adolescents ages 16 and older. 20 mg once daily for 4 to 8 wk.
Children ages 1 to 16 weighing 20 kg (44 lb) or more. 20 mg once daily for 4 to 8 wk.
Children ages 1 to 16 weighing 10 kg (22 lb) to less than 20 kg (44 lb). 10 mg once daily for 4 to 8 wk.
Children ages 1 to 16 weighing 5 kg (11 lb) to less than 10 kg (22 lb). 5 mg once daily for 4 to 8 wk.
Children ages 1 mo to less than 1 yr weighing 10 kg (22 lb) or more. 10 mg once daily up to 6 wk.
Children ages 1 mo to less than 1 yr weighing 5 kg (11 b) to less than 10 kg (22 lb). 5 mg once daily up to 6 wk.
Children ages 1 mo to less than 1 yr weighing 3 kg (6.6 lb) to less than 5 kg (11 lb). 2.5 mg once daily up to 6 wk.

∗ *To provide maintenance of healing of erosive esophagitis due to acid-mediated GERD*

D.R. CAPSULES, D.R. ORAL SUSPENSION

Adults and adolescents ages 16 and older. 20 mg once daily up to 12 mo.
Children ages 1 to 16 weighing 20 kg (44 lb) or more. 20 mg once daily up to 12 mo.
Children ages 1 to 16 weighing 10 kg (22 lb) to less than 20 kg (44 lb). 10 mg once daily up to 12 mo.

Children ages 1 to 16 weighing 5 kg (11 lb) to less than 10 kg (22 lb). 5 mg once daily for up to 12 mo.

±**DOSAGE ADJUSTMENT** For adult patients with hepatic impairment and Asian patients, dosage reduced to 10 mg once daily.

✱ *To provide short-term treatment of active benign gastric ulcer*

D.R. CAPSULES, D.R. ORAL SUSPENSION

Adults. 40 mg daily for 4 to 8 wk.

✱ *To treat active duodenal ulcer short-term*

D.R. CAPSULES, D.R. ORAL SUSPENSION

Adults. 20 mg once daily for 4 wk, with an additional 4 wk of therapy, as needed.

✱ *To eradicate* Helicobacter pylori *in order to reduce risk of duodenal ulcer recurrence*

D.R. CAPSULES, D.R. ORAL SUSPENSION

Adults. 40 mg once daily with clarithromycin 500 mg 3 times daily for 14 days. If ulcer present at start of therapy, 20 mg once daily for an additional 14 days. Alternatively, 20 mg twice daily with amoxicillin 1,000 mg twice daily, and clarithromycin 500 mg twice daily for 10 days. If ulcer is present at start of therapy, 20 mg once daily for an additional 18 days.

✱ *To provide long-term treatment of gastric hypersecretory conditions, such as multiple endocrine adenoma syndrome, systemic mastocytosis, and Zollinger-Ellison syndrome*

D.R. CAPSULES, D.R. ORAL SUSPENSION

Adults. 60 mg once daily, and increased as needed. For doses greater than 80 mg give in divided doses. *Maximum:* 120 mg 3 times daily.

Drug Administration

P.O.

- Give omeprazole before meals, preferably in the morning for once-daily dosing and before breakfast and dinner for twice-daily dosing. An antacid may also be given, as prescribed.
- Tablets (including ODT tablets) and capsules should be swallowed whole with water and not chewed, crushed, or split/opened. If patient has difficulty swallowing tablets or capsules, oral suspension form should be used.
- To prepare oral suspension form, empty powder into a container with 5 ml of water (2.5-mg packet) or 15 ml of water (10-mg packet). Stir. Let thicken for 2 to 3 min. Stir and administer within 30 min. If any material remains after patient drinks solution, add more water, stir, and have patient drink residual solution.
- To administer via a gastric or nasogastric tube, add 5 ml of water to a catheter-tipped syringe and then add contents of 2.5-mg packet (or 15 ml of water for 10-mg packet). Immediately shake the syringe and allow to thicken for 2 to 3 min. Shake syringe again and inject through tubing within 30 min. Refill syringe with equal amount of water, shake, and flush any remaining contents into tube.

Route	Onset	Peak	Duration
P.O.	1 hr	0.5–3.5 hr	72–96 hr

Half-life: 0.5–1 hr

Contraindications

Concurrent therapy with rilpivirine-containing products; hypersensitivity to omeprazole, substituted benzimidazoles, or their components

Interactions

DRUGS

atazanavir, nelfinavir, rilpivirine: Decreased plasma levels of these agents; promote drug resistance to these drugs
cilostazol diazepam, digoxin, phenytoin, tacrolimus: Increased exposure of these drugs
citalopram: Increased exposure of citalopram leading to increased risk of QT prolongation
clopidogrel: Reduced effectiveness of clopidogrel
CYP2C19 or CYP3A4 inducers, such as rifampin, St. John's wort: Decreased exposure of omeprazole
CYP2C19 or CYP3A4 inhibitors, such as voriconazole: Increased exposure of omeprazole
dasatinib, erlotinib, iron salts, itraconazole, ketoconazole, mycophenolate mofetil, nilotinib: Reduced absorption of these drugs
methotrexate: Possibly delayed methotrexate elimination and increased risk of toxicity
saquinavir: Increased plasma saquinavir level and risk of toxicity
St. John's wort, rifampin: Decreased plasma omeprazole level
warfarin: Possibly increased risk of abnormal bleeding

Mechanism of Action

Interferes with gastric acid secretion by inhibiting the hydrogen potassium adenosine triphosphatase (H+ K+ -ATPase) enzyme system, or proton pump, in gastric parietal cells. Remember that normally, the proton pump uses energy from hydrolysis of adenosine triphosphate to drive hydrogen (H^+) and chloride (Cl^-) out of parietal cells and into the stomach lumen in exchange for potassium (K^+), which leaves the stomach lumen and enters parietal cells. Following this exchange, H^+ and Cl^- combine in the stomach to form hydrochloric acid (HCl), as shown below left. Irreversibly blocks the exchange of intracellular H^+ and extracellular K^+, as shown below right. Preventing H^+ from entering the stomach lumen, omeprazole keeps additional HCl from forming.

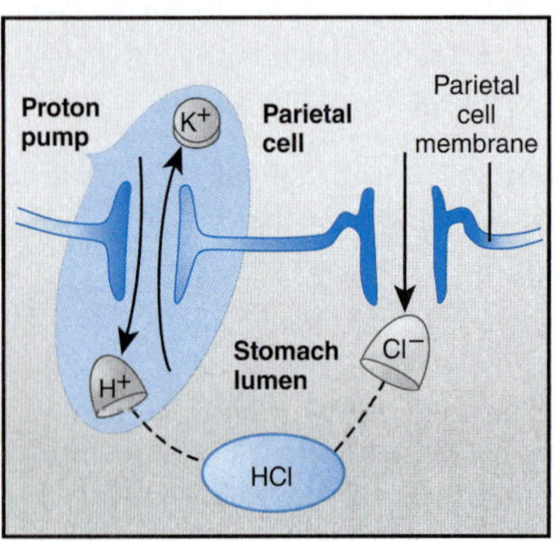

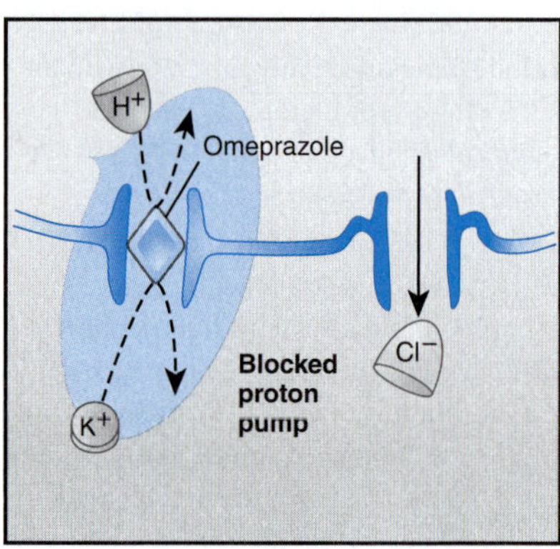

Adverse Reactions

CNS: Agitation, asthenia, dizziness, drowsiness, fatigue, fever, headache, malaise, psychic disturbance, somnolence
CV: Chest pain, hypertension, peripheral edema
EENT: Anterior ischemic, optic atrophy or neuritis, optic neuropathy, otitis media, stomatitis
ENDO: **Hypoglycemia**
GI: Abdominal pain, acid regurgitation, constipation, diarrhea, ***Clostridioides difficile*-associated diarrhea**, dyspepsia, elevated liver enzymes, flatulence, fundic gland polyps (long-term use), **hepatic dysfunction or failure**, indigestion, nausea, **pancreatitis**, vomiting
GU: Acute tubulointerstitial nephritis, elevated serum creatinine, erectile dysfunction, glycosuria, hematuria, interstitial nephritis, microscopic pyuria, proteeinuria, testicular pain, urinary frequency, UTI
HEME: **Agranulocytosis**, anemia, **hemolytic anemia**, **leukopenia**, leukocytosis, **neutropenia**, **pancytopenia**, **thrombocytopenia**
MS: Back pain, bone fracture, joint pain
RESP: **Bronchospasms**, cough, upper respiratory infection
SKIN: Acute generalized exanthematous pustulosis, alopecia, cutaneous lupus erythematosus, dry skin, **erythema multiforme**, hyperhidrosis, petechiae, photosensitivity, pruritus, purpura, rash, **Stevens-Johnson syndrome**, **toxic epidermal necrolysis**, urticaria
Other: **Anaphylaxis**, **angioedema**, **drug reaction with eosinophilia and systemic symptoms (DRESS)**, **hypocalcemia**, **hypokalemia**, **hypomagnesemia**, **hyponatremia**, systemic lupus erythematosus, vitamin B_{12} deficiency (long-term use), weight gain

Childbearing Considerations

PREGNANCY

- It is not known if drug causes fetal harm.
- Use with caution only if benefit to mother outweighs potential risk to fetus.

LACTATION

- Drug may be present in breast milk.
- Mothers should check with prescriber before breastfeeding.

Nursing Considerations

- Know that proton pump inhibitors, such as omeprazole, should not be prescribed longer than medically necessary.
- Know that both cutaneous and systemic lupus erythematosus have occurred within days to years after proton pump therapy, such as omeprazole, was initiated. The most common symptoms presented were arthralgia, cytopenia, and rash. Report such findings to prescriber.

! **WARNING** Monitor patient after drug administration for bronchospasms. If present, withhold drug and notify prescriber. Provide supportive care, as needed and ordered.

! **WARNING** Monitor patient for hypersensitivity reactions, which could become life-threatening such as anaphylaxis or angioedema. Also, monitor patient for severe cutaneous adverse reactions that may begin with a rash. (Know that DRESS may only initially present with a fever or swollen lymph nodes.). Be aware omeprazole should not be given to patients who have developed a hypersensitivity or serious skin reaction in the past. If present, notify prescriber, expect drug to be discontinued, and provide supportive care, as needed and ordered.

! **WARNING** Monitor patient for bronchospasms. If present, notify prescriber immediately, expect drug to be discontinued, and provide supportive care, as needed and ordered.

! **WARNING** Monitor patient's renal function closely because drug may cause adverse effects on the kidneys. If renal function deteriorates, notify prescriber and expect drug to be discontinued.

! **WARNING** Be aware that long-term use of omeprazole may increase the risk of gastric carcinoma and symptomatic response to omeprazole therapy does not rule out the presence of gastric tumors.

! **WARNING** Keep in mind that if omeprazole is given with antibiotics, watch for diarrhea from *Clostridioides difficile*, which may be mild or become life-threatening. If *C. difficile* is suspected, expect to obtain a stool specimen. If diagnosis is confirmed, notify prescriber and expect to withhold drug and treat with electrolytes, fluids, protein, and an antibiotic effective against *C. difficile*, as ordered.

! **WARNING** Monitor the patient, especially the patient on long-term therapy, for hypomagnesemia. Hypomagnesemia may lead to hypocalcemia and/or hypokalemia and may exacerbate underling hypocalcemia in patients at risk. If patient is to remain on omeprazole long term, expect to monitor the patient's serum magnesium level, as ordered, and if level becomes low, anticipate magnesium replacement therapy and omeprazole to be discontinued.

- Know that because drug can interfere with absorption of vitamin B_{12}, monitor patient for macrocytic anemia.
- Monitor patient for bone fracture, especially in patients receiving multiple daily doses for more than a year because proton pump inhibitors, such as omeprazole, increase risk for osteoporosis-related fractures of the hip, spine, or wrist.
- Know that omeprazole therapy may produce false elevations of serum chromogranin levels, used to help diagnosis presence of neuroendocrine tumors. If test results are high, withhold omeprazole therapy temporarily and repeat test, as ordered.

PATIENT TEACHING

- Instruct patient how to administer form of omeprazole prescribed.
- Encourage patient to avoid alcohol, aspirin products, ibuprofen, and foods that may increase gastric secretions during therapy. Tell the patient to notify all prescribers about prescription drug use.

! **WARNING** Alert patient that drug may cause bronchospasms. If patient develops difficulty breathing after drug is taken, tell patient to seek immediate medical care.

! **WARNING** Alert patient that drug may cause serious allergic and skin reactions that could be severe. At first sign of a fever, rash, or swollen lymph nodes, tell patient to stop drug and notify prescriber. If severe, tell patient to seek immediate medical care.

! **WARNING** Advise patient to notify prescriber if patient notices a decrease in the amount of urine voided or there is blood in the urine. Also, tell the patient to notify prescriber if new or worsening joint pain or a rash on his arms or cheeks that gets worse in the sun occurs.

! **WARNING** Advise patient to notify prescriber immediately about abdominal pain or diarrhea. Also, tell patient to stop taking omeprazole and notify prescriber if other persistent, serious, or unusual reactions occur.

ondansetron

Zuplenz

ondansetron hydrochloride

Class and Category

Pharmacologic class: Selective serotonin ($5\text{-}HT_3$) receptor antagonist
Therapeutic class: Antiemetic

Indications and Dosages

* *To prevent nausea and vomiting associated with highly emetogenic cancer chemotherapy*

DISINTEGRATING TABLETS, ORAL SOLUTION, ORAL SOLUBLE FILM (ZUPLENZ), TABLETS

Adults. 24 mg 30 min before chemotherapy. Films and disintegrating tablets given as three 8-mg doses (allowing each 8-mg film or disintegrating tablet to dissolve completely before another given).

I.V. INFUSION

Adults and children ages 6 mo to 18 yr. Three 0.15-mg/kg doses, starting with first dose given 30 min before chemotherapy and second and third doses given 4 and 8 hr after first dose. Infused over 15 min for each dose. *Maximum:* 16 mg given as three 0.15 mg/kg doses.

* *To prevent nausea and vomiting associated with moderately emetogenic cancer chemotherapy*

DISINTEGRATING TABLETS, ORAL SOLUTION, ORAL SOLUBLE FILM (ZUPLENZ), TABLETS

Adults and adolescents ages 12 and older. *Initial:* One 8-mg dose given 30 min before chemotherapy and one 8-mg dose given 8 hr after the first dose. Then, one 8-mg dose given every 12 hr for 1 to 2 days after completion of chemotherapy.
Children ages 4 to 11. *Initial:* One 4-mg dose given 30 min before chemotherapy with one 4-mg dose given 4 and 8 hr after the first dose. Then, one 4-mg dose given every 8 hr for 1 to 2 days after completion of chemotherapy.

* *To prevent nausea and vomiting associated with initial and repeat courses of emetogenic chemotherapy*

I.V. INFUSION

Adults and children ages 6 mo to 18 yr. Three 0.15-mg/kg doses, starting with first dose given 30 min before chemotherapy and second and third doses given 4 and 8 hr after first dose. I.V. infusion given over 15 min. *Maximum:* 16 mg per dose.

* *To prevent nausea and vomiting associated with radiotherapy in patients receiving either total body irradiation, single high-dose fraction to the abdomen, or daily fractions to the abdomen*

DISINTEGRATING TABLETS, ORAL SOLUTION, ORAL SOLUBLE FILM (ZUPLENZ), TABLETS

Adults receiving total body irradiation. 8-mg dose given 1 to 2 hr before each fraction of radiotherapy administered each day.
Adults receiving single high-dose fraction radiotherapy to the abdomen. 8-mg dose given 1 to 2 hr before radiotherapy, with subsequent 8-mg doses given every 8 hr after the first dose for 1 to 2 days after completion of radiotherapy.
Adults receiving daily fractionated radiotherapy to the abdomen. 8-mg dose given 1 to 2 hr before radiotherapy with subsequent 8-mg doses given every 8 hr after the first dose for each day radiotherapy is given.

* *To prevent postoperative nausea and vomiting*

DISINTEGRATING TABLETS, ORAL SOLUTION, TABLETS

Adults. 16 mg as a single dose 1 hr before anesthesia induction.

ORAL SOLUBLE FILM (ZUPLENZ)

Adults. 16 mg given as two 8-mg films (first 8-mg film allowed to dissolve completely before second 8-mg film given) 1 hr before induction of anesthesia.

I.V. INJECTION

Adults and children ages 12 and older. 4 mg injected undiluted over at least 30 sec but preferably over 2 to 5 min as a single dose just before anesthesia induction or if nausea or vomiting develops within 2 hr after surgery, providing no prophylactic antiemetics had been given preoperatively.

Children ages 1 mo to 12 yr weighing more than 40 kg (88 lb). 4 mg injected undiluted over at least 30 sec but preferably over 2 to 5 min as a single dose just before anesthesia induction or if nausea or vomiting develops within 2 hr after surgery, providing no prophylactic antiemetics had been given preoperatively.

Children ages 1 mo to 12 yr weighing 40 kg (88 lb) or less. 0.1 mg/kg injected undiluted over at least 30 sec but preferably over 2 to 5 min as a single dose just before or immediately after anesthesia induction or if nausea or vomiting develops within 2 hr after surgery, providing no prophylactic antiemetics had been given preoperatively.

I.M. INJECTION

Adults and children ages 12 and older. 4 mg undiluted as a single dose just before anesthesia induction or if nausea within 2 hr after surgery, providing no prophylactic antiemetics had been given preoperatively.

±**DOSAGE ADJUSTMENT** For patients with severe hepatic impairment, maximum dosage limited to 8 mg daily I.V. or P.O.

Drug Administration

P.O.

- For orally disintegrating tablet administration: With dry, gloved hands, open blister containing orally disintegrating tablet by peeling backing off. Don't push tablet through foil blister. Place on top of patient's tongue. It will dissolve in seconds. Then, have patient swallow with saliva. A drink afterward is not needed.
- For oral film administration: With dry, gloved hands, open film pouch and immediately place film on top of patient's tongue. It will dissolve in 4 to 20 sec. Then, have patient swallow with or without a beverage. If using more than 1 film, allow each film to dissolve completely before administering the next film.
- For oral solution administration: Use calibrated container or oral syringe to measure dose of oral solution. Store at room temperature and protect from light. Oral solution container should also be stored upright.

I.V.

- Drug may precipitate at the stopper/vial interface in vials stored upright. If this happens, resolubilize by shaking the vial vigorously.
- For I.V. infusion used to prevent nausea and vomiting related to chemotherapy: Dilute drug for adults in 50 ml of 0.9% Sodium Chloride Injection or 5% Dextrose in Water. In children, dilute drug in 10 to 50 ml of 0.9% Sodium Chloride Injection or 5% Dextrose in Water depending on fluid needs. Infuse over 15 min.
- After dilution, solution is stable at room temperature under normal lighting conditions for 48 hr if diluted with 0.9% Sodium Chloride Injection, 5% Dextrose Injection, 5% Dextrose combined with either 0.45% or 0.9% Sodium Chloride Injection, or 3% Sodium Chloride Injection.
- For I.V. injection used to prevent postoperative nausea and vomiting: Inject undiluted over at least 30 sec but preferably over 2 to 5 min.
- *Incompatibilities:* Alkaline solutions

I.M.

- Administer undiluted into a large muscle mass.

Route	Onset	Peak	Duration
P.O.	30 min	1–2 hr	Unknown
I.V.	5 min	10 min	Unknown
I.M.	Unknown	30 min	Unknown

Half-life: 3.1–5.8 hr

Mechanism of Action

Blocks serotonin receptors centrally in the chemoreceptor trigger zone and peripherally at vagal nerve terminals in the intestine to reduce nausea and vomiting by preventing serotonin release in the small intestine

N O

(probable cause of chemotherapy- and radiation-induced nausea and vomiting) and by blocking signals to the CNS. May also bind to other serotonin receptors and to mu-opioid receptors.

Contraindications

Concomitant use of apomorphine, hypersensitivity to ondansetron or its components

Interactions

DRUGS

5-HT_3 receptor antagonists, selective serotonin reuptake inhibitors, serotonin and noradrenaline reuptake inhibitors: Increased risk of serotonin syndrome
carbamazepine, phenytoin, rifampin: Possibly decreased ondansetron blood concentrations
tramadol: Possibly interference with pain control from tramadol

Adverse Reactions

CNS: Agitation, akathisia, anxiety, ataxia, dizziness, drowsiness, dystonia, fever, headache, **hypotension**, restlessness, seizures, **serotonin syndrome**, syncope, somnolence, thirst, weakness
CV: **Arrhythmias**, **cardiopulmonary arrest** (parenteral form), chest pain, **hypotension**, **myocardial ischemia**, palpitations, **prolonged QT interval**, **shock**, tachycardia, **torsades de pointes**
EENT: Accommodation disturbances, altered taste, blurred vision, dry mouth, **laryngeal edema**, **laryngospasm**, **stridor**, transient blindness
GI: Abdominal pain, anorexia, constipation, diarrhea, elevated liver enzymes, flatulence, indigestion, **intestinal obstruction**, masking of progressive gastric and ileus distention
RESP: **Bronchospasms**, **pulmonary embolism**, shortness of breath
SKIN: Flushing, hyperpigmentation, maculopapular rash, pruritus, **Stevens-Johnson syndrome**, **toxic epidermal necrolysis**, urticaria
Other: **Anaphylaxis**; **angioedema**; hiccups; injection-site burning, pain, and redness

Childbearing Considerations

PREGNANCY

- It is not known if drug causes fetal harm.
- Use with caution only if benefit to mother outweighs potential risk to fetus.

LACTATION

- Drug may be present in breast milk.
- Mothers should check with prescriber before breastfeeding.

Nursing Considerations

! WARNING Know that if hypokalemia or hypomagnesemia is present, these electrolyte imbalances should be corrected before ondansetron is administered because of increased risk for QT-interval prolongation, which could predispose the patient to develop torsades de pointes. Monitor patient's electrocardiogram, as ordered, and especially in patients with bradyarrhythmias, congestive heart failure, hypokalemia, or hypomagnesemia or in patients taking other medications known to prolong the QT interval. Be aware that no dosage greater than 16 mg should be given intravenously at any 1time due to increased risk of prolonged QT interval.

! WARNING Be aware that oral disintegrating tablets may contain aspartame, which is metabolized to phenylalanine and must be avoided in patients with phenylketonuria.

! WARNING Monitor patient for chest pain that may be caused by myocardial ischemia and which may appear immediately after administration of drug.

! WARNING Monitor patient closely for a hypersensitivity reaction, which could become life-threatening, such as anaphylaxis and bronchospasm. If present, discontinue drug, notify prescriber, and provide supportive care, as needed and ordered.

! WARNING Monitor patient closely for serotonin syndrome, which may include agitation, chills, confusion, diaphoresis, diarrhea, fever, hyperactive reflexes, poor coordination, restlessness, shaking, talking or acting with uncontrolled excitement, tremor, and twitching.

- Be aware that ondansetron may mask symptoms of adynamic progressive ileus or gastric distention after abdominal surgery. Monitor patient for decreased bowel activity, especially if patient has risk factors for GI obstruction.

PATIENT TEACHING

- Instruct patient how to administer form of ondansetron prescribed.

! **WARNING** Tell patient that oral disintegrating tablets may contain aspartame, which should be advoided in patients with phenylketonuria. However, inform patient each 4- and 8-mg orally disintegrating tablet contains less than 0.03 mg phenylalanine.

! **WARNING** Warn patient that drug may cause chest pain, which could occur immediately after drug is taken. If present, tell patient to seek immediate medical care.

! **WARNING** Advise patient drug may cause an allergic reaction, including difficulty breathing. If present, tell patient to notify prescriber and seek immediate medical care.

! **WARNING** Advise patient to notify prescriber if patient experiences persistent, serious, unusual, or worsening symptoms.

- Reassure patient with transient blindness that it will resolve within a few minutes to 48 hours.

opicapone

Ongentys

Class and Category

Pharmacologic class: Catechol-O-methyltransferase (COMT) inhibitor
Therapeutic class: Antiparkinsonian

Indications and Dosages

✳ *As adjunct to treat levodopa/carbidopa in patients with Parkinson's disease experiencing "off" episodes*

CAPSULES

Adults. 50 mg once daily at bedtime.

± **DOSAGE ADJUSTMENT** For patients with moderate hepatic impairment, dosage reduced to 25 mg once daily.

Drug Administration

P.O.

- Administer drug at bedtime.
- Patient should not eat food for 1 hr before and for at least 1 hr after taking drug.
- If a dose is missed, administer next dose at scheduled time.

Route	Onset	Peak	Duration
P.O.	Unknown	Unknown	< 24 hr

Half-life: 1–2 hr

Mechanism of Action

Prevents the breakdown of levodopa where it turns into dopamine in the brain to help maintain normal movement in Parkinson's disease.

Contraindications

Concomitant use of nonselective MAO inhibitors; hypersensitivity to opicapone or its components; presence of paraganglioma, pheochromocytoma, or other catecholamine-secreting neoplasms

Interactions

DRUGS

drugs metabolized by COMT, such as dobutamine, dopamine, epinephrine, isoproterenol, norepinephrine; nonselective MAO inhibitors, such as isocarboxazid, phenelzine, tranylcypromine: Increased levels of catecholamines, possibly leading to arrhythmias, excessive changes in blood pressure, and increased heart rate

Adverse Reactions

CNS: Agitation, aggressiveness, delusions, dizziness, dyskinesia, falling asleep during daytime, hallucinations, lack of impulse control, insomnia, somnolence, syncope
CV: Hypertension, **hypotension**
EENT: Dry mouth
GI: Constipation
Other: Elevated creatine kinase levels, weight loss

Childbearing Considerations

PREGNANCY

- It is not known if drug can cause fetal harm. However, animal studies suggest the possibility of fetal abnormalities.
- Use with caution only if benefit to mother outweighs potential risk to fetus.

LACTATION

- It is not known if drug is present in breast milk.
- Mothers should check with prescriber before breastfeeding.

Nursing Considerations

! **WARNING** Know that opicapone should not be given to patients with severe hepatic impairment.

! **WARNING** Be aware that opicapone should not be discontinued abruptly.

! **WARNING** Monitor patient's blood pressure because opicapone may cause both orthostatic and nonorthostatic hypotension. If hypotension occurs, notify prescriber, as drug may have to be discontinued or a dosage reduction in a concomitantly administered antihypertensive drug may be needed.

! **WARNING** Be aware that a symptom complex resembling neuroleptic malignant syndrome (altered consciousness, autonomic instability, elevated temperature, and muscular rigidity) has occurred when opicapone dosage has been rapidly reduced, drug is withdrawn, or changes are made in dosages of other drugs that increase central dopaminergic tone. When drug is discontinued, monitor patient closely for adverse effects and expect prescriber to make adjustment of other dopaminergic therapies, as needed.

- Provide safety measures for patients receiving opicapone because drug may cause patient to fall asleep during activities of daily living. Monitor patient for excessive drowsiness but know that patient may feel alert immediately prior to falling asleep. Notify prescriber of such problems, as drug may have to be discontinued. Also, if other drugs are being taken, such as other dopaminergic or sedating drugs, dosage of any of these drugs may have to be reduced.
- Monitor patient for the development of dyskinesia or exacerbation of preexisting dyskinesia, as this was the most common adverse reaction associated with drug. Notify prescriber if present.
- Monitor patient for hallucinations and psychotic-like behavior. If present, notify prescriber, as drug may have to be discontinued.

PATIENT TEACHING

- Instruct patient, family, or caregiver how to administer opicapone and what to do if a dose is missed.

! **WARNING** Urge patient not to discontinue opicapone suddenly.

- Alert patient and family or caregiver that falling asleep during activities of daily living may occur without warning. Caution patient to avoid driving, operating machinery, and other hazardous activity until effect of drug is known and resolved.
- Tell patient to rise from a lying or sitting position slowly to avoid fainting or light-headedness.
- Review adverse reactions with patient, family, or caregiver, especially abnormal movement of body parts, hallucinations, and psychotic-like behaviors; falling asleep suddenly; and/or experiencing intense urges to binge-eat, gamble, have sex, or spend money. If present, instruct patient to notify prescriber.

! **WARNING** Tell patient to call prescriber if symptoms of confusion, fever, or severe muscle stiffness occur.

! **WARNING** Tell patient to notify prescriber if other persistent, serious, or unusual adverse reactions occur.

- Inform patient and family or caregiver to tell all prescribers that opicapone is being taken as well as any other drugs, including dietary supplements, herbal products, and over-the-counter drugs.

oritavancin diphosphate

Kimyrsa, Orbactiv

Class and Category

Pharmacologic class: Lipoglycopeptide
Therapeutic class: Antibiotic

Indications and Dosages

* *To treat acute bacterial skin and skin structure infections caused by gram-positive microorganisms, such as* Enterococcus faecalis *(vancomycin-susceptible isolates only),* Staphylococcus aureus *(including methicillin-susceptible and methicillin-resistant isolates),* Streptococcus agalactiae, S. dysgalactiae, S. anginosus *group (*S. anginosus, S. constellatus, S. intermedius*), or* S. pyogenes

I.V. INFUSION

Adults. 1,200 mg infused over 1 hr as a 1-time dose.

Drug Administration

- Be aware that there are 2 oritavancin products that are different in the following ways: dose strengths, duration of infusion, reconstitution and dilution instructions, and compatible diluents. Be sure the correct product is being prepared and administered properly.

Kimyrsa

- Reconstitute drug by adding 40 ml of Sterile Water for Injection to 1 vial to provide a 30 mg/ml solution.
- Gently swirl contents to avoid foaming and ensure that all powder is completely dissolved. Solution should appear clear and colorless to pink.
- Dilute by withdrawing and discarding 40 ml from a 250-ml intravenous bag of either 0.9% Sodium Chloride Injection or 5% Dextrose in Water. Withdraw 40 ml of drug from vial and add to intravenous bag to bring volume back to 250 ml yielding 4.8 mg/ml.
- The combined storage time (reconstituted solution in the vial and diluted solution in the bag) and 1-hr infusion time should not exceed 4 hr at room temperature or 12 hr if refrigerated.
- Flush intravenous line with 0.9% Sodium Chloride Injection or 5% Dextrose in Water solution before and after administering drug.
- Infuse drug over 1 hr. If patient develops an infusion-related reaction, such as flushing, pruritus, or urticaria, slow or stop the infusion and notify prescriber.
- *Incompatibilities for Kimyrsa:* Drugs formulated at a basic or neutral pH or solutions other than 0.9% Sodium Chloride Injection or 5% Dextrose in Water, other drugs

Orbactiv

- Reconstitute drug by adding 40 ml of Sterile Water for Injection to each vial (3 vials are needed) to provide a 10-mg/ml solution per vial. Gently swirl to avoid foaming and to completely dissolve the powder. Solution should appear clear, colorless to pale yellow.
- Withdraw and discard 120 ml from a 1,000-ml intravenous bag of 5% Dextrose in Water (never use 0.9% Sodium Chloride Injection). Then, withdraw 40 ml from each of the 3 reconstituted vials and add to 5% Dextrose in Water intravenous bag to bring bag volume back to 1,000 ml. This will yield a concentration of 1.2 mg/ml.
- Once mixed in infusion bag, use within 6 hr when stored at room temperature or within 12 hr when refrigerated. Time to reconstitute solution, dilute solution, and 3-hr infusion time should not exceed the storage time.
- Flush intravenous line with 5% Dextrose in Water solution before and after administering drug.
- Infuse drug over 3 hr. If patient develops an infusion-related reaction, such as flushing, pruritus, or urticaria, slow or stop the infusion and notify prescriber.
- *Incompatibilities for Orbactiv:* 0.9% Sodium Chloride Injection solution, other solutions containing 0.9% Sodium Chloride Injection, other additives or drugs mixed in 0.9% Sodium Chloride Injection, drugs formulated with a basic or neutral pH (possibly)

Route	Onset	Peak	Duration
I.V.	Unknown	Unknown	Unknown

Half-life: 245 hr

Mechanism of Action

Kills bacteria by inhibiting cell wall synthesis.

Contraindications

Hypersensitivity to oritavancin and its components, intravenous unfractionated heparin sodium administration used within 5 days following oritavancin administration

Interactions

DRUGS

drugs with a narrow therapeutic window that are predominantly metabolized by CYP450 enzymes: Possibly decreased or increased concentration of these drugs

warfarin: Increased risk of bleeding

Adverse Reactions

CNS: Dizziness, headache
CV: Peripheral edema, tachycardia
ENDO: **Hypoglycemia**
GI: ***Clostridioides difficile*–associated diarrhea**, diarrhea, elevated liver enzymes, nausea, vomiting

HEME: Anemia, eosinophilia
MS: Myalgia, osteomyelitis, tenosynovitis
RESP: **Bronchospasm**, wheezing
SKIN: **Erythema multiforme**, leukocytoclastic vasculitis, pruritus, rash, urticaria
Other: **Anaphylaxis**; **angioedema**; antibodies to oritavancin; hyperuricemia; infusion reactions, such as back or chest pain, chills, erythema, flushing of the upper body, pruritus, tremor, or urticaria; infusion-site extravasation, induration, or phlebitis

Childbearing Considerations

PREGNANCY

- It is not known if drug causes fetal harm.
- Use with caution only if benefit to mother outweighs potential risk to fetus.

LACTATION

- Drug may be present in breast milk.
- Mothers should check with prescriber before breastfeeding.

Nursing Considerations

- Use oritavancin cautiously in patients with a history of hypersensitivity to glycopeptides because of the possibility of cross-sensitivity.

! **WARNING** Monitor patient for a hypersensitivity reaction, which may become life-threatening, such as anaphylaxis or angioedema. If present, discontinue infusion immediately, notify prescriber, and provide supportive care, as needed and ordered.

! **WARNING** Assess patient for signs of secondary infection, such as profuse, watery diarrhea. If such diarrhea develops, contact prescriber and expect to obtain a stool specimen to rule out pseudomembranous colitis caused by *Clostridioides difficile*. If confirmed, know that *C.difficile* infection may range from being mild to causing fatal colitis. Expect to withhold drug and treat with an antibiotic effective against *C. difficile*, as ordered. Also expect to give electrolytes, fluids, protein supplementation, as needed and ordered.

! **WARNING** Monitor patient closely for signs of bleeding, especially if patient is taking warfarin therapy because drug may artificially prolong and INR for up to 12 hours, making monitoring of the effectiveness of warfarin unreliable for at least 12 hours after the administration of oritavancin. Drug may also artificially prolong aPTT for up to 120 hours and activated clotting time (ACT) for up to 24 hours after a single 1,200-mg dose of oritavancin. If patient requires monitoring of anticoagulation effects, a nonphospholipid-dependent coagulation test, such as Factor Xa assay or an alternative anticoagulant not requiring aPTT monitoring, may be required.

- Monitor patient for osteomyelitis, as drug has been shown to produce more cases of osteomyelitis than vancomycin used to treat similar infections. If present, be prepared to institute appropriate alternative antibacterial therapy.

PATIENT TEACHING

- Instruct patient that oritavancin will be given intravenously as a one time dose.

! **WARNING** Alert patient that an allergic reaction can occur up to a day after oritavancin has been administered. Instruct the patient to notify staff during infusion or prescriber once home of any signs of an allergic reaction. If severe after returning home, tell patient to seek immediate medical care.

! **WARNING** Urge patient to tell prescriber if diarrhea develops, even 2 months or more after oritavancin ends as additional treatment may be needed.

! **WARNING** Advise patient to contact prescriber if persistent, serious, or unusual adverse effects occur after receiving drug.

oseltamivir phosphate

Tamiflu

Class and Category

Pharmacologic class: Selective neuraminidase inhibitor
Therapeutic class: Antiviral

Indications and Dosages

✱ *To treat acute uncomplicated illness due to* influenza A and B *infection in patients who have been symptomatic for no more than 48 hours*

CAPSULES, ORAL SUSPENSION

Adults and adolescents. 75 mg (12.5 ml) twice daily for 5 days.

Children ages 1 to 12 weighing more than 40.1 kg (88.22 lb). 75 mg (12.5 ml) twice daily.

Children ages 1 to 12 weighing 23.1 kg (50.82 lb) to 40 kg (88 lb). 60 mg (10 ml) twice daily.

Children ages 1 to 12 weighing 15.1 kg (33.22 lb) to 23 kg (50.6 lb). 45 mg (7.5 ml) twice daily.

Children ages 1 to 12 weighing 15 kg (33 lb) or less. 30 mg (5 ml) twice daily.

ORAL SUSPENSION

Infants 2 wk to less than 1 yr at any weight. 0.5 ml/kg twice daily.

✱ *To prevent* influenza A and B *infection*

CAPSULES, ORAL SUSPENSION

Adults and adolescents. 75 mg (12.5 ml) once daily for at least 10 days following close contact with an infected individual, up to 6 wk during a community outbreak, and up to 12 wk for immunocompromised patients.

Children ages 1 to 12 weighing more than 40.1 kg (88 lb). 75 mg (12.5 ml) once daily for at least 10 days following close contact with an infected individual, up to 6 wk during a community outbreak, and up to 12 wk for immunocompromised patients.

Children ages 1 to 12 weighing 23.1 kg (50.82 lb) to 40 kg (88 lb). 60 mg (10 ml) once daily for at least 10 days following close contact with an infected individual, up to 6 wk during a community outbreak, and up to 12 wk for immunocompromised patients.

Children ages 1 to 12 weighing 15.1 (33.22 lb) to 23 kg (50.6 lb). 45 mg (7.5 ml) once daily for at least 10 days following close contact with an infected individual, up to 6 wk during a community outbreak, and up to 12 wk for immunocompromised patients.

Children ages 1 to 12 weighing 15 kg (33 lb) or less. 30 mg (5 ml) once daily for at least 10 days following close contact with an infected individual, up to 6 wk during a community outbreak, and up to 12 wk for immunocompromised patients.

±**DOSAGE ADJUSTMENT** For adult patients with a creatinine clearance between 30 and 60 ml/min, dosage reduced to 30 mg (5 ml) twice daily for 5 days to treat influenza A and B infection and 30 mg (5 ml) once daily to prevent influenza A and B infection. For adult patients with a creatinine clearance of between 10 to 30 ml/min, dosage reduced to 30 mg (5 ml) once daily for 5 days to treat influenza A and B infection and 30 mg (5 ml) every other day to prevent influenza A and B infection. For adult patients with end-stage renal disease on hemodialysis, dosage reduced to 30 mg (5 ml) given immediately and then 30 mg (5 ml) after each hemodialysis cycle (treatment duration not to exceed 5 days) to treat influenza A and B infection and 30 mg (5 ml) given immediately and then 30 mg (5 ml) after alternate hemodialysis cycles to prevent influenza A and B infection. For patients with end-stage renal disease on continuous ambulatory peritoneal dialysis, dosage reduced to a single 30-mg (5 ml) dose administered immediately to treat influenza A and B infection and 30 mg (5 ml) given immediately and then 30 mg (5 ml) once weekly to prevent influenza A and B infection.

Drug Administration

P.O.

- Administer with or without food, but patient may tolerate drug better if given with food.
- Capsules should be swallowed whole and not chewed or crushed. However, for the patient who cannot swallow capsules, the capsules may be opened and mixed with sweetened liquids such as regular or sugar-free chocolate syrup, corn syrup, caramel topping, or light brown sugar (dissolved in water).
- To make oral suspension, tap closed bottle several times to loosen powder. Add 55 ml of water to drug bottle and shake closed bottle well for 15 sec.
- During an emergency and when oral suspension is not available or the age-appropriate strengths of oseltamivir capsules to mix with sweetened liquids are not available, the pharmacist can make an

emergency suspension preparation that contains 6 mg/ml using 75-mg capsules. It is only stable for 5 days at room temperature or 5 wk when stored in a refrigerator.
- Shake oral suspension well before using. Use the oral dispenser device that comes with the product to measure dosage.
- Manufactured oral suspension can be stored in the refrigerator for up to 17 days or 10 days if stored at room temperature; then discard. Avoid freezing.

Route	Onset	Peak	Duration
P.O.	Unknown	2.5–6 hr	Unknown

Half-life: 1–3 hr

Mechanism of Action

Inhibits influenza virus neuraminidase, affecting release of viral particles after conversion to its active form.

Contraindications

Hypersensitivity to oseltamivir phosphate or its components

Interactions

DRUGS

live-attenuated influenza vaccine (intranasal): Possibly decreased effectiveness

Adverse Reactions

CNS: Abnormal behavior, agitation, altered level of consciousness, anxiety, delirium, delusions, headache, **hypothermia**, nightmares, **seizures**
CV: **Arrhythmia**
ENDO: Aggravation of diabetes mellitus
GI: Diaper rash, diarrhea, elevated liver enzymes, **GI bleeding**, **hemorrhagic colitis**, **hepatitis**, nausea, vomiting
SKIN: Dermatitis, eczema, **erythema multiforme**, rash, **Stevens-Johnson syndrome**, **toxic epidermal necrolysis**, urticaria
Other: **Anaphylaxis**, **angioedema**, generalized pain

Childbearing Considerations

PREGNANCY

- It is not known if drug causes fetal harm.
- Use with caution only if benefit to mother outweighs potential risk to fetus.

LACTATION

- Drug is present in breast milk.
- Mothers should check with prescriber before breastfeeding.

Nursing Considerations

! **WARNING** Monitor patient for serious hypersensitivity reactions, which could become life-threatening, such as anaphylaxis and angioedema. Also, monitor patient for serious skin reactions such as erythema multiforme, Stevens-Johnson syndrome, and toxic epidermal necrolysis. If present, discontinue oseltamivir therapy immediately, notify prescriber, and be prepared to provide supportive care, as needed and ordered.

! **WARNING** Monitor patient for adverse GI reactions that could become life-threatening, such as GI bleeding, hemorrhagic colitis, or hepatitis. Monitor patient's liver enzymes, as ordered. If serious GI adverse reactions occur, notify prescriber immediately, expect drug to be discontinued and provide supportive care, as needed and ordered.

- Be aware that although uncommon, abnormal behavior and delirium have occurred after administration of oseltamivir, especially in children. While the onset is abrupt, rapid resolution usually occurs once oseltamivir is discontinued.

PATIENT TEACHING

- Instruct patient that for oseltamivir to be most effective, therapy should begin as soon as possible with the first appearance of flu symptoms (no later than 48 hours of onset of symptoms) and as soon as possible after exposure.
- Instruct patient how to administer form of oseltamivir prescribed.
- Alert patient that oral suspension contains above-normal maximum daily limits of sorbitol and may cause dyspepsia and diarrhea, especially in patients with hereditary fructose intolerance.

! **WARNING** Advise patient to seek immediate medical care if an allergic reaction, unusual or severe skin reactions, or serious GI reactions occur.

- Alert patient and family or caregiver that, although uncommon, abnormal behavior and delirium have occurred, especially in children. Notify prescriber if present and expect drug to be discontinued.

- Inform patient that oseltamivir is not a substitute for receiving an annual flu vaccination.

oteseconazole

Vivjoa

Class and Category

Pharmacologic class: Azole antifungal
Therapeutic class: Antifungal

Indications and Dosages

✱ *To reduce incidence of recurrent vulvovaginal candidiasis (RVVC) in women with a history of RVVC who are not of childbearing age*

CAPSULES

Adult females who are not of childbearing age. 600 mg on day 1, 450 mg on day 2, and then 150 mg every 7 days starting on day 14 for 11 wk.

✱ *As adjunct with fluconazole therapy to reduce incidence of recurrent vulvovaginal candidiasis (RVVC) in women with a history of RVVC who are not of childbearing age*

Adult females who are not of childbearing age. 150 mg on days 1, 4, and 7 followed by 150 mg on days 14 through 20, then 150 mg every 7 days starting on day 28 for 11 wk.

Drug Administration

P.O.

- Have patient swallow capsules whole and not chew, crush, dissolve, or open capsule.
- Administer with food.

Route	Onset	Peak	Duration
P.O.	Unknown	Unknown	Unknown

Half-life: 138 days

Mechanism of Action

Damages fungal cells by interfering with a cytochrome P-450 enzyme needed to convert lanosterol to ergosterol in essential part of the fungal cell membrane. Decreased ergosterol synthesis causes increased cell permeability, which allows cell contents to leak making fungal cells ineffective.

Contraindications

Females of childbearing age, hypersensitivity to oteseconazole or its components

Interactions

DRUGS

breast cancer resistance protein (BCRP) transporter substrates such as rosuvastatin: Possibly increased exposure of these substrates leading to increased risk of adverse reactions

Adverse Reactions

CNS: Headache including migraines and sinus
GI: Dyspepsia, nausea
GU: Dysuria; **genital, uterine, or vaginal hemorrhage**; menometrorrhagia; vulvovaginal irritation including burning, discomfort, and pain
SKIN: Hot flush
Other: Elevated blood creatine phosphokinase

Childbearing Considerations

PREGNANCY

- Drug causes embryo-fetal toxicity.
- Drug is contraindicated in females of childbearing age.

LACTATION

- It is not known if drug is present in breast milk.
- Drug is contraindicated in females of childbearing age.

REPRODUCTION

- Drug is contraindicated in females of childbearing age.

Nursing Considerations

! **WARNING** Ensure female patients are not of childbearing age before administering oteseconazole as drug causes embryo-fetal toxicity.

! **WARNING** Monitor patient for genital, uterine, or vaginal hemorrhage. If present, notify prescriber immediately.

PATIENT TEACHING

! **WARNING** Advise patient that oteseconazole is contraindicated in females of childbearing age because it may cause fetal harm. Breastfeeding is also contraindicated.

- Instruct patient how to administer oteseconazole.

! WARNING Tell patient to notify prescriber immediately if genital, uterine, or vaginal heavy bleeding occurs.

oxandrolone

Class, Category, and Schedule

Pharmacologic class: Androgen
Therapeutic class: Appetite stimulant
Controlled substance schedule: III

Indications and Dosages

✱ As adjunct to offset protein catabolism from prolonged use of corticosteroids; to provide relief of bone pain from osteoporosis

TABLETS

Adults. 2.5 to 20 mg in divided doses given 2 to 4 times daily for 2 to 4 wk; intermittent therapy repeated, as needed. *Maximum:* 20 mg daily.
Children. Less than 0.1 mg/kg daily; intermittent therapy repeated, as needed.

± DOSAGE ADJUSTMENT For elderly patients, dosage not to exceed 5 mg twice daily.

Drug Administration

P.O.

- Drug may be given with or without food.

Route	Onset	Peak	Duration
P.O.	Unknown	1 hr	Unknown

Half-life: 10–13 hr

Mechanism of Action

Promotes tissue-building processes and reverses catabolic or tissue-depleting processes by promoting protein anabolism.

Contraindications

Breast cancer (males); breast cancer with hypercalcemia (females); hypercalcemia; hypersensitivity to oxandrolone, anabolic steroids, or their components; nephrosis; pregnancy; prostate cancer

Interactions

DRUGS

ACTH, adrenal steroids: Increased risk of edema
oral hypoglycemic agents: Inhibited metabolism of these drugs
warfarin: Increased risk anticoagulant effect

Adverse Reactions

CNS: Depression, excitement, insomnia
CV: Decreased serum HDL level, edema, hyperlipidemia, hypertension
ENDO: Feminization in postpubertal males (epididymitis, gynecomastia, impotence, oligospermia, priapism, testicular atrophy), glucose intolerance, virilism in females (acne, clitoral enlargement, decreased breast size, deepened voice, diaphoresis, emotional lability, flushing, hirsutism, hoarseness, libido changes, male-pattern baldness, menstrual irregularities, nervousness, oily skin or hair, vaginal bleeding, vaginitis, weight gain), virilism in prepubertal males (acne, decreased ejaculatory volume, penis enlargement, prepubertal closure of epiphyseal plates, unnatural growth of body and facial hair)
GI: Diarrhea, elevated liver enzymes, **hepatocellular carcinoma**, jaundice, nausea, vomiting
GU: Benign prostatic hyperplasia, **prostate cancer**, urinary frequency, urine retention (elderly men)
HEME: Iron deficiency anemia, **leukemia**, **prolonged bleeding time**
Other: Fluid retention, **hypercalcemia** (females), physical and psychological dependence, sodium retention

Childbearing Considerations

PREGNANCY

- Drug may cause fetal harm.
- Drug is contraindicated during pregnancy.

LACTATION

- It is not known if drug is present in breast milk.
- A decision should be made to discontinue breastfeeding or the drug to avoid potential adverse reactions in the breastfed infant.

REPRODUCTION

- Females of childbearing age should use an effective contraceptive throughout drug therapy.

Nursing Considerations

- Use oxandrolone cautiously in patients with heart disease because drug has hypercholesterolemic effects.
- Provide adequate calories and protein, as ordered, to maintain a positive nitrogen balance during oxandrolone therapy.

! **WARNING** Anticipate an increased risk of fluid and sodium retention in patients with cardiac, hepatic, or renal dysfunction. Weigh patient daily to detect fluid retention. If patient has fluid retention, expect a sodium-restricted diet or diuretics to be ordered.

! **WARNING** Monitor patient for persistent, serious, or unusual adverse reactions because drug can cause cancer such as leukemia and liver or prostate cancer.

! **WARNING** Know that if patient takes an oral anticoagulant, INR or PT should be checked, as ordered. Monitor patient for bleeding. If present, notify prescriber immediately and institute measures to contain bleeding.

- Monitor blood glucose level frequently, especially in patients with diabetes, because drug can cause glucose intolerance.

PATIENT TEACHING

! **WARNING** Alert patient that drug may cause certain types of cancers before drug therapy begins.

- Advise patient to consume a diet high in calories and protein to achieve maximum therapeutic effect of oxandrolone.

! **WARNING** Advise females of childbearing age that she must use contraception during oxandrolone therapy and should notify prescriber immediately if pregnancy occurs.

! **WARNING** Urge patient to weigh daily during therapy and to report swelling or unexplained weight gain at once.

! **WARNING** Advise bleeding precautions (such as an electric shaver and soft toothbrush) if patient takes an oral anticoagulant. Tell patient to notify prescriber immediately if bleeding occurs.

- Explain that drug may alter libido.
- Inform females that drug may cause permanent physical changes, such as clitoral enlargement, deepened voice, and hair growth.
- Inform mothers breastfeeding should not be done during drug therapy.
- Review signs and symptoms of hyperglycemia with patient and to notify prescriber if present. Instruct diabetic patient to monitor blood glucose level frequently.

oxazepam

Class, Category, and Schedule

Pharmacologic class: Benzodiazepine
Therapeutic class: Anxiolytic
Controlled substance schedule: IV

Indications and Dosages

∗ *To treat anxiety*

CAPSULES

Adults and adolescents. *For mild to moderate anxiety:* 10 to 15 mg 3 times daily or 4 times daily. *For severe anxiety:* up to 30 mg 3 times daily or 4 times daily.

∗ *To help manage acute alcohol withdrawal symptoms*

CAPSULES

Adults. 15 to 30 mg 3 times daily or 4 times daily.

± **DOSAGE ADJUSTMENT** For elderly or debilitated patients, initial dose reduced to 10 mg 3 times daily increased cautiously to 15 mg 3 times daily or 4 times daily, as needed.

Drug Administration

P.O.

- Store at room temperature in a tight, light-resistant container.
- Capsules should be swallowed whole and not chewed, crushed, or opened.

Route	Onset	Peak	Duration
P.O.	30–60 min	2–3 hr	6–8 hr

Half-life: 6–15 hr

Mechanism of Action

May potentiate the effects of gamma-aminobutyric acid (GABA) and other inhibitory neurotransmitters by binding to specific benzodiazepine receptors in limbic and cortical areas of the CNS. Remember that GABA inhibits excitatory stimulation, which helps control emotional behavior. Remember also the limbic system contains highly dense areas of benzodiazepine receptors, which may explain oxazepam's antianxiety and alcohol withdrawal effects.

Contraindications

Hypersensitivity to oxazepam or its components, psychoses

Interactions

DRUGS

CNS depressants, opioids, other benzodiazepines: Increased risk of severe CNS and respiratory depression

ACTIVITIES

alcohol use: Increased risk of severe CNS and respiratory depression

Adverse Reactions

CNS: Anxiety (in daytime), ataxia, confusion, depression, dizziness, drowsiness, fatigue, headache, insomnia, nightmares, sleep disturbance, slurred speech, syncope, talkativeness, tremor, vertigo
GI: Nausea
Other: Drug tolerance, physical and psychological dependence, withdrawal symptoms

Childbearing Considerations

PREGNANCY

- Pregnancy exposure registry: 1-866-961-2388.
- Drug may cause fetal harm.
- Prolonged use of drug during pregnancy can result in neonatal sedation and withdrawal syndrome, which may be life-threatening if not recognized and treated.
- Maternal use of drug shortly before delivery may result in floppy infant syndrome.
- Drug should be avoided during pregnancy, if possible.

LABOR AND DELIVERY

- Drug is not recommended for use in pregnant women immediately before or during labor because it may produce respiratory depression in the neonate. Monitor neonate closely for signs of excess sedation and respiratory depression.
- An opioid antagonist, such as naloxone, must be available at the time of delivery in the event it is needed to reverse opioid-induced respiratory depression in the neonate.

LACTATION

- Drug is present in breast milk.
- Breastfeeding is not recommended during drug therapy. However, if breastfeeding occurs monitor infant for poor feeding and weight gain, sedation, and slowed respirations.

Nursing Considerations

! **WARNING** Be aware that excessive use of benzodiazepines, including oxazepam, may lead to abuse, addiction, misuse, overdose, and possibly death. Monitor patient's intake of drug closely and for evidence of physical and psychological dependence. Also, have naloxone readily available for emergency treatment of opioid overdose.

- Be aware that drug shouldn't be stopped abruptly after prolonged use; doing so may cause seizures or withdrawal symptoms, such as insomnia, irritability, and nervousness. Know that withdrawal symptoms can occur when therapy lasts only 1 or 2 weeks. Also, be aware that protracted withdrawal syndrome with withdrawal symptoms lasting weeks to more than 12 months can occur.

! **WARNING** Be aware that oxazepam should only be used concomitantly with opioid therapy in patients for whom other treatment options are inadequate. If prescribed together, expect dosing and duration of oxazepam to be limited. Monitor patient closely for signs and symptoms of a decrease in consciousness, including coma, profound sedation, and significant respiratory depression. Notify prescriber immediately and provide emergency supportive care, as death may occur. Monitor respiratory status in patients with pulmonary disease (such as severe COPD), respiratory depression, or sleep apnea; drug may worsen ventilatory failure.

! **WARNING** Be aware that drug may worsen acute intermittent porphyria or myasthenia gravis, and cause severe renal impairment.

- Expect an increased risk of falls among elderly patients from impaired cognition and motor function. Take safety precautions.

- Expect patient with late-stage Parkinson's disease to experience decreased cognition or coordination and, possibly, increased psychosis.

PATIENT TEACHING

- Instruct patient how to administer oxazepam.

! **WARNING** Instruct patient not to take oxazepam more often than prescribed and not to take it longer than absolutely needed because excessive or prolonged use can lead to abuse, addiction, misuse, overdose, and possibly death. Encourage patient and family to have naloxone available in the home in the event of an opioid overdose. Instruct family or caregiver how to recognize an opioid overdose such as severe respiratory depression and profound sedation and how to administer naloxone. Stress importance of immediately calling 911 after administering naloxone.

- Advise patient to avoid use of alcohol or other CNS-deppressant drugs during therapy with oxazepam.

! **WARNING** Alert patient to the drug interaction between oxazepam and opioids and not to combine the 2 unless directed to do so by a prescriber and only after prescriber has been informed of oxazepam therapy.

! **WARNING** Stress importance that oxazepam shouldn't be stopped abruptly after prolonged use; doing so may cause seizures or withdrawal symptoms, such as insomnia, irritability, and nervousness. Inform patient that withdrawal symptoms can occur when therapy lasts only 1 or 2 weeks. Also, alert patient that protracted withdrawal syndrome with withdrawal symptoms lasting weeks to more than 12 months may occur. Instead, urge patient to consult prescriber for any questions or concerns regarding oxazepam therapy.

! **WARNING** Instruct patient to keep drug in a safe place to prevent theft and out of the reach of children.

! **WARNING** Inform pregnant patients that prolonged use of drug during pregnancy may cause harm to the baby when born. Encourage patient to speak with prescriber about alternative drug therapy during pregnancy.

- Caution patient about possible drowsiness and reduced coordination. Tell patient to take safety precautions and to avoid performing hazardous activities that require alertness such as driving until resolved.
- Inform mothers breastfeeding is not recommended during oxazepam therapy. However, if breastfeeding occurs tell mothers to monitor their infant for poor feeding and weight gain, sedation, and slowed respirations.

oxcarbazepine

Oxtellar XR, Trileptal

Class and Category

Pharmacologic class: Carboxamide derivative
Therapeutic class: Anticonvulsant

Indications and Dosages

✱ As adjunct to treat partial seizures

ORAL SUSPENSION, TABLETS (TRILEPTAL)

Adults and adolescents over age 16. *Initial:* 300 mg twice daily. Dosage increased by 600 mg/day every wk. *Maintenance:* 1,200 mg daily in 2 divided doses. *Maximum:* 2,400 mg daily in 2 divided doses.
Children ages 4 to 16. *Initial:* 4 to 5 mg/kg (maximum 300 mg) twice daily to maximum initial dose of 600 mg daily. *Maintenance:* 900 mg daily for children weighing 20 to 29 kg (44 to 64 lb); 1,200 mg daily for those weighing 29.1 to 39 kg (65 to 86 lb); 1,800 mg daily for those weighing more than 39 kg.
Children ages 2 to 4 weighing 20 kg (44 lb) or more. *Initial:* 8 to 10 mg/kg in 2 divided doses not to exceed 600 mg daily. Dose increased as needed, over 2 to 4 wk to achieve maximum maintenance dose. *Maximum maintenance:* 60 mg/kg in 2 divided doses.
Children ages 2 to 4 weighing less than 20 kg (44 lb). *Initial:* 16 to 20 mg/kg daily in 2 divided doses, increased, as needed, over 2 to 4 wk to achieve maximum maintenance dose. *Maximum maintenance:* 60 mg/kg/day in 2 divided doses.

✱ As monotherapy to treat partial seizures

N O

ORAL SUSPENSION, TABLETS (TRILEPTAL)

Adults and adolescents over age 16. *Initial:* 300 mg twice daily. Dosage increased by 300 mg/day every 3 days, as needed. *Maintenance:* 1,200 mg daily. *Maximum:* 1,200 mg daily.

Children ages 4 to 16. *Initial:* 4 to 5 mg/kg twice daily, increased by 5 mg/kg daily every third day, as needed. *Maintenance:* Based on weight as follows: 70 kg (154 lb): 1,500 to 2,100 mg/day; 60 to 65 kg (132 to 143 lb): 1,200 to 2,100 mg/day; 50 to 55 kg (110 to 121 lb): 1,200 to 1,800 mg/day; 45 kg (99 lb): 1,200 to 1,500 mg/day; 35 to 40 kg (77 to 88 lb): 900 to 1,500 mg/day; 25 to 30 kg (55 to 66 lb): 900 to 1,200 mg/day; and 20 kg (44 lb): 600 to 900 mg/day.

* *To convert to monotherapy in treating partial seizures*

ORAL SUSPENSION, TABLETS (TRILEPTAL)

Adults and adolescents over age 16. *Initial:* 300 mg twice daily while reducing dose of concomitant anticonvulsant drug. Dosage increased by up to 600 mg daily every wk over 2 to 4 wk, as needed, while dosage of other anticonvulsant reduced to complete withdrawal over 3 to 6 wk. *Maintenance:* 1,200 mg daily. *Maximum:* 2,400 mg daily.

Children ages 4 to 16. *Initial:* 4 to 5 mg/kg twice daily while reducing dose of concomitant anticonvulsant drug. Dosage increased by up to 10 mg/kg daily in weekly increments, as needed, to maximum maintenance dosage while dosage of other anticonvulsant is reduced over 3 to 6 wk to complete withdrawal.

Maintenance: Based on weight as follows: 70 kg (154 lb): 1,500 to 2,100 mg/day; 60 to 65 kg (132 to 143 lb): 1,200 to 2,100 mg/day; 50 to 55 kg (110 to 121 lb): 1,200 to 1,800 mg/day; 45 kg (99 lb): 1,200 to 1,500 mg/day; 35 to 40 kg (77 to 88 lb): 900 to 1,500 mg/day; 25 to 30 kg (55 to 66 lb): 900 to 1,200 mg/day; and 20 kg (44 lb): 600 to 900 mg/day.

±**DOSAGE ADJUSTMENT** For patients receiving concomitantly strong CYP3A4 enzyme inducers or UGT inducers, dosage adjustment may be required. For patients with creatinine clearance less than 30 ml/min, usual initial dosage reduced by 50% and titration to maintenance dose done slowly.

* *To treat partial seizures*

XR TABLETS (OXTELLAR XR)

Adults and adolescents over age 16. *Initial:* 600 mg once daily for 1 wk, increased in 600 mg/day increments weekly to reach target dose. *Maintenance:* 1,200 to 2,400 mg once daily. *Maximum:* 2,400 mg once daily.

Children ages 6 to 17. *Initial:* 8 to 10 mg/kg once daily, not to exceed initial dose of 600 mg in first wk, then increased by 8 to 10 mg/kg in once-daily increments weekly, not to exceed dose of 600 mg daily. *Usual:* 1,800 mg daily for those weighing more than 39 kg (more than 86 lb); 1,200 mg daily for those weighing 29.1 to 39 kg (65 to 86 lb); 900 mg daily for children weighing 20 to 29 kg (44 to 64 lb).

±**DOSAGE ADJUSTMENT** For patients taking concurrent strong CYP3A4 enzyme inducers or UGT enzyme inducers, initial dosage increased to 900 mg once daily for adults and 12 to 15 mg/kg (not to exceed 900 mg in the first week) once daily for pediatric patients. For adult patients with a creatinine clearance less than 30 ml/min, initial dosage decreased by 50% with subsequent dosage increases made weekly in increments of 300 to 450 mg/day to achieve desired response. For elderly patients, initial dosage reduced to 300 to 450 mg/day with subsequent dosage increases made weekly in increments of 300 to 450 mg/day to achieve desired response.

Drug Administration

P.O.

- Administer XR tablets 1 hr before or 2 hr after a meal because adverse reactions are more likely to occur when taken with food. If patient has difficulty swallowing XR tablets, daily dosages can be achieved by using lower-strength tablets such as 150 mg.
- Be aware that in conversion of immediate-release form to extended-release form, higher dosages of extended-release form maybe necessary.
- Tablets should be swallowed whole and not chewed, crushed, or split.
- Shake suspension well before using. Withdraw prescribed amount using supplied oral dosing syringe. Mix dose in a small glass of water just before administering it, or patient can swallow

drug directly from syringe. Rinse syringe with warm water and let it dry thoroughly. Discard any unused oral suspension after 7 wk of first opening the bottle.
- Oral immediate-release tablets and oral suspension may be interchanged at equal doses.

Route	Onset	Peak	Duration
P.O.	Unknown	3–13 hr	Unknown
P.O./E.R.	Unknown	7 hr	Unknown

Half-life: 2–11 hr

Mechanism of Action

May prevent or halt seizures by blocking or closing sodium channels in neuronal cell membrane. Preventing sodium from entering the cell may slow nerve impulse transmission, thus decreasing the rate at which neurons fire.

Contraindications

Hypersensitivity to oxcarbazepine, eslicarbazepine acetate, or their components

Interactions

DRUGS

hormonal contraceptives: Rendered less effective by immediate-release oxcarbazepine
phenytoin: Possibly increased phenytoin levels with increased risk of adverse reactions
strong CYP3A4 or UGT inducers (carbamazepine, phenobarbital, phenytoin, rifampin): Decreased oxcarbazepine levels with decreased effectiveness

ACTIVITIES

alcohol use: Possibly additive CNS depressant effects

FOODS

all food (XR tablets): Increased risk of adverse effects

Adverse Reactions

CNS: Abnormal coordination or gait, agitation, amnesia, asthenia, ataxia, confusion, difficulty concentrating, dizziness, EEG abnormalities, emotional lability, fatigue, fever, headache, hypoesthesia, insomnia, language or speech problems, nervousness, psychomotor slowing, **seizures**, somnolence, **status epilepticus**, **suicidal ideation**, tremor, vertigo
CV: **AV block**, chest pain, **hypotension**, peripheral edema
EENT: Abnormal vision, diplopia, ear infection, earache, epistaxis, nystagmus, pharyngitis, rhinitis, sinusitis, taste perversion
ENDO: Hot flashes, hypothyroidism, syndrome of inappropriate antidiuretic hormone secretion
GI: Abdominal pain, anorexia, constipation, diarrhea, elevated liver or pancreatic enzymes, gastritis, indigestion, nausea, **pancreatitis**, vomiting
GU: Frequent urination, UTI, vaginitis
HEME: **Agranulocytosis**, **aplastic anemia**, eosinophilia, **leukopenia**, **pancytopenia**, purpura
MS: Arthralgia, back pain, decreased bone mineral density, dysarthria, fractures, muscle weakness, osteoporosis (long-term therapy with immediate-release form)
RESP: Bronchitis, cough, respiratory tract infection
SKIN: Acne, acute generalized exanthematous pustulosis, diaphoresis, **erythema multiforme**, maculopapular rash, rash, **Stevens-Johnson syndrome**, **toxic epidermal necrolysis**
Other: **Anaphylaxis**, **drug reaction with eosinophilia and systemic symptoms (DRESS)**, **hyponatremia**, lymphadenopathy, **multiorgan hypersensitivity**

Childbearing Considerations

PREGNANCY

- Pregnancy exposure registry: 1-888-233-2334 or http://www.aedpregnancyregistry.org.
- Drug may cause fetal harm such as an increased risk of congenital malformations, including oral clefts and ventricular septal defects.
- An increase in seizure activity may occur during pregnancy.
- Use with caution only if benefit to mother outweighs potential risk to fetus.

LACTATION

- Drug is present in breast milk.
- Mothers should check with prescriber before breastfeeding. If breastfeeding occurs, infant should be monitored for adverse effects.

REPRODUCTION

- Females of childbearing age using hormonal contraceptives containing ethinyl estradiol or levonorgestrel should use an additional or alternative nonhormonal contraceptive during drug therapy.

Nursing Considerations

- Monitor therapeutic oxcarbazepine levels during initiation and titration and expect to adjust dosage accordingly.

! **WARNING** Monitor patient for a hypersensitivity reaction, which could become life-threatening, such as anaphylaxis, DRESS, or multiorgan hypersensitivity. Know that patient with an hypersensitivity reaction to carbamazepine may have hypersensitivity to oxcarbazepine. Also, know patients carrying the HLA-B*1502 allele may be at increased risk for Stevens-Johnson syndrome or toxic epidermal necrolysis. If a hypersensitivity reaction occurs or at the first appearance of a rash or other skin reaction (DRESS may only initially exhibit as a fever or swollen lymph nodes), notify prescriber and expect to stop drug. Provide supportive care, as needed and ordered.

- Monitor serum sodium level for signs of hyponatremia, especially during first 3 months. Know that elderly patients may be at higher risk for hyponatremia because of age-related reductions in creatinine clearance.

! **WARNING** Implement seizure precautions, as needed. If seizures occur, expect oxcarbazepine to be discontinued.

! **WARNING** Monitor patient closely for evidence of suicidal thinking or behavior, especially when therapy starts or dosage changes.

- Monitor patient for CNS adverse reactions that may involve cognitive symptoms, coordination abnormalities, fatigue, and somnolence.

! **WARNING** Expect to discontinue oxcarbazepine gradually, as abrupt withdrawal may increase risk of seizure frequency and development of status epilepticus.

PATIENT TEACHING

- Instruct patient how to administer form of oxcarbazepine prescribed.
- Instruct patient not to drink alcohol during oxcarbazepine therapy.

! **WARNING** Warn patient not to stop taking oxcarbazepine abruptly, as an increase in seizure activity may occur and possibly lead to status epilepticus. Instead, encourage patient to discuss questions or concerns with prescriber.

! **WARNING** Tell patient to notify prescriber immediately if seizures occur despite oxcarbazepine therapy.

! **WARNING** Alert patient that drug may cause an allergic reaction or serious skin reactions. If present, tell patient to notify prescriber and, if severe, to seek immediate medical care.

! **WARNING** Urge family or caregiver to watch patient closely for evidence of suicidal tendencies, especially when therapy starts or dosage changes, and to report concerns to prescriber at once.

! **WARNING** Review signs and symptoms of a low sodium level with patient. Tell the patient to report signs and symptoms to prescriber, such as confusion, increase in severity of seizures, lack of energy, nausea, or tiredness.

! **WARNING** Inform patient that dizziness, double vision, and unsteady gait as well as other adverse CNS signs and symptoms may occur. Caution patient not to drive or perform any other hazardous activity if these effects occur and until they are resolved.

! **WARNING** Tell patient to notify prescriber if other persistent, serious, or unusual adverse reactions occur.

- Alert females of childbearing age that oxcarbazepine may render hormonal contraceptives containing ethinyl estradiol or levonorgestrel ineffective. Urge her to use an additional or a different contraceptive during oxcarbazepine therapy. Also, tell her to alert prescriber if pregnancy occurs as drug may cause fetal harm and seizure activity may increase during pregnancy.

- Inform mothers breastfeeding to monitor infant for adverse reactions.

oxybutynin

Oxytrol, Oxytrol for Women

oxybutynin chloride

Ditropan XL, Gelnique 10%

Class and Category

Pharmacologic class: Anticholinergic
Therapeutic class: Antispasmodic (urinary)

Indications and Dosages

✱ *To provide relief of symptoms of bladder instability associated with voiding in patients with reflex neurogenic bladder (dysuria, frequency, urge incontinence, urgency, or urinary leakage) or uninhibited neurogenic bladder*

SYRUP, TABLETS (OXYBUTYNIN)

Adults. 5 mg 2 or 3 times daily. *Maximum:* 5 mg 4 times daily.
Children over age 5. 5 mg twice daily. *Maximum:* 5 mg 3 times daily.

±**DOSAGE ADJUSTMENT** For frail, elderly adults, dosage reduced to 2.5 mg 2 or 3 times daily.

✱ *To treat overactive bladder with symptoms of frequency, urge urinary incontinence, or urgency*

E.R. TABLETS (DITROPAN XL)

Adults. *Initial:* 5 or 10 mg daily, adjusted by 5 mg/wk, as needed. *Maximum:* 30 mg daily.

TRANSDERMAL SYSTEM (OXYTROL, OXYTROL FOR WOMEN)

Adults. System supplying 3.9 mg daily, applied twice weekly.

TOPICAL GEL (GELNIQUE 10%)

Adults. 1 sachet or 1 actuation of the metered dose pump applied once daily.

✱ *To treat symptoms of detrusor muscle overactivity of bladder associated with a neurological condition, such as spina bifida*

E.R. TABLETS (DITROPAN XL)

Children ages 6 and older. *Initial:* 5 mg once daily, increased in 5 mg increments weekly, as needed. *Maximum:* 20 mg once daily.

Drug Administration

P.O.

- E.R. tablets should be swallowed whole and not chewed, crushed, or divided.
- Use a calibrated device when measuring syrup dosage. Store syrup at room temperature.

TRANSDERMAL

- Apply transdermal system to dry, intact, fold-free skin of abdomen, buttock, or hip immediately after removing from pouch preferably on the same two days of the week. Do not store patch outside of sealed pouch. Do not divide or cut patch into pieces and damaged patches should not be used.
- Avoid areas that are irritated or scraped or have been treated with lotions, oils, or powders.
- Apply by removing the first piece of the protective liner, placing the patch, adhesive side face down, and pressing firmly onto the skin. Bend the patch in half and gently roll the remaining part onto patient's skin using your fingertips. As patch is rolled in place, the second piece of protective liner should move off the patch. Apply firm pressure over the patch. Avoid touching the sticky adhesive side when putting on the patch, as this may cause the patch to fall off early.
- If patch partly or completely falls off, press it back in place. If it does not stay, replace with a new patch, but remove at scheduled time.
- Do not use same site for at least 7 days.
- Rotate sites.
- Remove old patch slowly and carefully to avoid damaging the skin. Once off, fold the patch in half with sticky sides together and discard.
- Store patches at room temperature, avoiding exposure to sunlight.
- Allow patient to bathe, exercise, or shower while wearing patch. Patient may also go swimming once home because contact with water will not alter effectiveness of patch.

TOPICAL

- Put on gloves, then apply gel to dry, intact skin on patient's abdomen, shoulders, thighs, or upper arms immediately after sachet is opened.
- Avoid applying to recently shaved skin surfaces.

- Have patient cover area if close skin-to-skin contact at application site is anticipated.
- Make sure patient does not bathe or shower for 1 hr after application.
- Rotate application sites.

Route	Onset	Peak	Duration
P.O./E.R.	Unknown	4–6 hr	24 hr
Topical	Unknown	Unknown	Unknown
Transdermal	Unknown	24–48 hr	96 hr

Half-life: 2–13 hr (P.O.); Unknown (topical/transdermal)

Mechanism of Action

Exerts antimuscarinic (atropine-like) and potent direct antispasmodic (papaverine-like) actions on smooth muscle in the bladder and decreases detrusor muscle contractions to increase bladder capacity and decrease the urge to void.

Contraindications

Angle-closure glaucoma, gastric retention, hypersensitivity to oxybutynin or its components, urine retention

Interactions

DRUGS

anticholinergics: Increased anticholinergic effects; possibly decreased absorption of some concomitantly administered drugs with major concern for those drugs with a narrow therapeutic index

antimycotic agents (itraconazole, miconazole), ketoconazole, macrolide antibiotics (erythromycin, clarithromycin): Increased plasma oxybutynin concentrations with increased risk of adverse reactions

carbamazepine concurrently with dantrolene: Increased risk of confusion, drowsiness, nystagmus, slurred speech, unsteadiness, and vomiting suggestive of carbamazepine toxicity

ACTIVITIES

alcohol use: Increased CNS effects

Adverse Reactions

CNS: **Abnormal behaviors**, **agitation**, asthenia, confusion, delirium, depression, dizziness, drowsiness, fatigue, hallucinations, headache, insomnia, memory impairment, nervousness, psychosis, restlessness, **seizures**, somnolence, thirst

CV: **Arrhythmias**, chest discomfort, edema, hypertension, **hypotension**, palpitations, peripheral edema, **QT-interval prolongation**, tachycardia, vasodilation

EENT: Abnormal or blurred vision; cycloplegia; dry eyes, mouth, nose, and throat; eye irritation; glaucoma; keratoconjunctivitis sicca; mydriasis; nasal congestion; nasopharyngitis; rhinitis; sinusitis

ENDO: Hot flashes, hyperglycemia, suppression of lactation

GI: Abdominal pain, anorexia, constipation, decreased GI motility, diarrhea, dysphagia, esophagitis, flatulence, gastroesophageal reflux, indigestion, nausea, vomiting

GU: Cystitis, dysuria, impotence, urinary hesitancy, urine retention, UTI

MS: Arthralgia, arthritis, back pain

RESP: **Asthma**, bronchitis, cough, dysphonia, upper respiratory tract infection

SKIN: Decreased sweating, dry skin, flushing, pruritus, rash, urticaria

Other: **Anaphylaxis**, **angioedema**, application-site reactions (anesthesia, dermatitis, erythema, irritation, papules, pruritus), flu-like symptoms, fungal infections, **heatstroke**

Childbearing Considerations

PREGNANCY

- It is not known if drug causes fetal harm.
- Use with caution only if benefit to mother outweighs potential risk to fetus.

LACTATION

- It is not known if drug is present in breast milk.
- Mothers should check with prescriber before breastfeeding.

Nursing Considerations

- Use oxybutynin cautiously in patients with diarrhea because it may signal incomplete GI obstruction, especially in patients with colostomy or ileostomy. Also, use cautiously in patients with dementia treated with cholinesterase inhibitors because drug may aggravate symptoms.
- Use cautiously in patients with autonomic neuropathy, myasthenia gravis, or Parkinson's disease, because drug may adversely affect these conditions. If exacerbation of symptoms occurs, notify prescriber and expect drug to be discontinued.

- Use cautiously in patients with benign prostatic hyperplasia, gastroesophageal reflux disease, or hyperthyroidism as drug may aggravate these conditions.
- Keep in mind that decreased GI motility can cause adynamic ileus; assess for abdominal pain and ileus. Also, use with caution in patients who have intestinal atony or ulcerative colitis because of decreased GI motility.
- Assess urinary symptoms before and after treatment to evaluate effectiveness.
- Monitor patient for anticholinergic CNS effects, such as agitation, confusion, hallucinations, and somnolence, especially in the first few months of therapy or when dosage is increased. If such effects occur, notify prescriber and expect dosage to be reduced or drug discontinued.

! **WARNING** Monitor patient for hypersensitivity reactions which may become life-threatening such as anaphylaxis or angioedema. If present, notify prescriber, stop oxybutynin therapy, as ordered, and provide supportive care, as needed and ordered.

! **WARNING** Watch for adverse cardiovascular reactions in patients with arrhythmias, coronary artery disease, heart failure, or hypertension because drug's antimuscarinic effects may increase their risk. Also, monitor patient's blood pressure for hypotension.

! **WARNING** Monitor patient for other adverse reactions that are persistent, serious, or unusual.

PATIENT TEACHING

- Instruct patient how to administer form of oxybutynin prescribed.
- Urge patient to avoid alcohol during therapy.

! **WARNING** Alert patient that drug may cause an allergic reaction. If present, tell patient to notify prescriber and, if severe, to seek immediate medical care.

- Warn of possible decreased alertness and advise patient against performing hazardous activities until drug's CNS effects are known and resolved.

! **WARNING** Tell patient to notify prescriber if other persistent, serious, or unusual adverse reactions occur.

- Caution patient to avoid excessive sun exposure and strenuous exercise because of increased risk of heatstroke.

! **WARNING** Remind patient to keep drug, including discarded patches out of the reach of children.

oxycodone

Xtampza ER

oxycodone hydrochloride

Oxaydo, OxyContin, Roxicodone, Roxybond, Supeudol (CAN)

Class, Category, and Schedule

Pharmacologic class: Opioid
Therapeutic class: Opioid analgesic
Controlled substance schedule: II

Indications and Dosages

✳ *To relieve pain severe enough to require opioid treatment and for which alternative treatment options such as nonopioid analgesics or opioid combination products are inadequate or not tolerated*

CAPSULES (OXYCODONE), ORAL SOLUTION (ROXICODONE), TABLETS (OXAYDO, ROXICODONE ROXYBOND)

Adults. 5 to 15 mg every 4 to 6 hr.

SUPPOSITORY (SUPEUDOL)

Adults. 1 suppository 3 to 4 times daily.

TABLETS (SUPEUDOL)

Adults. 5 to 10 mg every 6 hr.

✳ *To manage severe and persistent pain that requires an extended treatment period with a daily opioid analgesic and for which alternative treatment options are inadequate*

E.R. TABLETS (OXYCONTIN)

Adults who haven't received opioids before; adults converting from other opioids. *Initial:* 10 mg every 12 hr, increased every 1 to 2 days, as needed, to achieve desired pain control.

N O

Adults converting from other oral oxycodone formulations. Half the 24-hr oxycodone dose every 12 hr.
Adults converting from methadone. Highly individualized.
Adults converting from transdermal fentanyl. Highly individualized. *Usual:* 10 mg oxycodone for each 25 mcg/hr of fentanyl patch dosage every 12 hr, beginning 18 hr after removing patch.
Children ages 11 and older who are already receiving opioids for at least 5 consecutive days and requiring at least 20 mg of oxycodone daily. *Initial:* Highly individualized and based on the type of opioid taken prior to oxycodone dosing. For example, using the conversion factor of 0.9 for oral hydrocodone in manufacturer's guidelines, a total daily hydrocodone dosage of 50 mg is converted to 45 mg of oxycodone daily or 22.5 mg every 12 hr. After rounding down to the nearest available strength, the dosage would be 20 mg every 12 hr, increased every 1 to 2 days, as needed.

E.R. CAPSULES (XTAMPZA ER)

Adults who are opioid-naïve, not opioid tolerant, or converting from other opioids. 9 mg every 12 hr, increased, as needed, with dose adjusted to obtain balance between management of pain and opioid-related adverse reactions. *Maximum:* 288 mg daily in divided doses.
Adults converting from fentanyl transdermal patch. Highly individualized. *Usual:* 9 mg oxycodone for each 25 mcg/hr of fentanyl patch dosage every 12 hr, beginning 18 hr after removing patch.
Adults converting from other oral oxycodone formulations. Highly individualized. *Usual:* Half the 24-hr oxycodone dose every 12 hr.
Adults converting from methadone. Highly individualized.

±**DOSAGE ADJUSTMENT** For elderly patients, patients with hepatic impairment, or patients currently taking a CNS depressant, one-third to one-half the usual starting dose and then adjusted, as needed.

Drug Administration

P.O.

- Tablet should be swallowed whole and not broken, chewed, or crushed because of rapid release possibly causing a fatal overdose. Be aware that Roxybond tablets contain ingredients that make the tablet more difficult to manipulate for abuse and misuse even if tablet is subjected to physical manipulation and/or chemical extraction.
- Capsules should be swallowed whole without chewing or crushing. However, for patient who has difficulty swallowing E.R. capsules, capsule can be opened, contents sprinkled on soft foods or sprinkled into a cup, and then administered directly into patient's mouth. Give patient water to rinse mouth to ensure that all capsule contents have been swallowed.
- For patient with a gastrostomy or nasogastric tube, Xtampza ER capsules can be opened and carefully poured directly into the tube after the tube has been flushed with water. Do not pre-mix the capsule contents with the liquid used to flush them through the tube. After instilling capsule content into tube, draw up 15 ml of water into a syringe, insert syringe into the tube and flush the capsule content through the tube. Repeat flushing 2 more times, each with 10 ml of water, to ensure that no content is left in the tube. Milk or liquid nutritional supplement may be used in place of water to flush tube. Do not administer tablet form through a gastric, nasogastric or other feeding tubes as it may cause obstruction of the tube.
- Check to be sure the right oral solution strength is being used before measuring dose. It comes in 5 mg per 5 ml and 100 mg per 5 ml. The 100 mg per 5 ml concentration should only be used in patients who are opioid tolerant. Use a calibrated device when measuring oral solution dosage. The 100 mg per 5 ml oral solution comes with an oral syringe that should always be used to measure the dose.
- Administer E.R capsules with food. Have patient consume about the same amount of food for every dose in order to maintain consistent blood levels of drug. Administer other forms of oxycodone with or without food.
- Have patient swallow 1 E.R. tablet (OxyContin) at a time, with enough water to ensure complete swallowing immediately after patient places tablet in his mouth;

otherwise, choking on tablets or difficulty swallowing tablets may occur due to the swelling and hydrogelling property of tablet if left in the mouth too long.

- E.R. tablets and capsules are not interchangeable.

P.R.

- If suppository is soft, place in refrigerator for 30 min or run it under cold water while wrapped.

Route	Onset	Peak	Duration
P.O.	10–30 min	0.5–1 hr	3–6 hr
P.O./E.R.	Unknown	4–5 hr	12 hr
P.R.	Unknown	Unknown	Unknown

Half-life: 3–5 hr

Mechanism of Action

Alters perception of and emotional response to pain at spinal cord and higher levels of CNS by blocking release of inhibitory neurotransmitters, such as acetylcholine and gamma-aminobutyric acid.

Contraindications

Acute or severe bronchial asthma or hypercarbia in an unmonitored setting or in the absence of resuscitative equipment, GI obstruction, hypersensitivity to oxycodone or its components, paralytic ileus, significant respiratory depression

Interactions

DRUGS

5-HT$_3$ receptor antagonists, certain muscle relaxants (cyclobenzaprine, metaxalone), drugs that affect the serotonin neurotransmitter system (mirtazapine, tramadol, trazodone), MAO inhibitors, including I.V. methylene blue and linezolid, selective serotonin reuptake inhibitors, serotonin and norepinephrine reuptake inhibitors, tricyclic antidepressants, triptans: Increased risk of serotonin syndrome

anticholinergics: Possibly severe constipation and ileus; increased risk of urinary retention

anxiolytics, antipsychotics, benzodiazepines, generalized anesthetics, muscle relaxants, other CNS depressants, other opioids, sedating antihistamines, tranquilizers, tricyclic antidepressants: Increased risk of severe respiratory depression and significant sedation and somnolence

CYP3A4 inducers, such as carbamazepine, phenytoin, rifampin: Possibly decreased oxycodone levels making it less effective

CYP3A4 inhibitors, such as azole antifungal drugs, macrolide antibiotics, and protease inhibitors: Possibly increased plasma oxycodone levels and prolonged opioid effects with possible overdose effects

diuretics: Reduced effectiveness of diuretics

MAO inhibitors, such as linezolid, phenelzine, tranylcypromine: Increased risk of serotonin syndrome; increased risk of opioid toxicity

mixed agonist/antagonist and partial agonist opioid analgesics, such as buprenorphine, butorphanol, nalbuphine, pentazocine: Decreased analgesic effect of oxycodone and/or precipitation of withdrawal symptoms

muscle relaxants, such as cyclobenzaprine, metaxalone: Enhanced neuromuscular blocking action increasing degree of respiratory depression; increased risk of serotonin syndrome

ACTIVITIES

alcohol use: Additive CNS and respiratory depressive effects that may become severe

Adverse Reactions

CNS: Abnormal dreams, anxiety, asthenia, chills, dizziness, drowsiness, euphoria, excitation, headache, insomnia, nervousness, sedation, **seizures**, somnolence, syncope, twitching

CV: **Bradycardia**, chest pain, **hypotension**, orthostatic hypotension, palpitations

EENT: Blurred vision, **choking** or difficulty swallowing tablets (OxyContin), dry eyes or mouth, lens opacities, miosis

ENDO: **Adrenal insufficiency** (rare), **hypoglycemia**, syndrome of inappropriate antidiuretic hormone secretion

GI: Abdominal pain, anorexia, constipation, diarrhea, dyspepsia, dysphagia, elevated liver enzymes, gastritis, hiccups, ileus, nausea, vomiting

GU: Amenorrhea, decreased libido, erectile dysfunction, impotence, infertility, lack of menstruation, oliguria, urinary hesitancy, urine retention

RESP: Dyspnea, **respiratory depression**

SKIN: Diaphoresis, pruritus, rash

Other: **Anaphylaxis**, drug tolerance, **hyponatremia**, opioid-induced allodynia and hyperalgesia, physical and psychological dependence, withdrawal symptoms

Childbearing Considerations

PREGNANCY

- Drug may cause fetal harm.
- Prolonged use of drug during pregnancy can result in neonatal opioid withdrawal syndrome (NOWS), which may be life-threatening if not recognized and treated.
- Avoid prolonged use during pregnancy. Use with caution only if benefit to mother outweighs potential risk to fetus.

LABOR AND DELIVERY

- Drug is not recommended for use in pregnant women immediately before or during labor. Opioids may alter length of time of labor.
- Opioids cross the placental barrier and may produce respiratory depression and psycho-physiologic effects in the neonate. Monitor neonate closely for signs of excess sedation and respiratory depression.
- An opioid antagonist, such as naloxone, must be available at the time of delivery in the event it is needed to reverse opioid-induced respiratory depression in the neonate.

LACTATION

- Drug is present in breast milk.
- Mothers should check with prescriber before breastfeeding.
- If breastfeeding occurs, monitor infant for excess sedation and respiratory depression. Withdrawal can occur when mother ceases breastfeeding or opioid is discontinued.

REPRODUCTION

- Chronic use of opioids may reduce fertility.

Nursing Considerations

! **WARNING** Be aware that excessive use of opioids like oxycodone may lead to abuse, addiction, misuse, overdose, and possibly death. For this reason, a Risk Evaluation and Mitigation Strategy (REMS) is required for oxycodone to be prescribed. Monitor patient's intake of drug closely and for evidence of physical dependence. Also, have naloxone readily available for emergency treatment of opioid overdose.

! **WARNING** Use extreme caution when administering oxycodone to patients with conditions accompanied by hypoxia or decreased respiratory reserve, such as asthma, COPD, or cor pulmonale. This is because even with usual therapeutic dosages, oxycodone may decrease respiratory drive while simultaneously increasing airway resistance to the point of apnea. Monitor patient's respiratory status closely, especially in cachectic, debilitated, and elderly patients and in patients with chronic pulmonary disease. Respiratory depression may occur at any time, but it is most likely to occur during the initiation of therapy or following a dose increase. Have resuscitative equipment nearby.

! **WARNING** Use oxycodone with extreme caution in patients who may be at risk for carbon dioxide retention (e.g., those with increased intracranial pressure or brain tumors). Monitor for signs of sedation and respiratory depression, especially when initiating therapy. Oxycodone may reduce respiratory drive, and the resultant carbon dioxide retention can further increase intracranial pressure. Also, know that opioids like oxycodone may obscure signs and symptoms in a patient with a head injury.

- Assess patient's pain level regularly, and give drug as prescribed before pain becomes severe.
- Assess patient for possible paradoxical excitation during dosage titration.
- Monitor patient for a paradoxic increase in pain known as opioid-induced hyperalgesia or an increase in sensitivity to pain known as opioid-induced allodynia, especially when oxycodone dosage increases. Do not confuse this with tolerance, which is the need for increasing doses of opioids to maintain an effect. If opioid-induced allodynia and hyperalgesia is suspected, notify prescriber and expect dosage to be decreased or opioid rotation to be prescribed.

! **WARNING** Know that oxycodone should not be used for an extended period of time unless pain remains severe enough to require an opioid analgesic and alternative treatment options continue to be inadequate.

! **WARNING** Be aware that abuse of crushed controlled-release tablets poses a hazard of overdose and death. If you suspect abuse and determine that patient also is abusing alcohol or illicit substances, notify prescriber immediately because risk of overdose and death is increased. If you suspect parenteral abuse, be aware that tablet excipients, especially talc, may result in endocarditis, infection, local tissue necrosis, pulmonary granulomas, and valvular heart injury.

! **WARNING** Monitor patient for a hypersensitivity reaction, which could become life-threatening, such as anaphylaxis. If present, notify prescriber, expect drug to be switched to another analgesic, and provide supportive care, as needed and ordered.

- Monitor patient's blood pressure closely, especially when initiating oxycodone therapy and when titrating the dose because oxycodone may cause severe hypotension and syncope in ambulatory patients due to its vasodilatory effects. Risk of hypotension is greater in patients who already have been compromised by a reduced blood volume or concurrent administration of certain CNS depressant drugs, such as general anesthetics and phenothiazines.

! **WARNING** Monitor patients with seizure disorders closely because oxycodone may induce or aggravate seizure disorders.

! **WARNING** Monitor patient's blood glucose level, especially if diabetic, because opioids may cause hypoglycemia.

! **WARNING** Be aware that oxycodone should only be used concomitantly with benzodiazepine therapy or other CNS depressants in patients for whom other treatment options are inadequate. If prescribed together, expect dosing and duration of oxycodone to be limited. Monitor patient closely for signs and symptoms of a decrease in consciousness, including coma, profound sedation, and significant respiratory depression. Notify prescriber immediately and provide emergency supportive care, as death may occur.

! **WARNING** Be aware that oxycodone given concomitantly with CYP3A4 inhibitors (or if CYP3A4 inducers are discontinued) can result in a fatal overdose of oxycodone.

! **WARNING** Know that many drugs may interact with opioids like oxycodone to cause serotonin syndrome. Monitor patient closely for signs and symptoms, such as agitation, diaphoresis, diarrhea, fever, hallucinations, labile blood pressure, muscle twitching or stiffness, nausea, shakiness, shivering, tachycardia, trouble with coordination, or vomiting. Notify prescriber at once because serotonin syndrome may be life-threatening. Be prepared to discontinue drug, if possible and ordered, and provide supportive care.

! **WARNING** Monitor patient for adrenal insufficiency. Although rare, it can be life-threatening. Monitor patient for anorexia, dizziness, fatigue, hypotension, nausea, vomiting, or weakness. Notify prescriber if adrenal insufficiency is suspected and expect diagnostic testing to be done. If confirmed, expect to administer corticosteroids and wean patient off oxycodone, if possible.

! **WARNING** Monitor neonates born to mothers with chronic oxycodone use for NOWS. Know that it can be life-threatening if not recognized and treated appropriately. Monitor neonate for severe respiratory problems, seizures, and other severe adverse effects. Be prepared to provide emergency supportive care, as needed and ordered.

- Know that oxycodone can cause sleep-related breathing disorders, such as central sleep apnea (CSA) or sleep-related hypoxemia. Use of drug increases the risk of CSA in a dose-dependent way. Let prescriber know if patient experiences CSA and expect oxycodone dosage to possibly be reduced.
- Assess patient for abdominal pain because oxycodone may mask underlying GI disorders.
- Know that oxycodone therapy should not be stopped abruptly in a physically dependent patient.

PATIENT TEACHING

! **WARNING** Instruct patient how to administer form of oxycodone prescribed.

! **WARNING** Warn patient that oxycodone use can lead to abuse, addiction, misuse, overdose, and possibly death, even with normal dosing. Stress importance of patient not increasing dosage or frequency of administration without consulting prescriber. Encourage family or caregiver to obtain naloxone for home use; if and when it's needed, it will be readily available. Review signs and symptoms of an opioid overdose and how to administer naloxone. Stress importance of the need to call 911 if naloxone is administered.

! **WARNING** Warn patient not to consume alcohol or take a benzodiazepine or other CNS depressant without prescriber knowledge, as severe respiratory depression can occur and may lead to death.

! **WARNING** Warn patient not to stop oxycodone therapy abruptly after long-term use.

! **WARNING** Alert patient that drug may cause an allergic reaction. If present, tell patient to notify prescriber and, if severe, to seek immediate medical attention.

! **WARNING** Urge patient to alert prescriber if persistent, serious, or unusual adverse reactions occur.

! **WARNING** Warn patient to keep drug out of reach of children because ingestion of the drug by a child can be fatal.

! **WARNING** Caution pregnant patient not to increase dosage or take drug for a prolonged period, as adverse effects can cause infant to experience life-threatening withdrawal when born.

! **WARNING** Inform mothers who are breastfeeding to monitor the breastfed infant for excessive sedation and respiratory depression and to seek immediate medical care for infant, if present. Alert mother that infant may experience withdrawal symptoms when mother stops taking drug or stops breastfeeding. Encourage her to consult pediatrician before doing so.

- Caution patient to avoid hazardous activities such as driving during oxycodone therapy until CNS effects are known and resolved.
- Inform patient that long-term use of opioids like oxycodone may decrease sex hormone levels, causing decreased libido, erectile dysfunction, impotence, infertility, or lack of menstruation. Encourage patient to report any symptoms to prescriber.
- Instruct patient to notify all prescribers of opioid use.
- Instruct patient to dispose of unused drug by flushing down the toilet, if a drug take-back option is not readily available.

oxymorphone hydrochloride

Class, Category, and Schedule

Pharmacologic class: Opioid
Therapeutic class: Opioid analgesic
Controlled substance schedule: II

Indications and Dosages

✱ *To relieve pain severe enough to require opioid treatment and for which alternative treatment options such as nonopioid analgesics or opioid combination products are inadequate or not tolerated.*

TABLETS

Adults receiving an opioid for first time. *Initial:* 10 to 20 mg every 4 to 6 hr, as needed, with dosage adjusted based on patient response. *Maximum initial dose:* 20 mg.
Adults converting from other oral opioids. Highly individualized.

± **DOSAGE ADJUSTMENT** For patients with mild hepatic impairment or renal impairment (a creatinine clearance less than 50 ml/min) or who are elderly, initial dose reduced to 5 mg and titrated slowly. For patients receiving a CNS depressant, dosage begun at one-third to one-half usual initial dose.

E.R. TABLETS

Adults who are opioid-naïve or opioid nontolerant. *Initial:* 5 mg every 12 hr. Dosage adjusted based on patient's response.

Adults converting form other oral opioids. Half the patient's total daily dose every 12 hr.
Adults converting from other opioids. Highly individualized and dependent on prior oral opioid used
Adults converting from methadone. Highly individualized.

±**DOSAGE ADJUSTMENT** For patients who are opioid-naïve with mild hepatic impairment or renal impairment or who are elderly, initial dose kept at 5 mg and dosage titrated slowly. For patients on prior opioid therapy with mild hepatic impairment or renal impairment, initial dosage reduced by 50% and titration done slowly. For patients receiving a CNS depressant, dosage begun at one-third to one-half the usual initial dose.

Drug Administration

P.O.

- Administer tablets on an empty stomach at least 1 hr before or 2 hr after a meal.
- Tablets should be swallowed whole and not broken, chewed, crushed, or divided.

Route	Onset	Peak	Duration
P.O.	10–30 min	1–2 hr	3–6 hr

Half-life: 7–10 hr

Mechanism of Action

Alters perception of and emotional response to pain at spinal cord and higher levels of CNS by blocking release of inhibitory neurotransmitters, such as acetylcholine and gamma-aminobutyric acid.

Contraindications

Acute or severe bronchial asthma in an unmonitored setting or in the absence of resuscitative equipment; GI obstruction, including paralytic ileus; hypersensitivity to oxymorphone or its components; moderate or severe hepatic impairment; significant respiratory depression

Interactions

DRUGS

5-HT$_3$ receptor antagonists, certain muscle relaxants (cyclobenzaprine, metaxalone), drugs that affect the serotonin neurotransmitter system (mirtazapine, tramadol, trazodone), MAO inhibitors (such as I.V. methylene blue or linezolid), selective serotonin reuptake inhibitors, serotonin and norepinephrine reuptake inhibitors, tricyclic antidepressants, triptans: Increased risk of serotonin syndrome
anticholinergics: Increased risk of urine retention, severe constipation
anxiolytics, antipsychotics, benzodiazepines, general anesthetics, muscle relaxants, other CNS depressants, other opioids, sedating antihistamines, tranquilizers: Increased risk of severe respiratory depression and significant sedation and somnolence
diuretics: Decreased effectiveness of diuretics
MAO inhibitors: Increased risk of serotonin syndrome; increased risk of opioid toxicity
mixed agonist/antagonist and partial agonist opioid analgesics, such as buprenorphine, butorphanol, nalbuphine, pentazocine: Possibly reduced analgesic effect of oxymorphone
muscle relaxants: Enhanced neuromuscular blocking action increasing degree of respiratory depression

ACTIVITIES

alcohol use: Additive CNS and respiratory depressant effects which could be severe

Adverse Reactions

CNS: Agitation, asthenia, **CNS depression**, confusion, delusions, depersonalization, dizziness, drowsiness, euphoria, fatigue, hallucinations, headache, insomnia, lightheadedness, nervousness, nightmares, restlessness, **seizures**, somnolence, tiredness, tremor, weakness
CV: **Bradycardia**, hypertension, **hypotension**, palpitations, tachycardia
EENT: Blurred vision, diplopia, dry mouth, **laryngeal edema**, **laryngospasm**, miosis, tinnitus
ENDO: **Adrenal insufficiency**
GI: Abdominal cramps or pain, anorexia, biliary colic, constipation, elevated serum amylase level, **hepatotoxicity**, ileus, nausea, vomiting

GU: Decreased urine output, decreased libido, dysuria, erectile dysfunction, impotence, infertility, lack of menstruation, urinary frequency and hesitancy, urine retention
MS: Muscle rigidity (with large doses), uncontrolled muscle movements
RESP: **Apnea**, **atelectasis**, **bradypnea**, **bronchospasm**, dyspnea, **irregular breathing**, **respiratory depression**, wheezing
SKIN: Dermatitis, diaphoresis, erythema, flushing of face, pruritus, urticaria
Other: **Anaphylaxis**; **angioedema**; injection-site burning, pain, redness, and swelling; opioid-induced allodynia and hyperalgesia; psychological and physical dependence

Childbearing Considerations

PREGNANCY

- Drug may cause fetal harm.
- Prolonged use of drug during pregnancy can result in neonatal opioid withdrawal syndrome (NOWS), which may be life-threatening if not recognized and treated. NOWS occurs when a newborn has been exposed to opioid drugs like oxymorphone for a prolonged period while in utero and may cause severe respiratory problems, seizures, and other severe adverse effects.
- Avoid prolonged use during pregnancy. Use with caution only if benefit to mother outweighs potential risk to fetus.

LABOR AND DELIVERY

- Drug is not recommended for use in pregnant women immediately before or during labor. Opioids may alter length of time of labor.
- Opioids cross the placental barrier and may produce respiratory depression and psycho-physiologic effects in the neonate. Monitor neonate closely for signs of excess sedation and respiratory depression.
- An opioid antagonist, such as naloxone, must be available at the time of delivery in the event it is needed to reverse opioid-induced respiratory depression in the neonate.

LACTATION

- It is not known if drug is present in breast milk.
- Mothers should check with prescriber before breastfeeding.
- If breastfeeding occurs, monitor infant for excess sedation and respiratory depression.

REPRODUCTION

- Chronic use of opioids may reduce fertility.

Nursing Considerations

! WARNING Be aware that excessive use of opioids like oxymorphone may lead to abuse, addiction, misuse, overdose, and possibly death. Monitor patient's intake of drug closely and watch for evidence of physical dependence. Know that drug use now requires a Risk Evaluation and Mitigation Strategy (REMS) for a prescription.

! WARNING Use extreme caution when administering oxymorphone to patients with conditions accompanied by decreased respiratory reserve or hypoxia, such as asthma, COPD, or cor pulmonale. This is because oxymorphone, even with usual therapeutic dosages, may decrease respiratory drive while simultaneously increasing airway resistance to the point of apnea. Have naloxone readily available.

! WARNING Use oxymorphone with extreme caution in patients who may be at risk for carbon dioxide retention (e.g., those with brain tumors or increased intracranial pressure). Monitor for signs of respiratory depression and sedation, especially when initiating therapy. Oxymorphone may reduce respiratory drive, and the resultant carbon dioxide retention can further increase intracranial pressure. Also, know that opioids like oxymorphone may obscure signs and symptoms in a patient with a head injury.

- Use cautiously in patients with biliary tract disease because drug may cause spasm of sphincter of Oddi; mild hepatic impairment because drug is metabolized in liver; and impaired renal function because drug is excreted by kidneys.
- Use cautiously in patients receiving mixed agonist-antagonist opioid analgesics because these drugs may reduce analgesic effect of oxymorphone or may cause withdrawal symptoms.
- Use cautiously in elderly patients because plasma oxymorphone levels in the elderly are higher than in younger patients.

! **WARNING** Know that oral hydromorphone shouldn't be used "as needed" or for first 24 hours after surgery in patients not already taking opioids because of the risk of oversedation and respiratory depression.

- Assess patient's pain level regularly, and give drug as prescribed before pain becomes severe.
- Monitor patient for a paradoxic increase in pain known as opioid-induced hyperalgesia or an increase in sensitivity to pain known as opioid-induced allodynia, especially when oxymorphone dosage increases. Do not confuse this with tolerance, which is the need for increasing doses of opioids to maintain an effect. If opioid-induced allodynia and hyperalgesia is suspected, notify prescriber and expect dosage to be decreased or opioid rotation to be prescribed.

! **WARNING** Monitor patient for a hypersensitivity reaction, which could become life-threatening, such as anaphylaxis or angioedema. If present, notify prescriber, expect a different analgesic to be prescribed, and provide supportive care, as needed and ordered.

! **WARNING** Monitor patient's respiratory status closely for respiratory depression, especially in cachectic, debilitated, or elderly patients; when initiating or titrating dosages; or when other drugs that depress respiration are given together. Have resuscitative equipment nearby. Report respiratory depression immediately because severe respiratory depression may occur. Be prepared to provide supportive care.

! **WARNING** Monitor patient's blood pressure closely, especially when initiating oxymorphone therapy and when titrating the dose because oxymorphone may cause severe hypotension and syncope in ambulatory patients due to its vasodilatory effects. Risk of hypotension is greatest in patients who already have been compromised by a reduced blood volume or concurrent administration of certain CNS depressant drugs, such as general anesthetics and phenothiazines.

! **WARNING** Monitor patient for hypoglycemia, especially diabetics, because opioids like oxymorphone may lower blood glucose levels.

! **WARNING** Monitor patient for seizures, especially patient with a seizure history. Institute seizure precautions, as appropriate.

! **WARNING** Be aware that oxymorphone should only be used concomitantly with benzodiazepine therapy or other CNS depressants in patients for whom other treatment options are inadequate. If prescribed together, expect dosing and duration of oxymorphone to be limited. Monitor patient closely for signs and symptoms of a decrease in consciousness, including coma, profound sedation, and significant respiratory depression. Notify prescriber immediately and provide emergency supportive care, as death may occur.

! **WARNING** Know that many drugs may interact with opioids like oxymorphone to cause serotonin syndrome. Monitor patient closely for signs and symptoms, such as agitation, diaphoresis, diarrhea, fever, hallucinations, labile blood pressure, muscle twitching or stiffness, nausea, shakiness, shivering, tachycardia, trouble with coordination, or vomiting. Notify prescriber at once because serotonin syndrome may be life-threatening. Be prepared to discontinue drug, if possible and ordered, and provide supportive care.

! **WARNING** Monitor patient for adrenal insufficiency. Although rare, it can be life-threatening. Monitor patient for anorexia, dizziness, fatigue, hypotension, nausea, vomiting, or weakness. Notify prescriber if adrenal insufficiency is suspected and expect diagnostic testing to be done. If confirmed, expect to administer corticosteroids and wean patient off oxymorphone, if possible.

! **WARNING** Monitor bowel and urinary status; constipation may be so severe it causes ileus.

! **WARNING** Monitor neonates born to mothers with chronic oxymorphone use for NOWS. Know that it can be life-threatening if not recognized and treated appropriately. Monitor neonate for severe respiratory problems, seizures, and other severe adverse effects. Be prepared to provide emergency supportive care, as needed and ordered.

- Monitor patient for signs of excessive opioid-related adverse reactions. If present, notify prescriber and expect next dose to be reduced.
- Offer fluids to relieve dry mouth.
- Taper dosage, as ordered, before stopping therapy, to prevent withdrawal in physically dependent patients.

PATIENT TEACHING

- Instruct patient how to administer form of oxymorphone prescribed.

! **WARNING** Tell patient to take oxymorphone exactly as prescribed and not to stop abruptly; warn that drug can cause abuse, misuse, overdose, physical dependence, and possibly death. Encourage patient and family or caregiver to have naloxone on hand. Instruct family or caregiver on recognizing signs and symptoms of an opioid overdose, such as severe respiratory depression and profound sedation, and instruct on how to administer naloxone. Stress importance of calling 911 immediately if naloxone is administered.

- Emphasize importance of taking drug before pain becomes severe.
- Encourage patient to increase fluid and fiber intake during therapy to prevent constipation.

! **WARNING** Emphasize need to avoid alcohol, benzodiazepine therapy, and CNS depressants during therapy because of risk of severe life-threatening adverse reactions.

! **WARNING** Alert patient that drug can cause an allergic reaction. If present, tell patient to notify prescriber and, if severe, to seek immediate medical care.

! **WARNING** Tell patient to notify prescriber of any persistent, serious, or unusual adverse reactions.

! **WARNING** Warn patient to keep drug out of the reach of children, as accidental ingestion may be fatal.

! **WARNING** Caution pregnant patient not to increase dosage or take drug for a prolonged period, as adverse effects can cause infant to experience life-threatening withdrawal when born.

! **WARNING** Instruct mothers who are breastfeeding to monitor their infant for excessive sedation and respiratory depression. Warn them that the breastfed infant may experience withdrawal symptoms when mother stops taking oxymorphone or stops breastfeeding. Encourage her to consult with pediatrician before doing so.

- Caution patient to avoid potentially hazardous activities until drug's CNS effects are known and resolved.
- Inform patient that long-term use of opioids like oxymorphone may decrease sex hormone levels, causing decreased libido, erectile dysfunction, impotence, infertility, or lack of menstruation. Encourage patient to report any symptoms to prescriber.
- Instruct patient to notify all prescribers of opioid use.
- Instruct patient to dispose of unused drug by flushing down the toilet, if a drug take-back option is not readily available.
- Instruct patient not to stop taking oxymorphone abruptly as drug dosage must be tapered off.

ozanimod hydrochloride

Zeposia

Class and Category

Pharmacologic class: Sphingosine 1-phosphate receptor modulator
Therapeutic class: Immunosuppressant

Indications and Dosages

✶ *To treat relapsing forms of multiple sclerosis, including active secondary progressive disease, clinically isolated syndrome, and relapsing-remitting disease; to treat moderate to severe active ulcerative colitis*

CAPSULES

Adults. *Initial:* 0.23 mg once daily for days 1 through 4; increased to 0.46 mg once daily for days 5 through 7; increased to 0.92 mg once daily for day 8 and thereafter. *Maintenance:* 0.92 mg once daily.

±**DOSAGE ADJUSTMENT** For patients with mild to moderate chronic hepatic impairment, maintenance dosage reduced to 0.92 mg once every other day.

Drug Administration

P.O.

- Capsules should be swallowed whole and not chewed, crushed, or opened.
- Can be given with or without meals.
- If patient misses a dose during the first 2 weeks of treatment, titration regimen must be reinitiated. For patients who miss a dose after the first 2 weeks of treatment, noretitration is necessary.

Route	Onset	Peak	Duration
P.O.	Unknown	6–8 hr	Unknown

Half-life: 21 hr

Mechanism of Action

Binds to sphingosine 1-phosphate receptors 1 and 2 to block the capability of lymphocytes to leave lymph nodes thereby reducing the number of lymphocytes in the bloodstream. May reduce the lymphocyte migration into the central nervous system, which may help to reduce signs and symptoms of relapsing multiple sclerosis.

Contraindications

Experienced within the past 6 mo class III or IV heart failure, decompensated heart failure requiring hospitalization, MI, stroke, transient ischemic attack, or unstable angina; hypersensitivity to ozanimod or its components; presence of Mobitz type II second-degree or third-degree atrioventricular block, sick sinus syndrome, or sinoatrial block, unless a pacemaker is in place; severe, untreated sleep apnea; use within 14 days of MAO inhibitor therapy

Interactions

DRUGS

adrenergic and serotonergic drugs, such as nonselective MAO inhibitors, opioids (meperidine and its derivatives, methadone, tramadol), selective norepinephrine reuptake inhibitors, selective serotonin reuptake inhibitors, tricyclics, tyramine: Increased risk of serious adverse reactions, such as hypertensive crisis

antineoplastic, immune-modulating, or immunosuppressive drugs: Increased risk of additive immune effects

breast cancer resistance protein inhibitors: Increased exposure of active metabolites of ozanimod, which may increase risk of ozanimod adverse reactions

class Ia antiarrhythmics, such as procainamide, quinidine; class III antiarrhythmics, such as amiodarone, sotalol; QT-prolonging drugs with known arrhythmogenic properties: Possibly increased risk for torsades de pointes in patients with bradycardia

combined beta-blocker and calcium channel blocker: Possible additive effects on heart rate

CYP2C8 inducers (strong), such as rifampin: Reduced exposure of ozanimod active metabolites leading to reduced effectiveness

CYP2C8 inhibitors (strong), such as gemfibrozil: Increased expousure of ozanimod leading possibly to risk of ozanimod adverse effects

live-attenuated vaccines: Increased risk of infection

MAO inhibitors: Possibly decreased exposure of ozanimod; possibly inhibition of MAO inhibitor effects

vaccinations: Possibly less effective

FOODS

tyramine-rich foods, such as foods that are aged, cured, fermented, pickled, or smoked: Increased risk of hypertensive crisis

Adverse Reactions

CNS: **Posterior reversible encephalopathy syndrome**, **progressive multifocal leukoencephalopathy (PML)**

CV: **Atrioventricular conduction delays**, **bradyarrhythmia**, **bradycardia** (transient), hypertension, **hypertensive crisis**, orthostatic hypotension, peripheral edema

EENT: Macular edema

GI: Abdominal pain, elevated liver enzymes or total bilirubin, **hepatic dysfunction or failure**, **rectal adenocarcinoma**

GU: Cervical cancer, UTI

MS: Back pain

RESP: Decreased absolute forced expiratory volume over 1 sec (FEV_1), dyspnea, upper respiratory infections

N O

SKIN: **Basal cell or squamous cell carcinoma, melanoma,** rash, urticaria
Other: **Immunosuppression; infections** (may be serious or life-threatening); **malignancies, such as adenocarcinomas, breast cancer, or seminoma**

Childbearing Considerations

PREGNANCY

- Pregnancy exposure registry: 1-877-301-9314 or www.zeposiapregnancyregistry.com.
- It is not known if drug can cause fetal harm. However, animal studies suggest that a serious risk may exist.
- Use with caution only if benefit to mother outweighs potential risk to fetus.

LACTATION

- It is not known if drug is present in breast milk.
- Mothers should check with prescriber before breastfeeding.

REPRODUCTION

- Females of childbearing age should use an effective contraceptive method during treatment and for 3 mo after treatment is discontinued.

Nursing Considerations

! **WARNING** Know that ozanimod should not be administered to patients who have received alemtuzumab because of risk of additive immunosuppression. Also, use ozanimod cautiously in patients receiving other antineoplastic, immune-modulating, or immunosuppressive drugs.

- Expect to obtain results of the following tests and evaluations prior to starting ozanimod therapy: cardiac evaluation, CBC, liver function tests, and an ophthalmic evaluation. In addition, determine if patient is taking or has taken antineoplastic, immune-modulating, or immunosuppressive therapies or drugs that could slow atrioventricular conduction or slow heart rate because of increased risk for adverse reactions.
- Ensure that patient who has no history of having had chickenpox has been tested for antibodies to varicella-zoster virus before ozanimod therapy begins. Expect to administer varicella-zoster virus vaccine to antibody-negative patients. Know that live-attenuated vaccine immunizations should be administered at least 1 month prior to initiation of ozanimod.

! **WARNING** Monitor patient's respiratory status and notify prescriber if patient develops dyspnea because dose-dependent reductions in absolute forced expiratory volume over 1 second may occur with ozanimod therapy.

! **WARNING** Assess patient's blood pressure regularly, as an increase may occur. Although uncommon, a hypertensive crisis may also occur as a result of ozanimod therapy. Do not give patient foods containing very large amounts (i.e., more than 150 mg) of tyramine because of an increased sensitivity to tyramine as a result of ozanimod therapy.

! **WARNING** Monitor patient for signs and symptoms of infection because serious, life-threatening, or even fatal (rare) infections have occurred with ozanimod therapy. Know that therapy should be delayed in patients with an active infection until the infection is resolved. Ozanimod particularly increases the risk of herpes zoster, urinary tract, and viral upper respiratory tract infections. Be aware that therapy may have to be interrupted if a serious infection occurs. Continue monitoring patient for infection for at least 3 months after ozanimod therapy is discontinued.

! **WARNING** Assess patient's heart rate regularly because initiation of ozanimod may result in a transient decrease in heart rate or cause delays in atrioventricular conduction. If patient develops any of the following, expect prescriber to consult with a cardiologist: arrhythmias requiring treatment with class 1a or class III antiarrhythmic drugs; heart failure or ischemic heart disease; history of cardiac arrest, cerebrovascular disease, MI, second-degree Mobitz type II or higher AV block, sick sinus syndrome, sinoatrial heart block, or uncontrolled hypotension; or significant QT prolongation.

! **WARNING** Monitor patient's liver enzymes and total bilirubin, as ordered, because elevations may occur with ozanimod therapy. Notify prescriber if patient develops signs and symptoms of liver dysfunction, such as unexplained abdominal pain, anorexia, fatigue, jaundice, nausea, or vomiting as well as an AST or ALT value greater than 1.5 times upper-level normal. If present, expect drug to be discontinued if significant liver injury is confirmed.

! **WARNING** Be aware drug may cause cancer, including skin malignancies. Monitor patient closely for any abnormal or unusual adverse reactions.

! **WARNING** Monitor patient for posterior reversible encephalopathy syndrome or PML and report suspicions immediately to prescriber. Know that patients who experience PML also may experience immune reconstitution inflammatory syndrome, which can result in death. Expect ozanimod to be withheld until such disorders has been excluded. If confirmed, expect ozanimod to be discontinued and appropriate supportive care given, as needed and ordered.

- Monitor elderly patients for cardiac and hepatic adverse drug reactions because of decreased cardiac and hepatic function in this population.
- Assess patient for changes in vision, as ozanimod may cause macular edema. Patients at increased risk are those who have a history of uveitis or diabetes mellitus.
- Be aware that a severe increase in disability may occur when ozanimod is discontinued, though this is rare. If present, notify prescriber and expect appropriate treatment to be given, as prescribed.

PATIENT TEACHING

- Instruct patient how to administer ozanimode and what to do if a dose is missed.

! **WARNING** Review with patient foods that are rich in tyramine, such as foods that are aged, cured, fermented, pickled, or smoked, and stress importance of avoiding these foods while taking ozanimod.

! **WARNING** Warn females of childbearing age to use effective contraception during ozanimod therapy and for 3 months following discontinuation of drug because of potential fetal risk.

! **WARNING** Review signs and symptoms of infection and infection control measures to take while receiving ozanimod and for 3 months following drug discontinuation. Stress importance of notifying prescriber if an infection occurs.

! **WARNING** Review signs and symptoms of liver dysfunction with patient. Stress importance of patient alerting prescriber if any are present.

! **WARNING** Warn patient to notify prescriber immediately of any persistent, serious, or unusual adverse reactions such as neurological changes, changes in breathing or vision, or skin abnormalities.

- Inform patient that vaccines containing live virus should be avoided during ozanimod therapy and for 3 months after drug is discontinued or given at least 1 month prior to start of therapy.
- Tell patient to report any significant increase in disability after ozanimod is discontinued.

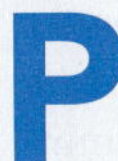

paliperidone

Invega

paliperidone palmitate

Erzofri, Invega Hafyera, Invega Sustenna, Invega Trinza

Class and Category

Pharmacologic class: Benzisoxazole derivative
Therapeutic class: Antipsychotic (atypical)

Indications and Dosages

✱ *To treat schizophrenia*

E.R. TABLETS (INVEGA)

Adults. *Initial:* 6 mg once daily; then increased or decreased in increments of 3 mg daily every 5 or more days, as needed. *Maximum:* 12 mg daily.

Adolescents ages 12 to 17. *Initial:* 3 mg once daily; then increased in increments of 3 mg daily every 5 or more days, as needed. *Maximum:* 12 mg once daily for adolescents weighing 51 kg (112.2 lb) or more; 6 mg for adolescents weighing less than 51 kg (112.2lb).

I.M. INJECTION (INVEGA SUSTENNA)

Adults. *Initial:* 234 mg on day 1 and 156 mg on day 8. *Maintenance:* 39 to 234 mg monthly. Maintenance dosage decreased or increased monthly according to patient's response and tolerance. *Maximum:* 234 mg monthly.

I.M. INJECTION (ERZOFRI)

Adults with established tolerability with oral paliperidone or oral risperidone. *Initial:* 351 mg followed by 39 mg to 234 mg 4 wk later with dose dependent on response and tolerability. *Maintenance:* 39 mg to 234 mg monthly. Maintenance dosage decreased or increased according to patient's response and tolerance. *Maximum:* 234 mg monthly.

I.M. INJECTION (INVEGA TRINZA)

Adults who have been adequately treated with Invega Sustenna for at least 4 mo. *Initial:* 273 mg if last monthly Sustenna dose was 78 mg; 410 mg if last monthly Sustenna dose was 117 mg; 546 mg if last monthly Sustenna dose was 156 mg; or 819 mg if last monthly Sustenna dose was 234 mg, administered within 7 days before or after next monthly Sustenna dose would have been given with dosage adjustment made thereafter every 3 mo, as needed. *Maintenance:* 273 to 819 mg every 3 mo. *Maximum:* 819 mg every 3 mo.

I.M. INJECTION (INVEGA HAFYERA)

Adults who have been adequately treated with Invega Sustenna for at least 4 mo. *Initial:* 1,092 mg if last paliperidone palmitate extended-release injectable suspension dose was 156 mg or 1,560 mg if last paliperidone palmitate extended-release injectable suspension dose was 234 mg, administered within 7 days before or after next monthly Sustenna dose would have been given with dosage adjustment made every 6 mo thereafter, as needed. *Maintenance:* 1,092 to 1.560 mg every 6 mo. *Maximum:* 1,560 mg every 6 mo.

Adults who have been adequately treated with Invega Trinza for at least one 3-mo injection cycle. *Initial:* 1,092 mg if last every 3-mo paliperidone palmitate extended-release injectable suspension dose was 546 mg or 1,560 mg if last every-3-mo paliperidone palmitate E.R. injectable suspension dose was 819 mg, administered within 14 days before or after next monthly Trinza dose would have been given with dosage adjustment made every 6 mo thereafter, as needed. *Maintenance:* 1,092 to 1.560 mg every 6 mo. *Maximum:* 1,560 mg every 6 mo.

✱ *To treat schizoaffective disorder*

E.R. TABLETS (INVEGA)

Adults. *Initial:* 6 mg once daily; then increased or decreased in increments of 3 mg daily every 4 or more days, as needed. *Maximum:* 12 mg daily.

I.M. INJECTION (INVEGA SUSTENNA)

Adults. *Initial:* 234 mg on day 1 and 156 mg on day 8. *Maintenance:* 78 to 234 mg monthly. Maintenance dosage decreased or increased monthly according to patient's response and tolerance. *Maximum:* 234 mg monthly.

I.M. INJECTION (ERZOFRI)

Adults with established tolerability with oral paliperidone or oral risperidone. *Initial:* 351 mg followed by 78 mg to 234 mg 4 wk later with dose dependent on response and tolerability. *Maintenance:* 78 mg to 234 mg monthly with each dose adjusted, as needed. *Maximum:* 234 mg monthly.

DOSAGE ADJUSTMENT For patients taking E.R. tablets with mild renal impairment (creatinine clearance 50 to 79 ml/min), initial dosage decreased to 3 mg daily then increased to maximum dosage 6 mg daily; moderate to severe renal impairment (creatinine clearance 10 ml/min to less than 50 ml/min), initial dose decreased to 1.5 mg daily, then increased to maximum dosage of 3 mg daily. For patients receiving Invega Sustenna with mild renal impairment (creatinine clearance equal to or greater than 50 ml/min but less than 80 ml/min), initial dosage decreased to 156 mg on day 1 and second dose given 1 wk later decreased to 117 mg, followed by 78 mg monthly. For patients receiving Erzofri with mild renal impairment (creatine clearance greater than 50 mg/ml to less than 80 ml/min), initial dose of 234 mg given followed by a dosage of 78 mg 4 wk later with monthly adjustments made thereafter and given as 39 mg, 78 mg, 117 mg, or 156 mg. Maximum dosage of Erzofri reduced to 156 mg monthly. Erzofri is not recommended in patients with moderate or severe renal impairment (creatinine clearance less than 50 ml/min). For patients receiving Invega Trinza with mild renal impairment (creatine clearance greater than 50 ml/min to less than 80 ml/min), patient stabilized using Invega Sustenna then transitioned to Invega Trinza. Invega Trinza is not recommended in patients with moderate or severe renal impairment (creatinine clearance less than 50 ml/min). For patients receiving Invega Hafyera with mild renal impairment (creatine clearance greater than 50 ml/min to less than 80 ml/min), patient stabilized with possible dosage adjustment using once-a-month formulation before transitioning to Invega Hafyera or dosage adjusted and stabilized before transitioning from once-a-month to once-every-three-months formulation. Invega Hafyera is not recommended in patients with moderate or severe renal impairment (creatinine clearance less than 50 ml/min). For elderly patients with any degree of renal impairment, Invega Hafyera should not be used; for all other formulations dosage reduced. For patients receiving a strong CYP3A4 inducer, such as carbamazepine, rifampin, or St. John's wort, these drugs should be avoided if patients are to receive an injectable form of paliperidone. If use of these drugs must continue, extended-release tablets (Invega) should be used instead of an injectable form.

Drug Administration

P.O.

- Administer with a liquid beverage.
- E.R. tablets must be swallowed whole and not chewed, crushed, or divided.

I.M.

- Do not administer by any other route.
- Drug is supplied in a prefilled syringe along with 2 different-size needles. Use only the needles provided with the product.
- Administer dose as a single injection.
- Do not mix with any product or diluent.
- Follow manufacturer guidelines when patient is being switched between long-acting products or to or from E.R. tablets.
- A patient must not receive an every-6-mo injection preparation unless patient has already been adequately treated with a once-a-month form for at least 4 mo or an every-3-mo form has been administered for at least one 3-mo cycle.
- Rotate sites.

Invega Sustenna

- Shake syringe vigorously for a minimum of 10 sec before administration.
- Select needle. For injection into the deltoid muscle for patient weighing less than 90 kg (198 lb), use the 1-inch, 23 G needle; for patient weighing 90 kg (198 lb) or more, use the 1.-inch, 22 G needle.
- When injecting into the gluteal muscle (upper outer quadrant), use the 1-inch, 22 G needle regardless of patient weight and after 2 doses have been given in the deltoid muscle.
- When initiating drug, inject the first two doses into the deltoid muscle.

- Prepare for administration by holding the syringe with the tip cap pointing up and removing cap with a gentle twisting motion.
- Peel back safety needle pouch half way open. Grasp needle sheath using the plastic peel pouch. Hold the syringe pointing up and attache needle using a gentle twisting motion to avoid needle hub cracks or damage. Pull needle sheath away from the needle with a straight pull. Do not twist the sheath as the needle may be loosened from the syringe.
- De-aerate the syringe.
- Inject slowly, deep into muscle.
- After injection use thumb or finger of one hand or a flat surface to activate the needle protection system. The system is fully activated when a click is heard.
- If target date for second initiation injection is missed or patient misses a maintenance dose, follow manufacturer's instructions.

Erzofri

- Peel needle pouch half way open and place on a clean surface.
- Shake syringe vigorously for a minimum of 10 sec. While holding syringe upright, remove the cap with an easy counterclockwise twisting motion. Do not touch syringe tip.
- Select needle for administration. For injections given in the deltoid muscle for patient who weighs 90 kg or more, use the 1½-inch 22 gauge needle (needle with gray colored hub); if patient weighs less than 90 kg, use the 1-inch 23 gauge needle (needle with blue colored hub). For subsequent injections that can be given in gluteal muscle, use the 1½-inch 22 gauge needle (needle with gray colored hub) regardless of patient's weight. Attach needle to syringe with an easy clockwise twisting motion. Do not remove the pouch until the syringe and needle are securely attached. Pull the needle sheath away from the needle with a straight pull. Do not twist the sheath as the needle may be loosened from the syringe.
- De-aerate the syringe by moving the plunger rod carefully forward.
- Administer first dose in deltoid muscle; Administer in the deltoid or gluteal for subsequent doses. Do not administer by any other route. Inject slowly and deeply.
- After injection, use either thumb or finger of one hand or a flat surface to activate the needle protection system. The system is fully activated when a click is heard.
- Monthly dose may be given up to 7 days before or after the monthly scheduled time. If a dose is missed, follow manufacturer instructions.

Invega Trinza

- Shake syringe vigorously for at least 15 sec to ensure a homogeneous suspension and that the needle does not get clogged during injection, which would deliver an incomplete dose. Once syringe has been shaken, inject drug within 5 min.
- Select the appropriate needle. Use only the thin-wall needles provided with the 3-mo product for the injection. Do not use needles from the 1-mo product or other commercially available needles, to reduce risk of blockage.
- When injecting into the deltoid muscle for patient weighing less than 90 kg (198 lb), use the 1-inch, 22 G needle; for patient weighing 90 kg (198 lb) or more, use the 1½-inch, 22 G needle.
- When injecting into the gluteal muscle, use the 1½-inch, 22 G needle regardless of patient weight.
- Prepare for administration by attaching needle to syringe with an easy clockwise twisting motion Do not remove the pouch until the syringe and needle are securely attached. Pull the needle sheath away from the needle with as straight pull. Do not twist the sheath as the needle maybe loosened from the syringe.
- De-aerate the syringe by moving the plunger rod carefully forward.
- Administer a deltoid injection into the center of the deltoid muscle; administer a gluteal injection in the upper outer quadrant.
- If an incomplete dose is administered, do not reinject the dose remaining in the syringe and do not administer another dose. Notify prescriber.
- May administer drug up to 2 wk before or after the 3-mo scheduled time.
- If 4 mo or more have elapsed since last dose, do not give scheduled dose; instead obtain an order to follow manufacturer's guidelines for reinitiation.

Invega Hafyera

- Shake syringe vigorously for at least 15 sec, rest briefly, and then shake again for 15 sec. Solution should appear uniform, thick, and milky white. Administer within 5 min. If more than a 5-min lapse occurs, the syringe will have to be shaken vigorously again for at least 30 sec.
- Open pouch cover. Place pouch with needle inside on a clean surface. Then hold syringe with cap pointing up and twist and pull off the cap.
- Attach the needle using only the needle provided with the drug. Do not interchange needles from other dosage forms or use any other commercially available needle.
- Attach the needle using a gentle twisting motion to avoid needle hub cracks or damage. Holding the syringe upright, gently pull back the plunger to clear the syringe tip of any solid product and remove air bubbles.
- Administer deeply into the upper-outer quadrant of the gluteal muscle only. Inject slowly (will take about 30 sec) and take care to avoid injection into a blood vessel. Resistance may be felt while administering drug, but this is normal. Confirm that the entire content of syringe has been injected before removing needle from muscle. After injection is complete, use thumb or a flat surface to secure the needle in the safety device. The needle is secure when a click is heard. After injection, hold pressure over the site; do not rub the injection site.
- If an incomplete dose is administered, do not reinject the dose remaining in the syringe and do not administer another dose. Notify prescriber.
- Follow manufacturer's guidelines if a dose is missed.

Route	Onset	Peak	Duration
P.O.	Unknown	24 hr	Unknown
I.M.	1 day	13 days	126 days

Half-life: 23 hr (P.O.); 25–49 hr (I.M.)

Mechanism of Action

Blocks serotonin and dopamine receptors selectively in mesocortical tract of CNS to suppress psychotic symptoms.

Contraindications

For all forms: History of cardiac arrhythmias, congenital heart disease, or congenital long-QT syndrome; hypersensitivity to paliperidone, risperidone, or its components
For oral form: Preexisting severe gastrointestinal narrowing

Interactions

DRUGS

alpha agonists, alpha-blockers, angiotensin-converting enzyme (ACE) inhibitors, angiotensin II receptor blockers (ARBs), beta-blockers, calcium channel blockers, diuretics (thiazide, nitrates, vasodilators): Increased risk of hypotension, including orthostatic
antiarrhythmics of class IA (such as quinidine, procainamide) and class III (such as amiodarone, sotalol), antibiotics (such as gatifloxacin, moxifloxacin), antipsychotics (such as chlorpromazine, thioridazine): Increased risk of QT-interval prolongation
CNS depressants: Additive CNS depression
CYP3A4 and P-gp strong inducers (carbamazepine, rifampin, St. John's wort): Decreased plasma paliperidone level and effectiveness
dopamine agonist, including levodopa: Possibly antagonized effects of dopamine agonist and other dopamine agonists

ACTIVITIES

alcohol use: CNS depression

Adverse Reactions

CNS: Agitation, akathisia, anxiety, asthenia, bradykinesia, catatonia, cogwheel rigidity, **CVA**, depression, disruption of body temperature regulation, dizziness, drooling, dyskinesia, dystonia, extrapyramidal disorder, fatigue, fever, headache, hyperkinesia, hypertonia, insomnia, lethargy, **neuroleptic malignant syndrome**, nightmares, nuchal rigidity, parkinsonism, psychomotor hyperactivity, psychosis, restlessness, **seizures**, sleep disorder, somnambulism, somnolence, syncope, tardive dyskinesia, transient ischemic attack, tremor, vertigo
CV: **Bradycardia**, bundle branch block, elevated cholesterol and triglyceride level, first-degree heart block, hypertension, ischemia, orthostatic hypotension,

palpitations, peripheral edema, **prolonged QT interval**, tachycardia, vascular ischemia, **venous thrombosis**
EENT: Blurred vision, dry mouth, eye movement disorder, inability to open mouth or jaw (trismus), nasal congestion, nasopharyngitis, oromandibular dystonia, pharyngolaryngeal pain, rhinitis, salivary hypersecretion, **swollen tongue**, tonsillitis, toothache
ENDO: Breast discharge, engorgement, pain, or tenderness; gynecomastia; hyperglycemia; hyperinsulinemia; hyperprolactinemia
GI: Abdominal discomfort or pain, change in appetite, constipation, diarrhea, dyspepsia, dysphagia, elevated liver enzymes, flatulence, ileus, nausea, **small intestinal obstruction**, upper abdominal pain, vomiting
GU: Cystitis, erectile dysfunction, menstrual abnormalities, priapism, retrograde ejaculation, urinary incontinence or retention, UTI
HEME: **Agranulocytosis**, **anemia**, **leukopenia**, **neutropenia**, **thrombocytopenia**, **thrombotic thrombocytopenic purpura**
MS: Arthralgia; back or limb pain; dysarthria; joint stiffness; muscle rigidity, spasms, tightness, or twitching; myalgia; torticollis
RESP: Cough, dyspnea, upper respiratory tract infection
SKIN: Drug eruption, eczema, pruritus, rash, urticaria
Other: **Anaphylaxis**, **angioedema**, generalized chest discomfort, injection-site reactions, weight gain or loss

Childbearing Considerations

PREGNANCY

- Pregnancy exposure registry: 1-866-961-2388 or http://womensmentalhealth.org/clinical-and-research-programs/pregnancyregistry/.
- Drug may cause fetal harm.
- Exposure to drug during the third trimester of pregnancy increases the risk for extrapyramidal and/or withdrawal symptoms following delivery.
- Use with caution only if benefit to mother outweighs potential risk to fetus.

LACTATION

- Drug is present in breast milk.
- Mothers should check with prescriber before breastfeeding.
- If breastfeeding occurs, advise mothers to monitor their infants for excess sedation, extrapyramidal symptoms (tremors and abnormal muscle movements), failure to thrive, and jitteriness.

REPRODUCTION

- Know that females of childbearing age may experience a decrease in fertility during drug therapy that is reversible when drug is discontinued.

Nursing Considerations

! **WARNING** Keep in mind paliperidone shouldn't be used to treat dementia-related psychosis in the elderly because of an increased mortality risk. Parenteral paliperidone is not recommended for patients with moderate to severe renal impairment.

! **WARNING** Know that drug shouldn't be given if patient has a condition that severely narrows GI tract because tablet doesn't change shape as it passes and could cause blockage.

- Use paliperidone cautiously in patients with cardiovascular disease because drug may cause orthostatic hypotension. Also, use cautiously in patients with Lewy bodies because these patients are more sensitive to antipsychotic drugs. Monitor patient for increased sensitivity manifested as confusion, extrapyramidal symptoms, postural instability with frequent falls, and obtundation.

! **WARNING** Monitor patient for a hypersensitivity reaction, which could become life-threatening, such as anaphylaxis or angioedema. If present, notify prescriber, expect drug to be discontinued, and provide supportive care, as needed.

! **WARNING** Check CBC often during first few months of therapy, especially if patient has low WBC count or history of drug-induced leukopenia or neutropenia. If WBC count declines, and especially if neutrophil count goes below 1,000/mm^3, expect to stop drug.

If neutropenia is significant, also watch for evidence of infection and provide appropriate treatment, as prescribed.

! **WARNING** Monitor blood glucose level because drug increases risk of hyperglycemia, which in turn may lead to hyperosmolar coma or ketoacidosis.

! **WARNING** Notify prescriber immediately and expect to stop drug if patient shows signs of neuroleptic malignant syndrome (altered mental status, autonomic instability, hyperpyrexia, muscle rigidity). Patients at risk for developing neuroleptic malignant syndrome are patients with dementia with Lewy bodies or Parkinson's disease because these patients can experience increased sensitivity to paliperidone.

- Monitor patient for involuntary, dyskinetic movements that may occur during therapy or after drug is discontinued. Notify prescriber, if present, and expect to stop therapy. In some cases, therapy may have to continue despite tardive dyskinesia.
- Institute fall measures because of potential for adverse CNS effects.

PATIENT TEACHING

- Instruct patient how to administer oral form of paliperidone.
- Stress importance of compliance with dosing schedule if drug is being administered intramuscularly.
- Advise patient to avoid alcohol while taking paliperidone.
- Explain that shell of tablet will be eliminated in stool but that this is a harmless effect.
- Stress importance of compliance with routine blood tests, if ordered.
- Advise patient to notify all prescribers of paliperidone therapy and not to take over-the-counter preparations, including herbal products, without consulting prescriber.

! **WARNING** Alert patient drug may cause an allergic reaction. If present, tell patient to notify prescriber and, if severe, to seek immediate medical care.

! **WARNING** Tell male patients that painful or prolonged penile erections can occur while taking paliperidone. Instruct him to seek immediate emergency medical attention if this occurs.

- Tell patient to contact prescriber if abnormal movements occur.
- Instruct patient with diabetes to monitor blood glucose level closely, as drug can affect glycemic control. Also, review signs and symptoms of hyperglycemia with all patients and tell them to notify prescriber if present.
- Alert the patient who experiences hyperprolactinemia as a result of paliperidone therapy that reproductive function may become impaired. Also, review signs and symptoms of amenorrhea or galactorrhea in females and erectile dysfunction or gynecomastia in males. If this is a concern for the patient, patient should consult prescriber.

! **WARNING** Instruct patient to alert prescriber immediately if he experiences any other persistent, severe, or unusual signs and symptoms.

- Urge patient to rise slowly from sitting or lying position to minimize orthostatic hypotension.
- Caution patient to avoid hazardous activities until CNS effects of drug are known and resolved. Review fall precautions with patient as well.
- Advise patient to avoid activities that may cause overheating, such as becoming dehydrated, being exposed to extreme heat, or exercising strenuously.
- Advise pregnant patients to alert prescriber when she is close to entering her third trimester because of potential harm to the fetus.
- Inform mothers to monitor their breastfed infant for abnormal muscle movements, excess sedation, failure to thrive, jitteriness, or tremors.

palonosetron hydrochloride

Class and Category

Pharmacologic class: Selective serotonin subtype 3 (5-HT_3) receptor antagonist
Therapeutic class: Antiemetic

Indications and Dosages

✱ To prevent acute and delayed nausea and vomiting from chemotherapy

I.V. INJECTION

Adults. 0.25 mg given over 30 sec about 30 min before start of chemotherapy.

I.V. INFUSION

Infants 1 mo of age to less than 17 yr. 20 mcg/kg infused over 15 min about 30 min before start of chemotherapy. *Maximum:* 1.5 mg as a single dose.

✱ To prevent postoperative nausea and vomiting for up to 24 hr after surgery

I.V. INJECTION

Adults. 0.075 mg given over 10 sec immediately before induction of anesthesia.

Drug Administration

I.V.

- Flush I.V. line with 0.9% Sodium Chloride Injection before and after giving drug.
- For I.V. injection, administer a 0.25-mg dose over 30 sec and a 0.075-mg dose over 10 sec.
- For I.V. infusion, administer over 15 min.
- Store at room temperature and protect from light.
- *Incompatibilities:* Other I.V. drugs

Route	Onset	Peak	Duration
I.V.	Unknown	Unknown	3–5 days

Half-life: 40 hr

Contraindications

Hypersensitivity to palonosetron or its components

Interactions

DRUGS

5-HT_3 receptor antagonists, selective serotonin reuptake inhibitors, serotonin and noradrenaline reuptake inhibitors: Increased risk of serotonin syndrome

Adverse Reactions

CNS: Anxiety, dizziness, drowsiness, dyskinesia, fatigue, headache, insomnia, **serotonin syndrome**, weakness

Mechanism of Action

Remember that chemotherapy may induce nausea and vomiting by irritating the small intestine's mucosa, causing mucosal enterochromaffin cells to release serotonin (5-HT_3) thereby stimulating sympathetic receptors on afferent vagal nerve endings to cause the vomiting reflex. Through blocking 5-HT_3 receptors to keep the vagus nerve from inducing the vomiting reflex, drug reduces or prevents nausea and vomiting. May block also 5-HT_3 receptors centrally in the brain's chemoreceptor trigger zone.

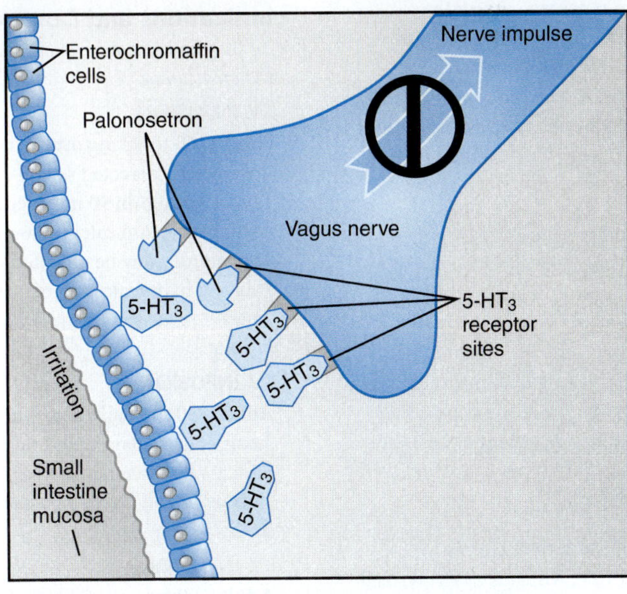

P

CV: **Bradycardia**, **hypotension**, **prolonged QT interval**, tachycardia
GI: Abdominal pain, constipation, diarrhea
SKIN: Dermatitis, pruritus, rash
Other: **Hyperkalemia**, **hypersensitivity reactions (anaphylaxis**, **angioedema**, **bronchospasm**, dyspnea, erythema, pruritus, rash, swelling), injection-site reaction (burning, discomfort, induration, pain)

Childbearing Considerations

PREGNANCY

- It is not known if drug can cause fetal harm.
- Use with caution only if benefit to mother outweighs potential risk to fetus.

LACTATION

- It is not known if drug is present in breast milk.
- A decision should be made to discontinue breastfeeding or to discontinue the drug if breastfeeding occurs.

Nursing Considerations

! **WARNING** Use palonosetron cautiously in patients who have or may develop prolonged cardiac conduction intervals—especially QT interval—such as those with congenital QT syndrome, hypokalemia, or hypomagnesemia; those taking an antiarrhythmic, a diuretic known to induce electrolyte abnormalities, or another drug that may prolong QT interval; and those who have received cumulative high-dose anthracycline therapy. With these patients, obtain a baseline ECG before giving palonosetron; repeat the ECG 15 minutes or 24 hours after giving drug, as ordered. Notify prescriber of any delayed conduction.

! **WARNING** Monitor patient for hypersensitivity reactions, especially patient hypersensitive to other selective serotonin receptor antagonists. Hypersensitivity reactions could become life-threatening, such as anaphylaxis, angioedema, or bronchospasms. If a reaction occurs, notify prescriber immediately, expect drug to be discontinued, and provide supportive care, as needed and ordered.

! **WARNING** Monitor patient closely for serotonin syndrome, which is characterized by agitation, coma, diarrhea, hallucinations, hyperreflexia, hyperthermia, incoordination, labile blood pressure, nausea, tachycardia, or vomiting. Notify prescriber immediately because serotonin syndrome may be life-threatening and provide supportive care, as needed and ordered.

PATIENT TEACHING

- Inform patient that drug will need to be administered intravenously.

! **WARNING** Instruct patient to immediately notify staff if patient suddenly does not feel well including experiencing difficulty breathing or tightness of throat.

- Advise patient to avoid hazardous activities after drug administration until drug's CNS effects are known and resolved.
- Tell mothers breastfeeding should not be undertaken during drug therapy; otherwise drug will have to be discontinued.

pamidronate disodium

Class and Category

Pharmacologic class: Bisphosphonate
Therapeutic class: Antiosteoporotic

Indications and Dosages

✱ *To treat moderate or severe cancer-induced hypercalcemia*

I.V. INFUSION

Adults. 60 to 90 mg over 2 to 24 hr as a single dose when corrected serum calcium level is 12 to 13.5 mg/dl; 90 mg over 2 to 24 hr when corrected serum calcium level is greater than 13.5 mg/dl. May be repeated, as needed, after 7 days if hypercalcemia recurs.

✱ *To treat moderate to severe Paget's disease of bone*

I.V. INFUSION

Adults. 30 mg daily over 4 hr on 3 consecutive days for a total dose of 90 mg. Repeated, as needed and tolerated.

✱ *To treat osteolytic bone metastases of breast cancer*

I.V. INFUSION

Adults. 90 mg over 2 hr every 3 to 4 wk.

✱ To treat osteolytic bone lesions of multiple myeloma

I.V. INFUSION

Adults. 90 mg over 4 hr every mo.

±**DOSAGE ADJUSTMENT** For patients with renal deterioration (normal baseline creatinine but an increase of 0.5 mg/dl or more or an abnormal baseline creatinine with an increase of 1 mg/dl or more) being treated for osteolytic bone metastases of breast cancer or osteolytic bone lesions of multiple myeloma, retreatment given only after creatinine has returned to within 10% of the baseline value.

Drug Administration

I.V.

- No more than 90 mg should be given at any one time because of increased risk of serious adverse effect on kidneys.
- For treatment of hypercalcemia of malignancy, dilute drug in 1,000 ml of 0.45% or 0.9% Sodium Chloride Injection or 5% Dextrose Injection and administer over at least 2 hr and up to 24 hr for the 60- and 90-mg doses. Solution is stable for up to 24 hr stored at room temperature.
- For treatment of Paget's disease, dilute drug in 500 ml of 0.45% or 0.9% Sodium Chloride Injection or 5% Dextrose Injection and infuse over 4 hr.
- For treatment of osteolytic bone metastases of breast cancer, dilute drug in 250 ml of 0.45% or 0.9% Sodium Chloride Injection or 5% Dextrose Injection and infuse over 2 hr.
- For treatment of osteolytic bone lesions of multiple myeloma, dilute 90 mg in 500 ml of 0.45% or 0.9% Sodium Chloride Injection or 5% Dextrose Injection and infuse over 4 hr.
- *Incompatibilities:* Calcium-containing solutions such as Ringer's solution, other drugs

Route	Onset	Peak	Duration
I.V.	24 hr	1 mo	Unknown

Half-life: 21–35 hr

Mechanism of Action

Inhibits bone resorption, possibly by impairing attachment of osteoclast precursors to mineralized bone matrix, thus reducing the rate of bone turnover in Paget's disease and osteolytic metastases. Reduces the flow of calcium also from resorbing bone into bloodstream.

Contraindications

Hypersensitivity to pamidronate, other bisphosphonates, or their components

Interactions

DRUGS

nephrotoxic drugs: Increased risk of nephrotoxicity

thalidomide: Increased risk of renal dysfunction in patients with multiple myeloma

Adverse Reactions

CNS: Confusion, fever, psychosis, visual hallucinations

CV: **Hypotension**

EENT: Conjunctivitis, ocular inflammation

GI: Abdominal cramps, anorexia, **GI bleeding**, indigestion, nausea, vomiting

GU: **Azotemia**, focal segmental glomerulonephropathies, glomerulosclerosis, hematuria, **nephritis**, **nephrotic syndrome**, **renal toxicity leading to failure**, renal tubular disorders

HEME: **Leukopenia**, **lymphopenia**

MS: Atypical fractures of femur; muscle spasms or stiffness; osteonecrosis (mainly of jaw); severe bone, joint, or muscle pain

RESP: **Adult respiratory distress syndrome**, dyspnea, **interstitial lung disease**

SKIN: Pruritus, rash

Other: **Anaphylaxis**, **angioedema**, flu-like symptoms, **hyperkalemia**, **hypernatremia**, **hypocalcemia**, **hypokalemia**, **hypomagnesemia**, **hypophosphatemia**, injection-site pain and swelling, reactivation of herpes simplex and herpes zoster

Childbearing Considerations

PREGNANCY

- Drug may cause fetal harm, such as skeletal and other abnormalities. This risk includes posttreatment if a female of childbearing age becomes pregnant.
- Drug is not recommended for use during pregnancy.

LACTATION

- It is not known if drug is present in breast milk.
- Mothers should check with prescriber before breastfeeding.

Nursing Considerations

- Make sure patient has had a dental checkup before invasive dental procedures during pamidronate therapy, especially if he has cancer; is receiving chemotherapy, a corticosteroid, or head or neck radiation; or has poor oral hygiene. Risk of osteonecrosis is increased in these patients.
- Obtain serum creatinine level before each treatment, as ordered. Notify prescriber of abnormal results because drug may have to be withheld or dosage adjusted until creatinine level returns to normal.

! **WARNING** Stay alert for patient possibly experiencing a fever during first 3 days of therapy, especially in patients receiving high doses. If fever develops, obtain CBC with differential, as ordered, and alert prescriber. Continue to monitor patient for adverse hematological adverse reactions such as anemia, leukopenia, or thrombocytopenia, especially during the first 2 weeks of therapy. Institute bleeding and infection control measures.

! **WARNING** Monitor patient for a hypersensitivity reaction, which could become life-threatening, such as anaphylaxis or angioedema. If present, notify prescriber immediately, expect drug to be discontinued, and provide supportive care, as needed and ordered.

! **WARNING** Monitor patient's vital signs closely as drug can cause hypotension and significant changes in respiratory function.

! **WARNING** Monitor patient for hypocalcemia, especially if patient has had thyroid surgery. Expect to administer calcium and vitamin D supplementation in the absence of hypercalcemia in patients with multiple myeloma or predominantly lytic bone metastases, patients who are at risk of calcium or vitamin D deficiency, or patients with Paget's disease of the bone.

! **WARNING** Monitor patient's serum electrolytes (including calcium, magnesium, and phosphate levels), as ordered throughout therapy because electrolyte abnormalities may occur.

! **WARNING** Monitor patient for other persistent, serious, or unusual adverse reactions.

PATIENT TEACHING

- Inform patient that drug will be administered intravenously.
- Emphasize need to comply with prescribed administration schedule for pamidronate.
- Review if calcium and vitamin D supplementation should be or not be used, which is dependent on patient's calcium level and indication being treated.

! **WARNING** Tell patient to notify staff or prescriber immediately if patient suddenly does not feel well, has difficulty breathing, or experiences other persistent, serious, or unusual adverse reactions such as pain in hip or thigh in the absence of trauma as drug may cause an allergic reaction and other significant adverse reactions.

- Instruct patient on proper oral hygiene and on need to notify prescriber about upcoming invasive dental procedures.
- Advise females of childbearing age to alert prescriber if pregnancy occurs.

pantoprazole sodium

Pantoloc (CAN), Protonix, Protonix I.V.

Class and Category

Pharmacologic class: Proton pump inhibitor
Therapeutic class: Antiulcer

Indications and Dosages

* *To treat erosive esophagitis associated with gastroesophageal reflux disease (GERD) short term*

D.R. ORAL SUSPENSION, D.R.TABLETS

Adults. 40 mg daily for up to 8 wk. Repeated for another 4 to 8 wk if healing doesn't occur.
Children ages 5 and older weighing 40 kg (88 lb) or more. 40 mg once daily for up to 8 wk.
Children ages 5 and older weighing 15 kg (33 lb) up to 40 kg (88 lb). 20 mg once daily for up to 8 wks.

* *To treat gastroesophageal reflux disease (GERD) in patients with a history of erosive esophagitis of up to 10 days in adults and up to 7 days in pediatric patients who are 3 months and older*

I.V. INFUSION, I.V. INJECTION

Adults. 40 mg once daily for 7 to 10 days, followed by oral doses. I.V. infusion infused over 15 min; I.V. injection injected over at least 2 min.

I.V. INFUSION

Children ages 1 to 17 weighing more than 40 kg (88 lb). 40 mg infused over 15 min once daily, switching to an oral formulation within 7 days.

Children ages 1 to 17 weighing more than 15 kg (33 lb) up to 40 kg (88 lb). 20 mg infused over 15 min once daily switching to an oral formulation within 7 days.

Children ages 1 to 17 weighing up to 15 kg (33 lb). 10 mg infused over 15 min once daily switching to an oral formulation within 7 days.

Children ages 3 mo to less than 1 yr. 0.8 mg/kg infused over 15 min once daily switching to an oral formulation within 7 days.

∗ *To maintain healing of erosive esophagitis and reduce relapse of daytime and nighttime symptoms in patients with GERD*

D.R. ORAL SUSPENSION, D.R. TABLETS

Adults. 40 mg daily for up to 12 mo.

∗ *To treat pathological hypersecretion conditions, including Zollinger-Ellison syndrome*

D.R. TABLETS

Adults. 40 mg twice daily. *Maximum:* 240 mg daily.

I.V. INFUSION, I.V. INJECTION

Adults. 80 mg every 12 hr adjusted based on patient's acid output measurements up to 80 mg every 8 hr. *Maximum:* 240 mg daily. I.V. infusion infused over 15 min; I.V. Injection injected over at least 2 min.

Drug Administration

P.O.

- D.R. tablets should be swallowed whole and not broken, chewed, or crushed.
- Administer D.R. oral suspension 30 min before a meal. When mixing with 1 teaspoon of applesauce, administer within 10 min and encourage patient to take repeated sips of water to make sure granules are washed down into the stomach. When mixing with apple juice, use only 1 teaspoon of apple juice to mix granules in, stir for 5 sec (granules will not dissolve) and give immediately to patient to drink. Do not mix with any other soft foods or juices because proper pH is needed for stability. After administration, rinse container once or twice with more apple juice and give to patient to drink to ensure that full dose has been given.
- Do not divide the 40 mg D.R. oral suspension packet to create a 20 mg dosage for children.
- To administer D.R. oral suspension via a nasogastric or gastrostomy tube, attach a 60-ml syringe after discarding plunger to a 16 French or larger tube. Hold syringe attached to the tubing as high as possible while giving the D.R. oral suspension to prevent any bending of the tubing. Empty granules into the barrel of a 60-ml syringe. Add 10 ml of apple juice and gently tap and/or shake barrel of syringe to help rinse the syringe and tube of the drug. Add 10 ml of apple juice to syringe and follow with another 10 ml of apple juice to ensure no granules remain in the syringe.

I.V.

- Flush I.V. line with 0.9% Sodium Chloride Injection, 5% Dextrose in Water, or Lactated Ringer's Injection before and after giving drug.
- Administer through a dedicated line or through a Y-site.
- When giving I.V. injection over 2 min, reconstitute with 10 ml of 0.9% Sodium Chloride Injection to a concentration of 4 mg/ml. Reconstituted solution may be stored up to 24 hr at room temperature.
- When giving I.V. infusion over 15 min for treatment of GERD, reconstitute with 10 ml 0.9% Sodium Chloride Injection. Then, further dilute with 100 ml (of 0.9% Sodium Chloride Injection or 5% Dextrose Injection for final concentration of 0.4 mg/ml) for adults and children ages 1 to 17. Reconstitute with 21 ml of 0.9% Sodium Chloride Injection (for final concentration of 1.3 mg/ml) for children ages 3 mo to less than 1 yr.
- When giving I.V. infusion over 15 min for treatment of pathological hypersecretion, including Zollinger-Ellison syndrome, reconstitute each vial with 10 ml of 0.9% Sodium Chloride. Then, combine contents of 2 vials and dilute with 80 ml of 0.9% Sodium Chloride Injection or 5% Dextrose

P

Injection (for a final concentration of 0.8 mg/ml).
- Reconstituted solution may be stored for up to 6 hr prior to dilution at room temperature; once diluted, solution can be stored at room temperature for up to 24 hr from the time of initial reconstitution.
- When giving through a Y-site, immediately stop administration if discoloration or precipitation occurs.
- Monitor patient for injection site reactions. Thrombophlebitis will require the I.V. site to be changed.
- Protect from light.
- *Incompatibilities:* Midazolam (Y-site administration), solutions other than 0.9% Sodium Chloride Injection or 5% Dextrose Injection, zinc-containing products

Route	Onset	Peak	Duration
P.O.	2.5 hr	2.5 hr	24 hr
I.V.	15–30 min	Unknown	24 hr

Half-life: 1 hr

Mechanism of Action

Interferes with gastric acid secretion by inhibiting the hydrogen-potassium-adenosine triphosphatase (H^+-K^+-ATPase) enzyme system, or proton pump, in gastric parietal cells. Remember that normally the proton pump uses energy from hydrolysis of ATPase to drive H^+ and chloride (Cl^-) out of parietal cells and into the stomach lumen in exchange for potassium (K^+), which leaves the stomach lumen and enters parietal cells. Following this exchange, H^+ and Cl^- combine in the stomach to form hydrochloric acid (HCl). Inhibiting the final step in gastric acid production by the drug blocking the exchange of intracellular H^+ and extracellular K^+ prevents H^+ from entering the stomach and additional HCl from forming.

Contraindications

Concurrent therapy with rilpivirine-containing products; hypersensitivity to pantoprazole, substituted benzimidazoles, or their components

Interactions

DRUGS

atazanavir, nelfinavir, rilpivirine: Significantly decreased plasma levels of these drugs reducing antiviral effect; possible increased risk of drug resistance

dasatinib, erlotinib, iron salts, itraconazole, ketoconazole, mycophenolate mofetil, nilotinib: Possible decreased absorption of these drugs and decreased effectiveness

methotrexate: Increased risk of methotrexate toxicities

saquinavir: Possibly increased risk of antiretroviral toxicity

warfarin: Increased INR, PT, and bleeding risk

Adverse Reactions

CNS: Anxiety, asthenia, confusion, depression, dizziness, fatigue, fever, hallucinations, headache, hypertonia, hypokinesia, insomnia, malaise, migraine, somnolence, speech disorder, vertigo

CV: Chest pain, elevated triglycerides, hypercholesterolemia, hyperlipidemia

EENT: Anterior ischemic optic neuropathy, blurred vision, dry mouth, increased salivation, otitis media, pharyngitis, rhinitis, sinusitis, taste disorder, tinnitus

ENDO: Hyperglycemia

GI: Abdominal pain, atrophic gastritis, ***Clostridioides difficile*–associated diarrhea**, constipation, diarrhea, elevated liver enzymes, flatulence, fundic gland polyps (long-term use), gastroenteritis, **hepatic failure**, **hepatitis**, **hepatotoxicity**, indigestion, jaundice, nausea, **pancreatitis**, vomiting

GU: Elevated serum creatinine level, erectile dysfunction, interstitial nephritis, tubulointerstitial nephritis

HEME: **Agranulocytosis**, **leukopenia**, **pancytopenia**, **thrombocytopenia**

MS: Arthralgia, back or neck pain, bone fracture, myalgia, **rhabdomyolysis**

RESP: Bronchitis, dyspnea, increased cough, upper respiratory tract infection

SKIN: Acute generalized exanthematous pustulosis, cutaneous lupus erythematosus, **erythema multiforme**, photosensitivity, pruritus, rash, **Stevens-Johnson syndrome**, **toxic epidermal necrolysis**

Other: **Anaphylaxis**, **angioedema**, **drug reaction with eosinophilia and systemic symptoms (DRESS)**, elevated creatine kinase and phosphokinase levels, flu-like symptoms, generalized pain, hyperuricemia, **hypocalcemia**, **hypokalemia**, **hypomagnesemia**, **hyponatremia**, infection, injection-site reaction (including thrombophlebitis), systemic lupus erythematosus, vitamin B_{12} deficiency, weight changes

Childbearing Considerations

PREGNANCY

- It is not known if drug can cause fetal harm.
- Use with caution only if benefit to mother outweighs potential risk to fetus.

LACTATION

- Drug is present in breast milk.
- Mothers should check with prescriber before breastfeeding.

Nursing Considerations

! WARNING Ensure the continuity of gastric acid suppression during transition from oral to I.V. pantoprazole (or vice versa) because even a brief interruption of effective suppression can lead to serious complications.

! WARNING Expect to check patient's calcium, magnesium and potassium levels before pantoprazole therapy begins. Hypomagnesemia may lead to hypocalcemia and/or hypokalemia and may exacerbate underlying hypocalcemia in at-risk patients. If patient is to remain on pantoprazole long term, expect to monitor the patient's serum magnesium level, as ordered. If level becomes low, anticipate magnesium replacement therapy to be ordered and pantoprazole to be discontinued.

- Be aware that a symptomatic response to the drug does not rule out the presence of a gastric tumor.
- Know that proton pump inhibitors such as pantoprazole should not be given longer than medically necessary.

! WARNING Monitor patient for severe cutaneous and hypersensitivity adverse reactions., which could become life-threatening, such as anaphylaxis, angioedema, and DRESS. At the first sign of a rash (DRESS may only initially present with a fever or swollen lymph nodes) or other hypersensitivity reactions, notify prescriber, expect drug to be discontinued, and provide supportive care as needed and ordered.

! WARNING Monitor patient for diarrhea from *Clostridioides difficile*, which can occur with or without antibiotics in patients taking pantoprazole and can range from being mild to fatal. If severe diarrhea occurs, notify prescriber and expect to obtain a stool specimen to confirm diagnosis. If confirmed, expect drug to be discontinued and administer an antibiotic effective against *C. difficile*, as ordered. Also, expect to administer electrolytes, fluids, and protein supplementation, as needed and ordered.

! WARNING Monitor patient's CBC and platelet count regularly, as ordered because drug can cause serious adverse hematological reactions. Monitor patient for bruising, bleeding, and infection. Institute bleeding and infection control measures. Expect to monitor prothrombin time or international normalized ratio during therapy if patient takes an oral anticoagulant.

- Monitor patient's urine output because pantoprazole may cause changes in renal function. Notify prescriber if urine output decreases or there is blood in the patient's urine.
- Monitor patient for bone fracture, especially in patients receiving multiple daily doses for more than a year because proton pump inhibitors, such as pantoprazole, increase risk of osteoporosis-related fractures of the hip, spine, or wrist.
- Know that both cutaneous and systemic lupus erythematosus have occurred within days to years after proton pump therapy such as pantoprazole was initiated. The most common symptoms presented were arthralgia, cytopenia, and rash. Report such findings to prescriber.

! WARNING Monitor patient for other persistent, serious, or unusual adverse reactions.

- Expect drug to be withheld for at least 14 days before assessment of serum chromogranin A levels is performed because levels increase when gastric acidity is decreased and thus interfere with diagnostic investigations for neuroendocrine tumors.

- Don't give pantoprazole within 4 weeks of testing for *Helicobacter pylori* because antibiotics, bismuth preparations, and proton pump inhibitors suppress *H. pylori* and may lead to false-negative results. Drug also may cause false-positive results in urine screening tests for tetrahydrocannabinol. Consult guidelines for pantoprazole use before testing.
- Be aware that pantoprazole may result in false-positive urine screening tests for tetrahydrocannabinol.
- Be aware that if therapy lasts more than 3 years, patient may not be able to absorb vitamin B_{12} because of achlorhydria or hypochlorhydria. Treatment for cyanocobalamin deficiency may be needed.

PATIENT TEACHING

- Instruct patient how to administer oral form of pantoprazole prescribed. Inform patient that sometimes drug is given intravenously.
- Advise patient to expect relief of symptoms within 2 weeks of starting therapy. Tell patient to notify prescriber if he has a suboptimal response to drug or an early symptomatic relapse.

! **WARNING** Alert patient that drug may cause severe adverse skin and hypersensitivity reactions. Tell patient to stop drug immediately at the first sign of a fever, rash, or swollen lymph nodes or allergic reaction and contact prescriber and, if severe, to seek immediate medical care.

! **WARNING** Instruct patient to notify prescriber if diarrhea occurs and becomes prolonged or severe as additional therapy may be needed to prevent condition from becoming worse.

! **WARNING** Review bleeding and infection control measures with patient. Tell patient to notify prescriber if bruising, unexplained bleeding, or infection occurs. Advise patient who takes warfarin to follow bleeding precautions and to notify prescriber immediately if bleeding occurs.

- Advise patient to notify prescriber if patient notices he is experiencing a decrease in the amount of urine voided or there is blood in his urine. Also, tell the patient to notify prescriber if he experiences new or worsening joint pain or a rash on his arms or cheeks that gets worse in the sun.

! **WARNING** Instruct patient to notify prescriber if other persistent, serious, or unusual signs and symptoms occur while taking pantoprazole.

- Remind patient to notify all prescribers of pantoprazole use and not to take any over-the-counter medication, including herbal supplements, without discussing with prescriber.
- Advise patient taking pantoprazole for longer than 3 years to alert prescriber if he experiences signs and symptoms of vitamin B_{12} deficiency, such as constipation or diarrhea, heart palpitations, mental problems (depression or memory loss), pale skin, or feeling light-headed, tired, or weak.

paroxetine hydrochloride

Paxil, Paxil CR

paroxetine mesylate

Brisdelle

Class and Category

Pharmacologic class: Selective serotonin reuptake inhibitor (SSRI)
Therapeutic class: Antianxiety, antidepressant, antiobsessional, antipanic, premenstrual analgesic

Indications and Dosages

✶ *To treat major depression*

C.R. TABLETS (PAXIL CR)

Adults. *Initial:* 25 mg daily, increased as tolerated by 12.5 mg daily every wk. *Maximum:* 62.5 mg daily.

ORAL SUSPENSION (PAXIL), TABLETS (PAXIL)

Adults. *Initial:* 20 mg daily, increased as tolerated by 10 mg daily every wk. *Maximum:* 50 mg daily.

✶ *To treat obsessive–compulsive disorder*

ORAL SUSPENSION (PAXIL), TABLETS (PAXIL)

Adults. *Initial:* 20 mg daily, increased as tolerated by 10 mg daily every wk. *Usual:* 20 to 60 mg daily. *Maximum:* 60 mg daily.

✱ *To treat panic disorder*

C.R. TABLETS (PAXIL CR)

Adults. *Initial:* 12.5 mg daily, increased by 12.5 mg daily every wk, as needed. *Maximum:* 75 mg daily.

ORAL SUSPENSION (PAXIL), TABLETS (PAXIL)

Adults. *Initial:* 10 mg daily, increased as tolerated by 10 mg daily every wk. *Usual:* 10 to 60 mg daily. *Maximum:* 60 mg daily.

✱ *To treat social anxiety disorder*

C.R. TABLETS (PAXIL CR)

Adults. *Initial:* 12.5 mg daily, increased by 12.5 mg daily every wk, as needed. *Maximum:* 37.5 mg daily.

ORAL SUSPENSION (PAXIL), TABLETS (PAXIL)

Adults. *Initial:* 20 mg daily, increased as tolerated by 10 mg daily every wk. *Usual:* 20 to 60 mg daily. *Maximum:* 60 mg daily.

✱ *To treat generalized anxiety disorder*

ORAL SUSPENSION (PAXIL), TABLETS (PAXIL)

Adults. *Initial:* 20 mg daily, increased as tolerated by 10 mg daily every wk. *Usual:* 20 to 50 mg daily. *Maximum:* 50 mg daily.

✱ *To treat posttraumatic stress disorder*

ORAL SUSPENSION, TABLETS (PAXIL)

Adults. *Initial:* 20 mg daily, increased as tolerated by 10 mg daily every wk. *Usual:* 20 to 50 mg daily. *Maximum:* 50 mg daily.

✱ *To treat premenstrual dysphoric disorder*

C.R. TABLETS (PAXIL CR)

Adults. *Initial:* 12.5 mg daily, increased, as needed, after 1 wk to 25 mg daily. Alternatively, 12.5 mg daily in the morning only during luteal phase of menstrual cycle (2-wk period before onset of menstrual cycle), increased, as needed, after 1 wk to 25 mg daily in the morning during luteal phase of menstrual cycle.

±**DOSAGE ADJUSTMENT** For patients with any of the above conditions who are debilitated, elderly, or have severe hepatic or renal dysfunction, initially 10 mg daily; maximum 40 mg daily. For these same patients who are taking C.R. tablets, initial dose is 12.5 mg, but dosage may have to be reduced and titration intervals increased, as needed. If these patients are being treated for major depressive disorder or panic disorder, dosage should not exceed 50 mg daily and for social anxiety disorder, dosage should not exceed 37.5 mg daily.

✱ *To treat moderate to severe vasomotor symptoms associated with menopause*

CAPSULES (BRISDELLE)

Adults. 7.5 mg once daily at bedtime.

Drug Administration

P.O.

- Capsules and tablets should be swallowed whole and not broken, chewed, crushed, or opened.
- Shake oral suspension well before administration. Use a calibrated device or oral syringe to measure oral suspension dosage.
- Give immediate-release tablets and oral suspension in the morning.
- Give capsules at bedtime.

Route	Onset	Peak	Duration
P.O.	1–2 wk	3–8 hr	Unknown
P.O./E.R.	Unknown	6–10 hr	Unknown

Half-life: 15–33.2 hr

Mechanism of Action

Exerts antianxiety, antidepressant, antiobsessional, and antipanic effects as well as relieves symptoms associated with premenstrual dysphoric disorder and hot flashes associated with menopause by potentiating serotonin activity in CNS and inhibiting serotonin reuptake at presynaptic neuronal membrane. Blocked serotonin reuptake increases levels and prolongs activity of serotonin at synaptic receptor sites.

Contraindications

Concomitant therapy with pimozide or thioridazine; hypersensitivity to paroxetine or its components; pregnancy (Brisdelle); use within 14 days of an MAO inhibitor, including linezolid or methylene blue I.V.

Interactions

DRUGS

amphetamines, buspirone, cisapride, fentanyl, isoniazid, linezolid, lithium, MAO inhibitors,

meperidine, methadone, methylene blue (I.V.), other selective serotonin reuptake inhibitors, other serotonin norepinephrine reuptake inhibitors, procarbazine, St. John's wort, tramadol, tricyclic antidepressants, triptans, tryptophan: Possibly increased risk of serotonin syndrome
anticoagulants such as warfarin, aspirin and other antiplatelet drugs, NSAIDs: Increased anticoagulant activity and risk of bleeding
atomoxetine; risperidone; other drugs metabolized by CYP2D6, such as amitriptyline, desipramine, fluoxetine, imipramine, phenothiazines, type IC antiarrhythmics: Increased plasma levels of these drugs
cimetidine: Possibly increased blood paroxetine level
digoxin: Possibly decreased digoxin effects
drugs highly protein bound: Increased adverse reactions of these drugs and paroxetine
fosamprenavir/ritonavir: Significantly decreased plasma levels of paroxetine
phenytoin: Possibly altered levels of both drugs
pimozide: Increased risk of prolonged QT interval, increased risk of extrapyramidal symptoms
procyclidine: Increased blood procyclidine level and anticholinergic effects
tamoxifen: Decreased tamoxifen effectiveness
theophylline: Possibly increased blood theophylline level and risk of toxicity
thioridazine: Increased thioridazine level, possibly leading to prolonged QT interval and life-threatening ventricular arrhythmias
tricyclic antidepressants: Increased blood antidepressant levels; increased risk of toxicity, including seizures

ACTIVITIES

alcohol use: Possibly altered psychomotor function

Adverse Reactions

CNS: Agitation, akathisia, asthenia, confusion, decreased concentration, dizziness, drowsiness, emotional lability, **Guillain-Barré syndrome**, hallucinations, headache, hypomania, insomnia, mania, **neuroleptic malignant syndrome**, paresthesia, psychomotor agitation, restlessness, restless leg syndrome, **seizures**, **serotonin syndrome**, somnolence, **status epilepticus**, **suicidal ideation**, tremor
CV: Palpitations, tachycardia, **torsades de pointes**, **vasculitic syndromes**, **ventricular fibrillation or tachycardia**
EENT: Angle-closure glaucoma, blurred vision, dry mouth, **laryngospasms**, optic neuritis, partial or total loss of smell, rhinitis, taste perversion
ENDO: Galactorrhea, prolactinemia, syndrome of inappropritate ADH secretion
GI: Abdominal cramps or pain, **acute pancreatitis**, anorexia, constipation, diarrhea, elevated liver enzymes, flatulence, nausea, **severe liver dysfunction**, vomiting
GU: **Acute renal failure**, decreased libido, absence or delayed orgasm (females), delayed or failed ejaculation, erectile dysfunction, impotence, sexual dysfunction, urine retention
HEME: **Agranulocytosis**, **aplastic anema**, **bleeding events**, **bone marrow aplasia**, **hemolytic anemia**
MS: Back pain, bone fracture, myalgia, myasthenia, myopathy
RESP: Allergic alveolitis, **pulmonary hypertension**
SKIN: Diaphoresis, rash, **Stevens-Johnson syndrome**, **toxic epidermal necrolysis**
Other: **Anaphylaxis**, **drug reaction with eosinophilia and systemic symptoms (DRESS)**, **hyponatremia**, porphyria, weight gain or loss

Childbearing Considerations

PREGNANCY

- Pregnancy exposure registry: 1-866-961-2388 or https://womensmentalhealth.org/clinical-and-researchprograms/pregnancyregistry/antidepressants.
- Drug causes fetal harm with congenital malformations, particularly cardiovascular malformations with exposure in first trimester.
- Premature birth may occur. When drug is used late in the third trimester, the neonate may develop complications requiring prolonged hospitalization, respiratory support, and tube feeding.
- Mother may develop eclampsia.
- Drug is not recommended for use in pregnant women and is contraindicated for treatment of vasomotor symptoms during pregnancy.

LABOR AND DELIVERY

- Use of drug in the month before delivery may increase risk of postpartum hemorrhage.

LACTATION

- Drug is present in breast milk.
- Mothers should check with prescriber before breastfeeding.
- Monitor infant who is breastfed for agitation, irritability, or poor feeding or weight loss.

REPRODUCTION

- Drug may affect sperm quality, which may affect fertility in some men.

Nursing Considerations

- Be aware that Brisdelle is not used to treat any psychiatric condition because it contains a lower dose of paroxetine.
- Watch for akathisia (inner sense of restlessness) and psychomotor agitation, especially during the first few weeks of therapy.

! **WARNING** Watch patient closely (especially young adults), for suicidal tendencies, particularly when therapy starts and dosage changes occur because depression may worsen temporarily during these times, possibly leading to suicidal ideation.

! **WARNING** Monitor patient for severe cutaneous and hypersensitivity adverse reactions, which could become life-threatening, such as anaphylaxis, angioedema, or DRESS. At the first sign of a rash (DRESS may only initially exhibit a fever or swollen lymph nodes) or other hypersensitivity reactions, notify prescriber, expect drug to be discontinued, and provide supportive care as needed and ordered.

! **WARNING** Monitor patient for seizures, especially patients with a seizure history. Institute seizure precautions, as appropriate.

! **WARNING** Monitor patient closely for evidence of bleeding, especially if patient also takes a drug known to cause bleeding, such as anticoagulants (warfarin), antiplatelets (aspirin), or a NSAID.

! **WARNING** Monitor patient closely for serotonin syndrome exhibited by agitation, coma, diarrhea, hallucinations, hyperreflexia, hyperthermia, incoordination, labile blood pressure, nausea, tachycardia, or vomiting. Notify prescriber immediately because serotonin syndrome may be life-threatening and provide supportive care, as needed. Be aware that serotonin syndrome in its most severe form may resemble neuroleptic malignant syndrome, which includes autonomic instability with possibly rapid changes in mental status and vital signs, hyperthermia, and muscle rigidity. Stop drug immediately and provide supportive care, as needed and ordered.

- Watch for mania, which may result from any antidepressant in a susceptible patient.
- Be aware that pathological fractures have been associated with antidepressant therapy. Monitor patient for unexplained bone pain, bruising, joint tenderness, or swelling.

! **WARNING** Monitor patient for other persistent, serious, or unusual adverse reactions as drug may adversely affect multiple body systems to cause mild to life-threatening adverse reactions.

- Expect to taper drug rather than stop it abruptly to minimize adverse reactions.

PATIENT TEACHING

- Advise patient that drug may cause mild pupillary dilation, which may lead to an episode of acute angle-closure glaucoma. Encourage patient to have eye exam before starting therapy to see if he is at risk.
- Instruct patient how to take form and product of paroxetine prescribed.
- Urge patient to avoid alcohol during therapy; effects with paroxetine are unknown.

! **WARNING** Tell family or caregiver to observe patient closely for suicidal tendencies, especially when therapy starts or dosage changes and especially if patient is a young adult.

- Explain that full effect may take 4 weeks. However, inform patient that episodes of acute depression may persist for months or longer requiring continued follow-up.
- Instruct patient not to stop drug abruptly but to taper dosage as instructed.

! **WARNING** Alert patient that drug may cause severe adverse skin and hypersensitivity reactions. Tell patient to stop drug immediately at the first sign of a fever, rash, or swollen lymph nodes or allergic reaction and contact prescriber and, if severe, to seek immediate medical care.

! **WARNING** Tell patient not to take aspirin or NSAIDs during therapy because they increase the risk of bleeding. Review bleeding precautions and tell patient to notify prescriber at once if bleeding occurs. Tell patient taking anticoagulants that risk of bleeding is also increased.

- Tell patient to notify prescriber if she develops unexplained bone pain, joint tenderness, or swelling of extremity.
- Instruct patient to speak with prescriber with concerns about sexual dysfunction. Alert male patient that drug may alter sperm quality, which may affect fertility.

! **WARNING** Urge patient to notify prescriber immediately if patient develops other persistent, serious, or unusual adverse reactions.

- Caution patient to alert all prescribers about paroxetine therapy because of potentially serious drug interactions.
- Suggest that patient avoid hazardous activities until drug's CNS effects are known and resolved.
- Alert females of childbearing age to use effective contraception during drug therapy and to notify prescriber if pregnancy occurs.
- Instruct mothers who are breast feeding to monitor their infant for agitation, irritability, poor feeding or weight loss. If present, tell mother to notify pediatrician.

pegfilgrastim
Neulasta

pegfilgrastim-apgf
Nyvepria

pegfilgrastim-bmez
Ziextenzo

pegfilgrastim-cbqv
Udenyca

pegfilgrastim-fpgk
Stimufend

pegfilgrastim-jmdb
Fulphila

pegfilgrastim-pbbk
Fylnetra

Class and Category

Pharmacologic class: Colony-stimulating factor
Therapeutic class: Hematopoietic

Indications and Dosages

* *To increase survival in patients acutely exposed to myelosuppressive doses of radiation.*

SUBCUTANEOUS INJECTION (NEULASTA, UDENYCA)

Adults and children weighing 45 kg (99 lb) or more. 6 mg as soon as possible after exposure, followed by 6 mg 1 wk later.
Children weighing between 31 and 44 kg (68.2–96.8 lb). 4 mg as soon as possible after exposure, followed by 4 mg 1 wk later.
Children weighing between 21 and 30 kg (46.2–66 lb). 2.5 mg as soon as possible after exposure, followed by 2.5 mg 1 wk later.
Children weighing between 10 and 20 kg (22–44 lb). 1.5 mg as soon as possible after exposure, followed by 2.5 mg 1 wk later.
Children weighing less than 10 kg (22 lb). 0.1 mg/kg as soon as possible after exposure, followed by 0.1 mg/kg 1 wk later.

* *To reduce the risk of infection, as manifested by febrile neutropenia, in patients with nonmyeloid malignancies receiving myelosuppressive chemotherapy*

SUBCUTANEOUS INJECTION (FULPHILA, FYLNETRA, NEULASTA, NYVEPRIA, STIMUFEND, UDENYCA, ZIEXTENZO)

Adults and children weighing more than 45 kg (99 lb). 6 mg once with each chemotherapy cycle but not administered between 14 days before and 24 hr after administration of cytotoxic chemotherapy. **Children weighing between 31 and 44 kg (68.2–96.8 lb).** 4 mg once with each chemotherapy cycle but not administered between 14 days before and 24 hr after administration of cytotoxic chemotherapy. **Children weighing between 21 and 30 kg (46.2–66 lb).** 2.5 mg once with each chemotherapy cycle but not administered between 14 days before and 24 hr after administration of cytotoxic chemotherapy. **Children weighing between 10 and 20 kg (22–44 lb).** 1.5 mg once with each chemotherapy cycle but not administered between 14 days before and 24 hr after administration of cytotoxic chemotherapy. **Children weighing less than 10 kg (22 lb).** 0.1 mg/kg once with each chemotherapy cycle but not administered between 14 days before and 24 hr after administration of cytotoxic chemotherapy.

Drug Administration

SUBCUTANEOUS

- Store drug in refrigerator and protect from freezing and light. If Fulphila or Fylnetra, become frozen, drug may be allowed to thaw one time in refrigerator before injection. Discard if either drug becomes frozen more than once.
- Needle cover for Neulasta and Stimufend contains dry natural rubber and should not be handled by persons with a latex allergy.
- Don't use prefilled syringe for doses less than 0.6 ml (6 mg) because syringe does not bear graduation marks for doses that small.
- Let drug warm to room temperature for 30 min before injection and protect from light.
- Don't shake solution.
- Do not use prefilled syringe if it has been dropped on a hard surface.
- Discard drug that contains particles, is discolored, or was stored more than 48 hr at room temperature for Neulasta or Udenyca; 72 hr for Fulphila, Fylnetra, and Stimufend; 120 hr for Ziextenzo; or 15 days for Nyvepria.
- Administer via a single-dose prefilled syringe for manual administration or use an on-body injector for Neulasta or Udenyca, which is co-packaged with a single-dose prefilled syringe. The on-body injector is not recommended for patients with hematopoietic subsyndrome of acute radiation syndrome or children.
- If using the on-body injector for Neulasta or Udenyca follow manufacturer's instructions closely. Notify prescriber immediately if the on-body injector malfunctions and a missed or partial dose occurs.
- If using a prefilled syringe, inject drug into intact, nonirritated areas of the abdomen, back of arm, thigh, or upper outer area of buttocks.
- Rotate sites.

Route	Onset	Peak	Duration
SubQ	Unknown	16–120 hr	14 days

Half-life: 15–80 hr

Mechanism of Action

Induces formation of neutrophil progenitor cells by binding to receptors on granulocytes, which then divide. Potentiates the effects of mature neutrophils also, thus reducing fever and the risk of infection from severe neutropenia. Know that drug is pharmacologically identical to human granulocyte colony-stimulating factor.

Contraindications

Hypersensitivity to filgrastim, pegfilgrastim, or their components; use of on-body injector if acrylic adhesive hypersensivity is present

Interactions

DRUGS

lithium: Increased neutrophil production

Adverse Reactions

CNS: Fever
CV: **Aortitis**, edema, **hypotension**
GI: Elevated liver enzymes, **splenic rupture**, splenomegaly
GU: **Glomerulonephritis**
HEME: **Acute myeloid leukemia (patients with breast or lung cancer)**, **capillary**

P

leak syndrome, **hemoconcentration**, leukocytosis, **sickle cell crisis**, **thrombocytopenia**
MS: Bone or extremity pain, myelodysplastic syndrome (patients with breast or lung cancer)
RESP: **Acute respiratory distress syndrome**, **alveolar hemorrhage**, dyspnea, **hypoxia**, **pulmonary infiltrates**
SKIN: Acute febrile neutrophilic dermatosis (Sweet's syndrome), contact dermatitis (on-body injector), cutaneous vasculitis, erythema, flushing, pruritus, rash, urticaria
Other: **Anaphylaxis**, **angioedema**, antibody formation to pegfilgrastim, application-site reactions with on-body injector (bruising, discomfort, erythema, hemorrhage, pain), elevated uric acid level, hypoalbuminemia, injection-site reactions (erythema, induration, pain)

Childbearing Considerations

PREGNANCY

- It is not known if drug can cause fetal harm.
- Use with caution only if benefit to mother outweighs potential risk to fetus.

LACTATION

- It is not known if drug is present in breast milk.
- Mothers should check with prescriber before breastfeeding.

Nursing Considerations

- Check CBC, hematocrit, and platelet count before and periodically during therapy.

! **WARNING** Monitor patient for signs of hypersensitivity, which may become life-threatening, such as anaphylaxis or angioedema. If present, notify prescriber immediately, expect drug to be discontinued, and provide supportive care, as needed and ordered.

- Be aware that the drug may cause local injection site skin reactions and the on-body injector may also cause application-site reactions, including contact dermatitis.

! **WARNING** Monitor patient for signs and symptoms of aortitis, such as abdominal pain, back pain, fever, increased inflammatory markers (C-reactive protein, WBC count), or malaise, as drug will have to be discontinued. Know that aortitis may occur as early as the first week after therapy is begun.

! **WARNING** Be aware that patients receiving filgrastim (parent drug) have had splenic rupture and acute respiratory distress syndrome, which may be life-threatening. Assess patient for fever, respiratory distress, and upper abdominal or shoulder tip pain and notify prescriber immediately, if present.

! **WARNING** Monitor patient for edema and hypotension that may indicate development of capillary leak syndrome. If present, notify prescriber and be prepared to provide supportive care, as ordered.

! **WARNING** Monitor patient's renal function, as ordered, because drug may cause glomerulonephritis. If renal dysfunction is suspected, notify prescriber and, if confirmed, expect drug to be withheld or dosage reduced.

! **WARNING** Monitor patient's platelet counts because of risk for thrombocytopenia.

- Assess patients with sickle cell disease for signs of sickle cell crisis; urge hydration. Know that drug should be discontinued if sickle cell crisis occurs.
- Be aware that transient positive bone imaging changes may occur because of increased hematopoietic activity of the bone marrow in response to pegfilgrastim therapy.
- Give nonopioid and opioid analgesics, as ordered, if patient experiences bone pain.

PATIENT TEACHING

- Teach patient who will self-administer drug using the prefilled syringe how to prepare, give, and store drug. Alert patient using Neulasta or Stimufend brand that needle cover on prefilled syringe contains dryg natural rubber and should not be handled if she has a latex allergy.
- Instruct patient how to use an on-body injector, if prescribed. Alert patient using the on-body injector that it uses acrylic adhesive, which can cause a significant reaction to those allergic to acrylic adhesive. Instruct patient to notify prescriber immediately if a dose is missed or only

partial given due to malfunction of the device. Tell patient to inform all healthcare workers of the presence of the on-body injector, as it should not be exposed to medical imaging studies (CT scan, MRI, ultrasound, or X-ray), oxygen-rich environments, or radiation treatment. Caution patient that instructions on use of device must be followed carefully.

- Advise patient to have family or caregiver nearby when he administers the first dose using the on-body injector and to avoid driving or operating heavy machinery during hours 26 to 29 following application of the device.
- Warn patient to keep the on-body injector at least 4 inches away from electrical equipment, such as cell phones, cordless telephones, microwaves, and other common appliances because of possible interference with its function.

! **WARNING** Alert patient that drug may cause serious allergic reactions. Tell patient to notify prescriber, if present, and to seek immediate emergency medical care, if severe.

! **WARNING** Urge patient to report promptly any persistent, serious, or unusual adverse reactions such as breathing difficulty, chest tightness, left upper abdominal pain, rash, shoulder tip pain and evidence of infection (chills, fever).

- Emphasize the importance of follow-up tests.

penicillin G benzathine

Bicillin L-A

penicillin G potassium

Pfizerpen

penicillin G procaine

penicillin G sodium

penicillin V potassium

Class and Category

Pharmacologic class: Penicillin
Therapeutic class: Antibiotic

Indications and Dosages

✶ *To treat systemic infections caused by gram-positive organisms (including* Bacillus anthracis, Corynebacterium diphtheriae, *enterococci,* Listeria monocytogenes, Staphylococcus aureus, *or* S. epidermidis*), gram-negative organisms (including* Neisseria gonorrhoeae, N. meningitidis, Pasteurella multocida, *or* Streptobacillus moniliformis *[rat-bite fever]), and gram-positive anaerobes (including* Actinomyces israelii *[actinomycosis],* Clostridium perfringens, C. tetani, Peptococcus *species,* Peptostreptococcus *species, or spirochetes, especially* Treponema carateum *[pinta],* T. pallidum, *and* T. pertenue *[yaws])*

I.M. INJECTION, I.V. INFUSION (PENICILLIN G POTASSIUM, PENICILLIN G SODIUM)

Adults and children. Highly individualized based on type and severity of infection. Dosage ranges from 1 to 24 million units daily in divided doses usually every 4 to 6 hr, although some infections such as meningococcal meningitis or septicemia may require divided dosing every 2 hr.

I.M. INJECTION (PENICILLIN G PROCAINE)

Adults and adolescents. Highly individualized based on severity and type of infection. Dosages range from 300,000 to 1,200,000 units daily and may be given in divided doses every 12 hr in some infections.

✶ *To treat Group A streptococcal respiratory infections*

I.M. INJECTION (PENICILLIN G BENZATHINE)

Adults and children weighing more than 45 kg (100 lb). 1.2 million units as a single injection.

Children weighing 27 to 45 kg (59 to 100 lb). 900,000 units as a single injection.
Infants and children weighing less than 27 kg (59 lb). 300,000 to 600,000 units as single injection.

∗ *To treat congenital syphilis*

I.M. INJECTION (PENICILLIN G BENZATHINE)

Children ages 2 to 12. Dosage adjusted based on adult dosing schedule.
Children under age 2. 50,000 units/kg as a single injection. *Maximum:* 2.4 million units/dose.

∗ *To treat primary, secondary, or latent syphilis*

I.M. INJECTION (PENICILLIN G BENZATHINE)

Adults. 2.4 million units as a single injection.

∗ *To treat late (neurosyphilis or tertiary) syphilis*

I.M. INJECTION (PENICILLIN G BENZATHINE)

Adults. 2.4 million units every wk for 3 wk.

∗ *To provide prophylaxis for glomerulonephritis and rheumatic fever*

I.M. INJECTION (PENICILLIN G BENZATHINE)

Adults. 1.2 million units once a mo or 600,000 units every 2 wk following an acute attack.

∗ *To treat bejel, pinta, and yaws caused by susceptible organisms*

I.M. INJECTION (PENICILLIN G BENZATHINE)

Adults. 1.2 million units as a single injection.

∗ *To treat mild to moderate severe upper respiratory tract streptococcal infections, including erysipelas and scarlet fever*

ORAL SOLUTION, TABLETS (PENICILLIN V POTASSIUM)

Adults and adolescents. 125 to 250 mg (200,000 to 400,000 units) every 6 to 8 hr for 10 days.

∗ *To treat mild to moderate pneumococcal infections; to treat mild skin and soft tissue staphylococcal infection; to treat mild to moderate staphylococcal (Vincent's) infection of the oropharynx*

ORAL SOLUTION, TABLETS (PENICILLIN V POTASSIUM)

Adults and adolescents. 250 to 500 mg (400,000 to 800,000 units) every 6 hr (pneumococcal infections) or 6 to 8 hr (for other infections).

∗ *To prevent recurrence following chorea and/or rheumatic fever*

ORAL SOLUTION, TABLETS (PENICILLIN V POTASSIUM)

Adults and adolescents. 125 mg to 250 mg (200,000 to 400,000 units) twice daily on a continuing basis.

±**DOSAGE ADJUSTMENT** For uremic patients receiving penicillin G potassium or penicillin G sodium with creatinine clearance greater than 10 ml/min, full loading dose given followed by one-half of the loading dose every 4 to 5 hours. For patients receiving penicillin G potassium or penicillin G sodium with creatinine clearance of less than 10 ml/min, full loading dose given followed by one-half of the loading dose every 8 to 10 hours.

Drug Administration

P.O.

- Administer tablets with a full glass of water on an empty stomach at least an hr before or 2 hr after eating.
- Reconstitute oral solution by tapping bottle until all powder flows freely. Slowly add 75 ml for 100-ml bottle size or 150 ml for a 200-ml bottle size by first partially filling bottle; replace cap and shake vigorously. Then, add remaining water and shake again. Solution will be red in color.
- Shake oral solution container well before using. Use calibrated device to measure dosage when using oral solution. Store oral solution in refrigerator. Discard after 14 days.

I.V.

- Only penicillin G potassium and penicillin G sodium are administered intravenously.
- Do not administer penicillin G potassium to children requiring less than 1 million units per dose.
- Drug may come as a premixed solution or in powder form requiring reconstitution and further dilution.
- If reconstituting drug for penicillin G potassium use Sterile Isotonic Sodium Chloride for Parenteral use and use 0.9% Sodium Chloride Injection or 5% Dextrose in Water for penicillin G sodium.
- Dilute by first loosening powder in vial. Then, hold vial horizontally and rotate it

while slowly directing the stream of diluent (amount of diluent to use is dependent on dose; see manufacturer's guidelines) against the wall of vial. Shake vial vigorously after all the diluent has been added.

- To make a continuous intravenous drip determine the volume of fluid and rate of its administration required by patient in a 24-hr period in the usual manner for fluid therapy. Then, add the appropriate daily dosage of diluted penicillin to this fluid. For example, if adult patient requires 2 liters of fluid over 24 hr and a daily dosage of 10 million units of penicillin, add 5 million units to each liter and adjust flow rate to infuse each liter over 12 hr.
- For intermittent I.V. infusion for adults using penicillin G sodium administer slowly over 1 to 2 hr. For children, each dose of penicillin G sodium given as an intermittent IV infusion slowly over 30 min.
- Administer penicillin at least 1 hr before other antibiotics.
- Store reconstituted solution for 7 days.
- *Incompatibilities:* Carbohydrate solutions at alkaline pH for penicillin G potassium; none reported by manufacturer for penicillin G sodium

I.M.

- If penicillin formulation requires reconstitution, use Sterile Water for Injection in a small amount.
- Inject deep into large muscle mass such as the upper, outer quadrant of the dorsogluteal or the ventrogluteal site. In neonates, infants, and small children, the midlateral aspect of the thigh is usually preferred.
- Inject at a slow, steady rate when administering penicillin G benzathine or penicillin G procaine because of the high concentration of suspended material.
- Apply ice to relieve pain.
- Injecting any penicillin into or near a nerve may result in permanent neurological damage.

Route	Onset	Peak	Duration
P.O.	Unknown	30–60 min	Unknown
I.V.	Unknown	Unknown	Unknown
I.M.	Unknown	Varies	Varies

Half-life: < 1.4 hr

Mechanism of Action

Inhibits final stage of bacterial cell wall synthesis by competitively binding to penicillin-binding proteins inside the cell wall as penicillin-binding proteins are responsible for various steps in bacterial cell wall synthesis. Binding to these proteins leads to cell wall lysis.

Contraindications

Hypersensitivity to penicillin or its components

Interactions

DRUGS

aspirin, ethacrynic acid, furosemide, indomethacin, phenylbutazone, probenecid, sulfonamides, thiazide diuretics: Possibly prolonged blood penicillin level

chloramphenicol, erythromycin, sulfonamides, tetracycline: Possibly interference with penicillin's bactericidal effect

Adverse Reactions

CNS: Confusion, dizziness, dysphasia, hallucinations, headache, lethargy, permanent neurological damage (inadvertent intravascular administration), sciatic nerve irritation (I.M. injection), **seizures**

CV: Labile blood pressure, palpitations

EENT: Black "hairy" tongue, oral candidiasis, stomatitis, taste perversion

GI: Abdominal pain, ***Clostridioides difficile*-associated diarrhea (CDAD)**, diarrhea, elevated liver enzymes (transient), indigestion, nausea, **pseudomembranous colitis**

GU: **Acute interstitial nephritis**, vaginal candidiasis

MS: Muscle twitching

SKIN: Acute generalized exanthematous pustulosis, Nicolau syndrome, rash, **Stevens-Johnson syndrome**, **toxic epidermal necrolysis**

Other: **Drug reaction with eosinophilia and systemic symptoms (DRESS)**; **electrolyte imbalances**; **hypersensitivity reactions**; injection-site necrosis, pain, or redness

Childbearing Considerations

PREGNANCY

- It is not known if drug causes fetal harm.
- Use with caution only if benefit to mother outweighs potential risk to fetus.

P

LACTATION

- Drug is present in breast milk.
- Mothers should check with prescriber before breastfeeding.

Nursing Considerations

- Obtain body tissue and fluid samples for culture and sensitivity tests as ordered before giving first dose. Expect to begin drug therapy before test results are known.

! **WARNING** Monitor patient for hypersensitivity reactions including severe cutaneous adverse reactions beginning with a rash (DRESS may only initially present as a fever or swollen lymph nodes). If present, notify prescriber, expect drug to be discontinued, and provide supportive care, as needed and ordered.

! **WARNING** Assess patient for signs of secondary infection, such as profuse, watery diarrhea. If such diarrhea develops, contact prescriber and expect to obtain a stool specimen to rule out pseudomembranous colitis caused by *Clostridioides difficile.* The infection can range from being mild to causing fatal colitis. If confirmed, expect to withhold penicillin and treat with an antibiotic effective against *C. difficile*, as ordered. Also, expect to administer electrolytes, fluids, and protein supplementation, as needed and ordered.

! **WARNING** Monitor serum sodium level and assess for early signs of heart failure in patients receiving high doses of penicillin G sodium. Be aware that each gram of penicillin G potassium also contains 1.02 mEq of sodium. This is especially important when giving penicillin G potassium to a patient at risk for fluid overload or hypertension.

! **WARNING** Monitor patient for seizures, especially patients with a seizure history. Institute seizure precautions, as appropriate.

PATIENT TEACHING

! **WARNING** Instruct patient to report previous allergies to penicillins before taking first dose of drug as a different antibiotic will have to be used.

- Instruct patient how to take the oral form of penicillin prescribed.
- Warn patient receiving penicillin as an I.M. injection that it may be painful but applying ice to the site may help to relieve the discomfort.

! **WARNING** Tell patient to notify prescriber immediately if an allergy occurs including skin reactions such as a fever, rash, or swollen lymph nodes. If present, tell patient to instruct patient to notify prescriber and, if severe, to seek immediate medical care.

! **WARNING** Urge patient to tell prescriber if diarrhea develops, even 2 months or more after penicillin therapy ends as additional therapy may be needed to prevent diarrhea from being worse.

! **WARNING** Tell patient to notify prescriber of any persistent, severe, or unusual adverse effects.

phentermine hydrochloride

Adipex-P, Lomaira

Class, Category, and Schedule

Chemical class: Sympathomimetic amine
Therapeutic class: Anorectic
Controlled substance schedule: IV

Indications and Dosages

* *As adjunct for short-term weight reduction in conjunction with behavioral modification, caloric restriction, and exercise in management of exogenous obesity in patients with an initial body mass index greater than or equal to 30 kg/m², or greater than or equal to 27 kg/m² in the presence of other risk factors, such as controlled hypertension, diabetes, or hyperlipidemia*

CAPSULES, TABLETS (ADIPEX-P)

Adults and adolescents ages 17 and older. *Initial:* 18.75 to 37.5 mg once daily and then dosage adjusted, as needed. Alternatively, 18.75 mg given twice daily and then dosage adjusted, as needed.

± **DOSAGE ADJUSTMENT** For patients with severe renal impairment (eGFR between

15 to 29 ml/min), dosage reduced to 15 mg daily.

TABLETS (LOMAIRA)

Adults and adolescents ages 17 and older. 8 mg 3 times daily.

Drug Administration

P.O.

- Tablet may be halved, as needed, but should be swallowed without chewing or crushing.
- Capsules should be swallowed whole and not chewed, crushed, or opened.
- Administer Lomaira half an hr before meals. Administer Adipex-P before breakfast or 1 to 2 hr after breakfast.
- Avoid administering in late evening, to prevent insomnia.

Route	Onset	Peak	Duration
P.O.	Unknown	3–4.4 hr	Unknown

Half-life: 20 hr

Mechanism of Action

Thought to be related to its ability to suppress appetite although its precise mechanism of action is unknown.

Contraindications

Agitated states; breastfeeding; during or 14 days after MAO inhibitor therapy; glaucoma; history of cardiovascular disease, such as arrhythmias, congestive heart failure, coronary artery disease, stroke, or uncontrolled hypertension; history of drug abuse; hypersensitivity to phentermine, other sympathomimetic amines, or their components; hyperthyroidism; pregnancy

Interactions

DRUGS

adrenergic neuron blocking drugs: Possibly decreased hypotensive effect of these drugs
insulin, oral hypoglycemic drugs: Possibly increased risk of hypoglycemia
MAO inhibitors: Increased risk of hypertensive crisis

ACTIVITIES

alcohol use: Possibly increased incidence of serious adverse reactions

Adverse Reactions

CNS: Dizziness, dysphoria, euphoria, headache, insomnia, overstimulation, psychosis, restlessness, tremor
CV: Hypertension, ischemic events, palpitations, **regurgitant cardiac valvular disease**, tachycardia
EENT: Dry mouth, unpleasant taste
GI: Constipation, diarrhea, other gastrointestinal disturbances
GU: Changes in libido, impotence
RESP: **Primary pulmonary hypertension**
SKIN: Urticaria
Other: Physical and psychological dependence

Childbearing Considerations

PREGNANCY

- Drug may cause fetal harm.
- Drug is contraindicated in pregnancy.

LACTATION

- It is not known if drug is present in breast milk.
- Drug is contraindicated during breastfeeding.

Nursing Considerations

! **WARNING** Be aware that phentermine is a controlled substance and may cause physical and psychological dependency. Monitor patient's intake of drug closely.

! **WARNING** Use cautiously in patients with even mild hypertension because drug can raise blood pressure. Monitor patient's blood pressure closely and report any persistent elevation.

! **WARNING** Monitor patient for anginal pain, dyspnea (most common), lower extremity edema, or syncope because a life-threatening disorder, primary pulmonary hypertension, has occurred in patients taking phentermine alone or concomitantly with dexfenfluramine or fenfluramine. If signs or symptoms develop, notify prescriber, expect drug to be discontinued, and assist with diagnostic testing to confirm presence of disorder.

! **WARNING** Assess patients with diabetes who are taking insulin or oral hypoglycemic agents for signs and symptoms of hypoglycemia. If persistent or serious hypoglycemia occurs, notify prescriber and expect to adjust the antidiabetic medication dosage, as ordered.

! **WARNING** Know that serious regurgitant cardiac valvular disease has occurred in otherwise healthy patients taking phentermine alone or in combination with dexfenfluramine or fenfluramine. Regularly evaluate patient's heart sounds for presence of murmurs, especially those associated with aortic, mitral, or tricuspid valvular disease.

PATIENT TEACHING

- Inform patient that phentermine therapy is not a substitute for behavioral changes, caloric restriction, and exercise.
- Instruct patient how to administer phentermine.

! **WARNING** Caution patient to take phentermine exactly as prescribed and not to increase dosage or dosage interval if tolerance to drug develops because drug may cause physical and/or psychological dependence. Remind patient drug is for short-term use only. Instead, instruct patient to notify prescriber if tolerance occurs, as drug will have to be discontinued.

- Instruct patient to avoid drinking alcoholic beverages while taking phentermine, as serious adverse reactions may occur.

! **WARNING** Warn patient not to combine phentermine therapy with other drug products for weight loss, including herbal products, over-the-counter drugs, and prescription drugs. Tell patient to inform all prescribers of phentermine use.

! **WARNING** Tell patient to keep drug out of reach of children and anyone who has a drug addiction and to take measures to prevent drug theft.

! **WARNING** Advise patients with diabetes who are taking medication to control their blood glucose levels to watch for low blood glucose reactions. If persistent or severe hypoglycemia occurs, instruct patient to notify prescriber, as dosage of the diabetic medication may have to be reduced.

! **WARNING** Instruct patient to discontinue phentermine therapy and notify prescriber if chest pain, decrease in exercise tolerance, difficulty breathing, lower extremity swelling, or shortness of breath develop during phentermine therapy. Also, advise patient with high blood pressure to monitor blood pressure regularly and to alert prescriber if a persistent and significant elevation occurs.

! **WARNING** Tell patient to notify prescriber immediately if other persistent, serious, or unusual adverse reactions occur.

- Caution patient to avoid hazardous activities, such as driving or operating machinery, until the nervous system effects of the drug are known and resolved.
- Tell females of childbearing age to notify prescriber immediately if pregnancy occurs, as drug will have to be discontinued immediately.
- Inform mothers who are breastfeeding that breastfeeding must be discontinued during phentermine therapy.

phenytoin

Dilantin-125, Dilantin Infatabs

phenytoin sodium

Dilantin, Phenytek

Class and Category

Pharmacologic class: Hydantoin derivative
Therapeutic class: Anticonvulsant

Indications and Dosages

✱ *To treat tonic–clonic or psychomotor (temporal) seizures*

CHEWABLE TABLETS, ORAL SUSPENSION (PHENYTOIN)

Adults who have received no previous treatment. *Initial:* 100-mg tablet or 125-mg (5 ml) suspension 3 times daily, adjusted every 7 to 10 days, as needed and tolerated. *Maximum:* 600-mg chewable tablets; 625-mg (25 ml) oral suspension
Children. *Initial:* 5 mg/kg daily in divided doses 2 or 3 times daily and adjusted, as needed and tolerated. *Maintenance:* 4 to 8 mg/kg daily in divided doses 2 or 3 times daily. *Maximum:* 300 mg daily.

∗ *To treat tonic–clonic or psychomotor (temporal) seizures; to prevent and treat seizures occurring during or following neurosurgery*

E.R. CAPSULES (PHENYTOIN SODIUM)

Adults who have received no previous treatment. *Initial:* 100 mg 3 times daily, adjusted every 7 to 10 days, as needed and tolerated. Once patient is stabilized on 100 mg 3 times daily, dosage regimen may be changed to 300 mg once daily. *Maintenance:* 100 mg 3 time daily (to treat seizures) or 4 times daily (for prophylaxis following neurosurgery), 200 mg 3 times daily, or 300 mg once daily.

±**DOSAGE ADJUSTMENT** For hospitalized patients without hepatic or renal disease, oral loading dose given initially consisting of 400 mg followed in 2 hours by 300 mg, and then followed in 2 more hours by another 300 mg, for a total of 1 g.

Children. *Initial:* 5 mg/kg daily in divided doses 2 or 3 times daily and adjusted, as needed and tolerated. *Maintenance:* 4 to 8 mg/kg daily in divided doses 2 or 3 times daily. *Maximum:* 300 mg daily.

∗ *To treat status epilepticus; to prevent or treat seizures during neurosurgery*

I.V. INFUSION (PHENYTOIN SODIUM)

Adults. *Loading dose:* 10 to 15 mg/kg not to exceed 50 mg/min. *Maintenance:* 100-mg I.V. or P.O. every 6 to 8 hr.

Children. *Loading dose:* 15 to 20 mg/kg not to exceed 3 mg/kg/min or 50 mg/min, whichever is slower. *Maintenance:* Highly individualized I.V. or P.O. every 6 to 8 hr.

±**DOSAGE ADJUSTMENT** For elderly patients, dosage reduced. For patients who are known to be intermediate or poor metabolizers of CYP2C9 substrates, dosage reduced.

Drug Administration

P.O.

- Administer with meals to minimize GI upset.
- Capsules should be swallowed whole with a glass of water and not chewed, crushed, or opened. Do not use capsules that are discolored.
- Chewable tablets may be chewed thoroughly before swallowing or tablet can be swallowed whole.
- Shake oral suspension container before use. Use a calibrated device to measure oral suspension dosage. Store oral suspension at room temperature.
- Dosage adjustment will be needed if patient switches to a different oral preparation. Oral preparations are not interchangeable mg per mg.

I.V.

- Can be initiated with either a loading dose or an infusion.
- If undiluted drug is refrigerated or becomes frozen, a precipitate might form; this will dissolve again after solution is allowed to stand at room temperature. A faint yellow coloration may develop but does not alter potency of drug.
- Check patency of I.V. catheter by testing with a flush of 0.9% Sodium Chloride Injection before administration. Repeat flush after administration.
- Administer directly into a central vein or large peripheral vein through a large-gauge catheter.
- For adult loading dose, infuse slowly at no more than 50 mg/min for adults (will take about 20 min for a 70-kg [150-lb] patient); for pediatric loading dose, infuse slowly at a rate not exceeding 3 mg/kg/min or 50 mg/min, whichever is slower.
- To prepare infusion, dilute drug in 0.9% Sodium Chloride Injection to a final concentration of no less than 5 mg/ml. Do not refrigerate diluted solution but administer immediately. Use an in-line filter (0.22 to 0.55 microns). Complete infusion within 1 to 4 hr.
- Assess I.V. site for signs of extravasation frequently because drug can cause tissue necrosis.
- *Incompatibilities:* Dextrose and dextrose-containing solutions, other drugs

I.M.

- Although I.M. injection is an FDA-approved route of administration for phenytoin sodium, it is not recommended due to erratic absorption, pain on injection, and serious injection-site reactions that may occur, such as necrosis.
- A different anticonvulsant should be used in place of using I.M. phenytoin sodium.

Route	Onset	Peak	Duration
P.O.	Unknown	1.5–3 hr	Unknown
P.O./E.R.	Unknown	4–12 hr	Unknown
I.V.	10–60 min	1–2 hr	Unknown

Half-life: 7–42 hr

Mechanism of Action

Limits the spread of seizure activity and the start of new seizures by regulating voltage-dependent calcium and sodium channels in neurons, inhibiting calcium movement across neuronal membranes, and enhancing sodium-potassium ATP activity in neurons and glial cells. Stabilizes the neurons from all these actions.

Contraindications

For all forms: Concurrent use with delavirdine or nonnucleoside reverse transcriptase inhibitors; history of prior acute hepatoxicity attributed to phenytoin; hypersensitivity to phenytoin, other hydantoins, or their components
For I.V. form: Adams-Stokes syndrome, second- and third-degree A-V block, sinoatrial block, sinus bradycardia

Interactions

DRUGS

albendazole, anticoagulants (apixaban, dabigatran, edoxaban, rivaroxaban), antiepileptics (carbamazepine, felbamate, lacosamide, lamotrigine, oxcarbazepine, topiramate), antilipidemic agents (atorvastatin, fluvastatin, simvastatin), antiplatelets (ticagrelor), antiviral agents (efavirenz, fosamprenavir when given alone, indinavir, lopinavir/ritonavir, nelfinavir, ritonavir, saquinavir), calcium channel blockers (nifedipine, nimodipine, verapamil), chlorpropamide, clozapine, cyclosporine, digoxin, disopyramide, folic acid, methadone, mexiletine, praziquantel, quetiapine: Decreased blood levels of these drugs by phenytoin
amiodarone, antidepressants (fluoxetine, fluvoxamine, sertraline), antiepileptic drugs (ethosuximide, felbamate, oxcarbazepine, topiramate), antineoplastic agents (capecitabine, fluorouracil), azoles (fluconazole, ketoconazole, itraconazole, miconazole, voriconazole), chloramphenicol, chlordiazepoxide, disulfiram, estrogen, fluvastatin, gastric acid reducing agents (H2antagonist, such as cimetidine, omeprazole), isoniazid, methylphenidate, phenothiazines, salicylates, sulfonamides (sulfadiazine, sulfamethizole, sulfamethoxazole-trimethoprim, sulfaphenazole), ticlopidine, tolbutamide, trazodone, warfarin: Possibly increased phenytoin serum levels
antiepileptics (carbamazepine, vigabatrin), antineoplastic agents usually in combination(bleomycin, carboplatin, cisplatin, doxorubicin, methotrexate), antiviral agents (fosamprenavir, nelfinavir, ritonavir), diazepam, diazoxide, folic acid, reserpine, rifampin, St. John's wort, theophylline: Possibly decreased phenytoin serum levels
antiepileptics (phenobarbital, valproate sodium, valproic acid): Possibly decreased or increased phenytoin serum levels
azoles (fluconazole, ketoconazole, itraconazole, posaconazole, voriconazole), antineoplastic agents (irinotecan, paclitaxel, teniposide), corticosteroids, delavirdine, doxycycline, estrogens, furosemide, neuromuscular blocking agents (cisatracurium, pancuronium, rocuronium, vecuronium), oral contraceptives, paroxetine, quinidine, rifampin, sertraline, theophylline, vitamin D, warfarin: Decreased effectiveness of these drugs by phenytoin
valproate: Increased risk of valproate-associated hyperammonemia

ACTIVITIES

alcohol use: Additive CNS depression, increased blood phenytoin levels with acute alcohol use; decreased blood phenytoin levels with chronic alcohol use

Adverse Reactions

CNS: Ataxia, cerebellar atrophy, confusion, depression, dizziness, drowsiness, excitement, fever, headache, involuntary motor activity, lethargy, nervousness, peripheral neuropathy, phenytoin-induced dyskinesias, restlessness, slurred speech, **suicidal ideation**, tremor, vertigo, weakness
CV: **Bradycardia**, **cardiac arrest**, **hypotension**, periarteritis nodosa, polyarteritis, vasculitis
EENT: Amblyopia, conjunctivitis, diplopia, earache, epistaxis, eye pain, gingival hyperplasia, hearing loss, loss of taste, nystagmus, pharyngitis, photophobia, rhinitis, sinusitis, taste perversion, tinnitus

ENDO: Gynecomastia, hyperglycemia
GI: Abdominal pain, **acute hepatic failure**, anorexia, constipation, diarrhea, epigastric pain, jaundice, hepatic dysfunction, **hepatic necrosis**, **hepatitis**, nausea, vomiting
GU: Glycosuria, Peyronie's disease, priapism, **renal failure**
HEME: Acute intermittent porphyria (exacerbation), **agranulocytosis**, anemia, eosinophilia, **granulocytopenia**, **leukopenia**, macrocytosis, **megaloblastic anemia**, **pancytopenia**, **pure red cell aplasia**, **thrombocytopenia**
MS: Arthralgia, arthropathy, bone fractures, decreased bone mineral density, muscle twitching, osteomalacia, polymyositis
RESP: **Apnea**, **asthma**, bronchitis, cough, dyspnea, **hypoxia**, increased sputum production, pneumonia, **pneumothorax**, **pulmonary fibrosis**
SKIN: Acute generalized exanthematous pustulosis, bullous dermatitis, **exfoliative dermatitis**, maculopapular or morbilliform rash, purpuric dermatitis, **Stevens-Johnson syndrome**, **toxic epidermal necrolysis**, unusual hair growth, urticaria
Other: **Angioedema**, benign lymph node hyperplasia, **drug reaction with eosinophilia and systemic symptoms (DRESS)**, facial feature coarsening or enlargement, **Hodgkin's disease**, immunoglobulin abnormalities, injection-site pain, lupus-like symptoms, lymphadenopathy, **lymphoma**, porphyria, weight gain or loss

Childbearing Considerations

PREGNANCY

- Pregnancy exposure registry: 1-888-233-2334 or http://www.aedpregnancyregistry.org/.
- Drug may cause fetal harm, such as congenital malformations, adverse developmental outcomes, and less common malignancies, including neuroblastoma in children whose mothers received phenytoin during pregnancy.
- Be aware that a potentially life-threatening bleeding disorder may occur in newborns exposed to drug in utero but can be prevented with vitamin K administration to the mother before delivery and to the neonate after birth.
- Use with extreme caution only if absolutely necessary and benefit to mother outweighs potential risk to fetus.
- Be aware that decreased serum concentrations of drug may occur during pregnancy requiring frequent monitoring of drug levels in mother throughout the pregnancy.

LACTATION

- Drug is present in breast milk.
- Mothers should check with prescriber before breastfeeding.

REPRODUCTION

- Females of childbearing age using an oral contraceptive should use an additional or alternative nonhormonal contraceptive during drug therapy.

Nursing Considerations

! WARNING Know that patients of Asian ancestry who have the genetic allelic variant HLA-B 1502 or are CYP2C9*3 carriers can develop serious and sometimes fatal dermatologic reactions 10 times more often than people without these genetic variants. Phenytoin shouldn't be used as a substitute for carbamazepine in these patients.

! WARNING Monitor blood pressure and ECG tracings continuously when administering I.V. phenytoin. Be aware that bradycardia and cardiac arrest have occurred in patients receiving recommended dosages, in addition to patients experiencing phenytoin toxicity. Most cases of cardiac arrest occurred in patients with underlying cardiac disease.

- Expect continuous enteral feedings to disrupt phenytoin absorption and, possibly, reduce blood phenytoin level. Discontinue tube feedings 1 hour before and after phenytoin administration, as prescribed. Anticipate giving increased phenytoin doses to compensate for reduced bioavailability during continuous tube feedings.
- Know that therapeutic phenytoin level ranges from 10 to 20 mcg/L. Expect to monitor phenytoin serum levels based on the unbound fraction in patients with hepatic or renal disease or those with hypoalbuminemia because the fraction of unbound phenytoin is increased in these patients.

! **WARNING** Monitor patient closely for elevated therapeutic levels because high serum levels that are sustained may cause cerebellar atrophy (rare), delirium, encephalopathy, irreversible cerebellar dysfunction, or psychosis. Expect to obtain serum levels if early signs of dose-related CNS toxicity develop in any patient because some patients may be slow metabolizers of phenytoin. If above therapeutic range levels are found, expect phenytoin dosage to be reduced. If symptoms persist, expect drug to be discontinued.

! **WARNING** Know that phenytoin should not be stopped abruptly, as status epilepticus may occur. Instead, expect drug to be discontinued gradually.

! **WARNING** Monitor patient closely for evidence of suicidal thinking or behavior, especially when therapy starts or dosage changes.

! **WARNING** Monitor patient closely for hypersensitivity or severe cutaneous reaction such as angioedema or DRESS. At first sign of a hypersensitivity reactions or rash (DRESS may only initially present with fever or swollen lymph nodes), notify prescriber, expect drug to be discontinued and another drug substituted, and provide supportive care, as needed and ordered.

! **WARNING** Monitor patient's hematologic status during therapy because phenytoin can cause blood dyscrasias. A patient with a history of agranulocytosis, leukopenia, or pancytopenia may have an increased risk of infection because phenytoin can cause myelosuppression.

- Anticipate that drug may worsen intermittent porphyria.
- Monitor blood glucose level of patient with diabetes mellitus frequently because drug can stimulate glucagon secretion and impair insulin secretion, either of which can raise blood glucose level.
- Monitor thyroid hormone levels in patient receiving thyroid replacement therapy because phenytoin may decrease circulating thyroid hormone levels and increase thyroid-stimulating hormone level. Also, know that drug may decrease dexamethasone or metyrapone test results or increase serum levels of alkaline phosphatase, gamma glutamyl transpeptidase (GGT), or glucose.
- Be aware that long-term phenytoin therapy may increase patient's requirements for folic acid or vitamin D supplements. However, keep in mind that a diet high in folic acid may decrease seizure control.

PATIENT TEACHING

- Instruct patient, family, or caregiver how to administer form of phenytoin prescribed.
- Advise patient to take drug exactly as prescribed; she should not change brands, dosage, or stop taking drug unless instructed by prescriber.
- Urge patient to avoid alcohol during therapy.

! **WARNING** Urge family or caregiver to watch patient closely for evidence of suicidal tendencies, especially when therapy starts or dosage changes, and to report concerns at once to prescriber.

! **WARNING** Alert patient that drug may cause an allergic reaction. If present, tell patient to notify prescriber and, if severe, to seek immediate medical care.

! **WARNING** Instruct patient to notify prescriber at the first sign of a fever, rash, or swollen lymph nodes or if persistent, severe, or other unusual skin reactions occur.

! **WARNING** Tell patient to report any signs of heart dysfunction, such as dizziness, feeling heart skipping beats, slow pulse, or tiredness.

! **WARNING** Inform females of childbearing age to notify prescriber immediately if pregnancy occurs, as phenytoin may cause fetal harm. Instruct females of childbearing age using an oral contraceptive to use an additional or alternative nonhormonal contraceptive during drug therapy.

- Caution patient to avoid hazardous activities until drug's CNS effects are known and resolved.
- Inform patient with diabetes mellitus about the increased risk of hyperglycemia and the possible need for increased antidiabetic

drug dosage during therapy. Advise her to check blood glucose level often.

- Emphasize the importance of good oral hygiene and encourage patient to inform her dentist that she's taking phenytoin.
- Encourage patient to wear medical identification that indicates her diagnosis and drug therapy.

pimavanserin

Nuplazid

Class and Category

Pharmacologic class: Serotonin 5-HT receptor inverse agonist and antagonist
Therapeutic class: Atypical antipsychotic

Indications and Dosages

✱ *To treat delusions and hallucinations associated with Parkinson's disease psychosis*

CAPSULES, TABLETS

Adults. 34 mg (two 17-mg tablets) once daily.

± **DOSAGE ADJUSTMENT** For patients taking strong CYP3A4 inhibitors, such as ketoconazole concurrently, dosage reduced to 10 mg once daily.

Drug Administration

P.O.

- Capsules may be swallowed whole or opened and contents sprinkled over a tablespoon of applesauce, pudding, yogurt, or a liquid nutritional supplement. Administer immediately and warn patient not to chew it before swallowing.

Route	Onset	Peak	Duration
P.O.	Unknown	6 hr	Unknown

Half-life: 57 hr

Mechanism of Action

Thought to mediate through a combination of inverse agonist and antagonist activity at serotonin 5-HT_{2A} receptors and to a lesser extent at serotonin 5-HT_{2C} receptors to eradicate delusions and hallucinations associated with Parkinson's disease psychosis.

Contraindications

Hypersensitivity to pimavanserin or its components

Interactions

DRUGS

antibiotics, such as gatifloxacin, moxifloxacin; antipsychotics, such as chlorpromazine, thioridazine, ziprasidone; class 1A antiarrhythmics, such as disopyramide, procainamide, quinidine; class III antiarrhythmics, such as amiodarone, sotalol: Possible prolonged QT interval, increasing risk of cardiac arrhythmias

carbamazepine, efavirenz, modafinil, nafcillin, phenytoin, rifampin, St. John's wort, thioridazine: Possibly reduced pimavanserin exposure, resulting in decreased effectiveness

clarithromycin, itraconazole, ketoconazole, indinavir: Increased pimavanserin exposure, leading to possible adverse reactions

Adverse Reactions

CNS: Aggression, agitation, confusion, fatigue, gait disturbance, hallucination, somnolence
CV: Peripheral edema, **QT prolongation interval**
EENT: Circumoral edema, **throat tightness, tongue swelling**
GI: Constipation, nausea
GU: UTI
RESP: Dyspnea
SKIN: Rash, urticaria
Other: **Angioedema**

Childbearing Considerations

PREGNANCY

- It is not known if drug can cause fetal harm.
- Use with caution only if benefit to mother outweighs potential risk to fetus.

LACTATION

- It is not known if drug is present in breast milk.
- Mothers should check with prescriber before breastfeeding.

Nursing Considerations

! **WARNING** Keep in mind that pimavanserin shouldn't be used to treat dementia-related psychosis in the elderly because of an increased mortality risk.

! **WARNING** Know that pimavanserin therapy should be avoided in patients with a history of cardiac arrhythmias, known QT prolongation, or in combination with other drugs known to prolong the

P

QT interval. Drug should also not be used in patients who are at risk for hypokalemia or hypomagnesemia or in the presence of congenital prolongation of the QT interval or symptomatic bradycardia. Monitor patient's ECG regularly for evidence of QT prolongation.

- Use cautiously in patients with renal impairment, including severe impairment and end-stage renal disease.

! WARNING Monitor patient for evidence of a hypersensitivity reaction which could become life-threatening such as angioedema. If present, notify prescriber, expect drug to be discontinued, and provide supportive care, as needed and ordered.

PATIENT TEACHING

- Instruct patient, family, or caregiver how to administer form of pimavanserin prescribed.

! WARNING Alert patient, family, or caregiver that drug may cause an allergic reaction. If present, tell them to notify prescriber and, if severe, to seek immediate medical care.

- Instruct patient and family or caregiver to alert all prescribers about pimavanserin therapy and not to take any over-the-counter drugs (including herbal preparations) without prescriber knowledge.

pioglitazone hydrochloride

Actos

Class and Category

Pharmacologic class: Thiazolidinedione
Therapeutic class: Antidiabetic

Indications and Dosages

✱ *To achieve glucose control in type 2 diabetes mellitus as monotherapy or as adjunct in combination with insulin, metformin, or a sulfonylurea*

TABLETS

Adults. *Initial:* 15 or 30 mg once daily, increased in increments of 15 mg, as needed, to maximum dose. *Maximum:* 45 mg daily.

±**DOSAGE ADJUSTMENT** For patients with congestive heart failure, starting dose is 15 mg once daily. For patients receiving concomitant gemfibrozil or other strong CYP2C8 inhibitors, maximum dose should not exceed 15 mg once daily. For patients taking insulin, insulin dosage decreased by 10% to 25% if hypoglycemia occurs.

Drug Administration

P.O.

- Drug may be given at any time of day but consistently at the same time of day.
- If a dose is missed, skip missed dose and resume dosing schedule the next day. Do not double dose to make up for missed dose.

Route	Onset	Peak	Duration
P.O.	30 min	2 hr	24 hr

Half-life: 3–7 hr

Mechanism of Action

Decreases insulin resistance by enhancing the sensitivity of insulin-dependent tissues, such as adipose tissue, the liver, and skeletal muscle, and reduces glucose output from the liver. Activates peroxisome proliferator-activated receptor-gamma (PPARg) receptors, which modulate transcription of insulin-responsive genes involved in glucose control and lipid metabolism thereby reducing hyperglycemia, hyperinsulinemia, and hypertriglyceridemia in patients with type 2 diabetes mellitus and insulin resistance. Requires endogenous insulin to work effectively because pioglitazone doesn't increase pancreatic insulin secretion.

Contraindications

Hypersensitivity to pioglitazone or its components, New York Heart Association (NYHA) class III or IV heart failure

Interactions

DRUGS

gemfibrozil and other strong CYP2C8 inhibitors: Increased pioglitazone effect
insulin, oral antidiabetic agents: Possibly increased risk of hypoglycemia
ketoconazole: Possibly decreased metabolism of pioglitazone
rifampin or other CYP2C8 inducers: Possibly altered glucose control

topiramate: Decreased exposure of pioglitazone and its active metabolites

Adverse Reactions

CNS: Headache
CV: **Congestive heart failure**, edema
EENT: Blurred vision, decreased visual acuity, macular edema, pharyngitis, sinusitis, tooth disorders
GI: Elevated liver enzymes, **hepatitis**, **hepatic failure**, jaundice
HEME: Decreased hemoglobin level and hematocrit
MS: Fractures (in women), myalgia
RESP: Upper respiratory tract infection
Other: Weight gain

Childbearing Considerations

PREGNANCY

- It is not known if drug can cause fetal harm.
- Use with caution only if benefit to mother outweighs potential risk to fetus.

LACTATION

- It is not known if drug is present in breast milk.
- Mothers should check with prescriber before breastfeeding.

REPRODUCTION

- Be aware that drug may result in ovulation in some anovulatory women, which increases the risk of an unintended pregnancy.

Nursing Considerations

! WARNING Be aware that pioglitazone isn't recommended for patients with symptomatic heart failure.

! WARNING Know that pioglitazone may increase the risk for bladder cancer and should only be used with extreme caution in patients with a history of bladder cancer.

! WARNING Know that pioglitazone should not be given to patients with active liver disease or who have an elevated alanine transaminase (ALT) values exceeding 2.5 times the upper limit of normal. Be prepared to monitor liver enzymes before therapy begins, every 2 months during first year, and annually thereafter, as ordered, because drug is extensively metabolized in the liver. Expect to stop drug if jaundice develops or ALT values exceed 2.5 times normal because drug may cause hepatitis or hepatic failure.

- Monitor glucose levels, as ordered, to evaluate effectiveness of therapy and monitor glycosylated hemoglobin level to assess drug's long-term effectiveness.

! WARNING Assess for signs and symptoms of hypoglycemia in diabetic patient, especially if patient is also taking another antidiabetic drug.

! WARNING Monitor patient for signs and symptoms of congestive heart failure, such as edema, rapid weight gain, or shortness of breath because pioglitazone can cause fluid retention that may lead to or worsen heart failure. Notify prescriber immediately of any deterioration in the patient's cardiac status, and expect to discontinue drug, as ordered.

PATIENT TEACHING

! WARNING Alert patient of the risk of bladder cancer before pioglitazone is administered. Review signs and symptoms of bladder dysfunction and tell patient, if present, to notify prescriber immediately.

- Emphasize the need for patient to continue diet control, exercise program, and weight management during pioglitazone therapy.
- Instruct the patient how to administer pioglitazone.

! WARNING Advise patient to notify prescriber immediately if she experiences fluid retention, shortness of breath, or sudden weight gain because drug may have to be discontinued.

! WARNING Warn patient with diabetes who is taking any additional antidiabetic drugs, to watch for hypoglycemia. Review how to treat hypoglycemia appropriately. If hypoglycemia occurs frequently or is severe, tell patient to notify prescriber.

- Urge patient to report vision changes promptly and expect to have an eye examination by an ophthalmologist, regardless of when the last examination occurred.
- Inform female patient that she may be at risk for fractures during pioglitazone therapy and urge her to take safety precautions to prevent falls and other injuries.

- Instruct patient to keep laboratory appointments for liver enzymes, as ordered, typically every 2 months during first year of therapy and annually thereafter.

pitavastatin calcium

Livalo

pitavastatin magnesium

Zypitamag

Class and Category

Pharmacologic class: HMG-CoA reductase inhibitor (statin)
Therapeutic class: Antilipemic

Indications and Dosages

✷ *As adjunct to diet to reduce low-density lipoprotein cholesterol (LDL-C) in patients with primary hyperlipidemia*

TABLETS (LIVALO, ZYPITAMAG)

Adults. 2 mg to 4 mg once daily. *Maximum:* 4 mg once daily

±**DOSAGE ADJUSTMENT** For patients with moderate to severe renal impairment (eGFR 15 to 59 ml/min) or patients receiving hemodialysis, initial dosage reduced to 1 mg once daily, with maximum of 2 mg once daily. For patients taking erythromycin, dosage shouldn't exceed 1 mg daily; for patients taking rifampin, dosage shouldn't exceed 2 mg daily.

✷ *As adjunct to diet to reduce LDL-C in patients with heterozygous familial hypercholesterolemia*

TABLETS (LIVALO)

Adults and children ages 8 and older. 2 mg to 4 mg once daily. *Maximum:* 4 mg once daily.

Drug Administration

P.O.

- Administer drug at any time of day but be consistent.
- Administer with or without food.

Route	Onset	Peak	Duration
P.O.	Unknown	1 hr	Unknown

Half-life: 12 hr

Mechanism of Action

Reduces plasma cholesterol and lipoprotein levels by inhibiting cholesterol and HMG-CoA reductase synthesis in the liver, thereby increasing number of LDL receptors on liver cells, and enhancing LDL uptake and breakdown. Sustained inhibition of cholesterol synthesis in the liver, decreases levels of very low-density lipoproteins.

Contraindications

Active liver disease (including unexplained persistent hepatic transaminase elevation) or decompensated cirrhosis, breastfeeding (Zypitamag), concurrent cyclosporine therapy, hypersensitivity to pitavastatin or its components

Interactions

DRUGS

colchicine, fibrates, such as gemfibrozil: Increased risk of myopathy, including rhabdomyolysis
cyclosporine, erythromycin, rifampin: Increased pitavastatin exposure; increased risk of myopathy and rhabdomyolysis
niacin (1 g or greater/day): Increased risk of adverse skeletal muscle effects

ACTIVITIES

alcohol: Increased risk of liver injury with heavy use

Adverse Reactions

CNS: Asthenia, cognitive impairment, confusion, depression, dizziness, fatigue, headache, hypoesthesia, insomnia, malaise, memory loss, peripheral neuropathy
EENT: Nasopharyngitis
ENDO: Elevated glycosylated hemoglobin level, hyperglycemia
GI: Abdominal discomfort or pain, constipation, diarrhea, dyspepsia, elevated liver enzymes, **hepatic failure**, **hepatitis**, jaundice, nausea
GU: **Acute renal failure**, erectile dysfunction, **myoglobinuria**
MS: Arthralgia, back or extremity pain, immune-mediated necrotizing myopathy (rare), muscle spasms, myalgia, myopathy, myositis, **rhabdomyolysis**
RESP: **Interstitial lung disease**
SKIN: Lichen planus, pruritus, rash, urticaria
Other: **Angioedema**, elevated creatine phosphokinase level, flu-like symptoms

Childbearing Considerations

PREGNANCY

- Drug may cause fetal harm.
- It is recommended drug be discontinued when pregnancy occurs but the ongoing therapeutic needs of the mother should be taken into account before doing so.

LACTATION

- It is not known if drug is present in breast milk.
- Drug is not recommended for use in mothers who are breastfeeding.

REPRODUCTION

- Advise females of childbearing age to use effective contraception during drug therapy.

Nursing Considerations

- Note that pravastatin, another HMG-CoA reductase inhibitor, sounds similar to pitavastatin and could be confusing. Make sure of correct drug before giving.

! WARNING Monitor liver enzymes, as ordered, before pitavastatin therapy starts and as indicated during therapy. Although increases usually appear soon after drug therapy is started, are transient, not accompanied by symptoms, and resolve or improve on continued therapy or after a brief interruption of therapy, fatal and non-fatal hepatic failure have rarely occurred. Know that patients who drink alcohol heavily and/or have a history of liver disease may be at increased risk for liver injury. If patient develops serious hepatic injury exhibited by hyperbilirubinemia or jaundice in addition to liver enzyme elevation, notify prescriber and expect pitavastatin to be immediately discontinued.

- Expect to monitor patient's lipid levels after 4 weeks of therapy to determine drug effectiveness and periodically thereafter, as ordered. Expect dosage to be adjusted if lipid levels remain elevated.

! WARNING Monitor patient for a hypersensitivity reaction, which could become life-threatening, such as angioedema. If present, notify prescriber immediately, expect drug to be discontinued, and provide supportive care, as needed and ordered.

! WARNING Monitor patients with risk factors for myopathy, such as concurrent use of colchicine, niacin-containing products (greater than 1 g daily), or fibrates. Also know that cyclosporine is a contraindication and gemfibrozil is not recommended during pitavastatin therapy. Additional risk factors include the elderly (over age 65), presence of renal impairment, or in patients who are being inadequately treated for hypothyroidism. Monitor patient throughout therapy for muscular complaints and an elevated blood creatine kinase level because myopathy may lead to the severe form of rhabdomyolysis which may cause renal failure and death. Notify prescriber if present and expect drug to be discontinued if patient's creatine kinase level becomes markedly elevated, or if myopathy is suspected or confirmed.

- Know that, although rare, immune-mediated necrotizing myopathy has been associated with statin therapy. Monitor patient for elevated serum creatine kinase levels and proximal muscle weakness, which persists despite discontinuation of the statin. Additional neuromuscular and serologic testing may be needed. Expect drug to be discontinued, if immune-mediated necrotizing myopathy is confirmed. Patient may need immunosuppressive therapy to treat it.
- Monitor patient's blood glucose levels and HbA1C in patients with diabetes because pitavastatin as a statin may increase blood glucose levels and alter control.

PATIENT TEACHING

- Emphasize that pitavastatin is an adjunct to, not a substitute for, a low-cholesterol diet.
- Instruct patient how to administer pitavastatin.

! WARNING Alert patient that drug may cause an allergic reaction. If present, tell patient to notify prescriber immediately and, if severe, to seek immediate medical care.

! WARNING Advise patient to limit alcohol ingestion while taking pitavastatin because alcohol-induced liver dysfunction may be difficult to differentiate from pitavastatin-induced liver dysfunction.

! WARNING Instruct patient to immediately report unexplained muscle pain, tenderness, or weakness, especially if accompanied by fever or malaise.

- Instruct patient to consult prescriber before taking over-the-counter products, especially niacin, because of increased risk of adverse muscle effects.
- Inform patient, especially diabetics, that pitavastatin may increase blood glucose levels and alter their control. Encourage patient to monitor their blood glucose levels closely throughout pitavastatin therapy.
- Tell females of childbearing age to notify prescriber if pregnancy occurs as drug is not recommended during pregnancy. Also advise patient to use effective contraception throughout drug therapy.
- Inform mothers breastfeeding is not recommended during pitavastatin therapy.

NEW!

pivmecillinam

Pivya

Class and Category

Pharmacologic class: Pencillin
Therapeutic class: Antibiotic

Indications and Dosages

∗ *To treat uncomplicated urinary tract infections in females caused by susceptible isolates of* Escherichia coli, Proteus mirabilis, *and* Staphylococcus saprophyticus

TABLETS

Females ages 18 yr and older. 185 mg 3 times daily for 3 to 7 days, as indicated.

Drug Administration

P.O.

- Administer drug with or without food.
- If a dose is missed, administer dose as soon as possible but do not double the dose to make up for the missed dose.

Route	Onset	Peak	Duration
P.O.	Unknown	60-120 min	Unknown

Half-life: 30-90 min

Mechanism of Action

Breaks down into its active antibacterial agent, mecillinam, to prevent susceptible bacteria from forming a cell wall, thus killing the microorganisms that cause UTIs.

Contraindications

Acute porphyria; carnitine deficiency; hypersensitivity to pivmecillinam, other beta-lactam antibacterial drugs such as cephalosporins and penicillins, or their components

Interactions

DRUGS

methotrexate: Reduced clearance of methotrexate from the body resulting in possible adverse reactions
valproate, valproic acid, other pivalate-generating drugs: Decreased carnitine concentrations in plasma, which may increase the risk of carnitine depletion-associated adverse reactions

Adverse Reactions

CNS: Dizziness, headache, vertigo
EENT: Mouth ulceration
GI: Abdominal pain, abnormal liver function, ***Clostridioides difficile*-associated diarrhea**, diarrhea, dyspepsia, esophageal ulcer, esophagitis, nausea, vomiting
GU: Genital pruritus, vulvovaginal candidiasis
HEME: **Acute porphyria**, **thrombocytopenia**
SKIN: Acute generalized exanthematous pustulosis (AGEP), pruritus, rash, **Stevens-Johnson Syndrome (SJS)**, **toxic epidermal necrolysis (TEN)**, urticaria
Other: **Anaphylaxis**, angioedema, **carnitine decreased**, **drug reactions with eosinophilia and systemic symptoms (DRESS)**

Childbearing Considerations

PREGNANCY

- Drug does not appear to cause fetal harm.
- Use with caution only if benefit to mother outweighs potential risk to fetus.
- Be aware treatment of a pregnant female with the drug prior to delivery may cause a false positive test for isovaleric acidemia in the newborn as part of newborn screening.

LACTATION

- It is not known if drug is present in breast milk.
- Mothers should check with prescriber before breastfeeding.

Nursing Considerations

! WARNING Do not administer pivmecillinam to a patient with primary or secondary carnitine deficiency due to inherited metabolic disorders known to cause carnitine depletion. Monitor patient for carnitine depletion throughout drug therapy exhibited by confusion, fatigue, hypoglycemia and muscle aches. Alert prescriber immediately if present and expect drug to be discontinued.

! WARNING Assess patient for previous hypersensitivity reactions to carbapenems, cephalosporins, penicillins, and other beta-lactams before administering pivmecillinam because cross sensitivity may occur. Also assess patient for a history of sensitivity to multiple allergens which may increase patient risk of experiencing a hypersensitivity to pivmecillinam. Monitor patient closely throughout drug therapy for a hypersensitivity or serious skin reaction, which could become life-threatening such as angioedema, anaphylaxis, or DRESS. If present or at first sign of rash (DRESS may only initially present with a fever or swollen lymph nodes), notify prescriber, expect drug to be discontinued, and provide supportive care, as needed and ordered.

! WARNING Monitor patient for *Clostridiodes difficile*–associated diarrhea even up to 2 months after drug therapy has been discontinued that may range in severity from mild diarrhea to fatal colitis. If suspected, obtain laboratory confirmation. If positive, expect drug to be discontinued, administer drug therapy for *C. difficile*, provide fluid and electrolyte therapy as well as protein supplement, as ordered. If severe, surgical intervention may be needed.

- Be aware that treatment of a pregnant female prior to delivery may cause a false positive test for isovaleric acidemia in the newborn as part of newborn screening. Ensure prompt follow-up of a positive screening result.

PATIENT TEACHING

! WARNING Tell patient to alert prescriber before taking pivmecillinam if patient takes valproate, valproic acid, or other pivalate-generating drugs as pivmecillinam may cause carintine depletion.

- Instruct patient how to administer pivmecillinam and what to do if a dose is missed. Stress importance of taking drug for entire time prescribed.

! WARNING Alert patient drug may cause an allergic reaction or severe skin reactions. If present, tell patient to notify prescriber, stop taking the drug, and, if severe, to seek immediate medical care.

! WARNING Alert patient that diarrhea may occur with pivmecillinam use, which could occur as late as 2 months after drug therapy is completed and may range from being mild to severe. If severe, tell patient to seek immediate medical attention.

plazomicin sulfate

Zemdri

Class and Category

Pharmacologic class: Aminoglycoside
Therapeutic class: Antibiotic

Indications and Dosages

✱ *To treat complicated urinary tract infections, including pyelonephritis, caused by* Enterobacter cloacae, Escherichia coli, Klebsiella pneumoniae, *or* Proteus mirabilis

I.V. INFUSION

Adults and adolescents ages 18 and older who have a creatinine clearance greater than or equal to 90 ml/min. 15 mg/kg infused over 30 min every 24 hr for 4 to 7 days.

±**DOSAGE ADJUSTMENT** For patients with a creatinine clearance less than 90 ml/min but equal to or greater than 60 ml/min, dosage remains at 15 mg/kg every 24 hours. For patients with a creatinine clearance less than 60 ml/min but greater than or equal to 30 ml/min, dosage reduced to 10 mg/kg every 24 hours. For patients with a creatinine clearance less than 30 ml/min but greater than or equal to 15 ml/min, dosage reduced to 10 mg/kg and dosage interval increased to every 48 hours. For all patients with a plasma trough level measured 30 min before second dose that is greater than or equal to 3 mcg/ml, dosing interval increased by 1.5-fold. For example, a dosing interval of every 24 hours

P

would be increased to every 36 hours or if every 48 hours the dosing interval would be increased to every 72 hours.

Drug Administration

I.V.

- Keep drug stored in refrigerator until ready to use.
- Each drug vial contains 500-mg plazomicin freebase in 10 ml Water for Injection, giving a concentration of 50 mg/ml.
- Dilute drug vial solution in 0.9% Sodium Chloride Injection or Lactated Ringer's Injection to achieve a final volume of 50 ml for intravenous infusion.
- After dilution, drug solution is stable for 24 hr at room temperature.
- Infuse each dose over 30 min.
- *Incompatibilities:* Other I.V. drugs

Route	Onset	Peak	Duration
I.V.	Unknown	Unknown	Unknown

Half-life: 3.5 hr

Mechanism of Action

Binds to bacterial 30S ribosomal subunit to inhibit protein synthesis, which exerts a bactericidal effect.

Contraindications

Hypersensitivity to plazomicin, other aminoglycosides, or their components

Interactions

DRUGS

None reported by manufacturer.

Adverse Reactions

CNS: Dizziness, headache, vertigo
CV: Hypertension, **hypotension**
EENT: Hearing loss, ototoxicity, tinnitus
GI: ***Clostridioides difficile*–associated diarrhea**, constipation, diarrhea, elevated liver enzymes, gastritis, nausea, vomiting
GU: Elevated serum creatinine, hematuria, impaired renal function, **nephrotoxicity**
RESP: Dyspnea
Other: **Hypersensitivity reactions**, **hypokalemia**

Childbearing Considerations

PREGNANCY

- Drug may cause fetal harm.
- Drug is not recommended during pregnancy.

LACTATION

- It is not known if drug is present in breast milk.
- Mothers should check with prescriber before breastfeeding.

Nursing Considerations

! **WARNING** Expect to assess creatinine clearance in all patients prior to first dose of plazomicin and daily during therapy. For patients with renal impairment with a creatinine clearance of 15 ml/min or greater but less than 90 ml/min, expect plasma trough concentrations to be below 3 mcg/ml. Plasma trough level should be measured about 30 min before administration of second dose. If level is greater than or equal to 3 mcg/ml, expect a dosage adjustment to be made by extending the dosing interval by 1.5-fold, for example, from every 24 hours to every 36 hours or from every 48 hours to every 72 hours. Know that patients at greater risk for nephrotoxicity are the elderly, patients with existing impaired renal function, and those who are receiving concomitant nephrotoxic drugs.

- Ensure patient maintains adequate hydration throughout therapy because dehydration may lead to renal impairment.

! **WARNING** Monitor patient for hypersensitivity reactions. If present, notify prescriber immediately and expect plazomicin to be discontinued. Provide supportive care, as needed and ordered.

! **WARNING** Monitor patient for adverse reactions associated with neuromuscular blockade because aminoglycosides such as plazomicin have been associated with neuromuscular blockade. Patients at high risk include patients with underlying neuromuscular disorders (including myasthenia gravis) or patients who are receiving concomitantly neuromuscular blocking drugs.

! **WARNING** Assess patient for signs of secondary infection, such as profuse, watery diarrhea. If such diarrhea develops, contact prescriber and expect to obtain a stool specimen to rule out pseudomembranous colitis caused by *Clostridioides difficile*. Know that CDAD may range from being mild to causing fatal colitis. If confirmed, notify prescriber and expect to withhold plazomicin and treat with an antibiotic effective against *C. difficile*, as ordered. Also, expect to administer electrolytes, fluids, and protein supplementation, as needed and ordered.

- Monitor patient for hearing loss, tinnitus, and/or vertigo because plazomicin may cause ototoxicity that may be irreversible and may not show up until after drug has been discontinued. Patients at higher risk include those with a family history of hearing loss, already have renal impairment, or are receiving higher doses and/or longer durations of therapy than recommended. Ototoxicity may also occur in patients with certain mitochondrial DNA variants.

PATIENT TEACHING

- Inform patient plazomicin is administered intravenously.

! **WARNING** Tell patient that it is important to keep hydrated during plazomicin therapy because dehydration increases the risk of kidney impairment.

! **WARNING** Instruct patient to report to staff any adverse reactions that might indicate an allergic reaction (such as hives, itching, and rash) because an allergic reaction can become serious.

! **WARNING** Alert patient that diarrhea is a common problem with antibacterial drugs. Tell patient that bloody or watery stools can occur up to more than 2 months after plazomicin therapy has been discontinued. Stress importance of reporting diarrhea to prescriber.

! **WARNING** Warn females of childbearing age to notify prescriber immediately if pregnancy occurs because aminoglycosides such as plazomicin can cause fetal harm and is not recommended during pregnancy.

! **WARNING** Inform patient with an underlying neuromuscular disease or patient who is receiving neuromuscular blocking agents that aggravation of muscle weakness has been reported with other aminoglycosides. Tell patient to report any muscle weakness that is abnormal for the patient to prescriber.

- Tell patient to report any changes in balance or hearing or if she experiences new onset or changes in preexisting buzzing or roaring in the ears, even after the course of plazomicin therapy has finished.

plecanatide

Trulance

Class and Category

Pharmacologic class: Guanylate cyclase-C agonist

Therapeutic class: Intestinal mobility agent

Indications and Dosages

✷ *To treat chronic idiopathic constipation or irritable bowel syndrome with constipation*

TABLETS

Adults. 3 mg once daily.

Drug Administration

P.O.

- Tablet should be swallowed whole.
- For patient who has difficulty swallowing tablets, crush tablet to a powder and mix with 1 teaspoon of room-temperature applesauce. Administer immediately. Do not store mixture for later use.
- Alternatively, drug may be administered in water by placing tablet in cup, adding 30 ml of room-temperature water, and gently swirling tablet/water mixture for at least 10 sec. Have patient swallow entire contents of tablet/water mixture immediately. If any portion of tablet is left in the cup, add another 30 ml of room-temperature water to the cup, swirl for at least 10 sec, and have patient swallow mixture immediately. Do not store the tablet/water mixture for later use.
- To administer drug through a gastric or nasogastric feeding tube, begin by placing tablet in a cup; then add 30 ml of room-temperature water. Gently swirl the tablet/water mixture for at least 15 sec. Flush the feeding tube with 30 ml of water. Draw up drug mixture using the same syringe and immediately administer via the

P

feeding tube. Do not reserve for future use. If any portion of tablet is left in the cup, add another 30 ml of room-temperature water, swirl for at least 15 sec. Using the same syringe, administer via the feeding tube. Follow by flushing the feeding tube with at least 10 ml of water.

- Store in a dry place at room temperature, keeping desiccant in bottle.
- If a dose is missed it should be skipped and drug administration resumed at the next regularly scheduled time. Do not double dose to make up for missed dose.

Route	Onset	Peak	Duration
P.O.	Unknown	Unknown	Unknown

Half-life: Unknown

Mechanism of Action

Acts locally on the luminal surface of the intestinal epithelium, resulting in an increase in both extracellular and intracellular concentrations of cyclic guanosine monophosphate (cGMP). Elevating intracellular cGMP stimulates secretion of bicarbonate and chloride into the intestinal lumen, which increases intestinal fluid and accelerates transit time to relieve constipation.

Contraindications

Children under age 6, hypersensitivity to plecanatide or its components, known or suspected mechanical gastrointestinal obstruction

Interactions

DRUGS

None reported by manufacturer.

Adverse Reactions

CNS: Dizziness
EENT: Nasopharyngitis, sinusitis
GI: Abdominal distention or tenderness, diarrhea, flatulence, elevated liver enzymes, nausea
GU: UTI
RESP: Upper respiratory tract infection
Other: Dehydration

Childbearing Considerations

PREGNANCY

- Drug is negligibly absorbed systemically following oral administration so drug exposure to fetus is minimal. However, it is not known if drug causes fetal harm.
- Use with caution only if benefit to mother outweighs potential risk to fetus.

LACTATION

- It is not known if drug is present in breast milk.
- Mothers should check with prescriber before breastfeeding.

Nursing Considerations

- Monitor patient's bowel movements to determine effectiveness of plecanatide.

! **WARNING** Monitor patient for diarrhea, which can become severe. If severe diarrhea occurs, withhold drug. Notify prescriber and expect to follow measures to rehydrate patient, as ordered.

PATIENT TEACHING

- Instruct patient how to administer plecanatide and what to do if a dose is missed.
- Caution patient not to exceed dosage, as severe dehydration may occur.

! **WARNING** Tell patient to stop taking drug and notify prescriber if severe diarrhea occurs.

! **WARNING** Warn patient to keep plecanatide out of the reach of children, especially those who are less than age 6.

ponesimod

Ponvory

Class and Category

Pharmacologic class: Sphingosine 1-phosphate receptor modulator
Therapeutic class: Immunomodulator

Indications and Dosages

* *To treat relapsing forms of multiple sclerosis (MS), to include active secondary progressive disease, clinically isolated syndrome, and relapsing-remitting disease*

TABLETS

Adults. *Initial:* 2 mg on days 1 and 2; 3 mg on days 3 and 4; 4 mg on days 5 and 6; 5 mg on day 7; 6 mg on day 8; 7 mg on day 9; 8 mg on day 10; 9 mg on day 11; 10 mg on days 12, 13, and 14 followed by 20 mg on day 15 and thereafter. *Maintenance:* 20 mg once a day.

Drug Administration

P.O.

- Ensure that therapies are readily available to treat symptomatic bradycardia before administering first dose.
- Expect to monitor patient with the following conditions for 4 hr or more after administering the first dose because drug can cause bradycardia: presence of first- or second-degree Mobitz II AV block or sinus bradycardia with a heart rate less than 55 beats/min or history of heart failure or MI that has occurred more than 6 mo prior to initiating drug therapy and patient is in stable condition.
- Check that an ECG has been done before administering drug and then repeated 4 hr after first dose is administered.
- Administer tablet whole without breaking or crushing tablet.
- Use starter pack when initiating drug therapy and follow titration schedule exactly, which helps reduce adverse cardiac reactions.
- Monitor patient for signs and symptoms of bradycardia. Assess patient's blood pressure and pulse at least hourly. Be aware that pulse rate may begin to decrease within an hr of administration but typically recovers to baseline levels 4–5 hr later.
- Additional monitoring of these patients is required if patient's heart rate postdose is less than 45 beats/min, it is at the lowest value postdose, or the patient's 4-hr postdose ECG shows new onset of second-degree or higher AV block. If abnormalities are present, initiate continuous ECG monitoring and other appropriate treatment (may include need to monitor patient overnight or need for cardiologist consult), as ordered, until abnormalities are resolved.
- If fewer than 4 consecutive doses are missed during titration, resume treatment with the first missed titration dose and resume the titration schedule at that dose and titration day.
- If fewer than 4 consecutive doses are missed during maintenance, resume treatment with maintenance dosage.
- If 4 or more consecutive doses are missed during titration or maintenance, treatment should be reinitiated with day 1 of the titration regimen.

Route	Onset	Peak	Duration
P.O.	Unknown	2–4 hr	Unknown

Half-life: 33 hr

Mechanism of Action

Binds to sphingosine 1-phosphate (S1P) receptors to block the release of lymphocytes from lymph nodes resulting in reducing the number of lymphocytes in peripheral blood and possibly reducing lymphocyte migration into the central nervous system.

Contraindications

Class III or IV heart failure, decompensated heart failure requiring hospitalization, MI, transient ischemic attack (TIA), or unstable angina within the last 6 mo; hypersensitivity to ponesimod or its components; presence of Mobitz type II second-degree, third-degree atrioventricular (AV) block, sick sinus syndrome, or sinoatrial block, unless a functioning pacemaker is in place

Interactions

DRUGS

antineoplastic, immune-modulating, or immunosuppressive drugs: Increased risk of additive immune effects during ponesimod therapy and for wk following administration
beta-blockers: Additive effects on lowering heart rate
CYP3A4 (strong) and UGT1A1 inducers, such as carbamazepine, phenytoin, rifampin: Possibly decreased systemic ponesimod levels, making drug less effective
live attenuated vaccines: Increased risk of infection during and for up to 2 wk after ponesimod is discontinued
vaccinations: Decreased effectiveness of vaccinations during and for up to 2 wk after ponesimod is discontinued

Adverse Reactions

CNS: Depression, dizziness, fatigue, fever, insomnia, migraine, **posterior reversible encephalopathy syndrome**, **seizures**, vertigo
CV: **Atrioventricular conduction delays**, **bradycardia**, chest discomfort,

hypercholesterolemia, hypertension, peripheral edema
EENT: Dry mouth, macular edema, rhinitis, sinusitis
GI: Dyspepsia, elevated liver enzymes, **hepatic injury**
GU: UTI
MS: Back or extremity pain, joint swelling
RESP: Cough, dyspnea, increased risk of upper respiratory infection
SKIN: **Cutaneous malignancies**
Other: **Immunosuppression**, **hyperkalemia**, increased C-reactive protein, infections, **lymphopenia**

Childbearing Considerations

PREGNANCY

- Drug may cause fetal harm based on animal studies.
- Use with caution only if benefit to mother outweighs potential risk to fetus.

LACTATION

- It is not known if drug is present in breast milk.
- Mothers should check with prescriber before breastfeeding.

REPRODUCTION

- Females of childbearing age should use an effective contraception during drug therapy and for 1 wk after drug is discontinued.

Nursing Considerations

! **WARNING** Know that ponesimod therapy is not recommended in patients with a history of cardiac arrest, cerebrovascular disease, severe untreated sleep apnea, or uncontrolled hypertension because a serious reduction in heart rate may not be well tolerated in these patients. Also, know that ponesimod should not be initiated after treatment with alemtuzumab.

! **WARNING** Know that drug therapy should not be initiated in a patient with an infection until it is resolved because drug decreases peripheral lymphocyte counts by as much as 40% of baseline values. Monitor patient for infections throughout ponesimod therapy, as life-threatening infections, such as cryptococcal meningitis, herpes simplex encephalitis, and varicella-zoster meningitis have occurred with other drugs in the same class as ponesimod. Know that taking immunosuppressants may increase patient's risk of infection. Notify prescriber if signs and symptoms of an infection occur, as drug may have to be withheld until infection is resolved.

- Administer ponesimod with caution to patients who are or have received antineoplastic, immune-modulating, or immunosuppressive therapies including corticosteroids because additive immune system effects may occur predisposing patient to infection. Be aware that ponesimod remains in the blood for up to 1 week after it is discontinued. Treatment with immunosuppressants during this time may cause additive effect on the immune system.
- Be aware that live attenuated vaccine immunizations should be administered at least 1 month prior to the patient starting ponesimod therapy.
- Ensure that the following has been assessed prior to administering the first dose of ponesimod: Cardiac evaluation (ECG and possible cardiologist consultation), complete blood count including lymphocyte count within past 6 months, liver function tests within last 6 months, drug therapy review (current or prior history of antineoplastic, immunosuppressive, or immune-modulating therapies and drugs that may slow atrioventricular conduction or heart rate), ophthalmic evaluation including the macula, presence of antibodies to varicella zoster virus if history or full course of vaccination against virus cannot be confirmed, skin examination, and a detailed vaccination history.

! **WARNING** Monitor patients with severe respiratory disease, such as asthma, chronic obstructive pulmonary disease, or pulmonary fibrosis because drug can adversely affect respiratory function, especially in the first month of drug therapy.

! **WARNING** Monitor patient for signs and symptoms of liver dysfunction, such as unexplained abdominal pain, anorexia, fatigue, nausea, vomiting, or yellowing of skin or dark urine. This is because ponesimod may cause liver injury. If signs and symptoms of liver dysfunction are present, notify prescriber, expect liver function studies to be done, and, if significant liver injury is present, for drug to be discontinued.

! WARNING Assess patient's skin periodically for abnormalities because ponesimod may cause skin cancer, including melanoma, especially in patients with risk factors for skin cancer.

! WARNING Monitor patient for progressive multifocal leukoencephalopathy (PML), an opportunistic viral infection of the brain, which has occurred with other drugs in the same class. Notify prescriber immediately if signs and symptoms occur during drug therapy (sudden onset of altered mental status, seizures, severe headache, or visual disturbances) because serious neurological complications or death, may occur. If confirmed, expect drug to be discontinued.

- Assess patient's blood pressure regularly during ponesimod therapy because drug may increase blood pressure.
- Monitor patient's vision throughout drug therapy because ponesimod may cause macular edema, especially in patients with a history of diabetes mellitus or uveitis. If a change in vision occurs, notify the prescriber and expect an ophthalmic evaluation to be done.
- Expect to monitor patient even after ponesimod is discontinued. This is because severe exacerbation of MS resulting in a significant increase in disability may occur, although rarely, after the drug is discontinued.

PATIENT TEACHING

- Instruct patient how to administer ponesimod.
- Inform patients that a first-dose 4-hour monitoring period may be required depending on medical history. If abnormalities develop, the monitoring may be extended and possibly include an overnight stay in a healthcare facility.
- Stress importance of patient following the titration schedule to reach maintenance dosing, as drug dosage may have to be reevaluated if more than 3 doses are missed.
- Advise patient to avoid live, attenuated vaccines while taking ponesimod. If necessary, tell patient to alert prescriber regarding planned immunization, as ponesimod therapy will have to be withheld 1 week prior and for 4 weeks after the vaccination.

! WARNING Alert patient that ponesimod increases risk of an infection during therapy and for up to 2 weeks after therapy is discontinued. Inform patient the most common infection is an upper respiratory infection, although other less common but more serious and possibly life-threatening infections could also occur. Review signs and symptoms of infection and tell patient to notify prescriber immediately, if present.

! WARNING Advise patient and family or caregiver to immediately notify the prescriber if patient develops a sudden onset of altered mental status, severe headache, seizure, or visual disturbances. Stress that a delay in reporting these symptoms could cause permanent neurologic deficits.

! WARNING Tell patient to notify prescriber if they experience new onset or worsening of dyspnea.

! WARNING Review signs and symptoms of hepatic dysfunction with patient and stress importance of notifying prescriber if present.

! WARNING Advise patient to assess the skin regularly. If any suspicious skin lesions appear, patient should have it assessed. Encourage patient to wear protective clothing and use a sunscreen with a high protection factor when outdoors and to avoid sunlight and ultraviolet light as much as possible.

- Alert patient that ponesimod may cause visual changes. If changes occur, patient should notify prescriber and expect to have an ophthalmic examination.
- Warn patient that severe disability, although rare, may occur when ponesimod therapy is discontinued. Tell them to report to the prescriber worsening symptoms of MS after drug has been discontinued.
- Advise females of childbearing age to use an effective contraceptive during ponesimod

therapy and for 1 week after drug has been discontinued. If pregnancy occurs, stress importance of notifying prescriber.

- Tell patient that drug continues to have effects for up to 2 weeks after the last dose.

posaconazole

Noxafil

Class and Category

Pharmacologic class: Triazole
Therapeutic class: Antifungal

Indications and Dosages

✷ *To prevent invasive* Aspergillus *and* Candida *infections in patients at high risk because of severe immunocompromise from such conditions as graft-versus-host disease with hematopoietic stem-cell transplant or hematologic malignancies with prolonged neutropenia from chemotherapy*

ORAL SUSPENSION

Adults and adolescents. 200 mg (5 ml) 3 times daily until recovery from immunosuppression or neutropenia.

D.R. ORAL SUSPENSION

Children ages 2 and older weighing between 36 kg (79.2 lb) and 40 kg (88 lb). *Loading dose:* 240 mg (8 ml) twice daily on day 1. *Maintenance:* 240 mg (8 ml) once daily starting on day 2.

Children ages 2 and older weighing 26 kg (57.2 lb) but less than 36 kg (79.2 lb). *Loading dose:* 210 mg (7 ml) twice daily on day 1. *Maintenance:* 210 mg (7 ml) once daily starting on day 2.

Children ages 2 and older weighing 21 kg (46.2 lb) but less than 26 kg (57.2 lb). *Loading dose:* 180 mg (6 ml) twice daily on day 1. *Maintenance:* 180 mg (6 ml) once daily starting on day 2.

Children ages 2 and older weighing 17 kg (37.4 lb) but less than 21 kg (46.2 lb). *Loading dose:* 150 mg (5 ml) twice daily day 1. *Maintenance:* 150 mg (5 ml) once daily starting on day 2.

Children ages 2 and older weighing 12 kg (26.4 lb) but less than 17 kg (37.4 lb). *Loading dose:* 120 mg (4 ml) twice daily on day 1. *Maintenance:* 120 mg (4 ml) once daily starting on day 2.

Children ages 2 and older weighing 10 kg (22 lb) but less than 12 kg (25.4 lb). *Loading dose:* 90 mg (3 ml) twice daily on day 1. *Maintenance:* 90 mg (3 ml) once daily starting on day 2.

D.R. TABLETS

Adults and children ages 2 and older weighing more than 40 kg (88 lb). *Loading dose:* 300 mg twice daily on day 1. *Maintenance:* 300 mg once daily starting on day 2 until recovery from immunosuppression or neutropenia.

I.V. INFUSION

Adults. *Loading dose:* 300 mg twice daily on day 1. *Maintenance:* 300 mg once daily starting on day 2 until recovery from neutropenia or immunosuppression. I.V. infused slowly over 90 min.

Children ages 2 and older. *Loading dose:* 6 mg/kg up to maximum of 300 mg twice daily on day 1. *Maintenance:* 6 mg/kg up to a maximum of 300 mg once daily starting on day 2 until recovery from immunosuppression or neutropenia. I.V. infused slowly over 90 min.

✷ *To treat invasive aspergillosis*

D.R. TABLETS, I.V. INFUSION

Adults and adolescents. *Loading dose:* 300 mg twice daily on day 1. *Maintenance dose:* 300 mg once daily starting on day 2 for 6 to 12 wks. I.V. infused slowly over 90 min.

✷ *To treat oropharyngeal candidiasis*

ORAL SUSPENSION

Adults and adolescents. *Initial:* 100 mg (2.5 ml) twice daily on day 1, followed by 100 mg (2.5 ml) once daily for 13 days.

✷ *To treat oropharyngeal candidiasis refractory to fluconazole and/or itraconazole*

ORAL SUSPENSION

Adults and adolescents. 400 mg (10 ml) twice daily with duration based on severity and clinical response.

± **DOSAGE ADJUSTMENT** For patients with renal dysfunction, no adjustment needed for oral dosing. For patients with a creatinine clearance of less than 50/ml/min, I.V. form should be avoided, unless necessary; if used and serum creatinine levels increase then I.V. form should be switched to oral form. For patients with acute myeloid leukemia, dose reduced across all dosing phases.

Drug Administration

P.O.

- Do not interchange D.R. tablet or D.R. oral suspension with immediate-release oral suspension because of differences in the dosing of each formulation.
- Shake immediate-release oral suspension well before administering. Use only the spoon provided in the package to measure dosage. Each dose should be administered during or immediately following (within 20 min) a full meal to enhance absorption. If patient cannot eat a full meal, administer drug with an acidic carbonated beverage such as ginger ale or a liquid nutritional supplement. Rinse dosing spoon with water after each use. Store at room temperature.
- Administer D.R. tablets with or without food. D.R. tablets should be swallowed whole and not chewed, crushed, or divided.
- Open packet of D.R. oral suspension immediately before preparation. Remove cap from mixing liquid and push bottle adapter into the neck of bottle. Once in place, leave bottle adapter there. Remove 9 ml of mixing liquid using the provided blue syringe. Put cap back on bottle. Do not use any other solution to mix drug. Use the provided mixing cup to combine the 9 ml of liquid and entire contents of one packet of drug and mix, which will provide a final concentration of about 30 mg/ml. Shake the mixing cup vigorously for 45 sec to mix powder and mixing liquid. The mixture should look cloudy and free of clumps when fully mixed. Administer D.R. oral suspension with food within 1 hr. Using only the provided notched tip syringes provided by manufacturer, use the green one if dose is 3 ml or less and blue one if dose is more than 3 ml. Discard any remaining suspension as not all the mixture in the mixing cup will be used. The maximum dose that can be accurately removed from the mixing cup after reconstitution is 240 mg (8 ml). Hand wash mixing cup and reuse or use a similar mixing cup with a lid for subsequent doses. The notched tip syringes may also be handwashed and reused. A separate box of notched tip syringes comes with the Noxafil Powder Mix kit. Store at room temperature.

I.V.

- Prepare drug by first removing vial from refrigerator and allowing it to warm to room temperature.
- Transfer 1 vial (16.7 ml) of the drug solution to an intravenous bag or bottle containing 0.45% or 0.9% Sodium Chloride Injection, 5% Dextrose in Water, 5% Dextrose Injection and 0.45% or 0.9% Sodium Chloride Injection, or 5% Dextrose Injection and 20 mEq Potassium Chloride to achieve a concentration between 1 mg/ml and 2 mg/ml. Solution should appear colorless to yellow. Variations of color within this range do not affect the quality of the drug.
- Once mixed, use immediately, or refrigerate for up to 24 hr. Discard any unused solution.
- Administer through a 0.22-micron polyethersulfone (PES) or polyvinylidene difluoride (PVD) filter using a central venous line.
- If a central venous line is not available, drug may be administered through a peripheral venous catheter only as a single dose in advance of a central venous line being placed or to bridge the period during which a central venous line is replaced or is in use for other treatment.
- Infuse slowly over 90 min through a central venous line or 30 min through a peripheral line.
- Never administer drug by bolus injection.
- *Incompatibilities:* 4.2% Sodium Bicarbonate solution, 5% Dextrose with Lactated Ringer's solution, or Lactated Ringer's solution; drugs other than amikacin sulfate, caspofungin, ciprofloxacin, daptomycin, dobutamine hydrochloride, famotidine, filgrastim, gentamicin sulfate, hydromorphone hydrochloride, levofloxacin, lorazepam, meropenem, micafungin, morphine sulfate, norepinephrine bitartrate, potassium chloride, vancomycin hydrochloride

Route	Onset	Peak	Duration
P.O.	Unknown	3–5 hr	Unknown
I.V.	Unknown	1.5 hr	Unknown

Half-life: 24.5–35 hr

P

Mechanism of Action

Blocks synthesis of ergosterol, an essential component of fungal cell membrane, by inhibiting 14 alpha-demethylase, an enzyme needed for conversion of lanosterol to ergosterol. Lacking ergosterol increases cellular permeability with cell contents leaking, making cells ineffective.

Contraindications

Concurrent therapy with atorvastatin, lovastatin, simvastatin, sirolimus; concurrent therapy with venetoclax in patients with chronic lymphocytic leukemia or small lymphocytic lymphoma; hypersensitivity to posaconazole, other azole antifungals, or their components; use with CYP3A4 substrates, such as pimozide and quinidine, or ergot alkaloids; use of D.R. oral suspension in patients with hereditary fructose intolerance

Interactions

DRUGS

alprazolam, triazolam: Increased plasma levels of these drugs which could potentiate and prolong hypnotic and sedative effects
calcium channel blockers (diltiazem, felodipine, nicardipine, nifedipine, verapamil): Increased plasma concentrations of these drugs with increased risk of adverse reactions
cimetidine (oral suspension only), efavirenz, esomeprazole (oral suspension only), fosamprenavir, metoclopramide (oral suspension only), phenytoin, rifabutin: Possibly decreased plasma level of posaconazole
cyclosporine, tacrolimus: Increased plasma levels of these drugs, with increased risk of adverse reactions, including leukoencephalopathy and nephrotoxicity
digoxin: Increased risk of digitalis toxicity
ergot alkaloids: Increased plasma ergot alkaloid level and increased risk of ergotism
HMG-CoA reductase inhibitors: Increased plasma statin level and increased risk of rhabdomyolysis
midazolam: Increased midazolam plasma concentrations by about 5-fold, which will prolong hypnotic and sedative effects
pimozide, quinidine: Increased plasma concentrations of these drugs, leading to QT prolongation and torsades de pointes
sirolimus: Increased sirolimus blood concentration with possible sirolimus toxicity
venetoclax: Increased risk of venetoclax toxicities such as neutropenia, serious infections, and tumor lysis syndrome
vinca alkaloids: Increased plasma vinca alkaloid level and increased risk of neurotoxicity

ACTIVITIES

alcohol: Faster release for oral delayed-release suspension

Adverse Reactions

CNS: Anxiety, asthenia, dizziness, fatigue, fever, headache, insomnia, rigors, tremor, weakness
CV: Edema, hypertension, **hypotension**, **QT-interval prolongation**, tachycardia
EENT: Blurred vision, epistaxis, herpes simplex, mucositis, pharyngitis, stomatitis, taste perversion
ENDO: Hyperglycemia, pseudoaldosteronism
GI: Abdominal pain, anorexia, bilirubinemia, constipation, diarrhea, dyspepsia, elevated liver enzymes, hepatomegaly, jaundice, nausea, **pancreatitis**, vomiting
GU: **Acute renal failure**, elevated blood creatinine level, **vaginal hemorrhage**
HEME: Anemia, **neutropenia (febrile)**, **thrombocytopenia**
MS: Arthralgia, back or musculoskeletal pain
RESP: Cough, dyspnea, pneumonia, **respiratory failure**, upper respiratory tract infection
SKIN: Diaphoresis, petechiae, pruritus, rash
Other: **Bacteremia**, cytomegalovirus infection, dehydration, **hypocalcemia**, **hypokalemia**, **hypomagnesemia**, **septic shock**, weight loss

Childbearing Considerations

PREGNANCY

- Drug may cause fetal harm, based on animal studies.
- Use with caution only if benefit to mother outweighs potential risk to fetus.

LACTATION

- It is not known if drug is present in breast milk.
- Mothers should check with prescriber before breastfeeding.

Nursing Considerations

! **WARNING** Determine sorbitol/fructose/sucrose exposure prior to administrating D.R. oral suspension because life-threatening hypoglycemia, hypophosphatemia, lactic acidosis, and hepatic failure may occur in patients with hereditary fructose intolerance (HFI). Keep in mind the diagnosis of HFI may not yet be established in pediatric patients.

! **WARNING** Know that posaconazole injection should be avoided, if possible, in patients with moderate or severe renal impairment (eGFR less than 50 ml/min). If not possible, expect to monitor serum creatinine levels, as ordered, and if increases occur, anticipate patient being switched to oral posaconazole therapy.

- Obtain baseline assessment of liver function and check periodically during therapy, as ordered. If elevations occur or patient has evidence of elevated liver enzymes, notify prescriber.
- Expect to obtain electrolytes and correct any disturbances, as prescribed before and routinely during posaconazole therapy.

! **WARNING** Know that cross-sensitivity may occur in patients who have had a hypersensitivity reaction to other azoles. Monitor patient closely for any hypersensitivity reactions. If present, notify prescriber, expect drug to be discontinued, and provide supportive care, as needed and ordered.

! **WARNING** Monitor patients with potentially proarrhythmic conditions because posaconazole may prolong QT interval.

- Monitor patient experiencing severe diarrhea or vomiting for breakthrough fungal infections.

! **WARNING** Monitor patient for other persistent, serious, or unusual adverse reactions.

PATIENT TEACHING

! **WARNING** Alert patient and family or caregiver before administering D.R. oral suspension that a life-threatening condition can occur with patients with hereditary fructose intolerance (HFI). If patient has HFI, tell patient and family or caregiver to notify prescriber.

- Instruct patient how to administer form of posaconazole prescribed.
- Tell patient to report severe diarrhea or vomiting because these conditions may interfere with drug effectiveness.

! **WARNING** Instruct patient to notify prescriber immediately if patient develops other persistent, serious, or unusual adverse reactions, including an allergic reaction.

potassium acetate

potassium bicarbonate

K+Care ET, Klor-Con/EF, K-Lyte

potassium bicarbonate and potassium chloride

Klorvess Effervescent Granules, Neo-K (CAN), Potassium Sandoz (CAN)

potassium bicarbonate and potassium citrate

Effer-K, K-Lyte DS

potassium chloride

K-10 (CAN), KCl 5% (CAN), K-Long (CAN), Klor-Con 10, Klor-Con Powder, Klor-Con/25 Powder, K-Norm, K-Sol, K-Tab

potassium citrate

Urocit-K

potassium gluconate

Glu-K, Potassium-Rougier (CAN)

potassium gluconate and potassium chloride

Kolyum

potassium gluconate and potassium citrate

Twin-K

trikates

Tri-K

Class and Category

Pharmacologic class: Electrolyte cation
Therapeutic class: Electrolyte replacement

Indications and Dosages

✱ *To prevent or treat hypokalemia in patients who can't ingest sufficient dietary potassium or who are losing potassium because of a condition, such as hepatic cirrhosis or prolonged vomiting or drug use such as potassium-wasting diuretics or certain antibiotics*

EFFERVESCENT TABLETS (POTASSIUM BICARBONATE)

Adults and adolescents. 25 to 50 mEq/g once or twice daily, as needed and tolerated. *Maximum:* 100 mEq daily.

EFFERVESCENT TABLETS (POTASSIUM BICARBONATE AND POTASSIUM CHLORIDE)

Adults and adolescents. 20, 25, or 50 mEq once or twice daily, as needed and tolerated. *Maximum:* 100 mEq daily.

EFFERVESCENT TABLETS (POTASSIUM BICARBONATE AND POTASSIUM CITRATE)

Adults and adolescents. 25 or 50 mEq once or twice daily, as needed and tolerated. *Maximum:* 100 mEq daily.

ELIXIR (POTASSIUM GLUCONATE)

Adults and adolescents. 20 mEq 2 to 4 times daily, as needed and tolerated. *Maximum:* 100 mEq daily.
Children. 2 to 3 mEq/kg daily in divided doses.

E.R. CAPSULES (POTASSIUM CHLORIDE)

Adults and adolescents. *For treatment:* 40 to 100 mEq daily in divided doses 2 or 3 times daily. *For prevention:* 16 to 24 mEq daily in divided doses 2 or 3 times daily. *Maximum:* 100 mEq daily.

E.R. TABLETS (POTASSIUM CHLORIDE)

Adults and adolescents. 6.7 to 20 mEq 3 times daily. *Maximum:* 100 mEq daily.

GRANULE PACKETS (POTASSIUM BICARBONATE AND POTASSIUM CHLORIDE)

Adults and adolescents. 20 mEq once or twice daily, as needed and tolerated. *Maximum:* 100 mEq daily.

GRANULES FOR ORAL SUSPENSION (POTASSIUM CHLORIDE)

Adults and adolescents. 20 mEq 1 to 5 times/day, as needed and tolerated. *Maximum:* 100 mEq daily.

ORAL SOLUTION (POTASSIUM CHLORIDE)

Adults and adolescents. 20 mEq 1 to 4 times daily, as needed and tolerated. *Maximum:* 100 mEq daily.
Children. 1 to 3 mEq/kg daily in divided doses.

ORAL SOLUTION (POTASSIUM GLUCONATE AND POTASSIUM CHLORIDE, POTASSIUM GLUCONATE, AND POTASSIUM CITRATE)

Adults and adolescents. 20 mEq 2 to 4 times daily, as needed and tolerated. *Maximum:* 100 mEq daily.
Children. 2 to 3 mEq/kg daily in divided doses.

POWDER PACKET FOR ORAL SOLUTION (POTASSIUM CHLORIDE)

Adults. 15 to 25 mEq 2 to 4 times daily, as needed and tolerated. *Maximum:* 100 mEq daily.
Children. 1 to 3 mEq/kg daily in divided doses, as needed and tolerated.

POWDER PACKET FOR ORAL SOLUTION (POTASSIUM GLUCONATE AND POTASSIUM CHLORIDE)

Adults and adolescents. 20 mEq 2 to 4 times daily, as needed and tolerated. *Maximum:* 100 mEq daily.
Children. 2 to 3 mEq/kg daily in divided doses.

ORAL TRIKATES SOLUTION (POTASSIUM ACETATE, POTASSIUM BICARBONATE, AND POTASSIUM CITRATE)

Adults and adolescents. 15 mEq 3 to 4 times daily, as needed and tolerated. *Maximum:* 100 mEq daily.
Children. 2 to 3 mEq/kg daily in divided doses.

TABLETS (POTASSIUM GLUCONATE)

Adults and adolescents. 5 to 10 mEq 2 to 4 times daily, as needed and tolerated. *Maximum:* 100 mEq daily.

✱ *To treat hypokalemia when oral replacement is not feasible*

I.V. INFUSION (POTASSIUM ACETATE)

Adults. Highly individualized. Infusion rate should not exceed 1 mEq/kg/hr.

I.V. INFUSION (POTASSIUM CHLORIDE)

Adults and adolescents with serum potassium level above 2.5 mEq/L. Up to 10 mEq/hr. *Maximum:* 200 mEq daily.
Adults and adolescents with serum potassium level below 2 mEq/L, ECG changes, or paralysis. Up to 40 mEq/hr. *Maximum:* 400 mEq daily.

±**DOSAGE ADJUSTMENT** For all patients, dosage adjusted based on patient's ECG patterns and serum potassium level.

✱ *To treat renal tubular acidosis with calcium stones, hypocitraturic calcium oxalate nephrolithiasis of any etiology, and uric acid lithiasis with or without calcium stones*

TABLETS (POTASSIUM CITRATE)

Adults. *For patients with mild to moderate hypocitraturia:* 10 mEq 3 times or 15 mEq 2 times daily with meals. *For patients with severe hypocitraturia:* 30 mEq 2 times daily or 20 mEq 3 times daily with meals.

±**DOSAGE ADJUSTMENT** For patients with cirrhosis or renal impairment, dosage started at the lower end of the dosing range for all formulations of potassium.

Drug Administration

P.O.

- Administer with or immediately after meals.
- Mix potassium chloride for oral solution or potassium gluconate elixir in cold water, orange juice, tomato juice (if patient isn't sodium restricted), or apple juice, and stir for 1 full min before administering.
- Mix potassium bicarbonate, potassium bicarbonate and potassium chloride, and potassium bicarbonate and potassium citrate effervescent tablets with cold water and allow to dissolve completely. Have patient sip solution slowly over a 5 to 10 min period with a meal.
- Ensure that powder form is completely dissolved before administering.
- E.R. forms should be swallowed whole and not chewed or crushed.

I.V.

- Use only when oral replacement is not feasible or life-threatening hypokalemia is present.
- Never directly inject undiluted potassium concentrate because it may be immediately fatal. Never administer as an intravenous push to avoid life-threatening hyperkalemia.
- Don't connect flexible plastic containers in series because of increased risk of residual air contained in the primary container that could cause an air embolism.
- Dilute potassium concentrate for injection with an adequate volume of solution before I.V. use following manufacturer's guidelines.
- Infuse potassium slowly at a controlled rate using a calibrated infusion device. Rate of infusion for an adult is dependent upon patient's needs.
- If possible, administer via a central intravenous route.
- High concentrations of potassium should only be given through a central line.
- *Incompatibilities:* None reported by manufacturer

Route	Onset	Peak	Duration
P.O.	Unknown	1–2 hr	Unknown
P.O./E.R.	Unknown	4 hr	8 hr
I.V.	Immediate	Unknown	Unknown

Half-life: Unknown

Mechanism of Action

Acts as the major cation in intracellular fluid, activating many enzymatic reactions essential for physiologic processes, including nerve impulse transmission and cardiac and skeletal muscle contraction. Helps to maintain electroneutrality in cells also by

P

controlling exchange of intracellular and extracellular ions and helps to maintain normal renal function and acid–base balance.

Contraindications

Acute dehydration, Addison's disease (untreated), concurrent use with amiloride or triamterene (potassium chloride), or potassium-sparing diuretics (all forms of potassium), crush syndrome, disorders that may delay drug passing through GI tract (potassium citrate), heat cramps, hyperkalemia, hypersensitivity to potassium salts or their components, peptic ulcer disease (potassium citrate), renal impairment with azotemia or oliguria, severe hemolytic anemia, UTI (potassium citrate)

Interactions

DRUGS

ACE inhibitors, aliskiren, amiloride, angiotensin II receptor antagonists, beta-blockers, blood products, corticosteroids, cyclosporine, eplerenone, heparin, NSAIDs, potassium-containing drugs, potassium-sparing diuretics, spironolactone, tacrolimus, triamterene: Increased risk of hyperkalemia that can become severe

amphotericin B, corticosteroids (glucocorticoids, mineralocorticoids), gentamicin, penicillins, polymyxin B: Possibly hypokalemia

anticholinergics, drugs with anticholinergic activity: Increased risk of GI ulceration, stricture, and perforation

antiepileptics, diuretics: Increased risk of hyponatremia when used with high concentration of potassium chloride

calcium salts (parenteral): Possibly arrhythmias

digoxin: Increased risk of digitalis toxicity

insulin, laxatives, sodium bicarbonate: Decreased serum potassium level

sodium polystyrene sulfonate: Possibly decreased serum potassium level and fluid retention

thiazide diuretics: Possibly hyperkalemia when diuretic is discontinued

FOODS

low-salt milk, salt substitutes: Increased risk of hyperkalemia

Adverse Reactions

CNS: Chills, confusion, fever, **hyponatremic encephalopathy (with use of high concentration of potassium chloride)**, paralysis, paresthesia, weakness

CV: **Arrhythmias**, **asystole**, **bradycardia**, **cardiac arrest**, chest pain, **ECG changes**, peripheral edema, **ventricular fibrillation**

EENT: Throat pain when swallowing

GI: Abdominal pain; **bloody stools**; diarrhea; flatulence; **GI bleeding**, **obstruction**, **perforation**, or ulceration; nausea; vomiting

RESP: Dyspnea, **pulmonary edema (with high concentration of potassium chloride)**

SKIN: Rash

Other: **Anaphylaxis**; **angioedema**; extravasation reactions, such as necrosis, nerve or tendon injury, ulcers, or vascular injury; **hyperkalemia**; hypervolemia (with high concentration of potassium chloride); **hypokalemia**; **hyponatremia (with use of high concentration of potassium chloride)**; infusion-site reactions, such as burning sensation, erythema, irritation, pain, phlebitis, pruritus, rash, or **thrombosis**

Childbearing Considerations

PREGNANCY

- It is not known if drug causes fetal harm but may if hyperkalemia occurs.
- Use with caution only if benefit to mother outweighs potential risk to fetus.

LACTATION

- Potassium is normally present in breast milk.
- Mothers should check with prescriber before breastfeeding.

Nursing Considerations

! WARNING Review patient's medical history before administering potassium chloride because there are many conditions that may predispose patient to develop hyperkalemia, which could become life-threatening and increase sensitivity to potassium.

! WARNING Monitor serum potassium level before and during administration of I.V. potassium. Be aware that mild or moderate hyperkalemia is asymptomatic and may be manifested only by increased serum potassium concentrations, and possibly by characteristic ECG changes. Monitor patient for signs of hyperkalemia, such as arrhythmias, confusion, dyspnea, and paresthesia, which may occur at any time during potassium therapy.

- Be aware that liquid form of oral potassium should be prescribed for patients with delayed gastric emptying, esophageal compression, or intestinal obstruction or stricture, as well as patients with dysphagia or swallowing disorders, to decrease the risk of tissue damage from solid forms of potassium that may remain in contact with the GI mucosa for a prolonged period of time.
- Monitor patient receiving tablet forms of potassium for abdominal pain or distention, GI bleeding, or severe vomiting, as this may indicate GI obstruction, perforation, or ulceration and should be reported immediately.

! WARNING Assess patient for signs of hypokalemia regularly, including arrhythmias, fatigue, and weakness indicating a need to increase potassium dosage.

! WARNING Monitor patient for a hypersensivity reaction which could become life-threatening, such as anaphylaxis or angioedema. Be aware that some forms of potassium contain tartrazine, which may cause an allergic reaction, such as asthma. If present, notify prescriber immediately, stop form of potassium being administered, and provide supportive care, as needed and ordered.

! WARNING Monitor patient for signs and symptoms of adverse GI reactions, which could become life-threatening, such as GI bleeding.

! WARNING Monitor serum creatinine level and urine output during administration because adequate renal function is needed for potassium supplementation. Notify prescriber about signs of decreased renal function because renal impairment may predispose patient to fluid overload and/or hyperkalemia. Also, know that some forms of potassium may contain aluminum, which may become toxic in a patient with impaired renal function.

! WARNING Monitor patient for any other persistent, serious, or unusual adverse reactions.

PATIENT TEACHING

- Instruct patient how to administer the oral form of potassium prescribed.
- Advise patient receiving drug intravenously to alert staff if injection site pain or swelling occurs.

! WARNING Review signs and symptoms of hyperkalemia and hypokalemia. Tell patient to notify prescriber if any occurs.

! WARNING Alert patient that drug may cause an allergic reaction. If present, tell patient to notify staff if receiving drug intravenously or prescriber if receiving drug orally and, if severe, to seek immediate medical care.

- Teach patient how to take her radial pulse and advise her to notify prescriber about significant changes in heart rate or rhythm.

! WARNING Advise patient to watch stools for changes in color and consistency and to notify prescriber immediately if they become black, tarry, or red or patient develops any other GI adverse reaction.

! WARNING Tell patient to notify prescriber if any other persistent, serious, or unusual adverse reactions occur.

- Inform patient that although she may see waxy form of E.R. tablet in stools, she has received all of the potassium.
- Urge patient to keep follow-up laboratory appointments as directed by prescriber to determine serum potassium level.

pramipexole dihydrochloride

Class and Category

Pharmacologic class: Nonergoline dopamine agonist
Therapeutic class: Antiparkinsonian

Indications and Dosages

✱ To treat Parkinson's disease

TABLETS

Adults. *Initial:* 0.125 mg 3 times daily for 1 wk, gradually increased every 5 to 7 days, as needed. Alternatively, can be increased weekly thereafter as follows: for wk 2, 0.25 mg 3 times daily; for wk 3, 0.5 mg 3 times daily; for wk 4, 0.75 mg 3 times daily; for wk 5, 1 mg 3 times day; for wk 6, 1.25 mg 3 times daily; and for wk 7, 1.5 mg 3 times daily. *Maintenance:* 1.5 to 4.5 mg daily in divided doses 3 times daily. *Maximum:* 4.5 mg daily.

±**DOSAGE ADJUSTMENT** For patients with renal impairment, dosage reduced as follows: for creatinine clearance greater than 50 ml/min, maximum dose limited to 1.5 mg 3 times daily; for creatinine clearance of 30 to 50 ml/min, initial dosage of 0.125 mg given twice daily and maximum dose limited to 0.75 mg 3 times daily; for creatinine clearance of 15 to less than 30 ml/min, initial dosage of 0.125 mg given once daily and maximum dose limited to 1.5 mg once a day. For patients with creatinine clearance of less than 15 ml/min, drug not given.

E.R. TABLETS

Adults. *Initial:* 0.375 mg once daily, increased every 5 to 7 days, first to 0.75 mg and then by 0.75-mg increments, as needed. *Maximum:* 4.5 mg daily.

±**DOSAGE ADJUSTMENT** For patients with moderate renal impairment (creatinine clearance between 30 and 50 ml/min), initial dosage taken every other day with dosage adjustment done after 1 week in increments of 0.375 mg weekly, as needed, to maximum dosage of 2.25 mg daily.

✱ To treat restless leg syndrome

TABLETS

Adults. *Initial:* 0.125 mg once daily 2 to 3 hr before bedtime. Increased in 4 to 7 days, as needed, to 0.25 mg once daily. Further increased in 4 to 7 days to 0.5 mg once daily, as needed.

±**DOSAGE ADJUSTMENT** For patients with moderate to severe renal impairment (creatinine clearance 20 to 60 ml/min), dosage interval for titration increased to 14 days, as needed.

Drug Administration

P.O.

- Administer with food if GI upset occurs.
- Tablets should be swallowed whole and not chewed, crushed, or divided.
- Give drug used to treat restless leg syndrome 2 to 3 hr before bedtime.
- Patient may be switched overnight from immediate-release tablets to E.R. tablets at the same daily dose, but dosage adjustment may be needed after monitoring effectiveness of switch.
- A retitration of therapy may be required if a significant interruption in therapy occurs.
- Store drug at room temperature.

Route	Onset	Peak	Duration
P.O.	Rapid	2 hr	8–12 hr
P.O./E.R.	Unknown	6 hr	Unknown

Half-life: 8–12 hr

Mechanism of Action

May stimulate dopamine receptors in the brain, thereby easing symptoms of Parkinson's disease, which is thought to be caused by a dopamine deficiency.

Contraindications

Hypersensitivity to pramipexole or its components

Interactions

DRUGS

butyrophenones, metoclopramide, phenothiazines, thioxanthenes: Decreased pramipexole effectiveness

Adverse Reactions

CNS: Abnormal behavior or thinking, amnesia, anxiety, asthenia, compulsive behaviors, such as pathological gambling or uncontrollable shopping or sexual activity, confusion, dream disturbances, drowsiness, dyskinesia, dystonia, fatigue, fever, hallucinations, headache, insomnia, malaise, paranoia, psychotic-like behavior, restlessness, syncope

CV: **Cardiac failure**, edema, orthostatic hypotension

EENT: Diplopia, dry mouth, rhinitis, vision changes

ENDO: Inappropriate antidiuretic hormone secretion (SIADH)

GI: Anorexia, constipation, dysphagia, eating disorders, nausea, vomiting
GU: Altered libido, hypersexuality, impotence, priapism, urinary frequency, urinary incontinence
MS: Arthralgia, myalgia, myasthenia, postural deformity, **rhabdomyolysis**
RESP: Pneumonia
SKIN: Diaphoresis, erythema, pruritis, rash, urticaria
Other: Weight gain or loss, withdrawal symptoms

Childbearing Considerations

PREGNANCY

- It is not known if drug can cause fetal harm.
- Use with caution only if benefit to mother outweighs potential risk to fetus.

LACTATION

- It is not known if drug is present in breast milk. However, lactation inhibition is likely to occur because drug inhibits prolactin secretion.
- Mothers should check with prescriber before breastfeeding.

Nursing Considerations

- Use pramipexole cautiously in patients with hypotension, or retinal problems (such as macular degeneration). Drug may worsen these conditions. Monitor patient's blood pressure and vision for changes.
- Know that some patients have reported worsening of their Parkinson's disease symptoms when tablet residue was visible in their stool. If this occurs, notify prescriber, as pramipexole therapy may have to be reevaluated.

! WARNING Avoid stopping pramipexole abruptly because doing so may cause a symptom complex resembling neuroleptic malignant syndrome consisting of altered level of consciousness, autonomic instability, hyperpyrexia, and muscle rigidity.

- Monitor patients with renal impairment because pramipexole elimination may be decreased.

! WARNING Assess patient for skin changes regularly because melanomas may occur at a higher rate in patients with Parkinson's disease. It isn't clear if this is a result of the disease or drugs used to treat it.

- Take safety precautions per facility policy until drug's CNS effects are known.
- Monitor patient for postural deformity (antecollis, bent spine syndrome, Pisa syndrome) that may occur several months after pramipexole therapy has been initiated or after increasing dose. If present, notify prescriber and expect dosage to be decreased or drug discontinued, which may improve condition.
- Monitor patient for hallucinations and psychotic-like behavior. Risk for hallucinations is higher if patient is older than 65 years. Changes in behavior or thinking may include aggressive behavior, agitation, confusion, delirium, delusions, disorientation, hallucinations, mania-like symptoms, paranoid ideation, and psychotic-like behavior.

! WARNING Monitor patient for withdrawal symptoms, which may occur during tapering or after drug is discontinued. Monitor patient for altered consciousness, fever, and muscular rigidity. If present, notify prescriber and expect to administer a low-dose dopamine agonist, if severe.

PATIENT TEACHING

- Instruct patient how to administer pramipexole for the condition prescribed.
- Inform patient that if drug is not taken for a period of time, the dosage may have to be retitrated when started again.
- Inform patient that improvement in motor performance and activities of daily living may take 2 to 3 weeks.
- Advise patient to contact prescriber if he observes residue in his stool, which may resemble a swollen original E.R. tablet or swollen pieces of the original tablet.

! WARNING Caution patient not to stop taking pramipexole abruptly.

! WARNING Advise patient to report unexplained muscle pain, tenderness, or weakness to prescriber.

- Caution patient about possible dizziness, drowsiness, or light-headedness which may result from orthostatic hypotension. Advise her not to rise quickly from a lying or sitting position to minimize these effects.

- Instruct patient to notify prescriber immediately about vision problems or urinary frequency or incontinence.
- Urge patient to have regular skin examinations by a dermatologist or other qualified health professional.
- Advise patient and family or caregiver to notify prescriber about onset of compulsive and intense urges, such as eating binges, compulsive shopping, hypersexuality, or pathological gambling. Dosage may have to be reduced or drug discontinued.
- Inform patient and family or caregiver that hallucinations and other psychotic-like behavior may occur, with elderly patients over age 65 more at risk. If present, notify prescriber.
- Tell patient to alert prescriber if posture changes that cannot be controlled occur, such as neck bending forward; bending forward at the waist; or tilting sideways when sitting, standing, or walking.

! **WARNING** Inform patient that withdrawal symptoms may occur during a dosage reduction or after drug is discontinued. Review withdrawal symptoms with patient and tell patient to notify prescriber if present.

pramlintide acetate

SymlinPen 60, SymlinPen 120

Class and Category

Pharmacologic class: Human amylin analogue
Therapeutic class: Antidiabetic

Indications and Dosages

* *As adjunct to achieve euglycemia in patients with type 1 diabetes who use mealtime insulin therapy but have not achieved desired glucose control*

SUBCUTANEOUS INJECTION

Adults. *Initial:* 15 mcg just before major meals up to 4 times daily with 50% reduced dosage of preprandial rapid-acting or short-acting insulin, including fixed-mix insulins. Dosage increased in increments of 15 mcg, as tolerated, but no less than every 3 days to minimize nausea. *Maintenance:* 30 to 60 mcg before major meals.

±**DOSAGE ADJUSTMENT** For patients experiencing nausea or if nausea persists at higher dosages, dosage decreased to 30 mcg before major meals.

* *As adjunct to achieve euglycemia in patients with type 2 diabetes who use mealtime insulin, with or without a sulfonylurea and/or metformin, and have not achieved desired glucose control*

SUBCUTANEOUS INJECTION

Adults. *Initial:* 60 mcg immediately before major meals up to 3 times daily combined with dosage reduction of preprandial rapid-acting or short-acting insulin, including fixed-mix insulins, by 50%. Dosage increased to 120 mcg before major meals if no significant nausea has occurred after at least 3 days.

±**DOSAGE ADJUSTMENT** For patients receiving a 120-mcg dosage before major meals and experiencing nausea or if nausea persists at 120 mcg before major meals, dosage decreased to 60 mcg before major meals.

Drug Administration

SUBCUTANEOUS

- Ensure that mealtime insulin dose has been reduced by 50% upon initiation of drug therapy.
- Allow drug to warm to room temperature before administering to avoid injection-site adverse reactions.
- Administer immediately prior to each major meal that contains 250 calories or more or 30 or more grams of carbohydrates. Dose should be skipped if meal is skipped or meal provides less than 250 calories or less than 30 g of carbohydrates.
- Inject drug into the abdomen or thigh. Do not inject into arm because absorption is variable from this site.
- Do not inject into same site as insulin.
- Rotate sites.
- Administer pramlintide and insulin in separate syringes, as drug should not be mixed with any type of insulin.
- Wait at least 3 days between dose titrations to minimize nausea.
- If drug is discontinued for illnesses or surgery, initiation protocol will have to be followed when drug is reinstituted.
- Store pens in refrigerator or at room temperature. Discard pens after 30 days, regardless of how they were stored.
- If a dose is missed, skip dose and resume scheduled dosing schedule.

Route	Onset	Peak	Duration
SubQ	Unknown	19–21 min	3 hr

Half-life: 8 min

Mechanism of Action

Slows the rate at which food is released from stomach to small intestine, thus reducing initial postprandial rise in serum glucose level. Suppresses glucagon secretion also and promotes satiety, thus furthering weight loss, which also lowers serum glucose level. Be aware that pramlintide is a synthetic analogue of amylin, a naturally occurring neuroendocrine hormone secreted with insulin by pancreatic beta cells. Reduction in or absence of the secretion of insulin and amylin occurs in diabetes.

Contraindications

Gastroparesis, hypersensitivity to pramlintide or its components, hypoglycemia unawareness

Interactions

DRUGS

drugs that alter GI motility (such as anticholinergics) or slow intestinal absorption of nutrients (such as alpha-glucosidase inhibitors): Altered effects of these drugs
insulin: Alters pharmacokinetic parameters of pramlintide if mixed in the same syringe. Pramlintide and insulin must not be mixed together and must be administered as separate injections.
oral drugs: Delayed absorption

Adverse Reactions

CNS: Dizziness, fatigue, headache
EENT: Blurred vision, pharyngitis
GI: Abdominal pain, anorexia, nausea, **pancreatitis**, vomiting
MS: Arthralgia
RESP: Coughing
SKIN: Diaphoresis
Other: **Hypersensitivity reactions**; local injection-site reaction, such as redness, swelling, or pruritus

Childbearing Considerations

PREGNANCY

- It is not known if drug can cause fetal harm.
- Use with caution only if benefit to mother outweighs potential risk to fetus.

LACTATION

- It is not known if drug is present in breast milk.
- Mothers should check with prescriber before breastfeeding.

Nursing Considerations

- Know that because of the risks involved with pramlintide therapy, insulin-using patients with type 1 or 2 diabetes must have failed to achieve adequate glycemic control despite individualized insulin management and must be receiving ongoing care with guidance from insulin prescriber and a diabetes educator before pramlintide is prescribed.

! WARNING Be aware pramlintide should not be prescribed for patients with poor compliance with current insulin regimen, poor compliance with monitoring blood glucose level, a glycosylated hemoglobin greater than 9%, recurrent severe hypoglycemia that required assistance during past 6 months, hypoglycemia unawareness, gastroparesis, concurrent therapy with drugs that stimulate GI motility, and pediatric patients.

- Monitor patient's premeal and postmeal blood glucose levels regularly to determine effectiveness of pramlintide and insulin therapy and to detect hypoglycemia.

! WARNING Monitor patient for a hypersensitivity reaction. If present, notify prescriber, expect drug to be discontinued, and provide supportive care, as needed and ordered.

! WARNING Be aware that although pramlintide doesn't cause hypoglycemia, its use with insulin increases the risk of insulin-induced severe hypoglycemia, which can result in loss of consciousness, coma, or seizures. Monitor patient for 3 hours after each dose of pramlintide, especially if patient is taking any other drugs that may cause hypoglycemia. Know that symptoms may occur with a rapid decrease in blood glucose level regardless of glucose values. If hypoglycemia occurs, provide supportive care, including glucagon, if prescribed, and notify prescriber. Expect insulin dosage accompanying pramlintide to be reduced. Expect pramlintide to be stopped if patient develops recurrent hypoglycemia that requires medical assistance, develops persistent nausea, or becomes noncompliant with therapy or follow-up visits.

- Know that early warning symptoms of hypoglycemia may be different or appear less severe if patient has had diabetes for a long time; has diabetic nerve disease; takes a beta-blocker, clonidine, guanethidine, or reserpine; or is under intensified diabetes control.

PATIENT TEACHING

- Instruct patient how to administer pramlintide subcutaneously using the Symlin Pen and what to do if a dose is missed.
- Emphasize need to monitor blood glucose level often, especially before and after eating to determine effectiveness of drug.
- Alert patient that she'll need close follow-up care, at least weekly until a target dose of pramlintide has been reached, she's tolerating the drug well, and her blood glucose level is stable.
- Inform patient that nausea is common with pramlintide; urge her to notify prescriber because dosage may have to be decreased.
- Explain that local injection-site reactions, such as itching, redness, or swelling, may occur but usually resolve in a few weeks.

! **WARNING** Tell patient drug may cause an allergic reaction. If present, tell patient to notify prescriber and, if severe, to seek immediate medical care.

! **WARNING** Alert patient and family or caregiver that insulin-induced hypoglycemia may occur within 3 hours of injecting pramlintide and could be quite severe. Review signs and symptoms and appropriate treatment. Advise patient to obtain a prescription for glucagon and provide instructions on its use. Tell patient to notify prescriber if hypoglycemia occurs because insulin dosage will have to be reduced.

- Caution patient to avoid hazardous activities that require mental alertness until effects of pramlintide are known and resolved.
- Instruct patient to never share the SymlinPen with anyone else, even if the needle has been changed because of a risk for transmission of blood-borne pathogens.

prasugrel hydrochloride

Effient

Class and Category

Pharmacologic class: $P2Y_{12}$ platelet inhibitor (thienopyridine)

Therapeutic class: Antiplatelet

Indications and Dosages

* *To reduce rate of thrombotic cardiovascular events (including stent thrombosis) in patients with acute coronary syndrome who will be managed with percutaneous coronary intervention (PCI) because of non-ST-elevation MI or unstable angina or in patients with ST-elevation MI managed with primary or delayed PCI*

TABLETS

Adults. *Loading:* 60 mg followed by maintenance dose. *Maintenance:* 10 mg once daily.

± **DOSAGE ADJUSTMENT** For patients weighing less than 60 kg (132 lb), daily maintenance dosage may be reduced to 5 mg once daily.

Drug Administration

P.O.

- Tablet should be swallowed whole and not broken, chewed, or crushed.
- Store at room temperature, keep desiccant in bottle at all times.
- Drug should be taken with aspirin 75 mg to 325 mg daily.

Route	Onset	Peak	Duration
P.O.	< 30 min	30 min	5–9 days

Half-life: 2–15 hr

Mechanism of Action

Binds irreversibly to ADP receptors on platelets after forming its active metabolite to inhibit platelet activation and aggregation for the lifetime of the platelet, which is 7 to 10 days. Prevents thrombus formation because without platelet activation and aggregation, thrombus cannot form.

Contraindications

Active bleeding, history of transient ischemic attack or stroke, hypersensitivity to prasugrel or its components

Interactions

DRUGS

fibrinolytic agents, NSAIDs (chronic use), warfarin: Increased risk of bleeding
opioids: Decreased or delayed prasugrel absorption

Adverse Reactions

CNS: Dizziness, fatigue, fever, headache, **intracranial hemorrhage**
CV: **Atrial fibrillation**, **bradycardia**, hypercholesterolemia, hyperlipidemia, hypertension, **hypotension**, peripheral edema
EENT: Epistaxis, retinal hemorrhage
GI: Diarrhea, **GI or retroperitoneal hemorrhage**, hepatic dysfunction, nausea
HEME: Anemia, **bleeding**, **leukopenia**, **severe thrombocytopenia**, **thrombotic thrombocytopenia purpura**
MS: Back or limb pain
RESP: Cough, dyspnea, **hemoptysis**
SKIN: Subcutaneous hematoma, rash
Other: **Anaphylaxis**, **angioedema**, **hypersensitivity reactions**, **malignancies**, noncardiac chest pain

Childbearing Considerations

PREGNANCY

- Drug may cause fetal harm due to risk of bleeding.
- Use with caution only if benefit to mother outweighs potential risk to fetus.

LACTATION

- It is not known if drug is present in breast milk.
- Mothers should check with prescriber once condition has stabilized before breastfeeding.

Nursing Considerations

- Be aware that patient should be receiving daily aspirin therapy (75 or 325 mg) throughout prasugrel therapy.

! WARNING Be aware that drug isn't recommended for patients ages 75 and older (except in high-risk situations, such as history of previous MI or presence of diabetes) or in patients who have active bleeding or a history of a transient ischemic attack or stroke.

! WARNING Know that prasugrel shouldn't be given to patients likely to undergo emergency coronary artery bypass graft (CABG) surgery because of increased bleeding risk. Drug should be discontinued at least 7 days before any surgery.

! WARNING Monitor patient for a hypersensitivity reaction, which could become life-threatening, such as anaphylaxis or angioedema. Know that patients who have had a serious hypersensitivity reaction to thienopyridines, such as clopidogrel or ticlopidine are at higher risk for serious hypersensivitiy reactions. Notify prescriber if present, expect drug to be discontinued, and provide supportive care, as needed and ordered.

! WARNING Monitor patient closely for bleeding because prasugrel can cause life-threatening hemorrhage. Monitor patients closely who have risk factors for bleeding, which include a body weight less than 60 kg, a history of bleeding, or concurrent therapy with drugs that increase risk of bleeding, such as chronic use of NSAIDs, fibrinolytic therapy, heparin, or warfarin. Be aware that because prasugrel inhibits platelet aggregation for the lifetime of the platelet, which is 7 to 10 days, withholding a dose is unlikely to be helpful in managing a bleeding event or the risk of bleeding associated with an invasive procedure. Expect to administer exogenous platelets but only 6 hours after prasugrel loading dose or 4 hours after maintenance dose was given.

! WARNING Report hypotension in patients who have recently undergone CABG surgery or other surgical procedures, coronary angiography, or percutaneous coronary intervention while taking drug. In this setting, expect therapy to continue because stopping prasugrel, especially in first few weeks after acute coronary syndrome, increases the risk of adverse cardiovascular effects.

! **WARNING** Monitor patient's CBC regularly, as ordered, watching for evidence of thrombotic thrombocytopenic purpura, such as abnormal blood counts, fever, neurologic abnormalities, or renal dysfunction. Notify prescriber immediately because condition can be fatal. Expect to implement emergency treatment, such as plasmapheresis.

PATIENT TEACHING

- Instruct patient how to administer prasugrel.
- Emphasize importance of taking prasugrel exactly as prescribed, without lapses in therapy, for drug to be effective and adverse reactions to be reduced.
- Instruct patient to take daily dose of aspirin as prescribed.

! **WARNING** Alert patient that drug may cause an allergic reaction. If present, tell patient to notify prescriber and, if severe, to seek immediate medical care.

! **WARNING** Caution patient that bleeding may last longer than usual. Instruct the patient to report unusual bleeding or bruising. Urge patient to take precautions against bleeding, such as using an electric shaver and a soft-bristled toothbrush. Also, discourage use of NSAIDs, including over-the-counter products, during prasugrel therapy because of risk of bleeding. Advise patient to avoid activities that could cause traumatic injury and bleeding.

! **WARNING** Tell patient to notify prescriber of any other persistent, serious, or unusual adverse reaction.

- Instruct patient to inform all healthcare providers that he takes prasugrel.

pravastatin sodium

Class and Category

Pharmacologic class: HMG-CoA reductase inhibitor (statin)
Therapeutic class: Antilipemic

Indications and Dosages

* *To prevent cardiovascular and coronary events in patients at risk; to treat hyperlipidemia, hypertriglyceridemia, or primary dysbetalipoproteinemia*

TABLETS

Adults. *Initial:* 40 mg to 80 mg once daily. *Maximum:* 80 mg once daily.

± **DOSAGE ADJUSTMENT** For patients with severe renal impairment, those taking cyclosporine, and elderly patients, initial dosage reduced to 10 mg once daily. (Another statin product will need to be prescribed because drug is no longer available in a 10 mg strength.) For elderly patients and those taking cyclosporine, maintenance dosage usually limited to 20 mg daily. For patients taking clarithromycin or erythromycin, dosage limited to 40 mg once daily.

* *To treat pediatric heterozygous familial hypercholesterolemia*

TABLETS

Adolescents ages 14 to 18. 40 mg once daily.
Children ages 8 to 13. 20 mg once daily.

Drug Administration

P.O.

- Administer drug consistently at about the same time every day.
- Give drug 1 hr before or 4 hr after giving a bile acid sequestrant such as cholestyramine or colestipol.

Route	Onset	Peak	Duration
P.O.	Unknown	60–90 min	Unknown

Half-life: 2.6–3.2 hr

Mechanism of Action

Inhibits cholesterol synthesis in liver by blocking the enzyme needed to convert hydroxymethylglutaryl-CoA (HMG-CoA) to mevalonate, a cholesterol precursor. Blocking cholesterol synthesis increases breakdown of LDL cholesterol in the liver.

Contraindications

Active hepatic disease or decompensated cirrhosis; hypersensitivity to pravastatin or its components

Interactions

DRUGS

cholestyramine, colestipol: Decreased exposure of pravastatin with decreased effectiveness
clarithromycin and other macrolide antibiotics, colchicine, cyclosporine,

gemfibrozil, niacin, other fibrates: Increased risk of rhabdomyolysis and acute renal failure

Adverse Reactions

CNS: Anxiety, asthenia, chills, confusion, cognitive impairment, cranial nerve dysfunction, depression, dizziness, fatigue, headache, malaise, memory loss, nervousness, nightmare, peripheral nerve palsy, sleep disturbance
CV: Angina pectoris, chest pain, vasculitis
EENT: Blurred vision, diplopia, rhinitis
ENDO: Abnormal thyroid function, elevated glycosylated hemoglobin levels and fasting glucose levels, gynecomastia, hyperglycemia
GI: Abdominal pain, cholestatic jaundice, cirrhosis, constipation, diarrhea, elevated liver enzymes, flatulence, **fulminant hepatic necrosis**, heartburn, **hepatic failure**, **hepatitis**, hepatoma, indigestion, nausea, **pancreatitis**, vomiting
GU: Dysuria, nocturia, urinary frequency
HEME: ESR elevation, **Hemolytic anemia**, positive ANA, purpura
MS: Arthralgia, immune-mediated necrotizing myopathy, musculoskeletal cramps or pain, myalgia, myopathy, polymyalgia rheumatica, **rhabdomyolysis**, tendon disorder
RESP: Cough, dyspnea, **interstitial lung disease**, upper respiratory tract infection
SKIN: Dermatomyositis, **erythema multiforme**, lichen planus, photosensitivity, rash, **Stevens-Johnson syndrome**, **toxic epidermal necrolysis**
Other: **Anaphylaxis**, **angioedema**, elevated creatine phosphokinase, flu-like symptoms, lupus-like syndrome

Childbearing Considerations

PREGNANCY

- Drug may cause fetal harm.
- Drug is not recommended in pregnant women.
- Drug should be discontinued immediately when pregnancy is known.

LACTATION

- Drug is present in breast milk.
- Drug is not recommended with breastfeeding.

REPRODUCTION

- Females of childbearing age should use a reliable contraceptive throughout pravastatin therapy.

Nursing Considerations

- Use pravastatin cautiously in patients with hepatic or renal impairment and in elderly patients.

! WARNING Monitor liver enzymes, as ordered, before pravastatin therapy starts and as indicated during therapy. Although increases usually appear soon after drug therapy is started, are transient, not accompanied by symptoms, and resolve or improve on continued therapy or after a brief interruption of therapy, fatal and non-fatal hepatic failure have rarely occurred. Know that patients who drink alcohol heavily and/or have a history of liver disease may be at increased risk for liver injury. If patient develops serious hepatic injury exhibited by hyperbilirubinemia or jaundice in addition to liver enzyme elevation, notify prescriber and expect pravastatin to be immediately discontinued.

- Monitor blood lipoprotein level, as indicated, to evaluate response to therapy.

! WARNING Monitor patient for a hypersensitivity reaction, which could become life-threatening, such as anaphylaxis or angioedema. If present, notify prescriber, expect drug to be discontinued, and provide supportive care, as needed and ordered.

! WARNING Monitor patient for unexplained muscle aches or weakness and significant increases in creatine kinase level. Report such findings to prescriber because, in rare instances, drug causes myopathy and rhabdomyolysis with acute renal failure caused by myoglobinuria. Rare fatalities have occurred. Risk factors include patients who are 65 years of age or older, patients receiving concurrent therapy with other drugs known to increase risk (cyclosporin, colchicine, fibrates, gemfibrozil, and niacin), or patients with renal impairment or uncontrolled hypothyroidism, Additional neuromuscular and serologic testing may be needed if immune-mediated necrotizing myopathy is suspected. Expect to stop drug and provide supportive care, as needed and ordered. Immunosuppressive drugs may be needed to treat immune-mediated necrotizing myopathy.

- Monitor patient's BUN and serum creatinine levels periodically for abnormal elevations.
- Monitor fasting blood glucose levels and HbA1c as elevations have occurred during pravastatin therapy.

! **WARNING** Monitor patient for other persistent, serious, or unusual adverse reactions.

PATIENT TEACHING

- Instruct patient how to administer pravastatin.
- Tell patients prescribed cholestyramine or colestipol to take pravastatin 1 hr before or 4 hr after taking cholestyramine or colestipol.
- Instruct patient not to stop taking pravastatin without consulting prescriber, even when cholesterol level returns to normal.

! **WARNING** Alert patient that pravastatin may cause an allergic reaction. If present, tell patient to notify prescriber and, if severe, to seek immediate medical care.

! **WARNING** Advise patient to notify prescriber at once about muscle pain, tenderness, weakness, and other evidence of myopathy.

! **WARNING** Urge females of childbearing age to use a reliable method of contraception during pravastatin therapy and to notify prescriber at once if pregnancy occurs.

! **WARNING** Instruct patient to notify prescriber immediately if other persistent, serious, or unusual adverse reactions occur.

- Caution patient not to perform hazardous activities, such as driving, until effects of drug are known and resolved.
- Advise mothers not to breastfeed while on pravastatin therapy.

prazosin hydrochloride

Minipress

Class and Category

Pharmacologic class: Alpha-blocker
Therapeutic class: Antihypertensive

Indications and Dosages

* *To manage hypertension as monotherapy or as adjunct with other antihypertensive drugs*

CAPSULES

Adults. *Initial:* 1 mg 2 or 3 times daily, increased slowly to maintenance dose. *Maintenance:* 6 to 15 mg daily in divided doses. *Maximum:* 40 mg daily in divided doses.

± **DOSAGE ADJUSTMENT** For patients having a diuretic or other antihypertensive agent added to prazosin therapy, dosage reduced to 1 or 2 mg 3 times daily and retitration done.

Drug Administration

P.O.

- Give drug at same times daily.

Route	Onset	Peak	Duration
P.O.	0.5–1.5 hr	2–4 hr	10–24 hr

Half-life: 2–3 hr

Mechanism of Action

Inhibits alpha$_1$-adrenergic receptors competitively and selectively to promote peripheral arterial and venous dilation and reduce peripheral vascular resistance, thereby lowering blood pressure.

Contraindications

Hypersensitivity to prazosin, other quinazolines, or their components

Interactions

DRUGS

antihypertensives, beta-blockers, diuretics, phosphodiesterase-5 inhibitors: Increased risk of hypotension and syncope

Adverse Reactions

CNS: Asthenia, dizziness, drowsiness, fatigue, headache, insomnia, malaise, nervousness, syncope
CV: Angina, **bradycardia**, edema, orthostatic hypotension, palpitations, vasculitis
EENT: Dry mouth, eye pain
ENDO: Gynecomastia
GI: Nausea
GU: Priapism, urinary frequency or incontinence
SKIN: Urticaria
Other: **Hypersensitivity reactions**

Childbearing Considerations

PREGNANCY

- It is not known if drug can cause fetal harm.

- Use with caution only if benefit to mother outweighs potential risk to fetus.

LACTATION

- Drug is present in breast milk.
- Mothers should check with prescriber before breastfeeding.

Nursing Considerations

- Monitor blood pressure regularly to evaluate effectiveness of therapy.

! **WARNING** Monitor patient for a hypersensitivity reaction. If present, notify prescriber, expect drug to be discontinued, and provide supportive care, as needed and ordered.

! **WARNING** Monitor patients with renal impairment because of increased sensitivity to prazosin's effects; in those with angina pectoris because drug may induce or aggravate angina; in those with narcolepsy because prazosin may worsen cataplexy; and in elderly patients because they're at increased risk for drug-induced hypotension.

PATIENT TEACHING

- Instruct patient how to administer prazosin.
- Emphasize need to take drug even if feeling well.
- Advise patient to avoid drinking alcohol, exercising in hot weather, or standing for long periods because these activities increase risk of orthostatic hypotension.
- Instruct patient not to take any drugs, including over-the-counter forms, without consulting prescriber, to avoid serious interactions.

! **WARNING** Alert patient that drug may cause an allergic reaction. If present, notify prescriber and, if severe, to seek immediate medical care.

! **WARNING** Instruct male patient that a prolonged erection may occur with prazosin therapy. If it lasts longer than 4 hours, stress importance of seeking immediate medical assistance.

! **WARNING** Advise patient to notify prescriber immediately about persistent, serious, or unusual adverse reactions, especially dizziness and fainting.

- Suggest rising slowly from lying or sitting position to minimize orthostatic hypotension.
- Urge patient to avoid hazardous activities until drug's CNS effects are known and resolved.

prednisolone

Delta-Cortef, Millipred

prednisolone sodium phosphate

Orapred ODT, Pediapred

Class and Category

Pharmacologic class: Glucocorticoid
Therapeutic class: Immunosuppressant

Indications and Dosages

* *To treat acute and chronic inflammatory and immunosuppressive disorders*

SYRUP, TABLETS (PREDNISOLONE); ORAL SOLUTION, ORALLY DISINTEGRATING TABLETS (PREDNISOLONE SODIUM PHOSPHATE)

Adults. Highly individualized. *Dosage range:* 5 to 60 mg daily or in divided doses.
Children. *Initial:* 0.14 to 2 mg/kg/day divided and given 3 or 4 times daily. Then, dosage adjusted, as needed. *Maintenance:* Gradual decrease in small decrements to lowest dose that maintains an adequate clinical response.

* *To treat acute exacerbations of multiple sclerosis*

SYRUP, TABLETS (PREDNISOLONE); ORAL SOLUTION, ORALLY DISINTEGRATING TABLETS (PREDNISOLONE SODIUM PHOSPHATE)

Adults. 200 mg daily for 1 wk, followed by 80 mg every other day for 1 mo.

* *To treat uncontrolled asthma in children taking inhaled corticosteroids and long-acting bronchodilators*

ORAL SOLUTION, ORALLY DISINTEGRATING TABLETS (PREDNISOLONE SODIUM PHOSPHATE)

Children. 1 to 2 mg/kg once daily or in 2 divided doses and continued for 3 to 10 days

P

or longer until child achieves a peak expiratory flow rate of 80% of personal best, or until symptoms resolve. *Maximum:* 60 mg daily.

∗ *To treat pediatric nephrotic syndrome*

ORAL SOLUTION, ORALLY DISINTEGRATING TABLETS, (PREDNISOLONE SODIUM PHOSPHATE)

Children. *Initial:* 60 mg/m^2/day in 3 divided doses for 4 wk, followed by 40 mg/m^2 once every other day for 4 wk.

Drug Administration

P.O.

- Administer once-daily dose in morning.
- Give with food to minimize GI upset.
- For oral solution, use the calibrated syringe that comes with it for measuring dosage. For syrup, use a calibrated device to measure dosage.
- For orally disintegrating tablets, do not remove tablet from blister pack until ready to administer. With dry, gloved hands, peel back the foil on the blister pack and carefully remove tablet. Do not push tablet through the foil because it can break easily. Place tablet on patient's tongue to dissolve completely. Patient may swallow after dissolution with saliva or with water.
- Tablets should not be broken, chewed, or crushed.

Route	Onset	Peak	Duration
P.O.	Rapid	1–2 hr	3–36 hr

Half-life: 2–3 hr

Mechanism of Action

Binds to intracellular glucocorticoid receptors and suppresses inflammatory and immune responses by:

- inhibiting neutrophil and monocyte accumulation at inflammation site and suppressing their phagocytic and bactericidal activity
- stabilizing lysosomal membranes
- suppressing antigen response of macrophages and helper T cells
- inhibiting synthesis of inflammatory response mediators, such as cytokines, interleukins, and prostaglandins.

Contraindications

Hypersensitivity to prednisolone or its components, systemic fungal infection

Interactions

DRUGS

aminoglutethimide: Possibly loss of induced adrenal suppression
amphotericin B, diuretics: Possibly severe hypokalemia
antacids, cholestyramine, colestipol: Decreased prednisolone absorption
anticholinesterase agents: Possibly severe weakness in patients with myasthenia gravis
barbiturates, phenytoin, rifampin: Decreased prednisolone effects
cyclosporine: Increased risk of seizures
digoxin: Possibly arrhythmias and digitalis toxicity from hypokalemia
estrogens, oral contraceptives: Decreased clearance, increased elimination half-life, and increased therapeutic and toxic effects of prednisolone
insulin, oral antidiabetics: Increased risk of hyperglycemia
isoniazid, salicylates: Decreased blood level of these drugs
ketoconazole, macrolide antibiotics: Possibly decreased prednisolone metabolism
live or inactivated vaccines, toxoids: Possibly diminished response to vaccines or toxoids
NSAIDs: Increased risk of GI ulceration and bleeding, possibly added therapeutic effect when NSAIDs are used to treat arthritis
warfarin: Possibly inhibition of warfarin effect

ACTIVITIES

alcohol use: Increased risk of GI ulceration and bleeding

FOODS

sodium-containing foods: Increased risk of edema and hypertension

Adverse Reactions

CNS: Euphoria, headache, insomnia, nervousness, psychosis, restlessness, **seizures**, vertigo
CV: Edema, **heart failure**, hypertension
EENT: Cataracts, exophthalmos, glaucoma, increased ocular pressure

ENDO: **Adrenal insufficiency**, Cushing's syndrome, growth suppression in children, hyperglycemia
GI: Anorexia, **GI bleeding** and ulceration, increased appetite, indigestion, **intestinal perforation**, nausea, **pancreatitis**, vomiting
GU: Menstrual irregularities
MS: Avascular necrosis of joints, bone fractures, muscle atrophy or weakness, myalgia, osteoporosis
SKIN: Acne; diaphoresis; ecchymosis; flushing; petechiae; striae; thin, fragile skin
Other: Delayed wound healing, **hypernatremia**, **hypokalemia**, **immunosuppression**, infections (bacterial, fungal, helminthic, protozoan, viral), injection-site scarring, **Kaposi's sarcoma**, negative nitrogen balance, risk of infection

Childbearing Considerations

PREGNANCY

- Drug can cause fetal harm such as orofacial clefts when used in first trimester.
- Drug should be used with caution during pregnancy only if benefit to mother outweighs potential risk to fetus.
- Monitor infant for hypoadrenalism if mother has received large doses of drug during pregnancy.

LACTATION

- Drug is present in breast milk and, in high doses, could interfere with endogenous corticosteroid production, suppress growth, or cause other adverse effects in the breastfed infant.
- The lowest dose possible is recommended to minimize exposure to breastfed infant.

Nursing Considerations

! **WARNING** Avoid using prednisolone in patients with a history of active tuberculosis because drug can reactivate the disease.

! **WARNING** Monitor patient for seizures, especially patient with a history of seizures. Institute seizure precautions, as appropriate.

! **WARNING** Assess patient regularly for evidence of adverse reactions, including heart failure and GI bleeding. Notify prescriber of any persistent, serious, or unusual adverse reactions. Also, monitor patient's intake, output, and daily weight.

! **WARNING** Be aware that prolonged use may cause hypothalamic-pituitary-adrenal suppression. Withdraw drug gradually, as ordered, if therapy lasts longer than 2 weeks. Stopping abruptly may cause acute adrenal insufficiency or, possibly, death.

- Be aware that patient may be at risk for emotional instability or psychic disturbance while taking prednisolone, especially if predisposed to them or taking high doses.
- Monitor growth pattern in children; prednisolone may retard bone growth.

PATIENT TEACHING

! **WARNING** Stress importance of childbearing females to alert prescriber of possiblility of being pregnant before prednisolone therapy begins because drug can cause fetal harm in the first trimester.

- Instruct patient how to administer form of oral prednisolone prescribed.
- Emphasize need to take drug exactly as prescribed because taking too much increases risk of serious adverse reactions.
- Urge patient to avoid alcohol during therapy because of increased risk of GI ulcers and bleeding.

! **WARNING** Review infection control measures with patient and family or caregiver. Urge patient and family or caregiver to notify prescriber if an infection is present. Advise patient to avoid people with contagious infections because drug has an immunosuppressant effect. Urge her to notify prescriber immediately about exposure to measles or chickenpox.

! **WARNING** Warn patient about receiving live virus vaccines during drug therapy. Also, caution about coming in contact with people who have recently received live vaccines.

! **WARNING** Instruct patient to notify prescriber immediately about joint pain, swelling, tarry stools, and visual disturbances or any other persistent, serious, or unusual adverse effects.

! WARNING Caution patient not to discontinue drug abruptly.

- Urge patient to avoid hazardous activities until drug's CNS effects are known and resolved.
- Instruct diabetic patient to check her blood glucose level often because prednisolone may cause hyperglycemia.
- Advise patient to comply with follow-up visits to assess drug's effectiveness and detect adverse reactions.
- Urge patient to carry medical identification revealing prednisolone therapy.

prednisone

Prednisone Intensol, Rayos, Winpred (CAN)

Class and Category

Pharmacologic class: Glucocorticoid
Therapeutic class: Immunosuppressant

Indications and Dosages

* *To treat adrenal insufficiency and acute and chronic inflammatory and immunosuppressive disorders*

D.R. TABLETS, ORAL SOLUTION, TABLETS

Adults and children. Highly individualized. *Range:* 5 to 60 mg daily as a single dose or in divided doses.

* *To treat acute exacerbations of multiple sclerosis*

D.R. TABLETS, ORAL SOLUTION, TABLETS

Adults. 200 mg daily for 1 wk, then 80 mg every other day for 1 mo.

Drug Administration

P.O.

- Administer once-daily doses in the morning to match body's normal cortisol secretion schedule.
- Administer drug with food or milk to minimize GI upset.
- Tablets should be swallowed whole and not broken, chewed, or crushed.
- For oral solution, use a calibrated device to measure dosage. Store at room temperature, protected from light. Discard 90 days after opening container of oral solution.

Route	Onset	Peak	Duration
P.O.	Unknown	2 hr	Unknown
P.O./E.R.	4 hr	6–6.5 hr	Unknown

Half-life: 2–3 hr

Mechanism of Action

Binds to intracellular glucocorticoid receptors and suppresses inflammatory and immune responses by:
- inhibiting neutrophil and monocyte accumulation at inflammation site and suppressing their phagocytic and bactericidal activity.
- stabilizing lysosomal membranes.
- suppressing antigen response of macrophages and helper T cells.
- inhibiting synthesis of inflammatory response mediators, such as cytokines, interleukins, and prostaglandins.

Contraindications

Hypersensitivity to prednisone or its components, systemic fungal infection

Interactions

DRUGS

aminoglutethimide: Possibly loss of corticosteroid-induced adrenal suppression
amphotericin B (parenteral): Possibly development of cardiac enlargement and congestive heart failure
anticholinesterase agents: Possibly severe weakness in patients with myasthenia gravis
cholestyramine: Increased clearance of prednisone
cyclosporine: Increased risk of seizures
CYP3A4 inducers (barbiturates, phenytoin, carbamazepine, rifampin): Increased metabolism of prednisone
CYP3A4 inhibitors (ketoconazole, macrolide antibiotics): Decreased prednisone metabolism
digoxin: Possibly arrhythmias and digitalis toxicity from hypokalemia
diuretics: Possibly decreased natriuretic and diuretic effects of diuretics, severe hypokalemia (with potassium-depleting diuretics)
estrogens, oral contraceptives: Decreased clearance, increased elimination half-life,

and increased therapeutic and toxic effects of prednisone
insulin, oral antidiabetic agents: Possibly less effective, causing increased blood glucose levels
isoniazid: Decreased blood isoniazid level
NSAIDs: Increased risk of GI ulceration and bleeding, possibly added therapeutic effect when NSAIDs are used to treat arthritis
toxoids, vaccines: Possibly loss of antibody response, increased risk of neurologic complications
warfarin: Increased risk of reduced effectiveness of warfarin

ACTIVITIES

alcohol use: Increased risk of GI ulceration and bleeding

FOODS

sodium-containing foods: Increased risk of edema and hypertension

Adverse Reactions

CNS: Euphoria, headache, insomnia, nervousness, psychosis, restlessness, **seizures**, vertigo
CV: Edema, **heart failure**, hypertension
EENT: Cataracts, exophthalmos, glaucoma, increased ocular pressure
ENDO: **Adrenal insufficiency**, Cushing's syndrome, growth suppression in children, hyperglycemia
GI: Anorexia, **GI bleeding** and ulceration, increased appetite, indigestion, **intestinal perforation**, nausea, **pancreatitis**, vomiting
GU: Menstrual irregularities
MS: Avascular necrosis of joints, bone fractures, muscle atrophy or weakness, myalgia, osteoporosis
SKIN: Acne; diaphoresis; ecchymosis; flushing; petechiae; striae; thin, fragile skin
Other: Delayed wound healing, **hypernatremia**, **hypokalemia**, **immunosuppression**, infections (bacterial, fungal, helminthic, protozoan, viral), **Kaposi's sarcoma**, negative **Kaposi's sarcoma**, nitrogen balance

Childbearing Considerations

PREGNANCY

- It is not known if drug can cause fetal harm, although animal studies suggest a higher risk for cleft palate.
- Drug should be used with caution during pregnancy only if benefit to mother outweighs potential risk to fetus.
- Monitor infant for hypoadrenalism if mother has received large doses of drug during pregnancy.

LACTATION

- Drug is present in breast milk and high doses could interfere with endogenous corticosteroid production, suppress growth, or cause other adverse effects in the breastfed infant.
- Lowest dose of drug used to minimize exposure to breastfed infant.

Nursing Considerations

! **WARNING** Avoid using prednisone in patients with a history of active tuberculosis because drug can reactivate the disease.

! **WARNING** Monitor patient for seizures, especially patient with a history of seizures. Institute seizure precautions, as appropriate.

! **WARNING** Monitor patient for infections, which can be mild but also can be severe and at times fatal. Be aware that the risk of infection related complications increases with increasing predisone dosages. Institute infection control measures.

! **WARNING** Assess patient regularly for evidence of adverse reactions, including heart failure and GI bleedings. Notify prescriber of any persistent, serious, or unusual adverse reactions. Also, monitor patient's intake, output, and daily weight.

! **WARNING** Be aware that prolonged use may cause hypothalamic-pituitary-adrenal suppression. Withdraw drug gradually, as ordered, if therapy lasts longer than 2 weeks. Stopping abruptly may cause acute adrenal insufficiency or, possibly, death.

- Be aware that patient may be at risk for emotional instability or psychic disturbance while taking prednisone, especially if predisposed to them or taking high doses.
- Monitor growth pattern in children; prednisone may retard bone growth.

PATIENT TEACHING

! **WARNING** Stress importance of childbearing females to alert prescriber of possiblility of being pregnant before prednisone therapy begins because drug may cause fetal harm in the first trimester.

- Instruct patient how to administer form of oral prednisone prescribed.
- Emphasize need to take drug exactly as prescribed because taking too much increases risk of serious adverse reactions.
- Urge patient to avoid alcohol during therapy because of increased risk of GI ulcers and bleeding.

! **WARNING** Review infection control measures with patient and family or caregiver. Urge patient and family or caregiver to notify prescriber if an infection is present. Advise patient to avoid people with contagious infections because drug has an immunosuppressant effect. Urge her to notify prescriber immediately about exposure to measles or chickenpox.

! **WARNING** Caution against receiving live virus vaccines during drug therapy. Also, caution about coming in contact with people who have recently received live vaccines.

! **WARNING** Instruct patient to notify prescriber immediately about joint pain, swelling, tarry stools, and visual disturbances or any other persistent, serious, or unusual adverse effects.

! **WARNING** Caution patient not to discontinue drug abruptly.

! **WARNING** Tell mothers high doses could interfere with endogenous corticosteroid production, suppress growth, or cause other adverse effects in the breastfed infant. Suggest mother discuss with prescriber about the possibility of using lowest dose of drug to minimize exposure to breastfed infant.

- Urge patient to avoid hazardous activities until drug's CNS effects are known and resolved.
- Instruct diabetic patient to check her blood glucose level often because prednisone may cause hyperglycemia.
- Advise patient to comply with follow-up visits to assess drug's effectiveness and detect adverse reactions.
- Urge patient to carry medical identification revealing prednisone therapy.

pregabalin

Lyrica, Lyrica CR

Class, Category, and Schedule

Pharmacologic class: Gamma-aminobutyric acid (GABA) analogue
Therapeutic class: Analgesic, anticonvulsant
Controlled substance schedule: V

Indications and Dosages

✱ *To relieve neuropathic pain associated with diabetic peripheral neuropathy*

CAPSULES, ORAL SOLUTION

Adults. *Initial:* 50 mg 3 times daily, increased to 100 mg 3 times daily, within 1 wk, as needed. *Maximum:* 300 mg daily.

E.R. TABLETS

Adults. *Initial:* 165 mg once daily after evening meal, then increased to 330 mg once daily within 1 wk, as needed and tolerated. *Maximum:* 330 mg once daily.

✱ *To relieve postherpetic neuralgia*

CAPSULES, ORAL SOLUTION

Adults. *Initial:* 75 mg twice daily or 50 mg 3 times daily, increased to 150 mg twice daily or 100 mg 3 times daily within 1 wk, as needed. Then, increased to 300 mg twice daily or 200 mg 3 times daily in 2 to 4 wk, as needed. *Maximum:* 600 mg daily.

E.R. TABLETS

Adults. *Initial* 165 mg once daily after evening meal, then increased to 330 mg once daily within 1 wk, as needed and tolerated. Dosage further increased to 660 mg once daily after 2 to 4 wk, as needed and tolerated. *Maximum:* 660 mg once daily.

✱ *As adjunct therapy to manage partial-onset seizures*

CAPSULES, ORAL SOLUTION

Adults and adolescents ages 17 and older. *Initial:* 150 mg daily in 2 or 3 divided doses, then increased, as needed. *Maximum:* 600 mg daily in 2 or 3 divided doses.

Children ages 4 and older weighing 30 kg (66 lb) or more. *Initial:* 2.5 mg/kg/day in 2 or 3 divided doses, then increased, as needed. *Maximum:* 10 mg/kg/day in 2 or 3 divided doses, not to exceed 600 mg/day.

Children ages 4 and older weighing less than 30 kg (66 lb). *Initial:* 3.5 mg/kg/day in 2 or 3 divided doses. *Maximum:* 14 mg/kg/day in 2 or 3 divided doses.

Infants and children ages 1 mo to 4 yr weighing less than 30 kg (66 lb). *Initial:* 3.5 mg/kg/day in 3 divided doses. *Maximum:* 14 mg/kg/day in 3 divided doses.

∗ *To manage fibromyalgia*

CAPSULES, ORAL SOLUTION

Adults. *Initial:* 75 mg twice daily, increased to 150 mg twice daily in 1 wk, as needed, and then to 225 mg twice daily in 1 wk, as needed. *Maximum:* 450 mg daily.

∗ *To manage neuropathic pain associated with spinal cord injury*

CAPSULES, ORAL SOLUTION

Adults. *Initial:* 75 mg twice daily, increased to 150 mg twice daily in 1 wk, as needed, and then to 300 mg twice daily after 2 to 3 wk, as needed. *Maximum:* 600 mg daily.

±**DOSAGE ADJUSTMENT** For adult patients with renal impairment with a creatinine clearance of 30 to 60 ml/min, daily dosage reduced by 50%. For adult patients with a creatinine clearance less than 30 ml/min, E.R. pregabalin not given. For adult patients with a creatinine clearance of 15 to 30 ml/min, daily dosage of immediate-release form reduced by 75% and frequency reduced to once or twice daily. For adult patients with a creatinine clearance less than 15 ml/min, daily dosage of immediate-release form reduced to as low as 25 mg daily. For adult patients receiving hemodialysis, daily dosage of immediate-release form is reduced and supplemental dose given immediately after every 4-hour hemodialysis session as follows: If reduced daily dosage is 25 mg daily, supplemental dose of 25 or 50 mg given; if reduced daily dosage is 25 to 50 mg daily, supplemental dose of 50 or 75 mg given; if reduced daily dosage is 50 to 75 mg daily, supplemental dose of 75 or 100 mg given; and if reduced daily dosage is 75 mg, supplemental dose of 100 or 150 mg given.

Drug Administration

P.O.

- Use calibrated device to measure dosage of oral solution.
- E.R. tablets and capsules should be swallowed whole and not chewed, crushed, or split.
- Administer E.R. tablets after evening meal.
- When converting patient from immediate-release formulation to E.R. formulation, administer morning dose of immediate-release pregabalin and then administer first dose of E.R. form in the evening on the day of the switch following manufacturer's guidelines for dosage conversion.
- Do not stop drug therapy abruptly; taper gradually over a minimum of 1 wk, as ordered.

Route	Onset	Peak	Duration
P.O.	Unknown	1.5–3 hr	Unknown
P.O./E.R.	Unknown	8–12 hr	Unknown

Half-life: 6.3 hr

Mechanism of Action

Binds to alpha$_2$-delta site, an auxiliary subunit of voltage calcium channels, in CNS tissue where it may reduce calcium-dependent release of several neurotransmitters, possibly by modulating calcium channel function. Decreased pain sensation and seizure activity occur with fewer neurotransmitters.

Contraindications

Hypersensitivity to pregabalin or its components

Interactions

DRUGS

CNS depressants: Increased risk of additive CNS adverse reactions, such as dizziness, respiratory depression, or somnolence

lorazepam, oxycodone: Additive effects on cognitive and gross motor function

opioid analgesics: Increased risk of constipation, intestinal obstruction, or paralytic ileus

ACTIVITIES

alcohol use: Additive effects on cognitive and gross motor function

Adverse Reactions

CNS: Abnormal gait, amnesia, anxiety, asthenia, ataxia, balance disorder, confusion, depression, difficulty concentrating, dizziness, euphoria, extrapyramidal syndrome, fatigue, fever, headache, hypertonia, hypesthesia, incoordination, **intracranial hypertension**, myoclonus,

nervousness, neuropathy, paresthesia, psychotic depression, schizophrenic reaction, somnolence, stupor, **suicidal ideation**, tremor, twitching, vertigo
CV: Chest pain, **heart failure**, peripheral edema, **ventricular fibrillation**
EENT: Amblyopia, blurred vision, conjunctivitis, decreased visual acuity, diplopia, dry mouth, nystagmus, otitis media, sinusitis, tinnitus, visual field defect
ENDO: Gynecomastia, **hypoglycemia**
GI: Abdominal distention or pain, constipation, diarrhea, flatulence, gastroenteritis, **GI hemorrhage**, increased appetite, nausea, vomiting
GU: **Acute renal failure**, anorgasmia, decreased libido, impotence, **nephritis**, urinary frequency, urinary incontinence, urine retention
HEME: **Leukopenia**, **thrombocytopenia**
MS: Arthralgia, back pain, elevated creatine kinase level, leg or muscle cramps, myalgia, myasthenia
RESP: **Apnea**, dyspnea, pneumonia, **respiratory depression (could be severe)**
SKIN: Bullous pemphigoid, ecchymosis, **exfoliative dermatitis**, pruritus, **Stevens-Johnson syndrome**
Other: **Anaphylaxis**, **angioedema**, **hypersensitivity reactions**, increased risk of viral infection, weight gain

Childbearing Considerations

PREGNANCY

- Pregnancy exposure registry: 1-888-233-2334 or http://www.aedpregnancyregistry.org/.
- Drug can cause fetal harm based on animal studies.
- Use with caution only if benefit to mother outweighs potential risk to fetus.

LACTATION

- Drug is present in breast milk.
- Breastfeeding is not recommended because of the potential risk of tumorigenicity in the breastfed infant.

REPRODUCTION

- Drug may cause a reduction in sperm concentration by 50% or more.

Nursing Considerations

! **WARNING** Monitor patient's symptoms for effectiveness of drug. Monitor patient for seizures, especially in patient with a history of seizures or taking drug to treat seizures.

! **WARNING** Monitor patient for a hypersensitivity reaction, which could become life-threatening, such as anaphylaxis or angioedema. If present, notify prescriber, expect drug to be discontinued, and give supportive care, as needed and ordered.

! **WARNING** Monitor patient's respiratory status closely because respiratory depression that can become life-threatening has occurred with drug administration. Increased risk includes patients who are also taking other CNS depressants, including opioids, or patient who has an existing respiratory impairment disorder. If patient shows signs of respiratory depression and sedation, notify prescriber and expect dosage to be decreased or drug discontinued.

! **WARNING** Monitor patient closely for evidence of suicidal behavior or thinking, especially when therapy starts or dosage changes.

! **WARNING** Monitor patient for hypoglycemia, especially diabetic patients taking antidiabetic agents. If present, treat according to institutional protocols and notify prescriber.

! **WARNING** Monitor patient closely for adverse reactions as drug can cause serious to life-threatening adverse reactions affecting multiple body systems. Notify prescriber if persistent, serious, or unusual adverse reactions occur. Be aware that children younger than 4 years have a higher change of experiencing pneumonia, somnolence, or viral infection.

! **WARNING** Know that pregabalin therapy should be stopped gradually over at least 1 week to decrease risk of seizure activity and avoid unpleasant symptoms, such as diarrhea, headache, insomnia, and nausea.

PATIENT TEACHING

! **WARNING** Tell females of childbearing age to alert prescriber of pregnancy status before pregabalin is administered because drug may cause fetal harm.

! **WARNING** Inform male patient who plans to father a child that drug could impair his fertility before drug is administered.

Encourage patient to discuss any concerns with prescriber before drug therapy is begun.

- Instruct patient how to administer form of pregabalin prescribed.

! **WARNING** Warn against stopping pregabalin abruptly. Tell patient that when pregabalin is no longer needed, the dosage should be tapered gradually over a minimum of 1 week before it is discontinued.

! **WARNING** Alert patient that drug may cause an allergic reaction. Tell patient to alert prescriber, if present, and to seek immediate medical care, if severe.

! **WARNING** Urge family or caregiver to watch patient closely for evidence of suicidal tendencies, especially when therapy starts or dosage changes and to report concerns at once to prescriber.

! **WARNING** Tell patient to notify prescriber if persistent, serious, or unusual adverse reactions occur as drug can cause various adverse reactions, some of which could be quite serious, needing immediate attention.

- Urge patient to avoid hazardous activities until she knows how drug affects her and effects are resolved.
- Instruct diabetic patients to inspect their skin while taking pregabalin because of possible development of skin sores or ulcers.

procainamide hydrochloride

Class and Category

Pharmacologic class: Sodium channel blocker of cardiomyocytes
Therapeutic class: Antiarrhythmic (class 1a)

Indications and Dosages

∗ *To treat life-threatening ventricular arrhythmias*

I.V. INFUSION OR INJECTION

Adults. *Initial loading dose:* 100 mg by I.V. injection every 5 min until arrhythmia is controlled or maximum total dose of 500 mg is reached and given at a rate not to exceed 50 mg/min. Dosing should not be resumed for at least 10 min or longer at this point. Alternatively, 20 mg/ml given at a constant rate of 1 ml/min for 25 to 30 min. *Maintenance:* 2 to 6 mg/min by continuous infusion. *Maximum:* 1 g.

∗ *To treat ventricular extrasystoles and arrhythmias associated with anesthesia and surgery*

I.M. INJECTION

Adults. 100 to 500 mg.

∗ *To treat less life-threatening arrhythmias in patients who are nauseated or vomiting, who are receiving nothing by mouth preoperatively, or who may have malabsorptive problems*

I.M. INJECTION

Adults. *Initial:* 50 mg/kg daily and divided into fractional doses of one-eighth to one-fourth given every 3 to 6 hr.

± **DOSAGE ADJUSTMENT** For elderly patients or those with hepatic or renal insufficiency, dosage possibly reduced or dosing intervals increased.

Drug Administration

- Place patient in a supine position before giving procainamide I.M. or I.V., to minimize hypotensive effects. Monitor blood pressure often and ECG tracings continuously during administration and for 30 min afterward.
- Inspect parenteral solution for particles and discoloration before giving drug; discard if particles are present or solution is darker than light amber.

I.V.

- For I.V. injection as a loading dose, dilute procainamide with 5% Dextrose Injection according to manufacturer's instructions and inject into a vein or tubing of an established I.V. line slowly at a rate not to exceed 50 mg/min.
- For I.V. infusion as a loading dose, dilute 1 g in 50 ml of 5% Dextrose Injection to a concentration of 20 mg/ml. Administer at a constant rate of 1 ml/min for up to 25 to 30 min.
- For I.V. infusion as a maintenance dose, dilute 1g of drug in 500 ml of 5% Dextrose Injection to a 2 mg/ml concentration and administer at a rate of 1 to 3 ml/min. However, if fluid intake must be limited, dilute 1 g of drug in 250 ml of 5% Dextrose

Injection to a 4 mg/ml concentration and infuse at a rate of 0.5 to 1.5 ml/min.
- Administer I.V. infusion with an infusion pump or other controlled-delivery device.
- Don't infuse or inject more than recommended amount per minute because heart block or cardiac arrest may occur.
- *Incompatibilities:* None reported by manufacturer

I.M.

- Use I.M. route only if I.V. route is not feasible because injection is painful.
- Inject deeply into a large muscle mass. Injection may be painful.
- Rotate injection sites.

Route	Onset	Peak	Duration
I.V.	Immediate	Immediate	Unknown
I.M.	10–30 min	15–60 min	Unknown

Half-life: 2.5–4.7 hr

Mechanism of Action

Prolongs recovery period after myocardial repolarization by inhibiting sodium influx through myocardial cell membranes, which prolongs refractory period, causing myocardial automaticity, conduction velocity, and excitability to decline.

Contraindications

Complete heart block, hypersensitivity to procainamide or its components, systemic lupus erythematosus, torsades de pointes

Interactions

DRUGS

antiarrhythmics: Additive cardiac effects
anticholinergics: Additive antivagal effects on A-V nodal conduction
neuromuscular blockers: Possibly increased or prolonged neuromuscular blockade

Adverse Reactions

CNS: Chills, disorientation, dizziness, lightheadedness
CV: **Heart block (second-degree)**, **hypotension**, **pericarditis**, **prolonged QT interval**, tachycardia
EENT: Bitter taste
GI: Abdominal distress, anorexia, diarrhea, nausea, vomiting
HEME: **Agranulocytosis**, **neutropenia**, **thrombocytopenia**
MS: Arthralgia, myalgia
RESP: Pleural effusion
SKIN: Pruritus, rash
Other: Drug-induced fever

Childbearing Considerations

PREGNANCY

- It is not known if drug can cause fetal harm.
- Use with caution only if benefit to mother outweighs potential risk to fetus.

LACTATION

- Drug is present in breast milk.
- Because drug is administered in a hospital setting, once patient is stabilized, prescriber should be consulted as to when, if at all, breastfeeding may resume to avoid potential serious adverse reactions in the breastfed infant.

Nursing Considerations

! **WARNING** Know that if drug is to be given I.M. and patient's platelet count is below 50,000/mm^3, notify prescriber at once because patient may develop bleeding, bruising, or hematomas from procainamide-induced bone marrow suppression and thrombocytopenia. Expect to give procainamide I.V.

! **WARNING** Monitor patient's cardiovascular status closely throughout procainamide therapy because drug can cause life-threatening adverse effects, such as heart block, hypotension, percarditis, or prolong QT interval.

- Anticipate that patient has reached maximum clinical response when ventricular tachycardia resolves, hypotension develops, or QRS complex is 50% wider than original width.

! **WARNING** Monitor patient's CBC because drug can cause serious hematologic adverse effects, such as agranulocytosis, neutropenia, and thrombocytopenia. Maintain bleeding and infection control measures.

PATIENT TEACHING

- Inform patient that drug must be given as an injection.

! **WARNING** Advise patient to notify staff immediately if patient suddenly doesn't feel well or develops persistent, serious, or unusual adverse reactions.

- Inform mothers whose condition has stabilized after procainamide therapy to check with prescriber as to when breastfeeding may be resumed, if possible, to avoid potential serious adverse reactions in infant.

prochlorperazine

Compro

prochlorperazine edisylate

prochlorperazine maleate

Class and Category

Pharmacologic class: Piperazine phenothiazine

Therapeutic class: Antiemetic

Indications and Dosages

∗ *To control nausea and vomiting related to surgery*

I.V. INFUSION OR INJECTION (PROCHLORPERAZINE EDISYLATE)

Adults. 5 to 10 mg at a rate not to exceed 5 mg/ml 15 to 30 min before anesthesia, as needed. Dosage repeated once, as needed. *Maximum:* 10 mg/dose, 40 mg daily.

I.M. INJECTION (PROCHLORPERAZINE EDISYLATE)

Adults. 5 to 10 mg 1 to 2 hr before anesthesia, as needed. Repeated once in 30 min, as needed. *Maximum:* 10 mg/dose, 40 mg daily.

∗ *To control severe nausea and vomiting*

TABLETS (PROCHLORPERAZINE MALEATE)

Adults and adolescents. 5 to 10 mg 3 or 4 times daily. *Maximum:* 40 mg daily.

Children ages 2 and older weighing 18 kg (40 lb) to 38.5 kg (85 lb). 2.5 mg 3 times daily or 5 mg 2 times daily. *Maximum:* 15 mg daily.

Children ages 2 and older weighing 13.5 kg (30 lb) to 17 kg (39 lb). 2.5 mg 2 or 3 times daily. *Maximum:* 10 mg daily.

Children ages 2 and older weighing 9 kg (20 lb) to 13 kg (29 lb). 2.5 mg once or twice daily. *Maximum:* 7.5 mg daily.

I.V. INFUSION OR INJECTION (PROCHLORPERAZINE EDISYLATE)

Adults. 2.5 to 10 mg at a rate not to exceed 5 mg/min. *Maximum:* 10 mg/dose; 40 mg daily.

I.M. INJECTION (PROCHLORPERAZINE EDISYLATE)

Adults and adolescents. 5 to 10 mg every 3 to 4 hr, as needed. *Maximum:* 40 mg daily.

Children ages 2 to 12. 0.132 mg/kg (0.06 mg/lb), then switched to oral form as soon as possible, usually after 1 dose.

SUPPOSITORIES (PROCHLORPERAZINE)

Adults. 25 mg twice daily.

∗ *To manage schizophrenia*

TABLETS (PROCHLORPERAZINE MALEATE)

Adults and adolescents with mild symptoms. 5 to 10 mg 3 or 4 times daily, increased gradually every 2 to 3 days, as needed and tolerated. *Maximum:* 150 mg daily.

Adults and adolescents with moderate symptoms. 10 mg 3 or 4 times daily, gradually increased every 2 to 3 days until symptoms are controlled or adverse reactions occur.

Children ages 2 to 12 weighing at least 9 kg (20 lb). *Initial:* 2.5 mg 2 or 3 times daily (maximum 10 mg on day 1), then increased, as needed. *Maximum for children ages 6 to 12:* total daily dose of 25 mg beginning day 2 and onward, *Maximum for children ages 2 to 6:* total daily dose of 20 mg beginning day 2 and onward.

I.M. INJECTION (PROCHLORPERAZINE EDISYLATE)

Adults and adolescents with severe symptoms. *Initial:* 10 to 20 mg, repeated every 2 to 4 hr (or in resistant cases every hr), as needed, to bring symptoms under control (usually 3 to 4 doses). Then, switched to oral dosing as soon as possible. *Maintenance:* If unable to switch to oral form, continue with 10 to 20 mg every 4 to 6 hr.

Children ages 2 to 12 weighing at least 9 kg (20 lb). 0.132 mg/kg (0.06 mg/lb) then switched to oral form as soon as possible, usually after 1 dose.

∗ *To treat nonpsychotic anxiety*

TABLETS (PROCHLORPERAZINE MALEATE)

Adults. 5 mg 3 or 4 times daily. *Maximum:* 20 mg daily for no longer than 12 wk.

±DOSAGE ADJUSTMENT For debilitated, elderly, and emaciated patients, initial dose usually reduced and subsequent dosage increased.

Drug Administration

P.O.

- Can be administered with or without food.

I.V.

- May be given undiluted as injection or diluted in 0.9% Sodium Chloride Injection when administered as an infusion.
- Administer slowly at no more than 5 mg/min as an injection or infusion.
- Never give as a I.V. bolus.
- Monitor patient for hypotension, as risk is higher with I.V. administration.
- Avoid contact between skin and solution because contact dermatitis could result.
- Protect drug from light.
- Parenteral solution may develop slight yellowing that won't affect potency. Don't use if discoloration is pronounced or precipitate is present.
- *Incompatibilities:* Other I.V. drugs

I.M.

- Inject slowly, deep into upper outer quadrant of buttocks.
- Rotate I.M. injection sites to prevent irritation and sterile abscesses.
- Avoid contact between skin and solution because contact dermatitis could result.

P.R.

- If too soft, refrigerate drug for 30 min or run under cold water while still wrapped.
- Moisten suppository with water before insertion.

Route	Onset	Peak	Duration
P.O.	30–40 min	Unknown	3–4 hr
I.V.	Unknown	30–60 min	Unknown
I.M.	1–20 min	Unknown	3–4 hr
P.R.	1 hr	Unknown	3–12 hr

Half-life: 6–10 hr

Mechanism of Action

Alleviates psychotic symptoms by blocking dopamine receptors, depressing release of selected hormones, and producing alpha-adrenergic blocking effect in the brain. Alleviates nausea and vomiting by centrally blocking dopamine receptors in the medullary chemoreceptor trigger zone and by peripherally blocking the vagus nerve in the GI tract. Anticholinergic effects and alpha-adrenergic blockade reduces anxiety through anticholinergic effects and alpha-adrenergic blockade, which decreases arousal and filtering of internal stimuli to the brain stem reticular activating system.

Contraindications

Age less than 2 years; coma; hypersensitivity to prochlorperazine, other phenothiazines or their components; pediatric surgery; severe CNS depression; use of large quantities of CNS depressants; weight less than 9 kg (20 lb)

Interactions

DRUGS

anticonvulsants: Possibly lowered seizure threshold by prochlorperazine
antihypertensives, such as guanethidine and related compounds: Possibly action of these drugs may be counteracted by prochlorperazine
CNS depressants: Possibly intensify or prolong action of these drugs
oral anticoagulants: Possibly diminished effects of oral anticoagulants
phenytoin: Possible interference with phenytoin metabolism leading to phenytoin toxicity
propranolol: Increased plasma levels of both drugs
thiazide diuretics: Possibly accentuate orthostatic hypotension

ACTIVITIES

alcohol use: Additive CNS depression

Adverse Reactions

CNS: Akathisia, altered temperature regulation, dizziness, drowsiness, extrapyramidal reactions (such as dystonia, pseudoparkinsonism, tardive dyskinesia)
CV: **Hypotension**, orthostatic hypotension, tachycardia
EENT: Blurred vision, dry mouth, nasal congestion, ocular changes, pigmentary retinopathy
ENDO: Galactorrhea, gynecomastia
GI: Constipation, epigastric pain, nausea, vomiting
GU: Dysuria, ejaculation disorders, menstrual irregularities, urine retention

SKIN: Decreased sweating, photosensitivity, pruritus, rash
Other: Weight gain

Childbearing Considerations

PREGNANCY

- Drug may cause fetal harm.
- Neonates exposed to drug during the third trimester of pregnancy are at risk for extrapyramidal and withdrawal symptoms after birth.
- Use with caution only if benefit to mother outweighs potential risk to fetus.

LACTATION

- Drug may be present in breast milk.
- Mothers should check with prescriber before breastfeeding.

Nursing Considerations

! **WARNING** Be aware that prochlorperazine shouldn't be used to treat dementia-related psychosis in the elderly because of increased mortality risk.

! **WARNING** Monitor patient's vital signs for signs of hypotension and tachycardia. Notify prescriber if present.

- Monitor patient closely for other adverse reactions that may be persistent, serious, or unusual.

PATIENT TEACHING

- Instruct patient how to administer oral form of prochlorperazine prescribed.

! **WARNING** Urge patient to avoid alcohol and over-the-counter drugs that may contain CNS depressants.

- Caution patient on long-term therapy not to stop prochlorperazine abruptly; doing so may lead to adverse reactions, such as nausea, trembling, and vomiting.
- Advise patient to rise slowly from lying and sitting positions to minimize effects of orthostatic hypotension.
- Urge patient to avoid hazardous activities because of the risk of drowsiness and impaired judgment and coordination until effects are known and resolved.
- Instruct patient to avoid excessive sun exposure and to wear sunscreen outdoors.
- Urge patient to notify prescriber about involuntary movements and restlessness.
- Advise pregnant patient to alert prescriber when entering her third trimester.

progestins

levonorgestrel

medroxyprogesterone acetate

Alti-MPA (CAN), Provera

megestrol acetate

Megace OS (CAN)

norethindrone acetate

progesterone

Crinone, PMS-Progesterone (CAN), Prometrium

Class and Category

Pharmacologic class: Progesterone hormone
Therapeutic class: Ovarian hormone replacement

Indications and Dosages

✷ *As adjunct to treat metastatic renal cancer*

I.M. INJECTION (MEDROXYPROGESTERONE)

Adults. *Initial:* 400 mg to 1 g every wk until improvement and stabilization. *Maintenance:* 400 mg or more every mo.

✷ *To treat metastatic breast cancer*

TABLETS (MEGESTROL)

Adults. 40 mg 4 times daily.

✷ *As adjunct to treat metastatic endometrial cancer*

TABLETS (MEGESTROL)

Adult females. 40 to 320 mg daily in divided doses.

P

I.M. INJECTION (MEDROXYPROGESTERONE)

Adults. *Initial:* 400 mg to 1 g every wk until improvement and stabilization. *Maintenance:* 400 mg or more every mo.

* *To treat anorexia, cachexia, or significant weight loss in patients who have AIDS*

SUSPENSION (MEGESTROL)

Adults. 625 mg (5 ml) daily.

* *To treat endometriosis*

TABLETS (NORETHINDRONE ACETATE)

Adult females. *Initial:* 5 mg once daily for 2 wk, increased by 2.5 mg daily at 2-wk intervals to total dose of 15 mg daily. *Maintenance:* 15 mg daily for 6 to 9 mo unless temporarily discontinued because of break through menstrual bleeding.

* *To treat secondary amenorrhea*

TABLETS (MEDROXYPROGESTERONE)

Adult females. 5 to 10 mg once daily for 5 to 10 days, starting anytime during menstrual cycle.

TABLETS (NORETHINDRONE ACETATE)

Adult females. 2.5 to 10 mg once daily for 5 to 10 days during last half of menstrual cycle.

CAPSULES, TABLETS (PROGESTERONE)

Adult females. 400 mg daily at bedtime for 10 days.

I.M. INJECTION (PROGESTERONE)

Adult females. 5 to 10 mg daily for 6 to 8 consecutive days.

VAGINAL GEL (PROGESTERONE)

Adult females. 45 mg (1 applicatorful of 4% vaginal gel) every other day for up to 6 doses. Dosage increased, as needed, to 90 mg (1 applicatorful of 8% vaginal gel) every other day for up to 6 doses.

* *To treat dysfunctional uterine bleeding*

TABLETS (MEDROXYPROGESTERONE)

Adult females. 5 to 10 mg daily for 5 to 10 days, starting on day 16 or 21 of menstrual cycle.

TABLETS (NORETHINDRONE ACETATE)

Adult females. 2.5 to 10 mg daily for 5 to 10 days during last half of menstrual cycle.

I.M. INJECTION (PROGESTERONE)

Adult females. 5 to 10 mg daily for 6 consecutive days.

* *To reduce endometrial hyperplasia in nonhysterectomized postmenopausal women receiving daily oral conjugated estrogen therapy*

TABLETS (MEDROXYPROGESTERONE)

Postmenopausal women with intact uterus. 5 to 10 mg for 12 to 14 consecutive days each mo, either beginning on day 1 of the cycle or day 16 of the cycle.

CAPSULES, TABLETS (PROGESTERONE)

Postmenopausal women with intact uterus. 200 mg once a day at bedtime for 12 consecutive days per 28-day cycle.

* *To prevent pregnancy (postcoital)*

TABLETS (LEVONORGESTREL)

Adult and adolescent females. 0.75 mg as soon as possible within 72 hr of intercourse. Second dose given 12 hr later.

Drug Administration

- Drug is a hazardous drug requiring safe handling and disposal precautions.
- Pregnant women should avoid exposure to drug.

P.O.

- Administer tablets and capsules with a full glass of water.
- Administer progesterone at night because it can make patient dizzy or drowsy.
- Shake container vigorously for at least 1 min for oral suspension form. Use a calibrated device to measure dose. Store at room temperature.

I.M.

- Shake suspension container vigorously for at least 1 min before withdrawing dose.
- Use a 1½-inch, 22 G needle for injection.
- Stretch the injection site with thumb and index finger and insert needle quickly using a rapid dart like motion into the upper-outer quadrant of the buttock. Inject slowly, over 5 to 7 sec. Pat site lightly after injection; don't rub it for medroxyprogesterone administration; massage area in a circular motion after progesterone administration.
- Rotate sites.

VAGINAL

- Remove applicator from sealed wrapper. Grip applicator firmly by thick end and shake it down like a thermometer to ensure that the contents are at the thin end.
- Twist tab off and discard.
- Insert thin end of applicator gently into the vagina while patient is in a sitting position or lying on her back with knees bent.

- Press thick end of applicator firmly to deposit gel.
- Remove applicator and discard.

Route	Onset	Peak	Duration
P.O.	Unknown	3 hr	Unknown
I.M.	Rapid	Unknown	3–4 hr
Vaginal	Unknown	Unknown	Unknown

Half-life: 5–20 min

Mechanism of Action

May diminish response to endogenous hormones in tumor cells by decreasing the number of steroid hormone receptors, causing a direct antiproliferative or cytotoxic effect on cell cycle growth and increased terminal cell differentiation. Decreases adrenal production of androstenedione and estradiol by some progestins given at higher dosages, which may decrease estrogen- or testosterone-sensitive tumors. Stimulation of appetite and metabolic effects by Megestrol promotes weight gain. Binding of progestins to cytosolic receptors that are loosely bound in cell nucleus also increases protein synthesis and improves cachexia.

Reduces availability or stability of hormone receptor complex, shuts off estrogen-responsive genes, or causes negative feedback mechanism that decreases number of functioning estrogen receptors through progestins effect on other hormones, especially estrogen. These actions allow menstrual cycle to function normally, alleviating amenorrhea and dysfunctional uterine bleeding and inducing menses. Acts also to transform proliferative uterine endometrium into a more differentiated, secretory one, which is the basis for using medroxyprogesterone to treat some types of amenorrhea. Remember that in a normal ovulatory cycle not resulting in pregnancy, decline in progesterone secretion caused by degeneration of corpus luteum in late luteal phase results in endometrial sloughing. A similar sloughing occurs after 5 to 10 days of medroxyprogesterone, provided that adequate estrogen-stimulated proliferation has occurred during follicular phase.

Inhibiting secretion of gonadotropins from the pituitary gland by levonorgestrel creates an atrophic endometrium, resulting in contraceptive effect.

Contraindications

Active thromboembolic disorder; disease; hypersensitivity to progestins, sesame oil/seeds (progesterone), or their components; known or suspected breast or genital cancer; missed abortion (progesterone); pregnancy; significant hepatic disease; thrombophlebitis; undiagnosed vaginal bleeding

Interactions

DRUGS

aminoglutethimide: Possibly decreased blood level of medroxyprogesterone

atazanavir, clarithromycin, indinavir, itraconazole, ketoconazole, nefazodone, nelfinavir, ritonavir, saquinavir, telithromycin, voriconazole: Possibly increased progestin level leading to potential for increased adverse reactions

barbiturates, including bosentan, carbamazepine, felbamate, griseofulvin, oxcarbazepine, phenytoin, primidone, rifampin, St. John's wort, topiramate: Possibly decreased effectiveness of progestin

CYP3A4 inhibitors, such as ketoconazole: Possibly increased bioavailability of progesterone

thyroid hormone: Decreased thyroid hormone effectiveness; increased thyroid hormonal levels

warfarin: Possibly increased INR

Adverse Reactions

CNS: Altered or reduced coordination or speech, depression, dizziness, drowsiness, fatigue, headache, irritability, migraine, mood changes, nervousness, postmenopausal dementia, syncope, unusual tiredness or weakness

CV: Fluid retention, **hypotension**, **thromboembolism**

ENDO: **Adrenal insufficiency or suppression**, **breast cancer**, breast pain or tenderness, Cushing's syndrome, decreased T_3 resin uptake, delayed return of fertility in women, elevated thyroid-binding globulin, galactorrhea, hyperglycemia

EENT: Gingival bleeding, swelling, or tenderness; vision changes or loss

GI: Abdominal cramps or pain, cholestatic jaundice, diarrhea, nausea, vomiting

GU: Amenorrhea, breakthrough bleeding or menometrorrhagia, changes in cervical erosion and secretions, decreased libido, hypermenorrhea, ovarian enlargement, or cysts

HEME: **Clotting and bleeding abnormalities**
MS: Back pain, decreased bone density, osteoporosis, osteoporotic fractures
RESP: **Acute eosinophilic pneumonia** (progesterone in sesame oil), dyspnea
SKIN: Acne, alopecia, dermal edema, hirsutism, melasma, pruritus, rash, urticaria
Other: **Anaphylaxis**; **angioedema**; hot flashes; injection-site irritation, pain, or redness; numbness or pain in arm, chest, or leg; weight gain or loss

Childbearing Considerations

PREGNANCY

- Drug may cause fetal harm.
- Drug is contraindicated in pregnancy. If pregnancy occurs, drug should be discontinued immediately.

LACTATION

- Drug is present in breast milk in small amounts.
- A decision may have to be made to discontinue breastfeeding or the drug to avoid potential serious adverse reactions in the breastfed infant.

Nursing Considerations

- Be aware that progestin/estrogen therapy shouldn't be used to prevent cardiovascular disease or dementia.

! **WARNING** Use progestins cautiously in patients with risk factors for arterial vascular disease, such as diabetes mellitus, hypercholesterolemia, hypertension, obesity, systemic lupus erythematosus, tobacco use, or a family or personal history of venous thromboembolism. Drug worsens these conditions. Monitor patient closely.

! **WARNING** Use progestins cautiously in patients who have CNS disorders, such as depression or seizures because progestins may worsen these conditions. Monitor patient closely.

! **WARNING** Monitor patient for a hypersensitivity reaction, which could become life-threatening, such as anaphylaxis or angioedema. If present, notify prescriber, expect drug to be discontinued, and provide supportive care, as needed and ordered.

! **WARNING** Be aware that acute eosinophilic pneumonia may occur in patients receiving progesterone in sesame oil intramuscularly. Monitor patient for dyspnea with hypoxic respiratory insufficiency and fever that may occur 2 to 4 weeks after patient starts progesterone in sesame oil therapy. If this reaction is suspected, notify prescriber and expect drug to be discontinued immediately.

! **WARNING** Notify prescriber immediately if patient develops signs of thrombotic events. Expect to discontinue progestin if such signs occur and provide emergency care, as ordered.

! **WARNING** Monitor patient for adrenal suppression, especially with megestrol therapy. If suspected, notify prescriber.

! **WARNING** Expect to stop progestin therapy in any woman who develops evidence of cancer; cardiovascular disease, such as CVA, MI, pulmonary embolism, or venous thrombosis; or dementia.

PATIENT TEACHING

! **WARNING** Explain risks of progestin therapy before therapy is begun, including breast, endometrial, or ovarian cancer; cardiovascular disease; dementia; and gallbladder disease, especially in postmenopausal women.

- Instruct patient how to use the oral form of progestin prescribed.

! **WARNING** Alert patient that drug may cause an allergic reaction. If an allergic reaction occurs, tell patient to notify prescriber immediately, and, if severe, to seek immediate medical care.

! **WARNING** Advise patient receiving progesterone intramuscularly that drug contains sesame oil, which can cause a serious respiratory condition. Tell patient this adverse reaction usually occurs 2 to 4 weeks after progesterone therapy is initiated. Urge patient to report difficulty breathing and fever to prescriber immediately.

- Instruct females of childbearing age to notify prescriber if uterine bleeding continues longer than 3 months or if menstruation is delayed by 45 days.

> **! WARNING** Warn females of childbearing age taking progestin for noncontraceptive purposes to use a contraceptive method to prevent pregnancy because drug may harm fetus. Stress importance of notifying prescriber immediately if she misses a period.

- Caution females of childbearing age who vomit within 1 hour of taking progestin for emergency contraception to contact prescriber about whether to repeat dose.

> **! WARNING** Instruct patient of the importance of seeking immediate medical care if patient experiences chest pain, coughing up blood, feeling faint or lightheaded, or has shortness of breath or develops pain, redness, and swelling in a lower extremity.

- Direct patient to alert all prescribers about progestin therapy because certain blood tests may be affected.
- Emphasize importance of good dental hygiene and regular dental checkups because elevated progestin level increases growth of normal oral flora, which may lead to gum tenderness, bleeding, or swelling.
- Encourage mothers wishing to breastfeed to discuss with prescriber before doing so as breastfeeding may adversely affect the breastfed infant.

promethazine hydrochloride

Promethegan

Class and Category

Pharmacologic class: Phenothiazine
Therapeutic class: Antiemetic, antihistamine, antivertigo, sedative-hypnotic

Indications and Dosages

✱ To prevent or treat motion sickness

SUPPOSITORIES, SYRUP, TABLETS

Adults. 25 mg 30 to 60 min before travel and repeated 8 to 12 hr later, as needed. Then, on succeeding days, 25 mg twice daily, once upon arising and again before evening meal, as needed.
Children ages 2 and older. 12.5 to 25 mg before travel and repeated every 12 hr, as needed.

✱ To prevent or treat nausea and vomiting in certain types of anesthesia and surgery

SYRUP, TABLETS

Adults. *Initial:* 12.5 to 25 mg every 4 to 6 hr, as needed. *Maximum:* 150 mg daily.
Children ages 2 and older. 1.1 mg/kg/dose (maximum 25 mg/dose) every 4 to 6 hr, as needed.

I.M. INJECTION, I.V. INFUSION

Adults. 12.5 to 25 mg every 4 to 6 hr, as needed. *Maximum:* 150 mg daily. I.V. infused slowly over 10 to 15 min.

I.M. INJECTION

Children ages 2 and older. 1.1 mg/kg (maximum half of adult dose), as needed.

SUPPOSITORIES

Adults. 12.5 to 25 mg every 4 to 6 hr, as needed. *Maximum:* 150 mg daily.
Children ages 2 and older. 1.1 mg/kg/dose (maximum half of adult dose) every 4 to 6 hr, as needed.

✱ To treat signs and symptoms of allergic response

SUPPOSITORIES, SYRUP, TABLETS

Adults and adolescents. 12.5 mg 4 times daily before meals and at bedtime, as needed. Or, 25 mg at bedtime, as needed.
Children ages 2 and older. 6.25 to 12.5 mg 3 times daily, as needed. Or, 25 mg at bedtime, as needed.

I.M. INJECTION, I.V. INFUSION

Adults. 25 mg repeated within 2 hr, as needed. I.V. infused slowly over 10 to 15 min.

✱ As an adjunct to analgesics for preoperative or postoperative sedation

I.M. INJECTION, I.V. INFUSION, SUPPOSITORIES, SYRUP, TABLETS

Adults. 25 to 50 mg as a single dose. I.V. infused slowly over 10 to 15 min.

SUPPOSITORIES, SYRUP, TABLETS

Children ages 2 and older. 1.1 mg/kg as a single dose. *Maximum:* 25 mg/dose.

I.M. INJECTION

Children ages 2 and older. 1.1 mg/kg (maximum half of adult dose) as a single dose.

✱ To relieve apprehension and promote nighttime sleep

I.M. INJECTION, SYRUP, TABLETS, SUPPOSITORIES

Adults. 25 to 50 mg at bedtime.

±**DOSAGE ADJUSTMENT** For elderly patients, dosage usually decreased.

✱ *To provide obstetric sedation*

I.M. INJECTION, I.V. INFUSION

Adult and adolescent females. 25 to 50 mg for early stages of labor; 25 to 75 mg after labor is established, repeated once or twice every 4 hr, as needed. *Maximum:* 100 mg/24 hr. I.V. infused slowly over 10 to 15 min.

Drug Administration

P.O.

- Administer with food if GI irritation occurs.
- Use calibrated device to measure dosage of syrup.

I.V.

- Determine dose and withdraw required volume from ampule or vial and transfer into an infusion bag. Use a filter needle when withdrawing drug from the ampule.
- For adults, dilute 12.5 mg , 25 mg or 50 mg in 50 ml of Sodium Chloride Injection; dilute 75 mg in 100 ml of same solution. Concentration should not exceed 25 mg/ml.
- For children, dilute up to 25 mg in 25 ml of 0.9% Sodium Chloride Injection and 25 to 50 mg doses in 50 ml of same solution. Concentration should not exceed 1 mg/ml.
- Gently invert infusion bag.
- Check patency of the I.V. access site before administration as extravasation can be harmful.
- Avoid inadvertent intra-arterial injection because it can cause arteriospasm.
- Infusion best infused through a central line. Infuse through a running I.V. line. Use the port that is farthest from the patient's vein if a peripherial vein must be used. Do not administer peripherally through a hand or wrist I.V; a large vein should be used.
- For adults, infuse over 20 to 40 min at a rate not to exceed 2.5 ml/min for 12.5 to 50 mg doses and 5 ml/min for a 75 mg dose.
- For children, infuse at a maximum rate of 1.25 ml/min.
- Severe chemical irritation and damage to tissues, including gangrene, may occur at infusion site. Stop infusion immediately if patient complains of pain at infusion site and notify prescriber immediately.
- *Incompatibilities:* Other drugs or solutions (except for 0.9% Sodium Chloride)

I.M.

- Preferred route of parenteral administration.
- Inject deep into large muscle mass.
- Rotate sites.
- Avoid injecting drug subcutaneously; severe tissue damage and gangrene may develop.

P.R.

- If suppository is too soft for administration, place in refrigerator for 30 min or run suppository under cold water before removing wrapper.
- Store in refrigerator.

Route	Onset	Peak	Duration
P.O.	15–60 min	Unknown	4–8 hr
I.V.	3–5 min	Unknown	4–8 hr
I.M., P.R.	20 min	Unknown	4–8 hr

Half-life: 10–19 hr

Mechanism of Action

Competes with histamine for H_1-receptor sites, thereby antagonizing many histamine effects and reducing allergy signs and symptoms. Prevents motion sickness, nausea, and vertigo by acting centrally on medullary chemoreceptive trigger zone and by decreasing vestibular stimulation and labyrinthine function in the inner ear. Promotes sedation and relieves anxiety by blocking receptor sites in CNS, directly reducing stimuli to the brain.

Contraindications

Children under the age of 2; comatose state; hypersensitivity to promethazine, other phenothiazines, or their components; intra-arterial or subcutaneous injection (parenteral)

Interactions

DRUGS

anticholinergics: Possibly intensified anticholinergic adverse effects

CNS depressants: Additive CNS depression

epinephrine: Reversed vasopressor effect of epinephrine; increased risk of hypotension

MAO inhibitors: Increased risk of extrapyramidal effects

ACTIVITIES

alcohol use: Additive CNS depression

Adverse Reactions

CNS: Akathisia, CNS stimulation, confusion, dizziness, drowsiness, dystonia, euphoria, excitation, fatigue, hallucinations, hysteria, incoordination, insomnia, irritability, nervousness, **neuroleptic malignant syndrome**, paradoxical stimulation, pseudoparkinsonism, restlessness, sedation, **seizures**, syncope, tardive dyskinesia, tremor
CV: **Bradycardia**, hypertension, **hypotension**, tachycardia
EENT: Blurred vision; diplopia; dry mouth, nose, and throat; nasal congestion; tinnitus; vision changes
ENDO: Hyperglycemia
GI: Anorexia, cholestatic jaundice, ileus, nausea, rectal burning or stinging (suppository form), vomiting
GU: Dysuria
HEME: **Agranulocytosis**, **leukopenia**, **thrombocytopenia**, **thrombocytopenic purpura**
RESP: **Apnea**, **respiratory depression**, tenacious bronchial secretions
SKIN: Dermatitis, diaphoresis, photosensitivity, rash, urticaria
Other: **Angioedema**, paradoxical reactions, severe injection site reactions (including gangrene)

Childbearing Considerations

PREGNANCY

- It is not known if drug can cause fetal harm. However, drug should not be used within 2 wk of delivery due to potential inhibition of platelet aggregation in the newborn.
- Use with caution only if benefit to mother outweighs potential risk to fetus.

LACTATION

- It is not known if drug is present in breast milk.
- A decision may have to be made to discontinue breastfeeding or the drug to avoid potential serious adverse reactions in the breastfed infant.

Nursing Considerations

! **WARNING** Use promethazine cautiously in children and elderly patients because they may be more sensitive to its effects, patients with cardiovascular disease or hepatic dysfunction because of potential adverse effects, patients with asthma because of anticholinergic effects, and patients with seizure disorders or those who take drugs that may affect seizure threshold because drug may lower seizure threshold.

! **WARNING** Monitor infusion or injection site closely because severe tissue injury, including gangrene can occur with parenteral administration. Stop infusion immediately if patient complains of pain at infusion site. Notify prescriber immediately of any abnormalities at infusion or injection site.

! **WARNING** Monitor patient for a hypersensivity reaction, which may become life-threatening, such as angioedema. If present, notify prescriber, expect drug to be discontinued, and provide supportive care, as needed and ordered.

! **WARNING** Monitor respiratory function because drug may suppress cough reflex and cause thickening of bronchial secretions, aggravating such conditions as asthma and COPD. Rarely, it may depress respirations and induce apnea.

! **WARNING** Monitor patient's hematologic status as ordered because promethazine may cause bone marrow depression, especially when used with other known marrow-toxic agents. Assess patient for signs and symptoms of infection or bleeding.

! **WARNING** Monitor patient for evidence of neuroleptic malignant syndrome, such as fever, hypertension or hypotension, involuntary motor activity, mental changes, muscle rigidity, tachycardia, and tachypnea. Be prepared to provide supportive treatment and drug therapy, as needed and ordered.

- Be aware that patient shouldn't have intradermal allergen tests within 72 hours of receiving promethazine because drug may significantly alter flare response.

PATIENT TEACHING

- Instruct patient how to administer oral form of promethazine prescribed. Tell patients receiving drug parenterally that it will be given either as an I.M. injection or I.V. infusion.
- Urge patient to avoid alcohol and other CNS depressants during therapy.

- Advise patient to avoid over-the-counter drugs unless approved by prescriber.
- Stress importance of patient alerting staff if pain occurs at I.V. site, if drug is administered intravenously.

! **WARNING** Alert patient drug may cause an allergic reaction. Tell patient to notify prescriber, if present, and, if severe, to seek immediate medical care.

! **WARNING** Stress importance of seeking immediate medical care if difficulty breathing occurs.

- Instruct patient to notify prescriber immediately if she has involuntary movements and restlessness.

! **WARNING** Tell patient to notify prescriber if other persistent, serious, or unusual adverse reactions occur.

- Instruct patient to avoid hazardous activities until drug's CNS effects are known and resolved.
- Suggest rinsing mouth and use of sugarless gum or hard candy to relieve dry mouth.
- Urge patient to avoid excessive sun exposure and to use sunscreen when outdoors.
- Inform mothers breastfeeding should not be undertaken while receiving drug or drug will have to be discontinued.

propafenone hydrochloride

Rythmol SR

Class and Category

Pharmacologic class: Sodium channel antagonist

Therapeutic class: Class IC antiarrhythmic

Indications and Dosages

* *To treat life-threatening ventricular arrhythmias; to prolong time of recurrence of paroxysmal supraventricular tachycardia associated with disabling symptoms in patients without structural heart disease*

TABLETS

Adults. *Initial:* 150 mg every 8 hr; after 3 or 4 days, increased to 225 mg every 8 hr as needed; after an additional 3 or 4 days, further increased to 300 mg every 8 hr, as needed. *Maximum:* 900 mg daily.

* *To prolong time of recurrence of symptomatic atrial fibrillation/flutter in patients with episodic (paroxysmal or persistent) atrial fibrillation who do not have structural heart disease*

TABLETS

Adults. Initial: 150 mg every 8 hr; after 3 or 4 days, increased to 225 mg every 8 hr, as needed; after an additional 3 or 4 days, further increased to 300 mg every 8 hr, as needed. *Maximum:* 900 mg daily.

E.R. CAPSULES

Adults. *Initial:* 225 mg every 12 hr, increased after 5 or more days to 325 mg every 12 hr, as needed, and further increased to 425 mg every 12 hr, as needed.

± **DOSAGE ADJUSTMENT** For patients with hepatic impairment, second- or third-degree AV block, or significant widening of the QRS complex, dosage may have to be reduced.

Drug Administration

P.O.

- E.R. capsules should be swallowed whole and not chewed, crushed, or opened.
- If a dose is missed, administer next dose at the normal scheduled time. Do not double dose to make up for missed dose.

Route	Onset	Peak	Duration
P.O.	Unknown	2–3.5 hr	Unknown
P.O./E.R.	Unknown	3–8 hr	Unknown

Half-life: 2–10 hr

Mechanism of Action

Prolongs recovery period after myocardial repolarization by inhibiting sodium influx through myocardial cell membranes and prolonging the refractory period, causing myocardial automaticity, excitability, and conduction velocity to decline.

Contraindications

Bronchospastic disorders, such as asthma; Brugada syndrome; cardiogenic shock; concurrent use of both a CYP2D6 inhibitor and a CYP3A4 inhibitor (Rythmol SR); electrolyte imbalances; heart failure (uncontrolled); hypersensitivity to propafenone or its components; severe hypotension or obstructive pulmonary disease; sinus bradycardia or AV conduction disturbances (without artificial pacemaker)

Interactions

DRUGS

amiodarone: Possibly altered cardiac conduction and repolarization
cimetidine, fluoxetine: Possibly increased blood propafenone level
CYP2D6 inhibitors and CYP3A4 inhibitors combined: Significantly increased concentration of propafenone, increasing risk of proarrhythmias and other adverse reactions
digoxin: Increased risk of digitalis toxicity
haloperidol, imipramine, venlafaxine: Possibly increased levels of these drugs
lidocaine: Possibly increased CNS adverse effects of lidocaine
metoprolol, propranolol: Increased blood level and half-life of these drugs
orlistat: Possibly decreased absorption of propafenone
quinidine: Decreased propafenone metabolism
rifampin: Possibly decreased propafenone level
warfarin: Increased blood warfarin level and risk of bleeding

FOODS

grapefruit juice: Possibly increased blood propafenone level

Adverse Reactions

CNS: Anxiety, depression, dizziness, fatigue, headache, somnolence, tremor, weakness
CV: Angina, **atrial flutter**, **AV block**, **bradycardia**, chest pain, edema, **heart failure**, **hypotension**, **irregular heartbeat**, palpitations, **prolonged QT interval**, tachycardia, **ventricular arrhythmias**, **worsened supraventricular arrhythmias**
EENT: Altered taste, blurred vision, dry mouth
GI: Constipation, diarrhea, flatulence, nausea, vomiting
GU: Decreased sperm count, hematuria
HEME: **Agranulocytosis**
MS: Muscle weakness
RESP: Dyspnea, rales, upper respiratory tract infection, wheezes
SKIN: Ecchymosis, rash
Other: Elevated blood alkaline phosphatase, exacerbation of myasthenia gravis, flu-like symptoms, positive ANA titers

Childbearing Considerations

PREGNANCY

- It is not known if drug can cause fetal harm. However, other antiarrhythmic agents have caused fetal/neonatal arrhythmias when given during pregnancy.
- Fetal/neonatal monitoring for arrhythmia is recommended during and after drug therapy in pregnant women.
- Use with caution only if benefit to mother outweighs potential risk to fetus.

LABOR AND DELIVERY

- Increased risk of arrhythmias during labor and delivery.

LACTATION

- Drug is present in breast milk.
- Mothers should check with prescriber before breastfeeding.

REPRODUCTION

- Drug may transiently impair spermatogenesis in male patients.

Nursing Considerations

- Assess patient for electrolyte imbalances, such as hyperkalemia, before starting propafenone. If present, expect to treat, as ordered, to reduce risk of adverse cardiac reactions.

! **WARNING** Use propafenone cautiously in patients with heart failure or myocardial dysfunction because drug may further depress myocardial contractility.

- Monitor ECG tracings, blood pressure, and pulse rate, particularly at start of therapy and with dosage increases. Expect propafenone to be discontinued if Brugada syndrome is confirmed with ECG changes.
- Anticipate fetal/neonatal monitoring for arrhythmia during and after drug therapy has been given to mother.

! **WARNING** Monitor patients with renal impairment closely because about 50% of the drug's metabolites are excreted in the urine, increasing risk of propafenone overdose.

! **WARNING** Monitor patient for signs of infection, such as chills, fever, or sore throat because propafenone may cause agranulocytosis, particularly during the initial 3 months of therapy. If present, notify prescriber.

PATIENT TEACHING

- Instruct patient how to administer form of propafenone prescribed and what to do if a dose is missed.
- Advise patient not to stop propafenone or change dosage without asking prescriber.

! WARNING Tell patient to notify prescriber promptly of any signs of infection, such as fever, sore throat, or chills.

! WARNING Tell patient to notify prescriber if persistent, severe, or unusual adverse reactions occur.

- Advise patient to avoid hazardous activities until drug's CNS effects are known and resolved.
- Urge patient to increase fluid intake and dietary fiber if she becomes constipated.
- Explain that drug may cause an unusual taste. Advise patient to notify prescriber if taste interferes with compliance.
- Urge patient to carry medical identification showing that she takes propafenone.

propofol
(disoprofol)
Diprivan

Class and Category
Pharmacologic class: Phenol derivative
Therapeutic class: Sedative-hypnotic

Indications and Dosages
∗ *To provide sedation for critically ill patients in intensive care who are intubated and mechanically ventilated*

I.V. INFUSION

Adults. *Initial:* 5 mcg/kg/min (0.3 mg/kg/hr), increased in increments of 5 to 10 mcg/kg/min (0.3 mg/kg/hr to 0.6 mg/kg/hr) greater than every 5 min until desired level of sedation is achieved. *Maintenance:* 5 to 50 mcg/kg/min (0.3 mg/kg/hr to 3 mg/kg/hr) or higher. *Maximum:* 4 mg/kg/hr.

Drug Administration
I.V.

- Consult prescriber about pretreating injection site with 1 ml of 1% lidocaine to minimize pain, burning, or stinging that may occur. If ordered, lidocaine shouldn't be added to propofol solution in quantities greater than 20 mg lidocaine/200 mg propofol because emulsion may become unstable.
- Give drug through a larger vein in forearm or antecubital fossa to minimize injection-site discomfort.
- Inspect drug for particulate matter and discoloration prior to administration. Don't use if drug appears to have excessive aggregation or creaming, if large droplets are visible, or if there are other forms of separation.
- Drug is provided as a ready-to-use formulation. However, if dilution is necessary, it should only be diluted with 5% Dextrose Injection and not diluted to a concentration less than 2 mg/ml because it is an emulsion. In diluted form, drug is more stable when in contact with glass rather than with plastic.
- Follow strict aseptic technique. Disinfect the vial rubber stopper with 70% isopropyl alcohol. Use a sterile vent spike and sterile tubing to administer drug. Keep number of I.V. manipulations to a minimum.
- Shake container well before using. Once vial has been spiked, administration should begin and must be completed within 12 hr. Discard tubing and any unused drug after 12 hr.
- Don't infuse drug through filter with a pore size of less than 5 microns; doing so could cause emulsion to break down.
- Use a drop counter syringe pump, or volumetric pump to safely control infusion rate.
- Protect solution from light.
- *Incompatibilities:* Blood and plasma, other I.V. drugs

Route	Onset	Peak	Duration
I.V.	15–30 sec	Unknown	3–10 min

Half-life: 2–10 min

Mechanism of Action
Decreases cerebral blood flow, cerebral metabolic oxygen consumption, and intracranial pressure and increases cerebrovascular resistance, which may play a role in propofol's hypnotic effects.

Contraindications

Hypersensitivity to propofol or its components, to eggs or egg products, or to soybeans or soy products

Interactions

DRUGS

CNS depressants, such as barbiturates, benzodiazepines, chloral hydrate, droperidol, fentanyl, meperidine, morphine: Additive CNS depressant, respiratory depressant, and hypotensive effects; possibly decreased emetic effects of opioids
nitrous oxide, opioids, potent inhalational agents (enflurane, halothane, isoflurane): Increased anesthetic, cardiorespiratory, or sedative effects of propofol
valproate: Increased blood levels of propofol increasing risk of cardiorespiratory depression and sedation

ACTIVITIES

alcohol use: Additive CNS depressant, respiratory depressant, and hypotensive effects

Adverse Reactions

CV: **Bradycardia**, **hypotension**
GI: Nausea, vomiting
MS: Involuntary muscle movement (transient)
RESP: **Apnea**
Other: **Anaphylaxis**, injection-site burning, pain, or stinging

Childbearing Considerations

PREGNANCY

- It is not known if drug can cause fetal harm but drug exposure during the third trimester may adversely affect brain development.
- Use with caution only if benefit to mother outweighs potential risk to fetus.

LABOR AND DELIVERY

- Drug is not recommended for obstetrics, including cesarean section deliveries because drug may cause neonatal nervous and respiratory system depression at birth.

LACTATION

- Drug is present in breast milk.
- Mothers should check with prescriber before breastfeeding after her condition has stabilized.

Nursing Considerations

! **WARNING** Know that repeated or lengthy (greater than 3 hours) use of sedation drugs, such as propofol should be avoided, if possible, in pregnant females during their third trimester because the combined use may affect the development of children's brains.

! **WARNING** Use propofol cautiously in patients with cardiac disease, peripheral vascular disease, impaired cerebral circulation, or increased intracranial pressure because drug may aggravate these disorders.

! **WARNING** Monitor patient for propofol infusion syndrome, especially with prolonged high-dose infusions. It may cause severe metabolic acidosis, hyperkalemia, lipemia, rhabdomyolysis, hepatomegaly and cardiac and renal failure. Alert prescriber at once and be prepared to provide emergency supportive care as needed and ordered.

! **WARNING** Monitor patient for a hypersensitivity reaction, which could become life-threatening, such as anaphylaxis. If present, notify prescriber immediately and provide supportive care, as needed and ordered.

! **WARNING** Know that dosage must be tapered before stopping therapy. Stopping abruptly will cause rapid awakening, anxiety, agitation, and resistance to mechanical ventilation. Do not abruptly discontinue drug prior to weaning or daily evaluation of sedation levels.

PATIENT TEACHING

- Urge patient (if feasible to do so) and family or caregiver to voice concerns and ask questions before propofol administration.
- Inform patient (if feasible) and family or caregiver propofol will be administered intravenously.
- Reassure patient and family or caregiver that patient will be monitored closely during administration and that vital functions will be supported, as needed.

propranolol hydrochloride

Hemangeol, Inderal LA, Inderal XL, InnoPran XL

Class and Category

Pharmacologic class: Beta-adrenergic blocker
Therapeutic class: Antianginal, antiarrhythmic, antihypertensive, anti-MI, antimigraine, antitremor, hypertrophic cardiomyopathy, and pheochromocytoma therapy adjunct

Indications and Dosages

✷ *To manage hypertension*

E.R. CAPSULES (INDERAL LA)

Adults. *Initial:* 80 mg once daily, increased to 120 mg or higher until blood pressure is adequately controlled. *Maintenance:* 120 to 160 mg once daily. *Maximum:* 640 mg once daily.

XL CAPSULES (INDERAL XL, INNOPRANXL)

Adults. *Initial:* 80 mg once daily, increased, as needed, to 120 mg once daily. *Maximum:* 120 mg daily.

ORAL SOLUTION, TABLETS

Adults. *Initial:* 40 mg twice daily, increased, as needed. *Maintenance:* 80–240 mg every 8 to 12 hr. *Maximum:* 640 mg daily.

✷ *To reduce angina frequency and increase exercise tolerance in patients with chronic angina*

E.R. CAPSULES (INDERAL LA)

Adults. *Initial:* 80 mg once daily, increased at 3- to 7-day intervals, as needed. *Usual:* 160 mg once daily. *Maximum:* 320 mg once daily.

ORAL SOLUTION, TABLETS

Adults. 80 to 320 mg daily in divided doses 2, 3, or 4 times daily. *Maximum:* 320 mg/day in divided doses.

✷ *To control ventricular rate in patients with atiral fibrillation and a rapid ventircular response*

ORAL SOLUTION, TABLETS

Adults. 10 to 30 mg 3 or 4 times daily and adjusted, as needed.

✷ *To treat life-threatening cardiac arrhythmias*

I.V. INJECTION

Adults. 1 to 3 mg administered no greater than 1 mg/ml; repeated after 2 min and again after 4 hr, as needed.

✷ *To control essential tremor*

ORAL SOLUTION, TABLETS

Adults. *Initial:* 40 mg twice daily and adjusted, as needed. *Maintenance:* 120 to 320 mg/day in 2 to 3 divided doses. *Maximum:* 320 mg daily.

✷ *To prevent vascular migraine headaches*

E.R. CAPSULES (INDERAL LA)

Adults. *Initial:* 80 mg once daily, increased gradually to achieve optimal migraine prophylaxis. *Usual:* 160 to 240 mg once daily.

ORAL SOLUTION, TABLETS

Adults. *Initial:* 20 mg 4 times daily, increased gradually, as needed. *Maximum:* 240 mg daily.

✷ *As adjunct to treat hypertrophic subaortic stenosis*

ORAL SOLUTION, TABLETS

Adults. 20 to 40 mg 3 or 4 times daily before meals and at bedtime.

E.R. CAPSULES (INDERAL LA)

Adults. 80 to 160 mg once daily.

✷ *As adjunct to manage pheochromocytoma*

ORAL SOLUTION, TABLETS

Adults. *For operable tumors:* 60 mg in divided doses for 3 days before surgery, concurrently with an alpha-blocker. *For inoperable tumors:* 30 mg daily in divided doses concurrently with an alpha-blocker.

✷ *To reduce cardiovascular mortality in patients who have survived the acute phase of MI and are clinically stable*

ORAL SOLUTION, TABLETS

Adults. *Initial:* 40 mg 3 times daily for 1 mo, then increased to 60–80 mg 3 times daily, as tolerated. *Maintenance:* 180 to 240 mg daily in 2 to 4 divided doses. *Maximum:* 240 mg daily.

✷ *To treat proliferating infantile hemangioma requiring systemic therapy*

ORAL SOLUTION (HEMANGEOL)

Infants age 5 wk to 5 mo. *Initial:* 0.6 mg/kg twice daily for 1 wk followed by 1.1 mg/kg twice daily for 1 wk followed by maintenance dose. *Maintenance:* 1.7 mg/kg twice daily for 6 mo.

± **DOSAGE ADJUSTMENT** For elderly patients and patients with liver impairment, dosage may need to be decreased.

Drug Administration

- Obtain apical pulse and blood pressure before administering. If abnormal, withhold drug and notify prescriber.

P.O.

- Administer immediate-release tablets on an empty stomach.
- Administer immediate-release tablets and oral solution given twice daily at least 9 hr apart.
- Administer immediate-release tablets and oral solution used to treat hypertrophic subaortic stenosis before meals and at bedtime.
- Administer Hemangeol oral solution doses used to treat proliferating infantile hemangioma at least 9 hr apart during or after feeding. Do not shake oral solution before use. Administer directly into the child's mouth using the oral dosing syringe. However, drug may be diluted in a small quantity of milk or fruit juice and given in a baby's bottle, as needed. If child spits up a dose or if you are not sure child has gotten all of the drug, do not give another dose. Wait until the next scheduled dose. Skip the dose if child is not eating or is vomiting. Discard any opened bottle of oral solution after 2 months. Monitor blood pressure and heart rate for 2 hr after first dose or after an increased dose.
- Administer E.R. capsules with or without food but be consistent. Administer at bedtime.
- Use a calibrated device to measure dosage of oral solution when giving oral solution other than Hemangeol oral solution. For Hemangeol oral solution use the oral dosing syringe that comes with the drug.
- Store drug at room temperature.

I.V.

- Be aware that I.V. dosage is much smaller than oral dosage.
- Give I.V. injection at no more than 1 mg/min. Do not administer as a continuous I.V. infusion.
- Monitor ECG continuously, as ordered, when giving I.V. injection. Have emergency drugs and equipment available in case of hypotension or cardiac arrest.
- Protect injection solution from light.
- *Incompatibilities:* None reported by manufacturer.

Route	Onset	Peak	Duration
P.O.	30 min	1–4 hr	6–12 hr
P.O./E.R.	Unknown	6–14 hr	24–27 hr
I.V.	Immediate	1 min	2–4 hr

Half-life: 3–6 hr

Mechanism of Action

Through beta-blocking action, propranolol:

- prevents arterial dilation and inhibits renin secretion, resulting in decreased blood pressure (in hypertension and pheochromocytoma) and relief of migraine headaches.
- decreases heart rate, which helps resolve tachyarrhythmias.
- improves myocardial contractility, which helps ease symptoms of hypertrophic cardiomyopathy.
- decreases myocardial oxygen demand, which helps prevent anginal pain and death of myocardial tissue.

In addition, peripheral beta-adrenergic blockade may play a role in propranolol's ability to alleviate tremor.

Contraindications

Bronchial asthma; cardiogenic shock; decompensated heart failure; greater than first-degree block, sick sinus syndrome, or sinus bradycardia unless a permanent pacemaker is in place; hypersensitivity to propranolol or any of its components

Interactions

DRUGS

alpha-blockers (prazosin): May cause prolongation of first dose hypotension and syncope
cholestyramine, colestipol: Significantly reduces plasma concentrations of propranolol, which may result in loss of effectiveness
clonidine: Possibly antagonized antihypertensive effects of clonidine
corticosteroids: Possibly increased risk of hypoglycemia
CYP1A2 inducers (montelukast, phenytoin), CYP2C19 inducers (rifampin): Decreased plasma levels of propranolol resulting in loss of effectiveness
CYP1A2 inhibitors (ciprofloxacin, enoximone, fluvoxamine), CYP2D6 inhibitors (bupropion, fluoxetine, paroxetine, quinidine): Increased

P

exposure to propranolol increasing risks of adverse reactions, such as bradycardia and hypotension
dobutamine: Reduced sensitivity to dobutamine stress echocardiography in patients undergoing evaluation for myocardial ischemia
MAO inhibitors, tricyclic antidepressants: Increased risk of significant hypertension
NSAIDs: Possibly decreased hypotensive effects
propafenone: Increased blood level and adverse reactions, such as bradycardia and postural hypotension
warfarin: Increased risk of bleeding

ACTIVITIES

alcohol: Possibly decreased or increased plasma propranolol level
nicotine chewing gum, smoking cessation, smoking deterrents: Possibly decreased therapeutic effects of propranolol

Adverse Reactions

CNS: Anxiety, depression, dizziness, drowsiness, fatigue, fever, insomnia, lethargy, nervousness, weakness
CV: **AV conduction disorders**, **bradycardia**, cold limbs, **heart failure**, **hypotension**
EENT: Dry eyes, **laryngospasm**, nasal congestion, pharyngitis
ENDO: **Hypoglycemia**
GI: Abdominal pain, constipation, diarrhea, nausea, vomiting
GU: Impotence, Peyronie's disease, sexual dysfunction
HEME: **Agranulocytosis**, nonthrombocytopenic purpura, **thrombocytopenic purpura**
MS: Muscle weakness, myopathy, myotonia
RESP: **Bronchospasm**, dyspnea, **respiratory distress**, wheezing
SKIN: Alopecia, **erythema multiforme**, erythematous rash, **exfoliative dermatitis**, psoriasiform rash, **Stevens-Johnson syndrome**, **toxic epidermal necrolysis**, urticaria
Other: **Anaphylaxis**, flu-like symptoms, systemic lupus-like reaction

Childbearing Considerations

PREGNANCY

- Drug may have the potential to cause fetal harm, such as congenital anomalies and intrauterine growth retardation.
- Use with caution only if benefit to mother outweighs potential risk to fetus.

LABOR AND DELIVERY

- Neonates born to mothers who received drug at parturition may exhibit bradycardia, hypoglycemia, and/or respiratory depression.
- Neonates need to be monitored closely for adverse effects.

LACTATION

- Drug is present in breast milk.
- Mothers should check with prescriber before breastfeeding.
- If breastfeeding occurs, monitor infant for low pulse rate or signs and symptoms of low blood glucose level as well as respiratory depression.

REPRODUCTION

- Drug may cause erectile dysfunction.

Nursing Considerations

! WARNING Use propranolol cautiously in patients with bronchospastic lung disease because it may induce asthmatic attack, and in patients with underlying skeletal muscle disease; isolated reports of myopathy and myotonia have occurred with propranolol use.

- Monitor blood pressure, apical and radial pulses, fluid intake and output, daily weight, respiration, and circulation in extremities before and during therapy.

! WARNING Know that because drug's negative inotropic effect can depress cardiac output, cardiac output should be monitored in patients with heart failure, particularly those with severely compromised left ventricular dysfunction.

! WARNING Monitor patient for a hypersensitivity reaction, which could become life-threatening, such as anaphylaxis. If present, notify prescriber, expect drug to be switched to another drug, and provide supportive care, as needed and ordered.

! WARNING Monitor patient for hypoglycemia, especially diabetic patient taking an antidiabetic drug because propranolol can prolong hypoglycemia or promote hyperglycemia. It also can mask signs of hypoglycemia, especially tachycardia, palpitations, and tremor, but it doesn't suppress diaphoresis or hypertensive response to hypoglycemia. When administering Hemangeol form to infant, monitor for signs and symptoms of hypoglycemia, which can occur at any time during treatment. Risk increased during poor oral food intake, presence of an infection, or vomiting or when glucose demands are increased such as during a cold, infection, or time of stress. If any of these situations occur, notify prescriber and expect to withhold drug. Treat hypoglycemia according to institutional protocol.

! WARNING Monitor patient for other persistent, severe, or unusual adverse reactions.

! WARNING Be aware that stopping drug abruptly, even for surgery, may cause MI, myocardial ischemia, severe hypertension, or ventricular arrhythmias, especially in patients with cardiac disease. However, be aware that the heart may not be able to respond to reflex adrenergic stimuli normally during surgery, which increases the risks of general anesthesia and surgical procedures. It also may cause increased intraocular pressure to return. Dosage should be reduced gradually.

! WARNING Know that propranolol can mask tachycardia in hyperthyroidism and that abrupt withdrawal in patients with hyperthyroidism or thyrotoxicosis can cause thyroid storm.

PATIENT TEACHING

- Instruct patient, family, or caregiver how to administer the propranolol product prescribed.
- Caution patient not to change dosage without consulting prescriber and not to stop taking drug abruptly.
- Advise smoker to notify prescriber immediately if she stops smoking because cessation may decrease drug metabolism, calling for dosage adjustments.

! WARNING Alert patient that drug may cause an allergic reaction. Tell patient to notify prescriber, if present, and to seek immediate medical care, if severe.

! WARNING Advise patient to notify prescriber immediately if she has shortness of breath, weight gain, or signs and symptoms of worsening heart failure.

! WARNING Instruct patient on signs and symptoms of hypoglycemia and how to treat, if present. Know that drug may mask signs and symptoms of hypoglycemia. Instruct family or caregiver administering Hemangeol form to infant to monitor for signs and symptoms of hypoglycemia, which can occur at any time during treatment. Warn family or caregiver that risk is increased during poor oral food intake, presence of an infection, or vomiting or when glucose demands are increased such as during a cold, infection, or time of stress. If any of these situations occur, family or caregiver should be told to withhold drug and notify prescriber.

! WARNING Stress importance of notifying prescriber of any other persistent, serious, or unusual adverse reactions.

! WARNING Tell breastfeeding mothers to monitor infant for low pulse rate or signs and symptoms of low blood glucose level as well as respiratory depression.

- Advise patient to consult prescriber before taking over-the-counter drugs, especially cold products.
- Urge patient to avoid hazardous activities until CNS effects of drug are known and resolved.
- Tell patient to notify prescriber if pregnancy occurs because drug may have to be discontinued.

pyridostigmine bromide

Mestinon, Mestinon-SR (CAN), Mestinon Timespans, Regonol

Class and Category

Pharmacologic class: Cholinesterase inhibitor
Therapeutic class: Muscle stimulant

Indications and Dosages

✶ *To treat symptoms of myasthenia gravis*

ORAL SOLUTION, TABLETS

Adults. Highly individualized. *Average dose:* 600 mg daily spaced to provide maximum relief when maximum strength is needed. *For mild symptoms:* 60 mg to 360 mg daily, spaced to provide maximum relief. *For severe symptoms:* As high as 1,500 mg daily, spaced to provide maximum relief.

E.R. TABLETS

Adults and adolescents. 180 to 540 mg once or twice daily (at least 6 hr between doses).

* *To reverse the effects of neuromuscular blockers*

I.V. INJECTION

Adults. 0.1 to 0.25 mg/kg no faster than 1 mg/min immediately before or with 0.6 to 1.2 mg of I.V. atropine.

± **DOSAGE ADJUSTMENT** For patients with renal impairment, dosage possibly reduced.

Drug Administration

P.O.

- Administer with a full glass of water or with food or milk if GI distress occurs.
- E.R. tablets should be swallowed whole and not chewed, crushed, or split.
- Use a calibrated device to measure dosage of oral solution.
- Store oral solution at room temperature. Store tablets in a dry place with silica gel enclosed.

I.V.

- Administer as an I. V. injection no faster than 1 mg/min.
- Keep atropine sulfate nearby for emergency use.
- *Incompatibilities:* Alkaline solutions

Route	Onset	Peak	Duration
P.O.	20–30 min	1–2 hr	3–4 hr
P.O. (E.R.)	30–60 min	1–2 hr	6–12 hr
I.V.	2–5 min	Unknown	2–4 hr

Half-life: 1–3 hr

Mechanism of Action

Improves muscle strength compromised by myasthenia gravis or neuromuscular blockade by competing with acetylcholine for its binding site on acetylcholinesterase thereby potentiating the effects of acetylcholine on skeletal muscle and the GI tract. Inhibited destruction of acetylcholine allows freer transmission of nerve impulses across the neuromuscular junction.

Contraindications

Hypersensitivity to pyridostigmine or its components, mechanical obstruction of GI or urinary tract

Interactions

DRUGS

4-aminopyridine: Delayed onset of action of pyridostigmine

aminoglycosides, bacitracin, colistin, magnesium salts, polymyxin B, sodium colistimethate, tetracyclines: Possible antagonized effects of pyridostigmine

quinidine: Possibly recurrent paralysis

Adverse Reactions

EENT: Increased salivation, lacrimation, miosis

GI: Abdominal cramps, diarrhea, increased peristalsis, nausea, vomiting

GU: Urinary frequency, incontinence, or urgency

MS: Fasciculations, muscle spasms or weakness

RESP: Increased tracheobronchial secretions

SKIN: Diaphoresis

Childbearing Considerations

PREGNANCY

- It is not known if drug may cause fetal harm.
- Use with caution only if benefit to mother outweighs potential risk to fetus.

LACTATION

- Drug may be present in breast milk.
- Mothers should check with prescriber before breastfeeding.

Nursing Considerations

! **WARNING** Maintain a rigid dosing schedule because a missed or late dose can precipitate myasthenic crisis.

- Observe for cholinergic reactions when administering drug I.V.

! **WARNING** Be aware that pyridostigmine overdose may obscure diagnosis of myasthenic crisis because main symptom in both is muscle weakness. Treat cholinergic crisis by stopping anticholinesterase, giving atropine as prescribed, and helping with endotracheal intubation and mechanical ventilation, if needed.

- Be aware that reversal of neuromuscular blockade usually occurs in 15 to 30 minutes. Be prepared to maintain patient airway and ventilation until normal voluntary respiration returns completely. Assess respiratory measurements and muscle tone with peripheral nerve stimulator device, as indicated.
- Monitor patients with renal disease because drug is mainly excreted unchanged by kidneys. Monitor BUN and serum creatinine levels.

PATIENT TEACHING

- Instruct patient how to administer oral form of pyridostigmine prescribed.

! **WARNING** Warn that a late or missed dose can precipitate a crisis. Suggest the use of a battery-operated alarm clock as a reminder.

- Ask patient to record pyridostigmine dosage, times taken, and drug effects to help determine optimal dosage and schedule.
- Urge patient to carry medical identification describing her condition and drug regimen.

Q R S

quetiapine fumarate

Seroquel, Seroquel XR

Class and Category

Pharmacologic class: Dibenzothiazepine derivative
Therapeutic class: Antipsychotic

Indications and Dosages

* *To treat schizophrenia*

TABLETS

Adults. *Initial:* 25 mg twice daily on day 1. Increased by 25 to 50 mg 2 or 3 times daily on days 2 and 3, then to 300 to 400 mg daily by day 4, in divided doses 2 or 3 times daily. Increased every 2 days or more in increments of 25 to 50 mg twice daily, as needed. *Usual:* 150 to 750 mg/day. *Maximum:* 750 mg daily.
Adolescents ages 13 to 17. *Initial:* 25 mg twice daily on day 1; 50 mg twice daily on day 2; 100 mg twice daily on day 3; 150 mg twice daily on day 4; and 200 mg twice daily on day 5. Increased further in increments no greater than 100 mg/day. *Usual:* 400 to 800 mg/day divided into 2 or 3 doses daily. *Maximum:* 800 mg daily.

E.R. TABLETS

Adults. *Initial:* 300 mg once daily. Dosage increased daily in increments up to 300 mg, as needed. *Usual:* 400 to 800 mg/day. *Maximum:* 800 mg once daily.
Adolescents ages 13 to 17. *Initial:* 50 mg once daily on day 1; 100 mg once daily on day 2; 200 mg once daily on day 3; 300 mg once daily on day 4; 400 mg once daily on day 5. Increased further in increments no greater than 100 mg/day, as needed. *Usual:* 400 to 800 mg/day. *Maximum:* 800 mg once daily.

* *To maintain schizophrenia therapy with monotherapy*

E.R. TABLETS

Adults. *Usual:* 400 to 800 mg daily after dosage has been titrated to usual dosage. *Maximum:* 800 mg daily.

* *To treat mania bipolar I as monotherapy or as an adjunct to lithium or divalproex*

TABLETS

Adults. *Initial:* 50 mg twice daily on day 1; 100 mg twice daily on day 2; 150 mg twice daily on day 3; and 200 mg twice daily on day 4. Increased in increments of no greater than 200 mg/day, as needed, by day 6. *Usual:* 400 to 800 mg/day. *Maximum:* 800 mg/day.

E.R. TABLETS

Adults. *Initial:* 300 mg once daily on day 1; 600 mg once daily on day 2; and between 400 and 800 mg once daily on day 3 and beyond. *Usual:* 400 to 800 mg once daily. *Maximum:* 800 mg once daily.

* *To treat mixed bipolar I disorder as monotherapy or as adjunct to lithium or divalproex*

E.R. TABLETS

Adults. *Initial:* 300 mg once daily on day1; 600 mg once daily on day 2; and between 400 and 800 mg once daily on day 3 and beyond. *Usual:* 400 to 800 mg once daily. *Maximum:* 800 mg once daily.

* *To treat pediatric mania bipolar I as monotherapy*

TABLETS

Children and adolescents ages 10 to 17. *Initial:* 25 mg twice daily on day 1; 50 mg twice daily on day 2; 100 mg twice daily on day 3; 150 mg twice daily on day 4, and 200 mg twice daily on day 5. Increased in no greater increments than 100 mg/day, as needed. *Usual:* 400 to 600 mg/day divided into 2 or 3 doses daily. *Maximum:* 600 mg/day.

E.R. TABLETS

Children and adolescents ages 10 to 17. *Initial:* 50 mg once daily on day 1; 100 mg once daily on day 2; 200 mg once daily on day 3; 300 mg once daily on day 4; and 400 mg once daily on day 5. *Usual:* 400 to 600 mg once daily. *Maximum:* 600 mg once daily.

* *To treat bipolar depression*

TABLETS

Adults. *Initial:* 50 mg on day 1; 100 mg on day 2; 200 mg on day 3; and 300 mg on day 4. *Maximum:* 300 mg/day.

E.R. TABLETS

Adults. *Initial:* 50 mg once daily on day 1; 100 mg once daily on day 2; 200 mg once daily on day 3; and 300 mg once daily on day 4. *Usual:* 300 mg once daily. *Maximum:* 300 mg once daily.

✶ *As adjunct to divalproex or lithium therapy as part of maintenance therapy for bipolar I disorder*

E.R. TABLETS, TABLETS

Adults. Continued on same dosage stabilized on with doses given twice daily totaling 400 to 800 mg once daily. *Maximum:* 800 mg once daily.

✶ *As adjunctive therapy with antidepressants to treat major depressive disorder*

E.R. TABLETS

Adults. *Initial:* 50 mg once daily on days 1 and 2 and 150 mg once daily on day 3. *Usual:* 150 to 300 mg once daily. *Maximum:* 300 mg once daily.

±**DOSAGE ADJUSTMENT** For patients with hepatic impairment, initial dosage no higher than 25 mg once daily for I.R. form and 50 mg once daily for E.R. form and increased in increments of 25 mg/day for I.R. form and 50 mg/day for E.R. form depending on response and tolerance. For elderly patients, initial dosage of either form reduced to 50 mg/day and dose increased in increments of 50 mg/day, as needed. For patients receiving CYP3A4 inducers (avasimibe, carbamazepine, phenytoin, rifampin, St. John's wort), dosage increased up to 5-fold of the original dose. When CYP3A4 inducer is discontinued, dosage reduced to original level within 7 to 14 days. For patients receiving CYP3A4 inhibitors (ketoconazole, indinavir, itraconazole, nefazodone, ritonavir), dosage reduced to one-sixth of original dose. When CYP3A4 drug is discontinued, dosage increased 6-fold.

Drug Administration

P.O.

- Administer I.R. tablets without regard to food intake; administer E.R. tablets without food or with a light meal of about 300 calories, preferably in the evening.
- E.R. tablets should be swallowed whole and not chewed, crushed, or divided.

Route	Onset	Peak	Duration
P.O.	Unknown	1.5 hr	Unknown
P.O./E.R.	Unknown	6 hr	Unknown

Half-life: 6–7 hr

Mechanism of Action

May produce antipsychotic effects by interfering with dopamine binding to dopamine type 2 (D_2)-receptor sites in the brain and by antagonizing serotonin 5-HT_2, dopamine type 1 (D_1), histamine H_1, and alpha$_1$-adrenergic and alpha$_2$-adrenergic receptors.

Contraindications

Hypersensitivity to quetiapine or its components

Interactions

DRUGS

anticholinergic drugs: Increased risk of severe gastrointestinal adverse reactions related to hypomotility
antihypertensives: Increased risk of hypotension
CNS depressants: Possibly increased CNS depression
CYP3A4 inducers (avasimibe, carbamazepine, phenytoin, rifampin, St. John's wort): Decreased exposure of quetiapine with decreased effectiveness
CYP3A4 inhibitors (ketoconazole, indinavir, itraconazole, nefazodone, ritonavir): Increased exposure of quetiapine increasing risk of adverse reactions
dopamine agonists, levodopa: Possibly antagonized effects of these drugs

ACTIVITIES

alcohol use: Possibly enhanced CNS depression

Adverse Reactions

CNS: Abnormal dreams, akathisia, anxiety, attention disturbance, confusion, depression, disorientation, dizziness, drowsiness, dystonia, extrapyramidal reactions, fatigue, hypertonia, **hypothermia**, irritability, lethargy, mental impairment, migraine, **neuroleptic malignant syndrome**, restless leg syndrome, motor and sensory instability, paresthesia, retrograde amnesia,

somnolence, **suicidal ideation**, tardive dyskinesia, tremor
CV: **Cardiomyopathy**, dyslipidemia, hypercholesterolemia, **hypotension**, increased heart rate, **myocarditis**, orthostatic hypotension, palpitations, **QT-interval prolongation**, tachycardia
EENT: Blurred vision, cataracts, dry mouth, ear pain, nasal congestion, pharyngitis, rhinitis, sinusitis
ENDO: Galactorrhea, hyperglycemia, **hyperosmolar coma**, hyperprolactinemia, hypothyroidism, **ketoacidosis**, syndrome of inappropriate ADH secretion
GI: Anorexia, constipation, dysphagia, **hepatitis**, ileus, indigestion, **intestinal obstruction**, **ischemic colon**, **liver necrosis or failure**, **pancreatitis**, vomiting
GU: Decreased libido, nocturnal enuresis, pollakiuria, UTI, urinary retention
HEME: **Agranulocytosis**, **leukopenia**, **neutropenia**, **thrombocytopenia**
MS: Back or neck pain, dysarthria, muscle spasms or weakness, myalgia, **rhabdomyolysis**
RESP: Cough, dyspnea, **sleep apnea**
SKIN: Acute generalized exanthematous pustulosis, cutaneous vasculitis, diaphoresis, **Stevens-Johnson syndrome**, **toxic epidermal necrolysis**
Other: **Anaphylaxis**, **drug reaction with eosinophilia and systemic symptoms (DRESS)**, flu-like symptoms, **hyponatremia**, weight gain

Childbearing Considerations

PREGNANCY

- Pregnancy exposure registry: 1-866 -961-2388 or http://womensmentalhealth.org/clinical-and-research-programs/pregnancyregistry/.
- Drug may cause fetal harm if exposed in the third trimester increasing risk for extrapyramidal and/or withdrawal symptoms following delivery.

LACTATION

- Drug is present in breast milk.
- Mothers should check with prescriber before breastfeeding.

REPRODUCTION

- Drug may increase prolactin levels, which may lead to a reversible reduction in fertility in female patients.

Nursing Considerations

! WARNING Know that quetiapine shouldn't be used for elderly patients with dementia-related psychosis because drug increases the risk of death in these patients.

! WARNING Know that quetiapine should not be given to patients who have a history of cardiac arrhythmias, such as bradycardia; patients with a family history of QT prolongation; or patients who experience hypokalemia or hypomagnesemia. The drug also should not be used with other drugs that prolong the QT interval or may cause an electrolyte imbalance or in a patient who has a congenital prolongation of the QT interval, congestive heart failure, or heart hypertrophy because quetiapine may increase the QT interval, which may increase the risk of torsades de pointes and/or sudden death. Be aware that elderly patients are also at a higher risk for QT interval to become prolonged.

! WARNING Monitor patients (particularly children and young adults) closely for suicidal tendencies, especially when therapy starts or dosage changes because depression may worsen temporarily during these times.

! WARNING Monitor patient for a hypersensitivity or severe skin reaction, which could become life-threatening, such as anaphylaxis or DRESS. If present (DRESS may only initially present with a fever or swollen lymph nodes), notify prescriber, expect drug to be discontinued, and provide supportive care, as needed and ordered.

- Monitor patient for prolonged abnormal muscle contractions, especially during the first few days of quetiapine therapy, in male patients and in younger patients.
- Monitor laboratory results during first 3 weeks of therapy for transient elevations in hepatic enzyme levels. Notify prescriber if they persist or worsen.

! WARNING Check CBC often during the first few months of therapy, as ordered, in patients with a low WBC count or a history of drug-induced hematologic problems. If counts drop or patient develops a fever or other signs of infection, notify prescriber, expect to discontinue drug, and provide supportive care.

! **WARNING** Monitor patient taking quetiapine for predisposing factors for neuroleptic malignant syndrome, such as dehydration, heat stress, organic brain disease, and physical exhaustion. Neuroleptic malignant syndrome includes altered mental status, autonomic instability (which may include arrhythmias, blood pressure abnormalities, diaphoresis, hyperpyrexia, irregular pulse, or tachycardia), and muscle rigidity.

- Monitor patient for signs of tardive dyskinesia, a potentially irreversible complication characterized by involuntary, dyskinetic movements of eyelids, face, jaw, mouth, or tongue. Notify prescriber if such signs develop because quetiapine therapy may have to be stopped.
- Monitor patient for orthostatic hypotension, especially during initial dosage titration period. Be prepared to correct underlying conditions, such as dehydration and hypovolemia, before starting quetiapine therapy, as prescribed. Also, monitor patient for an increase in blood pressure. Check blood pressure, especially in adolescents and children, at the beginning of and periodically during treatment.
- Assess patient for hypothyroidism because drug can cause dose-dependent decreases in total and free thyroxine (T_4) levels.
- Monitor patient's blood glucose and lipid levels routinely, as ordered, because drug increases the risk of hyperglycemia and hypercholesterolemia.

! **WARNING** Monitor patient for other persistent, serious, or unusual adverse reactions because drug can adversely affect many body systems.

- Institute fall precautions because patients receiving quetiapine have a greater risk of falling.
- Expect to gradually taper off quetiapine therapy when discontinued, as ordered, to avoid acute withdrawal symptoms such as insomnia, nausea, and vomiting.

PATIENT TEACHING

- Instruct patient how to administer form of quetiapine prescribed.
- Caution patient to avoid consuming alcoholic beverages because they can increase dizziness and drowsiness.
- Advise patient not to stop taking quetiapine suddenly because doing so may exacerbate his symptoms or produce withdrawal symptoms.

! **WARNING** Urge family or caregiver to watch patient closely for suicidal tendencies, especially when therapy starts or dosage changes and particularly if patient is a child or young adult.

! **WARNING** Alert patient that drug may cause an allergic reaction, including a serious skin reaction. At the first sign of a fever, rash, swollen lymph nodes, or other signs and symptoms of an allergy, tell patient to notify prescriber immediately and to seek immediate medical care.

! **WARNING** Urge patient to notify prescriber if a fever, flu-like symptoms, sore throat, or any other infection occurs, as drug may have to be discontinued and an evaluation for a potential infection be done.

! **WARNING** Advise patient to contact prescriber if his pulse rate becomes abnormally slow or irregular.

! **WARNING** Caution patient to avoid dehydration, exposure to extreme heat, or exercising strenuously because drug may disrupt body's ability to reduce body temperature.

- Inform patient that quetiapine therapy may cause dizziness or drowsiness. Advise him not to drive or perform other activities that require alertness until drug's full CNS effects are known and resolved. Also, review fall precautions with patient.
- Instruct patient to rise slowly from a lying or seated position to reduce the risk of dizziness or fainting.
- Encourage patient on long-term therapy to have regular eye examinations so that cataracts can be detected.

! **WARNING** Tell patient to alert prescriber of other persistent, serious, or unusual adverse ractions.

- Tell pregnant patients to alert prescriber when they are going to be entering their third trimester.
- Alert patient that a false-positive drug test for methadone or tricyclic antidepressants may occur with quetiapine use.

quinapril hydrochloride

Accupril

Class and Category

Pharmacologic class: Angiotensin-converting enzyme (ACE) inhibitor
Therapeutic class: Antihypertensive

Indications and Dosages

* *To treat hypertension*

TABLETS

Adults not on diuretics. *Initial:* 10 to 20 mg once daily, adjusted every 2 wk based on clinical response. *Maintenance:* 20 to 80 mg daily or in divided doses twice daily.
Adults on diuretics. *Initial:* 5 mg once daily, adjusted every 2 wk based on clinical response. *Maintenance:* 20 to 80 mg daily or in divided doses twice daily.

± **DOSAGE ADJUSTMENT** For patients with creatinine clearance of greater than 60 ml/min, initial dosage started at 10 mg daily. For patients with creatinine clearance of 30 to 60 ml/min, initial dosage reduced to 5 mg daily. For patients with creatinine clearance of 10 to 30 ml/min, initial dosage reduced to 2.5 mg daily. For elderly patients, initial dosage started at 10 mg once daily, then titrated slowly to optimal response.

* *As adjunct to manage heart failure*

TABLETS

Adults. *Initial:* 5 mg twice daily, increased, weekly, as needed and tolerated. *Maintenance:* 20 to 40 mg twice daily given in 2 equally divided doses.

± **DOSAGE ADJUSTMENT** For patients with creatinine clearance above 30 ml/min, initial dosage reduced to 5 mg daily. For patients with creatinine clearance of 10 to 30 ml/min, initial dosage reduced to 2.5 mg daily. If initial dosage is well tolerated, dosage increased to twice daily the following day with weekly dosage adjustments made, as needed.

Drug Administration

P.O.

- Administer with or without food but avoid giving with a high-fat meal because of decreased absorption.

Route	Onset	Peak	Duration
P.O.	1 hr	1–2 hr	24 hr

Half-life: 0.8–3 hr

Mechanism of Action

Blocks conversion of angiotensin I to angiotensin II, leading to vasodilation, and reduces aldosterone secretion, which prevents water retention. Reduces peripheral arterial resistance also. Reduction in blood pressure occurs as a result of these combined actions. Relieving fluid buildup in heart failure occurs as a result of a reduction of aldosterone secretion.

Contraindications

Aliskiren therapy in patients with diabetes; history of angioedema related to previous treatment with ACE inhibitor; hypersensitivity to quinapril or its components; use of a neprilysin inhibitor, such as sacubitril within 36 hr

Interactions

DRUGS

aliskiren (patients with diabetes and/or renal impairment), angiotensin receptor blockers, other ACE inhibitors: Increased risk of hyperkalemia, hypotension, and renal dysfunction
diuretics: Increased risk of hypotension
lithium: Possibly increased blood lithium level and risk of toxicity
mTOR inhibitors, such as temsirolimus; neprilysin inhibitors, such as sacubitril: Increased risk of angioedema
NSAIDs: Decreased antihypertensive effect of quinapril; increased risk of renal dysfunction in the elderly or patients who have preexisting renal dysfunction or are volume depleted
potassium preparations, potassium-sparing diuretics, potassium supplements: Increased risk of hyperkalemia
sodium aurothiomalate: Possibly nitritoid reactions, such as facial flushing, hypotension, nausea, vomiting
tetracyclines: Reduced tetracycline absorption

FOODS

foods high in potassium, such as milk or potatoes, potassium-containing salt substitutes: Increased risk of hyperkalemia

Adverse Reactions

CNS: **CVA**, depression, dizziness, drowsiness, fatigue, fever, headache, insomnia, lightheadedness, malaise, nervousness, paresthesia, sleep disturbance, somnolence, syncope, vertigo

CV: Angina pectoris, **arrhythmias**, **cardiogenic shock**, chest pain, edema, **heart failure**, **hypertensive crisis**, **hypotension**, orthostatic hypotension, **MI**, palpitations, tachycardia, vasodilation

EENT: Amblyopia, dry mouth or throat, loss of taste, pharyngitis

GI: Abdominal pain, constipation, diarrhea, dyspepsia, elevated liver enzymes, flatulence, **GI hemorrhage**, **hepatitis**, indigestion, nausea, **pancreatitis**, vomiting

GU: **Acute renal failure**, elevated blood urea nitrogen and creatinine, impotence, UTI, **worsening renal failure**

HEME: **Agranulocytosis**, **hemolytic anemia**, **thrombocytopenia**

MS: Arthralgia, back pain, myalgia

RESP: Cough, dyspnea, **eosinophilic pneumonitis**

SKIN: Alopecia, dermatopolymyositis, diaphoresis, **exfoliative dermatitis**, flushing, pemphigus, photosensitivity, pruritus, rash, urticaria

Other: **Anaphylaxis**, **angioedema**, **hyperkalemia**, **hyponatremia**

Childbearing Considerations

PREGNANCY

- Drug can cause fetal harm, especially if exposure occurs during the second or third trimester.
- Drug reduces fetal renal function, leading to anuria and renal failure, and increases fetal and neonatal morbidity and death. It can also cause fetal lung hypoplasia, hypotension, and skeletal deformations, such as skull hypoplasia.
- Drug is contraindicated in pregnant females and should be discontinued as soon as possible if pregnancy occurs.

LACTATION

- Drug is present in breast milk.
- Mothers should check with prescriber before breastfeeding.

Nursing Considerations

! **WARNING** Keep in mind patients with heart failure, hyponatremia, or severe salt or volume depletion; those who've recently received intensive diuresis or an increase in diuretic dosage; and those undergoing dialysis may be at risk for excessive hypotension. Monitor blood pressure often for first 2 weeks of therapy and whenever quinapril or diuretic dosage increases. If excessive hypotension occurs, notify prescriber immediately, place patient in a supine position, and, if prescribed, infuse normal saline solution, as ordered.

! **WARNING** Monitor patient for a hypersensitivity reaction, which could become life-threatening, such as anaphylaxis or angioedema. Know that patients with a history of angioedema unrelated to ACE inhibitor therapy may be at increased risk of angioedema while receiving quinapril. If a hypersensitivity reaction occurs, notify prescriber immediately, expect drug to be discontinued, and provide supportive care, as needed and ordered. Be aware that if angioedema involves the glottis, larynx, or tongue, airway obstruction is most likely to occur requiring epinephrine 1:1000 (0.3 to 0.5 ml) to be administered subcutaneously along with other supportive care.

- Monitor patient's vital signs and cardiopulmonary status often to assess drug's effectiveness.

! **WARNING** Monitor patients for signs and symptoms of hyperkalemia, especially in patients with diabetes mellitus, renal impairment, or patients taking concomitant therapy with drugs that raise potassium levels. Monitor serum potassium levels, as ordered.

! **WARNING** Monitor patient's CBC, as ordered and assess patient regularly for bruising, unexplained bleeding or infection because drug can cause serious adverse hematologic effects. Institute bleeding and infection control measures, as warranted.

! **WARNING** Monitor patient's BUN and creatinine levels, as ordered because drug can have an adverse effect on renal function. Notify prescriber of any persistent and significant abnormalities in renal function or test results.

! **WARNING** Monitor patient for other persistent, serious, or unusual adverse reactions because drug can adversely affect many body systems.

PATIENT TEACHING

- Instruct patient on how to administer quinapril.
- Explain that drug may cause dizziness and lightheadedness, especially for first few days of therapy. Advise patient to avoid hazardous activities until drug's CNS effects are known and resolved and to notify prescriber if he faints.

! **WARNING** Alert patient that drug may cause an allergic reaction. If present, tell patient to notify prescriber. Also, instruct patient to stop taking quinapril if he has difficulty breathing or swallowing or experiences swelling of the eyes, face, lips, or tongue and seek immediate medical care.

! **WARNING** Review signs and symptoms of hyperkalemia and hyponatremia with patient. And tell patient to notify prescriber, if present. Instruct patient to consult prescriber before using potassium supplements or salt substitutes that contain potassium. Stress importance of complying with ordered blood tests to check for an electrolyte imbalance.

! **WARNING** Review bleeding and infection measues with patient. Urge patient to notify prescriber if bruising, unexplained bleeding, or infection occurs.

! **WARNING** Tell patient to notify prescriber if other persistent, serious, or unusual adverse reactions occur.

- Inform females of childbearing age of risks of taking quinapril during pregnancy. Caution her to use effective contraception during drug therapy and to notify prescriber immediately if pregnancy occurs.
- Advise patient having surgery or receiving anesthesia to tell specialist that he takes quinapril.

rabeprazole sodium

AcipHex

Class and Category

Pharmacologic class: Proton pump inhibitor
Therapeutic class: Antiulcer

Indications and Dosages

* *To provide short-term treatment of erosive esophagitis or ulcerative gastroesophageal reflux disease (GERD)*

D.R. TABLETS

Adults. 20 mg once daily for 4 to 8 wk; course may be repeated if healing has not occurred at the end of 8 wk.

D.R. TABLETS

Adults and adolescents ages 12 and older. 20 mg daily for 4 wk (adults) and 8 wk (adolescents). Course may be repeated if symptoms aren't completely resolved (adults).

* *To provide maintenance treatment of erosive esophagitis or GERD*
* *To treat symptomatic GERD*

Indications and Dosages

* *To provide short-term treatment of erosive esophagitis or ulcerative gastroesophageal reflux disease (GERD)*

D.R. TABLETS

Adults. 20 mg once daily for no longer than 12 mo.

* *To promote healing of duodenal ulcer*

D.R. TABLETS

Adults. 20 mg once daily after the morning meal for up to 4 wk. Course may be repeated if symptoms aren't completely resolved.

* *As adjunct to reduce the risk of duodenal ulcer recurrence by eradicating* Helicobacter pylori

D.R. TABLETS

Adults. 20 mg twice daily with morning and evening meals in conjunction with amoxicillin 1,000 mg twice daily and clarithromycin 500 mg twice daily for 7 days.

* *To treat hypersecretory conditions, such as Zollinger-Ellison syndrome*

D.R. TABLETS

Adults. *Initial:* 60 mg once daily; may be increased, as needed, to 100 mg daily or 60 mg twice daily continuously for up to 1 yr.

Drug Administration

P.O.

- D.R. tablets are to be swallowed whole and not chewed, crushed, or divided; they can be administered with or without food. If used to heal a duodenal ulcer, D.R. tablets should be administered after morning meal; if used to eradicate *Helicobacter pylori*, administer before morning and evening meals.
- If a dose is missed and it is almost time for the next dose, skip the missed dose. Do not give 2 doses at the same time.

Route	Onset	Peak	Duration
P.O./D.R.	$<$ 1 hr	1–6.5 hr	24 hr

Half-life: 1–2 hr

Mechanism of Action

Decreases gastric acid secretion by suppressing its release at the secretory surface of gastric parietal cells. Increases gastric pH and decreases basal acid output also, which helps to heal ulcerated areas. Transforming to an active sulfonamide in the gastric parietal cells increases the clearance rate of *H. pylori.*

Contraindications

Concurrent therapy with rilpivirine-containing products; hypersensitivity to rabeprazole, other substituted benzimidazoles (lansoprazole, omeprazole), or their components

Interactions

DRUGS

atazanavir, nelfinavir, rilpivirine: Decreased exposure of these antiretrovirals with possible decreased antiviral effect and increased development of drug resistance
clarithromycin: Increased risk of serious adverse reactions, including possibly fatal arrhythmias
dasatinib, erlotinib, iron salts, itraconazole, ketoconazole, mycophenolate mofetil, nilotinib: Reduced absorption of these drugs decreasing effectiveness
digoxin: Increased risk of digitalis toxicity
methotrexate: Increased risk of methotrexate toxicities
saquinavir: Increased exposure resulting in possible increased toxicity
tacrolimus: Possibly increased exposure of tacrolimus, especially in transplant patients who are intermediate or poor metabolizers of CYP2C19
warfarin: Possibly increased prothrombin time (PT), international normalized ratio (INR)

Adverse Reactions

CNS: **Coma**, delirium, disorientation, dizziness, headache, malaise, vertigo
EENT: Blurred vision
ENDO: Elevated TSH levels
GI: Abdominal pain, ***Clostridioides difficile*-associated diarrhea**, diarrhea, fundic gland polyps, jaundice, nausea, vomiting
GU: Acute tubulointerstitial nephritis, erectile dysfunction
HEME: **Agranulocytosis, hemolytic anemia, leukopenia, pancytopenia, thrombocytopenia**
MS: Bone fracture, **rhabdomyolysis**
RESP: **Bronchospasm, interstitial pneumonia**
SKIN: Acute generalized exanthematous pustulosis (AGEP), cutaneous lupus erythematosus, bullous and other drug skin eruptions, **erythema multiforme**, rash, **Stevens-Johnson syndrome, toxic epidermal necrolysis**, urticaria
Other: **Anaphylaxis, angioedema, drug reaction with eosinophilia and systemic symptoms (DRESS), hyperammonemia, hypocalcemia, hypokalemia, hypomagnesemia, hypotnatremia**, systemic lupus erythematosus, vitamin B_{12} deficiency (long-term use)

Childbearing Considerations

PREGNANCY

- It is not known if drug can cause fetal harm.
- Use with caution only if benefit to mother outweighs potential risk to fetus.

LACTATION

- It is not known if drug is present in breast milk.
- Mothers should check with prescriber before breastfeeding.

Nursing Considerations

! WARNING Determine patient's magnesium level, as ordered, before drug therapy begins and during therapy if long-term therapy is expected or patient takes drugs that may cause hypomagnesemia such as diuretics. Hypomagnesemia may occur with rabeprazole therapy that has lasted longer than 3 months, although most cases have occurred after therapy had been given for more than a year. Notify prescriber if magnesium level drops below normal, as hypomagnesemia may cause arrhythmias, seizures, and tetany; may lead to hypocalcemia and/or hyperkalemia; and may exacerbate underlying hypocalcemia in at-risk patients such as patients with hypoparathyroidism. Expect patient to receive magnesium and/or calcium replacement and drug to be discontinued if patient does not respond well to replacement therapy.

! **WARNING** Monitor Japanese men receiving rabeprazole closely for adverse reactions because they're more likely than other patients to have increased blood drug levels.

! **WARNING** Monitor patient closely for hypersensitivity reactions, which may become life-threatening, such as anaphylaxis, angioedema, bronchospasm, or severe cutaneous reactions (DRESS may only initially present with a fever or swollen lymph nodes). Notify prescriber, if fever, rash, swollen lymph nodes, or other signs of a reaction is present, and expect drug to be discontinued. Provide supportive care, as needed and prescribed.

! **WARNING** Monitor patient for diarrhea because diarrhea, including *Clostridioides difficile*–associated diarrhea, may occur with rabeprazole therapy, especially in hospitalized patients and can range from being mild to fatal. Notify prescriber if persistent or severe diarrhea develops and expect to obtain a stool specimen to confirm diagnosis. If *C. difficile* is confirmed, expect drug to be discontinued and administer an antibiotic effective against *C. difficile*, as ordered. Also, expect to administer electrolytes, fluids, and protein supplementation, as needed and ordered.

- Monitor patient for impaired hepatic function exhibited by jaundice, especially in patients with a history of hepatic dysfunction.
- Monitor patient for bone fracture, especially in patient receiving multiple daily doses for more than a year because proton pump inhibitors like rabeprazole increase risk of osteoporosis-related fractures of the hip, wrist, and spine.
- Monitor patient for arthralgia and rash, as rabeprazole may cause either cutaneous or systemic lupus erythematosus in patients as a new onset or an exacerbation of the existing autoimmune disease. Know that proton pump inhibitors like rabeprazole should not be given longer than necessary. If patient becomes symptomatic, notify prescriber. If confirmed, expect drug to be discontinued. Know that most patients improve within 12 weeks after drug is discontinued.
- Expect to monitor serum gastrin level in long-term therapy to detect elevation.
- Be aware that symptomatic response to rabeprazole therapy does not preclude the presence of a gastric tumor. Expect patients who have a suboptimal response or an early symptomatic relapse after completing rabeprazole therapy to have further diagnostic testing done.
- Be aware that rabeprazole may produce false readings on the following tests: secretin stimulation test assessing for gastrinoma and serum chromogranin levels assessing for neuroendocrine tumors; these require rabeprazole to be withheld for at least 14 days before tests are performed. Urine tests for tetrahydrocannabinol may result in a false-positive result.

PATIENT TEACHING

- Instruct patient how to administer rabeprazole.
- Inform patients with hypersecretory conditions, such as Zollinger-Ellison syndrome, that treatment can last for a year or longer.

! **WARNING** Warn Japenese patients that they are at higher risk for adverse reactions.

! **WARNING** Alert patient that drug may cause an allergic reaction, including severe skin reactions. If a fever, rash, swollen lymph nodes, or other allergic reaction occurs, tell patient to stop drug, notify prescriber, and, if symptoms are severe, to seek immediate medical care.

! **WARNING** Review signs and symptoms of hypomagnesemia with the patient. Tell the patient to alert prescriber immediately if present. Alert patient he will probably need a blood test to confirm the abnormality. If confirmed, inform patient he may need to take magnesium and/or calcium replacement therapy and that drug may need to be discontinued.

! WARNING Advise patient to contact prescriber if he develops persistent or severe diarrhea that is accompanied by abdominal pain and fever.

- Instruct patient to notify prescriber immediately if he develops new or worsening joint pain or a rash on his arms or cheeks that gets worse in the sun.
- Tell patient to notify prescriber if he experiences a decrease in the amount of urine voided or if urine has blood in it.

! WARNING Instruct patient to notify prescriber of any other persistent, severe, or unusual adverse reactions.

- Tell patient to inform all prescribers of rabeprazole therapy.
- Inform patient that vitamin B_{12} deficiency may occur if drug is taken longer than 3 years.

raloxifene hydrochloride

Evista

Class and Category

Pharmacologic class: Selective estrogen receptor modulator (SERM)
Therapeutic class: Antiosteoporotic

Indications and Dosages

∗ *To prevent and treat osteoporosis in postmenopausal women; to reduce risk of invasive breast cancer in postmenopausal women with osteoporosis; to reduce risk of invasive breast cancer in postmenopausal women at high risk*

TABLETS

Adults. 60 mg daily.

Drug Administration

P.O.

- May be administered with or without food.
- Do not administer drug for at least 72 hr before and during prolonged immobilization. Expect to resume therapy after patient is fully mobile again.

Route	Onset	Peak	Duration
P.O.	Unknown	0.5–6 hr	24 hr

Half-life: 1–2 hr

Mechanism of Action

Prevents osteoporosis by binding to estrogen receptors, which decreases bone resorption and increases bone mineral density in postmenopausal women. May reduce risk of invasive breast cancer because of its binding effects on estrogen receptors.

Contraindications

Active or previous history of thromboembolic disease, hypersensitivity to raloxifene or its components, pregnancy

Interactions

DRUGS

cholestyramine: Decreased raloxifene absorption
diazepam, diazoxide, lidocaine, other highly protein-bound drugs: Possibly interference with binding sites
systemic estrogens: Safety not known
warfarin: Possibly decreased PT

Adverse Reactions

CNS: CVA, depression, fever, insomnia, migraine
CV: Chest pain, hot flashes, peripheral edema, **thromboembolism**, thrombophlebitis
EENT: Laryngitis, pharyngitis, sinusitis
ENDO: Hot flashes
GI: Abdominal pain, cholelithiasis, flatulence, indigestion, nausea, vomiting
GU: Cystitis, infertility, leukorrhea, UTI, vaginitis
MS: Arthralgia, arthritis, leg cramps or spasms, myalgia
RESP: Cough, pneumonia, **pulmonary embolism**
SKIN: Diaphoresis, rash
Other: Flu-like symptoms, weight gain

Childbearing Considerations

PREGNANCY

- Drug is not for use in females of childbearing age.

- Drug is contraindicated in pregnant females.

LACTATION

- It is not known if drug is present in breast milk.
- Drug is not for use in breastfeeding mothers.

Nursing Considerations

! **WARNING** Be aware that raloxifene should not be used in premenopausal females.

! **WARNING** Use cautiously in patients who smoke or have a history of atrial fibrillation, hypertension, stroke, or transient ischemic attack (TIA) because raloxifene may increase the risk of stroke.

! **WARNING** Monitor patient for signs and symptoms of a blood clot that could result in a CVA or pulmonary embolus. Expect prescriber to stop drug at least 72 hours before and during periods of prolonged immobilization because of increased risk for thromboembolism. Resume raloxifene therapy as prescribed after patient is fully ambulatory.

! **WARNING** Monitor patient's limbs for impaired circulation and pain (possible thromboembolism). Notify prescriber immediately, if impairment and pain are present.

- Use cautiously in patients with renal impairment because effects of raloxifene on renal system are unknown.

PATIENT TEACHING

- Instruct patient how to administer raloxifene.
- Advise patient that postmenopausal women require an average of 1,500 mg of elemental calcium and 400 to 800 international units of vitamin D daily. Vitamin D requirement is increased in women who are chronically ill or nursing-home bound, women with GI malabsorption syndromes, and women over age 70. Review dietary sources of calcium and vitamin D, and have patient discuss supplements with prescriber, as needed.
- Advise patient to avoid lengthy immobility during travel while taking raloxifene because of the increased risk of thromboembolism.

! **WARNING** Instruct patient to report adverse reactions to prescriber immediately, especially coughing up blood, leg pain or swelling, shortness of breath, sudden change in vision, or sudden chest pain.

- Emphasize the importance of compliance with long-term raloxifene therapy.

raltegravir potassium

Isentress, Isentress HD

Class and Category

Pharmacologic class: HIV integrase strand transfer inhibitor
Therapeutic class: Antiretroviral

Indications and Dosages

✷ *As adjunct to treat human immunodeficiency virus (HIV-1) infection*

CHEWABLE TABLETS, TABLETS

Adults who are treatment-naïve or who are virologically suppressed on an initial regimen of raltegravir of 400 mg twice daily. 1,200 mg once daily if using 600-mg film-coated tablets or 400 mg twice daily if using 400-mg film-coated tablets.
Adults who are treatment-experienced. 400 mg twice daily using 400-mg film-coated tablets.
Adults who are treatment-experienced or treatment-naïve and taking rifampin concomitantly. 800 mg twice daily using 400-mg film-coated tablets.
Children weighing at least 40 kg (88 lb) and are treatment-naïve or virologically suppressed on an initial regimen of raltegravir 400 mg twice daily. 1,200 mg once daily using 600-mg film-coated tablets, 400 mg twice daily using 400-mg film-coated tablets, or 300 mg twice daily using chewable tablets.
Children weighing at least 28 kg (61.6 lb) but less than 40 kg (88 lb). 400 mg twice daily using 400-mg film-coated tablets or 200 mg twice daily using chewable tablets.
Children weighing at least 25 kg (55 lb) but less than 28 kg (61.6 lb). 400 mg twice daily using 400-mg film-coated tablets or 150 mg twice daily using chewable tablets.

CHEWABLE TABLETS

Children ages 4 wk and older weighing 20 kg (44 lb) to less than 25 kg (55 lb). 150 mg twice daily.

CHEWABLE TABLETS, ORAL SUSPENSION

Children ages 4 wk and older weighing 14 kg (30.8 lb) to less than 20 kg (44 lb). 100 mg (10 ml) twice daily.
Children ages 4 wk and older weighing 10 kg (22 lb) to less than 14 kg (30.8 lb). 75 mg twice daily using chewable tablets or 80 mg (8 ml) twice daily using oral suspension.

ORAL SUSPENSION

Children at least 4 wk of age and weighing 8 kg (17.6 lb) to less than 10 kg (22 lb). 60 mg (6 ml) twice daily.
Children at least 4 wk of age and weighing 6 kg (13.2 lb) to less than 8 kg (17.6 lb). 40 mg (4 ml) twice daily.
Children at least age 4 wk of age and weighing 4 kg (8.8 lb) to less than 6 kg (13.2 lb). 30 mg (3 ml) twice daily.
Children at least age 4 wk of age and weighing 3 kg (6.6 lb) to less than 4 kg (8.8 lb). 25 mg (2.5 ml) twice daily.
Neonates ages 1 wk to 4 wk weighing 4 kg (8.8 lb) to less than 5 kg (11 lb). 15 mg (1.5 ml) twice daily.
Neonates ages 1 wk to 4 wk weighing 3 kg (6.6 lb) to less than 4 kg (8.8 lb). 10 mg (1 ml) twice daily.
Neonates ages 1 wk to 4 wk weighing 2 kg (4.4 lb) to less than 3 kg (6.6 lb). 8 mg (.08 ml) twice daily.
Neonates ages birth to 1 wk weighing 4 kg (8.8 lb) to less than 5 kg (11 lb). 7 mg (0.7 ml) once daily.
Neonates ages birth to 1 wk weighing 3 kg (6.6 lb) to less than 4 kg (8.8 lb). 5 mg (0.5 ml) once daily.
Neonates ages birth to 1 wk weighing 2 kg (4.4 lb) to less than 3 kg (6.6 lb). 4 mg (0.4 ml) once daily.

±**DOSAGE ADJUSTMENT** For mothers who have taken raltegravir 2 to 24 hours before delivery, neonates (ages birth to 4 weeks) are given the first dose between 24 and 28 hours after birth, regardless of weight.

Drug Administration

P.O.

- Chewable tablets and oral suspension cannot be substituted for the 400-mg or 800-mg film-coated tablets because the formulations have different pharmacokinetic profiles.
- Do not administer drug before dialysis because the extent to which the drug is dialyzable is unknown.
- Film-coated tablets must be swallowed whole and not chewed, crushed, or divided.
- Chewable tablets may be chewed or swallowed whole. Maximum dose is 300 mg twice daily. Chewable tablets can be crushed and added to 5 ml of breast milk, juice, or water. After 2 min, crush any remaining pieces of the tablet(s) with a spoon and administer immediately. Add 5 ml of liquid to cup again, swirl, and administer immediately to ensure that entire dose has been given.
- Mix oral suspension form using the provided mixing cup by pouring packet contents into 10 ml of water in the cup and mixing. Gently swirl the cup for 45 sec in a circular motion to mix powder. Do not shake. Once mixed, measure the recommended dose with a syringe and administer within 30 min of mixing. Discard any remaining suspension. Maximum daily dose is 100 mg twice daily.

Route	Onset	Peak	Duration
P.O.	Unknown	1.5–3 hr	24 hr

Half-life: 9 hr

Mechanism of Action

Inhibits HIV integrase by binding to the integrase active site and blocking the strand transfer step of retroviral DNA integration, which is needed for the HIV replication cycle.

Contraindications

Hypersensitivity to raltegravir or its components

Interactions

DRUGS

aluminum- and/or magnesium-containing antacids, calcium carbonate antacid, carbamazepine, etravirine, phenobarbital, phenytoin, rifampin: Decrease in plasma concentration of raltegravir and its effectiveness

Adverse Reactions

CNS: Abnormal dreams, asthenia, cerebellar ataxia, depression, dizziness, fatigue, fever, headaches, insomnia, malaise, nightmares, paranoia, **suicidal ideation**
CV: Elevated cholesterol and triglycerides
EENT: Conjunctivitis
ENDO: Hyperglycemia
GI: Abdominal pain, anorexia, bilirubin increase, diarrhea, dyspepsia, elevated liver and pancreatic enzymes, flatulence, gastritis, **hepatic failure**, **hepatitis**, nausea, vomiting
GU: Genital herpes, nephrolithiasis, **renal failure**
HEME: Decreased hemoglobin count, **neutropenia**, **thrombocytopenia**
MS: Elevated creatine kinase, myopathy, **rhabdomyolysis**
SKIN: Blisters, rash, **Stevens-Johnson syndrome**, **toxic epidermal necrolysis**
Other: **Angioedema and other hypersensitivity reactions**, **drug reaction with eosinophilia and systemic symptoms (DRESS)**, herpes zoster, **immune reconstitution syndrome**

Childbearing Considerations

PREGNANCY

- Pregnancy exposure registry: 1-800-258-4263.
- It is not known if drug can cause fetal harm.
- Use with caution only if benefit to mother outweighs potential risk to fetus.

LACTATION

- It is not known if drug is present in breast milk.
- The Centers for Disease Control and Prevention recommends that HIV-1 infected mothers not breastfeed to avoid risking postnatal transmission of HIV-1 infection to infants. They also do not recommend breastfeeding because of potential drug-induced adverse reactions in the infant.

Nursing Considerations

! **WARNING** Ask patient before starting raltegravir therapy if he has ever experienced an elevated creatine kinase level, myopathy, or rhabdomyolysis or is taking any drugs known to cause these conditions (such as fenofibrate, gemfibrozil, statins, or zidovudine) because drug may increase risk of developing these conditions.

! **WARNING** Monitor patient closely for a hypersensitivity or severe skin reactions, which could become life-threatening, such as angioedema and DRESS. Notify prescriber and expect raltegravir to be discontinued immediately if patient develops a hypersensitivity reaction, including a rash (DRESS may only initially present with a fever or swollen lymph nodes.). Be aware that a delay in discontinuing drug may result in a life-threatening situation. Provide supportive care, as ordered and needed.

! **WARNING** Monitor patient for changes in behavior or thinking that could result in suicidial ideation. Notify prescriber immediately, institute suicide precautions, and expect drug to be changed to a different drug.

! **WARNING** Be aware that immune reconstitution syndrome has occurred in patients treated with combination antiretroviral therapy, including raltegravir. The inflammatory response predisposes susceptible patients to opportunistic infections, such as cytomegalovirus, *Mycobacterium avium* infection, *Pneumocystis jiroveci* pneumonia, or tuberculosis. Autoimmune disorders such as Graves' disease, Guillain-Barré syndrome, or polymyositis have also occurred. Report sudden or unusual adverse reactions to prescriber.

! **WARNING** Monitor patient for other persistent, serious, or unusual adverse reactions because drug can affect many body systems and some of the adverse reactions could become life-threatening, such as hepatic or renal failure.

PATIENT TEACHING

- Instruct patient, family, or caregiver how to administer the form of raltegravir prescribed and what to do if a dose is missed.

! **WARNING** Warn patient, family, or caregiver to avoid missing doses of raltegravir, as it can result in the development of resistance to the drug.

! **WARNING** Alert patient and family or caregiver that chewable tablet form contains phenylalanine and can be harmful to patients with phenylketonuria.

! **WARNING** Alert patient, family, or caregiver that drug may cause an allergic or severe skin reaction. Tell them to notify prescriber immediately if a fever, rash, swollen lymph nodes, or other allergic reactions occur as drug will need to be switched to a different drug.

! **WARNING** Inform patient and family or caregiver that drug may cause abnormal behavior and thinking increasing risk of suicide and to watch patient closely. If present, prescriber should be notified immediately. Review suicide precautions with family or caregiver.

- Instruct patient, family, or caregiver to immediately report any unexplained muscle pain, tenderness, or weakness.

! **WARNING** Inform patient, family, or caregiver to notify prescriber if other persistent, severe, or unusual adverse reactions occur, including evidence of an infection.

- Inform mothers that breastfeeding is not recommended during raltegravir therapy.

ramelteon

Rozerem

Class and Category

Pharmacologic class: Melatonin receptor agonist
Therapeutic class: Hypnotic

Indications and Dosages

* *To treat insomnia in patients having difficulty falling asleep*

TABLETS

Adults. 8 mg once nightly within 30 min of bedtime.

Drug Administration

P.O.

- Administer drug 30 min before bedtime.
- Tablets should be swallowed whole and not chewed, crushed, or divided.
- Avoid giving with or after a high-fat meal.
- Be aware that drug should not be administered with fluvoxamine. Drug should be used with caution in patients taking other CYP1A2 inhibiting drugs.

Route	Onset	Peak	Duration
P.O.	30 min	0.5–1.5 hr	Unknown

Half-life: 1–2.6 hr

Mechanism of Action

Binds to melatonin receptors MT1 and MT2 in the suprachiasmatic nucleus (SCN) of the hypothalamus to induce sleep.

Contraindications

Concurrent therapy with fluvoxamine, history of angioedema with previous ramelteon treatment, hypersensitivity to ramelteon or its components

Interactions

DRUGS

benzodiazepines, melatonin, other sedative-hypnotics: Possible additive sedative effects
donepezil, doxepin, fluconazole, fluvoxamine, ketoconazole: Increased plasma ramelteon levels
rifampin: Decreased ramelteon effectiveness

ACTIVITIES

alcohol use: Possibly additive CNS effect

Adverse Reactions

CNS: Agitation, amnesia, anxiety, bizarre behavior, complex behaviors such as sleep driving, depression, dizziness, fatigue, hallucinations, headache, insomnia exacerbation, mania, somnolence, **suicidal ideation**
EENT: **Throat tightness**
ENDO: Decreased testosterone level, increased prolactin level
GI: Diarrhea, dysgeusia, nausea, vomiting
MS: Arthralgia, myalgia
RESP: Dyspnea, upper respiratory tract infection
Other: **Anaphylaxis**, **angioedema**

Childbearing Considerations

PREGNANCY

- It is not known if drug can cause fetal harm but animal studies suggest it might.
- Use with caution only if benefit to mother outweighs potential risk to fetus.

LACTATION

- It is not known if drug is present in breast milk.
- Mothers should check with prescriber before breastfeeding.
- It is recommended that mothers should interrupt breastfeeding and pump and discard breast milk during treatment and for 25 hr after last dose. If breastfeeding does occur, monitor the breastfed infant for feeding difficulties and somnolence.

REPRODUCTION

- Drug may affect reproductive hormones or cause problems with infertility.

Nursing Considerations

- Be aware that ramelteon therapy is not recommended for patients with COPD or severe sleep apnea because its effects have not been studied in these patient populations.
- Use cautiously in patients with mild-to-moderate hepatic dysfunction. Drug is contraindicated in severe hepatic dysfunction.
- Be aware that ramelteon is not classified as a controlled substance.

! **WARNING** Monitor patient closely for hypersensitivity reactions, which could become life-threatening, such as anaphylaxis or angioedema. If present, notify prescriber, expect drug to be discontinued, and provide supportive care, as needed and ordered.

! **WARNING** Watch patient closely for suicidal tendencies, particularly when therapy starts, because depression may worsen temporarily during this time, possibly leading to suicidal ideation.

PATIENT TEACHING

- Instruct patient how to administer ramelteon.
- Advise limiting alcohol during therapy.
- Tell patient to notify prescriber if insomnia worsens or new signs or symptoms occur.

! **WARNING** Alert patient that drug may cause an allergic reaction. If present, tell patient to notify prescriber and, if severe, to seek immediate medical care.

! **WARNING** Urge family or caregiver to watch patient closely for suicidal tendencies, especially when therapy starts.

- Caution patient to avoid potentially hazardous activities after taking ramelteon; drug's intended effect is to decrease alertness.
- Advise patient that drug may cause abnormal behaviors during sleep, such as driving a car, eating, having sex, or talking on the phone without any recall of the event. If family or caregiver notices any such behavior or patient sees evidence of such behavior upon awakening, prescriber should be notified.
- Inform patient that drug may affect reproductive hormones; urge patient to report cessation of menses (females), galactorrhea (females), decreased libido, or problems with infertility.
- Advise mothers to interrupt breastfeeding and pump and discard breast milk during treatment and for 25 hr after last dose. If breastfeeding does occur, tell mothers to monitor their breastfed infant for feeding difficulties and somnolence.

ramipril

Altace

Class and Category

Pharmacologic class: Angiotensin-converting enzyme (ACE) inhibitor
Therapeutic class: Antihypertensive

Indications and Dosages

✱ *To treat heart failure after MI*

CAPSULES

Adults. *Initial:* 2.5 mg twice daily with dose decreased to 1.25 mg twice daily if hypotension occurs. Dosage increased after 1 wk, as tolerated. Dosage further increased about every 3 wk to achieve maintenance dose. *Maintenance:* 5 mg twice daily.

± **DOSAGE ADJUSTMENT** For patients with renal impairment (creatinine clearance less than 40 ml/min), initial dose reduced to 1.25 mg once daily and then increased to 1.25 mg twice daily, and up to maximum dose of 2.5 mg twice daily, as needed.

✱ *To reduce risk of CVA or MI and death from cardiovascular causes*

CAPSULES

Adults ages 55 and older. *Initial:* 2.5 mg once daily for 1 wk, followed by 5 mg once daily for 3 wk, and then increased, as tolerated, to 10 mg once daily.

±**DOSAGE ADJUSTMENT** For patients who are hypertensive or recently post-MI, daily dosage may also be divided.

✱ *To treat hypertension*

CAPSULES

Adults not taking a diuretic. *Initial:* 2.5 mg once daily with dosage adjusted according to blood pressure response. *Maintenance:* 2.5 to 20 mg once daily or in divided doses twice daily.

±**DOSAGE ADJUSTMENT** For patients who have hypertension with renal impairment (creatinine clearance less than 40 ml/min), initial dose reduced to 1.25 mg once daily and then titrated upward till blood pressure is controlled or maximum total daily dose (not to exceed 5 mg) is reached. For patients with hypertension who experience a diminished drug effect toward end of dosing interval, dosage increased or daily dosage divided into 2 doses. For all patients regardless of indication being treated, if dehydrated from past or present diuretic use or who have renal artery stenosis, initial dosage reduced to 1.25 mg daily.

Drug Administration

P.O.

- Capsules should be swallowed whole and not chewed or crushed.
- If patient cannot swallow capsule, open and sprinkle contents onto about 4 ounces of applesauce or mix with 4 ounces of apple juice or water. If not administered immediately, mixture may be stored for 24 hr at room temperature or 48 hr in refrigerator.
- Expect to monitor patient being treated for heart failure post-MI for at least 2 hrs after initial dose and until blood pressure has stabilized for at least an additional hour.

Route	Onset	Peak	Duration
P.O.	1–2 hr	1–4 hr	24 hr

Half-life: 13–17 hr

Mechanism of Action

Blocks conversion of angiotensin I to angiotensin II, causing vasodilation, and reduces aldosterone secretion, which prevents water retention. Reduces peripheral arterial resistance also. Reduction of blood pressure occurs as a result of these combined actions.

Contraindications

Aliskiren therapy in patients with diabetes; hypersensitivity to ramipril, other ACE inhibitors or their components; use of neprilysin inhibitor, such as sacubitril, within 36 hr

Interactions

DRUGS

aliskiren (patients with diabetes and/or renal impairment), angiotensin receptor blockers, other ACE inhibitors: Increased risk of hyperkalemia, hypotension, and renal dysfunction
diuretics: Possibly hypotension
lithium: Increased risk of lithium toxicity
mTOR inhibitors, such as temsirolimus, neprilysin inhibitor such as sacubitril: Increased risk of angioedema
NSAIDs: Decreased antihypertensive effect of ramipril; increased risk of renal dysfunction in the elderly and patients with preexisting renal dysfunction or volume depletion
potassium preparations, potassium-sparing diuretics: Risk of hyperkalemia
sodium aurothiomalate: Increased risk of nitritoid reaction (facial flushing, hypotension, nausea, vomiting)

FOODS

potassium-rich foods, such as milk and potatoes, potassium-containing salt substitutes: Increased risk of hyperkalemia

Adverse Reactions

CNS: Depression, dizziness, drowsiness, fatigue, fever, headache, insomnia, lightheadedness, malaise, paresthesia, sleep disturbance, syncope, vertigo
CV: Chest pain, **hypotension**, orthostatic hypotension, palpitations, tachycardia

EENT: Amblyopia, dry mouth, loss of taste, pharyngitis
GI: Abdominal pain, constipation, diarrhea, elevated liver enzymes, jaundice, **hepatic failure**, **hepatitis**, nausea, vomiting
GU: **Acute renal failure**, elevated BUN and serum creatinine levels, impotence, oliguria, **progressive azotemia**
HEME: **Agranulocytosis**, anemia, **bone marrow depression**, **pancytopenia**
MS: Arthralgia, back pain, myalgia
RESP: Cough, dyspnea
SKIN: Alopecia, diaphoresis, flushing, onycholysis, pemphigoid, photosensitivity, pruritus, rash, **Stevens-Johnson syndrome**, **toxic epidermal necrolysis**, urticaria
Other: **Anaphylaxis**, **angioedema**, **hyperkalemia**

Childbearing Considerations

PREGNANCY

- Drug can cause fetal harm, especially if exposure occurs during the second or third trimester.
- Drug reduces fetal renal function leading to anuria and renal failure and increases fetal and neonatal morbidity and death. It can also cause fetal lung hypoplasia, hypotension, and skeletal deformations, such as skull hypoplasia.
- Drug is not recommended in pregnant females and should be discontinued as soon as possible if pregnancy occurs.

LACTATION

- It is not known if drug is present in breast milk.
- Drug is not recommended for use during breastfeeding.

Nursing Considerations

- Monitor blood pressure frequently during therapy to assess drug's effectiveness.

! WARNING Keep in mind patients with dehydration, heart failure, or hyponatremia; those who've recently received intensive diuresis or an increase in diuretic dosage; and those having dialysis may risk excessive hypotension. Monitor such patients closely the first 2 weeks of therapy and whenever ramipril or diuretic dosage increases. If excessive hypotension occurs, notify prescriber immediately, place patient in a supine position, and, if prescribed, infuse normal saline solution.

! WARNING Monitor patient for a hypersensitivity reaction, which could become life-threatening, such as angioedema. If present, notify prescriber, expect drug to be discontinued, and provide supportive care, as needed and ordered.

! WARNING Monitor patient's serum potassium level, as ordered, and assess often for signs and symptoms of hyperkalemia, especially in patients with diabetes mellitus or renal insufficiency and those taking concomitantly other drugs that raise serum potassium levels.

! WARNING Monitor patient's CBC and platelet count, as needed and ordered and patient for bruising, unexplained bleeding, or infection because drug can cause significant adverse hematologic reactions.

- Monitor patient's BUN and creatinine levels, as ordered, especially in patients with hepatic or renal impairment. If patient develops jaundice or marked elevations of hepatic enzymes, or BUN and creatinine become elevated, notify prescriber and expect ramipril to be discontinued.

PATIENT TEACHING

- Instruct patient how to administer form of ramipril prescribed.
- Explain that drug may cause dizziness and lightheadedness, especially during first few days of therapy. Instruct patient to notify prescriber immediately if a fainting episode occurs.

! WARNING Alert patient that drug may cause an allergic reaction. If present, advise patient to notify prescriber and, if severe, to seek immediate medical care.

! WARNING Review signs and symptoms of a high potassium level. Also, review bleeding and infection control measures with patient. Tell patient to alert prescriber if these or other adverse reactions occur.

- Urge patient to tell providers that ramipril therapy is being taken before having surgery or receiving anesthesia.
- Tell patient to ask prescriber before using supplements or salt substitutes that contain potassium.

- Inform females of childbearing age to notify prescriber immediately if pregnancy occurs as drug will have to be discontinued.
- Inform mothers breastfeeding is not recommended.

ranolazine

Ranexa

Class and Category

Pharmacologic class: Cardiac agent
Therapeutic class: Antianginal

Indications and Dosages

✶ *To treat chronic angina*

E.R. TABLETS, ORAL GRANULES

Adults. *Initial:* 500 mg twice daily, increased to 1,000 mg twice daily, as needed. *Maximum:* 1,000 mg twice daily.

± **DOSAGE ADJUSTMENT** For patients taking a moderate CYP3A inhibitor, such as diltiazem, erythromycin, or verapamil, maximum dosage reduced to 500 mg twice daily. For patients taking P-gp inhibitors, such as cyclosporine, E.R. tablet dosage may have to be reduced.

Drug Administration

P.O.

- Tablets should be swallowed whole and not chewed, crushed, or divided.
- Avoid administering drug with grapefruit juice.
- Sprinkle oral granules on 1 tablespoon of soft food and have patient consume immediately. Tell patient not to chew or crush the granules.
- To administer via a gastric or nasogastric tube, add the content of a sachet of oral granules to a plastic catheter tip syringe and add 50 ml of water for nasogastric administration and 30 ml for gastric tube administration. Gently shake syringe for about 15 sec before administering through a 12 French or larger tube. Rinse with 15 ml (nasogastic tube) or 20 ml (gastric tube) of additional water, if needed.

Route	Onset	Peak	Duration
P.O.	Unknown	2–5 hr	Unknown

Half-life: 7 hr

Mechanism of Action

Exerts antianginal and anti-ischemic effects by an unknown mechanism not dependent on reductions in blood pressure or heart rate. Inhibits cardiac late sodium current, but how this action inhibits angina symptoms is also unknown.

Contraindications

Hypersensitivity to ranolazine or its components, liver cirrhosis, use of CYP3A inducers or strong inhibitors

Interactions

DRUGS

CYP2D6 substrates, such as antipsychotics, tricyclic antidepressants: Increased plasma levels of these drugs
CYP3A inducers, such as carbamazepine, phenobarbital, phenytoin, rifabutin, rifampin, rifapentine, St. John's wort: Decreased blood ranolazine level and decreased effectiveness
CYP3A substrates, such as cyclosporine, lovastatin, simvastatin, sirolimus, tacrolimus: Possibly increased blood levels of these drugs
CYP3A inhibitors, such as clarithromycin, diltiazem, erythromycin, fluconazole, indinavir, itraconazole, ketoconazole, nefazodone, nelfinavir, ritonavir, saquinavir, verapamil: Increased blood ranolazine level and increased risk of adverse reactions
digoxin: Increased blood digoxin level
metformin: Increased metformin levels when ranolazine dosage reaches 1,000 mg twice daily

ACTIVITIES

grapefruit juice, grapefruit-containing products: Increased blood ranolazine level and increased risk of adverse reactions

Adverse Reactions

CNS: Abnormal coordination, asthenia, confusion, dizziness, hallucination, headache, hypoesthesia, myoclonus, paresthesia, syncope, tremor, vertigo
CV: **Bradycardia**, **hypotension**, orthostatic hypotension, palpitations, peripheral edema, **QT-interval prolongation**
EENT: Blurred vision, dry mouth, tinnitus
ENDO: **Hypoglycemia**
GI: Abdominal pain, anorexia, constipation, dyspepsia, nausea, vomiting
GU: Dysuria, elevated blood urea and creatinine levels, hematuria, **renal failure**, urinary retention

HEME: Eosinophilia, **leukopenia**, **pancytopenia**, **thrombocytopenia**
RESP: Dyspnea, **pulmonary fibrosis**
SKIN: Diaphoresis, pruritus, rash
Other: **Angioedema**

Childbearing Considerations

PREGNANCY

- It is not known if drug can cause fetal harm.
- Use with caution only if benefit to mother outweighs potential risk to fetus.

LACTATION

- It is not known if drug is present in breast milk.
- Mothers should check with prescriber before breastfeeding.

Nursing Considerations

- Assess effectiveness of ranolazine at preventing anginal pain.

! **WARNING** Monitor patient for a hypersensitivity reaction, which could become life-threatening, such as angioedema. If present, notify prescriber, expect drug to be discontinued, and provide supportive care, as needed and ordered.

! **WARNING** Expect to monitor's patient's ECG, as ordered for evidence of a prolonged QT interval, which increases in a dose-related manner.

! **WARNING** Know that acute renal failure may occur in some patients with severe renal impairment (creatinine clearance less than 30 ml/min) while taking drug. Monitor patient's serum creatinine levels and blood urea nitrogen after drug therapy begins and then periodically, as ordered. If elevations occur, notify prescriber and expect drug to be discontinued.

! **WARNING** Monitor patient's blood glucose level because ranolazine may cause hypoglycemia. Also, monitor patient's CBC and platelet count for abnormalities because drug may cause serious adverse hematological reactions. Assess patient for bruising, unexplained bleeding, or signs and symptoms of an infection.

- Monitor patient's serum magnesium, potassium, and liver enzyme levels.

PATIENT TEACHING

- Instruct patient how to administer ranolazine.
- Advise patient to avoid grapefruit and grapefruit juice while taking ranolazine.

! **WARNING** Alert patient that drug may cause an allergic reaction. If present, tell patient to notify prescriber and, if severe, to seek immediate medical care.

! **WARNING** Review signs and symptoms of hypoglycemia and how to treat if it occurs. Also, review bleeding and infection control measures.

! **WARNING** Advise patient to notify prescriber if other persistent, severe, or unusual adverse reactions occur.

- Instruct patient to notify all prescribers of ranolazine use.

rasagiline

Azilect

Class and Category

Pharmacologic class: Irreversible monoamine oxidase inhibitor (MAOI)
Therapeutic class: Antiparkinsonian

Indications and Dosages

∗ *To treat Parkinson's disease as monotherapy; as adjunct in patients not taking levodopa*

TABLETS

Adults. 1 mg once daily.

∗ *As adjunct with levodopa in treatment of Parkinson's disease*

TABLETS

Adults. 0.5 mg once daily increased to 1 mg once daily, as needed.

± **DOSAGE ADJUSTMENT** For patients with mild hepatic failure or taking ciprofloxacin or other CYP1A2 inhibitors, dosage shouldn't exceed 0.5 mg daily.

Drug Administration

P.O.

- Administer at about the same time each day.
- If a dose is missed, skip the missed dose and resume dosing schedule the next day. Do not double the dose to make up for the missed dose.

Route	Onset	Peak	Duration
P.O.	Unknown	1 hr	1 wk

Half-life: 1.5–3.5 hr

Mechanism of Action

Inhibits metabolic degradation of catecholamines and serotonin in the CNS and peripheral tissues, increasing extracellular dopamine level in the striatum. Increased dopamine levels help control alterations in voluntary muscle movement (such as rigidity and tremors) in Parkinson's disease because dopamine, a neurotransmitter, is essential for normal motor function. Stimulating central and peripheral dopaminergic 2 (D_2) receptors on postsynaptic cells, dopamine inhibits firing of striatal neurons (such as cholinergic neurons), which improves motor function.

Contraindications

Concurrent therapy with cyclobenzaprine, dextromethorphan, or St. John's wort; hypersensitivity to rasagiline or its components; use within 14 days of MAO inhibitors, meperidine, methadone, other selective MAO-B inhibitors, propoxyphene, or tramadol

Interactions

DRUGS

antipsychotics, metoclopramide: Possible diminished effectiveness of rasagiline
CYP1A2 inhibitors, such as ciprofloxacin: Increased plasma rasagiline concentrations
dextromethorphan: Increased risk of bizarre behavior or episodes of psychosis
MAO inhibitors, meperidine, selective MAO-B inhibitors: Increased risk of serious, sometimes fatal, adverse reactions
MAO inhibitors, sympathomimetics: Increased risk of hypertensive crisis
selective serotonin reuptake inhibitors; serotonin–norepinephrine reuptake inhibitors; tetracyclic, triazolopyridine, or tricyclic antidepressants: Increased risk of serotonin syndrome

FOODS

foods high in tyramine: Possibly significant increase in blood pressure

Adverse Reactions

CNS: Abnormal dreams, amnesia, anxiety, asthenia, ataxia, **cerebral ischemia**, **coma**, compulsive behaviors (binge eating, increased sexual urges, intense urges to spend money), confusion, **CVA**, daytime sleepiness, depression, difficulty thinking, dizziness, dyskinesia, dystonia, fever, hallucinations, headache, malaise, manic-depressive reaction, nightmares, paresthesia, psychotic-like behavior, **seizures**, **serotonin syndrome**, somnolence, stupor, syncope, vertigo
CV: Angina, bundle branch heart block, chest pain, **heart failure**, **MI**, **hypertensive crisis**, postural hypotension, thrombophlebitis, **ventricular fibrillation or tachycardia**
EENT: Blurred vision, conjunctivitis, dry mouth, epistaxis, gingivitis, **hemorrhage**, **laryngeal edema**, retinal detachment or hemorrhage, rhinitis
GI: Abdominal pain, anorexia, constipation, diarrhea, dyspepsia, dysphagia, elevated liver enzymes, gastroenteritis, **GI hemorrhage**, **intestinal obstruction or perforation**, nausea, vomiting
GU: **Acute renal failure**, albuminuria, decreased libido, hematuria, impotence, incontinence, priapism
HEME: Anemia, **leukopenia**, **thrombocytopenia**
MS: Arthralgia, arthritis, bone necrosis, bursitis, leg cramps, myasthenia, neck pain or stiffness, tenosynovitis
RESP: **Apnea**, **asthma**, cough, dyspnea, pleural effusion, **pneumothorax**, **interstitial pneumonia**
SKIN: Alopecia, **carcinoma**, diaphoresis, ecchymosis, **exfoliative dermatitis**, **melanoma**, pruritus, ulcer, vesiculobullous rash
Other: **Angioedema and other hypersensitivity reactions**, flu-like symptoms, **hypocalcemia**, weight loss

Childbearing Considerations

PREGNANCY

- It is not known if drug can cause fetal harm.
- Use with caution only if benefit to mother outweighs potential risk to fetus.

LACTATION

- It is not known if drug is present in breast milk.
- Mothers should check with prescriber before breastfeeding.

Nursing Considerations

! WARNING Monitor patient for a hypersensitivity reaction, which could become life-threatening, such as angioedema. If present, notify prescriber, expect drug to be discontinued, and provide supportive care, as needed and ordered.

! WARNING Monitor patient's respiratory function closely as drug may cause serious to life-threatening adverse reactions.

! WARNING Monitor patient's blood pressure closely throughout therapy. Notify prescriber immediately if patient has evidence of hypertensive crisis or signs and symptoms suggesting a stroke. Expect to stop drug immediately if these occur. Monitor patient closely for other adverse reactions, which could be quite serious such as acute renal failure, GI hemorrhage, or hypersensitivity reactions. Immediately notify prescriber, if adverse reactions occur. Be prepared to provide emergency care, as needed and ordered.

- Be aware that patient may experience orthostatic hypotension, especially in the first 2 months of rasagiline therapy and that it may also occur while patient is supine.

! WARNING Monitor patient for seizures, especially patients with a seizure history. Institute seizure precautions, as needed.

! WARNING Monitor patient closely for serotonin syndrome, a rare but serious adverse effect of rasagiline. Signs and symptoms include agitation, confusion, diaphoresis, diarrhea, fever, hyperactive reflexes, poor coordination, restlessness, shaking, talking or acting with uncontrolled excitement, tremor, and twitching. If symptoms occur, notify prescriber immediately, expect to discontinue drug, and provide supportive care.

- Monitor patient receiving rasagiline with levodopa for worsening of preexisting dyskinesia. If it occurs, notify prescriber and expect levodopa dosage to be decreased.

! WARNING Ensure that patient has regular skin assessments done because drug can cause skin cancer.

! WARNING Monitor patient for other persistent, serious, or unusual adverse reactions because drug can adversely affect many body systems.

PATIENT TEACHING

- Instruct patient how to administer rasagiline.
- Remind patient not to exceed the recommended dose because of risk of hypertension.

! WARNING Stress importance of avoiding tyramine-rich foods, such as aged cheese (e.g., Stilton), which may increase blood pressure greatly. If patient doesn't feel well soon after eating a suspected high-tyramine meal, he should contact prescriber immediately or seek immediate medical care.

! WARNING Alert patient that drug may cause an allergic reaction. If present, tell patient to notify prescriber and, if severe, to seek immediate medical care.

! WARNING Caution patient to avoid hazardous activities until CNS effects of drug are known and resolved. Some patients have fallen asleep without warning while engaged in activities of daily living, including driving.

- Suggest that patient change position slowly to minimize orthostatic hypotension.
- Alert patient that drug may cause changes in behavior that may be severe or hallucinations, especially at the initiation of drug therapy or when an increase in dosage occurs. If they occur, tell patient to notify prescriber promptly.
- Alert patient and family or caregiver that drug may cause compulsive or impulsive behaviors, such as binge eating, gambling, increased sexual activities, or spending money inappropriately. If any questionable behavior occurs, instruct patient and family or caregiver to notify prescriber, as dosage may have to be adjusted or drug discontinued.

! WARNING Advise patient and family or caregiver to notify prescriber if other persistent, serious, or unusual adverse reactions occur. If severe, urge patient to seek immediate medical care.

- Instruct patient to notify all prescribers of rasagiline therapy, especially if antidepressants or antibiotics such as ciprofloxacin or a similar drug are being considered, and to avoid taking any over-the-counter cold medications.

remdesivir

Veklury

Class and Category

Pharmacologic class: SARS-CoV-2 nucleotide analog RNA polymerase inhibitor
Therapeutic class: Antiretroviral

Indications and Dosages

✱ *To treat coronavirus disease 2019 (COVID-19) in patients with positive results of direct severe acute respiratory syndrome coronavirus 2 (SARS-CoV-2) viral testing and requiring hospitalization*

I.V. INFUSION

Adults and children weighing at least 40 kg (88 lb). *Loading dose:* 200 mg as a single dose on day 1. *Maintenance:* 100 mg once daily beginning on day 2 for 4 additional days for patients not requiring invasive mechanical ventilation and/or extracorporeal membrane oxygenation (ECMO) and who show signs of improvement or 9 additional days if patient does not demonstrate clinical improvement or patient requires invasive mechanical ventilation and/or ECMO.

I.V. INFUSION (USING ONLY INJECTION FORM SUPPLIED AS 100-MG LYOPHILIZED POWDER IN VIAL)

Infants 28 days and older weighing at least 3 kg (6.6 lb) to children weighing less than 40 kg (88 lb). *Loading dose*: 5 mg/kg as a single dose on day 1. *Maintenance:* 2.5 mg/kg once daily beginning on day 2 for 4 additional days for patients not requiring invasive mechanical ventilation and/or extracorporeal membrane oxygenation (ECMO) and who show signs of improvement or 9 additional days if patient does not demonstrate clinical improvement or patient requires invasive mechanical ventilation and/or ECMO.

Infants at least 28 days old weighing 1.5 kg (3.3 lb) to less than 3 kg (6.6 lb). *Loading dose:* 2.5 mg/kg as a single dose on day 1. *Maintenance:* 1.25 mg/kg once daily beginning on day 2 for 4 additional days for infants not requiring invasive mechanical ventilation and/or ECMO and who show signs of improvement or 9 additional days if infant does not demonstrate clinical improvement or requires invasive mechanical ventilation and/or ECMO.

Infants birth to less than 28 days old and weighing at least 1.5 kg (3.3 lb). *Loading dose:* 2.5 mg/kg as a single dose on day 1. *Maintenance:* 1.25 mg/kg once daily beginning on day 2 for 4 additional days for infants not requiring invasive mechanical ventilation and/or ECMO and who show signs of improvement or 9 additional days if infant does not demonstrate clinical improvement or requires invasive mechanical ventilation and/or ECMO.

✱ *To treat symptomatic coronavirus disease 2019 (COVID-19) within 7 days of symptom onset in nonhospitalized patients who have mild-to-moderate COVID-19, and are at high risk for progression to severe COVID-19, including hospitalization or death*

I.V. INFUSION

Adults and children weighing at least 40 kg (88 lb). *Loading dose:* 200 mg as a single dose on day 1. *Maintenance:* 100 mg once daily given on days 2 and 3.

I.V. INFUSION (USING ONLY INJECTION FORM SUPPLIED AS 100-MG LYOPHILIZED POWDER IN VIAL)

Infants 28 days and older weighing at least 3 kg (6.6 lb) to children weighing less than 40 kg (88 lb). *Loading dose:* 5 mg/kg as a single dose on day 1. *Maintenance:* 2.5 mg/kg once daily on days 2 and 3.

Infants at least 28 days old weighing 1.5 kg (3.3 lb) to less than 3 kg (6.6 lb). *Loading dose:* 2.5 mg/kg as a single dose on day 1. *Maintenance:* 1.25 mg/kg once daily for days 2 and 3.

Infants birth to less than 28 days old and weighing at least 1.5 kg (3.3 lb). *Loading dose:* 2.5 mg/kg as a single dose on day 1. *Maintenance:* 1.25 mg/kg once daily for days 2 and 3.

Drug Administration

I.V.

- Drug is available in 2 dosage forms: as a 100-mg lyophilized powder in a vial, which must be reconstituted, and as a 100-mg/20-ml solution.

- Solution or powder (when reconstituted) should appear clear, colorless to yellow and free of visible particles.
- Do not exceed infusion rate, to help prevent hypersensitivity reactions. Slower infusion rates, with a maximum infusion time of up to 120 min, can potentially prevent infusion-related hypersensitivity reactions.
- *Incompatibilities:* Other drugs or solutions other than 0.9% Sodium Chloride Injection

Lyophilized powder form

- Only use the 100-mg lyophilized powder in vial for pediatric patients birth and older and weighing at least 1.5 kg (3.3 lb) to children weighing less than 40 kg (88 lb). First, reconstitute with 19 ml of Sterile Water for Injection. Do not use any other solution to reconstitute drug. Discard vial if a vacuum does not pull the Sterile Water for Injection into the vial. Immediately shake vial for 30 sec. Allow contents to settle for 2 to 3 min. Solution should be clear after 3 min. If not, shake vial again for 30 sec and allow contents to settle for 2 to 3 min. Repeat as needed until contents of vial are completely dissolved. Discard vial if contents do not completely dissolve. Following reconstitution, each vial contains 100 mg/20 ml (5 mg/ml) of drug solution. Follow with dilution immediately.
- For pediatric patients birth and older and weighing at least 1.5 kg (3.3 lb) to children weighing less than 40 kg (88 lb), dilute reconstituted powder in 0.9% Sodium Chloride Injection to achieve a concentration of 1.25 mg/ml. Small 0.9% Sodium Chloride Injection infusion bags (e.g., 25, 50, or 100 ml) or an appropriately sized syringe should be used for pediatric dosing. After withdrawing the required volume of reconstituted solution from the vial into the bag or syringe, gently invert the bag or syringe 20 times to mix the solution. Do not shake. Infuse the prepared diluted solution immediately. A syringe and syringe pump may be used for infusion volumes less than 50 ml.
- For pediatric patients birth and older and weighing at least 1.5 kg (3.3 lb) to children weighing less than 40 kg (88 lb), infuse over 30 to 120 min with the rate of infusion (ml/min) calculated based on the total infusion volume and total infusion time.
- For adults and pediatric patients weighing 40 kg (88 lb) or more, dilute reconstituted powder in either a 100-ml or 250-ml 0.9% Sodium Chloride Injection infusion bag as follows: Withdraw and discard from infusion bag the volume of 0.9% Sodium Chloride Injection solution to be replaced by drug solution (40 ml for loading dose of 200 mg; 20 ml for maintenance dose of 100 mg). Withdraw the required volume of drug from vial and transfer to the selected infusion bag. Gently invert bag 20 times to mix solution. Do not shake. The prepared infusion solution is stable for 24 hr at room temperature or 48 hr if refrigerated.
- For adults and children weighing 40 kg (88 lb) or more, infuse over 30 to 120 min. If using a 250-ml infusion bag volume, rate should be 8.33 ml/min to deliver drug in 30 min; 4.17 ml/min to deliver drug in 60 min; and 2.08 ml/min to deliver drug in 120 min. If using a 100-ml infusion bag volume, rate should be 3.33 ml/min to deliver drug in 30 min; 1.67 ml/min to deliver drug in 60 min; and 0.83 ml/min to deliver drug in 120 min.

Solution form

- Do not use this form in pediatric patients weighing 1.5 kg (3.3 lb) to children weighing less than 40 kg (88 lb).
- Withdraw and discard volume of 0.9% Sodium Chloride Injection solution to be replaced by drug solution from a 250-ml infusion bag (40 ml for loading dose of 200 mg; 20 ml for maintenance dose of 100 mg). Do not use a 100-ml infusion bag. Withdraw the required volume of drug from vial by first pulling syringe plunger rod back to fill syringe with about 10 ml of air. Inject air into drug vial above the level of the solution. Invert vial and withdraw the required volume of drug solution into the syringe. The last 5 ml of solution requires more force to withdraw. Transfer the required volume of drug solution into the 250-ml infusion bag.
- Gently invert bag 20 times to mix solution in the bag. Do not shake. The prepared infusion solution is stable for 24 hr at room temperature or 48 hr if refrigerated.

- Infuse over 30 to 120 min. Rate should be 8.33 ml/min to deliver drug in 30 min; 4.17 ml/min to deliver drug in 60 min; and 2.08 ml/min to deliver drug in 120 min.

Route	Onset	Peak	Duration
I.V.	Unknown	Unknown	Unknown

Half-life: 1 hr

Mechanism of Action

Blocks the COVID-19 virus from copying itself, although how it does this is not known.

Contraindications

Hypersensitivity to remdesivir or its components

Interactions

DRUGS

chloroquine phosphate, hydroxychloroquine sulfate: Potential antagonism to remdesivir interfering with drug's effectiveness against COVID-19

Adverse Reactions

CNS: **Seizures**
CV: Decreased heart rate
ENDO: Increased blood glucose level
GI: Abdominal pain, elevated bilirubin and liver enzymes, diarrhea, nausea
GU: **Acute kidney injury**, decreased creatinine clearance and eGFR, elevated creatinine, proteinuria
HEME: Decreased hemoglobin, lymphocytes, or WBC count; **elevated activated partial thromboplastin clostting time (APPT)** or **prothrombin time (PT)**
SKIN: Rash
Other: **Altered potassium levels**; **anaphylaxis**, **angioedema**, **and other hypersensitivity reactions**; infusion reactions

Childbearing Considerations

PREGNANCY

- Pregnancy exposure registry: 1-800-616-3791 or https://covid-pr.pregistry.com.
- Drug may cause fetal harm.
- Use with caution only if benefit to mother outweighs potential risk to fetus.

LACTATION

- Drug is present in breast milk.
- Mothers should check with prescriber before breastfeeding.

Nursing Considerations

- Determine patient's eGFR, liver enzymes, and prothrombin time before starting remdesivir therapy and continue to monitor during therapy, as ordered, because drug may adversely alter these values causing adverse effects.

! **WARNING** Monitor patient closely during and after drug administration for hypersensitivity reactions that could include anaphylactic reactions or are infusion related. Assess patient for angioedema, bradycardia, diaphoresis, dyspnea, fever, hypertension, hypotension, hypoxia, nausea, rash, shivering, tachycardia, or wheezing. Slower infusion rates, with a maximum infusion time of up to 120 minutes, can potentially prevent these signs and symptoms. If signs and symptoms are serious, immediately discontinue infusion, notify prescriber, and provide supportive care, as needed and ordered.

! **WARNING** Notify prescriber if patient's alanine aminotransferase (ALT) levels increase to greater than 10 times the upper limit of normal, as drug may have to be discontinued. However, if patient exhibits signs or symptoms of liver inflammation that are accompanied by an ALT elevation, drug must be discontinued.

! **WARNING** Monitor patient for seizures, especially patients with a seizure disorder. Institute seizure precautions, as appropriate.

! **WARNING** Monitor patient for other persistent, serious, or unusual adverse reactions.

- Be aware that chloroquine phosphate or hydroxychloroquine sulfate should not be coadministered with remdesivir because remdesivir becomes less effective.

PATIENT TEACHING

! **WARNING** Tell females of childbearing age to alert prescriber if pregnant before drug is given because drug effects on fetus are unknown.

- Instruct patient to notify remdesivir prescriber of current chloroquine phosphate or hydroxychloroquine sulfate therapy before therapy begins.

- Inform patient that drug will be given intravenously.

! **WARNING** Review signs and symptoms of an allergic reaction and urge patient to report symptoms immediately to staff.

- Instruct patient to inform staff of any discomfort or adverse effects at infusion site during or after daily infusion.
- Tell patient to notify staff if any other adverse reactions are experienced.

repaglinide

Class and Category

Pharmacologic class: Meglitinide
Therapeutic class: Antidiabetic

Indications and Dosages

✱ *As adjunct to achieve glucose control in type 2 diabetes mellitus as monotherapy in patients whose glycosylated hemoglobin (HbA1C) level is less than 8%*

TABLETS

Adults. *Initial:* 0.5 mg daily 30 min before each meal. Dosage doubled, as needed, every wk until adequate glucose response obtained. *Maintenance:* 0.5 to 4 mg/dose up to 4 times daily. *Maximum:* 16 mg daily in divided doses of not more than 4 mg/dose.

✱ *As adjunct to achieve glucose control in type 2 diabetes mellitus as monotherapy in patients whose HbA1C is 8% or greater*

TABLETS

Adults. *Initial:* 1 or 2 mg daily 30 min before each meal. Dosage doubled, as needed, every wk until adequate glucose response obtained. *Maintenance:* 0.5 to 4 mg/dose up to 4 times daily. *Maximum:* 16 mg daily in divided doses of not more than 4 mg/dose.

± **DOSAGE ADJUSTMENT** For patients with severe renal impairment (creatinine clearance 20 to 40 ml/min), dosage initiated at 0.5 mg before each meal and then titrated gradually, as needed. Concomitant use with clopidogrel should be avoided but if not possible, dosage initiated at 0.5 mg and total daily dose not to exceed 4 mg. For patients taking concomitant strong CYP2C8 or CYP3A4 inducers or CYP2C8 or CYP3A4 inhibitors, individualized dosing adjustments needed. For patients receiving concomitant cyclosporine therapy, total daily dose of 6 mg should not be exceeded.

Drug Administration

P.O.

- Administer drug within 30 min of each meal.
- If a meal is skipped, also skip the scheduled dose for that meal.

Route	Onset	Peak	Duration
P.O.	15–60 min	1 hr	4–6 hr

Half-life: 1 hr

Mechanism of Action

Stimulates release of insulin from functioning pancreatic beta cells. Interaction with the adenosine triphosphatase (ATP)–potassium channel on the beta cell membrane prevents potassium from leaving the cell, which causes the beta cell to depolarize and the cell membrane's calcium channel to open resulting in calcium moving into the cell and insulin moving out to lower blood glucose level. Be aware that the extent of insulin release is glucose dependent; the lower the glucose level, the less insulin is secreted from the cell.

Contraindications

Concurrent therapy with gemfibrozil, hypersensitivity to repaglinide or its components

Interactions

DRUGS

ACE inhibitors, angiotensin II receptor blocking agents, disopyramide, fibrates, fluoxetine, monoamine oxidase inhibitors, nonsteroidal anti-inflammatory agents (NSAIDs), pentoxifylline, pramlintide, propoxyphene, salicylates, somatostatin analogues (e.g., octreotide), and sulfonamide antibiotics: Increased risk of hypoglycemia

atypical antipsychotics (clozapine, olanzapine), calcium channel blockers, corticosteroids, danazol, diuretics, estrogens, glucagon, isoniazid, niacin, oral contraceptives, phenothiazines, progestogens (in oral contraceptives), protease inhibitors, somatropin, sympathomimetics (albuterol,

epinephrine, terbutaline), thyroid hormones: Possibly decreased effectiveness of repaglinide; loss of glucose control
beta-blockers, clonidine, guanethidine, reserpine: Possibly blunt signs and symptoms of hypoglycemia
cyclosporine, CYP2C8 inhibitors (clopidogrel, deferasirox, gemfibrozil, montelukast, trimethoprim), CYP3A4 inhibitors (clarithromycin, erythromycin, ketoconazole, itraconazole): Increased blood repaglinide level, resulting in enhanced and prolonged blood glucose–lowering effects
CYP2C8 and CYP3A4 inducers: Decreased blood repaglinide level, resulting in decreased effectiveness

Adverse Reactions

CNS: Headache
CV: Angina
EENT: Rhinitis, sinusitis
ENDO: **Hypoglycemia**
GI: Diarrhea, elevated liver enzymes, **hepatitis**, nausea, **pancreatitis**
HEME: **Hemolytic anemia**, **leukopenia**, **thrombocytopenia**
MS: Arthralgia, back pain
RESP: Bronchitis, upper respiratory tract infection
SKIN: Alopecia, **Stevens-Johnson syndrome**
Other: **Anaphylaxis**

Childbearing Considerations

PREGNANCY

- It is not known if drug can cause fetal harm.
- Use with caution only if benefit to mother outweighs potential risk to fetus.

LACTATION

- It is not known if drug is present in breast milk.
- Drug is not recommended during breastfeeding because of the potential for hypoglycemia in the breastfed infant.

Nursing Considerations

! WARNING Be aware that repaglinide shouldn't be used with NPH insulin because the combination may increase the risk of serious cardiovascular adverse reactions such as angina.

- Expect to check HbA1C level every 3 months, as ordered, to assess patient's long-term control of blood glucose level.

! WARNING Monitor patient for a hypersensitivity reaction, which could become life-threatening, such as anaphylaxis. If present, notify prescriber, expect drug to be discontinued, and provide supportive care, as needed and ordered.

! WARNING Monitor patient for signs and symptoms of hypoglycemia. Severe hypoglycemia may cause seizures, be life-threatening, or even cause death. Be aware hypoglycemia may happen suddenly and symptoms may differ from patient to patient. Risk factors include changes in meal pattern, level of physical activity, prescribed drugs, or repaglinide use with other antidiabetic drugs. Patients with hepatic or renal impairment are also at higher risk for hypoglycemia. If hypoglycemia occurs, notify prescriber as dosage may need to be reduced and treat according to institutional protocol.

! WARNING Monitor patient for other persistent, serious, or unusual adverse reactions.

- During times of increased stress, such as from infection, surgery, or trauma, monitor blood glucose level often and assess need for additional insulin.

PATIENT TEACHING

- Explain that repaglinide is an adjunct to diet in managing type 2 diabetes mellitus.
- Instruct patient how to administer repaglinide.
- Tell patient to skip dose whenever a meal is skipped to decrease risk of hypoglycemia.
- Inform patient that changes in blood glucose level may cause blurred vision or visual disturbances, especially when repaglinide therapy starts. Reassure patient that these changes are usually transient.
- Inform patient that HbA1C level will be tested every 3 to 6 months until blood glucose level is controlled.

! WARNING Alert patient that drug may cause an allergic reaction. Tell patient to notify prescriber, if present, and, if severe, to seek immediate medical care.

! WARNING Teach patient how to monitor blood glucose level. Review signs and symptoms of hypoglycemia with patient and family or caregiver and how to treat hypoglycemia. Have patient obtain a prescription for glucagon to have at home for family or caregiver to use. Instruct family or caregiver how to administer glucagon if a hypoglycemic reaction becomes severe and to seek immediate emergency care for patient if patient does not respond to glucagon administration. If hypoglycemia occurs frequently or is severe, prescriber should be notified.

! **WARNING** Tell patient to notify prescriber of any other persistent, serious, or unusual adverse reactions.

- Inform mothers wishing to breastfeed that breastfeeding is not recommended during drug therapy.
- Advise patient to wear or carry identification indicating patient has diabetes. Encourage patient to carry candy or other simple carbohydrates with her to treat mild episodes of hypoglycemia.

reslizumab

Cinqair

Class and Category

Pharmacologic class: Interleukin-5 antagonist monoclonal antibody
Therapeutic class: Immunomodulator

Indications and Dosages

∗ *Adjunct for add-on maintenance treatment in patients with severe asthma who have an eosinophilic phenotype*

I.V. INFUSION

Adults. 3 mg/kg infused over 20 to 50 min every 4 wk.

Drug Administration

I.V.

- Remove drug from refrigerator and allow to come to room temperature.
- To minimize foaming, do not shake vial.
- Inspect for particulate matter and discoloration. Solution should be clear to slightly hazy/opalescent, colorless to slightly yellow. Know that because reslizumab is a protein, particles may be present that appear translucent to white and amorphous. Do not use if discolored or other foreign particulate matter is present.
- Withdraw proper volume for dosage based on weight and discard any unused portion.
- Inject drug slowly into an infusion bag containing 50 ml of 0.9% Sodium Chloride Injection to minimize foaming. Drug is compatible with polyvinylchloride (PVC) or polyolefin infusion bags.
- Gently invert the bag to mix the solution. Do not shake.
- If not administered immediately, diluted solution may be stored in refrigerator or at room temperature for up to 16 hr, which must include the time for administration. Store drug protected from light.
- Use an infusion set with an in-line, low- protein-binding filter (pore size of 0.2 micron). Drug is compatible with cellulose acetate, nylon, polyethesulfone (PES), and polyvinylidene fluoride (PVDF) in-line infusion filters.
- If diluted solution was stored in refrigerator allow solution to reach room temperature before infusing. Infuse drug over 20 to 50 min according to total volume to be infused and patient's weight. Do not infuse in the same intravenous line with other agents.
- Never administer drug by I.V. push.
- After infusion is complete, flush the intravenous line with 0.9% Sodium Chloride Injection.
- *Incompatibilities:* Other I.V. drugs or solution other than 0.9% Sodium Chloride Injection

Route	Onset	Peak	Duration
I.V.	Unknown	Unknown	Unknown

Half-life: 24 days

Mechanism of Action

Inhibits IL-5 activity (the major cytokine responsible for activation and survival, differentiation, growth, and recruitment of eosinophils) by blocking its binding to the IL-5 receptor complex found on the eosinophil cell surface. Remember that eosinophils are among many cell types involved in inflammation. By inhibiting IL-5 signaling, the production and survival of eosinophils are reduced, which then reduces inflammation present in asthma.

Contraindications

Hypersensitivity to reslizumab or its components

Interactions

DRUGS

None reported by manufacturer.

Adverse Reactions

EENT: Oropharyngeal pain
GI: Vomiting
MS: Elevated CPK levels; chest, extremity, or neck musculoskeletal pain; muscle fatigue or spasms; myalgia
RESP: **Decreased oxygen saturation**, dyspnea, wheezing
SKIN: Urticaria
Other: **Anaphylaxis**, antibodies to reslizumab, **malignancy**

Childbearing Considerations

PREGNANCY

- It is not known if drug can cause fetal harm although monoclonal antibodies are transported across the placental barrier in a linear fashion as pregnancy progresses; therefore, potential effects on a fetus increases as the pregnancy progresses.
- Use with caution only if benefit to mother outweighs potential risk to fetus.

LACTATION

- It is not known if drug is present in breast milk, although human IgG is present in breast milk.
- Mothers should check with prescriber before breastfeeding.

Nursing Considerations

! **WARNING** Know that reslizumab should not be used to treat acute asthma symptoms or acute exacerbations, including acute bronchospasm or status asthmaticus.

- Check to see that patient with an existing parasitic (helminth) infection has received treatment prior to starting reslizumab therapy because drug may interfere with resolving the infection. If patient becomes infected while receiving reslizumab and does not respond to antihelminth treatment, notify prescriber, as reslizumab will have to be discontinued until infection is resolved.

! **WARNING** Be aware that concurrent inhaled or systemic corticosteroid therapy should not be abruptly discontinued when reslizumab therapy is initiated, as systemic withdrawal symptoms may occur. Expect reductions to be done gradually, as ordered.

! **WARNING** Monitor patient for a hypersensitivity reaction, which could become life-threatening, such as anaphylaxis. These reactions most often occur during or within 20 minutes after completion of the infusion, although reactions have occurred before the second dose 4 weeks later. If severe symptoms, such as anaphylaxis, occur, stop infusion at once, notify prescriber, and provide supportive care, as needed and ordered. Know that if anaphylaxis occurs, drug should be permanently discontinued. Be aware that reslizumab-specific IgE antibodies may not be detected in patients who have had a previous experience of anaphylactic reactions to the drug.

! **WARNING** Be aware that, infrequently, malignancies of many different types have occurred within 6 months after patient's exposure to reslizumab. Report any persistent, severe, or unusual symptoms immediately to the prescriber.

PATIENT TEACHING

! **WARNING** Remind patient that reslizumab is not used to treat acute asthma symptoms or acute exacerbations. If asthma symptoms worsen or become acute, instruct patient to seek immediate emergency care.

! **WARNING** Tell patient not to change any concurrent inhaled or systemic corticosteroid dosage when starting reslizumab until instructed to do so by prescriber. Inform patient that if a dosage reduction is done, it will be done gradually to avoid withdrawal symptoms. Remind patient that corticosteroids should never be abruptly stopped.

! **WARNING** Inform patient that drug may cause an allergic reaction that could become life-threatening. If present, tell patient to notify prescriber and, if severe, to seek immediate medical care.

! **WARNING** Alert patient that drug may cause malignancies. Instruct patient to notify prescriber or seek immediate medical care if persistent, severe, or unusual symptoms occurs.

revefenacin

Yupelri

Class and Category

Pharmacologic class: Anticholinergic
Therapeutic class: Bronchodilator

Indications and Dosages

✱ *To provide maintenance therapy for patients with chronic obstructive pulmonary disease (COPD)*

ORAL INHALATION SOLUTION

Adults. 175 mcg once daily by nebulizer. *Maximum:* 175 mg once daily.

Drug Administration

INHALATION

- Remove unit-dose vial from foil pouch and open immediately before use.
- Administer by the orally inhaled route via a standard jet nebulizer connected to an air compressor and using a mouthpiece.
- Do not mix any other drugs in the nebulizer with revefenacin, as drug compatibility is unknown.

Route	Onset	Peak	Duration
Inhalation	45 min	14–41 min	24 hr

Half-life: 22–70 hr

Mechanism of Action

Inhibits muscarinic receptor M3 in smooth muscles of the airways to produce bronchodilation.

Contraindications

Hypersensitivity to revefenacin or its components

Interactions

DRUGS

OATP1B1 and OATP1B3 inhibitors, such as cyclosporine, rifampicin: Possibly increased systemic exposure of revefenacin leading to increased adverse reactions

other anticholinergics: Possible additive anticholinergic effects leading to increased adverse reactions

Adverse Reactions

CNS: Dizziness, headache
CV: Hypertension
EENT: Dry mouth, nasopharyngitis, oropharyngeal pain
MS: Back pain
RESP: Bronchitis, cough, **paradoxical bronchospasms**, upper respiratory infection
Other: **Immediate hypersensitivity reactions**

Childbearing Considerations

PREGNANCY

- It is not known if drug can cause fetal harm.
- Use with caution only if benefit to mother outweighs potential risk to fetus.

LACTATION

- It is not known if drug is present in breast milk.
- Mothers should check with prescriber before breastfeeding.

Nursing Considerations

! **WARNING** Be aware that revefenacin should not be initiated in patients during acutely deteriorating or potentially life-threatening episodes of COPD. It should also not be used to relieve acute bronchospasms; know that acute symptoms should be treated with an inhaled, short-acting beta$_2$-agonist.

! **WARNING** Monitor patient for an immediate hypersensitivity reaction or paradoxical bronchospasm that may become life-threatening. If this should occur following a nebulizer treatment with revefenacin, notify prescriber immediately; expect to administer an inhaled, short-acting bronchodilator, as ordered, for treatment of bronchospasms; and know that revefenacin should be discontinued immediately and alternative therapy substituted.

- Notify prescriber if revefenacin no longer controls symptoms of bronchoconstriction because this may indicate that patient's condition is deteriorating, and other forms of therapy may be required. The dosage or frequency of revefenacin should not be increased in this situation.

- Monitor patients with narrow-angle glaucoma because revefenacin may worsen the condition. Question patient frequently about presence of blurred vision, colored images, eye discomfort or pain, or visual halos in association with red eyes from conjunctival congestion and corneal edema. Notify prescriber immediately, if present.
- Monitor patients with urinary retention because revefenacin may worsen condition. Monitor patient for signs and symptoms of urinary retention, such as difficulty passing urine or painful urination, especially in patients with bladder-neck obstruction or prostatic hyperplasia.

PATIENT TEACHING

! **WARNING** Inform patient that revefenacin therapy is not meant to relieve acute symptoms of COPD and extra doses should never be used for that purpose. Instead, acute symptoms should be treated with an inhaled short-acting $beta_2$-agonist, such as albuterol.

- Teach patient how to administer drug using a standard jet nebulizer.
- Warn patient not to inhale more than 1 dose at any given time. Remind him the daily dosage should not exceed 1 unit-dose vial.

! **WARNING** Inform patient that drug may cause paradoxical bronchospasm. If present, patient should use an inhaled, short-acting bronchodilator immediately, stop taking revefenacin, and notify prescriber.

! **WARNING** Tell patient drug may cause allergic reactions that may occur after revefenacin has been administered. Instruct patient to notify prescriber, as drug will have to be discontinued, and to seek immediate medical care if reaction is severe.

! **WARNING** Stress importance of keeping plastic vials out of the reach of children because the vials' small size poses a choking danger if swallowed.

- Instruct patient to notify prescriber immediately if he experiences decreased effectiveness or needs more of his inhaled short-acting $beta_2$ agonist or experiences a decrease in lung function. Warn him not to stop taking revefenacin without consulting prescriber, as symptoms may reoccur or become worse.
- Instruct patient to report the presence of blurred vision, colored images, eye discomfort or pain, or visual halos in association with red eyes from conjunctival congestion and corneal edema.
- Tell patient, especially if he has bladder-neck obstruction or prostatic hyperplasia, to report difficulty passing urine or painful urination.

ribavirin

Virazole

Class and Category

Pharmacologic class: Nucleoside analogue
Therapeutic class: Antiviral

Indications and Dosages

✱ *As adjunct to treat chronic hepatitis C (CHC) infection in combination with interferon alfa-2b (pegylated and nonpegylated) in patients with compensated liver disease*

CAPSULES

Adults weighing more than 105 kg (231 lb). 600 mg in morning and 800 mg in evening for 24 wk (genotype 2 or 3) and 48 wk (genotype 1).
Adults weighing 81 to 105 kg (178 to 231 lb) and children ages 3 to 18 weighing more than 73 kg (162 lb). 600 mg in morning and 600 mg in evening for 24 wk (genotype 2 or 3) and 48 wk (genotype 1).
Adults weighing 66 to 80 kg (145 to 177 lb) and children ages 3 to 18 weighing 60 to 73 kg (132 to 162 lb). 400 mg in morning and 600 mg in evening for 24 wk (genotype 2 or 3) and 48 wk (genotype 1).
Adults weighing less than 66 kg (144 lb) and children ages 3 to 18 weighing 47 to 59 kg (103 to 131 lb). 400 mg in morning and 400 mg in evening for 24 wk (genotype 2 or 3) and 48 wk (genotype 1).
Children ages 3 to 18 weighing less than 47 kg (103 lb). 15 mg/kg/day divided and given in 2 doses for 24 wk (genotype 2 or 3) and 48 wk (genotype 1).

✱ *As adjunct to treat chronic hepatitis C (CHC) infection in combination with peginterferon alfa-2a in patients with compensated liver disease who have not been previously treated with interferon alpha*

TABLETS

Adults with genotypes 1 or 4 weighing 75 kg (165 lb) or more. 1200 mg in 2 divided doses for 48 wk.

Adults with genotypes 1 or 4 weighing less than 75 kg (165 lb). 1,000 mg in 2 divided doses for 48 wk.

Adults with genotypes 2 or 3. 800 mg in 2 divided doses for 24 wk.

Children ages 5 to 18 weighing 75 kg (165 lb) or more. 600 mg in morning and 600 mg in evening for 24 to 48 wk depending on genotype.

Children ages 5 to 18 weighing 60 to 74 kg (132 to 162.8 lb). 400 mg in morning and 600 mg in evening for 24 to 48 wk depending on genotype.

Children ages 5 to 18 weighing 47 to 59 kg (103.4 to 129.8 lb). 400 mg in morning and 400 mg in evening for 24 to 48 wk depending on genotype.

Children ages 5 to 18 weighing 34 to 46 kg (74.8 to 101.2 lb). 200 mg in morning and 400 mg in evening for 24 to 48 wk depending on genotype.

Children ages 5 to 18 weighing 23 to 33 kg (50.6 to 72.6 lb). 200 mg in morning and 200 mg in evening for 24 to 48 wk depending on genotype.

∗ *As adjunct to treat chronic hepatitis C (regardless of genotype) with HIV coinfection in combination with peginterferon alfa-2a*

TABLETS

Adults. 800 mg daily for 48 wk.

∗ *To treat hospitalized infants and young children with severe lower respiratory tract infections due to respiratory syncytial virus (RSV)*

INHALATION SOLUTION (VIRAZOLE)

Hospitalized infants and young children. 20 mg/ml administered by SPAG-2 unit with continuous aerosol for 12 to 18 hr daily for 3 to 7 days.

± **DOSAGE ADJUSTMENT** For patients with renal dysfunction and severe adverse reactions, dosage adjustment individualized.

Drug Administration

P.O.

- Drug is classified as a hazardous drug and has the potential for carcinogenicity and teratogenicity.
- Administer with food.
- Administer consistently at the same times daily, morning, and evening.
- Capsules and tablets should be swallowed whole and not chewed, crushed, or opened/split.
- If a dose is missed, administer it as soon as possible during the same day. Do not double the next dose.

INHALATION

- Use in children only.
- Do not mix with or simultaneously give with other aerosolized medications.
- Prepare powder for administration as a solution by reconstituting drug with a minimum of 75 ml of Sterile Water for Injection or Inhalation in the original 100-ml glass vial. Do not use Bacteriostatic Water. Shake well.
- Transfer solution to the clean, sterilized 500-ml SPAG-2 reservoir.
- Further dilute to a final volume of 300 ml with Sterile Water for Injection or Inhalation. Do not use Bacteriostatic Water. The final concentration should be 20 mg/ml.
- Discard solutions in the SPAG-2 unit at least every 24 hr and when the liquid level is low before adding newly reconstituted solution.

Route	Onset	Peak	Duration
P.O.	Unknown	1–2 hr	Unknown
Inhalation	Unknown	Unknown	Unknown

Half-life: 12 days

Mechanism of Action

May inhibit HCV polymerase or respiratory syncytial virus in a selective biochemical reaction as precise mechanism is unknown.

Contraindications

Autoimmune hepatitis (oral), coadministration with didanosine (oral), creatinine clearance less than 50 ml/min (oral), hemoglobinopathies (sickle cell anemia, thalassemia major [oral]), hypersensitivity to ribavirin or its components, men whose female partners are pregnant, pregnancy (oral)

Interactions

DRUGS

azathioprine: Increased risk of azathioprine-related myelotoxicity and severe pancytopenia

didanosine: Increased risk of didanosine-induced toxicities, such as hepatic failure, pancreatitis, peripheral neuropathy, and symptomatic hyperlactatemia/lactic acidosis
lamivudine, stavudine, zidovudine: Possibly decreased effectiveness of these drugs; increased risk of hepatic toxicity, anemia, and hepatic decompensation

Adverse Reactions

CNS: Aggression, agitation, anger, anxiety, asthenia, chills, **CVA**, depression, dizziness, emotional swings in mood, fatigue, fever, hallucinations, headache, impaired concentration, insomnia, irritability, lethargy, malaise, memory impairment, nervousness, peripheral neuropathy, psychosis, rigors, **suicidal ideation**, vertigo
CV: Angina, **bigeminy**, **bradycardia** (inhalation solution), **cardiac arrest**, chest pain, **hypotension** (inhalation solution)
EENT: Blurred vision, conjunctivitis, dry mouth, hearing impairment or loss, pharyngitis, retinal detachment or exudates, rhinitis, significant ophthalmologic disorders, sinusitis, taste perversion, transient blindness
ENDO: Hyperglycemia, hypothyroidism, growth retardation (children)
GI: Abdominal pain, anorexia, cholangitis, colitis, constipation, diarrhea, dyspepsia, elevated liver enzymes, fatty liver, **GI bleeding**, **hepatic decompensation**, hepatomegaly, hyperbilirubinemia, nausea, **pancreatitis**, peptic ulcer, vomiting
GU: Menstrual disorder
HEME: Anemia, **hemolytic anemia**, **leukopenia**, **neutropenia**, **pure red cell aplasia**, reticulocytosis (inhalation solution), **thrombocytopenia**, **thrombotic thrombocytopenic purpura**
MS: Arthralgia, back pain, extremity pain, musculoskeletal pain, myalgia, myositis
RESP: Cough, dyspnea, **pulmonary embolism or hypertension** (inhalation solution in children); **apnea**, **atelectasis**, bacterial pneumonia, **bronchospasm**, **cyanosis**, dyspnea, **hypoventilation**, **pneumothorax**, **pulmonary edema**, **ventilator dependence**, **worsening of respiratory status** (inhalation solution)
SKIN: Alopecia, dermatitis, diaphoresis, dry skin, eczema, erythroderma, flushing, pruritus, rash, **Stevens-Johnson syndrome**, **toxic epidermal necrolysis**, urticaria
Other: **Anaphylaxis**; **angioedema**; autoimmune disorders; bacterial, fungal, or viral infections; dehydration; flu-like symptoms; graft rejection (liver or renal); hyperuricemia; weight loss

Childbearing Considerations

PREGNANCY

- Pregnancy exposure registry: 1-800-593-2214.
- Drug can cause fetal harm with significant embryocidal and teratogenic effects.
- A negative pregnancy must be obtained immediately before drug therapy begins and periodic pregnancy tests done during treatment and for 9 mo following discontinuation of drug.
- Drug is contraindicated in females who are pregnant and in male partners of females who are pregnant. If pregnancy occurs, drug must be discontinued immediately.

LACTATION

- It is not known if drug is present in breast milk.
- A decision should be made to either discontinue the drug or breastfeeding.

REPRODUCTION

- Females of childbearing age should use effective contraception during drug therapy and for 9 mo after drug has been discontinued; male patients and their female partners of childbearing age should use effective contraception during drug therapy and for 6 mo after drug has been discontinued.
- Drug may impair male fertility.

Nursing Considerations

! WARNING Ensure females of childbearing age or partners of male patients who are of childbearing age have a negative pregnancy test before drug therapy begins and then monthly pregnancy tests from then on. Drug must be discontinued immediately with confirmation of pregnancy.

- Know that because ribavirin is used in conjunction with alpha interferons, serious and severe visual changes may occur. Know that patient should have a baseline ophthalmologic exam before therapy begins. Patients with preexisting ophthalmologic disorders, such as diabetic or hypertensive retinopathy, should receive periodic eye examinations throughout therapy or at any time ocular symptoms appear. Expect drug to be discontinued in patients who develop new or worsening ophthalmologic disorders.

- Know that patient requires the following tests to be performed before ribavirin therapy is started and then periodically thereafter, as ordered, to establish a baseline before treatment starts and allow early detection of adverse effects during treatment: ECG; standard hematologic tests, including hemoglobin; liver function tests; and TSH levels. Expect dosage to be temporarily withheld or discontinued, as ordered, if patient experiences severe adverse reactions or test abnormalities.

! WARNING Be aware that oral ribavirin therapy should not be given to patients with a creatinine clearance less than 50 ml/min because of risk of severe renal dysfunction. Also, know that ribavirin should not be given to patient with a history of significant or unstable cardiac disease because drug may cause a deterioration of cardiovascular status.

! WARNING Monitor patient for a hypersensitivity reaction, which could become life-threatening, such as anaphylaxis or angioedema. If present, notify prescriber, expect drug to be discontinued, and provide supportive care, as needed and ordered.

! WARNING Expect patient's lungs to be assessed regularly for evidence of pulmonary function impairment or pulmonary infiltrates because drug can cause serious or even life-threatening pulmonary adverse reactions. If either develops, expect ribavirin therapy to be discontinued.

! WARNING Monitor patients with impaired renal function and those over the age of 50 during therapy for anemia. Because anemia usually occurs early in treatment, expect to obtain a baseline of patient's hemoglobin and then assess at 2 and 4 weeks after therapy begins. Know that any patient who develops a decreased hemoglobin level below 10 g/dl should have dosage modified or drug discontinued, as ordered, because potentially fatal MIs have occurred from anemia induced by ribavirin therapy. For patients with a history of stable cardiovascular disease, expect a permanent dosage reduction to occur if the hemoglobin decreases by more than or equal to 2 g/dl during any 4-week period. If the hemoglobin remains less than 12 g/dl after 4 weeks of therapy on a reduced dose, expect drug to be discontinued. Also, monitor patient taking azathioprine concomitantly for pancytopenia and bone marrow suppression, which usually occurs within 3 to 7 weeks after concomitant administration of pegylated interferon/ribavirin and azathioprine. Expect drug to be discontinued if pancytopenia develops.

! WARNING Monitor patient for signs and symptoms of pancreatitis (abdominal pain and tenderness, anorexia, fever, nausea, vomiting). If present, notify prescriber and expect drug to be discontinued.

! WARNING Monitor patient closely for suicidal ideation. Suicidal ideation or attempts occur more frequently among pediatric patients, primarily adolescents, when compared to adult patients during treatment and off-therapy follow-up.

- Monitor patient closely with preexisting but stable cardiac disease. Expect that if there is any deterioration in cardiovascular status, ribavirin therapy will be discontinued.

! WARNING Monitor patient for other persistent, serious, or unusual adverse reactions because drug may adversely affect many body systems and has the potential to cause some life-threatening reactions.

PATIENT TEACHING

! WARNING Inform females of childbearing age or partners of male patients who are of childbearing age that a negative pregnancy test must be obtained before ribavirin therapy is begun. Also, tell them a pregnancy test must be performed monthly during ribavirin therapy and for 9 months (6 months if male partner has taken drug) after therapy is finished. Urge the use of a reliable form of contraception throughout treatment and for 9 months after drug has been discontinued (6 months if male partner has taken the drug). Stress importance of notifying prescriber immediately if pregnancy occurs or is suspected.

- Instruct patient how to administer oral or inhalation form of ribavirin prescribed and what to do if a dose is missed.
- Tell patient to maintain adequate hydration throughout ribavirin therapy.

! **WARNING** Alert patient that drug may cause an allergic reaction. If present, tell patient to notify prescriber and, if severe, to seek immediate medical care.

! **WARNING** Advise patient to alert prescriber immediately for any breathing difficulties and, if severe, to seek immediate medical care.

! **WARNING** Caution patient and family or caregiver to watch for changes in behavior or mood as ribavirin may cause suicidal ideation, especially in adolescent patients. If changes are noted, stress importance of contacting prescriber.

- Caution patient not to perform hazardous activities, such as driving, until effects of ribavirin on the nervous system are known and resolved.
- Inform family or caregiver that growth retardation often occurs with combination therapy that includes ribavirin. Reassure family or caregiver that following treatment, rebound growth and weight gain occur in most children.

! **WARNING** Tell patient to notify prescriber of any other persistent, serious, or unusual adverse reactions.

- Instruct patient to comply with dental checkups and to brush teeth thoroughly twice daily. If vomiting should occur, stress importance of rinsing out mouth thoroughly afterward.
- Inform mothers breastfeeding should not be undertaken during drug therapy or drug will have to be discontinued.
- Stress importance of complying with scheduled laboratory tests.

rifampin
(rifampicin)

Rifadin, Rifadin I.V., Rimactane, Rofact (CAN)

Class and Category

Pharmacologic class: Semisynthetic rifamycin
Therapeutic class: Antimycobacterial antitubercular

Indications and Dosages

∗ *As adjunct to treat tuberculosis caused by all strains of* Mycobacterium tuberculosis

CAPSULES, ORAL SUSPENSION, I.V. INFUSION

Adults. 10 mg/kg once daily with other antitubercular drugs for 4 mo. *Maximum:* 600 mg daily.
Children. 10 to 20 mg/kg once daily in combination with other antitubercular drugs for 4 mo. *Maximum:* 600 mg daily.

∗ *To eliminate meningococci from nasopharynx of asymptomatic carriers of* Neisseria meningitidis

CAPSULES, ORAL SUSPENSION, I.V. INFUSION

Adults. 600 mg every 12 hr for 2 days (total of 4 doses).
Infants ages 1 mo and older and children. 10 mg/kg every 12 hr for 2 days (total of 4 doses). *Maximum:* 600 mg/dose.
Infants under age 1 mo. 5 mg/kg every 12 hr for 2 days (total of 4 doses).

Drug Administration

P.O.

- Administer 1 hr before or 2 hr after a meal with a full glass of water.
- If patient is unable to swallow a capsule, have pharmacist prepare an oral suspension.
- Shake oral suspension well before measuring dose. Use a calibrated device when measuring dose of oral suspension.
- Store oral suspension at room temperature or in refrigerator for 4 wk, then discard.

I.V.

- Reconstitute by adding 10 ml Sterile Water for Injection to 600-mg vial. Swirl gently to dissolve to yield a concentration of 60 mg/ml.

- Reconstituted solution is stable at room temperature for up to 30 hr.
- Withdraw appropriate dose and add to 500 ml of 0.9% Sodium Chloride Injection or 5% Dextrose in Water (preferred solution) and infuse at a rate that will complete infusion by 3 hr. Or, withdraw appropriate dose and add to 100 ml of 0.9% Sodium Chloride Injection or 5% Dextrose in Water (preferred solution) and infuse over 30 min.
- Dilutions using 5% Dextrose Injection are stable at room temperature for up to 8 hr; after 8 hr precipitation of rifampin may occur. Dilutions using 0.9% Sodium Chloride Injection are stable at room temperature for up to 6 hr.
- *Incompatibilities:* Diltiazem hydrochloride, other I.V. solutions

Route	Onset	Peak	Duration
P.O.	Unknown	2–4 hr	Unknown
I.V.	Unknown	0.5 to 3 hr	Unknown

Half-life: 2–3 hr

Mechanism of Action

Inhibits bacterial and mycobacterial RNA synthesis by binding to DNA-dependent RNA polymerase, thereby blocking RNA transcription. Exhibits dose-dependent bactericidal or bacteriostatic action. Is highly effective against rapidly dividing bacilli in extracellular cavitary lesions, such as those found in the nasopharynx.

Contraindications

Concurrent use of atazanavir, darunavir, fosamprenavir, lurasidone, praziquantel, ritonavir/saquinavir, saquinavir, or tipranavir; hypersensitivity to rifampin, other rifamycins, or their components

Interactions

DRUGS

antacids: Possibly reduced rifampin absorption

antiarrhythmics (disopyramide, mexiletine, quinidine, propafenone, tocainide), anticonvulsants (phenytoin), antiestrogens (tamoxifen, toremifene), antifungals (fluconazole, itraconazole, ketoconazole), antipsychotics (haloperidol), antiretrovirals (atazanavir, darunavir, efavirenz, fosamprenavir, indinavir, saquinavir, tipranavir, zidovudine), benzodiazepines (diazepam), benzodiazepine-related drugs (zopiclone, zolpidem), beta-blockers (metoprolol, propranolol), calcium channel blockers (diltiazem, nifedipine, verapamil), caspofungin, chloramphenicol, clarithromycin, corticosteroids (prednisolone), dapsone, digoxin, doxycycline, enalapril, fluoroquinolones (moxifloxacin, pefloxacin), hepatitis C antiviral (daclatasvir, simeprevir, sofosbuvir, telaprevir), hypoglycemic agents oral (glipizide, glyburide), immunosuppressive agents (cyclosporine, tacrolimus), irinotecan, levothyroxine, losartan, lurasidone, methadone, mifepristone, narcotic analgesics (morphine, oxycodone), praziquantel, quinine, selective 5-HT$_3$ receptor antagonists (ondansetron), statins (simvastatin), systemic hormonal contraceptives (estrogens, progestins), telithromycin, theophylline, thiazolidinediones (rosiglitazone), ticagrelor, tricyclic antidepressants (nortriptyline), warfarin: Decreased exposure and effectiveness of these drugs

antihypertensives: Possibly interference of antihypertensive action of these drugs

atovaquone: Decreased concentration of atovaquone and increased concentration of rifampin, which may increase risk of toxicities

clopidogrel: Increased risk of bleeding

cotrimoxazole, probenecid: Increased rifampin concentration

halothane, isoniazid: Possibly hepatotoxicity

ritonavir/saquinavir: Increased risk of severe hepatotoxicity

ACTIVITIES

alcohol use: Increased risk of hepatotoxicity

Adverse Reactions

CNS: Ataxia, behavioral changes, chills, confusion, difficulty concentrating, dizziness, drowsiness, fatigue, fever, generalized numbness, headache, paresthesia, psychoses

CV: **Cardiac myopathy**, **chest pain**, **hypotension**, **thrombotic microangiopathy**, vasculitis

EENT: Conjunctivitis; discolored saliva, sputum, tears, and teeth; mouth or tongue soreness; periorbital edema; visual disturbances

ENDO: **Adrenal insufficiency** (rare), hyperglycemia or **hypoglycemia** (in patients with diabetes)
GI: Abdominal cramps, anorexia, cholestasis, diarrhea, discolored feces, elevated liver enzymes, epigastric discomfort, flatulence, heartburn, **hepatitis**, **hepatotoxicity**, jaundice, nausea, **pseudomembranous colitis**, **shock-like syndrome with hepatic involvement**, vomiting
GU: **Acute renal failure or tubular necrosis**, discolored urine, elevated BUN and serum uric acid, hematuria, **hemolytic uremia syndrome**, interstitial nephritis, menstrual disturbances, **renal insufficiency**
HEME: **Agranulocytosis** (rare), decreased hemoglobin, **disseminated intravascular coagulation (DIC)**, eosinophilia, **hemolytic anemia**, **leukopenia**, **neutropenia**, purpura, **thrombocytopenia** (rare), **thrombotic thrombocytopenic purpura**
MS: Arthralgia, extremity pain, muscle weakness, myalgia (rare)
RESP: **Acute bronchospasm**, cough, **pulmonary toxicity (interstitial lung disease)**, shortness of breath, wheezing
SKIN: Acute generalized exanthematous pustulosis, discolored skin and sweat, **erythema multiforme**, flushing, pemphigoid reaction, pruritus, rash, **Stevens-Johnson syndrome**, **toxic epidermal necrolysis**, urticaria
Other: **Anaphylaxis**, **angioedema**, **drug reaction with eosinophilia and systemic symptoms (DRESS)**, flu-like symptoms, lymphadenopathy, paradoxical drug reaction

Childbearing Considerations

PREGNANCY

- It is not known if drug causes fetal harm, but animal studies suggest it may as drug does cross the placental barrier. When given during the last few wk of pregnancy drug can cause postnatal hemorrhages in both mother and infant.
- Use with caution only if benefit to mother outweighs potential risk to fetus.

LACTATION

- Drug is present in breast milk.
- A decision should be made to discontinue breastfeeding or the drug to avoid potential serious adverse reactions.

REPRODUCTION

- Females of childbearing age using an oral hormonal contraceptive should use an additional contraceptive throughout therapy.

Nursing Considerations

! WARNING Be aware that rifampin should not be used to treat meningococcal infection because of the possibility of rapid emergence of resistant organisms.

- Obtain blood samples or other specimens for culture and sensitivity testing, as ordered, before giving rifampin and throughout therapy to monitor response to drug.

! WARNING Expect to obtain liver enzymes, as ordered, before and every 2 to 4 weeks during therapy. Immediately report abnormalities. Also, monitor patient for liver dysfunction, such as abdominal pain, darkened urine, loss of appetite, and yellowish discoloration of the eyes and skin. Know that drug can cause serious liver dysfunction that could become life-threatening.

! WARNING Monitor patient for hypersensitivity reactions, including severe skin reactions which could become life-threatening such as anaphylaxis, angioedema and DRESS. Notify prescriber if present, expect drug to be discontinued, and provide supportive care, as needed and ordered. Know that DRESS may only initially present with a fever or swollen lymph nodes although a rash is most common.

! WARNING Monitor patient for acute respiratory distress syndrome or respiratory failure because rifampin may cause pulmonary toxicity. If present, drug will have to be discontinued immediately and supportive care given, as needed and ordered.

! WARNING Be aware that rifampin can cause myelosuppression and increase risk of infection. Notify prescriber immediately if signs of infection, such as fever, develop. Also, monitor patient for unexplained bleeding or other serious hematologic adverse reactions and report immediately.

! **WARNING** Monitor patients with diabetes mellitus because rifampin therapy can cause hypoglycemia and may make diabetes management more difficult because of its effect on possibly raising blood glucose levels.

- Expect drug to discolor body fluids, skin, and teeth reddish orange to reddish brown.
- Be aware that paradoxical drug reaction (recurrence or appearance of new symptoms) may occur in patients who have shown improvement to drug therapy. It is usually transient and should not be misunderstood as treatment failure.

! **WARNING** Monitor patient for other persistent, serious, or unusual adverse reactions.

PATIENT TEACHING

- Instruct patient, parents, or caregiver how to administer rifampin.
- Emphasize the need to take drug exactly as prescribed. Explain that not completing the full course of therapy or skipping doses may decrease the effectiveness of the treatment and increase the chance that resistance to drug may develop, making it ineffective to treat an infection patient might develop in the future. Emphasize importance of compliance with the full course of therapy.
- Advise patient to avoid alcohol, herbal products, or any drug that adversely affects the liver (without prescriber consent) during rifampin therapy.

! **WARNING** Alert patient that an allergic reaction may occur with rifampin therapy. Review signs and symptoms with patient. Advise patient to alert prescriber if an allergic reaction occurs; if severe, stress importance of seeking immediate medical care. Also, instruct patient to notify prescriber immediately if fever, rash, swollen lymph nodes, or other skin abnormalities occur, as reaction may become severe and life-threatening.

! **WARNING** Urge patient to seek immediate medical care if difficulty breathing occurs.

! **WARNING** Urge patient to notify prescriber about anorexia, cough, darkened urine, fever, flu-like symptoms, joint pain or swelling, malaise, nausea, rash, shortness of breath, swollen lymph nodes, vomiting, wheezing, and yellowish eyes or skin. Also, advise patient to seek medical care immediately if symptoms worsen.

! **WARNING** Review bleeding and infection control measures. Tell patient to notify prescriber immediately, if present.

! **WARNING** Advise females of childbearing age who take an oral hormonal contraceptive to use an additional form of birth control during rifampin therapy. If pregnancy occurs, tell patient to alert prescriber. In addition, warn patient to alert prescriber when only a few weeks away from delivery to avoid potential bleeding issues in both patient and neonate.

! **WARNING** Inform patient with diabetes mellitus that rifampin therapy may affect blood glucose levels and to monitor blood glucose levels closely, especially for hypoglycemia. Make sure patient knows how to treat hypoglycemia appropriately and to notify prescriber if hypoglycemia occurs frequently or hyperglycemia is persistent. Tell patient to seek immediate medical care if hypoglycemia is severe.

- Alert patient that drug may discolor feces, saliva, skin, sputum, sweat, tears, teeth, and urine reddish brown to reddish orange or yellow. Discoloration of teeth and soft contact lenses may be permanent.
- Tell mothers breastfeeding should not be undertaken during rifampin therapy or drug will need to be discontinued.
- Tell patient to inform all prescribers of rifampin therapy.

rifaximin

Xifaxan

Class and Category

Pharmacologic class: Rifamycin
Therapeutic class: Antibiotic

Indications and Dosages

✶ *To treat irritable bowel syndrome with diarrhea (IBS-D)*

TABLETS

Adults. 550 mg 3 times daily for 14 days. May be repeated up to 2 times for reoccurrence.

∗ *To treat travelers' diarrhea caused by noninvasive strains of* Escherichia coli

TABLETS

Adults and children ages 12 and older. 200 mg 3 times daily for 3 days.

∗ *To reduce risk of overt hepatic encephalopathy*

TABLETS

Adults. 550 mg twice daily.

Drug Administration

P.O.

- Administer drug without regard to food.

Route	Onset	Peak	Duration
P.O.	Unknown	1 hr	Unknown

Half-life: 2–5 hr

Mechanism of Action

Inhibits bacterial RNA synthesis by binding to DNA-dependent RNA polymerase, thereby blocking RNA transcription to cause bacterial cell impairment or death.

Contraindications

Hypersensitivity to rifaximin, any of the rifamycin-class antimicrobial agents, or their components

Interactions

DRUGS

P-glycoprotein inhibitors, such as cyclosporine: Increased exposure to rifaximin leading to possible risk of increased adverse reactions
warfarin: Altered INR levels possibly requiring warfarin dosage adjustment

Adverse Reactions

CNS: Anxiety, depression, dizziness, fatigue, fever, headache, insomnia
CV: Peripheral edema
EENT: Nasal passage irritation, nasopharyngitis, taste loss
GI: Abdominal pain, anorexia, ascites, ***Clostridioides difficile*–associated colitis**, constipation, diarrhea, **dysentery**, elevated ALT liver enzyme, nausea, vomiting
GU: **Acute renal failure**, UTI
HEME: Anemia
MS: Arthralgia, muscle spasms, myalgia, **rhabdomyolysis**
RESP: Cough, dyspnea
SKIN: **Exfoliative dermatitis**, flushing, pruritus, rash, **Stevens-Johnson syndrome**, **toxic epidermal necrolysis**, urticaria
Other: **Anaphylaxis**, **angioedema**, elevated blood creatine phosphokinase, weight loss

Childbearing Considerations

PREGNANCY

- It is not known if drug can cause fetal harm, although some animal studies suggest it may cause fetal harm.
- Use with caution only if benefit to mother outweighs potential risk to fetus.

LACTATION

- It is not known if drug is present in breast milk.
- Mothers should check with prescriber before breastfeeding.

Nursing Considerations

! **WARNING** Be aware that rifaximin should not be used in patients with travelers' diarrhea complicated by blood in the stool, diarrhea due to pathogens other than *E. coli*, or in the presence of fever.

! **WARNING** Use extreme caution in patients with severe hepatic impairment because of increased rifaximin exposure in these patients which could lead to possible increased risk of adverse reactions.

! **WARNING** Monitor patient for signs and symptoms of hypersensitivity reactions, including severe skin reactions. Notify prescriber if rash or other adverse reactions are present, expect drug to be discontinued, and provide supportive care, as needed and ordered.

! **WARNING** Notify prescriber if diarrhea gets worse or persists for more than 48 hours in patients being treated for diarrhea or for a new onset of diarrhea in patients being treated for hepatic encephalopathy. The patient may be experiencing *C. difficile* colitis associated with antibiotic use which may be mild or become life-threatening. Expect to obtain a stool specimen for diagnositic purposes. If confirmed, expect, rifaximin to be discontinued and an antibiotic effective against *C. difficile* along with electrolytes, fluids, and protein supplementation therapy, to be administered, as needed and ordered.

PATIENT TEACHING

- Instruct patient how to administer rifampin.
- Stress importance of taking drug for length of time prescribed, even when feeling better.

! **WARNING** Alert patient that an allergic reaction may occur with rifampin therapy. Review signs and symptoms with patient. Advise patient to alert prescriber if an allergic reaction occurs; if severe, stress importance of seeking immediate medical care. Also, instruct patient to notify prescriber immediately if rash or other skin abnormalities occur, as skin reactions may become severe.

! **WARNING** Tell patient to report diarrhea that gets worse or persists for more than 48 hours or new onset or reoccurrence of diarrhea, as diarrhea may occur even after rifaximin has been discontinued, requiring additional treatment.

rilpivirine

Edurant, Edurant Ped

Class and Category

Pharmacologic class: Nonnucleoside reverse transcriptase inhibitor (NNRTI)
Therapeutic class: Antiretroviral

Indications and Dosages

* *As adjunct to treat human immunodeficiency virus type 1 (HIV-1) infection in antiretroviral treatment-naïve patients with HIV-1 RNA equal to or less than 100,000 copies/ml at the start of therapy*

TABLETS

Adults and children ages 2 and older weighing at least 25 kg (55 lb). 25 mg once daily with a meal.

TABLETS FOR ORAL SUSPENSION

Children ages 2 and older weighing 20 kg (44 lb) to less than 25 kg (55 lb). 15 mg once daily.
Children ages 2 and older weighing 14 kg (30.8 lb) to less than 20 kg (44 lb). 12.5 mg once daily.

± **DOSAGE ADJUSTMENT** For patients taking rifabutin concomitantly, dosage increased to 50 mg once daily.

* *To provide short-term treatment of HIV-1 infection in combination with cabotegravir in patients who are virologically suppressed (HIV-1 RNA less than 50 copies/ml) and on a stable antiretroviral regimen with no history of treatment failure and with no known or suspected resistance to either cabotegravir or rilpivirine as either an oral lead-in to assess the tolerability of rilpivirine prior to administration of the combination product Cabenuva (cabotegravir, rilpivirine E.R. injectable suspension) or to provide oral therapy for patients who will miss planned injection dosing with Cabenuva E.R. injectable suspension*

TABLETS

Adults requiring lead-in dosing. 25 mg rilpivirine with 30 mg oral cabotegravir once daily for at least 28 days with last oral dose given on the same day injections with Cabenuva are started.
Adults replacing planned missed Cabenuva injections. 25-mg rilpivirine with 30-mg oral cabotegravir once daily for up to 2 consecutive mo of missed Cabenuva injections and started 1 mo after last injection dose of Cabenuva and continued until the day injection dosing is restarted.

Drug Administration

P.O.

- Do not interchange tablets and tablets used for oral suspension as there is a difference in bioavailability between the 2 formulations.
- Administer drug with a meal; a protein drink is not adequate to count as a meal.
- Tablets (not used for oral suspension) should be swallowed whole and not chewed, crushed, or split.
- Tablet for oral suspension should only be given to children weighing at least 14 kg (30.8 lb) to less than 25 kg (55 lb).
- Tablets for oral suspension should not be chewed or swallowed whole. Instead, place tablets for oral suspension in a cup (do not crush) and add 5 ml of drinking water at room temperature. Swirl cup carefully for 1 to 2 min to disperse the tablets. The solution will begin to look cloudy. Administer the water solution or dilute further with 5 ml of drinking water, milk or orange juice or mix with applesauce. Swirl liquid and administer

immediately or use spoon to administer applesauce mixture immediately. Make sure the entire dose is taken. If needed, if some of the drug is still in the cup, add another 5 ml of drinking water (or alternative beverage or soft food) swirl and have patient drink again.

- If administering drug with cabotegravir, administer both drugs at the same time each day with a meal.
- The last oral dose of drug administered with oral cabotegravir should be given on the same day injections with Cabenuva are started or restarted.

Route	Onset	Peak	Duration
P.O.	Unknown	4–5 hr	Unknown

Half-life: 50 hr

Mechanism of Action

Inhibits HIV-1 replication by noncompetitive inhibition of HIV-1 reverse transcriptase.

Contraindications

Concomitant therapy with carbamazepine, dexamethasone (more than a single dose), esomeprazole, lansoprazole, omeprazole, oxcarbazepine, pantoprazole, phenobarbital, phenytoin, rabeprazole, rifampin, rifapentine, or St. John's wort; hypersensitivity to rilpivirine or its components

Interactions

DRUGS

aluminum- or magnesium-containing antacids, calcium carbonate, cimetidine, famotidine: Decreased rilpivirine concentration and significantly decreased effectiveness

atazanavir, atazanavir/ritonavir, clarithromycin, darunavir/ritonavir, delavirdine, erythromycin, fluconazole, fosamprenavir, fosamprenavir/ritonavir, indinavir, itraconazole, lopinavir/ritonavir, nelfinavir, posaconazole, saquinavir/ritonavir, telithromycin, tipranavir, voriconazole: Increased concentration of rilpivirine with possible prolonged action and risk of adverse reactions

carbamazepine, dexamethasone (more than a single dose), phenobarbital, phenytoin, proton pump inhibitors, rifampin, rifapentine, St. John's wort: Possibly significant decrease in rilpivirine plasma concentrations, resulting in loss of virologic response

drugs that prolong QT interval: Increased risk of torsades de pointes

ketoconazole: Decreased ketoconazole concentration and effectiveness and increased rilpivirine concentration with possible prolonged action and risk of adverse reactions

methadone: Possible decreased methadone concentration with increased risk of opiate withdrawal

other NNRTIs (efavirenz, etravirine, nevirapine), rifabutin: Decreased concentration of rilpivirine with possible decreased effectiveness

Adverse Reactions

CNS: Abnormal dreams, anxiety, depression, dizziness, dysphoria, fatigue, fever, headache, insomnia, mood changes, sleep disorders, somnolence, **suicidal ideation**

CV: Elevated cholesterol and triglycerides

EENT: Conjunctivitis, oral ulceration

ENDO: Cushingoid appearance, fat redistribution

GI: Abdominal discomfort or pain, anorexia, cholecystitis, cholelithiasis, diarrhea, elevated bilirubin or liver enzymes, **hepatitis**, **hepatotoxicity**, nausea, vomiting

GU: Elevated creatinine, **glomerulonephritis**, nephrolithiasis, **nephrotic syndrome**

HEME: Eosinophilia

SKIN: Blisters, rash

Other: **Angioedema**, **drug reaction with eosinophilia and systemic symptoms (DRESS)**, **immune reconstitution syndrome**, **immune reconstitution syndrome**

Childbearing Considerations

PREGNANCY

- Pregnancy exposure registry: 1-800-258-4263.
- Drug does not appear to cause fetal harm.
- Monitor viral loads more closely because pregnancy may cause a lower exposure of rilpivirine.
- Drug can be administered during pregnancy.

LACTATION

- It is not known if drug is present in breast milk.

- The Centers for Disease Control and Prevention recommends that HIV-1 infected mothers not breastfeed to avoid risking postnatal transmission of HIV-1 infection to infants. They also do not recommend breastfeeding because of potential drug-induced adverse reactions in the infant.

Nursing Considerations

! WARNING Know that drug should not be used in patients taking other medications with a known risk of torsades de pointes or in patients at higher risk of torsades de pointes because rilpivirine may cause QT prolongation.

! WARNING Obtain liver enzymes before therapy begins, as ordered, in patients with marked transaminase elevations, patients treated with other medications associated with liver toxicity, and patients with underlying hepatic disease, including hepatitis B or C viral infections. Also, monitor liver enzymes throughout therapy, as ordered, on all patients because rilpivirine may cause hepatotoxicity. Know that persistent elevations of serum transaminase levels may require rilpivirine therapy to be discontinued.

! WARNING Obtain BUN and creatinine levels before rilpivirine therapy begins, as ordered, and periodically thoughout treatment because drug may cause serious to life-threatening kidney dysfunction such as acute renal failure and glomerulonephritis.

- Obtain cholesterol and triglyceride levels before starting rilpivirine therapy and periodically throughout therapy because drug may cause an increase in total cholesterol and triglycerides.

! WARNING Monitor patient for a hypersensitivity or skin reaction, which could become life-threatening, such as angioedema or DRESS. Notify prescriber and expect rilpivirine to be discontinued immediately if patient develops a hypersensitivity or severe skin reaction, including a severe rash accompanied by blisters, conjunctivitis, eosinophilia, facial edema, fever, joint or muscle aches, lip swelling, malaise, or oral lesions. DRESS may only initially present with a fever or swollen lymph nodes. Be aware that a delay in discontinuing drug may result in a life-threatening situation. Provide supportive care, as needed and ordered.

! WARNING Monitor patient's emotional status and mood, as rilpivirine may cause significant depression, mood changes, and suicidal ideation. Report any changes to prescriber.

! WARNING Be aware that immune reconstitution syndrome has occurred in patients treated with combination antiretroviral therapy, including rilpivirine. The inflammatory response predisposes susceptible patients to opportunistic infections, such as cytomegalovirus, *Mycobacterium avium* infection, *Pneumocystis jiroveci* pneumonia, or tuberculosis. Autoimmune disorders such as Graves' disease, Guillain-Barré syndrome, or polymyositis have also occurred. Report sudden or unusual adverse reactions to prescriber.

PATIENT TEACHING

- Instruct patient, family, or caregiver how to administer rilpivirine.

! WARNING Advise patient that rilpivirine therapy may cause severe allergic or skin reactions. Tell her to report any signs of an allergic reaction or a rash, especially if it is accompanied by blisters, conjunctivitis, facial edema, fatigue, fever, joint or muscle aches, liver problems, or oral lesions and to seek immediate medical attention.

! WARNING Inform patient about severe liver disease that may occur with rilpivirine. Tell her to report signs and symptoms of liver disease, such as acholic stools, anorexia, fatigue, malaise, nausea, tenderness over liver area, or yellowing of skin or whites of the eyes and to seek immediate medical attention.

! WARNING Review signs and symptoms of renal dysfunction such as fatigue, decreased urine output, and leg edema. Tell patient to report any abnormalities to prescriber.

! **WARNING** Tell patient and family or caregiver to report any signs of depression, mood changes, sleep disorders, or suicidal thoughts to prescriber.

! **WARNING** Instruct patient to report any other persistent, severe, or unusual signs and symptoms.

- Inform patient that rilpivirine therapy may cause changes in her body appearance because of fat redistribution. Prepare her for the possibility of developing breast enlargement, central obesity, dorsocervical fat enlargement (buffalo hump), facial wasting, and peripheral wasting.
- Alert mothers that breastfeeding is not recommended during rilpivirine therapy.
- Tell patient to report all drugs being taken, including over-the-counter medications and herbals, as serious drug interactions may occur. Advise patient not to begin any new drug therapy without first checking with prescriber.
- Stress importance of being compliant with tests ordered to screen for adverse effects of rilpivirine therapy.

rimegepant

Nurtec ODT

Class and Category

Pharmacologic class: Calcitonin gene-related peptide (CGRP) receptor antagonist
Therapeutic class: Antimigraine

Indications and Dosages

∗ *To treat acute migraine*

ORALLY DISINTEGRATING TABLETS

Adults. 75 mg. *Maximum:* 75 mg in a 24-hr period and no more than 18 doses in a 30-day period.

± **DOSAGE ADJUSTMENT** For patients taking a moderate inhibitor of CYP3A4 or potent inhibitors of P-gp, length of time a second dose may be taken increased to every 48 hours.

∗ *To prevent episodic migraines*

ORALLY DISINTEGRATING TABLETS

Adults. 75 mg every other day.

Drug Administration

P.O.

- Using dry gloved hands, peel back foil covering of one blister and gently remove tablet. Do not push tablet through the foil.
- Administer immediately, without additional liquid, by placing tablet on or under patient's tongue.
- Do not store tablet outside the blister pack for future use.

Route	Onset	Peak	Duration
P.O.	Unknown	1.5 hr	Unknown

Half-life: 11 hr

Mechanism of Action

Blocks CGRP receptors to help stop inflammation, pain signals, and swelling of blood vessels that occur in the brain during a migraine headache.

Contraindications

Hypersensitivity to rimegepant or its components

Interactions

DRUGS

BCRP or P-gp inhibitors: Possibly increased exposure to rimegepant with possibly increased risk of adverse reactions
CYP3A4 moderate or strong inducers: Decreased rimegepant exposure with possible loss of effectiveness
CYP3A4 moderate or strong inhibitors: Increased (strong) or possible increased (moderate) rimegepant exposure with possibly increased risk of adverse reactions

Adverse Reactions

GI: Abdominal pain, dyspepsia, nausea
MS: Dyspnea
SKIN: Severe rash
Other: **Hypersensitivity reactions**

Childbearing Considerations

PREGNANCY

- Pregnancy exposure registry: 1-877-366-0324, web address: nurtecpregnancyregistry.com, or email: nurtecpregnancyregistry@ppd.com.
- It is not known if drug can cause fetal harm.

- Use with caution only if benefit to mother outweighs potential risk to fetus.
- Know that pregnant females with migraine may be at increased risk of gestational hypertension and preeclampsia.

LACTATION

- Drug is present in breast milk in low amounts.
- Mothers should check with prescriber before breastfeeding.

Nursing Considerations

! **WARNING** Know that rimegepant should not be administered to patients taking BCRP or P-gp inhibitors and moderate or strong CYP3A inducers because these drugs interfere with the effectiveness of rimegepant.

! **WARNING** Know that rimegepant should not be administered to patients taking strong CYP3A inhibitors because these drugs increase exposure of rimegepant and increase the risk of adverse reactions.

! **WARNING** Monitor patient for hypersensitivity reactions, including dyspnea and rash, which could become severe. Hypersensitivity has been known to occur days after administration and could be serious. If present, notify prescriber, expect drug to be discontinued, and provide supportive care given, as needed and ordered.

PATIENT TEACHING

- Instruct patient on how to administer rimegepant.

! **WARNING** Alert patient that drug may cause an allergic reaction. Remind patient that such reactions may occur days after taking drug. If an allergic reaction occurs, urge patient to contact prescriber or if severe to seek immediate medical care.

- Tell patient to report all drugs being taken, including over-the-counter medications and herbals, because drug interactions may occur. Advise patient not to begin any new drug therapy without first checking with prescriber.

risankizumab-rzaa

Skyrizi

Class and Category

Pharmacologic class: Monoclonal antibody
Therapeutic class: Anti-inflammatory, immunosuppressant

Indications and Dosages

* *To treat moderate to severe plaque psoriasis in patients who are candidates for systemic therapy or phototherapy; to treat active psoriatic arthritis as monotherapy or in combination with nonbiologic disease-modifying antirheumatic drugs (DMARDs)*

SUBCUTANEOUS INJECTION

Adults. *Initial:* 150 mg followed by 150 mg 4 wk later and then 150 mg every 12 wk thereafter.

* *To treat moderately to severely active Crohn's disease*

I.V. INFUSION, SUBCUTANEOUS INJECTION

Adults. *Induction:* 600 mg I.V. infused over at least 60 min and repeated at wk 4 and again at wk 8. *Maintenance:* 180 or 360 mg subcutaneously at wk 12 and every 8 wk thereafter.

* *To treat moderate to severe active ulcerative colitis*

I.V. INFUSION, SUBCUTANEOUS INJECTION

Adults. *Induction:* 1,200 mg I.V. infused over at least 2 hr and repeated at wk 4 and again at wk 8. *Maintenance:* 180 or 360 mg subcutaneously at wk 12 and every 8 wk thereafter.

Drug Administration

I.V.

- I.V. route used only for induction purposes to treat Crohn's disease and ulcerative colitis.
- Determine the dose and number of drug vials needed. 1 drug vial will be needed for Crohn's disease and 2 vials for ulcerative colitis.
- Do not shake drug vial. For induction doses to treat Crohn's disease, withdraw 10 ml from drug vial and inject into an

infusion bag or glass bottle containing 100 ml, 250 ml, or 500 ml 5% Dextrose Injection. For induction doses to treat ulcerative colitis, withdraw 10 ml from each of the 2 drug vials and inject into an infusion bag or glass bottle containing 250 ml or 500 ml 5% Dextrose Injection. Final concentration will be 1.2 mg/ml to 6 mg/ml depending on volume of dilution solution used. Do not shake drug solution.

- Infuse over at least 60 min (Crohn's disease) or over at least 2 hr (ulcerative colitis). Complete the infusion within 8 hr of dilution.
- Diluted solution may be refrigerated for up to 20 hr or 8 hr at room temperature; time must include time required for administration. If refrigerated, allow solution to warm to room temperature before infusing. Protect from light.
- *Incompatibilities:* Other drugs

SUBCUTANEOUS

Prefilled pen or syringe

- Use prefilled pen or syringe for drug administration to treat plaque psoriasis and psoriatic arthritis. Use only the prefilled syringe for maintenance doses for Crohn's disease and ulcerative colitis.
- Take drug carton out of refrigerator and allow drug to warm at room temperature keeping it out of direct sunlight (15 to 30 min for prefilled syringe; 30 to 90 min for prefilled pen) without removing the prefilled syringe or pen from carton.
- Visually inspect solution for particulate matter and discoloration (solution should be colorless to slightly yellow and clear to slightly opalescent).
- Do not shake and do not use if pen or syringe has been dropped or damaged.
- If using 2 separate 75-mg single-dose prefilled syringes for a 150-mg dose, inject in 2 different anatomical sites.
- Do not remove the cap until right before injection. Inject into the abdomen, thigh, or upper outer arm at a 45 degree angle using syringe or at a 90 degree angle using pen. Do not inject into an area that is affected by psoriasis, bruised, indurated, red, or tender.
- When injecting drug using the prefilled pen, hold the pen so the green activator button and inspection window are visible. It is normal to see 1 or more bubbles in the solution. Hold the pen with fingers on the gray hand grips. Push and keep pressing down against injection site before pressing the green activator button. Press the green activator button and hold the pen for 15 sec. A loud click will be heard meaning the injection has started. Keep pressing the pen until the pen has made a second click or the yellow indicator has filled the inspection window. This may take up to 15 sec. Then slowly pull the pen straight out from the skin. The white needle sleeve will cover the needle tip and make another click.
- When injecting drug using the prefilled syringe, do so in the same manner for giving any subcutaneous injection.
- Do not rub the site. Slight bleeding may occur at the injection site, but this is normal.
- If dose is missed, administer as soon as possible and then resume dosing at the regular scheduled time.

On-body injector with prefilled cartridge

- Use on-body injector with prefilled cartridges only for maintenance dosing for Crohn's disease and ulcerative colitis.
- Remove carton from refrigerator and allow to reach room temperature for about 45 to 90 min. Keep out of direct sunlight. Do not remove the prefilled cartridge or on-body injector from carton during this time and do not shake carton.
- Once drug is at room temperature, inspect the solution in the cartridge. It should appear clear to yellow and may contain tiny clear or white particles.
- Load the cartridge into the on-body injector and prepare injector for site placement following manufacturer's instructions. Do not touch the start button until it is placed unto the patient's skin and is ready to inject. Select injection site. If using abdomen, move and hold patient's abdominal skin to create a firm, flat surface for injection at least 2 in from the navel. This is not necessary if using anterior thigh for placement of injector. However, plan to position the injector so that the blue status light can be seen. When the blue light flashes, the injector is ready. Now place the injector onto the selected injection site with the status light visible. Press start button within 5 min of placing the on-body

injector on patient's skin. The start button can only be pressed once.

- The status light will then continuously flash green and a pumping sound may be heard during the injection. (If status light flashes red, do not continue injection and remove device from patient's skin. Notify prescriber as manufacturer will need to be called.)
- It may take up to 5 min to complete injection. The injector will stop on its own. Beeps will be heard and the status light will change to a solid green. Remove the injector from the injection site following manufacturer's instructions.
- Do not use injector or cartridge if either has been dropped or damaged. Do not reuse either component. The injector and cartridge are for 1-time use only. Do not let the injector get wet with water or any other liquids.
- Limit patient's physical activity during the injection. Moderate activities such as bending, reaching for something, or walking is permissible. Keep electronic devices including cell phones at least 12 inches from on-body injector until injection is complete.

Route	Onset	Peak	Duration
SubQ	Unknown	Unknown	Unknown

Half-life: 28 days

Mechanism of Action

Thought to block interleukin-23, which causes inflammation and swelling, reducing the signs and symptoms of active psoriatic arthritis and plaque psoriasis although exact mechanism is unknown.

Contraindications

Hypersensitivity to risankizumab-rzaa or its components

Interactions

DRUGS

immunosuppressants: Enhanced immunosuppressive effect
live vaccines: Possibly increased risk of infection

Adverse Reactions

CNS: Fatigue, fever, headache
CV: Elevated lipid levels
EENT: Allergic rhinitis
ENDO: Hyperglycemia
GI: Abdominal pain, elevated liver enzymes, **hepatotoxicity**
GU: UTI
HEME: Anemia
MS: Arthralgia, back pain, osteomyelitis
RESP: Pneumonia, upper respiratory infections
SKIN: Cellulitis, eczema, rash
Other: **Anaphylaxis**; **angioedema**; antibody formation to risankizumab-rzaa; infections, including herpes zoster and tinea; injection-site reactions, such as bruising, erythema, extravasation, hematoma, hemorrhage, infection, inflammation, irritation, pain, pruritus, swelling, warmth; **sepsis**

Childbearing Considerations

PREGNANCY

- Pregnancy exposure registry: 1-877-302-2161.
- It is not known if drug can cause fetal harm, but drug does cross the placental barrier and may cause immunosuppression in the exposed fetus. Live virus immunizations should be delayed for a minimum of 5 months after birth.
- Use with caution only if benefit to mother outweighs potential risk to fetus.

LACTATION

- It is not known if drug is present in breast milk.
- Mothers should check with prescriber before breastfeeding.

Nursing Considerations

! WARNING Know that risankizumab-rzaa should not be given to patient with an active infection until infection resolves or is adequately treated. Use risankizumab-rzaa cautiously in patients with chronic infection or a history of recurrent infection.

- Check to determine that patient is up to date on immunizations before initiating treatment with risankizumab-rzaa. Know that live vaccines should be avoided during drug therapy.
- Be sure patient has been evaluated for tuberculosis (TB) prior to initiating treatment with risankizumab-rzaa. Expect

TB treatment to be initiated in patients with a history of active or latent TB in whom an adequate course of treatment cannot be confirmed. Monitor patient for signs and symptoms of active TB during and after drug therapy. Know that risankizumab-rzaa should not be given to patients with active TB.

! **WARNING** Evaluate bilirubin and liver enzymes in patients being treated for Crohn's disease and ulcerative colitis before treatment begins, during the 12 weeks of induction, and then periodically thereafter, as ordered. Monitor patient for liver dysfunction, which could become severe causing hepatotoxicity. If present, notify prescriber and expect drug therapy to be interrupted until drug is determined to be or not be the cause of liver dysfunction. If confirmed, expect drug to be discontinued.

! **WARNING** Monitor patient for hypersensitivity reactions, which could be sever such as anaphylaxis or angioedema. If present, stop drug therapy, notify prescriber, and expect to provide emergency supportive care, as ordered.

! **WARNING** Institute infection control measures and monitor patient for signs and symptoms of infection throughout therapy. Notify prescriber if an infection is suspected or known and expect drug to be withheld until infection is resolved because an infection could develop into life-threatening sepsis.

PATIENT TEACHING

- Tell patient that the first dose of drug must be given under the supervision of a healthcare professional.
- Teach patient and family or caregiver how to administer risankizumab-rzaa as a subcutaneous injection and what to do if a dose is missed.

! **WARNING** Alert patient to possibility of an allergic reaction. Advise patient, if an allergic reaction occurs, to stop drug, notify prescriber, and seek immediate medical care if serious or severe symptoms occur.

! **WARNING** Review infection control measures with patient and family or caregiver. Urge patient to notify prescriber immediately if an infection is suspected or known.

! **WARNING** Caution patient receiving drug for Crohn's disease or ulcerative colitis to be alert for signs and symptoms of liver dysfunction such as abdominal pain, anorexia, dark urine, fatigue, jaundice, nausea, or vomiting.

- Advise patient to avoid vaccination with live vaccines and immediately prior to or after drug therapy. Tell them to alert all prescribers about risankizumab-rzaa therapy prior to any potential vaccination. Also, inform mothers to alert pediatrician of risankizumab-rzaa use during pregnancy because live virus immunizations should be delayed for a minimum of 5 months after birth.

risedronate sodium

Actonel, Atelvia

Class and Category

Pharmacologic class: Bisphosphonate
Therapeutic class: Antiosteoporotic

Indications and Dosages

* *To treat Paget's disease of bone*

TABLETS (ACTONEL)

Adults. 30 mg once daily for 2 mo. Repeated after 2 mo if relapse occurs or if serum alkaline phosphatase level fails to normalize.

* *To prevent or treat glucocorticoid-induced osteoporosis in patients taking a dose of 7.5 mg or more of prednisone or equivalent daily*

TABLETS (ACTONEL)

Adults. 5 mg once daily.

* *To prevent or treat postmenopausal osteoporosis*

TABLETS (ACTONEL)

Postmenopausal women. 5 mg daily. 35 mg once weekly, 75 mg taken on 2 consecutive days once a mo, or 150 mg once a mo.

* *To treat postmenopausal osteoporosis*

E.R. TABLETS (ATELVIA)

Postmenopausal women. 35 mg once weekly.

* *To treat osteoporosis in men*

TABLETS (ACTONEL)

Adult males. 35 mg once weekly.

Drug Administration

P.O.

- Administer I.R. tablet with 6 to 8 ounces of plain water (no supplements should be present in the water such as found in mineral water). Administer at least 30 min before the first beverage, food, or medication of the day. Tablet should be swallowed whole and not chewed or sucked on.
- Ensure patient does not eat or drink anything after drug has been administered for at least 30 min. Follow manufacturer's instructions for a missed dose.
- E.R. tablets should be swallowed whole and not chewed, crushed, or divided. Administer in the morning following breakfast with at least 4 ounces of plain water (no supplements added such as found in mineral water). If a dose is missed, administer on the morning after dose is missed and then return to original dosing schedule.
- Ensure that patient is in an upright position when drug is administered and does not lie down for 30 min afterward.

Route	Onset	Peak	Duration
P.O.	1 hr	1 hr	Unknown
P.O./E.R.	Unknown	3 hr	Unknown

Half-life: 1.5 hr, initial; terminal exponential, 480 hr

Mechanism of Action

Hinders excessive bone remodeling characteristic of Paget's disease by binding to bone and reducing the rate at which osteoclasts are resorbed by bone. Decreases elevated rate of bone turnover also that is typically seen in osteoporosis.

Contraindications

Esophageal abnormalities that delay esophageal emptying, such as achalasia or stricture; hypersensitivity to risedronate or its components; hypocalcemia; inability to sit or stand upright for at least 30 min

Interactions

DRUGS

angiogenesis inhibitors, chemotherapy, corticosteroids: Possibly increased risk of osteonecrosis of the jaw
aspirin, NSAIDs: Increased risk of GI irritation
calcium-containing preparations, including antacids: Impaired absorption of risedronate
histamine 2 blockers, proton pump inhibitors: Faster drug release of D.R. form of drug increasing drug exposure and possible adverse reactions

FOODS

all foods: Decreased risedronate bioavailability when taking Actonel form of drug

Adverse Reactions

CNS: Anxiety, asthenia, depression, dizziness, fatigue, headache, insomnia, sciatica, syncope, vertigo, weakness
CV: Chest pain, hypercholesterolemia, hypertension, peripheral edema, vasodilation
EENT: Amblyopia, cataract, dry eyes, eye inflammation, nasopharyngitis, painful swallowing, pharyngitis, rhinitis, sinusitis, tinnitus
GI: Abdominal pain, colitis, constipation, diarrhea, dyspepsia, dysphagia, eructation, esophagitis, esophageal or gastric ulcers, flatulence, gastritis, nausea, vomiting
GU: UTI
MS: Arthralgia; atypical femur fractures; back, limb, neck, or shoulder pain; jaw osteonecrosis; leg cramps or spasms; myasthenia; myalgia; osteoarthritis; retrosternal pain; severe incapacitating bone, joint, or muscle pain
RESP: **Asthma exacerbation**; bronchitis, cough, pneumonia, upper respiratory tract infection
SKIN: Bullous reaction, pruritus, rash, **Stevens-Johnson syndrome**, **toxic epidermal necrolysis**
Other: **Anaphylaxis**, **angioedema and other hypersensitivity reactions**; flu-like symptoms; **hypocalcemia**

Childbearing Considerations

PREGNANCY

- It is not known if drug can cause fetal harm.
- Know that there is a theoretical risk of fetal harm, especially skeletal, if a woman becomes pregnant after completing a course of bisphosphonate therapy. Time between cessation of drug therapy to conception, the

particular bisphosphonate used, and route of administration that may cause fetal harm are unknown.

- Use with caution only if benefit to mother outweighs potential risk to fetus.

LACTATION

- It is not known if drug is present in breast milk.
- A decision should be made to discontinue breastfeeding or the drug to avoid potential serious adverse reactions in the infant.

Nursing Considerations

! **WARNING** Be aware that risedronate isn't recommended for patients with severe renal impairment.

- Make sure patient has had a dental checkup before having invasive dental procedures during risedronate therapy, especially if patient has cancer; is receiving angiogenesis inhibitors, chemotherapy, corticosteroids, or head or neck radiation; or has poor oral hygiene because risk of jaw osteonecrosis is increased in these patients.
- Give supplemental calcium and vitamin D, as prescribed, during risedronate therapy if patient's dietary intake is inadequate.
- Give antacids and calcium supplements at different time of day than risedronate administration to avoid impaired drug absorption and altered effectiveness.

! **WARNING** Monitor patient for a hypersensitivity reaction, which could become life-threatening, such as anaphylaxis or angioedema. If present, notify prescriber, expect drug to be discontinued, and provide supportive care, as needed and ordered.

! **WARNING** Monitor patient's respiratory function and report abnormalities to prescriber, especially an asthma exacerbation which could become life-threatening.

! **WARNING** Monitor patient for any other persistent, serious, or unusual adverse reactions.

PATIENT TEACHING

- Instruct patient how to administer form of risedronate prescribed and what to do if a dose is missed.

! **WARNING** Alert patient that drug may cause an allergic reaction. If present, tell patient to notify prescriber and, if severe, to seek immediate medical care.

- Tell patient to take antacids or calcium supplements at different times than risedronate.

! **WARNING** Advise patient to stop taking risedronate and to notify prescriber if she develops dysphagia, new or worsening heartburn, or pain while swallowing (retrosternal pain).

! **WARNING** Tell patient experiencing difficulty breathing, especially if patient has a history of asthma, to stop taking drug and seek immediate medical care.

! **WARNING** Instruct patient to alert prescriber if other persistent, serious, or unusual adverse reactions occur.

! **WARNING** Urge females of childbearing age to tell prescriber if pregnancy is being planned or occurs because of risk to fetal skeleton.

- Alert patient that drug may cause severe bone, joint, or muscle pain or new groin or thigh pain that might be reflective of an atypical femur fracture. Prescriber should be notified.
- Tell mothers breastfeeding should not be undertaken during risedronate therapy or drug will need to be discontinued.
- Instruct patient about proper oral hygiene and about the need to notify prescriber about invasive dental procedures.

risperidone

Perseris, Risperdal, Risperdal Consta, Risvan, Rykindo, Uzedy

Class and Category

Pharmacologic class: Benzisoxazole derivative

Therapeutic class: Antipsychotic

Indications and Dosages

* *To treat schizophrenia*

ORAL SOLUTION, ORALLY DISINTEGRATING TABLETS, TABLETS

Adults. *Initial:* 2 mg once daily or divided and given as 1 mg twice daily, increased at intervals of 24 hr or longer in increments of 1 to 2 mg daily to target dose of 4 to 8 mg once daily or divided and given twice daily. *Effective dose range*: 4 to 16 mg once daily or divided and given twice daily. *Maximum:* 16 mg daily.

Adolescents ages 13 to 17. *Initial:* 0.5 mg once daily in the morning or evening, increased, as needed, every 24 hr or longer in 0.5- to 1-mg increments to target dose of 3 mg daily. *Effective dose range:* 1 to 6 mg once daily in the morning or evening. *Maximum:* 6 mg once daily.

I.M. INJECTION (RISPERDAL CONSTA, RYKINDO)

Adults. *Initial:* After tolerability established with oral risperidone, 25 mg every 2 wk, increased, as needed, every 4 wk to 37.5 or 50 mg. *Maximum:* 50 mg every 2 wk. Oral risperidone or another antipsychotic drug therapy continued after first I.M. injection for 3 wk (Risperdal Consta) or oral risperidone for 7 days (Rykindo).

I.M. INJECTION

Adults. *Initial:* After tolerability established with oral risperidone, 75 mg (if oral dose was 3 mg) or 100 mg (if oral dose was 4 mg) one day after the last oral dose and given once mo. *Maximum:* No more than 1 dose (75 mg or 100 mg) per mo.

SUBCUTANEOUS INJECTION (PERSERIS)

Adults. 90 mg or 120 mg injected into abdomen only once monthly. Tolerability should be established first with oral risperidone for patient who has never received drug before. If oral dose was 3 mg daily, 90 mg is administered subcutaneously 1 day after oral dose; if oral dose was 4 mg, 120 mg administered subutaneously 1 day after oral dose.

SUBCUTANEOUS INJECTION (UZEDY)

Adults who had been receiving 2 mg of oral risperidone daily. 50 mg once a mo or 100 mg once every 2 mo begun the day after the last dose of oral theapy give.

Adults who had been receiving 3 mg of oral risperidone daily. 75 mg once a mo or 150 mg once every 2 mo begun the day after the last dose of oral therapy given.

Adults who had been receiving 4 mg of oral risperidone daily. 100 mg once a mo or 200 mg once every 2 mo begun the day after the last dose of oral therapy given.

Adults who had been receiving 5 mg of oral risperidone daily. 125 mg once a mo or 250 mg once every 2 mo begun the day after the last dose of oral therapy given.

* *To treat bipolar mania as monotherapy*

ORAL SOLUTION, ORALLY DISINTEGRATING TABLETS, TABLETS

Adults. *Initial:* 2 or 3 mg daily, increased, as needed, by 1 mg every 24 hr or longer up to 6 mg. *Maximum:* 6 mg daily for no more than 3 wk.

Adolescents and children ages 10 to 17. *Initial:* 0.5 mg once daily in the morning or evening, increased, as needed, every 24 hr or longer in 0.5- to 1-mg increments to recommended dose of 1 to 2.5 mg daily. *Maximum:* 2.5 mg once daily for no more than 3 wk.

I.M. INJECTION (RISPERDAL CONSTA, RYKINDO)

Adults. After tolerability established with oral risperidone, 25 mg every 2 wk, increased, as needed, every 4 wk to 37.5 or 50 mg. *Maximum:* 50 mg every 2 wk. Oral risperidone or another antipsychotic drug therapy continued after first I.M. injection for 3 wk (Risperdal Consta) or oral risperidone for 7 days (Rykindo).

* *As adjunct to treat bipolar mania with lithium or valproate therapy*

ORAL SOLUTION, ORALLY DISINTEGRATING TABLETS, TABLETS

Adults. *Initial*: 2 to 3 mg daily, increased, as needed, by 1 mg every 24 hr or longer up to 6 mg. *Maximum:* 6 mg daily for no more than 3 wk.

I.M. INJECTION (RISPERDAL CONSTA, RYKINDO)

Adults. After tolerability established with oral risperidone, 25 mg every 2 wk, increased, as needed, every 4 wk to 37.5 or 50 mg. *Maximum:* 50 mg every 2 wk. Oral risperidone or another antipsychotic drug therapy continued after first I.M. injection for 3 wk (Risperdal Consta) or oral risperidone for 7 days (Rykindo).

* *To treat irritability associated with autistic disorder*

ORAL SOLUTION, ORALLY DISINTEGRATING TABLETS, TABLETS

Adolescents and children ages 5 and older weighing 20 kg (44 lb) or more. *Initial:* 0.5 mg daily, increased after 4 days to 1 mg daily. Dosage further increased, as needed, in 2-wk intervals in 0.5-mg increments.

Adolescents and children ages 5 and older weighing less than 20 kg (44 lb). *Initial:* 0.25 mg daily, increased after 4 days to 0.5 mg daily. Dosage further increased, as needed, in 2-wk intervals in 0.25-mg increments.

±**DOSAGE ADJUSTMENT** *For oral dosage:* For elderly patients and patients with severe hepatic or renal impairment or who are taking CYP2D6 inhibitors, starting doses reduced with maximum dose not exceeding 8 mg daily in adults. For patients taking CYP3A4 inducers, such as carbamazepine, phenobarbital, phenytoin, or rifampin, dosage may have to be increased up to double the patient's usual dose.

For I.M. doses: For patients with hepatic or renal impairment, initial dose of Risperdal Consta or Rykindo may have to be reduced to 12.5 mg kept at 75 mg or reduced from 100 mg to 75 mg for Risvan. For patients starting a CYP3A4 inducer during risperidone therapy, a dosage increase of risperidone may be needed. For patients starting a CYP2D6 inhibitor, a dosage decrease of risperidone may be needed.

For subcutaneous doses: For patients with hepatic or renal impairment, the lower dose of 90 mg once a month (Perseris) or 50 mg once a month (Uzedy) recommended for the initial dose. For patients receiving a CYP2D6 inhibitor, lowest dose of drug should be used with possible interruption of drug therapy, as needed. For patients receiving strong CYP3A4 inducers, dosage may have to be increased and additional oral risperidone may be needed.

Drug Administration

P.O.

- Administer oral solution directly from the oral dosing syringe or mix with coffee, orange juice, low-fat milk, or water but not with cola or tea. Store oral solution at room temperature.
- For orally disintegrating tablets, break open the blister unit with dry gloved hands by peeling the foil back to expose the tablet. Do not push tablet through the foil because this could damage tablet. Have patient place tablet immediately on the tongue, where it will dissolve within sec. Orally disintegrating tablet should not be chewed or spit out of mouth.

I.M.

Risperdal Consta

- Remove Risperdal Consta from refrigerator and allow it to come to room temperature for at least 30 min before reconstitution.
- Follow manufacturer's guidelines for reconstitution, following the illustrations closely, and use only the diluent supplied in the dose pack. After dilution, shake the vial vigorously while holding the plunger rod down for a minimum of 10 sec to ensure a homogeneous suspension. Suspension should appear milky, thick, and uniform. Transfer suspension to syringe.
- Just before injection, shake syringe vigorously again. Give using only the needle supplied in the dose pack. Within 2 min of reconstitution, inject entire contents of syringe into the upper outer quadrant of gluteal area using the 2-inch 20 G needle (longer needle with yellow colored hub) or into the deltoid muscle using the 1-inch 21 G needle (shorter needle with green-colored hub).
- Never combine 2 different dose strengths into a single injection.
- If drug can't be given right after reconstitution, shake the upright vial vigorously back and forth again until particles are resuspended before administration.
- Discard reconstituted drug if not used within 6 hr.
- Never administer I.M. form intravenously.

Rykindo

- Remove Rykindo from refrigerator and allow it to come to room temperature for at least 30 min before reconstitution.
- Follow manufacturer's guidelines for reconstitution, following the illustrations closely, and use only diluent supplied. After dilution, shake the vial vigorously for at least 30 sec. Then check the suspension, which should appear milky, thick, and uniform. Immediately proceed to the next step so suspension does not settle.

- Invert vial completely. Slowly pull plunger rod to withdraw entire contents from the vial into the syringe.
- Hold Luer-Lok adapter on the syringe and unscrew from vial adapter. Label syringe for identification purposes. Discard both vial and vial adapter.
- Holding the Luer-Lok adapter on the syringe, attach syringe to needle luer connection with a firm clockwise twisting motion until snug. Do not touch needle luer opening.
- Fully remove the blister pouch. Just before injection, shake syringe vigorously for 20 to 30 sec until there is no depositon of powder, as some settling will have occurred. Move the needle safety device back towards the syringe. Then hold the Luer-Lik adapter on syringe and carefully pull the transparent needle protector straight off. Do not twist transparent needle protector, as the luer connection may loosen.
- Hold syringe upright and tap gently to make any air bubles rise to the top. Slowly and carefully press plunger rod upward to remove air.
- Immediately inject entire contents of syringe intramuscularly into the upper-outer quadrant of the gluteal muscle of the patient.
- Using one hand, place needle safety device at a 45-degree angle on a hard, flat surface. Press down with a firm, quick motion until needle is fully engaged in safety device. Properly dispose syringe in approved sharps container.

Risvan

- Do not substitute any component of the drug kit.
- Ensure that solvent syringe contents flows normally as a liquid. The solvent freezes at 66 degrees F. If the solvent is frozen or partially frozen, warm it at room temperature until it flows normally.
- Follow manufacturer's guidelines for reconstitution and preparing injection syringe.
- Inject drug within 15 min after reconstitution. Use the proper needle. If injecting into the deltoid muscle, use the 21 G, 1-inch needle with green cap; if injecting into the gluteus muscle, use the 20 G, 2-inch needle with yellow cap. Remove excess air bubbles but do not expel any drops of the drug.
- Inject ONLY in the deltoid or gluteus muscle. Inject drug slowly and steadily as the drug is thick due to the viscosity of the drug. Wait a few sec before removing the needle.
- Cover the needle by pressing on the needle guard using a finger or a flat surface. Properly dispose syringe in approved sharps container.

SUBCUTANEOUS

- Drug by this route should only be given by a healthcare professional.
- Neither a loading dose nor supplemental oral risperidone doses are needed when giving drug as a subcutaneous injection. Tolerance to drug should be established first in patients who have never received risperidone.

Perseris

- Remove Perseris from refrigerator and allow it to come to room temperature for at least 15 min before preparing drug for administration. Only prepare drug when ready to administer the dose, not before.
- Wear gloves when preparing drug for administration.
- Follow manufacturer's guidelines for reconstitution, following the illustrations closely, and use only the diluent supplied in the dose pack.
- When fully mixed, drug should be a cloudy suspension that is uniform in color. It can vary from white to yellow-green. If any clear areas occur in the mixture, continue to mix it until the distribution of the color is uniform.
- Pinch the skin and inject ONLY into the abdomen or back of upper arm after removing excess air from syringe; inject drug slowly and steadily. Angle used to inject drug will depend on the amount of subcutaneous tissue present at site.
- Do not rub the injection site after the injection. If there is bleeding, apply a bandage but use minimal pressure.
- Can be stored in refrigerator; if stored at room temperature, drug will have to be discarded after 7 days.

Uzedy

- Remove Uzedy from refrigerator and allow it to come to room temperature for at least 30 min. (Be aware Uzedy is a solid at refrigerated temperatures and must reach room temperature prior to administration.) Do not warm any other way and keep drug protected from light.

- Uzedy kit contains one sterile single-dose, prefilled glass syringe and 1 sterile 21 G × 5/8-inch needle. Do not substitute any components of the kit for administration. The drug in the syringe should appear white to off-white, opaque in color and free from non-white particulate matter. Do not use if any component of the kit is damaged or expiration date has passed.
- When drug has reached room temperature, expose the safety needle hub by peeling back the paper tab of the needle pouch. Then set aside for later use.
- This step must be performed to ensure complete dosing as failure to move the bubble to the cap of the syringe could result in incomplete dosage. To do this, firmly hold the syringe by the white collar. Flick syringe with a forceful downward whipping motion of your full arm to move the bubble to the cap of the syringe. Repeat this action 3 times to ensure that the bubble is at the cap of the syringe. (Standing while doing this may help achieve the necessary force.) Check that the bubble is where it needs to be. If not, repeat flicking syringe forcefully until it is.
- Hold the syringe vertically by the white collar. Bend and snap off the cap. Do not touch the syringe tip. While holding the syringe vertically with the white collar at the top, push the green hub of the safety needle inside the white collar and rotate the safety needle while holding the white collar until secure and tight. Inspect the needle connection to check that the hub is not damaged.
- Inject the drug ONLY in the abdomen or back outer area of the upper arms. Do not inject into an area that is bruised, callused, hard, red, tattooed, tender, or has scars or stretch marks.
- To inject, remove the needle sheath. Do not expel any visible air bubble. Pinch at least 1 inch of the area of cleaned skin with your free hand. Insert the needle into the subcutaneous tissue (actual angle of injection will depend on the amount of subcutaneous tissue.) Do not apply pressure to the plunger while inserting the needle.
- Release the pinched skin once the needle is in the subcutaneous tissue and inject the drug by pushing the plunger slowly, firmly, and steadily until the entire dose is administered. Inject the entire dose at one time, without interruption. Check that the plunger stopper is at the white collar. (Drug is viscous so expect to feel resistance during injection. Do not use excessive force in an attempt to deliver the drug faster.)
- Wait 2 to 3 sec after the dose is delivered before removing the needle. Slowly pull the needle out from the injection site at the same angle of insertion.
- Activate the safety needle shield either by placing the needle shield on a flat surface and pulling the syringe backward until the needle shield covers the needle tip or press either your thumb or finger on the needle shield and push it forward until the needle shield covers the needle tip. Listen for an audible click when the needle safety shield is locked. Dispose of all syringe components in a sharps container.

Route	Onset	Peak	Duration
P.O.	Unknown	1 hr	Unknown
I.M.	3 wk	4–6 wk	7 wk
SubQ	Unknown	4–6 hr	Unknown

Half-life: 3–20 hr (P.O.); 3–6 days (I.M.); 9–11 days (SubQ)

Mechanism of Action

Blocks serotonin and dopamine receptors selectively in the mesocortical tract of the CNS to suppress psychotic symptoms.

Contraindications

Hypersensitivity to risperidone, paliperidone, or its components

Interactions

DRUGS

antihypertensives: Increased antihypertensive effects

clozapine: Decreased risperidone clearance with long-term concurrent use

CNS depressants: Additive CNS depression

CYP2D6 inhibtors such as fluoxetine, paroxetine: Increased plasma risperidone level

CYP3A4 inducers such as carbamazepine, phenobarbital, phenytoin, rifampin: Increased

risperidone clearance with decreased effectiveness
dopamine agonists, levodopa: Possibly antagonized effects of these drugs
methylphenidate: Increased risk of extrapyramidal symptoms

ACTIVITIES

alcohol use: Additive CNS depression

Adverse Reactions

CNS: Abnormal coordination, aggressiveness, agitation, akathisia, anxiety, asthenia, catatonia, confusion, decreased concentration, depression, dizziness, dream disturbances, drooling, drowsiness, dyskinesia, dystonia, fatigue, fever, headache, **hypothermia**, impaired motor skills, insomnia, lassitude, malaise, mania, memory loss, nervousness, **neuroleptic malignant syndrome**, paresthesia, parkinsonism, restlessness, **seizures**, shaking of head repeatedly, sleepwalking, somnambulism, somnolence, tardive dyskinesia, tremor, vertigo
CV: **Atrial fibrillation**, **bradycardia**, bundle branch block, **cardiopulmonary arrest**, chest pain, elevated triglyceride levels, first-degree AV block, hypercholesterolemia, orthostatic hypotension, palpitations, **QT-interval prolongation**, tachycardia
EENT: Conjunctivitis, decreased or increased salivation, dry mouth, ear pain, epistaxis, nasal congestion, pharyngitis, retinal artery occlusion, rhinitis, sinusitis, taste alteration, vision changes
ENDO: **Diabetic ketoacidosis** (patients with diabetes), elevated prolactin level, galactorrhea, hyperglycemia, hyperprolactinemia, **hypoglycemia**, inappropriate antidiuretic hormone secretion (SIADH), pituitary adenoma, precocious puberty, water intoxication
GI: Abdominal pain, anorexia, constipation, diarrhea, dysphagia, gastritis, ileus, indigestion, **intestinal obstruction**, jaundice, nausea, **pancreatitis**, vomiting
GU: Amenorrhea, decreased libido, delayed ejaculation, dysmenorrhea, dysuria, glucosuria, hypermenorrhea, incontinence, increased appetite, polyuria, priapism, sexual dysfunction, urinary incontinence or retention, UTI
HEME: **Agranulocytosis**, anemia, **leukopenia**, **neutropenia**, **thrombocytopenia**, **thrombotic thrombocytopenic purpura**
MS: Arthralgia; back, buttock, extremity, or neck pain; dysarthria; muscle weakness; myalgia
RESP: Cough, dyspnea, **pulmonary embolism**, **sleep apnea**, upper respiratory tract infection
SKIN: Alopecia, diaphoresis, dry skin, eczema, hyperpigmentation, photosensitivity, pruritus, rash, seborrhea, **Stevens-Johnson syndrome**, **toxic epidermal necrolysis**
Other: **Anaphylaxis**; **angioedema**; flu-like symptoms; infections; injection-site induration, pain, redness, or swelling; weight gain or loss

Childbearing Considerations

PREGNANCY

- Pregnancy exposure registry: 1-866-961-2388 or http://womensmentalhealth.org/clinical-and-research-programs/pregnancyregistry/.
- Drug may cause fetal harm.
- Neonates exposed to drug during the third trimester of pregnancy are at risk for extrapyramidal and withdrawal symptoms.
- Use with caution only if benefit to mother outweighs potential risk to fetus.

LACTATION

- Drug is present in human milk.
- Mothers should check with prescriber before breastfeeding.
- If breastfeeding occurs, monitor infant for signs of abnormal muscle movements, excess sedation, failure to thrive, jitteriness, and tremors.

REPRODUCTION

- Infertility may occur because of hyperprolactinemia but is reversible.

QRS

Nursing Considerations

! **WARNING** Be aware that risperidone should not be used to treat elderly patients with dementia-related psychosis because it increases risk of death in these patients.

- Assess patient for orthostatic hypotension that may cause dizziness, syncope (in some patients), and tachycardia, especially when initiating treatment, re-initiating treatment, or increasing the dose.
- Use risperidone cautiously in debilitated patients, elderly patients, and patients with

hepatic or renal dysfunction or hypotension because of their increased sensitivity to the drug.

! **WARNING** Monitor patient for a hypersensitivity reaction, which could become life-threatening, such as anaphylaxis or angioedema. If present, notify prescriber, expect drug to be discontinued, and provide supportive care, as needed and ordered.

! **WARNING** Monitor patient's vital signs regularly for abnormalites such as below normal temperature, breathing difficulties, irregular or slow pulse, or orthostatic hypotension.

! **WARNING** Monitor patient's CBC, as ordered, because serious adverse hematologic reactions may occur, such as agranulocytosis, leukopenia, or neutropenia. More frequent monitoring during the first few months of risperidone therapy is recommended for patients with a history of drug-induced leukopenia or neutropenia, or those who have had a significantly low WBC count in the past. If abnormalities occur during therapy, monitor patient for fever or other signs of infection, notify prescriber, and expect drug to be discontinued if severe.

! **WARNING** Monitor patient's blood glucose levels if patient is a diabetic because drug can adversely affect blood glucose control causing either hyperglycemia, which could become severe enough to cause diabetic ketoacidosis, or hypoglycemia. If present, notify prescriber and treat according to institutional protocol.

! **WARNING** Monitor patients, especially patients with a history of seizures, that seizures, although rare, may occur in those with schizophrenia.

! **WARNING** Assess patients with Lewy body dementia or Parkinson's disease for increased sensitivity to the drug, exhibited by confusion, extrapyramidal symptoms, frequent falls, obtundation, postural instability, and signs and symptoms of neuroleptic malignant syndrome (altered mental status, autonomic instability, hyperpyrexia, muscle rigidity), which can be fatal. Notify prescriber immediately if neuroleptic malignant syndrome is suspected and expect risperidone to be discontinued.

- Monitor patient's lipid levels as ordered because drug increases the risk of hypercholesterolemia.
- Monitor patient for tardive dyskinesia, especially in the elderly and particularly elderly women. Be aware it may occur even at low doses and after discontinuation of treatment. Alert prescriber, if present, as drug may have to be discontinued.

! **WARNING** Monitor patient for other persistent, severe, or unusual adverse reactions.

- Institute fall precautions.

PATIENT TEACHING

! **WARNING** Inform patient and family or caregiver that orally disintegrating tablets contain phenylalanine and should not be used if patient has been diagnosed with PKU.

- Instruct patient and family or caregiver how to administer oral form of risperidone.
- Inform patient receiving parenteral risperidone that injections must be administered by a healthcare professional. Alert patient receiving drug by subcutaneous injection that a lump may be felt for several weeks at injection site. Caution patient not to rub or massage the injection site and to be careful in the placement of any belts or clothing waistbands.
- Urge patient to avoid alcohol because of its additive CNS effects.
- Instruct patient to avoid overheating and becoming dehydrated during drug therapy.

! **WARNING** Alert patient and family or caregiver that drug may cause an allergic reaction. If present, tell patient to notify prescriber and, if severe, to seek immediate medical care.

! **WARNING** Instruct patient and family or caregiver to notify prescriber immediately if patient notices a below normal temperature, an irregular or slow pulse, or has difficulty breathing as well as feeling faint or lightheaded when sitting up or standing. Instruct patient that dizziness upon standing can be minimized by rising slowly from a sitting or lying position and to avoid sudden position changes.

! **WARNING** Review bleeding and infection control measures with patient and family or caregiver. Tell them to alert prescriber if bruising, unexplained bleeding, or an infection occurs.

! **WARNING** Alert diabetic patient and family or caregiver that drug may alter blood glucose control. Review signs and symptoms of high and low blood glucose levels and to notify prescriber immediately for persistent changes. Educate patient on how to properly treat hypoglycemia.

! **WARNING** Inform patient and family or caregiver that seizures, although rare, may occur, especially if patient has a history of seizures.

! **WARNING** Stress importance with male patient to seek emergency care if an erection becomes painful or lasts longer than usual.

- Caution patient and family or caregiver that risperidone may cause sleepwalking.
- Alert patient that drug may cause involuntary movements that may not be reversible. If present, stress importance of notifying prescriber immediately.
- Caution patient to avoid performing hazardous activities, such as driving, until CNS effects are known and resolved. Review fall precautions with patient.
- Inform patient that drug may cause amenorrhea or galactorrhea in females or erectile dysfunction or gynecomastia in men, and for patient and family or caregiver to alert prescriber, if present.

! **WARNING** Tell patient and family or caregiver to notify prescriber if other persistent, serious, or unusual adverse reaction occurs.

- Instruct patient and family or caregiver to inform all prescribers of risperidone therapy and not to take any new medication, including over-the-counter preparations, without discussing use with prescriber first.
- Advise pregnant patients to alert prescriber when they are approaching the third trimester.
- Instruct mothers who are breastfeeding while taking risperidone to monitor the infant for abnormal muscle movements, excess sedation, failure to thrive, jitteriness, or tremors.
- Stress importance of complying with ordered laboratory testing.

ritlecitinib

Liftulo

Class and Category

Pharmacologic class: Janus kinase (JAK) inhibitor

Therapeutic class: Anti-alopecia agent

Indications and Dosages

* *To treat severe alopecia areata*

CAPSULES

Adults and children ages 12 and older. 50 mg once daily.

± **DOSAGE ADJUSTMENT** For patients who develop a lymphocyte count less than 500/mm^3 during drug therapy, drug withheld and only restarted when the absolute lymphocyte count (ALC) reaches 500/mm^3 or greater. For patients who develop a platelet count of less than 50,000/mm^3, drug discontinued.

Drug Administration

P.O.

- Capsules may be taken with or without food but at about the same time daily.
- Capsules should be swallowed whole and not chewed, crushed, or split.
- For a missed dose, administer as soon as possible unless it is less than 8 hr before the next dose, which would require missed dose to be skipped.

Route	Onset	Peak	Duration
P.O.	Unknown	1 hr	Unknown

Half-life: 1.3–2.3 hr

Mechanism of Action

Blocks the adenosine triphosphate (ATP) binding site, which irreversibly inhibits Janus kinase 3 and tyrosine kinase activity. Also, irreversibly inhibits signaling of immune receptors dependent on (TEC) kinase family members. However, how the inhibition of specific Janus kinase and tyrosine kinase enzymes causes hair growth is not known.

Contraindications

Hypersensitivity to ritlecitinib or its components

Interactions

DRUGS

CYP3A inducers (strong) such as rifampin: Possibly reduced effectiveness of ritlecitinib
CYP1A2 and CYP3A substrates: Possibly increased risk of serious adverse reactions when small concentration changes are made

Adverse Reactions

CNS: Dizziness, fever, headache
CV: **Acute MI**
EENT: Retinal artery occlusion, stomatitis
GI: Diarrhea, elevated liver enzymes
HEME: **Decreased platelet count**, **decreased red blood cell count**, lymphopenia
RESP: **Pulmonary embolus**
SKIN: Acne, atopic dermatitis, folliculitis, **non-melanoma skin cancer**, rash, urticaria
Other: **Anaphylaxis**; elevated creatine phosphokinase levels; **malignancies including lymphomas**; serious infections including appendicitis, COVID-19 infection possibly complicated with pneumonia, TB; **sepsis**; viral reactivation including herpes zoster and possibly hepatitis B or C

Childbearing Considerations

PREGNANCY

- Pregnancy exposure registry: 1-877-390-2940.
- It is not known if drug can cause fetal harm although animal studies suggest it might.
- Use with caution only if benefit to mother outweighs potential risk to fetus.

LACTATION

- It is not known if drug is present in breast milk.
- Mothers should not breastfeed their infant during drug therapy and for about 14 hours after the last dose.

Nursing Considerations

! **WARNING** Expect patient to be screened for tuberculosis (TB) before ritlecitinib therapy begins and periodically during drug therapy because drug should not be given to patients with active TB. TB treatment should be started in patients prior to initiation of ritlecitinib therapy who are newly diagnosed with latent TB or previously did not receive treatment for latent TB. Also, know that it is recommended to initiate TB treatment in a patient with a negative latent TB test before drug is administered if patient is at high risk for developing TB during treatment with ritlecitinib

! **WARNING** Screen patient for viral reactivation such as hepatitis and herpes zoster, as ordered, before ritlecitinib is started. Know that drug is not recommended for use in patients with hepatitis B or hepatitis C and drug should be temporarily withheld if patient develops herpes zoster during drug therapy until the episode resolves.

- Ensure that patient is up to date on recommended immunizations prior to ritlecitinib therapy. Expect live attenuated vaccines to be avoided during drug therapy.

! **WARNING** Be aware that ritlecitinib is not recommended for use in patients with severe hepatic impairment because drug may increase impairment.

! **WARNING** Know that ritlecitinib should be avoided in patients with an active serious infection. Monitor patient throughout drug therapy for signs and symptoms of infection. If an opportunistic or serious infection occurs, expect drug to be temporarily withheld, a prompt and complete diagnostic testing appropriate for an immunocompromised patient done, and antimicrobial therapy prescribed. Ritlecitinib therapy can be resumed once the infection is under control.

- Expect to obtain a lymphocyte count and a platelet count before ritlecitinib therapy is begun and then again at 4 weeks into therapy and then periodically thereafter because drug will need to be temporarily withheld if the absolute lymphocyte count (ALC) drops below 500/mm^3 and not restarted until the ALC is at 500/mm^3 or higher. If the patient's platelet count drops below 50,000 mm^3 expect drug to be discontinued.

! **WARNING** Monitor patient closely for a hypersensitivity reaction, which could become life-threatening, such as anaphylaxis. If present, notify prescriber, expect drug to be discontinued, and provide supportive care, as needed and ordered

! **WARNING** Be aware that another JAK inhibitor given to patients with rheumatoid arthritis who were 50 years of age and older with at least one cardiovascular risk factor had a higher rate for thromboembolic events such as deep vein thrombosis and pulmonary embolism as well as major cardiovascular events, including sudden cardiovascular death and non-fatal CVA and MI. Monitor patient closely because ritlecitinib is also a JAK inhibitor.

! **WARNING** Monitor patient for other persistent, serious, or unusual adverse reactions because ritlecitinib therapy has also caused malignancy and lymphoproliferative disorders. Periodic skin examinations are recommended for patients at increased risk for skin cancer.

PATIENT TEACHING

- Instruct patient how to take ritlecitinib and what to do if a dose is missed.

! **WARNING** Alert patient that drug may cause an allergic reaction. If present, instruct patient to notify prescriber and, if severe, to seek immediate medical care and to stop taking drug.

! **WARNING** Review infection control measures with patient and family or caregiver. Tell patient and family or caregiver to notify prescriber if any signs and symptoms of an infection occur, including herpes zoster.

! **WARNING** Advise patient that ritlecitinib therapy increases the risk for a blood clot. Review the signs and symptoms of thrombosis with the patient and family or caregiver and emphasis importance of seeking immediate medical care if any signs and symptoms of a thrombosis occur.

! **WARNING** Warn patient that ritlecitinib may increase the risk of developing certain cancers. Advise patient to notify prescriber of any persistent, serious, or unusual signs and symptoms. Also, stress importance of having a periodic skin examination while taking ritlecitinib.

- Inform patient that blood tests will need to be performed before and during ritlecitinib therapy. Stress importance of compliance with having the tests done.
- Reassure patient that if drug is temporarily interrupted for less than 6 weeks, regrown scalp hair loss is not expected to occur.
- Warn patient not to receive any vaccinations with a live vaccine during ritlecitinib therapy and to inform all prescribers of ritlecitinib therapy before any vaccination is done.
- Advise mothers not to breastfeed during ritlecitinib therapy and for about 14 hours after the last dose of the drug is taken.

ritonavir

Norvir

Class and Category

Pharmacologic class: Protease inhibitor
Therapeutic class: Antiretroviral

Indications and Dosages

* *As adjunct to treat human immunodeficiency viral type 1 (HIV-1) infection*

TABLETS

Adults. *Initial:* 300 mg twice daily, increased by 100 mg twice daily every 2 to 3 days until maximum dose reached. *Maximum:* 600 mg twice daily.
Children old enough to swallow tablets. *Initial:* 250 mg/m^2 twice daily, increased by 50 mg/m^2 twice daily every 2 to 3 days until a maintenance dosage is reached. *Maintenance:* 350 to 400 mg/m^2 twice daily. *Maximum:* 600 mg twice daily.

ORAL POWDER

Adults. *Initial:* 300 mg twice daily, increased by 100 mg twice daily every 2 to 3 days until maximum dose reached. *Maximum:* 600 mg twice daily.
Children older than 1 mo. *Initial:* 250 mg/m^2 twice daily, increased by 50 mg/m^2 twice daily every 2 to 3 days until a maintenance dosage is reached. *Maintenance:*

350 to 400 mg/m² twice daily. *Maximum:* 600 mg twice daily.

±**DOSAGE ADJUSTMENT** For patients taking other protease inhibitors, such as atazanavir, darunavir, fosamprenavir, saquinavir, or tipranavir, dosage reduced.

Drug Administration

P.O.

- Administer drug with meals.
- Tablets should be swallowed whole and not chewed, crushed, or divided.
- Be aware that oral powder form of ritonavir should only be used for dosing increments of 100 mg. If the dose is less than 100 mg or the dose falls between 100-mg intervals, other forms should be used instead of the powder.
- Mix oral powder form with soft food, such as applesauce or vanilla pudding, or mix with liquid, such as chocolate milk, 4 ounces of infant formula, or water. Use a calibrated dosing syringe to measure dosage, especially for infants and children. Once mixed, use within 2 hr or discard.
- Know that the oral powder (mixed with water) or solution form may be given via a feeding tube.

Route	Onset	Peak	Duration
P.O.	Unknown	2–4 hr	Unknown

Half-life: 3–5 hr

Mechanism of Action

Inhibits HIV protease to render the enzyme incapable of processing the Gag-Pol polyprotein precursor, which leads to the production of noninfectious immature HIV particles.

Contraindications

Concomitant therapy with other protease inhibitors, potent CYP3A inducers, or therapy that is highly dependent on CYP3A for drug clearance and for which elevated plasma concentrations have resulted in serious and/or life-threatening reactions (alfuzosin, amiodarone, cisapride, colchicine, dihydroergotamine, dronedarone, ergotamine, flecainide, lomitapide, lovastatin, lurasidone, methylergonovine, midazolam [oral], pimozide, propafenone, quinidine, ranolazine, St. John's wort, sildenafil [when used for treatment of pulmonary arterial hypertension], simvastatin, triazolam, voriconazole); hypersensitivity to ritonavir or its components; use of potent CYP3A inducers where significantly reduced ritonavir plasma concentrations may be associated with the potential loss of virologic response and possible resistance and cross-resistance, such as anticancer agents (apalutamide) or herbal products (St. John's wort)

Interactions

DRUGS

amprenavir, atazanavir, atorvastatin, bedaquiline, bosentan, buspirone, carbamazepine, clarithromycin, clonazepam, clorazepate, colchicine, corticosteroids, cyclosporine, darunavir, dasatinib, desipramine, diazepam, diltiazem, disopyramide, dronabinol, estazolam, ethinyl estradiol, ethosuximide, fentanyl, fluoxetine, flurazepam, ibrutinib, indinavir, itraconazole, ketoconazole, lidocaine, lomitapide, maraviroc, methamphetamine, metoprolol, mexiletine, midazolam (parenteral), nefazodone, nifedipine, nilotinib, paroxetine, perphenazine, propoxyphene, quetiapine, quinine, rifabutin, risperidone, rosuvastatin, salmeterol, saquinavir, simeprevir, sirolimus, tacrolimus, thioridazine, timolol, tipranavir, trazodone, tricyclic antidepressants, venetoclax, verapamil, zolpidem: Increased concentration of these drugs with possible risk of prolonged action and adverse reactions

atovaquone, bupropion, divalproex, lamotrigine, phenytoin, raltegravir, rifampin, theophylline, voriconazole: Decreased concentration of these drugs with possible decreased efficacy

avanafil, sildenafil, tadalafil, vardenafil: Increased concentration of PDE5 inhibitors with possible increased risk of adverse reactions, including hypotension, prolonged erection, syncope, visual changes

delavirdine: Increased concentration of ritonavir with possible risk of prolonged action and adverse reactions

digoxin: Increased concentration of digoxin with possible increased risk of digitalis toxicity

disulfiram, metronidazole: Increased risk of adverse reactions, especially "hangover" symptoms because ritonavir contains ethanol
methadone: Decreased concentration of methadone with increased risk of opiate withdrawal symptoms
meperidine: Increased concentrations of the metabolite of meperidine with possible risk of prolonged action and adverse reactions
rivaroxaban: Increased concentration of rivaroxaban with possible increased risk of bleeding
vinblastine, vincristine: Increased concentration of these drugs with increased risk of significant gastrointestinal or hematologic adverse reactions
warfarin: Altered INR in either direction requiring possible dosage adjustments

Adverse Reactions

CNS: Asthenia, attention disturbance, confusion, dizziness, fatigue, paresthesia, peripheral neuropathy, **seizures**, syncope
CV: **AV block**, elevated cholesterol and triglycerides, hypertension, **hypotension**, orthostatic hypotension, peripheral edema, right bundle branch block
EENT: Blurred vision, oral paresthesia, oropharyngeal pain
ENDO: Cushingoid appearance, fat redistribution, hot flashes
GI: Abdominal pain, bilirubin increase, diarrhea, dysgeusia, dyspepsia, elevated liver and pancreatic enzymes, flatulence, gastroesophageal reflux disease, **GI hemorrhage**, **hepatitis**, **hepatotoxicity**, jaundice, nausea, **pancreatitis**, vomiting
GU: Increased urination, nephrolithiasis, **renal insufficiency**
HEME: Anemia, decreased red blood cells, **leukopenia**, **neutropenia**, **thrombocytopenia**
MS: Arthralgia, back pain, elevated creatine phosphokinase, myalgia, myopathy, peripheral coldness
RESP: **Bronchospasm**, coughing
SKIN: Acne, facial edema, flushing, pruritus, rash, skin eruptions, **Stevens-Johnson syndrome**, **toxic epidermal necrolysis**, urticaria
Other: **Anaphylaxis**, **angioedema**, dehydration, **electrolyte imbalances**, gout, **immune reconstitution syndrome**, lipodystrophy (acquired)

Childbearing Considerations

PREGNANCY

- Pregnancy exposure registry: 1-800-258-4263.
- It is not known if drug can cause fetal harm.
- Be aware that the oral solution form is not recommended during pregnancy because there is no known safe level of ethanol exposure during pregnancy.
- Use other forms with caution only if benefit to mother outweighs potential risk to fetus.

LACTATION

- Drug is present in breast milk.
- The Centers for Disease Control and Prevention recommends that HIV-1 infected mothers not breastfeed to avoid risking postnatal transmission of HIV-1 infection to infants. They also do not recommend breastfeeding because of potential drug-induced adverse reactions in the infant.

REPRODUCTION

- Females of childbearing age using a hormonal form of contraception should use an additional or alternative form during drug therapy.

Nursing Considerations

! WARNING Know that dihydroergotamine or ergotamine should not be coadministered with ritonavir because acute ergot toxicity may occur, exhibited by ischemia of the extremities and other tissues, including the central nervous system and vasospasm.

! WARNING Be aware that adrenal suppression and Cushing's syndrome may occur when ritonavir is coadministered with budesonide or fluticasone propionate. Monitor patient closely because adrenal suppression may become life-threatening, especially during times of stress such as infections.

- Use cautiously in patients with cardiomyopathies, ischemic heart disease, preexisting conduction system abnormalities, or structural heart disease because ritonavir may prolong patient's PR interval.

- Expect to check patient's cholesterol and triglyceride levels prior to starting ritonavir therapy and then periodically throughout therapy. Notify prescriber if elevated and expect patient to be treated for the lipid disorder.

! **WARNING** Assess patient regularly for signs of hypersensitivity reactions, which could become life-threatening, such as anaphylaxis or angioedema. Report any abnormal findings to prescriber, expect ritonavir to be discontinued, and provide supportive care, as needed and ordered.

! **WARNING** Monitor patients with hepatitis (especially B and C), liver enzyme abnormalities, or preexisting liver disease because of the increased risk of hepatotoxicity during ritonavir therapy. Expect to monitor liver enzymes, as ordered, in these patients more frequently during the first 3 months of ritonavir therapy.

! **WARNING** Assess patient's skin regularly because ritonavir may cause serious to life-threatening skin reactions. Notify prescriber if abnormalities are observed.

! **WARNING** Monitor patient for pancreatitis, such as the presence of abdominal pain, abnormal serum amylase or lipase values, nausea, or vomiting. If suspected, notify prescriber and expect ritonavir to be discontinued, if confirmed.

! **WARNING** Be aware that immune reconstitution syndrome has occurred in patients treated with combination antiretroviral therapy, including ritonavir. The inflammatory response predisposes susceptible patients to opportunistic infections, such as cytomegalovirus, *Mycobacterium avium* infection, *Pneumocystis jiroveci* pneumonia, or tuberculosis. Autoimmune disorders, such as Graves' disease, Guillain-Barré syndrome, or polymyositis have also occurred. Report sudden or unusual adverse reactions to prescriber.

! **WARNING** Monitor patients with hemophilia for increased bleeding because spontaneous skin hemarthrosis and hematomas have occurred in these patients while taking ritonavir. Provide supportive care, as needed and ordered.

- Monitor patient's blood glucose levels throughout ritonavir therapy because some patients have experienced an exacerbation of diabetes mellitus or have developed hyperglycemia or new-onset diabetes mellitus with protease inhibitor therapy.
- Observe patient for redistribution of body fat, including breast enlargement, central obesity, development of buffalo hump, facial wasting, and peripheral wasting, which may produce a cushingoid-type appearance.

! **WARNING** Monitior patient for other persistent, serious, or unusual adverse reactions.

PATIENT TEACHING

- Instruct patient how to take form of ritonavir prescribed.

! **WARNING** Instruct patient to report any signs of an allergic reaction or skin abnormalities immediately to the prescriber.

! **WARNING** Inform patients with hemophilia of increased risk of bleeding and the need to seek immediate medical attention if bleeding occurs.

! **WARNING** Tell patient to inform prescriber of any other persistent, serious, or unusual adverse reaction.

- Alert patient that fat distribution may occur with ritonavir therapy, altering appearance.
- Warn patient to alert all prescribers of ritonavir therapy because serious drug interactions can occur.
- Alert female of childbearing age using oral contraceptives or patch contraceptives containing ethinyl estradiol that alternative methods of contraception should be used.
- Instruct mothers not to breastfeed while receiving ritonavir therapy.

rituximab
Rituxan

rituximab-abbs
Truxima

rituximab-arrx
Riabni

rituximab-pvvr
Ruxience

Class and Category

Pharmacologic class: Monoclonal antibody
Therapeutic class: Anti-inflammatory, immunosuppressant

Indications and Dosages

∗ *To treat rheumatoid arthritis*

I.V. INFUSION (RIABNI, RITUXAN, RUXIENCE, TRUXIMA)

Adults. Two 1,000-mg infusions separated by 2 wk. Subsequent courses administered every 24 wk or based on clinical evaluation, but no sooner than every 16 wk.

∗ *To treat moderate to severe pemphigus vulgaris*

I.V. INFUSION (RITUXIMAB)

Adults. *Induction:* Two 1,000-mg infusions separated by 2 wk. *Maintenance:* 500-mg infusion at mo 12 and every 6 mo thereafter or based on clinical evaluation.
Adults who have relapsed. 1,000-mg infusion on relapse. Subsequent infusions given no sooner than 16 wk following previous infusion.

∗ *To treat non-Hodgkin lymphoma (NHL)*

I.V. INFUSION (RIABNI, RITUXIMAB, RUXIENCE, TRUXIMA)

Adults with relapsed or who have refractory, low-grade, or follicular CD20-positive, B-cell NHL. 375 mg/m^2 once a wk for 4 to 8 doses.
Adults receiving retreatment for relapsed or refractory, low-grade, or follicular CD20-positive, B-cell NHL. 375 mg/m^2 once a wk for 4 doses.
Adults with previously untreated follicular, CD20-positive, B-cell NHL. 375 mg/m^2 administered on day 1 of each cycle of chemotherapy for up to 8 doses. *Maintenance:* If complete or partial response occurs after chemotherapy, 375 mg/m^2 every 8 wk for 12 doses.
Adults with nonprogressing, low-grade, CD20-positive, B-cell NHL after first-line CVP chemotherapy. Following completion of 6 to 8 cycles of CVP chemotherapy, 375 mg/m^2 once weekly for 4 doses at 6-mo intervals to a maximum of 16 doses.
Adults with diffuse large B-cell NHL. 375 mg/m^2 on day 1 of each cycle of chemotherapy for up to 8 infusions.

I.V. INFUSION (RITUXAN)

Children ages 6 mo and older with previously untreated, advanced stage, CD20-positive diffuse large B-cell lymphoma, Burkitt lymphoma, or Burkitt-like lymphoma. 375 mg/m^2 for 6 infusions (2 doses during each of the induction courses, COPDAM1 and COPDAM2, and 1 dose during each of the 2 consolidation courses of CYM/CYVE). Infusion initiated at a rate of 0.5 mg/kg/hr (maximum 50 mg/hr) and if no infusion toxicity, infusion rate increased by 0.5 mg/kg/hr every 30 min to a maximum of 400 mg/hr. For subsequent infusions in the absence of infusion toxicity, infused at 1 mg/kg/hr (maximum 50 mg/hr) and if no infusion toxicity develops, infusion rate increased by 1 mg/kg/hr every 30 min to a maximum of 400 mg/hr.

∗ *To treat chronic lymphocytic leukemia (CLL)*

I.V. INFUSION (RIABNI, RITUXAN, RUXIENCE, TRUXIMA)

Adults. 375 mg/m^2 on day prior to initiation of FC chemotherapy, then 500 mg/m^2 on day 1 of cycles 2–6 (every 28 days).

∗ *To treat granulomatosis with polyangiitis (Wegener's granulomatosis) and microscopic polyangiitis*

I.V. INFUSION (RIABNI, RITUXAN, RUXIENCE, TRUXIMA)

Adults. *Induction:* 375 mg/m^2 once a wk for 4 wk. *Maintenance:* Two 500-mg infusions separated by 2 wk, followed by a 500-mg infusion every 6 mo based on clinical evaluation.

I.V. INFUSION (RITUXAN)

Children ages 2 and older. *Induction:* 375 mg/m² once a wk for 4 wk. *Maintenance:* Two 250-mg/m² infusions separated by 2 wk, followed by a 250-mg/m² infusion every 6 mo based on clinical evaluation.

* *To treat mature B-cell acute leukemia in children*

I.V. INFUSION (RITUXAN)

Children ages 6 mo and older with previously untreated mature B-cell acute leukemia. *Induction:* 375 mg/m² once a wk for 4 wk. *Maintenance:* Two 250-mg/m² infusions separated by 2 wk, followed by a 250-mg/m² infusion every 6 mo based on clinical evaluation.

±**DOSAGE ADJUSTMENT** For all patients, dosage adjustments made following manufacturer's guidelines for each indication and the additional drugs given concomitantly.

Drug Administration

I.V.

- Premedicate patient with acetaminophen and an antihistamine prior to each infusion, as ordered, to prevent or lessen severity of an infusion reaction. If glucocorticoid therapy is part of patient's regimen, it should also be administered about 30 min prior to infusion, as ordered.
- Prepare infusion by withdrawing the necessary amount of drug and dilute to a final concentration of 1 mg/ml to 4 mg/ml in an infusion containing either 0.9% Sodium Chloride Injection or 5% Dextrose Injection. Gently invert bag to mix the solution. Do not mix or dilute with other drugs. Discard any unused portion left invial.
- Diluted solutions may be stored refrigerated for 24 hr.
- For adults, unless otherwise specified in manufacturer's guidelines, infuse first infusion at 50 mg/hr. If no infusion toxicity noted, infusion rate increased by 50-mg/hr increments every 30 min to a maximum of 400 mg/hr. For subsequent infusions, initiate infusion rate at 100 mg/hr, and if no infusion toxicity noted, rate increased by 100-mg/hr increments at 30-min intervals to a maximum of 400 mg/hr.
- For children, unless otherwise specified in manufacturer's guidelines, initiate infusion at a rate of 0.5 mg/kg/hr (maximum 50 mg/hr) and if no infusion toxicity, infusion rate increased by 0.5 mg/kg/hr every 30 min to a maximum of 400 mg/hr. For subsequent infusions in the absence of infusion toxicity, infused at 1 mg/kg/hr (maximum 50 mg/hr) and if no infusion toxicity develops, infusion rate increased by 1 mg/kg/hr every 30 min to a maximum of 400 mg/hr.
- Severe infusion reactions most often occur within 30 to 120 min of beginning the first infusion. Patients at higher risk include patients with preexisting cardiac or pulmonary conditions, those who experienced prior cardiopulmonary adverse reactions, and those with high numbers of circulating malignant cells (25,000/mm³ or greater). Depending on the severity of the infusion reaction, stop infusion or slow infusion rate as some could be life-threatening, such as angioedema, bronchospasms, and hypotension. Know that reaction may resolve with slowing or interruption of the infusion and with supportive care (acetaminophen, diphenhydramine, and intravenous saline). If warranted, expect to resume infusion upon improvement of symptoms by continuing infusion at one-half the previous rate.
- Never administer drug as an I.V. bolus or give as an intravenous push.
- *Incompatibilities:* Other drugs; other solutions except for 0.9% Sodium Chloride Injection or 5% Dextrose Injection

Route	Onset	Peak	Duration
I.V.	7–56 days	Unknown	Unknown

Half-life: 14–62 days

Mechanism of Action

Targets the CD20 antigen expressed on the surface of pre-B and mature B lymphocytes. Binding to CD20 causes drug-mediated B-cell lysis to occur. Remember that B cells are believed to play a role in the pathogenesis of rheumatoid arthritis and associated chronic synovitis. In rheumatoid arthritis, B cells may be acting at multiple sites in the autoimmune/inflammatory process, including through antigen presentation, production of rheumatoid factor and other auto-antibodies, proinflammatory cytokine production, and T-cell activation. Improvement of rheumatoid arthritis signs and symptoms may occur when B-cell lysis occurs.

Contraindications

Hypersensitivity to rituximab or its components

Interactions

DRUGS

immunosuppressants: Enhanced immunosuppressive effects
vaccines (live): Possibly increased risk of infection

Adverse Reactions

CNS: Anxiety, asthenia, chills, depression, dizziness, fatigue, fever, headache, insomnia, irritability, migraine, paresthesia, peripheral sensory neuropathy, **progressive multifocal leukoencephalopathy (PML)**, **posterior reversible encephalopathy syndrome**, **reversible posterior leukoencephalopathy syndrome**
CV: **Cardiogenic shock**, **fatal cardiac failure**, hypertension, **hypotension**, increased LDH, **MI**, peripheral edema, systemic vasculitis, tachycardia, **ventricular fibrillation**
EENT: Conjunctivitis, epistaxis, optic neuritis, rhinitis, sinusitis, throat irritation, uveitis
ENDO: Hyperglycemia, hypophosphatemia, weight gain
GI: Abdominal pain, **bowel obstruction and perforation**, diarrhea, dyspepsia, elevated liver enzymes, nausea, vomiting
GU: UTI
HEME: **Anemia**, **bone marrow hypoplasia**, **febrile neutropenia**, **hyperviscosity syndrome in Waldenstrom macroglobulinemia**, **leukopenia**, **lymphopenia**, **neutropenia**, **prolonged hypogammaglobulinemia**, **prolonged pancytopenia**, **thrombocytopenia**
MS: Arthralgia, back pain, muscle spasms, musculoskeletal pain, myalgia, polyarticular arthritis
RESP: **Bronchospasm**, dyspnea, **fatal bronchiolitis obliterans and interstitial lung disease**, increased cough, pleuritis, upper respiratory infections
SKIN: Alopecia, flushing, lichenoid or vesiculobullous dermatitis, night sweats, **paraneoplastic pemphigus (blistering of mucous membranes and skin)**, pruritus, pyoderma gangrenosum (large, painful sores), rash, skin papilloma, **Stevens-Johnson syndrome**, **toxic epidermal necrolysis**, urticaria
Other: **Angioedema**, antibody formation to rituximab, **disease progression of Kaposi's sarcoma**, generalized pain, herpes simplex or zoster, **HIV-associated lymphoma (fatal)**, infections (bacterial, fungal, viral), infusion reactions (**angioedema**, **bronchospasm**, chills/rigors, dizziness, fever, headache, myalgia, nausea, pruritus, rash, urticaria, vomiting), lupus-like syndrome, serum sickness, **tumor lysis** (**acute renal failure**, **hyperkalemia**, **hyperphosphatemia**, **hyperuricemia**, **hypocalcemia**), vasculitis with rash

Childbearing Considerations

PREGNANCY

- Drug can cause fetal harm, such as B-cell lymphocytopenia.
- Use with caution only if benefit to mother outweighs potential risk to fetus.
- If drug used during pregnancy, neonate should be observed for signs of infection.

LACTATION

- It is not known if drug is present in breast milk.
- Breastfeeding is not recommended during drug therapy and for 6 mo following last dose.

REPRODUCTION

- Advise females of childbearing age to use effective contraception during drug treatment and for at least 12 mo after last dose.

Nursing Considerations

! WARNING Screen all patients for hepatitis B virus (HBV) by measuring hepatitis B surface antigen (HbsAg) and hepatitis B core antibody (anti-HBc) before initiating rituximab, as ordered, because HBV reactivation can occur and can result in severe liver dysfunction or even death. Patient will need to be monitored for up to 24 months after completion of rituximab therapy. Also, obtain complete blood count

(CBC), including platelets, prior to first dose. Once treatment is begun, obtain CBC with differential and platelet counts prior to each drug course in patients with lymphoid malignancies. During treatment with chemotherapy, obtain CBC with differential and platelet counts at weekly to monthly intervals and more frequently in patients who develop cytopenia.

- Ensure that patient is up to date on immunizations before rituximab is started because immunization with live-virus vaccines is not recommended before or during rituximab therapy. Nonlive vaccines should be administered at least 4 weeks before a course of rituximab is given.

! **WARNING** Be prepared to perform cardiac monitoring during and after all infusions of rituximab for patients who develop clinically significant arrhythmias or who have a history of angina or arrhythmia. This is because life-threatening cardiac adverse reactions, such as cardiogenic shock, MI, or ventricular fibrillation, may occur with rituximab therapy.

! **WARNING** Monitor patient for hypersensitivity or severe mucocutaneous reactions., which could become life-threatening, such as angioedema or Stevens-Johnson syndrome. If present, notify prescriber, expect drug to be discontinued, and provide supportive care, as needed and ordered.

! **WARNING** Monitor patient for new-onset neurological manifestations that may be suggestive of progressive multifocal leukoencephalopathy (PML), which can occur with rituximab therapy. Know that most cases are diagnosed within 12 months of the last infusion of drug. If suspected, expect an MRI and lumbar puncture to be obtained. If confirmed, expect rituximab to be discontinued.

- Obtain CBC with differential and platelet counts at 2- to 4-month intervals for patients with granulomatosis with polyangiitis, microscopic polyangiitis, and rheumatoid arthritis. Continue to monitor all patients throughout rituximab therapy for cytopenia and after final dose and until resolution if present.

! **WARNING** Institute infection control measures and monitor patient for signs and symptoms of infection, as serious infections, including fatal bacterial, fungal, and new or reactivated viral infections, can occur. If infection is serious, expect rituximab to be discontinued and appropriate anti-infective therapy instituted. Know that prophylaxis treatment for *Pneumocystis jirovecii* pneumonia and herpes virus infections may be given during treatment with rituximab and in some cases up to 6 or 12 months following last infusion.

! **WARNING** Monitor patient's serum creatinine level and patient for oliguria if being treated for NHL with rituximab because renal toxicity may occur. Renal toxicity may occur with tumor lysis syndrome but also in patients receiving cisplatin. Be aware that concomitant administration of cisplatin and rituximab is not an approved treatment regimen. In addition, patient treated for NHL is also at risk for bowel obstruction and perforation. If patient develops abdominal pain or repeated vomiting, notify prescriber at once.

! **WARNING** Monitor patient being treated for non-Hodgkin lymphoma for tumor lysis syndrome (acute renal failure, hyperkalemia, hyperphosphatemia, and hypocalcemia), which can sometimes be fatal and usually occurs within 12 to 24 hours after the first infusion. Patients at higher risk include patients with high number of circulating malignant cells (25,000/mm^3 or greater) or high tumor burden. If present, expect to provide aggressive intravenous hydration and antihyperuricemic therapy in patients at high risk, as ordered. Expect electrolyte abnormalities to be corrected and renal function and fluid balance monitored, as ordered. Also, provide supportive care that may include dialysis, as ordered.

! **WARNING** Monitor patient for any other persistent, serious, or unusual adverse reactions.

PATIENT TEACHING

- Inform patient that drug will be administered intravenously.

! **WARNING** Instruct patient on the signs and symptoms of an hypersensitivity or infusion reaction. Urge patient to report any signs or symptoms immediately to staff, if present.

! **WARNING** Tell patient or family or caregiver to monitor the skin for abnormal effects. If blisters, painful sores, or ulcers appear in the mouth, or if peeling skin, pustules, or rash develops, tell patient to contact prescriber immediately.

! **WARNING** Review other signs and symptoms that should be reported to prescriber, including persistent, severe, or unusual reactions that may warrant immediate attention, such as those that may occur with the cardiovascular system, hepatitis B virus reaction, progressive multifocal leukoencephalopathy, and tumor lysis syndrome.

- Instruct patient and family or caregiver on infection control measures, including avoiding people who are ill.
- Advise females of childbearing age to use effective contraception while receiving rituximab and for 12 months after last dose. However, if pregnancy occurs during drug therapy, tell mothers to observe their neonate for an infection.
- Instruct mothers not to breastfeed during treatment with rituximab and for at least 6 months after last dose.

rivaroxaban

Xarelto

Class and Category

Pharmacologic class: Factor Xa inhibitor
Therapeutic class: Anticoagulant

Indications and Dosages

∗ *To reduce the risk of stroke and systemic embolism in patients with nonvalvular atrial fibrillation*

TABLETS

Adults with creatinine clearance greater than 50 ml/min. 20 mg once daily with evening meal.

Adults with creatinine clearance between 15 and 50 ml/min. 15 mg once daily with evening meal.

∗ *To prevent deep vein thrombosis, which may lead to pulmonary embolism following hip or knee replacement surgery*

TABLETS

Adults with creatinine clearance of 15 ml/min or greater. 10 mg once daily begun 6 to 10 hr after surgery once hemostasis has been established and given for 12 days after knee replacement surgery; 35 days after hip replacement surgery.

∗ *To treat deep vein thrombosis or pulmonary embolism*

TABLETS

Adults with creatinine clearance of 15 ml/min or greater. 15 mg twice daily for 21 days, followed by 20 mg once daily.

∗ *To reduce risk of recurrence of deep vein thrombosis or pulmonary embolism in patients at continued risk*

TABLETS

Adults with a creatinine clearance of 15 ml/min or greater. 10 mg once daily after at least 6 mo of standard anticoagulant therapy.

∗ *To prevent venous thromboembolism in acutely ill medical patients at risk for thromboembolic complications not at high risk of bleeding*

TABLETS

Adults with a creatinine clearance of 15 mg/ml or greater. 10 mg once daily, for a total of 31 to 39 days.

∗ *To reduce risk of major cardiovascular events in patients with chronic coronary artery disease or peripheral artery disease*

TABLETS

Adults regardless of creatinine clearance level. 2.5 mg twice daily with 75- or 100-mg aspirin once daily.

∗ *To reduce risk of major thrombotic vascular events in patients with peripheral artery disease (PAD), including patients after lower extremity revascularization due to symptomatic PAD*

TABLETS

Adults regardless of creatinine clearance level. 2.5 mg twice daily with 75- or 100-mg aspirin once daily. For lower extremity revascularization, therapy started once hemostasis has been established.

∗ *To treat venous thromboembolism and reduce risk of recurrent venous thromboembolism in pediatric patients*

ORAL SUSPENSION, TABLETS

Children less than age 18 weighing 50 kg (110 lb) or greater. 20 mg once daily with food about 24 hr apart following at least 5 days of parenteral anticoagulation therapy.

Children less than age 18 weighing between 30 kg (66 lb) and 49.9 kg (109.78 lb). 15 mg once daily with food about 24 hr apart following at least 5 days of parenteral anticoagulation therapy.

ORAL SUSPENSION

Children less than age 18 weighing 12 kg (26.4 lb) to 29.9 kg (65.78 lb). 5 mg twice daily about 12 hr apart with food following at least 5 days of parenteral anticoagulation therapy. *Maximum:* 10 mg daily.

Children less than age 18 weighing 10 kg (22 lb) to 11.9 kg (26.18 lb). 3 mg 3 times daily about 8 hr apart with food following at least 5 days of parenteral anticoagulation therapy. *Maximum:* 9 mg daily.

Children less than age 18 weighing 9 kg (19.8 lb) to 9.9 kg (21.78 lb). 2.8 mg 3 times daily about 8 hr apart with food following at least 5 days of parenteral anticoagulation therapy. *Maximum:* 8.4 mg daily.

Children weighing 8 kg (17.6 lb) to 8.9 kg (19.58 lb). 2.4 mg 3 times daily about 8 hr apart with food following at least 5 days of parenteral anticoagulation therapy. *Maximum:* 7.2 mg daily.

Children weighing 7 kg (15.4 lb) to 7.9 kg (17.38 lb). 1.8 mg 3 times daily about 8 hr apart with feeding following at least 5 days of parenteral anticoagulation therapy. *Maximum:* 5.4 mg daily.

Children weighing 5 kg (11 lb) to 6.9 kg (15.18 lb). 1.6 mg 3 times daily about 8 hr apart with feeding following at least 5 days of parenteral anticoagulation therapy. *Maximum*: 4.8 mg daily.

Children weighing 4 kg (8.8 lb) to 4.9 kg (10.78 lb). 1.4 mg 3 times daily about 8 hr apart with feeding following at least 5 days of parenteral anticoagulation therapy. *Maximum:* 4.2 mg daily.

Children weighing 3 kg (6.6 lb) to 3.9 kg (8.58 lb). 0.9 mg 3 times daily about 8 hr apart with feeding following at least 5 days of parenteral anticoagulation therapy. *Maximum:* 2.7 mg daily.

Children weighing 2.6 kg (5.72 lb) to 2.9 g (6.38 lb). 0.8 mg 3 times daily about 8 hr apart with feeding following at least 5 days of parenteral anticoagulation therapy. *Maximum:* 2.4 mg daily.

±**DOSAGE ADJUSTMENT** For infants less than 6 months of age, the infants must have been at least 37 weeks of gestation at birth, have had at least 10 days of oral feeding, and weight was 2.6 kg or greater at the time of dosing. For children with thrombosis, therapy continued for at least 3 months but may be extended up to 12 months, except for children less than 2 with catheter-related thrombosis. For children less than 2 with catheter-related thrombosis, therapy continued for at least 1 month but may be extended up to 3 months, as needed. For children ages 1 and older with mild renal impairment (creatinine 50 to 80 ml/min), no dosage adjustment necessary; drug should not be used if renal impairment is more severe. For children less than 1, drug should be avoided in children with serum creatinine results above 97.5 percentile (see manufacturer's guidelines for chart).

∗ *To prevent thromboembolism in children with congenital heart disease after the Fontan procedure*

ORAL SUSPENSION, TABLETS

Children ages 2 and older weighing 50 kg (110 lb) or more. 10 mg once daily about 24 hr apart. *Maximum:* 10 mg daily.

ORAL SUSPENSION

Children ages 2 and older weighing 30 kg (66 lb) to 49.9 kg (109.78 lb). 7.5 mg once daily about 24 hr apart. *Maximum:* 7.5 mg daily.

Children ages 2 and older weighing 20 kg (44 lb) to 29.9 kg (65.78 lb). 2.5 mg 2 times daily about 12 hr apart. *Maximum:* 5 mg.

Children ages 2 and older weighing 12 kg (26.4 lb) to 19.9 kg (43.78 lb). 2 mg twice daily about 12 hr apart. *Maximum:* 4 mg.

Children ages 2 and older weighing 10 kg (22 lb) and 11.9 kg (26.18 lb). 1.7 mg twice daily about 12 hr apart. *Maximum:* 3.4 mg daily.

Children ages 2 and older weighing 8 kg (17.6 lb) to 9.9 kg (21.78 lb). 1.6 mg twice

daily about 12 hr apart. *Maximum:* 3.2 mg daily.
Children ages 2 and older weighing 7 kg (15.4 lb) to 7.9 kg (17.38 lb). 1.1 mg twice daily about 12 hr apart. *Maximum:* 2.2 mg daily.

Drug Administration

P.O.

- Follow manufacturer's guidelines when patient is being switched to and from rivaroxaban and when a dose is missed.
- Be aware that oral suspension can be used with PVC, polyurethane, or silicone NG tubing.

Adults

- Give 15- or 20-mg tablets with food; 2.5- or 10-mg tablets need not be taken with food.
- For nonvalvular atrial fibrillation, give drug with the evening meal.
- For adults unable to swallow tablets, crush tablets and mix with applesauce immediately prior to administration and if dose is 15 mg or 20 mg, follow with food.
- Administering drug via a nasogastric tube or gastric feeding tube requires tablets to be crushed and suspended in 50 ml of water. Following administration, flush tube with water, and give enteral feeding immediately if dose is 15 mg or 20 mg.
- Drug is stable in water or in applesauce for up to 4 hr.

Children

- For reduction of recurrent venous thromboembolism or treatment of venous thromboembolism, all doses should be given with a feeding or food to enhance absorption. Feedings or food are not necessary for thromboprophylaxis in children with congenital heart disease after the Fontan procedure.
- Measure child's weight routinely because dosage is based upon weight.
- Oral suspension is prepared by a pharmacist and can be stored at room temperature. Use the calibrated syringe provided with drug to measure dosage.
- If infant or child vomits or spits up the dose within 30 min after administration, give a new dose. If it is more than 30 min, do not administer another dose and give the next dose as scheduled.
- Tablets must be swallowed whole and not chewed, crushed, or split.
- Administering drug via a nasogastric tube or gastric feeding tube requires tablets to be crushed and suspended in 50 ml of water or oral suspension to be used. After administration, flush the tube with water. Also, following administration, enteral feeding should be given immediately if child is being treated for venous thromboembolism or reduction of recurrent venous thromboembolism.

Route	Onset	Peak	Duration
P.O.	Unknown	2–4 hr	Unknown

Half-life: 5–9 hr

Mechanism of Action

Blocks the active site of factor Xa selectively, which plays a central role in the cascade of blood coagulation. Impairment of blood clotting occurs when the action of factor Xa is absent.

Contraindications

Active pathological bleeding, hypersensitivity to rivaroxaban or its components

Interactions

DRUGS

anticoagulants, aspirin, clopidogrel, dual antiplatelet therapy, fibrinolytic therapy, heparin, NSAIDs, other antithrombotic agents or platelet aggregation inhibitors, selective serotonin reuptake inhibitors, serotonin–norepinephrine reuptake inhibitors, warfarin: Possibly increased bleeding risk
combined strong CYP3A and P-glycoprotein (P-gp) inducers, such as carbamazepine, phenytoin, rifampin, St. John's wort: Decreased effectiveness of rivaroxaban
combined CYP3A4 and P-gp inhibitors, such as conivaptan, diltiazem, dronedarone, erythromycin, fluconazole, indinavir/ritonavir, itraconazole, ketoconazole, lopinavir/ritonavir, ritonavir, verapamil: Increased rivaroxaban exposure resulting in increased bleeding risk

Adverse Reactions

CNS: Anxiety, **cerebral hemorrhage**, depression, dizziness, epidural hematoma, fatigue, hemiparesis, insomnia, **subdural hematoma**, syncope
EENT: Epistaxis, intraocular bleeding

GI: Abdominal pain, cholestasis, **cytolytic hepatitis, GI bleeding, hepatitis**, jaundice, **retroperitoneal hemorrhage, vomiting**
GU: Anticoagulant-related nephropathy
HEME: Agranulocytosis, decreased hemoglobin, **excessive bleeding, hemorrhage, thrombocytopenia**
MS: Back or extremity pain, intra-articular bleeding, muscle spasm
RESP: Cough, **eosinophilic pneumonia, pulmonary hemorrhage** with or without bronchiectasis
SKIN: Blister formation, pruritus, rash, **Stevens-Johnson syndrome**
Other: Anaphylactic shock, anaphylaxis, angioedema, drug reaction with eosinophilia and systemic symptoms (DRESS)

Childbearing Considerations

PREGNANCY

- Drug has the potential to cause fetal harm as a result of bleeding at any site in the fetus and/or neonate from drug use during pregnancy.
- Use with caution only if benefit to mother outweighs potential risk to fetus.

LABOR AND DELIVERY

- Drug may increase the risk of bleeding for both mother and fetus/neonate during labor and delivery.

LACTATION

- Drug is present in breast milk.
- Mothers should check with prescriber before breastfeeding.

REPRODUCTION

- Females of childbearing age should discuss pregnancy planning with prescriber because of potential for significant uterine bleeding that may require surgery to stop bleeding.

Nursing Considerations

! **WARNING** Know that rivaroxaban should not be given to patients with moderate or severe hepatic impairment, to patients with any hepatic disease associated with coagulopathy, and to patients with a creatinine clearance that is less than 15 ml/min. Monitor patient's hepatic and renal function, as ordered, throughout rivaroxaban therapy. Expect rivaroxaban to be discontinued if hepatitis or other serious hepatic dysfunction or acute renal failure occurs.

! **WARNING** Know that rivaroxaban should not be given to acutely ill medical patients at high risk of bleeding to prevent a venous thrombosis event. High-risk conditions include active cancer; gastroduodenal ulcer in the 3 months prior to treatment; or a history of bronchiectasis, bleeding in the 3 months prior to treatment, dual antiplatelet therapy, or pulmonary cavitation or hemorrhage.

! **WARNING** Do not expect to give rivaroxaban to patients with triple-positive antiphospholipid syndrome because of increased rates of recurrent thrombotic events.

! **WARNING** Be aware that rivaroxaban should not be given to patients with prosthetic heart valves or as an alternative to unfractionated heparin in patients with pulmonary embolism who are hemodynamically unstable or who may receive pulmonary embolectomy or thrombolysis.

- Be aware that manufacturer's guidelines should be followed when patient is switching from or to other anticoagulants. For example, when patient is switching from warfarin to rivaroxaban therapy, expect warfarin to be discontinued and rivaroxaban started when the international normalized ratio (INR) is below 3. For patients currently receiving an anticoagulant other than warfarin, such as low-molecular-weight heparin or nonwarfarin oral anticoagulant, expect to start rivaroxaban therapy within 2 hours of the next scheduled evening administration of the drug, and plan to omit administration of the other anticoagulant, as ordered. For unfractionated heparin being administered by continuous infusion, expect to stop the infusion and start rivaroxaban therapy at the same time. For patients currently taking rivaroxaban and transitioning to an anticoagulant with rapid onset, expect rivaroxaban to be discontinued and the first dose of the other anticoagulant given at the time the next rivaroxaban would have been given.

! **WARNING** Know that if patient has an epidural catheter inserted, it should not be removed any earlier than 18 hours for younger patients (less than 45 years) and 26 hours for older patients (60 years and older) after the last rivaroxaban dose was administered. Obtain specific guidelines for catheter removal from prescriber for patients between the ages of 45 and 60. The next rivaroxaban dose should not be administered any earlier than 6 hours after removal of the catheter because an epidural or spinal hematoma can occur and can result in long-term or permanent paralysis. If traumatic puncture occurs, know that rivaroxaban should be withheld for 24 hours.

- Expect rivaroxaban to be discontinued 24 hours before an invasive procedure or surgery, if possible and restarted after adequate hemostasis has been established after the invasive surgery or procedure.

! **WARNING** Monitor patient closely for signs and symptoms of a hypersensitivity or skin reaction, which can become life-threatening such as anaphylaxis, angioedema, or DRESS (DRESS may initially only present with a fever or swollen lymph nodes although rash is a common reaction). If present, notify prescriber immediately, expect drug to be switched to a different drug, and provide supportive care, as needed and ordered.

! **WARNING** Monitor patient closely for bleeding, as rivaroxaban therapy may cause life-threatening bleeding. Expect to administer the antidote available to reverse the anti-factor Xa activity of rivaroxaban if bleeding is significant. Be aware that bleeding risks are higher in elderly patients.

! **WARNING** Monitor patient for other persistent, serious, or unusual adverse reactions as drug can affect many body systems adversely with some reactions becoming life-threatening.

! **WARNING** Be aware that if rivaroxaban is discontinued and adequate alternative anticoagulation is not present, the risk for thrombosis increases. Monitor patient closely.

PATIENT TEACHING

- Instruct patient how to administer form of rivaoxaban prescribed.
- Emphasize the importance of taking rivaroxaban exactly as prescribed.

! **WARNING** Warn patient not to stop taking rivaroxaban without first consulting prescriber.

! **WARNING** Advise females of childbearing age to notify prescriber immediately if pregnancy occurs. Alert females of childbearing age to discuss pregnancy planning because of the potential risk of significant bleeding with the drug that may require gynecological surgical intervention.

! **WARNING** Alert patient that drug may cause an allergic or severe skin reaction and to alert prescriber if present or seek immediate medical care, if severe.

! **WARNING** Advise patient to report any unusual bleeding or bruising to prescriber. Inform patient that it may take longer for him to stop bleeding and to take bleeding precautions, such as avoiding the use of a razor and using a soft-bristle toothbrush.

! **WARNING** Instruct patient who has had spinal anesthesia or puncture to watch for back pain, muscle weakness, numbness (especially in the lower limbs), stool or urine incontinence, or tingling. If present, stress importance of notifying prescriber immediately.

- Tell patient to alert all prescribers to use of rivaroxaban therapy before any invasive procedure, including dental work, is scheduled.
- Caution patient not to take any prescription or nonprescription medication, including over-the-counter and herbal medicines, without first consulting with prescriber.

rivastigmine

Exelon Patch

Class and Category

Pharmacologic class: Cholinesterase inhibitor
Therapeutic class: Antidementia

Indications and Dosages

✱ *To treat mild, moderate, and severe Alzheimer's disease*

TRANSDERMAL

Adults. *Initial:* 4.6 mg/24 hr. *For patients with mild to moderate Alzheimer's disease:* After 4 wk, increased to 9.5 mg/24 hr. When therapeutic effect begins to decrease and with at least 4 wk from last dosage increase, dosage increased to 13.3 mg/24 hr. *For patients with severe Alzheimer's disease:* After 4 wk, increased to 9.5 mg/24 hr. and after another 4 wk, increased to 13.3 mg/24 hr. *Maximum:* 13.3 mg/24 hr.

✱ *To treat mild-to-moderate dementia in Parkinson's disease*

TRANSDERMAL

Adults. *Initial:* 4.6 mg/24 hr. After 4 wk, increased to 9.5 mg/24 hr. When therapeutic effect begins to decrease, dosage increased to 13.3 mg/24 hr. *Maximum:* 13.3 mg/24 hr.

± **DOSAGE ADJUSTMENT** For patients with mild-to-moderate hepatic impairment, 4.6 mg/24 hr patch used for both initial and maintenance dose. For patients with low body weight of less than 50 kg (110 lb) and experiencing excessive nausea and vomiting, maintenance dose of patch reduced to 4.6 mg/24 hr.

Drug Administration

TRANSDERMAL

- Do not use patch if pouch seal is broken or the patch is cut, damaged, or changed in any way.
- Apply patch to clean, dry, hairless, intact skin in a location, such as the back, which won't be likely to be removed by patient, rubbed by tight clothing and won't be affected by cream, lotion, or powder. However, if back is not possible, upper arm or chest may be used. Do not apply to skin that is cut, irritated, or red or skin where cream, lotion, or powder has recently been applied.
- Press firmly into place for about 30 sec until the edges are adhered to skin.
- Remove the old patch before applying a new one and use a new application site daily. Do not reuse the same site for 14 days.
- If patch falls off or a dose is missed, apply a new patch immediately, and then replace this patch the following day at the usual application time.
- Wash hands with soap and water after removing patch. Place used patches in previously saved pouch and discard.

Route	Onset	Peak	Duration
P.O.	Unknown	1 hr	8–10 hr
Transdermal	Unknown	8–16 hr	24 hr

Half-life: 1.5–3 hr

Mechanism of Action

May slow the decline of cognitive function by increasing acetylcholine concentration at cholinergic transmission sites, which prolongs and exaggerates the effects of acetylcholine that are otherwise blocked by toxic levels of anticholinergics. Declining cognitive function is partially related to cholinergic deficits along neuronal pathways projecting from the basal forebrain to the cerebral cortex and hippocampus that are involved in attention, cognition, learning, and memory.

Contraindications

History of application-site reactions suggestive of allergic contact dermatitis (for patch form); hypersensitivity to carbamate derivatives, rivastigmine, or their components

Interactions

DRUGS

anticholinergics: Possibly decreased effectiveness of anticholinergics
beta-blockers: Possible additive bradycardic effects resulting in syncope
metoclopramide: Increased risk of additive extrapyramidal adverse reactions
other cholinomimetic drugs: Possibly increased cholinergic effects

Adverse Reactions

CNS: Aggression, anxiety, asthenia, confusion, depression, dizziness, extrapyramidal movements, fatigue, fever, hallucinations, headache, insomnia, malaise, nightmares, **seizures**, somnolence, tremor, worsening of parkinsonism
CV: Hypertension, **QT prolongation**, tachycardia, **torsades de pointes**
EENT: Rhinitis
GI: Abdominal pain, anorexia, constipation, diarrhea, duodenal ulcers, elevated liver enzymes, flatulence, **hepatitis**, indigestion, nausea, vomiting

GU: UTI
SKIN: Allergic or disseminated dermatitis, increased sweating, reaction at patch application site (papule or vesicle formation, pruritus, redness, swelling), **Stevens-Johnson syndrome**, urticaria
Other: Dehydration, flu-like symptoms, **hypersensivity reactions**, weight loss

Childbearing Considerations

PREGNANCY

- It is not known if drug can cause fetal harm.
- Use with caution only if benefit to mother outweighs potential risk to fetus.

LACTATION

- It is not known if drug is present in breast milk.
- Mothers should check with prescriber before breastfeeding.

Nursing Considerations

! **WARNING** Be aware that rivastigmine should be started at lowest recommended dosage and adjusted to effective maintenance dosage because initial therapy at high dosage can cause serious adverse GI reactions, including anorexia, nausea, and weight loss. Also, a higher-than-recommended starting dosage may cause severe vomiting and possibly esophageal rupture. If treatment is interrupted for longer than several days, expect to restart at lowest recommended dosage.

- Be aware that drug shouldn't be stopped abruptly because doing so may increase behavioral disturbances and precipitate a further decline in cognitive function.

! **WARNING** Monitor patient closely for hypersensitivity including skin reactions regardless of route of administration. If suspected, notify prescriber, expect drug to be discontinued, and provide supportive care, as needed and ordered.

! **WARNING** Monitor respiratory status of patients with pulmonary disease, including asthma, chronic bronchitis, and emphysema because rivastigmine has a weak affinity for peripheral cholinesterase, which may increase bronchoconstriction and bronchial secretions.

! **WARNING** Monitor patient for seizures, especially patients with a seizure disorder. Institute seizure precautions, as appropriate.

! **WARNING** Montior patient's liver function, including liver enzymes, as ordered, throughout therapy because drug can cause hepatic dysfunction and hepatitis.

- Monitor patient for adequate urine output because cholinomimetics, such as rivastigmine, may induce or exacerbate bladder or urinary tract obstruction.
- Monitor patients with Parkinson's disease for exaggerated parkinsonian symptoms, which may result from drug's increased cholinergic effects on CNS.

PATIENT TEACHING

- Explain to patient and family or caregiver that rivastigmine can't cure Alzheimer's or Parkinson's disease but may slow the progressive deterioration of memory and improve patient's ability to perform activities of daily living.
- Teach patient and family or caregiver how to administer rivastigmine patch.
- Instruct family or caregiver to supervise patient's use of rivastigmine.
- Urge family or caregiver to contact prescriber and to withhold drug if patient stops taking it for more than several days.

! **WARNING** Alert patient that drug may cause an allergic reaction. Emphasize importance of inspecting skin for signs of an allergic reaction, such as presence of hives, itching, rash, or redness. If present, instruct family or caregiver to notify prescriber, as drug will have to be discontinued. If reaction is severe, tell patient, family, or caregiver to seek immediate medical care.

! **WARNING** Tell family or caregiver to notify prescriber if other persistent, serious, or unusual adverse reactions occur.

roflumilast

Daliresp

Class and Category

Pharmacologic class: Selective phosphodiesterase 4 inhibitor

Therapeutic class: Antipulmonic obstructive agent

Indications and Dosages

∗ *To reduce the risk of COPD exacerbations in patients with severe COPD associated with chronic bronchitis and a history of exacerbations*

TABLETS

Adults. *Initial:* 250 mcg once daily for 4 wk, then increased to maintenance dose of 500 mcg daily.

Drug Administration

P.O.

- Administer at same time daily.
- Administer with or without food.

Route	Onset	Peak	Duration
P.O.	Unknown	0.5–2 hr	Unknown

Half-life: 17–30 hr

Mechanism of Action

Increases intracellular cyclic AMP in lung cells by inhibiting a major cyclic AMP-metabolizing enzyme in lung tissue to improve pulmonary function

Contraindications

Hypersensitivity to roflumilast or its components, moderate to severe liver impairment

Interactions

DRUGS

CYP450 inducers, such as carbamazepine, phenobarbital, phenytoin, rifampicin: Decreased effectiveness of roflumilast

CYP450 inhibitors or dual inhibitors (both CYP1A2 and CYP3A4), such as cimetidine, enoxacin, erythromycin, fluvoxamine, ketoconazole; oral contraceptives containing gestodene and ethinyl estradiol: Increased roflumilast exposure with increased risk of adverse effects

Adverse Reactions

CNS: Anxiety, depression, dizziness, headache, insomnia, **suicidal ideation**, tremor
CV: **Atrial fibrillation**
EENT: Rhinitis, sinusitis
ENDO: Gynecomastia
GI: Abdominal pain, **acute pancreatitis**, anorexia, diarrhea, dyspepsia, gastritis, nausea, vomiting
GU: **Acute renal failure**, UTI
MS: Back pain, muscle spasms
SKIN: Rash, urticaria
Other: **Angioedema**, flu-like symptoms, weight loss

Childbearing Considerations

PREGNANCY

- It is not known if drug can cause fetal harm.
- Use with caution only if benefit to mother outweighs potential risk to fetus.

LABOR AND DELIVERY

- Drug should not be used during labor and delivery, as animal studies showed drug disrupts the labor and delivery process.

LACTATION

- It is not known if drug is present in breast milk.
- Breastfeeding is not recommended during drug therapy.

Nursing Considerations

! **WARNING** Be aware that drug is not to be used for relief of acute bronchospasm.

- Monitor effectiveness of roflumilast to reduce COPD exacerbations.

! **WARNING** Monitor patient for a hypersensitivity reaction, which may become life-threatening, such as angioedema. If present, notify prescriber, expect drug to be discontinued, and provide supportive care, as needed and ordered.

! **WARNING** Watch patient closely for suicidal tendencies because roflumilast has been associated with an increase in psychiatric adverse reactions, such as depression and insomnia, as well as suicidal ideation.

! **WARNING** Monitor patient for other persistent, serious, or unusual adverse reactions.

- Monitor patient's weight and notify prescriber if significant weight loss occurs.

PATIENT TEACHING

! **WARNING** Warn patient that roflumilast is not a bronchodilator and should not be used to relieve acute bronchospasm.

- Instruct patient how to administer roflumilast.
- Tell patient to alert prescriber if episodes of COPD increases indicating drug is not as effective.

! **WARNING** Alert patient that drug may cause an allergic reaction. If present, tell patient to notify prescriber and, if severe, to seek immediate medical attention.

! **WARNING** Tell family or caregiver to monitor patient for suicidal tendencies because drug may worsen depression during roflumilast therapy and increase suicidal thinking.

! **WARNING** Instruct patient to alert prescriber if other persistent, severe, or unusual adverse reactions occur such as significant weight loss.

- Inform mothers breastfeeding is not recommended during roflumilast therapy.

rolapitant hydrochloride

Varubi

Class and Category

Pharmacologic class: Substance P and neurokinin-1 receptor antagonist
Therapeutic class: Antiemetic

Indications and Dosages

* *As adjunct to prevent delayed nausea and vomiting associated with initial and repeat courses of emetogenic cancer chemotherapy*

TABLETS

Adults receiving cisplatin-based highly emetogenic cancer chemotherapy; adults receiving moderately emetogenic cancer chemotherapy and combinations of anthracycline and cyclophosphamide.
180 mg in combination with dexamethasone and a 5-HT_3 receptor antagonist within 2 hr prior to chemotherapy.

Drug Administration

P.O.

- Administer within 2 hr prior to chemotherapy.
- Administer again only after at least 2 wk have passed.

Route	Onset	Peak	Duration
P.O.	30 min	4 hr	Unknown

Half-life: 169–183 hr

Mechanism of Action

Crosses the blood–brain barrier to occupy brain P/NK1 receptors, which prevents nerve transmission of signals that cause nausea and vomiting.

Contraindications

Children less than 2 years of age; concurrent therapy with CYP2 d6 substrates with a narrow therapeutic index, such as pimozide and thioridazine; hypersensitivity to rolapitant or its components

Interactions

DRUGS

dextromethorphan and other CYP2D6 substrates: May increase plasma concentrations of these drugs
digoxin and other P-gp substrates with a narrow therapeutic index; irinotecan, methotrexate, topotecan, and other BCRP substrates with a narrow therapeutic index: Increased plasma concentrations of these drugs, which increases risk of adverse reactions
pimozide, thioridazine, and other CYP2D6 substrates with a narrow therapeutic index: Increased plasma concentrations of these drugs, which can result in QT prolongation and torsades de pointes
rifampin and other strong CYP3A4 inducers: Decreased plasma concentrations and effectiveness of rolapitant

Adverse Reactions

CNS: Dizziness
EENT: Stomatitis
GI: Abdominal pain, anorexia, dyspepsia, hiccups
GU: UTI
HEME: Anemia, **neutropenia**

Childbearing Considerations

PREGNANCY

- It is not known if drug can cause fetal harm.
- Use with caution only if benefit to mother outweighs potential risk to fetus.

LACTATION

- It is not known if drug is present in breast milk.
- Mothers should check with prescriber before breastfeeding.

REPRODUCTION

- Drug may impair fertility in females in a reversible fashion, according to animal studies.

Nursing Considerations

! **WARNING** Know that rolapitant should not be given to patients with severe hepatic impairment but in the event its use cannot be avoided, monitor patient closely for rolapitant-related adverse reactions.

- Make sure dexamethasone and a 5-HT_3 receptor antagonist have also been prescribed and are on hand ready to be given, as directed.

! **WARNING** Monitor patient's CBC with differential, as ordered because drug may cause neutropenia. If present, monitor patient for infection.

PATIENT TEACHING

- Review with patient when rolapitant is to be administered in conjunction with the patient's chemotherapy. Also, instruct patient when to take dexamethasone if it is prescribed after his chemotherapy.

! **WARNING** Review signs and symptoms of an infection and stress importance of alerting prescriber immediately, if present.

- Tell patient to inform all prescribers of rolapitant therapy.

romosozumab-aqqg

Evenity

Class and Category

Pharmacologic class: Monoclonal antibody
Therapeutic class: Antiosteoporotic

Indications and Dosages

* *To treat osteoporosis in postmenopausal women at risk for fracture or who have failed or are intolerant to other available osteoporosis therapy*

SUBCUTANEOUS INJECTION

Postmenopausal women. 210 mg (two 105-mg injections) once a mo for 12 mo.

Drug Administration

SUBCUTANEOUS

- Administer by injecting 2 consecutive 105-mg injections to complete the 210-mg dose.
- Remove 2 prefilled syringes from carton kept in refrigerator by grasping the syringe barrel when removing from the tray. Do not grasp the plunger or gray needle cap and do not remove gray needle cap until ready to give injection.
- Visually inspect the solution in each syringe. It should be clear to opalescent, colorless to light yellow.
- Allow solution to sit at room temperature for at least 30 min before injecting. Do not warm in any other way.
- Inject each injection for the monthly dose in 2 separate locations, (abdomen, outer area of upper arm, or thigh). Do not inject where skin is bruised, hard, red, or tender, and avoid injecting into areas with scars or stretch marks. Repeat steps with second syringe.
- Administer a missed dose as soon as possible and reschedule remaining monthly doses from date of last dose.

Route	Onset	Peak	Duration
SubQ	2 wk	5 days	Unknown

Half-life: 12.8 days

Mechanism of Action

Inhibits the action of sclerostin, a regulatory factor in bone metabolism, which increases bone formation and, to a lesser extent, decreases bone resorption.

Contraindications

Hypersensitivity to romosozumab-aqqg or its components, uncorrected hypocalcemia

Interactions

DRUGS

None reported by manufacturer.

Adverse Reactions

CNS: Asthenia, CVA, headache, insomnia, paresthesia
CV: MI, peripheral edema
MS: Arthralgia, atypical subtrochanteric and diaphyseal femoral fractures, muscle spasms, neck pain, osteonecrosis of the jaw

SKIN: Dermatitis, **erythema multiforme**, rash, urticaria
Other: **Angioedema**, antibody formation to romosozumab, **hypocalcemia**, injection-site reactions (erythema, pain)

Childbearing Considerations

PREGNANCY

Drug is not indicated for use in females of childbearing age.

LACTATION

- Drug is not indicated for use in females of childbearing age.

Nursing Considerations

! **WARNING** Know that romosozumab-aqqg should not be administered to patients who have had a CVA or MI within the preceding year. Additionally, romosozumab-aqqg should be discontinued if CVA or MI occurs during therapy.

! **WARNING** Ensure that preexisting hypocalcemia is corrected prior to initiating romosozumab-aqqg therapy. Monitor patient's calcium level throughout therapy because drug may cause hypocalcemia. Patients at greater risk are those with severe renal impairment or who are receiving dialysis. Ensure that patient is taking adequate amounts of calcium and vitamin D supplements.

- Check to see if patient has had a routine oral exam and any abnormalities taken care of before starting romosozumab-aqqg therapy because drug can cause osteonecrosis of the jaw, which could occur spontaneously with tooth extraction and/or local dental infection with delayed healing. Patients should be counseled to maintain good oral hygiene.

! **WARNING** Monitor patient for hypersensitivity reactions that could be life-threatening, such as angioedema or severe skin reactions such as erythema multiforme. If signs and symptoms occur, notify prescriber, expect drug to be discontinued, and provide supportive care, as needed and ordered.

! **WARNING** Monitor patient's cardiac status throughout romosozumab therapy because drug increases the risk of major adverse cardiac events. If patient develops any abnormality, notify prescriber immediately. If confirmed, expect drug to be discontinued.

- Monitor patient for other persistent, serious, or unusual adverse reactions such as groin, hip, or thigh pain and limitation of movement that could be indicative of a drug-induced fracture.

PATIENT TEACHING

- Inform patient that romosozumab-aqqg therapy will be given by a healthcare professional monthly for 12 months and requires 2 consecutive subcutaneous injections to achieve the dose each month.
- Instruct patient to take a calcium and vitamin supplement while taking romosozumab.

! **WARNING** Instruct patient on the signs and symptoms of a heart attack or stroke. Urge patient to seek immediate medical attention if present.

! **WARNING** Alert patient that drug may cause an allergic or skin reaction. Tell patient to notify prescriber and to seek immediate medical care, if severe.

! **WARNING** Review signs and symptoms of hypocalcemia with patient. Tell patient to notify prescriber immediately, if present, and to seek immediate medical care, if severe.

- Tell patient to alert prescriber if dull, aching thigh pain occurs or if new or unusual groin, hip, or thigh pain is present or if any other persistent, serious, or unusual adverse reactions occur.
- Tell patient to inform dentist of romosozumab-aqqg therapy before any dental work is done, especially invasive dental procedures.

ropinirole hydrochloride

Class and Category

Pharmacologic class: Nonergot alkaloid dopamine agonist
Therapeutic class: Antiparkinsonian

Indications and Dosages

✱ *To treat signs and symptoms of Parkinson's disease*

TABLETS

Adults. *Initial:* 0.25 mg 3 times daily. Dosage titrated upward every wk according to the following schedule: 0.25 mg 3 times daily in wk 1; 0.5 mg 3 times daily in wk 2; 0.75 mg 3times daily in wk 3; 1 mg 3 times daily in wk 4. After wk 4, as needed, dosage increased by 1.5 mg daily every wk up to 9 mg daily, then by 3 mg/day up to 24 mg daily. *Maximum:* 24 mg/day in 3 divided doses.

E.R. TABLETS

Adults. *Initial:* 2 mg once daily for 1 to 2 wk, increased, as needed, in increments of 2 mg/day at 1 wk or longer intervals. *Maintenance for patients with early Parkinson's disease:* 12 mg daily or lower. *Maintenance for patients with advanced Parkinson's disease:* 8 mg daily or lower.

✱ *To treat moderate to severe primary restless legs syndrome*

TABLETS

Adults. *Initial:* 0.25 mg daily 1 to 3 hr before bedtime. Dosage increased, as needed, on day 3 to 0.5 mg and then to 1 mg at beginning of wk 2 (day 8). Dosage further increased in 0.5-mg increments every wk for 4 wk, as needed, followed by a 1-mg increase for wk 7, as needed. *Maximum:* 4 mg daily.

± **DOSAGE ADJUSTMENT** For patients with end-stage renal disease on hemodialysis, dosage titration of immediate-release tablets is based on tolerability and need for efficacy, with recommended maximum total daily dose reduced to 18 mg/day for treatment of Parkinson's disease and 3 mg daily for patients with restless legs syndrome receiving regular dialysis. For patients with end-stage renal disease on hemodialysis and taking extended-release tablets, initial dose is 2 mg daily with dosage titration based on tolerability and need for efficacy, with recommended maximum total daily dose limited to 18 mg/day in patients receiving regular dialysis.

Drug Administration

P.O.

- Administer drug with food if adverse GI effects occur.
- Extended-release tablets should be swallowed whole and not chewed, crushed, or divided.
- Administer drug to treat restless legs syndrome 1 to 3 hr before bedtime.
- If a dose is missed administer it as soon as possible on the same day; if not, skip dose and resume regular scheduled dosing the next day. Do not double dose to make up for missed dose.

Route	Onset	Peak	Duration
P.O.	Unknown	1–2 hr	6 hr
P.O./E.R.	Unknown	6–10 hr	Unknown

Half-life: 6 hr

Mechanism of Action

Stimulates directly postsynaptic dopamine type 2 (D_2) receptors within the brain and acts as an agonist at peripheral D_2 receptors to inhibit the firing of striatal cholinergic neurons, thus helping to control alterations in voluntary muscle movement (such as rigidity and tremors) associated with Parkinson's disease and restless legs syndrome.

Contraindications

Hypersensitivity to ropinirole or its components

Interactions

DRUGS

ciprofloxacin, other CYP1A2 inhibitors: Altered drug clearance and increased blood level of immediate-release ropinirole tablets

CYP1A2 inducers; dopamine antagonists, such as butyrophenones, metoclopramide, phenothiazines, thioxanthenes: Possibly decreased effectiveness of ropinirole

ethinyl estradiol (higher doses associated with hormone replacement therapy): Possibly reduced clearance of ropinirole

ACTIVITIES

smoking: Increased clearance of ropinirole with decreased effectiveness

Adverse Reactions

CNS: Abnormal dreaming, aggression, agitation, amnesia, anxiety, asthenia, compulsive behaviors, confusion, delirium, delusions, disorientation, dizziness, dyskinesia, falling asleep during activities of daily living, fatigue, hallucinations, headache, hypoesthesia, hypokinesia, insomnia, malaise, mania, nervousness,

neuralgia, paranoid ideation, paresis, paresthesia, psychotic-like behaviors, rigors, somnolence, syncope, transient ischemic attack, tremor, vertigo
CV: **Acute coronary syndrome**, angina, **bradycardia**, **cardiac failure**, chest pain, hypertension, **MI**, orthostatic hypotension, palpitations, peripheral edema, **sick sinus syndrome**, tachycardia
EENT: Abnormal vision, diplopia, dry mouth, increased salivation, nasal congestion, nasopharyngitis, rhinitis, toothache
GI: Abdominal pain, constipation, diarrhea, dyspepsia, dysphagia, flatulence, **gastric hemorrhage**, gastroenteritis, indigestion, **intestinal obstruction**, **ischemic hepatitis**, nausea, **pancreatitis**, vomiting
GU: Elevated BUN level, erectile dysfunction, pyuria, urinary incontinence, UTI
HEME: Anemia
MS: Arthralgia; arthritis; back pain; exacerbation of limb pain (restless legs syndrome); muscle cramps, spasms, or stiffness; myalgia; neck pain; osteoarthritis; tendinitis
RESP: **Asthma**, bronchitis, cough, dyspnea, upper respiratory tract infection
SKIN: Diaphoresis, flushing, hot flashes, **melanoma**, night sweats, pruritus, rash, urticaria
Other: **Angioedema**, elevation of serum creatine phosphokinase (CPK), flu-like symptoms, viral infection, weight loss, withdrawal symptoms

Childbearing Considerations

PREGNANCY

- It is not known if drug can cause fetal harm, but animal studies suggest harm may occur.
- Use with caution only if benefit to mother outweighs potential risk to fetus.

LACTATION

- It is not known if drug is present in breast milk.
- Inhibition of lactation is likely because drug inhibits the secretion of prolactin.
- Mothers should check with prescriber before breastfeeding.

Nursing Considerations

- Know that when ropinirole is given as adjunct to levodopa, expect concurrent dosage of levodopa to be gradually decreased as tolerated.

! WARNING Monitor patient for a hypersensitivity reaction, which could become life-threatening, such as angioedema. If present, notify prescriber, expect drug to be discontinued, and provide supportive care, as needed and ordered.

! WARNING Assess patient for skin changes regularly because risk of melanoma is higher in patients with Parkinson's disease. It isn't clear whether this results from disease or from the drugs used to treat it.

- Watch for orthostatic hypotension, especially in patient with early Parkinson's disease. Orthostatic hypotension can occur more than 4 weeks after start of therapy or after a dosage reduction because ropinirole may impair systemic regulation of blood pressure.
- Monitor patient for excessive sedation periodically during therapy. Excessive, acute drowsiness may arise as late as 1 year after starting therapy. Avoid giving CNS depressants, other CNS-interacting drugs, and sleep aids during ropinirole therapy because they increase the risk of somnolence.
- Monitor patient for hallucinations or other psychotic-like behavior, especially if patient has Parkinson's disease, is elderly, or takes levodopa.
- Monitor patient for worsening of preexisting dyskinesia; ropinirole may potentiate dopaminergic adverse effects of levodopa.

! WARNING Watch for altered mental status during drug withdrawal. Rapid dose reduction may lead to a symptom complex resembling neuroleptic malignant syndrome that includes altered level of consciousness, autonomic instability, fever, and muscle rigidity. Instead, expect to stop ropinirole therapy gradually over 8 days, as follows: over first 4 days, dosage reduced from 3 times daily to twice daily; during last 3 days, dosage reduced to once daily, followed by complete withdrawal of drug. Watch for withdrawal symptoms (anxiety, apathy, depression, fatigue, pain, and sweating) during and after drug is discontinued. Be aware that these symptoms do not usually respond to levodopa. Instead, in cases of severe withdrawal symptoms expect a trial of readministration of a dopamine agonist at the lowest effective dose.

PATIENT TEACHING

- Inform patient with Parkinson's disease that ropinirole helps to improve muscle control and movement but doesn't cure Parkinson's disease.
- Instruct how to administer ropinirole and what to do if a dose is missed.
- Urge patient to avoid consuming alcohol and other sedating drugs (such as sleep aids) during therapy because they may increase drug's CNS depressant effects.
- Inform patient that smoking may decrease effectiveness of ropinirole. If smoking is started or stopped during therapy, patient should notify prescriber.

! **WARNING** Caution patient not to stop taking ropinirole abruptly. If concerns arise over ropinirole therapy, encourage her to speak with prescriber. Remind patient that withdrawal symptoms (anxiety, apathy, depression, fatigue, pain, and sweating) can occur during dosage reduction or after discontinuation of drug or if dosage decreased rapidly (altered consciousness, fever, and muscular rigidity). In either case, instruct patient to notify prescriber immediately.

! **WARNING** Instruct patient to notify prescriber if allergic reactions occur. If present, tell patient to notify prescriber and, if severe, to seek immediate medical care.

! **WARNING** Alert patient that skin cancer may occur although it is unknown if the risk is related to the disease or the drug. Encourage patient to have regular skin check-ups.

- Caution patient to avoid hazardous activities until CNS effects of drug, including sedation, are known and resolved.
- Tell the patient that if she falls asleep during normal activities, she should notify prescriber.
- Urge patient to stand up slowly from a lying or sitting position to avoid feeling dizzy, faint, nauseated, or sweaty.
- Alert patient and family or caregiver that drug may cause hallucinations and other psychotic-like behavior. Also, warn patient that drug may cause involuntary movements. Tell patient to notify prescriber right away, if present.
- Explain to patient with restless legs syndrome that symptoms might appear in early morning or have an earlier onset in the evening or even the afternoon during ropinirole therapy and could be worse or spread to other limbs. Urge patient to notify prescriber if this occurs.
- Advise patient and family or caregiver to notify prescriber about intense urges (as for gambling or sex) because dosage may have to be reduced or drug discontinued.
- Tell patient to inform all prescribers of ropinirole therapy.

rosuvastatin calcium

Crestor, Ezallor Sprinkle

Class and Category

Pharmacologic class: HMG-CoA reductase inhibitor
Therapeutic class: Antilipemic

Indications and Dosages

∗ *As adjunct to treat hyperlipidemia, mixed dyslipidemia, hypertriglyceridemia, and primary dysbetalipoproteinemia (type III hyperlipoproteinemia); to slow the progression of atherosclerosis*

TABLETS (CRESTOR), CAPSULES (EZALLOR SPRINKLE)

Adults. Individualized based on patient's LDL-C level and risk for CV events. *Dosage range:* 5 to 40 mg once daily.

∗ *To prevent primary cardiovascular disease (reduce the risk of MI, stroke, or need for arterial revascularization procedures) in patients without clinically evident coronary artery disease (CAD) but with increased risk factors of cardiovascular disease, such as age (men ages 50 and older; women ages 60 and older), high-sensitivity C-reactive protein (hsCRP) of 2 mg/l or greater, and the presence of at least one additional cardiovascular disease risk factor, such as hypertension, low HDL-C, smoking, or a family history of premature CAD*

TABLETS (CRESTOR), CAPSULES (EZALLOR SPRINKLE)

Adults. Individualized based on patient's LDL-C level and risk for CV events. *Dosage range:* 5 to 40 mg once daily.

∗ *As adjunct to treat homozygous familial hypercholesterolemia*

TABLETS (CRESTOR), CAPSULES (EZALLOR SPRINKLE)

Adults. Individualized based on patient's LDL-C level and risk for CV events. *Dosage range:* 5 to 40 mg once daily.
Children ages 7 to 17. 20 mg once daily.

∗ *As adjunct to treat pediatric heterozygous familial hypercholesterolemia*

TABLETS (CRESTOR)

Children ages 10 to 17. 5 to 20 mg once daily. *Maximum:* 20 mg daily.
Children ages 8 to younger than 10. 5 to 10 mg daily. *Maximum:* 10 mg daily.

±**DOSAGE ADJUSTMENT** For Asian patients, initial dosage reduced to 5 mg once daily and maximum dose limited to 20 mg once daily. For patients with severe renal impairment (creatinine clearance less than 30 ml/min) and not on dialysis, initial dose kept at 5 mg once daily and maximum dosage not to exceed 10 mg. For dosage adjustments related to multiple drug interactions, manufacturer's guidelines followed.

Drug Administration

P.O.

- Capsules and tablets should be swallowed whole and not chewed or crushed.
- Capsules can be opened for patients who cannot swallow capsules and contents sprinkled on soft food, such as applesauce or pudding. Stir mixture for 10 to 15 sec. Drug mixture should be swallowed within 1 hr and not stored for future use.
- Capsules can be used to administer drug via a nasogastric tube (16-French or greater). Open capsule and empty content into a 60-ml catheter-tipped syringe, add 40 ml of water, replace plunger, and shake syringe vigorously for 15 sec. Insert syringe into nasogastric tube and administer drug. Afterward, flush nasogastric tube with 20 ml of additional water. Do not use any other liquid except water. Once mixed in syringe, use immediately and do not store for future use.
- Space drug administration at least 2 hr apart when antacids are also administered.
- If dose is missed, resume treatment with the next dose. Do not double dose to make up for missed dose.

Route	Onset	Peak	Duration
P.O.	1 wk	3–5 hr	Unknown

Half-life: 19 hr

Mechanism of Action

Inhibits the enzyme, 3-hydroxy-3-methylglutaryl-coenzyme A (HMG-CoA) reductase, which reduces lipid levels by increasing the number of hepatic low-density lipoprotein (LDL) receptors on the cell surface to increase uptake and catabolism of LDL. Inhibits hepatic synthesis of very-low-density lipoprotein (VLDL) also, which decreases the total number of VLDL and LDL particles.

Contraindications

Active liver disease, decompensated cirrhosis, hypersensitivity to rosuvastatin or its components

Interactions

DRUGS

antacids (aluminum and magnesium hydroxide combination): Decreased blood rosuvastatin level if given within 2 hr of rosuvastatin reducing rosuvastatin effectiveness
atazanavir/ritonavir, capmatinib, colchicine, cyclosporine, darolutamide, dasabuvir/ombitasvir/paritaprevir/ritonavir, elbasvir/grazoprevir, enasidenib, febuxostat, fenofibrates, fostamatinib, gemfibrozil, glecaprevir/pibrentasvir, ledipasvir/sofosbuvir, lopinavir/ritonavir, niacin (equal to or greater than 1 g/day), other lipid-lowering drugs, regorafenib, simeprevir, sofosbuvir/velpatasvir, sofosbuvir/velpatasvir/voxilaprevir, tafamidis, teriflunomide, ticagrelor: Increased rosuvastatin level and risk of myopathy and rhabdomyolysis
warfarin: Increased INR significantly

ACTIVITIES

alcohol: Increased rosuvastatin exposure with increased risk of hepatic injury

QRS

Adverse Reactions

CNS: Asthenia, cognitive impairment, confusion, depression, dizziness, headache, hypertonia, insomnia, memory loss, nightmares, paresthesia, peripheral neuropathy
CV: Chest pain, hypertension, peripheral edema
EENT: New-onset or exacerbation of ocular myasthenia, pharyngitis, rhinitis, sinusitis
ENDO: Elevated fasting glucose and glycosylated hemoglobin levels, gynecomastia, hyperglycemia, thyroid function abnormalities
GI: Abdominal pain, constipation, diarrhea, elevated liver enzymes, gastroenteritis, **hepatic dysfunction or failure**, **hepatitis**, jaundice, nausea, **pancreatitis**
GU: **Acute renal failure**, hematuria, proteinuria, UTI
HEME: **Thrombocytopenia**
MS: Arthralgia, arthritis, back pain, immune-mediated necrotizing myopathy, myalgia, myopathy, **rhabdomyolysis**
RESP: Bronchitis, increased cough, **interstitial lung disease**
SKIN: Lichenoid drug eruption, rash, urticaria
Other: **Angioedema**, **drug reaction with eosinophilia and systemic symptoms (DRESS)**, flu-like symptoms, generalized pain, infection, new-onset or exacerbation of myasthenia gravis

Childbearing Considerations

PREGNANCY

- Drug may cause fetal harm.
- Drug should be discontinued as soon as pregnancy is known or extreme caution used if drug therapy continues during the pregnancy.

LACTATION

- Drug is present in breast milk.
- Drug is not recommended in mothers who are breastfeeding.

REPRODUCTION

- Females of childbearing age should use effective contraception during drug therapy.

Nursing Considerations

- Monitor serum lipoprotein level, as ordered, to evaluate response to therapy.

! **WARNING** Obtain baseline liver enzymes and expect to monitor them thereafter, as ordered. Know that if alanine transaminase (ALT) or aspartate transferase (AST) levels increase to more than 3 times the normal range, expect dosage to be reduced or drug discontinued. Patients at increased risk for hepatic injury include patients who consume large quantities of alcohol or who have a history of liver disease.

! **WARNING** Obtain a BUN and creatinine level before therapy starts and then periodically, as ordered, because drug can cause acute renal failure. Notify prescriber if proteinuria or hematuria appears in patient's routine urinalysis because rosuvastatin dosage may have to be reduced or drug discontinued.

! **WARNING** Monitor patient for a hypersensitivity or severe skin reaction, which could become life-threatening, such as angioedema or DRESS. Be aware that DRESS may initially only present with a fever or swollen lymph nodes. If present, notify prescriber, expect drug to be discontinued, and provide supportive care, as needed and ordered.

! **WARNING** Monitor patients with risk factors for myopathy, such as patients 65 years and older or patients with hypothyroidism, or renal impairment. Expect drug to be temporarily withheld if patient develops any condition that may be related to myopathy or that predisposes her to renal failure, such as hypotension; major surgery; sepsis; severe electrolyte, endocrine, or metabolic disorders; trauma; or uncontrolled seizures. Expect rosuvastatin to be discontinued if patient develops markedly elevated creatine kinase levels, or if myopathy is diagnosed because the more severe and life-threatening form rhabdomyolysis may develop.

- Monitor patient's fasting blood glucose levels and HbA1C levels routinely, as ordered, especially if patient is a diabetic because drug may cause hyperglycemia.

! **WARNING** Notify prescriber if any other persistent, serious, or unusual adverse reactions occur.

PATIENT TEACHING

- Instruct patient how to take the form of rosuvastatin prescribed and what to do if a dose is missed.
- Encourage patient to follow a low-fat, low-cholesterol diet.
- Tell patient who takes antacids to wait at least 2 hours after taking rosuvastatin.

! **WARNING** Alert patient that drug may cause an allergic reaction or severe skin reactions. If present, including a fever, rash, swollen lymph nodes, or other signs and symptoms, tell patient to notify prescriber immediately and, if severe, to seek immediate medical care.

! **WARNING** Review signs and symptoms of liver dysfunction such as anorexia, dark urine, fatigue, jaundice, or right upper abdominal discomfort. Tell patient to notify prescriber immediately, if present.

! **WARNING** Instruct patient to notify prescriber immediately about muscle pain, tenderness, or weakness, especially if accompanied by fever or malaise. He should also tell prescriber if these symptoms occur even after drug is discontinued.

- Inform patient that drug may increase blood glucose levels, especially if patient is a diabetic. Review signs and symptoms of hyperglycemia. Encourage patient to have blood glucose levels and HbA1C levels checked routinely.

! **WARNING** Tell patient to notify prescriber of any other persistent, serious, or unusual adverse reactions.

- Tell patient to inform all prescribers of rosuvastatin therapy and not take any new drugs, including over-the-counter drugs, without consulting prescriber of rosuvastatin first.
- Tell females of childbearing age about the need to use reliable contraceptive method while taking drug. Instruct her to notify prescriber at once if pregnancy occurs to discuss if drug should be discontinued.
- Remind mothers breastfeeding is not recommended during rosuvastatin therapy.

safinamide mesylate

Xadago

Class and Category

Pharmacologic class: Monoamine oxidase type B (MAO-B) inhibitor
Therapeutic class: Antiparkinsonian

Indications and Dosages

✷ *As adjunct to levodopa/carbidopa treatment in patients with Parkinson's disease experiencing "off" episodes*

TABLETS

Adults. *Initial:* 50 mg once daily, increased after 2 wk to 100 mg once daily, as needed and tolerated.

± **DOSAGE ADJUSTMENT** For patients with moderate hepatic impairment, maximum dosage kept at 50 mg once daily.

Drug Administration

P.O.

- Administer drug consistently at about the same time each day.
- If a dose is missed, administer the next dose at the same time it's due the next day.
- Store at room temperature.

Route	Onset	Peak	Duration
P.O.	Unknown	1.8–2.8 hr	Unknown

Half-life: 20–26 hr

Mechanism of Action

Inhibits monoamine oxidase B activity through blocking the catabolism of dopamine leading to increased dopamine levels, which in turn increases dopaminergic activity in the brain. Increased dopaminergic activity in the brain is thought to improve Parkinson's disease symptoms although precise mechanism is unknown.

Contraindications

Concurrent use with amphetamine and their derivatives, cyclobenzaprine, dextromethorphan, linezolid, methylphenidate, opioid drugs (meperidine and its derivatives, methadone, propoxyphene, or tramadol), other MAO inhibitors or other drugs that are potent inhibitors of MAOs, serotonin–norepinephrine reuptake inhibitors, St. John's wort, tetracyclic, triazolopyridine, or tricyclic antidepressants; hypersensitivity to safinamide or its components; severe hepatic impairment

Interactions

DRUGS

amphetamine, antidepressants (tetracyclic, triazolopyridine, tricyclic), cyclobenzaprine, methylphenidate, opioid drugs, serotonin–norepinephrine reuptake inhibitors, St. John's wort: Increased risk of life-threatening serotonin syndrome
antipsychotics, metoclopramide: Possibly decreased effectiveness of safinamide; exacerbation of Parkinson's disease symptoms
dextromethorphan: Increased risk of abnormal behavior or psychosis
isoniazid, other MAO inhibitors, other drugs that are potent inhibitors of MAO, sympathomimetics, tyramine: Increased risk of hypertensive crisis

Adverse Reactions

CNS: Anxiety, compulsive behaviors, confusion, dyskinesia, falling asleep during activities of daily living, fever, hallucinations, headache, insomnia, lack of impulse control, **serotonin syndrome**
CV: Hypertension, orthostatic hypotension
EENT: Gingival swelling, retinal pathology, **tongue swelling**
GI: Dyspepsia, elevated liver enzymes, nausea
RESP: Cough, dyspnea
SKIN: Rash
Other: Hypersensitivity reactions

Childbearing Considerations

PREGNANCY

- It is not known if drug may cause fetal harm, but animal studies suggest harm may occur.
- Use with caution only if benefit to mother outweighs potential risk to fetus.

LACTATION

- It is not known if drug is present in breast milk.
- Mothers should check with prescriber before breastfeeding.

Nursing Considerations

- Be aware that safinamide therapy should not be used in patients with a major psychotic disorder because drug may exacerbate the psychosis.

! WARNING Monitor patient for hypersensitivity reactions, which may become life-threatening, such as swelling of tongue. Notify prescriber immediately, expect drug to be discontinued, and provide supportive care, as needed and ordered.

! WARNING Monitor patient's blood pressure closely because safinamide may cause hypertension or exacerbate existing hypertension. Be aware that although dietary restriction is not necessary during treatment with recommended doses, certain foods that are very high in tyramine (more than 150 mg) may cause severe hypertension.

! WARNING Monitor patient closely for serotonin syndrome, a rare but serious adverse effect of MAO inhibitors, such as safinamide. Signs and symptoms include agitation, confusion, diaphoresis, diarrhea, fever, hyperactive reflexes, poor coordination, restlessness, shaking, talking or acting with uncontrolled excitement, tremor, and twitching. If symptoms occur, notify prescriber immediately, expect to discontinue drug, and provide supportive care.

- Monitor patient for dyskinesia because safinamide may cause dyskinesia or exacerbate preexisting dyskinesia. Notify prescriber because reducing the patient's daily levodopa dosage or the dosage of another dopaminergic drug may lessen the dyskinesia.
- Monitor patient for hallucinations or psychotic behavior. If present, expect dosage to be reduced or drug discontinued.
- Monitor patient for visual changes, especially in patients with a history of certain eye disorders, such as active retinopathy, albinism, family history of hereditary retinal disease, inherited retinal conditions, macular or retinal degeneration, retinitis pigmentosa, or uveitis. This is because retinal degeneration and loss of photoreceptor cells may occur with safinamide therapy.

! WARNING Be aware that 100-mg dose should be tapered to 50 mg for 1 week before safinamide is discontinued. This is because a symptom complex resembling neuroleptic malignant syndrome, exhibited by altered consciousness, autonomic instability, elevated temperature, and muscular rigidity has occurred with rapid dose reduction, withdrawal of, or changes in drugs that increase central dopaminergic tone.

PATIENT TEACHING

- Instruct patient how to administer safinamide and what to do if a dose is missed.

! **WARNING** Instruct patient to avoid foods very high in tyramine such as alcoholic beverages (beer, red wine, sherry, some liqueurs, vermouth), aged cheeses, citrus and tropical fruits, cured or processed meats, fermented or pickled vegetables because consuming such may cause very high blood pressure.

- Stress importance of not stopping drug abruptly. If patient has concerns about safinamide therapy, advise him to speak with prescriber.

! **WARNING** Alert patient that allergic reactions, such as difficulty breathing or swelling of tongue may occur. If present, instruct patient to seek immediate medical care.

- Advise patient to avoid performing hazardous activities, as drug may cause daytime sleepiness or episodes of falling asleep during activities that require full attention, such as driving. Tell patient to notify prescriber of any such occurrence.
- Tell patient and family or caregiver drug may cause patient to experience intense urges to perform compulsive behaviors such as binge eating, gambling excessively, having sex frequently, or spending money uncontrollably. If present, prescriber should be notified, as dosage may have to be reduced or drug discontinued.
- Advise patient to inform all prescribers of safinamide therapy.

! **WARNING** Instruct patient and family or caregiver to notify prescriber if other persistent, severe, or unusual adverse effects occur.

salmeterol xinafoate

Serevent Diskus

Class and Category

Pharmacologic class: Long-acting beta$_2$ agonist (LABA)
Therapeutic class: Bronchodilator

Indications and Dosages

* *To treat asthma and prevent bronchospasm in patients with reversible obstructive airway disease, including symptoms of nocturnal asthma, who are currently using an inhaled corticosteroid*

ORAL INHALATION POWDER

Adults and children ages 4 and older. 1 inhalation (50 mcg) every 12 hr in the morning and evening.

* *To provide maintenance treatment of bronchospasm associated with chronic obstructive pulmonary disease (COPD)*

ORAL INHALATION POWDER

Adults. 1 inhalation (50 mcg) every 12 hr in the morning and evening.

* *To prevent exercise-induced bronchospasm in patients who do not have persistent asthma or, if persistent asthma present, used in conjunction with an inhaled corticosteroid*

ORAL INHALATION POWDER

Adults and children ages 4 and older. 1 inhalation (50 mcg) at least 30 min before exercise. *Maximum:* No more than 1 inhalation (50 mcg) every 12 hr.

Drug Administration

INHALATION

- Administer twice-daily doses 12 hr apart, morning and evening.
- Administer at least 30 min before exercise if used to prevent exercise-induced bronchospasm.
- Do not use a spacer device when administering drug.
- Remove diskus from foil pouch when administering for the first time and write date on label. Hold the diskus in left hand and place thumb of right hand in thumb grip. Push the thumb grip as far as it will go until the mouthpiece shows and snaps into place. Have patient hold the diskus in a level, flat position with the mouthpiece

toward patient. Have patient slide the lever away from the mouthpiece as far as it will go until a click is heard. Then, patient should exhale and then place mouthpiece to his lips and inhale quickly and deeply through his mouth, not his nose. After removing mouthpiece from his mouth, patient should hold his breath for at least 10 sec, and exhale slowly. To close diskus, place thumb in the thumb grip and slide it back as far as it will go.

- Have patient rinse mouth with water after each dose to minimize dry mouth.
- Store drug in a dry place away from heat and sunlight in the unopened foil pouch until ready for use.
- Discard diskus 6 wk after removing it from overwrap or when dose indicator reads zero.

Route	Onset	Peak	Duration
Inhalation	0.5–2 hr	20 min	12 hr

Half-life: 5.5 hr

Mechanism of Action

Attaches to $beta_2$ receptors on bronchial cell membranes, stimulating the intracellular enzyme adenylate cyclase to convert adenosine triphosphate to cAMP. Increased intracellular cAMP level inhibits histamine release, relaxes bronchial smooth-muscle cells, and stabilizes mast cells.

Contraindications

Hypersensitivity to salmeterol, its components, or to milk proteins (severe); primary treatment of status asthmaticus or other acute episodes of asthma or COPD where intensive measures are required; treatment of asthma without use of an inhaled corticosteroid

Interactions

DRUGS

atazanavir, clarithromycin, indinavir, itraconazole, ketoconazole, nefazodone, nelfinavir, ritonavir, saquinavir, telithromycin: Possibly increased risk of adverse cardiovascular effects

beta-blockers: Blocked pulmonary effect of salmeterol; possibly produce severe bronchospasms

loop or thiazide diuretics: Increased risk of hypokalemia and potentially life-threatening arrhythmias

MAO inhibitors, tricyclic antidepressants: Potentiated adverse vascular effects, such as hypertensive crisis

Adverse Reactions

CNS: Dizziness, fever, headache, nervousness, paresthesia, tremor

CV: Palpitations, tachycardia

EENT: Dry mouth, nose, and throat; sinus problems

GI: Nausea

MS: Arthralgia

RESP: Cough, **paradoxical bronchospasm**

SKIN: Contact dermatitis, eczema, rash, urticaria

Other: **Angioedema**, generalized aches and pains

Childbearing Considerations

PREGNANCY

- It is not known if drug can cause fetal harm.
- Use with caution only if benefit to mother outweighs potential risk to fetus.

LABOR AND DELIVERY

- Drug use should be restricted to patients only if the benefit clearly outweighs the risk because drug may interfere with uterine contractions.

LACTATION

- It is not known if drug is present in breast milk.
- Mothers should check with prescriber before breastfeeding.

Nursing Considerations

! **WARNING** Be aware that salmeterol shouldn't be used to relieve bronchospasm quickly because of its prolonged onset of action and that patients already taking drug twice daily shouldn't take additional doses for exercise-induced bronchospasm.

! **WARNING** Be aware that a study suggests that asthma-related deaths may increase in asthmatics receiving salmeterol. Know that salmeterol should not be used in patients whose asthma is adequately controlled on low- or medium-dose inhaled corticosteroids and it should only be used as additional therapy for patients with asthma who are currently taking but are not adequately controlled on an inhaled corticosteroid. Salmeterol should never be used as monotherapy in the treatment of asthma. Monitor this patient population closely throughout salmeterol therapy and notify prescriber immediately of any changes in patient's respiratory status. Expect to discontinue use as soon as possible.

! WARNING Stop salmeterol immediately and notify prescriber if patient develops paradoxical bronchospasm. Risk is greatest with first use of a new canister.

! WARNING Monitor patient for a hypersensitivity reaction, which could become life-threatening, such as angioedema. If present, notify prescriber, expect drug to be switched to another drug, and provide supportive care, as needed and ordered.

! WARNING Watch for arrhythmias and changes in blood pressure after use in patients with cardiovascular disorders, including arrhythmias, hypertension, and ischemic cardiac disease because of drug's beta-adrenergic effects.

- Monitor patient's compliance. Expect adults with poor compliance and children and adolescents who require the addition of a long-acting beta agonist, such as salmeterol, to be prescribed a combination product containing both an inhaled corticosteroid and a long-acting beta agonist to increase compliance.

PATIENT TEACHING

! WARNING Inform patients with asthma that salmeterol must be taken with an inhaled corticosteroid because a life-threatening reaction may occur if drug is taken alone.

- Instruct patient how to administer salmeterol.
- Tell patient to take drug exactly as prescribed and not to increase dosage or frequency of use. Advise patient with asthma or COPD against using drug more than every 12 hours.
- Instruct patient to notify prescriber if patient needs 4 or more oral inhalations of rapid-acting inhaled bronchodilator a day for 2 or more consecutive days, or if patient uses more than one canister of rapid-acting bronchodilator in an 8-week period.

! WARNING Instruct patient to seek immediate medical attention if after taking salmeterol breathing problems, a fast or irregular heartbeat, high blood glucose level, or any persistent, severe, or unusual side effect develops.

! WARNING Alert patient that drug may cause an allergic reaction. If present, tell patient to notify prescriber and, if severe, to seek immediate medical care.

- Caution patient not to use other drugs to treat his underlying respiratory condition without consulting prescriber and to let all prescribers know salmeterol is being taken.

! WARNING Caution patient to keep salmeterol diskus out of the reach of children. Also, tell patient not to give the diskus to other people, even if they have the same symptoms because it may harm them.

- Stress importance of compliance with the prescribed drug therapy.

sarilumab

Kevzara

Class and Category

Pharmacologic class: Monoclonal antibody
Therapeutic class: Antiarthritic

Indications and Dosages

✱ *To treat moderate to severe active rheumatoid arthritis in patients who have had an inadequate response or intolerance to one or more disease-modifying antirheumatic drugs (DMARDs) as monotherapy or in combination with methotrexate or other conventional DMARDs*

SUBCUTANEOUS INJECTION

Adults. 200 mg once every 2 wk.

✱ *To treat patients with polymyalgia rheumatica who have had an inadequate response to corticosteroids or who cannot tolerate corticosteroid taper as monotherapy following discontinuation of corticosteroids*

SUBCUTANEOUS INJECTION

Adults. 200 mg once every 2 wk, in combination with a tapering course of

QRS

systemic corticosteroids followed by monotherapy when corticosteroids are discontinued.

✶ *To treat active polyarticular juvenile idiopathic arthritis.*

SUBCUTANEOUS INJECTION

Children weighing 63 kg (138.6 lb) or more. 200 mg once every 2 wk using only the prefilled syringe.

±**DOSAGE ADJUSTMENT** For patients with neutropenia or thrombocytopenia, dosage reduced to 150 mg once every 2 weeks. For patients experiencing an absolute neutrophil count (ANC) between 500 to 1,000 cells/mm^3, sarilumab withheld until ANC becomes greater than 1,000 cells/mm^3. Dosage restarted at 150 mg every 2 wk and then dosage increased to 200 mg and given every 2 wk, when clinically appropriate. For patients experiencing an ANC less than 500 cells/mm^3, drug discontinued. For patients experiencing a low platelet count between 50,000 to 100,000 cells/mm^3, drug withheld until platelets become greater than 100,000 cells/mm^3. Dosage restarted at 150 mg every 2 wk and then dosage increased to 200 mg every 2 wk, when clinically appropriate. For patients experiencing a platelet count less than 50,000 cells/mm^3 and confirmed with repeat testing, drug discontinued. For patients experiencing an elevated alanine transaminase (ALT) or aspartate transaminase (AST) greater than upper level normal (ULN) to 3 times ULN or less, dosage may have to be modified on an individual basis. For patients experiencing an ALT or AST greater than 3 times ULN to 5 times ULN or less, drug withheld until ALT or AST is less than 3 times ULN. Dosage restarted at 150 mg every 2 wk and then dosage increased to 200 mg every 2 wk, as clinically appropriate. For patients experiencing an ALT or AST greater than 5 times ULN, drug discontinued.

Drug Administration

SUBCUTANEOUS

- Use only the prefilled syringe when administering drug to children.
- Remove drug from refrigerator, place on a flat surface, and allow prefilled syringe to sit at room temperature for 30 min and the prefilled pen for 60 min prior to administering the injection. Do not warm drug any other way.
- Inspect the solution in the syringe/pen. Solution should be clear and colorless to pale yellow. If solution is cloudy, discolored, or contains particles, discard it and use a new prefilled syringe or pen.
- Do not inject drug into areas of skin that appear bruised, damaged, tender, or has scars.
- To administer drug using the prefilled syringe, do not get rid of any air bubbles in the syringe. Pinch the skin and inject into abdomen or back of upper arm at a 45 degree angle. Inject slowly until plunger is as far as it will. Before removing needle, check to be sure syringe is empty.
- To administer drug using the prefilled pen, the window should be clear indicating the pen has not been used. If the window is a solid yellow, discard and get a new pen. Twist off the orange cap and place the yellow needle cover on patient's abdomen, anterior aspect of thigh, or upper outer arms at a 90 degree angle. Press down and hold the pen firmly against the patient's skin. A click will be heard when injection starts and the window will start to turn solid yellow. The injection can take up to 15 sec. When a second click is heard, entire window should be a solid yellow. Remove pen from skin.
- Do not rub injection site following injection with either pen or syringe.
- Rotate sites.
- Store drug in refrigerator in original carton and protect from light. However, if stored at room temperature, discard after 14 days.

Route	Onset	Peak	Duration
SubQ	Unknown	2–4 days	28–43 days

Half-life: 8–10 days

Mechanism of Action

Binds to IL-6 receptors to inhibit IL-6 mediated signaling of inflammatory processes, which occurs in rheumatoid arthritis. Without IL-6 mediated signaling, IL-6, as a proinflammatory cytokine, cannot be produced by endothelial and synovial cells in joints to help relieve inflammation present in rheumatoid arthritis.

Contraindications

Hypersensitivity to sarilumab or its components

Interactions

DRUGS

atorvastatin, lovastatin, oral contraceptives: Possibly decreased effectiveness of these drugs
CYP450 substrates with narrow therapeutic index, such as theophylline, warfarin: Possibly altered dosage requirements
live vaccines: Increased risk of vaccine-related infection

Adverse Reactions

CNS: Fatigue
CV: Elevated cholesterol and triglyceride levels
EENT: Nasopharyngitis
GI: Constipation, elevated liver enzymes, **GI perforation**
GU: UTI
HEME: **Decreased platelet count**, **neutropenia**, **thrombocytopenia**
MS: Myalgia
RESP: Upper respiratory infections
SKIN: Pruritic rash, urticaria
Other: **Anaphylaxis**; anti-sarilumab antibody formation; herpes zoster reactivation; **immunosuppression**; infections such as bacterial, invasive fungal, mycobacterial, tuberculosis, viral, or other opportunistic infections; injection-site erythema, pruritis, rash; **malignancies**

Childbearing Considerations

PREGNANCY

- Pregnancy exposure registry: 1-877-311-8972.
- Drug may affect immune system of fetus/neonate in mothers exposed to drug during pregnancy because monoclonal antibodies cross the placental barrier.
- Use with caution only if benefit to mother outweighs potential risk to fetus.
- Be aware that administration of live vaccines may decrease response in infants exposed to the drug during pregnancy.

LACTATION

- It is not known if drug is present in breast milk.
- Mothers should check with prescriber before breastfeeding.

Nursing Considerations

! WARNING Be aware that sarilumab therapy should not be started in patients who have an elevated ALT or AST above 1.5 times the upper limit of normal, an absolute neutrophil count (ANC) less than 2,000/mm^3, or platelet count less than 150,000/mm^3.

! WARNING Know that sarilumab should not be used with biological DMARDs because of increased immunosuppression and increased risk of infection.

! WARNING Know that patients with active hepatic disease or hepatic impairment are not candidates for sarilumab therapy because drug can have adverse effects on liver, as evidenced by elevation in liver enzymes.

! WARNING Be aware that sarilumab should be avoided in patients with active infections. Monitor patient for signs and symptoms of infection because of sarilumab's immunosuppressant action. Serious and sometimes fatal infections due to bacterial, invasive fungal, mycobacterial, viral, or other opportunistic pathogens have occurred with sarilumab therapy. Be aware that patients 65 years and older are at higher risk for developing serious infections. If infection occurs, notify prescriber, expect drug to be withheld for serious infections until infection is eradicated, and administer prescribed treatment for the infection.

- Expect patient to be tested for latent tuberculosis (TB) before sarilumab therapy is started. If result is positive, patient will need to be treated before sarilumab is initiated. In patient who has a history of active or latent TB and for whom an adequate course of treatment cannot be confirmed, or results are negative, but patient has risk factors for TB infection, patient may need to be treated before beginning sarilumab therapy.
- Ensure patient is up to date with current immunization guideline. Avoid administering live vaccines to patient during treatment because of increased risk of infection caused by the vaccine.
- Monitor patient for response to sarilumab therapy. If a decreased response to

sarilumab occurs after it was shown to be effective this may indicate the formation of antibodies against the drug has occurred.

! **WARNING** Monitor patient for hypersensitivity reactions, which could become life-threatening, such as anaphylaxis. If present, notify prescriber, expect drug to be withheld, and provide supportive care, as needed and ordered.

! **WARNING** Monitor patient closely for GI perforation, which is a life-threatening condition. Patients taking concurrent therapy with corticosteroids or NSAIDs or who have diverticulitis are at increased risk. Alert prescriber at once if patient complains of abdominal issues, especially sudden abdominal pain.

- Expect to monitor patient's ANC and platelet counts regularly. Institute bleeding and infection control measures. Expect dosage modifications or drug withholding until target levels are met or patient exhibits bruising, unexplained bleeding, or signs and symptoms of an infection.

PATIENT TEACHING

- Instruct patient how to administer sarilumab with either the prefilled pen or prefilled syringe as a subcutaneous injection. Alert family or caregiver that only the prefilled syringe should be used for a child.
- Instruct patient not to receive any live vaccines while taking sarilumab.

! **WARNING** Warn patient that allergic reactions can occur with sarilumab therapy. Tell patient to alert prescriber if present, and to seek immediate medical care, if severe.

! **WARNING** Instruct patient on bleeding and infection precautions. Warn patient to avoid taking unprescribed aspirin or NSAIDs. Also patient should avoid people with an active infection. Tell patient to report bruising, unexplained bleeding or any evidence of an infection to prescriber immediately.

! **WARNING** Instruct patient to notify prescriber and seek immediate emergency medical attention if abdominal signs and symptoms, such as sudden pain, occur.

- Inform mothers to alert pediatrician if sarilumab was administered during pregnancy because of decreased response in the infant when given live vaccines.
- Inform patient that frequent blood tests will have to be performed to monitor for adverse effects. Stress importance of patient compliance with these appointments.

saxagliptin hydrochloride

Onglyza

Class and Category

Pharmacologic class: Dipeptidyl peptidase-4 (DPP-4) inhibitor

Therapeutic class: Antidiabetic

Indications and Dosages

∗ *As adjunct to diet and exercise to improve blood glucose control in type 2 diabetes mellitus*

TABLETS

Adults. 2.5 or 5 mg once daily.

± **DOSAGE ADJUSTMENT** For patients with moderate or severe renal impairment (eGFR less than 45 ml/min), patients with end-stage renal disease, patients having hemodialysis, and patients receiving strong CYP3A4/5 inhibitors (atazanavir, clarithromycin, indinavir, itraconazole, ketoconazole, nefazodone, nelfinavir, ritonavir, saquinavir, telithromycin), dosage not to exceed 2.5 mg once daily.

Drug Administration

P.O.

- Tablets should be swallowed whole and not chewed, crushed, or divided.
- Tablets may be taken at any time of day regardless of meals but consistently.
- If a dose is missed, administer it as soon as possible unless it is time for the next dose. Do not double next dose to make up for missed dose.

Route	Onset	Peak	Duration
P.O.	Unknown	2 hr	24 hr

Half-life: 2.5 hr

Mechanism of Action

Remember incretin hormones, such as glucose-dependent insulinotropic polypeptide (GIP) and glucagon-like peptide-1 (GLP-1), are released into bloodstream from small intestine in response to meals, where they stimulate pancreatic beta cells to release insulin. Inactivation of incretin hormones by the enzyme, dipeptidyl peptidase-4 causes blood glucose levels to rise within minutes. Inhibition of this enzyme by saxagliptin provides more time for incretin hormones to increase insulin levels and blunt glucagon secretion, which leads to more insulin and less hepatic glucose production to lower blood glucose levels. Preventing inactivation of the incretin hormone, GLP-1, also reduces glucagon secretion. from pancreatic alpha cell, which in turn, reduces glucose production in the liver.

Contraindications

Hypersensitivity to saxagliptin or its components

Interactions

DRUGS

insulin, sulfonylureas: Increased risk of hypoglycemia
strong CYP3A4/5 inhibitors, such as atazanavir, clarithromycin, indinavir, itraconazole, ketoconazole, nefazodone, nelfinavir, ritonavir, saquinavir, telithromycin: Increased plasma saxagliptin level
insulin, sulfonylureas: Increased risk of hypoglycemia

Adverse Reactions

CNS: Headache
CV: **Heart failure**, peripheral edema
EENT: Sinusitis, nasopharyngitis
ENDO: **Hypoglycemia**
GI: Abdominal pain, **acute pancreatitis**, gastroenteritis, vomiting
GU: Elevated plasma creatinine level, UTI
HEME: **Lymphopenia**
MS: Arthralgia (disabling, severe), **rhabdomyolysis**
RESP: Upper respiratory tract infection
SKIN: Bullous pemphigoid, **exfoliative skin conditions**, rash, urticaria
Other: **Anaphylaxis**, **angioedema**

Childbearing Considerations

PREGNANCY

- It is not known if drug can cause fetal harm.
- Use with caution only if benefit to mother outweighs potential risk to fetus.

LACTATION

- It is not known if drug is present in breast milk.
- Mothers should check with prescriber before breastfeeding.

Nursing Considerations

! WARNING Know that saxagliptin shouldn't be used to treat type 1 diabetes mellitus or diabetic ketoacidosis.

- Evualte patient's renal function by obtaining an eGFR, as ordered, before starting saxagliptin therapy and then periodically thereafter to monitor patient's renal function.
- Monitor patient's blood glucose level and glycosalated hemoglobin to assess effectiveness of saxagliptin therapy.

! WARNING Monitor patient closely for hypersensitivity and severe skin reactions, especially within the first 3 months of therapy beginning with first dose. These reactions can become life-threatening, such as anaphylaxis, angioedema, and exfoliative skin conditions. Use cautiously in patients who have experienced angioedema with another dipeptidyl peptidase-4 inhibitor because it is not known if a cross-sensitivity reaction may occur with saxagliptin. If present, notify prescriber immediately, expect to discontinue drug, and provide supportive care, as needed and ordered.

! WARNING Monitor patient for signs and symptoms of heart failure during saxagliptin therapy because drug may increase risk. If present, notify prescriber, expect drug to be discontinued, and provide supportive care, as ordered.

! WARNING Monitor patient for signs and symptoms of acute pancreatitis such as severe, sharp pain in the upper abdominal accompanied by fever, nausea, and vomiting. If present, notify prescriber, expect to stop saxagliptin, as ordered, and provide supportive care, as needed.

! **WARNING** Watch for hypoglycemia in patients taking insulin or other antidiabetics, such as sulfonylureas. Expect dosage of insulin or other antidiabetics, such as sulfonylureas, to be decreased to reduce risk of hypoglycemia.

! **WARNING** Monitor patient for other persistent, serious, or unusual adverse reactions.

PATIENT TEACHING

- Emphasize that saxagliptin isn't a replacement for diet and exercise therapy.
- Instruct patient how to administer saxagliptin.
- Instruct patient to notify prescriber if fever, illness, infection, surgery, trauma, or other stress occurs because blood glucose control may not be well controlled with saxagliptin therapy alone and may require temporary insulin therapy.
- Explain importance of self-monitoring glucose levels during saxagliptin therapy.

! **WARNING** Tell patient drug may cause an allergic reaction as well as severe skin reactions. Advise patient to watch for the development of blisters or breakdown of the outer layer of skin. If an allergic or skin reaction occurs, tell patient to notify prescriber immediately and to seek immediate medical care, if severe.

! **WARNING** Review signs and symptoms of heart failure with patient, such as difficulty breathing; swelling of feet, hands, or legs; or unexplained weight gain. Tell patient to notify prescriber immediately, if present.

! **WARNING** Tell patient to report signs and symptoms of acute pancreatitis such as severe, sharp pain in the upper abdominal area accompanied by fever, nausea, and vomiting.

! **WARNING** Review with patient who has diabetes and is taking insulin or other antidiabetics how to recognize hypoglycemia and how to treat it if it should occur. Urge patient to carry glucose at all times in case hypoglycemia occurs. Advise patient to notify prescriber if hypoglycemia occurs frequently or is severe.

- Advise patient to seek medical attention if severe joint pain occurs. Tell patient that joint pain may develop within a day of taking saxagliptin or may develop years later.

scopolamine transdermal system

Transderm Scop

Class and Category

Pharmacologic class: Belladonna alkaloid
Therapeutic class: Antiemetic

Indications and Dosages

✱ *To prevent nausea and vomiting associated with motion sickness or recovery from anesthesia and/or opiate analgesia and surgery*

TRANSDERMAL SYSTEM

Adults and adolescents. 1 transdermal system (1 mg) applied behind ear before antiemetic effect is required as follows: 4 hr before event known to cause motion sickness, evening before surgery, or 1 hr before caesarian section. Patch removed 24 hr postsurgical procedure. Patch may remain in place up to 3 days for prevention of motion sickness and may be replaced, as needed.

Drug Administration

TRANSDERMAL

- Wear gloves and apply patch on hairless area behind ear.
- Do not apply more than 1 patch.
- Do not cut patch.
- Once the patch is in place, ensure patient does not touch or apply pressure to the patch while it is being worn because pressure exerted on it may cause scopolamine to ooze out at the edge.
- If patch becomes displaced, remove it and apply a new one.

- Wash hands after application and also wash hands and application site with soap and water after the patch is removed.
- When removing the old patch, fold the used patch in half with the sticky side together and discard.
- Remove patch before patient undergoes an MRI, as skin burns may occur if left in place.
- Store pouches at room temperature in an upright position and do not bend or roll the pouches.

Route	Onset	Peak	Duration
Transdermal	4 hr	24 hr	72 hr

Half-life: 9.5 hr

Mechanism of Action

Blocks neural pathways in the inner ear to relieve motion sickness.

Contraindications

Angle-closure glaucoma; hypersensitivity to scopolamine, other belladonna alkaloids, or their components

Interactions

DRUGS

anticholinergics (other): Possibly intensified anticholinergic effects, including CNS adverse reactions, intestinal obstruction, and/or urinary retention
CNS depressants: Possibly potentiated effects of either drug, resulting in additive sedation
oral drugs absorbed in stomach: Possibly delayed absorption of oral drugs

ACTIVITIES

alcohol use: Additive CNS effects

Adverse Reactions

CNS: Agitation, amnesia, attention disturbance, confusion, coordination abnormalities, delusions, dizziness, drowsiness, euphoria, exacerbation of psychosis, hallucinations, headache, insomnia, memory loss, paradoxical stimulation, paranoia, restlessness, speech disorder, **seizures**, somnolence, vertigo
CV: Palpitations, tachycardia
EENT: Acute angle-closure glaucoma; amblyopia; blurred vision; dry eyes, mouth, nose, and throat; eyelid irritation; increased intraocular pressure; itchy eyes; mydriasis; pharyngitis
GI: Constipation, decreased GI motility, dysphagia
GU: Dysuria, urinary hesitancy, urine retention
SKIN: Decreased sweating, dry skin, erythema, flushing, rash, skin irritation
Other: Application site (blistering, burning, pruritus, or rash), withdrawal symptoms upon removal of patch

Childbearing Considerations

PREGNANCY

- It is not known if drug can cause fetal harm.
- Drug should be avoided in pregnant females experiencing severe preeclampsia because of increased risk for eclamptic seizures.
- Use with caution only if benefit to mother outweighs potential risk to fetus in other circumstances.

LACTATION

- Drug is present in breast milk.
- Mothers should check with prescriber before breastfeeding.

Nursing Considerations

- Assess effectiveness of scopolamine to relieve nausea and vomiting.
- Monitor heart rate for transient tachycardia, which may occur with high doses of drug. Rate should return to normal within 30 minutes.

! **WARNING** Monitor patient for psychiatric reactions. If present, remove patch immediately and notify prescriber.

! **WARNING** Monitor patient closely for seizure activity. If present, notify prescriber immediately, institute seizure precautions, and expect drug to be discontinued.

- Monitor for pain. In presence of pain, drug may act as a stimulant and produce delirium if used without meperidine or morphine.
- Assess for bladder distention and monitor urine output because drug's antimuscarinic effects can cause urine retention. Patients at risk include patients suspected of having intestinal obstruction, patients with pyloric obstruction or patients with impeded flow of urine from disease of the prostate

or urinary bladder neck obstruction, and patients receiving other anticholinergic drugs. Expect to remove patch if patient experiences difficulty urinating.

- Monitor bowel sounds as drug may decrease GI motility.
- Monitor patient for other persistent, serious, or unusual adverse reactions.
- Monitor patient who has worn the patch for several days for withdrawal symptoms, which usually occur 24 hours or more after the patch has been removed.

PATIENT TEACHING

- Instruct patient how to apply a scopolamine transdermal patch.

! **WARNING** Instruct patient to fold the used patch in half with the sticky side together and discard in a manner that prevents accidental contact or ingestion by children or pets.

- Instruct patient to avoid alcohol while wearing the scopolamine patch.

! **WARNING** Instruct patient to remove patch if undergoing an MRI, as skin burns can occur if left in place.

! **WARNING** Advise patient to immediately remove the transdermal system and contact prescriber if experiencing blurred vision, eye pain or discomfort, or halos or colored images in association with red eyes from conjunctival congestion and corneal edema. Also tell patient to remove patch immediately if cognitive or psychiatric adverse reactions occur and notify prescriber. If these adverse reactions are severe, tell patient to seek immediate medical care. Suggest to patient who complains of dry eyes to use lubricating drops.

- Advise patient to avoid hazardous activities until drug's CNS effects are known and resolved.
- Tell patient to notify prescriber if other persistent, serious, or unusual adverse reactions occur.
- Tell patient wearing patch for more than a couple of days to be alert for signs of withdrawal when patch is discontinued. If severe, patient should contact prescriber.

selegiline hydrochloride

Zelapar

selegiline transdermal system

Emsam

Class and Category

Pharmacologic class: Monoamine oxidase inhibitor (MAOI)
Therapeutic class: Antidepressant (Emsam), antidyskinetic

Indications and Dosages

✷ *As adjunct to carbidopa-levodopa therapy to treat Parkinson's disease in patients whose response to therapy has deteriorated*

ORALLY DISINTEGRATING TABLETS (ZELAPAR)

Adults. *Initial:* 1.25 mg once daily and given for at least 6 wk before breakfast and without a drink; then increased to 2.5 mg once daily, as needed.

± **DOSAGE ADJUSTMENT** For patients with mild-to-moderate hepatic dysfunction, dosage kept at 1.25 mg once daily.

✷ *To treat depression*

TRANSDERMAL SYSTEM (EMSAM)

Adults. *Initial:* 6 mg/24 hr daily. Increased every 2 wk in increments of 3 mg/24 hr, as needed. *Maximum:* 12 mg/24 hr.

± **DOSAGE ADJUSTMENT** For elderly patients (65 years and older), dosage not to exceed 6 mg/24 hr daily.

Drug Administration

P.O.

- Administer before breakfast without any liquid.
- Do not push tablet through the foil on the blister pack but instead peel back the foil with dry gloved hands and gently remove tablet.
- Immediately place tablet on top of patient's tongue and let it disintegrate.
- Do not have patient drink or ingest any food for 5 min before and after drug administration.

- Store blister tablets in sachet pouch at room temperature. Discard unused tablets 3 mo after opening pouch.

TRANSDERMAL

- Apply patch at about the same time daily.
- Wash area gently and thoroughly with soap and warm water, then rinse until all soap is removed. After drying area, patch is ready to be applied.
- Apply patch to outer surface of upper arm, upper torso below the neck and above the waist, or upper thigh. Do not apply patch to broken, calloused, hairy, irritated, oily, or scarred skin. Also, patch should not be placed where clothing may rub patch off of site.
- Do not cut patch.
- Wash hands well after application.
- Only one patch may be worn at a time.
- If a patch falls off, apply a new patch to a new site and resume previous schedule.

Route	Onset	Peak	Duration
P.O.	5 min	15–40 min	Unknown
Transdermal	Unknown	Unknown	24 hr

Half-life: 1.3–10 hr

Mechanism of Action

Reduces dopamine metabolism by noncompetitively inhibiting the brain enzyme, monoamine oxidase type B, to increase the amount of dopamine available to relieve symptoms of parkinsonism. Enhanced dopamine transmission may occur because of selegiline's metabolites ability to inhibit its reuptake at synapses.

Contraindications

For all forms: Hypersensitivity to selegiline or its components
For oral form: Concurrent therapy with cyclobenzaprine, dextromethorphan, or St. John's wort; use of MAO inhibitors or meperidine or other opioids within 14 days of therapy
For transdermal form: Children less than 12 years, concomitant therapy within 2 weeks with carbamazepine, dextromethorphan, dual serotonin, and norepinephrine reuptake inhibitors (duloxetine, venlafaxine), opiate analgesics (meperidine, methadone, pentazocine, propoxyphene, tramadol), oxcarbazepine, selective serotonin reuptake inhibitors (fluoxetine [use within 5 wk], paroxetine, sertraline), tricyclic antidepressants (clomipramine, imipramine); pheochromocytoma

Interactions

DRUGS

amphetamines, buspirone, sympathomimetic amines: Increased risk of severe hypertension
carbamazepine: Increased risk of hypertensive crisis
dextromethorphan: Increased risk of brief episodes of bizarre behavior or psychosis, increased risk of serotonin syndrome
dopamine antagonists, such as antipsychotics, metoclopramide: Possibly decreased effectiveness of selegiline
MAO inhibitors, including linezolid: Increased risk for hypertensive crisis
serotonergic drugs, such as opiate analgesics (meperidine, methadone, pentazocine, propoxyphene, tramadol), selective serotonin reuptake inhibitors (fluoxetine, paroxetine, sertraline), serotonin and norepinephrine reuptake inhibitors (duloxetine, venlafaxine), tricyclic antidepressants (clomipramine, imipramine): Increased risk of serotonin syndrome

ACTIVITIES

alcohol use, such as tap beer and beers not pasteurized: Increased risk of hypertension

FOODS

foods that contain tyramine or other high-pressor amines: Increased risk of sudden and severe hypertension

Adverse Reactions

CNS: Anxiety, ataxia, chills, compulsive behaviors, such as intense urges to perform certain activities (such as gambling or sex), confusion, depression, dizziness, drowsiness, dyskinesia, euphoria, extrapyramidal reactions, falling asleep during activities of daily living, fatigue, hallucinations, headache, insomnia, irritability, lethargy, memory loss, mood changes, nervousness, paresthesia, precipitation of manic/mixed episodes, restlessness, **serotonin syndrome**, somnolence, **suicidal ideation**, syncope, tremor, weakness
CV: **Arrhythmias**, **chest pain**, hypertension, orthostatic hypotension, palpitations, peripheral edema

EENT: Altered taste, blepharospasm, blurred vision, burning lips or mouth, diplopia, dry mouth, pharyngitis, rhinitis, sinusitis, stomatitis, tinnitus, tooth disorder
GI: Abdominal pain, anorexia, constipation, diarrhea, dyspepsia, dysphagia, flatulence, **GI bleeding**, heartburn, nausea, vomiting
GU: Dysuria, urinary hesitancy, urinary urgency, urine retention
MS: Arthralgia, back and leg pain, leg cramps, muscle fatigue and spasms, myalgia, neck stiffness
RESP: **Asthma**, **dyspnea**
SKIN: Dermatitis, diaphoresis, dry skin, ecchymosis, hypertrophy, photosensitivity, pruritus, rash, ulcers, urticaria
Other: Application site reactions (Emsam), **hypokalemia**

Childbearing Considerations

PREGNANCY

- It is not known if drug can cause fetal harm.
- Use with caution only if benefit to mother outweighs potential risk to fetus.

LACTATION

- It is not known if drug is present in breast milk.
- Mothers should check with prescriber before breastfeeding if using oral form.
- Breastfeeding not recommended during treatment with transdermal form and for 5 days after the final dose.

Nursing Considerations

- Expect to screen patient for a family or personal history of bipolar disorder, hypomania, or mania before selegiline therapy is begun because drug may precipitate manic/mixed episodes.

! **WARNING** Be aware oral form contains phenylalanine and should not be given to patients with phenylketonuria (PKU).

- Monitor for decreased symptoms of Parkinson's disease to evaluate drug's effectiveness.

! **WARNING** Ensure patient receiving 9 mg/24 hr or 12 mg/24 hr avoids tyramine-rich foods and for 2 weeks after a dose reduction to 6 mg/24 hr.

! **WARNING** Monitor patient's serum potassium level, as ordered because drug can cause hypokalemia.

! **WARNING** Monitor patient for changes in behavior, moods, and thinking because drug can worsen conditions such as dementia, severe pyschosis, tardive dyskinesia, and tremor. Also, it may cause suicidal tendencies, especially when therapy starts or dosage changes.

! **WARNING** Assess patient for skin changes regularly because risk of melanoma is increased in patients with Parkinson's disease. It isn't clear whether increase results from disease or drugs used to treat it.

! **WARNING** Monitor patient for serotonin syndrome, which can be life-threatening. Signs and symptoms to watch for include autonomic instability, gastrointestinal symptoms, mental status changes, neuromuscular changes, and seizures. If present, stop selegiline therapy immediately (remove transdermal system, if present), notify prescriber, and provide supportive care, as ordered.

- Be aware that drug can reactivate gastric ulcers because it prevents breakdown of gastric histamine. Assess for related signs and symptoms, such as abdominal pain.

! **WARNING** Monitor patient for other persistent, serious, or unusual adverse reactions.

PATIENT TEACHING

! **WARNING** Alert patient that oral form contains phenylalanine and tell patient to alert prescriber if patient has phenylketonuria (PKU).

- Instruct patient how to take form of selegiline prescribed.

! **WARNING** Caution patient to take only prescribed amount because increased dosage may cause severe adverse reactions.

- Advise patient to avoid taking oral selegiline in the late afternoon or evening because it may interfere with sleep.

! **WARNING** Urge patient to avoid tyramine-rich foods and beverages during and for 2 weeks after stopping selegiline therapy unless patient is prescribed the lowest dosage of transdermal system (6 mg/24 hours), which doesn't require diet modification. Review which foods are considered tyramine-rich. Stress importance of seeking immediate medical attention if the following acute symptoms occur: heart racing or palpitations, neck stiffness, severe headache, or other sudden or unusual symptoms.

! **WARNING** Caution patient to avoid exposing transdermal patch to sources of direct heat, such as electric blankets, heat lamps, heating pads, hot tubs, prolonged sunlight exposure, or saunas.

! **WARNING** Instruct patient to notify prescriber if symptoms develop that could indicate an overdose, including muscle twitching and eye spasms.

! **WARNING** Urge family or caregiver to monitor patient closely for suicidal tendencies, especially when therapy starts or dosage changes.

! **WARNING** Alert patient to the risk for melanoma. Urge patient to have regular skin examinations done by a dermatologist or other qualified healthcare professional.

- Urge patient to avoid hazardous activities until drug's CNS effects are known and resolved.
- Advise patient to change positions slowly to minimize the effects of orthostatic hypotension.
- Suggest that patient elevate his legs when sitting to reduce ankle swelling.
- Urge patient to avoid excessive sun exposure.
- Urge patient to notify prescriber if dry mouth lasts longer than 2 weeks. Advise him to have routine dental checkups.
- Tell patient to inform prescriber of any new medications, including prescription drugs, over-the-counter drugs, and also including herbal preparations.
- Advise patient and family or caregiver to notify prescriber about intense urges (as for gambling or sex) because dosage may have to be reduced or drug discontinued.
- Inform mothers that breastfeeding is not recommended during treatment with the transdermal form of selegiline and for 5 days after final dose.

semaglutide

Ozempic, Rybelsus, Wegovy

Class and Category

Pharmacologic class: Glucagon-like peptide-1 (GLP-1) receptor agonist
Therapeutic class: Antidiabetic

Indications and Dosages

✶ *As adjunct to diet and exercise to improve glycemic control in type 2 diabetes mellitus*

TABLETS (RYBELSUS)

Adults using formulation R1. 3 mg on an empty stomach once daily at least 30 min before anything taken by mouth for 30 days, then increased to 7 mg once daily for 30 days, and then further increased to 14 mg once daily, as needed.

Adults using formulation R2. *Initial:* 1.5 mg on an empty stomach once daily at least 30 min before anything taken by mouth for 30 days, then increased to 4 mg once daily for 30 days, and then further increased to 9 mg once daily, as needed.

SUBCUTANEOUS INJECTION (OZEMPIC)

Adults. *Initial:* 0.25 mg once a wk for 4 wk, then increased to 0.5 mg once a wk. Dosage further increased to 1 mg once a wk, as needed, after another 4 wk with dosage further increased to 2 mg once a wk, as needed, after another 4 wk. *Maximum:* 2 mg once a wk.

✶ *To reduce risk of major adverse cardiovascular events (cardiovascular death, CVA, or non-fatal MI) in patients with type 2 diabetes mellitus and established cardiovascular disease*

SUBCUTANEOUS INJECTION (OZEMPIC)

Adults. *Initial:* 0.25 mg once a wk for 4 wk, then increased to 0.5 mg once a wk. Dosage further increased to 1 mg once a wk, as needed, after another 4 wk with dosage further increased to 2 mg once a wk, as needed, after another 4 wk. *Maximum:* 2 mg once a wk.

✶ *To reduce risk of major adverse cardiovascular events (cardiovascular death or non-fatal CVA or MI) in patients with established cardiovascular disease and either being obese or overweight*

SUBCUTANEOUS INJECTION (WEGOVY)

Adults. *Initial:* 0.25 mg once weekly for 4 wk. Dosage then increased as follows:

0.5 mg once weekly for wk 5–8, 1 mg once weekly for wk 9–12, 1.7 mg once weekly for wk 13–16 to achieve maintenance dose. *Maintenance:* 1.7 mg or 2.4 mg once weekly.

✱ *To reduce excess body weight and maintain weight reduction long-term in patients with obesity or overweight patients in the presence of at least one weight-related comorbid condition*

SUBCUTANEOUS INJECTION (WEGOVY)

Adults and children ages 12 and older. *Initial:* 0.25 mg once weekly for 4 wk. Dosage then increased as follows: 0.5 mg once weekly for wk 5–8, 1 mg once weekly for wk 9–12, 1.7 mg once weekly for wk 13–16. *Maintenance:* 1.7 mg or 2.4 mg once weekly.

± **DOSAGE ADJUSTMENT** For patients unable to tolerate the 2.4 mg once-weekly maintenance dosage, maintenance dosage reduced to 1.7 mg once weekly. For patients who cannot tolerate the 1.7 mg once-weekly dosage, drug discontinued.

Drug Administration

- Expect possible reduction in concomitantly administered insulin secretagogue or insulin to reduce the risk of hypoglycemia.

P.O.

- There are 2 formulations (formulation R1 and formulation R2) with different recommended dosages. Be sure the correct formulation and dose is being administered as the two formulations are not interchangeable.
- Administer tablet at least 30 min before first food, beverage, or other drug administration of the day and give with no more than 4 ounces of plain water.
- Tablets should be swallowed whole and not chewed, crushed, or divided.
- Use only 14-mg tablet to administer a 14-mg dose; do not use two 7-mg tablets to achieve a 14-mg dose.

SUBCUTANEOUS

- Inspect solution. It should be clear and colorless. Do not use if particles are present or solution is colored.
- Administer once weekly on the same day each wk, without regard to meals. However, when administering Ozempic, day of weekly administration may be changed as long as the time between the 2 doses is at least 48 hr apart.
- Follow manufacturer guidelines on how to use pen injector to administer drug.
- Inject into patient's abdomen, thigh, or upper arm.
- Rotate sites.
- If Ozempic dose is missed, administer as soon as possible within 5 days of missed dose.
- If a Wegovy dose is missed and the next scheduled dose is more than 2 days away, administer dose as soon as possible. If one dose is missed and the next scheduled dose is less than 2 days away, skip the missed dose. If 2 or more consecutive doses of Wegovy are missed, dosing may be resumed as scheduled or, if needed, retitrated to reduce GI symptoms.
- Store unused pen in refrigerator with cap on, avoiding excessive heat and sunlight. Once first dose is given for Ozempic, pen can be stored at room temperature for up to 56 days. Store Wegovy pens in refrigerator or for 28 days if kept at room temperature.
- When administering with insulin, administer as separate injections; never mix the 2 drugs. Insulin can be injected into the same area as semaglutide but not adjacent to each other.

Route	Onset	Peak	Duration
P.O.	Unknown	1 hr	Unknown
SubQ	Unknown	1–3 days	Unknown

Half-life: 1 wk

Mechanism of Action

Binds selectively to and activates the GLP-1 receptor to regulate appetite, thereby lowering body weight through decreased caloric intake. Binding of GLP-1 receptors also reduces blood glucose through a mechanism that stimulates insulin secretion and lowers glucagon secretion, both in a glucose-dependent manner. Lowering of glucose may also occur in a minor way through the delay in gastric emptying in the early postprandial phase.

Contraindications

Family or personal history of medullary thyroid carcinoma, hypersensitivity to semaglutide or its components, multiple endocrine neoplasia syndrome type 2 (MEN2)

Interactions

DRUGS

insulin, insulin secretagogues, such as sulfonylureas: Increased risk of hypoglycemia
oral drugs: Delayed absorption of these drugs

Adverse Reactions

CNS: Anxiety, dizziness, fatigue, headache, syncope
CV: **Hypotension**, increase in resting heart rate (Wegovy)
EENT: Diabetic retinopathy complications, distortion of taste, nasopharyngitis, sinusitis
ENDO: **Hypoglycemia**
GI: Abdominal distention or pain, acute gallbladder disease, **acute pancreatitis (including necrotizing)**, anorexia, cholecystitis, cholelithiasis, constipation, diarrhea, dyspepsia, elevated liver or pancreatic enzymes, eructation, flatulence, gastroesophageal reflux disease, gastritis, ileus, nausea, **severe GI disorders**, vomiting
GU: **Acute kidney injury**, **worsening of chronic renal failure**, UTI
MS: Ligament sprain
RESP: **Pulmonary aspiration** (during deep sedation or general anesthesia)
SKIN: Alopecia, rash, urticaria
Other: **Anaphylaxis**, **angioedema**, anti-semaglutide antibodies, flu-like symptoms, injection-site reactions (discomfort, erythema, induration, inflammation, irritation, pruritus)

Childbearing Considerations

PREGNANCY

- Pregnancy exposure registry: 1-877-390-2760 or www.wegovypregnancyregistry.com (for Wegovy exposure).
- Drug may cause fetal harm, based on animal studies.
- Use not recommended in pregnancy when using Wegovy and drug should be discontinued if pregnancy occurs; use with caution for other brands only if benefit to mother outweighs potential risk to fetus.

LACTATION

- It is not known if drug is present in breast milk.
- Mothers should check with prescriber before breastfeeding if taking Ozempic or Wegovy; breastfeeding is not recommended during Rybelsus therapy.

REPRODUCTION

- Females of childbearing age require an alternative drug at least 2 mo before a planned pregnancy.

Nursing Considerations

! **WARNING** Know that semaglutide should not be given to patients with a history of pancreatitis because effects are unknown. Monitor all patients for signs and symptoms of pancreatitis, such as persistent severe abdominal pain, which sometimes may radiate to the back and which may or may not be accompanied by vomiting. If pancreatitis is suspected, expect drug to be discontinued.

! **WARNING** Be aware semaglutide has caused GI adverse reactions, sometimes severe. Drug should not be given to patients with severe gastroparesis.

! **WARNING** Monitor patient for a hypersensitivity reaction, which could become life-threatening, such as anaphylaxis and angioedema. If present, notify prescriber, expect drug to be discontinued, and provide supportive care, as needed and prescribed.

! **WARNING** Monitor patient's blood pressure for hypotension. Also, monitor patient taking Wegovy brand for an increase in resting heart rate.

! **WARNING** Monitor patient closely for renal dysfunction, especially when initiating or escalating the dose of semaglutide because drug can cause acute kidney injury or worsen chronic renal failure.

! **WARNING** Monitor patient for hypoglycemia if patient is taking Wegovy brand to treat conditions other than diabetes mellitus or patient is also taking insulin or an insulin secretagogue, such as a sulfonylurea, as dosage of these drugs may need to be reduced. Know that hypoglycemia may become severe. Treat according to institutional protocol and notify prescriber.

! **WARNING** Be aware that because semaglutide delays gastric emptying, pulmonary aspiration may occur during elective procedures or surgeries if patient receives deep sedation or general anesthesia.

- Monitor patient for acute gallbladder disease such as clay-colored stools, fever, jaundice, and upper abdominal pain. If present, notify prescriber.
- Monitor patient with a history of diabetic retinopathy for progression of the disorder.
- Monitor elderly patients, especially if 75 or older, because of an increased risk of experiencing more serious adverse reactions.

PATIENT TEACHING

- Instruct patient how to administer form of semaglutide prescribed, including how to administer a subcutaneous injection, if appliable, and what to do if a dose is missed.
- Tell patient who is administering drug subcutaneously along with insulin to administer the 2 drugs as separate injections and never to mix them. The 2 injections can be administered in the same body region, but injections should not be adjacent to each other.
- Remind patient never to share the semaglutide pen with anyone else, even if the needle has been changed because of an increased risk of transmitting bloodborne pathogens.

! **WARNING** Alert patient drug may cause an allergic reaction. If present, tell patient to notify prescriber and, if severe to seek immediate medical care.

! **WARNING** Review signs and symptoms of hypoglycemia with patient and how to treat if it should occur. Tell patient to notify prescriber if hypoglycemia occurs often or is severe. If severe, urge patient to seek immediate medical care.

! **WARNING** Tell patient to report acute GI adverse reactions, severe abdominal pain that may or may not radiate to the back and possibly be accompanied by vomiting. Also tell patient to report signs and symptoms of a gallbladder attack such as clay-colored stools, fever, pain in upper abdomen, or yellowing of eyes or skin.

- Tell patient to report any visual changes to prescriber.

! **WARNING** Advise patient to alert prescriber if other persistent, serious, or unusual adverse reactions occur.

- Advise females of childbearing age to notify prescriber if pregnancy occurs. Alert patient taking Wegovy that drug is not recommended during pregnancy and will need to be discontinued. If patient is taking other brands of semaglutide, prescriber will need to determine if continuation of the drug during pregnancy is warranted in her situation. Also, tell patient to alert prescriber 2 months in advance if pregnancy is being planned.
- Tell patient to inform all prescribers of semaglutide use, especially before undergoing procedures or surgery that requires deep sedation or general anesthesia.

sertraline hydrochloride

Zoloft

Class and Category

Pharmacologic class: Selective serotonin reuptake inhibitor (SSRI)
Therapeutic class: Antianxiety, antidepressant, antiobessive-compulsant, antipanic, antiposttraumatic stress, antipremenstrual dysphoric

Indications and Dosages

✱ *To treat major depression*

ORAL SOLUTION, TABLETS

Adults. *Initial:* 50 mg daily, increased in increments of 25 to 50 mg daily every wk, as needed. *Maximum:* 200 mg daily.

✱ *To treat obsessive–compulsive disorder*

ORAL SOLUTION, TABLETS

Adults and adolescents. *Initial:* 50 mg daily, increased in increments of 25 to 50 mg daily every wk, as needed.
Maximum: 200 mg daily.
Children ages 6 to 12. *Initial:* 25 mg daily, increased in increments of 25 mg every wk, as needed. *Maximum:* 200 mg daily.

✱ *To treat panic disorder, with or without agoraphobia; to treat posttraumatic stress disorder; to treat social anxiety disorder*

ORAL SOLUTION, TABLETS

Adults. *Initial:* 25 mg daily, increased by 25 to 50 mg daily every wk, as needed. *Maximum:* 200 mg daily.

* *To treat premenstrual dysphoric disorder (PMDD)*

ORAL SOLUTION, TABLETS

Adult females of childbearing age. *Initial:* 50 mg daily throughout menstrual cycle. Alternatively, 50 mg daily during luteal phase of menstrual cycle only (starting 14 days prior to menses and continuing through onset of menses). Dosage increased each menstrual cycle in 50-mg increments up to 150 mg daily, or each luteal phase up to 100 mg daily, as needed. If 100-mg daily dosage given for each luteal phase, dosage regimen given as 50 mg daily for first 3 days followed by 100 mg daily during remaining dosage cycle. *Maximum:* 150 mg daily for dosing throughout menstrual cycle, or 100 mg daily for dosing during luteal phase only.

±**DOSAGE ADJUSTMENT** For patients with mild hepatic dysfunction, all dosages reduced by 50%.

Drug Administration

P.O.

- Use the supplied calibrated dropper to measure oral solution dose. However, don't use if allergic to latex, as dropper contains dry natural rubber.
- Mix oral solution with 4 ounces of ginger ale, lemon/lime soda, lemonade, orange juice, or water. Do not mix with any other solutions. Stir. A slight haze may appear but is normal.
- Administer oral solution immediately after mixing.
- Store oral solution and tablets at room temperature.

Route	Onset	Peak	Duration
P.O.	1–2 wk	4.5–8.8 hr	Unknown

Half-life: 26 hr

Mechanism of Action

Inhibits reuptake of the neurotransmitter serotonin by CNS neurons, thereby increasing the amount of serotonin available in nerve synapses to possibly elevate mood and reduce depression. May also relieve symptoms of premenstrual dysphoric disorder or other psychiatric conditions attributed to serotonin deficiency.

Contraindications

Concurrent use of disulfiram (oral solution) or pimozide; hypersensitivity to sertraline or its components; use within 14 days of an MAO inhibitor, including intravenous methylene blue and linezolid.

Interactions

DRUGS

antibiotics (erythromycin, gatifloxacin, moxifloxacin, sparfloxacin), antipsychotics (chlorpromazine, droperidol, iloperidone, mesoridazine, ziprasidone), class 1A antiarrhythmics (procainamide, quinidine), class III antiarrhythmics (amiodarone, sotalol), dolasetron, halofantrine, levomethadyl, mefloquine, methadone, pentamidine, pimozide, probucol, tacrolimus: Increased risk of QT-interval prolongation and/or ventricular arrhythmias

aspirin, clopidogrel, heparin, NSAIDs, warfarin: Increased anticoagulant activity and risk of bleeding

atomoxetine, desipramine, dextromethorphan, flecainide, metoprolol, nebivolol, perphenazine, phenytoin, propafenone, thioridazine, tolterodine, venlafaxine: Possibly increased blood levels of these drugs, leading to increased risk of arrhythmias

buspirone, fentanyl, lithium, MAO inhibitors (I.V. methylene blue, linezolid, selegiline, tranylcypromine), other selected serotonin reuptake inhibitors, serotonin–norepinephrine reuptake inhibitors, St. John's wort, tricyclic antidepressants, triptans, tryptophan: Increased risk of potentially fatal serotonin syndrome

disulfiram: May interact with oral solution that contains alcohol

highly bound drugs to plasma protein: Increased free concentrations of sertraline, increasing risk of adverse reactions

Adverse Reactions

CNS: Abnormal dreams, aggressiveness, agitation, amnesia, anxiety, apathy, ataxia, **cerebrovascular spasm**, **coma**, confusion, delusions, depression, dizziness, drowsiness, emotional lability, euphoria, extrapyramidal symptoms, fatigue, fever, hallucination, headache, hyperkinesia, hypoesthesia, insomnia, lethargy, malaise, nervousness,

neuroleptic malignant syndrome-like reaction, paranoid reaction, paresthesia, psychomotor hyperactivity, psychosis, **seizures**, **serotonin syndrome**, somnolence, **suicidal ideation**, syncope, tremor, weakness, yawning
CV: **Atrial arrhythmias**, **AV block**, **bradycardia**, hypertension, palpitations, **prolonged QT interval**, **torsades de pointes**, vasculitis, vasodilation, **ventricular tachycardia**
EENT: Abnormal accommodation, acute angle-closure glaucoma, blindness, cataract, conjunctivitis, dry mouth, earache, epistaxis, eye pain, optic neuritis, rhinitis, sinusitis, teeth grinding, tinnitus, vision changes
ENDO: Galactorrhea, hyperglycemia, hyperprolactinemia, hypothyroidism, syndrome of inappropriate ADH secretion
GI: Abdominal cramps or pain, anorexia, constipation, diarrhea, elevated liver enzymes, flatulence, hepatic dysfunction, **hepatic failure**, **hepatitis**, increased appetite, indigestion, jaundice, nausea, **pancreatitis**, vomiting
GU: **Acute renal failure**; anorgasmia (females); decreased libido; ejaculation disorders; erectile dysfunction; enuresis; hematuria; impotence; leucorrhea; menstrual disorders; priapism; polyuria; urinary frequency, incontinence, or retention; vaginal hemorrhage
HEME: **Agranulocytosis**, **altered platelet function**, **aplastic anemia**, **hemorrhage**, **leukopenia**, **pancytopenia**, **thrombocytopenia**
MS: Arthralgia, dystonia, lockjaw, muscle cramps or weakness, myalgia, **rhabdomyolysis**
RESP: **Bronchospasm**, coughing, dyspnea, **eosinophilic pneumonia**, **pulmonary hypertension**
SKIN: Alopecia, dermatitis including bullous, diaphoresis, flushing, photosensitivity, pruritus, purpura, rash, severe cutaneous disorders, **Stevens-Johnson syndrome**, **toxic epidermal necrolysis**, urticaria
Other: **Anaphylaxis**, **angioedema**, **hyponatremia**, lupus-like syndrome, serum sickness, weight loss

Childbearing Considerations

PREGNANCY

- Drug may cause fetal harm, especially if given in late pregnancy, as drug exposure increases risk of multiple neonatal complications after birth, including feeding difficulties, persistent pulmonary hypertension, respiratory complications, and seizures of the newborn.
- Use with caution only if benefit to mother outweighs potential risk to fetus.
- Oral solution contains 12% alcohol and is not recommended during pregnancy.

LACTATION

- Drug is present in breast milk.
- Mothers should check with prescriber before breastfeeding.

Nursing Considerations

! **WARNING** Be aware that sertraline should not be given to patients with bradycardia, congenital long-QT syndrome, hypokalemia or hypomagnesemia, recent acute MI, or uncompensated heart failure because of increased risk of prolonged QT interval and torsades de pointes. It should also not be given to patients who are taking other drugs that prolong the QT interval. Expect hypokalemia and hypomagnesemia to be corrected before sertraline therapy is begun.

- Ensure patient has been screened for a family or personal history of bipolar disorder, hypomania, or mania before initiating sertraline therapy for depression. This is because effective antidepressant therapy can promote development of mania in predisposed people. If mania develops, notify prescriber immediately and expect to withhold sertraline.

! **WARNING** Monitor patient for a hypersensitivity reaction, which could become life-threatening, such as anaphylaxis or angioedema. If present, notify prescriber, expect drug to be switched to a different drug, and provide supportive care, as needed and ordered.

! **WARNING** Watch closely for suicidal tendencies, especially when therapy starts and dosage changes and especially in children and adolescents.

! **WARNING** Monitor patient closely for evidence of serotonin syndrome, such as agitation, coma, diarrhea, hallucinations, hyperthermia, hyperreflexia, incoordination, labile blood pressure, nausea, tachycardia, and vomiting. Serotonin syndrome in its most severe form can resemble neuroleptic malignant syndrome, which includes autonomic instability, hyperthermia, mental status changes, muscle rigidity, and possibly rapid changes in vital signs. Notify prescriber immediately because serotonin syndrome reactions that resemble neuroleptic malignant syndrome may be life-threatening. Be prepared to provide supportive care, as needed and ordered.

! WARNING Monitor patient for hypo-osmolarity of serum and urine and for hyponatremia, which may indicate sertraline-induced syndrome of inappropriate ADH secretion.

! WARNING Monitor patient for seizure activity. If present, notify prescriber immediately and institute seizure precautions.

! WARNING Monitor patient closely for evidence of GI bleeding, especially if patient takes a drug known to cause it, such as aspirin, an NSAID, or warfarin.

! WARNING Monitor liver enzymes in patients with hepatic dysfunction, as ordered. Also, montitor BUN and serum creatinine levels in patients with renal dysfunction, as ordered. This is important because drug may cause hepatic or renal failure.

! WARNING Monitor patient for any other persistent, serious, or unusual adverse reactions because drug can affect many body systems and, in some instances, cause life-threatening adverse reactions.

! WARNING Be aware drug should not be discontinued abruptly; instead, dosage should be tapered when discontinuation is the goal.

PATIENT TEACHING

- Advise patient that drug may cause mild pupillary dilation, which may lead to an episode of acute angle-closure glaucoma. Encourage patient to have an eye exam before starting therapy to see if he is at risk.

! WARNING Warn patient that oral solution contains alcohol and should not be taken with disulfiram or during pregnancy. Advise patient to ask prescriber for a different form of the drug.

- Instruct patient how to take form of sertraline prescribed.

! WARNING Advise patient with a latex sensitivity to use an alternate dispenser if oral solution is prescribed because the supplied dropper dispenser contains dry natural rubber.

! WARNING Caution patient not to stop taking drug abruptly. Explain that gradual tapering helps to avoid withdrawal symptoms.

! WARNING Alert patient that drug may cause an allergic reaction. If present, tell patient to notify prescriber and, if severe, to seek immediate medical care.

! WARNING Warn family or caregiver to watch patient closely for evidence of suicidal thinking or behavior, especially when therapy starts or dosage changes, and especially if patient is a child or adolescent.

! WARNING Alert patient that drug may cause seizure activity. If a seizure occurs, tell patient to notify prescriber immediately.

! WARNING Tell patient that sertraline increases the risk of serotonin syndrome and reactions that resemble neuroleptic malignant syndrome, rare but serious complications, when taken with some other drugs. Teach patient how to recognize signs and symptoms of these disorders and advise him to notify prescriber immediately if they occur.

! WARNING Inform patient that use of certain drugs, such as aspirin, NSAIDs, other antiplatelet drugs, warfarin, or other anticoagulants, with sertraline may increase his risk for bleeding. Advise patient to consult prescriber before taking any over-the-counter products, especially aspirin products or NSAIDs.

- Advise patient to avoid hazardous activities until drug's CNS effects are known and resolved.
- Encourage patient to discuss concerns about sexual dysfunction, if present.

! **WARNING** Tell patient to alert prescriber of any other persistent, serious, or unusual adverse reactions as some may become severe.

- Alert patient that false-positive urine testing for benzodiazepines may occur while taking sertraline, requiring a more sensitive test to be performed.

sevelamer carbonate

Renvela

sevelamer hydrochloride

Renagel

Class and Category

Pharmacologic class: Polymeric phosphate binder

Therapeutic class: Phosphate binder

Indications and Dosages

✱ *To control serum phosphate level in patients with chronic kidney disease on dialysis*

TABLETS (RENAGEL)

Adults not taking a phosphate binder. *Initial for serum phosphorus level greater than 5.5 to less than 7.5 mg/dl:* 800 mg 3 times daily with meals. *Initial for serum phosphorus level of 7.5 mg/dl or greater:* 1,600 mg 3 times daily with meals.

±**DOSAGE ADJUSTMENT** For all patients, dosage adjusted based on the serum phosphorus concentration with goal of lowering serum phosphorus to 5.5 mg/dl or less and increased or decreased by 800 mg/meal at 2-week intervals, as needed. If serum phosphorus level is greater than 5.5 mg/dl, dosage increased by 800 mg/meal at 2-week intervals; if serum phosphorus level is between 3.5 and 5.5 mg/dl, dosage remains unchanged; and if serum phosphorus level is less than 3.5 mg/dl, dosage decreased by 800 mg/meal at 2-week intervals. For adult patients being switched from calcium acetate to sevelamer carbonate, 800 mg of sevelamer can be substituted for every 667 mg of calcium acetate being taken.

POWDER FOR ORAL SUSPENSION (RENVELA), TABLETS (RENVELA)

Adults not taking a phosphate binder. *Initial for serum phosphorus level greater than 5.5 to less than 7.5 mg/dl:* 800 mg 3 times daily with meals. *Initial for serum phosphorus level of 7.5 mg/dl or greater:* 1,600 mg 3 times daily with meals. Dosage increased or decreased by 800 mg/meal at 2-wk intervals, as needed.

Children ages 6 and older not taking a phosphate binder. *Initial for body surface area of 0.75 m^2 to less than 1.2 m^2:* 800 mg 3 times daily with meals, then dosage titrated every 2 wk by 400 mg/meal, as needed. *Initial for body surface area of 1.2 m^2 or greater:* 1,600 mg 3 times daily with meals and dosage titrated every 2 wk by 800 mg/meal, as needed.

±**DOSAGE ADJUSTMENT** For adult patients being switched from calcium acetate to sevelamer carbonate, 800 mg of sevelamer can be substituted for every 667 mg of calcium being taken.

Drug Administration

P.O.

- Administer with meals.
- Tablets should be swallowed whole with water and not broken, chewed, or crushed.
- When using powder to make oral suspension for dose increments of 0.4 g, use one-half of a 0.8-g packet.
- Mix with 30 ml of water for a 0.4-g or 0.8-g dose; 60 ml for a 2.4-g dose. More than one packet can be mixed together.
- Stir mixture vigorously, even though it does not dissolve, and have patient drink entire preparation immediately or restir prior to administration if taken up to 30 min after being mixed.
- As an alternative to water, packet may be premixed with a small amount of food or beverage and administered within 30 min as part of the meal.

- Do not heat powder mixture or add to heated foods or liquids.
- If patient is also taking ciprofloxacin, administer at least 2 hr before or 6 hr after sevelamer. If patient is also taking mycophenolate mofetil, administer at least 2 hr before sevelamer.

Route	Onset	Peak	Duration
P.O.	1–2 wk	Unknown	Unknown

Half-life: Unknown

Mechanism of Action

Inhibits phosphate absorption in the intestine by binding dietary phosphate, thereby lowering serum phosphorus level.

Contraindications

Bowel obstruction; hypersensitivity to sevelamer carbonate, sevelamer hydrochloride, or their components

Interactions

DRUGS

oral drugs, such as ciprofloxacin, cyclosporine, levothyroxine, mycophenolate mofetil, tacrolimus: Possible decreased bioavailability of oral drugs requiring separate administration times

Adverse Reactions

CNS: Headache, fever
CV: Hypertension, **hypotension**, **thrombosis**
EENT: Nasopharyngitis
GI: Abdominal pain, **bleeding GI ulcers**, colitis, constipation (severe), diarrhea, dysphagia, fecal impaction, flatulence, **GI necrosis**, ileus, indigestion, **intestinal obstruction or perforation**, nausea, vomiting
RESP: Bronchitis, dyspnea, increased cough, upper respiratory tract infection
MS: Arthralgia, back or limb pain
SKIN: Pruritus, rash
Other: **Hypersensitivity reactions**, **hypophosphatemia**, infection

Childbearing Considerations

PREGNANCY

- Drug is not absorbed systemically and so is not expected to result in fetal exposure.
- Drug may decrease serum levels of fat-soluble vitamins and folic acid in pregnant females.
- Use with caution only if benefit to mother outweighs potential risk to fetus.

LACTATION

- Drug is not absorbed systemically and so is not expected to be in breast milk.
- Mother should check with prescriber before breastfeeding.

Nursing Considerations

! **WARNING** Suggest suspension form be used in patients with swallowing disorders because tablet may get stuck in the esophagus in these individuals, and they may require hospitalization and emergency intervention to remove it.

- Monitor serum phosphorus level to determine drug's effectiveness.

! **WARNING** Monitor patient for hypersensitivity reactions. If present, notify prescriber, expect drug to be discontinued, and provide supportive care, as needed and ordered.

! **WARNING** Monitor blood pressure frequently for hypotension. Also, monitor patient for signs and symptoms of a thrombosis.

! **WARNING** Monitor patient closely for adverse GI reactions as some may become life-threatening, such as GI bleeding ulcers or necrosis, intestinal obstruction, and perforation.

! **WARNING** Be aware that severe hypophosphatemia may occur in patient with dysphagia, major GI tract surgery, or severe GI motility disorder (including severe constipation) because drug prevents phosphate absorption.

PATIENT TEACHING

- Instruct patient how to take form of sevelamer prescribed.
- Inform patient of potential need for fat-soluble vitamins and folic acid supplements, especially if patient is pregnant.

! **WARNING** Alert patient that drug may cause an allergic reaction. If present tell patient to notify prescriber and to seek immediate medical care, if severe.

! **WARNING** Review signs and symptoms of a thrombosis and advise patient to seek immediate medical attention, if present.

! **WARNING** Review signs and symptoms of adverse GI reactions such as sudden onset of abdominal pain or new onset of bloody stool. Warn patient to notify prescriber immediately, if present. Also, instruct patient to report new onset or worsening of existing constipation to prescriber.

! **WARNING** Review signs and symptoms of hypophosphatemia in patients with dysphagia, major GI tract surgery, or severe GI motility disorder (including severe constipation) and to notify prescriber immediately, if present.

sildenafil citrate

Revatio, Viagra

Class and Category

Pharmacologic class: Phosphodiesterase 5 (PDE5) inhibitor
Therapeutic class: Antihypertensive (pulmonary arterial), erectile dysfunction agent

Indications and Dosages

* *To treat erectile dysfunction*

TABLETS (VIAGRA)

Men younger than 65. *Initial:* 50 mg taken 30 min to 4 hr before sexual activity although best if taken 1 hr before sexual activity; decreased or increased, as needed, based upon response. *Usual range:* 25 to 100 mg. *Maximum:* Once per day with dosage not exceeding 100 mg.

± **DOSAGE ADJUSTMENT** For male patients over age 65 with hepatic dysfunction or severe renal insufficiency (creatinine clearance less than 30 ml/min), and those taking an alpha-blocker or potent CYP3A4 inhibitors (erythromycin, itraconazole, ketoconazole, saquinavir) or ritonavir, initial dose 25 mg. Maximum dosage for patients taking ritonavir is 25 mg within a 48-hr period.

* *To treat pulmonary arterial hypertension in order to improve exercise ability and delay clinical worsening of condition in patients classified as group 1 by the World Health Organization*

ORAL SUSPENSION, TABLETS (REVATIO)

Adults. 20 mg 3 times daily and titrated upward to maximum dose, as needed. *Maximum:* 80 mg 3 times daily.

I.V. INJECTION (REVATIO)

Adults. 10 mg as an I.V. bolus 3 times daily.

* *To treat pulmonary arterial hypertension in order to improve exercise ability in pediatric patients classified as group I by the World Health Organization and, in pediatric patients too young to perform standardized exercise testing, pulmonary hemodynamics thought to underlie improvements in exercise*

ORAL SUSPENSION, TABLETS (REVATIO)

Children ages 1 to 17 weighing 45 kg (99 lb) or more. 20 mg 3 times daily and increased, as needed, in children weighing more than 45 kg (99 lb) to 40 mg 3 times daily. *Maximum:* 40 mg 3 times daily for children weighing more than 45 kg (99 lb).
Children ages 1 to 17 weighing 20 kg (44 lb) to 45 kg (99 lb). 20 mg 3 times daily.
Children ages 1 to 17 weighing 20 kg (44 lb) or less. 10 mg 3 times daily.

± **DOSAGE ADJUSTMENT** For patients taking concomitant moderate-to-strong CYP3A inducers such as bosentan, dosage may need to be increased when initiating treatment with these inducers and reduced when moderate-to-strong CYP3A inducers are discontinued.

Drug Administration

P.O.

Revatio

- Reconstitute powder for oral suspension by tapping bottle to release the powder; then remove the cap. Accurately measure out 60 ml of water and pour the water into bottle, replace cap, and shake bottle vigorously for a minimum of 30 sec. Then, add another 30 ml of water to bottle. Replace cap and shake bottle vigorously again for a minimum of 30 sec. Solution should be clear and colorless and contain 10-mg sildenafil per ml. Press bottle adaptor into the neck of the bottle. The adaptor should be used so the oral syringe can be filled with the drug from the bottle. Replace cap on the bottle.
- Do not mix with any other drug or additional flavoring agent.

- Store reconstituted oral suspension at room temperature or in refrigerator.
- Discard any remaining oral suspension 60 days after reconstitution.

I.V.

- Used for patients unable to take oral medication.
- Drug supplied as a ready-to-use solution in a single-use glass vial.
- Inspect solution before administering. It should be clear and colorless.
- Administer as an I.V. bolus.
- *Incompatibilities:* None reported by manufacturer

Route	Onset	Peak	Duration
P.O.	30–60 min	30–120 min	4 hr
I.V.	Unknown	Unknown	Unknown

Half-life: 4 hr

Mechanism of Action

Enhances the effect of nitric oxide released in the penis by stimulation to increase cGMP level, relaxed smooth muscle, and increase blood flow to the corpus cavernosum, thus producing an erection.

Preventing breakdown of cyclic guanosine monophosphate by phosphodiesterase, levels increase, leading to smooth-muscle relaxation of the pulmonary vasculature and subsequently, vasodilation. Decreased pressure within the pulmonary vasculature then occurs, which improves tolerance to exercise and delays worsening of pulmonary arterial hypertension.

Contraindications

Concomitant use with riociguat, a guanylate cyclase stimulator; continuous or intermittent nitrate therapy in any form; hypersensitivity to sildenafil or its components

Interactions

DRUGS

alpha-blockers, amlodipine, nitrates: Possible additive blood pressure-lowering effects
CYP3A moderate to strong inducers such as bosentan: Decreased sildenafil exposure with decreased effectiveness
CYP3A4 strong inhibitors such as erythromycin, itraconazole, ketoconazole, ritonavir, saquinavir: Significantly increased systemic exposure of sildenafil, increasing risk of adverse reactions

Adverse Reactions

CNS: **CVA**, dizziness, headache, **intracerebral and subarachnoid hemorrhages**, migraine, **seizures**, syncope, transient global amnesia, transient ischemic attack
CV: **Heart failure**, hypertension, **hypotension, myocardial infarction or ischemia**, orthostatic hypotension, palpitations, **sudden cardiac death**, tachycardia, vaso-occlusive crisis (presence of pulmonary hypertension coupled with sickle cell disease), **ventricular arrhythmias**
EENT: Blurred vision; change in color perception; diplopia; epistaxis; hearing loss; increased intraocular pressure; nasal congestion; nonarteritic anterior ischemic optic neuropathy (NAION); ocular burning, pressure, redness, or swelling; paramacular edema; photophobia; retinal vascular bleeding or disease; tinnitus; visual decrease or temporary vision loss; vitreous detachment
ENDO: Uncontrolled diabetes mellitus
GI: Diarrhea, dyspepsia
GU: Cystitis, dysuria, painful erection, priapism, UTI
MS: Arthralgia, back or extremity pain, myalgia
RESP: **Pulmonary hemorrhage**, upper respiratory tract infection
SKIN: Flushing, photosensitivity rash, urticaria

Childbearing Considerations

PREGNANCY

- Trade name, Viagra, is not indicated for use in females.
- It is not known if Revatio, can cause fetal harm.
- Use Revatio with caution only if benefit to mother outweighs potential risk to fetus.

LACTATION

- Trade name, Viagra, is not indicated for use in females.
- Revatio appears to be present in breast milk.
- Mothers should check with prescriber before breastfeeding if prescribed Revatio.

Nursing Considerations

! WARNING Do not administer drug to patients who take nitrates.

! **WARNING** Know that sildenafil is not recommended to be used in patients with retinitis pigmentosa because patient is at higher risk for significant adverse effects on vision. Monitor vision, especially in patients over age 50; who have coronary artery disease, diabetes, hypertension, or hyperlipidemia; or who smoke because, although rare, sildenafil may cause nonarteritic anterior ischemic optic neuropathy (NAION) that may lead to decreased vision or permanent vision loss. Patients at higher risk for NAION include those who have already experienced it in the past and those who have a low cup to optic disc ratio or retinitis pigmentosa.

! **WARNING** Be aware that concomitant use of Revatio with strong CYP3A inhibitors is not recommended. CYP3A inhibitors also should be used with extreme caution with Viagra because drug increases blood levels of sildenafil.

! **WARNING** Use sildenafil with extreme caution in the elderly and patients with hepatic or renal dysfunction, and men with penile abnormalities that may predispose them to priapism. In addition, use cautiously in patients who have suffered a life-threatening arrhythmia, CVA, or MI within the last 6 months or in patients with cardiac failure, coronary artery disease causing unstable angina, hypertension (blood pressure greater than 170/110), related anemias, resting hypotension (blood pressure less than 90/50), retinitis pigmentosa, or sickle cell, as sildenafil therapy has not been studied in these patient groups.

- Use cautiously in patients with left ventricular outflow obstruction, such as aortic stenosis and idiopathic hypertrophic subaortic stenosis, and those with severely impaired autonomic control of blood pressure because these conditions increase patient's sensitivity to vasodilators, such as sildenafil.
- Assess patient's blood pressure and heart rate and rhythm before drug therapy begins and monitor often throughout drug therapy for abnormalities.

! **WARNING** Monitor patient being treated for pulmonary hypertension secondary to sickle cell disease for vaso-occlusive crisis (severe pain and change in color and temperature if extremity is involved) that may become severe enough to require hospitalization. Notify prescriber immediately and prepare to provide supportive care.

! **WARNING** Monitor patient for other persistent, serious, or unusual adverse reactions as drug can affect many body systems and has the potential to cause life-threatening adverse reactions such as pulmonary hemorrhage or ventricular arrhythmias.

PATIENT TEACHING

- Instruct patient, family, or caregiver how to administer brand and form of sildenafil prescribed.
- Explain that sildenafil used to treat erectile dysfunction may be taken up to 4 hours before sexual activity, but that taking it 1 hour beforehand provides the most effective results.

! **WARNING.** Advise male patient taking Revatio used to treat pulmonary hypertension not to take Viagra or other PDE-5 inhibitors to treat erectile dysfunction.

! **WARNING** Warn patient not to take sildenafil if he also takes any form of organic nitrate, either continuously or intermittently, or other PDE5 inhibitors because profound hypotension and death could result. Also, caution patient to inform prescriber of all medications taken, as dosage may have to be decreased if a drug, such as an alpha-blocker has also been prescribed.

! **WARNING** Tell patient to stop taking drug and contact prescriber if sudden loss of vision in one or both eyes occurs or if he has a loss of hearing and possibly occurring with dizziness or tinnitus.

! **WARNING** Urge patient to notify prescriber immediately if a painful erection occurs or an erection lasts longer than 4 hours, to avoid possible penile damage and permanent loss of erectile function.

! **WARNING** Tell patient to notify prescriber immediately if any other persistent, serious, or unusual adverse reactions occur. Urge patient to seek immediate medical care, if severe.

- Instruct diabetic patient to monitor his blood glucose level frequently because drug may affect glucose control.
- Advise patient taking sildenafil for erectile dysfunction to seek sexual counseling to enhance the drug's effects.
- Tell mothers wishing to breastfeed their infant to consult prescriber of Revatio first.

silodosin

Rapaflo

Class and Category

Pharmacologic class: Alpha-adrenergic blocker
Therapeutic class: Benign prostatic antihyperplasia agent

Indications and Dosages

∗ *To treat symptomatic benign prostatic hyperplasia*

CAPSULES

Adult males. 8 mg once daily with a meal. *Maximum:* 8 mg daily.

±**DOSAGE ADJUSTMENT** For patients with moderate renal impairment (creatinine clearance between 30 and 50 ml/min), dosage reduced to 4 mg daily.

Drug Administration

P.O.

- Administer drug with a meal.
- For patient who can't swallow capsules, open capsule and sprinkle contents on a tablespoonful of cool or room-temperature applesauce. Administer within 5 min. Patient should not chew mixture. Follow with an 8-ounce glass of cool water. Don't store mixture for future use.

Route	Onset	Peak	Duration
P.O.	2–6 hr	6–7 hr	9–15 hr

Half-life: 13 hr

Mechanism of Action

Binds to postsynaptic $alpha_1$ adrenoreceptors located in the bladder base and neck, prostate gland, and prostatic capsule and urethra. Blocking action at these adrenoreceptor sites causes relaxation of smooth muscle in the local area, which improves urine flow and reduces other benign prostatic hyperplasia symptoms.

Contraindications

Hypersensitivity to silodosin and its components, severe hepatic insufficiency (Child-Pugh score 10 or above), severe renal insufficiency (creatinine clearance less than 30 ml/min), use with alpha-blockers (doxazosin, prazosin, terazosin) or strong CYP3A4 inhibitors (clarithromycin, ketoconazole, itraconazole, and ritonavir)

Interactions

DRUGS

alpha-blockers: Possibly increased risk of orthostatic hypotension
antihypertensives: Increased risk of dizziness and orthostatic hypotension
CYP3A4 inhibitors, such as clarithromycin, diltiazem, erythromycin, itraconazole, ketoconazole, ritonavir; strong P-glycoprotein inhibitors, such as cyclosporine: Increased serum silodosin levels and risk of adverse reactions

Adverse Reactions

CNS: Asthenia, dizziness, headache, insomnia, syncope
CV: Orthostatic hypotension
EENT: Nasal congestion, nasopharyngitis, rhinorrhea, sinusitis
GI: Abdominal pain, diarrhea, elevated liver enzymes, impaired hepatic function, jaundice
GU: Elevated prostate specific antigen level, retrograde ejaculation
SKIN: Pruritus, purpura, rash, **toxic skin eruption**, urticaria
Other: **Angioedema**

Childbearing Considerations

PREGNANCY

- Drug is not indicated for use in women.

LACTATION

- Drug is not indicated for use in women.

REPRODUCTION

- Male infertility is possible and may be reversible if it occurs.

Nursing Considerations

- Use silodosin cautiously in patients with impaired hepatic or renal impairment.

- Monitor effectiveness of drug to control symptoms of prostatic hyperplasia.

! WARNING Monitor patient for a hypersensitivity or severe skin reaction, which could become life-threatening, such as angioedema or toxic skin eruptions. If present, notify prescriber, expect drug to be discontinued, and provide supportive care, as needed and ordered.

- Monitor patient's blood pressure for reduction, especially if he takes an antihypertensive with silodosin.

PATIENT TEACHING

- Instruct patient how to administer silodosin.

! WARNING Tell patient drug may cause an allergic reaction or a severe skin reaction. If present, tell patient to notify prescriber and, if severe, to seek immediate medical care.

- Advise patient to avoid hazardous activities until drug's CNS effects are known and resolved.
- Tell patient to rise slowly from a lying or sitting position to prevent lightheadedness.
- Advise patient planning cataract surgery or other ocular procedure to tell ophthalmologist that he takes silodosin or has taken it in the past because of potential adverse reactions.

simvastatin

FloLipid, Zocor

Class and Category

Pharmacologic class: HMG-CoA reductase inhibitor (statin)
Therapeutic class: Antilipemic

Indications and Dosages

* *To reduce risk of total mortality by reducing risk of coronary heart disease death, non-fatal MI and CVA, and the need for coronary and non-coronary revascularization procedures in patients with established cerebrovascular disease, coronary heart disease, diabetes, and/or peripheral vascular disease, who are at high risk of coronary heart disease events; as adjunct to diet to reduce low-density lipoprotein cholesterol (LDL-C) in patients with primary hyperlipidemia or heterozygous familial hypercholesterolemia; as adjunct to diet to treat patients with hypertriglyceridemia or primary dysbetalipoproteinemia*

ORAL SUSPENSION, TABLETS

Adults. 20 mg to 40 mg once daily in the evening. *Maximum:* 40 mg daily (80 mg only for patient who has been taking 80 mg daily chronically for 12 mo or more without evidence of muscle toxicity).

* *As adjunct to treat homozygous familial hypercholesterolemia*

TABLETS (ZOCOR)

Adults. *Initial:* 20 to 40 mg once daily in the evening. *Maximum:* 40 mg once daily.

ORAL SUSPENSIOIN (FLOLIPID)

Adults. 40 mg once daily in the evening on an empty stomach.

* *As adjunct to treat adolescent heterozygous familial hypercholesterolemia*

TABLETS (ZOCOR)

Children ages 10 to 17 with girls at least 1 yr postmenarche. *Initial:* 10 mg once daily in the evening. Adjusted every 4 wk, as needed, to achieve target LDL-cholesterol level. *Maintenance:* 10 to 40 mg once daily in the evening. *Maximum:* 40 mg once daily.

ORAL SUSPENSION (FLOLIPID)

Children ages 10 to 17 with girls at least 1 yr postmenarche. 5 to 40 mg once daily in the evening on empty stomach.

±**DOSAGE ADJUSTMENT** For patients with severe renal impairment, initial dosage reduced to 5 mg daily. For patients taking diltiazem, dronedarone, or verapamil, daily dosage should not exceed 10 mg; for patients taking amiodarone, amlodipine, or ranolazine, daily dosage should not exceed 20 mg. For patients taking lomitapide, daily dosage reduced by 50% and maximum dosage should not exceed 20 mg (40 mg once daily for patients previously taking 80 mg daily chronically while taking lomitapide). For patients at high risk of coronary artery disease event due to existing CHD, diabetes, peripheral vessel disease, or history of CVA or other cerebrovascular disease and taking oral suspension, initial dosage started and maintained at 40 mg once daily.

Drug Administration

P.O.

- Administer drug in the evening with or without food for tablet form and on an empty stomach for oral suspension.
- Do not administer drug with grapefruit juice.
- Give drug 1 hr before or 4 hr after giving bile acid sequestrant, cholestyramine, or colestipol.
- Shake oral suspension bottle well for at least 20 sec before using.
- Use a calibrated device to measure oral suspension dosage.
- Store oral suspension at room temperature and protect from heat. Discard within 30 days after opening.

Route	Onset	Peak	Duration
P.O.	>3 wk	1.3–2.4 hr	Unknown

Half-life: 1–2 hr

Mechanism of Action

Interferes with the hepatic enzyme, hydroxymethylglutaryl-coenzyme A reductase, thereby reducing the formation of mevalonic acid, a cholesterol precursor, which, in turn, interrupts the pathway necessary for cholesterol synthesis. Declining cholesterol levels in hepatic cells causes LDLs to be consumed, which reduces the levels of circulating total cholesterol and serum triglycerides.

Contraindications

Active hepatic disease; concurrent use with strong CYP3A4 inhibitors, such as boceprevir, clarithromycin, cobicistat-containing products, erythromycin, HIV protease inhibitors, itraconazole, ketoconazole, nefazodone, posaconazole, telaprevir, or telithromycin; concurrent use with cyclosporine, danazol, or gemfibrozil; hypersensitivity to simvastatin or its components

Interactions

DRUGS

amiodarone, antiretroviral protease inhibitors boceprevir, calcium channel blockers (amlodipine, diltiazem, verapamil), cobicistat-containing products, clarithromycin, colchicine, cyclosporine, danazol, daptomycin, dronedarone, erythromycin, gemfibrozil and other fibrates, itraconazole, ketoconazole, nefazodone, niacin (1 g daily or more), posaconazole, ranolazine, telaprevir, telithromycin, voriconazole: Increased risk of myopathy or rhabdomyolysis
digoxin: Possibly slight elevation in blood digoxin level
lomitapide: Increased simvastatin levels increasing risk of adverse reactions
oral anticoagulants: Increased bleeding or prolonged PT

FOODS

grapefruit juice (1 or more quarts daily): Increased risk of myopathy or rhabdomyolysis

Adverse Reactions

CNS: Asthenia, cognitive impairment, dizziness, fatigue, headache, insomnia, vertigo
CV: **Atrial fibrillation**, chest pain, edema
EENT: Cataracts, ocular myasthenia, rhinitis, sinusitis
ENDO: Elevated HbA1C levels, hyperglycemia
GI: Abdominal pain, constipation, diarrhea, elevated liver enzymes, flatulence, gastritis, heartburn, **hepatic failure**, indigestion, nausea, **pancreatitis**, vomiting
GU: Erectile dysfunction, UTI
MS: Immune-mediated necrotizing myopathy, myalgia, myopathy, **rhabdomyolysis**
RESP: Bronchitis, **interstitial lung disease**, upper respiratory tract infection
SKIN: Alopecia, eczema, **erythema multiforme**, flushing, lichen planus, photosensitivity, pruritus, purpura, rash, skin and nail changes (discoloration, dryness, nodules), **Stevens-Johnson syndrome**, **toxic epidermal**, urticaria
Other: Exacerbation or new myasthenia gravis

Childbearing Considerations

PREGNANCY

- Drug may cause fetal harm.
- Drug is not recommended during pregnancy.
- Drug should be discontinued when pregnancy becomes known.

LACTATION

- It is not known if drug is present in breast milk.
- Breastfeeding is not recommended during drug therapy.

REPRODUCTION

- Females of childbearing age should use effective contraception throughout drug therapy.

Nursing Considerations

! **WARNING** Be aware concurrent therapy with niacin (greater than 1 g daily) and simvastatin is not recommended for use with Chinese patients because of increased risk of myopathy.

- Use simvastatin cautiously in elderly patients and those with hepatic or renal impairment.
- Expect to obtain liver enzymes prior to initiation of simvastatin therapy and then thereafter, as needed because drug may adversely affect liver function.
- Know that 80 mg of simvastatin is used rarely, since it is associated with a high risk of myopathy. If 40 mg of simvastatin is not sufficiently efficacious, know that an alternative agent should replace simvastatin, as ordered.
- Monitor serum lipoprotein level, as ordered, to evaluate response to therapy.

! **WARNING** Monitor patient for elevated CPK level (as ordered) or for muscle pain, tenderness, or weakness and other symptoms of myopathy; if left unchecked, the more serious form—rhabdomyolysis—may occur, which may lead to renal failure. Risk factors for myopathy include being 65 years or older, of female gender, taking 80 mg dose daily, and having renal impairment or uncontrolled hypothyroidism. If CPK level is significantly elevated or patient has symptoms of myopathy, notify prescriber and expect to withhold drug, as ordered.

- Monitor patient for signs and symptoms of hyperglycemia because drug may elevate fasting serum glucose levels and increase HbA1C levels even in nondiabetics.

! **WARNING** Monitor patient for other persistent, serious, or unusual adverse reactions.

PATIENT TEACHING

- Instruct patient how to administer form of simvastatin prescribed
- Advise patient to avoid grapefruit juice to decrease risk of drug toxicity.
- Instruct patient to follow low-fat, cholesterol-lowering diet explaining that drug therapy will help but not replace lifestyle changes needed to lower cholesterol levels.

! **WARNING** Urge patient to notify prescriber immediately about muscle pain, tenderness, or weakness and other symptoms of myopathy and symptoms of abnormal liver function, such as anorexia, dark urine, fatigue, right upper abdominal discomfort, or yellowing of skin.

- Inform patient, especially if patient has diabetes, that drug may raise blood glucose levels. Review signs and symptoms of hyperglycemia and tell patient to notify prescriber if present. Instruct patients with diabetes of need to test blood sugar regularly and to obtain an HbA1C periodically.
- Encourage family or caregiver to notify prescriber if patient develops or exhibits confusion, forgetfulness, and worsening memory loss.

! **WARNING** Instruct patient to inform prescriber if other persistent, serious, or unusual adverse reactions occur while taking simvastatin.

- Inform females of childbearing age of need to use a reliable contraceptive method while taking drug. Instruct patient to notify prescriber at once if pregnancy occurs as drug is not recommended during pregnancy.
- Tell mothers breastfeeding is not recommended during simvastatin therapy.

siponimod fumaric acid

Mayzent

Class and Category

Pharmacologic class: Sphingosine-1-phosphate (S1P) receptor modulator
Therapeutic class: Anti-inflammatory

Indications and Dosages

✷ *To treat relapsing forms of multiple sclerosis, including active secondary progressive disease, clinically isolated syndrome, and relapsing-remitting disease*

TABLETS

Adults with CYP2C9 genotypes *1/*1, *1/*2, or *2/*2. *Initial titration:* 0.25 mg once daily on days 1 and 2; 0.5 mg once daily on day 3; 0.75 mg once daily on day 4; and 1.25 mg once daily on day 5, followed by maintenance dose. *Maintenance:* 2 mg once daily beginning on day 6.
Adults with CYP2C9 genotypes *1/*3 and *2/*3. *Initial titration:* 0.25 mg once daily on days 1 and 2; 0.5 mg once daily on day 3; and 0.75 mg once daily on day 4, followed by maintenance dose. *Maintenance:* 1 mg once daily beginning on day 5.

±**DOSAGE ADJUSTMENT** For all patients, if 1 initial titration dose is missed for more than 24 hours, treatment reinitiated with day 1 of the titration regimen. For all patients, if maintenance treatment is interrupted for 4 or more consecutive daily doses, treatment reinitiated with day 1 of titration regimen.

Drug Administration

P.O.

- Tablets should be swallowed whole and not chewed, crushed, or divided.
- Expect to monitor patient for 6 hr or more after first dose according to manufacturer's guidelines.
- Store unopened containers of drug in refrigerator.
- Open bottles and blister pack may be stored at room temperature for 3 mo. Do not refrigerate after opening container.

Route	Onset	Peak	Duration
P.O.	Unknown	4 hr	Unknown

Half-life: 30 hr

Mechanism of Action

Binds with high affinity to S1P receptors 1 and 5, to block the capacity of lymphocytes to egress from lymph nodes, thereby reducing the number of lymphocytes in peripheral blood and lymphocyte migration into the central nervous system.

Contraindications

CVA; CYP2C9 *3/*3 genotype; decompensated heart failure requiring hospitalization; history within past 6 mo of class III or IV heart failure; hypersensitivity to siponimod or its components; MI, TIA, or unstable angina; presence of Mobitz type II second-degree AV block, third-degree AV block, or sick sinus syndrome, unless a functioning pacemaker is in place

Interactions

DRUGS

class 1A (procainamide, quinidine), class III (amiodarone, sotalol), drugs that decrease heart rate (digoxin, diltiazem, ivabradine, verapamil), QT prolongation drugs: Increased risk of bradycardia or torsades de pointes
antineoplastics, immune-modulating agents, immunosuppressants: Increased risk of additive immune effects
beta-blockers: Additive lowering of heart rate
CYP2C9 inducers, CYP3A4 inducers: Significant decrease in siponimod exposure
CYP2C9 inhibitors, CYP3A4 inhibitors: Significant increase in siponimod exposure, increasing risk of adverse reactions
live attenuated vaccines: Increased risk of infection
nonlive vaccines: Possibly diminished therapeutic effect of vaccine

Adverse Reactions

CNS: Asthenia, **CVA (ischemic)**, dizziness, falling, headache, **posterior reversible encephalopathy**, **progressive multifocal leukoencephalopathy**, **(PML) seizures**, tremor

CV: AV block (first or second degree), **bradycardia**, hypertension, **MI**, peripheral edema
EENT: Macular edema
GI: Diarrhea, elevated liver enzymes, nausea
HEME: **Lymphopenia**
MS: Extremity pain
RESP: Decreased pulmonary function, **pulmonary embolism**
SKIN: **Cutaneous malignancies such as basal cell carcinoma, malignant melanoma, and squamous cell carcinoma**
Other: **Immune reconstitution inflammatory syndrome**, herpes zoster, serious infections

Childbearing Considerations

PREGNANCY

- Pregnancy exposure registry: 1-877-311-8972; email: MotherToBaby@health.ucsd.edu; or www.mothertobaby.org/join-study.
- Drug may cause fetal harm, according to animal studies.
- Use with caution only if benefit to mother outweighs potential risk to fetus.

LACTATION

- It is not known if drug is present in breast milk.
- Mothers should check with prescriber before breastfeeding.

REPRODUCTION

- Females of childbearing age should use an effective contraceptive throughout siponimod therapy and for 10 days following drug discontinuation.

Nursing Considerations

- Ensure that all of the following have been assessed before the initiation of siponimod therapy: complete blood count, CYP2C9 genotype determination, and liver function studies (bilirubin and transaminase levels within past 6 months). Also, ensure that patient has had a cardiac examination, including an ECG to determine whether preexisting conduction abnormalities are present as well as an ophthalmic evaluation (including an evaluation of the fundus and the macula). Check current or prior medications taken by patient such as drugs that could slow heart rate or affect atrioventricular conduction; exposure to antineoplastics, immunosuppressives, or immune-modulating therapies that could cause additive immunosuppressive effects; and vaccinations (patient tested for antibodies to varicella-zoster virus, with negative test results requiring vaccination prior to starting therapy).

! WARNING Evaluate patient for signs and symptoms of an infection before siponimod therapy begins. Review patient's recent CBC results. Know that drug should not be started in patients with a severe active infection until the infection is resolved. Also, be aware that patients should continue to be monitored for infection until at least 3 to 4 weeks after drug is discontinued. Provide treatment for an infection, as prescribed, and expect drug to be temporarily withheld if a serious infection develops. Know that life-threatening infections, such as cryptococcal meningitis and disseminated cryptococcal infections have occurred, along with cases of herpes viral infection that may lead to varicella-zoster meningitis. Although progressive multifocal leukoencephalopathy has not occurred with siponimod therapy, it has occurred in similar treatment modalities in patients with multiple sclerosis.

! WARNING Assess patient's skin regularly for abnormalities beginning before drug is initiated because drug may cause cutaneous malignancies such as basal cell carcinoma, malignant melanoma, or squamous cellcarcinoma. Be aware that Kaposi's sarcoma and Merkel cell carcinoma have occurred in patients treated with other S1P receptor modulators.

- Know that with the first dose, 6-hour monitoring should be done, especially in patients with sinus bradycardia (heart rate less than 55 beats/min) or first- or second-degree AV block and in patients with a history of heart failure or MI. First dose should be administered in a setting to manage symptomatic bradycardia. Monitor patient for 6 hours after administering dose, with hourly blood pressure and pulse measurements. Obtain an ECG at the end of day 1. After day 1, determine if patient has any of the following abnormalities (even in the absence of symptoms) and continue monitoring patient, if present, until the abnormality resolves: heart rate 6 hours postdose is less than 45 beats/min, heart rate 6 hours postdose is at the lowest value postdose, or ECG 6 hours postdose shows new-onset second-degree or higher AV block. If postdose symptomatic bradycardia, bradyarrhythmia, or conduction-related symptoms occur, if ECG 6 hours postdose shows new-onset second-degree or higher AV block, or QTc is greater than or equal to 500 msec, expect to initiate appropriate management, as ordered. Begin continuous ECG monitoring and continue monitoring patient until symptoms have resolved. If drug treatment is required, expect patient to be monitored overnight and the 6-hour monitoring period repeated after the second dose. Also, expect a consultation with a cardiologist to be ordered.

! **WARNING** Be aware of the possibility that posterior reversible encephalopathy syndrome or progressive multifocal leukoencephalopathy (PML) may occur with siponimod therapy. Be aware that longer treatment duration increases the risk of PML. Report any unexpected neurological or psychiatric signs and symptoms to prescriber. If either disorder is confirmed expect drug to be discontinued. Be aware that immune reconstitution syndrome has occurred within a few months in patients treated with siponimod who developed PML and subsequently discontinued treatment. The inflammatory response seen in immune reconstitution syndrome predisposes susceptible patients to opportunistic infections, such as cytomegalovir, *Mycobacterium avium* infection, *Pneumocystiss jiroveci* pneumonia, or tuberculosis. Autoimmune disorders, such as Graves' disease, Guillain-Barré syndrome or polymyositis, have also occurred.

- Be aware that patients with a history of uveitis or who have diabetes mellitus are at increased risk of macular edema during siponimod therapy. Monitor patient for any visual changes.
- Monitor patient's liver enzymes, as ordered. Assess patient for signs and symptoms of liver dysfunction, such as abdominal pain, anorexia, dark urine, fatigue, jaundice, nausea, rash, and vomiting. Patients with history of liver dysfunction are at higher risk to developing liver dysfunction with siponimod. Report findings to prescriber.

! **WARNING** Monitor patient for any other persistent, serious, or unusual adverse reactions.

! **WARNING** Monitor patient for severe increased disability after siponimod therapy has been discontinued. Although rare, stopping siponimod therapy may exacerbate multiple sclerosis and cause a disease rebound.

- Be aware that it may take up to 4 weeks after siponimod therapy is discontinued for the pharmacodynamic effects on the patient's immune system to end. During this time, caution should be used in prescribing immunosuppressants.

PATIENT TEACHING

- Prepare patient for the 6-hour monitoring period required for the first dose.
- Instruct patient how to administer siponimod and what to do if a dose is missed, including the possible need for a repeat of a first-dose 6-hour monitoring period.
- Stress importance of taking siponimod exactly as prescribed. Advise patient not to stop taking drug without first discussing concerns with prescriber.
- Advise patient to avoid receiving live attenuated vaccines while taking siponimod and for 4 weeks after drug is discontinued.

! **WARNING** Review infection control measures with patient. Caution patient to avoid anyone with an infection. Tell patient to notify prescriber if infection occurs.

! **WARNING** Instruct patient to inspect skin regularly for abnormalities and report any such findings to prescriber. Tell patient to limit exposure to sunlight and ultraviolet light. Also, tell patient to wear protective clothing and use a sunscreen with a high protection factor.

! **WARNING** Tell patient, family, or caregiver to be alert for changes in patient's neurological status and to notify prescriber immediately if changes are observed.

! **WARNING** Inform females of childbearing age of the possibility of fetal harm with drug therapy; instruct them to use effective contraception throughout therapy and for 10 days after drug is discontinued. Stress importance of reporting pregnancy to prescriber immediately.

- Stress importance of having regular eye examinations during siponimod therapy and tell patient to report any visual changes to prescriber immediately.
- Advise patient to contact prescriber if new-onset or worsening dyspnea occurs.
- Review signs and symptoms of liver dysfunction with patient and tell patient to contact prescriber if present.

! **WARNING** Tell patient to notify prescriber of any other persistent, serious, or unusual adverse reactions.

- Tell patient that upon discontinuation of drug, a rebound effect may occur, exhibited by an exacerbation of the condition.
- Advise patient that drug effects last for up to 4 weeks after drug is discontinued.

sirolimus
(rapamycin)
Rapamune

Class and Category
Pharmacologic class: Macrocyclic lactone
Therapeutic class: Immunosuppressant

Indications and Dosages
✱ *To prevent rejection of kidney transplantation*

ORAL SOLUTION, TABLETS

Adults at high-immunologic risk. *Initial:* Up to 15-mg loading dose on day 1 post-transplantation. *Maintenance:* 5 mg daily beginning on day 2, with dosage adjusted based on trough level taken between days 5 and 7, as needed, with further adjustments made, as needed, every 7 to 14 days. *Maximum:* 40 mg daily.
Adults and adolescents weighing 40 kg (88 lb) or more at low- to moderate-immunologic risk. *Initial:* 6-mg loading dose. *Maintenance:* 2 mg daily, with dosage adjusted according to trough levels, every 7 to 14 days, as needed. *Maximum:* 40 mg daily.
Adolescents weighing less than 40 kg (88 lb) at low- to moderate-immunologic risk. *Initial:* 3-mg/m^2 loading dose. *Maintenance:* 1 mg/m^2 daily.

✱ *To treat lymphangioleiomyomatosis*

ORAL SOLUTION, TABLETS

Adults. 2 mg daily, dosage adjusted according to trough level 10 to 20 days later, then every 7 to 14 days, as needed, until a stable maintenance dose achieved.

± **DOSAGE ADJUSTMENT** For patients with mild-to-moderate impaired hepatic function, maintenance dosage adjustment reduced by one-third; for patients with severe impaired hepatic function, maintenance dosage adjustment reduced by one-half. For patients discontinuing concomitant cyclosporine therapy, maintenance dosage increased.

Drug Administration
P.O.

- Give initial dose as soon after transplantation as possible, as ordered, and daily dose 4 hr after cyclosporine, as ordered.
- Administer drug consistently either with or without food to prevent changes in absorption rate. However, do not administer with grapefruit juice.
- Tablets should be swallowed whole and not chewed, crushed, or divided.
- If oral suspension is stored in refrigerator, a slight haze may be present. If so, bring solution to room temperature and then shake gently until haze disappears. Use only the amber oral dose syringe supplied to withdraw prescribed amount of drug from bottle after fitting the oral syringe adapter to the neck of drug bottle. Mix oral solution with at least 2 ounces (60 ml) of orange juice or water in a glass or plastic container but not Styrofoam. Don't dilute drug in grapefruit juice or any other liquid. Stir vigorously and have patient drink solution immediately. Then, rinse glass with at least 4 ounces (120 ml) of additional liquid, stir vigorously, and have patient drink that liquid to make sure that all of drug is taken.
- Oral solution is usually stored in refrigerator but may be left at room

temperature for no more than 15 days; if stored in oral amber syringe, it may be stored at room temperature for 24 hr.
- Discard oral solution after 1 mo.
- When storing tablets or oral solution, protect from light.
- Avoid direct contact with skin or mucous membranes; if it occurs, wash area thoroughly with soap and water; rinse eyes with plain water.

Route	Onset	Peak	Duration
P.O.	Unknown	1–6 hr	Unknown

Half-life: 46–78 hr

Mechanism of Action

Inhibits activation and proliferation of T-lymphocytes and antibody production. Inhibits cell cycle progression from the G_1 to the S phase also, possibly by inhibiting a key regulatory kinase believed to suppress cytokine-driven T-cell proliferation. Interferes with the body rejecting the transplanted kidney and abnormal growth of muscle-like cells that occur in lymphangioleiomyomatosis as a result of these actions.

Contraindications

Hypersensitivity to sirolimus or its components, malignancy

Interactions

DRUGS

cannabidiol; cyclosporine; strong CYP3A4 and P-gp inhibitors, such as clarithromycin, erythromycin, itraconazole, ketoconazole, telithromycin, voriconazole; weak or moderate CYP3A4 and P-gp inhibitors, such as bromocriptine, cimetidine, cisapride, clotrimazole, danazol, diltiazem, fluconazole, letermovir, metoclopramide, nicardipine; protease inhibitors such as boceprevir, indinavir, ritonavir, telaprevir, troleandomycin: Increased sirolimus concentrations, increasing risk of adverse reactions

strong CYP3A4 and P-gp inducers, such as rifabutin, rifampin; weak to moderate CYP3A4 and P-gp inducers, such as carbamazepine, phenobarbital, phenytoin, rifapentine, St. John's wort: Decreased sirolimus concentrations, decreasing effectiveness

live vaccines: Vaccination may be less effective

verapamil: Increased concentrations of verapamil and sirolimus

FOODS

grapefruit juice: Possibly decreased metabolism of sirolimus

Adverse Reactions

CNS: Asthenia, dizziness, fever, headache, insomnia, **posterior reversible encephalopathy syndrome**, **progressive multifocal leukoencephalopathy (PML)**, tremor

CV: **Atrial fibrillation**, chest pain, **deep vein thrombosis**, hyperlipidemia, hypersensitivity vasculitis, hypertension, hypertriglyceridemia, **pericardial effusion**, peripheral edema, **tachycardia**

EENT: **Epistaxis**, **nasopharyngitis**, **stomatitis**

ENDO: Hyperglycemia

GI: Abdominal pain, ascites, constipation, diarrhea, elevated liver enzymes, **hepatic artery thrombosis** (liver transplant), **hepatotoxicity**, nausea, **pancreatitis**, vomiting

GU: Azoospermia, BK viral nephritis, elevated serum creatinine level, focal segmental glomerulosclerosis, **hemolytic uremic syndrome**, menstrual disorders, **nephrotic syndrome**, ovarian cysts, proteinuria, **pyelonephritis**, UTI

HEME: Anemia, **leukopenia**, **neutropenia**, **pancytopenia**, **thrombocytopenia**, **thrombocytopenic purpura**

MS: Arthralgia, bone necrosis, low back or flank pain, joint abnormality, myalgia

RESP: Alveolar proteinosis, **bronchial anastomotic dehiscence** (lymphangioleiomyomatosis after lung transplant), dyspnea on exertion, **interstitial lung disease**, pleural effusion, pneumonia, **pulmonary embolism or hemorrhage**, upper respiratory tract infection

SKIN: Acne, **cancer**, **including melanoma and Merkel cell carcinoma**, **exfoliative dermatitis**, rash

Other: **Anaphylaxis**; **angioedema**; cytomegalovirus; delayed wound healing; Epstein-Barr virus; herpes simplex or zoster; **hypokalemia**; **hypophosphatemia**; increased susceptibility to infection, including opportunistic infections such as tuberculosis and activation of latent viral infections;

lymphedema; lymphocele; **lymphoma**; **sepsis**; weight gain or loss

Childbearing Considerations

PREGNANCY

- Drug can cause fetal harm.
- Drug should be discontinued immediately when pregnancy is known.

LACTATION

- It is not known if drug is present in breast milk but due to drug's mechanism of action it may cause serious adverse effects in breastfed infants.
- A decision should be made to discontinue breastfeeding or the drug to avoid potential serious adverse reactions in the breastfed infant.

REPRODUCTION

- Females of childbearing age should use effective contraception throughout drug therapy and for 12 wk after drug has been discontinued.
- Both female and male fertility may be affected by drug use; females may develop menstrual disorders (including amenorrhea and menorrhagia) and ovarian cysts and males may develop azoospermia.

Nursing Considerations

! WARNING Be aware that sirolimus isn't recommended in liver or lung transplant patients.

- Know that when using trough level to determine drug's effectiveness, dosage adjustment should be made only after other factors are taken into account, such as signs, symptoms, and tissue biopsy findings. Keep in mind that interpretation methods vary among laboratories and values aren't interchangeable.
- Monitor whole blood sirolimus concentrations, as ordered, in patients receiving concentrated form of drug, patients with hepatic impairment, patients weighing less than 40 kg (88 lb), and those receiving potent CYP3A4 inducers or inhibitors concurrently.

! WARNING Monitor patient for a hypersensitivity reaction, which could become life-threatening such as anaphylaxis or angioedema. If present, notify prescriber, expect drug to be switched to a different drug, and provide supportive care, as needed and ordered.

! WARNING Monitor serum creatinine level, as ordered, because BK virus-associated nephropathy has occurred with sirolimus therapy. In addition, patients receiving sirolimus and cyclosporine may develop impaired renal function. Notify prescriber of any increases in serum creatinine level because sirolimus or cyclosporine dosage may have to be adjusted or drug discontinued. Monitor patients who are receiving other drugs known to adversely affect renal function, such as aminoglycosides and amphotericin B; together, they may further decrease renal function. Expect to monitor patient's urinary excretion, as ordered. If protein appears in urine, notify prescriber as sirolimus may need to be discontinued.

! WARNING Monitor patient for signs and symptoms of infection and check CBC results, as ordered, to detect sirolimus-induced blood dyscrasias or changes in neutrophil count, which may indicate infection. Monitor patients with recent exposure to chickenpox or measles. If infection develops, notify prescriber immediately and monitor patient for worsening symptoms because they have an increased risk of developing severe generalized disease while taking sirolimus.

! WARNING Monitor patient's skin for changes because sirolimus may cause skin cancer or life-threatening exfoliative dermatitis.

- Monitor patients with wounds who are taking sirolimus because drug may impair or delay wound healing, especially in patients with a body mass index greater than 30 kg/m^2.
- Explain to a patient with hyperlipidemia the potential need to institute dietary changes, an exercise program, and a lipid-lowering drug regimen if blood cholesterol or triglyceride levels increase because drug may aggravate hyperlipidemia.

! WARNING Monitor patient for other persistent, serious, or unusual adverse reactions because drug can affect many body systems and may cause some reactions that could become life-threatening, such as electrolyte imbalances, pancreatitis, or sepsis.

PATIENT TEACHING

- Instruct patient how to administer form of sirolimus prescribed.

! **WARNING** Warn patient not to take drug with grapefruit juice.

- Instruct patient not to receive live vaccines during sirolimus therapy.

! **WARNING** Alert patient that drug may cause an allergic reaction. If present, tell patient to notify prescriber and, if severe, to seek immediate medical care.

! **WARNING** Review signs and symptoms of infection and infection control measures to take during sirolimus therapy. Urge patient to avoid people with colds, flu, or other infections because immunosuppression makes him more vulnerable. Tell patient to notify prescriber immediately if exposed to chicken pox or measles.

! **WARNING** Inform patient that sirolimus therapy may increase risk of skin cancer. Tell patient to avoid prolonged sun exposure, sun lamps, and tanning booths. He should use a sunscreen with a high protection factor and wear protective clothing when outdoors. Advise patient to have regular skin examinations done and to notify prescriber immediately if he notices any skin changes.

! **WARNING** Instruct patient to alert prescriber if other persistent, serious, or unusual adverse reactions occur.

- Tell patient to inform all prescribers of sirolimus therapy because sirolimus interacts with many drugs, including over-the-counter drugs.
- Advise females of childbearing age that sirolimus may be harmful to unborn child. Stress importance of using an effective contraceptive before therapy starts, throughout therapy, and for 12 weeks after therapy is ended. If pregnancy does occur, instruct patient to notify prescriber immediately.
- Inform mothers breastfeeding should not be undertaking during sirolimus therapy or drug will need to be discontinued.
- Advise patient to keep follow-up appointments for blood tests, as ordered.

sitagliptin phosphate

Januvia, Zituvio

Class and Category

Pharmacologic class: Dipeptidyl peptidase-4 (DPP-4) inhibitor
Therapeutic class: Antidiabetic

Indications and Dosages

* *As adjunct to achieve control of glucose level in type 2 diabetes mellitus*

TABLETS

Adults. 100 mg once daily.

± **DOSAGE ADJUSTMENT** For patients with moderate renal insufficiency (eGFR of 30 ml/min to less than 45 ml/min), dosage reduced to 50 mg once daily; for patients with severe renal insufficiency (eGFR less than 30 ml/min) or end-stage renal disease requiring hemodialysis or peritoneal dialysis, dosage reduced to 25 mg once daily.

Drug Administration

P.O.

- Administer tablets at about same time daily to maintain consistency.
- Can be given with or without food.
- Tablets should be swallowed whole and not chewed, crushed, or divided.

Route	Onset	Peak	Duration
P.O.	Unknown	1–4 hr	Unknown

Half-life: 12.4 hr

Mechanism of Action

Inhibits the dipeptidyl peptidase-4 enzyme to slow inactivation of incretin hormones, which are released by the intestine throughout the day but increase in response to a meal to increase insulin synthesis and release from pancreatic beta cells. Be aware that one type of incretin hormone, glucagon-like peptide (GLP-1), also lowers glucagon secretion from pancreatic alpha cells, which reduces hepatic glucose production. Decreased blood glucose level in type 2 diabetes results from these combined actions.

Contraindications

Hypersensitivity to sitagliptin or its components

Interactions

DRUGS

digoxin: Slightly increased plasma digoxin level

insulin or insulin secretagogue, such as sulfonylureas: Possibly increased hypoglycemic effects

Adverse Reactions

CNS: Headache

CV: **Heart failure**

EENT: Mouth ulceration, nasopharyngitis, stomatitis

GI: Abdominal pain; **acute pancreatitis**, including **necrotizing** and non-fatal hemorrhagic; constipation; diarrhea; elevated liver enzymes; nausea, vomiting

GU: **Acute renal failure**, tubulointerstitial nephritis, worsening renal function

RESP: Upper respiratory tract infection

MS: Arthralgia (disabling, severe), back or extremity pain, myalgia, **rhabdomyolysis**

SKIN: Bullous pemphigoid, cutaneous vasculitis, pruritus, rash, **Stevens-Johnson syndrome**, urticaria

Other: **Anaphylaxis**, **angioedema**

Childbearing Considerations

PREGNANCY

- Pregnancy exposure registry: 1-800-986-8999.
- It is not known if drug can cause fetal harm.
- Use with caution only if benefit to mother outweighs potential risk to fetus.

LACTATION

- It is not known if drug is present in breast milk.
- Mothers should check with prescriber before breastfeeding.

Nursing Considerations

! **WARNING** Assess patient's renal function before starting sitagliptin therapy, as ordered, and periodically thereafter as drug may cause acute renal failure. In moderate to severe renal dysfunction, expect dosage to be reduced and frequency of assessing renal function increased. Also, know that renal function should be assessed more frequently in elderly patients because aging can be associated with reduced renal function.

- Monitor patient's blood glucose level, as ordered, to determine effectiveness of sitagliptin therapy.

! **WARNING** Monitor patient for a hypersensitivity reaction, which could become life-threatening, such as anaphylaxis or angioedema. If present, notify prescriber, expect sitagliptin to be discontinued, and provide supportive care, as needed and ordered.

! **WARNING** Be aware that heart failure has occurred with 2 other drugs in the same class as sitagliptin. Monitor patient for signs and symptoms of heart failure and if present report immediately to prescriber; provide care according to standard protocols, as ordered; and know that sitagliptin may have to be discontinued.

! **WARNING** Monitor patient for hypoglycemia if drug is used in combination with insulin or insulin secretagogues, such as sulfonylureas.

! **WARNING** Monitor patient for other persistent, serious, or unusual adverse reactions because drug can affect many body systems and has the potential to cause life-threatening adverse reactions, such pancreatitis, rhabdomyolysis, or Stevens-Johnson syndrome.

PATIENT TEACHING

- Instruct patient how to administer sitagliptin.
- Emphasize the need to follow diet control and exercise programs during sitagliptin therapy.
- Teach patient how to monitor blood glucose level and when to report changes. Inform patient that periodic blood tests will be done to determine effectiveness of drug such as a fasting blood glucose and glycosylated hemoglobin and to

assess kidney function. Urge patient to be compliant with laboratory appointments.

! **WARNING** Alert patient that drug may cause an allergic reaction. If present, tell patient to notify prescriber and, if severe, to seek immediate medical care.

! **WARNING** Review signs and symptoms of heart failure, such as rapid weight increase, shortness of breath, or swelling in feet. Instruct patient to immediately report such to prescriber.

! **WARNING** Instruct patient to stop taking sitagliptin and report persistent, severe abdominal pain, possibly radiating to the back and accompanied by vomiting.

! **WARNING** Alert patient also taking insulin or insulin secretagogues, such as a sulfonylurea, that hypoglycemia may occur. Instruct patient how to recognize and treat hypoglycemia and to notify prescriber if it occurs.

! **WARNING** Tell patient to notify prescriber immediately if other persistent, serious, or unusual adverse reactions occur.

- Instruct patient to contact prescriber if he develops other illnesses, such as infection, or experiences surgery or trauma because his diabetes medication may require adjustment.
- Advise patient to carry identification indicating that she has diabetes.

sodium ferric gluconate complex

(contains 62.5 mg elemental iron per 5 ml)
Ferrlecit

Class and Category

Pharmacologic class: Iron salt, mineral
Therapeutic class: Hematinic

Indications and Dosages

✶ *To treat iron deficiency anemia in patients receiving hemodialysis and supplemental epoetin therapy*

I.V. INFUSION OR INJECTION

Adults. 10 ml (125 mg of elemental iron) infused over 1 hr per dialysis session. I.V. injection given undiluted slowly at a rate of up to 12.5 mg/min for each dialysis session. *Maximum:* 125 mg per dose. *Usual:* Minimum cumulative dose of 1-g elemental iron given over 8 sequential dialysis treatments. Dosage repeated at lowest dosage needed to maintain target levels of hemoglobin and hematocrit and acceptable limits of blood iron level.

I.V. INFUSION

Children ages 6 and older. 0.12 ml/kg (1.5 mg/kg of elemental iron) infused over 1 hr per dialysis session. *Maximum:* 125 mg per dose.

Drug Administration

I.V.

- For I.V. injection for adults, administer undiluted slowly at a rate of up to 12.5 mg/min per dialysis session.
- For I.V. infusion in adults, dilute in 100 ml of 0.9% Sodium Chloride Injection and infuse immediately over 1 hr per dialysis session.
- For I.V. infusion in children, dilute in 25 ml of 0.9% Sodium Chloride Injection and infuse immediately over 1 hr.
- *Incompatibilities:* Other I.V. drugs or solutions (other than 0.9% Sodium Chloride Injection), parenteral nutrition

Route	Onset	Peak	Duration
I.V.	Unknown	Varies	Unknown

Half-life: 1 hr

Mechanism of Action

Acts to replenish iron stores lost during hemodialysis as a result of increased blood loss or increased iron utilization from epoetin therapy. Normalizes RBC production also by binding with hemoglobin or being stored as ferritin in reticuloendothelial cells of the bone marrow, liver, and spleen.

Contraindications

Hypersensitivity to sodium ferric gluconate or its components

Interactions

DRUGS

oral iron preparations: Possibly reduced absorption of oral iron supplements

Adverse Reactions

CNS: Asthenia, dizziness, fatigue, fever, headache, hypertonia, hypoesthesia, loss of consciousness, nervousness, paresthesia, **seizures**, syncope
CV: **Acute myocardial ischemia (with in-stent thrombosis)**, chest pain, generalized edema, hypertension, **hypotension**, phlebitis, **shock**, tachycardia
EENT: Dry mouth, taste altered
GI: Abdominal pain, diarrhea, nausea, vomiting
HEME: **Hemorrhage**
MS: Back pain, leg cramps
RESP: Cough, dyspnea, upper respiratory tract infection, wheezing
SKIN: Diaphoresis, discoloration, pallor, pruritus, skin discoloration
Other: **Anaphylaxis and other hypersensitivity reactions**, generalized pain, **hyperkalemia**, infusion or injection-site reaction, including superficial thrombophlebitis, **shock**

Childbearing Considerations

PREGNANCY

- Drug can cause fetal harm under certain circumstances, especially in the second and third trimesters. For instance, drug may cause circulatory failure in mother, which in turn causes bradycardia in the fetus.
- Be aware that drug also contains benzyl alcohol, which does not appear to have an effect on fetus through maternal drug administration; however, even though it is not given to neonates and infants, if it were it can cause serious adverse events and death when administered intravenously.

LACTATION

- It is not known if drug is present in breast milk. However, benzyl alcohol is possibly present in breast milk and may be transferred to neonate during breastfeeding.
- Alternative iron replacement therapies without benzyl alcohol recommended for mothers who are breastfeeding.

Nursing Considerations

- Expect to monitor blood hemoglobin level, hematocrit, serum ferritin level, and transferrin saturation, as ordered, before, during, and after sodium ferric gluconate therapy. Make sure serum iron level is tested 48 hours after last dose. To prevent iron toxicity, notify prescriber and expect to end therapy if blood iron level is normal or elevated.

! **WARNING** Determine if patient has had any previous history of reactions to parenteral iron products before therapy begins. Monitor patient for a hypersensitivity reaction, which could become life-threatening, such as anaphylaxis. If present, notify prescriber immediately, expect drug to be discontinued, and provide supportive care, as needed and ordered.

- Be aware that most patients need a minimum cumulative dose of 1 g of elemental iron administered over eight sequential dialysis treatments.

! **WARNING** Assess blood pressure often after drug administration because hypotension may occur and may be related to infusion rate or total cumulative dose. Avoid rapid infusion and be prepared to provide I.V. fluids for volume expansion.

! **WARNING** Monitor patient for possible iron overload, characterized by bleeding in GI tract and lungs, decreased activity, pale conjunctivae, and sedation.

! **WARNING** Monitor patient for any other persistent, serious, or unusual adverse reactions and notify prescriber, if present.

PATIENT TEACHING

- Inform patient drug is given intravenously.
- Warn patient not to take any oral iron preparations during sodium ferric gluconate therapy without first consulting prescriber.

! **WARNING** Alert patient that drug may cause an allergic reaction. Tell patient to notify prescriber if an allergic reaction is present and to seek immediate medicare care, if severe.

! **WARNING** Advise patient to report any persistent, serious (such as chest pain), or unusual adverse reactions to prescriber.

- Tell females of childbearing age to notify prescriber if pregnancy occurs before second trimester occurs.

sodium zirconium cyclosilicate

Lokelma

Class and Category

Pharmacologic class: Potassium binder
Therapeutic class: Potassium reducer

Indications and Dosages

✱ *To treat hyperkalemia in nonlife-threatening situations*

ORAL SUSPENSION

Adults. *Initial:* 10 g 3 times daily for up to 48 hr. *Maintenance:* 10 g once daily. Dosage increased during maintenance in increments of 5 g at weekly or longer intervals, as needed, based on serum potassium. *Usual maintenance dosage range:* 5 g every other day to 15 g daily.

±**DOSAGE ADJUSTMENT** For patients on chronic hemodialysis, initial dose reduced to 5 mg once daily on nondialysis days. Initial dose of 10 mg on nondialysis days may be given if patient's serum potassium level is greater than 6.5 mEq/L. Usual maintenance dose range is 5 to 15 mg once daily, on nondialysis days.

Drug Administration

P.O.

- Empty entire contents of packet(s) into a drinking glass containing about 3 tablespoons of water or more if patient desires. Stir well and administer immediately. If powder remains in the drinking glass, add more water, stir, and have patient drink immediately. Repeat until no powder remains, to ensure that entire dose has been given.
- Administer other oral drugs at least 2 hr before or after sodium zirconium cyclosilicate.

Route	Onset	Peak	Duration
P.O.	1 hr	1.2 hr	Unknown

Half-life: Unknown

Mechanism of Action

Increases fecal potassium excretion through binding of potassium in the lumen of the gastrointestinal tract to reduce the concentration of free potassium in the gastrointestinal lumen, thereby lowering serum potassium levels.

Contraindications

Hypersensitivity to sodium zirconium cyclosilicate or its components

Interactions

DRUGS

oral drugs that have pH-dependent solubility: Altered absorption of these drugs, possibly causing altered efficacy or safety

Adverse Reactions

CV: Edema
GI: Constipation
Other: **Hypokalemia**

Childbearing Considerations

PREGNANCY

- Drug is not absorbed systemically and is not expected to affect the fetus.

LACTATION

- Drug is not absorbed systemically and is not expected to be present in breast milk.

Nursing Considerations

! **WARNING** Know that sodium zirconium cyclosilicate should not be given to patients with abnormal postoperative bowel motility disorders, bowel impaction or obstruction, or severe constipation because drug may be ineffective or even worsen these GI conditions.

! **WARNING** Monitor patient for signs and symptoms of hypokalemia. If suspected, obtain laboratory confirmation, as ordered. Also monitor patients on hemodialysis for acute illnesses associated with decreased oral intake or diarrhea that can increase the risk of hypokalemia during drug therapy.

- Monitor patient for edema, especially patients who should restrict their sodium intake or are prone to fluid retention, such as those with heart failure or renal disease.
- Be aware that drug has radiopaque properties and may give the appearance of an imaging agent during abdominal X-ray procedures.

PATIENT TEACHING

- Instruct patient how to administer sodium zirconium cyclosilicate.

- Instruct patient to take other oral drugs at least 2 hours before or after sodium zirconium cyclosilicate administration, to prevent other drugs from not being absorbed properly.

! WARNING Review signs and symptoms of hypokalemia and notify prescriber immediately, if suspected. Tell patient to seek immediate medical care for confirmation and treatment, as needed.

- Advise patient to limit dietary sodium intake, as needed, and to notify prescriber if fluid retention occurs.
- Instruct patient to notify prescriber if an acute illness that restricts intake or causes diarrhea occurs, as dosage of drug may have to be adjusted.
- Tell patient to notify prescriber of sodium zirconium cyclosilicate use prior to an abdominal X-ray.

sofosbuvir

Sovaldi

Class and Category

Pharmacologic class: NS5B polymerase inhibitor
Therapeutic class: Antiviral

Indications and Dosages

∗ *As adjunct to treat chronic hepatitis C virus (HCV) infection in patients with genotype 1 or 4 who are without cirrhosis or who have compensated cirrhosis and used in combination with pegylated interferon and ribavirin*

TABLETS

Adults who are treatment-naïve. 400 mg once daily for 12 wk.

±**DOSAGE ADJUSTMENT** For patients with genotype 1 who are ineligible to receive an interferon-based regimen, concomitant drug therapy with ribavirin for 24 wks may be considered.

∗ *As adjunct to treat chronic hepatitis C virus (HCV) infection in patients with genotype 2 or 3 who are without cirrhosis or who have compensated cirrhosis and used in combination with ribavirin*

ORAL PELLETS, TABLETS

Adults and children ages 3 and older weighing at least 35 kg (77 lb). 400 mg once daily for 12 wk for genotype 2 and 24 wk for genotype 3.
Children ages 3 and older weighing 17 kg (37.4 lb) to less than 35 kg (77 lb). 200 mg once daily for 12 wk for genotype 2 and 24 wk for genotype 3.
Children ages 3 and older weighing less than 17 kg (37.4 lb). 150 mg once daily for 12 wk for genotype 2 and 24 wk for genotype 3.

∗ *As adjunct to treat chronic hepatitis C virus (HCV) infection in patients with hepatocellular carcinoma waiting for a liver transplant in combination with ribavirin*

TABLETS

Adults. 400 mg once daily for 48 wk or until liver transplant becomes available.

Drug Administration

P.O.

- Administer at about the same time daily to maintain consistency. Give with or without food.
- Oral pellet can be administered directly into mouth without chewing or with food. To administer with food at or below room temperature, sprinkle the pellets on one or more spoonfuls of nonacidic foods, such as chocolate syrup, ice cream, mashed potato, or pudding and gently mix.
- The mixture should be consumed within 30 min and not chewed to avoid a bitter aftertaste.

Route	Onset	Peak	Duration
P.O.	Unknown	0.5–2 hr	Unknown

Half-life: 0.4 hr

Mechanism of Action

Undergoes intracellular metabolism to form an active uridine analogue triphosphate, which is then incorporated into HCV RNA by the NS5B polymerase and acts as a chain terminator.

Contraindications

Hypersensitivity to sofosbuvir or its components

Interactions

DRUGS

amiodarone: Possibly development of serious symptomatic bradycardia *carbamazepine, oxcarbazepine, phenobarbital, phenytoin, rifabutin, rifampin, rifapentine, St. John's wort, tipranavir/ritonavir:* Possibly decreased sofosbuvir plasma concentration, leading to reduced effectiveness

Adverse Reactions

CNS: Asthenia, chills, depression (severe), fatigue, fever, headache, insomnia, irritability, **suicidal ideation**
GI: Anorexia, diarrhea, elevated pancreatic enzymes, hyperbilirubinemia, nausea
HEME: Anemia, **neutropenia**, **pancytopenia**, **thrombocytopenia**
MS: Elevated creatine kinase, myalgia
SKIN: Pruritus, rash (sometimes with blisters or angioedema-like swelling)
Other: **Angioedema**, flu-like symptoms

Childbearing Considerations

PREGNANCY

- It is not known if drug can cause fetal harm. However, because drug is given in combination with ribavirin or peginterferon alfa and ribavirin, drug combinations can cause fetal harm and are contraindicated in pregnant females and in men whose female partners are pregnant.
- Females of childbearing age and female partners of childbearing age of male patients must have a negative pregnancy test prior to drug therapy being initiated.

LACTATION

- It is not known if drug is present in breast milk.
- Breastfeeding is contraindication in mothers taking drug combinations with ribavirin or peginterferon alfa and ribavirin.

REPRODUCTION

- Be aware that females of childbearing age and female partners of childbearing age of male patients must use at least 2 effective methods of contraception during combination treatment and for at least 6 mo after drugs are discontinued.
- Females of childbearing age and female partners of childbearing age of male patients must undergo monthly pregnancy tests.

Nursing Considerations

! WARNING Ensure that females of childbearing age and partners of male patients of childbearing age have a negative pregnancy test before sofosbuvir therapy begins. Expect test to be repeated monthly.

! WARNING Ensure that all patients have been tested for current or prior hepatitis B virus (HBV) infection before sofosbuvir therapy begins because in patients coinfected with HBV and HCV there is risk of hepatitis B virus reactivation that may result in fulminant hepatitis, hepatic failure, or even death. If patient tests positive for HBV, monitor patient closely for clinical and laboratory signs, as ordered, of hepatitis flare or HBV reactivation during treatment with sofosbuvir and during posttreatment follow-up. Expect treatment for HBV infection to be given, as needed and ordered.

! WARNING Know that reducing the dosage of sofosbuvir or interrupting treatment should be avoided to prevent treatment failure. Also, be aware that if other drugs used in combination with sofosbuvir are discontinued, sofosbuvir should also be discontinued.

! WARNING Monitor patient for a hypersensitivity reaction, which could become life-threatening, such as angioedema. If present, notify prescriber, expect drug to be switched to another drug, and provide supportive care, as needed and ordered.

! WARNING Monitor patient for changes in mood and worsening depression as drug may cause suicidal ideation.

! WARNING Obtain a CBC analysis periodically during therapy, as ordered, because drug may cause serious to life-threatening hematological adverse reactions. Monitor patient for bleeding and infection.

! WARNING Monitor patient also receiving amiodarone with sofosbuvir for symptomatic bradycardia that may be severe enough to require pacemaker intervention. Be aware that bradycardia may occur up to 2 weeks after sofosbuvir therapy has begun. Patients at risk include those taking beta-blockers or those with underlying advanced liver disease or cardiac disorders. Expect patient to be hospitalized for cardiac monitoring for the first 48 hours of sofosbuvir therapy. Notify prescriber if bradycardia occurs and expect drug to be discontinued. Know that bradycardia generally disappears after drug is discontinued.

PATIENT TEACHING

- Instruct patient how to administer form of sofosbuvir prescribed.
- Tell patient to take sofosbuvir exactly as ordered and not to discontinue it without prescriber knowledge.

! **WARNING** Teach patient how to take a pulse and to report immediately a sudden decrease in pulse rate or signs and symptoms of serious bradycardia, such as chest pain, confusion, dizziness, excessive tiredness, fainting or near-fainting, malaise, memory problems, shortness of breath, or weakness.

! **WARNING** Alert patient that drug may cause an allergic reaction. If present, tell patient to notify prescriber and, if severe, to seek immediate medical care.

! **WARNING** Advise females of childbearing age and female partners of childbearing age of male patients to notify prescriber immediately if pregnancy occurs because the combination of drugs used with sofosbuvir therapy may cause fetal harm. If patient is also taking ribavirin with sofosbuvir, tell patient to use 2 reliable contraceptives during treatment and for at least 6 months after stopping ribavirin.

! **WARNING** Tell family or caregiver that drug may alter patient's mood and worsen depression to point of causing suicidal thoughts. If present, tell them to notify prescriber immediately and institute suicidal precautions until drug effects are gone.

! **WARNING** Review bleeding and infection control measues with patient. Tell him to notify prescriber if bruising, unexplained bleeding or infection occurs.

- Tell patient who is also taking amiodarone hospitalization for cardiac monitoring for the first 48 hours of sofosbuvir therapy will be needed.
- Tell patient to inform all prescribers of sofosbuvir therapy because drug reacts with many different drugs, which may cause reduced effectiveness or increased risk of adverse reactions.
- Tell mothers breastfeeding should not be undertaken during drug therapy.

solifenacin succinate

VESIcare, VESIcare LS

Class and Category

Pharmacologic class: Antimuscarinic
Therapeutic class: Bladder antispasmodic

Indications and Dosages

* *To treat overactive urinary bladder with symptoms of frequency, urge incontinence, and urgency*

TABLETS

Adults. 5 mg once daily; if tolerated well, increased to 10 mg daily.

± **DOSAGE ADJUSTMENT** For patients with severe renal impairment (creatinine clearance less than 30 ml/min) or moderate hepatic impairment or patients taking ketoconazole or other potent CYP3A4 inhibitors, dosage limited to 5 mg daily.

* *To treat neurogenic detrusor overactivity in pediatric patients*

ORAL SUSPENSION (VESICARE LS)

Children ages 2 and older weighing 60 kg (132 lb) or more. *Initial:* 5 ml (5 mg) once daily, increased, as needed. *Maximum:* 10 ml (10 mg) once daily.
Children ages 2 and older weighing more than 45 kg (121 lb) to 60 kg (132 lb). *Initial:* 4 ml (4 mg) once daily, increased, as needed. *Maximum:* 8 ml (8 mg) once daily.
Children ages 2 and older weighing more than 30 kg (66 lb) to 45 kg (121 lb). *Initial:* 3 ml (3 mg) once daily, increased, as needed. *Maximum:* 6 ml (6 mg) once daily.
Children ages 2 and older weighing more than 15 kg (33 lb) to 30 kg (66 lb). *Initial:* 3 ml (3 mg) once daily, increased, as needed. *Maximum:* 5 ml (5 mg) once daily.

Children ages 2 and older weighing 9 kg (19.8 lb) to 15 kg (33 lb). *Initial:* 2 ml (2 mg) once daily, increased, as needed. *Maximum:* 4 ml (4 mg) once daily.

± **DOSAGE ADJUSTMENT** For children with severe renal impairment (creatinine clearance less than 30 ml/min) or moderate hepatic impairment or patients taking ketoconazole or other potent CYP3A4 inhibitors and taking oral suspension, starting dose should not be exceeded.

Drug Administration

P.O.

- Tablets should be swallowed whole with a full glass of water and not chewed, crushed, or divided.
- Do not administer oral suspension at same time as with food or other drinks, as this may result in a bitter taste. Shake oral suspension well before using. Use a calibrated device to measure dosage. Follow administration with water or milk. Store at room temperature and discard after 28 days of first opening.
- If a tablet dose is missed, skip the dose and resume scheduled dosing the next day. If a dose of oral supension is missed, administer it as soon as possible, unless more than 12 hr have passed since the missed dose. If more than 12 hr have passed, missed dose is skipped and next dose taken at usual time.

Route	Onset	Peak	Duration
P.O.	Unknown	3–8 hr	Unknown

Half-life: 45–68 hr

Mechanism of Action

Antagonizes the effect of acetylcholine on muscarinic receptors in detrusor muscle, decreasing the muscle spasms that cause inappropriate bladder emptying, thereby resulting in increased bladder capacity and volume, which relieves the sensation of frequency and urgency and enhances bladder control.

Contraindications

Gastric retention, hypersensitivity to solifenacin or its components, uncontrolled angle-closure glaucoma, urine retention

Interactions

DRUGS

CYP3A4 inducers: Possibly decreased concentration of solifenacin and its effectiveness

ketoconazole, other potent CYP3A4 inhibitors: Increased serum concentrations of solifenacin and increased risk of adverse effects

Adverse Reactions

CNS: Confusion, delirium, depression, dizziness, fatigue, hallucinations, headache, somnolence

CV: **Atrial fibrillation**, hypertension, palpitations, peripheral edema, **prolonged QT interval**, tachycardia, **torsades de pointes**

EENT: Blurred vision, distortion of sense of taste, dry eyes or mouth, glaucoma, nasal dryness, pharyngitis, sialadenitis

GI: Abdominal pain, anorexia, **colonic or intestinal obstruction**, constipation, elevated liver enzymes, fecal impaction, gastroesophageal reflux disease, ileus, indigestion, nausea, vomiting

GU: Renal impairment, UTI, urinary retention

MS: Muscle weakness

RESP: **Airway obstruction from angioedema**, cough, dysphonia

SKIN: Dry skin, **erythema multiforme**, **exfoliative dermatitis**, pruritus, rash, urticaria

Other: **Anaphylaxis**, **angioedema**, flu-like symptoms, **hyperkalemia**

Childbearing Considerations

PREGNANCY

- It is not known if drug can cause fetal harm.
- Use with caution only if benefit to mother outweighs potential risk to fetus.

LACTATION

- It is not known if drug is present in breast milk.
- Mothers should check with prescriber before breastfeeding.

Nursing Considerations

- Use cautiously in patients with intestinal atony, myasthenia gravis, or ulcerative colitis because solifenacin may decrease

GI motility; in patients with significant bladder outflow obstruction because solifenacin may cause urine retention; in patients with hepatic impairment because solifenacin is metabolized in the liver; and in patients with renal impairment because solifenacin excretion may be impaired.

! **WARNING** Monitor patient closely, even after first dose, for a hypersensitivity reaction, which could become life-threatening, such as anaphylaxis or angioedema. Although uncommon, if a hypersensitivity reaction occurs, notify prescriber, expect drug to be discontinued, and provide supportive care, as needed and ordered.

- Monitor patient for signs of anticholinergic CNS adverse reactions, especially after treatment started or dosage increased.
- Monitor elderly patients, especially those ages 75 and older, for adverse reactions because they're at increased risk for solifenacin-induced adverse reactions.

! **WARNING** Monitor patient for other persistent, serious, or unusual adverse reactions such as cardiac arrhythmias or colonic or intestinal obstruction.

PATIENT TEACHING

- Instruct patient how to administer form of solifenacin prescribed and what to do if a dose is missed.
- Inform patient that alcohol may cause drowsiness. Urge patient to limit or avoid alcoholic beverages while taking solifenacin.

! **WARNING** Tell patient to report allergic reaction to prescriber; if serious, instruct patient to seek immediate medical care and stop taking drug.

! **WARNING** Caution patient to avoid exertion in a warm or hot environment because sweating may be delayed, which could increase body temperature and increase risk of heatstroke.

- Advise patient to avoid potentially hazardous activities until drug's CNS effects are known and resolved.

! **WARNING** Tell patient to notify prescriber if other persistent, serious, or unusual adverse reactions occur.

solriamfetol hydrochloride

Sunosi

Class, Category, and Schedule

Pharmacologic class: Dopamine and norepinephrine reuptake inhibitor
Therapeutic class: Analeptic
Controlled substance schedule: IV

Indications and Dosages

✱ *To improve wakefulness in patients with excessive daytime sleepiness associated with narcolepsy*

TABLETS

Adults. 75 mg once daily, increased after at least 3 days to 150 mg once daily, as needed. *Maximum:* 150 mg daily.

✱ *To improve wakefulness in patients with excessive daytime sleepiness associated with obstructive sleep apnea*

TABLETS

Adults. 37.5 mg once daily, then doubled at intervals of at least 3 days to maximum dose, as needed. *Maximum:* 150 mg daily.

± **DOSAGE ADJUSTMENT** For patients with moderate renal impairment (eGFR between 30 and 59 ml/min), initial dose reduced or kept at 37.5 mg once daily, with dose increased to a maximum of 75 mg once daily after at least 7 days. For patients with severe renal impairment (eGFR between 15 and 29 ml/min), dosage reduced or kept at 37.5 mg once daily with no titration.

Drug Administration

P.O.

- For patients taking a 37.5 mg dose, split a 75 mg tablet in half at the score line.
- Administer drug when patient wakes in morning. Avoid administering drug within 9 hr of planned sleep because drug may interfere with sleep if taken too late in the day.

Route	Onset	Peak	Duration
P.O.	Unknown	2 hr	9 hr

Half-life: 7.1 hr

Mechanism of Action

Thought to be related to its activity as a dopamine and norepinephrine reuptake inhibitor but precise mechanism of action is unknown.

Contraindications

Hypersensitivity to solriamfetol or its components, use within 14 days of MAO inhibitors

Interactions

DRUGS

dopaminergic drugs: Possibly altered pharmacodynamic effects
drugs that increase blood pressure: Increased risk of hypertension
MAO inhibitors: Increased risk of hypertensive crisis

Adverse Reactions

CNS: Agitation, anxiety, bruxism, disturbances in attention, dizziness, feeling jittery, headache, insomnia, irritability, panic attack, restlessness, thirst, tremor
CV: Chest discomfort or pain, hypertension, palpitations, tachycardia
EENT: Dry mouth
GI: Abdominal pain, anorexia, constipation, diarrhea, nausea, vomiting
RESP: Cough, dyspnea
SKIN: Erythematous rash, excessive diaphoresis, rash, urticaria
Other: **Hypersensitivity reactions**, weight loss

Childbearing Considerations

PREGNANCY

- Pregnancy exposure registry: 1-877-283-6220 or https://sunosipregnancyregistry.com/.
- It is not known if drug can cause fetal harm.
- Use with caution only if benefit to mother outweighs potential risk to fetus.

LACTATION

- It is not known if drug is present in breast milk.
- Mothers should check with prescriber before breastfeeding.
- If breastfeeding occurs, mother should monitor infant for agitation, anorexia, insomnia, and reduced weight gain.

Nursing Considerations

! WARNING Obtain patient's blood pressure prior to beginning solriamfetol therapy; blood pressure must be adequately controlled before drug is given, as hypertension increases risk of adverse cardiovascular events, including cardiovascular death, CVA, or MI. Monitor patient's blood pressure and heart rate throughout solriamfetol therapy. Notify prescriber if elevations occur. Expect new-onset hypertension or exacerbations of preexisting hypertension to be treated. Know that if patient experiences increase in blood pressure or heart rate that cannot be managed with a dosage reduction of drug or other appropriate measures, drug will likely be discontinued.

- Use solriamfetol cautiously in patients with risk factors for major adverse cardiovascular events, especially patients with known cardiovascular and cerebrovascular disease, preexisting hypertension, and patients with advanced age. Also, use caution if patient is taking other drugs that increase blood pressure and heart rate.
- Use solriamfetol cautiously in patients with bipolar disorders or psychosis. Be aware that patients with moderate or severe renal impairment may be at higher risk of psychiatric symptoms because of the prolonged half-life of the drug.

! WARNING Monitor patient for hypersensitivity reactions, such as erythematous rash, rash, and urticaria. If present, notify prescriber, expect drug to be discontinued, and provide supportive care, as needed and ordered.

- Monitor patient for possible emergence or exacerbation of psychiatric symptoms, such as anxiety, insomnia, and irritability, which may occur with solriamfetol therapy. If any occur, notify prescriber and expect dosage to be reduced or drug discontinued.

PATIENT TEACHING

- Instruct how to take solriamfetol.
- Instruct patient to avoid taking drug within 9 hours of planned sleep because drug

may interfere with sleep if taken too late in the day.

! **WARNING** Teach patient and family or caregiver how to take a blood pressure and pulse rate. Provide guidelines for when to call prescriber if elevated. Also, tell patient and family or caregiver to seek emergency care if signs or symptoms of a heart attack or stroke are present.

! **WARNING** Alert patient that drug may cause an allergic reaction, such as hives or a rash. If present, tell patient to notify prescriber. If severe, urge patient to seek immediate medical care.

- Inform patient that anxiety, insomnia, and irritability may occur with drug use. If troublesome, tell patient to discuss with prescriber.
- Tell mothers who are breastfeeding to monitor infant for agitation, anorexia, insomnia, and reduced weight gain.

sotagliflozin

Inpefa

Class and Category

Pharmacologic class: Dual sodium-glucose co-transporter 1 (SGLT1) and 2 (SGLT2) inhibitors

Therapeutic class: Cardiovascular support, heart failure agent

Indications and Dosages

∗ *To reduce risk of cardiovascular death, hospitalization for heart failure, and urgent heart failure visits in patients with heart failure or who have type 2 diabetes mellitus, chronic kidney disease, and other cardiovascular risk factors*

TABLET

Adults. 200 mg once daily and after 2 wk increased to 400 mg once daily, as tolerated.

Drug Administration

P.O.

- Administer not more than 1 hr before first meal of the day.
- Tablets should be swallowed whole and not chewed, crushed, or split.
- If dose is missed by more than 6 hr, administer next dose the following day.

Route	Onset	Peak	Duration
P.O.	Unknown.	2.5–4 hr	Unknown

Half-life: 5-10 hr

Mechanism of Action

Reduces intestinal absorption and renal reabsorption of glucose and sodium, which may lower both pre- and afterload of the heart. It also downregulates sympathetic activity. These actions help to reduce heart failure severity. The drug's role in reducing risk of cardiovascular death is unknown.

Contraindications

Hypersensitivity to sotagliflozin or its components

Interactions

DRUGS

digoxin: Increased exposure of digoxin increasing risk for digitalis toxicity

insulin, insulin secretagogues: Increased risk of hypoglycemia

lithium: Possibly decrease serum lithium concentrations reducing lithium effectiveness

uridine 5'-diphospho-glucoronosyltransferase (UGT) enzyme inducers such as rifampin: May significantly reduce sotagliflozin exposure decreasing sotaglitflozin effectiveness

FOODS

high-caloric meals: Increased sotagliflozin exposure increasing risk of adverse reactions

Adverse Reactions

CNS: Dizziness

ENDO: **Hypoglycemia, ketoacidosis**

GI: Diarrhea

GU: Decreased estimated glomerular filtration rate, elevated serum creatinine levels, genital mycotic infections, **necrotizing fasciitis of perineum (Fournier's gangrene)**, positive urine glucose tests, **pyelonephritis**, **urosepsis**, UTI

Other: **Volume depletion**

Childbearing Considerations

PREGNANCY

- Drug may cause adverse renal effects on developing fetus according to animal studies.
- Drug is not recommended for use during the second and third trimester of pregnancy.

LACTATION

- It is not known if drug is present in breast milk.
- Mothers should not breastfeed while taking drug because kidney maturation continues through the first 2 years of life.

Nursing Considerations

! **WARNING** Assess patient's volume status and correct, if needed and as prescribed, prior to starting sotagliflozin therapy because drug can cause intravascular volume contraction leading to symptomatic hypotension and acute kidney injury. Continue to monitor patient throughout therapy for dehydration and renal dysfunction. Obtain a serum creatinine level, as ordered, prior to starting drug and then periodically, as ordered. Patients at highest risk for intravascular volume contraction include the elderly and patients with chronic renal insufficiency, congestive heart failure, and hypovolemia or patients who take diuretics. Notify prescriber immediately if patient has fluid losses or reduced oral intake as acute kidney injury may occur. Expect drug to be temporarily withheld until fluid balance is restore.

! **WARNING** Monitor patient closely for ketoacidosis that have occurred in patients with diabetes taking sotagliflozin. Be aware that ketoacidosis can become life-threatening quickly even when blood glucose levels are less than 250 mg/dl. Expect to monitor ketones in patients with type 2 diabetes mellitus and in others at risk for ketoacidosis. Notify prescriber immediately if ketoacidosis is suspected and expect drug to be discontinued. Be prepared to treat patient's ketoacidosis, as ordered. Be aware that patients at higher risk include patients with a history of alcohol abuse or who have a pancreatic insulin deficiency from any cause or have reduced caloric intake. Expect drug to be temporarily discontinued if patient must undergo prolonged fasting due to acute illness or for at least 3 days prior to surgery.

! **WARNING** Be aware that patients receiving insulin or insulin secretagogues may require a lower dose of these agents because sotagliflozin used in combination increases the risk of hypoglycemia. Monitor patient closely for hypoglycemia. If present, treat according to institutional protocol and notify prescriber.

! **WARNING** Monitor patient for a rare but life-threatening necrotizing infection of the perineum called Fournier's gangrene. Notify prescriber immediately if patient develops erythema, pain, swelling or tenderness in the genital or perineal area, along with fever or malaise. Expect treatment with broad-spectrum antibiotics and, if needed, surgical debridement of the area. Expect sotagliflozin to be discontinued. and an alternative treatment for glycemic control.

- Monitor patients for genital mycotic infections or urinary tract infections, especially those with a history of such. If present, notify prescriber and treat, as ordered.
- Be aware sotagliflozin increases urinary glucose excretion and will lead to positive urine glucose tests. Use only blood tests to monitor glucose control. Also, know that measurements using 1,5-AG assay is not recommended because it is unreliable in the presence of SGLT2 inhibitors such as sotagliflozin. Other methods should be used to monitor the patient's glycemic control.

PATIENT TEACHING

- Instruct patient how to administer sotagliflozin and what to do if a dose is missed.

! **WARNING** Advise patient to maintain adequate fluid intake throughout sotagliflozin therapy. However, tell patient to notify prescriber if he is unable to take a normal amount of daily fluids due to fasting or illness or experiences an excessive loss of fluids from perspiration or gastrointestinal illnesses as drug may need to be temporarily withheld. Stress importance of paying attention to signs of dehydration and seeking medical attention quickly, if present.

! **WARNING** Review signs and symptoms of ketoacidosis with patient and urge him to seek immediate medical attention, if present, even if blood glucose level is less than 250 mg/dl. Teach patient how to check for ketones in urine, if appropriate.

! **WARNING** Educate patient also taking insulin or insulin secretagogues on the signs and symptoms of hypoglycemia and emergency treatment. Advise patient to notify prescriber if hypoglycemia occurs frequently or is severe.

- Tell patient to monitor blood glucose level using blood tests instead of urine tests because drug increases urinary glucose excretion and will lead to positive urine glucose tests.
- Advise female patients of childbearing age to notify prescriber if pregnancy occurs as the drug is not recommended during the second and third trimester of pregnancy.
- Alert mothers that breastfeeding should not be undertaken.

sotalol hydrochloride

Betapace, Betapace AF, Sorine, Sotacor (CAN), Sotylize

Class and Category

Pharmacologic class: Nonselective beta-blocker
Therapeutic class: Class III antiarrhythmic

Indications and Dosages

* *To treat life-threatening ventricular arrhythmias*

TABLETS, ORAL SOLUTION (SOTYLIZE)

Adults. *Initial:* 80 mg twice daily, increased, as needed, in increments of 80 mg every 3 days provided patient's QT interval is less than 500 msec. *Maintenance:* 160 to 320 mg daily in divided doses twice daily or 3 times daily. *Maximum:* 320 mg daily; 640 mg daily for refractory life-threatening arrhythmias.
Children ages 2 and older with normal renal function: *Initial:* 1.2 mg/kg 3 times daily; may be titrated up to maximum of 2.4 mg/kg 3 times daily allowing at least 36 hr between dose increments.

ORAL SOLUTION (SOTYLIZE)

Children under age 2 with normal renal functions. Highly individualized.

I.V. INFUSION (SOTALOL I.V.)

Adults. *Loading dose:* Highly individualized and dependent on the creatinine clearance and target oral dose. *Maintenance:* 75 mg when substituted for 80-mg oral dose; 112.5 mg when substituted for 120-mg oral dose; and 150 mg when substituted for 160-mg oral dose. Dosage frequency same as for oral dosage. Loading doses infused over 1 hr and maintenance doses infused over 5 hr.

* *To delay recurrence of atrial fibrillation and atrial flutter in patients currently in sinus rhythm*

TABLETS, ORAL SOLUTION (SOTYLIZE)

Adults. *Initial:* 80 mg twice daily, increased every 3 days in 80-mg increments daily provided QTc interval is less than 500 msec. *Usual:* 120 mg twice daily. *Maximum:* 320 mg daily.
Children ages 2 and older with normal renal function: *Initial:* 1.2 mg/kg 3 times daily; may be titrated up to maximum of 2.4 mg/kg 3 times daily allowing at least 36 hr between dosage increments.

I.V. INFUSION (SOTALOL I.V.)

Adults. *Loading dose:* Highly individualized and dependent on the creatinine clearance and target oral dose. *Maintenance:* 75 mg when substituted for 80-mg oral dose; 112.5 mg when substituted for 120-mg oral dose; and 150 mg when substituted for 160-mg oral dose. Dosage frequency same as for oral dosage. Loading doses infused over 1 hr and maintenance doses infused over 5 hr.

± **DOSAGE ADJUSTMENT** For adult patients with renal impairment, dosage reduced or dosage interval increased as follows: a creatinine clearance between 30 and 59 ml/min, oral dosage interval increased to every 24 hours; creatinine clearance between 10 and 29 ml/min, oral dosage interval increased to 36 or 48 hours; and if creatinine clearance is less than 10 ml/min, oral dosage individualized. For children with renal impairment, dosage reduced or dosage interval increased although specific adjustments hasn't been investigated.

Drug Administration

P.O.

- Administer consistently at the same time(s) daily.
- Give 2 hr before or after antacids containing aluminum oxide or magnesium hydroxide.

- Oral solution strength is 5 mg/ml. To administer an 80-mg dose, 16 ml are required; for 120-mg dose, 24 ml are required; for 160-mg dose, 32 ml are required; for 240-mg dose, 48 ml are required; and for a 320-mg dose, 64 ml are required.
- Use a calibrated device to measure oral solution dosage.
- Store drug at room temperature.

I.V.

- Dilute drug with 0.9% Sodium Chloride Injection, 5% Dextrose in Water, or Lactated Ringer's solution using a volume consistent with fluid restriction.
- Use a volumetric infusion pump for administration.
- Infuse loading dose over 1 hr and maintenance doses over 5 hr each.
- When storing drug at room temperature, protect from light.
- *Incompatibilities:* None reported by manufacturer

Route	Onset	Peak	Duration
P.O.	1–2 hr	2.5–4 hr	Unknown
I.V.	5–10 min	1 hr	Unknown

Half-life: 12 hr

Mechanism of Action

Combines class II and class III antiarrhythmic activity to increase sinus cycle length, decrease AV nodal conduction, and increase AV nodal refractoriness. Suppression of SA node automaticity and AV node conductivity decreases atrial and ventricular ectopy.

Contraindications

Acquired or congenital QT syndromes (QT interval greater than 450 ms); bronchial asthma or related bronchospastic conditions; cardiogenic shock; decompensated heart failure; hypersensitivity to sotalol or its components; second- or third-degree AV block, sick sinus syndrome, or sinus bradycardia (less than 50 beats/min) without functioning pacemaker; serum potassium less than 4 mEq/L

Interactions

DRUGS

antacids: Altered sotalol effectiveness
beta-agonists, such as albuterol, isoproterenol, terbutaline: Decreased effects of these drugs
calcium channel blockers: Additive effects on atrioventricular conduction or ventricular function resulting in bradycardia and hypotension
catecholamine-depleting agents, such as guanethidine, reserpine; negative chronotropes, such as beta-blockers, digitalis glycosides, diltiazem, verapamil: Possibly excessive reduction of resting sympathetic nervous tone resulting in marked bradycardia and/or hypotension causing syncope
class I and III antiarrhythmias; other drugs known to cause QT prolongation: Prolonged refractoriness possibly resulting in prolonged QT interval
clonidine: Increased risk of bradycardia; increased risk of rebound hypertension when clonidine discontinued
insulin, oral antidiabetic drugs: Impaired glucose control, increased risk of hyperglycemia, and masked hypoglycemia

Adverse Reactions

CNS: Anxiety, clouded sensorium (slight), depression, dizziness, drowsiness, emotional liability, fatigue, fever, headache, incoordination, insomnia, lethargy, nervousness, paralysis, weakness
CV: **AV conduction disorders**, **bradycardia**, **heart failure**, hyperlipidemia, **hypotension**, peripheral vascular insufficiency, **prolonged QT interval**, sinus arrest or pauses, **torsades de pointes**, **ventricular arrhythmias**
EENT: Nasal congestion
ENDO: Hyperglycemia, **hypoglycemia**
GI: Abdominal pain, constipation, diarrhea, nausea, vomiting
GU: Sexual dysfunction
HEME: Eosinophilia, **leukopenia**, **thrombocytopenia**
MS: Muscle weakness, myalgia
RESP: **Bronchospasm**, dyspnea, **pulmonary edema**, wheezing
SKIN: Alopecia, hyperhidrosis, photosensitivity, pruritus, rash, urticaria
Other: **Anaphylaxis**

Childbearing Considerations

PREGNANCY

- Drug may cause fetal harm, such as growth restriction, hyperbilirubinemia, hypoglycemia, increased risk of prolonged

QT interval, transient fetal bradycardia, and possible intrauterine death.
- Use with caution only if benefit to mother outweighs potential risk to fetus.
- Breakthrough arrhythmias, including ventricular tachycardia, are increased during pregnancy.

LABOR AND DELIVERY
- Risk of arrhythmias increases during labor and delivery requiring continuous monitoring.

LACTATION
- Drug is present in breast milk.
- Breastfeeding should not be done during drug therapy.

REPRODUCTION
- Drug may cause erectile dysfunction.

Nursing Considerations

! **WARNING** Know that sotalol as a beta-blocker should be avoided, if possible, in patients with bronchospastic disease. If sotalol is ordered, expect the smallest effective dose to be used.

! **WARNING** Expect to obtain baseline QT interval before starting sotalol and periodically throughout therapy, as ordered. This is because drug can cause life-threatening ventricular arrhythmias associated with QT interval prolongation. Know that if patient has been taking amiodarone and it is being discontinued, sotalol shouldn't be started until QT interval has returned to baseline because of possible adverse cardiac effects. Intravenous sotalol should not be initiated if the baseline QTc is longer than 450 ms. If QTc prolongs to 500 ms or greater, notify prescriber at once and expect dose to be reduced or drug discontinued. Be aware that sotalol-induced bradycardia increases the risk of torsades de pointes, especially after cardioversion, and may require emergency pacemaker insertion, especially in children.

! **WARNING** Be aware that stopping sotalol abruptly may cause life-threatening reactions, such as exacerbations of angina pectoris and MI. Expect to gradually reduce dosage over a period of 1 to 2 weeks, as ordered when discontinuing long-term sotalol therapy. For this reason, chronic beta-blocker therapy, such as sotalol, is not routinely withheld prior to major surgery. However, be aware that the impaired ability of the heart to respond to reflex adrenergic stimuli may increase the risks of general anesthesia and surgical procedures.

- Monitor apical and radial pulses, blood pressure, circulation in extremities, daily weight, fluid intake and output, and respiratory rate, before and during sotalol therapy.

! **WARNING** Monitor patient for a hypersensitivity reaction, which may become life-threatening, such as anaphylaxis. Know that a patient with a history of anaphylactic reaction to a variety of allergens may have a more severe reaction when taking sotalol and may be unresponsive to the usual doses of epinephrine used to treat the allergic reaction. If present, notify prescriber, expect drug to be switched to a different drug, and provide supportive care, as needed and ordered.

! **WARNING** Monitor patient for heart failure that can occur or worsen during initiation or titration of sotalol because of its beta-blocking effects.

! **WARNING** Monitor patient closely for hypoglycemia. Know that early warning signs of hypoglycemia, such as tachycardia may be prevented by sotalol therapy increasing risk for prolonged or severe hypoglycemia that can occur at any time, especially in children, patients with diabetes or patients who are fasting because of not eating regularly, having surgery, or vomiting. Notify prescriber if hypoglycemia occurs and treat according to institutional protocol.

! **WARNING** Monitor serum electrolyte levels because drug can increase risk of torsades de pointes in patients with electrolyte imbalances, especially hypokalemia or hypomagnesemia.

! **WARNING** Assess patient carefully for thyroid abnormalities because drug may mask certain clinical signs of hyperthyroidism. Avoid abrupt withdrawal of sotalol, which may cause an exacerbation of symptoms of hyperthyroidism, including thyroid storm.

- Be aware that falsely elevated levels of urinary metanephrine may occur during sotalol therapy when levels are measured by fluorimetric or photometric methods.

PATIENT TEACHING

- Instruct patient how to administer oral form of sotalol prescribed.

! **WARNING** Caution patient not to abruptly stop taking sotalol, as life-threatening effects may occur.

- Advise patient to take drug 2 hours before or after antacids containing aluminum oxide or magnesium hydroxide.

! **WARNING** Teach patient how to take a pulse and blood pressure and to weigh himself daily. Tell him to alert prescriber of any persistent and significant changes such as difficulty breathing or a slow or erratic pulse.

! **WARNING** Tell females of childbearing age to notify prescriber immediately if pregnancy occurs as drug may cause fetal harm. Also, tell patient to notify prescriber if pulse becomes irregular during pregnancy.

! **WARNING** Review signs and symptoms of hypoglycemia with patient. Teach him how to test his own blood glucose level because drug may mask early signs of hypoglycemia with the potential for prolonged or severe hypoglcyemia occurring. Also, review how to treat hypoglycemia and to seek immediate medical care if prolonged or severe. Advise patient to avoid fasting, if possible, but to alert prescriber if vomiting occurs or surgery is scheduled.

- Urge patient to avoid hazardous activities until drug's CNS effects are known and resolved.

! **WARNING** Tell patient to alert prescriber if any other persistent, serious, or unusual adverse reactions occur.

- Urge patient to consult prescriber before taking over-the-counter drugs, especially cold remedies, which may decrease sotalol's effectiveness.
- Advise mothers that breastfeeding should not be undertaken while taking sotalol.

spironolactone

Aldactone, CaroSpir

Class and Category

Pharmacologic class: Potassium-sparing diuretic
Therapeutic class: Diuretic

Indications and Dosages

* *As adjunct to increase survival, manage edema, and to reduce need for hospitalization for heart failure when used in addition to standard therapy in patients with severe heart failure (NYHA class III–IV) and reduced ejection fraction*

TABLETS (ALDACTONE)

Adults with serum potassium of 5.0 mEq/L or less and eGFR greater than 50 ml/min. *Initial:* 25 mg once daily. Dosage increased to 50 mg once daily, as needed.

ORAL SUSPENSION (CAROSPIR)

Adults with a serum potassium of 5.0 mEq/L or less and eGFR greater than 50 ml/min. *Initial:* 20 mg (4 ml) once daily, increased to 37.5 mg (7.5 ml) once daily, as needed.

± **DOSAGE ADJUSTMENT** For heart failure patients developing hyperkalemia while receiving a dose of 25 mg (tablet) or 20 mg (4 ml) (oral suspension) daily, dosage reduced to 25 mg (tablet) or 20 mg (4 ml) (oral suspension) every other day. For heart failure patients with an eGFR between 30 to 50 ml/min taking tablet form, initial dosage interval increased to every other day. For heart failure patients with an eGFR between 30 and 50 ml/min taking oral suspension, initial dosage reduced to 10 mg (2 ml) once daily.

* *As adjunct to treat hypertension*

TABLETS (ALDACTONE)

Adults. *Initial:* 25 to 100 mg daily as a single dose or in divided doses for at least 2 wk; gradually adjusted every 2 wk, as needed, if initial dose is less than 100 mg, to control blood pressure. *Maximum:* 100 mg daily.

ORAL SUSPENSION (CAROSPIR)

Adults. *Initial:* 20 mg (4 ml) to 75 mg (15 ml) daily as a single dose or in divided doses for at least 2 wk; gradually adjusted every 2 wk, as needed, if initial dose less than 75 mg (15 ml). *Maximum:* 75 mg (15 ml) daily.

∗ *To treat edema associated with nephrotic syndrome*

TABLETS (ALDACTONE)

Hospitalized adults. *Initial:* 100 mg daily as a single dose or in divided doses but may range from 25 mg to 200 mg. When given as the only agent for diuresis, dosage may be increased only after at least 5 days. *Maximum:* 200 mg daily.

∗ *To treat edema associated with hepatic cirrhosis*

ORAL SUSPENSION (CAROSPIR)

Hospitalized adults. *Initial:* 75 mg (15 ml) daily as a single dose or in divided doses, for at least 5 days before increasing dosage, as needed. *Maximum:* 100 mg (20 ml) daily.

TABLETS (ALDACTONE)

Hospitalized adults. *Initial:* 100 mg daily as a single dose or in divided doses but may range from 25 mg to 200 mg. When given as the only agent for diuresis, dosage may be increased only after at least 5 days. *Maximum:* 200 mg daily.

∗ *To treat primary hyperaldosteronism*

TABLETS (ALDACTONE)

Adults waiting for surgery. 100 to 400 mg daily.

Adults unable to have surgery. Highly individualized with lowest effective dosage given to manage condition.

Drug Administration

P.O.

- Administer drug with or without food but be consistent.
- Shake oral suspension well before use and use a calibrated device to measure dosage. Store at room temperature.
- Do not interchange oral suspension for tablet form, as the 2 formulations are not interchangeable.

Route	Onset	Peak	Duration
P.O.	2–4 hr	2.5–5 hr	2–3 days

Half-life: 1–2 hr

Contraindications

Addison's disease, concomitant use of eplerenone, hyperkalemia, hypersensitivity to spironolactone or its components

Interactions

DRUGS

abiraterone: Possibly increased prostate-specific antigen levels in presence of prostate cancer

ACE inhibitors, aldosterone blockers, angiotensin II antagonists, heparin and low-molecular-weight heparin, NSAIDs, other potassium-sparing diuretics, potassium-containing drugs, potassium supplements, trimethoprim: Increased risk of severe hyperkalemia

acetylsalicylic acid: Possibly reduced effectiveness of spironolactone

cholestyramine: Increased risk of hyperkalemic metabolic acidosis

CYP2C8 substrates (repaglinide), CYP3A substrates (midazolam, sirolimus, tacrolimus): Possibly increased exposure of these drugs

digoxin: Possibly increased half-life of digoxin, increasing exposure to digoxin

lithium: Possibly lithium toxicity

NSAIDs: Decreased antihypertensive effect of spironolactone

FOODS

high potassium diet, low-salt milk, salt substitutes: Increased risk of severe hyperkalemia

Adverse Reactions

CNS: Ataxia, confusion, dizziness, drowsiness, **encephalopathy**, fatigue, fever, headache, lethargy, somnolence

CV: **Hypotension**, vasculitis

EENT: Increased intraocular pressure, nasal congestion, tinnitus, vision changes

ENDO: Breast or nipple pain, gynecomastia, hyperglycemia

GI: Abdominal cramping or pain, anorexia, constipation, diarrhea, flatulence, **gastric bleeding** or ulceration, gastritis, **mixed cholestatic/hepatocellular toxicity**, nausea, vomiting

GU: Amenorrhea, decreased libido, impotence, irregular menses, postmenopausal bleeding, **renal failure**, worsening renal function

HEME: **Agranulocytosis**, **aplastic anemia**, **leukopenia**, **neutropenia**, **thrombocytopenia**

MS: Arthralgia, back and leg pain, leg cramps, muscle weakness, myalgia

RESP: Cough, dyspnea
SKIN: Alopecia, erythematous or maculopapular cutaneous eruptions, pruritus, **Stevens-Johnson syndrome**, **toxic epidermal necrolysis**, urticaria
Other: **Anaphylaxis**, dehydration, **drug reaction with eosinophilia and systemic symptoms (DRESS)**, **hyperkalemia**, hyperuricemia, **hypocalcemia**, **hypochloremic metabolic alkalosis**, **hypomagnesemia**, **hyponatremia**

Childbearing Considerations

PREGNANCY

- Drug may cause fetal harm affecting sex differentiation of the male fetus.
- Drug should be avoided in pregnant females.

LACTATION

- Drug is not present in breast milk, but an active metabolite has been found in breast milk.
- Mothers should check with prescriber before breastfeeding.

REPRODUCTION

- Females of childbearing age should use effective contraceptive measures throughout drug therapy.

Nursing Considerations

- Expect to evaluate patient's serum potassium level within 1 week after spironolactone therapy begins and regularly thereafter or as ordered. Notify prescriber if level exceeds 5 mEq/L or patient's renal function deteriorates (serum creatinine level exceeding 4 mg/dl).
- Evaluate spironolactone's effectiveness by assessing blood pressure and presence and degree of edema.

! WARNING Monitor patient for a hypersensitivity or severe skin reaction, which may become life-threatening such as anaphylaxis or DRESS. Be aware that DRESS may only initially present as a fever or swollen lymph nodes although rash is the most common sign. If present, notify prescriber, expect drug to be discontinued, and provide supportive care, as needed and ordered.

! WARNING Monitor patients for excessive diuresis, which may cause dehydration, hypotension, and worsening renal function, especially in patients who are salt-depleted or those taking ACE inhibitors or angiotensin II receptor blockers. Renal function may worsen if patient is also taking nephrotoxic

Mechanism of Action

Remember that normally aldosterone attaches to receptors on the walls of distal convoluted tubule cells, causing sodium (Na^+) and water (H_2O) reabsorption in the blood, as shown at left. Spironolactone competes with aldosterone for these receptors, thereby preventing sodium and water reabsorption and causing their excretion through the distal convoluted tubules, as shown below right. Increased urinary excretion of sodium and water reduces blood volume and blood pressure.

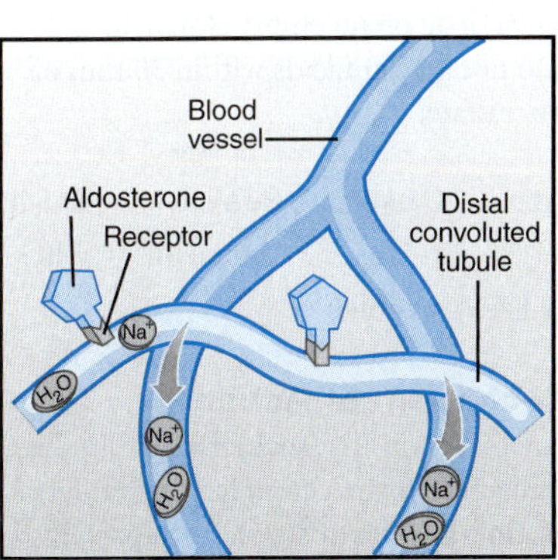

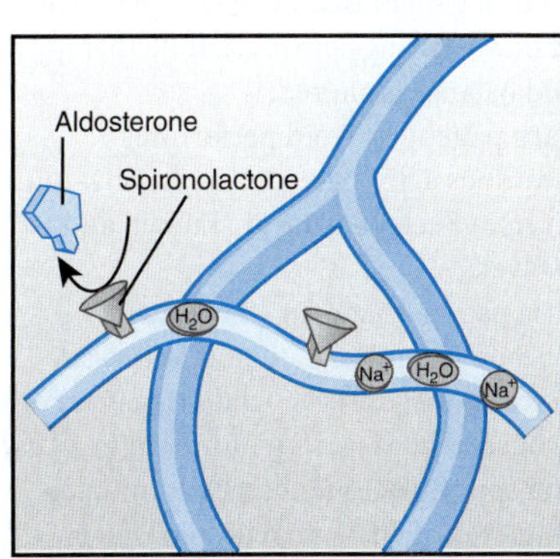

QRS

drugs such as aminoglycosides, cisplatin, and NSAIDs. Monitor patient's fluid status and renal function periodically, as ordered.

! **WARNING** Monitor patient for electrolyte and metabolic abnormalities such as hyperglycemia, hyperkalemia, hypocalcemia, hypochloremic alkalosis, hypomagnesemia, or hyponatremia. Know that hyperuricemia can also occur. Report any abnormalities to prescriber and expect to confirm with laboratory testing.

! **WARNING** Monitor patient for other persistent, serious, or unusual adverse reactions because some can be quite serious such as encephalopathy and hematological reactions.

PATIENT TEACHING

- Instruct patient how to administer form of spironolactone prescribed.
- Teach patient who takes spironolactone for hypertension how to measure his blood pressure. Urge patient to monitor it regularly and report a pressure that is consistently higher than normal.

! **WARNING** Alert patient that drug may cause an allergic or severe skin reaction. If a fever, rash, swollen lymph nodes,or other signs and symptoms of an allergic or skin reaction occurs, tell patient to notify prescriber and to seek immediate medical care.

! **WARNING** Review bleeding and infection control precautions with patient. Tell patient to alert prescriber if bruising, unexplained bleeding, or infection occurs.

- Caution patient that he may experience dizziness during spironolactone therapy if fluid balance is altered.
- Warn patient to avoid performing hazardous activities, such as driving, until adverse effects of drug are known and resolved.
- Alert patient that drug may cause gynecomastia. Tell patient that the risk increases in a dose-dependent manner with an onset that may occur 1 month to 1 year after spironolactone therapy is initiated. Reassure patient that gynecomastia is usually reversible.

! **WARNING** Tell patient to notify prescriber immediately if other persistent, serious, or unusual adverse reactions occur.

! **WARNING** Advise females of childbearing age to report pregnancy immediately to prescriber as drug will need to be discontinued. Encourage patient to use effective contraceptive measures throughout spironolactone therapy to avoid pregnancy.

- Instruct patient to inform prescriber of any new condition or new drug therapy, including over-the-counter medications, so that prescriber can evaluate if the patient is at increased risk for hyperkalemia.

sucralfate

Carafate

Class and Category

Pharmacologic class: GI protectant
Therapeutic class: Antiulcer

Indications and Dosages

∗ *To treat active duodenal ulcer*

ORAL SUSPENSION, TABLETS

Adults. 1 g (10 ml) 4 times daily for 4 to 8 wk, possibly less.

∗ *To prevent reoccurrence of duodenal ulcer*

TABLETS

Adults and adolescents. 1 g twice daily for up to 1 yr.

± **DOSAGE ADJUSTMENT** For elderly patients, dosage started at lower end of dosing range.

Drug Administration

P.O.

- Give drug on an empty stomach.
- Do not give antacids within 30 min of sucralfate.

Route	Onset	Peak	Duration
P.O.	1–2 hr	Unknown	6 hr

Half-life: Unknown

Mechanism of Action

May react with hydrochloric acid in the stomach to form a complex that buffers acid by adhering electrostatically to proteins on the ulcer's surface to create a protective barrier at the ulcer site. Inhibits back-diffusion of hydrogen ions and adsorbs bile acids and pepsin also to promote healing of an existing duodenal ulcer and prevent reoccurring ulcer formation.

Contraindications

Hypersensitivity to sucralfate or its components

Interactions

DRUGS

cimetidine, ciprofloxacin, digoxin, fluoroquinolone antibiotics, ketoconazole, l-thyroxine, phenytoin, quinidine, tetracycline, theophylline: Decreased bioavailability of these drugs

Adverse Reactions

CNS: Dizziness, drowsiness, headache, insomnia, lightneadedness, vertigo
EENT: Dry mouth
ENDO: Hyperglycemia
GI: Constipation, diarrhea, indigestion, nausea, vomiting
MS: Back pain
RESP: **Bronchospasm**, dyspnea
SKIN: Pruritus, rash, urticaria
Other: **Anaphylaxis**, **angioedema**

Childbearing Considerations

PREGNANCY

- It is not known if drug can cause fetal harm.
- Use with caution only if benefit to mother outweighs potential risk to fetus.

LACTATION

- It is not known if drug is present in breast milk.
- Mothers should check with prescriber before breastfeeding.

Nursing Considerations

! WARNING Monitor patient for a hypersensitivity reaction, which could become life-threatening, such as anaphylaxis or angioedema. If present, notify prescriber, expect drug to be discontinued, and provide supportive care, as needed and ordered.

! WARNING Watch patient carefully for bronchospasms after drug is administered.

! WARNING Monitor patients with chronic renal failure because of increased risk of aluminum toxicity.

- Monitor diabetic patient's blood glucose level closely because sucralfate may cause hyperglycemia significant enough to require an adjustment of antidiabetic drug therapy prescribed.

PATIENT TEACHING

- Instruct patient how to administer form of sucralfate prescribed.
- Caution patient not to take antacids within 30 minutes of taking sucralfate and to check with prescriber before taking any other drugs within 2 hours of sucralfate.

! WARNING Alert patient that drug may cause an allergic reaction. If present, tell patient to notify prescriber and, if severe, to seek immediate medical care.

! WARNING Tell patient to alert prescriber and seek immediate medical care if difficulty breathing occurs after taking drug. Stress importance of stopping sucralfate therapy.

! WARNING Review signs and symptoms of aluminium toxicity with patient who has chronic renal failure.

- Stress importance of diabetic patient monitoring blood glucose levels closely as drug may alter blood glucose control. If persistent changes occur, have patient notify prescriber.

sucroferric oxyhydroxide

Velphoro

Class and Category

Pharmacologic class: Polynuclear iron (III) oxyhydroxide
Therapeutic class: Phosphate binder

Indications and Dosages

∗ *To control serum phosphorus levels in patients with chronic kidney disease on dialysis*

CHEWABLE TABLETS

Adults and children ages 12 and older. *Initial:* 500 mg 3 times daily with meals, increasing or decreasing dosage in 500-mg increments weekly, as needed. *Usual maintenance:* 1,500 to 2,000 mg daily. *Maximum:* 3,000 mg daily.

Children ages 9 to 12. 500 mg twice daily with meals, increasing or decreasing dosage in 500-mg increments weekly, as needed. *Usual maintenance:* 1,500 daily. *Maximum:* 3,000 mg daily.

Drug Administration

P.O.

- Give drug with meals and administer all other oral drugs prescribed for patient at a different time because absorption of the other drugs may be affected.
- Chewable tablets must be chewed or crushed and not swallowed whole.
- Chewable tablets do not have to be taken with water or other liquid.
- Drug can stain teeth.
- If a dose is missed, skip the missed dose and resume regularly scheduled dosing regimen.

Route	Onset	Peak	Duration
P.O.	Unknown	Unknown	Unknown

Half-life: 6 hr

Mechanism of Action

Absorbs dietary phosphate in the GI tract and eliminates bound phosphate through feces, which prevents phosphate from being absorbed into the blood and thereby causing both calcium phosphorus product levels and serum phosphorus levels to decrease.

Contraindications

Hypersensitivity to sucroferric oxyhydroxide or its components

Interactions

DRUGS

acetylsalicylic acid, cephalexin, doxycycline, levothyroxine: Absorption of these drugs may be affected

Adverse Reactions

EENT: Abnormal drug distaste, tooth discoloration
GI: Dark-colored feces, diarrhea, nausea
SKIN: Rash

Childbearing Considerations

PREGNANCY

- Drug is not absorbed systemically and not expected to result in fetal exposure.

LACTATION

- Drug is not absorbed systemically and not expected to result in fetal exposure.

Nursing Considerations

- Monitor patient's serum phosphorus levels regularly, as ordered, to determine drug effectiveness and need for dosage adjustments.

> **! WARNING** Monitor patient for a hypersensitivity reaction exhibited by a rash. If present, notify prescriber and expect drug to be discontinued.

- Monitor patients who have a history of hemochromatosis or other diseases characterized by iron accumulation, patients who develop peritonitis during peritoneal dialysis, and patients with significant gastric or hepatic disorders or following major GI surgery because sucroferric oxyhydroxide effects on these conditions are not known.
- Be aware that drug can cause discolored stool possibly masking GI bleeding.

PATIENT TEACHING

- Instruct patient how to administer form of sucroferric oxyhydroxide prescribed and what to do if a dose is missed.
- Instruct patient to take any concomitant drug therapy at least 2 hours before sucroferric oxyhydroxide.

> **! WARNING** Alert patient that drug may cause an allergic reaction exhibited as a rash. Tell patient to report any rash to prescriber and to stop taking drug.

- Inform patient that drug may cause discolored (black) stool, but this effect is usually harmless. However, if patient experiences other GI signs and symptoms with the discolored stool, patient should notify prescriber. Inform patient that drug may also stain teeth.

sufentanil

Dsuvia

Class, Category, and Schedule

Pharmacologic class: Opioid agonist
Therapeutic class: Opioid analgesic
Controlled substance schedule: II

Indications and Dosages

✱ *To relieve acute pain in a hospital setting, which is severe enough to require an opioid analgesic and for which alternative treatments are inadequate in a medically supervised healthcare setting*

SUBLINGUAL TABLETS

Adults. 30 mcg, as needed, with a minimum of 1 hr between doses. *Maximum:* 360 mcg or 12 tablets in 24 hr, and not for use for more than 72 hr.

Drug Administration

P.O.

- Drug is a biohazard drug. Take appropriate precautions.
- Administered only in a hospital setting.
- If patient has a dry mouth, give patient ice chips prior to administering drug.
- Put on gloves and tear open the notched pouch only when ready to administer drug. Be aware that the pouch contains one clear plastic single-dose applicator (SDA) that houses a single, blue-colored tablet in the tip.
- Remove the white lock from the green pusher by squeezing the sides together and detaching from pusher. To avoid accidentally ejecting the tablet, avoid touching the green pusher before placing the SDA in patient's mouth for administration.
- To administer, tell patient to open mouth and touch the tongue to the roof of the mouth, if possible. Rest the SDA lightly on patient's lips or lower teeth. Place the SDA tip under the tongue and aim at the floor of patient's mouth or sublingual space. Avoid direct mucosal contact with the SDA tip. Gently depress the green pusher to deliver the tablet to patient's sublingual space.
- Tablet should be allowed to dissolve under the tongue and not chewed or swallowed.
- Visually confirm tablet placement. If tablet is not in patient's mouth, it must be retrieved and disposed of according to institutional CII waste procedures.
- Discard the used SDA in biohazard waste container after administration.
- Patient should not eat or drink, and should minimize talking, for 10 min after receiving drug.

Route	Onset	Peak	Duration
P.O.	> 10 min	1 hr	2.3–3.8 hr

Half-life: 164 min

Mechanism of Action

Binds to and activates selective mu-opioid receptors found throughout the central nervous system to produce pain relief.

Contraindications

Acute or severe bronchial asthma in an unmonitored setting or in the absence of resuscitative equipment; GI obstruction, including paralytic ileus; hypersensitivity to sufentanil or its components; significant respiratory depression

Interactions

DRUGS

5-HT$_3$ inhibitors (used to treat psychiatric disorders), linezolid, methylene blue (intravenous), selective serotonin reuptake inhibitors, serotonin and norepinephrine reuptake inhibitors, tricyclic antidepressants, triptans: Increased risk of serotonin syndrome

anticholinergic drugs: Possibly increased risk of urinary retention and/or severe constipation, which may lead to paralyticileus

benzodiazepines and other CNS depressants: Increased risk of serious adverse reactions, such as coma, hypotension, profound sedation, and severe respiratory depression

CYP3A4 inducers, such as carbamazepine, phenytoin, rifampin: Decreased plasma concentration of sufentanil, resulting in decreased efficacy or possible withdrawal symptoms in patients who have developed physical dependence to sufentanil

CYP3A4 inhibitors, such as azole-antifungal agents (ketoconazole), macrolide antibiotics (erythromycin), and protease inhibitors (ritonavir): Increased plasma concentration of sufentanil, resulting in increased or prolonged effects

diuretics: Reduced efficacy of diuretics

MAO inhibitors: Increased risk of serotonin syndrome; increased risk of opioid toxicity

mixed agonist/antagonist or partial agonist opioid analgesics, such as buprenorphine, butorphanol, nalbuphine, pentazocine: Possibly reduced analgesic effect of sufentanil and possible precipitation of withdrawal symptoms *muscle relaxants:* Possibly enhanced neuromuscular blocking action of skeletal muscle relaxants; increased degree of respiratory depression

ACTIVITIES

alcohol use: Increased risk of serious adverse reactions, such as coma, hypotension, profound sedation, and severe respiratory depression

Adverse Reactions

CNS: Agitation, anxiety, confusion, disorientation, dizziness, euphoric mood, hallucination, headache, hemiparesis, insomnia, lethargy, memory impairment, mental status changes, **seizures**, **serotonin syndrome**, somnolence, syncope
CV: **Bradycardia (severe)**, **electrocardiogram abnormalities**, hypertension, **hypotension (severe)**, orthostatic hypotension, tachycardia
EENT: Oral hypoesthesia
ENDO: **Adrenal insufficiency**
GI: Abdominal distention or pain, belching, constipation, diarrhea, dyspepsia, elevated liver enzymes or serum amylase levels, flatulence, gastritis, nausea, postoperative ileus, spasm of the sphincter of Oddi, vomiting
GU: Decreased urine output, oliguria, **renal failure**, urinary hesitation or retention
MS: Muscle spasms
RESP: **Apnea**, **atelectasis**, **bradypnea**, **decreased oxygen saturation and respiratory rate**, **hypoventilation**, **hypoxia**, **life-threatening respiratory depression**, **respiratory distress or failure**
SKIN: Diaphoresis, flushing, pruritus, rash
Other: **Anaphylaxis**, opioid-induced allodynia and hyperalgesia, physiological and physical dependence

Childbearing Considerations

PREGNANCY

- Drug may cause fetal harm.
- Prolonged use of drug during pregnancy can result in neonatal opioid withdrawal syndrome (NOWS), which may be life-threatening if not recognized and treated.
- Use with caution only if benefit to mother outweighs potential risk to fetus.

LABOR AND DELIVERY

- Drug is not recommended for use in pregnant females immediately before or during labor. Opioids may alter length of time of labor.
- Opioids cross the placenta and may produce respiratory depression and psychophysiologic effects in the neonate. Monitor neonate closely for signs of excess sedation and respiratory depression.
- An opioid antagonist, such as naloxone, must be available at the time of delivery in the event it is needed to reverse opioid-induced respiratory depression in the neonate.

LACTATION

- Drug is present in breast milk.
- Mothers should check with prescriber before resuming breastfeeding.
- Infants exposed to drug through breast milk should be monitored for excess sedation and respiratory depression.

REPRODUCTION

- Although drug is given for no more than 72 hr, be aware that chronic use of opioids may reduce fertility in females and males.

Nursing Considerations

! **WARNING** Be aware that excessive use of sufentanil may lead to abuse, addiction, misuse, overdose, and possibly death even in the short time sufentanil is given. Know that sufentanil is available only through a restricted Risk Evaluation and Mitigation Strategy (REMS) program. Monitor patient's intake of drug closely. Alert prescriber if patient has a history of dependence on other opioids.

! **WARNING** Use extreme caution when administering sufentanil to patients with significant chronic obstructive pulmonary disease or cor pulmonale, and to patients having a substantially decreased respiratory reserve, hypercapnia, hypoxia, or preexisting respiratory depression, especially when initiating or titrating therapy. These patients may develop respiratory depression, even with usual therapeutic doses because sufentanil may decrease patient's respiratory drive to the point of apnea.

- Use sufentanil cautiously in cachectic, debilitated, or elderly patients, especially when initiating and titrating therapy, as these patients are at increased risk for adverse effects, especially respiratory depression.

- Monitor effectiveness of sufentanil in relieving pain; consult prescriber as needed.
- Monitor patient for a paradoxic increase in pain known as opioid-induced hyperalgesia or an increase in sensitivity to pain known as opioid-induced allodynia, especially when sufentanil dosage increases. Do not confuse this with tolerance, which is the need for increasing doses of opioids to maintain an effect. If opioid-induced allodynia and hyperalgesia is suspected, notify prescriber and expect opioid rotation to be prescribed.

! WARNING Monitor patient for a hypersensitivity reaction, which could become life-threatening, such as anaphylaxis. If present, notify prescriber immediately, expect drug to be discontinued, and provide supportive care, as needed and ordered.

! WARNING Monitor patient for respiratory depression that could become life-threatening quickly, especially when drug is initiated or if patient is accidently exposed to drug. However, know that respiratory depression may occur at any time during sufentanil use and may occur even when used as recommended. If patient develops respiratory depression, expect to give naloxone.

! WARNING Monitor patient's vital signs closely. Know that in addition to respiratory depression, sufentanil may cause severe hypotension, especially in patients whose blood pressure is already compromised by a depleted blood volume or after concurrent administration of drugs that decrease blood pressure. Also, be aware that drug may cause bradycardia in some patients.

! WARNING Know that sufentanil may cause sleep-related disorders, including central sleep apnea and sleep-related hypoxemia increasing the risk in a dose-dependent fashion. If patient develops central sleep apnea, know that sufentanil dose may have to be decreased.

! WARNING Monitor patients closely who may be susceptible to the intracranial effects of carbon dioxide retention from respiratory depression caused by sufentanil therapy, such as patients with head injuries or those who have a preexisting elevation in intracranial pressure.

! WARNING Be aware that sufentanil may increase the frequency of seizures in patients with seizure disorders and may increase risk of seizures in the presence of other conditions associated with seizures. Monitor patient closely.

! WARNING Be aware that prolonged use of opioids like sufentanil should not be given to pregnant females immediately before labor and delivery, and while in labor as newborn may experience neonatal opioid withdrawal syndrome (NOWS). This syndrome may exhibit as excessive or high-pitched crying, poor feeding, rapid breathing, or trembling. If not recognized and treated appropriately, it can become life-threatening.

! WARNING Monitor patient for adrenal insufficiency. Although rare, it can be life-threatening. Monitor patient for anorexia, dizziness, fatigue, hypotension, nausea, vomiting, or weakness. Notify prescriber if adrenal insufficiency is suspected and expect diagnostic testing to be done. If diagnosis is confirmed, expect to administer corticosteroids and discontinue sufentanil.

- Monitor patient for decreased bowel motility in postoperative patients receiving sufentanil, as drug may obscure the development of acute abdominal conditions.
- Assess patient for constipation and provide a high-fiber diet and adequate fluid intake, if not contraindicated, because constipation can become severe.

! WARNING Notify prescriber if patient develops other persistent, serious, or unusual adverse reactions.

! WARNING Be aware that concomitant use with CYP3A4 inhibitors or discontinuation of CYP3A4 inducers can result in a fatal overdose of sufentanil.

! WARNING Be aware that sufentanil should only be used concomitantly with benzodiazepine therapy in patients for whom other treatment options are inadequate. If prescribed together, expect dosing and duration of sufentanil to be limited. Monitor patient closely for signs and symptoms of a decrease in consciousness, including coma, profound sedation, and significant respiratory depression. Notify prescriber immediately and provide emergency supportive care, as death may occur.

! **WARNING** Know that many drugs may interact with opioids like sufentanil to cause serotonin syndrome. Monitor patient closely for signs and symptoms, such as agitation, diaphoresis, diarrhea, fever, hallucinations, labile blood pressure, muscle twitching or stiffness, nausea, shakiness, shivering, tachycardia, trouble with coordination, or vomiting. Notify prescriber at once because serotonin syndrome may be life-threatening. Be prepared to discontinue drug, if possible and ordered, and provide supportive care.

PATIENT TEACHING

- Inform patient sufentanil will be administered by healthcare staff in a hospital setting.
- Advise patient not to drink or eat and to minimize talking for 10 minutes after each dose of the drug.

! **WARNING** Stress importance of requesting drug before pain is severe. Also, tell him not to take it longer than absolutely needed because excessive or prolonged use can lead to abuse, addiction, misuse, overdose, and possibly death. However, advise patient that if pain sensitivity develops despite drug use to alert staff.

! **WARNING** Caution patient to avoid having alcohol or other drugs brought to the healthcare setting because ingesting alcohol, including medications containing alcohol, increases the risk of overdose, respiratory depression, and death, as does taking other types of depressants, including benzodiazepines, together with sufentanil therapy.

! **WARNING** Alert patient that respiratory depression may occur with sufentanil use, especially when drug is first given, and to report any breathing difficulties immediately.

! **WARNING** Tell patient drug may cause an allergic reaction. If patient does not feel well or experiences being itchy or experiences a rash to notify staff immediately.

- Instruct patient to rise slowly from a lying or sitting position and to lie or sit down if he experiences lightheadedness. If effect is frequent or severe, tell him to notify prescriber.
- Urge patient to consume plenty of fluids and high-fiber foods, if not contraindicated, to prevent constipation.

! **WARNING** Tell patient to alert staff if any persistent, serious, or unusual adverse reactions occur.

! **WARNING** Inform pregnant patients that prolonged use of drug during pregnancy can cause neonatal harm at birth.

- Alert mothers who were breastfeeding before drug given to check with prescriber before breastfeeding is resumed. If breastfeeding occurs, tell mother to monitor infant closely for excess sedation and respiratory depression.
- Caution patient to avoid performing harzardous activities such as driving after being released from hospital until CNS effects of the drug are known and resolved.

sulfasalazine

Azulfidine, Azulfidine EN-Tabs, Salazopyrin (CAN), Salazopyrin EN-Tabs (CAN)

Class and Category

Pharmacologic class: Salicylate-sulfonamide
Therapeutic class: Anti-inflammatory

Indications and Dosages

∗ *To treat mild-to-moderate ulcerative colitis; as adjunct to treat severe ulcerative colitis; to prolong remission period between acute attacks of ulcerative colitis*

D.R. TABLETS, TABLETS

Adults. *Initial:* 3 to 4 g daily in evenly divided doses every 8 hr and increased, as needed. *Maintenance:* 500 mg every 6 hr.

Children ages 6 and older. *Initial:* 40 to 60 mg/kg daily in 3 to 6 divided doses. *Maintenance:* 30 mg/kg daily in 4 divided doses.

✱ To treat rheumatoid arthritis in patients who have not responded to salicylates or other NSAIDs

D.R. TABLETS

Adults. *Initial:* 500 mg daily during wk 1, increased by 500 mg daily every wk, as needed, up to 2,000 mg daily in 2 divided doses. If no response after 12 wk, increased to 3,000 mg daily. *Maintenance:* 1,000 mg every 12 hr. *Maximum:* 3,000 mg daily.

✱ To treat juvenile rheumatoid arthritis in patients who have not responded to salicylates or other NSAIDs

D.R. TABLETS

Children ages 6 and older. 30 to 50 mg/kg daily in divided doses twice daily. *Maximum:* 2 g daily.

±**DOSAGE ADJUSTMENT** For patients with ulcerative colitis, initial dosage may be reduced in half if GI intolerance occurs and then gradually increased. If GI intolerance continues, drug may be temporarily withheld for 5 to 7 days and then restarted at a lower daily dose. For adult patients with rheumatoid arthritis as a means to reduce possible GI intolerance, initial dosage may be reduced to 0.5 to 1 g daily and then increased weekly, as needed. For children with juvenile rheumatoid arthritis as a means to reduce possible GI intolerance, initial dosage may be reduced to one-quarter to one-third of expected maintenance dose and then gradually increased weekly to reach maintenance dose.

Drug Administration

P.O.

- Administer drug with meals (I.R.) or after meals (D.R.).
- Give drug with a full glass of water.
- D.R. tablets should be swallowed whole and not chewed, crushed, or divided.

Route	Onset	Peak	Duration
P.O.	Unknown	3–12 hr	Unknown
P.O./D.R.	Unknown	6 hr	Unknown

Half-life: 6–14 hr

Mechanism of Action

Be aware that as a prodrug of sulfapyridine and 5-aminosalicylic acid (mesalamine), more sulfapyridine and mesalamine is delivered to the colon than either metabolite could provide alone. Provides antibacterial action along the intestinal wall with mesalamine inhibiting cyclooxygenase, thereby decreasing the production of arachidonic acid metabolites and reducing colonic inflammation. Reduces also joint inflammation locally caused by rheumatoid arthritis.

Contraindications

Hypersensitivity to salicylates, sulfasalazine or its metabolites, sulfonamides, or their components; intestinal or urinary obstruction; porphyria

Interactions

DRUGS

digoxin: Possibly inhibited absorption and decreased blood level of digoxin
folic acid (vitamin B_9): Decreased folic acid absorption
methotrexate: Increased incidence of GI adverse reactions, especially nausea

Adverse Reactions

CNS: Ataxia, chills, depression, fatigue, fever, **Guillain-Barré syndrome**, headache, insomnia, **meningitis**, peripheral neuropathy, **seizures**, vertigo, weakness
CV: **Myocarditis**, **pericarditis**, vasculitis
EENT: Hearing loss, orange-yellow tears, oropharyngeal pain, pharyngitis, tinnitus
GI: Abdominal pain, anorexia, **cirrhosis**, diarrhea, elevated liver enzymes, **hepatitis**, **hepatotoxicity**, indigestion, jaundice, nausea, **pancreatitis**, ulcerative colitis exacerbation, vomiting
GU: Crystalluria, decreased ejaculatory volume, deteriorating renal function, discoloration of urine (orange-yellow) male infertility, **nephritis**, nephrolithiasis, **nephrotic syndrome**, orange-yellow urine, **toxic nephrosis**
HEME: **Agranulocytosis**, **aplastic anemia**, **hemolytic anemia**, **hematophagic histiocytosis**, **leukopenia**, **neutropenia**, **thrombocytopenia**, **unusual bleeding** or bruising
MS: Arthralgia, **rhabdomyolysis**
RESP: **Cyanosis**, **eosinophilic infiltration**, **idiopathic pulmonary fibrosis**, **lymphocytic interstitial pneumonitis**, pleuritis pneumonia

SKIN: Acute generalized exanthematous pustulosis (AGEP), alopecia, discoloration of skin (orange-yellow), **erythema multiforme**, **exfoliative dermatitis**, photosensitivity, pruritus, purpura, rash, **Stevens-Johnson syndrome**, **toxic epidermal necrolysis**, urticaria
Other: **Anaphylaxis**, **angioedema**, **drug rash with eosinophilia and systemic symptoms (DRESS)**, folate deficiency, infections (serious), lupus erythematosus-like syndrome, mononucleosis-like syndrome, **sepsis**, serum sickness syndrome

Childbearing Considerations

PREGNANCY

- It is not known if drug can cause fetal harm. However, drug does pass the placental barrier, increasing risk of kernicterus in the neonate.
- Use with caution only if benefit to mother outweighs potential risk to fetus.

LACTATION

- Drug is present in breast milk.
- Infants less than 2 mo of age should not be breastfed because of risk of kernicterus. Mothers should check with prescriber before breastfeeding older infants.
- Be aware that studies are mixed regarding drug causing bloody stools and/or diarrhea in breastfed infants.

REPRODUCTION

- Infertility and oligospermia have been reported in male patients; reversal usually occurs when drug is discontinued.

Nursing Considerations

! **WARNING** Be aware that patients with hematologic toxicity or hepatic or renal dysfunction who are given sulfasalazine may develop serious to life-threatening adverse reactions. Assess patient for fever, jaundice, pallor, purpura, or sore throat prior to drug being given. Monitor BUN and serum creatinine levels, CBC, and liver enzymes, before and periodically during sulfasalazine therapy. Expect drug to be withheld while awaiting laboratory results in patients experiencing symptoms of hematologic, hepatic, or renal dysfunction. Expect drug to be discontinued if renal function deteriorates during sulfasalazine therapy.

! **WARNING** Use sulfasalazine cautiously in patients with a history of recurring or chronic infections because drug may predispose patient to infections that could lead to sepsis. Monitor patients for new infections throughout therapy. If present, notify prescriber.

! **WARNING** Be aware that sulfasalazine doses over 4 g or a blood level over 50 mcg/ml increase the risk of adverse and toxic reactions.

! **WARNING** Monitor patient, especially during the first month of sulfasalazine therapy, for hypersensitivity or skin reactions that may become life-threatening, such as anaphylaxis or DRESS. Be aware that DRESS may only initially present with a fever or swollen lymph nodes although rash is most common. At first sign of hypersensitivity, or skin reaction notify prescriber, expect drug to be discontinued, and provide supportive care, as needed and ordered.

! **WARNING** Monitor patient for other persistent, serious, or unusual adverse reactions because drug can affect many body systems and can cause potentially life-threatening adverse reactions such as severe hematological reactions, myocarditis, or pancreatitis.

- Monitor fluid intake and output and urine color, consistency, and pH. Acidic urine may require alkalization to prevent crystalluria.
- Be aware that measurements, by liquid chromatography, of urinary normetanephrine may cause a false-positive test result.

PATIENT TEACHING

- Instruct patient how to administer form of sulfasalazine prescribed.
- Advise patient and family or caregiver that it is important for patient to drink a full glass of water when drug is taken. In addition, patient should drink at least 64 ounces of fluid per day to prevent crystalluria.
- Instruct patient and family or caregiver to administer drug around the clock.
- Inform patient that symptom relief may take 2 to 5 days for ulcerative colitis and 4 to 12 weeks for rheumatoid arthritis.

! **WARNING** Alert patient that drug may cause an allergic or serious skin reaction. If a fever, rash, swollen lymph nodes or other signs and symptoms are present, instruct patient to notify prescriber and, if severe, to seek immediate medical care.

! **WARNING** Review bleeding and infection control measures with patient. Tell patient to notify prescriber if bruising, unexplained bleeding, or infection occurs as treatment may be needed to prevent more serious reactions.

- Alert patient that drug may turn skin and urine orange-yellow.
- Advise contact lens wearer to consider wearing glasses during therapy because drug can permanently stain contact lenses yellow.
- Instruct patient to avoid prolonged sun exposure and to wear protective clothing and sunscreen when outdoors.
- Instruct mothers who are breastfeeding to stop taking sulfasalazine or stop breastfeeding immediately if their infant develops bloody stools or diarrhea, and to notify pediatrician. Also, inform mothers that breastfeeding is not recommended for infants under 2 months of age.
- Urge patient to comply with laboratory tests and follow-up visits to monitor drug's effect.

sumatriptan

Imitrex Nasal Spray, Tosymra Nasal Spray

sumatriptan succinate

Imitrex, Imitrex STAT dose, Onzetra Xsail, Zembrace SymTouch

Class and Category

Pharmacologic class: Serotonin 5-HT_1 receptor agonist
Therapeutic class: Antimigraine

Indications and Dosages

✱ *To relieve acute migraine attacks, with or without aura*

TABLETS (IMITREX)

Adults. 25, 50, or 100 mg as a single dose as soon as possible after onset of symptoms, repeated after at least 2 hr, as needed. *Maximum:* 200 mg daily.

± **DOSAGE ADJUSTMENT** For patients with mild-to-moderate hepatic dysfunction, 50 mg is maximum single dose.

SUBCUTANEOUS INJECTION (ZEMBRACE SYMTOUCH)

Adults. *Initial:* 3 mg, repeated after 1 hr, as needed. *Maximum:* 4 (3-mg) injections/24 hr with dosages separated by at least 1 hr.

SUBCUTANEOUS INJECTION (IMITREX)

Adults. *Initial:* 1 to 6 mg depending on severity of headache, repeated after at least 1 hr, as needed. *Maximum:* 12 mg (two 6-mg injections) in 24 hr with doses separated by at least 1 hr.

NASAL SPRAY (IMITREX)

Adults. 5 mg, 10 mg, or 20 mg given as a single spray in 1 nostril or 10 mg given as a single 5-mg spray in each nostril. One additional dose may be taken if migraine not resolved or another attack occurs after at least 2 hr. *Maximum:* 40 mg daily; treatment of 4 headaches/30 day.

NASAL SPRAY (TOSYMRA)

Adults. 10 mg given as a single spray in 1 nostril. Dose repeated after at least 1 hr if migraine not resolved or another attack occurs. Alternatively, 10 mg given as a single spray in 1 nostril and, if migraine not relieved after 1 hr, another sumatriptan product may be administered. *Maximum:* 30 mg daily with each 10-mg dose separated by at least 1 hr.

NASAL POWDER (ONZETRA XSAIL)

Adults. 22 mg (11 mg in each nostril). One additional dose given after 2 hr if migraine not resolved or another attack occurs. *Maximum:* 44 mg (2 doses) in 24 hr or 22 mg plus 1 dose of another sumatriptan product, separated by at least 2 hr, in 24 hr.

✱ *To relieve cluster headaches*

SUBCUTANEOUS INJECTION (IMITREX)

Adults. *Initial:* 6 mg, repeated after 1 or 2 hr, as needed. *Maximum:* 2 (6-mg) injections/24 hr with dosages separated by at least 1 hr.

Drug Administration

- Administer drug as soon as symptoms of migraine or cluster headaches occur.

P.O.

- Tablets should be swallowed whole and not chewed, crushed, or divided.
- Administer with fluids to help disguise unpleasant taste.

SUBCUTANEOUS

- Needle shield of prefilled syringe and pen contains dry natural rubber, which may cause an allergic reaction if latex sensitive.
- Never administer by any other route.
- Rotate sites.
- Store at room temperature protected from light.
- Inject only in the abdomen or thigh if using an autoinjector.

Imitrex Autoinjector

- Imitrex can be used with an autoinjector device for 4-mg and 6-mg doses only.
- Use device only if adequate skin and subcutaneous thickness of at least 1/4 inch is present.
- To use, open lid of the carrying case, tear off tamper-evident seal, and open the lid over the syringe cartridge. Hold pen by the ridges at the top. Take pen out of the carrying case. Check to make sure the white priming rod is not sticking out from the lower end of the pen. If it is, put pen back into the carrying case and press down firmly until a click is felt. Take pen out of the carrying case again.
- Put pen in the open cartridge pack and turn to the right until it will not turn any more (about a half a turn). Hold the loaded pen by the ridges and pull it straight out. It may be hard to pull on the pen but this is normal. Do not press the blue button yet. The pen is not ready to use.
- Select injection site, which may be injected into side of the upper arm or thigh.
- Release safety catch by pressing pen firmly against the skin until the gray part of the barrel slides against the blue part and cannot be pressed any further. The gray part of the barrel must stay in contact with the blue part while injecting drug. When injecting, hold pen against the skin for at least 5 sec.
- After each use, put pen back into the carrying case to reset the white priming rod before the next use.

Zembrace SymTouch Autoinjector

- Hold device in one hand and pull red cap off with the other hand, being careful not to put or press thumb, fingers, or hand over the yellow needle guard.
- Select injection site, which may be injected into upper arm or thigh. Place the autoinjector at a 90-degree angle with the yellow needle guard end gently pressed against patient's skin. Press and hold autoinjector down against the skin. A click will be heard as injection starts. Continue to hold the device down until a second click is heard. Wait 5 sec before removing autoinjector. The yellow needle guard will drop down and lock over the needle. Check that the red plunger rod has filled the drug viewing window, which means the full dose has been given.
- Do not reuse the autoinjector. Discard.

INTRANASAL POWDER

- Administer by using one 11-mg nosepiece in each nostril.
- To use nosepiece, remove clear device cap from the reusable delivery device, remove a disposable nosepiece from its foil pouch, and click nosepiece into the device body.
- Fully press and promptly release the white piercing button on the device body to pierce the capsule inside the nosepiece. Press piercing button only once and release prior to administration to each nostril.
- Have patient insert nosepiece into the nostril so that it makes a tight seal. Keeping the nosepiece in the nose, have patient rotate device to place mouthpiece into the mouth.
- Have patient blow forcefully through the mouthpiece to deliver the powder into the nasal cavity. Listen for a rattling sound, which indicates patient has blown forcefully.
- After drug is administrated, have patient remove and discard the nosepiece.
- Use same process using a second 11-mg nosepiece in the other nostril to complete the 22-mg dose.

INTRANASAL SPRAY

- Have patient blow nose before administering drug.
- Have patient hold head in an upright position, while gently closing one nostril. Patient should breathe gently out through mouth.
- Hold drug container with thumb supporting container at bottom and index and middle fingers on either side of the nozzle.
- Insert nozzle into open nostril about ½ inch. While patient gently takes a breath

in through the nose, press the blue plunger firmly to release dose.

- After removing nozzle, have patient gently breathe in through the nose and out through the mouth for 10 to 20 sec. Patient should not breathe deeply.
- After use, rinse tip of bottle with hot water (don't suction water into bottle) and dry with a clean tissue. Replace cap after cleaning.

Route	Onset	Peak	Duration
P.O.	30 min	2–2.5 hr	Unknown
SubQ	10 min	12 min	9–24 hr
Nasal spray	15–30 min	5–23 min	Unknown
Nasal powder	Unknown	45 min	Unknown

Half-life: 2–2.5 hr

Mechanism of Action

May stimulate 5-HT_1 receptors, causing selective vasoconstriction of dilated and inflamed cranial blood vessels in carotid circulation, thus decreasing carotid arterial blood flow and relieving acute migraines and cluster headaches.

Contraindications

Coronary artery disease; history of basilar or hemiplegic migraine, CVA, or transient ischemic attack; hypersensitivity to sumatriptan or its components; ischemic bowel disease; peripheral vascular disease; recent use (within 24 hr) of ergotamine-containing medication, ergot-type medication (such as dihydroergotamine or methysergide), or another 5-hydroxytryptamine 1 (5-HT_1) agonist; severe hepatic impairment; uncontrolled hypertension; use of a MAO inhibitor within 14 days; Wolff-Parkinson-White syndrome or arrhythmias associated with other cardiac accessory conduction pathway disorders

Interactions

DRUGS

antidepressants, lithium: Increased risk of serious adverse effects
ergotamine-containing drugs: Possibly additive or prolonged vasoconstrictive effects, including serotonin syndrome
fluoxetine, fluvoxamine, paroxetine, sertraline: Possibly hyperreflexia, incoordination, and weakness
MAO inhibitors: Risk of decreased sumatriptan clearance, increased risk of serious adverse effects
other triptans: Additive vasospastic effects; increased risk of serotonin syndrome
selective serotonin reuptake inhibitors, serotonin–norepinephrine reuptake inhibitors, tricyclic antidepressants: Increased risk of serotonin syndrome

Adverse Reactions

CNS: Anxiety, atypical sensations, dizziness, drowsiness, fatigue, fever, headache, malaise, sedation, **serotonin syndrome**, **seizures**, vertigo, weakness
CV: **Arrhythmias**; chest heaviness, pain, pressure, or tightness; **coronary artery vasospasm**; **ECG changes**; hypertension; **hypotension**; palpitations; peripheral vascular ischemia
EENT: Abnormal vision, blindness or partial vision loss, jaw or mouth discomfort, nasal burning or irritation, nose or throat discomfort, photophobia (P.O., subcutaneous), taste perversion (nasal), tongue numbness or soreness
GI: Abdominal discomfort, **bloody diarrhea**, **colonic ischemia**, dysphagia
MS: Muscle cramps, myalgia, neck pain or stiffness
SKIN: Diaphoresis, erythema, flushing, pallor, photosensitivity (P.O., subcutaneous), pruritus, rash, urticaria
Other: **Anaphylaxis**; **angioedema**; injection-site burning, erythema, hemorrhage, induration, irritation, pain, paresthesia, pruritis, swelling, and urticaria

Childbearing Considerations

PREGNANCY

- It is not known if drug can cause fetal harm.
- Use with caution only if benefit to mother outweighs potential risk to fetus.

LACTATION

- Drug is present in breast milk following subcutaneous administration.
- Mothers should check with prescriber before breastfeeding.
- If mother decides to breastfeed, breastfeeding should be avoided for 12 hr after mother takes drug, regardless of form used.

Nursing Considerations

- Be aware that sumatriptan shouldn't be given to elderly patients because they're more likely to have coronary artery disease (CAD) and more pronounced blood pressure increases.

! **WARNING** Don't give sumatriptan within 24 hours of another 5-HT_1 receptor agonist, such as naratriptan, rizatriptan, or zolmitriptan with the exception of a single dose of another sumatriptan product, provided the doses are separated by at least 1 to 2 hours depending on brand used. Don't give an ergotamine-containing or ergot-type drug within 24 hours of sumatriptan therapy. Doing so increases risk of serious adverse interactions and effects.

! **WARNING** Monitor patient closely for a hypersensitivity reaction, which could become life-threatening, such as anaphylaxis and angioedema. If present, notify prescriber immediately, expect drug to be discontinued, and provide supportive care, as needed and ordered.

! **WARNING** Assess patient for arrhythmias, chest pain, or other signs of heart disease and monitor blood pressure in patients with CAD before and for at least 1 hour after sumatriptan administration.

! **WARNING** Know that for patients with seizure disorder, seizure precautions should be instituted according to facility policy because sumatriptan may lower seizure threshold.

! **WARNING** Monitor patient closely for serotonin syndrome exhibited by agitation, coma, diarrhea, hyperreflexia, hyperthermia, incoordination, labile blood pressure, nausea, tachycardia, or vomiting. Notify prescriber immediately because serotonin syndrome may be life-threatening and provide supportive care.

! **WARNING** Monitor patient for other persistent, serious, or unusual adverse reactions.

PATIENT TEACHING

! **WARNING** Urge patient to contact prescriber and avoid taking sumatriptan if headache symptoms aren't typical.

- Instruct patient how to administer form of sumatriptan prescribed.
- Tell patient to take drug as soon as possible after the onset of migraine symptoms.
- Instruct patient not to take a second dose if first dose doesn't provide significant relief.
- Remind patient not to exceed prescribed daily dosage. Inform patient that overuse of the drug for 10 or more days per month may lead to exacerbation of headache and may require detoxification. If use of the drug increases, advise patient to notify his prescriber.
- Tell patient injecting drug subcutaneously to alert prescriber if an allergy to latex exists, as the needle cap of the prefilled syringe is made of a latex derivative. Advise patient never to share the medication with another person even if they have the same symptoms, as cross-contamination and severe adverse reactions could occur. Inform patient that burning, pain, and redness may be experienced for 10 to 30 minutes after subcutaneous injection. Suggest applying ice to relieve pain and redness.
- Encourage patient to lie down in a dark, quiet room after taking drug to help relieve migraine.

! **WARNING** Instruct patient to seek emergency care for chest, jaw, or neck tightness after drug use because drug may cause coronary artery vasospasm; subsequent doses may require ECG monitoring.

! **WARNING** Tell patient to notify prescriber if an allergic reaction occurs and if severe to seek immediate medical care

! **WARNING** Alert patient with seizure disorder that drug may lower seizure threshold.

! **WARNING** Urge patient to inform all prescribers of sumatriptan therapy because of potentially dangerous drug interactions.

- Advise patient to avoid potentially hazardous activities until drug's CNS effects are known and resolved.
- Encourage yearly ophthalmologic examinations for patients who require prolonged drug therapy.
- Inform mothers who are breastfeeding that breastfeeding should be avoided for 12 hours after treatment with sumatriptan to minimize infant exposure to drug.

suvorexant

Belsomra

Class, Category, and Schedule

Pharmacologic class: Orexin receptor antagonist
Therapeutic class: Hypnotic
Controlled substance schedule: IV

Indications and Dosages

✷ To treat insomnia characterized by difficulties with sleep onset and/or sleep maintenance

TABLETS

Adults. 10 mg once nightly within 30 min of bedtime, increased, as needed, to 20 mg once daily. *Maximum:* 20 mg once daily at night.

±**DOSAGE ADJUSTMENT** For patients taking moderate CYP3A inhibitors, dosage reduced to 5 mg once per night, with maximum dosage not exceeding 10 mg once per night. For patients taking CNS depressants concurrently, dosage may have to be decreased.

Drug Administration

P.O.

- Administer within 30 min of bedtime, preferably on an empty stomach because food can delay drug's effects.
- Administer when patient has at least 7 hr remaining for sleep.

Route	Onset	Peak	Duration
P.O.	30 min	2 hr	Unknown

Half-life: 12 hr

Mechanism of Action

Antagonism of orexin receptors blocks the binding of wake-promoting neuropeptides orexin A and orexin B to produce sleep.

Contraindications

Hypersensitivity to suvorexant and its components, narcolepsy

Interactions

DRUGS

CNS depressants: Additive CNS and respiratory depression; increased risk of abnormal behavior and thinking
CYP3A inducers: Decreased effectiveness of suvorexant
CYP3A inhibitors: Increased effect of suvorexant and incidence of adverse reactions
digoxin: Increased serum digoxin levels

ACTIVITIES

alcohol use: Additive CNS depression; increased risk of abnormal behavior and thinking

Adverse Reactions

CNS: Abnormal dreams, amnesia, anxiety, cataplexy-like behaviors (mild), complex sleep behaviors (sleepwalking, engaging in activities while not fully awake), dizziness, hallucinations, headache, impaired daytime wakefulness, leg weakness (temporary), psychomotor hyperactivity, sleep paralysis (temporarily), somnolence, **suicidal ideation**, worsening of depression
CV: Palpitations, tachycardia
EENT: Dry mouth
GI: Diarrhea, nausea, vomiting
RESP: Cough, upper respiratory tract infection
SKIN: Pruritus
Other: Physical and psychological dependence

Childbearing Considerations

PREGNANCY

- It is not known if drug can cause fetal harm.
- Use with caution only if benefit to mother outweighs potential risk to fetus.

LACTATION

- It is not known if drug is present in breast milk.
- Mother should check with prescriber before breastfeeding.
- If breastfeeding takes place, mother should monitor infant for excessive sedation.

Nursing Considerations

! **WARNING** Use suvorexant with extreme caution in patients with a history of alcohol or drug abuse because of risk of addiction.

- Use suvorexant cautiously in debilitated or elderly patients and those with depression or impaired respiratory function.

! **WARNING** Monitor respiratory status, especially in patients with respiratory compromise, who are at increased risk for respiratory depression.

! **WARNING** Watch patient closely for suicidal tendencies, particularly when therapy starts and dosage changes because depression may worsen temporarily during these times, possibly leading to suicidal ideation.

- Monitor obese patients and women closely for adverse effects because these patients are at increased risk. Be aware that there is a dosage relationship to development of adverse reactions in general.
- Institute fall precautions because drug causes drowsiness.

PATIENT TEACHING

! **WARNING** Alert patient that drug is a controlled substance and can cause addiction. Instruct patient to take drug exactly as prescribed and not to increase dosage or frequency of use without consulting prescriber.

- Instruct patient how to administer suvorexant.
- Tell patient to notify prescriber if insomnia worsens or new signs or symptoms occur.
- Advise patient to avoid alcohol while taking suvorexant.

! **WARNING** Urge family or caregiver to watch patient closely for suicidal tendencies, especially when therapy starts or dosage changes.

- Caution patient to avoid potentially hazardous activities after taking suvorexant; drug's intended effect is to decrease alertness. Tell patient that CNS depressant effects may persist in some patients for up to several days after drug is discontinued.
- Advise patient that drug may cause abnormal behaviors during sleep that extend into daytime, causing wakefulness impairment, including driving a car, eating, talking on the phone, or having sex without any recall of the event. If family or caregiver notices any such behavior or patient sees evidence of such behavior upon awakening, drug should be withheld, and prescriber notified.
- Review fall precautions with patient.
- Tell mothers who are breastfeeding to monitor infant for excessive sedation.

T

tacrolimus

Astagraf XL, Envarsus XR, Prograf

Class and Category

Pharmacologic class: Calcineurin inhibitor
Therapeutic class: Immunosuppressant

Indications and Dosages

* *To prevent organ rejection in patients undergoing allogeneic heart, kidney, or liver transplantation*

CAPSULES (PROGRAF)

Adults having kidney transplantation in combination with azathioprine. 0.2 mg/kg/day given in 2 equally divided doses every 12 hr with first dose begun between 6 and 24 hr post-transplant but only after renal function has recovered.
Adults having kidney transplantation in combination with mycophenolate mofetil (MMF)/IL-2 receptor antagonist therapy. 0.1 mg/kg/day given in 2 equally divided doses every 12 hr with first dose begun between 6 and 24 hr post-transplant but only after renal function has recovered.
Adults having liver transplantation with corticosteroids only. 0.10 to 0.15 mg/kg/day given in 2 equally divided doses every 12 hr. First dose administered 6 hr after transplantation.
Adults having heart or lung transplantation with azathioprine or MMF. 0.075 mg/kg/day given in 2 equally divided doses every 12 hr. First dose administered 6 hr after transplantation.

CAPSULES, ORAL SUSPENSION (PROGRAF)

Children having kidney transplantation. 0.3 mg/kg/day given in 2 equally divided doses every 12 hr.
Children having liver transplantation. 0.15 to 0.2 mg/kg/day (capsules) or 0.2 mg/kg/day (oral suspension) given in 2 equally divided doses every 12 hr. First dose administered 6 hr after transplantation.
Children having heart transplantation. 0.3 mg/kg/day (0.1 mg/kg/day if antibody induction treatment is administered) given in 2 equally divided doses every 12 hr.
Children having lung transplantation. 0.3 mg/kg/day given in 2 equally divided doses every 12 hr.

I.V. INFUSION (PROGRAF)

Adults having kidney or liver transplantation. 0.03 to 0.05 mg/kg/day beginning no sooner than 6 hr after transplantation.
Adults having heart transplantation. 0.01 mg/kg/day beginning no sooner than 6 hr after transplantation.
Adults having a lung transplantation. 0.01 to 0.03 mg/kg/day beginning no sooner than 6 hr after transplantation.
Children having liver transplantation. 0.03 to 0.05 mg/kg/day beginning no sooner than 6 hr after transplantation.

± **DOSAGE ADJUSTMENT** For patients with hepatic or renal impairment, dosage kept at lower end of range with possible need for further reduction. For kidney transplant patients with postoperative oliguria, drug therapy may be delayed until renal function shows signs of recovery. For African American adults taking capsule form and patients with cystic fibrosis with lung transplantation using either capsules or oral suspension, higher doses may be needed to attain trough concentrations.

* *To prevent organ rejection in patients undergoing kidney transplantation*

E.R. CAPSULES (ASTAGRAF XL)

Adults taking MMF and steroids with basiliximab. *Initial:* 0.15 to 0.2 mg/kg once daily prior to reperfusion or within 48 hr of completion of transplant procedure. Dosage then adjusted to achieve target trough concentration range.
Adults taking MMF and steroids without basiliximab. *Preoperatively:* 0.1 mg/kg as a single dose within 12 hr prior to reperfusion. *Postoperatively:* 0.2 mg/kg as the second dose given at least 4 hr after the preoperative dose and within 12 hr after reperfusion, then adjusted to achieve target trough concentration ranges.
Children with basiliximab MMF and steroids. 0.3 mg/kg once daily administered within 24 hr following reperfusion.

±**DOSAGE ADJUSTMENT** For African American patients, higher doses may be needed to attain trough concentrations comparable to those of Caucasian patients. For patients with severe hepatic impairment, lower dosage may be required. For patients taking CYP3A inducers or inhibitors, dosage may have to be adjusted.

* *To prevent organ rejection in patients undergoing kidney transplantation and are converting from a tacrolimus immediate-release product*

XR TABLETS (ENVARSUS XR)

Adults in combination with other immunosuppressants. *Initial:* 80% of total daily dose of immediate-release product given once daily, then adjusted to achieve target whole blood trough concentration range of 4 to 11 ng/ml.

* *To prevent organ rejection in de novo kidney transplant patients*

XR TABLETS (ENVARSUS XR)

Adults in combination with other immunosuppressants. *Initial:* 0.14 mg/kg/day, then titrated, as needed.

±**DOSAGE ADJUSTMENT** For African American patients, higher doses may be needed to attain trough concentrations comparable to those of Caucasian patients. For patients with severe hepatic impairment, lower dosage may be required. For patients receiving CYP3A inducers or inhibitors concomitantly, dosage may have to be adjusted.

Drug Administration

P.O.

- Do not interchange Astagraf XL (E.R. capsules) or substitute for E.R. tablets, I.R. capsules, or oral suspension. Do not interchange Envarsus XR (E.R. tablets) or substitute with E.R. capsules, I.R. capsules, or oral suspension. Do not interchange Prograf capsules and granules or substitute for other E.R. products.
- Keep in mind when converting patient from parenteral to oral therapy, expect to give oral form 8 to 12 hr after infusion is discontinued.
- To prepare oral suspension, empty the entire contents of each Prograf granules packet into a glass cup. Add 15 to 30 ml of room-temperature drinking water to the cup. Mix and administer entire contents of cup immediately. Granules will not completely dissolve. For younger patients, the suspension can be drawn up via a non-PVC oral syringe that is dispensed with drug. Refill the cup or syringe with 15 to 30 ml of water and give to patient to ensure that all the medication is taken. Do not sprinkle Prograf granules on food.
- Administer Prograf, 12 hr apart, at same time each day with or without food but administer consistently.
- Administer E.R. form of drug once daily in the morning either 1 hr before a meal or 2 hr after a meal on an empty stomach.
- Capsules and tablets should be swallowed whole and not chewed, crushed, or divided.
- Do not administer with grapefruit juice.

I.V.

- Be aware that I.V. tacrolimus therapy should only be given if patient can't tolerate oral tacrolimus. Patient should be switched to oral therapy as soon as possible.
- Solution prepared by pharmacist.
- Once diluted, drug should be stored in glass or polyethylene containers (not PVC containers because of decreased stability and possible extraction of phthalates).
- Use a PVC-free tubing to administer drug, if situation warrants, such as in pediatric dosing.
- Infuse as a continuous infusion.
- Monitor patient closely for anaphylaxis during I.V. administration. Make sure emergency equipment and drugs, such as aqueous solution of epinephrine and oxygen, are immediately available.
- Discard after 24 hr if not used.
- *Incompatibilities:* Solutions of pH 9 or greater such as acyclovir or ganciclovir; PVC containers

Route	Onset	Peak	Duration
P.O.	Unknown	1.5–3 hr	Unknown
P.O./E.R.	Unknown	6 hr	Unknown
I.V.	Rapid	1–2 hr	Unknown

Half-life: 12 hr

Mechanism of Action

Inhibits T-lymphocyte activation, possibly by binding to an intracellular protein,

FKBP-12 to cause a formation of a complex of tacrolimus-FKBP-12, calcineurin, calcium, and calmodulin, which inhibits phosphatase activity of calcineurin. This inhibition may prevent dephosphorylation and translocation of nuclear factor of activated T-cells, a nuclear component thought to initiate gene transcription for the formation of lymphokines. Inhibiting T-lymphocyte activation produces immunosuppression.

Contraindications

Hypersensitivity to tacrolimus or its components, hypersensitivity to polyoxyl 60 hydrogenated castor oil (parenteral form)

Interactions

DRUGS

amiodarone, boceprevir, bromocriptine, cannabidiol, chloramphenicol, cimetidine, cisapride, clarithromycin, clotrimazole, cyclosporine, danazol, diltiazem, erythromycin, ethinyl estradiol, fluconazole, ganciclovir, itraconazole, ketoconazole, lansoprazole, letermovir, magnesium-aluminum-hydroxide, methylprednisolone, metoclopramide, nefazodone, nelfinavir, nicardipine, nifedipine, omeprazole, protease inhibitors, ritonavir, Schisandra sphenanthera extracts, telaprevir, troleandomycin, verapamil, voriconazole and other CYP3A inhibitors: Possibly increased blood tacrolimus level; increased risk of serious adverse reactions, such as neurotoxicity or QT prolongation

carbamazepine, caspofungin, methylprednisolone, phenobarbital, phenytoin, prednisone, rifabutin, rifampin, St. John's wort and other CYP3A4 inducers: Possibly decreased blood tacrolimus level

CYP3A inhibitors, nephrotoxic drugs (aminoglycosides, amphotericin B, cisplatin, ganciclovir, nucleotide reverse transcriptase inhibitors, protease inhibitors): Increased vasoconstrictive effect on renal vasculature, toxic tubulopathy, and tubulointerstitial effects leading to an increased risk for nephrotoxicity

mycophenolic acid: Possibly increased plasma mycophenolic acid level

sirolimus: Increased risk of thrombotic microangiopathy

vaccines (live or killed): Possibly suppressed immune response and increased adverse effects of vaccine

ACTIVITIES

alcohol use (Astagraf XL, Envarsus XR): Increased rate of release of tacrolimus; increased risk of serious adverse reactions, such as neurotoxicity or QT prolongation

FOODS

grapefruit, grapefruit juice: Possibly increased blood tacrolimus trough levels in liver transplant patients

Adverse Reactions

CNS: Asthenia, **coma**, **CVA**, delirium, dizziness, fever, headache, hemiparesis, insomnia, jittery feeling, **leukoencephalopathy**, mental changes, motor and sensory dysfunction, mutism, **neurotoxicity**, paresthesia, **posterior reversible encephalopathy syndrome**, **progressive multifocal leukoencephalopathy**, **seizures**, speech disorder, syncope, tremor

CV: **Atrial and ventricular arrhythmias**, **cardiac arrest**, chest pain, hypercholesterolemia, hyperlipemia, hypertension, hypertriglyceridemia, myocardial hypertrophy, **MI**, **myocardial ischemia**, **pericardial effusion**, peripheral edema, **QT-interval prolongation**, **T wave abnormality on ECG**, **torsades de pointes**, **venous thrombosis**

EENT: Blindness, cortical blindness, deafness, hearing loss, optic atrophy or neuropathy, photophobia

ENDO: Cushingoid features, diabetes mellitus (new onset), hot flashes, hyperglycemia

GI: Abdominal pain, anorexia, ascites, bile duct stenosis, cholangitis, **cirrhosis**, colitis, constipation, diarrhea, dyspepsia, enterocolitis, fatty liver, gastric ulcer, gastroenteritis, gastroesophageal reflux disease, **GI perforation**, **hepatic cytolysis or failure**, **hepatic impairment or toxicity**, **hepatitis**, impaired gastric emptying, jaundice, nausea, **liver necrosis**, **pancreatitis (including hemorrhagic or necrotizing)**, **veno-occlusive liver disease**, vomiting

GU: BK virus nephropathy, elevated creatinine and BUN levels, hemorrhagic cystitis, **hemolytic uremic syndrome**, micturition abnormality, **nephrotoxicity**, oliguria, **renal failure**, renal impairment, UTI

HEME: **Agranulocytosis**, anemia, **decreased blood fibrinogen**, **disseminated intravascular coagulation (DIC)**, **febrile neutropenia**, **hemolytic anemia**, leukocytosis, **leukopenia**, **neutropenia**, **pancytopenia**, **prolonged activated partial thromboplastin time**, **pure red cell aplasia**, **thrombocytopenia**, **thrombocytopenic purpura**, **thrombotic microangiopathy**, **thrombotic thrombocytopenic purpura**
MS: Arthralgia, back pain, extremity pain including calcineurin inhibitor–induced pain syndrome
RESP: **Acute respiratory distress syndrome**, **atelectasis**, **bronchiolitis obliterans syndrome**, bronchitis, cough, dyspnea, **interstitial lung disease**, **lung infiltration**, pleural effusion, pneumonia, **pulmonary embolism or hypertension**, **respiratory distress or failure**
SKIN: Flushing, hyperpigmentation, **malignancy**, photosensitivity, pruritus, rash, **Stevens-Johnson syndrome**, **toxic epidermal necrolysis**
Other: **Anaphylaxis**, cytomegalovirus infection, **hyperkalemia**, **hypokalemia**, **hypomagnesemia**, **hypophosphatemia**, impaired wound healing, infections, **lymphoproliferative or malignant disorders**, **multiorgan failure**, opportunistic infections (including activation of latent viral infections), primary graft dysfunction, weight loss

Childbearing Considerations

PREGNANCY

- Pregnancy exposure registry: 1-877-955-6877 or https://www.transplantpregnancyregistry.org/.
- Drug can cause fetal harm such as congenital abnormalities and fetal distress, as well as low birth weight, renal dysfunction, and transient neonatal hyperkalemia at birth.
- Use with caution only if benefit to mother outweighs potential risk to fetus.

LABOR AND DELIVERY

- There is an increased risk for premature delivery (less than 37 wk) following maternal exposure to drug.

LACTATION

- Drug is present in breast milk.
- Mothers should check with prescriber before breastfeeding.

REPRODUCTION

- Females of childbearing age need to use a reliable method of contraception before drug therapy is begun and throughout drug therapy.
- Female and male fertility may be affected by drug therapy.

Nursing Considerations

! WARNING Know that tacrolimus should not be given to patients with congenital long QT syndrome because of increased risk of life-threatening ventricular arrhythmias.

! WARNING Know that sirolimus should not be administered with tacrolimus because of the potential for severe adverse reactions.

- Know that tacrolimus therapy should not be started within 24 hours of cyclosporine, and vice versa. If tacrolimus or cyclosporine blood levels are elevated beyond 24 hours of either drug being discontinued, know that the other drug should not be started until elevation is resolved.
- Check to be sure patient is up to date on all immunizations according to the standard schedule. If possible, live vaccines should be avoided.
- Expect to give drug with corticosteroid therapy.
- Be aware that children usually need higher doses of tacrolimus than adults.
- Monitor patient's blood tacrolimus trough levels regularly, as ordered. Higher trough levels increase risk of toxicity, especially nephrotoxicity and neurotoxicity.

! WARNING Monitor patient for a hypersensitivity reaction, which could become life-threatening, such as anaphylaxis. If present, notify prescriber, expect drug to be switched to another drug, and provide supportive care, as needed and ordered.

! WARNING Watch for evidence of neurotoxicity, especially in patients receiving high doses of drug. Evidence of encephalopathy includes headache, impaired consciousness, loss of motor function, psychiatric disturbance, seizures, and tremors.

! WARNING Monitor patient's ECG and electrolytes, as ordered, periodically throughout tacrolimus therapy because drug may prolong the QT interval, especially in patients with bradyarrhythmias, congestive heart failure, electrolyte disturbances, and concomitant use of certain antiarrhythmic drugs.

! **WARNING** Be aware that tacrolimus therapy increases the risk of patient developing serious infections and malignancies. Monitor patient closely, as patient may need to be hospitalized because of life-threatening severity.

! **WARNING** Monitor patient for thrombotic microangiopathy, including hemolytic uremic syndrome and thrombotic thrombocytopenic purpura, which may occur with tacrolimus therapy. Know that risk factors include graft-verus host disease, human leukocyte antigen mismatch, severe infections, and use of calcineurin inhibitors and mTOR inhibitors. If thrombotic microangiopathy is suspected, notify prescriber at once.

! **WARNING** Monitor results of liver and renal function tests, as ordered, to detect signs of decreased function. Changes in liver function may affect effectiveness of tacrolimus or increase risk of adverse effects. Expect to decrease dosage if severe liver impairment or decreased renal impairment occurs or temporary interrupt tacrolimus therapy if acute renal impairment associated with tacrolimus toxicity occurs, as ordered.

- Monitor blood pressure, especially in patients with history of hypertension, because drug can worsen this condition.
- Know that tacrolimus may increase serum cholesterol, lipid, and triglyceride levels.
- Monitor patient's blood glucose level closely because tacrolimus may cause post-transplant hyperglycemia with the need for insulin therapy, especially in African American and Hispanic patients.
- Monitor patient's serum potassium level, as ordered, because drug can alter it.

PATIENT TEACHING

! **WARNING** Advise females of childbearing age to use effective contraceptive measures before starting drug and continuing throughout therapy. If pregnancy occurs, tell her to alert prescriber immediately.

- Tell patient to inspect the tacrolimus medication when a new prescription is received and before taking it. If it looks different or dosage instructions have changed, tell patient to alert prescriber, because tacrolimus products are not interchangeable.
- Instruct patient how to administer form and brand of tacrolimus prescribed.
- Tell patient to avoid consuming alcohol or grapefruit juice or eating grapefruit while taking tacrolimus.
- Advise patient not to stop taking drug without consulting prescriber.
- Teach patient how to take a blood pressure and provide guidelines for when blood pressure readings should be reported to prescriber.
- Instruct patient not to receive live virus vaccines during therapy because of possible adverse effects and inactivated vaccines may not be as effective if administered during tacrolimus therapy. Urge patient to avoid people who have received such vaccines or to wear a protective mask when around them.

! **WARNING** Alert patient that drug may cause an allergic reaction. Tell patient to notify prescriber if an allergic reaction is present and, if severe, to seek immediate medical care.

! **WARNING** Review infection control measures. Caution patient to avoid having contact with people who have infections during therapy because tacrolimus causes immunosuppression. Stress importance of notifying prescriber if an infection occurs, as it can become severe. Tell patient to report chills; cough; fever; flu-like symptoms; muscle aches; or painful, red, or warm areas on the skin.

! **WARNING** Warn patient that tacrolimus may cause cancer because of its immunosuppressant action. Tell patient to report any unexplained or unusual signs and symptoms to prescriber.

! **WARNING** Warn patient that drug can cause blood clotting disorders. Urge patient to seek immediate medical attention if bruises, confusion, decreased urination, fatigue, fever, petechia, or yellowing of eyes or skin occurs.

- Inform patient that tacrolimus therapy may result in insulin-dependent diabetes. Tell patient to report frequent urination or an increase in fatigue, hunger, or thirst.

! **WARNING** Tell patient to notify prescriber of any other persistent, serious, or unusual adverse reactions.

- Instruct patient to limit exposure to direct sunlight and to wear protective clothing and use broad-spectrum sunscreen when exposure can't be avoided.
- Instruct patient to alert all prescribers to tacrolimus therapy and not to take any over-the-counter drugs, including herbal products, without consulting prescriber first.
- Emphasize the importance of having repeated laboratory tests while taking tacrolimus and urge compliance.

tadalafil

Adcirca, Alyq, Cialis, Tadliq

Class and Category

Pharmacologic class: Phosphodiesterase-5 (PDE5) inhibitor
Therapeutic class: Benign prostatic antihyperplasia agent, erectile dysfunction agent, vasodilator

Indications and Dosages

* *To treat erectile dysfunction*

TABLETS (CIALIS)

Men. *Initial:* 10 mg at least 30 min before sexual activity; dosage decreased to 5 mg or increased to 20 mg, based on clinical response. Alternatively, 2.5 mg once daily without regard to timing of sexual activity, increased to 5 mg once daily, as needed.

± **DOSAGE ADJUSTMENT** For patients who take drug on an as-needed basis and are taking potent CYP3A4 inhibitors, such as ketoconazole or ritonavir, dosage shouldn't exceed 10 mg every 72 hr. For patients taking potent CYP3A4 inhibitors and drug once daily, the maximum recommended dose shouldn't exceed 2.5 mg daily. For patients who take drug on an as-needed basis and have a creatinine clearance of 30 to 50 ml/min, initial dosage decreased to 5 mg daily and maximum dosage not to exceed 10 mg every 48 hr. For patients who take drug on an as-needed basis and have a creatinine clearance of less than 30 ml/min or who are on hemodialysis, maximum dose should not exceed 5 mg every 72 hr. For patients who take drug once daily and have a creatinine clearance of less than 30 ml/min, once-daily dosing is not recommended. For patients who take drug on an as-needed basis and have mild to moderate hepatic dysfunction, dosage should not exceed 10 mg once every day.

* *To treat benign prostatic hyperplasia (BPH)*

TABLETS (CIALIS)

Men. 5 mg once daily.

± **DOSAGE ADJUSTMENT** For patients taking potent CYP3A4 inhibitors, such as ketoconazole or ritonavir, dosage reduced to 2.5 mg daily. For patients with a creatinine clearance of 30 to 50 mg/ml, initial dosage reduced to 2.5 mg once daily with possible increase to 5 mg, based upon individual response. For patients with a creatinine clearance less than 30 ml/min, drug use is not recommended for this indication.

* *To treat BPH and erectile dysfunction*

TABLETS (CIALIS)

Men. 5 mg once daily without regard to timing of sexual activity.

± **DOSAGE ADJUSTMENT** For patients taking potent CYP3A4 inhibitors, such as ketoconazole or ritonavir, dosage reduced to 2.5 mg daily. For patients with a creatinine clearance of 30 to 50 mg/ml, initial dosage reduced to 2.5 mg once daily with possible increase to 5 mg, based upon individual response. For patients with a creatinine clearance less than 30 ml/min, drug use is not recommended for this indication.

* *To treat pulmonary arterial hypertension in order to improve exercise ability in patients classified as group 1 by the World Health Organization*

ORAL SUSPENSION (TADLIQ), TABLETS (ADCIRCA, ALYQ)

Adults. 40 mg once daily.

± **DOSAGE ADJUSTMENT** For patients with mild to moderate hepatic or renal impairment or who have already taken ritonavir for at least 1 week, initial dosage of 20 mg once daily and then increased as tolerated. For patients already taking tadalafil and being prescribed ritonavir, tadalafil temporarily discontinued for at least 24 hours before ritonavir starts. Then, after at least 1 week of ritonavir, tadalafil restarted at 20 mg once daily and then increased to 40 mg once daily, as tolerated.

Drug Administration

P.O.

- Drug should not be administered concurrently with nitrates.
- Drug used to treat erectile dysfunction on an as-needed basis should be administered at least 30 min before sexual activity.
- Drug prescribed daily should be administered at about the same time every day.
- Shake bottle of oral suspension for 30 sec before measuring dose. Use a calibrated measuring device to measure dose. Store oral suspension at room temperature.

Route	Onset	Peak	Duration
P.O.	< 45 min	1.5–6 hr	< 36 hr

Half-life: 17.5 hr

Mechanism of Action

Enhances the effect of nitric oxide released in the penis during sexual stimulation. Remember that nitric oxide activates the enzyme guanylate cyclase, which causes increased levels of cGMP in the corpus cavernosum. This leads to increased blood flow to the penis, thus producing an erection. Although the mechanism of action is unknown in the treatment of BPH, it is known that the enzyme, phosphodiesterase type 5, is present in the bladder and prostate and is thought to possibly be involved in reducing the symptoms of BPH.
Preventing breakdown of cyclic guanosine monophosphate by phosphodiesterase, levels increase, which leads to smooth muscle relaxation of the pulmonary vasculature and subsequently, vasodilation. Vasodilation causes the pressure within the pulmonary vasculature to decrease, which improves tolerance to exercise and delays worsening of pulmonary arterial hypertension.

Contraindications

Concomitant guanylate cyclase stimulator therapy, such as riociguat; continuous or intermittent nitrate therapy; hypersensitivity to tadalafil or its components

Interactions

DRUGS

alpha-blockers (alfuzosin, doxazosin, tamsulosin), antihypertensives, nitrates: Increased risk of hypotension, which could become severe
antacids (aluminum hydroxide/magnesium hydroxide): Reduction in rate of absorption of tadalafil
CYP3A4 inducers, such as rifampin: Possibly decreased tadalafil exposure
CYP3A4 inhibitors, such as ketoconazole, HIV protease inhibitor (ritonavir): Possible increased tadalafil exposure

ACTIVITIES

alcohol use: Potentiated blood pressure–lowering effects

FOODS

grapefruit juice: Possibly prolonged tadalafil effects

Adverse Reactions

CNS: Asthenia, **CVA**, dizziness, fatigue, headache, hypesthesia, insomnia, migraine, paresthesia, **seizures**, somnolence, syncope, transient global amnesia, vertigo
CV: Angina pectoris, chest pain, hypertension, **hypotension**, **MI**, palpitations, peripheral edema, postural hypotension, **sudden cardiac death**, tachycardia
EENT: Blurred vision, changes in color vision, conjunctivitis, dry mouth, epistaxis, eyelid swelling, eye pain, hearing or visual loss, increased lacrimation, nasal congestion, nasopharyngitis, nonarteritic anterior ischemic optic neuropathy (NAION), pharyngitis, retinal artery or vein occlusion, tinnitus, visual field defects
GI: Diarrhea, dysphagia, dyspepsia, elevated liver enzymes, esophagitis, gastritis, gastroesophageal reflux, nausea, upper abdominal pain, vomiting
GU: Priapism, spontaneous penile erection, UTI
MS: Arthralgia, back or neck pain, extremity pain, myalgia
RESP: Bronchitis, cough, dyspnea, upper respiratory tract infection
SKIN: Diaphoresis, **exfoliative dermatitis**, flushing, pruritus, rash, **Stevens-Johnson syndrome**, urticaria
Other: **Angioedema and other hypersensitivity reactions**, flu-like symptoms

Childbearing Considerations

PREGNANCY

- Cialis is not indicated in female patients.
- Pregnant women with pulmonary arterial hypertension are at risk for heart failure,

stroke, preterm delivery, and maternal and fetal death.

- It is not known if Adcirca, Alyq, or Tadliq can cause fetal harm.
- Use Adcirca, Alyq, or Tadliq with caution only if benefit to mother outweighs potential risk to fetus.

LACTATION

- Cialis is not indicated in female patients.
- It is not known if Adcirca, Alyq, or Tadliq is present in breast milk.
- Mothers should check with prescriber before breastfeeding when prescribed Adcirca, Alyq, or Tadliq.

REPRODUCTION

- Sperm count may be decreased with drug therapy.

Nursing Considerations

! WARNING Know that patients with hereditary degenerative retinal disorders, including retinitis pigmentosa, should not receive tadalafil because of the risk of serious ophthalmic adverse reactions.

! WARNING Be aware that patients with severe hepatic or renal impairment should not receive tadalafil because its effects in these patients are unknown.

! WARNING Know that patients taking any form of nitrates should not receive drug because the combination can cause severe hypotension and possibly death.

- Monitor blood pressure and heart rate and rhythm before and during therapy.

! WARNING Monitor patient for a hypersensitivity reaction, which may become life threatening such as angioedema. If present, notify prescriber, expect drug to be discontinued, and provide supportive care, as needed and ordered.

! WARNING Monitor patients closely who have left ventricular outflow obstructon, such as aortic stenosis and idiopathic hypertrophic subaortic stenosis, and those with severely impaired autonomic control of blood pressure because these conditions increase sensitivity to vasodilators, such as tadalafil. Also, monitor patient for signs and symptoms of an MI because MIs have occurred with tadalafil therapy. Know that drug also has been associated with sudden cardiac death. Be prepared to treat a cardiac emergency.

! WARNING Monitor patients for priapism. Patients at higher risks include patients with leukemia, multiple myeloma, penile deformities (such as angulation, cavernosal fibrosis, or Peyronie's disease), or sickle cell anemia. If present, notify prescriber immediately.

! WARNING Monitor patient for other persistent, serious, or unusual adverse reactions as drug can affect many body systems.

PATIENT TEACHING

! WARNING Tell patient not to take tadalafil if any form of organic nitrate, either continuously or intermittently is taken, because profound hypotension and death could result.

- Instruct patient how to administer drug for the condition and brand of drug prescribed.
- Advise patient to avoid alcohol or grapefruit juice consumption while taking tadalafil.
- Tell male patients taking tadalafil for pulmonary arterial hypertension not to take another form of tadalafil under the brand name of Cialis or any other PDE5 inhibitors to treat erectile dysfunction.

! WARNING Alert patient that drug may cause an allergic reaction. If present, tell patient to notify prescriber and, if severe, to seek immediate medical care.

! WARNING Urge patient to notify prescriber immediately if erection is painful or lasts longer than 4 hours, to avoid possible penile damage and permanent loss of erectile function.

! WARNING Tell patient to seek immediate medical attention if hearing loss is experienced that may be accompanied by dizziness or tinnitus or a sudden loss of vision in one or both eyes.

- Advise patient taking tadalafil to treat erectile dysfunction to obtain sexual counseling to help enhance the drug's effects.

tamoxifen citrate

Soltamox

Class and Category

Pharmacologic class: Selective estrogen receptor modulator (SERM)
Therapeutic class: Anti-estrogen agent

Indications and Dosages

* *To treat estrogen receptor–positive metastatic breast cancer in men and women*

ORAL SOLUTION, TABLETS

Adults. 20 to 40 mg daily. Dosages greater than 20 mg divided and administered twice daily (morning and evening).

* *As adjuvant treatment of patients with early-stage estrogen receptor–positive breast cancer; to reduce occurrence of contralateral breast cancer when used as adjuvant therapy for the treatment of breast cancer*

ORAL SOLUTION, TABLETS

Adults. 20 mg daily for 5 to 10 yr.

* *To reduce the risk of invasive breast cancer in women with ductal carcinoma in situ (DCIS) after radiation and surgery; to reduce the risk of breast cancer in women at high risk*

ORAL SOLUTION, TABLETS

Adults. 20 mg daily for 5 yr.

Drug Administration

P.O.

- Tablets should be swallowed whole and not chewed, crushed, or divided. Tablets should be taken with water.
- Use the dosing cup that comes with drug when measuring dosage of oral solution. Store at room temperature and protect from light. Discard 3 mo after opening.

Route	Onset	Peak	Duration
P.O.	Unknown	5 hr	Unknown

Half-life: 5–7 days

Mechanism of Action

May block the effects of estrogen on breast tissue by competing with estrogen for estrogen receptor binding sites to prevent estrogen from possibly stimulating the growth of cancer cells.

Contraindications

Hypersensitivity to tamoxifen or its components; women at high risk for breast cancer and women with DCIS and a history of deep vein thrombosis or pulmonary embolus or who need coumarin-type anticoagulant therapy

Interactions

DRUGS

bromocriptine: Possibly increased blood tamoxifen level
CYP2D6 inducers: Possibly decreased plasma concentrations of tamoxifen
CYP2D6 inhibitors: Possibly altered tamoxifen efficacy
cytotoxic agents: Increased risk of thromboembolic events
warfarin and other coumarin-type anticoagulants: Increased anticoagulant effect of these drugs

Adverse Reactions

CNS: Confusion, **CVA**, depression, dizziness, fatigue, headache, lightheadedness, somnolence, weakness
CV: Edema, hyperlipidemia, **thrombosis**
EENT: Keratopathy, ocular toxicity (including cataracts), optic neuritis, retinopathy
GI: Elevated liver enzymes, **hepatotoxicity**, nausea, vomiting
GU: **Endometrial cancer**, endometrial hyperplasia, endometrial polyps, genital itching, menstrual irregularities, ovarian cysts, vaginal discharge (females); impotence, decreased libido (males)
HEME: Anemia, **leukopenia**, **thrombocytopenia**
MS: Transient bone or tumor pain
RESP: **Pulmonary embolism**
SKIN: Bullous pemphigoid, dry skin, **erythema multiforme**, rash, **Stevens-Johnson syndrome**, thinning hair
Other: **Angioedema**, hot flashes, **hypercalcemia**, weight gain

Childbearing Considerations

PREGNANCY

- Drug may cause fetal harm.
- Drug is not recommended during pregnancy.
- A negative pregnancy test must be obtained before drug therapy is begun.

LACTATION

- It is not known if drug is present in breast milk.
- Breastfeeding should not be done during drug therapy and for 3 mo following the last dose.

REPRODUCTION

- Females of childbearing age should use barrier or other nonhormonal contraceptive method if sexually active before starting drug, throughout drug therapy, and for 9 mo after drug has been discontinued.
- Male patients with female partners of childbearing age should use effective contraception during drug therapy and for 6 months following the last dose.

Nursing Considerations

! **WARNING** Be aware that women with ductal carcinoma in situ and those at high risk for breast cancer are more likely to develop pulmonary emboli, stroke, or uterine cancer than others receiving tamoxifen.

! **WARNING** Ensure that females of childbearing age have a negative pregnancy test before tamoxifen therapy is begun.

- Know that if patient is premenopausal, drug therapy should begin in the middle of menstruation; if patient's menstrual cycles are irregular, a negative pregnancy test before therapy starts will be used when therapy can safely start.
- Expect patient to undergo an ophthalmic examination before and periodically during tamoxifen therapy. Also, expect to monitor patient for adverse ocular reactions, such as cataracts.

! **WARNING** Obtain liver function tests, as ordered, before drug therapy begins as a baseline and then periodically throughout therapy. Monitor patient for liver function dysfunction throughout therapy because drug can cause hepatotoxicity.

! **WARNING** Monitor patient for a hypersensitivity reaction, which could become life-threatening, such as angioedema. If present, notify prescriber, expect drug to be discontinued, and provide supportive care, as needed and ordered.

! **WARNING** Monitor blood calcium level and assess patient for signs and symptoms of hypercalcemia, such as nausea, thirst, and vomiting; tamoxifen may cause hypercalcemia in breast cancer patients with bone metastasis within a few weeks of starting treatment.

! **WARNING** Assess patient for signs and symptoms of thromboembolic events, such as change in mental status, leg pain, or shortness of breath. Notify prescriber immediately if signs and symptoms suggestive of a thromboembolic event is present, and provide supportive care, as needed and ordered.

- Monitor patient's cholesterol and triglyceride levels and platelet and WBC counts periodically, as ordered.

! **WARNING** Monitor patient for other persistent, serious, or unusual adverse reactions as some may be quite serious such as endometrial cancer or pulmonary embolus.

PATIENT TEACHING

! **WARNING** Make sure that patient has been informed about serious or potentially life-threatening adverse effects associated with tamoxifen before therapy begins.

- Instruct patient how to take form of tamoxifen prescribed.

! **WARNING** Alert patient that tamoxifen may cause an allergic reaction. Tell patient to notify prescriber if an allergic reaction is present and, if severe, to seek immediate medical care.

- Inform patient of the most common side effects: hot flashes, irregular menses, and vaginal discharge.

! **WARNING** Advise patient to notify prescriber if she experiences calf swelling or leg pain during tamoxifen therapy because they may indicate a blood clot.

! **WARNING** Instruct patient to report signs of hepatotoxicity, such as flu-like symptoms, nausea, tiredness, or yellow color to eyes or skin.

! **WARNING** Urge patient to consult prescriber if adverse reactions, such as nausea and vomiting, are interfering with dosage schedule. These symptoms may be a sign of hypercalcemia.

! **WARNING** Advise patient to have regular gynecologic examinations and to notify prescriber about abnormal symptoms, including abdominal or pelvic pain and unusual vaginal bleeding or discharge suggestive of endometrial cancer. Urge patients who are taking tamoxifen for prophylaxis to have regular mammograms because tamoxifen doesn't prevent all breast cancers. Also, tell patient to inform prescriber of any new breast lumps.

! **WARNING** Stress importance of females of childbearing age or female partner of childbearing age of a male patient to use a barrier or other nonhormonal contraceptive method if sexually active before starting drug and throughout drug therapy. Females of childbearing age taking tamoxifen should continue the additional contraception for 9 months after drug has been discontinued and females of childbearing age whose partners are taking the drug to continue the additional contraception for 6 months. The prescriber should be notified immediately if pregnancy occurs as drug will need to be discontinued.

- Inform mothers that breastfeeding should not be undertaken during tamoxifen therapy and for 3 months after drug is discontinued.

tamsulosin hydrochloride

Flomax

Class and Category

Pharmacologic class: Alpha-adrenergic antagonist

Therapeutic class: Benign prostatic hyperplasia (BPH) agent

Indications and Dosages

∗ *To treat BPH*

CAPSULES

Adults. *Initial:* 0.4 mg daily 30 min after same meal of each day for 2 to 4 wk, increased to 0.8 mg daily if no response to initial dosage. *Maximum:* 0.8 mg daily.

± **DOSAGE ADJUSTMENT** For patients taking 0.4 mg strength, drug should not be used in combination with strong CYP3A4 inhibitors such as ketoconazole.

Drug Administration

P.O.

- Administer 30 min after same meal each day.
- Capsules should be swallowed whole and not chewed, crushed, or opened.
- Know that if drug is given on an empty stomach, patient's blood pressure should be monitored because of the increased risk of orthostatic hypotension.
- Be aware that if patient doesn't take drug for several days, therapy should be resumed at 0.4 mg/dose, as prescribed, and then increased, as needed.

Route	Onset	Peak	Duration
P.O.	4–8 hr	4–8 hr	9–15 hr

Half-life: 9–13 hr

Mechanism of Action

Blocks $alpha_1$-adrenergic receptors in the prostate to inhibit smooth muscle contraction in the bladder neck and prostate, prostatic capsule, and prostatic urethra, which improves the rate of urine flow and reduces symptoms of BPH.

Contraindications

Hypersensitivity to tamsulosin or its components

Interactions

DRUGS

alpha-blockers: Additive effects of both drugs

cimetidine: Risk of decreased tamsulosin clearance

CYP2D6 inhibitors, such as paroxetine and terbinafine; CYP3A4 inhibitors, such as erythromycin, ketoconazole: Possibly increased plasma tamsulosin level

phosphodiesterase-5 inhibitors: Increased risk of hypotension

Adverse Reactions

CNS: Asthenia, dizziness, drowsiness, headache, insomnia, syncope, vertigo

T

CV: **Arrhythmia**, **atrial fibrillation**, chest pain, orthostatic hypotension, palpitations, tachycardia
EENT: Amblyopia, diplopia, dry mouth, epistaxis, intraoperative floppy iris syndrome (during cataract and glaucoma surgery), pharyngitis, rhinitis, visual impairment
GI: Constipation, diarrhea, nausea, vomiting
GU: Decreased libido, ejaculation disorders, priapism
MS: Back pain
RESP: Dyspnea, **respiratory impairment**
SKIN: Desquamation, **erythema multiforme**, **exfoliative dermatitis**, pruritus, rash, **Stevens-Johnson syndrome**, urticaria
Other: **Angioedema**

Childbearing Considerations

PREGNANCY

- Drug is not indicated for female patients.

LACTATION

- Drug is not indicated for female patients.

Nursing Considerations

! **WARNING** Be aware that prostate cancer should be ruled out before tamsulosin therapy begins.

! **WARNING** Monitor patient for a hypersensitivity reaction, which could become life-threatening, such as angioedema. If present, notify prescriber, expect drug to be discontinued, and provide supportive care, as needed and ordered.

! **WARNING** Assess patient's skin regularly for abnormalities, some of which could be severe.

! **WARNING** Monitor patient's vital signs closely throughout therapy. Notify prescriber if patient develops dyspnea, an irregular or rapid pulse, or significant changes in blood pressure.

PATIENT TEACHING

- Instruct patient how to administer tamsulosin and what to do if a dose is missed.

! **WARNING** Alert patient that drug may cause an allergic reaction. Tell patient to notify prescriber if an allergic reaction occurs and, if severe, to seek immediate medical care.

! **WARNING** Advise patient to seek immediate medical care if dyspnea or an irregular or rapid pulse rate develops.

- Advise patient to avoid potentially hazardous activities until drug's CNS effects are known and resolved. Mention the need for caution if dosage is increased.
- Advise patient to change position slowly, especially after initial dose and each dosage increase, to minimize effects of orthostatic hypotension.
- Tell patient to inform ophthalmologist of tamsulosin therapy because drug may increase risk for complications with cataract surgery.

telavancin hydrochloride

Vibativ

Class and Category

Pharmacologic class: Lipoglycopeptide
Therapeutic class: Antibiotic

Indications and Dosages

∗ *To treat complicated skin and skin structure infections caused by gram-positive organisms such as* Enterococcus faecalis *(vancomycin-susceptible isolates only),* Staphylococcus aureus, Streptococcus agalactiae, S. anginosus *group (includes* S. anginosus, S. constellatus, *and* S. intermedius*), or* S. pyogenes

I.V. INFUSION

Adults. 10 mg/kg every 24 hr for 7 to 14 days.

∗ *To treat hospital-acquired and ventilator-associated bacterial pneumonia caused by* S. aureus *when alternative treatments are not suitable*

I.V. INFUSION

Adults. 10 mg/kg every 24 hr for 7 to 21 days.

± **DOSAGE ADJUSTMENT** For patients with creatinine clearance of 30 to 50 ml/min, dosage reduced to 7.5 mg/kg every 24 hours. For patients with creatinine clearance of at least 10 but less than 30 ml/min, 10 mg/kg every 48 hours.

Drug Administration

I.V.

- Reconstitute 750-mg vial with 45 ml of a diluent such as 0.9% Sodium Chloride

Injection, 5% Dextrose Injection, or Sterile Water for Injection to obtain a concentration of 15 mg/ml. To prevent foaming during reconstitution, allow the vacuum of the vial to pull the diluent from the syringe into the vial. Do not forcefully inject diluent into vial. Discard vial if vacuum did not pull the diluent into the vial. Do not shake vial or final infusion solution. Although reconstitution usually takes under 2 min, it can sometimes take as long as 20 min for drug vial contents to be dissolved completely.

- Dilute doses of 150 to 800 mg in 100 to 250 ml of 0.9% Sodium Chloride Injection, 5% Dextrose Injection, or Lactated Ringer's Injection before infusing. Doses less than 150 mg or greater than 800 mg should be further diluted in a volume that yields a final concentration of 0.6 to 0.8 mg/ml.
- Use reconstituted solution within 12 hr if stored at room temperature or 7 days if refrigerated. Use diluted solution within 12 hr if stored at room temperature, 7 days if refrigerated, or 32 days if frozen (includes reconstitution time). The total time in the vial after reconstitution plus time in the infusion bag after dilution must be counted toward these storage times. Discard if time limit exceeds these parameters.
- If same I.V. line is used to infuse other drugs, flush line before and after infusion of telavancin with 0.9% Sodium Chloride Injection, 5% Dextrose Injection, or Lactated Ringer's Injection.
- Infuse over 60 min.
- Monitor patient for a reaction like red-man syndrome, which causes flushing of upper body, pruritus, rash, or urticaria. If present, stop or slow infusion to resolve and notify prescriber.
- *Incompatibilities:* Other I.V. drugs

Route	Onset	Peak	Duration
I.V.	Unknown	Unknown	Unknown

Half-life: 8 hr

Mechanism of Action

Inhibits cell wall synthesis and alters the permeability of bacterial membranes, causing cell wall lysis and cell death.

Contraindications

Hypersensitivity to telavancin or its components, intravenous unfractionated heparin sodium

Interactions

DRUGS

ACE inhibitors, loop diuretics, NSAIDs: Increased risk of nephrotoxicity

drugs known to prolong the QT interval, such as clarithromycin, disopyramide, erythromycin, quinidine: Increased risk of prolonged QT interval

Adverse Reactions

CNS: Dizziness, rigors
CV: **Prolonged QT interval**
EENT: Taste disturbance
GI: Abdominal pain, anorexia, diarrhea, ***Clostridioides difficile*–associated diarrhea**, nausea, vomiting
GU: Elevated creatinine level, foamy urine, **nephrotoxicity**
HEME: **Abnormal coagulation**
SKIN: Pruritus, rash
Other: **Anaphylaxis**, infusion-related reactions, such as erythema or pain

Childbearing Considerations

PREGNANCY

- Pregnancy exposure registry: 1-877-484-2700.
- Drug may cause fetal harm such as digital and limb malformations.
- Females of childbearing age should have pregnancy status verified before drug is initiated.
- Drug should not be used in pregnancy unless benefit to mother outweighs potential risk to fetus.

LACTATION

- It is not known if drug is present in breast milk.
- Mothers should check with prescriber before breastfeeding.

REPRODUCTION

- Females of childbearing age should use an effective contraceptive during drug therapy and for 2 days after the final dose.
- Drug may impair male fertility.

Nursing Considerations

! **WARNING** Know that telavancin isn't recommended for patients with congenital long QT syndrome, severe left ventricular hypertrophy, uncompensated heart failure or who currently have a prolonged QT interval because drug may prolong the QT interval, causing life-threatening complications.

! **WARNING** Know that use of intravenous unfractionated heparin sodium is contraindicated with telavancin because the APTT test results may be falsely prolonged for up to 18 hours after telavancin administration.

- Use cautiously in patients taking drugs known to prolong the QT interval because of increased risk of a prolonged QT interval. Monitor QT interval regularly during therapy, as ordered.

! **WARNING** Obtain baseline serum creatinine level before telavancin therapy starts because preexisting moderate to severe renal impairment may increase mortality in the presence of telavancin therapy and is not recommended in such patients unless the benefit outweighs the potential risk. Expect to monitor patient's serum creatinine level throughout therapy, as ordered, because drug may cause nephrotoxicity, especially in patients with congestive heart failure, diabetes mellitus, hypertension, or preexisting renal disease and in patients taking nephrotoxic drugs, such as ACE inhibitors, loop diuretics, and NSAIDs. If renal function declines, notify prescriber and expect to discontinue telavancin.

! **WARNING** Ensure females of childbearing age have a negative pregnancy test result before telavancin therapy begins.

! **WARNING** Monitor patient for a hypersensitivity reaction, which could become life-threatening, such as anaphylaxis. If present, notify prescriber, expect drug to be discontinued, and provide supportive care, as needed and ordered.

! **WARNING** Monitor patient for diarrhea, which may range from mild to severe and may occur more than 2 months after antibiotic is discontinued. Report diarrhea and, if *Clostridioides difficile* is suspected, expect a stool sample to be ordered. If *C. difficile* is confirmed, provide supportive care, such as antibiotic therapy to treat *C. difficile*, electrolyte and fluid replacement, protein supplementation, and possibly surgical intervention, as needed and ordered.

- Be aware that while telavancin doesn't interfere with coagulation, it does interfere with certain tests used to monitor coagulation, such as activated clotting time, APTT, coagulation-based factor Xa tests, INR, and PT. Collect blood samples for coagulation tests as close as possible to administration of next dose of telavancin to minimize interference.

PATIENT TEACHING

- Inform patient that telavancin will be administered intravenously.

! **WARNING** Inform females of childbearing age that a negative pregnancy test result must be obtained before telavancin therapy can begin. Also, instruct patient to use effective contraception during telavancin therapy and for 2 days after the last dose.

! **WARNING** Alert patient that drug may cause an allergic reaction. Tell patient to notify staff if difficulty breathing or other signs of a hypersensitivity reaction occur.

! **WARNING** Caution patient that diarrhea may occur more than 2 months after antibiotic has been discontinued and to report any persistent or severe episodes to prescriber as further treatment may be needed.

- Tell patient that drug may cause taste to be altered. Also, alert patient that urine will be foamy.
- Advise patient to alert all prescribers that telavancin is being taken because some drugs may interact with it, causing serious adverse effects.
- Instruct patient to notify staff or prescriber of any other persistent, severe, or unusual adverse effects that may occur during drug therapy.

telmisartan

Micardis

Class and Category

Pharmacologic class: Angiotensin II receptor blocker (ARB)
Therapeutic class: Antihypertensive

Indications and Dosages

✱ *To manage hypertension, alone or with other antihypertensives*

TABLETS

Adults. *Initial:* 40 mg daily. *Maintenance:* 20 to 80 mg daily. *Maximum:* 80 mg daily.

✱ *To reduce risk of MI, stroke, or death from cardiovascular causes in patients at high risk who are unable to take ACE inhibitors*

TABLETS

Adults ages 55 and older. 80 mg once daily.

Drug Administration

P.O.

- Do not remove tablets from blister until immediately before administration.
- Administer with or without food.

Route	Onset	Peak	Duration
P.O.	1–2 hr	30–60 min	24 hr

Half-life: 24 hr

Mechanism of Action

Blocks angiotensin II from binding to receptor sites in many tissues, including adrenal glands and vascular smooth muscle causing inhibition of the aldosterone-secreting and vasoconstrictive effects of angiotensin II, which reduces blood pressure.

Contraindications

Concurrent aliskiren therapy in patients with diabetes, hypersensitivity to telmisartan or its components

Interactions

DRUGS

aliskiren: Increased risk of hyperkalemia, hypotension, and renal dysfunction
digoxin: Increased peak blood digoxin level and risk of digitalis toxicity
lithium: Increased serum lithium levels and toxicity
NSAIDs: Increased risk of renal dysfunction in elderly patients and those with volume depletion and existing renal dysfunction; increased risk of hypotension
potassium-sparing diuretics, potassium supplements: Increased risk of hyperkalemia

FOOD

salt substitutes containing potassium: Increased risk of hyperkalemia

Adverse Reactions

CNS: Asthenia, dizziness, fatigue, headache, syncope, weakness
CV: **Atrial fibrillation**, **bradycardia**, chest pain, **congestive heart failure**, edema, hypertension, **hypotension**, **MI**, orthostatic hypotension, peripheral edema
EENT: Pharyngitis, sinusitis
ENDO: **Hypoglycemia** (in diabetics)
GI: Abdominal pain, diarrhea, elevated liver enzymes, indigestion, hepatic dysfunction, nausea, vomiting
GU: **Acute renal failure**, erectile dysfunction, renal dysfunction, UTI
HEME: Anemia, eosinophilia, **thrombocytopenia**
MS: Back pain, leg or muscle cramps, leg edema, myalgia, **rhabdomyolysis**, tendinitis, tendon pain, tenosynovitis
RESP: Cough, upper respiratory tract infection
SKIN: Diaphoresis, erythema, rash, **toxicoderma**, urticaria
Other: **Anaphylaxis**, **angioedema**, elevated creatine kinase or uric acid level, flu-like symptoms, **hyperkalemia**, **hyponatremia**, hypovolemia

Childbearing Considerations

PREGNANCY

- Drug can cause fetal harm, especially if exposure occurs during the second or third trimester.
- Drug reduces fetal renal function, leading to anuria and renal failure, and increases fetal and neonatal morbidity and death. It can also cause fetal lung hypoplasia, hypotension, and skeletal deformations, such as skull hypoplasia.
- Drug is contraindicated in pregnant women and should be discontinued as soon as possible if pregnancy occurs.

LACTATION

- It is not known if drug is present in breast milk.
- Breastfeeding is not recommended because of potential serious adverse reactions, including hyperkalemia, hypotension, and renal impairment in the breastfed infant.

Nursing Considerations

! WARNING Be aware that telmisartan should not be given to pregnant women during the

T

second and third trimesters because drug can increase the risk of fetal harm.

- Give telmisartan cautiously to patients with dehydration or hyponatremia.
- Expect prescriber to add a diuretic to regimen if patient's blood pressure isn't well controlled by telmisartan.
- Check patient's blood pressure regularly to assess effectiveness of telmisartan therapy. Be prepared to treat symptomatic hypotension by placing patient in supine position and giving normal saline solution, as ordered.

! **WARNING** Monitor patient for a hypersensitivity reaction, which could become life-threatening, such as anaphylaxis or angioedema. If present, notify prescriber, expect drug to be discontinued, and provide supportive care, as needed and ordered.

! **WARNING** Monitor BUN and serum creatinine levels and urine output in patients with impaired renal function because they're at increased risk for oliguria, progressive azotemia, and possibly acute renal failure.

! **WARNING** Monitor liver enzymes, as appropriate, and assess for evidence of drug toxicity in patients with severe hepatic disease because they're at increased risk for toxicity from increased drug accumulation.

PATIENT TEACHING

- Instruct patient how to administer telmisartan.
- Advise patient not to use potassium supplements or salt substitutes that contain potassium without checking with prescriber first.

! **WARNING** Alert patient that drug may cause an allergic reaction. If present, tell patient to notify prescriber and, if severe, to seek immediate medical care.

! **WARNING** Review signs and symptoms of kidney and liver dysfunction with patient. Stress importance of notifying prescriber if either dysfunction is suspected and expect confirmation to be done with laboratory analysis.

- Advise patient to avoid hazardous activities until telmisartan's CNS effects are known and resolved.
- Instruct patient to change position slowly to minimize effects of orthostatic hypotension.
- Advise patient to drink adequate amounts of fluid during hot weather and when exercising.
- Instruct patient to consult prescriber before taking any new drug.

! **WARNING** Advise females of childbearing age to notify prescriber immediately if pregnancy occurs as drug will need to be discontinued.

- Inform mothers not to breastfeed their infant during telmisartan therapy.

temazepam

Restoril

Class, Category, and Schedule

Pharmacologic class: Benzodiazepine
Therapeutic class: Sedative-hypnotic
Controlled substance schedule: IV

Indications and Dosages

∗ *To provide short-term management of insomnia*

CAPSULES

Adults. 7.5 mg, 15 mg, or 30 mg nightly. *Maximum:* 30 mg daily for no longer than 10 consecutive days.

± **DOSAGE ADJUSTMENT** For elderly or debilitated patients, dosage kept at 7.5 mg nightly with maximum not exceeding 15 mg daily for no longer than 10 consecutive days.

Drug Administration

P.O.

- Administer drug 30 min before bedtime.
- Do not administer more than 10 consecutive days.

Route	Onset	Peak	Duration
P.O.	10–20 min	1.5 hr	Unknown

Half-life: 3.5–18.4 hr

Mechanism of Action

May potentiate the effects of gamma-aminobutyric acid (GABA) and other inhibitory neurotransmitters by binding to specific benzodiazepine receptor sites in cortical and limbic areas of the CNS. Binding to these receptor sites increases GABA's inhibitory effects and blocks cortical and limbic arousal.

Contraindications

Hypersensitivity to temazepam, other benzodiazepines, or their components; pregnancy

Interactions

DRUGS

opioids, other benzodiazepines: Increased risk of respiratory depression that could become severe, profound sedation

ACTIVITIES

alcohol use: Increased CNS and respiratory depression that could be severe

Adverse Reactions

CNS: Aggressiveness, anxiety (in daytime), ataxia, complex behaviors (such as sleep driving), confusion, decreased level of consciousness or concentration, depression, dizziness, drowsiness, euphoria, fatigue, headache, insomnia, nightmares, slurred speech, **suicidal ideation**, syncope, talkativeness, tremor, vertigo, wakefulness during last third of night
CV: Palpitations, tachycardia
EENT: Abnormal or blurred vision, increased salivation, **throat tightness**
GI: Abdominal pain, constipation, diarrhea, hepatic dysfunction, jaundice, nausea, thirst, vomiting
GU: Decreased libido
HEME: **Agranulocytosis**, anemia, **leukopenia**, **neutropenia**, **thrombocytopenia**
MS: Muscle spasm or weakness
RESP: Dyspnea, increased bronchial secretions
SKIN: Diaphoresis, flushing, pruritus, rash
Other: **Acute or protracted withdrawal syndrome**, **anaphylaxis**, **angioedema**, physical and psychological dependence

Childbearing Considerations

PREGNANCY

- Pregnancy exposure registry: 1-866-961-2388 or https://womensmentalhealth.org/pregnancyregistry/.
- Drug may cause fetal harm because of potential for increased risk of congenital malformations as well as neonatal CNS depression when drug is given during last few weeks of pregnancy.
- A pregnancy test should be performed before drug therapy is begun.
- Drug is contraindicated in females of childbearing age who are or may become pregnant.

LACTATION

- It is not known if drug is present in breast milk.
- Mothers should check with prescriber before breastfeeding.

REPRODUCTION

- Females of childbearing age should use effective contraception during drug therapy.

Nursing Considerations

! **WARNING** Be aware temazepam is contraindicated in pregnant patients. Ensure that a negative pregnancy test is obtained before administering drug to females of childbearing age.

! **WARNING** Assess patient for history of abuse, misuse, and addiction as well as prior dependence and withdrawal reactions to benzodiazepine use because drug can cause physical and psychological dependence. Monitor patient's use of drug closely throughout therapy. Alert prescriber if abuse, misuse, or addiction is suspected.

! **WARNING** Monitor patient for a hypersensitivity reaction, which could become life threatening such as anaphylaxis or angioedema. If present, notify prescriber, expect drug to be discontinued, and provide supportive care, as needed and ordered.

! **WARNING** Assess patients with respiratory depression, severe COPD, or sleep apnea for signs of respiratory failure.

! **WARNING** Watch patient closely for suicidal tendencies, particularly when therapy starts and dosage changes, because depression may worsen temporarily during these times and could lead to suicidal ideation.

! **WARNING** Be aware that temazepam can aggravate acute intermittent porphyria, myasthenia gravis, and severe renal impairment. Monitor patient closely.

! **WARNING** Know that opioids and other CNS depessants should only be used concomitantly with benzodiazepine therapy in patients for whom other treatment options are inadequate. If prescribed together, expect dosing and duration of the opioid to be limited. Monitor patient closely for signs and symptoms of a decrease in consciousness, including coma, profound sedation, and significant respiratory depression. Notify prescriber immediately and provide emergency supportive care, as needed and ordered, as death may occur without treatment.

- Implement safety precautions, according to facility policy, especially in elderly patients, because they're more sensitive to drug's CNS effects and at higher risk for falls.
- Know that temazepam may cause deterioration of cognition or coordination in patients with late-stage Parkinson's disease or worsening psychosis.

! **WARNING** Be aware that drug shouldn't be discontinued abruptly, even after only 1 to 2 weeks of therapy, because doing so may cause an acute withdrawal syndrome that could become life-threatening or a protracted withdrawal syndrome that could last weeks to more than 12 months. Expect to taper dosage slowly for discontinuation purposes.

PATIENT TEACHING

! **WARNING** Warn females of childbearing age temazepam should not be taken during pregnancy because it can cause fetal harm and that a negative pregnancy test will be required before temazepam therapy can begin. Stress importance of using effective contraception throughout drug therapy. Advise these patients to immediately report pregnancy.

- Instruct patient how to administer temazepam.
- Tell patient to take temazepam exactly as prescribed and not to stop or change dosage without consulting prescriber. Warn patient not to take drug for more than 10 consecutive days because of the potential for physical and psychological dependence.

! **WARNING** Advise patient to avoid consuming alcohol because it increases drug's sedative effects and the risk of such abnormal behaviors as sleep driving. Also, tell patient that combining alcohol or a benzodiazepine such as temazepam with an opioid could result in severe respiratory depression and even death.

! **WARNING** Stress importance of not stopping drug abruptly. Explain the risks associated with abrupt cessation, including abdominal cramps, acute sense of hearing, confusion, depression, nausea, numbness, perceptual disturbances, photophobia, sweating, tachycardia, tingling, trembling, and vomiting. Tell patient acute withdrawal syndrome could become life-threatening. Also, warn patient that abrupt cessation may cause protracted withdrawal syndrome that could last weeks to more than 12 months.

! **WARNING** Alert patient that temazepam may cause an allergic reaction. Tell patient to notify prescriber if an allergic reaction occurs and, if severe, to seek immediate medical attention.

! **WARNING** Urge family or caregiver to watch patient closely for suicidal tendencies, especially when therapy starts or dosage changes.

- Caution patient about possible drowsiness. Advise to avoid potentially hazardous activities until drug's CNS effects are known and resolved and to take fall precautions.
- Advise patient that drug may cause abnormal behaviors during sleep, such as driving a car, eating, talking on the phone, or having sex without any recall of the event. If family notices any such behavior or patient sees evidence of such behavior upon awakening, the prescriber should be notified.
- Instruct patient to inform all prescribers of temazepam use, especially when pain medication may be prescribed.

tenapanor

Ibsrela, Xphozah

Class and Category

Pharmacologic class: Sodium/hydrogen exchanger 3 (NHE3) inhibitor
Therapeutic class: GI agent, phosphorus reduction agent

Indications and Dosages

* *To treat irritable bowel syndrome with constipation*

TABLETS (IBSRELA)

Adults. 50 mg twice daily immediately before first meal of the day and immediately before dinner.

* *As adjunct to reduce serum phosphorus in patients with chronic kidney disease on diaysis as add-on therapy in patients who have an inadequate response to phosphate binders or who are intolerant of any dose of phosphate binder therapy*

TABLETS (XPHOZAH)

Adults. 30 mg twice daily immediately before first meal of the day and immediately before evening meal.

Drug Administration

P.O.

- Administer drug immediately before breakfast or first meal of the day and immediately before dinner.
- Do not administer Xphozah right before a hemodialysis session but instead administer right before the next meal following dialysis.
- Separate administration of drug and sodium polystyrene sulfonate by at least 3 hr.
- Store tenapanor at room temperature; keep in original container and protect from moisture. Desiccant should not be removed from bottle, nor should drug be subdivided or repackaged.
- If a dose is missed, the missed dose should be skipped.

Route	Onset	Peak	Duration
P.O.	Unknown	Unknown	Unknown

Half-life: Unknown

Mechanism of Action

Reduces absorption of sodium from the small intestine and colon by inhibiting sodium/hydrogen exchanger 3 (NHE3) on the apical surface of the enterocytes, resulting in an increase in water secretion into the intestinal lumen to accelerate intestinal transit time, which then causes a softer stool consistency. Reduces abdominal pain associated with irritable bowel syndrome with constipation by decreasing visceral hypersensitivity and decreasing intestinal permeability. Inhibition of NHE3 also decreases phosphate absorption by reducing phosphate permeability through the paracellular pathway.

Contraindications

Children less than 6 yr of age, hypersensitivity to tenapanor or its components, known or suspected mechanical GI obstruction

Interactions

DRUGS

OATP2B1 substates: Possibly reduced exposure for OAT2B1 substrates reducing effectiveness

sodium polystyrene sulfonate: Binds to tenapanor decreasing tenapanor's ability to be effective

Adverse Reactions

CNS: Dizziness

GI: Abdominal pain, abnormal GI sounds, diarrhea that could be severe, flatulence, **rectal bleeding**

Other: **Hyperkalemia**

Childbearing Considerations

PREGNANCY

- Drug is minimally absorbed systemically and not expected to result in fetal exposure.

LACTATION

- It is not known if drug is present in breast milk.
- Drug is minimally absorbed systemically and not expected to result in relevant exposure to breastfed infants.

Nursing Considerations

! **WARNING** Monitor patient's serum potassium level, as ordered, because drug may cause hyperkalemia.

- Monitor patient for diarrhea. If severe, notify prescriber, suspend dosing, and rehydrate patient, as needed and ordered.

PATIENT TEACHING

- Instruct patient how to administer tenapanor and what to do if a dose is missed.
- Remind patient not to use laxatives or stool softeners during tenapanor therapy.

! **WARNING** Also, remind patient to store drug securely and out of the reach of children, as accidental ingestion, especially by children younger than 6 years of age, may cause severe diarrhea and dehydration.

! **WARNING** Tell patient to stop taking tenapanor and notify prescriber if severe diarrhea occurs.

tenecteplase

TNKase

Class and Category

Pharmacologic class: Tissue plasminogen activator (tPA)
Therapeutic class: Thrombolytic

Indications and Dosages

* *To reduce mortality associated with acute ST elevation MI (STEMI)*

I.V. INJECTION

Adults weighing 90 kg (198 lb) or more. 50 mg (10 ml) injected rapidly over 5 sec.
Adults weighing 80 kg (176 lb) to 90 kg (198 lb). 45 mg (9 ml) injected rapidly over 5 sec.
Adults weighing 70 kg (154 lb) to 80 kg (176 lb). 40 mg (8 ml) injected rapidly over 5 sec.
Adults weighing 60 kg (132 lb) to 70 kg (154 lb). 35 mg (7 ml) injected rapidly over 5 sec.
Adults weighing less than 60 kg (132 lb). 30 mg (6 ml) injected rapidly over 5 sec.

* *To treat acute ischemic stroke*

I.V. INJECTION

Adults weighing 90 kg (198 lb) or more. 25 mg (5 ml) injected rapidly over 5 sec.
Adults weighing 80 kg (176 lb) to 90 kg (198 lb). 22.5 mg (4.5 ml) injected rapidly over 5 sec.
Adults weighing 70 kg (154 lb) to 80 kg (176 lb). 20 mg (4 ml) injected rapidly over 5 sec.
Adults weighing 60 kg <132 lb) to 70 kg (154 lb). 17.5 mg (3.5 ml) injected rapidly over 5 sec.
Adults weighing less than 60 kg (132 lb). 15 mg (3 ml) injected rapidly over 5 sec.

Drug Administration

I.V.

- Reconstitute immediately before use because drug contains no antibacterial preservatives.
- Use the supplied 10-ml syringe pre-filled with Sterile Water for Injection and dual cannula device to reconstitute and administer drug.
- Use 5.2 ml of the Sterile Water for Injection provided for 25 mg vial; 10 ml for 50 mg vial.
- Using a sterile syringe, aseptically withdraw the Sterile Water for Injection from the diluent vial and reconstitute the TNNKase vial by directing the stream into the lyophilized powder to obtain a final concentration of 5 mg/ml.
- Gently swirl—don't shake—vial until contents are completely dissolved. If slight foaming occurs during reconstitution, allow drug to stand undisturbed for a few minutes to allow large bubbles to dissipate. Solution should be colorless to pale yellow and transparent.
- Withdraw prescribed dose from reconstituted drug in vial, using supplied syringe. Discard any unused solution. If reconstituted solution is not used immediately, refrigerate vial and if not used within 8 hr, discard reconstituted solution.
- Flush any dextrose-containing I.V. lines with 0.9% Sodium Chloride Injection before and after administering drug.
- Administer as a single I.V. bolus rapidly over 5 sec.
- *Incompatibilities:* Dextrose-containing solutions

Route	Onset	Peak	Duration
I.V.	Immediate	Unknown	20–24 min

Half-life: 90–130 min

Mechanism of Action

Binds to fibrin and converts plasminogen to plasmin to break down fibrin, fibrinogen, and other clotting factors, resulting in dissolution of a coronary artery thrombus.

Contraindications

Active internal bleeding, aneurysm, arteriovenous malformation, bleeding disorders, brain tumor, history of cerebrovascular accident, hypersensitivity to tenecteplase or its components, intracranial or intraspinal surgery or trauma within past 2 mo, severe uncontrolled hypertension

Interactions

DRUGS

abciximab, aspirin, clopidogrel, dipyridamole, heparin, oral anticoagulants, ticlopidine: Possibly increased risk of bleeding

thrombolytics: Increased risk of thrombo-embolic events

Adverse Reactions

CNS: **Intracranial hemorrhage**

CV: Arrhythmias (accelerated idioventricular rhythm, ventricular premature depolarizations, ventricular tachycardia), bradycardia, cholesterol embolism, thromboembolic events

EENT: Epistaxis, gingival bleeding, **laryngeal edema**, pharyngeal bleeding

GI: GI and retroperitoneal bleeding

GU: Genitourinary bleeding, prolonged or heavy menstrual bleeding

HEME: Bleeding, hematoma

RESP: Hemoptysis

SKIN: Bleeding at puncture sites, surgical incision sites, or venous cutdown sites; rash; urticaria

Other: Anaphylaxis, angioedema

Childbearing Considerations

PREGNANCY

- It is not known if drug can cause fetal harm, although maternal hemorrhage may result in fetal death.
- Use with caution only if benefit to mother outweighs potential risk to fetus.

LACTATION

- It is not known if drug is present in breast milk.
- Mothers should check with prescriber before breastfeeding.

Nursing Considerations

! **WARNING** Be aware that patients undergoing a planned percutaneous coronary intervention (PCI) for STEMI receiving tenecteplase therapy are at increased risk of heart failure and recurrent ischemia. In patients with large ST segment elevation MI, expect prescriber to choose either thrombolysis or PCI as primary treatment for reperfusion.

! **WARNING** Expect patient to be monitored for arrythmias that may become life threatening such as bradycardia and ventricular tachycardia. Have anti-arrhythmic therapy available to treat bradycardia and/or ventricular irritability, if needed.

- Assess tenecteplase injection site for signs and symptoms of hematoma, including dark, deep purple bruises under skin and itching, pain, redness, or swelling. Also, monitor patient for delayed bleeding at puncture sites, bleeding from surgical incisions, and superficial bleeding.
- Avoid I.M. injections and nonessential handling of patient, if possible, for first few hours after drug administration.
- Know that if arterial puncture becomes necessary during first few hours after tenecteplase administration, expect to use an upper extremity that's accessible to manual compression. Apply pressure for at least 30 minutes after procedure, use a pressure dressing, and frequently monitor puncture site for signs of bleeding.

! **WARNING** Monitor patient for a hypersensitivity reaction, which could become life-threatening, such as anaphylaxis or angioedema during and for several hours after tenecteplase has been administered. If present, notify prescriber and provide supportive care, as needed and ordered.

! **WARNING** Assess for signs and symptoms of GI bleeding (such as bloody or black tarry stools, bloody or coffee-ground vomitus, and severe stomach pain; genitourinary bleeding (such as hematuria), intracranial bleeding (such as decreased level of consciousness), respiratory tract bleeding (such as hemoptysis), or retroperitoneal bleeding (such as abdominal pain or swelling or back pain). Notify prescriber immediately if patient develops any of these signs or symptoms.

! **WARNING** Expect to discontinue concomitant heparin or oral antiplatelet therapy immediately, if serious bleeding (not controllable by local pressure) occurs.

! **WARNING** Monitor patients at higher risk for thromboembolism, including patients with atrial fibrillation or mitral stenosis, while receiving a thrombolytic, such as tenecteplase because these patients are at high risk to develop a left heart thrombus.

- Be aware that during tenecteplase therapy, coagulation tests and/or measures of fibrinolytic activity may be unreliable unless laboratory takes specific precautions because drug can cause degradation of fibrinogen in blood samples removed for analysis.

PATIENT TEACHING

- Inform patient that drug will be given intraveneously.
- Instruct patient to limit physical activity after tenecteplase administration to reduce the risk of bleeding or injury.

! **WARNING** Stress importance of notifying staff immediately if any signs of an allergic reaction occur, including difficulty breathing.

! **WARNING** Advise patient to immediately report any bleeding, including from gums or nose. Also, tell patient to alert staff of any other persistent, serious, or unusual adverse reaction.

tenofovir alafenamide

Vemlidy

Class and Category

Pharmacologic class: Nucleoside analog reverse transcriptase inhibitor
Therapeutic class: Antiretroviral

Indications and Dosages

∗ *To treat chronic hepatitis B virus (HBV) infection in patients with compensated liver disease*

TABLETS

Adults and children ages 6 and older weighing at least 25 kg (55 lb). 25 mg once daily with food.

±**DOSAGE ADJUSTMENT** For adult patients taking carbamazepine concomitantly, dosage doubled.

Drug Administration

- Administer drug at about the same time daily.
- Give drug with food.
- Administer drug to patients receiving chronic hemodialysis after hemodialysis.

Route	Onset	Peak	Duration
P.O.	Unknown	0.5 hr	Unknown

Half-life: 0.5 hr

Mechanism of Action

Inhibits the activity of HBV reverse transcriptase by competing with the natural substrate, deoxyadenosine 5' triphosphate, and, after incorporation into DNA, by DNA chain termination.

Contraindications

Hypersensitivity to tenofovir alafenamide or its components

Interactions

DRUGS

acyclovir, aminoglycosides, cidofovir, ganciclovir, multiple NSAIDs, valacyclovir, valganciclovir: Increased risk of reduced renal function, increasing tenofovir alafenamide concentrations, which may lead to increased risk of adverse reactions
BCRP and P-gp inhibitors: Possibly increased absorption of tenofovir alafenamide
P-gp inducers, such as carbamazepine, oxcarbazepine, phenobarbital, phenytoin, rifabutin, rifampin, rifapentine, St. John's wort: Decreased absorption of tenofovir alafenamide

Adverse Reactions

CNS: Fatigue, headache
CV: Elevated LDL-cholesterol levels
GI: Abdominal pain, diarrhea, dyspepsia, elevated liver or pancreatic enzymes, flatulence, nausea, **pancreatitis**, **severe acute exacerbation of hepatitis B**, **severe hepatomegaly with steatosis**, vomiting
GU: **Acute renal failure**, **acute tubular necrosis**, **Fanconi syndrome**, glycosuria, renal impairment (new onset or worsening), proximal renal tubulopathy

MS: Back pain, bone density loss, elevated creatine kinase levels
RESP: Arthralgia, cough
SKIN: Rash, urticaria
Other: **Angioedema**, **lactic acidosis**

Childbearing Considerations

PREGNANCY

- Pregnancy exposure registry: 1-800-258-4263.
- It is not known if drug can cause fetal harm.
- Use with caution only if benefit to mother outweighs potential risk to fetus.

LACTATION

- It is not known if drug is present in breast milk.
- Mothers should check with prescriber before breastfeeding.

Nursing Considerations

- Know that HIV-1 antibody testing should be done on all HBV-infected patients before initiating therapy with tenofovir, alafenamide to avoid the development of HIV-1 resistance.

! **WARNING** Be aware that tenofovir alafenamide should not be used in combination with any other drug containing tenofovir or adefovir dipivoxil. Also, know that tenofovir alafenamide should not be administered with nephrotoxic agents, such as high-dose or multiple NSAIDs because of increased risk of renal dysfunction.

! **WARNING** Obtain an estimated creatinine clearance, serum creatinine, urine glucose, and urine protein in all patients prior to initiating tenofovir alafenamide therapy and periodically throughout, as ordered, because drug is principally eliminated by the kidneys. Also, know that patient's serum phosphorus level should be assessed before and during therapy if patient has chronic kidney disease. Monitor patient for life-threatening renal adverse reactions such as acute renal failure, acute tubular necrosis, and Fanconi syndrome throughout therapy.

! **WARNING** Monitor patient for a hypersensitivity reaction, which may become life-threatening, such as angioedema. If present, notify prescriber, expect drug to be switched to a different drug, and provide supportive care, as needed and ordered.

! **WARNING** Monitor patient for signs and symptoms, as well as laboratory findings, of lactic acidosis or pronounced hepatotoxicity that may develop with tenofovir alafenamide therapy. Know that hepatomegaly and steatosis may occur even in the absence of marked transaminase elevations.

- Notify prescriber if patient develops a fracture and/or muscle pain or weakness, persistent or worsening bone pain, or pain in extremities, as these symptoms require further evaluation.
- Be aware that patients who have a history of pathologic bone fracture or other risk factors for bone loss or osteoporosis should be assessed regularly for bone density loss. Patient may benefit from calcium and vitamin D supplementation.

! **WARNING** Monitor patient upon discontinuation of tenofovir alafenamide for several months because severe acute exacerbations of hepatitis have occurred when drug has been stopped. Monitoring should include not only an assessment for signs and symptoms of hepatitis, but also laboratory studies, such as liver enzymes, as ordered.

PATIENT TEACHING

- Instruct patient how to administer tenofovir alafenamide. Stress importance of not missing doses because doing so can result in the development of resistance to the drug.
- Tell patient to avoid high-dose or multiple NSAIDs while taking tenofovir alafenamide because of the risk of renal dysfunction.

! **WARNING** Warn patient not to stop taking drug without prescriber knowledge.

! **WARNING** Alert patient that drug may cause an allergic reaction. If present, tell patient to notify prescriber and, if severe, to seek immediate medical care.

! **WARNING** Caution patient to report any persistent, severe, or unusual adverse reactions to prescriber.

- Tell patient to inform all prescribers of tenofovir alafenamide therapy, as other drugs containing tenofovir should not be prescribed during therapy.

- Inform patient that bone density scanning may be ordered during tenofovir alafenamide therapy.

! **WARNING** Inform patients who are discontinuing tenofovir alafenamide to seek medical attention if signs and symptoms of hepatitis reappear. This is because severe acute exacerbations of hepatitis may occur for many months after drug has been discontinued. Encourage patient to comply with regular blood tests performed for several months after drug is discontinued.

tenofovir disoproxil fumarate

Viread

Class and Category

Pharmacologic class: Nucleoside reverse transcriptase inhibitor (NRTI)
Therapeutic class: Antiretroviral

Indications and Dosages

* *As adjunct to treat human immunodeficiency virus type 1 (HIV-1) infection; to treat chronic hepatitis B virus (HBV)*

TABLETS

Adults and children weighing at least 35 kg (77 lb). 300 mg once daily.
Children ages 2 and older weighing 28 kg (61.6 lb) to less than 35 kg (77 lb) and able to swallow a tablet. 250 mg once daily.
Children ages 2 and older weighing 22 kg (48.4 lb) to less than 28 kg (61.6 lb) and able to swallow a tablet. 200 mg once daily.
Children ages 2 and older weighing 17 kg (37.4 lb) to less than 22 kg (48.4 lb) and able to swallow a tablet. 150 mg once daily.

ORAL POWDER

Adults and children ages 2 and older weighing less than 35 kg (77 lb) but at least 10 kg (22 lb) who are unable to swallow a tablet. 8 mg/kg once daily. *Maximum:* 300 mg once daily.

± **DOSAGE ADJUSTMENT** For adult patients with a creatinine clearance between 30 and 49 ml/min, dosage interval increased to every 48 hours. For adult patients with a creatinine clearance between 10 and 29 ml/min, dosage interval increased to every 72 to 96 hours. For hemodialysis adult patients, dosage interval increased to every 7 days or after a total of approximately 12 hours of dialysis. There are no specific recommendations for children with renal dysfunction given by manufacturer.

Drug Administration

P.O.

- Weigh patient regularly for dosage adjustment, as needed.
- Measure oral powder using only the supplied dosing scoop. One level scoop delivers 1 g of powder, which contains 40 mg of tenofovir disoproxil fumarate. Mix with 2 to 4 ounces of soft food not requiring chewing, such as applesauce, baby food, or yogurt. Administer mixture immediately to avoid a bitter taste.
- Do not mix powder in a liquid because the powder may float on top of the liquid even after stirring.
- Administer tablets without regard to food intake.

Route	Onset	Peak	Duration
P.O.	Unknown	1–2 hr	Unknown

Half-life: 17 hr

Mechanism of Action

Inhibits the activity of HIV-1 reverse transcriptase and HBV reverse transcriptase by competing with the natural substrate deoxyadenosine 5' triphosphate and, after incorporation into DNA, by DNA chain termination.

Contraindications

Hypersensitivity to tenofovir disoproxil fumarate or its components

Interactions

DRUGS

atazanavir: Decreased atazanavir concentration decreasing drug effectiveness
atazanavir/ritonavir, darunavir/ritonavir, ledipasvir/sofosbuvir, lopinavir/ritonavir, sofosbuvir/velpatasvir/voxilaprevir: Increased tenofovir concentration with increased risk of adverse reactions
didanosine: Increased concentration of didanosine with increased risk of adverse reactions

drugs affecting renal function, such as aminoglycosides, acyclovir, cidofovir, ganciclovir, high-dose or multiple NSAIDs use, valacyclovir, valganciclovir: Possibly increased concentration of tenofovir and/or increased concentration of other renally eliminated drugs

Adverse Reactions

CNS: Anxiety, asthenia, depression, dizziness, fatigue, fever, headache, insomnia, peripheral neuropathy
CV: Chest pain, elevated cholesterol and triglycerides
EENT: Nasopharyngitis, sinusitis
ENDO: Hyperglycemia
GI: Abdominal pain, **acute hepatitis (severe)**, anorexia, diarrhea, dyspepsia, elevated liver and pancreatic enzymes, flatulence, **hepatomegaly with steatosis (severe)**, nausea, **pancreatitis**, vomiting
GU: **Acute renal failure**, **acute tubular necrosis**, elevated creatinine, **Fanconi syndrome**, hematuria, interstitial nephritis, **renal impairment**
HEME: Anemia, **neutropenia**
MS: Arthralgia, back pain, decreased bone density, elevated bone specific alkaline phosphatase and creatine kinase, muscular weakness, myalgia, myopathy, osteomalacia, **rhabdomyolysis**
RESP: Dyspnea, pneumonia, upper respiratory infections
SKIN: Diaphoresis, maculopapular rash, pruritus, pustular rash, rash, urticaria, vesiculobullous rash
Other: **Angioedema**, **hypokalemia**, **hypophosphatemia**, **immune reconstitution syndrome**, **lactic acidosis**, lipodystrophy, pain, weight loss

Childbearing Considerations

PREGNANCY

- Pregnancy exposure registry: 1-800-258-4263.
- Studies show no increase in fetal harm when drug is taken during the first and third trimesters.
- Use with caution only if benefit to mother outweighs potential risk to fetus.

LACTATION

- Drug is present in breast milk.
- The Centers for Disease Control and Prevention recommends that HIV-1 infected mothers not breastfeed to avoid risking postnatal transmission of HIV-1 infection to infants. They also do not recommend breastfeeding because of potential drug-induced adverse reactions in the infant.
- Mothers taking drug to treat hepatitis B viral infection should check with prescriber before breastfeeding.

Nursing Considerations

- Know that HIV-1 antibody testing should be done on all HBV-infected patients before initiating therapy with tenofovir disoproxil fumarate, to avoid the development of HIV-1 resistance.

! WARNING Be aware that tenofovir disoproxil fumarate should not be used in combination with any other drug containing tenofovir or adefovir dipivoxil. Also, know that tenofovir disoproxil fumarate should not be administered with nephrotoxic agents, such as high-dose or multiple NSAIDs because of increased risk of renal dysfunction.

! WARNING Obtain an estimated creatinine clearance, serum creatinine, urine glucose, and urine protein in all patients prior to initiating tenofovir disoproxil fumarate therapy and periodically throughout, as ordered, because drug is principally eliminated by the kidneys. Also, know that patient's serum phosphorus level should be assessed before and during therapy. Monitor patient for life-threatening renal adverse reactions such as acute renal failure, acute tubular necrosis, and Fanconi syndrome throughout therapy.

! WARNING Monitor patient for a hypersensitivity reaction, which could become life threatening such as angioedema. If present, notify prescriber, expect drug to be switched to a different drug, and provide supportive care, as needed and ordered.

! WARNING Monitor patient for signs and symptoms, as well as laboratory findings, of lactic acidosis or pronounced hepatotoxicity that may develop with tenofovir therapy. Know that hepatomegaly and steatosis may occur even in the absence of marked transaminase elevations.

! **WARNING** Be aware that immune reconstitution syndrome has occurred in patients treated with combination antiretroviral therapy, including tenofovir disoproxil fumarate. The inflammatory response predisposes susceptible patients to opportunistic infections, such as cytomegalovirus, *Mycobacterium avium* infection, *Pneumocystis jiroveci* pneumonia, or tuberculosis. Autoimmune disorders such as Graves' disease, Guillain-Barré syndrome, or polymyositis have also occurred. Report sudden or unusual adverse reactions to prescriber.

- Know that patients who have a history of pathologic bone fracture or other risk factors for bone loss or osteoporosis should be assessed regularly for bone density loss. Patient may benefit from calcium and vitamin D supplementation. Inform patient that bone density scanning may be ordered during tenofovir disoproxil fumarate therapy.

! **WARNING** Monitor patient being treated for hepatitis B upon discontinuation of tenofovir disoproxil fumarate for several months because severe acute exacerbations of hepatitis have occurred when drug has been stopped. Monitoring should include not only an assessment for signs and symptoms of hepatitis, but also laboratory studies, such as liver enzymes, as ordered.

PATIENT TEACHING

- Instruct patient how to administer form of tenofovir disoproxil fumarate prescribed. Stress importance of not missing doses because doing so can result in the development of resistance to the drug.
- Stress importance to take tenofovir disoproxil fumarate exactly as prescribed.

! **WARNING** Warn patient not to discontinue the drug without consulting prescriber.

- Tell patient to avoid high-dose or multiple NSAIDs while taking tenofovir disoproxil fumarate because of the risk of renal dysfunction.

! **WARNING** Alert patient that drug may cause an allergic reaction. If present, tell patient to notify prescriber and, if severe, to seek immediate medical care.

! **WARNING** Caution patient to report any persistent, severe, or unusual adverse reactions to prescriber.

- Inform patient that bone density scanning may be ordered during tenofovir disoproxil fumarate therapy. Also tell patient to consult prescriber about possible need for calcium and vitamin D supplementation.
- Tell patient to inform all prescribers of tenofovir disoproxil fumarate therapy, as other drugs containing tenofovir should not be prescribed during therapy.
- Inform mothers with HIV not to breastfeed during tenofovir disoproxil fumarate therapy.

! **WARNING** Inform patients who are discontinuing tenofovir disoproxil fumarate after being treated for hepatitis B virus to seek medical attention if signs and symptoms of hepatitis reappear. This is because severe acute exacerbations of hepatitis may occur for many months after drug has been discontinued.

terazosin hydrochloride

Tezruly

Class and Category

Pharmacologic class: Alpha-adrenergic blocker
Therapeutic class: Antihypertensive, benign prostatic hyperplasia (BPH) agent

Indications and Dosages

✱ *To manage hypertension*

CAPSULES ORAL SOLUTION

Adults. *Initial:* 1 mg nightly and increased, as needed. *Maintenance:* 1 to 5 mg daily as a single dose nightly or in divided doses every 12 hr. *Maximum:* 20 mg daily.

✱ *To treat symptomatic BPH*

CAPSULES, ORAL SOLUTION

Adults. *Initial:* 1 mg once at bedtime, increased in stepwise fashion to 2 mg, then 5 mg, and then 10 mg once nightly, as needed, for a minimum of 4 to 6 wk before dosage increased to 20 mg, as needed. *Maximum:* 20 mg daily.

Drug Administration

P.O.

- Administer once-daily dose at bedtime.
- Use a calibrated measuring device when measuring oral solution dose. Store at room temeprature.
- Capsules should be swallowed whole and not opened.
- Dosage will have to be retitrated if consecutive doses are missed for several days.

Route	Onset	Peak	Duration
P.O.	15 min	1 hr	24 hr

Half-life: 12 hr

Mechanism of Action

Blocks postsynaptic $alpha_1$-adrenergic receptors in many tissues, including the bladder neck, the prostate, and vascular smooth muscle to promote vasodilation, which reduces blood pressure and improves urine flow.

Contraindications

Hypersensitivity to terazosin or its components

Interactions

DRUGS

phosphodiesterase-5 inhibitors, verapamil: Additive blood pressure–lowering effects and symptomatic hypotension

Adverse Reactions

CNS: Asthenia, dizziness, headache, lethargy, nervousness, paresthesia, somnolence, syncope, vertigo
CV: Chest pain, **hypotension**, orthostatic hypotension, palpitations, peripheral edema, sinus tachycardia
EENT: Blurred vision, dry mouth, intraoperative floppy iris syndrome, nasal congestion, sinusitis
GI: Constipation, diarrhea, nausea, vomiting
MS: Arthralgia, back pain
Other: Flu-like symptoms, weight gain

Childbearing Considerations

PREGNANCY

- It is not known if drug can cause fetal harm.
- Use with caution only if benefit to mother outweighs potential risk to fetus.

LACTATION

- It is not known if drug is present in breast milk.
- Mothers should check with prescriber before breastfeeding.

Nursing Considerations

! **WARNING** Be aware that prostate cancer should be ruled out before giving terazosin for BPH.

- Monitor drug effectiveness.

! **WARNING** Monitor blood pressure 2 to 3 hours after initial dose because of possible first-dose hypotension and again after 24 hours to evaluate patient's response.

! **WARNING** Be aware that elderly patients may have exaggerated hypotension and other adverse reactions.

- Expect prescriber to reduce terazosin dosage if a diuretic or another antihypertensive is added to patient's regimen.

PATIENT TEACHING

- Instruct patient how to administer form of terazosin prescribed.

! **WARNING** Warn patient about possible first-dose hypotension. Tell patient to take safety precautions until first-dose effect is gone.

- Instruct patient to notify prescriber if several doses are missed in a row; caution against resuming therapy at previous dose without consulting prescriber.
- Advise patient to avoid hazardous activities until drug's CNS effects are known and resolved.
- Advise patient to change position and rise slowly to prevent syncope early in therapy. Suggest lying down or sitting if dizziness or lightheadedness occurs.
- Advise patient to avoid alcohol use, excessive exercise, exposure to hot weather, or prolonged standing because these activities can worsen orthostatic hypotension.
- Emphasize the importance of regular follow-up visits with prescriber to evaluate patient's response to drug.

terbinafine hydrochloride

Class and Category

Pharmacologic class: Allylamine derivative
Therapeutic class: Antifungal

Indications and Dosages

* *To treat onychomycosis of fingernails and toenails due to dermatophytes (tinea unguium)*

TABLETS

Adults. 250 mg once daily for 6 wk for fingernail onychomycosis and 12 wk for toenail onychomycosis.

Drug Administration

P.O.

- Administer drug without regard to food.
- Protect tablets from light.

Route	Onset	Peak	Duration
P.O.	Unknown	< 2 hr	Unknown

Half-life: 36 hr

Mechanism of Action

Inhibits the conversion of squalene mono-oxygenase to squalene epoxidase, a key enzyme in fungal biosynthesis with the resulting squalene accumulation weakening cell membranes and creating a deficiency of ergosterol, the fungal membrane component necessary for normal fungal growth.

Contraindications

Active or chronic liver disease, hypersensitivity to terbinafine or its components

Interactions

DRUGS

beta-blockers; class 1C antiarrhythmics, such as flecainide and propafenone; MAO inhibitors (type B); selective serotonin reuptake inhibitors; tricyclic antidepressants: Possibly increased blood levels of these drugs
cimetidine, other hepatic enzyme inhibitors: Significantly decreased terbinafine clearance, possibly increased adverse reactions
cyclosporine: Increased clearance of cyclosporine and decreased effectiveness of cyclosporine
CYP2C9 and CYP3A4 inhibitors, such as amiodarone and ketoconazole: Possibly increased systemic exposure of terbinafine
hepatotoxic drugs: Increased risk of hepatotoxicity
rifampin: Increased clearance and decreased effectiveness of terbinafine
warfarin: Possibly altered prothrombin time

ACTIVITIES

alcohol use: Increased risk of hepatic dysfunction

FOODS

caffeine: Decreased caffeine clearance

Adverse Reactions

CNS: Anxiety, depression, fatigue, fever, headache, hypoesthesia, malaise, paresthesia, vertigo
CV: **Myocarditis**, **pericarditis**, **thrombotic microangiopathy**, vasculitis
EENT: Hearing impairment, loss of smell, reduced visual acuity, taste loss or perversion (possibly severe), tinnitus, visual field defect
GI: Abdominal pain, anorexia, cholestasis, diarrhea, elevated liver enzymes, flatulence, **hepatic failure**, **hepatitis**, **hepatotoxicity**, indigestion, jaundice, nausea, **pancreatitis**, vomiting
GU: **Hemolytic uremic syndrome**, **nephritis**
HEME: **Agranulocytosis**, anemia, **neutropenia (severe)**, **pancytopenia**, **thrombocytopenia**, **thrombotic thrombocytopenic purpura**
MS: Arthralgia, myalgia, **rhabdomyolysis**
RESP: **Pneumonitis**
SKIN: Acute generalized exanthematous pustulosis, alopecia, bullous dermatitis, cutaneous lupus erythematosus, **erythema multiforme**, exacerbation of psoriasis, **exfoliative dermatitis**, photosensitivity, psoriasiform eruptions, pruritus, rash, **Stevens-Johnson syndrome**, **toxic epidermal necrolysis**, urticaria
Other: **Anaphylaxis**, **angioedema**, **drug reaction with eosinophilia and systemic symptoms (DRESS)**, elevated blood creatine phosphokinase, influenza-like illness, serum sickness-like reaction, systemic lupus erythematosus

Childbearing Considerations

PREGNANCY

- It is not known if drug can cause fetal harm.
- Drug therapy is not recommended to begin during pregnancy because treatment can be postponed until after delivery.

LACTATION

- Drug is present in breast milk.
- Breastfeeding is not recommended during drug therapy.

Nursing Considerations

- Know that because terbinafine has been linked to serious adverse hepatic effects, expect to send nail specimens for laboratory testing to confirm onychomycosis before starting therapy. Also, expect to check liver enzymes, as ordered, prior to starting therapy to rule out preexisting liver disease.

! **WARNING** Monitor patient for serious hypersensitivity or skin reactions, such as anaphylaxis, angioedema, or DRESS. Know that DRESS may also involve one or more organs and may initially only present with a fever or swollen lymph nodes although rash is most common. If a hypersensitivity or severe skin reaction is present, notify prescriber, expect drug to be discontinued, and provide supportive care, as needed and ordered.

! **WARNING** Monitor patient for hepatic failure (anorexia, dark urine, fatigue, jaundice, nausea, pale stools, right-upper abdominal pain, and vomiting). Know that periodic monitoring of liver enzymes should be done throughout therapy because hepatotoxicity may also occur in patients without preexisting liver disease. Expect to stop drug and obtain liver enzyme tests if these problems develop.

! **WARNING** Monitor patient's CBC, as ordered and patient for signs and symptoms of bleeding or infection. Know that thrombotic microangiopathy has occurred with terbinafine use and can be life-threatening. Notify prescriber promptly of any abnormalities, especially unexplained anemia and thrombocytopenia. If thrombotic microangiopathy is confirmed, expect drug to be discontinued.

! **WARNING** Monitor patient for other persistent, serious, or unusual adverse reactions.

PATIENT TEACHING

- Instruct patient how to administer terbinafine.
- Emphasize the need to complete the full course of terbinafine therapy to prevent relapse of infection.
- Discourage consumption of alcohol during therapy.

! **WARNING** Alert patient that drug may cause an allergic or skin reaction. Tell patient to contact prescriber at the first sign of an allergic reaction or fever, rash, swollen lymph nodes, or other signs and symptoms. If reaction is serious or severe, stress importance of seeking immediate medical care.

- Tell patient to contact prescriber if onychomycosis doesn't improve in a few weeks.

! **WARNING** Instruct patient to notify prescriber if persistent anorexia, dark urine, fatigue, jaundice, nausea, pale stools, or right-upper abdominal pain develops. Stress importance of stopping terbinafine therapy immediately if any of these symptoms occur and contacting prescriber.

! **WARNING** Review bleeding and infection control measures with patient. Instruct patient to inform prescriber of any unexplained bleeding or bruising that may occur as well as an infection. Also, warn patient that drug may cause tiny blood clots that could become life-threatening. Tell patient to seek immediate medical attention if changes in mental status or difficulty breathing occurs.

! **WARNING** Tell patient to alert prescriber of any other persistent, serious, or unusual adverse reactions.

- Advise patient to alert prescriber if loss or perversion of taste occurs and becomes severe enough to cause anxiety, depression, or weight loss.

- Instruct patient to avoid direct sunlight or UV light and to wear sunscreen when outdoors.
- Inform females of childbearing age contemplating pregnancy that drug should not be started during pregnancy.
- Tell mothers breastfeeding should not be undertaken during terbinafine therapy.

teriflunomide

Aubagio

Class and Category

Pharmacologic class: Pyrimidine synthesis inhibitor
Therapeutic class: Immunomodulator

Indications and Dosages

* *To treat relapsing forms of multiple sclerosis, including active secondary progressive disease, clinically isolated syndrome, and relapsing-remitting disease*

TABLETS

Adults. 7 or 14 mg once daily.

Drug Administration

P.O.

- Administer tablets with or without regard to food.

Route	Onset	Peak	Duration
P.O.	Unknown	1–4 hr	Unknown

Half-life: 18–19 days

Mechanism of Action

Inhibits dihydroorotate dehydrogenase, a mitochondrial enzyme involved in de novo pyrimidine synthesis to possibly reduce the number of activated lymphocytes in the central nervous system responsible for the signs and symptoms of multiple sclerosis.

Contraindications

Concurrent therapy with leflunomide; females of childbearing age not using reliable contraception; hypersensitivity to teriflunomide, leflunomide, or their components; pregnancy; severe hepatic impairment

Interactions

DRUGS

BCRP and organic anion transporting polypeptide B1 and B3 (OATP1B1/1B3) substrates, such as atorvastatin, nateglinide, pravastatin, repaglinide, rosuvastatin, simvastatin: Increased concentrations of these drugs
CYP1A2 substrates, such as alosetron, duloxetine, theophylline, tizanidine: Reduced effectiveness of these drugs
CYP2C8 substrates, such as paclitaxel, pioglitazone, repaglinide, rosiglitazone: Possibly increased exposure of these drugs with potential for leading to adverse effects
live vaccines: Increased risk of infection
oral contraceptives containing ethinyl estradiol or levonorgestrel: Increased systemic exposure of these drugs, increasing risk of adverse reactions
organic anion transporter 3 (OAT3) substrates, such as cefaclor, cimetidine, ciprofloxacin, furosemide, ketoprofen, methotrexate, penicillin G, zidovudine: Increased exposure of these drugs with possibly increased risk of adverse reactions
warfarin: Decreased peak international normalized ratio

Adverse Reactions

CNS: Anxiety, burning sensation, headache, paresthesia, peripheral neuropathy, sciatica
CV: Hypertension, palpitations
EENT: Blurred vision, conjunctivitis, oral herpes, sinusitis, toothache
GI: Abdominal distention, colitis, diarrhea, elevated liver enzymes, gastroenteritis, **hepatic dysfunction or failure**, **hepatotoxicity**, nausea, **pancreatitis**, upper abdominal pain
GU: **Acute renal failure**, acute uric acid nephropathy, cystitis, elevated serum creatinine levels
HEME: **Leukopenia**, **neutropenia**, **thrombocytopenia**
MS: Manifestation of carpal tunnel syndrome, musculoskeletal pain, myalgia
RESP: **Acute interstitial pneumonitis**, bronchitis, cough, dyspnea, **interstitial lung disease**, upper respiratory infection

SKIN: Acne, alopecia, pruritus, psoriasis or worsening of psoriasis (including pustular psoriasis), **Stevens-Johnson syndrome**, **toxic epidermal necrolysis**, urticaria
Other: **Anaphylaxis**, **angioedema**, **drug reaction with eosinophilia and systemic symptoms (DRESS)**, flu-like symptoms, **hyperkalemia**, infections such as tuberculosis, onset of seasonal allergies, weight loss

Childbearing Considerations

PREGNANCY

- Pregnancy exposure registry: 1-800-745-4447, option 2.
- Drug has the potential to cause fetal harm.
- Drug is contraindicated in pregnancy and in females of childbearing age not using effective contraception.
- A negative pregnancy test must be obtained before drug therapy is begun.
- If pregnancy occurs during drug therapy, drug must be discontinued immediately. Instituting an accelerated drug elimination procedure as soon as pregnancy is detected may decrease the risk to the fetus.

LACTATION

- It is not known if drug is present in breast milk.
- Breastfeeding should not be undertaken during drug therapy.

REPRODUCTION

- Females of childbearing age must use effective contraception during drug therapy, as it is essential that pregnancy be avoided during therapy. Females of childbearing age receiving drug who wish to become pregnant must discontinue drug with prescriber consent and undergo an accelerated drug elimination procedure. Contraceptive measures must continue after drug has been discontinued until plasma concentrations of drug are less than 0.02 mg/L (0.02 mcg/ml).
- Drug is present in semen. Therefore, men or their female partner of childbearing age must use effective contraception as well. If male patient wishes to father a child, drug must be discontinued, and an accelerated elimination procedure done or verification that the plasma concentration of drug is less than 0.02 mg/L (0.02 mcg/ml) before attempting to father a child.

Nursing Considerations

! WARNING Know that teriflunomide isn't recommended for patients with bone marrow dysplasia, severe immunodeficiency, or severe, uncontrolled infections because of its immunosuppressant effect. It is also not recommended for patients with liver disease or those with a serum alanine aminotransferase level greater than 2 times the upper-level normal prior to initiation of therapy because drug may worsen liver dysfunction.

! WARNING Obtain a pregnancy test on all females of childbearing age, as ordered, prior to starting teriflunomide therapy. Know that drug should not be started if pregnancy is confirmed or in women who refuse to use a reliable contraceptive. Be aware that if pregnancy occurs even within 2 years of the last dose of the drug, it should be reported through the pregnancy exposure registry.

- Test patient for latent tuberculosis before starting teriflunomide, as ordered. If positive, expect standard medical treatment to be given before teriflunomide therapy starts.
- Obtain baseline blood pressure before starting teriflunomide and monitor periodically thereafter because drug may cause hypertension.

! WARNING Know that patients with active acute or chronic infections should not begin drug treatment with teriflunomide until infection is resolved. Notify prescriber if patient develops a serious infection or skin condition during drug therapy because drug may have to be interrupted and charcoal or cholestyramine given to eliminate drug rapidly.

! WARNING Ensure that a CBC has been done within the past 6 months prior to starting teriflunomide therapy to use as a baseline. Repeat CBC, as ordered, thereafter if signs and symptoms of bone marrow suppression occur.

! WARNING Assess liver enzyme (ALT and AST) levels at start of therapy, monthly during first 6 months, and if stable, every 6 to 8 weeks thereafter, as ordered because drug can cause severe liver dysfunction. If levels become elevated greater than 3-fold upper-level normal, notify prescriber and expect teriflunomide therapy to be withheld until underlying cause is determined. If the elevation is thought to be teriflunomide induced, expect to start cholestyramine washout, as ordered, and monitor liver test weekly until normalized. If another cause is found for the elevation, expect to resume teriflunomide therapy.

! **WARNING** Monitor patient for a hypersensitivity or serious skin reaction, which could become life-threatening, such as anaphylaxis, angioedema, or DRESS. Know that DRESS may initially only present with a fever or swollen lymph nodes although a rash is most common. If present, notify prescriber, expect drug to be discontinued, and provide supportive care, as needed and ordered.

! **WARNING** Monitor patient's respiratory function closely because drug may cause interstitial lung disease that could become life-threatening. If patient develops a cough and dyspnea, notify prescriber; drug may have to be stopped, and patient may need charcoal or cholestyramine to eliminate drug rapidly.

! **WARNING** Check patient's serum potassium level, as ordered, if symptoms of acute renal failure or hyperkalemia occur.

- Monitor patients who are over 60 years of age, patients with diabetes, or in patients taking concomitant neurotoxic drugs, because of an increased risk of developing peripheral neuropathy. If peripheral neuropathy occurs during teriflunomide therapy, notify prescriber and expect drug to be discontinued and possibly cholestyramine washout ordered.

PATIENT TEACHING

! **WARNING** Caution females of childbearing potential not to become pregnant while taking drug because of the high risk of birth defects. Emphasize importance of using reliable forms of birth control and to notify prescriber immediately if pregnancy is suspected. Also, advise men and their female partner of childbearing age to use effective contraception to minimize possibility of pregnancy.

- Instruct patient how to administer teriflunomide.
- Advise patient to avoid live vaccines during teriflunomide therapy.

! **WARNING** Alert patient that drug may cause an allergic or serious skin reaction. If present, tell patient to notify prescriber, and, if severe, to seek immediate medical care.

! **WARNING** Review bleeding and infection control measures with patient. Tell patient to notify prescriber if bruising, unexplained bleeding, or an infection occurs.

! **WARNING** Tell patient to immediately report signs of respiratory dysfunction, such as cough and dyspnea.

- Instruct patient to notify prescriber if signs and symptoms of peripheral neuropathy develops.

! **WARNING** Tell patient to notify prescriber if patient experiences any other persistent, serious, or unusual adverse reactions.

- Inform mothers breastfeeding should not be undertaken during drug therapy.

tetracycline hydrochloride

Class and Category

Pharmacologic class: Tetracycline
Therapeutic class: Antibiotic

Indications and Dosages

* *To treat infections caused by gram-negative or gram-positive organisms*

CAPSULES

Adults. 250 mg 4 times daily or 500 mg twice daily. *For severe infections or those not responding to lower doses:* 500 mg 4 times daily. When used to treat streptococcal infections, therapy continued for 10 days. **Children ages 9 and older.** 25 to 50 mg/kg daily in 4 equally divided doses. When used to treat streptococcal infections, therapy continued for 10 days.

* *To treat moderate to severe acne vulgaris in patients requiring long-term treatment*

CAPSULES

Adults. *Initial:* 1,000 mg daily in divided doses until improvement occurs (usually in 3 wk); then dosage reduced gradually. *Maintenance:* 125 to 500 mg daily, every other day, or intermittently.

* *To treat brucellosis caused by susceptible organisms*

CAPSULES

Adults. 500 mg 4 times daily for 3 wk, given with streptomycin.

* *To treat gonorrhea caused by* Neisseria gonorrhoeae

CAPSULES

Adults. 500 mg 4 times daily for 7 days.

* *To treat syphilis in patients allergic to penicillin*

CAPSULES

Adults. 500 mg 4 times daily for 15 days (for early syphilis of less than 1 yr duration) or 30 days (for late syphilis with more than 1 yr duration except for neurosyphilis).

* *To treat uncomplicated endocervical, rectal, or urethral infections caused by* Chlamydia trachomatis

CAPSULES

Adults. 500 mg 4 times daily for at least 7 days.

±**DOSAGE ADJUSTMENT** For patients with renal impairment, dosage reduced or time intervals increased between doses.

Drug Administration

P.O.

- Never administer outdated drug because of increased risk of renal toxicity and Fanconi syndrome.
- Administer drug at least 1 hr before meals or 2 hr after meals because dairy products and some foods may interfere with absorption.
- Administer each dose with a full glass of water while patient is in an upright position and avoid bedtime administration to avoid esophageal or GI irritation.
- Avoid administering other drugs, including antacids, within 3 hr of tetracycline.

Route	Onset	Peak	Duration
P.O.	Unknown	2–4 hr	Unknown

Half-life: 6–12 hr

Mechanism of Action

Exerts a bacteriostatic effect against a wide variety of gram-negative and gram-positive organisms by passing through the bacterial lipid bilayer, where it binds reversibly to 30S ribosomal subunits. Blocking the binding of aminoacyl transfer RNA to messenger RNA inhibits bacterial protein synthesis.

Contraindications

Hypersensitivity to tetracycline or its components

Interactions

DRUGS

aluminum-, calcium-, or magnesium-containing antacids; iron supplements (oral); magnesium-containing laxatives; magnesium salicylate; multivitamins (containing manganese or zinc salts); sodium bicarbonate: Possibly impaired absorption of oral tetracycline and formation of nonabsorbable complexes

digoxin: Possibly increased digoxin level

methoxyflurane: Possibly nephrotoxicity

oral anticoagulants: Decreased plasma prothrombin activity

oral contraceptives (containing estrogen): Possibly reduced contraceptive reliability and increased risk of breakthrough bleeding (with long-term tetracycline use)

penicillins: Possibly decreased bactericidal effect of penicillins

FOODS

dairy products and other foods: Possibly impaired absorption of oral tetracycline

Adverse Reactions

CNS: Dizziness, lightheadedness, unsteadiness

EENT: Darkened or discolored tongue, enamel hypoplasia, glossitis, oral candidiasis, tooth discoloration (in children)

GI: Abdominal pain, anorexia, diarrhea, dysphagia, **enterocolitis**, esophageal ulceration, esophagitis, **hepatotoxicity**, **liver failure**, nausea, rectal candidiasis, vomiting

GU: Elevated BUN, vaginal candidiasis

HEME: Eosinophilia, **hemolytic anemia**, **neurtropenia**, **thrombocytopenia**, **thrombocytopenic purpura**

SKIN: Erythrematous and maculopapular rashes, **exfoliative dermatitis**, photosensitivity, urticaria

T

Other: **Anaphylaxis, angioedema**, exacerbation of sytemic lupus erythematosus, serum sickness-like reactions

Childbearing Considerations

PREGNANCY

- Drug can cause fetal harm such as adverse effects on skeletal and tooth development.
- The use of drug during last half of pregnancy may cause permanent discoloration of the child's teeth.
- Drug should not be used during pregnancy unless there is no alternative and benefit to mother outweighs potential risk to fetus.
- Pregnant women with renal disease may be more prone to develop drug-induced liver failure.

LACTATION

- Drug is present in breast milk.
- A decision should be made to discontinue breastfeeding or the drug to avoid potential serious adverse reactions in the breastfed infant.

REPRODUCTION

- Females of childbearing age who use oral contraceptives containing estrogen need to use another method of contraception while taking tetracycline because estrogen-containing contraceptives may be less effective.

Nursing Considerations

! WARNING Know that tetracycline should be avoided in children ages 8 and younger because drug may cause permanent brown or yellow tooth discoloration and enamel hypoplasia.

! WARNING Be aware that citric acid in tetracycline preparations may accelerate drug deterioration and that using outdated drug may cause Fanconi syndrome, characterized by multiple defects in renal tubular function. Symptoms include acidosis, bicarbonate wasting, glycosuria, hypokalemia, osteomalacia, and phosphaturia.

! WARNING Monitor patient for a hypersensitivity reaction, which could become life-threatening such as anaphylaxis or angioedema. If present, notify prescriber, expect drug to be discontinued, and provide supportive care, as needed and ordered.

! WARNING Monitor patient's liver enzymes and patient for signs and symptoms of liver dysfunction because tetracycline can cause hepatotoxicity. Pregnant women with renal disease may be more prone to develop drug-induced liver failure.

- Assess for photosensitivity, which can develop within a few minutes or up to several hours after exposure to sunlight or other ultraviolet (UV) light. Effects may last for 1 to 2 days after discontinuation of drug

PATIENT TEACHING

- Instruct patient how to administer tetracycline.
- Advise patient to avoid taking other drugs, including over-the-counter antacids and other preparations, within 3 hours of tetracycline.
- Urge patient to complete entire course of tetracycline therapy even if feeling better.
- Caution patient to avoid direct sunlight or UV light and to wear sunscreen when outdoors.
- Advise females of childbearing age who use oral contraceptives containing estrogen to use another method of contraception while taking tetracycline because contraceptives may be less effective. Tell patient to notify prescriber immediately if pregnancy occurs.
- Alert mothers that breastfeeding should not be undertaken while taking tetracycline or drug will need to be discontinued.
- Encourage patient to take safety precautions if she experiences dizziness or other adverse CNS reactions until resolved.

! WARNING Emphasize the need to discard outdated tetracycline because of the risk of toxic effects.

tezepelumab-ekko

Tezspire

Class and Category

Pharmacologic class: Thymic stromal lymphopoietin (TSLP) blocker, human monoclonal antibody
Therapeutic class: Antiasthmatic

Indications and Dosages

✱ As adjunct add-on maintenance treatment for patients with severe asthma

SUBCUTANEOUS INJECTION

Adults and children ages 12 and older. 210 mg once every 4 wk.

Drug Administration

SUBCUTANEOUS

- Each pre-filled pen, pre-filled syringe, and vial contain a single dose of the drug.
- Remove from refrigerator at least 60 min before administration to allow drug to reach room temperature. Do not shake, and do not expose to heat. Do not return to refrigerator once drug has reached room temperature. Do not use device from cartons with broken security seals.
- Drug solution is clear to opalescent, colorless to light yellow. Discard if solution is cloudy, discolored, or large particles are visible.
- Do not use if pen, syringe, or vial is dropped or damaged.
- Inject subcutaneously into the abdomen (except for the 2 inches around the navel), thigh, or upper arm. Do not inject in an area where skin is bruised, erythematous, hardened, or tender. Rotate sites.
- If a dose is missed, administer it as soon as possible and resume scheduled dosing. However, if it is close to the time of the next scheduled dose, skip the missed dose and administer next scheduled dose as planned.

Pre-filled pen

- Do not remove the cap until ready to inject drug.
- Grab the middle of the pre-filled pen body to remove it from the tray.
- Be aware the pen may contain small air bubbles. Do not expel the air bubbles prior to administration.
- To remove the cap, hold the pen with 1 hand and carefully pull the cap straight off with other hand. Do not touch needle or push the orange needle guard with a finger.
- Never replace the cap back on the pen once it has been removed.
- Inject subcutaneously either gently pinching the skin at the injection site or not pinching the skin. Place the orange needle guard flat against the skin at a 90-degree angle. Ensure viewing window can be seen on the pen. Press down firmly until the orange needle guard is no longer visible. A click will be heard indicating the injection has started. The orange plunger will move down in the viewing window during the injection.
- Continue to hold firmly for about 15 sec. A second click should then occur indicating the injection is done. The orange plunger will fill the viewing window. Pull the pen straight up. The orange needle guard will slide down and lock into place over the needle. Discard the pen into a sharps container.

Pre-filled syringe

- Do not remove the cap until ready to inject drug.
- Grab the syringe body to remove it from the tray. Do not grab it by the plunger.
- Be aware the syringe may contain small air bubbles. Do not expel the air bubbles prior to administration.
- To remove the cap, hold the syringe body and remove the needle cover by pulling straight off. A drop of solution may appear at the end of the needle. This is normal and does not need to be removed.
- Inject subcutaneously by gently pinching the skin at the injection site and inserting needle at a 45-degree angle. Then push the plunger all the way until the plunger head is completely between the needle guard activation clips.
- After injection, maintain pressure on the plunger head and remove needle from the skin. Release pressure on the plunger head to allow the needle guard to cover the needle. Do not re-cap the used pre-filled syringe. Discard the syringe into a sharps container.

Single-dose vial

- Withdraw dose from drug vial. No reconstitution is needed.
- Select injection site.
- Administer drug subcutaneously.

Route	Onset	Peak	Duration
SubQ	Unknown	3–10 days	Unknown

Half-life: 26 days

Mechanism of Action

Binds to human thymic stromal lymphopoietin (TSLP) to block its interaction with the TSLP receptor. Although the precise action of the drug is unknown in asthma, blocking TSLP action at the receptor site may reduce biomarkers and cytokines associated with airway inflammation to improve breathing.

Contraindications

Hypersensitivity to tezepelumab-ekko or its components

Interactions

None reported by manufacturer.

Adverse Reactions

EENT: Conjunctivitis, pharyngitis
MS: Arthralgia, back pain
SKIN: Rash
OTHER: **Anaphylaxis**, injection site reactions (erythema, pain, swelling)

Childbearing Considerations

PREGNANCY

- It is not known if drug can cause fetal harm although placental transfer of monoclonal antibodies occurs during the third trimester of pregnancy.
- Use with caution only if benefit to mother outweighs potential risks to fetus.

LACTATION

- It is not known if drug is present in breast milk.
- Mothers should check with prescriber before breastfeeding.

Nursing Considerations

- Anticipate patient with known helminth infection to be treated before tezepelumab therapy is begun because it is unknown if drug interferes with helminth treatment.

! **WARNING** Know that tezepelumab-ekko should never be used to relieve acute bronchospasm or status asthmaticus because drug effects are not immediate.

! **WARNING** Expect to continue systemic or inhaled corticosteroid therapy when tezepelumab-ekko is begun. Abrupt cessation of corticosteroid therapy may precipitate withdrawal symptoms. Instead, expect corticosteroid therapy to be gradually reduced.

! **WARNING** Monitor patient for a hypersensitivity reaction, which may become life-threatening, such as anayphylaxis. Reactions have occurred within hours of the drug being administered or as a delayed reaction days later. If present, notify prescriber, expect drug to be discontinued, and provide supportive care, as needed and ordered.

- Do not administer live attenuated vaccines to patient during tezepelumab-ekko therapy.

PATIENT TEACHING

- Tell patient, family, or caregiver how to administer tezepelumab-ekko as a subcutaneous injection using the pre-filled pen only.

! **WARNING** Stress importance of not abruptly stopping systemic or inhaled corticosteroid therapy when tezepelumab-ekko is begun but to follow prescriber's instructions.

! **WARNING** Warn patient not to use tezepelumab-ekko to treat acute bronchospasms or a severe asthma attack. Instead, tell patient to seek immediate medical attention.

- Advice patient to notify prescriber if asthma remains uncontrolled or worsens during tezepelumab-ekko therapy.

! **WARNING** Alert patient that drug may cause an allergic reaction. If present, tell patient to notify prescriber and, if severe, to seek immediate medical care.

- Instruct patient not to receive live attenuated vaccines while receiving tezepelumab-ekko therapy.

tiagabine hydrochloride

Gabitril

Class and Category

Pharmacologic class: Gamma-aminobutyric acid (GABA) reuptake inhibitor
Therapeutic class: Anticonvulsant

Indications and Dosages

✶ As adjunct to treat partial seizures

TABLETS

Adults already taking enzyme-inducing antiepileptic drugs. *Initial:* 4 mg once daily; increased by 4 to 8 mg/wk until desired response occurs, given in 2 to 4 divided doses daily. *Usual:* 32 to 56 mg daily. *Maximum:* 56 mg daily in 2 to 4 divided doses.
Children ages 12 to 18 already taking enzyme-inducing antiepileptic drugs. *Initial:* 4 mg once daily for 1 wk, then increased to 8 mg, followed a wk later by increases of 4 to 8 mg/wk until desired response occurs and given in 2 to 4 divided doses daily. *Maximum:* 32 mg daily in 2 to 4 divided doses.

±**DOSAGE ADJUSTMENT** For patients taking only non-enzyme-inducing antiepileptic drugs, dosage reduced and possibly a slower titration schedule required. For patients with impaired hepatic function, dosage individualized and reduced, or dosing interval increased, as needed.

Drug Administration

P.O.

- Administer drug with food.
- If more than 1 dose is missed, consult prescriber, as retitration of dose may be required.

Route	Onset	Peak	Duration
P.O.	Rapid	45 min	7–9 hr

Half-life: 7–9 hr

Mechanism of Action

Appears to inhibit neuronal and glial uptake of gamma-aminobutyric acid (GABA), the major inhibitory neurotransmitter in the CNS making more GABA available in the CNS to open chloride channels in postsynaptic membranes, thereby leading to membrane hyperpolarization and preventing transmission of nerve impulses.

Contraindications

Hypersensitivity to tiagabine or its components

Interactions

DRUGS

benzodiazepines, CNS depressants: Possibly additive CNS depression
carbamazepine, phenobarbital, phenytoin: Possibly decreased tiagabine effectiveness
St. John's wort: Possibly enhanced metabolism of tiagabine

ACTIVITIES

alcohol use: Possibly additive CNS depression

Adverse Reactions

CNS: Amnesia, anxiety, asthenia, ataxia, confusion, depression, dizziness, drowsiness, EEG abnormalities, hostility, impaired cognition, insomnia, lightheadedness, paresthesia, **seizures**, **status epilepticus**, **suicidal ideation**, tremor, weakness
EENT: Blurred vision, pharyngitis, stomatitis
GI: Abdominal pain, diarrhea, increased appetite, nausea, vomiting
GU: UTI
MS: Dysarthria
SKIN: Bullous dermatitis, ecchymosis, rash

Childbearing Considerations

PREGNANCY

- Pregnancy exposure registry: 1-888-233-2334 or http://www.aedpregnancyregistry.org/.
- Drug may cause fetal harm, based on animal studies.
- Use with caution only if benefit to mother outweighs potential risk to fetus.

LACTATION

- It is not known if drug is present in breast milk.
- Mothers should check with prescriber before breastfeeding.

Nursing Considerations

! **WARNING** Expect to taper dosage gradually, as prescribed, because stopping drug abruptly may increase seizure frequency or development of status epilepticus.

! **WARNING** Monitor patient for break through seizure activity. Institute seizure precautions, as needed and alert prescriber if seizures occur.

! **WARNING** Watch patient closely for evidence of suicidal tendencies, especially when therapy starts or dosage changes, and report concerns at once.

PATIENT TEACHING

- Instruct patient how to administer drug and what to do if a dose is missed.

! **WARNING** Instruct patient not to stop taking tiagabine abruptly. Explain that prescriber usually tapers dosage over 4 weeks to reduce the risk of withdrawal seizures.

- Urge patient to avoid alcohol use.

! **WARNING** Urge family or caregiver to watch patient closely for evidence of suicidal tendencies, especially when therapy starts or dosage changes, and to report concerns immediately.

- Advise patient to avoid hazardous activities until drug's CNS effects are known and resolved.
- Inform patient who takes a CNS depressant that drug may increase depressant effect.

ticagrelor

Brilinta

Class and Category

Pharmacologic class: $P2Y_{12}$ platelet inhibitor
Therapeutic class: Antiplatelet

Indications and Dosages

∗ *To reduce the rate of thrombotic cardiovascular events, such as cardiovascular death, MI, and stroke in patients with acute coronary syndrome (ACS) or history of MI; to reduce rate of stent thrombosis in patients who have been stented for treatment of ACS*

TABLETS

Adults. *Loading dose:* 180 mg. *Maintenance:* 90 mg given 6 to 12 hr after the loading dose, followed by 90 mg twice daily for 1 yr and then 60 mg twice daily thereafter along with aspirin 75 mg to 100 mg daily, if indicated.

∗ *To reduce the risk of a first MI or stroke in patients with coronary artery disease at high risk for such events*

TABLETS

Adults. 60 mg twice daily along with aspirin 75 mg to 100 mg daily.

∗ *To reduce the risk of stroke in patients with acute ischemic stroke (NIH Stroke Scale score 5 or less) or high-risk transient ischemic attack*

TABLETS

Adults. *Loading dose:* 180 mg along with 300 to 325 mg aspirin, followed by 90 mg given 6 to 12 hr after loading dose. *Maintenance:* 90 mg twice daily for up to 30 days along with 75 mg to 100 mg aspirin daily.

Drug Administration

P.O.

- Do not administer with another oral $P2Y_{12}$ platelet inhibitor.
- Crush tablets and mix with water for patients who are unable to swallow tablets whole. Know that the mixture can also be administered via a nasogastric tube.
- If a dose is missed, dose should be skipped.

Route	Onset	Peak	Duration
P.O.	30 min	1.5 hr	24 hr

Half-life: 7–9 hr

Mechanism of Action

Interacts reversibly with the platelet $P2Y_{12}$ ADP-receptor to prevent platelet activation.

Contraindications

Active pathological bleeding, history of intracranial hemorrhage, hypersensitivity to ticagrelor or its components

Interactions

DRUGS

aspirin (daily doses above 100 mg): Reduced effectiveness of ticagrelor
CYP3A inducers, such as carbamazepine, phenobarbital, phenytoin, rifampin: Reduces ticagrelor exposure, decreasing effectiveness
CYP3A inhibitors, such as atazanavir, clarithromycin, indinavir, itraconazole, ketoconazole, nefazodone, nelfinavir, ritonavir, saquinavir, voriconazole: Substantially increases ticagrelor exposure and risk of adverse reactions such as bleeding and dyspnea
digoxin: Altered blood digoxin levels
lovastatin, rosuvastatin, simvastatin: Increased serum levels of these drugs
opioids: Delayed or reduced absorption of ticagrelor

Adverse Reactions

CNS: Dizziness, fatigue, headache, **intracranial bleeding**

CV: **Atrial fibrillation**, **bradycardia including AV block**, chest pain, hypertension, **hypotension (may be severe)**, **intracardiac bleed with cardiac tamponade**
EENT: Epistaxis, intraocular bleeding with permanent vision loss
ENDO: Gynecomastia
GI: Diarrhea, nausea
GU: Elevated serum creatinine level
HEME: Minor or **major bleeding**, **thrombotic thrombocytopenic purpura**
MS: Back or noncardiac chest pain
RESP: **Central sleep apnea**, **Cheyne-Stokes respirations**, cough, dyspnea
SKIN: Bruising, rash
Other: **Angioedema**, elevated uric acid, **hypovolemic shock**

Childbearing Considerations

PREGNANCY

- It is not known if drug can cause fetal harm.
- Use with caution only if benefit to mother outweighs potential risk to fetus.

LACTATION

- It is not known if drug is present in breast milk.
- Breastfeeding is not recommended during drug therapy.

Nursing Considerations

! **WARNING** Be aware that ticagrelor shouldn't be given to patients with active pathological bleeding or who have a history of intracranial hemorrhage. It should also not be started in patients who are undergoing urgent coronary artery bypass graft (CABG) surgery or who have severe hepatic impairment.

! **WARNING** Know that patients with a history of bradycardia-related syncope not protected by a pacemaker, second- or third-degree AV block, or sick sinus syndrome may be at a higher risk of developing bradyarrhythmias with ticagrelor.

! **WARNING** Avoid abrupt interruption of ticagrelor therapy because doing so increases the risk of MI, stent thrombosis, and death.

- Be aware that maintenance doses of aspirin above 100 mg may decrease effectiveness of ticagrelor and should be limited to 75 to 100 mg daily.

! **WARNING** Monitor patient for a hypersensitivity reaction, which could become life-threatening, such as angioedema. If present, notify prescriber, expect drug to be switched to a different drug, and provide supportive care, as needed and ordered.

! **WARNING** Monitor patient closely for bleeding tendencies. Know that risk of bleeding increases with ticagrelor use in older patients as well as patients with a history of bleeding disorders or performance of percutaneous invasive procedures. Risk of bleeding also increases with concomitant use of drugs such as anticoagulant and fibrinolytic therapy, chronic use of nonsteroidal anti-inflammatory drugs, and higher doses of aspirin.

! **WARNING** Be suspicious of bleeding in a patient who becomes hypotensive and has recently undergone coronary angiography, CABG, PCI, or other surgical procedures, even if the patient does not have any signs of bleeding. Notify prescriber immediately if patient becomes hypotensive and expect to provide supportive care, as needed and ordered. Be aware that attempts to manage bleeding should be made without discontinuing drug, if possible, because stopping ticagrelor increases risk of subsequent cardiovascular events.

- Monitor patient for dyspnea that may occur with ticagrelor therapy. If dyspnea is determined to be caused by drug, expect to continue therapy, as no specific treatment is needed and it often resolves on its own. Also, monitor patient for central sleep apnea. If suspected, notify prescriber and expect further testing to be done to confirm disorder.
- Be prepared to discontinue ticagrelor therapy, as ordered, 5 days before surgery, if possible. However, drug should be restarted as soon as possible after surgery because of increased risk of MI, stroke, and even death.
- Be aware that ticagrelor can give false negative functional tests for heparin-induced thrombocytopenia (HIT) or false negative results in platelet functional tests for patients with HIT.

PATIENT TEACHING

- Instruct patient how to administer ticagrelor and what to do if a dose is missed.

! **WARNING** Warn patient not to discontinue ticagrelor therapy abruptly because of increased risk of life-threatening adverse effects.

- Caution patient to limit maintenance doses of aspirin to no more than 100 mg daily.

! **WARNING** Alert patient drug may cause an allergic reaction. If present, tell patient to notify prescriber and, if severe, to seek immediate medical care.

! **WARNING** Instruct patient to take bleeding precautions, such as avoiding the use of a razor and brushing teeth with a soft-bristled toothbrush. Advise patient to seek immediate emergency care if bleeding occurs and is serious.

- Caution patient that difficulty breathing may occur but that it is usually mild to moderate and often resolves with continued treatment. If bothersome or appears serious, tell patient to notify prescriber as drug may need to be discontinued.
- Tell patient to alert all prescribers and dentists of ticagrelor therapy.
- Advise mothers breastfeeding is not recommended during ticagrelor therapy.

tiotropium bromide

Spiriva HandiHaler, Spiriva Respimat

Class and Category

Pharmacologic class: Anticholinergic
Therapeutic class: Bronchodilator

Indications and Dosages

∗ *To provide long-term maintenance treatment of asthma*

ORAL INHALATION (SPIRIVA RESPIMAT)

Adults and children ages 6 and older. 2.5 mcg (2 inhalations of 1.25 mcg each) once daily. *Maximum:* 2.5 mcg every 24 hr.

∗ *To provide long-term maintenance treatment of bronchospasm associated with COPD, including chronic bronchitis and emphysema; to reduce COPD exacerbations*

ORAL INHALATION (SPIRIVA HANDIHALER)

Adults. 18 mcg (2 inhalations from one 18 mcg capsule) once daily. *Maximum:* 18 mcg every 24 hr.

ORAL INHALATION (SPIRIVA RESPIMAT)

Adults. 5 mcg (2 inhalations of 2.5 mcg each) once daily. *Maximum:* 5 mcg every 24 hr.

Drug Administration

INHALATION

HandiHaler

- After removing HandiHaler device from pouch, open the dust cap (lid) by pressing the green piercing button. Pull the dust cap upwards away from the base to expose the mouth piece. Open the mouthpiece by pulling the mouthpiece ridge up and away from the base so the center chamber is showing.
- Do not expose capsules to air until ready for use.
- Once the HandiHaler device is ready, remove a capsule from the blister pack, open the foil only as far as the stop line, to avoid exposing the rest of the capsules in the blister pack to air. Discard capsules if they are inadvertently exposed to air and won't be used immediately.
- Place capsule into the center chamber of HandiHaler device. Close the mouthpiece firmly against the gray base until a click is heard. Leave the dust cap open. Hold the HandiHaler device with the mouthpiece pointed up. Then press and release the green button on the side of inhalation device to pierce capsule. Then, have patient exhale completely, close her lips around the mouthpiece, inhale slowly and deeply, and then hold her breath for as long as is comfortable. Patient will need to repeat breathing procedure another time from the same capsule to get the full dose.
- Do not use device to give any other drug. The tiotropium capsule must be taken only using the device and never swallowed.
- Have patient rinse mouth after each treatment to help minimize throat dryness and irritation.

Respimat

- When using for the first time, press the safety catch while firmly pulling off the clear base, being careful not to touch the piercing element. Write the date to discard by on label (3 mo from the date cartridge is being inserted). Insert narrow end of cartridge into the inhaler. Place inhaler on a firm surface and push down firmly until it clicks in place. Then, put the clear base back into place and turn the base in the direction of the arrows on the label until it clicks (half a turn).

- Prime the device by first opening the cap until it snaps fully open and then actuating inhaler (pointed toward the ground) until an aerosol cloud is visible; then repeat the process 3 more times. If inhaler is not used for more than 3 days, inhaler should be actuated once prior to use; if not used for more than 21 days, inhaler should be activated 3 times prior to use.
- Open the cap until it snaps fully open. Have patient breathe out slowly and fully and then hand inhaler to patient asking patient to close lips around the mouthpiece without covering the air vents and pointing inhaler toward back of throat. While having patient take a slow, deep breath through the mouth, have patient press the dose-release button and continue to breathe in. Patient should hold breath for 10 sec or for as long as it is comfortable. Repeat procedure for second puff. Have patient remove inhaler from mouth and then close cap on inhaler.
- Only clean mouthpiece, including the metal part inside mouthpiece, with a damp cloth or tissue at least 1 time each wk.
- The Respimat inhaler should not be used to take any other drug.
- Have patient rinse mouth after each treatment to help minimize throat dryness and irritation.

Route	Onset	Peak	Duration
Inhalation	30 min	1–4 hr	> 24 hr

Half-life: 25–44 hr

Mechanism of Action

Prevents acetylcholine from attaching to muscarinic receptors on membranes of smooth muscle cells, thereby blocking acetylcholine's effects in the bronchi and bronchioles to relax smooth muscles and causes bronchodilation.

Contraindications

Hypersensitivity to tiotropium or its components

Interactions

DRUGS

anticholinergics: Possibly increased anticholinergic effects

Adverse Reactions

CNS: **CVA**, depression, difficulty speaking, dizziness, insomnia, paresthesia
CV: Angina, **atrial fibrillation**, chest pain, hypercholesterolemia, hypertension, palpitations, peripheral edema, **supraventricular tachycardia**, tachycardia
EENT: Application-site irritation (glossitis, mouth ulceration, pharyngolaryngeal pain), blurred vision, cataract, dry mouth, dysphonia, epistaxis, eye pain, glaucoma, glossitis, hoarseness, increased intraocular pressure, laryngitis, oral candidiasis, pharyngitis, rhinitis, sinusitis, stomatitis, throat irritation, visual halos
ENDO: Hyperglycemia
GI: Abdominal pain, constipation, diarrhea, dysphagia, gastroesophageal reflux, indigestion, **intestinal obstruction**, ileus, vomiting
GU: Difficulty urinating, urine retention, UTI
MS: Arthritis, leg or skeletal pain, myalgia
RESP: Cough, **paradoxical bronchospasm**, upper respiratory tract infection
SKIN: Pruritus, rash, urticaria
Other: **Anaphylaxis**, **angioedema**, candidiasis, dehydration, flu-like symptoms, **hypersensitivity reaction (immediate)**, infection

Childbearing Considerations

PREGNANCY

- It is not known if drug can cause fetal harm.
- Use with caution only if benefit to mother outweighs potential risk to fetus.

LACTATION

- It is not known if drug is present in breast milk.
- Mothers should check with prescriber before breastfeeding.

Nursing Considerations

! **WARNING** Be aware that tiotropium should never be used to relieve acute bronchospasm.

! **WARNING** Know that patients with a hypersensitivity to atropine should not receive tiotropium because tiotropium is a derivative of atropine. Also, use tiotropium cautiously in patients who have severe hypersensitivity to milk proteins.

- Use tiotropium cautiously in patients with angle-closure glaucoma, benign prostatic hyperplasia, or bladder neck obstruction.
- Know that when tiotropium is used for maintenance therapy in patients with asthma, it may take up to 8 weeks to realize maximum benefits.
- Monitor patient's pulmonary function, as ordered, to evaluate the effectiveness of tiotropium.

! **WARNING.** Monitor patient closely after giving first dose of tiotropium for immediate hypersensitivity reactions, which could become life-threatening such as anaphylaxis, angioedema, or paradoxical bronchospasms. If reaction occurs, notify prescriber and expect to stop tiotropium and provide supportive care, as needed and ordered.

- Monitor patient's renal function, as ordered, especially in patients with moderate to severe renal impairment, because tiotropium is excreted mainly by the kidneys. Monitor patient with renal dysfunction closely for anticholinergic effects.

! **WARNING** Monitor patient for other persistent, serious, or unusual adverse reactions because some of them could be quite serious such as arrhythmias, CVA, or intestinal obstruction.

PATIENT TEACHING

! **WARNING** Caution patient not to use tiotropium to treat acute bronchospasm and that drug should not be used more often than every 24 hours.

- Instruct patient on the proper use of the HandiHaler or Respimat inhalation device.
- Inform patient with asthma that when tiotropium is used for maintenance therapy, it may take up to 8 weeks to realize maximum benefits.

! **WARNING** Alert patient that drug may cause an allergic reaction. If present, tell patient to notify prescriber and, if severe, to seek immediate medical care.

- Advise patient to tell prescriber about decreased response to tiotropium as well as difficulty urinating, eye pain, palpitations, and vision changes.

! **WARNING** Tell patient to notify prescriber of any other persistent, serious, or unusual adverse reactions.

tirzepatide

Mounjaro, Zepbound

Class and Category

Pharmacologic class: Dual glucose-dependent insulinotropic polypeptide (GIP) and glucagon-like peptide-1 (GLP-1) receptor agonist
Therapeutic class: Antidiabetic

Indications and Dosages

∗ *As adjunct to diet and exercise to improve glycemic control in patients with type 2 diabetes mellitus*

SUBCUTANEOUS INJECTION (MOUNJARO)

Adults. *Initial:* 2.5 mg once weekly, increased after 4 wk to 5 mg once weekly. Further increased in increments of 2.5 mg with at least 4 wk between each adjustment, as needed. *Maximum:* 15 mg once a week.

∗ *As adjunct to a reduced calorie diet and increased physical activity for chronic weight management in patients with obesity in the presence of at least one weight-related comorbid condition; to treat moderate to severe obstructive sleep apnea (OSA) in patients with obesity*

SUBCUTANEOUS INJECTION (ZEPBOUND)

Adults. *Initial:* 2.5 mg once weekly, increased, after 4 wks to 5 mg once weekly. Then dosage increased in 2.5 mg increments after at least 4 wk on current dose, as needed, to reach maintenance dosage. *Maintenance:* 5 mg, 10 mg, or 15 mg once weekly (weight reduction) or 10 mg or 15 mg once weekly (OSA). *Maximum:* 15 mg once weekly.

Drug Administration

SUBCUTANEOUS

- Administer once weekly at any time of day and without regards to meals.
- Solution should appear clear and colorless to slightly yellow. Discard if solution is discolored or particulate matter is present.
- Inject into the patient's abdomen, thigh, or upper arm.
- When administering insulin concurrently, inject as a separate injection. Both injections may be given in the same body region but injections should not be adjacent to each other.
- Day of weekly administration may be changed as long as the time between the two doses is at least 3 days or 72 hours.
- Administer a missed dose as soon as possible within 4 days or 96 hours after the time of the missed dose. If more than 4 days has passed, skip missed dose and administer next dose on the regular scheduled day.
- Mounjaro and Zebound are available as a single-dose pen or single-dose vial.
- To administer the pen, pull off the gray base cap making sure pen is locked. Place clear base on skin, then unlock by turning the lock ring. Press the purple injection button and hold up to 10 sec. Listen for the first click indicating injection has started. Listen for second click along with making sure gray plunger is visible indicating injection is complete.
- To administer drug from the vial, first draw up the drug solution into the syringe. Then inject as a subcutaneous injection.
- Store pre-filled pens in refrigerator in original carton to protect from light.
- Pens and vials also can be stored at room temperature for up to 21 days.

Route	Onset	Peak	Duration
SubQ	Unknown	8–72 hr	Unknown

Half-life: 5 days

Mechanism of Action

Lowers glucose concentration by increasing first-second-phase insulin secretion and reducing glucagon levels in a glucose-dependent manner. It does this by selectively binding to and activating both the GIP and GLP-1 receptors. The drug also reduces body weight by decreasing appetite in patients with type 2 diabetes mellitus.

Contraindications

Family or personal history of medullary thyroid carcinoma (MTC), hypersensitivity to tirzepatide or its components, presence of multiple endocrine neoplasia syndrome type 2 (MEN2)

Interactions

DRUGS

insulin, insulin secretagogue such as sulfonylureas: Increased risk of hypoglycemia
oral drugs: Possibly impaired absorption of concomitantly administered oral drugs.
oral hormonal contraceptives: Possibly decreased effectiveness of hormonal contraceptives

Adverse Reactions

CNS: Depression, dysesthesia, fatigue, **suicidal ideation**
CV: **Hypotension**
EENT: Abnormal taste, dry mouth
ENDO: **Hypoglycemia**
GI: Abdominal pain or distention, acute gallbladder disease, anorexia, constipation, diarrhea, dyspepsia, elevated amylase and lipase levels, eructation, flatulence, gastroesophageal reflux disease, ileus, nausea, **pancreatitis (fatal hemorrhagic or necrotizing)**, **severe gastroparesis and other severe GI adverse reactions**, vomiting
GU: **Acute kidney injury**, **worsening of chronic renal disease**
RESP: **Pulmonary aspiration** (during deep sedation or general anesthesia)
SKIN: Alopecia, eczema, urticaria
Other: **Anaphylaxis**, **angioedema**, anti-tirzepatide antibodies, injection site reactions

Childbearing Considerations

PREGNANCY

- It is not known if drug can cause fetal harm although animal studies suggest it may.
- Use with caution only if benefit to mother outweighs potential risk to fetus.

LACTATION

- It is not known if drug is present in breast milk.
- Patient should check with prescriber before breastfeeding.

REPRODUCTION

- Women using oral hormonal contraceptives should switch to a non-oral contraceptive method or add a barrier method of contraception for 4 weeks after drug is begun and for 4 weeks after each dosage increase.

Nursing Considerations

! **WARNING** Be aware that tirzepatide should be avoided in patients with active suicidal ideation or a history of suicidal attempts.

! **WARNING** Know that tirzepatide is not recommended to be coadministered with other tirzepatide-containing products or any GLP-1 receptor agonist because of risk of serious adverse reactions.

- Be aware that tirzepatide is not recommended for patients with severe gastroparesis because of drug's potential adverse effects on the GI tract.

! **WARNING** Monitor patient for a hypersensitivity reaction, which could become life-threatening, such as anaphylaxis or angioedema. If present, notify prescriber, expect drug to be discontinued, and provide supportive care, as needed and ordered.

! **WARNING** Monitor patient for adverse GI reactions such as diarrhea, nausea, and vomiting during dosage adjustments. Be aware that these symptoms, if severe, could lead to dehydration and subsequently to acute kidney injury or worsening of chronic renal failure. However, know that renal dysfunction has occurred with tirzepatide use in patients with no known renal disease. Expect to monitor patient's renal function, as ordered, if dehydration occurs.

! **WARNING** Monitor patient closely for evidence of medullary thyroid cancer because tirzepatide use increases risk. Report to prescriber any patient complaints of dysphagia, dyspnea, or persistent hoarseness as well as the presence of a neck mass.

! **WARNING** Monitor patient for signs and symptoms of hypoglycemia, especially if patient is receiving insulin or insulin secretagogues concomitantly because risk of hypoglycemia is increased. Notify prescriber if hypoglycemia occurs and treat according to institutional protocol. If patient is also taking insulin or insulin secretagogues, expect dosage of these drugs to be adjusted.

! **WARNING** Know that acute pancreatitis, including fatal hemorrhagic or necrotizing pancreatitis has occurred with tirzepatide use. Monitor patient for signs and symptoms such as persistent severe abdominal pain that may radiate to the back and may be accompanied with vomiting. Expect drug to be discontinued, if confirmed, and provide supportive care, as ordered.

! **WARNING** Monitor patient for depression either new onset or worsening because suicidal ideation may occur.

! **WARNING** Be aware that drug may cause pulmonary aspiration during procedures or surgeries that require deep sedation or general anesthesia.

- Monitor patient with a history of diabetic retinopathy for progression.
- Monitor patient for acute gallbladder disease. If cholelithiasis is suspected, expect diagnostic studies to be done to confirm.

PATIENT TEACHING

- Instruct patient on how to administer tirzepatide as a subcutaneous injection and what to do if a dose is missed.
- Stress importance when administering insulin concurrently to inject both drugs as separate injections. However, tell patient both injections may be given in the same body region but injections should not be adjacent to each other.
- Tell patient day of weekly administration may be changed as long as the time between the two doses is at least 3 days or 72 hours.

! **WARNING** Alert patient that drug may cause an allergic reaction. If present, tell patient to notify prescriber and, if severe, to seek immediate medical care.

! **WARNING** Inform patient that GI adverse reactions could lead to dehydration and if severe, dehydration could lead to acute kidney injury. Tell patient to take precautions to avoid dehydration and if dehydration occurs, to alert prescriber for further hydration treatment.

! **WARNING** Alert patient that tirzepatide increases risk for medullary thyroid cancer. Stress importance of reporting dysphagia, dyspnea, presence of a neck mass, or persistent hoarseness.

! **WARNING** Review signs and symptoms of hypoglycemia with patient and how to treat. Inform patient taking concomitantly insulin or insulin secretagogues that risk of hypoglycemia is increased.

! **WARNING** Stress importance of notifying prescriber if patient experiences persistent severe abdominal pain that may radiate to the back and may be accompanied with vomiting.

! **WARNING** Inform patient and family or caregiver that drug may alter mood and possibly lead to depression or even suicidal behavior or thinking. Tell family or caregiver to notify prescriber immediately if changes in mood occurs as drug will need to be discontinued. Review suicidal precautions with family or caregiver to keep patient safe.

! **WARNING** Instruct patient to inform all prescribers of tirzepatide use, especially prescribers performing procedures or surgeries that require deep sedation or general anesthesia.

- Tell patient to alert prescriber if changes in vision occurs.
- Instruct patient on signs and symptoms of gallbladder disease and to notify prescriber if suspected
- Instruct females of child bearing age using oral hormonal contraceptives to switch to a non-oral contraceptive method or add a barrier method of contraception for 4 weeks after drug is begun and for 4 weeks after each dosage increase because drug delays gastric emptying which is greatest after the first dose and diminishes over time.

tizanidine hydrochloride

Zanaflex

Class and Category

Pharmacologic class: Alpha$_2$-adrenergic agonist
Therapeutic class: Antispasmodic

Indications and Dosages

✱ *To treat spasticity*

CAPSULES, TABLETS

Adults. *Initial:* 2 mg every 6 to 8 hr, as needed, for maximum of 3 doses in 24 hr and then increased gradually by 2 to 4 mg/dose after 1 to 4 days, as needed. *Maximum:* 36 mg daily; 16 mg/dose.

± **DOSAGE ADJUSTMENT** For patients with hepatic dysfunction or renal insufficiency (creatinine clearance less than 25 ml/min), dosage reduced during titration. If higher doses are required, dosages rather than dosing frequency should be increased.

Drug Administration

P.O.

- Administer capsules or tablets consistently at about the same time of day.
- Do not switch capsules for tablets and vice versa. While both forms are bioequivalent to each other under fasting conditions (more than 3 hr after a meal), they are not under fed conditions (within 30 min of meal). Maintain a consistent schedule of drug administered in a fasting or fed state.

Route	Onset	Peak	Duration
P.O.	Unknown	1–2 hr	3–6 hr

Half-life: 2.5 hr

Mechanism of Action

Reduces spasticity by decreasing the release of excitatory amino acids thereby increasing presynaptic inhibition of spinal motor neurons, with the greatest effects on polysynaptic pathways.

Contraindications

Hypersensitivity to tizanidine or its components; use with strong CYP1A2 inhibitors such as ciprofloxacin or fluvoxamine

Interactions

DRUGS

alpha$_2$-adrenergic agonists, antihypertensives: Possibly significant hypotension
CNS depressants: Increased additive effects such as excess sedation
moderate or weak CYP1A2 inhibitors, such as acyclovir, amiodarone, cimetidine, famotidine, fluoroquinolones other than strong CYP1A2 inhibitors, mexiletine, oral contraceptives, propafenone, ticlopidine, verapamil, zileuton: Possibly increased plasma tizanidine level; increased risk of bradycardia, hypotension, and sedation
oral contraceptives: Increased risk of bradycardia, excessive drowsiness, or hypotension
strong CYP1A2 inhibitors such as ciprofloxacin, fluvoxamine: Significantly decreased blood pressure and increased drowsiness and psychomotor impairment

ACTIVITIES

alcohol use: Increased adverse effects of tizanidine, additive CNS depression

Adverse Reactions

CNS: Anxiety, delusions, depression, dizziness, drowsiness, dyskinesia, fatigue, fever, hallucinations, nervousness, paresthesia, psychotic-like symptoms, sedation, **seizures**, slurred speech somnolence, tremors, weakness
CV: **Bradycardia**, hypotension, orthastatic hypotension, **ventricular tachycardia**
EENT: Blurred vision, dry mouth, pharyngitis, rhinitis
GI: Abdominal pain, anorexia, constipation, diarrhea, dyspepsia, elevated liver enzymes, **hepatic failure or liver injury**, **hepatitis**, **hepatomegaly**, jaundice, nausea, vomiting
GU: Urinary frequency, UTI
MS: Arthralgia, back pain, muscle weakness or spasms, myasthenia
RESP: **Respiratory compromise**
SKIN: Diaphoresis, **exfoliative dermatitis**, rash, **Stevens Johnson syndrome**, ulceration, urticaria
Other: **Anaphylaxis**, **angioedema**, infections, withdrawal symptoms (hypertonia, rebound hypertension, tachycardia)

Childbearing Considerations

PREGNANCY

- It is not known if drug can cause fetal harm.
- Use with caution only if benefit to mother outweighs potential risk to fetus.

LACTATION

- It is not known if drug is present in breast milk.
- Mothers should check with prescriber before breastfeeding.

Nursing Considerations

! WARNING Be aware that extreme caution is required if tizanidine is prescribed for a patient with hepatic impairment because drug is extensively metabolized in the liver. Monitor aminotransferase levels at baseline and 1 month after maximum dose is achieved, as ordered. Then monitor hepatic function periodically thereafter, as needed, if hepatic injury is suspected.

- Know that tizanidine should be reserved for activities of daily living and times when relief of spasticity is most important because of the short duration of therapeutic effects.

! WARNING Monitor patient for hypersensitivity reactions, which may become life-threatening such as anaphylaxis or angioedema. If present, notify prescriber, expect drug to be discontinued, and provide supportive care, as needed and ordered.

! WARNING Monitor patient closely for hypotension because syncope has occurred in patients taking tizanidine. Know that risk of hypotension can be minimized by dose titration. Monitor patient's blood pressure and signs and symptoms of hypotension during dosage titration. Be careful when moving patients from a supine to a fixed upright position. In addition, monitor patient receiving concurrent antihypertensive therapy. Know that drug is contraindicated with concomitant use with strong CYP1A2 because of significant hypotension.

- Monitor patients with renal impairment closely because they are at increased risk of developing common adverse reactions that may become more severe.

! WARNING Be aware that tizanidine should be stopped slowly by decreasing dosage by 2 mg to 4 mg daily to prevent rebound hypertension, tachycardia, and hypertonia as well as withdrawal. Know this is especially important for patients who have been receiving high doses (20 to 28 mg daily) for long periods (9 weeks or more) or who may be on concomitant treatment with narcotics.

- Monitor patient for hallucinations. If present notify prescriber as drug may need to be discontinued.
- Expect prolonged drug use to inhibit saliva.

PATIENT TEACHING

- Instruct patient how to administer form of tizanidine prescribed.
- Tell patient to take drug exactly as prescribed and not to switch between capsules and tablets.
- Urge patient to avoid alcohol (and other CNS depressants, if possible) during drug therapy because of additive CNS effects.

! **WARNING** Alert patient that drug may cause an allergic reaction. If present, tell patient to notify prescriber and, if severe, to seek immediate medical care.

! **WARNING** Caution patient not to stop taking tizanidine suddenly, to prevent adverse effects.

- Advise patient to change positions slowly to minimize effects of orthostatic hypotension.
- Instruct patient to avoid hazardous activities until drug's CNS effects are known and resolved. Tell patient to take fall precautions.
- Tell patient to notify dentist or prescriber if dry mouth lasts longer than 2 weeks.
- Instruct patient to inform all pharmacists and prescribers about any drug he starts or stops taking.

tobramycin sulfate

Bethkis, Kitabis Pak, Tobi, Tobi Podhaler, Tobramycin

Class and Category

Pharmacologic class: Aminoglycoside
Therapeutic class: Antibiotic

Indications and Dosages

✱ *To treat serious bacterial infections caused by susceptible strains of microorganisms as follows: bone, skin, and skin structure infections caused by* Enterobacter *species,* Escherichia coli, Klebsiella *species,* Pseudomonas aeruginosa, Proteus *species, or* Staphylococcus aureus; *CNS infections (meningitis) caused by susceptible organisms; complicated and recurrent urinary tract infections caused by* Citrobacter *species,* Enterobacter *species,* E. coli, Klebsiella *species,* Proteus *species,* Providencia, P. aeruginosa, Serratia *species, or* S. aureus; *intra-abdominal infections (including peritonitis) caused by* Enterobacter *species,* E. coli, *or* Klebsiella *species; lower respiratory tract infections caused by* Enterobacter *species,* E. coli, Klebsiella *species,* P. aeruginosa, Serratia *species, or* S. aureus; *or septicemia caused by* E. coli, Klebsiella *species, or* P. aeruginosa

I.V. INFUSION, I.M. INJECTION (TOBRAMYCIN)

Adults with serious infection. 1 mg/kg every 8 hr. I.V. infused over 20 to 60 min.
Adults with life-threatening infections. Up to 5 mg/kg daily in 3 to 4 divided doses, reduced as soon as clinically appropriate to 3 mg/kg daily in 3 equally divided doses and given every 8 hr. I.V. infused over 20 to 60 min.
Children and neonates ages 7 days and older. 2 to 2.5 mg/kg every 8 hr or 1.5 mg/kg to 1.89 mg/kg every 6 hr I.V. infused over 20 to 60 min.
Premature or full-term neonates ages 7 days or less. Up to 2 mg/kg every 12 hr. I.V. infused over 20 to 60 min.

± **DOSAGE ADJUSTMENT** For patients with renal impairment, dosage reduced and given every 8 hr or dosage interval increased with normal dosage. For obese patients dosage calculated by using the patient's estimated lean body weight plus 40% of the excess as the basic weight on which to figure mg/kg.

✱ *To treat pulmonary infection caused by* P. aeruginosa *in patients with cystic fibrosis*

I.M. INJECTION, I.V. INFUSION (TOBRAMYCIN)

Adults and children with severe cystic fibrosis. 2.5 mg/kg every 6 hr; dosage adjusted to achieve peak blood drug level of 8 to 12 mcg/ml and trough blood drug level below 2 mcg/ml I.V. infused over 20 to 60 min.

INHALATION (BETHKIS, KITABIS PAK, TOBI)

Adults and children ages 6 and older. 1 ampule (300 mg) twice daily 12 hr apart in alternating periods of 28 days on and 28 days off.

INHALATION (TOBI PODHALER)

Adults and children ages 6 and older. Four 28-mg capsules inhaled using Podhaler every 12 hr in alternating periods of 28 days on and 28 days off.

±**DOSAGE ADJUSTMENT** For patients with cystic fibrosis receiving parenteral therapy, dosage adjustments made based on serum levels of tobramycin.

Drug Administration

I.V.

- Dilute drug by adding 50 to 100 ml of 0.9% Sodium Chloride Injection or 5% Dextrose Injection for adults and a lesser amount for children.
- Infuse over 20 to 60 min. Do not infuse for less than 20 min because peak serum concentrations may exceed 12 mcg/ml.
- Flush I.V. line with 0.9% Sodium Chloride Injection or 5% Dextrose Injection after drug is administered.
- *Incompatibilities:* Other drugs

I.M.

- Withdraw dose directly from drug vial.
- Rotate sites.

INHALATION

- Administer dosages as close to 12 hr apart as possible. Do not administer less than 6 hr apart.
- Administer last, if other inhaled medications are being administered.
- Inhalation capsules should never be administered orally.
- Capsules for inhalation should be stored in the blister pack and each capsule removed immediately before use.
- Always administer capsules with Podhaler device. Use a new Tobi Podhaler device every 7 days.
- Don't expose ampules for inhalation solution to intense light. Refrigerate them or store at room temperature for up to 28 days.
- Do not use inhalation solution if it is cloudy.
- Have patient sit up or stand up and breathe normally through the mouthpiece of the nebulizer to deliver the inhalation solution. Nose clips may help patient breathe through the mouth.
- Administer nebulizer solution over 15 min or until sputtering from the output of the nebulizer has occurred for at least 1 min using the handheld reusable nebulizer with manufacturer recommended air compressor.
- Never dilute nebulizer solution or mix it with dornase alfa or other medication in the nebulizer.

Route	Onset	Peak	Duration
I.V.	Immediate	30 min	8 hr
I.M.	Unknown	30–60 min	8 hr
Inhalation	Unknown	60 min	Unknown

Half-life: 2–4 hr

Mechanism of Action

Inhibits bacterial protein synthesis by binding irreversibly to 1 of 2 aminoglycoside-binding sites on the 30S ribosomal subunit, resulting in bacteriostatic effects. May cause bactericidal effects from drug accumulating within cells so that the intracellular drug level exceeds the extracellular level.

Contraindications

Hypersensitivity to tobramycin, other aminoglycosides, or their components

Interactions

DRUGS

diuretics: Increased risk of aminoglycoside toxicity
general anesthetics, neuromuscular blockers: Possibly increased neuromuscular blockade
other drugs with nephrotoxic, neurotoxic, or ototoxic potential including systemic aminoglycosides: Increased risk of nephrotoxicity, neurotoxicity, and ototoxicity

Adverse Reactions

CNS: Confusion, dizziness, headache, inability to speak, lethargy, malaise, **neurotoxicity**, vertigo
EENT: Hearing loss, laryngitis, oropharyngeal pain, ototoxicity, pharyngitis (inhalation form), taste perversion, tinnitus, voice alteration (inhalation form)
GI: Anorexia, ***Clostridioides difficile*–associated diarrhea**, diarrhea, elevated liver enzymes, nausea, vomiting

GU: Elevated BUN and serum creatinine levels, **nephrotoxicity**, oliguria, proteinuria, **renal failure**
HEME: Anemia, leukocytosis, **leukopenia**, **neutropenia**, **thrombocytopenia**
MS: Myalgia
RESP: **Bronchospasm**, cough (inhalation form), decreased lung function (inhalation form), discolored sputum, dyspnea, hemoptysis (inhalation form), increased sputum production (inhalation form), wheezing
SKIN: **Exfoliative dermatitis**, pruritus, rash, urticaria
Other: **Hypersensitivity reactions**, **hypocalcemia**, **hypokalemia**, **hypomagnesemia**, **hyponatremia**, injection-site pain

Childbearing Considerations

PREGNANCY

- It is not known if drug can cause fetal harm. However, other aminoglycosides have caused fetal harm, such as irreversible bilateral congenital deafness.
- Use with extreme caution only if benefit to mother outweighs potential risk to fetus.

LACTATION

- Drug may be present in breast milk.
- A decision should be made to discontinue breastfeeding or the drug to avoid potential serious adverse reactions in the breastfed infant when administering parenteral form of drug.
- Mothers should check with prescriber about breastfeeding if inhaled form is taken.
- If breastfeeding occurs with inhaled form, mothers should monitor infant for bloody or loose stools and candidiasis (diaper rash, thrush).

Nursing Considerations

! WARNING Know that tobramycin can cause bilateral and irreversible hearing loss, especially in patients who have a maternal history of ototoxicity due to aminoglycoside use or a known mitochondrial DNA variant. Be aware tobramycin should not be given to these patients unless severity of infection and lack of safe and effective alternative therapies outweighs the risk of permanent hearing loss. Also, know ototoxicity has occurred in some patients even when aminoglycoside serum levels were normal. Assess for early signs of cochlear and vestibular ototoxicity, including ataxia, dizziness, high-frequency hearing loss, tinnitus, and vertigo. If present, expect an audiogram to be ordered. Drug may have to be discontinued.

! WARNING Be aware that prolonged respiratory paralysis may occur in patients receiving concomitant neuromuscular blocking agents. Also, monitor patients with muscular disorders because tobramycin may aggravate muscle weakness. High-risk patients include those with myasthenia gravis or Parkinson's disease.

- Expect the serum concentration of tobramycin to be monitored only through venipuncture, as a finger-stick sample may lead to falsely increased measurements of serum levels of the drug, which cannot be completely avoided with handwashing before testing is done. Monitor patients receiving concomitant inhaled and parenteral form of aminoglycoside therapy for toxicities. Obtain regular serum tobramycin levels, as ordered.

! WARNING Monitor patient for bronchospasms and wheezing after drug has been administered. Notify prescriber immediately, if present, and be prepared to treat, as ordered.

! WARNING Monitor patient for a hypersensitivity reaction. If present, notify prescriber, expect drug to be discontinued, and provide supportive care, as needed and ordered.

! WARNING Monitor patient closely for diarrhea, which may indicate pseudomembranous colitis caused by *Clostridioides difficile*, which could be mild or become life-threatening. If diarrhea occurs, notify prescriber and expect to obtain a stool specimen. If *C. difficile* is confirmed, expect tobramycin to be discontinued, and treat with an antibiotic effective against *C. difficile*, as ordered. Also, expect to administer electrolytes, fluids, and protein supplementation, as needed and ordered.

! **WARNING** Watch for signs of nephrotoxicity, such as elevated BUN and serum creatinine levels. Be aware that patients with renal dysfunction or who are taking nephrotoxic drugs should have measurements of serum concentrations of tobramycin and renal function done periodically, as ordered by prescriber. Expect dehydration to increase the risk of nephrotoxicity. Alert prescriber if patient experiences dehydration. If nephrotoxicity occurs, drug may have to be discontinued.

! **WARNING** Monitor serum calcium, magnesium, potassium, and sodium levels to detect electrolyte imbalances.

PATIENT TEACHING

- Instruct patient on how to administer drug by inhalation. If drug is not administered by inhalation, inform patient drug will be administered by a healthcare professional as an intramuscular injection or intravenously.

! **WARNING** Advise patient to immediately notify prescriber if shortness of breath or wheezing occurs after administration of tobramycin inhalation solution and, if severe, to seek immediate medical care.

! **WARNING** Alert patient that drug may cause an allergic reaction. If present, tell patient to notify prescriber or, if serious, to seek immediate medical care.

! **WARNING** Urge patient to tell prescriber about diarrhea that's severe or lasts longer than 2 days. Remind patient that watery or bloody stools may occur 2 or more months after antibiotic therapy and may be serious, requiring prompt treatment.

! **WARNING** Urge patient to immediately report high-frequency hearing loss and vertigo.

- Alert females of childbearing age to notify prescriber immediately if pregnancy occurs.
- Advise mothers who are breastfeeding that breastfeeding should not occur while receiving drug through an injection or intravenous route. If receiving drug through inhalation, mothers should check with prescriber. If mothers can breastfeed, tell them to monitor their infants for bloody or loose stools and for diaper rash or thrush.
- Remind patient to alert all prescribers about tobramycin therapy because drug interacts with many other drugs.

tocilizumab

Actemra

tocilizumab-bavi

Tofidence

tocilizumab-aazg

Tyeene

Class and Category

Pharmacologic class: Monoclonal antibody (interleukin-6 receptor inhibitor)
Therapeutic class: Antiarthritic (disease-modifying antirheumatic drug [DMARD])

Indications and Dosages

✳ *To treat moderate to severe active rheumatoid arthritis as monotherapy in patients who have had an inadequate response to one or more disease-modifying antirheumatic drugs (DMARDs) or as adjunct with methotrexate or other nonbiologic DMARDs*

I.V. INFUSION (ACTEMRA, TOFIDENCE, TYENNE)

Adults. 4 mg/kg infused over 60 min every 4 wk, increased, as needed, to 8 mg/kg infused over 60 min every 4 wk. *Maximum:* 800 mg per infusion.

SUBCUTANEOUS INJECTION (ACTEMRA, TYENNE)

Adults weighing 100 kg (220 lb) or more. 162 mg every wk.
Adults weighing less than 100 kg (220 lb). 162 mg every other wk, followed by increased dosage frequency to every wk, as needed.

✳ *To treat active systemic juvenile idiopathic arthritis as monotherapy or as adjunct with methotrexate*

I.V. INFUSION (ACTEMRA, TOFIDENCE, TYENNE)

Children ages 2 and older weighing 30 kg (66 lb) or more. 8 mg/kg infused over 60 min every 2 wk.

Children ages 2 and older weighing less than 30 kg (66 lb). 12 mg/kg infused over 60 min every 2 wk.

SUBCUTANEOUS INJECTION (ACTEMRA, TYENNE)

Children ages 2 and older weighing 30 kg (66 lb) or more. 162 mg once every wk.
Children ages 2 and older weighing less than 30 kg (66 lb). 162 mg every 2 wk.

✱ *To treat active polyarticular juvenile idiopathic arthritis*

I.V. INFUSION (ACTEMRA, TOFIDENCE, TYENNE)

Children ages 2 and older weighing 30 kg (66 lb) or more. 8 mg/kg infused over 60 min every 4 wk.
Children ages 2 and older weighing less than 30 kg (66 lb). 10 mg/kg infused over 60 min every 4 wk.

SUBCUTANEOUS INJECTION ACTEMRA, TYENNE)

Children ages 2 and older weighing 30 kg (66 lb) or more. 162 mg once every 2 wk.
Children ages 2 and older weighing less than 30 kg (66 lb). 162 mg once every 3 wk.

✱ *To treat giant cell arteritis*

I.V. INFUSION (ACTEMRA, TOFIDENCE, TYENNE)

Adults. 6 mg/kg infused over 60 min every 4 wk in combination with a tapering course of glucocorticoids. *Maximum*: 600 mg per infusion.

SUBCUTANEOUS INJECTION (ACTEMRA, TYENNE)

Adults. 162 mg once wk in combination with a tapering course of glucocorticoids. Alternatively, 162 mg once every other week in combination with a tapering course of glucocorticoids.

✱ *To treat chimeric antigen receptor T-cell-induced severe or life-threatening cytokine release syndrome*

I.V. INFUSION (ACTEMRA, TYENNE)

Adults and children ages 2 and older weighing 30 kg (66 lb) or more. 8 mg/kg infused over 60 min with up to 3 more doses administered with at least 8 hr between doses, as needed. *Maximum:* 800 mg per infusion.
Adults and children ages 2 and older weighing less than 30 kg (66 lb). 12 mg/kg infused over 60 min with up to 3 more doses administered at least 8 hr between doses, as needed. *Maximum:* 800 mg per infusion.

✱ *To treat systemic sclerosis–associated interstitial lung disease (SSc-ILD)*

SUBCUTANEOUS INJECTION (ACTEMRA)

Adults. 162 mg once a wk.

✱ *To treat coronavirus disease 2019 (COVID-19) in hospitalized patients who are receiving systemic corticosteroids and require extracorporeal membrane oxygenation (ECMO), noninvasive or invasive mechanical ventilation, or supplemental oxygen.*

I.V. INFUSION (ACTEMRA, TOFIDENCE, TYENNE)

Adults. 8 mg/kg infused over 60 min. If symptoms do not improve, a second dose of 8 mg/kg infused at least 8 hr later. *Maximum:* 800 mg per infusion.

± **DOSAGE ADJUSTMENT** For all patients, dosage reduction or interruption of dosing may be needed to manage dose-related laboratory abnormalities, including elevated liver enzymes, neutropenia, and thrombocytopenia. See manufacturer's guidelines for specific recommendations for dosage adjustments.

Drug Administration

I.V.

- Dilute using either a 100-ml infusion bag or bottle for patients weighing 30 kg or more or a 50-ml infusion bag or bottle for patients weighing less than 30 kg. Diluents to use include 0.45% (Actemra, Tyenne) or 0.9% Sodium Chloride Injection (Actemra, Tofidence, Tyenne).
- From the infusion bag, withdraw volume of solution equal to the volume of tocilizumab solution that will be added to infusion bag and discard.
- Slowly add drug from vial(s) into infusion bag or bottle and gently invert bag to mix while avoiding foaming.
- Discard any unused drug left in vial(s).
- Actemra solution diluted with 0.9% Sodium Chloride Injection may be refrigerated or stored at room temperature for up to 24 hr. Actemra diluted with 0.45% Sodium Chloride Injection, solution may be refrigerated for up to 24 hr or stored at room temperature for up to 4 hr. Tofidence diluted with 0.9% Sodium Chloride Injection may be refrigerated for up to 24 hr or room

temperature for up to 12 hr. Tyenne diluted with 0.9% or 0.45% Sodium Chloride Injection may be refrigerated for up to 24 hr or stored at room temperature for up to 4 hr. Tofidence diluted with 0.9% Sodium Chloride Injection may be refrigerated for up to 24 hr or room temperature for up to 12 hr. Tyenne diluted with 0.9% or 0.45% Sodium Chloride Injection may be refrigerated for up to 24 hr or stored at room temperature for up to 4 hr. Protect from light.

- If stored in refrigerator, allow solution to reach room temperature prior to infusion.
- Infuse drug with an infusion set, and never give as I.V. push or a bolus.
- Infuse over 60 min.
- *Incompatibilities:* Other drugs

SUBCUTANEOUS

- When transitioning from intravenous therapy to subcutaneous therapy, the first subcutaneous dose should be given instead of next scheduled intravenous dose.
- Administer Actemra using the pre-filled ACTPen autoinjector or pre-filled syringe. However, do not use the Actemra autoinjector for treatment of SSc-ILD. Administer Tyenne using the pre-filled pen autoinjector or pre-filled syringe.
- Inspect solution. It should be clear and colorless to pale yellow; do not use if cloudy, discolored, or contains particulate matter.
- Inject only in healthy skin areas; do not give into areas where skin is bruised, hard, red, tender or not intact. Also, do not inject into moles or scars.
- Rotate sites.

Route	Onset	Peak	Duration
I.V.	Unknown	Unknown	Unknown
SubQ	Unknown	3–4.5 days	Unknown

Half-life: 5–13 days

Mechanism of Action

Binds to interleukin 6 (IL-6) receptors to interrupt signaling through them. Remember that IL-6 is a proinflammatory cytokine produced by various cells, such as B- and T-cells, fibroblasts, lymphocytes, and monocytes. It is also produced by endothelial and synovial cells, leading to local production of IL-6 in joints affected by inflammatory processes, such as polyarticular juvenile idiopathic arthritis, rheumatoid arthritis, and systemic juvenile idiopathic arthritis. Binding of IL-6 receptors prevents inflammation-related signals from being relayed, which reduces inflammatory response and relieves signs and symptoms of inflammatory-related arthritis, giant cell arteritis, and cytokine release syndrome.

Contraindications

Hypersensitivity to tocilizumab or its components

Interactions

DRUGS

atorvastatin; cytochrome P-450 substrates with a narrow therapeutic index, such as cyclosporine, theophylline, warfarin; CYP3A4 substrates, such as lovastatin, oral contraceptives, simvastatin; omeprazole: Possibly decreased plasma levels of these drugs with decreased effectiveness

live vaccines: Increased risk of adverse vaccine effects

Adverse Reactions

CNS: Anxiety, demyelinating disorders, dizziness, headache, insomnia

CV: Elevated lipid levels, hypertension

EENT: Nasopharyngitis, oral ulceration

GI: Constipation, diarrhea, diverticulitis, elevated liver enzymes, gastritis, gastroenteritis, hepatic impairment, **hepatic failure**, **hepatitis**, **hepatotoxicity**, jaundice, nausea, **pancreatitis**, **perforation**, upper abdominal pain

GU: UTI

HEME: **Neutropenia**, **thrombocytopenia**

MS: Bacterial arthritis

RESP: Bronchitis, pneumonia, upper respiratory tract infection

SKIN: Cellulitis, generalized erythema, pruritus, rash, **Stevens-Johnson syndrome**, urticaria

Other: **Anaphylaxis**, anti-tocilizumab antibodies, herpes zoster, **drug reaction with eosinophilia and systemic symptoms (DRESS)**, **hypokalemia**, **immunosuppression**, infections, including activation of latent infections, injection-site reactions (erythema, pain, pruritus, swelling), **malignancies**, **sepsis**, tuberculosis with pulmonary or extrapulmonary disease

Childbearing Considerations

PREGNANCY

- Pregnancy exposure registry: 1-877-311-8972.

- It is not known if drug causes fetal harm. However, drug is increasingly transported across the placental barrier as pregnancy progresses, with the largest amount occurring during the third trimester, which may adversely fetal immune system.
- Use with caution only if benefit to mother outweighs potential risk to fetus because infants exposed to drug in utero may be at risk for adverse reactions or limited effectiveness when administered live or live attenuated vaccines.

LACTATION

- It is not known if drug is present in breast milk.
- Mothers should check with prescriber before breastfeeding.

Nursing Considerations

! **WARNING** Know that tocilizumab isn't recommended for patients with active liver disease or impairment because drug may adversely affect liver function because serious cases of hepatic injury have occurred with tocilizumab therapy, some of which resulted in need for liver transplant or death. Monitor patient's liver enzymes, as ordered, and patient for signs of dysfunction, such as abdominal discomfort (upper right), anorexia, dark urine, fatigue, or jaundice. Know that dosage may have to be reduced or drug withheld or discontinued depending on the specific liver enzyme abnormalities present.

- Make sure patient has a tuberculin skin test before therapy starts except for patients with COVID-19. If skin test is positive, tuberculosis (TB) treatment will have to be started before tocilizumab therapy can begin. Even patients who have tested negative for TB may develop TB during therapy. Monitor patient for low-grade fever, persistent cough, and wasting or weight loss; report such findings to prescriber.
- Ensure patient is up to date on immunizations before tocilizumab is begun. Do not administer live vaccines during drug therapy.

! **WARNING** Know that if patient has evidence of an active infection when drug is prescribed, therapy shouldn't start until infection has been treated except in the treatment of COVID-19. In patients with COVID-19 infection, monitor for new infections during and after drug therapy. Monitor all patients for infections, including invasive fungal infections, such as aspergillosis, candidiasis, or pneumocystis; or bacterial, mycobacterial, protozoal, or viral opportunistic infections during and after therapy, especially patients who are taking immunosuppressants. If a serious infection develops, expect prescriber to interrupt drug therapy until infection is controlled. However, know that the risks and benefits of treatment with tocilizumab in COVID-19 patients who have another concurrent infection will have to be weighed as to what is best for the patient.

- Use tocilizumab cautiously in patients with recurrent infection or increased risk of infection, patients who live in regions where histoplasmosis and TB are endemic, and patients with a history of CNS demyelinating disorders because they may occur, although rarely, during tocilizumab therapy.

! **WARNING** Obtain a baseline of patient's absolute neutrophil count, liver enzymes, and platelet count before starting tocilizumab therapy, as ordered. For patients with giant cell arteritis, rheumatoid arthritis, and systemic sclerosis-associated interstitial lung disease, therapy shouldn't begin if patient's absolute neutrophil count is below 2,000/mm^3 (less than 1,000/mm^3 for COVID-19 patients), ALT or AST level is above 1.5 times the upper limit of normal (10 times the upper limit of normal for COVID-19 patients), or platelet count is below 100,000/mm^3. Monitor these values, as ordered, every 4 to 8 weeks for the first 6 months after drug is initiated and then every 3 months after that, and report abnormalities. Dosage adjustment may be required, or drug may have to be discontinued if abnormalities occur. For example, drug should be discontinued if absolute neutrophil count drops below 500per mm^3.

! **WARNING** Monitor patient for a hypersensitivity or severe skin reaction, which could become life threatening such as

T

anaphylaxis or DRESS. Know that DRESS may initially only present with a fever or swollen lymph nodes although rash is the most common presentation. If present, notify prescriber, expect drug to be discontinued, and provide supportive care, as needed and ordered.

! **WARNING** Monitor patient for other persistent, serious, or unusual adverse reactions as some may be quite serious such as malignancies and pancreatitis.

- Assess patient's lipid parameters about 4 to 8 weeks after drug therapy is begun because tocilizumab can cause increases in patient's lipid profile. If elevated, expect patient to be managed per clinical guidelines.

PATIENT TEACHING

- Instruct patient, family, or caregiver on how to administer drug subcutaneously, if prescribed. Inform all other patients that drug will be administered intravenously.
- Caution against receiving live-virus vaccines while taking tocilizumab

! **WARNING** Review the signs and symptoms of an allergic or skin reaction and tell patient to notify prescriber if an allergic reaction occurs and, if severe, to seek immediate medical care.

- Inform patient that infections, including activation of latent infections such as TB, may occur during tocilizumab therapy. Review signs and symptoms of infections with patient as well as infection control measures to take. Advise patient to avoid people with infections.

! **WARNING** Instruct patient to seek immediate medical care if persistent, severe abdominal pain occurs. Also, report accompanying loss of appetite, fatigue, dark urine, or yellow skin because this could indicate a liver problem.

! **WARNING** Inform patient that risk of developing a malignancy is higher in patients taking tocilizumab, but it is still rare. Emphasize importance of follow-up visits and reporting any sudden or unusual signs or symptoms.

- Advise patient to inform all healthcare providers about tocilizumab use and to inform prescriber about any over-the-counter medications being taken, including herbal remedies and mineral and vitamin supplements.
- Urge females of childbearing age who becomes pregnant while receiving tocilizumab to contact prescriber.
- Inform mothers to alert pediatrician of tocilizumab use during pregnancy before live or live attenuated vaccines are given to the infant.
- Stress importance of complying with ordered blood tests during drug therapy.

tofacitinib citrate

Xeljanz, Xeljanz XR

Class and Category

Pharmacologic class: Janus kinase inhibitor
Therapeutic class: Antirheumatic (disease-modifying antirheumatic drug [DMARD])

Indications and Dosages

* *To treat active ankylosing spondylitis, active psoriaric arthritis, or moderate to severe active rheumatoid arthritis in patients who have had an inadequate response or intolerance to one or more tumor necrosis factor (TNF) blockers*

TABLETS

Adults. 5 mg twice daily.

E.R. TABLETS

Adults. 11 mg once daily.

± **DOSAGE ADJUSTMENT** For patients with moderate hepatic impairment or moderate or severe renal insufficiency, or patients taking concomitant strong CYP3A4 inhibitors, such as ketoconazole, or concomitant use with 1 or more drugs that result in both potent inhibition of CYP2C19, including fluconazole and moderate inhibition of CYP3A4, dosage of either I.R. or E.R. tablets reduced to 5 mg once daily and administered as an I.R. tablet. For patients with absolute neutrophil count (ANC) of 500 to 1,000 cells/mm^3, dosing interrupted until ANC is greater than 1,000 cells/mm^3, then dosage resumed at 5 mg twice daily for I.R. tablets and 11 mg once daily for E.R. tablets. For patients with a hemoglobin less than 8 g/dl or a decrease of more than 2 g/dl, dosing interrupted until hemoglobin values have normalized. For patients with a lymphocyte count less than 500 cells/mm^3 and confirmed with repeat testing or patients with a ANC less than 500 cells/mm^3, dosing discontinued.

* *To treat moderate to severe active ulcerative colitis in patients who have had an inadequate response or who are intolerant to TNF blockers*

TABLETS

Adults. *Induction:* 10 mg twice daily for 8 wk followed by 10 mg twice daily for another 8 wk, depending on therapeutic response. *Maintenance:* 5 mg twice daily, increased to 10 mg twice daily, if loss of response occurs, for shortest duration possible before returning to 5 mg twice daily.

E.R. TABLETS

Adults. *Initial:* 22 mg once daily for 8 wk followed by 22 mg once daily for another 8 wk, depending on therapeutic response. *Maintenance:* 11 mg once daily, increased to 22 mg once daily, if loss of response occurs, for shortest duration possible before returning to 11 mg once daily.

±**DOSAGE ADJUSTMENT** *For I.R. tablets*: For patients with moderate hepatic impairment or moderate or severe renal insufficiency, or patients taking a strong CYP3A4 inhibitor, such as ketoconazole or a moderate CYP3A4 inhibitor with a strong CYP2C19 inhibitor, such as fluconazole, dosage reduced to 5 mg twice daily if patient was taking 10 mg twice daily, and dosage reduced to 5 mg once daily if patient was taking 5 mg twice daily. For patients with an ANC between 500 and 1,000 cells/mm^3, dosage reduced to 5 mg twice daily if patient was taking 10 mg twice daily and dosage increased back to 10 mg twice daily when ANC is greater than 1,000. If patient was taking 5 mg twice daily, dosing interrupted until ANC is greater than 1,000 and then dosage resumed at 5 mg twice daily. For patients with a hemoglobin less than 8 g/dl or for patients who experience a decrease of more than 2 g/dl, drug therapy interrupted until hemoglobin values have normalized. For patients who experience an ANC or lymphocyte count less than 500 cells/mm^3, drug discontinued.
For E.R. tablets: For patients taking a strong CYP3A4 inhibitor, such as ketoconazole or a moderate CYP3A4 inhibitor with a strong CYP2C19 inhibitor, such as fluconazole and for patients with moderate hepatic impairment or moderate to severe renal impairment, dosage reduced to 11 mg once daily if patient was taking 22 mg once daily, and dosage reduced to 5 mg as I.R. form once daily if patient was taking 11 mg once daily. For patients with an ANC between 500 and 1,000 cells/mm^3, dosage reduced to 11 mg once daily if patient was taking 22 mg once daily and dosage increased back to 22 mg once daily when ANC is greater than 1,000. For patients taking 11 mg once daily, dosing interrupted and then resumed at 11 mg once daily when ANC is greater than 1,000. For patients with a hemoglobin less than 8 g/dl or for patients who experience a decrease of more than 2 g/dl, drug therapy interrupted until hemoglobin values have normalized. For patients who experience an ANC or lymphocyte count less than 500 cells/mm^3, drug discontinued.

* *To treat polyarticular juvenile idiopathic arthritis*

ORAL SOLUTION, TABLETS

Children ages 2 and older weighing 40 kg (88 lb) or more. 5 mg (5 ml) twice daily.

ORAL SOLUTION

Children ages 2 and older weighing 20 kg (44 lb) to less than 40 kg (88 lb). 4 mg (4 ml) twice daily.

Children ages 2 and older weighing 10 kg (22 lb) to less than 20 kg (44 lb). 3.2 mg (3.2 ml) twice daily.

±**DOSAGE ADJUSTMENT** For patients with moderate to severe renal impairment, moderate hepatic impairment, or who are receiving strong CYPA4 inhibitors, such as ketoconazole or a moderate CYP3A4 inhibitor with a strong CYP2C19 inhibitor, such as fluconazole, dosage interval reduced to once daily. For patients with a hemoglobin less than 8 g/dl or for patients who experience a decrease of more than 2 g/dl, drug therapy interrupted until hemoglobin values have normalized. For patients with an ANC between 500 and 1,000 cells/mm^3, dosage interrupted until ANC is greater than 1,000 cells/mm^3 or discontinued if ANC becomes less than 500 cells/mm^3. For patients with confirmed lymphocyte count less than 500 cells/mm^3, dosing discontinued.

Drug Administration

P.O.

- Tablets and oral solution are interchangeable but not with E.R. tablet form.
- For patients undergoing hemodialysis, administer drug after the dialysis session on dialysis days. If drug was taken before dialysis procedure, do not administer a supplemental dose after dialysis.
- Administer oral solution using the included press-in bottle adapter and oral dosing syringe. Push down on cap to remove. Do not shake. Insert press-in bottle adapter for first time use only. After removing air from dosing syringe, insert syringe tip into upright bottle through the opening of the press-in bottle adapter until it is firmly in place. Turn bottle upside down, withdraw dose. If bubbles appear in syringe, fully push plunger in so solution flows back into bottle and withdraw again. Turn bottle upright and place on flat surface. Remove syringe by pulling straight up on the oral dosing syringe barrel. Administer by placing the tip of the syringe into the inside of patient's cheek. Slowly push plunger all the way down. Make sure patient swallows the oral solution. Rinse plunger and barrel after use and allow to air-dry.
- E.R. tablets and I.R. tablets should be swallowed whole and not broken, chewed, or crushed.
- Drug may be taken with or without food.
- Store oral solution in original bottle at room temeprature and discard after 60 days from time bottle was opened for the first time. Protect from light.

Route	Onset	Peak	Duration
P.O.	Unknown	0.5–1 hr	Unknown
P.O./E.R.	Unknown	4 hr	Unknown

Half-life: 3–6 hr

Mechanism of Action

Modulates the signaling pathway by inhibiting the enzyme, Janus kinase (JAK). JAK is an intracellular enzyme that transmits signals arising from cytokine or growth factor–receptor interactions on the cellular membrane to influence cellular processes of hematopoiesis and immune cell function. Inhibiting the phosphorylation and activation of Signal Transducers and Activator of Transcription (STATs) needed to influence cellular processes lessens some of the signs and symptoms of conditions being treated.

Contraindications

Hypersensitivity to tofacitinib or its components

Interactions

DRUGS

CYP3A4 potent inducers, such as rifampin: Possibly loss or reduced effectiveness of tofacitinib

CYP3A4 potent inhibitors, such as ketoconazole, moderate CYP3A4 inhibitors/ potent CYP2C19 inhibitors, such as fluconazole: Increased tofacitinib exposure and adverse reactions

immunosuppressive drugs, such as azathioprine, cyclosporine, tacrolimus: Potentiated immunosuppression

live vaccines: Increased risk of infection

Adverse Reactions

CNS: **CVA**, fatigue, fever, headache, insomnia, paresthesia

CV: Elevated lipid levels, hypertension, **MI**, peripheral edema, **thrombosis (arterial or deep vein thrombosis)**

EENT: Esophageal candidiasis, nasopharyngitis, sinus congestion

GI: Abdominal pain, diarrhea, diverticulitis, dyspepsia, elevated liver enzymes, gastritis, hepatic steatosis, liver injury, nausea, vomiting

GU: Elevated serum creatinine levels, UTI

HEME: Anemia, **lymphopenia**, **neutropenia**

MS: Arthralgia, elevated creatine phosphokinase, joint swelling, musculoskeletal pain, tendinitis

RESP: Cough, dyspnea, **interstitial lung disease**, pneumonia, **pneumocystosis**, **pulmonary embolism**, upper respiratory infection

SKIN: Acne, cellulitis, erythema, **melanoma**, multidermatomal herpes zoster, **nonmelanoma skin cancers**, rash, pruritus, urticaria

Other: **Angioedema**, bacteria, mycobacterial, invasive fungal, viral, or other opportunistic infections, such as tuberculosis and other BK viral, cytomegalovirus, cryptococcus, or mycobacterial infections; dehydration; herpes zoster; **lymphoproliferative disorder**; **malignancies, such as breast, colorectal,**

gastric, lung, lymphoma, malignant melanoma, prostate, and renal cell

Childbearing Considerations

PREGNANCY

- Pregnancy exposure registry: 1-877-311-8972.
- It is not known if drug causes fetal harm, but animal studies suggest it may.
- Use with caution only if benefit to mother outweighs potential risk to fetus.

LACTATION

- Drug is present in breast milk.
- Breastfeeding is not recommended during drug therapy and for at least 18 hr after the last dose of I.R. tablets or oral solution or 36 hr after the last dose of E.R. tablets.

REPRODUCTION

- Females of childbearing should use effective contraception throughout drug therapy.
- Drug may reduce female fertility.

Nursing Considerations

! **WARNING** Know that tofacitinib should not be given to patients with severe hepatic impairment. Screen patient for viral hepatitis, as ordered, prior to starting tofacitinib therapy. Monitor the patient's liver enzymes routinely, as ordered, to detect liver dysfunction. Alert prescriber of any abnormalities and expect drug to be withheld during the investigation as to the cause of the elevated liver enzymes. If no other cause can be found, expect prescriber to discontinue drug.

! **WARNING** Be aware tofacitinib should not be given to patients with hemoglobin levels less than 9 g/dl because drug may cause hemoglobin to decrease further increasing the severity of anemia. Obtain a baseline of hemoglobin level, as ordered, and expect to monitor hemoglobin level after 4 to 8 weeks and then every 3 months.

! **WARNING** Be aware tofacitinib therapy should not be given to a patient who has an active infection, including localized infections. Also, tofacitinib should not be initiated in patients with a lymphocyte count less than 500 cells/mm^3 or an absolute neutrophil count (ANC) less than 1,000 cells/mm^3.

- Obtain patient's baseline of neutrophils and lymphocytes counts, as ordered. Once the baseline is established, expect prescriber to order a lymphocyte level every 3 months; an ANC level after 4 to 8 weeks of therapy and then every 3 months. These test results will guide the prescriber in making modifications in the patient's treatment plan. Monitor patient for signs and symptoms of infection during and after tofacitinib therapy. Patients at higher risk for infection include patients with a history of chronic or recurrent infections, exposure to TB, history of a serious infection or an opportunistic infection, have resided or traveled in areas of endemic mycoses or endemic TB, or have underlying conditions that may predispose them to infection. Notify prescriber if an infection develops and expect to obtain a complete blood count, if ordered. Be aware that drug should be discontinued if the patient has an ANC count or lymphocyte count less than 500 cells/mm^3. If the patient has an ANC level between 500 and 1,000 cells/mm^3, expect drug therapy to be interrupted until the ANC levels have returned to target range.
- Check to be sure that the patient has been tested for latent or active tuberculosis (TB) before tofacitinib therapy begins. Antituberculosis therapy might be prescribed for patients with a history of active or latent TB if completion of treatment cannot be verified. Also, patients who have a negative test for latent TB may also be prescribed antituberculosis therapy if they have risk factors for TB.
- Check with patient to be sure past immunizations received are in line with current immunization guidelines before starting tofacitinib therapy. If the patient needs further immunizations, ensure that it is done before drug therapy begins.
- Use caution when administering nondeformable E.R. form of drug to patients with preexisting severe GI narrowing. Rare reports of obstructive symptoms in patients with known strictures have occurred with other drugs utilizing a nondeformable E.R. formula.

! **WARNING** Monitor patient for a hypersensitivity reaction, which could become life threatening such as angioedema.

If present, notify prescriber, expect drug to be discontinued, and provide supportive care, as needed and ordered.

! **WARNING** Monitor patient for thrombosis, including arterial thrombosis, deep venous thrombosis, or pulmonary embolism, which may occur with tofacitinib therapy. Patients at increased risk are patients with rheumatoid arthritis taking 5 or 10 mg twice daily and are 50 years or older and have at least one cardiovascular risk factor.

! **WARNING** Be aware that patients 50 years and older with at least 1 cardiovascular risk factor treated with twice daily dosing of immediate-release tablets have a higher rate of all-cause mortality, including non-fatal MI or stroke or sudden cardiovascular death, compared to those treated with TNF blockers. Know that dosage is limited to once a day in patients 50 years and older who have at least 1 cardiovascular risk factor.

! **WARNING** Be aware that tofacitinib therapy increases risk of cancer. Monitor patient closely for persistent, serious, or unusual adverse reactions. The prescriber may choose to discontinue drug in patients who develop a malignancy during tofacitinib therapy.

! **WARNING** Monitor patients who may be at increased risk for GI perforation, such as a patient with a history of diverticulitis. Monitor patient closely throughout tofacitinib therapy. Notify prescriber if patient experiences new-onset abdominal symptoms suggestive of perforation.

- Know that viral reactivation, including herpes virus reactivation (herpes zoster), has occurred with tofacitinib therapy.
- Expect prescriber to order a lipid profile on the patient 4 to 8 weeks after tofacitinib therapy has begun because the drug has caused increases in lipid parameters generally within the first 6 weeks of therapy. Expect to manage hyperlipidemia, if present, according to clinical guidelines, as prescribed.

PATIENT TEACHING

! **WARNING** Make sure patient understands the serious adverse reactions associated with tofacitinib, such as the development of malignancies, before therapy begins. Advise patient at increased risk for skin cancer to have a periodic skin examination.

- Instruct patient how to administer form of tofacitinib prescribed.
- Alert patient that an inert tablet shell may be passed in the stool or via colostomy. If present, reassure patient that the active medication has already been absorbed by the time patient sees the shell.

! **WARNING** Warn patient to avoid live vaccines while taking tofacitinib.

! **WARNING** Alert patient that an allergic reaction may occur with drug use. Tell patient to notify prescriber, if present, and to seek immediate medical care, if serious.

! **WARNING** Review infection control measures with patient as well as the signs and symptoms of an infection. If an infection occurs, tell patient to notify prescriber immediately because the infection can become serious.

! **WARNING** Urge patient to seek immediate emergency care if patient experiences chest pain that worsens with breathing, leg pain or tenderness, red or discolored skin in the affected arm or leg, sudden shortness of breath, or swelling of arm or leg.

! **WARNING** Tell patient to notify prescriber of any other persistent, serious, or unusual adverse reaction.

- Stress importance for females of childbearing age to use effective contraception during treatment. Tell patient to notify prescriber if pregnancy occurs. Also, alert patient that drug may reduce fertility.
- Make mothers aware that breastfeeding should not be done while taking tofacitinib and for at least 18 hours after the last dose of I.R. tablets or oral solution or 36 hours after the last dose of E.R. tablets.

- Encourage patient to comply with laboratory blood tests needed to monitor patient's reaction to tofacitinib.

tolterodine tartrate

Detrol, Detrol LA

Class and Category

Pharmacologic class: Cholinergic receptor blocker
Therapeutic class: Antispasmodic

Indications and Dosages

* *To treat overactive bladder with urinary frequency, urgency, or urge incontinence*

TABLETS

Adults. 2 mg twice daily. Reduced to 1 mg twice daily based on patient response and tolerance.

± **DOSAGE ADJUSTMENT** For patients with significant hepatic or renal dysfunction (creatinine clearance between 10 and 30 ml/min) and for patients who are also receiving potent CYP3A4 inhibitors, such as clarithromycin, ketoconazole, or ritonavir, dosage reduced to 1 mg twice daily.

E.R. CAPSULES

Adults. 4 mg once daily. Reduced to 2 mg daily based on individual response and tolerance.

± **DOSAGE ADJUSTMENT** For patients with mild to moderate hepatic dysfunction, severe renal dysfunction (creatinine clearance between 10 to 30 ml/min), and for patients receiving potent CYP3A4 inhibitors, such as clarithromycin, ketoconazole, or ritonavir, dosage reduced to 2 mg once daily.

Drug Administration

P.O.

- Capsules and tablets should be swallowed whole and not chewed, crushed, or opened.

Route	Onset	Peak	Duration
P.O.	Unknown	1–2 hr	Unknown
P.O./E.R.	Unknown	2–6 hr	Unknown

Half-life: 2–6.9 hr

Mechanism of Action

Exerts antimuscarinic (atropine-like) and potent direct antispasmodic (papaverine-like) actions on smooth muscle in the bladder, which decreases detrusor muscle contractions thereby helping to reduce urinary frequency and urgency as well as urge-related incontinence.

Contraindications

Gastric retention; hypersensitivity to tolterodine tartrate, its components, or to fesoterodine fumarate E.R. tablets; uncontrolled angle-closure glaucoma; urine retention

Interactions

DRUGS

fluoxetine: Possibly decreased tolterodine metabolism increasing immediate-release tolterodine blood concentration
other anticholinergics: Increased risk of anticholinergic adverse effects such as blurred vision, constipation, dry mouth, and somnolence
potent CYP3A4 inhibitors, such as clarithromycin, itraconazole, ketoconazole, ritonavir: Possibly increased blood tolterodine level

Adverse Reactions

CNS: Confusion, disorientation, dizziness, drowsiness, fatigue, hallucinations, headache, memory impairment, somnolence, worsening of dementia
CV: Chest pain, edema, hypertension, palpitations, **QT prolongation**, tachycardia
EENT: Abnormal vision, blurred vision, dry eyes, dry mouth
GI: Abdominal pain, constipation, diarrhea, flatulence, indigestion, nausea
GU: Dysuria, urine retention, UTI
Other: **Anaphylaxis**, **angioedema**, flu-like symptoms

Childbearing Considerations

PREGNANCY

- It is not known if drug can cause fetal harm.
- Use with caution only if benefit to mother outweighs potential risk to fetus.

LACTATION

- It is not known if drug is present in breast milk.
- A decision should be made to discontinue breastfeeding or drug to avoid potential

serious adverse reactions in the breastfed infant.

Nursing Considerations

- Use cautiously in patients with decreased GI motility, myasthenia gravis, or narrow-angle glaucoma because tolterodine could make these conditions worse.

! WARNING Monitor patient for a hypersensitivity reaction, which could become life threatening such as anaphylaxis or angioedema. If present, notify prescriber, expect drug to be discontinued, and provide supportive care, as needed and ordered.

- Monitor patients with a history of bladder outflow obstruction for bladder distention or decreased urine output because tolterodine poses a risk of urine retention.
- Monitor patients for abdominal bloating or distention or patients with a history of GI obstructive disorders, such as pyloric stenosis, because of increased risk of gastric retention.
- Be aware that drug's antimuscarinic effects may produce blurred vision, dizziness, and drowsiness. If these occur, institute fall precautions according to facility policy.

PATIENT TEACHING

- Instruct patient how to administer form of tolterodine prescribed.

! WARNING Tell patient drug may cause an allergic reaction. If present, tell patient to notify prescriber and, if severe, to seek immediate medical care.

- Instruct patient taking tolterodine to notify prescriber of any difficulty urinating or infrequent urination.
- Advise patient not to drive or perform activities that require high alertness until drug's CNS and vision effects are known and resolved. Instruct patient to notify prescriber if blurred vision, dizziness, or drowsiness persists.
- Encourage patient to use sugarless candy, gum, or ice to relieve dry mouth. Advise patient to notify prescriber or dentist if dry mouth persists or worsens over 2 weeks.
- Inform mothers breastfeeding should not be undertaken or drug will have to be discontinued.

tolvaptan

Jynarque, Samsca

Class and Category

Pharmacologic class: Vasopressin receptor antagonist
Therapeutic class: Vasopressin antagonist

Indications and Dosages

✶ *To treat significant hypervolemic and euvolemic hyponatremia (serum sodium level less than 125 mEq/L or symptomatic but less-marked hyponatremia that has resisted correction with fluid restriction), including patients with heart failure or syndrome of inappropriate antidiuretic hormone (SIADH)*

TABLETS (SAMSCA)

Adults. *Initial:* 15 mg once daily, increased after at least 24 hr, to 30 mg once daily, and further increased to 60 mg once daily after at least 24 hr, as needed. *Maximum:* 60 mg once daily or given for no more than 30 days.

✶ *To slow kidney function decline in patients at risk of rapidly progressing autosomal dominant polycystic kidney disease*

TABLETS (JYNARQUE)

Adults. *Initial:* 45 mg upon waking followed with 15 mg 8 hr later for a total daily dose of 60 mg. Dosage titrated at least a wk later to 60 mg upon waking followed with 30 mg 8 hr later for a total daily dose of 90 mg. Dosage further titrated to target dose after another wk with 90 mg upon waking followed with 30 mg 8 hr later for a total daily dose of 120 mg and thereafter.

± DOSAGE ADJUSTMENT

For Jynarque: For patients taking concomitant moderate CYP3A inhibitors, initial dosage of 45 mg followed by 15 mg reduced to 15 mg and 15 mg 8 hours later; initial dosage of 60 mg followed by 30 mg reduced to 30 mg and 15 mg 8 hours later; and initial dosage of 90mg followed by 30 mg reduced to 45 mg and 15 mg 8 hours later.

Drug Administration

P.O.

- Administer without regard to food.
- Administer first dose of Jynarque when patient awakes in morning and second dose 8 hr later.

- Avoid administering drug with grapefruit or grapefruit juice.
- If a dose of Samsca is missed, administer missed dose as soon as possible unless it it almost time for next dose. If a dose of Jynarque is missed, skip dose and resume dosing at next regularly scheduled time.

Route	Onset	Peak	Duration
P.O.	2–4 hr	2–4 hr	Unknown

Half-life: 3–12 hr

Mechanism of Action

Raises serum sodium levels by decreasing urine osmolality and increasing urine output. Does this by preventing attachment of vasopressin-to-vasopressin V2 receptors on cell membranes in the nephron's collecting duct. Without vasopressin activity, urinary water excretion increases.

Contraindications

Acute need to raise serum sodium urgently; anuria; concomitant use of strong CYP3A inhibitors, such as clarithromycin, indinavir, itraconazole, ketoconazole, nefazodone, nelfinavir, ritonavir, saquinavir, telithromycin; hypovolemic hyponatremia; hypersensitivity to tolvaptan or its components; inability of patient to sense or respond appropriately to thirst; significant liver impairment or injury (Jynarque); uncorrected abnormal blood sodium concentrations or urinary outflow obstruction (Jynarque); use in patients with autosomal dominant polycystic kidney disease outside of FDA-approved REMS (Samsca)

Interactions

DRUGS

ACE inhibitors, angiotensin receptor blockers, potassium-sparing diuretics, potassium supplements: Increased risk of hyperkalemia
CYP3A inducers, such as barbiturates, carbamazepine, phenytoin, rifabutin, rifampin, rifapentine, St. John's wort: Decreased serum tolvaptan level and decreased effectiveness
CYP3A inhibitors, such as aprepitant, clarithromycin, diltiazem, erythromycin, fluconazole, ketoconazole, indinavir, itraconazole, nefazodone, nelfinavir, ritonavir, saquinavir, telithromycin, verapamil; P-gp inhibitors such as cyclosporine: Increased serum tolvaptan level and risk of adverse reactions
desmopressin: Possibly altered desmopressin activity
digoxin: Increased digoxin level

FOODS

grapefruit juice: Increased serum tolvaptan level

Adverse Reactions

CNS: Asthenia, **CVA**, fever, **osmotic demyelination syndrome**, thirst
CV: **Deep vein thrombosis, intracardiac thrombus, ventricular fibrillation**
EENT: Dry mouth
ENDO: **Diabetic ketoacidosis,** hyperglycemia
GI: Anorexia, constipation, **GI bleeding**, hepatic dysfunction, **hepatic injury**, **ischemic colitis**, nausea
GU: Nocturia, polyuria, **urethral or vaginal hemorrhage**
HEME: **Disseminated intravascular coagulation (DIC), prolonged prothrombintime**
MS: **Rhabdomyolysis**
RESP: **Pulmonary embolism, respiratory failure**
SKIN: Rash
Other: **Anaphylaxis**, dehydration, **hyperkalemia, hypernatremia, hyponatremia**, hypovolemia

Childbearing Considerations

PREGNANCY

- It is not known if drug can cause fetal harm.
- Use with caution only if benefit to mother outweighs potential risk to fetus.

LACTATION

- It is not known if drug is present in breast milk.
- Breastfeeding is not recommended during drug therapy.

Nursing Considerations

! **WARNING** Know that Jynarque brand is only available through a restricted program called the Jynarque REMS Program. Ensure that patient has been enrolled and has agreed to comply with ongoing monitoring requirements.

! **WARNING** Be aware that drug should not be given to patients with underlying liver disease, including cirrhosis, because drug can cause serious and potentially fatal liver injury. Expect patients prescribed Jynarque brand to have bilirubin and liver enzymes evaluated prior to starting Jynarque therapy, again after 2 and 4 weeks of therapy, then monthly for 18 months and every 3 months thereafter because of increased risk of serious liver injury. Expect patients prescribed Samsca brand to also have bilirubin and liver enzymes evaluated prior to starting Samsca therapy. Be aware that Samsca duration of therapy should be limited to 30 days because of the potential for liver injury. Monitor patient regardless of brand of tolvaptan taken for liver dysfunction. If present, notify prescriber and expect drug to be discontinued.

- Be aware that tolvaptan should not be given to patients with a creatine clearance of less than 10 ml/min because no benefit can be expected in patients who are anuric.

! WARNING Give Samsca brand of tolvaptan, initially or if reintroduced, in a hospital setting because too-rapid correction of hyponatremia (more than 12 mEq/L in 24 hour) causes osmotic demyelination (affective changes, coma, dysarthria, dysphagia, lethargy, mutism, spastic quadriparesis, seizures, death). If present, notify prescriber immediately and expect to stop tolvaptan and give hypotonic fluids.

! WARNING Monitor fluid and electrolyte balance regularly, especially when starting tolvaptan and adjusting dosage, as ordered. If patient develops hypernatremia, notify prescriber and expect to decrease dose or withhold drug and modify the patient's free-water infusion or intake, as ordered.

- Don't restrict patient's fluids during first 24 hours of Samsca therapy because doing so may increase the risk of overly rapid correction of dehydration, hypovolemia, and serum sodium.
- Use of hypertonic saline during Samsca therapy isn't recommended because effects are unknown.

! WARNING Monitor patient for a hypersensitivity reaction, which could become life threatening such as anaphylaxis. If present, notify prescriber, expect drug to be discontinued, and provide supportive care, as needed and ordered.

! WARNING Monitor patient for other persistent, serious, or unusual adverse reactions because drug can affect many body systems and has the potential to cause serious to life threatening adverse reactions.

PATIENT TEACHING

- Instruct patient how to administer brand of drug prescribed.
- Inform patient prescribed Samsca brand that the initial dose will need to be administered in a hospital setting and again if drug needs to be re-initiated.
- Instruct patient to consume fluids according to thirst during first 24 hours of therapy and not to try to limit fluid intake.

! WARNING Alert patient that drug may cause an allergic reaction. If present, tell patient to notify prescriber, and, if severe, to seek immediate medical care.

! WARNING Tell patient to notify prescriber if dark urine or yellowing of eyes and skin, fatigue, loss of appetite, or right upper abdominal pain are experienced.

! WARNING Urge patient to notify prescriber or seek immediate medical care if other persistent, serious, or unusual adverse reactions occur.

- Stress to patient receiving Jynarque the need to comply with frequent blood tests to monitor for adverse liver reactions.
- Inform mothers that breastfeeding is not recommended during drug therapy.
- Tell patient to resume fluid restriction and continued monitoring of sodium level and fluid status when drug is discontinued.

topiramate

Eprontia, Qudexy XR, Topamax, Topamax Sprinkle, Trokendi XR

Class and Category

Pharmacologic class: Sulfamate-substituted monosaccharide
Therapeutic class: Anticonvulsant

Indications and Dosages

✱ To treat partial-onset or primary generalized tonic–clonic seizures

CAPSULES (TOPAMAX SPRINKLE), ORAL SOLUTION (EPRONTIA), TABLETS (TOPAMAX)

Adults and children ages 10 and older. *Initial:* 25 mg twice daily in morning and evening for wk 1; 50 mg twice daily in morning and evening for wk 2; 75 mg twice daily in morning and evening for wk 3; 100 mg twice daily in morning and evening for wk 4; 150 mg twice daily in morning and evening for wk 5; and 200 mg twice daily in morning and evening for wk 6. *Maintenance:* 200 mg twice daily in morning and evening.

Children ages 2 to 10. *Initial:* 25 mg once daily in evening for wk 1. Increased to 25 mg twice daily in morning and evening for wk 2. Increased thereafter by 25 to 50 mg/day each subsequent wk, as tolerated, to reach minimum maintenance dose over the next 5 to 7 wk. *Maintenance:* For children weighing up to 11 kg (up to 24.2 lb), 75 to 125 mg twice daily; for children weighing 12 to 22 kg (26.4 to 48.4 lb), 100 to 150 mg twice daily; for children weighing 23 to 31 kg (50.6 to 68.2 lb), 100 to 175 mg twice daily; for children weighing 32 to 38 kg (70.4 to 83.6 lb), 125 to 175 mg twice daily; and for children weighing more than 38 kg (more than 83.6 lb), 125 to 200 mg twice daily. *Maximum:* Highest maintenance dosage for weight.

E.R. CAPSULES (QUDEXY XR, TROKENDI XR)

Adults and children ages 10 and older. *Initial:* 50 mg once daily for wk 1; 100 mg once daily for wk 2; 150 mg once daily for wk 3; 200 mg once daily for wk 4; 300 mg once daily for wk 5; and 400 mg once daily for wk 6 and beyond. *Maintenance:* 400 mg once daily.

Children ages 2 to less than 10 (Qudexy XR) and children ages 6 to less than 10 (Trokendi XR). *Initial:* 25 mg once daily at night for wk 1; 50 mg once daily at night for wk 2; then increased weekly in increments of 25 to 50 mg until minimum maintenance dose reached, usually within 5 to 7 wk. Additional increases in increments of 25 to 50 mg made weekly to maximum maintenance dose, as needed. *Maintenance:* For children weighing up to 11 kg (24.2lb), 150 to 250 mg once daily at night; for children weighing 12 to 22 kg (26.4 to 48.4lb), 200 to 300 mg once daily at night; for children weighing 23 to 31 kg (50.6 to 68.2 lb), 200 to 350 mg once daily at night; for children weighing 32 to 38 kg (70.4 to 83.6 lb), 250 to 350 mg once daily at night; and for children weighing more than 38 kg (83.6 lb), 250 to 400 mg once daily at night. *Maximum:* Highest maximum maintenance dose for weight.

✱ As adjunct to treat partial seizures, primary generalized tonic–clonic seizures, and seizures associated with Lennox-Gastaut syndrome

CAPSULES (TOPAMAX SPRINKLE), ORAL SOLUTION (EPRONTIA), TABLETS (TOPAMAX)

Adults and adolescents ages 17 and older. *Initial:* 25 to 50 mg daily in divided doses twice daily for 1 wk. Increased by 25 to 50 mg daily every wk thereafter until maintenance dose is reached. *Maintenance:* 200 to 400 mg daily in divided doses twice daily for partial-onset seizures and Lennox-Gastaut syndrome and 400 mg daily in divided doses twice daily for primary generalized tonic–clonic seizures.

Children ages 2 to 16. *Initial:* 1 mg/kg/day to 3 mg/kg daily at night for 1 wk. Increased every 1 to 2 wk by 1 to 3 mg/kg daily in divided doses twice daily until maintenance dose is reached. *Maintenance:* 5 to 9 mg/kg daily in divided doses twice daily.

E.R. CAPSULES (QUDEXY XR, TROKENDI XR)

Adults and adolescents ages 17 and older. *Initial:* 25 to 50 mg once daily, increased weekly in increments of 25 to 50 mg once daily, as needed. *Maximum:* 200 mg to 400 mg once daily (partial-onset seizures or Lennox-Gastaut syndrome) or 400 mg once daily (primary generalized tonic-clonic seizures).

Children ages 2 to less than 17 (Qudexy XR) and children ages 6 to less than 17 (Trokendi XR). *Initial:* 1 to 3 mg/kg/day once daily at night for 1 wk, increased every 1 to 2 wk in increments of 1 to 3 mg/kg/day, as needed. *Maximum:* 9 mg/kg/day or 400mg daily.

✱ To prevent migraine headache

CAPSULES (TOPAMAX SPRINKLE), ORAL SOLUTION (EPRONTIA), TABLETS (TOPAMAX)

Adults and children ages 12 and older. *Initial:* 25 mg daily in evening for wk 1; then 25 mg twice daily morning and evening for wk 2; then 25 mg in morning and 50 mg in evening for wk 3, then 50 mg twice daily in morning and evening for wk 4. *Maintenance:* 50 mg twice daily.

E.R. CAPSULES (QUDEXY XR, TROKENDI XR)

Adults and children ages 12 and older. *Initial:* 25 mg once daily for wk 1; 50 mg once daily for wk 2; 75 mg once daily for wk 3; and 100 mg once daily for wk 4. *Maintenance:* 100 mg once daily.

±**DOSAGE ADJUSTMENT** For patients with renal impairment (creatinine clearance less than 70 ml/min), dosage reduced by 50%. For patients undergoing hemodialysis, a supplemental dose may be required during a prolonged period of dialysis.

Drug Administration

P.O.

- Drug may be taken with or without food.
- Do not break tablets because of the bitter taste.
- Topamax Sprinkle and Qudexy XR capsules may be swallowed whole or opened and sprinkled onto a teaspoon of soft food. Mixture should be swallowed immediately and not chewed or crushed, nor should it be stored.
- Trokendi XR capsules should be swallowed whole and not chewed, crushed, or opened.
- Use a calibrated measuring device to measure and administer oral solution. Discard unused portion of oral solution after 90 days of first opening the bottle.

Route	Onset	Peak	Duration
P.O.	Unknown	1–4 hr	Unknown
P.O./E.R.	Unknown	20–24 hr	Unknown

Half-life: 21–56 hr

Mechanism of Action

May block the spread of seizures by reducing the length and frequency of excitatory transmission.

Contraindications

Hypersensitivity to topiramate or its components, recent alcohol use defined as within 6 hr prior to and 6 hr after taking topiramate (Trokendi XR)

Interactions

DRUGS

amitriptyline: Possibly high increase in amitriptyline blood concentration increasing risk of adverse reactions
antihistamines, barbiturates, benzodiazepines, CNS depressants, opioid analgesics, skeletal muscle relaxants, tricyclic antidepressants: Additive CNS depression
carbamazepine, phenytoin: Decreased blood topiramate level
hydrochlorothiazide: Possibly increased blood topiramate levels
lithium: Increased risk of lithium toxicity
oral contraceptives: Increased risk of breakthrough bleeding, decreased contraceptive efficacy
other carbonic anhydrase inhibitors, such as acetazolamide, zonisamide: Increased risk of kidney stone formation; increased severity of metabolic acidosis
pioglitazone: Possibly decreased exposure of pioglitazone with decreased effectiveness
valproic acid: Increased risk of hyperammonemia, with or without encephalopathy; increased risk of hypothermia

ACTIVITIES

alcohol use: Additive CNS depression

Adverse Reactions

CNS: Abnormal coordination, aggression, agitation, anxiety, aphasia, apathy, asthenia, ataxia, confusion, cognitive-related dysfunction, decreased concentration, depersonalization, depression, dizziness, dysphasia, emotional lability, **encephalopathy**, fatigue, fever, gait abnormality, hallucinations, headache, hyperkinesia, hyperthermia, hypoesthesia, hyporeflexia, insomnia, irritability, language problems, memory alterations or loss, mood changes, nervousness, neurosis, paresthesia, personality disorder, psychomotor slowing, psychosis, rigors, **seizures**, slurred or other abnormalities of speech, somnolence, stupor, **suicidal ideation**, syncope, thirst, tremor, vertigo

CV: **Bradycardia**, **cardiac arrest**, chest pain, edema, hypertension, **hypotension**, palpitations, vasodilation
EENT: Acute myopia and secondary angle-closure glaucoma syndrome, blurred vision, conjunctivitis, diplopia, dry mouth, edema of the pharynx, epistaxis, gingivitis, glossitis, gum hyperplasia, hearing loss, increased saliva, laryngitis, maculopathy, myopia, nystagmus, otitis media, periorbital pain, pharyngitis, rhinitis, secondary angle-closure glaucoma with acute myopia, sinusitis, taste loss or perversion, tinnitus, tongue edema, vision changes, including visual field defects
ENDO: Breast pain, hot flashes, hyperglycemia, **hypoglycemia**, hypothyroidism
GI: Abdominal pain, anorexia, constipation, diarrhea, dyspepsia, elevated gamma GGT levels, fecal incontinence, flatulence, gastroenteritis, gastroesophageal reflux, **hepatic failure**, **hepatitis**, increased appetite, indigestion, nausea, **pancreatitis**, vomiting
GU: Cystitis, decreased libido, dysmenorrhea, dysuria, elevated BUN and serum creatinine levels, frequent urination, hematuria, impotence, kidney stones, leukorrhea, menstrual irregularities, nephrocalcinosis, nocturia, premature ejaculation, prostatic disorder, renal calculi, renal tubular acidosis, urinary frequency or incontinence, UTI, **vaginal hemorrhage**, vaginitis
HEME: Anemia, **bleeding events**, **increased prothrombin time**, **elevated platelet count**, **leukopenia**, purpura, **thrombocytopenia**
MS: Arthralgia, back pain, decreased bone mineral density (children), dysarthria, involuntary muscle contractions, leg cramps or pain, muscle weakness, myalgia, skeletalpain
RESP: Bronchitis, cough, dyspnea, pneumonia, **pulmonary embolism**, upper respiratory tract infection
SKIN: Abnormal hair growth, acne, alopecia, bullous skin reactions, decreased or increased sweating, dermatitis, **erythema multiforme**, eczema, flushing, pallor, pemphigus, pruritus, rash, seborrhea, skin discoloration, **Stevens-Johnson syndrome**, **toxic epidermal necrolysis**
Other: Body odor, chronic metabolic acidosis, **decreased serum bicarbonate levels**, decreased height and weight (children), dehydration, elevated serum alkaline phosphatase or uric acid, flu-like symptoms, **hyperammonemia**, **hyperchloremia**, **hypersensitivity reactions**, **hyponatremia**, **hypophosphatemia**, increased susceptibility to infection, **metabolic acidosis**, moniliasis, weight gain or loss

Childbearing Considerations

PREGNANCY

- Pregnancy exposure registry: 1-888-233-2334 or http://www.aedpregnancyregistry.org/.
- Drug can cause fetal harm such as increased risk for major congenital malformations not limited to cleft lip or palate and being small for gestational age.
- Use with caution only if benefit to mother outweighs potential risk to fetus.

LABOR AND DELIVERY

- Drug may cause preterm labor and premature delivery.
- There is a potential for the development of drug-induced metabolic acidosis in the mother and/or in the fetus, which might affect the fetus's ability to tolerate labor.
- Neonates should be monitored for transient metabolic acidosis following birth if mother received drug.

LACTATION

- Drug is present in breast milk.
- Mothers should check with prescriber before breastfeeding.
- If breastfeeding occurs, monitor breastfed infant for diarrhea and somnolence.

REPRODUCTION

- Females of childbearing age should use an effective contraceptive throughout drug therapy. Contraceptives containing only estrogen or only progestin may be less effective and increases risk of breakthrough bleeding.

Nursing Considerations

- Obtain baseline serum bicarbonate level before topiramate therapy and monitor periodically throughout therapy, as ordered. Be aware that chronic, untreated metabolic acidosis may increase risk for nephrocalcinosis or nephrolithiasis and may cause rickets in children and/or osteoporosis increasing risk for fractures.
- Obtain baseline height and weight in children before drug therapy begins, and

then periodically, as drug may have negative effects on growth.

! **WARNING** Use topiramate cautiously in patients with impaired hepatic function, or inborn errors of metabolism, or those who are taking valproic acid; these patients may be at higher risk for hyperammonemia, with or without encephalopathy, while taking topiramate. In addition, hypothermia may occur in patients taking valproic acid concomitantly. If present, notify prescriber and expect topiramate or valproic acid therapy to be discontinued.

! **WARNING** Monitor patient for hypersenstivity reactions. If present, notify prescriber, expect drug to be switched to another drug, and provide supportive care, as needed and ordered.

! **WARNING** Monitor patient for break through seizure activity. Anticipate an increase in seizure activity if topiramate therapy for seizures stops abruptly. Take seizure precautions, as appropriate. Expect drug to be withdrawn gradually if time permits.

! **WARNING** Assess patient's skin frequently, as serious skin reactions may occur. If blisters or a rash develops, notify prescriber and expect drug to be discontinued.

! **WARNING** Monitor patient for bleeding events, especially patients who have conditions that increase risk of bleeding, who take drugs that cause thrombocytopenia such as other antiepileptic drugs, or who take drugs that affect platelet function or coagulation, such as anticoagulants, aspirin, NSAIDs, or selective serotonin reuptake inhibitors.

! **WARNING** Monitor patient for mood changes or worsening depression as topiramate can cause suicidal ideation that can begin as early as 1 week after drug therapy begins and can persist for the duration of therapy. If present, notify prescriber and institute suicide precautions.

! **WARNING** Keep in mind that if patient reports ocular pain or decreased visual acuity, notify prescriber immediately; topiramate may cause increased intraocular pressure and secondary angle-closure glaucoma as well as visual field defects. Expect to stop drug immediately.

- Monitor patient for cognitive-related dysfunction, especially patients who are started on a higher initial dose or have a rapid titration rate.
- Assess for signs of renal calculi, especially if patient has a history of this condition. Ensure patient is adequately hydrated to reduce risk of new stone formation.

! **WARNING** Monitor patient for other persistent, serious, or unusual adverse reactions as drug can affect many body systems and has the potential to cause serious to life-threatening adverse reactions such as encephalopathy, hypoglycemia, hypotension, and pancreatitis.

PATIENT TEACHING

! **WARNING** Advise females of childbearing age to use effective contraceptives because drug may cause congenital abnormalities if taken in the first trimester and may cause newborn to be small for gestational age. If patient takes an oral contraceptive, encourage patient to use another form of contraception during therapy because of possible decreased contraceptive effectiveness, especially if taking estrogen only or progestin only contraceptive. Tell patient to notify prescriber immediately if pregnancy occurs. Also, tell patient to alert prescriber if any significant change in menstrual bleeding pattern occurs.

- Instruct patient how to administer form of topiramate prescribed.
- Tell patient to alert prescriber if break through seizure activity occurs. Instruct patient to maintain seizure precautions.

! **WARNING** Caution patient not to stop taking topiramate abruptly because seizures may occur. Instead, patient should expect drug to be withdrawn gradually if it must be discontinued.

- Instruct patient to avoid alcohol use completely within 6 hours before and after taking topiramate.

- Tell patient to maintain adequate fluid intake to minimize the risk of developing kidney stones.

! **WARNING** Alert patient that drug may cause an allergic reaction. If present, tell patient to notify prescriber and, if severe, to seek immediate medical care.

! **WARNING** Alert patient that drug may cause serious skin reactions. If blistering or a rash appears, tell patient to notify prescriber immediately.

! **WARNING** Urge family or caregiver to watch patient closely for evidence of suicidal tendencies, especially when topiramate therapy starts or dosage changes, and to report concerns at once to prescriber.

! **WARNING** Tell patient to alert prescriber and to seek immediate medical care if unexpected or unexplained significant bleeding occurs, including heavy vaginal bleeding.

! **WARNING** Instruct patient to seek immediate medical care for blurred vision, other visual disturbances, or periorbital pain.

! **WARNING** Advise patient to watch for decreased sweating and significantly increased body temperature, especially during hot weather, and to notify prescriber immediately if they occur.

- Urge patient to avoid potentially hazardous activities until drug's CNS effects are known and resolved.
- Alert family or caregiver that drug can have a negative effect on growth and decrease bone mineral density in children. Encourage family or caregiver to discuss any concerns with prescriber.

! **WARNING** Tell patient to be alert for any other persistent, serious, or unusual adverse reactions and to notify prescriber immediately, if present. Urge patient to seek immediate medical care, if severe.

- Instruct mothers wishing to breastfeed to monitor infant for diarrhea and somnolence.

torsemide

Soaanz

Class and Category

Pharmacologic class: Loop diuretic
Therapeutic class: Antihypertensive, diuretic

Indications and Dosages

* *To treat edema in heart failure*

TABLETS

Adults. *Initial:* 10 or 20 mg once daily, adjusted by doubling dose each time to achieve desired effect. *Maximum:* 200 mg daily.

* *To treat edema in chronic renal failure*

TABLETS

Adults. *Initial:* 20 mg once daily adjusted by doubling dose each time to achieve desired effect. *Maximum:* 200 mg daily.

* *As adjunct to treat edema in hepatic cirrhosis with an aldosterone antagonist or a potassium-sparing diuretic*

TABLETS

Adults. *Initial:* 5 or 10 mg once daily, adjusted by doubling dose each time, as needed, to achieve desired effect. *Maximum:* 40 mg daily.

* *To manage hypertension*

TABLETS

Adults. *Initial:* 5 mg once daily, increased to 10 mg daily after 4 to 6 wk, if response is inadequate. *Maximum:* 10 mg daily.

Drug Administration

P.O.

- Administer daily dose in morning to prevent nocturia.

Route	Onset	Peak	Duration
P.O.	1 hr	1–2 hr	6–8 hr

Half-life: 3.5 hr

Mechanism of Action

Blocks active chloride and sodium reabsorption in the ascending loop of Henle by promoting rapid excretion of chloride, sodium, and water. Increases the production of renal prostaglandins, increasing the plasma renin level and renal vasodilation, which causes blood pressure to fall thereby reducing preload and afterload.

T

Contraindications

Anuric patients; hepatic coma; hypersensitivity to torsemide, povidone, or their components

Interactions

DRUGS

ACE inhibitors, angiotensin receptor blockers, antihypertensives: Additive hypotension; increased risk of renal impairment
ACTH, corticosteroids: Possibly increased risk of hypokalemia
aminoglycoside antibiotics, ethacrynic acid: Increased risk of ototoxicity
cholestyramine: Possibly decreased absorption of orally administered torsemide
CYP2C9 inducers, such as rifampin: Decreased plasma concentrations of torsemide, possibly decreasing effectiveness
CYP2C9 inhibitors, such as amiodarone, fluconazole, miconazole, oxandrolone: Increased plasma concentrations of torsemide and possibly increased risk of adverse reactions
CYP2C9 substrates, such as celecoxib or substrates with a narrow therapeutic range, such as phenytoin, warfarin: Possibly decreased effectiveness and safety of these drugs
digoxin: Increased risk of arrhythmias and digitalis toxicity due to hypokalemia or hypomagnesemia
indomethacin: Possibly decreased antihypertensive and diuretic effects of torsemide
lithium: Possibly lithium toxicity
nephrotoxic drugs such as aminoglycosides, cisplatin, NSAIDs: Increased risk of worsening renal function
NSAIDS, salicylates: Increased risk of nephrotoxicity and salicylate toxicity
probenecid, other organic anion drugs: Possibly decreased diuretic effect of torsemide
radiocontrast agents: Increased risk of renal toxicity

Adverse Reactions

CNS: Confusion, dizziness, drowsiness, fatigue, headache, insomnia, lethargy, nervousness, paresthesia, restlessness, thirst, weakness
CV: Chest pain, **ECG abnormalities**, edema, **hypotension**, tachycardia
EENT: Dry mouth, hearing loss, ototoxicity, pharyngitis, rhinitis, tinnitus, visual impairment
ENDO: Hyperglycemia
GI: Abdominal pain, anorexia, constipation, diarrhea, elevated liver enzymes, indigestion, nausea, **pancreatitis**, vomiting
GU: **Azotemia**, elevated blood urea creatinine and nitrogen levels, oliguria, urinary frequency or retention, worsening renal function
HEME: Anemia, **leukopenia**, **thrombocytopenia**
MS: Muscle spasms, myalgia
RESP: Cough
SKIN: Photosensitivity, pruritus, **Stevens-Johnson syndrome**, **toxic epidermal necrolysis**
Other: Elevated uric acid levels, **hypocalcemia**, hypochloremic alkalosis, **hypokalemia**, **hypomagnesemia**, **hyponatremia**, hypovolemia, thiamine (vitamin B1) deficiency

Childbearing Considerations

PREGNANCY

- It is not known if drug can cause fetal harm.
- Use with caution only if benefit to mother outweighs potential risk to fetus.

LACTATION

- It is not known if drug is present in breast milk.
- Mothers should check with prescriber before breastfeeding, as drug may suppress lactation.

Nursing Considerations

! WARNING Monitor patient's serum electrolyte levels and fluid intake and output to detect hypovolemia because dehydration can worsen renal function, causing acute renal failure. Patients at higher risk include patients who are taking renin-angiotensin aldosterone inhibitors or other nephrotoxic drugs or who are salt-depleted. Expect to monitor renal function in patients throughout drug therapy.

! WARNING Monitor patient with hepatic disease who has ascites or cirrhosis because a sudden shift in fluid and electrolyte balance may precipitate hepatic coma. Diuretic therapy can also contribute to a variety of disorders, such as azotemia, hypokalemia, hyponatremia, hypovolemia, or metabolic alkalosis in these patients, which can cause or worsen hepatic encephalopathy. Know that if this occurs, drug should be withheld or discontinued.

! **WARNING** Expect torsemide-induced electrolyte imbalances, such as hypokalemia and hypomagnesemia, to increase the risk of toxicity and fatal arrhythmias in a patient who takes a digitalis glycoside. Hypokalemia also potentiates the neuromuscular blockade effects of nondepolarizing neuromuscular blockers.

- Monitor blood glucose levels with diabetic patients because drug can raise blood glucose levels.

! **WARNING** Monitor patient for other persistent, serious, or unusual adverse reactions during drug therapy as drug may cause many and some could be quite serious.

PATIENT TEACHING

- Instruct patient how to administer torsemide.
- Tell patient to maintain an adequate fluid intake and to be aware that diarrhea, excessive perspiration, or vomiting can lower blood pressure, possibly causing fainting as well as decrease renal function. Advise patient to change position slowly to minimize the effects of orthostatic hypotension. Instruct patient to notify prescriber if excessive fluid loss or fainting occurs.
- Tell patient not to take any over-the-counter NSAIDs without consulting prescriber first.

! **WARNING** Instruct patient to notify prescriber at once about persistent, serious, or unusual adverse reactions that occur.

- Advise diabetic patient to monitor blood glucose level often because drug may raise it.

tralokinumab-ldrm

Adbry

Class and Category

Pharmacologic class: Interleukin-13 Antagonist
Therapeutic class: Monoclonal antibody

Indications and Dosages

∗ *To treat moderate-to-severe atopic dermatitis with or without topical corticosteroids in patients not adequately controlled with topical prescription therapies or when those therapies are not advisable*

SUBCUTANEOUS INJECTION

Adults and adolescents ages 18 and older. *Initial loading dose:* 600 mg (four 150-mg injections using prefilled syringe; two 300 mg injections using autoinjector). *Maintenance:* 300 mg (two 150-mg injections using pre-filled syringe; one 300 mg injection using autoinjector) every other wk and after 16 wk of treatment in which clear or almost clear skin is achieved, dosage frequency increased to every 4 wk.

Children ages 12 to 17. *Initial loading dose:* 300 mg (two 150-mg injections using pre-filled syringe). *Maintenance:* 150 mg using pre-filled syringe every other wk.

Drug Administration

SUBCUTANEOUS

- Pre-filled syringe can be used in both adults and childen ages 12 yr and older. Autoinjector is used only in adults.
- Remove the number of pre-filled syringes or autoinjectors needed for the dose to be administered from the refrigerator and allow to reach room temperature (25°C or 86°F), which will take about 30 min for the 150 mg/ml pre-filled syringes and 45 min for the autoinjector. Do not remove the needle cap while drug is reaching room temperature.
- If drug is not administered immediately, the syringes and autoinjectors may be kept at room temperature for up to 14 days and then discarded if not used.
- Drug solution should be clear to opalescent, colorless to pale yellow. Discard if solution is discolored or cloudy or contains visible particulate matter.
- When administering dose, administer the injections at different injection sites within the abdomen, thigh, or upper arm.
- Do not inject the drug into skin that is bruised, damaged, scarred, or tender.
- To use the pre-filled syringe, inject the drug at the selected site at a 45 degree angle.
- To use the autoinjector, place the needle guard of the autoinjector flat against the

T

patient's skin making sure viewing window is visible. Press the autoinjector down firmly on the injection site and hold in place. A click will be heard indicating injection has started and the yellow plunger will start to move. It will take about 15 sec to inject the full dose. A second click will be heard when the yellow plunger fills the viewing window. Keep pressing for another 5 sec, then remove the autoinjector.

- Do not rub the injection site.
- Rotate the body area used for the injection(s) with each subsequent set of injections.
- If a dose is missed, administer the dose as soon as possible. Then resume dosing at the regular scheduled time.

Route	Onset	Peak	Duration
SubQ	Unknown.	5–8 days	Unknown

Half-life: 3 wk

Mechanism of Action

Binds to human interleukin-13 (IL-13) to inhibit its interaction with selected IL-13 receptors. This action inhibits the release of proinflammatory cytokines, chemokines, and IgE to reduce inflammation found with atopic dermatitis.

Contraindications

Hypersensitivity to tralokinumab-ldrm or its components

Interactions

live vaccines: Possibly increased risk of infection

Adverse Reactions

EENT: Conjunctivitis, keratitis, nasopharyngitis, pharyngitis
HEME: Elevated eosinophil count, eosinophilia
RESP: Upper respiratory infections
OTHER: **Anaphylaxis**, **angioedema**, antibody formation against tralokinumab-ldrm, injection site reactions (erythema, pain, swelling)

Childbearing Considerations

PREGNANCY

- Pregnancy exposure registry: 1-877-311-8972 or https://mothertobaby.org/ongoing-study/adbry-tralokinumab/.
- It is not known if drug can cause fetal harm. However, human IgG antibodies cross the placental barrier with the potential for the drug to be transmitted from the mother to the developing fetus.
- Use with caution only if benefit to mother outweighs potential risk to fetus.

LACTATION

- It is not known if drug is present in breast milk.
- Patient should check with prescriber before breastfeeding.

Nursing Considerations

- Expect patients with preexisting helminth infections to be treated for the infection before tralokinumab-ldrm is begun. Be aware that if patient develops a helminth infection during drug therapy and does not respond to treatment, tralokinumab-ldrm will need to be withheld until the infection is irradicated.
- Ensure that patient is up to date on all immunizations before tralokinumab-ldrm therapy is begun because drug alter patient's immune response.

! WARNING Monitor patient closely for a hypersensitivity reaction, which may become life threatening such as anaphylaxis or angioedema. If present, notify prescriber immediately, expect drug to be discontinued, and provide supportive care, as needed and ordered.

PATIENT TEACHING

- Instruct patient, family member or caregiver how to administer tralokinumab-ldrm as a subcutaneous injection if injection will be administered at home.

! WARNING Alert patient that drug may cause an allergic reaction. If an allergic reaction is present, tell patient to notify prescriber and, if severe, to seek immediate medical care.

- Advise patient to report new onset or worsening eye symptoms to prescriber.
- Tell patient not to receive vaccinations using live vaccines during tralokinumab-ldrm therapy. Also, tell patient to inform prescriber of tralokinumab-ldrm therapy before non-live vaccines are administered.

tramadol hydrochloride

ConZip, Qdolo, Zytram XL (CAN)

Class, Category, and Schedule

Pharmacologic class: Opioid agonist
Therapeutic class: Opioid analgesic
Controlled substance schedule: IV

Indications and Dosages

* *To relieve pain severe enough to require opioid-like treatment and for which alternative treatment options such as nonopioid analgesics or opioid combination products are inadequate or not tolerated*

ORAL SOLUTION, TABLETS

Adults with chronic pain not requiring rapid onset of analgesic effect. *Initial:* 25 mg daily in morning, then titrated every 3 days in 25-mg increments in separate doses to reach 100 mg daily given as 25 mg 4 times daily. Then, if further analgesia is needed, total daily dose increased by 50 mg every 3 days to reach 200 mg daily given as 50 mg 4 times daily. After titration, 50 to 100 mg given, as needed, every 4 to 6 hr. *Maximum:* 400 mg daily.

Adults requiring rapid pain relief. 50 to 100 mg every 4 to 6 hr, as needed. *Maximum:* 400 mg daily.

±**DOSAGE ADJUSTMENT** For patients with creatinine clearance less than 30 ml/min, dosing interval increased to 12 hours with maximum daily dosage not to exceed 200 mg. For patients with severe hepatic dysfunction, dosage reduced to 50 mg every 12 hours. For elderly patients over age 75, total daily dosage reduced to 300 mg/day. For patients already receiving a benzodiazepine or other CNS depressant, initial dose of I.R. forms may be reduced and then titrated more slowly.

E.R. CAPSULES, E.R. TABLETS

Adults not currently treated with I.R. form of tramadol. 100 mg once daily, increased in 100-mg increments once daily every 5 days, as needed. *Maximum:* 300 mg once daily.

Adults maintained on tramadol I.R. form. Dosage calculated using the 24-hr I.R. dosage rounded down to the next lowest 100-mg increment. Dosage then adjusted, as needed. *Maximum:* 300 mg once daily.

Drug Administration

P.O.

- I.R. and E.R. capsules and tablets should be swallowed whole and not chewed, crushed, or opened/broken.
- Use a calibrated device to measure oral solution dosage. Store at room temperature.

Route	Onset	Peak	Duration
P.O.	1 hr	2–3 hr	Unknown
P.O./E.R.	Unknown	4–12 hr	Unknown

Half-life: 6–10 hr

Mechanism of Action

Binds with mu receptors and inhibits the reuptake of norepinephrine and serotonin, which may account for tramadol's analgesic effect.

Contraindications

Acute or severe bronchial asthma in the absence of resuscitative equipment or unmonitored setting; children under the age of 12; hypersensitivity to tramadol, opioids, or their components; known or suspected GI obstruction, including paralytic ileus; postoperative management in children ages 12 to 18 following adenoidectomy and/or tonsillectomy; significant respiratory depression; use within 14 days of MAO inhibitor therapy

Interactions

DRUGS

5-HT$_3$ receptor antagonists, certain muscle relaxants (cyclobenzaprine, metaxalone), drugs that affect the serotonin neurotransmitter system (mirtazapine, trazodone), selective serotonin reuptake inhibitors, serotonin and norepinephrine reuptake inhibitors, tricyclic antidepressants, triptans: Increased risk of serotonin syndrome

anticholinergics: Increased risk of urinary retention and/or severe constipation, which may lead to paralytic ileus

CYP2D6 inhibitors (bupropion, fluoxetine, paroxetine, quinidine): Decreased analgesia or increased tramadol exposure leading to increased risk for serious adverse events, including seizures and serotonin syndrome.

antipsychotics, anxiolytics, benzodiazepines, CNS depressants, general anesthetics, muscle

relaxants, other opioids, sedatives/hypnotics, tranquilizers: Increased risk of severe respiratory depression and possibly death
CYP3A4 inducers, such as carbamazepine, phenytoin, rifampin: Decreased plasma concentration of tramadol and effectiveness with possible onset of withdrawal
CYP3A4 inhibitors, such as azole antifungal agents, macrolide antibiotics, protease inhibitors: Increased plasma concentration of tramadol and risk of adverse reactions, such as seizures and serotonin syndrome and adverse reactions related to opioid toxicity
digoxin: Possible digoxin toxicity
diuretics: Reduced effectiveness of diuretics
mixed agonist/antagonist, partial agonist opioid analgesics: Possible reduced analgesic effect and/or precipitation of withdrawal symptoms
MAO inhibitors, such as linezolid, phenelzine, tranylcypromine: Increased risk of serotonin syndrome, opioid toxicity
muscle relaxants: Enhanced neuromuscular blocking action of skeletal muscle relaxants, increased degree of respiratory depression
warfarin: Possibly altered warfarin effects

ACTIVITIES

alcohol use: Additive CNS depression and respiratory depression that may become severe

Adverse Reactions

CNS: Agitation, anxiety, asthenia, depression, dizziness, emotional lability, euphoria, fatigue, fever, hallucinations, headache, hypertonia, hypoesthesia, insomnia, lethargy, nervousness, paresthesia, restlessness, rigors, **seizures**, **serotonin syndrome**, somnolence, **suicidal ideation**, tremor, vertigo, weakness
CV: Chest pain, orthostatic hypotension, **prolonged QT interval**, **torsades de pointes**, vasodilation
EENT: Blurred vision, dry mouth, nasal or sinus congestion, sore throat, vision changes
ENDO: **Adrenal insufficiency**, **hypoglycemia**, hot flashes
GI: Abdominal pain, anorexia, constipation, diarrhea, indigestion, nausea, vomiting
GU: Androgen deficiency, decreased libido, erectile dysfunction, impotence, infertility, lack of menstruation, urinary frequency, urine retention
MS: Arthralgia; back, limb, or neck pain
RESP: Cough, dyspnea, **respiratory depression (severe)**
SKIN: Diaphoresis, dermatitis, flushing, pruritus, rash
Other: **Anaphylaxis**, flu-like illness, **hyponatremia**, physical and psychological dependence

Childbearing Considerations

PREGNANCY

- Drug may cause fetal harm such as seizures and fetal death.
- Prolonged use of drug during pregnancy can result in neonatal opioid withdrawal syndrome (NOWS), which may be life-threatening if not recognized and treated.
- Avoid prolonged use during pregnancy. Use with caution only if benefit to mother outweighs potential risk to fetus.

LABOR AND DELIVERY

- Drug is not recommended for use in pregnant women immediately before or during labor. Opioids may alter length of time of labor.
- Opioids cross the placental barrier and may produce respiratory depression and psycho-physiologic effects in the neonate as well as seizure activity. Monitor neonate closely.
- An opioid antagonist, such as naloxone, must be available at the time of delivery in the event it is needed to reverse opioid-induced respiratory depression in the neonate.

LACTATION

- Drug is present in breast milk.
- Breastfeeding is not recommended during drug therapy because drug can cause excessive sedation and respiratory depression as well as withdrawal symptoms when drug or breastfeeding is discontinued.

REPRODUCTION

- Chronic use of opioids may reduce fertility in females and males.
- Drug may also produce adverse effects on male reproductive hormones and tissues, according to animal studies.

Nursing Considerations

! **WARNING** Be aware that tramadol shouldn't be given to patients with a history of anaphylactoid reactions to codeine or other opioids. Also, know that tramadol should be avoided in patients with acute abdominal conditions because it may mask signs and symptoms and alter assessment findings of the abdomen. Also, drug should not be given to children.

! **WARNING** Know that excessive use of tramadol may lead to abuse, addiction, misuse, overdose, and possibly death. Monitor patient's intake of drug closely and for evidence of physical dependence. Alert prescriber if patient has a history of dependence on other opioids. Be aware that a Risk Evaluation and Mitigation Strategy (REMS) is required before tramadol can be prescribed.

- Monitor patient for paradoxic increase in pain known as opioid-induced hyperalgesia or an increase in sensitivity to pain known as allodynia, especially when tramadol dosage increases. Do not confuse this with tolerance, which is the need for increasing doses of opioids to maintain an effect. If opioid-induced allodynia or hyperalgesia is suspected, notify prescriber and expect dosage to be decreased or opioid rotation to be prescribed.

! **WARNING** Be aware that elderly patients may have increased sensitivity to tramadol with drug decreasing cardiac, hepatic, or renal function more often. Expect dosage to be started at the low end of the dosing range and titrated slowly. Also monitor the elderly for more frequent signs of CNS and respiratory depression.

! **WARNING** Monitor patient for hyponatremia (confusion, disorientation), especially in females over the age of 65 and within the first week of therapy. Know that decreased serum sodium levels are often less than 120 mmol/L, which could be life-threatening. Confirm with a serum sodium level and, if present, discontinue drug and initiate appropriate treatment such as fluid restriction, as ordered.

! **WARNING** Monitor patient for a hypersensitivity reaction after giving first dose of tramadol, which could become life threatening such as anaphylaxis or angioedema. If present, notify prescriber, expect drug to be discontinued, and provide supportive care, as needed and ordered.

! **WARNING** Monitor patient closely for evidence of suicidal thinking or behavior, especially when therapy starts or dosage changes.

! **WARNING** Monitor patient for respiratory depression that could become life-threatening quickly, especially when drug is initiated, or dosage is increased. If patient develops respiratory depression, expect to give naloxone. Watch for seizures because naloxone may increase this risk.

! **WARNING** Monitor patients closely with conditions accompanied by hypercapnia, hypoxia, or decreased respiratory reserve, such as asthma, chronic obstructive pulmonary disease (COPD), or cor pulmonale. This is because even with usual therapeutic doses, tramadol may decrease respiratory drive while simultaneously increasing airway resistance to the point of apnea. Monitor patient's respiratory status closely, especially during the initiation of therapy or following a dose increase.

! **WARNING** Assess respiratory status often if patient has head injury or increased intracranial pressure because of possible increased carbon dioxide retention and CSF pressure, either of which may cause respiratory depression. Also, be aware that tramadol may constrict pupils, obscuring evidence of intracranial complications.

! **WARNING** Monitor patients with sleep-related breathing disorders because tramadol increases the risk of central sleep apnea in a dose-dependent fashion. If patient has central sleep apnea, know that tramadol dosage may have to be reduced.

! **WARNING** Watch for seizures in patients with epilepsy, a history of seizures, or an increased risk of seizures, such as those with alcohol or drug withdrawal, CNS infection, head injury, or metabolic disorder. Take seizure precautions.

! **WARNING** Monitor patient for hypoglycemia, especially if diabetic. If suspected, obtain a blood glucose level and, if confirmed, treat appropriately. Notify prescriber as tramadol may have to be discontinued.

! **WARNING** Monitor patient for adrenal insufficiency. Although rare, it can be life-threatening. Monitor patient for anorexia, dizziness, fatigue, hypotension, nausea, vomiting, or weakness. Notify prescriber if adrenal insufficiency is suspected and expect diagnostic testing to be done. If confirmed, expect to administer corticosteroids and wean patient off tramadol, if possible.

! **WARNING** Know that chronic maternal use of tramadol during pregnancy can result in neonatal opioid withdrawal syndrome (NOWS), which may be life-threatening if not recognized and treated appropriately. NOWS occurs when a newborn has been exposed to tramadol for a prolonged period while in utero.

! **WARNING** Be aware that tramadol should only be used concomitantly with benzodiazepine therapy in patients for whom other treatment options are inadequate. If prescribed together, expect dosing and duration of tramadol to be limited. Monitor patient closely for signs and symptoms of a decrease in consciousness, including coma, profound sedation, and significant respiratory depression. Notify prescriber immediately and provide emergency supportive care, as needed and ordered, as death may occur.

! **WARNING** Know that many drugs may interact with tramadol to cause serotonin syndrome. Monitor patient closely for signs and symptoms, such as agitation, diaphoresis, diarrhea, fever, hallucinations, labile blood pressure, muscle twitching or stiffness, nausea, shakiness, shivering, tachycardia, trouble with coordination, or vomiting. Notify prescriber at once because serotonin syndrome may be life-threatening. Be prepared to discontinue drug, if possible and ordered, and provide supportive care.

! **WARNING** Be aware that concomitant use of tramadol with CYP2D6 inhibitors may increase risk for opioid toxicity, opioid withdrawal, seizures and serotonin syndrome, opioid toxicity. Also, be aware that concomitant use of tramadol with CYP3A inducers or inhibitors may cause similar adverse reactions.

- Expect to taper tramadol rather than stopping it abruptly to avoid acute withdrawal symptoms, such as anxiety, diarrhea, insomnia, nausea, pain, panic attacks, paresthesias, piloerection, rigors, sweating, tremor, and upper respiratory symptoms.

PATIENT TEACHING

- Instruct patient how to administer form of tramadol prescribed.

! **WARNING** Urge patient to follow prescribed dose limits and dosing intervals to prevent respiratory depression. Warn patient that excessive or prolonged use can lead to abuse, addiction, misuse, overdose, and possibly death. Encourage patient and family or caretaker to have naloxone on hand in the event of an accidental overdose. Instruct family or caregiver on signs and symptoms of an opioid overdose and how to use naloxone. Stress importance of calling 911 immediately if naloxone is administered.

- Caution patient not to stop tramadol abruptly.

! **WARNING** Warn patient not to consume alcohol or take a benzodiazepine without prescriber knowledge, as severe respiratory depression can occur and may lead to death.

! **WARNING** Alert patient that drug can cause an allergic reaction. If present, tell patient to notify prescriber and, if severe, to seek immediate medical care.

! **WARNING** Urge family or caregiver to watch patient closely for evidence of suicidal tendencies, especially when therapy starts or dosage changes, and to report concerns at once to prescriber.

! **WARNING** Instruct patients with diabetes to monitor blood glucose closely because drug can cause hypoglycemia. Review appropriate treatment for hypoglycemia and tell patient to inform prescriber if hypoglycemia occurs frequently.

! **WARNING** Inform patient that seizure activity may occur with tramadol use and to notify prescriber immediately if a seizure occurs.

- Instruct patient to avoid hazardous activities until drug's CNS effects are known and resolved.
- Warn patient that tramadol may cause severe constipation. Advise patient to maintain adequate hydration, increase fiber in diet, and to seek treatment instructions from prescriber if constipation occurs and is not relieved soon after onset.
- Inform patient that long-term use of tramadol may decrease sex hormone levels, causing decreased libido, erectile dysfunction, impotence, infertility, or lack of menstruation. Encourage patient to report any symptoms to prescriber.

! **WARNING** Tell patient to notify prescriber immediately if he develops any other persistent, severe, sudden, or unusual adverse reactions.

! **WARNING** Caution patient to keep tramadol out of the reach of children because even 1 dose could result in a fatal overdose in a child.

- Instruct patient to inform all prescribers of tramadol therapy because of potential drug interactions.
- Urge females of childrearing age to notify prescriber if pregnancy occurs.
- Tell mothers wishing to breastfeed that it is not recommended during drug therapy.
- Instruct patient how to dispose of unused tramadol in accordance with local state guidelines and/or regulations.

trazodone hydrochloride

Class and Category

Pharmacologic class: Triazolopyridine derivative
Therapeutic class: Antidepressant

Indications and Dosages

∗ *To treat major depression*

TABLETS

Adults. 150 mg in divided doses daily, increased by 50 mg/day every 3 to 4 days. *Maximum for outpatients:* 400 mg daily in divided doses. *Maximum for inpatients experiencing more severe depression:* 600 mg daily in divided doses.

Drug Administration

P.O.

- Give drug after a meal or light snack to reduce dizziness.
- Give larger portion of daily dose at bedtime if drowsiness occurs.
- Tablets should be swallowed and not chewed or crushed. Tablet should only be broken along the score lines.

Route	Onset	Peak	Duration
P.O.	Unknown	1–2 hr	Unknown

Half-life: 5–9 hr

Mechanism of Action

Blocks serotonin reuptake along the presynaptic neuronal membrane, causing an antidepressant effect. Exerts also an alpha-adrenergic blocking action to produce a modest histamine blockade, causing a sedative effect. Inhibits the vasopressor response to norepinephrine, which reduces blood pressure.

Contraindications

Hypersensitivity to trazodone or its components, use within 14 days of an MAO inhibitor including intravenous methylene blue and linezolid

Interactions

DRUGS

antibiotics (gatifloxacin), antipsychotics (chlorpromazine, thioridazine, ziprasidone), class IA antiarrhythmics (disopyramide, procainamide, quinidine), class III antiarrhythmics (amiodarone, sotalol): Increased risk of prolonged QT interval and cardiac arrhythmia
anticoagulants, such as clopidogrel, dabigatran, rivaroxaban, warfarin; antiplatelets, such as aspirin: Increased risk of bleeding

barbiturates and other CNS depressants: Enhanced effect of CNS depressants
CYP3A4 inducers (strong), such as carbamazepine, phenytoin, rifampin, St. John's wort: Decreased exposure of trazodone decreasing effectiveness
CYP3A4 inhibitors (strong), such as clarithromycin, indinavir, itraconazole, ketoconazole, and ritonavir: Possibly increased plasma trazodone levels with increased risk of adverse reactions
digoxin, phenytoin: Possibly increased blood levels of these drugs and increased risk of toxicity
MAO inhibitors; other serotonergic drugs, such as buspirone, fentanyl, lithium, serotonin uptake inhibitor antidepressants, St. John's wort, tramadol, tricyclic antidepressants, triptans, tryptophan: Increased serotonin effects

ACTIVITIES

alcohol use: Increased CNS depression, risk of hypotension and respiratory depression

Adverse Reactions

CNS: Abnormal coordination or dreams, agitation, anxiety, aphasia, ataxia, balance disorder, chills, confusion, **CVA**, dizziness, drowsiness, extrapyramidal symptoms, fatigue, hallucinations, headache, insomnia, lightheadedness, memory impairment, migraine, nervousness, paresthesia, paranoid reaction, psychosis, **seizures**, **serotonin syndrome**, somnolence, stupor, **suicidal ideation**, syncope, tardive dyskinesia, tremor, vertigo, weakness
CV: **Arrhythmias**, **congestive heart failure**, edema, **hypotension**, orthostatic hypotension, palpitations, **prolonged QT interval**, vasodilation
EENT: Angle-closure glaucoma, blurred vision, diplopia, dry mouth
ENDO: Inappropriate ADH syndrome
GI: Abdominal pain, cholestasis, constipation, diarrhea, elevated bilirubin or liver enzymes, indigestion, jaundice, nausea, vomiting
GU: Anorgasmia; ejaculation disorders; decreased libido; priapism; urinary incontinence, retention, or urgency
HEME: **Hemolytic anemia**, leukocytosis
MS: Back pain, myalgia
RESP: **Apnea**, dyspnea
SKIN: Alopecia, hirsutism, night sweats, pruritus, psoriasis, rash, urticaria
Other: **Hyponatremia**

Childbearing Considerations

PREGNANCY

- Pregnancy exposure registry: 1-844-405-6185 or https:/womensmentalhealth.org/clinical-and-research-programs/pregnancyregistry/antidepressants/.
- It is not known if drug can cause fetal harm.
- Use with caution only if benefit to mother outweighs potential risk to fetus.

LACTATION

- Drug may be present in breast milk.
- Mothers should check with prescriber before breastfeeding.

Nursing Considerations

! **WARNING** Use trazodone cautiously in patients with cardiac disease because drug can cause arrhythmias.

- Expect most patients who respond to trazodone to do so by the end of the second week of therapy.

! **WARNING** Monitor patient's vital signs for significant changes such as hypotension, irregular pulse, and decreased to absent respirations. Notify prescriber immediately, if present, and be prepared to provide emergency intervention, as needed and ordered.

! **WARNING** Monitor patient for hypersensitivity reactions such as pruritis, rash, and urticaria. If present, notify prescriber, expect drug to be discontinued, and provide supportive care, as needed and ordered.

! **WARNING** Monitor patient's serum sodium level and patient for signs and symptoms of hyponatremia. Also, monitor patient's CBC and patient for evidence of hemolytic anemia.

! **WARNING** Closely monitor depressed patients for suicidal thoughts and tendencies. Notify prescriber if they occur and take suicide precautions according to facility policy.

! **WARNING** Be aware that trazodone therapy may increase the risk of priapism.

! **WARNING** Monitor patient closely for serotonin syndrome exhibited by agitation, coma, diarrhea, hallucinations, hyperreflexia, hyperthermia, incoordination, labile blood pressure, nausea, tachycardia, and vomiting. Notify prescriber immediately because serotonin syndrome may be life-threatening; provide supportive care.

- Be aware that adverse CNS reactions usually improve after patient completes a few weeks of therapy.

! **WARNING** Monitor patient for other persistent, serious, or unusual adverse reactions.

PATIENT TEACHING

- Advise patient that drug may cause mild pupillary dilation, which may lead to an episode of acute angle-closure glaucoma. Encourage patient to have an eye exam before starting therapy to see if he is at risk.
- Instruct patient how to administer trazodone.
- Urge patient to avoid taking trazodone on an empty stomach because doing so may increase the risk of dizziness or lightheadedness.
- Advise patient not to fast during trazodone therapy because of possible adverse CNS reactions.
- Caution patient not to take aspirin or NSAIDs without first discussing use with the prescriber.
- Instruct patient not to stop trazodone therapy abruptly.

! **WARNING** Alert patient drug may cause an allergic reaction. Tell patient to notify prescriber immediately, if present, and to seek immediate medical care, if severe.

! **WARNING** Inform patient and family or caregiver that drug can adversely affect mood to the point of causing suicidal thoughts. Tell family or caregiver to notify prescriber immediately and to institute suicidal precautions.

! **WARNING** Instruct male patient to notify prescriber immediately if an erection is painful or lasts longer than 4 hours.

- Caution patient to avoid potentially hazardous activities during therapy until nervous system effects are known and resolved.

! **WARNING** Instruct patient to notify prescriber if other persistent, serious, or unusual adverse reactions occur.

triamcinolone

triamcinolone acetonide

Kenalog-10, Kenalog-40, Kenalog-80, Nasacort Allergy 24 Hour, Zilretta

Class and Category

Pharmacologic class: Glucocorticoid
Therapeutic class: Corticosteroid

Indications and Dosages

✱ To treat a multitude of disorders exhibiting severe inflammation or need for immunosuppression

I.M. INJECTION (KENALOG-40, KENALOG-80)

Adults. 20 to 100 mg daily depending on specific disease entity being treated. *Suggested initial dosage:* 60 mg daily, increased or decreased according to response and duration of relief. *Usual:* 40 to 80 mg, but lower or higher doses may be needed. Dosage adjusted, as needed.
Children. *Initial:* 0.11 to 1.6 mg/kg daily in 3 or 4 divided doses. Dosage adjusted, as needed.

✱ To treat hay fever or pollen asthma in patients not responding to pollen administration and other conventional therapy

I.M. INJECTION (KENALOG-40, KENALOG-80)

Adults. 40 to 100 mg as a single dose for the pollen season.

✱ To treat acute exacerbations of multiple sclerosis

T

I.M. INJECTION (KENALOG-40, KENALOG-80)

Adults. 160 mg for 1 wk, followed by 64 mg every other day for 1 month.

✱ *To relieve inflammation caused by acute gouty arthritis, acute nonspecific tenosynovitis, acute or subacute bursitis, epicondylitis, rheumatoid arthritis, and synovitis*

INTRA-ARTICULAR INJECTION (KENALOG-10, KENALOG-40)

Adults. 2.5 to 5 mg for smaller joints and 5 to 15 mg for larger joints, as needed; dosage increased up to 10 mg for smaller joints; up to 40 mg for larger joints, as needed (Kenalog-40).

✱ *To relieve osteoarthritis pain of the knee*

E.R. INTRA-ARTICULAR INJECTION (ZILRETTA)

Adults. 32 mg injected as a single dose in the knee.

✱ *To relieve symptoms of perennial and seasonal allergic rhinitis*

NASAL SPRAY (NASACORT ALLERGY 24 HOUR)

Adults and children ages 12 and older. *Initial:* 220 mcg (2 sprays of 55 mcg in each nostril) once daily until symptoms improve. *Maintenance:* 110 mcg (1 spray of 55 mcg in each nostril) once a day.

Children ages 6 to 12. *Initial:* 110 mcg (1 spray of 55 mcg in each nostril) once a day, increased to 220 mcg (2 sprays of 55 mcg in each nostril) once a day, as needed, with dosage reduced when symptoms improve. *Maintenance:* 110 mcg (1 spray of 55 mcg in each nostril) daily. *Maximum:* 220 mcg or 4 sprays of 55 mcg daily.

Children ages 2 to 6. 110 mcg (1 spray of 55 mcg in each nostril) daily.

Drug Administration

I.M.

- Shake vial before withdrawing to ensure a uniform suspension.
- Inspect suspension for clumping or granular appearance. If present, do not use.
- Inject immediately after withdrawing from vial and inject deeply into the gluteal muscle.
- A longer needle length may be required in obese patients.
- Rotate sites.

INTRA-ARTICULAR

Kenalog

- Shake vial before withdrawing to ensure a uniform suspension.
- Inspect suspension for clumping or granular appearance. If present, do not use.
- Prescriber should inject immediately after drug is withdrawn from vial.

Zilretta

- Drug is supplied as a single-dose kit.
- Use only diluent supplied in the kit and follow manufacturer's guidelines for preparation.
- Once diluted, expect prescriber to inject drug immediately to avoid settling of the suspension, or store drug in vial for up to 4 hr at room temperature. Gently swirl vial to resuspend suspension prior to withdrawing drug from vial.
- Do not interchange drug with other formulations of injectable triamcinolone acetonide.

NASAL

- Shake container well before each use.
- Prime container by pressing and releasing spray nozzle until a fine mist is produced before first use. If drug not used for 2 wk or more, reprime.
- Have patient gently blow nose before administration.
- Insert nozzle into nostril, pointing away from the septum. Hold other nostril closed and have patient sniff gently while spraying.
- Do not have patient blow nose for at least 15 min after administration.

Route	Onset	Peak	Duration
I.M.	24–48 hr	Unknown	30–40 days
Intra-articular	> 12 hr	7 hr	28–42 days
Nasal	Unknown	1.5 hr	Unknown

Half-life: 88 min

Mechanism of Action

Triamcinolone:

- decreases peribronchial edema and mucus secretion by inhibiting the binding of allergens to immunoglobulin E antibodies on the surface of mast cells, thereby inactivating the release of chemotactic substances.
- decreases inflammation by interfering with leukocyte adhesion to capillary walls.

- inhibits the release of leukocytic acid hydrolases, preventing macrophage accumulation at the infection site.
- inhibits histamine and kinin release, preventing the formation of scar tissue.

Contraindications

Hypersensitivity to triamcinolone or its components, idiopathic thrombocytopenic purpura (I.M. injection)

Interactions

DRUGS

aminoglutethimide: Possible loss of corticosteroid-induced adrenal suppression
amphotericin B, potassium-depleting agents, such as diuretics: Increased risk of hypokalemia
aspirin, NSAIDs: Increased risk of gastrointestinal adverse effects
cholestyramine: Possible increased clearance of corticosteroids
cholinesterase inhibitors: Increased risk of severe muscle weakness in patients with myasthenia gravis
cyclosporine: Possible additive effects of both drugs' activity; increased risk of seizures
CYP3A4 inhibitors, such as atazanavir, clarithromycin, cobicistat-containing products, indinavir, itraconazole, ketoconazole, nefazodone, nelfinavir, ritonavir, saquinavir, telithromycin: Decreased triamcinolone clearance, increased risk of adverse effects
digitalis glycosides: Increased risk of arrhythmias and digitalis toxicity
estrogens, including oral contraceptives: Increased triamcinolone effects
hepatic enzyme inducers, such as barbiturates, carbamazepine, phenytoin, insulin, oral antidiabetic drugs: Increased blood glucose level
isoniazid: Possible decreased concentrations of isoniazid and its effectiveness
macrolide antibiotics: Significant decrease in corticosteroid clearance
toxoids, vaccines: Decreased response to toxoids and vaccines
warfarin: Possible inhibition of response to warfarin

Adverse Reactions

CNS: Depression, dizziness, emotional lability, exacerbated psychosis, fatigue, headache, **increased intracranial pressure with papilledema (pseudotumor cerebri)**, insomnia, malaise, neuritis, neuropathy, paresthesia, personality changes, psychiatric disorders, restlessness, **seizures**, vertigo
CV: Edema, **heart failure**, hypertension
EENT: Altered sense of smell or taste, cataracts, dry mouth, epistaxis (nasal form), glaucoma, hoarseness, nasal congestion, nasal irritation (nasal form), nasal septal perforation (nasal form), oropharyngeal candidiasis, pharyngitis, posterior subcapsular cataracts, rhinorrhea, secondary ocular infection, sinusitis, sneezing
ENDO: **Adrenal insufficiency**, cushing's syndrome, diabetes mellitus, growth retardation (children)
GI: Abdominal pain, constipation, diarrhea, dyspepsia, esophageal ulceration, gastritis, nausea, vomiting
GU: Altered motility and number of spermatozoa, cystitis, postmenopausal **vaginal hemorrhage**, renal disease, UTI, vaginitis
MS: Bone mineral density loss, bursitis, muscle wasting or weakness, myalgia, osteoporosis, tenosynovitis
RESP: **Asthma**, bronchitis, chest congestion, dyspnea, increased cough
SKIN: Ecchymosis, petechiae (parenteral form), photosensitivity, pruritus, rash, striae, urticaria
Other: **Anaphylaxis**; **angioedema**; flu-like symptoms; herpes infection; hiccups; immunosuppression, impaired wound healing; infections such as bacterial, fungal, helminthic, protozoan, and viral; injection-site atrophy, induration, pain, soreness, and sterile abscess; moon face; weight gain

Childbearing Considerations

PREGNANCY

- It is not known if drug can cause fetal harm.
- Use with caution only if benefit to mother outweighs potential risk to fetus.
- Infants born to mothers receiving drug during pregnancy should be monitored for hypoadrenalism.

LACTATION

- Drug is present in breast milk.
- Mothers should check with prescriber before breastfeeding because drug could interfere with endogenous corticosteroid production, suppress growth, or cause other adverse reactions.

Nursing Considerations

! **WARNING** Be aware that high doses of corticosteroids, such as triamcinolone aren't recommended for patients with cranial trauma who don't require a corticosteroid for another condition because they increase risk of death.

! **WARNING** Know that triamcinolone should be administered with extreme caution, if at all, in patients who have active or quiescent tuberculosis (TB) infection of the respiratory tract, ocular herpes simplex, systemic parasitic or viral infection, or untreated bacterial or fungal infection because drug can make these infections worse and at times fatal. Know that rate of infectious complications increases with increasing corticosteroid dosages such as triamcinolone. Be aware that triamcinolone may reactivate TB in patients who have a history of it. Assess patient for signs and symptoms of infection during drug therapy because steroid therapy such as triamcinolone increases risk of susceptibility to infections, especially with higher dosages.

! **WARNING** Use cautiously in patients with active or latent peptic ulcer, diverticulitis, fresh intestinal anastomoses, and nonspecific ulcerative colitis; there is increased risk of a perforation for these patients. Be aware that signs of peritoneal irritation following GI perforation in patients receiving steroid therapy may be minimal or absent.

- Monitor patient with cirrhosis carefully for an enhanced drug effect because increased metabolism of steroids may occur in the presence of cirrhosis.

! **WARNING** Monitor patients taking high doses, which may result in toxicity evidenced by life-threatening hypotension and metabolic acidosis.

- Adjust triamcinolone dosage, as ordered, in patients with changes in thyroid status because metabolic clearance of corticosteroids is decreased in hypothyroid patients and increased in hyperthyroid patients.

! **WARNING** Monitor patient for a hypersensitivity reaction, which could become life-threatening, such as anaphylaxis or angioedema. Although rare, triamcinolone has caused anaphylaxis that ended in death. If present, notify prescriber immediately, expect to discontinue triamcinolone therapy, and provide supportive care, as needed and ordered.

! **WARNING** Know that patients on corticosteroid therapy require an increased dosage of rapidly acting corticosteroids when unusual stress is anticipated, during the stressful event, and for a period after the stressful situation. Assess patient for signs and symptoms of adrenal insufficiency (fatigue, hypotension, lassitude, nausea, vomiting, and weakness) during times of stress, such as infection, surgery, or trauma. Notify prescriber immediately if you detect these signs and symptoms because adrenal insufficiency may be life-threatening. Drug-induced secondary adrenocortical insufficiency may be minimized by gradual reduction of dosage.

- Be aware that, although rare, bone mineral density loss and osteoporosis may occur, which may increase risk of fractures, especially in patients on prolonged triamcinolone therapy.

PATIENT TEACHING

- Instruct patient how to administer nasal spray, if prescribed. Otherwise tell patient drug will be administered by a health care professional either as an intramuscular injection or injected directly into the joint, depending on condition being treated.
- Advise patient to follow dosage recommendations when using the nasal spray over-the-counter preparation.
- Inform patient that maximum benefit of triamcinolone therapy may not occur for up to 2 weeks.

! **WARNING** Alert patient that drug may cause an allergic reaction. Advise patient to notify prescriber if present and if serious to seek immediate medical care.

! **WARNING** Caution patient to avoid exposure to people who have chickenpox or measles, as well as other contagious infections, throughout triamcinolone therapy and for 12 months afterward because triamcinolone induced immunosuppression can make any infection worse.

! **WARNING** Instruct patient to notify prescriber if unusual stress is anticipated or occurs as adrenal insufficiency (fatigue, hypotension, lassitude, nausea, vomiting, and weakness) may occur during times of stress, such as infection, surgery, or trauma. Tell patient to notify prescriber immediately if a stressful situation occurs.

- Advise patient to have periodic eye examinations during long-term therapy because triamcinolone can cause glaucoma or ocular nerve damage.

! **WARNING** Tell patient to notify prescriber if other persistent, severe, or unusual adverse reactions occur during triamcinolone therapy.

triazolam

Halcion

Class, Category, and Schedule

Pharmacologic class: Benzodiazepine
Therapeutic class: Sedative-hypnotic
Controlled substance schedule: IV

Indications and Dosages

✶ *To provide short-term management (usually 7 to 10 days) for insomnia*

TABLETS

Adults. 0.25 mg once nightly at bedtime. *Maximum:* 0.5 mg once nightly at bedtime (for patients with inadequate response to usual dose).

± **DOSAGE ADJUSTMENT** For elderly or debilitated patients or patients with low body weight, initial dosage not to exceed 0.125 mg and maximum dosage limited to 0.25 mg daily.

Drug Administration

P.O.

- Administer at bedtime.
- Do not administer with grapefruit juice.

Route	Onset	Peak	Duration
P.O.	15–30 min	0.5–2 hr	6–7 hr

Half-life: 1.5–5.5 hr

Mechanism of Action

Potentiates effects of the inhibitory neurotransmitter gamma-aminobutyric acid, which increases inhibition of the ascending reticular activating system and produces varying levels of CNS depression, including anticonvulsant activity, coma, hypnosis, sedation, and skeletal muscle relaxation.

Contraindications

Concurrent therapy with strong CYP3A inhibitors (itraconazole, ketoconazole, lopinavir, nefazodone, ritonavir); hypersensitivity to triazolam, other benzodiazepines, or their components

Interactions

DRUGS

CNS depressants, other benzodiazepines including anticonvulsants, antihistamines, psychotropic drugs: Additive depressant effects that could become severe, especially respiratory depression and severe sedation
CYP3A inducers: Decreased plasma concentration of triazolam significantly decreasing effectiveness
CYP3A inhibitors, such as cimetidine, clarithromycin, erythromycin, indinavir, isoniazid, itraconazole, ketoconazole, lopinavir, nefazodone, nelfinavir, oral contraceptives, saquinavir: Increased triazolam concentrations, increased risk of adverse reactions
opioids: Increased risk of respiratory depression or significant worsening of opioid-related respiratory depression

ACTIVITIES

alcohol use: Increased sedation, respiratory depression that could become severe

FOODS

grapefruit juice: Increased blood triazolam level and adverse reactions

Adverse Reactions

CNS: Abnormal behavior, aggression, agitation, anterograde amnesia, altered state of consciousness, anxiety, ataxia, complex

T

behaviors (such as sleep driving), confusion, coordination disorders, delusion, depression, dizziness, drowsiness, dystonia, euphoria, fatigue, grogginess, hallucination, headache, insomnia, irritability, lightheadedness, mania, memory impairment, nervousness, nightmares, restlessness, sedation, somnambulism, somnolence, syncope, talkativeness, tremor, vertigo
CV: Chest pain, tachycardia
EENT: Blepharitis, glossitis, stomatitis, taste disturbance, **throat tightness**, tongue discomfort, visual disturbances
GI: Abdominal distress, anorexia, constipation, jaundice, nausea, vomiting
GU: Bladder disorders, libido disorder, menstruation irregularity, urinary incontinence or retention
MS: Aching limbs; backache; dysarthria; muscle cramps, pain, spasticity
RESP: Dyspnea
SKIN: Pruritis
Other: **Anaphylaxis**, **angioedema**, paradoxical drug reaction, physical and psychological dependence, protracted withdrawal syndrome

Childbearing Considerations

PREGNANCY

- Pregnancy exposure registry: 1-866-961-2388 or https://womensmentalhealth.org/pregnancyregistry/.
- Drug may cause fetal harm if given during the later stages of pregnancy, such as feeding problems, respiratory depression, sedation, and withdrawal at birth.
- Use with caution only if benefit to mother outweighs potential risk to fetus.

LACTATION

- It is not known if drug is present in breast milk.
- Breastfeeding is not recommended during treatment and for 28 hr after last dose.
- If breastfeeding takes place during drug therapy, monitor infant for feeding problems, respiratory depression, sedation, and withdrawal symptoms (when drug therapy is stopped).

Nursing Considerations

! **WARNING** Evaluate patient's risk for abuse, addiction, and misuse before administering drug for the first time. Notify prescriber of any concerns. Assess patient for signs of physical and psychological dependence during therapy and notify prescriber if any occur.

- Use drug cautiously in patients with acute intermittent porphyria, myasthenia gravis, and severe renal impairment because it may aggravate these conditions.
- Use drug cautiously in patients with advanced Parkinson's disease because it may worsen cognition, coordination, and psychosis.

! **WARNING** Monitor patient closely for a hypersensitivity reaction, which could become life-threatening, such as anaphylaxis or angioedema. If present, notify prescriber, expect drug to be switched to a different drug, and provide supportive care, as needed and ordered.

! **WARNING** Monitor patient's arterial blood gas (ABG) results and respiratory depth and rate, as appropriate, because drug may worsen ventilatory failure in patient with pulmonary disease, such as respiratory depression, severe COPD, or sleep apnea.

- Take safety precautions for elderly patients because triazolam may impair cognitive and motor function and increase the risk for falls.

! **WARNING** Be aware that opioids should only be used concomitantly with benzodiazepine therapy, such as triazolam in patients for whom other treatment options are inadequate. If prescribed together, expect dosing and duration of the opioid to be limited. Monitor patient closely for signs and symptoms of a decrease in consciousness, including coma, profound sedation, and significant respiratory depression. Notify prescriber immediately and provide emergency supportive care, as needed and ordered because death may occur if not recognized and treated as an emergency.

! **WARNING** Be aware that triazolam shouldn't be discontinued abruptly, even with usual course of therapy of 7 to 10 days. Doing so can cause withdrawal symptoms that could be life-threatening. Monitor patient for abdominal cramps, confusion, depression, diaphoresis, hyperacusis, insomnia, irritability, nausea, nervousness, paresthesia, perceptual disturbances, photophobia, tachycardia, tremor, and vomiting and alert prescriber immediately, if present.

PATIENT TEACHING

- Instruct patient how to administer triazolam.

! **WARNING** Warn patient to take triazolam exactly as prescribed because drug can cause physical and psychological dependency.

- Advise patient to avoid grapefruit juice, as it may increase triazolam levels and increase risk of adverse reactions.
- Tell patient not to stop taking it abruptly because of the risk of withdrawal symptoms. Alert patient that a protracted withdrawal syndrome lasting weeks to more than 12 months may occur in some patients if drug is abruptly stopped.

! **WARNING** Urge patient to avoid alcohol consumption and opioid use because these increase drug's sedative effects, including respiratory depression which can become severe.

! **WARNING** Alert patient that drug may cause an allergic reaction. If an allergic reaction occurs, tell patient to notify prescriber and, if serious, to seek immediate medical care.

- Advise patient and family or caregiver that drug may cause abnormal behaviors during sleep, such as driving a car, eating, having sex, or talking on the phone without any recall of the event. If any such behavior occurs or patient sees evidence of such behavior upon awakening, the prescriber should be notified.
- Caution patient about possible drowsiness during therapy and to avoid performing hazardous activities, if present, until resolved. Also, tell patient to take fall precautions.
- Advise patient to notify prescriber about excessive drowsiness, third-semester pregnancy, and nausea.
- Instruct patient to inform all prescribers of triazolam use, especially when pain medication may be prescribed.
- Inform mothers breastfeeding is not recommended during treatment and for 28 hr after last dose. However, if breastfeeding takes place during drug therapy, monitor infant for feeding problems, respiratory depression, sedation, and withdrawal symptoms (when drug therapy is stopped).

trospium chloride

Trosec (CAN)

Class and Category

Pharmacologic class: Antimuscarinic
Therapeutic class: Bladder antispasmodic

Indications and Dosages

∗ *To treat overactive bladder with symptoms of urge or mixed urinary frequency, incontinence, or urgency*

TABLETS

Adults. 20 mg twice daily on an empty stomach at least 1 hr before meals.

± **DOSAGE ADJUSTMENT** For patients with severe renal insufficiency (creatinine clearance less than 30 ml/min), dosage reduced to 20 mg and administered at bedtime. For patients ages 75 an older, dosage reduced to 20 mg once daily.

Drug Administration

P.O.

- Administer with water on an empty stomach 1 hr before meals.

Route	Onset	Peak	Duration
P.O.	Unknown	5–6 hr	Unknown

Half-life: 20–35 hr

Mechanism of Action

Antagonizes the effect of acetylcholine on muscarinic receptors in the bladder; it's parasympatholytic action reduces the tonus of smooth muscle in the bladder. These actions increase maximum cystometric bladder capacity and volume with the first detrusor contraction, which relieves the sensation of frequency and urgency and enhances bladder control.

Contraindications

Gastric retention, hypersensitivity to trospium or its components, uncontrolled angle-closure glaucoma, urine retention

Interactions

DRUGS

anticholinergics: Increased frequency or severity of adverse effects
metformin: Decreased systemic exposure of trospium
morphine, pancuronium, procainamide, tenofovir, vancomycin: Possibly increased plasma concentration of all these drugs as well as trospium
orally administered drugs: Possibly altered absorption of some of these drugs

Adverse Reactions

CNS: Confusion, delirium, dizziness, drowsiness, fatigue, fever, hallucinations, headache, insomnia, lightheadedness, syncope
CV: Chest pain, **hypertensive crisis**, palpitations, tachycardia
EENT: Blurred vision; dry eyes, mouth, or throat; visual abnormalities
GI: Abdominal distention or pain, constipation, flatulence, gastritis, indigestion, vomiting
GU: Urine retention
MS: Rhabdomyolysis
SKIN: Decreased sweating, dry skin, flushing, rash, **Stevens-Johnson syndrome**
Other: Anaphylaxis, angioedema

Childbearing Considerations

PREGNANCY

- It is not known if drug can cause fetal harm.
- Use with caution only if benefit to mother outweighs potential risk to fetus.

LACTATION

- It is not known if drug is present in breast milk.
- Mothers should check with prescriber before breastfeeding.

Nursing Considerations

- Use trospium cautiously in patients with intestinal atony, myasthenia gravis, or ulcerative colitis because drug may decrease GI motility; patients with significant bladder outflow obstruction because drug may cause urine retention; patients with hepatic impairment because drug's effects on the liver are unknown; and patients with renal impairment because drug excretion may be impaired.

! **WARNING** Monitor patient for hypersensitivity reactions, which may become life-threatening, such as anaphylaxis or angioedema. Notify prescriber immediately, if present, expect drug to be discontinued, and provide supportive care, as needed and ordered.

! **WARNING** Monitor patient's blood pressure closely because drug can induce a hypertensive crisis. Alert prescriber immediately if blood pressure suddenly rises or is persistently above normal.

! **WARNING** Monitor patient for intense muscle aching or swelling, muscle stiffness or weakness or feeling utterly exhausted as drug can cause life threatening rhabdomyolysis.

- Monitor elderly patients carefully, especially those ages 75 or older, for adverse reactions because elderly patients have an increased risk of trospium-induced adverse reactions.
- Monitor patient for anticholinergic CNS adverse effects, such as confusion, dizziness, hallucinations, and somnolence. If present, notify prescriber and expect a dose reduction or drug to be discontinued.

PATIENT TEACHING

- Instruct patient how to administer trospium.

! **WARNING** Alert patient that drug may cause an allergic reaction. If an allergic reaction occurs, tell patient to notify prescriber and, if severe, to seek immediate medical care.

! **WARNING** Stress importance of informing prescriber if blood pressure is persistently above normal or patient suddenly does not feel well, has intense headache, or develops visual changes.

! **WARNING** Tell patient to inform prescriber immediately if muscle signs and symptoms occur such as achiness, stiffness, swelling or weakness in addition to feeling exhausted.

! WARNING Caution patient to avoid performing activities in a warm or hot environment because sweating may be delayed, which could cause a sudden increase in body temperature and heatstroke.

- Advise patient to avoid hazardous activities until drug's CNS effects are known and resolved.
- Advise patient, family, or caregiver to notify prescriber if patient develops confusion, dizziness, hallucinations, or somnolence, as dosage may have to be altered or drug discontinued.

U V W

ublituximab-xiiy

Briumvi

Class and Category

Pharmacologic class: CD20-directed cytolytic antibody
Therapeutic class: Anti-multiple sclerotic

Indications and Dosages

∗ *To treat relapsing forms of multiple sclerosis (MS), to include active secondary progressive disease, clinically isolated syndrome, and relapsing-remitting disease*

I.V. INFUSION

Adults. *Initial:* 150 mg followed by 450 mg 2 wk later. *Maintenance:* 450 mg given 24 wk after first infusion and every 24 wk thereafter.

Drug Administration

IV

- Ensure that females of childbearing age have a negative pregnancy test prior to administering every infusion.
- Expect to premedicate patient with methylprednisolone (or equivalent) 100 mg about 30 min before each infusion to reduce frequency and severity of infusion reactions. Expect also to premedicate patient with an antihistamine given either orally or intravenously about 30 to 60 min before each infusion to help further reduce adverse reactions. Additionally, an antipyretic such as acetaminophen may be prescribed prior to each infusion.
- Inspect drug solution prior to dilution. Solution should be clear to opalescent, colorless to slightly yellow. If solution is discolored or particulate matter is observed, discard vial and obtain a new one.
- Dilute drug in 250 ml of 0.9% Sodium Chloride Injection solution prior to administration by first removing 6 ml for first dose and 18 ml for second and subsequent doses from infusion bag prior to adding drug. Gently invert infusion bag to mix diluted solution. Do not shake. Do not use any other solution to dilute drug.
- Infuse through a dedicated line immediately after preparation. If unable to do so, diluted solution may be refrigerated for up to 24 hr. Never freeze. If the diluted solution was refrigerated, allow solution to come to room temperature prior to administration, which may take about 2 hr. The diluted solution can be stored for another 8 hr at room temperature accounting for both the equilibration time and infusion time.
- Administer diluted solution through a dedicated line.
- Infuse first infusion over 4 hr as follows: 10 ml/hr for first 30 min, increased to 20 ml/hr over next 30 min, then increased to 35 ml/hr for the next hr. Finally, infusion rate increased to 100 ml/hr for remaining 2 hr. Infuse second infusion given 2 wk later and subsequent infusions given every 24 wk after first infusion over 1 hr as follows: 100 ml/hr for 30 min then increased to 400 ml/hr for the remaining 30 min.
- Monitor patient for at least 1 hr after each of the first 2 infusions (and subsequent infusions, if necessary) for hypersensitivity and infusion reactions. Stop infusion for life-threatening hypersensitivity reactions and expect drug to be discontinued.
- For severe life-threatening infusion reactions, interrupt infusion immediately, notify prescriber, and expect to administer appropriate supportive care, as needed and ordered. Expect infusion to be restarted after all infusion related adverse reactions have resolved, restarting infusion at half the infusion rate at the time of the onset of reactions. If tolerated, rate may be increased to normal infusion rate for remainder of infusion.
- Reduce infusion rate for mild to moderate infusion related reactions to half the rate at the onset of the reaction(s) and maintain the reduced rate for at least 30 min. If tolerated, increase rate to normal infusion rate for the remainder of infusion.
- Expect a delayed or missed dose to be administered as soon as possible. Drug should not be held until the next scheduled infusion. Know that the infusion schedule will then be reset 24 wk after the missed infusion is administered. Ensure that infusions are separated by at least 5 mo.

- *Incompatibilities:* None listed by manufacturer

Route	Onset	Peak	Duration
I.V.	Unknown	Unknown	Unknown

Half-life: 22 days

Mechanism of Action

Unknown mechanism of action but it is thought to involve binding to CD20, a cell surface antigen present on pre-B and mature B lymphocytes. Binding results in cell lysis through antibody-dependent cellular cytolysis and complement-mediated cytolysis.

Contraindications

Active hepatitis B virus infection, history of life-threatening infusion reactions, hypersensitivity to ublituximab-xiiy or its components

Interactions

DRUGS

immunosuppressive drugs such as corticosteroids: Increased risk of infection
live-attenuated or live vaccines: Increased risk of adverse effects

Adverse Reactions

CNS: Fatigue, insomnia, **progressive multifocal leukoencephalopathy (PML)**
GI: **Hepatitis B virus (HBV) reactivation**
GU: UTI
HEME: Decreased neutrophil level
MS: Extremity pain
RESP: Respiratory infections
Other: **Hypersensitivity reactions**, immunoglobulin reduction, infections (bacterial, fungal, new or reactivated viral), infusion reactions (chills, headache, flu-like symptoms, pyrexia)

Childbearing Considerations

PREGNANCY

- Pregnancy exposure registry: 1-877-411-4546 or www.briumvipregnancyregistry.com.
- It is unknown if drug causes fetal harm, but animal studies suggest that fetal harm can occur due to fetal B-cell lymphopenia and reduced antibody response.
- Females of childbearing age require a negative pregnancy test prior to each infusion.
- Use with caution only if benefit to mother outweighs potential risk to fetus.

LACTATION

- It is not known if drug is present in breast milk.
- Mothers should check with prescriber before breastfeeding.

REPRODUCTION

- Females of childbearing age should use effective contraception during drug therapy and for 6 mo after drug is discontinued.

Nursing Considerations

- Ensure that all immunizations, according to immunization guidelines, have been administered to patient at least 4 weeks prior to starting ublituximab-xiiy for live or live-attenuated vaccines, and whenever possible, at least 2 weeks before for inactivated vaccines.

! **WARNING** Ensure that patient has a negative pregnancy test before each dose of ublituximab-xiiy is administered.

! **WARNING** Determine that screenings for HBV and quantitative serum immunoglobulins have been done before first dose is given. Therapy with ublituximab-xiiy is contraindicated in the presence of HBV. Therapy may have to be withheld in patients with low serum immunoglobulins until levels are higher.

! **WARNING** Expect to delay initiation of therapy if patient has an active infection until infection is resolved. Be aware patient is at risk for infections, including serious bacterial, fungal, and new or reactivated viral infections during therapy. Some infections may become life-threatening. Monitor patient for infections and institute infection control measures. Notify prescriber if an infection is suspected.

! **WARNING** Monitor patient for a hypersensitivity reaction. If present, notify prescriber, expect drug to be discontinued, and provide supportive care, as needed and ordered.

! **WARNING** Be aware that progressive multifocal leukoencephalopathy (PML) has the potential to occur with ublituximab-xiiy therapy. Notify prescriber at the first sign of PML, withhold drug, and expect patient to undergo a diagnostic workup to confirm diagnosis. Signs and symptoms to be alert for include changes in thinking, memory, and orientation that lead to confusion; disturbances of vision; personality changes; and progressive clumsiness or weakness on 1 side of the body. Be aware that these changes can gradually occur over days to weeks. Expect drug to be discontinued if PML is confirmed.

PATIENT TEACHING

! **WARNING** Alert females of childbearing age that a negative pregnancy test must be obtained before each dose of ublituximab-xiiy will be given. Stress importance of using an effective contraception during drug therapy and for 6 months after drug has been discontinued. If pregnancy should occur, tell patient to notify prescriber immediately.

- Inform patient that ublituximab-xiiy will be administered intravenously.
- Review signs and symptoms of an infusion reaction with patient and stress importance of reporting any that occur immediately. Tell patient some medication will be given prior to each infusion to reduce the frequency and risk of infusion reactions. Inform patient infusion reactions predominately occur after the first infusion but can occur up to 24 hours after receiving ublituximab-xiiy therapy and should be reported.
- Tell patient that if a dose is missed, it should be given as soon as possible without waiting until the next scheduled dose.

! **WARNING** Alert patient that drug may cause an allergic reaction. If present, tell patient to notify staff or prescriber (if it occurs at home) and, if severe, to seek immediate medical care.

! **WARNING** Review signs and symptoms of infection and infection control measures. Stress importance of notifying prescriber if an infection occurs, as it can become quite serious.

- Inform patient that vaccines should not be received during ofatumumab therapy. Inform mothers who were treated with drug during pregnancy not to have their infants receive live or live-attenuated vaccines until pediatrician indicates it is safe to do so.

ubrogepant

Ubrelvy

Class and Category

Pharmacologic class: Calcitonin gene-related peptide (CGRP) receptor antagonist
Therapeutic class: Antimigraine

Indications and Dosages

∗ *To treat acute migraine*

TABLETS

Adults. 50 mg or 100 mg followed by a second dose at least 2 hr after initial dose, if needed. *Maximum:* 200 mg/24 hr; treatment of 8 migraines in a 30-day period.

± **DOSAGE ADJUSTMENT** For patients taking concomitant moderate or weak CYP3A4 inducers, all doses kept at 100 mg. For patient taking strong CYP3A4 inducers, concomitant use needs to be avoided. For patients taking concomitant moderate or weak CYP3A4 inhibitors, BCRP and/or P-gp inhibitors, or who has severe hepatic or renal impairment, all doses kept at 50 mg and for patients taking a moderate CYP3A4 inhibitor, first dose kept at 50 mg and a second dose should be avoided for 24 hours.

Drug Administration

P.O.

- Do not administer tablets with grapefruit juice.

Route	Onset	Peak	Duration
P.O.	Unknown	1.5 hr	Unknown

Half-life: 5–7 hr

Mechanism of Action

Blocks CGRP, a protein released during a migraine attack, from binding to its receptors, thereby relieving migraine pain.

Contraindications

Concomitant therapy with strong CYP3A4 inhibitors, hypersensitivity to ubrogepant or its components

Interactions

DRUGS

BCRP and/or P-gp inhibitors, such as carvedilol, curcumin, eltrombopag, quinidine; CYP3A4 inhibitors (moderate), such as ciprofloxacin, cyclosporine, fluconazole, fluvoxamine; CYP3A4 inhibitors (strong), such as clarithromycin, itraconazole, ketoconazole, verapamil: Significant increase in exposure of ubrogepant and increased risk of adverse reactions

CYP3A4 inducers (strong), such as barbiturates, phenytoin, rifampin, St. John's wort: Significant reduction of ubrogepant exposure and decreased effectiveness

FOODS

grapefruit, grapefruit juice: Increased ubrogepant levels with increase in nausea and sleepiness

Adverse Reactions

CNS: Fatigue, somnolence
EENT: Dry mouth, **facial and throat edema**
GI: Nausea
RESP: Dyspnea
SKIN: Pruritus, rash, urticaria
Other: **Anaphylaxis**, **angioedema**

Childbearing Considerations

PREGNANCY

- Pregnancy exposure registry: 1-833-277-0206 or http://empresspregnancyregistry.com.
- It is not known if drug can cause fetal harm.
- Use with caution only if benefit to mother outweighs potential risk to fetus.
- Women with migraine may be at increased risk of gestational hypertension and preeclampsia during pregnancy.

LACTATION

- It is not known if drug is present in breast milk.
- Mothers should check with prescriber before breastfeeding.

Nursing Considerations

- Be aware that ubrogepant is not indicated for prevention of migraine.
- Use caution when administering drug to elderly patients.

! **WARNING** Monitor patient for a hypersensitivity reaction, which could become life-threatening, such as anaphylaxis or angioedema. If present, notify prescriber, expect drug to be discontinued, and provide supportive care, as needed and ordered.

PATIENT TEACHING

- Instruct patient how to administer ubrogepant.
- Tell patient to take ubrogepant exactly as prescribed and not to exceed the maximum dosage.
- Advise patient to avoid grapefruit or grapefruit juice intake because of increased risk of nausea and sleepiness. However, instruct patient not to take a second tablet within 24 hours if grapefruit or grapefruit juice was consumed or any of the following medications have been taken; ciprofloxacin, cyclosporine, fluconazole, fluvoxamine, or verapamil.

! **WARNING** Alert patient that drug may cause an allergic reaction. If an allergic reaction occurs, tell patient to notify prescriber and, if severe, to seek immediate medical care.

- Tell patient to inform all prescribers of ubrogepant therapy as well as use of over-the-counter medications or herbal products because of potential for drug interactions.

umeclidinium bromide

Incruse Ellipta

Class and Category

Pharmacologic class: Anticholinergic
Therapeutic class: Bronchodilator

Indications and Dosages

* *To provide maintenance treatment for chronic obstructive pulmonary disease (COPD)*

ORAL INHALATION

Adults. 62.5 mcg (1 inhalation) daily. *Maximum:* 62.5 mcg in a 24-hr period.

Drug Administration

INHALATION

- Administer drug at the same time of day.
- Open cover of inhaler only when ready to administer drug. If inhaler is opened and closed without drug being inhaled, the dose will be lost. It is not possible to accidentally take a double dose or an extra dose in 1 inhalation.
- Slide the cover down to expose mouthpiece. A click should be heard. No need to shake inhaler.
- Hand inhaler to patient and have patient breathe out fully while holding inhaler away from mouth. Then, have patient put inhaler into mouth and close lips firmly around it, fitting over the curved shape of the mouthpiece. Have patient take 1 long, steady, deep breath in through the mouth, not the nose.
- Ensure patient does not block the air vent with fingers.
- Have patient remove inhaler and hold breath for about 3 to 4 sec. Then, have patient breathe out slowly and gently.
- Inhaler may be cleaned using a dry tissue before closing the cover, although routine cleaning is not required. Slide the cover up and over the mouthpiece as far as it will go.
- When inhaler has fewer than 10 doses remaining, the left half of the counter will become red as a reminder to get a refill. When last dose in the inhaler is taken the counter will show "0."

Route	Onset	Peak	Duration
Inhalation	Unknown	5–15 min	Unknown

Half-life: 11 hr

Mechanism of Action

Inhibits the muscarinic M_3 receptor in smooth muscle to cause bronchodilation.

Contraindications

Hypersensitivity to umeclidinium or its components, severe hypersensitivity to milk proteins

Interactions

DRUGS

anticholinergics: Possibly additive effects

Adverse Reactions

CNS: Depression, dizziness, headache, vertigo
CV: **Atrial fibrillation**, **idioventricular rhythm**, supraventricular extrasystole, tachycardia
EENT: Abnormal voice, blurred vision, eye pain, glaucoma, nasopharyngitis, oropharyngeal pain, pharyngitis, rhinitis, worsening of narrow-angle glaucoma
GI: Abdominal pain (upper), diarrhea, dyspepsia, nausea
GU: Dysuria, urinary retention, UTI, worsening of urinary retention
MS: Arthralgia; back, extremity, or neck pain; myalgia
RESP: Cough, **paradoxical bronchospasm**, respiratory tract infection
SKIN: Pruritus, rash, urticaria
Other: **Anaphylaxis**, **angioedema**

Childbearing Considerations

PREGNANCY

- It is not known if drug can cause fetal harm.
- Use with caution only if benefit to mother outweighs potential risk to fetus.

LACTATION

- It is not known if drug is present in breast milk.
- Mothers should check with prescriber before breastfeeding.

Nursing Considerations

! **WARNING** Know that umeclidinium should not be initiated in patients who are experiencing a rapidly deteriorating or potentially life-threatening episode of COPD.

! **WARNING** Do not administer umeclidinium for relief of acute symptoms. Drug is not a rescue inhaler. Instead, acute symptoms should be treated with an inhaled, short-acting beta$_2$-agonist, as ordered.

! **WARNING** Be aware that patients with a severe milk protein allergy should not receive umeclidinium therapy because after inhaling other powder products containing lactose, some patients with a severe milk protein allergy have developed serious hypersensitivity reactions.

! **WARNING** Monitor patient for a hypersensitivity reaction, which could become life-threatening, such as anaphylaxis or angioedema. If present, notify prescriber, expect drug to be discontinued, and provide supportive care, as needed and ordered.

- Use with caution in patients with narrow-angle glaucoma or urinary retention because these conditions may worsen with umeclidinium therapy.

! **WARNING** Monitor patient's respiratory status for paradoxical bronchospasm. Because of its life-threatening nature, notify prescriber immediately; expect drug to be discontinued; and prepare to treat patient with an inhaled, short-acting bronchodilator, as ordered.

! **WARNING** Monitor patient for a fast and irregular pulse that may be suggestive of atrial fibrillation or an idioventricular arrhythmia.

PATIENT TEACHING

- Instruct patient how to administer umeclidinium.
- Tell patient not to use drug more than once in a 24-hour period.

! **WARNING** Remind patient that umeclidinium cannot be used to relieve acute symptoms of COPD. Instead, tell patient to treat acute symptoms with a prescribed inhaled, short-acting beta$_2$-agonist, such as albuterol, as prescribed.

! **WARNING** Urge patient to notify prescriber if symptoms worsen, if umeclidinium becomes less effective, or if there is a need for more inhalations of prescribed short-acting beta$_2$-agonist than usual. This may indicate that patient's condition is worsening.

- Instruct patient not to stop taking umeclidinium without prescriber knowledge because symptoms may recur.

! **WARNING** Inform patient that drug may cause paradoxical bronchospasms. If present, tell patient to discontinue drug and notify prescriber. If severe, tell patient to seek immediate medical care.

! **WARNING** Alert patient that drug may cause an allergic reaction. Tell patient to notify prescriber if an allergic reaction occurs. If the reaction is serious, patient should seek immediate medical care.

! **WARNING** Tell patient to notify prescriber immediately if she develops blurred vision, colored images in association with red eyes, eye discomfort, pain, or visual halos.

- Advise patient to notify prescriber if patient develops any difficulty passing urine or painful urination, especially if male patient has prostatic hyperplasia.

ustekinumab
Stelara

ustekinumab-aauz
Otulfi

ustekinumab-aekn
Selarsdi

ustekinumab-auub
Wezlana

ustekinumab-kfce
Yesintek

ustekinumab-srlf
Imuldosa

ustekinumab-stba
Steqeyma

ustekinumab-ttwe
Pyzchiva

Class and Category
Pharmacologic class: Monoclonal antibody
Therapeutic class: Immunomodulator

Indications and Dosages

* *To treat moderate to severe plaque psoriasis in patients who are candidates for phototherapy or systemic therapy*

SUBCUTANEOUS INJECTION

Adults and children ages 6 to 17 weighing more than 100 kg (220 lb). *Initial:* 90 mg followed by 90 mg 4 wk later and then 90 mg every 12 wk.
Adults weighing 100 kg (220 lb) or less and children ages 6 to 17 weighing 60 kg (132 lb) to 100 kg (220 lb). *Initial:* 45 mg followed by 45 mg 4 wk later and then 45 mg every 12 wk.

SUBCUTANEOUS INJECTION (PYZCHIVA, STELARA, WEZLANA, YESINTEK)

Children ages 6 to 17 weighing less than 60 kg (132 lb). 0.75 mg/kg, followed by 0.75 mg/kg 4 wk later and then 0.75 mg/kg every 12 wk.

* *To treat active psoriatic arthritis as monotherapy or in combination with methotrexate*

SUBCUTANEOUS INJECTION (STELARA, WEZLANA, YESINTEK)

Adults and children ages 6 to 17 weighing 60 kg (132 lb) or more. *Initial:* 45 mg, followed by 45 mg 4 wk later, and then 45 mg every 12 wk.
Children ages 6 to 17 weighing less than 60 kg (132 lb). 0.75 mg/kg, followed by 0.75 mg/kg 4 wk later and then 0.75 mg/kg every 12 wk.

SUBCUTANEOUS INJECTION (IMULDOSA,OTULFI, SELARSDI, STEQEYMA)

Adults. *Initial:* 45 mg followed by 45 mg 4 wk later, and then 45 mg every 12 wk.
Children ages 6 to 17 weighing 60 kg (132 lb) or more. *Initial:* 45 mg followed by 45 mg 4 wk later, and then 45 mg every 12 wk.

SUBCUTANEOUS INJECTION (PYZCHIVA)

Adults and children ages 6 to 17 weighing 60 kg (132 lb) or more. *Initial:* 45 mg followed by 45 mg 4 wk later, and then 45 mg every 12 wk.
Children ages 6 to 17 weighing less than 60 kg (132 lb). 0.75 mg/kg, followed by 0.75 mg/kg 4 wk later, and then 0.75 mg/kg every 12 wk.

± **DOSAGE ADJUSTMENT** For patients who weigh more than 100 kg (220 lb) and also have coexistent moderate to severe plaque psoriasis in addition to psoriatic arthritis, initial dosage increased to 90 mg followed by 90 mg 4 weeks later, and then 90 mg every 12 weeks.

* *To treat moderate to severe active Crohn's disease; to treat moderate to severe active ulcerative colitis*

I.V. INFUSION

Adults weighing more than 85 kg (187 lb). *Initial:* 520 mg infused over at least 60 min as a single infusion.
Adults weighing more than 55 kg (121 lb) but less than 85 kg (187 lb). *Initial:* 390 mg infused over at least 60 min as a single infusion.
Adults weighing 55 kg (121 lb) or less. *Initial:* 260 mg infused over at least 60 min as a single infusion.

SUBCUTANEOUS INJECTION

Adults. *Maintenance:* 90 mg 8 wk after initial intravenous dose, then every 8 wk thereafter.

Drug Administration

- Vials should be stored upright in refrigerator and protected from light.
- Do not shake vials before administration.
- Drug should be colorless to light yellow and may contain a few small translucent or white particles. Discard if solution is cloudy, discolored, or contains other particulate matter.

I.V.

- Calculate the dose and number of vials needed (may be based on patient weight).
- Withdraw volume equal to dosage volume from a 250-ml bag of 0.9% Sodium Chloride Injection. Brands except for Selarsdi may also use a 250-ml bag of 0.45% Sodium Chloride Injection. Add drug solution volume to bag and mix gently.
- Check specific manufacturer for brand being used for how long diluted solution may be stored before it is administered.
- Use only an infusion set with an in-line 0.2 micrometer, nonpyrogenic, low-protein-binding filter for infusion. Otulfi also requires using only polypropylene or polyvinyl chloride infusion sets.
- Infuse over at least 60 min.
- Do not infuse in the same I.V. line with other agents.
- *Incompatibilities:* Other drugs

SUBCUTANEOUS

- Needle cover on the prefilled syringe of Stelara brand contains dry natural rubber and should not be handled if allergic to latex.
- When using the prefilled syringe remember to prevent activating the needle safety guard prematurely by not touching the needle guard activation clips at any time during use. Hold the body and remove the needle cover. Do not hold the plunger or plunger head while removing the needle cover or the plunger may move.
- Use a 1-ml syringe with a 27 G, ½-inch needle when using the single-dose vial instead of the prefilled syringe.
- Do not use the prefilled syringe if it has been dropped without the needle cover in place.
- Inject into any quadrant of abdomen, gluteal region, thighs, or upper arms. Injection of entire prefilled syringe contents is necessary to activate the needle guard. After injection with the prefilled syringe, maintain pressure on the plunger head and remove the needle from the skin. Slowly take thumb off the plunger head to allow the empty syringe to move up until the entire needle is covered by the needle guard.
- Rotate sites, and avoid areas that are bruised, erythematous, indurated, or tender.

Route	Onset	Peak	Duration
SubQ	Unknown	7–13.5 days	Unknown
I.V.	Unknown	Unknown	Unknown

Half-life: 14–45.5 days

Mechanism of Action

Binds to p40 protein subunit used by interleukin (IL)-12 and IL-23 cytokines. These specific cytokines are involved in inflammatory and immune responses, such as natural killer cell activation and $CD4^+$ T-cell differentiation and activation. By disrupting signaling mediated by IL-12 and IL-23, signs and symptoms caused by inflammatory and immune responses are diminished or relieved.

Contraindications

Hypersensitivity to ustekinumab or its components

Interactions

DRUGS

live-virus vaccines: Increased risk of adverse vaccine effects

Adverse Reactions

CNS: Depression, dizziness, fatigue, fever, headache, **reversible posterior leukoencephalopathy syndrome (rare)**
EENT: Nasopharyngitis, pharyngolaryngeal pain, sinusitis
GI: Abdominal pain, diarrhea, diverticulitis, gastroenteritis, nausea
GU: UTI
MS: Back pain, myalgia, osteomyelitis
RESP: **Cryptogenic organizing pneumonia**; **eosinophilic pneumonia**; **interstitial pneumonia**; respiratory tract infections, including opportunistic fungal infections and tuberculosis
SKIN: Cellulitis, cutaneous small vessel vasculitis, erythrodermic psoriasis, pruritus, pustular psoriasis, rash, urticaria
Other: **Anaphylaxis**, **angioedema**, anti-ustekinumab antibodies, flu-like symptoms, injection-site reactions (bruising, erythema, hemorrhage, induration, irritation, pain, pruritus, swelling), **malignancies (breast, colorectal, head and neck, kidney, melanoma and nonmelanoma disorders of skin, prostate, or thyroid)**, serious infection (including bacterial, fungal, and viral infections), and reactivation of latent infections

Childbearing Considerations

PREGNANCY

- Pregnancy exposure registry: 1-877-311-8972.
- It is not known if drug can cause fetal harm. However, human IgG antibody crosses the placenta at an increased rate as pregnancy progresses and peaks during the third trimester so drug may be transferred to the fetus. Live attenuated vaccines should not be administered to infants exposed in utero for a minimum of 6 months after birth.
- Use with caution only if benefit to mother outweighs potential risk to fetus.

LACTATION

- Drug may be present in breast milk.
- Mothers should check with prescriber before breastfeeding.

Nursing Considerations

- Make sure patient has a tuberculin skin test before therapy starts. If skin test is positive, treatment of latent tuberculosis (TB) should start before ustekinumab therapy starts. Also, expect antituberculosis therapy to start if patient has a history of latent or active TB but adequate therapy can't be confirmed or if patient has a negative test for latent TB but has risk factors for TB. Monitor patients closely who live in regions where TB is endemic.
- Ensure patient is current with all immunizations before starting ustekinumab therapy because patient shouldn't receive live vaccines during treatment. BCG vaccines shouldn't be given for 1 year before or 1 year after ustekinumab therapy.
- Use caution when administering ustekinumab to a patient undergoing allergen immunotherapy because drug may decrease the protective effect of allergen immunotherapy, which in turn may increase the risk of an allergic reaction to a dose of allergen immunotherapy.

! WARNING Know that if patient has evidence of an active infection when drug is prescribed, therapy shouldn't start until infection has been treated. Monitor all patients for infection during therapy, especially those receiving immunosuppressants. Be on the alert for cough, dyspnea, and interstitial infiltrates following 1 to 3 doses that may suggest pneumonia has developed. If a serious infection, an opportunistic infection, or sepsis develops, expect prescriber to stop ustekinumab and start appropriate antimicrobial therapy. Monitor patient closely with a history of recurrent infection or increased risk of infection or who live in a region where histoplasmosis is prevalent.

! WARNING Monitor patient for a hypersensitivity reaction, which could become life-threatening, such as anaphylaxis or angioedema. At first sign of hypersensitivity, notify prescriber, expect drug to be discontinued, and provide supportive care, as needed and ordered.

! WARNING Be aware that patients with a history of cancer or who have genetic deficiencies in IL-12 or IL-23 should be thoroughly evaluated before ustekinumab therapy starts because various cancers have occurred in patients being treated with ustekinumab. Monitor patients throughout therapy for persistent, severe, or unusual signs and symptoms.

! WARNING Inspect patient's skin regularly for evidence of abnormalities because rapid appearance of multiple cutaneous squamous cell carcinoma has occurred in patients who had preexisting risk factors for nonmelanoma skin cancer. Patients who are over 60 years of age, have a medical history of prolonged immunosuppressant therapy, and those with a history of psoralen plus ultraviolet radiation using UVA bands (PUVA) treatment should be closely monitored.

! WARNING Monitor patient for confusion, headache, seizures, and vision disturbances, which may signal reversible posterior leukoencephalopathy syndrome, a rare neurologic disorder that may occur with ustekinumab therapy. If present, notify prescriber, expect ustekinumab therapy to be discontinued, and provide supportive care, as needed and ordered.

- Know that comparison of the incidence of antibodies to ustekinumab with the incidence of antibodies to other products may be misleading.

PATIENT TEACHING

- Teach patient or family or caregiver how to administer drug subcutaneously if self-administration is ordered by prescriber.
- Instruct patient to store drug vials standing up straight in refrigerator protected from light.
- Caution against receiving live-virus vaccines while taking ustekinumab; doing so may adversely affect the immune system. Inform mothers exposed to drug during pregnancy to alert pediatrician of drug exposure so that infant does not receive any live vaccines for the first six months.

! WARNING Alert patient that drug may cause an allergic reaction. Tell patient to notify prescriber immediately, if present, and to seek immediate medical care, if severe.

! **WARNING** Review infection control measures to follow during ustekinumab therapy. Teach patient to recognize and report evidence of infection. Advise patient to avoid people with infections and to have all ordered laboratory tests performed. Inform patient that TB may occur during ustekinumab therapy. Instruct him to report low-grade fever, persistent cough, or wasting or weight loss to prescriber.

! **WARNING** Inform patient that the risk of developing certain kinds of cancer is higher in patients taking ustekinumab. Emphasize importance of follow-up visits and reporting any persistent, sudden-onset, or unusual signs or symptoms. Also, encourage patient to have regular skin assessments done.

- Urge patient to inform all healthcare providers about ustekinumab use and to inform prescriber about all over-the-counter medications being taken, including herbal remedies and mineral and vitamin supplements.

valproate sodium

valproic acid

divalproex sodium

Depakote, Depakote ER, Depakote Sprinkle, Epival (CAN)

Class and Category

Pharmacologic class: Carboxylic acid derivative
Therapeutic class: Anticonvulsant

Indications and Dosages

* *To treat as monotherapy or as adjunct complex partial seizures that occur in isolation or associated with other types of seizures*

CAPSULES, D.R. SPRINKLE CAPSULES, D.R. TABLETS, E.R. CAPSULES, E.R. TABLETS, I.V. INFUSION (VALPROIC ACID, VALPROATE SODIUM, DIVALPROEX SODIUM)

Adults and children ages 10 and older. *Initial:* 10 to 15 mg/kg/day, increased by 5 to 10 mg/kg daily every wk, as needed. I.V. infusion administered over no less than 60 min. *Maximum:* 60 mg/kg daily.

* *To treat as monotherapy or as adjunct simple and complex absence seizures; as adjunctive therapy to treat multiple seizure types that include absence seizures*

CAPSULES, D.R. SPRINKLE CAPSULES, D.R. TABLETS, E.R. CAPSULES, E.R. TABLETS, I.V. INFUSION (VALPROIC ACID, VALPROATE SODIUM, DIVALPROEX SODIUM)

Adults and children ages 10 and older. *Initial:* 10 to 15 mg/kg/day, increased by 5 to 10 mg/kg daily every wk, as needed. I.V. infusion given over no less than 60 min. *Maximum:* 60 mg/kg/day.

* *To treat acute manic phase of bipolar disorder*

D.R. TABLETS (DIVALPROEX SODIUM)

Adults. *Initial:* 750 mg daily in divided doses. *Maximum:* 60 mg/kg daily.

E.R. TABLETS (DIVALPROEX SODIUM)

Adults. *Initial:* 25 mg/kg/day once daily, increased as rapidly as possible to achieve therapeutic dose. *Maximum:* 60 mg/kg/day.

* *To prevent migraine headache*

D.R. TABLETS (DIVALPROEX SODIUM)

Adults. *Initial:* 250 mg every 12 hr, increased as needed. *Maximum:* 1 g daily.

E.R. TABLETS (DIVALPROEX SODIUM)

Adults. *Initial:* 500 mg daily for 1 wk, increased up to 1 g daily, as needed. *Maximum:* 1 g daily.

Drug Administration

P.O.

- Administer with food to minimize GI irritation, if needed.
- Administer drug at least 2 hr before or 6 hr after cholestyramine.
- D.R. or E.R. tablets should be swallowed whole and not chewed, crushed, or divided.
- Capsules may be swallowed whole or contents sprinkled on a small amount (1teaspoon) of soft food such as applesauce or pudding just before administration. Administer immediately and ensure that patient does not chew mixture.

I.V.

- Dilute drug with at least 50 ml of 0.9% Sodium Chloride Injection, 5% Dextrose in Water, or Lactated Ringer's solution.

- Diluted solution may be stored for 24 hr.
- Infuse over 60 min at a rate not to exceed 20 mg/min. Rapid administration increases risk of adverse reactions and should be avoided.
- Know that patient should be switched from I.V. to P.O. form as soon as possible.
- *Incompatibilities:* None listed by manufacturer

Route	Onset	Peak	Duration
P.O.	Unknown	15–60 min	Unknown
I.V.	Unknown	Unknown	Unknown

Half-life: 4–16 hr

Mechanism of Action

Decreases possibly seizure activity by blocking reuptake of gamma-aminobutyric acid (GABA), the most common inhibitory neurotransmitter in the brain. GABA suppresses the rapid firing of neurons by inhibiting voltage-sensitive sodium channels.

Contraindications

Hepatic impairment; hypersensitivity to valproic acid, valproate sodium, divalproex sodium, or their components; mitochondrial disease caused by POLG mutations; pregnancy or females of childbearing age who are not using effective contraception (for prevention of migraine headaches); suspected POLG-related disorder in children under 2 yr of age; urea cycle disorders

Interactions

DRUGS

amitriptyline, nortriptyline: Increased plasma levels of these drugs
aspirin: Increased valproic acid level with possible increased risk of adverse reactions
cannabidiol: Increased risk of elevated liver enzymes
carbamazepine: Altered concentrations of carbamazepine
carbapenem antibiotics (ertapenem, imipenem, meropenem): Reduced serum valproic acid level, causing loss of seizure control
chlorpromazine: Increased trough plasma levels of valproate
cholestyramine: Decreased bioavailability of valproic acid
clonazepam: Increased risk of absence seizures
CNS depressants: Increased CNS depression
diazepam: Inhibited diazepam metabolism
estrogen-containing hormonal contraceptives: Possibly increased clearance of valproate, which may decrease effectiveness and increase risk of seizures
ethosuximide: Unpredictable blood ethosuximide level
felbamate: Impaired valproic acid metabolism and increased valproate level
lamotrigine: Decreased lamotrigine clearance
methotrexate: Possibly decreased valproate levels; potentially increased frequency of bipolar symptoms or seizures
phenobarbital, primidone: Possible increased phenobarbital concentrations resulting in CNS depression that could become severe
phenytoin: Increased risk of phenytoin toxicity, loss of seizure control
propofol: Possibly increased blood levels of propofol
rufinamide: Increased rufinamide concentrations
topiramate: Increased risk of hyperammonemia with or without encephalopathy
zidovudine: Clearance decreased for zidovudine resulting in increased concentrations

ACTIVITIES

alcohol use: Additive CNS depression

Adverse Reactions

CNS: Abnormal dreams or thinking, aggression, agitation, amnesia, apathy, asthenia, ataxia, attention disturbance, behavioral deterioration, catatonic reaction, cerebral pseudoatrophy, chills, cognitive decline, confusion, depression, dizziness, drowsiness, emotional upset, **encephalopathy**, euphoria, fever, gait abnormality, hallucinations, headache, hostility, hyperactivity, hyperesthesia, hypertonia, hypokinesia, **hypothermia**, increased reflexes, insomnia, irritability, lack of coordination, learning disorder, lethargy, **loss of seizure control**, malaise, nervousness, **paradoxical seizures**, paresthesia, parkinsonism, psychomotor hyperactivity, psychosis, sedation, speech disorder, somnolence, **suicidal ideation**,

tardive dyskinesia, tremor, twitching, vertigo, weakness
CV: **Bradycardia**, chest pain, edema, hypertension, **hypotension**, orthostatic hypotension, palpitations, peripheral edema, tachycardia, vasodilation
EENT: Amblyopia, conjunctivitis, diplopia, dry eyes, ear or eye pain, glossitis, hearing loss, nystagmus, parotid gland swelling, pharyngitis, rhinitis, sinusitis, spots before eyes, stomatitis, taste perversion, tinnitus
ENDO: Breast enlargement, elevated testosterone level, galactorrhea, hyperandrogenism, hyperglycemia, inappropriate ADH secretion, parotid gland swelling
GI: Abdominal pain, anorexia, constipation, diarrhea, dyspepsia, elevated liver enzymes, fecal incontinence, flatulence, gastroenteritis, **hepatotoxicity**, increased appetite, indigestion, jaundice, nausea, **pancreatitis**, vomiting
GU: Aspermia, azoospermia, cystitis, decreased sperm count or spermatozoa motility, dysuria, enuresis, male infertility, menstrual irregularities, polycystic ovary disease, **tubulointerstitial nephritis**, urinary incontinence, UTI, **vaginal hemorrhage**
HEME: Acquired Pelger-Huet anomaly, **agranulocytosis**, anemia, **aplastic anemia**, **bone marrow suppression**, eosinophilia, hematoma, **hypofibrinogenemia**, **leukopenia**, lymphocytosis, macrocytosis, **pancytopenia**, porphyria (acute, intermittent), **prolonged bleeding time**, **thrombocytopenia**
MS: Arthralgia, arthrosis, back pain, bone pain, decreased bone mineral density, dysarthria, fractures, leg cramps, myalgia, neck pain or rigidity, osteopenia, osteoporosis
RESP: Dyspnea, increased cough
SKIN: Alopecia, cutaneous vasculitis, diaphoresis, discoid lupus erythematosus, dry skin, ecchymosis, **erythema multiforme**, furunculosis, hair color or texture changes, hirsutism, maculopapular rash, nail and nail bed disorders, petechiae, photosensitivity, pruritus, rash, seborrhea, **Stevens-Johnson syndrome**, **toxic epidermal necrolysis**
Other: **Anaphylaxis**, decreased carnitine concentration, developmental delay (children), **drug reaction with eosinophilia and systemic symptoms (DRESS)**, **hyperammonemia**, **hyponatremia**, injection-site pain, weight gain or loss

Childbearing Considerations

PREGNANCY

- Pregnancy exposure registry: 1-888-233-2334 or https://www.aedpregnancyregistry.org.
- Drug causes fetal harm such as decreased IQ, major congenital malformations, and neurodevelopmental disorders. Drug may also cause fatal hepatic failure in fetus. In addition, drug may also increase risk of attention deficit/hyperactivity disorder and autism spectrum disorders.
- Drug is contraindicated in pregnant females and in females of childbearing age who are not using effective contraception for treatment of migraines.
- Use with extreme caution only if no alternate is effective in controlling bipolar disorder or epilepsy and the benefit to mother outweighs potential risk to fetus.
- Drug should not be discontinued abruptly if pregnancy occurs during drug therapy for epilepsy, as this can precipitate status epilepticus with resulting maternal and fetal hypoxia and threat to life.

LACTATION

- Drug is present in breast milk.
- Mothers should check with prescriber before breastfeeding.
- If breastfeeding occurs, monitor infant for jaundice or unusual bleeding or bruising.

REPRODUCTION

- Females of childbearing age should use effective contraception and be counseled regularly of its importance throughout drug therapy. This is especially important for females of childbearing age planning to become pregnant and at the onset of puberty for girls.
- Drug may cause male infertility.

Nursing Considerations

! **WARNING** Use caution when administering drug to children or patients with congenital metabolic disorders, organic brain disease, or severe seizure disorder accompanied by mental retardation; patients with history of hepatic disease; and patients receiving multiple anticonvulsants because they may be at increased risk for developing hepatotoxicity.

! WARNING Ensure that liver enzymes have been done prior to starting therapy and at frequent intervals after that because drug may cause hepatotoxicity that could be fatal. Watch for evidence of decreased hepatic function, including anorexia, facial edema, jaundice, lethargy, loss of seizure control, malaise, vomiting, and weakness, especially during the first 6 months of treatment. Notify prescriber immediately if hepatotoxicity is suspected and, if confirmed, expect drug to be discontinued immediately.

! WARNING Keep in mind hyperammonemia may occur even if liver function test results are normal. Monitor ammonia levels, as ordered. If patient develops unexplained lethargy, vomiting, or changes in mental status with an increase in ammonia level; if asymptomatic ammonia elevations are detected and persist; or if patient develops hypothermia even without hyperammonemia, expect to discontinue valproic acid.

! WARNING Monitor patient for a hypersensitivity reaction, including severe skin reactions which could become life-threatening, such as anaphylaxis or DRESS. If present including a rash or other serious skin manifestations (DRESS may only initially present with a fever or swollen lymph nodes although rash is most common), notify prescriber, expect drug to be switched to another drug, and provide supportive care, as needed and ordered.

! WARNING Watch patient closely for suicidal tendencies, particularly when therapy starts and dosage changes because depression may worsen temporarily during these times, possibly leading to suicidal ideation.

! WARNING Be aware that patient with hypoalbuminemia or another protein-binding deficiency is at increased risk for valproic acid toxicity.

! WARNING Monitor platelet count, as ordered, for signs of thrombocytopenia and patient for unexplained bruising or bleeding. Notify prescriber if abnormalities occur.

! WARNING Monitor patient for other persistent, serious, or unusual adverse reactions.

- Monitor patient's drug level, as ordered, especially early in therapy and if patient takes other drugs, because interactions can alter the blood level.
- Be aware drug may alter urine ketone test and thyroid function tests.

PATIENT TEACHING

! WARNING Urge females of childbearing age, including girls beginning the onset of puberty, to avoid pregnancy because drug can cause fetal harm. Instruct these patients to use effective contraception while taking drug and to notify prescriber immediately if pregnancy occurs.

- Instruct patient how to administer oral form of drug prescribed.
- Advise patient to take drug at least 2 hours before or 6 hours after cholestyramine, if prescribed.
- Inform patient to notify prescriber that if medication residue is seen in stools, plasma valproate levels may have to be checked and possibly an alternative treatment prescribed.
- Urge patient to avoid alcohol during therapy

! WARNING Alert patient that drug may cause an allergic reaction that may involve serious skin reactions. Tell patient to notify prescriber immediately if an allergic reaction including a fever, rash, swollen lymph nodes, or other skin reactions occur and, if severe, to seek immediate medical care.

! WARNING Urge family or caregiver to watch patient closely for suicidal tendencies, especially when therapy starts or dosage changes.

! WARNING Tell patient to alert prescriber if signs and symptoms of liver or pancreas dysfunction occurs such as abdominal pain, anorexia, nausea, and vomiting. Also, look for jaundice if liver dysfunction is suspected.

- Advise patient to avoid hazardous activities during therapy because drug may affect mental and motor performance.
- Advise patient to notify prescriber if tremor develops during therapy; it may be dose-related.

! **WARNING** Tell patient to notify prescriber of any other persistent, serious, or unusual adverse reactions.

- Advise mothers who are breastfeeding to monitor their infant for jaundice or unusual bleeding or bruising.

valsartan

Diovan

Class and Category

Pharmacologic class: Angiotensin II receptor blocker (ARB)

Therapeutic class: Antihypertensive

Indications and Dosages

* *To manage hypertension, alone or with other antihypertensives*

ORAL SUSPENSION, TABLETS

Adults. *Initial:* 80 or 160 mg once daily, increased, as needed. *Maximum:* 320 mg/day. **Children ages 1 to 16.** *Initial:* 1 mg/kg (up to 40 mg total) once daily, increased as needed and prescribed. Alternatively, 2 mg/kg may be initially given when a greater reduction of blood pressure is needed. *Maximum:* 4 mg/kg (up to 160 mg) daily.

ORAL SOLUTION

Adults. *Initial:* 40 or 80 mg twice daily, increased, as needed. *Maximum:* 320 mg/day. **Children ages 6 to 16.** *Initial:* 0.65 mg/kg (up to 40 mg total daily dose) twice daily, increased, as needed. *Maximum:* 1.35 mg/kg twice daily.

* *To treat New York Heart Association (NYHA) class II to IV heart failure*

ORAL SOLUTION, TABLETS

Adults. *Initial:* 40 mg twice daily, increased to 80 mg twice daily and then 160 mg twice daily, as needed. *Maximum:* 320 mg daily in 2 divided doses.

* *To reduce cardiovascular mortality in stable patients with left ventricular failure or dysfunction following an MI*

ORAL SOLUTION, TABLETS

Adults. *Initial:* 20 mg twice daily starting as early as 12 hr after MI, increased to 40 mg twice daily within 7 days, followed by subsequent adjustments to 160 mg twice daily as tolerated. *Maximum:* 160 mg twice daily.

Drug Administration

P.O.

- Tablets, oral solution, and oral suspension are not interchangeable on a milligram-per-milligram basis. Do not combine the dosage forms to achieve a total dose.
- An oral suspension can be prepared from tablets by the pharmacist for children who cannot swallow tablets. Oral suspension should be shaken for at least 10 sec before measuring dose. Use a calibrated device to measure dosage. Store oral suspension at room temperature for 30 days or store in refrigerator for 75 days.
- Oral solution should not be given to children under the age of 6.
- Oral solution form is available in a concentration of 4 mg/ml. Use a calibrated device to measure dosage. Store solution at controlled room temperature.

Route	Onset	Peak	Duration
P.O.	2 hr	2–4 hr	24 hr

Half-life: 6 hr

Mechanism of Action

Blocks the hormone angiotensin II from binding to receptor sites in adrenal glands, vascular smooth muscle, and other tissues. This action inhibits aldosterone-secreting and vasoconstrictive effects of angiotensin II, thereby reducing blood pressure. It also reduces renal reabsorption of sodium, which helps to reduce fluid retention that occurs in heart failure.

Contraindications

Concurrent aliskiren therapy in diabetic patients, hypersensitivity to valsartan or its components

Interactions

DRUGS

ACE inhibitors, aliskiren, other angiotensin receptor blockers: Increased risk of hyperkalemia, hypotension, and renal dysfunction
antihypertensives, diuretics: Additive hypotensive effect
lithium: Possibly increased serum lithium concentration and toxicity
NSAIDs: Increased risk of renal dysfunction, especially in the elderly and patients with or existing renal dysfunction or volume depletion; decreased hypertensive effect of valsartan
potassium salts, potassium-sparing diuretics, potassium supplements: Possibly hyperkalemia; increased serum creatinine in heart-failure patients

FOODS

high-potassium foods such as bananas or potatoes, potassium-containing salt substitutes: Possibly hyperkalemia

Adverse Reactions

CNS: Dizziness, fatigue, headache, insomnia, syncope, vertigo
CV: Edema, **hypotension**, orthostatic hypotension, vasculitis
EENT: Blurred vision, pharyngitis, rhinitis, sinusitis
GI: Abdominal pain, diarrhea, elevated liver enzymes, **hepatitis**, indigestion, nausea, vomiting
GU: **Acute renal failure**, increased blood creatinine level
HEME: **Thrombocytopenia**
MS: Arthralgia, back pain, **rhabdomyolysis**
RESP: Cough, upper respiratory tract infection
SKIN: Alopecia, bullous dermatitis, rash
Other: **Angioedema**, **hyperkalemia**, increased incidence of viral infection

Childbearing Considerations

PREGNANCY

- Drug can cause fetal harm. Drug given during the second or third trimester reduces fetal renal function and increases fetal and neonatal morbidity and death. Resulting oligohydramnios can lead to fetal anuria, renal failure, hypotension, lung hypoplasia, and skeletal malformations as well as fetal death.
- Drug is contraindicated in pregnant women. If pregnancy occurs, drug should be discontinued as soon as possible and an alternative drug given instead.

LACTATION

- It is not known if drug is present in breast milk.
- Breastfeeding is not recommended during drug therapy.

REPRODUCTION

- Females of childbearing age need to use an effective contraceptive during drug therapy and to report any suspected or known pregnancy immediately to prescriber.

Nursing Considerations

! **WARNING** Know that valsartan shouldn't be given to patients who are taking a diuretic or have hypovolemia because there is increased risk of severe hypotension from volume depletion. If severe hypotension occurs, place patient in a supine position, notify prescriber, and expect to give an intravenous infusion of normal saline.

! **WARNING** Be aware that valsartan shouldn't be given to pregnant patients because drug can cause fetal harm.

! **WARNING** Check patient's blood pressure often during therapy to determine effectiveness of drug and to detect hypotension.

- Be aware that maximal blood pressure reduction typically occurs after 4 weeks during therapy.

! **WARNING** Monitor patient for a hypersensitivity reaction, which could become life-threatening, such as angioedema. If present, notify prescriber, expect drug to be discontinued, and provide supportive care, as needed and ordered.

! **WARNING** Monitor serum potassium level because drug may elevate potassium level by blocking aldosterone secretion. Be aware that hyperkalemia occurs more often in children with underlying chronic kidney disease.

! **WARNING** Obtain a serum creatinine level periodically, as ordered, because changes in renal function can occur during valsartan therapy. Know that patients who are at high risk for renal dysfunction are patients with chronic kidney disease, renal artery stenosis, severe congestive heart failure, or who are volume-depleted. Notify prescriber of an elevated serum creatinine level and changes in voiding patterns because renal dysfunction could lead to acute renal failure.

! **WARNING** Monitor patient's liver enzymes, as ordered and patient for signs and symptoms of hepatic dysfunction because drug can cause hepatotoxicity.

! **WARNING** Monitor patient for any other persistent, serious, or unusual adverse reactions.

PATIENT TEACHING

- Instruct patient how to administer form of valsartan prescribed.
- Tell patient that lightheadedness can occur with valsartan therapy, especially during the first days of therapy. If fainting should occur, advise patient to stop taking valsartan and to notify prescriber. Remind patient that diarrhea, excessive perspiration, inadequate fluid intake, or vomiting can lower blood pressure and cause fainting.
- Advise patient to avoid using potassium-containing salt substitutes without consulting prescriber.

! **WARNING** Alert patient that drug may cause an allergic reaction. If present, tell patient to notify prescriber and, if severe, to seek immediate medical care.

! **WARNING** Instruct females of childbearing age to use reliable birth control during therapy and to notify prescriber at once if pregnancy occurs because valsartan may cause fetal harm. Drug will need to be discontinued.

! **WARNING** Review signs and symptoms of a high potassium level as well as kidney and liver dysfunction. Urge patient to notify prescriber, if present.

- Advise patient to avoid hazardous activities until drug's CNS effects are known and resolved.
- Inform mothers that breastfeeding should not be undertaken during drug therapy.

! **WARNING** Tell patient to notify prescriber if any other persistent, serious, or unusual adverse reaction occurs.

- Tell patients to inform all prescribers of valsartan therapy and any other drug therapy they are taking, including drugs known as NSAIDs, such as ibuprofen and naproxen.
- Urge patient to keep follow-up appointments to monitor progress.

vancomycin hydrochloride

Firvanq, Vancocin

Class and Category

Pharmacologic class: Glycopeptide
Therapeutic class: Antibiotic

Indications and Dosages

* *To treat pseudomembranous colitis caused by* Clostridioides difficile

CAPSULES, ORAL SOLUTION

Adults. 125 mg every 6 hr for 10 days.
Children. 40 mg/kg daily in 3 or 4 divided doses for 7 to 10 days. *Maximum:* 2 g daily.

* *To treat staphylococcal enterocolitis caused by* Staphylococcus aureus

CAPSULES, ORAL SOLUTION

Adults. 500 mg to 2 g daily in 3 or 4 divided doses for 7 to 10 days.
Children. 40 mg/kg daily in 3 or 4 divided doses for 7 to 10 days. *Maximum:* 2 g daily.

* *To treat serious or severe infections such as bone infections, infective endocarditis, lower respiratory infection, skin and skin structure infections, or septicemia caused by susceptible strains of methicillin-resistant* Staphylococcus aureus *(MRSA); to treat infections that are resistant to other antimicrobial drugs such as cephalosporins or penicillins*

I.V. INFUSION

Adults. 500 mg every 6 hr or 1 g every 12 hr infused over at least 60 min.
Children ages 1 mo and older. 10 mg/kg every 6 hr infused over at least 60 min.

Neonates ages 1 wk to 1 mo. *Initial:* 15 mg/kg followed by 10 mg/kg every 8 hr infused over at least 60 min.
Neonates under age 1 wk. *Initial:* 15 mg/kg followed by 10 mg/kg every 12 hr infused over at least 60 min.

±**DOSAGE ADJUSTMENT** For patients receiving I.V. vancomycin who has any degree of renal impairment, initial dose should be no less than 15 mg/kg and then dosage adjusted depending on renal function, as needed. For patients who are anephric, initial I.V. dose of 15 mg/kg given to achieve prompt therapeutic serum concentrations. Then vancomycin serum concentration measured after 24 hr of first dose to guide further I.V. therapy.

Drug Administration

P.O.

- Capsules should be swallowed whole and not chewed, crushed, or opened.
- Have pharmacist prepare oral solution if patient cannot swallow capsules. Shake oral solution well before measuring dose. Use a calibrated device to measure dosage of oral solution. Refrigerate solution when not in use. Discard after 14 days or if oral solution appears hazy or contains particulates.

I.V.

- Thaw frozen containers at room temperature or under refrigeration. Do not thaw by immersion in water baths or by microwave irradiation. Do not force thaw. Once thawed, check for minute leaks by squeezing the bag firmly. Do not use if leaks are detected. Agitate bag after solution has reached room temperature. If solution remains cloudy or insoluble precipitate is present or any seal is broken, discard. Thawed solution is stable for 72 hr at room temperature or 30 days refrigerated. Do not refreeze.
- Reconstitute 500-mg vial with 10 ml of Sterile Water for Injection, then further dilute with 100 ml of compatible solution; 750-mg vial with 15 ml of Sterile Water for Injection and further dilute with 150 ml of compatible solution; 1-g vial with 20 ml of Sterile Water for Injection and further dilute with 200 ml of compatible solution; and 1.5-g vial with 30 ml of Sterile Water for Injection and further dilute with 300 ml of compatible solution. Final concentration after dilution should be 5 mg/ml. In patients requiring fluid restriction, a concentration up to 10 mg/ml may be used.
- Compatible solutions to use for dilution include 0.9% Sodium Chloride Injection, 5% Dextrose Injection, 5% Dextrose Injection and 0.9% Sodium Chloride Injection, *Lactated* Ringer's Injection, and Lactated Ringer's and 5% Dextrose Injection.
- After dilution with 0.9% Sodium Chloride Injection or 5% Dextrose Injection, diluted solution may be stored in refrigerator for 14 days; after dilution with other compatible solutions previously listed, diluted solution may be stored in refrigerator for 96 hr.
- Infuse at no more than 10 mg/min or over at least 60 min, whichever is longer. Avoid rapid delivery because it may cause life-threatening effects such as cardiac arrest, chest pain, dyspnea, shock, urticaria, or wheezing. These reactions may be more severe in children and in patients receiving concomitant muscle relaxant anesthetics. Rapid infusion may also cause "vancomycin infusion reaction," characterized by erythema and pruritus involving the face, neck and upper torso. Infusion reactions most commonly occurs with higher drug concentrations (should be no more than 10 mg/ml) and/or rate of infusion is given less than 60 min although reactions may occur at any concentration or rate. Stop infusion if a reaction occurs and notify prescriber.
- Flush intravenous lines before and after administration if other antibacterial drugs are also being administered to patient in the same I.V. line.
- Observe I.V. infusion site for evidence of extravasation, including necrosis, pain, tenderness, and thrombophlebitis. If extravasation occurs, discontinue infusion immediately and notify prescriber.
- *Incompatibilities:* Beta-lactam antibiotics and other drugs (due to vancomycin's low pH)

Route	Onset	Peak	Duration
P.O.	Unknown	Unknown	Unknown
I.V.	Unknown	End of infusion	Unknown

Half-life: 4–6 hr

Mechanism of Action

Inhibits bacterial RNA and cell wall synthesis; alters permeability of bacterial membranes, causing cell wall lysis and cell death.

Contraindications

Hypersensitivity to corn or corn products when given with dextrose solutions, hypersensitivity to vancomycin or its components

Interactions

DRUGS

aminoglycosides (amikacin, gentamicin, tobramycin), amphotericin B, bacitracin (parenteral), cisplatin, colistin, polymyxin B, viomycin: Additive nephrotoxicity or neurotoxicity

anesthetic agents: Increased risk of erythema and histamine-like flushing

Adverse Reactions

CNS: Chills, depression, dizziness, fatigue, fever, headache, insomnia, vertigo

CV: **Hypotension**, peripheral edema, vasculitis

EENT: Hemorrhagic occlusive retinal vasculitis, ototoxicity

GI: Abdominal pain, constipation, ***Clostridioides difficile*–associated diarrhea (CDAD)**, diarrhea, flatulence, nausea, vomiting

GU: **Acute kidney injury**, interstitial nephritis, **nephrotoxicity**, UTI

HEME: Anemia, eosinophilia, **neutropenia**, **thrombocytopenia**

MS: Back pain

RESP: Dyspnea, wheezing

SKIN: **Acute generalized exanthematous pustulosis (AGEP)**; **exfoliative dermatitis**; extravasation with pain, tenderness, thrombophlebitis, and tissue necrosis; linear IgA bullous dermatosis (LABD); pruritus; rash; **Stevens-Johnson syndrome**; **toxic epidermal necrolysis**; urticaria

Other: **Anaphylaxis**, **drug reaction with eosinophilia and systemic symptoms (DRESS)**, drug-induced fever, **hypokalemia**, **infusion reactions (cardiac arrest**, **chest pain**, **dyspnea**, **shock**, **urticaria**, or **wheezing)**, injection-site inflammation, superinfection, vancomycin I.V. infusion reaction (erythema and urticaria of upper body)

Childbearing Considerations

PREGNANCY

- It is not known if oral drug can cause fetal harm.
- Know that vancomycin injection that contains excipients polyethylene glycol (PEG400) and N-acetyl D-alanine (NADA) should not be used during the first or second trimester of pregnancy because of increased risk of fetal spinal malformations, according to animal studies. Other formulations of vancomycin should be used instead.
- Use with caution only if benefit to mother outweighs potential risk to fetus.

LACTATION

- Drug is present in breast milk.
- Mothers should not breastfeed, or drug will need to be discontinued.

Nursing Considerations

! **WARNING** Know that vancomycin is not indicated for prophylaxis of endophthalmitis, nor should it be administered intracamerally or intravitreally, especially during or after cataract surgery because it may cause hemorrhagic occlusive retinal vasculitis that may result in permanent vision loss.

! **WARNING** Be aware that vancomycin injection that contains excipients polyethylene glycol (PEG400) and N-acetyl D-alanine (NADA) should not be used during the first or second trimester of pregnancy because of increased risk of fetal spinal malformations, according to animal studies. Other formulations of vancomycin should be used instead.

- Know that oral vancomycin is only used for GI *Clostridioides difficile* and staphylococcal infections. Patients cannot be converted from I.V. to oral vancomycin for other infections.
- Expect to monitor blood vancomycin concentrations frequently. Higher trough concentrations of 15 to 20 mg/L are commonly targeted now, though they are associated with more nephrotoxicity than the lower trough concentrations previously used. Monitoring vancomycin concentrations in patients with colitis or

renal impairment is especially important because significant increases in blood drug level have occurred in such patients taking multiple oral doses of vancomycin. Assess patient often for adverse reactions because vancomycin absorption may be increased in these conditions.

! **WARNING** Assess patient for hypersensitivity reactions, including severe skin reactions, which could become life-threatening, such as anaphylaxis and DRESS. DRESS may initially only present wtih a fever or swollen lymph nodes although a rash is most common. At the first sign of a hypersensitivity or severe skin reaction, notify prescriber immediately, expect drug to be discontinued, and provide supportive care, as needed and ordered.

! **WARNING** Monitor patient closely for diarrhea when receiving intravenous form of vancomycin because it may indicate pseudomembranous colitis caused by *C. difficile*, a risk with many antibiotics. Diarrhea may be mild to life-threatening. If diarrhea occurs during therapy, notify prescriber and expect to obtain a stool specimen. If confirmed, expect to withhold drug and treat with an antibiotic effective against *C. difficile*, as ordered. Also, expect to administer electrolytes, fluids, and protein supplementation, as needed and ordered.

! **WARNING** Monitor patient's blood pressure as drug can cause hypotension.

! **WARNING** Check CBC results and BUN and serum creatinine levels during therapy, especially if patient has renal impairment or takes an aminoglycoside because systemic vancomycin may cause acute kidney injury.

! **WARNING** Assess hearing during therapy. Transient or permanent ototoxicity may occur if patient receives an excessive amount of drug, has an underlying hearing loss, or receives concurrent aminoglycosides.

! **WARNING** Monitor patient for other persistent, severe, or unusual adverse reactions.

PATIENT TEACHING

! **WARNING** Tell females of childbearing age to alert prescriber before drug is given intravenously if pregnant because of potential harm to fetus.

- Instruct patient how to take oral form of vancomycin prescribed.
- Instruct patient to complete full course of oral vancomycin, as prescribed. However, advise patient to notify prescriber if no improvement occurs after a few days.

! **WARNING** Alert patient that drug may cause allergic reactions, including severe skin reactions. Tell patient to notify prescriber if an allergic or skin reaction occurs, including a fever, rash, swollen lymph nodes, or other skin abnormalities. If severe, instruct patient to seek immediate medical care.

! **WARNING** Instruct patient to notify prescriber if she develops persistent or severe diarrhea as further treatment may be needed.

! **WARNING** Tell patient to notify prescriber immediately if patient notices a decrease in hearing or any other persistent, serious, or unusual adverse reaction.

- Instruct patient to keep follow-up appointments during and after treatment.
- Inform mothers breastfeeding is not recommended during vancomycin therapy or if breastfeeding occurs, drug will need to be discontinued.

vardenafil hydrochloride

Class and Category

Pharmacologic class: Phosphodiesterase type 5 (PDE-5) inhibitor
Therapeutic class: Anti-impotence agent

Indications and Dosages

∗ *To treat erectile dysfunction*

ORALLY DISINTEGRATING TABLETS

Adults. 10 mg taken 1 hr before sexual activity. *Maximum:* 10 mg within 24-hr period.

TABLETS

Adults. 10 mg taken 1 hr before sexual activity; increased to 20 mg or decreased to 5 mg, as needed. *Maximum:* 20 mg and once-daily limit regardless of dosage.

±**DOSAGE ADJUSTMENT** For patients taking cobicistat or ritonavir, vardenafil dosage shouldn't exceed 2.5 mg in 72 hours. For patients taking atazanavir, clarithromycin, indinavir, itraconazole 400 mg daily, ketoconazole 400 mg daily, saquinavir, or another potent CYP3A4 inhibitor, vardenafil dosage shouldn't exceed 2.5 mg in 24 hours. For patients taking erythromycin, itraconazole 200 mg daily, or ketoconazole 200 mg daily, vardenafil dosage shouldn't exceed 5 mg in 24 hours. For patients 65 or over, initial dosage should be reduced to 5 mg. For patients on stable alpha-blocker therapy, starting dose limited to 5 mg. For patients with moderate hepatic impairment, starting dose limited to 5 mg and maximum dose should not exceed 10 mg.

Drug Administration

P.O.

- Tablets are not interchangeable with oral disintegrating tablets.
- Don't remove orally disintegrated tablet from blister pack until ready to use. Have patient place orally disintegrating tablet on his tongue immediately after removing it from the blister package and allow it to dissolve. It should not be chewed, crushed, or split, or not taken with any liquid.

Route	Onset	Peak	Duration
P.O.	60 min	0.5–2 hr	4 hr

Half-life: 4–6 hr

Mechanism of Action

Enhances effect of nitric oxide (released in the penis by sexual stimulation) and inhibits phosphodiesterase type 5, which increases cGMP level, relaxes smooth muscle, increasing blood flow into the corpus cavernosum to produce an erection.

Contraindications

Concurrent administration of guanylate cyclase stimulators (riociguat), concurrent intermittent or regular nitrate therapy and nitric oxide donors, hypersensitivity to vardenafil or its components

Interactions

DRUGS

alpha-blockers, antihypertensives, guanylate cyclase stimulators, nitrates, and nitric oxide donors: Profound hypotension
CYP3A4 inhibitors (moderate to strong), such as cobicistat, erythromycin, indinavir, ketoconazole, ritonavir, and other CYP3A4 inhibitors: Increased vardenafil effects
indinavir, ritonavir: Reduced blood levels of indinavir and ritonavir
p-glycoprotein substrates such as dabigatran: Possibly inhibits therapeutic effects of these drugs

FOODS

grapefruit juice: Possibly increased vardenafil effect

Adverse Reactions

CNS: Dizziness, headache, **seizures**, transient global amnesia
CV: **Hypotension**, **prolonged QT interval**
EENT: Decreased vision, hearing loss, loss of vision in one or both eyes, nasal congestion, nonarteritic anterior ischemic optic neuropathy (NAION), rhinitis, sinusitis, tinnitus
GI: Indigestion, nausea
GU: Priapism
MS: Back pain
SKIN: Flushing
Other: Flu-like symptoms

Childbearing Considerations

PREGNANCY

- Drug is not for use in females.

LACTATION

- Drug is not for use in females.

Nursing Considerations

! **WARNING** Know that vardenafil shouldn't be used by men taking class IA (procainamide, quinidine) or class III (amiodarone, sotalol) antiarrhythmics or by men who have congenital prolonged QT interval. Drug may potentiate prolonged QT interval. It should also not be used in men who have hypotension (resting systolic blood pressure of less than 90 mm Hg), MI (within last 6 months), presence of life-threatening arrhythmia, recent history of stroke, severe cardiac failure, uncontrolled hypertension (greater than 170/110 mm Hg), or unstable angina because drug use could worsen these conditions.

! **WARNING** Do not administer any form of nitrates to patient taking vardenafil because of profound hypotension possibly occurring.

If nitrates are necessary, vardenafil should be discontinued.

! **WARNING** Monitor blood pressure and heart rate before and after giving drug, especially if patient takes an alpha-blocker because of increased risk of symptomatic hypotension. Know that 4 hours should elapse after patient takes an alpha-blocker before administering vardenafil to avoid profound hypotension.

! **WARNING** Monitor patients closely with left ventricular outflow obstruction, such as aortic stenosis, and those with severely impaired autonomic control of blood pressure. These conditions increase sensitivity to vasodilators, such as vardenafil.

! **WARNING** Monitor men with penile abnormalities that may predispose them to priapism, or men with mild hepatic impairment or renal dysfunction (although it should not be used if patient is on dialysis).

- Monitor patient's vision, especially if he's over age 50; has coronary artery disease, diabetes, hyperlipidemia, or hypertension; or smokes because vardenafil rarely leads to nonarteritic ischemic optic neuropathy and vision that is decreased, possibly permanently.
- Monitor patient's hearing. Sudden decrease or loss, possibly with dizziness and tinnitus, may occur with vardenafil use. Report such changes immediately and expect drug to be discontinued.

PATIENT TEACHING

! **WARNING** Alert patient that orally disintegrating tablets contain phenylalanine and should not be taken by patients with phenylketonuria. It also contains sorbitol and should not be taken if patient has hereditary problems with fructose intolerance.

! **WARNING** Tell patient not to take vardenafil if he takes an organic nitrate, continuously or intermittently, or within 4 hours of taking an alpha-blocker because profound hypotension and death could result.

- Instruct patient how to administer vardenafil.
- Tell patient to take drug 1 hour before anticipated sexual activity for best results.

! **WARNING** Caution patient not to take vardenafil more than once daily or to exceed 20 mg daily for oral tablet or 10 mg for orally disintegrating tablet. Tell patient to call prescriber or go to the emergency department immediately if more than vardenafil prescribed is accidentally taken.

! **WARNING** Urge patient to notify prescriber at once if erection is painful or lasts longer than 4 hours, to avoid possible penile damage and permanent loss of erectile function.

- Tell patient to stop taking vardenafil and notify prescriber if sudden hearing loss, sudden loss of vision in one or both eyes, or trouble remembering things occurs.
- Advise patient to seek sexual counseling to enhance drug's effects. Inform patient taking orally disintegrating tablets that some form of sexual stimulation is needed for an erection to happen.
- Instruct patient to alert all prescribers of vardenafil use.

varenicline tartrate

Class and Category

Pharmacologic class: Nicotinic receptor partial agonist
Therapeutic class: Nicotinic blocker

Indications and Dosages

✷ As adjunct to smoking cessation treatment

TABLETS

Adults. *Initial:* 0.5 mg once daily for 3 days; then increased to 0.5 mg twice daily for 4 days, and then increased to 1 mg twice daily for a total of 12 wk of therapy. If effective, an additional 12 wk of therapy may be given.

± **DOSAGE ADJUSTMENT** For patients with severe renal impairment (creatinine clearance less than 30 ml/min), initial dose kept at 0.5 mg once daily then increased to maximum dose of 0.5 mg twice daily. For patients undergoing hemodialysis for end-stage renal disease, maximum dosage not to exceed 0.5 mg daily.

Drug Administration

P.O.

- Administer after eating and with a full glass of water.

- Drug may be initiated 1 wk before patient's set date to stop smoking. Alternatively, drug may be initiated, and then patient quits smoking between day 8 and day 35.

Route	Onset	Peak	Duration
P.O.	Unknown	3–4 hr	24 hr

Half-life: 24 hr

Mechanism of Action

Blocks nicotine from activating alpha$_4$beta$_2$ receptors by binding to them. This inhibits nicotine stimulation of the central nervous mesolimbic dopamine system, which is the area that produces pleasure in and reinforcement of smoking.

Contraindications

Hypersensitivity to varenicline or its components

Interactions

DRUGS

insulin, theophylline, warfarin: May alter pharmacodynamics or pharmacokinetics in these drugs
nicotine (transdermal): Increased adverse reactions

ACTIVITIES

alcohol use: May decrease alcohol tolerance, increasing intoxicating effects of alcohol, including aggressive behavior and sometimes amnesia of event

Adverse Reactions

CNS: Abnormal dreams, aggression, agitation, anxiety, asthenia, attention difficulties, behavior changes, **CVA**, delusions, depression, dizziness, dysgeusia, fatigue, hallucinations, headache, **homicidal ideation**, hostility, insomnia, irritability, lethargy, loss of consciousness, malaise, mania, mental impairment, panic, paranoia, psychosis, restlessness, **seizures**, sensory disturbances, sleep disorder, sleepwalking, somnambulism, somnolence, **suicidal ideation**, thirst
CV: Angina, chest pain, edema, hypertension, **MI**, peripheral ischemia, **thrombosis**, **ventricular extrasystole**
EENT: Dry mouth, epistaxis, gingivitis, rhinorrhea
ENDO: Hot flashes, hyperglycemia
GI: Abdominal pain, **acute pancreatitis**, anorexia, constipation, diarrhea, dyspepsia, flatulence, gastroesophageal reflux disease, **GI hemorrhage**, increased appetite, liver enzyme abnormalities, nausea, splenomegaly, vomiting
GU: **Acute renal failure**, polyuria, urine retention
HEME: Leukocytosis, **thrombocytopenia**
MS: Arthralgia, back pain, muscle cramp, musculoskeletal pain, myalgia
RESP: **Asthma**, dyspnea, **pulmonary embolism**
SKIN: Diaphoresis, **erythema multiforme**, pruritus, rash, **Stevens-Johnson syndrome**, urticaria
Other: **Angioedema and other hypersenstivity reactions**, flu-like syndrome, **hyperkalemia**, **hypokalemia**, lymphadenopathy

Childbearing Considerations

PREGNANCY

- It is not known if drug can cause fetal harm.
- Use with caution only if benefit to mother outweighs potential risk to fetus.

LACTATION

- It is not known if drug is present in breast milk.
- Mothers should check with prescriber before breastfeeding.
- If breastfeeding occurs, monitor the breastfed infant for excessive vomiting and seizures.

Nursing Considerations

- Know that varenicline is not recommended for use in children 16 years of age and younger.
- Use cautiously in patients with renal disease because varenicline is substantially excreted by the kidneys.

! WARNING Monitor patient for a hypersensitivity reaction, which could become life-threatening, such as angioedema. If present, notify prescriber immediately, expect to stop varenicline therapy, and provide supportive care, as needed and ordered.

! WARNING Monitor patient for seizures, especially within the first month of therapy, and in patients with a history of seizures or other factors that could lower their seizure threshold. Institute seizure precautions.

! WARNING Know that serious neuropsychiatric adverse effects have occurred with varenicline use, even in patients with no prior psychiatric history. Also, drug can worsen underlying psychiatric disorders. Aggressive or unusual behavior directed to self or others may be exhibited. Observe patient closely. If present, stop drug therapy immediately, notify prescriber, and provide safety measures to protect patient and others. Watch patient closely for suicidal tendencies, particularly when therapy starts and dosage changes because depression may worsen temporarily during these times, possibly leading to suicidal ideation.

- Know that even with varenicline therapy, nicotine withdrawal symptoms may occur with smoking cessation. If present, notify prescriber.

! WARNING Monitor patient for other persistent, serious, or unusual adverse reactions because drug can affect multiple body systems with the potential for life-threatening adverse reactions such as asthma, GI hemorrhage, pancreatitis, and thrombus.

PATIENT TEACHING

- Instruct patient how to administer varenicline after setting a date to quit smoking or starting therapy and then quitting smoking between days 8 and 35 of treatment.
- Inform patient and family or caregiver that nicotine withdrawal can occur even with varenicline use.
- Tell patient varenicline can be taken for an additional 12 weeks of therapy after smoking has stopped, as needed.
- Encourage patient to continue trying to stop smoking even if an early relapse occurs during varenicline therapy.
- Inform patient that the most common adverse reactions to varenicline therapy are insomnia and nausea, which are usually transient. If they persist, patient should notify prescriber; dosage reduction may help, if prescribed.

! WARNING Inform patient and family or caregiver that aggressive or unusual behavior can occur in patients with or without a history of mental illness. Tell them that if patient has an existing mental illness, varenicline therapy may worsen it. Inform them that sometimes these behaviors may become serious and can be directed to self or others and may be worsened by concomitant use of alcohol. Advise patient to avoid alcohol during varenicline therapy and urge family or caregiver to monitor patient closely for suicidal or homicidal tendencies, especially when therapy starts or dosage changes. Advise patient, family, or caregiver to notify prescriber about abnormal thinking or behavior and to stop taking drug immediately if this occurs.

! WARNING Alert patient that drug can cause an allergic reaction. If present, tell patient to notify prescriber and, if severe, to seek immediate medical care.

! WARNING Instruct patient to seek immediate medical care if a seizure or new or worsening symptoms of cardiovascular disease such as calf pain when walking, chest pain, shortness of breath, or sudden onset of difficulty speaking, numbness, or weakness is experienced.

- Caution patient to avoid hazardous activities until CNS effects of drug are known and resolved.
- Explain to patient, family, or caregiver that strange, unusual, or vivid dreams may occur during therapy. Also inform patient that sleepwalking may occur that can lead to behavior that may be harmful to self, others, or property. If sleepwalking occurs, tell patient to stop taking drug and notify prescriber.

! WARNING Tell patient to notify prescriber if other persistent, serious, or unusual adverse reactions occur.

- Advise mothers who are breastfeeding while taking varenicline to monitor infant for excessive vomiting and seizures. If present, tell patient to stop taking varenicline and have infant seen by a pediatrician.

vasopressin

Vasostrict

Class and Category

Pharmacologic class: Posterior pituitary hormone
Therapeutic class: Antidiuretic hormone

Indications and Dosages

* *To increase blood pressure in patients in vasodilatory shock (post-cardiotomy shock or sepsis) who remain hypotensive despite administration of catecholamines and fluids*

I.V. INFUSION

Adults. *Initial:* 0.01 units/min (septic shock) or 0.03 units/min (post-cardiotomy shock), titrated up by 0.005 units/min at 10- to 15-min intervals, as needed. After target blood pressure has been maintained for 8 hr without the use of catecholamines, dosage tapered by 0.005 units/min every hr, as tolerated, to maintain target blood pressure. *Maximum:* 0.07 units/min (septic shock); 0.1units/min (post-cardiotomy shock).

Drug Administration

I.V.

- If using a single-dose vial that requires dilution or a multiple-dose vial, dilute to a concentration of 0.1 units/ml using 0.9% Sodium Chloride Injection or 5% Dextrose in Water by diluting 50 units in 500 ml; if fluid restriction is present, dilute 100 units in 100 ml to yield a concentration of 1 unit/ml. Drug may also come as premixed in dextrose in a single dose vial that does not require further dilution prior to administration.
- Store diluted drug at room temperature for up to 18 hr or refrigerated for up to 24 hr.
- Use an infusion pump to administer drug.
- Infuse continuously starting with 0.03 units/min for post-cardiotomy shock or 0.01 units/min for septic shock. Titrate up by 0.005 units/min at 10- to 15-min intervals, as needed. Do not exceed 0.1 units/min for post-cardiotomy shock and 0.07 units/min for septic shock.
- After initial entry into the 10-ml multidose vial, vial must be refrigerated. Discard multidose 10-ml vial after 30 days from first puncture.
- *Incompatibilities:* None listed by manufacturer

Route	Onset	Peak	Duration
I.V.	Rapid	15 min	20 min

Half-life: < 10 min

Mechanism of Action

Be aware that vasoconstrictive effects are mediated by vascular V_1 receptors that are directly coupled to phospholipase C, resulting in release of calcium. This leads to vasoconstriction. In addition, vasopressin stimulates antidiuresis via stimulation of V_2 receptors that are coupled to adenyl cyclase. Both of these actions help to raise blood pressure.

Contraindications

Hypersensitivity to vasopressin or its components, hypersensitivity to 8-L-arginine vasopressin, hypersensitivity to chlorobutanol found in the 10-ml multiple-dose vial but not in the 1-ml single-dose vial

Interactions

DRUGS

catecholamines: Additive effect on mean arterial blood pressure and other hemodynamic parameters
drugs suspected of causing diabetes insipidus (clozapine, demeclocycline, foscarnet, lithium): Decreased diuretic and pressor effects of vasopressin
drugs suspected of causing SIADH (chlorpropamide, cyclophosphamide, enalapril, felbamate, haloperidol, ifosfamide, methyldopa, pentamidine, selected serotonin reuptake inhibitors, tricyclic antidepressants): Possibly increased diuretic and pressor effects of vasopressin
furosemide: Increased effect of vasopressin on osmolar clearance and urine flow
ganglionic blocking agents: Increased effect on mean arterial blood pressure
indomethacin: Possibly prolonged effect of vasopressin on cardiac index and systemic vascular resistance

Adverse Reactions

CV: **Atrial fibrillation**, **bradycardia**, **decreased cardiac index**, **myocardial ischemia**, **right heart failure**
EENT: Circumoral pallor

ENDO: Reversible diabetes insipidus
GI: Elevated bilirubin levels, mesenteric ischemia
GU: **Acute renal insufficiency**
HEME: **Decreased platelets**, **hemorrhagic shock**, **intractable bleeding**
MS: Distal limb ischemia
SKIN: Pruritus, rash, urticaria
Other: **Hypersensitivity reactions**, **hyponatremia**

Childbearing Considerations

PREGNANCY

- It is not known if drug can cause fetal harm. However, drug can produce tonic uterine contractions, which could threaten pregnancy continuation.
- Use with caution only if benefit to mother outweighs potential risk to fetus. Be aware that dosage increase may be needed in the second or third trimester.

LACTATION

- It is not known if drug is present in breast milk.
- Once condition is stabilized, mothers should check with prescriber before breastfeeding.

Nursing Considerations

! **WARNING** Use cautiously in patients with impaired cardiac response because vasopressin may worsen cardiac output. Also, be aware that a decrease in cardiac index may occur with the use of vasopressin, indicating worsening of cardiac function. Monitor patient closely for other cardiovascular adverse reactions such as atrial fibrillation, bradycardia, myocardial ischemia, or right heart failure and alert prescriber immediately, if present.

! **WARNING** Monitor patient for hypersensitivity reactions, which could be severe. Notify prescriber immediately, if present, and expect to provide supportive care, as needed and ordered.

! **WARNING** Monitor patient's BUN and creatinine level, as ordered, because drug can cause acute renal insufficiency. Also, monitor patient's platelet level, as ordered, because drug can cause a decrease in platelet count. Also, monitor patient for signs and symptoms of serious hematologic adverse reactions such as intractable bleeding. Notify prescriber immediately, if bleeding occurs or a significant drop in patient's platelet count occurs.

- Monitor patient for reversible diabetes insipidus after treatment of vasopressin is completed. Signs to be alert for include dilute urine, hypernatremia, and polyuria. Also monitor patient's serum electrolytes, fluid status, and urine output after vasopressin has been discontinued. Be aware that some patients may require readministration of vasopressin or administration of desmopressin to correct fluid and electrolyte shifts.

PATIENT TEACHING

- Inform patient, if alert, that drug will be administered intravenously.
- Tell patient to notify staff if discomfort occurs at the infusion site, if patient is able.

! **WARNING** Advise patient to immediately report any adverse reactions experienced, especially allergic reactions, such as difficulty breathing or swallowing, hives, or swelling of face or tongue.

venlafaxine hydrochloride

Effexor XR

venlafaxine besylate

desvenlafaxine

desvenlafaxine succinate

Class and Category

Pharmacologic class: Selective serotonin and norepinephrine reuptake inhibitor (SSNRI)
Therapeutic class: Antidepressant

Indications and Dosages

✱ *To treat and prevent relapse of major depression*

E.R. CAPSULES (EFFEXOR XR)

Adults. 75 mg once daily (for some patients, 37.5 mg once daily for 4 to 7 days before increasing to 75 mg daily); then increased by 75 mg daily every 4 days or longer, as needed. *Maximum:* 225 mg daily.

E.R. TABLETS (DESVENLAFAXINE)

Adults. 50 mg once daily. *Maximum:* 50 mg once daily.

E.R. TABLETS (VENLAFAXINE BESYLATE)

Adults who have received at least 75 mg/day of another venlafaxine E.R. product for at least 4 days. *Initial:* 112.5 mg once daily, Dosage increased in increments of up to 75 mg daily, as needed, using another venlafaxine E.R. product at intervals of 4 days or more. *Maximum:* 225 mg once daily.

✱ *To treat generalized anxiety disorder*

E.R. CAPSULES (EFFEXOR XR)

Adults. 75 mg once daily (for some patients, 37.5 mg once daily for 4 to 7 days before increasing to 75 mg once daily); then increased by 75 mg daily every 4 days or longer, as needed. *Maximum:* 225 mg daily.

E.R. TABLETS (VENLAFAXINE BESYLATE)

Adults who have received at least 75 mg/day of another venlafaxine E.R. product for at least 4 days. *Initial:* 112.5 mg once daily. Dosage increased in increments of up to 75 mg daily, as needed, using another venlafaxine E.R. product at intervals of 4 days or more. *Maximum:* 225 mg once daily.

✱ *To treat social anxiety disorder*

E.R. CAPSULES (EFFEXOR XR), E.R. TABLETS (VENLAFAXINE)

Adults. 75 mg once daily. *Maximum:* 75 mg once daily.

✱ *To treat panic disorder*

E.R. CAPSULES (EFFEXOR XR)

Adults. *Initial:* 37.5 mg once daily for 7 days, increased to 75 mg once daily, as needed; then increased by 75 mg daily every 4 days or more, as needed. *Maximum:* 225 mg daily.

± **DOSAGE ADJUSTMENT** *Effexor XR, venlafaxine besylate:* For patients with mild to moderate renal impairment, initial daily dose decreased by 25% to 50%. For patients undergoing dialysis or who have severe renal impairment, daily dose reduced by 50%. For patients with mild to moderate hepatic failure, dose reduced by 50%; for patients with severe hepatic impairment or hepatic cirrhosis, dosage may have to be reduced more than 50%. *Desvenlafaxine:* For patients with severe renal impairment and end-stage renal disease, maximum dose is 25 mg daily or 50 mg every other day.

Drug Administration

P.O.

- Administer venlafaxine products with food; desvenlafaxine with or without food and give with a full glass of water.
- Administer drug at the same time each day—morning or evening.
- Capsules and tablets should be swallowed whole and not chewed or crushed.
- If patient has trouble swallowing capsules, open capsule, sprinkle contents on a spoonful of applesauce, and have patient swallow immediately without chewing, followed by a glass of water.

Route	Onset	Peak	Duration
P.O./E.R.	1 2 wk	5.5–9 hr	Unknown

Half-life: 3–7 hr

Mechanism of Action

Inhibits neuronal reuptake of norepinephrine and serotonin, along with its active metabolite, *O*-desmethylvenlafaxine. These actions raise norepinephrine and serotonin levels at nerve synapses, elevating mood and reducing anxiety, depression, and panic.

Contraindications

Hypersensitivity to desvenlafaxine, venlafaxine, or their components; use of an MAO inhibitor within 14 days, including intravenous methylene blue and linezolid

Interactions

DRUGS

aspirin, NSAIDs, warfarin, and other anticoagulants: Increased risk of bleeding
CYP2D6 substrates, such as atomoxetine, desipramine, dextromethorphan, metoprolol, nebivolol, perphenazine, tolterodine: Increased risk of toxicity of these drugs
serotonergic drugs, such as amphetamines, buspirone, fentanyl, lithium, MAO inhibitors, other selected serotonin reuptake inhibitors,

other serotonin–norepinephrine reuptake inhibitors, St. John's wort, tramadol, tricyclic antidepressants, triptans, tryptophan: Possibly serotonin syndrome

ACTIVITIES

alcohol use: Increased CNS effects

Adverse Reactions

CNS: Abnormal dreams, agitation, amnesia, anxiety, asthenia, attention disturbance, bruxism, **cerebral ischemia**, chills, confusion, delirium, delusions, depersonalization, depression, dizziness, dream disturbances, drowsiness, dyskinesia, extrapyramidal disorder, fatigue, fever, hallucinations, headache, hypesthesia, hypomania, impaired balance and coordination, insomnia, irritability, mania, migraine, mood changes, nervousness, **neuroleptic malignant syndrome**, paresthesia, **seizures**, **serotonin syndrome**, somnolence, **suicidal ideation**, syncope, tardive dyskinesia, tremor, vertigo
CV: **Arrhythmias**, **AV block**, chest pain, **congestive heart failure**, elevated cholesterol and triglyceride levels, edema, **extrasystoles**, hypertension, **hypotension**, **MI**, palpitations, **prolonged QT interval**, sinus tachycardia, **Takotsubo cardiomyopathy**, thrombophlebitis, **torsades de pointes**, vasodilation, **ventricular fibrillation or tachycardia**, worsening of peripheral vascular disease
EENT: Abnormal vision, accommodation abnormality, angle-closure glaucoma, blurred vision, dry mouth, mucous membrane bleeding, mydriasis, pharyngitis, rhinitis, taste alteration, tinnitus
ENDO: Elevated blood prolactin levels, hot flashes, hyperglycemia, syndrome of inappropriate ADH secretion
GI: Abdominal pain, anorexia, colitis, constipation, diarrhea, elevated liver enzymes, flatulence, **GI hemorrhage**, **hepatic failure or necrosis**, **hepatitis**, indigestion, nausea, **pancreatitis**, vomiting
GU: Anorgasmia (women), decreased libido, ejaculation disorder, erectile dysfunction, **renal failure**, urinary incontinence or urgency, urine hesitancy or retention
HEME: **Abnormal bleeding**, **agranulocytosis**, anemia, **aplastic anemia**, leukocytosis, **leukopenia**, **neutropenia**, **pancytopenia**, **prolonged bleeding time**, **thrombocytopenia**
MS: Neck pain, musculoskeletal stiffness, **rhabdomyolysis**
RESP: Cough, **eosinophilic pneumonia**, increased dyspnea, **interstitial lung disease**
SKIN: Diaphoresis, ecchymosis, **erythema multiforme**, pruritus, rash, **Stevens-Johnson syndrome**, **toxic epidermal necrolysis**
Other: **Anaphylaxis**, **angioedema**, **and other hypersensitivity reactions**; discontinuation syndrome; **hyponatremia**; lymphadenopathy; weight gain or loss

Childbearing Considerations

PREGNANCY

- Pregnancy exposure registry: 1-844-405-6185 or https://womensmentalhealth.org/clinical-and-research-programs/pregnancyregistry/antidepressants/.
- Drug may cause fetal harm, especially if exposure occurs late in third trimester. At birth, neonate may possibly require prolonged hospitalization, respiratory support, and tube feeding.
- Use with caution only if benefit to mother outweighs potential risk to fetus.

LABOR AND DELIVERY

- Drug given within 1 month of delivery increases risk of postpartum hemorrhage.

LACTATION

- Drug is present in breast milk.
- Mothers should check with prescriber before breastfeeding.

Nursing Considerations

- Be aware that desvenlafaxine and venlafaxine should not be given to patients with bradycardia, congenital long QT syndrome, hypokalemia or hypomagnesemia, recent acute MI, or uncompensated heart failure because of increased risk of prolonged QT interval and torsades de pointes. It should also not be given to patients who are taking other drugs that prolong the QT interval. Expect hypokalemia and hypomagnesemia to be corrected before drug therapy is begun.

! WARNING Know that drug should not be given to pregnant patients who are in the latter half of the third trimester of pregnancy because it can adversely affect the neonate at birth and if given within 1 month of delivery mother's risk of postpartum hemorrhage is increased.

- Use cautiously in patients with a history of mania because desvenlafaxine and venlafaxine therapy may worsen condition.

! **WARNING** Know that drug shouldn't be stopped abruptly because doing so may cause multiple adverse effects, including asthenia, dizziness, flu-like symptoms, headache, insomnia, and nervousness. Notify prescriber if patient experiences aggression, suicidal thoughts, or violent behavior as well as visual changes and increased blood pressure during dosage reduction or discontinuation. Know that discontinuation may have to occur over several months.

! **WARNING** Watch patient for suicidal tendencies, especially when therapy starts and dosage changes.

! **WARNING** Monitor patient for a hypersensitivity reaction, which could become life-threatening, such as anaphylaxis or angioedema. If present, notify prescriber, expect drug to be switched to a different drug, and provide supportive care, as needed and ordered.

! **WARNING** Monitor patients for seizures, especially with patients who have a history of seizures. Institute seizure precautions, as appropriate.

! **WARNING** Monitor patients who have medical conditions that might be made worse by an increased heart rate, as in heart failure, hyperthyroidism, or recent MI.

! **WARNING** Monitor patient closely for abnormal bleeding that may range from ecchymosis to life-threatening hemorrhage. Know that concomitant use of desvenlafaxine, or venlafaxine with drugs known to affect bleeding or coagulation increases the risk of bleeding.

! **WARNING** Be aware that serotonin syndrome in its most severe form may resemble neuroleptic malignant syndrome, which includes autonomic instability with possibly rapid changes in vital signs, hyperthermia, mental status changes, and muscle rigidity. Withhold drug until prescriber has been notified and provide supportive care. Expect drug to be discontinued.

- Monitor blood pressure often during therapy because it may cause dose-related sustained increase in supine diastolic pressure. Notify prescriber if increase develops.

! **WARNING** Assess patient's electrolyte balance, as ordered, because drug can cause hyponatremia, especially in elderly patients and in patients who take diuretics or are volume-depleted. If patient has evidence of hyponatremia (confusion, headache, trouble concentrating, unsteadiness, weakness), notify prescriber. If imbalance is confirmed, give supportive care, as prescribed.

! **WARNING** Notify prescriber if patient develops other persistent, serious, or unusual adverse reactions.

- Be aware that false-positive urine immunoassay screening tests for amphetamine and phencyclidine (PCP) have been found in patients taking desvenlafaxine or venlafaxine. Expect different testing to be done to distinguish drug from PCP and amphetamine.

PATIENT TEACHING

- Encourage patient to have an eye exam before starting therapy to see if he is at risk for an episode of acute angle-closure glaucoma that may occur with drug use.

! **WARNING** Inform pregnant patients to alert prescriber when entering their third trimester as drug can adversely affect neonate when born. Also, tell these patients that drug should be avoided within 1 month of delivery.

- Instruct patient how to administer form of drug prescribed.
- Advise patient to avoid alcohol during desvenlafaxine or venlafaxine therapy.

! **WARNING** Caution patient not to stop taking drug abruptly, as serious adverse reactions could occur. Tell patient to notify prescriber during a dosage reduction or discontinuation of the drug if aggression, anxiety, irritability, suicidal thoughts, tremor, visual changes, or feelings of violence occur.

! **WARNING** Urge caregivers to monitor patient closely for suicidal tendencies, especially when therapy starts or dosage changes.

! **WARNING** Alert patient that drug may cause an allergic reaction. If present, tell patient to notify prescriber and, if severe, to seek immediate medical care.

- Encourage patient to discuss sexual dysfunction if present.

! **WARNING** Tell patient to report other persistent, severe, or unusual symptoms.

- Tell patient to inform all prescribers of desvenlafaxine or venlafaxine therapy and not to take any over-the-counter medications, including herbal preparations, without prescriber knowledge. Also, caution patient to avoid aspirin and NSAIDs, if possible, while taking desvenlafaxine or venlafaxine.
- Inform patient that urine screening tests for amphetamine and phencyclidine (PCP) may produce a false-positive for several days following discontinuation of desvenlafaxine or venlafaxine therapy, but that other tests may be done to distinguish drug from amphetamine and PCP.

verapamil hydrochloride

Calan SR, Verelan, Verelan PM

Class and Category

Pharmacologic class: Calcium channel blocker
Therapeutic class: Antianginal, antiarrhythmic, antihypertensive

Indications and Dosages

* *To treat angina at rest, including unstable (crescendo, pre-infarction) angina or vasospastic (Prinzmetal's variant) angina*

TABLETS

Adults. 80 mg to 120 mg 3 times daily.

± **DOSAGE ADJUSTMENT** For patients who may have an increased response such as being elderly or having decreased hepatic function, dosage reduced to 40 mg 3 times daily then increased daily or weekly, as needed.

* *To manage hypertension*

S.R. CAPSULES (VERELAN)

Adults. *Initial:* 180 mg once daily in the morning and then titrated, as needed, according to the following schedule: 240 mg once daily in the morning; then 360 mg once daily in the morning; and then 480 mg once daily in the morning.

± **DOSAGE ADJUSTMENT** For elderly and low-weight patients, initial dosage reduced to 120 mg once daily and then titrated, as needed, beginning with 180 mg once daily.

S.R. TABLETS (CALAN SR)

Adults. *Initial:* 180 mg once daily in the morning increased, as needed, to 240 mg once daily in the morning. Alternatively, titrated to 180 mg twice daily or 240 mg in the morning and 120 mg in the evening with further increase to 240 mg twice daily, as needed.

± **DOSAGE ADJUSTMENT** For elderly and low-weight patients, initial dosage reduced to 120 mg once daily.

TABLETS

Adults. *Initial:* 80 mg daily given in 3 divided doses and increased, as needed. *Maximum*: 480 mg daily.

± **DOSAGE ADJUSTMENT** For the elderly or people of small stature, initial dose reduced to 40 mg in 3 divided doses.

E.R. CAPSULES (VERELAN PM)

Adults. *Initial:* 200 mg nightly, increased to 300 mg nightly, then to 400 mg nightly, if needed.

± **DOSAGE ADJUSTMENT** For patients with an increased response to verapamil such as patients with impaired hepatic or renal function, elderly patients, and low-weight patients, initial dose reduced to 100 mg nightly and then titrated, as needed.

* *To treat supraventricular tachyarrhythmias, including atrial fibrillation or flutter*

TABLETS

Adults digitalized with chronic atrial fibrillation. 240 to 320 mg daily in divided 3 or 4 doses.

I.V. INJECTION (VERAPAMIL HYDROCHLORIDE)

Adults and adolescents ages 15 and older. *Initial:* 5 to 10 mg given as an I.V. bolus over at least 2 min (over at least 3 min for older patients); then 10 mg, as needed, if response isn't adequate after 30 min.

Children ages 1 to 15. *Initial:* 0.1 to 0.3 mg/kg given as an I.V. bolus over at least 2 min (usual single-dose range: 2 to 5 mg); then dosage repeated as needed, if response isn't adequate after 30 min. *Maximum:* 5 mg as the initial dose; 10 mg as a repeat dose.

Infants up to age 1. *Initial:* 0.1 to 0.2 mg/kg given as an I.V. bolus over at least 2 min (usual single-dose range: 0.75 to 2 mg); then dosage repeated, as needed, if response isn't adequate after 30 min.

∗ *To prevent paroxysmal supraventricular tachycardia*

TABLETS

Non-digitalized adults. 240 to 480 mg daily in divided 3 to 4 doses.

Drug Administration

P.O.

- Capsules should be swallowed whole and not chewed or crushed. Capsules may be opened and sprinkled on a spoonful of applesauce. Mixture should be swallowed immediately without chewing and followed with a glass of cool water. Administer Verelan PM capsules at bedtime.
- Do not store mixture for later use.
- Tablets should be swallowed whole and not chewed, crushed, or divided.
- Do not administer drug with grapefruit juice.

I.V.

- Maintain continuous ECG monitoring and keep emergency resuscitative equipment and drugs readily available during I.V. therapy.
- Inspect solution before administration; should be clear.
- Administer directly through free-flowing I.V. line with compatible solutions, including 0.9% Sodium Chloride Injection, 5% Dextrose in Water, or Ringer's Injection.
- Inject slowly over at least 2 min; at least 3 min for elderly patients.
- *Incompatibilities:* Albumin, amphotericin B, hydralazine hydrochloride, Sodium Lactate Injection in polyvinyl chloride bags, solutions with a pH above 6.0, trimethoprim with sulfamethoxazole

Route	Onset	Peak	Duration
P.O.	1–2 hr	1–2 hr	8–10 hr
P.O./E.R.	30 min	5–9 hr	24 hr
I.V.	1–5 min	10–15 min	0.5–1 hr

Half-life: 5–12 hr (P.O.); 2–5 hr (I.V.)

Mechanism of Action

Inhibits calcium movement into coronary and vascular smooth-muscle cells by blocking slow calcium channels in cell membranes. The resulting decrease in intracellular calcium level has the following effects:

- inhibits smooth-muscle cell contractions.
- decreases myocardial oxygen demand by relaxing coronary and vascular smooth muscle, reducing peripheral vascular resistance, and decreasing systolic and diastolic pressures.
- slows AV conduction time and prolongs AV nodal refractoriness.
- interrupts reentry circuit in AV nodal reentrant tachycardias.

Contraindications

Cardiogenic shock, concomitant use of beta-blockers (with I.V. verapamil), hypersensitivity to verapamil or its components, hypotension, severe heart failure unless secondary to supraventricular tachycardia that responds to verapamil, severe left ventricular dysfunction, sick sinus syndrome or second- or third-degree heart block unless artificial pacemaker is in place, use in atrial fibrillation or flutter and an accessory bypass tract is present such as Lown-Ganong-Levine or Wolff-Parkinson-White syndromes (with I.V. verapamil), ventricular tachycardia (with I.V. verapamil)

Interactions

DRUGS

antihypertensives: Hypotensive effects
aspirin: Increased bleeding time
beta-blockers: Increased risk of heart failure, hypotension, and severe bradycardia
carbamazepine, cyclosporine, theophylline: Increased risk of toxicity from these drugs
cimetidine: Decreased metabolism and increased blood level of verapamil
clonidine: Increased risk of severe sinus bradycardia

dantrolene: Increased risk of hyperkalemia and myocardial depression
digoxin: Increased blood digoxin level and risk of digitalis toxicity
disopyramide, flecainide: Additive negative inotropic effects
erythromycin, ritonavir: Increased blood verapamil level
HMG-CoA reductase inhibitors, such as atorvastatin, lovastatin, and simvastatin: Increased risk of myopathy and rhabdomyolysis
ivabradine: Increased exposure to ivabradine with possible exacerbation of bradycardia and conduction disturbances
lithium: Altered serum lithium levels
mTOR inhibitors, such as everolimus, sirolimus, temsirolimus: Increased plasma levels of mTOR inhibitors and verapamil
neuromuscular blockers: Prolonged recovery from neuromuscular blockade
paclitaxel: Decreased paclitaxel clearance
phenobarbital: Increased verapamil clearance
quinidine: Increased risk of quinidine toxicity, increased QT interval, additive negative inotropic effects
rifampin: Decreased bioavailability of oral verapamil
telithromycin: Increased risk of bradyarrhythmia, hypotension

ACTIVITIES

alcohol use: Increased blood alcohol level and prolonged CNS effects

FOODS

grapefruit juice: Increased verapamil level

Adverse Reactions

CNS: Asthenia, confusion, **CVA**, disequilibrium, dizziness, equilibrium disorders, extrapyramidal reactions, fatigue, headache, insomnia, paresthesia, psychosis, shakiness, somnolence, syncope
CV: **Abnormal ECG**, angina, **AV conduction disorders**, **bradycardia**, claudication, **heart failure**, hypertension, **hypotension**, **MI**, palpitations, peripheral edema, tachycardia, vasculitis
EENT: Blurred vision, dry mouth, tinnitus
ENDO: Gynecomastia, hyperprolactinemia
GI: Constipation, diarrhea, elevated liver enzymes, GI distress, nausea
GU: Galactorrhea, impotence, increased urination, menstrual irregularities
MS: Arthralgia, muscle spasms
RESP: Dyspnea, **pulmonary edema**
SKIN: Alopecia, diaphoresis, ecchymosis, **erythema multiforme**, exanthema, flushing, hyperkeratosis, pruritis, rash, **Stevens-Johnson syndrome**, urticaria
Other: **Angioedema** (rare)

Childbearing Considerations

PREGNANCY

- It is not known if drug causes fetal harm, although it does cross the placental barrier.
- Use with caution only if benefit to mother outweighs potential risk to fetus.

LACTATION

- Drug is present in breast milk.
- Breastfeeding should be discontinued during drug therapy.

Nursing Considerations

- Know that disopyramide or flecainide shouldn't be given within 48 hr before or 24 hr after verapamil because additive negative inotropic effects can result.

! WARNING Monitor patient for a hypersensitivity reaction or severe skin reaction, which could become life-threatening, such as angioedema and Stevens-Johnson syndrome. If present, notify prescriber, expect drug to be discontinued, and provide supportive care, as needed and ordered.

! WARNING Monitor patient with hypertrophic cardiomyopathy or idiopathic hypertrophic subaortic stenosis closely for early development of hypotension and pulmonary edema because second-degree AV block and sinus arrest can result.

! WARNING Notify prescriber if blood pressure or heart rate declines significantly.

! WARNING Monitor patient for other persistent, serious, or unusual adverse reactions.

- Institute measures to prevent constipation, including a high-fiber diet and a stool softener, as prescribed.

PATIENT TEACHING

- Direct patient to check pulse before taking verapamil and to notify prescriber if it's below 50 beats/min or as instructed by prescriber.

- Instruct patient how to administer oral form of verapamil prescribed.

! **WARNING** Alert patient that drug may cause an allergic reaction. If present, tell patient to notify prescriber and, if serious, to seek immediate medical care.

- Inform patient that adverse skin reactions may subside with continued verapamil use. Advise her to notify prescriber if rash persists.
- Caution patient about possible dizziness and the need to avoid potentially hazardous activities until drug's CNS effects are known and resolved.

! **WARNING** Instruct patient to notify prescriber of any other persistent, serious, or unusual adverse reactions, some of which could be quite serious such as heart failure or pulmonary edema.

- Encourage patient to increase dietary fiber intake to help prevent constipation. Advise her to notify prescriber if problem becomes persistent or severe.
- Inform mothers breastfeeding is not recommended during drug therapy.

vericiguat

Verquvo

Class and Category

Pharmacologic class: Soluble guanylate cyclase (sGC) stimulator
Therapeutic class: Vasodilator

Indications and Dosages

∗ *To reduce the risk of cardiovascular death and heart failure hospitalization following a hospitalization for heart failure or need for outpatient I.V. diuretics in adults with symptomatic chronic heart failure and ejection fraction less than 45%*

TABLETS

Adults. *Initial:* 2.5 mg once daily with food. Dose doubled every 2 wk to reach target maintenance dose of 10 mg, as tolerated. *Maintenance:* 10 mg once daily.

Drug Administration

P.O.

- Ensure that a pregnancy test has been done and is negative in females of childbearing age before administering the first dose.
- Administer drug with food.
- Tablet should be swallowed whole. However, for patients unable to swallow the tablet, crush and mix with water immediately before administering drug.

Route	Onset	Peak	Duration
P.O.	Unknown	Unknown	Unknown

Half-life: 30 hr

Mechanism of Action

Stimulates soluble guanylate cyclase (sGC), which is an enzyme in the nitric oxide signaling pathway. When nitric oxide binds to this enzyme, it catalyzes the synthesis of intracellular cyclic guanosine monophosphate (cGMP). cGMP helps to regulate cardiac contractility, cardiac remodeling, and vascular tone. By stimulating sGC, vericiguat increases levels of intracellular cGMP, which causes smooth muscles to relax and vasodilation to occur.

Contraindications

Concomitant therapy with other soluble guanylate cyclase stimulators, hypersensitivity to vericiguat or its components, pregnancy

Interactions

DRUGS

PDE-5 inhibitors: Potential for hypotension
other soluble guanylate cyclase stimulators: Additive effects leading to possibility of serious cardiovascular adverse reactions

Adverse Reactions

CV: Hypotension
HEME: Anemia

Childbearing Considerations

PREGNANCY

- Pregnancy exposure registry: 1-877-888-4231 or https://pregnancyreporting.verquvo-us.com.
- Drug may cause fetal harm such as heart and major blood vessel malformations, according to animal studies.
- Drug is contraindicated during pregnancy.

LACTATION

- It is not known if drug is present in breast milk.
- Breastfeeding is not recommended during drug therapy.

REPRODUCTION

- Females of childbearing age should use an effective method of contraception during drug therapy and for 1 mo after the final dose.

Nursing Considerations

! **WARNING** Ensure females of childbearing age has a negative pregnancy test result before administering the first dose as drug can cause fetal harm. Tell these patients to use an effective method of contraception during drug therapy and for 1 month after the final dose.

! **WARNING** Monitor patient's blood pressure for signs of hypotension.

- Assess patient for signs and symptoms of anemia, such as fatigue and pallor. Expect to monitor patient's hemoglobin and hematocrit, as well.

PATIENT TEACHING

! **WARNING** Alert females of childbearing age that vericiguat is contraindicated in pregnancy. Tell these patients that a negative pregnancy test will be required before drug therapy is started. Stress importance of notifying prescriber if pregnancy occurs during drug therapy.

- Instruct patient how to administer vericiguat.

! **WARNING** Instruct patient how to measure blood pressure and to alert prescriber if low blood pesssure readings occur.

- Advise patient to alert prescriber if signs and symptoms of anemia occurs such as fatigue and pallor.
- Tell mothers not to breastfeed their infant.

vibegron

Gemtesa

Class and Category

Pharmacologic class: Beta$_3$-adrenergic agonist

Therapeutic class: Bladder muscle relaxant

Indications and Dosages

✱ *To treat overactive bladder with symptoms of urge urinary incontinence, urgency, and urinary frequency; to treat overactive bladder with symptoms of urge urinary incontinence, urgency, and urinary frequency in males on pharmacological therapy for benign prostatic hyperplasia*

TABLETS

Adults. 75 mg once daily.

Drug Administration

P.O.

- Administer with a glass of water.
- Tablets may be crushed and mixed with a tablespoon of applesauce and ingested immediately. Follow immediately with a glass of water.

Route	Onset	Peak	Duration
P.O.	Unknown	1–3 hr	Unknown

Half-life: 30.8 hr

Mechanism of Action

Relaxes the detrusor smooth muscle during bladder filling to increase bladder capacity, which reduces overactive bladder symptoms.

Contraindications

Hypersensitivity to or its components

Interactions

DRUGS

digoxin: Increased serum digoxin concentrations

Adverse Reactions

CNS: Headache

EENT: Dry mouth, nasopharyngitis

GI: Constipation, diarrhea, nausea

GU: Increased residual urine volume, urinary retention, UTI

RESP: Bronchitis, upper respiratory infection

SKIN: Drug eruption, eczema, hot flush, pruritus, rash, urticaria

Other: **Angioedema**

Childbearing Considerations

PREGNANCY

- It is not known if drug can cause fetal harm.
- Use with caution only if benefit to mother outweighs potential risk to fetus.

LACTATION

- It is not known if drug is present in breast milk.

- Mothers should check with prescriber before breastfeeding.

Nursing Considerations

! WARNING Monitor patient for urinary retention, especially if patient has bladder outlet obstruction or is also taking a muscarinic antagonist drug for overactive bladder. If urinary retention develops, notify prescriber and expect drug to be discontinued.

- Monitor effectiveness of drug therapy to ease patient's symptoms.

! WARNING Monitor patient for a hypersensitivity reaction, which could become life-threatening such as angioedema. If present, notify prescriber expect drug to be discontinued and provide supportive care, as needed and ordered.

- Monitor patient for any other adverse reactions that may occur with drug use.

PATIENT TEACHING

- Instruct patient how to administer vibegron.

! WARNING Advise patient to notify prescriber immediately if urinary retention occurs and expect drug to be discontinued.

! WARNING Alert patient that drug may cause an allergic reaction. If present, tell patient to notify prescriber and, if severe. to seek immediate medical care.

- Review other adverse reactions that may occur with drug use. If any occur, tell patient to notify prescriber.

vigabatrin

Sabril, Vigadrone, Vigafyde

Class and Category

Pharmacologic class: Gamma-aminobutyric acid (GABA) transaminase inhibitor
Therapeutic class: Anticonvulsant

Indications and Dosages

✱ *As adjunct therapy for refractory complex partial seizures in patients with inadequate response to several alternative treatments and for whom potential benefits outweigh the risk of vision loss*

ORAL SOLUTION (VIGADRONE), TABLETS (SABRIL, VIGADRONE)

Adults, adolescents ages 17 and older, and children ages 2 to 16 weighing more than 60 kg (132 lb). *Initial:* 500 mg twice daily, increased weekly in 500-mg increments, as needed. *Maintenance:* 1.5 g twice daily.
Children ages 2 to 16 weighing more than 25 kg (55 lb) to less than 60 kg (132 lb). *Initial:* 250 mg twice daily, increased weekly, as needed. *Maintenance:* 1 g twice daily.
Children ages 2 to 16 weighing more than 20 kg (44 lb) to less than 25 kg (55 lb). *Initial:* 250 mg twice daily, increased weekly, as needed. *Maintenance:* 750 mg twice daily.
Children ages 2 to 16 weighing more than 15 kg (33 lb) to less than 20 kg (44 lb). *Initial:* 225 mg twice daily, increased weekly, as needed. *Maintenance:* 650 mg twice daily.
Children ages 2 to 16 weighing at least 10 kg (22 lb) to 15 kg (33 lb). *Initial:* 175 mg twice daily, increased weekly, as needed. *Maintenance:* 525 mg twice daily.

± **DOSAGE ADJUSTMENT** For adult patients and children 2 years or older with a creatinine clearance between 51 to 80 ml/min, dose reduced by 25%; a creatinine clearance between 31 to 50 ml/min, dose reduced by 50%; and a creatinine clearance between 11 to 30 ml/min, dose reduced by 75%.

✱ *As monotherapy for pediatric patients with infantile spasms for whom potential benefits outweigh risk of vision loss*

ORAL SOLUTION (VIGADRONE, VIGAFYDE)

Infants and children ages 1 mo to 2 yr. *Initial:* 50 mg/kg/day given in 2 divided doses, increased every 3 days by 25 to 50 mg/kg/day, as needed. *Maximum:* 150 mg/kg/day given in 2 divided doses.

Drug Administration

P.O.

- Tablets should be swallowed whole and not chewed, crushed, or split.
- Ensure that correct oral solution and strength of oral solutionis being used. Sabril and Vigadrone, once constituted supplies 50 mg/ml. Vigafyde is already in liquid form

that does not require constitution supplying 100 mg/ml.

- Mix Sabril and Vigadrone powder for oral solution by emptying the entire contents of each 500-mg packet needed into a clean cup; dissolve in 10 ml of cold or room-temperature water per packet to a final concentration of 50 mg/ml. Discard if final solution is not clear, colorless, or free of particles. Administer resulting solution immediately using the 3-ml or 10-ml oral syringe supplied by pharmacy.
- Vigafyde oral solution already comes in liquid form and does not require reconstitution. Administer Vigafyde with a calibrated measuring device.
- Drug may be given with or without food.
- Taper drug used to treat refractory complex partial seizures slowly as follows: For adults, decrease daily dose 1000/day on a weekly basis; for pediatric patients, decrease daily dose by one third every wk for 3 wk. For infants and children used to treat infantile spasms, dosage decreased at a rate of 25 mg/kg to 50 mg/kg every 3 to 4 days.

Route	Onset	Peak	Duration
P.O.	Unknown	1–2 hr	Unknown

Half-life: 10.5 hr

Mechanism of Action

Inhibits the action of gamma-aminobutyric acid transaminase (GABA-T), the enzyme responsible for metabolism of the inhibitory neurotransmitter GABA. This increases GABA level in the CNS, which may play a role in suppression of seizure activity. The mechanism of action for infantile spasms is unknown.

Contraindications

Hypersensitivity to vigabatrin and its components

Interactions

DRUGS

clonazepam: Increased risk of clonazepam-associated adverse reactions
phenytoin: Decreased serum phenytoin level

Adverse Reactions

CNS: Abnormal behavior or dreams, abnormal magnetic resonance imaging (MRI) in children age 6 and under, acute psychosis, anxiety, apathy, asthenia, attention disturbance, confusion, coordination abnormality, delirium, depression, dizziness, dystonia, **encephalopathy**, expressive language disorder, fatigue, fever, gait disturbance, headache, hyperreflexia, hypertonia, hypoesthesia, hypomania, hyporeflexia, hypotonia, insomnia, intramyelinic edema (infants), irritability, lethargy, malaise, **malignant hyperthermia**, memory loss, myoclonus, nervousness, paresthesia, peripheral neuropathy, postictal state, **seizures**, sensory disturbance, somnolence, **status epilepticus**, **suicidal ideation**, thirst, tremor, vertigo
CV: Chest pain, edema, peripheral edema
EENT: Asthenopia, blurred vision, deafness, diplopia, eye pain, **laryngeal edema**, nasopharyngitis, nystagmus, optic neuritis, pharyngolaryngeal pain, **stridor**, tinnitus, toothache, tunnel vision, vision loss (permanent and severe), visual field defect
ENDO: Delayed puberty
GI: Abdominal or stomach pain, cholestasis, constipation, decreased liver enzymes, diarrhea, distention, dyspepsia, esophagitis, **GI hemorrhage**, nausea, vomiting
GU: Dysmenorrhea, erectile dysfunction, UTI
HEME: Anemia
MS: Arthralgia; back or limb pain; dysarthria; muscle spasticity, spasms, or twitching
RESP: Bronchitis, cough, **pulmonary edema**, **respiratory failure**, upper respiratory infection
SKIN: Alopecia, maculopapular rash, pruritus, **Stevens-Johnson syndrome**, **toxic epidermal necrolysis**
Other: **Angioedema**, flu-like symptoms, **multiorgan failure**, weight gain

Childbearing Considerations

PREGNANCY

- Pregnancy exposure registry: 1-888-233-2334 or https://www.aedpregnancyregistry.org/.
- Drug may cause fetal harm, based on animal studies.
- Use with caution only if benefit to mother outweighs potential risk to fetus.

LACTATION

- Drug is present in breast milk.
- Breastfeeding is not recommended during drug therapy.

Nursing Considerations

! WARNING Monitor patient's vision, and make sure patient has been examined by an ophthalmic professional in which visual fields and retinal examination has been performed no later than 4 weeks after vigabatrin therapy has begun and then every 3 months throughout therapy and 3 to 6 months after therapy has been discontinued because drug can cause progressive and permanent bilateral concentric visual field constriction and severely reduce visual acuity. Be aware that while risk increases with total dose and duration of therapy, all patients are at risk for visual abnormalities even after drug has been stopped. Because of the risk of permanent and possibly severe vision loss, drug can be prescribed and obtained only through the REMS distribution program. Report any visual abnormalities immediately and expect drug to be discontinued.

! WARNING Monitor patient's temperature closely because drug can cause malignant hyperthermia.

! WARNING Monitor patient for a hypersensitivity reaction, which could become life-threatening, such as angioedema. If present, notify prescriber, expect drug to be switched to a different drug, and provide supportive care, as needed and ordered.

! WARNING Monitor patient for seizure activity that could become life-threatening, causing status epilepticus, especially in patients with a history of a seizure disorder. Notify prescriber immediately of any seizure like activity and be prepared to provide immediate supportive care, as needed and ordered. Institute seizure precautions.

! WARNING Monitor patient for suicidal ideation throughout therapy but especially when therapy starts or dosage changes.

- Know that abnormal MRI results have been noted in children 6 years and younger receiving vigabatrin.
- Monitor patient for evidence of peripheral neuropathy, such as numbness or tingling in feet or toes, progressive loss of reflexes, starting at the ankles, or reduced distal lower limb position sense or vibration. Alert prescriber if abnormalities are present.
- Assess patient routinely for edema, including peripheral edema.

! WARNING Monitor patient for other persistent, serious, or unusual adverse reactions as some can be quite serious such as GI hemorrhage and multiorgan failure.

PATIENT TEACHING

! WARNING Explain the risk of possibly permanent vision loss that may occur as blurred vision or tunnel vision before patient starts vigabatrin. Stress the importance of having vision checked every 3 months throughout therapy and 3 to 6 months after drug is discontinued even if patient is an infant. However, inform patient that vision testing may be insensitive and may not detect vision loss before it is severe and has become permanent.

- Instruct patient how to administer form of vigabatrin prescribed.

! WARNING Warn patient not to stop taking vigabatrin abruptly; the drug will need to be weaned off gradually over several weeks.

! WARNING Advise patient and family or caregiver to notify prescriber if patient has unusual behaviors or feelings, especially if related to suicidal ideation and particularly at the beginning of therapy and during dosage adjustments.

! WARNING Instruct patient to notify prescriber if temperature rises for no known reason.

! WARNING Alert patient that drug may cause an allergic reaction. Tell patient to notify prescriber, if present, and to seek immediate medical care, if severe.

! WARNING Inform patient that drug may cause seizure activity. Tell patient to seek immediate medical care if a seizure occurs.

- Caution patient not to perform hazardous activities such as operating equipment until CNS effects of drug are known and resolved.
- Alert patient to monitor his weight because drug may cause weight gain.

> ! **WARNING** Instruct patient to notify prescriber if any other persistent, serious, or unusual adverse reaction occurs.

- Advise females of childbearing age to report pregnancy to prescriber.
- Inform mothers that breastfeeding is not recommended during drug therapy.

vilazodone hydrochloride

Viibryd

Class and Category

Pharmacologic class: Selective serotonin reuptake inhibitor (SSRI)
Therapeutic class: Antidepressant

Indications and Dosages

✱ *To treat major depressive disorder*

TABLETS

Adults. *Initial:* 10 mg once daily for 7 days, followed by 20 mg once daily for 7 days, then increased to 40 mg once daily after 7 days, as needed.

± **DOSAGE ADJUSTMENT** For patients taking a strong CYP3A4 inhibitor (clarithromycin, itraconazole, voriconazole), dosage should not exceed 20 mg daily. For patients taking a strong CYP3A4 inducer (carbamazepine, phenytoin, rifampin) for more than 14 days, dosage may be increased up to twofold over 1 to 2 weeks but not exceed 80 mg daily.

Drug Administration

P.O.

- Administer drug with food.

Route	Onset	Peak	Duration
P.O.	Unknown	4–5 hr	Unknown

Half-life: 25 hr

Mechanism of Action

Exerts antidepressant effects by potentiating serotonin activity in CNS and inhibiting serotonin reuptake at the presynaptic neuronal membrane. Blocked serotonin reuptake increases levels and prolongs activity of serotonin at synaptic receptor sites.

Contraindications

Hypersensitivity to vilazodone or its components, use within 14 days of an MAO inhibitor therapy

Interactions

DRUGS

amphetamines, buspirone, fentanyl, lithium, MAO inhibitors, serotonin–norepinephrine reuptake inhibitors, serotonin reuptake inhibitors, St. John's wort, tramadol, tricyclic antidepressants, triptans, tryptophan: Increased risk of life-threatening adverse effects, such as serotonin syndrome
aspirin, NSAIDs, warfarin, and other anticoagulants: Increased risk of bleeding
CYP3A4 inhibitors, such as clarithromycin, itraconazole, voriconazole: Increased blood vilazodone levels with increased risk of adverse effects
digoxin: Possible increased risk of digoxin concentrations

Adverse Reactions

CNS: Abnormal dreams, dizziness, fatigue, feeling jittery, hallucinations, insomnia, irritability, mania, migraine, **neuroleptic malignant syndrome-like reactions**, panic attack, paresthesia, restlessness, **seizures**, **serotonin syndrome**, sleep paralysis, **suicidal ideation**, tremor
CV: Palpitations, **prolonged QT interval**, **torsades de pointes**, **ventricular extrasystoles**
EENT: Angle-closure glaucoma, blurred vision, cataracts, dry eyes or mouth
GI: **Acute pancreatitis**, anorexia, diarrhea, dyspepsia, flatulence, gastroenteritis, **GI bleeding**, increased appetite, nausea, vomiting
GU: Absent or delayed orgasm (females), decreased libido, delayed ejaculation, erectile dysfunction, pollakiuria
HEME: **Bleeding events**
MS: Arthralgia
SKIN: Diaphoresis, drug eruption, night sweats, rash, urticaria

Childbearing Considerations

PREGNANCY

- Pregnancy exposure registry: 1-844-405-6185 or https://womensmentalhealth.org/research/pregnancyregistry/antidepressants.
- Drug may cause fetal harm, especially if exposure occurs late in third trimester. Neonate exposed to drug in utero may require prolonged hospitalization, respiratory support, and tube feeding as a result of persistent pulmonary hypertension of the newborn and drug discontinuation syndrome.
- Use with caution only if benefit to mother outweighs potential risk to fetus.

LABOR AND DELIVERY

- If drug is given within 1 month of delivery mother is at increased risk of postpartum hemorrhage.

LACTATION

- It is not known if drug is present in breast milk.
- Mothers should check with prescriber before breastfeeding.

Nursing Considerations

! WARNING Be aware that vilazodone should not be given to patients with bradycardia, congenital long QT syndrome, hypokalemia or hypomagnesemia, recent acute MI, or uncompensated heart failure because of increased risk of prolonged QT interval and torsades de pointes. It should also not be given to patients who are taking other drugs that prolong the QT interval. Expect hypokalemia and hypomagnesemia to be corrected before vilazodone therapy is begun.

! WARNING Know that vilazodone should not be administered to pregnant women late in their third trimester because of potential neonatal complications at birth. Know that use of drug in the month before delivery may increase risk of postpartum hemorrhage.

- Use vilazodone cautiously in a patient with a seizure disorder because drug effect has not been studied in patients with seizures.

! WARNING Watch patient closely for suicidal tendencies, particularly when therapy starts and dosage changes because depression may worsen temporarily during these times, possibly leading to suicidal ideation.

! WARNING Monitor patient closely for evidence of GI bleeding, especially if patient also takes a drug known to cause GI bleeding, such as aspirin, NSAID, or warfarin.

! WARNING Monitor patient's serum sodium level, as ordered, especially in the elderly and patients with volume depletion because selective serotonin reuptake inhibitors, the class of drugs vilazodone belongs to, have caused hyponatremia. If patient develops confusion, difficulty concentrating, headache, memory impairment, unsteadiness, weakness, and sodium level has decreased, notify prescriber. Be prepared to provide supportive care, as needed and ordered.

! WARNING Monitor patient closely for serotonin syndrome exhibited by agitation, coma, diarrhea, hallucinations, hyperreflexia, hyperthermia, incoordination, labile blood pressure, nausea, tachycardia, or vomiting. Notify prescriber immediately because serotonin syndrome may be life-threatening; provide supportive care, as needed and ordered.

! WARNING Be aware that serotonin syndrome in its most severe form may resemble neuroleptic malignant syndrome, which includes autonomic instability with possibly rapid changes in mental status and vital signs, hyperthermia, and muscle rigidity. Notify prescriber immediately and provide supportive care, as needed and ordered.

- Watch for mania, which may result from any antidepressant in a susceptible patient.

! WARNING Monitor patient for other persistent, serious, or unusual adverse reactions, some of which could be quite serious such as QT prolongation and pancreatitis.

- Expect to taper vilazodone therapy gradually when drug is no longer required; abrupt discontinuation can precipitate withdrawal symptoms.

PATIENT TEACHING

- Encourage patient to have an eye exam before starting therapy to see if he is at risk for an episode of acute closure glaucoma that may be drug induced.

! WARNING Inform pregnant patients that vilazodone should not be administered late in their third trimester because of potential neonatal complications at birth. Also, tell these patients drug should not be given within 1 month of delivery.

- Instruct patient how to administer vilazodone.

! WARNING Tell family or caregiver to observe patient closely for suicidal tendencies, especially when therapy starts or dosage changes.

! WARNING Tell patient not to take aspirin or NSAIDs during therapy because they increase the risk of bleeding. If patient takes warfarin, tell patient to use bleeding precautions and to notify prescriber at once if bleeding occurs.

- Encourage patient to address sexual dysfunction with prescriber, if concerned.

! WARNING Advise patient to notify prescriber of any other persistent, severe, or unusual adverse reactions.

- Caution patient to alert all prescribers about vilazodone therapy because of potentially serious drug interactions.

viloxazine

Qelbree

Class and Category

Pharmacologic class: Selective norepinephrine reuptake inhibitor
Therapeutic class: Anti-ADHD agent

Indications and Dosages

* *To treat attention deficit hyperactivity disorder (ADHD)*

E.R. CAPSULES

Adults. *Initial:* 200 mg once daily increased in increments of 200 mg weekly, as needed. *Maximum:* 600 mg once daily.
Children ages 12 to 17. *Initial:* 200 mg once daily increased to 400 mg once daily after 1 wk, as needed. *Maximum:* 400 mg once daily.
Children ages 6 to 11. *Initial:* 100 mg once daily increased in increments of 100 mg weekly, as needed. *Maximum:* 400 mg once daily.

± **DOSAGE ADJUSTMENT** For patients with severe renal failure (eGFR less than 30 ml/min), initial dosage reduced to 100 mg once daily followed by weekly dosage increases of 50 to 100 mg once daily, as needed, with maximum dosage not to exceed 200 mg once daily.

Drug Administration

P.O.

- Capsules should be swallowed whole and not chewed, crushed, or cut.
- For patient who cannot swallow capsules, open and sprinkle entire contents over a teaspoonful or tablespoonful of applesauce or pudding. Mixture should be administered within 15 min if mixed with pudding and within 2 hr if mixed with applesauce. Mixture should not be stored for future use.
- Administer capsules with or without food.

Route	Onset	Peak	Duration
P.O.	Unknown	3–9 hr	Unknown

Half-life: 7 hr

Mechanism of Action

Unknown although it is thought to be related to the inhibition of the reuptake of norepinephrine to cause a calming effect in ADHD.

Contraindications

Concurrent use of sensitive CYP1A2 or CYP1A2 substrates with a narrow therapeutic range, hypersensitivity to viloxazine or its components, use within 14 days of MAO inhibitor therapy

Interactions

DRUGS

CYP1A2 substrates, CYP1A2 substrates with a narrow therapeutic range, CYP2D6 substrates, CYP3A4 substrates: Increased total exposure of these drugs, which may increase risk of adverse reactions
MAO inhibitors: Possibly development of life-threatening hypertensive crisis

Adverse Reactions

CNS: Dizziness, fatigue, fever, headache, hypomania or mania activation, insomnia, irritability, somnolence, **suicidal ideation**
CV: Increased diastolic blood pressure, tachycardia
EENT: Dry mouth, nasopharyngitis, pharyngitis, sinusitis
GI: Abdominal pain, anorexia, constipation, gastroesophageal reflux disease, nausea, vomiting

Childbearing Considerations

PREGNANCY

- Pregnancy exposure registry: 1-866-961-2388 or www.womensmentalhealth.org/preg.
- Drug may cause fetal harm according to animal studies.
- Use with caution only if benefit to mother outweighs potential risk to fetus.

LACTATION

- It is not known if drug is present in breast milk.
- Patient should check with prescriber before breastfeeding

Nursing Considerations

- Assess patient's vital signs, especially blood pressure and heart rate, before administering viloxazine, after a dosage increase, and periodically throughout therapy because drug can increase diastolic blood pressure as well as cause tachycardia.

! **WARNING** Determine if patient has a history of or family history of bipolar disorder, depression, or suicidal ideation before administering drug. Alert prescriber if present. Monitor patient closely for evidence of suicidal thinking and behavior as well as signs and symptoms of activation of hypomania or mania. If present, notify prescriber.

- Monitor patient's weight because viloxazine may cause anorexia.

PATIENT TEACHING

- Instruct patient, family, or caregiver how to administer viloxazine.

! **WARNING** Tell family or caregiver to notify prescriber if patient exhibits signs and symptoms of activation of hypomania or mania as well as suicidal thinking or behavior.

- Caution patient to avoid hazardous activities until the drug's CNS effects are known and resolved.
- Instruct patient to monitor weight and report any significant changes to prescriber.
- Tell patient of childbearing age to notify prescriber if pregnancy occurs.

vorapaxar

Zontivity

Class and Category

Pharmacologic class: Protease activated receptor-1 (PAR-1) inhibitor
Therapeutic class: Antiplatelet

Indications and Dosages

✱ *As adjunct with aspirin and/or clopidogrel to reduce thrombotic cardiovascular events in patients with a history of MI or peripheral arterial disease*

TABLETS

Adults. 2.08 mg once daily.

Drug Administration

P.O.

- Administer tablet with or without food.

Route	Onset	Peak	Duration
P.O.	1 wk	1–2 hr	Unknown

Half-life: 5–13 days

Mechanism of Action

Inhibits thrombin-induced and thrombin receptor agonist peptide-induced platelet aggregation.

Contraindications

Active pathologic bleeding; history of intracranial hemorrhage, stroke, or transient ischemic attack; hypersensitivity to vorapaxar or its components

Interactions

DRUGS

strong CYP3A inducers, such as carbamazepine, phenytoin, rifampin, St. John's wort: Decreased vorapaxar effectiveness *strong CYP3A inhibitors, such as boceprevir, clarithromycin, conivaptan, indinavir, itraconazole, ketoconazole, nefazodone, nelfinavir, posaconazole, ritonavir, saquinavir, telaprevir, telithromycin:* Increased vorapaxar exposure and adverse reactions

Adverse Reactions

CNS: Depression, **intracranial hemorrhage**
EENT: Diplopia, oculomotor disturbance, retinal disorder (including retinopathy)
GI: **GI bleeding**
HEME: Anemia, **bleeding events that may become severe**, iron deficiency
SKIN: Eruptions, exanthema, rash

Childbearing Considerations

PREGNANCY

- It is not known if drug can cause fetal harm.
- Drug should be discontinued when pregnancy occurs and expect to administer an alternative therapy with a shorter duration of action.

LACTATION

- It is not known if drug is present in breast milk.
- Breastfeeding is not recommended during drug therapy.

Nursing Considerations

! **WARNING** Know that drug should not be administered during pregnancy.

! **WARNING** Know that vorapaxar should not be given to patients with a history of intracranial hemorrhage, stroke, or transient ischemic attack because of an increased risk for intracranial hemorrhage. Drug should be discontinued in a patient who experiences a stroke while taking vorapaxar.

! **WARNING** Assess patient's bleeding risk before beginning vorapaxar therapy because vorapaxar increases the risk of bleeding in proportion to the patient's underlying bleeding risk. Factors that may increase the patient's risk of bleeding include the use of certain concomitant drugs, such as anticoagulants, chronic NSAIDs use, fibrinolytic therapy, selective serotonin reuptake inhibitors, or serotonin–norepinephrine reuptake inhibitors; history of bleeding disorders; low body weight; older age; or reduced hepatic or renal function. Know that vorapaxar should not be given to patients with severe hepatic impairment because of increased risk for bleeding. Know that drug increases the risk of fatal bleeding.

! **WARNING** Monitor patient for bleeding throughout vorapaxar therapy. Suspect bleeding in patient who is hypotensive and has recently undergone coronary angiography, coronary artery bypass graft surgery, percutaneous coronary intervention, or other surgical procedures. Stop vorapaxar therapy and notify prescriber immediately of suspected or known bleeding. Prepare to support patient according to standard of care, as there is no known treatment to reverse the antiplatelet effect of drug because of its long half-life. Significant inhibition of platelet aggregation has been known to persist for at least 4 weeks after drug has been discontinued.

- Monitor patient for a rash. If present notify prescriber.

PATIENT TEACHING

! **WARNING** Inform females of childbearing age drug should not be taken during pregnancy. If pregnancy occurs, tell patient to notify prescriber immediately.

- Instruct patient how to administer vorapaxar.
- Tell patient to take vorapaxar exactly as prescribed and not to discontinue drug without discussing it with prescriber.
- Inform patient that drug is usually prescribed along with other drugs, such as aspirin and/or clopidogrel.

! **WARNING** Inform patient that he may bleed or bruise more easily. Stress importance of promptly reporting any excessive, prolonged, or unanticipated bleeding, or blood in the stool or urine. Review safety precautions to avoid bleeding events, such as using an electric razor and soft toothbrush.

- Tell patient drug may cause a rash. If present, instruct patient to notify prescriber.
- Remind patient to inform all dentists and physicians of vorapaxar use prior to any dental procedure or surgery. Emphasize that the dentist or doctor performing the

procedure should talk to prescriber before stopping drug.

- Tell patient to keep prescriber informed of all dietary supplements, over-the-counter drugs, or prescription drugs he takes.

voriconazole

Vfend

Class and Category

Pharmacologic class: Triazole
Therapeutic class: Antifungal

Indications and Dosages

✶ *To treat invasive aspergillosis; to treat serious fungal infections caused by* Scedosporium apiospermum *and* Fusarium *species, including* Fusarium solani *in patients intolerant of or refractory to other therapy*

I.V. INFUSION

Adults, adolescents ages 15 and older regardless of body weight, and adolescents ages 12 to 14 weighing 50 kg (110 lb) or more. *Loading dose:* 6 mg/kg every 12 hr for 2 doses and infused at no more than 3 mg/kg/hr. *Maintenance:* 4 mg/kg every 12 hr and infused at no more than 3 mg/kg/hr for at least 7 days before being switched to oral form.

I.V. INFUSION

Children ages 12 to 14 weighing less than 50 kg (110 lb), children ages 2 to 12. *Loading dose:* 9 mg/kg every 12 hr for 2 doses and infused at no more than 3 mg/kg/hr. *Maintenance:* 8 mg/kg every 12 hr and infused at no more than 3 mg/kg/hr with dosage decreased or increased in 1 mg/kg steps, as needed, and given for at least 7 days before being switched to oral form.

±DOSAGE ADJUSTMENT For patients unable to tolerate I.V. maintenance dose of 4 mg/kg dose every 12 hr, dosage reduced to 3 mg/kg every 12 hr.

ORAL SUSPENSION, TABLETS

Adults weighing 40 kg (88 lb) or more, adolescents ages 15 and older regardless of body weight, and adolescents ages 12 to 14 weighing 50 kg (110 lb) or more. *After 7 days of I.V. therapy:* 200 mg every 12 hr, increased to 300 mg every 12 hr, as needed.
Adults weighing less than 40 kg (88 lb). *After 7 days of I.V. therapy:* 100 mg every 12 hr, increased to 150 mg every 12 hr, as needed.

ORAL SUSPENSION, TABLETS

Children age 2 to less than 12, adolescents ages 12 to 14 weighing less than 50 kg (110 lb). *After 7 days of I.V. therapy:* 9 mg/kg every 12 hr with dosage decreased or increased by 1 mg/kg, as needed. *Maximum:* 350 mg every 12 hr.

✶ *To treat candidemia in non-neutropenic patients and other deep-tissue disseminated* Candida *infections involving the abdomen, bladder wall, kidney, skin, or a wound*

I.V. INFUSION

Adults, adolescents ages 15 and older regardless of body weight, and adolescents ages 12 to 14 weighing 50 kg (110 lb) or more. *Loading dose:* 6 mg/kg every 12 hr for 2 doses and infused at no more than 3 mg/kg/hr. *Maintenance:* 3 to 4 mg/kg every 12 hr and infused at no more than 3 mg/kg/hr. I.V. therapy given for at least 14 days after symptoms resolve or last positive culture, whichever takes longer.
Children age 2 to less than age 12, adolescents ages 12 to 14 weighing less than 50 kg (110 lb). *Loading dose:* 9 mg/kg every 12 hr for 2 doses and infused at no more than 3 mg/kg/hr. *Maintenance:* 8 mg/kg every 12 hr infused at no more than 3 mg/kg/hr and then switched to oral form when feasible and significant improvement has occurred.

ORAL SUSPENSION, TABLETS

Adults weighing 40 kg (88 lb) or more, adolescents ages 15 and older regardless of weight, and adolescents ages 12 to 14 weighing 50 kg (110 lb) or more. *After I.V. therapy:* 200 mg every 12 hr and given for at least 14 days after symptoms resolve or last positive culture, whichever takes longer.
Adults weighing less than 40 kg (88 lb). *Maintenance:* 100 mg every 12 hr, increased to 150 mg every 12 hr, as needed, and given for at least 14 days after symptoms resolve or last positive culture, whichever takes longer.
Children age 2 to less than age 12, adolescents ages 12 to 14 weighing less than 50 kg (110 lb). *After I.V. therapy:* 9 mg/kg every 12 hr with dosage increased or decreased in 1 mg/kg steps, as needed. *Maximum:* 350 mg every 12 hr.

✶ *To treat esophageal candidiasis*

I.V. INFUSION

Children age 2 to less than age 12, adolescents ages 12 to 14 weighing less than 50 kg (110 lb). *Initial:* 4 mg/kg every 12 hr and infused at no more than 3 mg/kg/hr. Dosage increased or decreased in 1 mg/kg steps, as needed. After at least 5 days of therapy and only after there is significant improvement, therapy switched to oral form.

ORAL SUSPENSION, TABLETS

Adults weighing 40 kg (88 lb) or more, adolescents ages 15 and older regardless of weight, and adolescents ages 12 to 14 weighing 50 kg (110 lb) or more. 200 mg every 12 hr for at least 14 days and at least 7 days after signs and symptoms resolve.
Adults weighing less than 40 kg (88 lb). 100 mg every 12 hr for at least 14 days and at least 7 days after signs and symptoms resolve.
Children age 2 to less than 12, adolescents ages 12 to 14 weighing less than 50 kg (110 lb). *Maintenance:* 9 mg/kg every 12 hr with dosage increased or decreased, as needed, in 1 mg/kg steps. *Maximum:* 350 mg every 12 hr.

±**DOSAGE ADJUSTMENT** For adult use with efavirenz or phenytoin, maintenance dose increased. For adult patients with mild to moderate hepatic impairment, maintenance dosage reduced. For adult patients with mild to moderate hepatic cirrhosis, maintenance dosage reduced by 50%. For adult patients with moderate to severe renal impairment (creatinine clearance less than 50 ml/min), only oral drug should be given. No dosage guidelines for children are given by manufacturer.

Drug Administration

P.O.

- Administer at least 1 hr before or 1 hr after a meal.
- Shake oral suspension for about 10 sec before each use. Use oral dispenser supplied to measure dosage. Store at room temperature and discard after 14 days.

I.V.

- Reconstitute powder with 19 ml Sterile Water for Injection to obtain a volume of 20 ml with a concentrate of 10 mg/ml. Solution should be clear. It is recommended to use a standard 20-ml nonautomated syringe to ensure that exact amount of Sterile Water for Injection is dispensed. Discard vial if the vacuum does not pull solution into the vial.
- Shake vial until all powder is dissolved.
- Dilute to final concentration of 5 mg/ml or less using 0.9% Sodium Chloride Injection, 5% Dextrose Injection, or Lactated Ringer's solution (see manufacturer's guidelines for other appropriate solutions). This requires withdrawing and discarding at least an equal volume of diluent from infusion bag or bottle before instillation of drug concentrate. Final concentration should not be less than 0.5 mg/ml nor greater than 5 mg/ml.
- Discard partially used vials after mixing. If infusion isn't administered immediately, store in refrigerator for no longer than 24 hr.
- Administer I.V. infusion over 1 to 3 hr at a concentration of 5 mg/ml or less and no more than 3 mg/kg/hr. Never administer as an I.V. bolus.
- Observe patient receiving I.V. voriconazole closely for anaphylactoid-type reactions, such as chest tightness, dyspnea, faintness, fever, flushing, nausea, pruritus, rash, sweating, and tachycardia, which may occur immediately after starting infusion. Stop infusion if these reactions occur and notify prescriber immediately.
- *Incompatibilities:* 4.2% Sodium Bicarbonate infusion, I.V. solutions other than recommended by manufacturer, other I.V. drugs

Route	Onset	Peak	Duration
P.O./I.V.	Unknown	1–2 hr	12 hr

Half-life: Dose-dependent

Mechanism of Action

Prevents fungal ergosterol biosynthesis by inhibiting fungal cytochrome P-450–mediated 14 alpha-lanosterol demethylation. The loss of ergosterol in the fungal cell wall renders the fungal cell inactive.

Contraindications

Coadministration with long-acting barbiturates, carbamazepine, CYP3A4 substrates (astemizole, cisapride, ivabradine, pimozide, or quinidine), efavirenz (doses of 400 mg every 24 hr or higher), ergot alkaloids, lurasidone (IV infusion), naloxegol, rifabutin, rifampin, ritonavir (400 mg every 12 hr), sirolimus, St. John's wort, tolvaptan, venetoclax: hypersensitivity to voriconazole or its components

Interactions

DRUGS

alfentanil: Increased plasma alfentanil level and increased risk of adverse reactions
benzodiazepines: Possibly prolonged sedative effect of benzodiazepines
calcium channel blockers; HMG-CoA reductase inhibitors, such as lovastatin; omeprazole; rifabutin; sirolimus;, tyrosine kinase inhibitors (axitinib, bosutinib, cabozantinib, certinib, cobimetinib, dabrafenib, dasatinib, nilotinib, sunitinib, ibrutinib, ribociclib): Possibly increased plasma levels of these drugs, leading to increased risk of adverse reactions and toxicity
carbamazepine, long-acting barbiturates, rifabutin, rifampin, ritonavir, St. John's wort: Decreased plasma voriconazole concentration
cyclosporine, sirolimus, tacrolimus: Increased serum concentrations of these drugs and risk of toxicity, especially nephrotoxicity
CYP2C9, CYP2C19, and CYP3A4 inducers: Decreased voriconazole levels, decreasing effectiveness
CYP2C9, CYP2C19, and CYP3A4 inhibitors: Increased plasma levels of voriconazole, which may lead to prolonged QT interval and, rarely, torsades de pointes
CYP450 isoenzymes: Increased plasma concentrations of these drugs
efavirenz: Possibly significant decreased plasma voriconazole levels and increased plasma efavirenz levels
ergot alkaloids (dihydroergotamine, ergotamine): May increase plasma level of ergot alkaloids, leading to ergotism
everolimus, fluconazole, oral contraceptives: Increased plasma voriconazole level and risk of toxicity
fentanyl and other long-acting opiates metabolized by CYP3A4, such as oxycodone: Increased plasma level of fentanyl and other long-acting opiates with increased risk of adverse reactions
HIV protease inhibitors (amprenavir, nelfinavir, ritonavir, saquinavir), non-nucleoside reverse transcriptase inhibitors (delavirdine): Possibly inhibited metabolism of voriconazole leading to increased plasma voriconazole levels and plasma levels of these drugs
methadone: Increased plasma level of methadone, possibly leading to toxicity, including QT-interval prolongation
methotrexate: Increased risk of skin toxicity
NSAIDs: Increased plasma NSAID levels leading to possible increased adverse reactions, including toxicity
oral contraceptives: Increased plasma voriconazole level and risk of toxicity; increased plasma levels of oral contraceptives and risk of adverse reactions
phenytoin: Decreased plasma level of voriconazole and increased plasma level of phenytoin
sulfonylureas: Possibly increased plasma level of sulfonylureas and increased risk of hypoglycemia
vinca alkaloids: Possibly increased risk of neurotoxicity
warfarin: Possibly increased PTT

Adverse Reactions

CNS: Affect lability, agitation, anxiety, asthenia, ataxia, chills, depression, dizziness, fever, hallucinations, headache, hypothermia, insomnia, lethargy, paresthesia, **seizures**, syncope, vertigo
CV: **Arrhythmias**, **bradycardia**, **cardiac arrest**, chest pain, hypertension, **hypotension**, palpitations, peripheral edema, **prolonged QT interval**, **supraventricular tachycardia**, tachycardia, **torsades de pointes**, vasodilation, **ventricular tachycardia**
EENT: Abnormal or blurred vision, altered or enhanced visual perception, change in color perception, chromatopsia, dry eyes or mouth, eye hemorrhage, keratitis, nasal congestion, nystagmus, optic neuritis, papilledema, photophobia, tinnitus, visual disturbances that could be prolonged
ENDO: **Adrenal insufficiency**, **Cushing's syndrome**, **hypoglycemia**
GI: Abdominal pain or tenderness, cholestasis, cholestatic jaundice, diarrhea, dyspepsia, elevated liver enzymes, **fulminant hepatic failure**, **hepatitis**, hyperbilirubinemia, jaundice, nausea, **pancreatitis**, vomiting
GU: Abnormal kidney function **or toxicity**, **acute renal failure**, elevated serum creatinine level

HEME: Anemia, **leukopenia**, **pancytopenia**, **thrombocytopenia**
MS: Arthralgia, fluorosis, myalgia, periostitis, skeletal pain
RESP: Respiratory disorders, **respiratory failure**, tachypnea
SKIN: Alopecia, cheilitis, cutaneous lupus erythematosus, dermatitis (allergic or contact), diaphoresis, dry skin, eczema, **erythema multiforme**, **exfoliative dermatitis**, fixed drug eruption, flushing, furunculosis, maculopapular rash, **melanoma**, photosensitivity, pruritus, pseudoporphyria, psoriasis, rash, skin discoloration, **squamous cell carcinoma**, **Stevens-Johnson syndrome**, **toxic epidermal necrolysis**, urticaria
Other: **Anaphylaxis**, **angioedema**, **drug reaction with eosinophilia and systemic symptoms (DRESS)**, elevated alkaline phosphatase, herpes simplex, **hypercalcemia**, **hypermagnesemia**, **hyperphosphatemia**, **hypersensitivity reactions**, **hypokalemia**, **hypomagnesemia**, infusion reactions, such as phlebitis, **sepsis**

Childbearing Considerations

PREGNANCY

- Drug may cause fetal harm, based on animal studies.
- Use with caution only if benefit to mother outweighs potential risk to fetus.

LACTATION

- It is not known if drug is present in breast milk.
- Patient should check with prescriber before breastfeeding.

REPRODUCTION

- Females of childbearing age should use effective contraception during drug therapy.

Nursing Considerations

! **WARNING** Determine if patient has any problems with galactose intolerance, glucose–galactose malabsorption, or Lapp lactase deficiency before starting therapy because voriconazole tablets contain lactose and shouldn't be given to patients with these conditions.

- Obtain specimens for fungal culture and other relevant laboratory studies (including histopathology), as ordered, before giving first dose. Expect to begin drug before test results are known.

! **WARNING** Use voriconazole cautiously in patients hypersensitive to other azoles and in patients at risk for proarrhythmic events (such as those receiving cardiotoxic chemotherapy or concomitant drug therapy known to prolong QT interval, or those who have acquired or congenital QT prolongation, cardiomyopathy, hypokalemia, sinus bradycardia, or symptomatic arrhythmias [existing]) because drug may prolong the QT interval. Know that calcium, magnesium, and potassium imbalances should be corrected before starting voriconazole therapy as well as any time an imbalance occurs during voriconazole therapy. Monitor patient's electrolyte balance closely.

! **WARNING** Assess patient's liver function (including bilirubin), as ordered, at the start of voriconazole therapy and at least weekly for the first month of treatment. Then, monthly assessments thereafter because although it is uncommon, drug has caused serious hepatic reactions, including fatalities. Know that a higher frequency of elevated liver enzymes has been noted in children. Be aware that drug may be discontinued if liver abnormalities occur.

! **WARNING** Monitor patient for a hypersensitivity or serious skin reaction, which may become life-threatening, such as anaphylaxis, angioedema, or DRESS. If present, notify prescriber, expect voriconazole to be discontinued, and provide supportive care, as needed and ordered.

! **WARNING** Assess patient's skin regularly because drug can cause skin cancer. Know that if patient develops pre-malignant skin lesions, drug should be discontinued.

! **WARNING** Monitor diabetic patients also taking sulfonylureas closely for hypoglycemia, and check blood glucose levels regularly. Be prepared to treat hypoglycemia according to institutional protocol, if present.

! **WARNING** Monitor patient closely for pancreatitis, especially if patient is a child or has risk factors for acute pancreatitis, such as recent chemotherapy or hematopoietic stem cell transplantation.

! **WARNING** Monitor renal function, especially serum creatinine level, when giving I.V. form of voriconazole because drug may accumulate in body when creatinine clearance is less than 50 ml/min, increasing the risk of adverse reactions, including acute renal failure or renal toxicity.

- Assess patient's visual function, including color perception, visual acuity, and visual field, if voriconazole therapy continues longer than 28 days.
- Report skeletal pain to prescriber and expect skeletal x-rays to be done. If fluorosis or periostitis is found, anticipate voriconazole therapy to be discontinued.

PATIENT TEACHING

! **WARNING** Inform patient with galactose intolerance, glucose–galactose malabsorption, or Lapp lactase deficiency that voriconazole tablets contain lactose.

- Instruct patient how to administer oral voriconazole.
- Tell patient that frequent blood tests will have to be performed and importance of compliance with schedule.

! **WARNING** Alert patient that an allergic reaction or skin reaction may occur with drug therapy. Stress importance of alerting staff at the first sign of an allergic reaction (especially of a rash). Tell patient experiencing an allergic reaction at home to notify prescriber and to seek immediate medical care, if serious.

! **WARNING** Instruct patients with diabetes mellitus who are also taking a sulfonylurea to check blood glucose regularly and to monitor self for hypoglycemia, as drug increases risk of hypoglycemia. Review appropriate treatment for hypoglycemia with patient and family or caregiver.

! **WARNING** Urge patient to have regular skin examinations. Advise patient including child to avoid exposure to direct sunlight or UV light and to wear protective clothing and high sun protection factor sunscreen when outdoors. Tell patient or family or caregiver to notify prescriber if a severe sun reaction occurs as patient will need to see a dermatologist and the drug may possibly need to be discontinued. Long-term follow-up with a dermatologist also may be needed.

! **WARNING** Caution patient to report any other persistent, serious, or unusual signs and symptoms to staff (if drug given I.V.) or to prescriber.

- Caution patient not to drive at night and to avoid hazardous activities because drug may cause visual disturbances, including blurring or photophobia.
- Instruct females of childbearing age to use effective contraception during therapy and to notify prescriber immediately if pregnancy is suspected.
- Tell patient to alert all prescribers of voriconazole therapy.

vortioxetine hydrobromide

Trintellix

Class and Category

Pharmacologic class: Serotonin modulator
Therapeutic class: Antidepressant

Indications and Dosages

* *To treat major depressive disorder (MDD)*

TABLETS

Adults. *Initial:* 10 mg once daily, then increased to 20 mg once daily, as tolerated. *Maximum:* 20 mg once daily.

± **DOSAGE ADJUSTMENT** For patients who cannot tolerate higher doses, dosage may be decreased down to 5 mg once daily. For patients taking strong CYP inducers, such as carbamazepine, phenytoin, or rifampin concurrently for longer than 14 days, dosage increased up to 3 times the original dose and when inducer is discontinued, dosage decreased to original level within 14 days. For patients taking strong CYP2D6 inhibitors, such as bupropion, fluoxetine, paroxetine, or quinidine concurrently, dosage reduced by one-half, and when inhibitor is discontinued, dosage increased to original level within 14 days. For patients who are known

CYP2D6 poor metabolizers, maximum dosage is 10 mg once daily.

Drug Administration

P.O.

- Administer at about same time daily.
- May be taken with or without food.

Route	Onset	Peak	Duration
P.O.	1–2 wk	7–11 hr	Unknown

Half-life: 66 hr

Mechanism of Action

Enhances serotonergic activity in the central nervous system through inhibiting the reuptake of serotonin. Enhanced serotonergic activity is thought to relieve symptoms of depression.

Contraindications

Hypersensitivity to vortioxetine or its components; use within 14 days of an MAO inhibitor

Interactions

DRUGS

amphetamines, buspirone, fentanyl, lithium, MAO inhibitors, SNRIs, SSRIs, St. John's wort, tramadol, tricyclic antidepressants, triptans, tryptophans: Increased risk of serotonin toxicity

aspirin, NSAIDs, warfarin, and other anticoagulants and antiplatelets: Increased risk of bleeding

CYP2D6 inducers (strong), such as carbamazepine, phenytoin, rifampin: Decreased plasma vortioxetine levels with possible decreased effectiveness

CYP2D6 inhibitors (strong), such as bupropion, fluoxetine, paroxetine, and quinidine: Increased plasma vortioxetine levels with increased risk of adverse reactions

drugs that are highly protein bound, such as warfarin: May increase free concentrations of vortioxetine or other tightly bound drugs in plasma

Adverse Reactions

CNS: Abnormal dreams, activation of hypomania/mania, aggression, agitation, anger, dizziness, headache, hostility, irritability, **seizures**, **serotonin syndrome**, **suicidal ideation**, vertigo

EENT: Altered taste, angle-closure glaucoma, dry mouth

ENDO: Hyperprolactinemia

GI: **Acute pancreatitis**, constipation, diarrhea, dyspepsia, flatulence, nausea, vomiting

GU: Absent or delayed orgasm (females), decreased libido, ejaculatory delay or failure, erectile dysfunction, sexual performance, or sexual satisfaction difficulties

HEME: **Abnormal bleeding**

RESP: Difficulty breathing

SKIN: Flushing, hyperhidrosis, pruritus, rash, urticaria

Other: **Anaphylaxis and other hypersensitivity reactions**, **discontinuation disorder**, false-positive urine results for methadone, **hyponatremia**, weight gain

Childbearing Considerations

PREGNANCY

- Pregnancy exposure registry: 1-844-405-6185 or https://womensmentalhealth.org/clinical-and-research-programs/pregnancyregistry/antidepressants/.
- Drug may cause fetal harm, especially if exposed to drug late in third trimester, which may require prolonged hospitalization, respiratory support, and tube feeding as a result of persistent pulmonary hypertension of the newborn and drug discontinuation syndrome.
- Use with caution only if benefit to mother outweighs potential risk to fetus.

LABOR AND DELIVERY

- Drug may increase risk of postpartum hemorrhage if given within 1 month of delivery.

LACTATION

- It is not known if drug is present in breast milk.
- Mothers should check with prescriber before breastfeeding.

Nursing Considerations

! **WARNING** Know that vortioxetine should not be administered to a pregnant patient within 1 month of delivery as neonatal harm may occur at birth and mother may be at increased risk for postpartum hemorrhage.

! **WARNING** Be aware that at least 14 days should elapse between discontinuing an MAO inhibitor used to treat psychiatric disorders and initiation of vortioxetine therapy to avoid risk of patient developing serotonin syndrome. Also, know that at least 21 days should elapse after vortioxetine is discontinued and therapy with an MAO inhibitor used to treat a psychiatric disorder is begun.

- Screen patient for bipolar disorder before vortioxetine therapy is begun. Monitor patient for mania, which may result from use of drug in a susceptible patient, especially patients with bipolar disorder.

! **WARNING** Monitor patient for a hypersensitivity reaction, which could become life-threatening, such as anaphylaxis. If present, notify prescriber, expect drug to be switched to another drug, and provide supportive care, as needed and ordered.

! **WARNING** Watch patient closely for suicidal tendencies, particularly when therapy starts and dosage changes because depression may worsen temporarily during these times, possibly leading to suicidal ideation.

! **WARNING** Monitor patient for seizure activity, especially in a patient with a seizure disorder.

! **WARNING** Monitor patient closely for evidence of increased bleeding, such as GI bleeding, especially if patient also takes a drug known to cause GI bleeding, such as aspirin, a NSAID, warfarin, or other anticoagulants.

! **WARNING** Monitor patient's serum sodium level because hyponatremia has occurred with use of serotonergic drugs, including vortioxetine. Patients at greater risk include the elderly and patients taking diuretics or who are volume-depleted. Report signs and symptoms of hyponatremia, such as confusion, difficulty concentrating, headache, memory impairment, unsteadiness, or weakness. If left untreated, coma, death, hallucinations, respiratory arrest, seizures, or syncope may occur.

! **WARNING** Monitor patient closely for serotonin syndrome exhibited by agitation, coma, diarrhea, hallucinations, hyperreflexia, hyperthermia, incoordination, labile blood pressure, nausea, or vomiting. Notify prescriber immediately because serotonin syndrome may be life-threatening and provide supportive care.

! **WARNING** Monitor patient for any other persistent, serious, or unusual adverse reactions.

- Expect dosage to be decreased to 10 mg once daily for 1 week before vortioxetine is discontinued to avoid patient experiencing dizziness, headaches, mood swings, including muscle tension, runny nose, or sudden outbursts of anger that may occur in the first week of abrupt discontinuation of drug.

PATIENT TEACHING

! **WARNING** Tell pregnant patient to alert prescriber when she is within 1 month of deliver.

- Encourage patient to have an eye exam before starting therapy to see if at risk for an episode of acute angle-closure glaucoma that may be drug induced.
- Instruct patient how to administer vortioxetine.
- Tell patient to take drug exactly as prescribed, be consistent with daily administration time, and alert prescriber with concerns.
- Warn patient not to discontinue drug abruptly, as serious adverse reactions may occur.
- Inform patient that nausea is the most common side effect of vortioxetine therapy, and it commonly occurs within the first week of treatment.

! **WARNING** Alert patient that drug may cause an allergic reaction. If an allergic reaction occurs, tell patient to notify prescriber and, if severe, to seek immediate medical attention.

! **WARNING** Tell family or caregiver to observe patient closely for suicidal tendencies, especially when therapy starts or dosage changes and when drug is given to young adults.

- Advise patient to inform all prescribers of vortioxetine therapy.

! **WARNING** Alert patients about risk of bleeding when taking drugs known to increase risk of bleeding, such as aspirin, blood thinners, or NSAIDs.

! **WARNING** Inform elderly patient or patient who is taking drugs, such as diuretics, that cause dehydration of the risk of a low sodium level; tell patient to alert prescriber if new or sudden onset of symptoms are experienced.

! **WARNING** Emphasize importance of reporting any other persistent, severe, or sudden symptoms to prescriber.

- Encourage patient to discuss sexual difficulties with prescriber, if present.
- Tell patient to inform all prescribers of vortioxetine therapy and not to take any over-the-counter medications, including herbal products, without prescriber knowledge.

warfarin sodium

Jantoven

Class and Category

Pharmacologic class: Coumarin derivative
Therapeutic class: Anticoagulant

Indications and Dosages

∗ *To prevent and treat venous thrombosis and its extension, pulmonary embolism; to prevent and treat thromboembolic complications associated with atrial fibrillation and/or cardiac valve replacement; to reduce risk of death, recurrent MI, and thromboembolic events, such as stroke or systemic embolization after MI*

TABLETS

Adults. Highly individualized, based on age, body weight, comorbidities, concomitant medications, race, and sex and adjusted based on INR checked every 1 to 4 wk. *Usual initial:* 2 to 5 mg daily for 2 to 4 days. *Maintenance:* 2 to 10 mg daily based on target INR and PT results. Treatment should be given for length of time for these specific conditions as follows: 3 mo for patients with a deep venous thrombosis (DVT) or pulmonary embolism (PE) secondary to a transient reversible risk factor or for at least 3 mo for an unprovoked DVT or PE; at least 3 mo after an MI; long-term for 2 episodes of unprovoked DVT or PE; first 3 mo after bioprosthetic valve insertion in the mitral valve location; and long-term for atrial fibrillation and mitral stenosis or atrial fibrillation and prosthetic heart valves.

± **DOSAGE ADJUSTMENT** For Asian, debilitated, or elderly patients and patients with CYP2C9 or VKORC1 genotypes, initial and maintenance dosages reduced and then adjusted based on INR and PT results.

Drug Administration

P.O.

- Administer drug at the same time each evening.
- Drug dosages will be adjusted according to INR values.
- Avoid I.M. injections during warfarin therapy, if possible, because they can result in bleeding, bruising, and hematoma.
- If a dose is missed, administer as soon as possible on the day dose was missed. If not, do not double dose the next day to make up for a missed dose.

Route	Onset	Peak	Duration
P.O.	< 24 hr	1.5–3 days	2–5 days

Half-life: 20–60 hr

Mechanism of Action

Interferes with the liver's ability to synthesize vitamin K–dependent clotting factors, depleting clotting factors II (prothrombin), VII, IX, and X. This action, in turn, interferes with the clotting cascade. By depleting vitamin K–dependent clotting factors and interfering with the clotting cascade, warfarin prevents coagulation.

Contraindications

Bacterial endocarditis; bleeding or hemorrhagic tendencies such as active ulceration or overt bleeding of the GI, genitourinary, or respiratory tract as well as CNS hemorrhage, including cerebral aneurysms and dissecting aorta; blood dyscrasias; cerebral or dissecting aneurysm; cerebrovascular hemorrhage; eclampsia, preeclampsia, or threatened abortion; hypersensitivity to warfarin or its components; major lumbar or regional block anesthesia; malignant hypertension; mental state or condition that leads to lack of patient cooperation, or unsupervised situation; pericardial effusion; pericarditis; pregnancy except in women with mechanical heart valves, who are at high risk of thromboembolism; recent or planned neurosurgery, ophthalmic surgery, or traumatic surgery resulting in large open surfaces; spinal puncture and other diagnostic or therapeutic procedures with potential for uncontrollable bleeding

Interactions

DRUGS

acyclovir, allopurinol, alprazolam, amiodarone, amlodipine, amprenavir, aprepitant, atorvastatin, atazanavir, bicalutamide, capecitabine, cilostazol, cimetidine, ciprofloxacin, clarithromycin, conivaptan, cotrimoxazole, cyclosporine, darunavir/ritonavir, diltiazem, disulfiram, erythromycin, enoxacin, etravirine, famotidine, fluconazole, fluoxetine, fluvastatin, fluvoxamine, fosamprenavir, imatinib, indinavir, isoniazid, itraconazole, ketoconazole, lopinavir/ritonavir, methoxsalen, metronidazole, miconazole, mexiletine, nalidixic acid, nefazodone, nelfinavir, nilotinib, norfloxacin, NSAIDs, oral contraceptives, oxandrolone, phenylpropanolamine, posaconazole, propafenone, propranolol, ranolazine, ritonavir, saquinavir, sulfinpyrazone, terbinafine, telithromycin, thiabendazole, ticlopidine, tigecycline, tipranavir, verapamil, voriconazole, zafirlukast, zileuton: Increased anticoagulant effect of warfarin, increased risk of bleeding

armodafinil, amprenavir, aprepitant, bosentan, carbamazepine, efavirenz, etravirine, modafinil, montelukast, moricizine, nafcillin, phenobarbital, phenytoin, pioglitazone, prednisone, rifampin, rufinamide: Decreased anticoagulant effect of warfarin

herbal remedies (including garlic, ginkgo biloba, ginseng): Increased anticoagulant effect of warfarin, increased risk of bleeding

other herbal remedies (including co-enzyme Q10, ginseng, St. John's wort): Decreased anticoagulant effect

ACTIVITIES

alcohol use: Increased risk of hypoprothrombinemia

smoking, smoking cessation aids: Altered response to warfarin

Adverse Reactions

CNS: **Coma**, **intracranial hemorrhage**, loss of consciousness, syncope, weakness

CV: Angina, calcium uremic arteriolopathy (calciphylaxis), chest pain, **hypotension**

EENT: Epistaxis, intraocular hemorrhage

GI: Abdominal cramps and pain, diarrhea, **hepatitis**, jaundice, nausea, vomiting

GU: Hematuria, vaginal bleeding (abnormal)

HEME: Anemia, **potentially fatal hemorrhage**

SKIN: Alopecia, ecchymosis, petechiae, pruritus, purple-toe syndrome, tissue necrosis

Other: **Anaphylaxis**

Childbearing Considerations

PREGNANCY

- Drug can cause fetal harm, such as severe fetal abnormalities as well as fatal hemorrhage.
- Drug is contraindicated in pregnancy (except in pregnant women with mechanical heart valves).
- A pregnancy test should be performed before drug is begun.

LACTATION

- It is not clear if drug is present in breast milk.
- Mothers should check with prescriber before breastfeeding.
- If breastfeeding is undertaken, monitor infant for unusual bleeding or bruising.

REPRODUCTION

- Females of childbearing age should use effective contraception during treatment and for 1 mo after last dose of drug.

Nursing Considerations

! **WARNING** Ensure that females of childbearing age have a negative pregnancy test result before warfarin therapy is initiated. Inform patient that warfarin is contraindicated during pregnancy except if mother has mechanical heart values. Tell patient to alert prescriber immediately if pregnancy occurs.

- Expect to give another parenteral anticoagulant, such as enoxaparin or heparin, with oral warfarin for at least 3 days, or until desired response occurs, before giving warfarin only.

- Monitor INR (daily in acute care setting) and assess for therapeutic effects, as prescribed. Therapeutic INR levels are 2.0 to 3.0 for bioprosthetic heart valve, nonvalvular atrial fibrillation, and venous thromboembolism, and 2.5 to 3.5 after MI and for mechanical heart valve.

! **WARNING** Monitor patient for a hypersensitivity reaction, which can become life-threatening, such as anaphylaxis. If present, notify prescriber, expect drug to be switched to a different anticoagulant, and provide supportive care, as needed and ordered.

! **WARNING** Monitor patient with hepatic impairment closely for bleeding because hepatic impairment decreases metabolism of warfarin and impairs synthesis of clotting factors. Expect to monitor patient's INR more frequently.

! **WARNING** Be aware of the increased risk for intracranial hemorrhage if patient has cerebral ischemia (such as recent transient ischemic attack or minor ischemic stroke) and INR of 3 to 4.5. As ordered, withhold next warfarin dose and give vitamin K, as ordered, if INR exceeds 4 because of the risk of bleeding.

! **WARNING** Assess for occult bleeding if patient receives I.V. lipid emulsion or other medical product that contains soybean oil. Such products can decrease vitamin K absorption and increase warfarin's anticoagulant effect.

! **WARNING** Monitor patient for persistent, severe, sudden, or unusual signs and symptoms, as warfarin therapy may cause many adverse reactions, including calciphylaxis, a syndrome of blood clots, calcification of blood vessels, and skin necrosis. If diagnosed, expect warfarin therapy to be discontinued and alternative anticoagulation therapy prescribed.

PATIENT TEACHING

! **WARNING** Inform females of childbearing age to notify prescriber immediately if pregnancy occurs as drug is contraindicated in pregnancy except in mothers with mechanical valves. Instruct these patients to use an effective contraceptive during warfarin therapy and for at least 1 month after warfarin has been discontinued.

- Explain that warfarin therapy aims to prevent thrombosis by decreasing clotting ability while avoiding the risk of spontaneous bleeding.
- Instruct patient how to administer warfarin and what to do if a dose is missed.
- Urge patient to keep weekly follow-up appointments for blood tests after discharge until PT and INR levels are stabilized.
- Advise patient to avoid alcohol during warfarin therapy.
- Advise patient to avoid drastic changes in dietary habits, such as eating large amounts of leafy, green vegetables. Explain that dark green, leafy vegetables contain vitamin K that counteracts the effects of warfarin.

! **WARNING** Alert patient that drug may cause an allergic reaction. If present, tell patient to notify prescriber and, if severe, to seek immediate medical care.

! **WARNING** Advise patient to take precautions against bleeding, such as using an electric shaver and a soft-bristled toothbrush. Also, caution patient to avoid activities that could cause traumatic injury and bleeding. Advise patient to continue these precautions for 2 to 5 days after therapy stops, as directed, because anticoagulant effect may persist during this time. Urge patient to notify prescriber immediately about unusual bleeding and unexplained symptoms, such as abnormal vaginal bleeding; dizziness; easy bruising; gum bleeding; headache; nosebleeds; prolonged bleeding from cuts; red, black, or tarry stool; red or dark brown urine; swelling; and weakness.

! **WARNING** Tell mothers who are breastfeeding to monitor infant for bleeding or bruising and to notify prescriber immediately if either occurs.

! **WARNING** Tell patient to contact prescriber immediately if pain and discoloration of the skin mostly on areas of the body with a high fat content, such as abdomen, breasts, buttocks, hips, and thighs or any unusual symptoms are experienced. Explain that drug may cause reversible purple-toe syndrome but that this syndrome isn't harmful.

- Advise patient to consult prescriber before taking any other drugs, including over-the-counter drugs and herbal remedies during therapy. Also, instruct patient not to discontinue any drug, including over-the-counter drugs and herbal products taken regularly without consulting prescriber.
- Urge patient to carry medical identification that reveals patient is taking warfarin.
- Tell patient to inform all dentists and healthcare professionals about warfarin therapy, especially before any procedure or surgery, including dental, is performed.

X Y Z

zafirlukast

Accolate

Class and Category

Pharmacologic class: Leukotriene receptor antagonist
Therapeutic class: Antiasthmatic

Indications and Dosages

∗ *To prevent or treat chronic asthma*

TABLETS

Adults and children ages 12 and older. 20 mg twice daily.
Children ages 5 to 11. 10 mg twice daily.

Drug Administration

P.O.

- Administer drug at same times daily.
- Give drug on an empty stomach at least 1 hr before or 2 hr after meals.

Route	Onset	Peak	Duration
P.O.	1 wk	3 hr	12 hr

Half-life: 10 hr

Mechanism of Action

Inhibits the selective binding of cysteinyl leukotrienes (arachidonic acid derivatives that usually mediate inflammation in asthma and other inflammatory disorders) by competitively blocking receptor sites. This action causes bronchial relaxation and decreases bronchial hyperresponsiveness, eosinophil movement, mucus secretion, and vascular leakage.

Contraindications

Hepatic impairment, including hepatic cirrhosis, hypersensitivity to zafirlukast or its components

Interactions

DRUGS

aspirin: Increased blood zafirlukast level
carbamazepine, tolbutamide: Possibly increased levels of these drugs and, possibly, additive adverse effects
erythromycin: Decreased response to zafirlukast
fluconazole: Increased plasma zafirlukast levels
theophylline: Decreased zafirlukast level; possibly increased theophylline levels
warfarin: Prolonged PT

Adverse Reactions

CNS: Asthenia, depression, dizziness, fever, headache, insomnia, malaise
CV: Edema, vasculitis
GI: Abdominal pain, diarrhea, edema, elevated liver enzymes, **hepatic failure**, **hepatitis**, hyperbilirubinemia, indigestion, nausea, vomiting
HEME: **Agranulocytosis**, **bleeding**, eosinophilia
MS: Arthralgia, back pain, myalgia
RESP: **Eosinophilic pneumonia**
SKIN: Bruising, pruritus, rash, urticaria
Other: **Angioedema and other hypersensitivity reactions**, generalized pain, infections

Childbearing Considerations

PREGNANCY

- It is not known if drug can cause fetal harm.
- Use with caution only if benefit to mother outweighs potential risk to fetus.

LACTATION

- Drug is present in breast milk.
- Breastfeeding is not recommended during drug therapy.

Nursing Considerations

! WARNING Know that zafirlukast shouldn't be used to treat bronchospasm during an acute asthma attack or status asthmaticus; it can't relieve symptoms quickly enough.

- Assess respiratory depth, quality, and rate, as well as breath sounds, before and during treatment to evaluate response to therapy.

! WARNING Be aware that if patient is being weaned from corticosteroids while taking zafirlukast, patient should be monitored for Churg-Strauss syndrome—a rare allergic reaction characterized by eosinophilia, fever, myalgia, and weight loss—for cardiac complications, neuropathy, and worsening pulmonary symptoms.

! WARNING Monitor patient for a hypersensitivity reaction, which could become life-threatening, such as angioedema. If present, notify prescriber, expect drug to be discontinued, and provide supportive care, as needed and ordered.

! **WARNING** Monitor patient for liver dysfunction and expect to monitor liver enzyme levels, as ordered because drug can cause hepatic failure or hepatitis. Notify prescriber immediately if patient develops any evidence of liver dysfunction, such as anorexia, fatigue, flu-like symptoms, jaundice, lethargy, nausea, right upper-quadrant abdominal pain, or pruritus.

! **WARNING** Tell patient to report any other persistent, serious, or unusual adverse reactions, some of which could be serious such as hematological adverse reactions.

PATIENT TEACHING

! **WARNING** Urge patient to continue using prescribed rescue inhalants for acute asthma attacks. Stress importance of zafirlukast not being used to treat bronchospasm during an acute asthma attack or status asthmaticus. Explain that it can't relieve symptoms quickly enough.

- Instruct patient, family, or caregiver how to administer zafirlukast.
- Tell patient to take drug exactly as prescribed, in evenly spaced doses, every day, even during acute exacerbations and symptom-free periods.
- Teach patient how to use peak-flow meter to monitor pulmonary function.

! **WARNING** Alert patient that drug can cause an allergic reaction. If present, stress importance of notifying prescriber and, if severe, to seek immediate medical care.

! **WARNING** Tell patient to report immediately any evidence of liver dysfunction, such as anorexia, fatigue, flu-like symptoms, jaundice, lethargy, nausea, right upper-quadrant abdominal pain, or pruritus.

! **WARNING** Tell patient to notify prescriber of any other persistent, serious, or unusual adverse reactions.

- Inform mothers breastfeeding should not be undertaken during zafirlukast therapy.

zaleplon

Sonata

Class, Category, and Schedule

Pharmacologic class: Pyrazolopyrimidine
Therapeutic class: Hypnotic
Controlled substance schedule: IV

Indications and Dosages

* *Short-term treatment of insomnia*

CAPSULES

Adults up to age 65. 10 mg at bedtime as needed, for up to 35 days. *Usual:* 10 mg at bedtime for 7 to 10 days. *Maximum:* 20 mg at bedtime.

± **DOSAGE ADJUSTMENT** For patients who are debilitated or elderly, dosage reduced to 5 mg daily and maximum dosage reduced to 10 mg at bedtime. For patients who have hepatic impairment or low weight, or take cimetidine, dosage reduced to 5 mg at bedtime.

Drug Administration

P.O.

- Administer immediately before bedtime or after patient has gone to bed and has difficulty falling asleep.
- Avoid giving with or after a heavy, high-fat meal because decreased absorption may reduce drug's effects.

Route	Onset	Peak	Duration
P.O.	30 min	1 hr	3–4 hr

Half-life: 1 hr

Mechanism of Action

Binds selectively with type 1 benzodiazepine (BZ1 or omega$_1$) receptors on the gamma-aminobutyric acid-A receptor complex. This binding produces muscle relaxation and sedation as well as antianxiety and anticonvulsant effects.

Contraindications

Hypersensitivity to zaleplon or its components; past experience of complex sleep behaviors during zaleplon therapy

Interactions

DRUGS

carbamazepine, phenobarbital, phenytoin, rifampin: Reduced zaleplon effects
cimetidine: Increased blood zaleplon level

CNS depressants, diphenhydramine, imipramine, thioridazine: Additive CNS effects
erythromycin, ketoconazole: Increased zaleplon concentration
flumazenil: Reversal of zaleplon's sedation
promethazine: Possibly decreased plasma zaleplon concentration

ACTIVITIES

alcohol use: Increased CNS depression

FOODS

high-fat foods: Prolonged absorption time and reduced effectiveness of zaleplon

Adverse Reactions

CNS: Amnesia, anxiety, complex behaviors (such as sleep driving), depression, dizziness, drowsiness, fever, hallucinations, hypertonia, insomnia, nightmares, paresthesia, **seizures**, **suicidal ideation**, tremor, vertigo
EENT: Dry mouth, gingivitis, glossitis, mouth ulcers, stomatitis, **throat tightness**
GI: Anorexia, colitis, constipation, eructation, esophagitis, flatulence, gastritis, gastroenteritis, increased appetite, indigestion, **melena**, nausea, **rectal bleeding**, vomiting
MS: Back pain
RESP: Dyspnea
SKIN: Photosensitivity, pruritus, rash
Other: **Anaphylaxis**, **angioedema**, physical and psychological dependence

Childbearing Considerations

PREGNANCY

- It is not known if drug can cause fetal harm.
- Drug is not recommended for use in pregnant women because effects are unknown.

LACTATION

- Drug is present in breast milk in small amounts.
- Breastfeeding is not recommended during drug therapy.

Nursing Considerations

! **WARNING** Be aware zaleplon can cause physical and psychological dependency, which could lead to abuse, misuse, and addiction because drug has an abuse potential similar to that of benzodiazepines and benzodiazepine-like hypnotics. Monitor patient closely for signs of drug abuse and notify prescriber of any indications of abuse, misuse, or addiction.

! **WARNING** Watch patient closely for suicidal tendencies, particularly when therapy starts and dosage changes because depression may worsen temporarily during these times, possibly leading to suicidal ideation.

! **WARNING** Monitor patient closely for a hypersensitivity reaction, which could become life-threatening, such as anaphylaxis or angioedema. If present, immediately, notify prescriber, expect drug to be discontinued, and provide supportive care, as needed and ordered.

! **WARNING** Monitor patient for seizure activity, especially patients with a history of seizures. Institute seizure precautions, as appropriate.

! **WARNING** Assess patient regularly for signs and symptoms of GI dysfunction such as melana and rectal bleeding.

PATIENT TEACHING

! **WARNING** Explain that zaleplon is intended for short-term use. Warn patient that drug can cause physical and psychological dependency. Advise against using it for any condition other than insomnia and caution patient not to exceed prescribed dosage.

- Instruct patient how to administer zaleplon.
- Warn patient not to take drug with less than a full night of sleep remaining (7 or 8 hours) because of the risk of next-day psychomotor impairment, including impaired driving.
- Urge patient to avoid alcohol during zaleplon therapy because it increases risk of abnormal behaviors, such as sleep driving.
- Advise patient to consult prescriber before taking other CNS depressants.

! **WARNING** Alert patient that drug may cause an allergic reaction. Warn patient that zaleplon contains FD & C Yellow No. 5 (tartrazine), which can cause an allergic reaction, especially in those with an aspirin sensitivity. Instruct patient to notify prescriber immediately if an allergic reaction occurs and, if severe, to seek immediate medical care.

! **WARNING** Urge family or caregiver to watch patient closely for suicidal tendencies, especially when therapy starts or dosage changes. If present, tell family or caregiver to notify prescriber immediately. Review suicide precautions to take, if needed.

! **WARNING** Inform patient drug may cause seizure activity. Tell patient to seek immediate medical care if a seizure occurs. Review seizure precautions, as appropriate.

- Caution patient about performing hazardous activities, such as driving, until the effects of zaleplon are known and resolved because it can cause dizziness and drowsiness. Also, warn patient to take fall precautions.
- Explain that drug may cause abnormal behaviors during sleep, such as driving a car, eating, having sex, or talking on the phone without any recall of the event. If family or caregiver notices any such behavior or patient sees evidence of such behavior upon awakening, prescriber should be notified.

! **WARNING** Tell patient to alert prescriber of any other persistent, serious, or unusual adverse reactions.

- Tell females of childbearing age to notify prescriber if pregnancy occurs.
- Inform mothers breastfeeding is not recommended during zaleplon therapy.

zavegepant

Zavzpret

Class and Category

Pharmacologic class: Calcitonin gene-related peptide receptor antagonist
Therapeutic class: Antimigraine

Indications and Dosages

∗ *To treat acute migraine*

NASAL SPRAY

Adults. 10 mg as a single spray in one nostril, as needed. *Maximum:* 10 mg in a 24-hr period; 8 migraines in 30-day period.

Drug Administration

NASAL SPRAY

- Each unit-dose device delivers a single spray of 10 mg.
- Do not test spray, prime, or press the plunger before use.
- Have patient blow nose before using spray. Have patient close one nostril.
- Gently insert bottle tip into the one open nostril, keeping patient's head upright and mouth closed. Have patient breathe in slowly while squeezing the bottle. Do not let the nozzle come out while pressing the plunger. Then remove tip from nostril and discard device.
- Have patient keep head level for 20 sec. Also have patient breathe in through the nose and out through the mouth for 10 to 20 sec.
- If a drip from the nose occurs, have patient gently sniff.
- Store drug at room temperature.

Route	Onset	Peak	Duration
Nasal spray	Unknown	30 min	Unknown

Half-life: 6.55 hr

Mechanism of Action

Binds to calcitonin gene-related peptide ligand to block its binding to the receptor, which is thought to play a role in pain relief although the precise mechanism is unknown.

Contraindications

Hypersensitivity to zavegepant or its components

Interactions

DRUGS

intranasal decongestants: Possibly decreased absorption of zavegepant, which could decrease effectiveness of zavegepant
OATP1B3 and NTCP inducers: Possibly decreased zavegepant exposure, which could decrease effectiveness of zavegepant
OATP1B3 and NTCP inhibitors: Possibly increased zavegepant exposure, which could increase adverse reactions

Adverse Reactions

CV: Hypertension, Raynaud's phenomenon
EENT: Nasal discomfort, taste alteration
GI: Nausea, vomiting
SKIN: Urticaria
Other: **Angioedema**

Childbearing Considerations

PREGNANCY

- It is not known if drug can cause fetal harm.
- Use with caution only if benefit to mother outweighs potential risk to fetus.

- Know that women with migraines may be at increased risk for preeclampsia during pregnancy.

LACTATION

- It is not known if drug is present in breast milk.
- Mothers should check with prescriber before breastfeeding.

Nursing Considerations

- Be aware that zavegepant is not indicated to prevent migraines, only treat them.
- Plan to administer intransasal decongestants, if ordered, at least 1 hour after zavegepant administration because intranasal decongestants may decrease the absorption of zavegepant.

! WARNING Monitor patient for a hypersensitivity reaction, which could become life-threatening, such as angioedema. If present, notify prescriber immediately, expect drug to be discontinued, and provide supportive care, as needed and ordered.

PATIENT TEACHING

- Inform patient that zavegepant is prescribed to treat migraines, not prevent them.
- Instruct patient how to administer zavegepant as a nasal spray.
- Caution patient to take any prescribed intranasal decongestants at least 1 hour after zavegepant administration.

! WARNING Alert patient that drug can cause an allergic reaction. If present, tell patient to notify prescriber and, if severe, to seek immediate medical care.

- Instruct patient to notify all prescribers of zavegepant therapy and not to take any over-the-counter drugs, including herbal products, without alerting prescriber.

zidovudine

Retrovir

Class and Category

Pharmacologic class: Nucleoside reverse transcriptase inhibitor
Therapeutic class: Antiretroviral

Indications and Dosages

∗ *As adjunct to treat human immunodeficiency viral type (HIV-1) infection*

CAPSULES, ORAL SOLUTION

Adults. 300 mg twice daily.
Children at least 4 wk old to less than 18 years weighing 30 kg (66 lb) or more. 300 mg twice daily or 200 mg 3 times daily. Alternatively, 240 mg/m^2 body surface area (BSA) twice daily or 160 mg/m^2 BSA 3 times daily. *Maximum:* 600 mg daily divided into 2 or 3 doses.
Infants at least 4 wk old and children less than 18 years weighing 9 kg (19.8 lb) to less than 30 kg (66 lb). 9 mg/kg twice daily or 6 mg/kg 3 times daily. Alternatively, 240 mg/m^2 BSA twice daily or 160 mg/m^2 BSA 3 times daily. *Maximum:* 18 mg/kg/day divided into 2 or 3 doses.
Infants at least 4 wk old and weighing at least 4 kg (8.8 lb) but less than 9 kg (19.8 lb). 12 mg/kg twice daily or 8 mg/kg 3 times daily. Alternatively, 240 mg/m^2 BSA twice daily or 160 mg/m^2 BSA 3 times daily. *Maximum:* 24 mg/kg/day divided into 2 or 3 doses.

I.V. INFUSION

Adults. 1 mg/kg infused over 1 hr every 4 hr until oral dosage can be initiated.

∗ *To prevent maternal-fetal HIV-1 transmission*

CAPSULES, ORAL SOLUTION

Pregnant women at greater than 14 wk of pregnancy. 100 mg 5 times daily until start of labor.

I.V. INFUSION

Pregnant women during labor and delivery. *Initial:* 2 mg/kg infused over 1 hr followed by 1 mg/kg/hr until umbilical cord is clamped.

ORAL SOLUTION

Neonate within 12 hr after birth. 2 mg/kg every 6 hr for 6 wk.

I.V. INFUSION

Neonate within 12 hr after birth. 1.5 mg/kg infused over 30 min every 6 hr for 6 wk or until oral administration can be initiated.

± **DOSAGE ADJUSTMENT** For adult patients on dialysis or who have a creatinine clearance of less than 15 ml/min, oral dosage reduced to 100 mg every 6 to 8 hours and the intravenous dosage maintained at 1 mg/kg but dosing interval increased to every 6 to 8 hours. For adult patients whose hemoglobin falls to less than 7.5 g/dl or the reduction is greater than 25% of baseline and/or granulocyte count falls to less than 750 cells/mm^3 or the reduction is greater than 50% of baseline, drug withheld until marrow recovery occurs.

Drug Administration

P.O.

- Use calibrated device to measure syrup dosage; for neonates, use a syringe with 0.1-ml markings to ensure accurate dosage.
- Store capsules in a cool, dry environment.
- A missed dose should be administered as soon as possible. Never double the next dose to make up for the missed dose.

I.V.

- Drug vial stopper contains natural rubber latex and should not be handled by someone with a latex allergy.
- Dilute drug with 5% Dextrose Injection to achieve a concentration no greater than 4 mg/ml.
- Use diluted solution within 8 hr if left at room temperature and 48 hr if refrigerated.
- Infuse at a constant rate of 1 mg/kg slowly over 1 hr for adults and 30 min for neonates. If given to a pregnant woman during labor, follow initial infusion given over 1 hr by a continuous infusion at a rate of 1 mg/kg/hr until umbilical cord is clamped.
- Drug should never be given as a bolus injection or by rapid infusion, nor should it be administered intramuscularly.
- *Incompatibilities:* None listed by manufacturer

Route	Onset	Peak	Duration
P.O./I.V.	Unknown	30–90 min	Unknown

Half-life: 1–3 hr

Mechanism of Action

Be aware that after it is phosphorylated to its active metabolite, the metabolite inhibits the DNA- and RNA-dependent polymerase activities of HIV-1 reverse transcriptases via DNA chain termination after incorporation of the nucleotide analogue into viral DNA. This destroys activity of the HIV-1 viruses.

Contraindications

Hypersensitivity to zidovudine or its components

Interactions

DRUGS

bone marrow suppressive or cytotoxic agents, such as ganciclovir, interferon alfa, ribavirin: Possibly increased hematologic toxicity of zidovudine

doxorubicin, nucleoside analogues affecting DNA replication, such as ribavirin, stavudine: Antagonistic relationship between the 2 drugs

Adverse Reactions

CNS: Anxiety, asthenia, chills, confusion, decreased reflexes, depression, dizziness, fatigue, headache, insomnia, irritability, loss of mental acuity, malaise, mania, nervousness, neuropathy, paresthesia, **seizures**, somnolence, syncope, tremor, vertigo

CV: **Cardiomyopathy**, chest pain, **congestive heart failure**, **ECG abnormalities**, edema, left ventricular dilation, vasculitis

EENT: Amblyopia; ear discharge, erythema, pain, or swelling; hearing loss; macular edema; mouth ulcers; nasal congestion or discharge; oral mucosa pigmentation; photophobia; rhinitis; sinusitis; stomatitis; taste perversion

ENDO: Cushingoid appearance, fat redistribution, gynecomastia

GI: Abdominal cramps or pain, anorexia, constipation, diarrhea, dyspepsia, dysphagia, elevated liver or pancreatic enzymes, flatulence, **hepatic decompensation**, **hepatitis**, hyperbilirubinemia, jaundice, nausea, **pancreatitis**, **severe hepatomegaly with steatosis**, splenomegaly, vomiting

GU: Hematuria, urinary frequency or hesitancy

HEME: Anemia, **aplastic anemia**, **granulocytopenia**, **hemolytic anemia**, **leukopenia**, macrocytosis, **neutropenia**, **pancytopenia with marrow hypoplasia**, **pure red cell aplasia**, **thrombocytopenia**

MS: Arthralgia, back pain, musculoskeletal pain, muscle spasm, myalgia, myopathy, myositis, **rhabdomyolysis**

RESP: Abnormal breath sounds, cough, dyspnea, wheezing

SKIN: Diaphoresis, pigmentation changes in nails and skin, pruritus, rash, **Stevens-Johnson syndrome**, **toxic epidermal necrolysis**, urticaria

Other: **Anaphylaxis**, **angioedema**, elevated CPK and LDH levels, flu-like symptoms, generalized pain, **immune reconstitution syndrome**, intravenous site irritation or pain, **lactic acidosis**, lymphadenopathy, weight loss

Childbearing Considerations

PREGNANCY

- Pregnancy exposure registry: 1-800-258-4263.
- Drug does not appear to cause fetal harm.
- Use with caution only if benefit to mother outweighs potential risk to fetus, especially in the second and third trimesters.

LACTATION

- Drug is present in breast milk.
- The Centers for Disease Control and Prevention recommend that HIV-1 infected mothers not breastfeed to avoid risking postnatal transmission of HIV-1 infection to infants. They also do not recommend breastfeeding because of potential drug-induced adverse reactions in the infant.

Nursing Considerations

- Know that pediatric dosage is based upon body weight in kg or alternatively on BSA. In some cases, the dosage calculated by body weight will not be the same as that calculated by BSA.

! **WARNING** Monitor patient for a hypersensitivity reaction, which could become life-threatening, such as anaphylaxis or angioedema. If present, alert prescriber, expect drug to be discontinued, and provide supportive care, as needed and ordered.

! **WARNING** Monitor patients with hepatic dysfunction closely, including liver cirrhosis, because of potential for hepatic decompensation. Know that lactic acidosis and severe hepatomegaly with steatosis have occurred with zidovudine therapy, and death has occurred in some patients. Risk factors include presence of obesity, prolonged nucleoside exposure, and being a woman. However, know that lactic acidosis and severe hepatomegaly with steatosis have also occurred in patients with no known risk factors. Expect drug to be discontinued in any patient who develops clinical or laboratory findings suggestive of lactic acidosis or pronounced hepatotoxicity, even in the absence of marked transaminase elevations.

! **WARNING** Be aware that prolonged therapy increases the risk of myopathy and myositis, which could lead to life-threatening rhabdomyolysis. Monitor patient closely for adverse muscle signs and symptoms.

! **WARNING** Be aware that immune reconstitution syndrome has occurred in patients treated with combination antiretroviral therapy, including zidovudine. The inflammatory response predisposes susceptible patients to opportunistic infections, such as cytomegalovirus, *Mycobacterium avium* infection, *Pneumocystis jiroveci* pneumonia, or tuberculosis. Autoimmune disorders, such as Graves' disease, Guillain-Barré syndrome, or polymyositis have also occurred. Report sudden or unusual adverse reactions to prescriber.

! **WARNING** Monitor patients closely who are receiving interferon alfa and/or ribavirin in addition to zidovudine for treatment-associated toxicities, especially anemia, hepatic decompensation, and neutropenia. Dosage reduction or discontinuation of interferon alfa, ribavirin, or both may be required if zidovudine toxicities become serious.

- Know that coadministration of ribavirin and zidovudine exacerbates the development of zidovudine-induced anemia. For a patient who had developed severe anemia and/or neutropenia and required drug to be withheld until marrow recovered, adjunctive supportive measures such as epoetin alfa might be required when zidovudine therapy is restarted.
- Observe patient for redistribution of body fat, including breast enlargement, central obesity, development of buffalo hump, facial wasting, and peripheral wasting, which may produce a cushingoid-type appearance.

! **WARNING** Monitor patient for other persistent, serious, or unusual adverse reactions.

PATIENT TEACHING

- Instruct patient, family, or caregiver how to administer oral zidovudine and what to do if a dose is missed.

! **WARNING** Stress importance of taking extra care when administering drug to infants and children to avoid dosage errors.

! **WARNING** Alert patient, family, or caregiver that drug may cause an allergic reaction.

If present, tell patient to notify prescriber and, if severe, to seek immediate medical care.

! **WARNING** Inform patient that zidovudine may cause lactic acidosis, which if not treated, could be fatal. Tell patient to seek immediate medical attention if breathing difficulty, cold or numb feeling in arms and legs, dizziness, fast or uneven heart rate, muscle pain or weakness, nausea, vomiting, or any other unexpected or unusual signs or symptoms develops.

! **WARNING** Alert patient that severe conditions may develop while taking zidovudine. Encourage patient to notify prescriber and seek immediate medical care if any persistent, severe, or unusual symptoms are experienced. If toxicity develops, inform patient that transfusions may be needed or zidovudine discontinued.

- Inform patient that periodic laboratory studies will have to be performed and that compliance with these appointments is essential for early detection of adverse reactions.
- Alert patient that fat accumulation and redistribution may occur during zidovudine therapy.
- Advise patient to inform all prescribers of zidovudine therapy.
- Tell mothers that breastfeeding should not be done during zidovudine therapy.

zinc acetate

Galzin

zinc chloride

zinc gluconate

Orazinc

zinc sulfate

Orazinc 110, Orazinc 220, Verazinc, Zinc, Zinc-220, Zinca-Pak, Zincate

Class and Category

Pharmacologic class: Trace element, mineral
Therapeutic class: Nutritional supplement

Indications and Dosages

* *To prevent zinc deficiency based on recommended daily allowances*

CAPSULES, E.R. TABLETS, LOZENGES, TABLETS

Men ages 19 and older. 11 mg daily.
Women ages 19 and older. 8 mg daily.
Pregnant women. 11 mg daily.
Breastfeeding women. 12 mg daily.
Pregnant adolescents ages 14 to 18. 12 mg daily.
Breastfeeding adolescents ages 14 to 18. 13 mg daily.
Male adolescents ages 14 to 18. 11 mg daily.
Female adolescents ages 14 to 18. 9 mg daily.
Children ages 9 to 13. 8 mg daily.
Children ages 4 to 8. 5 mg daily.
Children ages 1 to 3. 3 mg daily.
Infants ages 7 mo to 12 mo. 3 mg daily.
Newborns to 6 mo. 2 mg daily.

* *To treat zinc deficiency*

CAPSULES, E.R. TABLETS, LOZENGES, TABLETS

Adults and children. Dosage individualized based on severity of deficiency.

I.V. INFUSION (ZINC CHLORIDE)

Metabolically stable adults receiving TPN. 2.5 to 4 mg daily.
Adults in acute catabolic state. 4.5 to 5 mg daily.
Adults with fluid loss from small bowel. 2.5 to 4 mg daily plus an additional 12.2 mg/liter to make up for 12. 2 mg/liter of small bowel fluid loss.
Adults with fluid loss from ileostomy output or liquid stool. 2.5 to 4 mg daily plus an additional 17.1 mg/kg of ileostomy output or liquid stool.

I.V. INFUSION (ZINC SULFATE)

Adults and adolescents. 3 mg daily.
Children weighing 10 kg (22 lb) or more. 50 mcg/kg (up to 3 mg/day) daily.
Children weighing 5 kg (11 lb) to less than 10 kg (22 lb). 100 mcg/kg daily.
Term neonates weighing 3 kg (6.6 lb) to less than 5 kg (11 lb). 250 mcg/kg daily.
Preterm neonates weighing less than 3 kg (6.6 lb). 400 mcg/kg daily.

* *To provide maintenance treatment for patients with Wilson's disease who have been initially treated with a chelating agent*

CAPSULES (GALZIN)

Adults. 50 mg 3 times daily.

Pregnant women. 25 mg 3 times daily, increased to 50 mg 3 times daily if drug effectiveness decreases.

Children ages 10 and older. 25 mg 3 times daily, increased to 50 mg 3 times daily if drug effectiveness decreases.

Drug Administration

P.O.

- Administer zinc supplements with a full glass of water and with food if GI upset occurs.
- Have patient let zinc lozenge dissolve in mouth slowly and completely and not to swallow it whole or chew it.
- Capsules and E.R. tablets should be swallowed whole and not chewed, crushed, or divided/opened.

I.V.

- Don't give I.V. zinc preparations that contain benzyl alcohol to neonates or premature infants because this preservative may cause a fatal toxic syndrome.
- I.V. zinc preparations are not for direct intravenous infusion but must be used as an admixture in parenteral nutrition solutions.
- Zinc must be diluted before administering intravenously.
- Prepare final admixture of zinc and parenteral nutrition solution according to manufacturer's guidelines.
- Visually inspect solution for precipitates and that the emulsion has not separated if lipid emulsion has been added. Separation of the emulsion is visible by a yellowish streak or accumulation of yellowish droplets in the admixed emulsion. Discard if any precipitates are noted.
- Protect admixture parenteral nutrition solution from light.
- *Incompatibilities:* Some additives may be incompatible with a particular mixture and must be determined to be compatible before adding to solution containing zinc.

Route	Onset	Peak	Duration
P.O.	Unknown	2 hr	Unknown

Half-life: 11 days

Mechanism of Action

Be aware zinc is needed for proper function of more than 200 metalloenzymes (those with tightly bound zinc atoms as an integral part of their structure), including alcohol dehydrogenase, alkaline phosphatase, carbonic anhydrase, carboxypeptidase A, and RNA polymerase. Zinc also helps maintain cell membrane, nucleic acid, and protein structure and is essential for certain physiologic functions, including cell growth and division, dark adaptation and night vision, host immunity, sexual maturation and reproduction, taste acuity, and wound healing. This mineral also provides cellular antioxidant protection by scavenging free radicals.

In addition, zinc acetate interferes with intestinal absorption of copper and produces a protein that binds with copper, preventing its transfer to blood. Bound copper is then excreted in stools, thus decreasing copper toxicity in Wilson's disease.

Contraindications

Hypersensitivity to zinc or its components

Interactions

DRUGS

copper supplements: Impaired copper absorption (with large doses of zinc)

oral iron supplements, oral phosphate salts, phosphorus-containing drugs: Decreased zinc absorption

quinolones, tetracyclines: Decreased absorption and possibly decreased effectiveness of these antibiotics

thiazide diuretics: Increased urinary excretion of zinc

zinc-containing preparations: Increased blood zinc level

FOODS

fiber- or phylate-containing foods (such as bran, cereals, whole-grain breads), phosphorus-containing foods (including milk, poultry): Decreased zinc absorption

Adverse Reactions

CNS: Neurologic deterioration

GI: Elevated alkaline phosphate, amylase, and lipase; gastric irritation or ulcer; nausea; vomiting

Other: Aluminum toxicity, copper deficiency

Childbearing Considerations

PREGNANCY

- It is not known if drug can cause fetal harm.
- Use with caution only if benefit to mother outweighs potential risk to fetus.
- Be aware that the recommended dosage allowance is increased during pregnancy.

LACTATION

- Drug is present in breast milk.
- Mothers should check with prescriber before breastfeeding.

Nursing Considerations

- Monitor blood alkaline phosphatase level monthly, as ordered; it may increase.

! **WARNING** Be aware that zinc chloride contains aluminum, which may accumulate to the point of toxicity if patient's kidney function is impaired. Assess kidney function regularly.

! **WARNING** Monitor patient for changes in neurological function. Notify prescriber immediately if changes occur.

! **WARNING** Monitor patient with preexisting copper deficiency for exacerbation of this condition; zinc can decrease serum copper level. For example, monitor patient receiving long-term zinc therapy for sideroblastic anemia, which may result from zinc-induced copper deficiency and is characterized by anemia, bone marrow problems, granulocytopenia, leukopenia, and neutropenia. Be aware that these effects are reversible after zinc is discontinued.

! **WARNING** Monitor patients taking oral zinc long-term for the development of gastric ulcers that could result in complications of anemia and gastric ulcer perforation with peritonitis. If patient exhibits signs and symptoms of gastric ulcer, notify prescriber, expect zinc therapy to be discontinued, and provide supportive care, as needed and ordered.

! **WARNING** Notify prescriber if patient develops an elevated serum alkaline phosphatase, amylase, and lipase that may last weeks to months possibly indicating the presence of pancreatitis. Know that levels return to high normal within the first one or two years of zinc therapy.

PATIENT TEACHING

- Explain the need for a zinc supplement.
- Instruct patient how to administer form of zinc prescribed.

! **WARNING** Alert family or caregiver that zinc therapy may cause neurological deterioration. If changes occur, prescriber should be notified.

! **WARNING** Tell patient, family, or caregiver to notify prescriber if other persistent, serious, or unusual adverse reactions occur.

ziprasidone hydrochloride

Geodon, Zeldox (CAN)

ziprasidone mesylate

Geodon for Injection

Class and Category

Pharmacologic class: Benzisoxazole
Therapeutic class: Antipsychotic

Indications and Dosages

✱ *To treat schizophrenia*

CAPSULES

Adults. *Initial:* 20 mg twice daily. Dosage increased as indicated every 2 or more days. *Usual:* 20 to 80 mg twice daily. *Maximum:* 80 mg twice daily.

✱ *To treat acute agitation in schizophrenic patients*

I.M. INJECTION

Adults. *Initial:* 10 to 20 mg. 10-mg dose may be given every 2 hr up to maximum dose; 20-mg dose may be given every 4 hr up to maximum dose. *Maximum:* 40 mg daily for no longer than 3 consecutive days.

✱ *To treat acute manic or mixed episodes of bipolar disorder*

CAPSULES

Adults. *Initial:* 40 mg twice daily on day 1; then increased to 60 or 80 mg on day 2 with further adjustments as needed.

✱ *As adjunct to lithium or valproate for maintenance treatment of bipolar I disorder*

CAPSULES

Adults. Same dose patient was initially stabilized on that falls within 40 to 80 mg twice daily.

Drug Administration

P.O.

- Capsules should be swallowed whole and not chewed, crushed, or opened.
- Administer drug with food.

I.M.

- Protect ziprasidone vials from light.
- Reconstitute by adding 1.2 ml Sterile Water for Injection to vial; shake vigorously until drug is dissolved. Each ml of reconstituted solution contains 20-mg ziprasidone and appears colorless to pale pink. Do not use any other diluent except Sterile Water for Injection. Discard any unused portion.
- Inject only as an I.M. injection.
- Reconstituted drug may be stored for up to 24 hr at room temperature protected from light or up to 7 days if refrigerated and protected from light.

Route	Onset	Peak	Duration
P.O.	Unknown	6–8 hr	12 hr
I.M.	Unknown	1 hr	Unknown

Half-life: 2–7 hr

Mechanism of Action

Blocks dopamine and serotonin receptors selectively in the mesocortical tract of the CNS, thereby suppressing psychotic symptoms.

Contraindications

Concurrent use of other drugs that prolong QT interval, history of arrhythmia or prolonged QT interval, hypersensitivity to ziprasidone or its components, recent acute MI, uncompensated heart failure

Interactions

DRUGS

carbamazepine: Possibly decreased blood ziprasidone level

drugs that prolong QT interval (including dofetilide, pimozide, quinidine, sotalol, sparfloxacin, and thioridazine): Increased risk of prolonged QT interval, torsades de pointes, and sudden death

ketoconazole: Possibly increased blood ziprasidone level

Adverse Reactions

CNS: Agitation, akathisia, amnesia, anxiety, asthenia, **CVA**, depression, dizziness, dystonia, extrapyramidal reactions, headache, hypertonia, hypomania, insomnia, mania, **neuroleptic malignant syndrome**, paresthesia, personality or speech disorder, **serotonin syndrome**, somnolence, **suicidal ideation**, syncope, tardive dyskinesia, tremor
CV: **Bradycardia**, chest pain, hypercholesterolemia, hypertension, orthostatic hypotension, **prolonged QT interval**, tachycardia, thrombophlebitis, vasodilation
EENT: Abnormal vision, dry mouth, increased salivation, rhinitis, **tongue swelling**
ENDO: Dysmenorrhea, hyperglycemia, hyperprolactinemia
GI: Abdominal pain, anorexia, constipation, diarrhea, dysphagia, indigestion, nausea, **rectal bleeding**, vomiting
GU: Priapism, urinary incontinence
HEME: **Agranulocytosis**, **leukopenia**, **neutropenia**
MS: Arthralgia, back pain, dysarthria, myalgia
RESP: Cough, **pulmonary embolism**, upper respiratory tract infection
SKIN: Allergic dermatitis, diaphoresis, **exfoliative dermatitis**, furunculosis, rash, **Stevens-Johnson syndrome**, urticaria
Other: **Angioedema**, **drug reaction with eosinophilia and systemic symptoms (DRESS)**, flu-like symptoms, injection-site pain, weight gain

Childbearing Considerations

PREGNANCY

- Pregnancy exposure registry: 1-866-961-2388 or http://womensmentalhealth.org/clinical-and-research-programs/pregnancyregistry/.
- Drug may cause fetal harm, especially during third trimester, as neonates are at increased risk for extrapyramidal and/or withdrawal symptoms following delivery.
- Use with caution only if benefit to mother outweighs potential risk to fetus.

LACTATION

- Drug is present in breast milk.
- Mothers should check with prescriber before breastfeeding.
- If breastfeeding occurs, mothers should monitor infant for excess sedation,

extrapyramidal symptoms, irritability, and poor feedings.

REPRODUCTION

- Drug may increase serum prolactin levels, which may lead to a reversible reduction in fertility in females of childbearing age.

Nursing Considerations

! **WARNING** Know that ziprasidone shouldn't be used to treat elderly patients with dementia-related psychosis because drug increases the risk of death in these patients.

! **WARNING** Monitor patient for a hypersensitivity or severe skin reaction, which could become life-threatening, such as angioedema or DRESS. DRESS may initially only present with a fever or swollen lymph nodes although rash is the most common presentation. If present, notify prescriber, expect drug to be discontinued, and provide supportive care, as needed and ordered.

! **WARNING** Monitor patient closely for evidence of suicidal thinking or behavior, especially when therapy starts or dosage changes.

! **WARNING** Assess cardiac rhythm in patients with hypokalemia or hypomagnesemia. Dizziness, palpitations, and syncope may indicate life-threatening torsades de pointes. Be prepared to stop ziprasidone if QT interval is greater than 500 milliseconds.

! **WARNING** Monitor patient's CBC, as ordered, because serious adverse hematologic reactions may occur, such as agranulocytosis, leukopenia, and neutropenia. Monitor more frequently during first few months of therapy if patient has a history of drug-induced leukopenia, neutropenia, or significantly low WBC count. If abnormalities occur during ziprasidone therapy, watch for fever and other evidence of infection, notify prescriber, and expect to discontinue drug if severe.

! **WARNING** Report evidence of neuroleptic malignant syndrome immediately, a rare but potentially fatal adverse reaction, including acute renal failure, altered mental status, arrhythmia, blood pressure changes, diaphoresis, hyperpyrexia, irregular pulse, muscle rigidity, myoglobinuria (rhabdomyolysis), and tachycardia.

- Monitor patient's blood glucose and lipid levels routinely, as ordered, because drug increases risk of hypercholesterolemia and hyperglycemia.
- Monitor patient, especially elderly women, for involuntary movements, which may become irreversible tardive dyskinesia. If symptoms develop, notify prescriber immediately and be prepared to stop drug.
- Know that long-standing hyperprolactinemia caused by ziprasidone therapy may cause decreased bone density if associated with hypogonadism.
- Institute fall precautions.

PATIENT TEACHING

! **WARNING** Advise pregnant patients entering their third trimester to discuss continued use of drug during the remainder of pregnancy as drug may cause adverse reactions in the infant upon birth.

- Instruct patient how to oral administer ziprasidone.

! **WARNING** Alert patient that drug may cause an allergic or severe skin reaction. If present such as a fever, rash, or swollen lymph nodes, tell patient to notify prescriber and, if severe, to seek immediate medical care.

! **WARNING** Tell family or caregiver to monitor patient closely for suicidal tendencies; patients with bipolar disorder or psychotic illness are at greater risk.

- Advise patient to avoid hazardous activities until CNS effects are known and resolved. Review fall precautions with patient and family or caregiver.
- Urge patient to rise slowly from lying or seated position to minimize orthostatic hypotension.

! **WARNING** Urge patient to notify prescriber immediately if he develops other persistent, serious, or unusual adverse reactions. If severe, tell him to seek immediate medical care.

- Advise mothers who are breastfeeding to monitor infant for excess sedation, extrapyramidal symptoms, irritability, and poor feedings.

zoledronic acid

Reclast

Class and Category

Pharmacologic class: Bisphosphonate
Therapeutic class: Antiosteoporotic

Indications and Dosages

∗ *To treat postmenopausal osteoporosis in women; to treat osteoporosis in men; to treat and prevent glucocorticoid-induced osteoporosis in patients receiving daily prednisone doses of 7.5 mg or greater for at least 12 months*

I.V. INFUSION

Adults. 5 mg infused over at least 15 min once yearly.

∗ *To prevent osteoporosis in postmenopausal women*

I.V. INFUSION

Postmenopausal women. 5 mg infused over at least 15 min every 2 yr.

∗ *To treat Paget's disease of the bone*

I.V. INFUSION

Adults. 5 mg infused over at least 15 min followed by 1,500 mg elemental calcium daily in divided doses and 800 international units of vitamin D daily, especially in the 2 wk following zoledronic acid administration.

Drug Administration

I.V.

- Ensure that patient is hydrated prior to administering drug.
- Expect to administer acetaminophen, if not contraindicated, following zoledronic acid therapy to reduce adverse reactions.
- Reclast comes as a ready-to-infuse solution.
- Drug may be refrigerated if not administered immediately for 24 hr after opening. Allow solution to come to room temperature before administration.
- Infuse over no less than 15 min.
- Give drug through a separate vented infusion line. Follow infusion by flushing I.V. line with 10 ml of 0.9% Sodium Chloride Injection.
- *Incompatibilities:* Calcium or other divalent cation-containing solutions, such as Lactated Ringer's solution

Route	Onset	Peak	Duration
I.V.	4–7 days	Unknown	32 days

Half-life: 146 hr

Mechanism of Action

Inhibits resorption of mineralized bone and cartilage by osteoclasts and induces osteoclast breakdown. In cancer-related hypercalcemia, hyperactive osteoclasts cause bone resorption and release of calcium into blood, which causes polyuria, GI disruption, progressive dehydration, and decreasing GFR. This, in turn, increases renal calcium resorption and worsens hypercalcemia. Zoledronic acid interrupts this process.

Contraindications

Acute renal impairment, creatinine clearance less than 35 ml/min (Reclast); hypersensitivity to zoledronic acid or its components; hypocalcemia (Reclast)

Interactions

DRUGS

aminoglycosides, calcitonin: Possibly additive serum calcium lowering effect
loop diuretics, such as furosemide: Possibly increased risk of hypocalcemia
nephrotoxic drugs, NSAIDs: Increased risk of nephrotoxicity

Adverse Reactions

CNS: Anxiety, asthenia, chills, confusion, depression, dizziness, fatigue, fever, headache, hyperesthesia, hypoesthesia, insomnia, malaise, paresthesia, tremor, vertigo, weakness
CV: **Atrial fibrillation**, **bradycardia**, chest pain, hypertension, **hypotension**, peripheral edema
EENT: Blurred vision, conjunctivitis, dry mouth, episcleritis, iritis, orbital edema or inflammation, osteonecrosis of external auditory canal, scleritis, sore throat, stomatitis, taste disturbance, uveitis
GI: Abdominal pain, anorexia, constipation, diarrhea, dyspepsia, nausea, vomiting
GU: **Acquired Fanconi syndrome**, elevated serum creatinine level, hematuria, proteinuria, **renal insufficiency or failure**, UTI
HEME: Anemia, **neutropenia**, **thrombocytopenia**
MS: Arthralgia; atypical subtrochanteric and diaphyseal femoral fractures; incapacitating bone, joint, or muscle pain; muscle cramps

or spasms; myalgia; osteonecrosis of the jaw, femur, or hip
RESP: **Bronchospasm**, cough, dyspnea, **exacerbation of asthma**, **interstitial lung disease**, upper respiratory tract infection
SKIN: Alopecia, dermatitis, diaphoresis, flushing, **Stevens-Johnson syndrome**, **toxic epidermal necrolysis**, urticaria
Other: **Aggravated malignant neoplasm**, **anaphylaxis**, **angioedema**, flu-like illness, **hyperkalemia**, **hypernatremia**, **hypersensitivity reactions**, **hypocalcemia**, **hypomagnesemia**, **hypophosphatemia**, infusion-site redness and swelling, weight gain

Childbearing Considerations

PREGNANCY

- Drug can cause fetal harm because there is a theoretical risk, especially skeletal and other abnormalities in fetus, if a woman becomes pregnant after completing a course of bisphosphonate therapy. Time between cessation of drug therapy to conception, the particular bisphosphonate used, and route of administration causing fetal harm are unknown.
- Drug should not be used during pregnancy or in women contemplating a future pregnancy.
- Pregnancy status should be verified before drug is administered.

LACTATION

- It is not known if drug is present in breast milk.
- Drug should not be given during breastfeeding.

REPRODUCTION

- Females of childbearing age should use an effective contraceptive during drug therapy and thereafter.
- Female fertility may be impaired, based on animal studies.

Nursing Considerations

- Be aware that zoledronic acid isn't indicated for hypercalcemia from hyperparathyroidism or other conditions that can cause hypercalcemia.

! **WARNING** Verify pregnancy status of females of childbearing age before zoledronic acid therapy is initiated. Be aware that drug should not be given during pregnancy because drug may cause fetal harm. Drug should also not be given to females of childbearing age contemplating a future pregnancy because drug can affect female fertility and has the potential to cause fetal harm if drug was administered in the past.

! **WARNING** Know that hypocalcemia and mineral metabolism disorders must be treated before zoledronic acid therapy begins. Monitor patient's serum calcium, magnesium, and phosphate levels, as ordered, during zoledronic acid therapy. If hypocalcemia, hypomagnesemia, or hypophosphatemia occurs, expect to give short-term supplemental therapy.

- Make sure patient has had a dental checkup before zoledronic acid therapy starts because risk of jaw osteonecrosis is increased in these patients, and invasive dental procedures during zoledronic acid therapy may worsen osteonecrosis.

! **WARNING** Assess patient's renal function, as ordered, before and during zoledronic acid therapy to detect renal deterioration.

! **WARNING** Monitor patient for dehydration. If present, notify prescriber and expect drug to be withheld until dehydration has been corrected. Expect to aggressively hydrate hypercalcemic patient with I.V. normal saline solution before and during zoledronic acid therapy, as prescribed, to achieve and maintain urine output of about 2 liters daily. However, assess patient frequently during hydration process, especially if patient has heart failure, for evidence of life-threatening over-hydration.

! **WARNING** Monitor patient for a hypersensitivity reaction, which could become life-threatening, such as anaphylaxis or angioedema. If present, notify prescriber, expect drug to be discontinued, and provide supportive care, as needed and ordered.

! **WARNING** Assess aspirin-sensitive asthma patients for worsening of respiratory symptoms during zoledronic acid therapy because other bisphosphonates have caused bronchoconstriction in these patients.

- Monitor patient closely for severe and occasionally incapacitating bone, joint, and/or muscle pain. If present, notify prescriber and expect to provide supportive care, as ordered, for pain relief.

! **WARNING** Monitor patient for other persistent, serious, or unusual adverse reactions, some of which could be life-threatening, such as aggravated malignancy neoplasm or hypotension.

PATIENT TEACHING

! **WARNING** Warn females of childbearing age that drug can cause fetal harm. Stress importance of using effective contraception during and after zoledronic acid therapy and to notify prescriber immediately if pregnancy occurs because drug will have to be stopped. Tell females of childbearing age to discuss drug use with prescriber before therapy begins if patient is contemplating a future pregnancy because drug may also impair female fertility and has the potential to cause fetal harm even when drug was given in the past.

! **WARNING** Inform patient not to take other bisphosphonates concurrently.

- Inform patient that drug will be administered intravenously. Instruct patient to drink at least two glasses of fluid within a few hours before receiving zoledronic acid intravenously.

! **WARNING** Alert patient that drug may cause an allergic reaction. If present, tell patient to notify staff or prescriber and, if severe, to seek immediate medical care.

! **WARNING** Tell aspirin-sensitive asthma patients to be on the alert for worsening of respiratory symptoms during zoledronic acid therapy because other bisphosphonates have caused bronchoconstriction in these patients. If present, tell patient to seek immediate medical care.

! **WARNING** Tell patient to notify prescriber if blood or other changes in urine, a change in amount of urine voided, or change in frequency of voiding pattern occurs. Stress importance of compliance in having regular blood tests that have been ordered to check kidney function.

- Advise patient to alert prescriber about bone, joint, or muscle pain or new or worsening groin, hip, or thigh pain.

! **WARNING** Instruct patient to notify prescriber of any other persistent, serious, or unusual adverse reactions.

- Teach patient the importance of eating a nutritious diet, including adequate amounts of calcium and vitamin D.
- Instruct patient on proper oral hygiene and on need to notify prescriber before undergoing invasive dental procedures.
- Inform these mothers that breastfeeding is not recommended during zoledronic acid therapy.

zolmitriptan

Zomig

Class and Category

Pharmacologic class: Selective 5-hydroxytryptamine agonist
Therapeutic class: Antimigraine

Indications and Dosages

* *To treat acute migraine headache with or without aura*

TABLETS

Adults. *Initial:* 1.25 or 2.5 mg, repeated in 2 hr as needed. *Maximum:* 5 mg as a single dose, 10 mg in 24 hr, or 3 headaches/mo.

ORAL DISINTEGRATING TABLETS

Adults. *Initial:* 2.5 mg, repeated in 2 hr, as needed. *Maximum:* 5 mg as a single dose, 10 mg in 24 hr, or 3 headaches/mo.

NASAL SPRAY

Adults and children ages 12 and older. *Initial:* 2.5 mg (1 spray) repeated in 2 hr as needed. Dosage increased to 5 mg/episode, as needed. *Maximum:* 5 mg as single dose; 10 mg/24 hr; or 4 headaches/mo.

± **DOSAGE ADJUSTMENT** For patients with moderate to severe hepatic impairment, initial oral dosage using tablet form should not be higher than 1.25 mg and maximum dose should not exceed 5 mg in 24 hours. Nasal spray or oral disintegrating tablets are not recommended for these patients. For patients receiving cimetidine concurrently, single dosage should not exceed 2.5 mg and the maximum dosage should not exceed 5 mg in a 24-hour period.

Drug Administration

P.O.

- Do not remove disintegrating tablet from blister pack until just before giving the tablet. Peel foil to open pack; do not push tablet through foil. Have patient put tablet on tongue and let dissolve and then swallow. Do not break orally disintegrating tablet.
- I.R. tablet may be broken in half, if needed to achieve correct dose.

NASAL

- Have patient blow nose before use.
- Don't test or prime spray before use, as it is a single-dose device.
- Have patient insert device into one nostril and close the other nostril with finger.
- Have patient press plunger device while breathing gently in through the nose. Device then removed and patient should then breathe gently through mouth for 5 to 10 sec.

Route	Onset	Peak	Duration
P.O.	Unknown	1.5–3 hr	Unknown
Nasal	5 min	3 hr	Unknown

Half-life: 2.8–3.7 hr

Mechanism of Action

Constricts dilated and inflamed cranial blood vessels in the carotid circulation and inhibits production of proinflammatory neuropeptides by binding to receptors on intracranial blood vessels and sensory nerves in the trigeminal-vascular system to stimulate negative feedback, which halts the release of serotonin.

Contraindications

History of basilar or hemiplegic migraine, stroke, or transient ischemic attack; hypersensitivity to zolmitriptan or its components; ischemic coronary artery or bowel disease; peripheral vascular disease; recent use (within 24 hr) of another 5-HT_1 agonist, ergotamine-containing medication, or ergot-type medication (such as dihydroergotamine or methysergide); uncontrolled hypertension; use of a MAO inhibitor within past 14 days; Wolff-Parkinson-White syndrome or arrhythmias associated with other cardiac accessory conduction pathway disorders

Interactions

DRUGS

5-HT_1 agonists: Increased risk of additive vasospastic reactions
cimetidine: Doubled blood zolmitriptan levels; prolonged zolmitriptan half-life
ergot alkaloids: Prolonged vasoconstriction effects
MAO inhibitors: Increased zolmitriptan effects
naratriptan, rizatriptan, sumatriptan: Prolonged zolmitriptan effects
selective serotonin reuptake inhibitors and serotonin norepinephrine reuptake inhibitors: Increased risk of developing serotonin syndrome

Adverse Reactions

CNS: Asthenia, dizziness, hyperesthesia, paresthesia, somnolence, vertigo
CV: Angina, **coronary artery vasospasm**, hypertension, **MI**, palpitations, transient myocardial ischemia, **ventricular fibrillation and tachycardia**
EENT: Dry mouth, vision disturbance
GI: Abdominal pain, **bloody diarrhea**, dysphagia, **GI or splenic infarction**, indigestion, **ischemic colitis**, nausea, vomiting
MS: Myalgia; myasthenia; pain, pressure, or tightness in jaw, neck, or throat
SKIN: Diaphoresis, flushing
Other: **Anaphylaxis**, **angioedema**

Childbearing Considerations

PREGNANCY

- It is not known if drug can cause fetal harm.
- Use with caution only if benefit to mother outweighs potential risk to fetus.
- Be aware that women with migraine may be at increased risk for preeclampsia during pregnancy.

LACTATION

- It is not known if drug is present in breast milk.
- Mothers should check with prescriber before breastfeeding.

Nursing Considerations

! **WARNING** Monitor patient for a hypersensitivity reaction, which could become life-threatening, such as anaphylaxis or angioedema. If present, notify prescriber, expect drug to be discontinued, and provide supportive care, as needed and ordered.

! **WARNING** Monitor patient for signs and symptoms of vasoconstriction, which may lead to colonic and vascular ischemia with abdominal pain and bloody diarrhea, especially if patient has ischemic bowel disease or peripheral vascular disease (including Raynaud's phenomenon).

! **WARNING** Monitor patient closely for signs and symptoms of angina. If patient develops chest pain, notify prescriber.

! **WARNING** Monitor patient closely for signs and symptoms of serotonin syndrome, which may include agitation, coma, diarrhea, hallucinations, hyperreflexia, hyperthermia, incoordination, labile blood pressure, nausea, tachycardia, and vomiting. Notify prescriber immediately because serotonin syndrome may be life-threatening. Be prepared to provide supportive care and discontinue zolmitriptan.

- Monitor elderly patients and those with hepatic impairment for increased blood pressure and notify prescriber if present.

! **WARNING** Monitor patient for other persistent, serious, or unusual adverse reactions, some of which could be life-threatening, such as an MI or splenic infarct.

PATIENT TEACHING

- Instruct patient how to administer form of zolmitriptan prescribed.
- Tell patient to take drug exactly as prescribed. Advise patient also not to take more than 10 mg in any 24-hour period, nor should drug be taken for more than recommended number of times per month because overuse of drug may lead to exacerbation of headache. Tell patient to be alert for migraine-like daily headaches developing or marked increase in frequency of migraine headaches that signals overuse may be occurring. Instruct patient to notify prescriber, as drug may no longer be as effective and drug withdrawal may be needed.

! **WARNING** Instruct patient not to take zolmitriptan within 24 hours of other drugs in the same class.

! **WARNING** Alert patient drug may cause an allergic reaction. If present, tell patient to notify prescriber and, if serious, to seek immediate medical care.

! **WARNING** If patient develops chest pain, tell patient to seek immediate medical care.

- Urge patient to notify prescriber about other persistent, serious, or unusual adverse reactions.
- Tell patient to inform all prescribers of zolmitriptan therapy because serious drug interactions may occur.

zolpidem tartrate

Ambien, Ambien CR, Edluar

Class, Category, and Schedule

Pharmacologic class: Imidazopyridine
Therapeutic class: Hypnotic
Controlled substance schedule: IV

Indications and Dosages

✱ *To provide short-term treatment of insomnia characterized by difficulties with sleep initiation and/or sleep maintenance*

S.L. TABLETS, TABLETS

Adult males. 5 or 10 mg at bedtime for 7 to 10 days; increased to 10 mg at bedtime if 5 mg ineffective. *Maximum:* 10 mg at bedtime.
Adult females. 5 mg at bedtime for 7 to 10 days, increased to 10 mg at bedtime, as needed. *Maximum:* 10 mg daily at bedtime.

± **DOSAGE ADJUSTMENT** For elderly or debilitated patients and patients with mild to moderate hepatic impairment, dosage reduced to 5 mg at bedtime for both men and women.

E.R. TABLETS

Adult males. 6.25 or 12.5 mg once nightly at bedtime; increased to 12.5 mg at bedtime if 6.25 mg ineffective. *Maximum:* 12.5 mg at bedtime.

Adult females. 6.25 mg once nightly at bedtime, increased to 12.5 mg at bedtime, as needed. *Maximum:* 12.5 mg at bedtime.

±**DOSAGE ADJUSTMENT** For elderly or debilitated patients and those with mild to moderate hepatic impairment, dosage reduced to 6.25 mg at bedtime for both men and women.

Drug Administration

P.O.

- Administer on an empty stomach at bedtime for faster sleep onset, but only administer if patient has 7 to 8 hr of sleep time remaining.
- E.R. tablets and I.R. tablets should be swallowed whole and not chewed, crushed, or divided.
- S.L. tablets should be placed under the tongue to dissolve; not swallowed or administered with water.

Route	Onset	Peak	Duration
P.O.	< 30 min	30–120 min	6–8 hr
P.O./E.R.	< 30 min	30–120 min	6–8 hr

Half-life: 1.5–3 hr

Mechanism of Action

May potentiate the effects of gamma-aminobutyric acid (GABA) and other inhibitory neurotransmitters. By binding to specific benzodiazepine receptors in the limbic and cortical areas of the CNS, zolpidem increases GABA's inhibitory effects, blocks cortical and limbic arousal, and preserves deep sleep (stages 3 and 4).

Contraindications

Development of complex sleep behaviors after taking zolpidem, hypersensitivity to zolpidem or its components

Interactions

DRUGS

barbiturates, chlorpromazine, general anesthetics, opioid agonists, other CNS depressants, phenothiazines, tramadol, tricyclic antidepressants: Possibly increased CNS depression and reduced psychomotor function
CYP3A4 inducers, such as rifampin, St. John's wort: Decreased effectiveness of zolpidem
CYP3A4 inhibitors, such as ketoconazole: Increased risk of zolpidem-induced adverse reactions
sertraline: Increased exposure to zolpidem

Adverse Reactions

CNS: Abnormal thinking, aggressiveness, amnesia, asthenia, ataxia, behavioral changes, complex behaviors (such as sleep driving), confusion, decreased level of consciousness or inhibition, dizziness, drowsiness, euphoria, hallucinations, headache, insomnia, lethargy, paradoxical CNS stimulation (including agitation, euphoria, hallucinations, hyperactivity, and nightmares), **suicidal ideation**, vertigo, worsening of depression
EENT: Application-site reactions from sublingual dose form (blisters, mucosal inflammation, oral ulcers), blurred vision, diplopia, **throat tightness**, visual abnormality
GI: Constipation, diarrhea, elevated liver enzymes, **hepatic injury**, hiccups, indigestion, jaundice, nausea, vomiting
GU: UTI
MS: Arthralgia, myalgia
RESP: Dyspnea, **respiratory depression**, upper or lower respiratory infection
Other: **Anaphylaxis**, **angioedema**, withdrawal symptoms

Childbearing Considerations

PREGNANCY

- Drug can cause fetal harm, as drug used late in third trimester may cause neonates at birth to experience hypotonia, respiratory depression, and sedation.
- Use with caution only if benefit to mother outweighs potential risk to fetus.

LACTATION

- Drug is present in breast milk.
- Mothers should check with prescriber before breastfeeding.
- If breastfeeding occurs, infant should be monitored for excess sedation, hypotonia, and respiratory depression. Mothers may interrupt breastfeeding by pumping and discarding breast milk during treatment and for 23 hr after last dose.

Nursing Considerations

! **WARNING** Know that zolpidem shouldn't be administered to pregnant women late in their third trimester because zolpidem may cause hypotonia, respiratory depression, and sedation in the newborn.

- Use zolpidem cautiously in patients with additional disorders because it isn't known if zolpidem therapy might aggravate these conditions, especially conditions with respiratory impairment.

- Be aware that zolpidem is a controlled substance. Expect patient to receive no more than a 1-month supply of zolpidem for outpatient therapy, with treatment being as short as possible.

! **WARNING** Monitor patient closely for suicidal tendencies, particularly when therapy starts or dosage increases because depression may worsen temporarily during these times, possibly leading to suicide.

! **WARNING** Monitor patient closely for a hypersensitivity reaction, which could become life-threatening, such as anaphylaxis or angioedema. If present, notify prescriber, expect drug to be discontinued, and provide supportive care, as needed and ordered.

! **WARNING** Monitor patients for respiratory depression, especially patients with compromised respiratory function such as may occur in myasthenia gravis or sleep apnea and patients who are taking concomitant opioids or other CNS depressants. Know that if patient takes opioids or other CNS depressants, expect lower dosages of opioids or other CNS depressants to be prescribed. Notify prescriber if patient exhibits a significant decrease in respiratory rate or difficulty breathing and expect drug to be discontinued.

- Know that zolpidem should not be withdrawn abruptly, especially after prolonged therapy, because patient may experience withdrawal symptoms, such as abdominal cramps or discomfort, fatigue, flushing, inconsolable crying, light-headedness, nausea, nervousness, panic attack, rebound insomnia, and vomiting.

PATIENT TEACHING

! **WARNING** Stress importance of pregnant patients late in their third trimester to discuss with prescriber continued use because of potential harm to the newborn.

- Instruct patient how to administer form of zolpidem prescribed.
- Caution patient to take drug exactly as prescribed and not to increase dosage unless directed by prescriber.

! **WARNING** Tell family or caregiver to observe patient closely for suicidal tendencies, especially when therapy starts or dosage changes.

! **WARNING** Alert patient that drug may cause an allergic reaction. If an allergic reaction occurs, tell patient to notify prescriber and, if severe, to seek immediate medical care.

! **WARNING** Warn patient that drug may cause respiratory depression, especially if patient uses opioids and other CNS depressants during zolpidem therapy because serious additive effects may occur that could become life-threatening. Advise patient to avoid opioid or other CNS depressant use while taking zolpidem. Tell patient to seek immediate medical care if patient has trouble breathing or respirations become slower than normal.

- Advise patient, family, or caregiver that zolpidem may produce abnormal behaviors during sleep, such as driving a car, eating, talking on the phone, or having sex without any recall of the event. If patient, family, or caregiver notices any such behavior or if patient sees evidence of such behavior upon awakening, prescriber should be notified.
- Tell patient that drug may cause drowsiness or decreased level of consciousness and even next-morning impairment from zolpidem use despite feeling fully awake. Advise patient to get a good night's sleep of at least 7 or 8 hours to help minimize this adverse effect. Tell patient to take precautions against falling and not to perform any hazardous activity, such as driving, especially after taking the drug and during the morning hours.
- Advise mothers breastfeeding during zolpidem therapy to monitor the infant for excess sedation, hypotonia, and slower-than-normal breathing because the drug passes through into breast milk. Encourage mothers to interrupt breastfeeding, pump, and then discard breast milk during zolpidem therapy and for 23 hours after

drug administration to minimize drug exposure of the breastfed infant, if possible.
- Advise patient not to abruptly stop taking zolpidem because withdrawal signs and symptoms may occur such as abdominal cramps or discomfort, fatigue, flushing, inconsolable crying, lightheadedness, nausea, nervousness, panic attack, and vomiting. Tell patient to notify prescriber, if withdrawal signs and symptoms occur.

zonisamide

Zonegran, Zonisade

Class and Category

Pharmacologic class: Sulfonamide
Therapeutic class: Anticonvulsant

Indications and Dosages

✶ *As adjunct to treat partial seizures in patients with epilepsy*

CAPSULES (ZONEGRAN)

Adults and adolescents over age 16. *Initial:* 100 mg once daily or divided and given twice daily. Dosage increased by 100 mg daily every 2 wk, as needed. *Usual:* 200 to 400 mg once daily or divided and given twice daily. Dosage may be further increased to 600 mg once daily or divided and given twice daily, as needed. *Maximum:* 600 mg once daily or divided and given twice daily.

ORAL SUSPENSION (ZONISADE)

Adults and adolescents ages 16 and older. *Initial:* 100 mg (5 ml) once daily or divided and given twice daily. Dosage increased by 100 mg (5 ml) daily every 2 wk, as needed. *Usual:* 200 (10 ml) to 400 mg (20 ml) once daily or divided and given twice daily. Dosage may be further increased to 600 mg (30 ml) once daily or divided and given twice daily, as needed. *Maximum:* 600 mg (30 ml) once daily or in 2 divided doses daily.

± **DOSAGE ADJUSTMENT** For patients with hepatic or renal dysfunction, a slower titration may be required. Drug should not be given to patients with an eGFR less than 50 ml/min.

Drug Administration

P.O.

- Drug is considered a hazardous drug that may require safe handling guidance.
- Capsules should be swallowed whole and not chewed, crushed, or opened.
- Oral suspension concentration is 100 mg/5 ml. Shake oral suspension bottle well before measuring each dose with a calibrated device. Administer the oral suspension directly into the patient's mouth. Store at room temperature. Discard 30 days after first opening bottle.

Route	Onset	Peak	Duration
P.O.	Unknown	2–6 hr	Unknown

Half-life: 63–69 hr

Mechanism of Action

May stop seizures and suppress their foci by blocking sodium channels and reducing voltage-dependent, inward currents from calcium channels. This action stabilizes neuronal membranes and suppresses synchronized neuronal hyperactivity.

Contraindications

Hypersensitivity to zonisamide, other sulfonamides, or their components

Interactions

DRUGS

CNS depressants: Additive CNS depressant effects
other carbonic anhydrase inhibitors: Increased risk of hyperammonemia and severity of metabolic acidosis; increased risk of kidney stone formation
topiramate, valproic acid: Increased risk of metabolic acidosis

ACTIVITIES

alcohol: Additive CNS depressant effects

FOODS

grapefruit juice: Possibly decreased metabolism of zonisamide

Adverse Reactions

CNS: Abnormal gait, agitation, anxiety, asthenia, ataxia, confusion, depression, difficulty concentrating, dizziness, **encephalopathy**, fatigue, headache, incoordination, insomnia, irritability, memory loss, nervousness, paresthesia, schizophrenia, **seizures**, somnolence, speech abnormalities, **suicidal ideation**, tremor
CV: Chest pain
EENT: Acute myopia, amblyopia, blurred vision, diplopia, dry mouth, increased

intraocular pressure (possibly leading to permanent vision loss), nystagmus, periorbital pain, pharyngitis, rhinitis, secondary closure angle glaucoma, taste alteration, tinnitus, visual disturbances
GI: Abdominal pain, **acute pancreatitis**, anorexia, constipation, diarrhea, dyspepsia, nausea, vomiting
GU: Renal calculi, transient decrease in estimated glomerular filtration rate (eGFR)
HEME: Anemia, **leukopenia**, **thrombocytopenia**
MS: Elevated creatine phosphokinase levels, **rhabdomyolysis**
RESP: Increased cough
SKIN: Ecchymosis, pruritus, rash
Other: **Angioedema**, **drug reaction with eosinophilia and systemic symptoms (DRESS)**, flu-like symptoms, **hyperammonemia (with or without encephalopathy)**, **metabolic acidosis**, weight loss

Childbearing Considerations

PREGNANCY

- Pregnancy exposure registry: 1-888-233-2334 or https://www.aedpregnancyregistry.org/.
- Drug may cause serious fetal harm.
- Use with caution only if benefit to mother outweighs potential risk to fetus.
- Neonates of mothers treated with drug should be monitored for metabolic acidosis.

LACTATION

- Drug is present in breast milk.
- Mothers should check with prescriber before breastfeeding.
- If breastfeeding occurs, infants should be monitored for decreased muscle tone, elevated temperature, excess sedation, poor feeding, and weight loss.

REPRODUCTION

- Females of childbearing age should use effective contraception during drug therapy and for one month after last dose.
- Drug may impair fertility in females.

Nursing Considerations

! WARNING Obtain a serum bicarbonate level before starting zonisamide and then periodically during therapy, as prescribed, because drug may cause metabolic acidosis, especially in patients with predisposing conditions or therapies or who are younger in age.

- Be aware that patients receiving doses of 300 mg daily or more are at increased risk for adverse CNS reactions, including decreased concentration, drowsiness, fatigue, and impaired speech.

! WARNING Be aware that zonisamide shouldn't be discontinued abruptly because doing so may increase frequency of seizures.

! WARNING Monitor patient for hypersensitivity and severe skin reactions, which could become life-threatening, such as angioedema or DRESS. Be aware that DRESS may initially only present with a fever or swollen lymph nodes although rash is the most common presentation. Notify prescriber immediately if a hypersensitivity or skin reaction occurs, expect drug to be switched to a different drug, and provide supportive care, as needed and ordered.

! WARNING Monitor patient closely for evidence of suicidal thinking or behavior, especially when therapy starts or dosage changes.

! WARNING Monitor patient for symptoms of hyperammonemia, such as lethargy, unexplained change in mental status, or vomiting. If suspected, obtain serum ammonia levels, as ordered. Know that drug-induced hyperammonemia may resolve or decrease in severity with a decrease of the daily dose.

! WARNING Monitor results of patient's CBC and other laboratory tests for signs of blood dyscrasias because zonisamide is a sulfonamide. Systemic absorption may result in life-threatening reactions, including agranulocytosis, aplastic anemia, and other blood dyscrasias.

- Monitor BUN and serum creatinine levels for signs of abnormally decreased eGFR. Expect some decrease in eGFR during first 4 weeks of treatment and a return to baseline within 2 to 3 weeks after drug is discontinued.
- Monitor patient for signs and symptoms of renal calculi.

! **WARNING** Monitor patient for other persistent, serious, or unusual adverse reactions.

PATIENT TEACHING

- Inform patient that zonisamide is usually prescribed with other anticonvulsants and that patient should continue to take all drugs as prescribed.
- Instruct patient how to administer form of zonisamide prescribed.
- Encourage patient to drink 6 to 8 glasses of water each day to prevent kidney stones, unless contraindicated.

! **WARNING** Stress importance of notifying prescriber if seizure activity occurs. Inform patient that prescriber may have to adjust zonisamide dosage over several weeks or months before stable dose is achieved.

! **WARNING** Warn patient not to abruptly stop taking the drug because doing so may increase frequency of seizures.

! **WARNING** Alert patient that drug may cause an allergic or serious skin reaction. If present, tell patient to notify prescriber and, if severe, to seek immediate medical care.

! **WARNING** Urge family or caregiver to watch closely for evidence of suicidal tendencies, especially when therapy starts or dosage changes, and to report concerns immediately to prescriber.

- Advise patient to use caution when driving or performing other activities that are hazardous or require mental alertness until adverse effects are known and resolved because zonisamide commonly causes decreased concentration, dizziness, and somnolence, particularly during first month of therapy.
- Advise patient to rise slowly from a lying or seated position to reduce the risk of dizziness.
- Instruct females of childbearing age to use an effective contraceptive throughout drug therapy. Tell these patients to notify prescriber immediately if pregnancy occurs.
- Alert mothers that if breastfeeding occurs, to monitor the infant for decreased muscle tone, elevated temperature, excess sedation, poor feeding, and weight loss. Tell patient to stop breastfeeding if any of these adverse effects occur and notify pediatrician immediately.
- Advise patient to wear a medical identification bracelet or necklace or carry medical identification with information about seizure disorder.

! **WARNING** Instruct patient to notify prescriber of other persistent, serious, or unusual adverse reactions occur.

Appendices

Abbreviations

The following abbreviations, which are common to nursing practice, may be used throughout the text.

ABG	arterial blood gas
ACE	angiotensin-converting enzyme
ADH	antidiuretic hormone
AIDS	acquired immunodeficiency syndrome
ALT	alanine aminotransferase
ANA	antinuclear antibodies
APTT	activated partial thromboplastin time
AST	aspartate aminotransferase
ATP	adenosine triphosphate
AV	atrioventricular
beat/min	beats per minute
BUN	blood urea nitrogen
°C	degrees Celsius
cAMP	cyclic adenosine monophosphate
(CAN)	Canadian drug trade name
cap	capsule
CBC	complete blood count
cGMP	cyclic guanosine monophosphate
CK	creatine kinase
Cl	chloride
cm	centimeter
CMV	cytomegalovirus
CNS	central nervous system
COPD	chronic obstructive pulmonary disease
CSF	cerebrospinal fluid
CV	cardiovascular I would delete this as CV can also mean cerebrovascular.
CVA	cerebrovascular accident
D_5LR	dextrose 5% in lactated Ringer's solution
D_5NS	dextrose 5% in normal saline solution
D_5/0.2NS	dextrose 5% in quarter-normal saline solution
D_5/0.45NS	dextrose 5% in half-normal saline solution
D_5W	dextrose 5% in water
D_{10}W	dextrose 10% in water
D_{50}W	dextrose 50% in water
dl	deciliter
DNA	deoxyribonucleic acid
D.R.	delayed release
DS	double-strength
DVT.	deep venous thrombosis
EC	enteric-coated
ECG	electrocardiogram
EEG	electroencephalogram
EENT	eyes, ears, nose, and throat
ENDO	endocrine
E.R.	extended release
EUAs	Emergency Use Authorizations
°F	degrees Fahrenheit
FDA	Food and Drug Administration
g	gram
GABA	gamma aminobutyric acid
eGFR	estimated glomerular filtration rate
GI	gastrointestinal
gtt	drop
GU	genitourinary
H_1	histamine$_1$
H_2	histamine$_2$
HDL	high-density lipoprotein
HEME	hematologic
HIV	human immunodeficiency virus
HMG-CoA	hydroxymethylglutaryl-coenzyme A
HPV	human papilloma virus
hr	hour/hours
HSV	herpes simplex virus
HZV	herpes zoster virus
ICP	intracranial pressure
I.D.	intradermal
IgA	immunoglobulin A
IgE	immunoglobulin E
I.M.	intramuscular
INR	international normalized ratio
I.R.	immediate-acting
I.V.	intravenous
IVPB	intravenous piggyback
kg	kilogram
KIU	kallikrein inactivator units
L	liter
LA	long-acting
lb	pound
LD	lactate dehydrogenase
LDL	low-density lipoprotein
LOC	level of consciousness
LR	lactated Ringer's solution
M	molar
m^2	square meter
MAO	monoamine oxidase
MAT	medication-assisted treatment
mcg	microgram
mEq	milliequivalent
mEq/L	milliequivalent per liter
mg	milligram
MI	myocardial infarction
min	minute/minutes
ml	milliliter
mm	millimeter
mm^3	cubic millimeter
mmol	millimole
mo	month
MS	musculoskeletal
msec	millisecond
Na	sodium
NaCl	sodium chloride
NG	nasogastric
ng	nanogram
NPH	human isophane insulin
NPO	nothing by mouth
NS	normal saline solution
0.225NS	quarter-normal saline (0.225%) solution
0.45NS	half-normal saline (0.45%) solution
NSAID	nonsteroidal anti-inflammatory drug

NYHA	New York Heart Association
ODT	orally disintegrating tablet(s)
OTC	over the counter
OUD	Opioid Use Disorder
PCA	patient-controlled analgesia
PE	pullmonary embolism
P.O.	by mouth
P.R.	by rectum
PSVT	paroxysmal supraventricular tachycardia
PT	prothrombin time
PTCA	percutaneous transluminal coronary angioplasty
PTT	partial thromboplastin time
PVC	premature ventricular contraction
RBC	red blood cell
REM	rapid eye movement
RESP	respiratory
RNA	ribonucleic acid
RSV	respiratory syncytial virus
SA	sinoatrial
sec	second
S.L.	sublingual
S.R.	sustained release
stat	immediately
SubQ	subcutaneous
supp	suppository
tab	tablet
T_3	triiodothyronine
T_4	thyroxine
USP	United States Pharmacopeia
UTI	urinary tract infection
VLDL	very-low-density lipoprotein
WBC	white blood cell
wk	week/weeks
yr	year/years

Data from Food and Drug Administration Opioid Medications (2021). Retrieved from https://www.fda.gov/drugs/information-drug-class/opioid-medications;
Data from Healthy Innovation, Safer Families: FDA's 2018 Strategic Policy Roadmap (2018). Retrieved from https://www.fda.gov/media/110587/download

Opioid Agents: Equianalgesic Doses

An equianalgesic dose of a synthetic opioid agonist is the dose that produces the same level of analgesia as 10 mg of I.M. or SubQ morphine, the principal opioid obtained from opium poppies. If your patient is switched from one opioid to another, expect to use the equianalgesic dose to decrease the risk of adverse reactions while increasing the likelihood of adequate pain relief. The chart below compares equianalgesic doses (oral and parenteral) for adults and children who weigh 50 kg (110 lb) or more.

OPIOID	ORAL DOSE	PARENTERAL DOSE
codeine	200 mg (not recommended)	120 to 130 mg
hydrocodone	30 mg	Not applicable
hydromorphone	7.5 mg	1.5 mg
meperidine	300 mg	75 to 100 mg
morphine (around-the-clock dosing)	30 mg	10 mg
morphine (single or intermittent dosing)	60 mg	10 mg
oxycodone	30 mg	Not applicable

Opioid Use: Safety Guidelines

Pain relief has been a long-standing goal in health care for patients with pain. Patients may experience short-term pain because of an illness, injury, or medical or surgical procedure. Others experience chronic or persistent pain, defined as pain that lasts longer than 3 months or beyond normal tissue healing, which can drastically alter quality of life.

Opioids are powerful pain-reducing drugs, and their efficacy has made them increasingly popular for both short- and long-term pain management. However, opioids are also addictive, especially when used inappropriately. This has led to their abuse and misuse in society, along with a sharp increase in recent years of opioid-related overdoses and deaths.

To address the opioid crisis in the United States, the Food and Drug Administration (FDA) has formulated and implemented a plan called the *FDA's Opioid Policy Work Plan*. This plan details eight measures the FDA is using to combat this problem and includes:

- Re-examining and updating the FDA's framework for evaluating the pre- and post-market safety of opioids based on risk and benefit considerations, including the potential risks for abuse or illicit use.
- Addressing inappropriate practices for prescribing opioids with new modifications to the Risk Evaluation and Mitigation Strategy (REMS) program to provide for the need for more training for healthcare professionals on the use of nonopioid pain alternatives, the safe use of I.R. opioid formulations, and how to manage pain appropriately.
- Supporting the development of more abuse-deterrent opioid formulations.
- Having naloxone available as an OTC preparation, which quickly provides the first step in the management of an opioid overdose in the home setting by the family or caregiver.
- Exploring new ways to regulate, package, and prescribe opioids to reduce overall exposure to opioid drugs and their abuse and misuse.
- Developing more products of nonaddictive pain remedies as well as the development of improved medication-assisted treatment (MAT).
- Implementing new approaches for oversight of illicit controlled substances and foreign unapproved drugs imported into the U.S. through international mail facilities.
- Launching a public campaign geared towards adopting MAT, including new steps to address the stigma and other challenges for more widespread availability and prescribing of MAT.

As a result of the FDA's Opioid Policy Work Plan, drug companies are now required to address several safety issues in their opioid drug labels (package inserts). Changes to individual sections of the drug label reflective of these safety issues are summarized here:

- **Boxed Warning**—Now includes warnings about addiction, abuse, and misuse; accidental ingestion; life-threatening respiratory depression; neonatal opioid withdrawal syndrome (NOWS); and any significant drug product-specific interactions that could raise the risk of adverse reactions associated with opioid use. In addition, the real danger for an opioid overdose and need for naloxone administration is addressed.
- **Indications and Usage**—Modified to emphasize that opioids are to be reserved for the management of pain only if alternative treatment options such as nonopioid analgesics cannot be used or are ineffective and the pain is severe enough to require an opioid analgesic.
- **Contraindications**—Includes patients with significant respiratory depression and patients with acute or severe bronchial asthma in an unmonitored setting or in the absence of resuscitative equipment.
- **Warning and Precautions**—Addresses each of the components found in the boxed warning as well as risks associated with concurrently administered CNS depressants; life-threatening respiratory depression in patients with chronic pulmonary disease; use in the elderly or patients who are cachectic or debilitated; and the potential development of adrenal insufficiency with opioid use. In addition, the FDA's recommendation to all prescribers to co-prescribe naloxone for patients at increased risk of opioid overdose is addressed, regardless of whether they are receiving a prescription for an opioid pain reliever or drugs to treat an opioid use disorder (OUD).
- **Drug Interactions**—Includes any significant drug-specific interactions that would increase the opioid effect as well as interactions between opioids and CNS depressants, including alcohol and between opioids and serotonergic drugs and the possibility of an interaction leading to an opioid overdose.
- **Adverse Reactions**—Lists all the serious adverse reactions addressed in the "Warnings and Precautions" section of the drug label as well as adding adrenal insufficiency and serotonin syndrome to the post marketing section that may occur as a result of opioid use.
- **Specific Populations**—Additional information is included regarding NOWS and potential for neonatal respiratory depression during delivery or with breastfeeding if mother is addicted to opioids; potential risk for infertility with chronic use; and increased risk for respiratory depression in the elderly.
- **Drug Abuse and Dependence**—Details information about opioid abuse and dependence is given.

- **Overdosage**—Adds or modifies information to address seriousness and current treatment of opioid overdose, including the use of naloxone to treat an opioid overdose as an immediate emergency measure.
- **Patient Counseling**—Includes information to be given to the patient on addiction, abuse, and misuse of opioids; risk of life-threatening respiratory depression or accidental ingestion; interactions with alcohol and other CNS depressants; risk of an opioid overdose and emergent treatment by the family's or caregiver's use of naloxone in the home; potential for adrenal insufficiency and serotonin syndrome and what to report; potential for development of NOWS and embryo-fetal toxicity during pregnancy, respiratory depression in infants during delivery and with breastfeeding if mother is addicted to opioids; how to dispose of the unused opioid; and the addition of a medication guide.

In addition to the changes listed above, the FDA is now requiring that all opioid drug label contains the following information:

- the risk of overdose increases as the dosage increases for all opioid pain medicines;
- immediate releasing (IR) opioids should not be used for an extended period of time unless a patient's pain remains severe enough to require them and alternative treatment options continue to be inadequate;
- many acute pain conditions treated in the outpatient setting require no more than a few days of an opioid pain medicine; and
- it is recommended to reserve extended release (ER) or long acting (LA) opioid pain medicines for severe and persistent pain that requires an extended treatment period with a daily opioid pain medicine and for which alternative treatment options are inadequate.

In addition, on August 25, 2023, the American Dental Association released a new guideline that recommends children under the age of 12 having short-term dental pain from extractions or toothache should not be prescribed opioids. Instead, the pain should be managed with OTC ibuprofen and/or acetaminophen.

The Centers for Disease Control (CDC) has also released recommendations for use of opioids in treating chronic pain. These recommendations exclude patients who are in active cancer treatment, palliative care, or end-of-life care.

The CDC recommends that opioids not be used as first-line therapy in the treatment of chronic pain. Instead, nonpharmacologic therapies, such as cognitive behavioral therapy, exercise, or nonopioid pharmacologic therapies, including NSAIDs, should be tried first. If opioids are prescribed, the CDC recommends that they be combined with nonpharmacologic or nonopioid pharmacologic therapy to provide greater benefits and lower opioid dosage requirements.

When opioids are used, the lowest possible effective dosage should be prescribed, and therapy should start with I.R. opioids rather than E.R. or long-acting opioids. In addition, the quantity prescribed should not go beyond the expected need for pain relief.

Closer follow-up is also recommended, with regular monitoring of patients to determine effectiveness of the prescribed pain measures. It is especially important to ascertain that the opioid is not causing harm and that naloxone is present for use in the home by the family or caregiver in the event of an opioid overdose. If benefits do not outweigh harm, it is recommended that the opioid dosage be reduced and then discontinued, as needed.

It is important that the patient's response to pain relief measures be accurately measured and assessed. Only then can the goal to provide effective pain relief, without causing the patient harm, be achieved. Although opioid therapy has its place in pain management, it is important to understand that opioids are not always necessary and, if used inappropriately, can cause much harm, not only to the patient but to society in general.

Data from Food and Drug Administration Opioid Medications (2021). Retrieved from https://www.fda.gov/drugs/information-drug-class/opioid-medications;
Data from Healthy Innovation, Safer Families: FDA's 2018 Strategic Policy Roadmap (2018). Retrieved from https://www.fda.gov/media/110587/download;
Data from Food and Drug Administration Drug Safety Communication dated April 13, 2023. Retrieved from www.fda.gov/media/167058/download;
American Dental Association, news release, August 25, 2023.

Parenteral Insulin Preparations

For each category of insulin, the following table lists the types of insulin according to the timing of their action: onset, peak, and duration for each type; common trade names along with the species; and key nursing considerations. Be alert for hyperglycemia or hypoglycemia that may occur when changes are made in the patient's insulin regimen. Do not repeatedly inject insulin subcutaneously into areas of lipodystrophy or localized cutaneous amyloidosis because hyperglycemia may occur; and a sudden change in the injection site to an unaffected area may cause hypoglycemia.

CATEGORY, SPECIES, AND TRADE NAMES	KEY NURSING CONSIDERATIONS
Rapid-acting insulin	
Onset: 10–20 min	**Peak:** 30–90 min **Duration:** 2–5 hr
Human ▪ Admelog (insulin lispro) ▪ Apidra (insulin glulisine) ▪ Fiasp (insulin aspart) ▪ Humalog (insulin lispro) ▪ Lyumjev (insulin lispro-aabc) ▪ NovoLog (insulin aspart) ▪ NovoRapid (insulin aspart) (CAN) **Concentrated** ▪ Humalog U-200 ▪ Lyumjev U-200 (insulin lispro-aabc)	▪ Only mix with NPH (intermediate-type) insulin, if needed, except for Humalog U-200, which should not be mixed with any other insulin. Administer immediately after mixing. ▪ When mixing rapid-acting insulin with a longer-acting insulin, always draw the rapid-acting insulin into the syringe first to avoid dosage errors. ▪ Be aware that Lyumjev comes in 2 strengths: U-100 and U-200. The U-200 prefilled pen contains 2 times as much insulin per 1 ml as standard U-100 insulin. ▪ When giving SubQ, give Admelog within 15 min before a meal or immediately after a meal; give Apidra up to 15 to 20 min before a meal, give Fiasp up to 2 min before a meal or up to 20 min after starting a meal; give Humalog up to 15 min before a meal or immediately after a meal; give Lyumjev at the start of a meal or up to within 20 min after starting a meal; and give NovoLog and NovoRapid 5 to 10 min before a meal. When giving rapid-acting insulin via an insulin pump, do not dilute or mix with any other insulin and change the insulin in the reservoir at least every 48 hr (Apidra), 6 days (Fiasp, NovoLog, NovoRapid), or 7 days (Humalog). Change the infusion sets and insertion site at least every 3 days or according to pump manual. ▪ Be aware that 1 unit of rapid-acting insulin has the same glucose-lowering ability as 1 unit of short-acting insulin. ▪ Rapid-acting insulin is available as a cartridge. Make sure to use the correct device for the brand of insulin prescribed, and don't add any other insulin to the cartridge. Change Fiasp PumpCart cartridge at least every 4 days or according to pump manual, whichever is shorter. ▪ Assess patient taking insulin concurrently with a thiazolidinedione for signs and symptoms of heart failure. If heart failure develops, provide supportive care and expect the thiazolidinedione to be discontinued or dosage reduced. ▪ Know that Fiasp's onset is 5–10 min and Lyumjev duration is 6 hr, which differs from other rapid-acting insulins. ▪ Admelog and Lyumjev (U-100 only) may also be given as a continuous subcutaneous infusion without being diluted and not mixed with other insulins when given in the insulin pump. Either may also be given as an intravenous infusion but only after dilution. Fiasp can also be used in insulin infusion pumps and has been approved to treat pediatric patients.

(continues)

Parenteral Insulin Preparations *(continued)*

CATEGORY, SPECIES, AND TRADE NAMES	KEY NURSING CONSIDERATIONS
Short-acting insulin	
Onset: 30–60 min **Peak:** 1.5–4 hr	**Duration:** 5–8 hr
Human ▪ Humulin-R ▪ Novolin ge Toronto (CAN) ▪ Novolin R ▪ ReliOn/Novolin R **Concentrated** ▪ Humulin-R U-500	▪ Don't use short-acting insulin if it's cloudy, discolored, or unusually viscous. ▪ Expect the U-500 strength to be used only to treat insulin resistance. Be very careful to use conversion chart if U-500 strength is being administered using U-100 syringes. Also, make sure the right strength of the short-acting insulin is being administered, as severe hypoglycemia and death have occurred because of administration, dispensing, and prescribing errors. ▪ Mix short-acting insulin with other insulin types, as needed. Always draw the short-acting insulin into the syringe first to avoid dosage errors. ▪ Do not repeatedly inject insulin into areas of lipodystrophy or localized cutaneous amyloidosis because hyperglycemia may occur; and a sudden change in the injection site to an unaffected area may cause hypoglycemia. ▪ Administer SubQ, I.M., or I.V., as prescribed. Use a continuous SubQ infusion pump, if ordered. The catheter tubing and reservoir insulin should be changed every 48 hr or as specified by the pump's manufacturer. ▪ When giving SubQ or I.M. injections, give the short-acting insulin 15 to 30 min before a meal or bedtime snack. ▪ Assess patient taking insulin concurrently with a thiazolidinedione for signs and symptoms of heart failure. If heart failure develops, provide supportive care and expect the thiazolidinedione to be discontinued or dosage reduced.
Intermediate-acting insulin	
Onset: 1–3 hr **Peak:** 4–12 hr	**Duration:** 12–24 hr
Human ▪ Humulin N ▪ Novolin ge NPH (CAN) ▪ Novolin N ▪ ReliOn/Novolin N	▪ Don't use intermediate-acting insulin if it contains precipitate that is clumped, granular, or clings to the side of the vial. ▪ Roll the vial gently between hands to mix; don't shake it. Also, gently turn the prefilled syringe up and down several times before using to achieve a uniform mixture. ▪ Administer by SubQ injection only, 30 min before a meal or bedtime snack. ▪ Be aware that intermediate-acting insulin rarely produces a blood glucose level that's as close to normal as possible. Expect to mix it with a rapid-acting or short-acting insulin, as prescribed, for optimum blood glucose control. ▪ Assess patient taking insulin concurrently with a thiazolidinedione for signs and symptoms of heart failure. If heart failure develops, provide supportive care and expect the thiazolidinedione to be discontinued or dosage reduced.

CATEGORY, SPECIES, AND TRADE NAMES	KEY NURSING CONSIDERATIONS
Long-acting insulin	
Onset: 1–1.5 hr **Peak:** None **Duration:** 24–28 hr	
Human ▪ Basaglar (insulin glargine) ▪ Detemir (insulin detemir) (CAN) ▪ Glargine (insulin glargine) (CAN) ▪ Lantus (insulin glargine) ▪ Levemir (insulin detemir) ▪ Rezvoglar (insulin glargine-aglr) ▪ Semglee (insulin glargine-yfgn)	▪ Don't use long-acting insulin if it contains precipitate that is clumped, granular, or that clings to the side of the vial. ▪ Do not mix insulin detemir or insulin glargine with another insulin or solution. ▪ Roll the vial gently between hands to obtain a uniform mixture; don't shake it. ▪ Administer by the SubQ route only. Inject insulin glargine once daily at any time, keeping the daily injection time consistent. Inject insulin detemir prescribed once daily with the evening meal or at bedtime; inject insulin detemir as prescribed twice daily with the morning meal and with the evening meal given at bedtime or 12 hr after the morning dose. ▪ Give insulin glargine at bedtime, if possible, so that additional insulin can be given while patient is awake if effects decline before 24 hr passes. If insulin glargine is given in the morning and its effects don't last 24 hr, hyperglycemia may occur while patient sleeps. ▪ Assess patient taking insulin concurrently with a thiazolidinedione for signs and symptoms of heart failure. If heart failure develops, provide supportive care and expect the thiazolidinedione to be discontinued or dosage reduced.
Ultra-long-acting insulin	
Onset: 1–6 hr **Peak:** None **Duration:** 36–42 hr	
▪ Tresiba (insulin degludec) **Concentrated** ▪ Toujeo U-300 (insulin glargine) ▪ Tresiba U-200 (insulin degludec)	▪ Don't use ultra-long-acting insulin if it contains precipitate that is clumped, granular, or clings to the side of the vial. ▪ Roll the vial gently between hands to obtain a uniform mixture; don't shake it. ▪ Be aware that Toujeo contains 3 times as much insulin (300 units/ml) in 1 ml as standard insulin (100 units/ml) and is not for use in children. Toujeo Max SoloStar holds 900 units of insulin glargine—more than any other long-acting insulin pen in the United States—and provides up to 160 units/ml in a single injection and allows for 2-unit increment adjustment. In comparison, Toujeo Solo Star pen contains 450 units of insulin glargine with a maximum dose of 80 units per injection, and dosage must be adjusted in 1-unit increments. ▪ Know that Tresiba is now approved for use in children ages 1 yr and older. ▪ Administer by the SubQ route only. Inject once daily at any time of day but keep time consistent. ▪ Assess patient taking insulin concurrently with a thiazolidinedione for signs and symptoms of heart failure. If heart failure develops, provide supportive care and expect the thiazolidinedione to be discontinued or dosage reduced. ▪ Be aware that recovery from hypoglycemia may take longer compared to shorter-acting insulins.

(continues)

Parenteral Insulin Preparations *(continued)*

CATEGORY, SPECIES, AND TRADE NAMES	KEY NURSING CONSIDERATIONS

Combination insulin

Onset: 30 min **Peak:** 1–12 hr **Duration:** 18–24 hr

Human

Intermediate-acting/rapid acting
- Humalog Mix 25 (CAN)
- Humalog Mix 50 (CAN)
- Humalog Mix 75/25
- Humalog Mix 50/50
- NovoLog Mix 50/50
- NovoLog Mix 70/30

Intermediate-acting/short-acting
- Humulin 30/70 (CAN)
- Humulin 70/30
- Novolin 70/30
- Novolin ge 30/70 (CAN)
- Novolin ge 40/60 (CAN)
- Novolin ge 50/50 (CAN)
- NovoMix 30 (CAN)
- ReliOn Novolin 70/30

Ultra-long-acting/rapid-acting
Ryzodeg 70/30

- Don't use combination insulin if it contains precipitate that is clumped or granular.
- Roll the vial gently between hands to mix; don't shake it. Also, gently turn the prefilled syringe up and down several times before using to achieve a uniform mixture.
- Administer combination insulin by the SubQ route only, 30 min before a meal.
- Be aware that Canadian and American products contain the same insulin ratio but express it differently. For example, the Canadian Humulin 30/70 and the American Humulin 70/30 both contain 30 units of a short-acting insulin and 70 units of an intermediate-acting insulin. Canadian products list the short-acting insulin first; American products list it second.
- Know that Ryzodeg 70/30 is composed of 70% long-acting insulin and 30% rapid-acting insulin. It is now approved for use in children ages 1 yr and older.
- Assess patient taking insulin concurrently with a thiazolidinedione for signs and symptoms of heart failure. If heart failure develops, provide supportive care and expect the thiazolidinedione to be discontinued or dosage reduced.

Combination insulin and glucagon-like peptide-1 (GLP-1) receptor agonist

Onset: 4–6 hr **Peak:** 8–20 hr **Duration:** 24–28 hr

Long-acting insulin/GLP-1 receptor agonist
- Xultophy 100/3.6 (insulin degludec/liraglutide)
- Soliqua 100/33 (insulin glargine/lixisenatide)

- Know that onset, peak, and duration are determined by the insulin contained in the combination.
- Expect the same adverse reactions that occur with the individual drugs making up the combination product. For example, liraglutide and lixisenatide may cause pulmonary aspiration during deep sedation or general anesthesia even when administered as in an insulin combination.
- Monitor for hypoglycemia that may become life-threatening, especially with lifestyle or medication changes. Know that hypoglycemia may be more difficult to recognize in elderly patients.
- Monitor renal function in patients with renal impairment or severe GI adverse reactions, as acute kidney injury can occur.
- Evaluate patient's serum potassium level, as ordered, because severe hypokalemia has occurred.
- Assess patient concurrently taking a thiazolidinedione for signs and symptoms of heart failure. If heart failure develops, provide supportive care and expect dosage to be reduced or drug discontinued.
- Monitor patient for signs and symptoms of pancreatitis.
- Be aware that recovery from hypoglycemia may take longer compared to shorter-acting insulins.

Suggested Pediatric Immunizations

Immunizations have come a long way since the first vaccine was discovered for smallpox by Edward Jenner in 1796. It took a little more than 100 years to pass before Dr. Louis Pasteur was able to prove that disease could be prevented by infecting humans with weakened germs when he used a vaccine to successfully prevent rabies in a boy bitten by a rabid dog. By the mid-20th century, Dr Jonas Salk and Dr. Albert Sabin developed the inactivated polio vaccine and live polio vaccine, respectively. With that and subsequent ones developed, vaccines have prevented the spread of serious childhood infectious diseases, which has saved countless lives and has prevented children from having to live with long-term health issues such as blindness, deafness, loss of limbs, or paralysis that may occur with some of these childhood infections.

Pediatric immunizations are vital to the health of a child. Following is a chart that lists common pediatric immunizations. The chart is formatted in chronological order from birth to 18 years of age and lists the recommended immunization for each age group. It also lists what the immunization protects against and the possible sequelae if the child is not immunized. Last, the chart also provides nursing considerations that include how the bacteria or virus is spread, which is helpful when teaching parents and caregivers preventative measures to keep children healthy, and important information that pertains only to a specific immunization. Monitor all pediatric patients for common reactions that may occur after the immunization has been given. These reactions are usually mild and resolve quickly such as local reactions at the injection site (burning, itching, pain, redness, or swelling) or a mild fever.

AGE	IMMUNIZATION	PROTECTION AGAINST	DANGERS OF NOT BEING VACCINATED	NURSING CONSIDERATIONS
Birth	**RSV antibody** (Respiratory syncytial virus)	Contagious viral infection of the nose, throat, and sometimes lung	▪ RSV infection is especially dangerous in infants and young children. ▪ Can cause severe inflammation of the airways and lungs possibly requiring hospitalization and mechanical ventilation	▪ Spread through air and direct contact ▪ Depends on mother's RSV vaccine status: CDC recommends a single dose of RSV vaccine for pregnant women during wk 32 to wk 36 of pregnancy to prevent RSV in infants less than 6 mo. If mother did not receive RSV vaccination during pregnancy, infant may receive preventive antibodies in the form of the vaccine.
	HepB (Hepatitis B vaccine)—first dose	Contagious viral infection of the liver	▪ Can cause chronic liver infection, liver failure, or liver cancer and possibly death	▪ Spread through contact with infected body fluids ▪ Given within 12 to 24 hr of birth ▪ Low-birth-weight infants given at 1 mo or when discharged from hospital ▪ If child never received immunization, first dose of HepB can be given at any age.

(continues)

Suggested Pediatric Immunizations *(continued)*

AGE	IMMUNIZATION	PROTECTION AGAINST	DANGERS OF NOT BEING VACCINATED	NURSING CONSIDERATIONS
1–2 mo	**HepB** (Hepatitis B vaccine)—2nd dose	See HepB above	See HepB above	▪ Second dose should be given 1 to 2 mo after the first dose.
2 mo	**DTaP** (Diphtheria, tetanus, and acellular pertussis vaccine)—1st dose	Contagious bacterial infection of the nose, throat, and sometimes lungs (diphtheria), lungs and airway (pertussis), and brain and nerves possibly causing lockjaw (tetanus)	▪ Diphtheria may cause swelling of the heart muscle, heart failure, coma, paralysis, and death. ▪ Tetanus may cause seizures, broken bones, difficulty breathing, and death. ▪ Pertussis may cause infection of the lungs and is especially dangerous for infants.	▪ Diphtheria and pertussis spread through air and direct contact. ▪ Tetanus spreads through spores found in soil and dust everywhere that enter body through broken skin.
	Hib (*Haemophilus influenzae* type b vaccine)	Contagious bacterial infection of the brain, lungs, spinal cord, or bloodstream	▪ Depends on body part infected but may cause brain damage, hearing loss, loss of extremity, or death	▪ Spread through air and direct contact
	IPV (Inactivated poliovirus vaccine)	Contagious viral infection of nerves and brain	▪ Causes paralysis and possibly death	▪ Spread through the mouth from stool on contaminated hands, food, or liquid, and by air and direct contact
	PCV (Pneumococcal conjugate vaccine)	Bacterial infection of ears, sinuses, lungs, and blood stream	▪ Depends on body part infected but may cause lung infection, septicemia, infection of the lining of the brain and spinal cord, and possibly death	▪ Spread through direct contact with respiratory droplets like saliva or mucus ▪ Can be given to older children ages 2 and older who have immune deficiency disorders such as asplenia or HIV infections or other conditions such as chronic heart or lung disease or who has a cochlear implant

AGE	IMMUNIZATION	PROTECTION AGAINST	DANGERS OF NOT BEING VACCINATED	NURSING CONSIDERATIONS
	RV (Rotavirus vaccine)	Contagious viral infection of the intestines	▪ Causes severe diarrhea and dehydration and possibly death	▪ Spread through the mouth from hands and food contaminated with stool
4 mo	**DTaP**—2nd dose	See DTaP above	See above	See above
	Hib—2nd dose	See Hib above	See Hib above	See Hib above
	IPV—2nd dose	See IPV above	See IPV above	See IPV above
	PCV—2nd dose	See PCV above	See PCV above	See PCV above
	RV—2nd dose	See RV above	See RV above	See RV above
6 mo	**DTaP**—3rd dose	See DTaP above	See DTaP above	See DTaP above
	Hib—Possible 3rd dose	See Hib above	See Hib above	▪ 3rd dose may be needed based on brand of vaccine given in previous Hib immunizations.
	PCV—3rd dose	See PCV above	See PCV above	See PCV above
	RV—Possible 3rd dose	See RV above	See RV above	▪ 3rd dose may be needed based on brand of vaccine given in previous RV immunizations.
	Influenza (Flu vaccine)	Contagious viral infection of the nose, throat, and sometimes lungs	▪ May cause infection of the lungs, sinus and ear infections, worsening of underlying heart or lung conditions, and possibly death	▪ Spread through air and direct contact ▪ Recommended every year for children 6 mo and older ▪ Children younger than 9 yr receiving flu vaccine for the first time or given only 1 dose before July 2023 will require 2 separate doses at least a month apart.

(continues)

Suggested Pediatric Immunizations *(continued)*

AGE	IMMUNIZATION	PROTECTION AGAINST	DANGERS OF NOT BEING VACCINATED	NURSING CONSIDERATIONS
				▪ Children younger than 9 yr receiving flu vaccine and have had at least 2 doses of flu vaccine before July 2023 will require only 1 dose. ▪ Given by injection or nasal spray. Nasal spray is only for healthy children and should NOT be given for children with weak immune systems or presence of chronic health conditions such as asthma, heart problems, diabetes, HIV, or sickle cell disease.
6 mo–18 yr	**COVID-19** vaccine	Contagious viral infection of the nose, throat, or lungs that may feel like a cold or flu	▪ May cause lung infection; blood clots; liver, heart, or kidney damage; long-term COVID-19; and possibly death	▪ Spread through air and direct contact ▪ Recommendations varies with manufacturer but first dose recommended to be initiated at 6 mo of age ▪ Number of doses dependent on if either unvaccinated or have had received previous doses of a particular manufacturer ▪ The updated 2023–2024 COVID-19 vaccine protects against the most common variants.
6–18 mo	**HepB**	See HepB above	See HepB above	See HepB above
	IPV	See IPV above	See IPV above	See IPV above
12–15 mo	**Hib**	See Hib above	See Hib above	See Hib above
	MMR (Measles, mumps, rubella) vaccine	Contagious viral infection that causes high fever, cough, red eyes, runny nose and rash (measles and rubella), and fever, tiredness, swollen cheeks, and tender swollen jaw (mumps)	▪ Measles may cause brain swelling, infection of the lungs, and possibly death	▪ Spread through air and direct contact ▪ Sometimes given together with varicella and is called MMRV

AGE	IMMUNIZATION	PROTECTION AGAINST	DANGERS OF NOT BEING VACCINATED	NURSING CONSIDERATIONS
			▪ Rubella (German measles) is very dangerous in pregnancy as it can cause miscarriage or still birth, premature delivery, and severe birth defects. ▪ Mumps can cause brain swelling, painful and swollen testicles or ovaries, deafness, and possibly death.	▪ May be given to infants as young as 6 mo if they will be traveling internationally. A second dose may be given as soon as 4 wk after the first dose if they are still traveling and are at risk. However, they should still be revaccinated at 12–15 mo and 4–6 yr of age.
	PCV	See PCV above	See PCV above	See PCV above
	Varicella (chickenpox) vaccine	Contagious viral infection that causes fever, headache, and an itchy, blistering rash	▪ May cause infected sores, brain swelling, lung infection, and possibly death	▪ Spread through air and direct contact
12–23 mo	**HepA** (Hepatitis A vaccine)	Contagious viral infection of the liver	▪ May cause liver failure and possibly death	▪ Spread through contaminated food or drink or close contact with an infected person ▪ Given as 2 injections at least 6 mo apart ▪ May be given as early as 6 mo to infants who will be in a place where hepatitis A is common. However, the child will still need to be revaccinated after their first birthday.
15–18 mo	**DTaP**	See DTaP above	See DTaP above	See DTaP above
4–6 yr	**DTaP**	See DTaP above	See DTaP above	See DTaP above
	MMR	See MMR above	See MMR above	See MMR above
	IPV	See IPV above	See IPV above	See IPV above
	Varicella	See Varicella above	See Varicella above	See Varicella above

(continues)

Suggested Pediatric Immunizations *(continued)*

AGE	IMMUNIZATION	PROTECTION AGAINST	DANGERS OF NOT BEING VACCINATED	NURSING CONSIDERATIONS
9–16 yr	**Dengue** vaccine	Contagious viral infection	▪ Most cases are mild and are resolved in about a week on their own. ▪ Severe cases can cause serious bleeding, shock, and possible death.	▪ Spreads from mosquitoes to people ▪ Given in 3 doses to children who already had dengue fever and live in areas where it is common (American Samoa, Puerto Rico, U.S. Virgin Islands)
11–12 yr	**HPV** (Human papillomavirus) vaccine	Contagious viral infection	▪ Can cause some types of cancer ▪ Causes genital warts	▪ Spread most commonly during anal or vaginal sex. It may also spread through close skin-to-skin touching during sex. ▪ Given as 2 injections over a 6- to 12-mo period ▪ Can be given as early as age 9 ▪ For teens and young adults ages 15 to 26, given as 3 injections over 6 mo
	TDaP (Tetanus, diphtheria, and pertussis booster)	See TDaP above	See TDaP above	▪ See TDaP for how disease is spread. ▪ Tetanus, diptheria, and pertussis booster
	MenACWY (Meningococcal vaccine for types A, C, W, and Y)	Contagious bacteria infection of meningococcal bacteria types A, C, W, and Y	▪ Causes infection of the brain and spinal cord as well as blood infections ▪ May result in permanent disability (deafness, brain damage, loss of limbs, or seizures) and possibly death	▪ Spread through throat and respiratory secretions from coughing or coming into close or lengthy contact with a person who carries the bacteria by kissing, sharing drinks, or living together with the infected person ▪ A booster dose is recommended at age 16. ▪ Recommended for all children ▪ May be given as early as 8 wk old (depending on vaccine brand) in infants and young children who are at risk for a meningococcal infection such as presence of some immune disorders, live or travel to countries where meningitis is common, or during an outbreak

AGE	IMMUNIZATION	PROTECTION AGAINST	DANGERS OF NOT BEING VACCINATED	NURSING CONSIDERATIONS
16–18 yr	**MenB** (Meningococcal vaccine for type B)	Contagious bacteria infection of the meningococcal bacterium type B	▪ May cause infection of the membrane of the brain and spinal cord as well as septicemia	▪ Spread through throat and respiratory secretions from couging or coming into close or lengthy contact with a person who carries the bacteria by kissing, sharing drinks, or living together with the infected person ▪ Given to children and teens in 2 to 3 doses depending on the brand ▪ Only recommended as routine for children ages 10 and older who have conditions that weaken the immune system, or during an outbreak

Data from Centers for Disease Control and Prevention. (2024). Child and adolescent immunization schedule by age, United States, 2024. Retrieved from https://www.cdc.gov/vaccines/schedules/hcp/imz/child-adolescent.html;
Data from Centers for Disease Control and Prevention. (2024). What diseases do these vaccines protect against? Retrieved from https://www.cdc.gov/vaccines/schedules/easy-to-read/child-easyread.html;
Data from Centers for Disease Control and Prevention. (2024). What disease do these vaccines protect against? Retrieved from https://www.cdc.gov

Selected Antihypertensive Combinations

Antihypertensive drugs are used along with lifestyle changes to manage hypertension. Antihypertensive combinations, which commonly include 1 or 2 antihypertensives and a diuretic, are used to simplify patients' drug regimens and, in some cases, to enhance drug actions.

The following table lists the generic and trade names; functional classes; usual adult

ANTIHYPERTENSIVE COMBINATION TRADE NAMES	ANTIHYPERTENSIVE GENERIC NAMES	DIURETIC GENERIC NAMES
Aldoril-15	methyldopa 250 mg	hydrochlorothiazide (HCTZ) 15 mg
Aldoril-25	methyldopa 250 mg	HCTZ 25 mg
Aldoril D30	methyldopa 500 mg	HCTZ 30 mg
Aldoril D50	methyldopa 500 mg	HCTZ 50 mg
Amturnide 150/5/12.5	aliskiren 150 mg, amlodipine 5 mg	HCTZ 12.5 mg
Amturnide 300/5/12.5	aliskiren 300 mg, amlodipine 5 mg	HCTZ 12.5 mg
Amturnide 300/5/25	aliskiren 300 mg, amlodipine 5 mg	HCTZ 25 mg
Amturnide 300/10/12.5	aliskiren 300 mg, amlodipine 10 mg	HCTZ 12.5 mg
Amturnide 300/10/25	aliskiren 300 mg, amlodipine 10 mg	HCTZ 25 mg
Apresazide 25/25	hydralazine hydrochloride (HCL) 25 mg	HCTZ 25 mg
Apresazide 50/50	hydralazine HCl 50 mg	HCTZ 50 mg
Apresazide 100/50	hydralazine HCl 100 mg	HCTZ 50 mg
Atacand HCT 16/12.5	candesartan cilexetil 16 mg	HCTZ 12.5 mg
Atacand HCT 32/12.5	candesartan cilexetil 32 mg	HCTZ 12.5 mg
Atacand HCT 32/25	candesartan cilexetil 32 mg	HCTZ 25 mg
Avalide-150	irbesartan 150 mg	HCTZ 12.5 mg
Avalide-300	irbesartan 300 mg	HCTZ 12.5 mg
Azor 5/20	amlodipine 5 mg, olmesartan 20 mg	None
Azor 5/40	amlodipine 5 mg, olmesartan 40 mg	
Azor 10/20	amlodipine 10 mg, olmesartan 20 mg	
Azor 10/40	amlodipine 10 mg, olmesartan 40 mg	
Benicar HCT 20/12.5	olmesartan medoxomil 20 mg	HCTZ 12.5 mg
Benicar HCT 40/12.5	olmesartan medoxomil 40 mg	HCTZ 12.5 mg
Benicar HCT 40/25	olmesartan medoxomil 40 mg	HCTZ 25 mg
Capozide 25/15	captopril 25 mg	HCTZ 15 mg
Capozide 25/25	captopril 25 mg	HCTZ 25 mg
Capozide 50/15	captopril 50 mg	HCTZ 15 mg
Capozide 50/25	captopril 50 mg	HCTZ 25 mg
Diovan HCT 80/12.5	valsartan 80 mg	HCTZ 12.5 mg
Diovan HCT 160/12.5	valsartan 160 mg	HCTZ 12.5 mg
Diovan HCT 160/25	valsartan 160 mg	HCTZ 25 mg
Diovan HCT 320/12.5	valsartan 320 mg	HCTZ 12.5 mg
Diovan HCT 320/25	valsartan 320 mg	HCTZ 25 mg
Dyazide 37.5/25	triamterene 37.5 mg	HCTZ 25 mg

dosages; and onset, peak, and duration for commonly used antihypertensive combinations. For information about the mechanisms of action, interactions, adverse reactions, and nursing considerations related to antihypertensive combinations, review the entries for the specific antihypertensives and diuretics that they contain.

FUNCTIONAL CLASSES	USUAL ADULT DOSAGES	ONSET, PEAK, AND DURATION
Centrally acting antiadrenergic and thiazide diuretic	1 tab 2 or 3 times daily 1 tab twice daily 1 tab daily 1 tab daily	**Onset:** Unknown **Peak:** 4–6 hr **Duration:** 12–24 hr
Direct renin inhibitor, calcium channel blocker, and thiazide diuretic	1 tab once daily 1 tab once daily 1 tab once daily 1 tab once daily 1 tab once daily	**Onset:** Unknown **Peak:** 3–8 hr **Duration:** Unknown
Peripherally acting arterial dilator and thiazide diuretic	1 cap once or twice daily 1 cap once or twice daily 1 cap once or twice daily	**Onset:** 20–30 min **Peak:** 1–2 hr **Duration:** 2–4 hr
Angiotensin II receptor antagonist and thiazide diuretic	1 tab once or twice daily 1 tab daily 1 tab daily	**Onset:** 1–2 wk **Peak:** Within 4 wk **Duration:** Unknown
ACE inhibitor and thiazide diuretic	1 tab daily 1 tab daily	**Onset:** Unknown **Peak:** Unknown **Duration:** Unknown
Calcium channel blocker and angiotensin II receptor antagonist	1 tab daily 1 tab daily 1 tab daily 1 tab daily	**Onset:** Unknown **Peak:** 1–6 hr **Duration:** 24 hr
Angiotensin II receptor antagonist and thiazide diuretic	1 tab daily 1 tab daily 1 tab daily	**Onset:** Unknown **Peak:** Unknown **Duration:** Unknown
ACE inhibitor and thiazide diuretic	1 tab daily to 3 times daily 1 tab once or twice daily 1 tab once daily to 3 times daily 1 tab once or twice daily	**Onset:** 15–60 min **Peak:** 60–90 min **Duration:** 6–12 hr
Angiotensin II receptor blocker and thiazide diuretic	1 or 2 tabs daily 1 tab daily 1 tab daily 1 tab daily 1 tab daily	**Onset:** 2 hr **Peak:** 6 hr **Duration:** 24 hr
Potassium-sparing diuretic and thiazide diuretic	1 or 2 caps or tabs daily	**Onset:** 2–4 hr **Peak:** 1 day **Duration:** 7–9 hr

(continues)

Selected Antihypertensive Combinations *(continued)*

ANTIHYPERTENSIVE COMBINATION TRADE NAMES	ANTIHYPERTENSIVE GENERIC NAMES	DIURETIC GENERIC NAMES
Edarbyclor 40/12.5	azilsartan 40 mg	chlorthalidone 12.5 mg
Edarbyclor 40/25	azilsartan 40 mg	chlorthalidone 25 mg
Exforge 5/160	amlodipine 5 mg, valsartan 160 mg	None
Exforge 10/160	amlodipine 10 mg, valsartan 160 mg	
Exforge 5/320	amlodipine 5 mg, valsartan 320 mg	
Exforge 10/320	amlodipine 10 mg, valsartan 320 mg	
Exforge HCT 5/160/12.5	amlodipine 5 mg, valsartan 160 mg	HCTZ 12.5 mg
Exforge HCT 10/160/12.5	amlodipine 10 mg, valsartan 160 mg	HCTZ 12.5 mg
Exforge HCT 5/160/25	amlodipine 5 mg, valsartan 160 mg	HCTZ 25 mg
Exforge HCT 10/160/25	amlodipine 10 mg, valsartan 160 mg	HCTZ 25 mg
Exforge HCT 10/320/25	amlodipine 10 mg, valsartan 320 mg	HCTZ 25 mg
Hyzaar 50/12.5	losartan potassium 50 mg	HCTZ 12.5 mg
Hyzaar 100/12.5	losartan potassium 100 mg	HCTZ 12.5 mg
Hyzaar 100/25	losartan potassium 100 mg	HCTZ 25 mg
Inderide 40/25	propranolol HCL 40 mg	HCTZ 25 mg
Inderide 80/25	propranolol HCl 80 mg	HCTZ 25 mg
Inderide LA 80/50	propranolol HCl 80 mg	HCTZ 50 mg
Inderide LA 120/50	propranolol HCl 120 mg	HCTZ 50 mg
Inderide LA 160/50	propranolol HCl 160 mg	HCTZ 50 mg
Lopressor HCT 50/25	metoprolol tartrate 50 mg	HCTZ 25 mg
Lopressor HCT 100/25	metoprolol tartrate 100 mg	HCTZ 25 mg
Lopressor HCT 100/50	metoprolol tartrate 100 mg	HCTZ 50 mg
Lotensin HCT 5/6.25	benazepril HCl 5 mg	HCTZ 6.25 mg
Lotensin HCT 10/12.5	benazepril HCl 10 mg	HCTZ 12.5 mg
Lotensin HCT 20/12.5	benazepril HCl 20 mg	HCTZ 12.5 mg
Lotensin HCT 20/25	benazepril HCl 20 mg	HCTZ 25 mg
Lotrel 2.5/10	amlodipine 2.5 mg, benazepril HCl 10 mg	None
Lotrel 5/10	amlodipine 5 mg, benazepril HCl 10 mg	None
Lotrel 5/20	amlodipine 5 mg, benazepril HCl 20 mg	None
Lotrel 5/40	amlodipine 5 mg, benazepril 40 mg	None
Lotrel 10/20	amlodipine 10 mg, benazepril HCl 20 mg	None
Lotrel 10/40	amlodipine 10 mg, benazepril 40 mg	None
Maxzide-25 37.5/25	triamterene 37.5 mg	HCTZ 25 mg
Maxzide 75/50	triamterene 75 mg	HCTZ 50 mg
Micardis HCT 40/12.5	telmisartan 40 mg	HCTZ 12.5 mg
Micardis HCT 80/12.5	telmisartan 80 mg	HCTZ 12.5 mg
Micardis HCT 80/25	telmisartan 80 mg	HCTZ 25 mg

FUNCTIONAL CLASSES	USUAL ADULT DOSAGES	ONSET, PEAK, AND DURATION
ACE inhibitor and thiazide-like diuretic	1 tab daily 1 tab daily	**Onset:** Unknown **Peak:** 6 hr **Duration:** 24 hr
Calcium channel blocker and angiotensin II receptor blocker	1 or 2 tabs daily 1 tab daily 1 tab daily 1 tab daily	**Onset:** Unknown **Peak:** 6–12 hr **Duration:** 24 hr
Calcium channel blocker, angiotensin II receptor blocker, and thiazide diuretic	1 tab daily 1 tab daily 1 tab daily 1 tab daily 1 tab daily	**Onset:** Unknown **Peak:** 2–6 hr **Duration:** Unknown
Angiotensin II receptor blocker and thiazide diuretic	1 or 2 tabs daily 1 tab daily 1 tab daily	**Onset:** Unknown **Peak:** 6 hr **Duration:** 24 hr or more
Beta-blocker and thiazide diuretic	1 or 2 tabs twice daily 1 or 2 tabs twice daily 1 cap daily 1 cap daily 1 cap daily	**Onset:** Unknown **Peak:** 1–1.5 hr **Duration:** Unknown
Beta-blocker and thiazide diuretic	2 tabs daily or 1 tab twice daily 1 or 2 tabs daily or 1 tab twice daily 2 tabs daily or 1 tab twice daily	**Onset:** 1 hr **Peak:** 1–2 hr **Duration:** Unknown
ACE inhibitor and thiazide diuretic	1 tab daily 1 tab daily 1 tab daily 1 tab daily	**Onset:** 1 hr **Peak:** 2–4 hr **Duration:** 24 hr
Calcium channel blocker and ACE inhibitor	1 or 2 caps daily 1 cap daily 1 cap daily 1 cap daily 1 cap daily 1 cap daily	**Onset:** Unknown **Peak:** Unknown **Duration:** 24 hr
Potassium-sparing diuretic and thiazide diuretic	1 tab daily 1 tab daily	**Onset:** 2–4 hr **Peak:** 1 day **Duration:** 7–9 hr
Angiotensin II receptor antagonist and thiazide diuretic	1 tab once or twice daily 1 tab once or twice daily 1 tab once daily	**Onset:** Within 3 hr **Peak:** In 4 wk **Duration:** Several days to 1 wk

(continues)

Selected Antihypertensive Combinations *(continued)*

ANTIHYPERTENSIVE COMBINATION TRADE NAMES	ANTIHYPERTENSIVE GENERIC NAMES	DIURETIC GENERIC NAMES
Moduretic	amiloride 5 mg	HCTZ 50 mg
Prinzide 10/12.5 Prinzide 20/12.5	lisinopril 10 mg lisinopril 20 mg	HCTZ 12.5 mg HCTZ 12.5 mg
Tekamlo 150/5 Tekamlo 150/10 Tekamlo 300/5 Tekamlo 300/10	aliskiren 150 mg, amlodipine 5 mg aliskiren 150 mg, amlodipine 10 mg aliskiren 300 mg, amlodipine 5 mg aliskiren 300 mg, amlodipine 10 mg	None None None None
Tekturna HCT 150/12.5 Tekturna HCT 150/25 Tekturna HCT 300/12.5 Tekturna HCT 300/25	aliskiren 150 mg aliskiren 150 mg aliskiren 300 mg aliskiren 300 mg	HCTZ 12.5 mg HCTZ 25 mg HCTZ 12.5 mg HCTZ 25 mg
Timolide 10/25	timolol maleate 10 mg	HCTZ 25 mg
Tribenzor 20/5/12.5 Tribenzor 40/5/12.5 Tribenzor 40/5/25 Tribenzor 40/10/12.5 Tribenzor 40/10/25	amlodipine 5 mg, olmesartan 20 mg amlodipine 5 mg, olmesartan 40 mg amlodipine 5 mg, olmesartan 40 mg amlodipine 10 mg, olmesartan 40 mg amlodipine 10 mg, olmesartan 40 mg	HCTZ 12.5 mg HCTZ 12.5 mg HCTZ 25 mg HCTZ 12.5 mg HCTZ 25 mg
Twynsta 40/5 Twynsta 40/10 Twynsta 80/5 Twynsta 80/10	telmisartan 40 mg, amlodipine 5 mg telmisartan 40 mg, amlodipine 10 mg telmisartan 80 mg, amlodipine 5 mg telmisartan 80 mg, amlodipine 10 mg	None None None None
Uniretic 7.5/12.5 Uniretic 15/12.5 Uniretic 15/25	moexipril HCL 7.5 mg moexipril 15 mg moexipril HCl 15 mg	HCTZ 12.5 mg HCTZ 12.5 mg HCTZ 25 mg
Valturna 150/160 Valturna 300/320	aliskiren 150 mg, valsartan 160 mg aliskiren 300 mg, valsartan 320 mg	None None
Vaseretic 10/25	enalapril maleate 10 mg	HCTZ 25 mg
Zestoretic 10/12.5 Zestoretic 20/12.5 Zestoretic 20/25	lisinopril 10 mg lisinopril 20 mg lisinopril 20 mg	HCTZ 12.5 mg HCTZ 12.5 mg HCTZ 25 mg
Ziac 2.5/6.25 Ziac 5/6.25 Ziac 10/6.25	bisoprolol fumarate 2.5 mg bisoprolol fumarate 5 mg bisoprolol fumarate 10 mg	HCTZ 6.25 mg HCTZ 6.25 mg HCTZ 6.25 mg

FUNCTIONAL CLASSES	USUAL ADULT DOSAGES	ONSET, PEAK, AND DURATION
Potassium-sparing diuretic and thiazide diuretic	1 or 2 tabs daily	**Onset:** 2 hr **Peak:** 6–10 hr **Duration:** 24 hr
ACE inhibitor and thiazide diuretic	1 or 2 tabs daily 1 or 2 tabs daily	**Onset:** 1 hr **Peak:** 6 hr **Duration:** 24 hr
Direct renin inhibitor and calcium channel blocker	1 or 2 tabs daily 1 tab daily 1 tab daily 1 tab daily	**Onset:** Unknown **Peak:** 3–8 hr **Duration:** 24 hr
Direct renin inhibitor and thiazide diuretic	1 tab daily 1 tab daily 1 tab daily 1 tab daily	**Onset:** Unknown **Peak:** 1–2.5 hr **Duration:** Unknown
Beta-blocker and thiazide diuretic	2 tabs daily or 1 tab twice daily	**Onset:** Unknown **Peak:** 1–2 hr **Duration:** Unknown
Angiotensin II receptor antagonist, calcium channel blocker, and thiazide diuretic	1 tab daily 1 tab daily 1 tab daily 1 tab daily 1 tab daily	**Onset:** Unknown **Peak:** 1–6 hr **Duration:** 24 hr
Angiotensin II receptor antagonist and calcium channel blocker	1 tab daily 1 tab daily 1 tab daily 1 tab daily	**Onset:** Unknown **Peak:** 1–6 hr **Duration:** Unknown
Potassium-sparing diuretic and thiazide diuretic	1 tab daily 1 tab daily 1 tab daily	**Onset:** 1 hr **Peak:** 3–6 hr **Duration:** 24 hr
Direct renin inhibitor and angiotensin II antagonist	1 tab daily 1 tab daily	**Onset:** Unknown **Peak:** 1–3 hr **Duration:** Unknown
ACE inhibitor and thiazide diuretic	1 tab once or twice daily	**Onset:** 1 hr **Peak:** 4–6 hr **Duration:** 24 hr
ACE inhibitor and thiazide diuretic	1 or 2 tabs daily 1 or 2 tabs daily 1 or 2 tabs daily	**Onset:** 1 hr **Peak:** 6 hr **Duration:** 24 hr
Beta-blocker and thiazide diuretic	1 or 2 tabs daily 1 or 2 tabs daily 1 or 2 tabs daily	**Onset:** Unknown **Peak:** Unknown **Duration:** Unknown

Selected Combination Antiviral Drugs

Combination antiviral drugs are used to treat viral infections, such as human immunodeficiency virus (HIV) and hepatitis C infections.

The following table lists the generic and trade names, FDA-approved indications, and usual adult dosages for some commonly used combination antivirals. Although you must individualize your care for a patient who receives an antiviral, be sure to include these general interventions in your plan of care:

- Avoid administering HIV drugs all at once.
- If patient takes an antacid, administer it 1 hour before or 2 hours after an antiviral because antacids may reduce antiviral absorption.
- Monitor hepatic enzyme levels to detect elevations and help prevent hepatotoxicity.
- Monitor BUN and serum creatinine levels to detect signs of impaired renal function.
- Monitor I.V. injection site for pain or phlebitis, which may result from the high pH of reconstituted solutions.
- Assess the immunosuppressed patient for opportunistic infections during antiviral therapy.
- Inform females of childbearing age that oral contraceptives may be ineffective when taken with HIV drugs. Suggest alternate contraceptive methods.

GENERIC AND TRADE NAMES	INDICATIONS	USUAL ADULT DOSAGES
Antivirals used for HIV infection		
abacavir sulfate, dolutegravir sodium, and lamivudine Triumeq	*To treat HIV-1 infection*	600 mg abacavir, 50 mg dolutegravir, and 300 mg lamivudine (1 tablet) P.O. once daily.
abacavir sulfate and lamivudine Epzicom	*As adjunct to treat HIV-1 infection*	600 mg abacavir and 300 mg lamivudine (1 tablet) P.O. daily.
abacavir sulfate, lamivudine, and zidovudine Trizivir	*As adjunct or as monotherapy to treat HIV-1 infection*	300 mg abacavir, 150 mg lamivudine, and 300 mg zidovudine (1 tablet) P.O. twice daily.
atazanavir sulfate and cobicistat Evotaz	*As adjunct to treat HIV-1 infection*	300 mg atazanavir and 150 mg cobicistat (1 tablet) P.O. once daily.
bictegravir sodium, emtricitabine, and tenofovir alafenamide fumarate Biktarvy	*To treat HIV-1 infection in patients with no antiretroviral treatment history or to replace current antiretroviral regimen*	50 mg bictegravir, 200 mg emtricitabine, and 25 mg tenofovir alafenamide (1 tablet) P.O. once daily.
cabotegravir and rilpivirine sodium Cabenuva	*To treat HIV-1 infection in adults and adolescents weighing at least 35 kg (77 lb)*	*Initial:* 600 mg of cabotegravir and 900 mg of rilpivirine I.M. given on last day of current antiretroviral therapy or oral lead-in, if used. *Maintenance:* 400 mg of cabotegravir and 600 mg of rilpivirine I.M. monthly. Alternatively, 600 mg cabotegravir and 900 mg rilpivirine I.M. given 1 mo apart for 2 consecutive months followed by same dosage every 2 months.
darunavir ethanolate and cobicistat Prezcobix	*As adjunct to treat HIV-1 infection*	800 mg darunavir and 150 mg cobicistat (1 tablet) P.O. once daily.

GENERIC AND TRADE NAMES	INDICATIONS	USUAL ADULT DOSAGES
Antivirals used for HIV infection *(continued)*		
darunavir ethanolate, cobicistat, emtricitabine, and tenofovir alafenamide fumarate Symtuza	*To treat HIV-1 infection*	800 mg darunavir, 150 mg cobicistat, 200 mg emtricitabine, and 10 mg tenofovir alafenamide (1 tablet) P.O. once daily.
dolutegravir sodium and lamivudine Dovato	*To treat HIV-1 infection in adults and adolescents with no antiretroviral treatment history or to replace current antiretroviral regimen weighing at least 25 kg ((55 lb)*	50 mg dolutegravir and 300 mg lamivudine (1 tablet) P.O. once daily.
dolutegravir sodium and rilpivirine hydrochloride Juluca	*To treat HIV-1 infection*	50 mg dolutegravir and 25 mg rilpivirine (1 tablet) P.O. once daily with a meal.
doravirine, lamivudine, and tenofovir disoproxil fumarate Delstrigo	*To treat HIV-1 infection*	100 mg doravirine, 300 mg lamivudine, and 300 mg tenofovir disoproxil fumarate (1 tablet) P.O. once daily.
efavirenz, emtricitabine, and tenofovir disoproxil fumarate Atripla	*As adjunct or monotherapy to treat HIV-1 infection in adults weighing at least 40 kg (88 lb) or more*	600 mg efavirenz, 200 mg emtricitabine, and 300 mg tenofovir disoproxil fumarate (1 tablet) P.O. once daily, at bedtime.
efavirenz, lamivudine, and tenofovir disoproxil fumarate Symfi Symfi Lo	*To treat HIV-1 infection in patients weighing at least 40 kg (88 lb) or more* *To treat HIV-1 infection in adults and children weighing at least 35 kg (77 lb)*	600 mg efavirenz, 300 mg lamivudine, and 300 mg tenofovir disoproxil fumarate (1 tablet) P.O. once daily. 400 mg efavirenz, 300 mg lamivudine, and 300 mg tenofovir disoproxil fumarate (1 tablet) P.O. once daily.
elvitegravir, cobicistat, emtricitabine, tenofovir alafenamide fumarate Genvoya	*To treat HIV-1 infection*	150 mg elvitegravir, 150 mg cobicistat, 200 mg emtricitabine, and 10 mg tenofovir alafenamide (1 tablet) once daily.
elvitegravir, cobicistat, emtricitabine, tenofovir disoproxil fumarate Stribild	*To treat HIV-1 infection*	150 mg elvitegravir, 150 mg cobicistat, 200 mg emtricitabine, 300 mg tenofovir (1 tablet) P.O. once daily with food.
emtricitabine, rilpivirine hydrochloride, tenofovir disoproxil fumarate Complera	*To treat HIV-1 infection*	200 mg emtricitabine, 25 mg rilpivirine, 300 mg tenofovir (1 tablet) P.O. daily with meal.
emtricitabine, rilpivirine hydrochloride, tenofovir alafenamide fumarate Odefsey	*To treat HIV-1 infection*	200 mg emtricitabine, 25 mg rilpivirine, and 25 mg tenofovir alafenamide (1 tablet) P.O. once daily.

(continues)

Selected Combination Antiviral Drugs *(continued)*

GENERIC AND TRADE NAMES	INDICATIONS	USUAL ADULT DOSAGES
Antivirals used for HIV infection *(continued)*		
emtricitabine and tenofovir alafenamide fumarate Descovy	*To treat HIV-1 infection*	200 mg emtricitabine and 25 mg tenofovir alafenamide (1 tablet) P.O. once daily in combination with other antiretrovirals.
emtricitabine and tenofovir disoproxil fumarate Truvada	*As adjunct to treat HIV-1 infection in patients weighing 17 kg (37.4 lb) or more*	*Weighing at least 35 kg (77 lb):* 200 mg emtricitabine and 300 mg tenofovir disoproxil fumarate (1 tablet) P.O. once daily. *Weighing 28 kg (61.6 lb) to less than 35 kg (77 lb):* 167 mg emtricitabine and 250 mg tenofovir disoproxil fumarate (1 tablet) P.O. once daily. *Weighing 22 kg (48.4 lb) to less than 28 kg (61.6 lb):* 133 mg emtricitabine, 200 mg tenofovir disoproxil fumarate (1 tablet) P.O. once daily. *Weighing 17 kg (37.4 lb) to less than 22 (48.4 lb):* 100 mg emtricitabine and 150 mg tenofovir disoproxil fumarate (1 tablet) P.O. once daily.
lamivudine and raltegravir potassium Dutrebis	*As adjunct to treat HIV-1 infection*	150 mg lamivudine and 300 mg raltegravir (1 tablet) P.O. twice daily.
lamivudine and tenofovir disoproxil fumarate Cimduo	*As adjunct to treat HIV-1 infection in patients weighing 35 kg (77 lb) or more*	300 mg lamivudine and 300 mg tenofovir disoproxil fumarate (1 tablet) P.O. once daily.
lamivudine and zidovudine (3 tC/AZT, 3 tC/ZDV) Combivir	*As adjunct to treat HIV-1 infection in patients who weigh 50 kg (110 lb) or more*	150 mg of lamivudine and 300 mg of zidovudine P.O. twice daily.
lopinavir and ritonavir Kaletra	*As adjunct to treat HIV-1 infection*	800 mg lopinavir and 200 mg ritonavir once daily or 400 mg lopinavir and 100 mg ritonavir P.O. twice daily.
Antivirals used for hepatitis C virus (HCV) infection		
dasabuvir sodium, ombitasvir, paritaprevir, and ritonavir Viekira XR	*To treat chronic HCV genotype 1b infection without cirrhosis or with compensated cirrhosis*	600 mg dasabuvir, 24.99 mg ombitasvir, 150 mg paritaprevir, and 99.99 mg ritonavir (3 E.R. tablets) P.O. once daily.
elbasvir and grazoprevir Zepatier	*To treat chronic HCV with genotype 1 or 4*	50 mg elbasvir and 100 mg grazoprevir (1 tablet) P.O. once daily.

GENERIC AND TRADE NAMES	INDICATIONS	USUAL ADULT DOSAGES
Antivirals used for hepatitis C virus (HCV) infection *(continued)*		
glecaprevir and pibrentasvir Mavyret	*To treat chronic HCV genotype 1, 2, 3, 4, 5, or 6 without cirrhosis or with compensated cirrhosis; to treat HCV genotype 1 infection in patients previously treated with a regimen containing an HCV NS5A inhibitor or an NS3/4A protease inhibitor, but not both*	300 mg glecaprevir and 120 mg pibrentasvir (3 tablets) P.O. once daily for 8 wk (HCV genotype 1, 2, 3, 4, 5, or 6 with no cirrhosis or compensated cirrhosis); 12 wk (HCV genotype 1 with previous treatment with an NS3/4/4A protease inhibitor without prior treatment with an NS5A inhibitor); 16 wk (HCV genotype 1 with an NS5A inhibitor without prior treatment with an NS3/4A protease inhibitor).
ledipasvir and sofosbuvir Harvoni	*To treat chronic HCV genotype 1, 4, 5, or 6 in patients without cirrhosis or with compensated cirrhosis; as adjunct to treat chronic hepatitis C genotype 1 in patients with decompensated cirrhosis or genotype 1 or 4 in liver transplant recipients without cirrhosis or compensated cirrhosis*	90 mg ledipasvir and 400 mg sofosbuvir (1 tablet) P.O. once daily.
ombitasvir, paritaprevir, and ritonavir Technivie	*As adjunct to treat chronic HCV genotype 4 in patients without cirrhosis*	25 mg ombitasvir, 150 mg paritaprevir, and 100 mg ritonavir (2 tablets) P.O. once daily in morning.
sofosbuvir and velpatasvir Epclusa	*To treat chronic HCV genotype 1, 2, 3, 4, 5, or 6 in patients with compensated cirrhosis or without cirrhosis, or with decompensated cirrhosis when used in combination with ribavirin*	400 mg sofosbuvir and 100 mg velpatasvir (1 tablet) P.O. once daily for 12 wk (adults); dosage based on weight and given once daily for 12 wk (children ages 3 and older).
sofosbuvir, velpatasvir, and voxilaprevir Vosevi	*To treat chronic HCV genotype 1, 2, 3, 4, 5, or 6 in patients with compensated cirrhosis or without cirrhosis in patients previously treated with an HCV regimen containing an NS5A inhibitor or genotype 1a or 3 infections previously treated with an HCV regimen containing sofosbuvir without an NS5A inhibitor*	400 mg sofosbuvir, 100 mg velpatasvir, and 100 mg voxilaprevir (1 tablet) P.O. once daily.

Selected Ophthalmic Drugs

Although less commonly prescribed than oral drugs, drugs instilled into the eyes are frequently brought into the clinical setting by patients with chronic conditions. In most cases, the patient, family, or caregiver has administered these preparations at home. Your patient teaching should include a review of proper administration and storage of these drugs. Have the patient, family, or caregiver demonstrate proper use of the drug to make sure it will be administered correctly at home. Use this time to reassess the patient's ability to continue self-medication. Also, instruct him to report any changes in the condition being treated, either negative or positive. A properly educated patient not only ensures safe drug administration, but also is more likely to detect adverse reactions that require a dosage reduction or drug discontinuation, thus preventing the development of more serious health problems.

The following chart lists the generic and trade names, FDA-approved indications, and usual adult dosages for those ophthalmic preparations you're most likely to see in your practice setting. The drugs are divided according to therapeutic use.

GENERIC AND TRADE NAMES	INDICATIONS	USUAL ADULT DOSAGES
Ophthalmic antibiotics		
azithromycin 1% AzaSite	*To treat bacterial conjunctivitis due to susceptible organisms*	1 gtt in affected eye(s) twice daily (8–12 hr apart) for first 2 days; then 1 gtt in affected eye(s) once daily for next 5 days.
bacitracin AK-Tracin	*To treat surface bacterial infections affecting the conjunctiva and cornea*	1/4-in to 1/2-in strip of ointment applied to conjunctival sac, 1 to 3 times daily or as needed.
besifloxacin 0.6% Besivance	*To treat bacterial conjunctivitis due to susceptible organisms*	1 gtt in affected eye(s) 3 times daily 4 to 14 hr apart for 7 days.
chloramphenicol 1% Diochloram, Pentamycetin/HC, Sopamycetin (CAN)	*To treat severe surface bacterial infections affecting the conjunctiva and cornea*	Apply small amount of ointment to lower conjunctival sac every 3 to 6 hr and, as needed, for at least 48 hr after eye resumes normal appearance.
ciprofloxacin hydrochloride0.3% Ciloxan	*To treat corneal ulcers due to* Pseudomonas aeruginosa, Staphylococcus aureus, S. epidermidis, Streptococcus pneumoniae, *or possibly* Serratia marcescens *or* S. viridans	2 gtt in affected eye every 15 min for first 6 hr, then 2 gtt every 30 min for rest of first day; on day 2, 2 gtt in affected eye every hr; on days 3 to 14, 2 gtt in affected eye every 4 hr.
	To treat bacterial conjunctivitis due to Haemophilus influenzae, S. aureus, S. epidermidis, S. pneumoniae, *or* S. viridans	1 or 2 gtt in conjunctival sac of affected eye every 2 hr while awake for first 2 days and then 1 or 2 gtt every 4 hr while awake for next 5 days; or 1/2-in strip of ointment in affected eye 3 times daily for 2 days, then twice daily for next 5 days.
erythromycin Ilotycin	*To treat superficial eye infections involving conjunctiva and/or cornea*	1 cm (0.39 in) of ointment applied in infected eye up to 6 times/day, depending on severity of infection.
	As adjunct to prevent ophthalmia neonatorum due to Neisseria gonorrhoeae *or* Chlamydia trachomatis	1 cm (0.39 in) of ointment applied in each eye.

GENERIC AND TRADE NAMES	INDICATIONS	USUAL ADULT DOSAGES
Ophthalmic antibiotics *(continued)*		
gatifloxacin 0.5% Zymaxid	*To treat bacterial conjunctivitis due to* Staphylococcus aureus, S. epidermidis, Streptococcus mitis, S. pneumoniae, *or* Haemophilus influenzae	1 gtt in affected eye every 2 hr while awake, up to 8 times daily on day 1; then 1 gtt 2 to 4 times daily while awake on days 2 to 7.
gentamicin sulfate Garamycin, Genoptic, Gentacidin, Gentak	*To treat bacterial infections, such as blepharitis, blepharoconjunctivitis, conjunctivitis, corneal ulcers, dacryocystitis, keratoconjunctivitis, or meibomianitis due to susceptible organisms*	1 or 2 gtt every 4 hr or, for severe infection, up to 2 gtt/hr; alternatively, 1/2-in strip of ointment applied to lower conjunctival sac twice daily or 3 times daily.
levofloxacin 0.5% Quixin	*To treat bacterial conjunctivitis due to susceptible organisms*	On days 1 and 2: 1 or 2 gtt every 2 hr while awake, up to 8 times/day; on days 3 to 7: 1 or 2 gtt every 4 hr while awake, up to 4 times/day.
moxifloxacin 0.5% Vigamox Moxeza 0.5%	*To treat bacterial conjunctivitis due to* Staphylococcus aureus, S. epidermidis, S. haemolyticus, S. hominis, Streptococcus pneumoniae, S. viridans *group,* Haemophilus influenzae, *or* Chlamydia trachomatis	1 gtt 3 times daily for 7 days.
ofloxacin 0.3% Ocuflox	*To treat conjunctivitis due to* Staphylococcus aureus, S. epidermidis, Streptococcus pneumoniae, Enterobacter cloacae, Haemophilus influenzae, Proteus mirabilis, *or* Pseudomonas aeruginosa	1 or 2 gtt in conjunctival sac every 2 to 4 hr for first 2 days; then 1 to 2 gtt 4 times daily for up to 5 more days.
	To treat bacterial corneal ulcers due to S. aureus, S. epidermidis, S. pneumoniae, E. cloacae, H. influenzae, Propionibacterium mirabilis, Propionibacterium aeruginosa, Serratia marcescens, *or* Propionibacterium acnes	1 or 2 gtt every 30 min while awake and 1 or 2 gtt every 4 to 6 hr after retiring for 2 days; then 1 or 2 gtt/hr while awake for up to 7 more days; then 1 to 2 gtt 4 times daily until end of treatment.
sulfacetamide sodium 10% Bleph-10, Ocusol 10, Ocusol 15, Ocusol 30, Sodium Sulamyd, Sulf-10, Sulfac 10%	*To treat conjunctivitis and other superficial eye infections due to susceptible organisms*	1 or 2 gtt solution in lower conjunctival sac every 2 to 3 hr initially, with dosage tapered by increasing time interval between doses as condition improves for up to 10 days; or 1/4-in to 1/2-in strip of ointment in conjunctival sac 4 times daily and bedtime.

(continues)

Selected Ophthalmic Drugs *(continued)*

GENERIC AND TRADE NAMES	INDICATIONS	USUAL ADULT DOSAGES
Ophthalmic antibiotics *(continued)*		
sulfacetamide sodium ointment 10%, solution 15% Isopto Cetamide	*As adjunct to treat trachoma*	2 gtt in lower conjunctival sac every 2 hr.
tobramycin Tobrasol 0.3%, Tobrex, Tomycine (CAN)	*To treat external superficial ocular infections and its adnexa due to susceptible organisms*	1 to 2 gtt every 1 to 4 hr, depending on severity of infection; or 1/2-in strip of ointment applied to lower conjunctival sac every 8 to 12 hr for mild to moderate infections or every 3 to 4 hr for severe infections.
tobramycin 0.3% (3 mg) and dexamethasone 0.1% (1 mg) TobraDex	*To treat steroid-responsive inflammatory ocular conditions for which a corticosteroid is indicated and where superficial bacterial ocular infection or a risk of bacterial ocular infection exists*	1 to 2 gtt every 4 to 6 hr; during first 24 to 48 hr, dosage may be increased to 1 to 2 gtt every 2 hr; or 1/2-in strip of ointment applied into the conjunctival sac up to 4 times daily.
Ophthalmic antiviral drugs		
acyclovir 3% Avaclyr	*To treat acute herpetic keratitis (dendritic ulcers) in patients with herpes simplex virus*	1-cm ribbon of ointment into the lower cul-de-sac of the affected eye 5 times daily (about 3 hr apart while awake) until corneal ulcer heals and then 1-cm ribbon 3 times daily for 7 days.
ganciclovir gel 0.15% Zirgan	*To treat acute herpes keratitis (dendritic ulcers)*	1 gtt 5 times daily (about every 3 hr while awake) until corneal ulcer heals; then 1 gtt 3 times daily for 7 days.
Ophthalmic anti-inflammatory drugs		
bromfenac 0.09% Xibrom (0.09%)	*To treat postoperative inflammation and reduce ocular pain after cataract extraction*	1 gtt in operative eye twice daily starting 24 hr after cataract surgery and continuing through first 2 wk of postoperative period.
Bromday (0.09%) Prolensa (0.07%)	*To treat postoperative inflammation and reduce ocular pain after cataract extraction*	1 gtt in operative eye once daily, starting 24 hr before cataract surgery and continuing through first 2 wk of postoperative period.
BromSite	*To treat postoperative inflammation and prevent ocular pain associated with cataract extraction*	1 gtt in operative eye twice daily (morning and evening) 1 day before surgery, day of surgery, and 14 days postoperatively.
cetirizine hydrochloride 0.24% Zerviate	*To treat ocular itching associated with allergic conjunctivitis*	1 gtt in affected eye(s) twice daily.

GENERIC AND TRADE NAMES	INDICATIONS	USUAL ADULT DOSAGES
Ophthalmic anti-inflammatory drugs *(continued)*		
dexamethasone Maxidex **dexamethasone sodium phosphate 0.1%** AK-Dex	*To treat allergic conjunctivitis; corneal injury from chemical or thermal burns or from penetration of foreign bodies; inflammatory conditions of the anterior segment of globe, conjunctiva, cornea, or eyelids; iridocyclitis; suppression of graft rejection after keratoplasty; and uveitis*	1 or 2 gtt of suspension or solution every hr during day and every 2 hr at night initially. When response occurs, 1 gtt every 4 hr; or apply 1/2-in to 1-in strip of ointment up to 4 times daily, then tapered to once daily.
diclofenac sodium 0.1% Voltaren, Voltaren Ophtha (CAN)	*To treat postoperative inflammation after removal of cataract*	1 gtt in conjunctival sac 4 times daily, starting 24 hr after surgery through first 2 postoperative wk.
	To provide temporary relief of pain and photophobia in corneal refractive surgery	1 or 2 gtt in operative eye 1 hr before surgery. Then, 1 or 2 gtt 15 min after surgery. Then, 1 gtt 4 times daily, starting 4 to 6 hr after surgery for up to 3 days, as needed.
difluprednate 0.05% Durezol	*To treat inflammation and pain associated with ocular surgery*	1 gtt in conjunctival sac of affected eye(s) 4 times daily for 2 wk starting 24 hr after surgery. Then, 1 gtt twice daily for 1 wk.
	To treat endogenous anterior uveitis	1 gtt into conjunctival sac of affected eye 4 times daily for 14 days, then tapered, as needed.
fluorometholone 0.1% Fluor-Op, FML Forte, FML Liquifilm, FML S.O.P.	*To treat corticosteroid-responsive inflammation of the anterior segment of the globe, bulbar and palpebral conjunctiva, and cornea*	1 gtt in conjunctival sac 2 to 4 times daily or, in severe conditions, up to every 4 hr during first 1 to 2 days, as needed; or 1.5-in strip of ointment in conjunctival sac once daily to 3 times daily.
fluorometholone acetate Eflone, Flarex		1 or 2 gtt in conjunctival sac 4 times daily or, in severe conditions, up to every 2 hr during first 1or 2 days, as needed.
ketorolac tromethamine Acular 0.5%	*To relieve ocular itching due to seasonal allergic conjunctivitis*	1 gtt in conjunctival sac of each eye 4 times daily.
	To treat postoperative inflammation in patients who have undergone cataract extraction	1 gtt in operative eye 4 times daily, starting 24 hr after surgery through first 2 postoperative wk.
Acuvail 0.45%	*To relieve pain and treat postoperative inflammation in patients who have undergone cataract extraction*	1 gtt in affected eye twice daily, starting 1 day before surgery, continuing through day of surgery and first 2 wk of postoperative period.
Acular LS 0.4%	*To reduce ocular burning/stinging and pain following corneal refractive surgery*	1 gtt in affected eye 4 times daily for up to 4 days following procedure.

(continues)

Selected Ophthalmic Drugs *(continued)*

GENERIC AND TRADE NAMES	INDICATIONS	USUAL ADULT DOSAGES
Ophthalmic anti-inflammatory drugs *(continued)*		
loteprednol etabonate Alrex 0.2%	*To relieve seasonal allergic conjunctivitis*	1 gtt of 0.2% suspension in affected eyes 4 times daily.
Lotemax 0.5% Inveltys 1%	*To treat postoperative inflammation following ocular surgery*	1 or 2 gtt in conjunctival sac of operated eye 4 times daily, beginning 24 hr after surgery and continuing through first 2 wk of postoperative period.
	To treat steroid-responsive inflammatory conditions of the anterior segment of the globe, bulbar and palpebral conjunctiva, and cornea	1 or 2 gtt in conjunctival sac of affected eye 4 times daily. Initially, dosage may be increased during first wk to 1 gtt every hr, as needed.
medrysone 1.0% HMS Liquifilm	*To treat allergic conjunctivitis, episcleritis, epinephrine sensitivity, and vernal conjunctivitis*	1 gtt into conjunctival sac up to every 4 hr.
olopatadine hydrochloride 0.1% Patanol	*To treat signs and symptoms of allergic conjunctivitis*	1 gtt twice daily at 6- to 8-hr intervals.
olopatadine hydrochloride 0.7% Pazeo	*To treat ocular itching associated with allergic conjunctivitis*	1 gtt into conjunctival sac in each affected eye once daily.
prednisolone acetate suspension 1% Econopred Plus, Omnipred, Pred Forte, Pred Mild **prednisolone sodium phosphate solution 1%** AK-Pred, Prednisol	*To treat steroid-responsive inflammation of the anterior segment of globe, cornea, and bulbar and palpebral conjunctiva; to treat corneal injury from chemical, radiation, or thermal burns, or penetration of foreign bodies*	1 or 2 gtt in conjunctival sac 2 to 4 times daily (suspension) or 1 gtt in conjunctival sac every 4 hr (solution) unless severe, then initially every hr during day and every 2 hr at night until response noted, then decreased to 1 gtt every 4 hr.
rimexolone 1% Vexol	*To treat anterior uveitis*	1 or 2 gtt in conjunctival sac every hr while awake in first wk; 1 gtt every 2 hr while awake in second wk; then tapered until uveitis resolves.
	To treat postoperative inflammation after ocular surgery	1 or 2 gtt in conjunctival sac of affected eye 4 times daily, starting 24 hr after surgery and continuing through first 2 postoperative wk.
Ophthalmic cycloplegic mydriatics		
atropine sulfate 1% Isopto Atropine, Minims	*To treat acute iritis or uveitis*	Small strip of ointment applied to conjunctival sac up to twice daily.
Atropine (CAN)	*To produce dilation for cycloplegic refraction*	1 gtt 40 min before refraction. *Maximum:* 2 gtt.

GENERIC AND TRADE NAMES	INDICATIONS	USUAL ADULT DOSAGES
Ophthalmic cycloplegic mydriatics *(continued)*		
cyclopentolate hydrochloride 0.5%, 1%, 2% AK-Pentolate, Cyclogyl, Minims Cyclopentolate (CAN), Pentolair	*To produce mydriasis and cycloplegia required in specific diagnostic procedures*	1 or 2 gtt of 0.5%, 1%, or 2% solution in each eye; then 1 or 2 gtt in 5 to 10 min, as needed.
homatropine hydrobromide 2%, 5% Isopto Homatropine, Minims Homatropine (CAN)	*To dilate pupils for cycloplegic refraction*	1 or 2 gtt in each eye, repeated in 5 to 10 min, as needed.
	To treat uveitis	1 or 2 gtt in affected eye(s) every 3 to 4 hr.
phenylephrine 2.5%, 10%	*To dilate pupil*	1 gtt per eye at 3- to 5-min intervals up to maximum of 3 drops per eye.
tropicamide 0.5%, 1% Mydriacyl, Opticyl, Tropicacyl	*To produce mydriasis*	1 to 2 gtt of 1% solution, repeated in 5 min, as needed.
	To dilate pupils for cycloplegic funduscopic exam	1 to 2 gtt of 0.5% solution in eyes 15 to 20 min before exam, repeated every 30 min, as needed.
Ophthalmic miotics		
acetylcholine chloride Miochol-E	*To produce papillary miosis in cataract surgery, penetrating keratoplasty, iridectomy, and other anterior segment surgery*	0.5 to 2 ml gently into anterior chamber before or after sutures secured or after lens placement in cataract surgery.
carbachol 0.01% Carbastat, Miostat	*To produce papillary miosis in ocular surgery; to reduce intensity of intraocular pressure elevation in first 24 hr after cataract surgery*	0.5 ml (solution) into anterior chamber before or after sutures secured or after lens placement in cataract surgery.
carbachol 0.75%, 1.5%, 2.25%, 3% Carboptic, Isopto Carbachol	*To treat open-angle glaucoma*	1 or 2 gtt up to 3 times daily.
flurbiprofen sodium 0.03% Ocufen	*To inhibit intraoperative miosis*	1 gtt in affected eye every 30 min, beginning 2 hr before surgery, up to total of 4 gtt.
phentolamine mesylate 0.75% Ryzumvi	*To reverse pharmacologicically induced mydriasis*	1 or 2 gtt in each dilated eye following ophthalmic examination or procedure.

(continues)

Selected Ophthalmic Drugs *(continued)*

GENERIC AND TRADE NAMES	INDICATIONS	USUAL ADULT DOSAGES
Ophthalmic miotics *(continued)*		
pilocarpine 1%, 2%, 4% Akarpine, Isopto Carpine, Miocarpine (CAN), Pilocar, Pilopine HS, Pilostat	*To treat primary open-angle glaucoma*	1 gtt up to 4 times daily; or 1-cm (0.39-in) ribbon of 4% gel at bedtime.
pilocarpine hydrochloride Akarpine, Isopto Carpine, Minocarpine (CAN), Pilocar, Pilopine HS, Pilostat	*To treat acute angle-closure glaucoma as emergency therapy*	1 gtt of 2% solution every 15 to 60 min for up to 4 doses.
pilocarpine nitrate 1% Minims Pilocarpine (CAN)	*To treat mydriasis due to mydriatic or cycloplegic drug therapy*	1 gtt of 1% solution.
pilocarpine hydrochloride 1.25% Vuity	*To treat presbyopia*	1 gtt in each eye once daily. One additional drop in each eye may be given 3 to 6 hr after first dose, as needed.
pilocarpine hydrochloride 0.4% Qlosi	To treat presbyopia	1 gtt in each eye, repeated after 2 to 3 hr, as needed. May be given daily or as needed up to twice daily.
Miscellaneous ophthalmic drugs		
alcaftadine 0.25% Lastacaft	*To prevent itching associated with allergic conjunctivitis*	1 gtt in each eye once daily.
apraclonidine hydrochloride 0.5% Iopidine	*As adjunct in patients on maximally tolerated medical therapy who require additional intraocular pressure (IOP) reduction*	1 or 2 gtt in affected eye(s) 3 times daily.
azelastine hydrochloride 0.05% Optivar	*To treat itching of the eye associated with allergic conjunctivitis*	1 gtt in affected eye twice daily.
bepotastine besilate 1.5% Bepreve	*To treat itching of the eye associated with allergic conjunctivitis*	1 gtt in affected eye twice daily.
betaxolol hydrochloride Betoptic 0.5%, Betoptic S 0.25%	*To treat chronic open-angle glaucoma or ocular hypertension*	1 or 2 gtt of 0.5% solution twice daily or 1 gtt of 0.25% solution twice daily.
bimatoprost 0.01%, 0.03% Lumigan	*To reduce elevated IOP in patients with open-angle glaucoma or ocular hypertension*	1 gtt in affected eye daily in evening.
brimonidine tartrate Alphagan 0.2%, Alphagan P 0.1%, 0.15%	*To reduce IOP in open-angle glaucoma or ocular hypertension*	1 gtt in affected eye 3 times daily, about 8 hr apart.
brimonidine tartrate 0.025% Lumify	*To remove eye redness*	1 gtt in affected eye(s) every 6 to 8 hr.

GENERIC AND TRADE NAMES	INDICATIONS	USUAL ADULT DOSAGES
Miscellaneous ophthalmic drugs *(continued)*		
brinzolamide 1% Azopt	*To reduce IOP in ocular hypertension or open-angle glaucoma*	1 gtt 3 times daily.
brinzolamide 1% and brimonidine tartrate 0.2% Simbrinza	*To reduce IOP in open-angle glaucoma or ocular hypertension*	1 gtt in affected eye 3 times daily.
carteolol hydrochloride 1% Ocupress	*To treat chronic open-angle glaucoma or intraocular hypertension*	1 gtt in conjunctival sac of affected eye twice daily.
cenegermin-bkbj 0.002% Oxervate	*To treat neurotrophic keratitis*	1 gtt in affected eye(s) 6 times daily at 2-hr intervals for 8 wk.
chloroprocaine hydrochloride 3% Iheezo	*To provide ocular surface anesthesia*	3 gtt to ocular surface of the planned procedure; reapplied, as needed.
cyclosporine 0.09% cyclosporine emulsion 0.05% Restasis	*To increase tear production in keratoconjunctivitis sicca*	1 gtt every 12 hr.
cyclosporine 0.1% Vevye	*To treat signs and symptoms of dry eye disease*	1 gtt in each eye twice daily about 12 hr apart.
cysteamine 0.44% Cystaran	*To treat corneal cystine crystal accumulation in patients with cystinosis*	1 gtt in each eye, every waking hr.
cysteamine 0.37% Cystadrops	*To treat corneal cystine crystal accumulation in patients with cystinosis*	1 gtt in each eye 4 times daily during waking hr.
dipivefrin hydrochloride 0.1% Propine	*To reduce IOP in chronic open-angle glaucoma*	1 gtt every 12 hr.
dorzolamide hydrochloride 2% Trusopt	*To treat increased IOP in ocular hypertension or open-angle glaucoma*	1 gtt in conjunctival sac of affected eye 3 times daily.
echothiophate iodide Phospholine Iodide	*To reduce elevated IOP*	1 gtt twice daily (morning and evening/bedtime). Alternatively, 1 gtt once daily or once every other day (at bedtime).
	To diagnose pediatric accommodative esotropia	1 gtt in both eyes once daily at bedtime for 2 or 3 wk.
	To treat pediatric accommodative esotropia	1 gtt in both eyes every other day *Maximum:* 1 gtt in both eyes every day.
emedastine difumarate Emadine	*To treat allergic conjunctivitis*	1 gtt in affected eye up to 4 times daily.

(continues)

Selected Ophthalmic Drugs *(continued)*

GENERIC AND TRADE NAMES	INDICATIONS	USUAL ADULT DOSAGES
Miscellaneous ophthalmic drugs *(continued)*		
ketotifen fumarate 0.025%, 0.035% Alaway, Zaditor	*To treat allergic conjunctivitis*	1 gtt in affected eye twice daily every 8 to 12 hr, but no more than twice daily.
latanoprost 0.005% Iyuzeh, Xalatan, Xelpros	*To reduce IOP in ocular hypertension or open-angle glaucoma*	1 gtt in conjunctival sac of affected eye daily in evening.
latanoprostene bunod 0.024% Vyzulta	*To reduce IOP in ocular hypertension or open-angle glaucoma*	1 gtt in affected eye(s) once daily in evening.
levobunolol hydrochloride AKBeta, Betagan, Novo-Levobunolol (CAN)	*To treat chronic open-angle glaucoma or ocular hypertension*	1 or 2 gtt of 0.5% solution once daily or 0.25% solution twice daily.
levocabastine hydrochloride 0.05% Livostin	*To treat signs and symptoms of seasonal allergic conjunctivitis*	1 gtt 4 times daily.
lifitegrast 5% Xiidra	*To treat dry eye disease*	1 gtt twice daily (about 12 hr apart) in each eye.
lotilaner 0.25% Xdemvy	*To treat Demodex blepharitis*	1 gtt twice daily (about 12 hr apart) in each eye for 6 wk.
metipranolol 0.3% OptiPranolol	*To reduce IOP in ocular hypertension or open-angle glaucoma*	1 gtt in affected eye twice daily.
naphazoline hydrochloride Ak-Con 0.1%, Albalon 0.1%, Clear Eyes 0.012%, Naphcon A 0.025%, Vasocon 0.05%	*To treat ocular congestion, irritation, or itching*	1 gtt of 0.1% solution every 3 to 4 hr; or 1 gtt of 0.012% to 0.03% solution up to 4 times daily for no more than 72 hr.
nedocromil sodium 2% Alocril	*To treat itching associated with both seasonal and perennial allergic conjunctivitis*	1 or 2 gtt twice daily.
netarsudil 0.02% Rhopressa	*To reduce IOP in ocular hypertension or open-angle glaucoma*	1 gtt in affected eye(s) once daily in evening.
netarsudil 0.02% and latanoprost 0.005% Rocklatan	*To reduce IOP in open-angle glaucoma or ocular hypertension*	1 gtt in affected eye(s) once daily in evening.
oomidenepag isopropyl 0.002% Omlonti	*To reduce IOP in open-angle glaucoma or ocular hypertension*	1 gtt in affected eye(s) once daily in the evening.

GENERIC AND TRADE NAMES	INDICATIONS	USUAL ADULT DOSAGES
Miscellaneous ophthalmic drugs *(continued)*		
oxymetazoline hydrochloride	*To provide relief from eye redness due to minor eye irritations*	1 or 2 gtt in conjunctival sac 4 times daily (at least 6 hr apart) for no more than 72 hr.
oxymetazoline hydrochloride 0.1% Uplifted	*To treat acquired blepharoptosis*	1 gtt in ptotic eye(s) once daily.
perfluorohexyloctane Miebo	*To treat dry eye disease*	1 gtt in each eye four times daily.
proparacaine hydrochloride 0.5% AK-Taine, Alcaine, Ophthetic, Parcaine	*To provide deep anesthesia during cataract extraction* *To provide anesthesia during removal of eye sutures* *To provide anesthesia during removal of foreign bodies* *To provide anesthesia during tonometry*	1 gtt every 5 to 10 min for 5 to 7 doses. 1 or 2 gtt 2 to 3 min before procedure. 1 or 2 gtt in affected eye before surgery. 1 or 2 gtt immediately before measurement.
sodium chloride, hypertonic Altachlore, Muro-128 2%, Muro-128 5%, Muroptic-5	*To provide temporary relief from corneal edema*	1 or 2 gtt every 3 to 4 hr; or ¼ in of ointment applied every 3 to 4 hr.
tafluprost 0.0015% Zioptan	*To reduce IOP in ocular hypertension or open-angle glaucoma*	1 gtt in conjunctival sac in affected eye(s) once daily in evening.
tetracaine 0.5% Pontocaine	*To provide eye anesthesia (short term)*	1 or 2 gtt, as needed.
tetrahydrozoline hydrochloride 0.05% Eye-Sine, Murine Plus, Optigene 3, Tetrasine, Visine	*To treat allergic conditions, conjunctival congestion, and irritation*	1 gtt up to 4 times daily or as directed.
timolol hemihydrate 0.25%, 0.5% Betimol **timolol maleate 0.25%, 0.5%** Apo-Timop (CAN), Timoptic **timolol maleate extended-release gel solution 0.25%, 0.5%** Timoptic-XE	*To reduce IOP in ocular hypertension or open-angle glaucoma*	1 gtt of 0.25% solution in affected eye twice daily, increased to 1 gtt of 0.5% solution, as needed; then 1 gtt daily; or 1 gtt E.R. gel solution in affected eye daily.
travoprost 0.003% Izba **travoprost 0.004%** Travatan	*To reduce elevated IOP in patients with open-angle glaucoma or ocular hypertension*	1 gtt in affected eye daily in evening.

Selected Topical Drugs

Topical drugs consist of an active drug prepared in a specified medium that promotes absorption through the skin. Media commonly are chosen based on drug solubility; rate of drug release; ability to hydrate the outer skin layer; ability to enhance penetration; drug stability; and interactions between the chosen medium, skin, and active ingredient.

Topical media include aerosols, creams, gels, lotions, ointments, powders, tinctures, and wet dressings. Aerosols, gels, lotions, and tinctures are convenient for application to the scalp and other hairy areas. Acutely inflamed areas are best treated with drying preparations, such as lotions, tinctures, and wet dressings. Chronic inflammation does well with applications of lubricating preparations, including creams and ointments.

Because of its physical properties, the skin can act as a holding area for many drugs, allowing slow penetration and prolonged duration of action. (This characteristic makes it important to understand the patient's allergies.) However, when administering topical or transdermal drugs that aren't prescribed for a specific location, keep in mind that penetration properties may vary in different areas of the body. For example, the axillae, face, scalp, and scrotum are more permeable than the limbs, and ventral surfaces typically are more permeable than dorsal surfaces.

Topical Drug Types

Topical drugs are classified as antibacterials, antifungals, antivirals, corticosteroids, retinoids, and other miscellaneous preparations.

- Antibacterials may be useful in the early treatment of minor skin infections and wounds. Minor skin infections may respond well to topical drugs applied at the infection site. Minor wounds should be treated at the site and in the immediately surrounding area to prevent other pathogens from colonizing the area.
- Antifungals usually are used to treat mucocutaneous infections, such as tineas, primarily ringworm and athlete's foot. Systemic use of antifungals is limited by their potentially toxic adverse effects, most commonly hepatic or renal damage. All fungi are completely resistant to conventional antibacterial drugs.
- Antivirals are used to inhibit viral replication. They work by targeting any one of the steps involved in viral replication: penetration into susceptible host cells; uncoating of the viral nucleic acid; synthesis of regulatory proteins, RNA and DNA, and structural proteins; assembly of viral particles; and release of the virus from the cell. Topical antivirals, such as penciclovir, can shorten the duration of herpetic lesions, lessen lesion pain, and minimize viral shedding.
- Corticosteroids reduce the signs and symptoms of inflammation. Topical corticosteroids cause vasoconstriction, probably by suppressing cell degranulation. They also cause decreased cell permeability by reducing histamine release from basal and mast cells.
- Retinoids, typically derivatives of vitamin A, are very effective in treating acne vulgaris, although the acne may appear to worsen before it improves. Retinoids are also useful for reducing wrinkles. When applied to the skin, retinoids remain primarily in the dermis; less than 10% of the drug is absorbed into the circulation. Prolonged use of retinoids promotes new dermal growth, new blood vessel formation, and thickening of the epidermis. Because these drugs are absorbed systemically and may have teratogenic effects, they shouldn't be used by pregnant women.
- Miscellaneous topical drugs are used to treat a variety of topical skin conditions, including dry skin, ichthyosis, parasitic infestations, psoriasis, and unwanted hair growth.

Administration Tips

Before applying a topical drug, clean the site and let it dry. Use gloves or a finger cot during application to prevent the drug from being absorbed through your own skin. Inform your patient of any expected discomfort, such as temporary burning or stinging. After application, cover the site only if required; some topical drugs shouldn't be covered with an occlusive dressing.

Be sure to teach the patient and family or caregiver the. correct administration technique. Also, review possible adverse reactions, highlighting those that should be reported to the prescriber. Stress the importance of complying with the drug regimen because some topical drugs require weeks or months of therapy to eradicate the underlying condition.

The following table includes the generic and trade names of many commonly prescribed topical drugs as well as their FDA-approved indications and usual adult dosages.

GENERIC AND TRADE NAMES	INDICATIONS	USUAL ADULT DOSAGES
Antibacterials		
azelaic acid cream 20% Azelex	*To treat mild to moderate inflammatory acne vulgaris*	Gently massage thin film into affected area twice daily (morning and evening).
azelaic acid foam 15% Finacea Foam **azelaic acid gel 15%** Finacea Gel	*To treat inflammatory papules and pustules of mild to moderate rosacea*	Apply thin layer to entire facial area twice daily (morning and evening).
bacitracin zinc	*To treat topical infections; to prevent infection in minor skin wounds, such as abrasions, minor burns, and cuts*	Apply light dusting of powder or thin film of ointment to affected area once daily to 3 times daily up to 1 wk.
benzoyl peroxide Benzac AC 2.5%/5%, Brevoxyl 4%, Desquam-E 2.5%-10%	*To treat mild to moderate inflammatory acne vulgaris*	Apply to affected area once daily, gradually increasing to 2 or 3 times daily.
Epsolay 5%	*To treat inflammatory lesions of rosacea*	Apply a pea-sized amount once daily in a thin layer to each area of the face affected.
clindamycin and benzoyl peroxide Acanya 1.2%/2.5%, Duac 1.2%/5%, Onexton 1.2%/3.75%	*To treat acne vulgaris*	Apply once daily (evening) to affected areas.
Benzaclin 1%/5%	*To treat acne vulgaris*	Apply twice daily (morning and evening) to affected areas.
clindamycin 1.2% and tretinoin 0.025% Veltin Gel, Ziana Gel	*To treat acne vulgaris*	Apply pea-sized amount to affected areas once daily in evening.
clindamycin phosphate Cleocin 1%, Clinda-Derm 1%, Clindagel 1%, Clindesse 2%, Clindets 1%, Dalacin T Topical Solution 1% (CAN), Evoclin 1%	*To treat inflammatory acne vulgaris* *To treat bacterial vaginosis*	Apply to affected area once or twice daily (morning and evening). 1 applicatorful (100 mg) intravaginally at bedtime for 7 days.
Xaciato 2%	*To treat bacterial vaginosis*	1 applicatorful (100 mg) intravaginally as a single dose at any time of day.
dapsone gel 7.5% Aczone	*To treat acne vulgaris*	Apply pea-sized amount in thin layer to entire face or other affected areas once daily.
dapsone gel 5% Aczone	*To treat acne vulgaris*	Apply pea-sized amount in thin layer to entire face or other affected areas twice daily.
erythromycin 1.5%, 2% Akne-Mycin, A/T/S, Ery-Derm, Erygel, Erythrogel, ETS (CAN), Sans-Acne (CAN), Staticin	*To treat inflammatory acne vulgaris*	Apply to affected areas once or twice daily (morning and evening).

(continues)

Selected Topical Drugs *(continued)*

GENERIC AND TRADE NAMES	INDICATIONS	USUAL ADULT DOSAGES
Antibacterials *(continued)*		
erythromycin 3% and benzoyl peroxide 5% Benzamycin	*To treat moderate inflammatory acne vulgaris*	Apply to affected areas twice daily (morning and evening).
gentamicin sulfate Garamycin, G-myticin	*To prevent or treat superficial skin infections due to susceptible bacteria; to treat superficial burns*	Apply small amount to skin in affected area 3 or 4 times daily.
mafenide acetate Sulfamylon	*As adjunct to treat second- and third-degree burns*	Apply 1/16-in layer aseptically to affected areas once or twice daily.
metronidazole 0.75%, 1% MetroCream, MetroGel, MetroLotion, Noritate	*To treat inflammatory papules and pustules of acne rosacea*	Apply thin film to affected area once or twice daily (morning and evening).
MetroGel-Vaginal	*To treat bacterial vaginosis*	1 applicatorful (37.5 mg) intravaginally at bedtime or twice daily for 5 days.
Nuvessa 1.3%	*To treat bacterial vaginosis*	1 applicatorful (65 mg) intravaginally as a single dose at bedtime.
minocycline 1.5% Zilxi	*To treat inflammatory lesions of rosacea*	Apply topical foam over all areas of the face once daily, gently rub into skin.
mupirocin 2% Bactroban, Bactroban Cream, Bactroban Nasal, Bactroban Ointment, Centany Nasal	*To treat impetigo due to* Staphylococcus aureus *or* Streptococcus pyogenes	Apply to affected areas 3 times daily up to 10 days.
	To treat secondary infections of traumatic skin lesions due to S. aureus *or* S. pyogenes	Apply thin film and cover with a gauze dressing 3 times daily for 10 days.
	To eradicate nasal colonization of methicillin-resistant S. aureus	Apply half of the contents of a unit-dose tube to each nostril twice daily for 5 days.
neomycin sulfate Myciguent	*To prevent or treat superficial bacterial infections*	Rub fingertip-size dose into affected area once daily to 3 times daily for no more than 1 wk.
ozenoxacin Xepi	*To treat impetigo due to* Staphylococcus aureus *or* Streptococcus pyogenes	Apply thin layer to affected area (not exceeding 100 cm^2) twice daily for 5 days.
povidone-iodine 0.75%, 10% Betadine, Betadine Cream, Betadine Spray	*To disinfect wounds and burns*	Apply or spray to affected area, as needed.
	To prepare skin for surgical incision	Wet skin with water, then apply 1 cc/20–30 sq in using 7.5% solution. Lather and scrub site for 5 min, then rinse. Follow with 10% solution painted on skin and allowed to dry.

GENERIC AND TRADE NAMES	INDICATIONS	USUAL ADULT DOSAGES
Antibacterials *(continued)*		
silver sulfadiazine 1% Flamazine (CAN), Silvadene, Thermazene	*To prevent and treat wound sepsis in second- and third-degree burns*	Apply 1/16-in layer aseptically once to twice daily to clean debrided burns; reapply promptly if removed.
sulfacetamide sodium 10% Klaron	*To treat acne vulgaris*	Apply thin film twice daily.
Antifungals		
butenafine hydrochloride 1% Lotrimin Ultra, Mentax	*To treat tinea corporis, tinea cruris, or tinea versicolor*	Apply to affected surrounding area once daily for 2 wk.
Lotrimin Ultra, Mentax	*To treat interdigital tinea pedis due to* Epidermophyton floccosum, Trichophyton mentagrophytes, *or* T. rubrum	Apply to affected and immediately surrounding area once daily for 4 wk or twice daily for 1 wk.
butoconazole nitrate 2% Femstat 3	*To treat vulvovaginal mycotic infections caused by* Candida *species*	1 applicatorful (100 mg) intravaginally at bedtime for 3 days.
Gynazole-1	*To treat vulvovaginal infections caused by* Candida albicans	1 applicatorful (100 mg) intravaginally once anytime day or night; may repeat course for total of 6 days in pregnant females (second and third trimester only).
ciclopirox olamine Loprox Cream 0.77% Loprox Shampoo 1%	*To treat candidiasis, tinea corporis, tinea cruris, tinea pedis, and tinea versicolor*	Massage gently into affected and surrounding area twice daily (morning and evening).
ciclopirox olamine 8% Penlac	*To treat seborrheic dermatitis*	Apply 5 ml to scalp (10 ml for long hair), lather and leave on scalp for 3 min, then rinse. Repeat twice weekly for 4 wk with minimum of 3 days between applications.
	To treat onychomycosis of the fingernails and toenails	Apply evenly to entire nail surface and surrounding 5 mm of skin at bedtime for up to 48 wk.
clotrimazole Canesten (CAN), Desenex, Femcare, FungiCURE, Fungoid, Gyne-Lotrimin, Lotrimin, Mycelex, Trivagizole	*To treat superficial fungal infections (tinea corporis, tinea cruris, tinea pedis, tinea versicolor, candidiasis)*	Apply thin film and massage into affected and surrounding area twice daily (morning and evening) for 2 to 8 wk.
	To treat vulvovaginal candidiasis	Insert 100-mg vaginal tablet at bedtime for 7 days; or 500-mg vaginal tablet at bedtime for 1 day; or 1 applicatorful intravaginally at bedtime for 7 days (or 3 days if using Trivagizole).
	To treat oropharyngeal candidiasis	Dissolve oral troche over 15 to 30 min 5 times/day for 14 days.
	To prevent oropharyngeal candidiasis	Dissolve oral troche over 15 to 30 min 3 times daily for duration of chemotherapy or until corticosteroid dosage is reduced to maintenance levels.

(continues)

Selected Topical Drugs *(continued)*

GENERIC AND TRADE NAMES	INDICATIONS	USUAL ADULT DOSAGES
Antifungals *(continued)*		
econazole nitrate 1% Ecostatin (CAN) Ecoza	*To treat tinea corporis, tinea cruris, tinea pedis, tinea versicolor*	Rub into affected area once or twice daily for at least 2 wk (4 wk for tinea pedis).
	To treat cutaneous candidiasis	Rub into affected area twice daily (morning and evening) for 2 wk.
	To treat interdigital tinea pedis	Apply to affected areas once daily for 4 wk.
efinaconazole 10% Jublia	*To treat onychomycosis of the toenail(s) due to* Trichophyton rubrum *or* Trichophyton mentagrophytes	Apply solution to affected toenail(s) once daily for 48 wk using the integrated flow-through brush applicator.
gentian violet 1%, 2%	*To treat candidiasis*	Apply 1% solution to affected area 2 or 3 times daily for 3 days.
	To help protect against skin infection in minor burns, cuts, or scrapes	Apply small amount of 2% solution to affected area once to 3 times daily.
ketoconazole 1%, 2% Ketoconazole, Nizoral	*To treat tinea corporis, tinea cruris, tinea pedis, and tinea versicolor due to susceptible organisms; to treat cutaneous candidiasis*	Apply thin film to affected and immediately surrounding area daily for at least 2 wk (6 wk for tinea pedis).
Ketoconazole Shampoo 2%, Nizoral AD Shampoo 1%	*To treat tinea versicolor*	Apply Nizoral AD Shampoo 1% to wet hair, lather, massage for 1 min, leave drug on scalp for 3 min, then rinse and repeat 2 times/wk for 4 up to 8 wk (with at least 3 days between shampoos), then intermittently, as needed. Alternatively, apply Ketoconazole Shampoo 2% only 1 time to wet hair, lather, massage for 1 min, leave drug on scalp for 5 min, then rinse.
Extina 2%, Xolegel 2%	*To treat seborrheic dermatitis*	Apply to affected and immediately surrounding area twice daily for 4 wk.
luliconazole 1% Luzu	*To treat interdigital tinea pedis*	Apply to affected area and about 1 in of the immediate surrounding area(s) once daily for 2 wk.
	To treat tinea cruris and tinea corporis	Apply to affected area and about 1 in of the immediate surrounding area(s) once daily for 1 wk.

GENERIC AND TRADE NAMES	INDICATIONS	USUAL ADULT DOSAGES
Antifungals *(continued)*		
miconazole nitrate 2% Fungoid, Micatin, ZeasorbAF	*To treat tinea corporis, tinea cruris, tinea pedis; cutaneous candidiasis; and common dermatophyte infections*	Apply cream sparingly (or powder or spray liberally) over affected area twice daily for 2 wk (4 wk for tinea corporis and tinea pedis).
	To treat tinea versicolor	Apply sparingly to affected area daily for 2 wk.
	To treat onychomycosis	Brush tincture on affected areas of nail surface, beds, and edges and under nail surface once or twice daily for up to several months; or spray on clean, dry, affected nails, holding actuator down for 1 or 2 sec once or twice daily.
Monistat 1, Monistat 3, Monistat 7,	*To treat vulvovaginal candidiasis*	Insert into vaginal canal at bedtime for 7 days (100 mg), repeated, as needed; insert 200-mg strength into vaginal canal at bedtime for 3 days; or insert 1,200-mg strength into vaginal canal as a single treatment.
naftifine hydrochloride 2% Naftin	*To treat tinea corporis, tinea cruris, and interdigital tinea pedis*	Apply to affected area and 1/2-in margin surrounding area once daily for 2 wk.
nystatin Nadostine (CAN), Nilstat, Nystop	*To treat cutaneous and mucocutaneous infections due to* Candida albicans	Apply cream to affected area twice daily or as indicated; or apply powder 2 or 3 times daily.
oxiconazole nitrate Oxistat, Oxizold (CAN)	*To treat tinea corporis, tinea cruris, and tinea pedis*	Apply to affected and surrounding area once or twice daily for 2 wk (4 wk for tinea pedis).
	To treat tinea versicolor	Apply cream to affected and surrounding area daily for 2 wk.
selenium sulfide 1%, 2.5% Selsun, Versel (CAN)	*To treat tinea versicolor*	Apply to scalp, lather with small amount of water, wait 10 min, then rinse, once daily for 7 days.
	To treat dandruff and seborrheic scalp dermatitis	Massage into wet scalp, wait 2 to 3 min, rinse, and repeat 2 times/wk for 2 wk, then once daily for 2, 3, or 4 wk.
sertaconazole nitrate 2% Ertaczo	*To treat interdigital tinea pedis caused by* Epidermophyton floccosum, Trichophyton mentagrophytes, *or* Trichophyton rubrum	Apply to affected areas both between the toes and the immediately surrounding healthy skin twice daily for 4 wk.
sulconazole nitrate 1% Exelderm	*To treat tinea corporis, tinea cruris, and tinea versicolor*	Massage small amount gently into affected and surrounding areas once or twice daily (tinea pedis) for 3 wk.

(continues)

Selected Topical Drugs *(continued)*

GENERIC AND TRADE NAMES	INDICATIONS	USUAL ADULT DOSAGES
Antifungals *(continued)*		
tavaborole Kerydin	*To treat onychomycosis of the toenails due to* Trichophyton mentagrophytes *or* Trichophyton rubrum	Apply to affected toenails, including under the tip of each toenail, once daily for 48 wk.
terbinafine hydrochloride 1% Lamisil	*To treat tinea versicolor*	Apply to affected area twice daily for 1 or 2 wk.
	To treat tinea corporis and tinea cruris	Apply thin film to affected area once or twice daily for 1 wk.
	To treat interdigital tinea pedis	Apply between the toes twice daily for 1 wk (interdigital tinea pedis) or to affected area daily for 1 wk.
	To treat tinea pedis involving bottom or sides of feet	Apply to affected area twice daily (morning and evening) for 2 wk.
terconazole 0.4%, 0.8% Terazol 3, Terazol 7	*To treat vulvovaginal candidiasis*	Insert 1 applicatorful (20 mg) intravaginally at bedtime for 3 days (0.4%) or 1 applicatorful (40 mg) for 7 days (0.8%); or insert 80-mg vaginal suppository at bedtime for 3 consecutive days.
tioconazole GyneCure Ovules (CAN), Vagistat-1	*To treat vulvovaginal candidiasis*	Insert 1 applicatorful (300 mg) or 1 suppository (300 mg) intravaginally at bedtime as a single dose.
tolnaftate 1% Absorbine Footcare, Aftate for Athlete's Foot, Aftate for Jock Itch, Dr. Scholl's Athlete's Foot, Genaspore, NP-27, PiTtrex, Quinsana Plus, Tinactin, Ting, Zeasorb AF	*To treat tinea corporis, tinea cruris, tinea manuum, tinea pedis, and tinea versicolor*	Apply to affected and surrounding areas twice daily (morning and evening), for 4 wk (2 wk for tinea cruris); continue for 2 wk after symptoms subside or up to 6 wk.
Antivirals		
acyclovir 5% Zovirax	*To treat initial genital herpes and selectively for non-life-threatening mucocutaneous herpes simplex in immunocompromised patients*	Apply ointment every 3 hr (6 times/day) for 7 days. Use finger cot, rubber glove, or applicator stick for both forms to prevent herpetic whitlow.
	To treat herpes labialis in immunocompetent patients	Apply cream to affected area 5 times daily for 4 days.
docosanol 10% Abreva	*To treat recurrent herpes labialis of lips and face*	Apply cream gently and completely to affected area 5 times daily, starting with first visible sign of lesion and continuing until lesion is healed.
penciclovir 1% Denavir	*To treat recurrent herpes labialis of lips and face*	Apply every 2 hr while awake for 4 days.

GENERIC AND TRADE NAMES	INDICATIONS	USUAL ADULT DOSAGES
Corticosteroids		
alclometasone dipropionate 0.05% Aclovate	*To relieve inflammatory and pruritic manifestations of corticosteroid-responsive dermatoses*	Apply thin film to affected area and massage 2 to 3 times daily.
amcinonide 0.01% Cyclocort	*To relieve inflammatory and pruritic manifestations of corticosteroid-responsive dermatoses*	Apply thin film to affected area and massage twice daily (lotion) or 2 to 3 times daily (cream, ointment).
betamethasone benzoate 0.05% Beben (CAN), Uticort	*To relieve inflammatory and pruritic manifestations of corticosteroid-responsive dermatoses*	Apply thin film or a few drops to affected area once or twice daily up to 45 g/wk (ointment, cream), 50 g/wk (gel), or 50 ml (lotion).
betamethasone dipropionate 0.05% Diprolene, Diprolene AF, Diprosone, Topilene (CAN)	*To relieve inflammatory and pruritic manifestations of corticosteroid-responsive dermatoses*	Apply thin film or a few drops to affected area once or twice daily.
betamethasone valerate 0.1% Betatrex, Beta-Val, Luxiq, Valisone	*To relieve inflammatory and pruritic manifestations of corticosteroid-responsive dermatoses*	Apply foam to scalp, and massage until foam disappears, twice daily (morning and evening). Apply thin film of cream or ointment 1 to 3 times daily. Apply a few drops of lotion twice daily (morning and evening).
clobetasol propionate 0.025% Impoyz	*To treat moderate to severe plaque psoriasis*	Apply thin layer to affected skin and rub in gently twice daily, up to 50 g/wk for 2 wk.
clobetasol propionate 0.05% Dermovate (CAN), Embeline, Temovate Olux	*To relieve inflammatory and pruritic manifestations of corticosteroid-responsive dermatoses* *To relieve moderate to severe inflammatory and pruritic manifestations of corticosteroid-responsive dermatoses of scalp*	Apply thin film to affected area and rub in gently twice daily (morning and evening), up to 50 g/wk, for 2 wk. Apply to affected area of scalp twice daily (once in morning and once in the evening), up to 50 g/wk, for 2 wk.
desonide 0.05% DesOwen, Tridesilon, Verdeso	*To relieve inflammatory and pruritic manifestations of corticosteroid-responsive dermatoses*	Apply thin film to affected area 2 to 4 times daily.
desoximetasone 0.05% Topicort **desoximetasone 0.25%** Topicort spray	*To relieve inflammatory and pruritic manifestations of corticosteroid-responsive dermatoses* *To treat plaque psoriasis*	Apply thin film to affected skin areas twice daily. Spray a thin film on to affected skin areas twice daily (rub in gently) for no more than 4 wk.

(continues)

Selected Topical Drugs *(continued)*

GENERIC AND TRADE NAMES	INDICATIONS	USUAL ADULT DOSAGES
Corticosteroids *(continued)*		
diflorasone diacetate 0.05% Florone, Psorcon	*To relieve inflammatory and pruritic manifestations of corticosteroid-responsive dermatoses*	Apply thin film to affected area once daily to 4 times daily.
fluocinolone acetonide 0.01% Derma Smooth FS, Fluoderm (CAN), Fluolar (CAN), Fluonid (CAN), Synalar, Synamol (CAN)	*To relieve inflammatory and pruritic manifestations of corticosteroid-responsive dermatoses*	Apply thin film to affected area 2 to 4 times daily.
	To treat seborrheic dermatoses	Use shampoo on scalp daily.
	To treat scalp psoriasis	Apply oil to affected areas on scalp and leave overnight.
fluocinonide 0.05% Lidemol (CAN), Lidex	*To relieve inflammatory and pruritic manifestations of corticosteroid-responsive dermatoses*	Apply thin film to affected area 2 to 4 times daily.
flurandrenolide Cordran 0.05%, Cordran Tape, Drenison 0.05% (CAN)	*To relieve inflammatory and pruritic manifestations of corticosteroid-responsive dermatoses*	Apply thin film to affected area and massage 2 to 3 times daily; or apply tape every 12 to 24 hr.
fluticasone propionate 0.05% Cutivate	*To treat atopic dermatitis; to relieve inflammatory and pruritic manifestations of corticosteroid-responsive dermatoses*	Apply thin film once or twice daily (atopic dermatitis) or twice daily (dermatoses).
halcinonide 0.1% Halog	*To relieve inflammatory and pruritic manifestations of corticosteroid-responsive dermatoses*	Apply sparingly and massage 2 to 3 times daily.
halobetasol propionate 0.05% Lexette, Ultravate	*To treat plaque psoriasis*	Apply thin film to affected area and rub in gently twice daily, up to 50 g/wk, for 2 wk.
halobetasol propionate 0.01% Bryhali		Apply thin layer to affected area and rub in gently once daily, up to 50 g/wk and for no longer than 8 wk.
halobetasol propionate 0.01% and tazarotene 0.045% Duobrii	*To treat plaque psoriasis*	Apply thin layer once daily to cover only affected areas and rub in gently.

GENERIC AND TRADE NAMES	INDICATIONS	USUAL ADULT DOSAGES
Corticosteroids *(continued)*		
hydrocortisone 0.25% Cetacort **hydrocortisone 0.5%** Cetacort, Cortate (CAN), Delacort, Dermtex HC, Emo Cort (CAN), Hydro-Tex **hydrocortisone 1%** Ala-Cort, Cort-Dome, Cortizone 10, Emo-Cort (CAN), Nutracort, Synacort **hydrocortisone 2%** Ala-Scalp HP, Dermasorb HC **hydrocortisone 2.5%** Anusol-HC, Emo-Cort (CAN), Hytone, Nutracort, Stie-Cort, Synacort, Texacort **hydrocortisone acetate 0.1%** Corticreme (CAN) **hydrocortisone acetate 0.5%** Corticaine, Cortacet (CAN), Cortoderm (CAN), Hyderm, Lanacort, Novo-Hydrocort (CAN)	*To relieve inflammatory and pruritic manifestations of corticosteroid-responsive dermatoses*	Apply thin film (aerosol foam, cream, lotion, ointment, solution) to affected area once daily to 4 times daily.
hydrocortisone acetate 1%, 2%, 2.5% Cortaid, Corticreme (CAN), Cortoderm (CAN), Hyderm (CAN), Maximum Strength Cortaid, Micort HC-Lipocream, Novo-Hydrocort (CAN) **hydrocortisone acetate 1% and pramoxine hydrochloride 1% topical aerosol foam** Epifoam	*To relieve inflammatory and pruritic manifestations of corticosteroid-responsive dermatoses*	Apply thin film (aerosol foam, cream, lotion, ointment, solution) to affected area once daily to 4 times daily.
hydrocortisone butyrate 0.1% Locoid		Apply to affected area 2 to 3 times daily.
hydrocortisone probutate 0.1% Pandel		Apply to affected area once or twice daily.
hydrocortisone valerate 0.2% Westcort		Apply to affected area 2 to 3 times daily.

(continues)

Selected Topical Drugs *(continued)*

GENERIC AND TRADE NAMES	INDICATIONS	USUAL ADULT DOSAGES
Corticosteroids *(continued)*		
hydrocortisone acetate, polymyxin B sulfate, and neomycin sulfate Cortisporin	*To treat corticosteroid-responsive dermatoses (short term) with mild bacterial infection*	Apply sparingly and massage 2 to 4 times daily.
mometasone furoate 0.1% Elocom (CAN), Elocon	*To relieve inflammatory and pruritic manifestations of corticosteroid-responsive dermatoses*	Apply thin film or a few drops to affected area daily.
prednicarbate 0.1% Dermatop	*To relieve inflammatory and pruritic manifestations of corticosteroid-responsive dermatoses*	Apply thin film to affected area twice daily.
triamcinolone acetonide 0.025%, 0.5% Aristocort, Aristocort A, Aristocort D (CAN), Kenalog, Triacet, Triaderm (CAN), Trianide Mild (CAN)	*To relieve inflammatory and pruritic manifestations of corticosteroid-responsive dermatoses*	Apply thin film of 0.025% to affected area 2 to 4 times daily; apply 0.1% or 0.5% 2 to 3 times daily.
triamcinolone acetonide 0.1% Aristocort, Aristocort A, Aristocort R (CAN), Delta-Tritex, Flutex, Kenac, Kenalog, Kenalog-H, Triacet, Triaderm (CAN), Trianide Regular (CAN) **triamcinolone acetonide 0.5%** Aristocort, Aristocort A, Aristocort C (CAN), Flutex, Kenalog, Triacet	*To relieve inflammatory and pruritic manifestations of corticosteroid-responsive dermatoses*	Apply thin film (cream) to affected area 2 to 4 times daily; 0.025% lotion or ointment once or twice daily; 0.1% lotion or ointment once daily; or 0.5% ointment once daily.
triamcinolone acetonide topical aerosol 0.2% Kenalog	*To relieve inflammatory and pruritic manifestations of corticosteroid-responsive dermatoses*	Spray affected area 3 times daily to 4 times daily.
Retinoids		
adapalene 0.1% Differin	*To treat acne vulgaris*	Apply thin film to affected area at bedtime.
tazarotene 0.1% Avage	*As adjunct to treat mitigation of facial fine wrinkling, facial mottled hyper- and hypopigmentation, and benign facial lentigines*	Apply pea-size amount to affected area at bedtime.

GENERIC AND TRADE NAMES	INDICATIONS	USUAL ADULT DOSAGES
Retinoids *(continued)*		
tazarotene 0.05%, 0.1% Avage, Tazorac	*To treat acne; to treat mild to moderately severe facial acne vulgaris*	Apply thin film to affected area at bedtime.
tazarotene 0.1% Fabior	*To treat acne vulgaris*	Apply thin layer to affected areas of the face and upper trunk once daily in the evening.
tazarotene 0.045% Arazlo	*To treat moderate to severe acne vulgaris*	Apply a thin layer to affected areas once daily.
tretinoin 0.025% Avita, Renova, Retin-A, Retin-A Micro, Stieva-A (CAN), Tretin-X **tretinoin 0.05%** Altreno	*To treat acne vulgaris*	Apply pea-size amount to clean, dry affected area at bedtime.
tretinoin and benzoyl peroxide 0.1%, 3% Twyneo	*To treat acne vulgaris*	Apply a thin layer to affected areas once daily.
trifarotene 0.005% Aklief	*To treat acne vulgaris*	Apply thin layer to affected areas of the face and/or trunk once daily in the evening.
Miscellaneous topical drugs		
abametapir 0.74% Xeglyze	*To treat head lice*	Apply to dry hair in amount sufficient to coat the hair and scalp thoroughly; leave on for 10 min, then rinse off with water.
adapalene 0.1% and benzoyl peroxide 2.5% gel Epiduo **adapalene 0.3% and benzoyl peroxide 2.5% gel** Epiduo Forte	*To treat acne vulgaris*	Apply pea-size amount to each clean, dry affected area once daily.
adapalene 0.15%, benzoyl peroxide 3.1%, and clindamycin phosphate 1.2 % Cabtreo	*To treat acne vulgaris*	Apply a thin layer to the affected areas once daily.
aminolevulinic acid hydrochloride 10% Ameluz	*As adjunct to treat mild to moderate severity of actinic keratoses on face and scalp with red light photodynamic therapy*	Apply gel with spatula or gloved fingertips about 1 mm thick and include about 5 mm of surrounding skin in conjunction. Allow to dry (about 10 min) before occlusive dressing applied. After 3 hr, remove dressing and gel and illuminate area with red light photodynamic therapy.

(continues)

Selected Topical Drugs *(continued)*

GENERIC AND TRADE NAMES	INDICATIONS	USUAL ADULT DOSAGES
Miscellaneous topical drugs *(continued)*		
ammonium lactate 12% Lac-Hydrin	*To treat dry, scaly skin and ichthyosis vulgaris*	Apply to affected area and rub in twice daily.
anacaulase-bcdb 8.8% NexoBrid	*To remove eschar from deep partial thickness and/or full thickness thermal burns*	Apply to an area up to 15% body surface area (BSA) followed by second application 24 hr later. Total treated area for both applications must not exceed 20% BSA.
anthralin Anthranol 1 (CAN), Anthranol 2 (CAN), Anthranol 3 (CAN), Anthrascalp (CAN), Drithocreme, Dritho-Scalp, Psoriatec, Zithranol, Zithranol-RR	*To treat chronic psoriasis*	Apply sparingly and massage into affected lesions daily.
	To treat chronic scalp psoriasis	Apply to lesions daily for 1 wk.
becaplermin Regranex	*To treat lower-extremity diabetic neuropathic ulcers that extend into the subcutaneous tissue or beyond and that have an adequate blood supply*	Amount applied to ulcers daily calculated based on size of ulcer.
berdazimer 10.3% Zelsuvmi	*To treat molluscum contagiosum*	Mix tube A and B in equal amounts and immediately apply a thin even layer once daily to each lesion for up to 12 wk.
brimonidine 0.33% Mirvaso	*To treat rosacea*	Apply pea-sized amount onto each of the 5 areas of the face once daily. Do not apply to eyes or lips.
calcipotriene 0.005% Dovonex, Sorilux	*To treat plaque psoriasis*	Apply cream or scalp lotion in a thin layer twice daily up to 8 wk
calcipotriene hydrate 0.005% and betamethasone dipropionate 0.064% Taclonex		Apply suspension to affected areas and rub in gently once daily for up to 8 wk.
Taclonex Scalp	*To treat moderate to severe plaque psoriasis of the scalp*	Apply suspension to affected scalp areas and rub in gently once daily for 2 to 8 wk or until skin clears.
cantharidin 0.7% Ycanth	*To treat molluscum contagiosum*	Apply a single application directly to each lesion every 3 wk, as needed.
capsaicin 0.025%, 0.075%, 0.1% Capsin, Zostrix	*To provide temporary pain relief from rheumatoid arthritis and osteoarthritis; to relieve neuralgias from pain following shingles (herpes zoster) infection*	Apply to affected area no more than 4 times daily.

GENERIC AND TRADE NAMES	INDICATIONS	USUAL ADULT DOSAGES
Miscellaneous topical drugs *(continued)*		
chlorhexidine gluconate 4% Betasept, Hibiclens	*To clean skin wounds*	Rinse area, apply minimal amount to cover, then wash and rinse thoroughly.
	To prepare skin for surgical incision	Apply liberally to surgical site and swab for at least 2 min. Dry with sterile towel and repeat once.
clascoterone 1% Winlevi	*To treat acne vulgaris*	Apply thin uniform layer of cream twice daily (morning and evening) to affected areas.
clotrimazole and betamethasone dipropionate 0.05%/1% Lotrisone	*To treat symptomatic inflammatory tinea corporis, tinea cruris, and tinea pedis*	Apply thin layer and massage cream gently into affected and surrounding skin areas twice daily for 2 wk (tinea corporis, tinea cruris) or for 4 wk (tinea pedis).
coal tar Denorex, Pentrax, Zetar, Zetar Shampoo	*To treat psoriasis*	Add 15 to 20 ml to lukewarm bath, immerse affected area for 15 to 20 min, and rinse thoroughly 3 to 7 times/wk.
	To treat dandruff or scalp seborrhea	Massage into wet scalp, rinse, repeat application and wait 5 min, then rinse again.
crisaborole 2% Eucrisa	*To treat mild to moderate atopic dermatitis*	Apply thin layer of ointment twice daily to affected areas.
crotamiton 10% Eurax	*To treat scabies*	Massage into cleansed body from chin to soles of feet and reapply after 24 hr; change bed linens next day, and bathe 48 hr after second dose; repeat in 7 to 10 days if new lesions appear.
	To treat symptomatic pruritic skin	Massage gently into affected areas until absorbed. Repeat as needed.
desoximetasone 0.05% Topicort	*To relieve inflammatory and pruritic manifestations of corticosteroid-responsive dermatoses*	Apply thin film twice daily to affected areas.
diclofenac sodium 1% Voltaren	*To treat osteoarthritis pain*	Apply 2.25 in (2 g) for upper body areas and 4.5 in (4 g) for lower body area of gel to affected area 4 times daily, every day.
diclofenac sodium 3% Solaraze	*To treat actinic keratoses*	Massage gel gently onto affected lesion areas twice daily for 60 to 90 days.

(continues)

Selected Topical Drugs *(continued)*

GENERIC AND TRADE NAMES	INDICATIONS	USUAL ADULT DOSAGES
Miscellaneous topical drugs *(continued)*		
doxepin hydrochloride 5% Zonalon	*To treat moderate pruritus associated with atopic dermatitis and chronic lichen simplex*	Apply thin film to affected area 4 times daily (every 3 to 4 hr) for up to 8 days.
eflornithine hydrochloride 13.9% Vaniqa	*To retard unwanted hair growth*	Apply thin film to affected area of face and chin twice daily (at least 8 hr apart); don't wash treated area for at least 4 hr.
fluocinolone acetonide 0.01%, hydroquinone 4%, tretinoin 0.05% TRI-LUMA Cream	*To treat severe facial melasma*	Apply a thin film lightly and uniformly to hyperpigmented areas of melasma, including about 1/2 in of skin surrounding each lesion daily at least 30 min before bedtime.
fluorouracil cream Carac 0.5% Efudex 2%, 5% Fluoroplex 1%	*To treat actinic and solar keratoses of face and anterior scalp*	Apply to lesions twice daily for 4 wk.
	To treat actinic or solar keratosis	Apply to lesions twice daily for 2 to 4 wk.
	To treat superficial basal cell carcinoma	Apply 5% preparation twice daily in sufficient amounts to cover lesions for up to 12 wks.
	To treat actinic or solar keratosis	Apply to lesions twice daily for 2 to 6 wk.
glycopyrronium 2.4% Qbrexza	*To treat primary axillary hyperhidrosis*	Apply once daily to both axillae using a single cloth.
hexachlorophene 3% Phisohex	*To use as a surgical scrub*	Wet hands and forearms with water, apply 5 ml of solution and rub into a copious lather for 3 min, then rinse; repeat once.
	To use for bacteriostatic cleansing	Wet hands with water, pour 5 ml into palm and work up a lather, then apply to area to be cleaned. Rinse thoroughly.
hydrocortisone acetate 1%, polymyxin B sulfate, bacitracin zinc, and neomycin sulfate Cortisporin	*To treat corticosteroid-responsive dermatoses associated with secondary bacterial infection*	Apply small amount to affected areas 2 to 4 times daily for up to 7 days.
hydroquinone Claripel 4%, Eldopaque 2%, Eldoquin 2% and 4%, Melanex 3%	*To treat hyperpigmentation and melanin*	Apply twice daily to the affected areas for no longer than 2 mo.

GENERIC AND TRADE NAMES	INDICATIONS	USUAL ADULT DOSAGES
Miscellaneous topical drugs *(continued)*		
imiquimod 2.5%, 3.75% Zyclara	*To treat facial or scalp actinic keratoses*	Apply 2.5% or 3.75% to affected area daily for two 2-wk treatment cycles separated by a 2-wk no-treatment period.
	To treat external genital and perianal warts	Apply 3.75% cream to the external genital and perianal warts until total clearance or up to 8 wk.
imiquimod 5% Aldara	*To treat external genital and perianal warts*	Apply thin layer to affected area and rub in 3 times/wk at bedtime for up to 16 wk; remove with soap and water after 6 to 10 hr.
	To treat actinic keratosis on face and scalp	Apply to affected area on face or scalp (but not both concurrently) for 16 wk.
	To treat superficial basal cell carcinoma	Apply to affected area 5 times per wk for 6 wk prior to bedtime and leave on skin for about 8 hr, then wash area with mild soap and water.
ingenol mebutate 0.015%, 0.05% Picato	*To treat actinic keratosis*	Apply 0.015% gel to face and scalp once daily for 3 consecutive days; apply 0.05% gel to trunk and extremities once daily for 2 consecutive days.
ivermectin 0.5% Sklice	*To treat head lice*	Apply to dry hair in amount sufficient to coat the hair and scalp thoroughly; leave on for 10 min, then rinse off with water.
ivermectin 1% Soolantra	*To treat inflammatory lesions of rosacea*	Apply pea-sized amount for each affected area of the face (chin, each cheek, forehead) once daily.
lidocaine 2.5% and prilocaine 2.5% EMLA	*For local anesthesia*	Apply 1 disk or thick layer of 2- to 2.5-g cream and cover with an occlusive dressing for at least 1 hr before the start of routine procedure or 2 hr before the start of painful procedure.
malathion 0.5% Ovide	*To treat pediculus humanus capitis (head lice and their ova) of scalp hair*	Apply to dry hair in amount just sufficient to wet the hair and scalp thoroughly; then let hair dry naturally. After 8 to 12 hr, shampoo and rinse hair and use a fine-toothed comb to remove dead lice and eggs. If lice are still present after 7 to 9 days, repeat application.

(continues)

Selected Topical Drugs *(continued)*

GENERIC AND TRADE NAMES	INDICATIONS	USUAL ADULT DOSAGES
Miscellaneous topical drugs *(continued)*		
mequinol 2%, tretinoin 0.01% Solage	*To treat solar lentigines*	Apply solution twice daily (morning and evening), at least 8 hr apart. Avoid application to surrounding skin, and do not bathe for 6 hr after application.
nitroglycerin 0.4% Rectiv	*To treat moderate to severe pain associated with chronic anal fissure*	Apply 1 in of ointment intra-anally every 12 hr for up to 3 wk.
oxybutynin chloride 10% Gelnique	*To treat overactive bladder with symptoms of urge urinary incontinence, urgency, and frequency*	Apply 1 sachet of gel or 1 activation of metered-dose pump once daily to clean, dry, intact skin on abdomen, upper arms/shoulders, or thighs.
permethrin 1% Nix	*To prevent or treat head lice*	Wash and dry hair, saturate scalp, leave on hair for 10 min, then rinse; remove nits with provided comb; repeat in 7 days if living mites are still present.
permethrin 5% Acticin, Elimite	*To treat scabies*	Massage into skin from head to soles of feet and remove after 8 to 10 hr; repeat in 14 days if living mites are still present.
pimecrolimus 1% Elidel	*To treat mild to moderate atopic dermatitis as a second-line therapy*	Apply to affected areas twice daily for up to 6 wk.
podofilox 0.5% Condylox	*To treat anogenital warts (gel)*	Apply gel to anogenital warts for 3 days, then withhold for 4 days; repeat cycle up to 4 times.
	To treat external genital warts (gel or solution)	Apply gel or solution to external genital warts every 12 hr in the morning and evening for 3 days, then withhold for 4 days; repeat cycle up to 4 times.
pyrethrin and piperonyl butoxide Licide, Pronto, RID	*To treat body, head, and pubic lice*	Apply to dry hair or affected body area. Massage through all hairy areas until hair is wet. Leave on hair for 10 min; then wash with warm water and rinse thoroughly. Repeat in 7 to 10 days.
roflumilast 0.3% Zoryve	*To treat plaque psoriasis, including intertriginous areas; to treat seborrheic dermatitis*	Apply to affected areas once daily and rub in completely.
roflumilast 0.15%	*To treat mild to moderate atopic dermatitis*	Apply to affected areas once daily and rub in completely.

GENERIC AND TRADE NAMES	INDICATIONS	USUAL ADULT DOSAGES
Miscellaneous topical drugs *(continued)*		
ruxolitinib 1.5% Opzelura	*To treat mild to moderate atopic dermatitis in non-immunocompromised patients*	Apply thin layer to affected areas of up to 20% body surface area. *Maximum:* 60 g/wk.
sirolimus 0.2% Hyftor	*To treat facial angiofibroma associated with tuberous sclerosis*	Apply 2.5 cm (800 mg) to facial area affected with angiofibroma twice daily (morning and bedtime).
sofpironium 12.45% Sofdra	*To treat primary axillary hyperhidrosis*	Apply 1 pump of gel at bedtime to first underarm and spread around area using provided applicator; repeat with second underarm. Let gel dry for 5 min.
spinosad 0.9% Natroba	*To treat head lice*	Apply to dry scalp and hair using only the amount needed to cover the scalp and hair. Rinse off with warm water after 10 min. Repeat in 7 days if live lice are still seen.
tacrolimus 0.03% and 0.1% Protopic	*To treat moderate to severe atopic dermatitis in patients unresponsive to other therapies*	Apply thin layer to affected areas twice daily, rubbing in gently and completely.
tapinarof 1% Vtama	*To treat plaque psoriasis; to treat atopic dermatitis*	Apply a thin layer to affected areas once daily.
tirbanibulin 1% Klisyri	*To treat actinic keratosis of face or scalp*	Apply to affected area(s) once daily for 5 consecutive days.
urea 41%, 45% Utopic	*To treat hyperkeratotic conditions*	Apply to affected area twice daily and rub in.

Syringe Drug Compatibility

The table below lets you know at a glance whether particular drugs are compatible for at least 15 minutes when mixed together in a syringe for immediate administration. However, keep in mind that drugs listed as compatible when mixed in a syringe may not be compatible when prepared for other routes of administration. Drug combinations prepared for immediate administration usually require a more concentrated solution than those prepared for infusion.

Key: C = Compatible; I = Incompatible; n/a = Compatibility information not available, no recommendations can be given.

	ATROPINE	CHLORPROMAZINE	DEXAMETHASONE	DIAZEPAM	DIPHENHYDRAMINE	DROPERIDOL	FUROSEMIDE	GLYCOPYRROLATE	HALOPERIDOL
atropine		C	n/a	n/a	C	C	n/a	C	I
chlorpromazine	C		n/a	n/a	C	C	n/a	C	n/a
dexamethasone	n/a	n/a		n/a	I	n/a	n/a	n/a	n/a
diazepam	n/a	n/a	n/a		n/a	n/a	n/a	I	n/a
diphenhydramine	C	C	I	n/a		C	n/a	C	I
droperidol	C	C	n/a	n/a	C		I	C	n/a
furosemide	n/a	n/a	n/a	n/a	n/a	I		n/a	n/a
glycopyrrolate	C	C	I	C	C	C	n/a		C
haloperidol	n/a	n/a	n/a	n/a	C	n/a	n/a	n/a	
heparin	C	I	n/a	I	n/a	I	C	n/a	I
hydromorphone	C	C	n/a	n/a	C	n/a	n/a	C	C
hydroxyzine	C	C	n/a	n/a	C	C	n/a	C	I
ketorolac	n/a	n/a	n/a	I	n/a	n/a	n/a	n/a	I
lidocaine	n/a	n/a	n/a	n/a	n/a	n/a	n/a	C	n/a
lorazepam	n/a	n/a	n/a	n/a	n/a	n/a	n/a	n/a	n/a
meperidine	C	C	n/a	C	C	C	n/a	C	n/a
metoclopramide	C	C	n/a	n/a	C	C	I	n/a	n/a
midazolam	C	C	n/a	n/a	C	n/a	n/a	C	C
morphine	C	C	n/a	n/a	C	C	n/a	C	I
pentobarbital	C	I	n/a	n/a	I	I	n/a	I	n/a
prochlorperazine	C	n/a	n/a	n/a	C	C	n/a	C	n/a
scopolamine	C	C	n/a	n/a	C	C	n/a	C	n/a

HEPARIN	HYDROMORPHONE	HYDROXYZINE	KETOROLAC	LIDOCAINE	LORAZEPAM	MEPERIDINE	METOCLOPRAMIDE	MIDAZOLAM	MORPHINE	PENTOBARBITAL	PROCHLORPERAZINE	SCOPOLAMINE
n/a	C	C	n/a	n/a	n/a	C	C	C	C	C	C	C
I	C	C	n/a	n/a	n/a	C	C	C	I	I	C	C
n/a	C	n/a	n/a	n/a	n/a	n/a	C	n/a	n/a	n/a	n/a	n/a
I	n/a	n/a	I	n/a	n/a	n/a	n/a	n/a	n/a	n/a	n/a	n/a
n/a	C	C	n/a	n/a	n/a	C	C	C	C	I	C	C
I	n/a	C	n/a	n/a	n/a	C	C	C	C	I	C	C
C	n/a	n/a	n/a	n/a	n/a	n/a	I	n/a	n/a	n/a	n/a	n/a
n/a	C	C	n/a	C	n/a	C	n/a	C	C	I	C	C
I	C	I	I	n/a	n/a	n/a	n/a	n/a	I	n/a	n/a	n/a
	n/a	n/a	n/a	C	n/a	I	C	n/a	C	n/a	n/a	n/a
n/a		C	I	n/a	C	n/a	n/a	C	n/a	C	I	C
n/a	C		I	C	n/a	C	C	C	C	I	C	C
n/a	I	I		n/a	n/a	n/a	n/a	n/a	n/a	n/a	I	n/a
C	n/a	C	n/a		n/a	n/a	C	n/a	n/a	n/a	n/a	n/a
n/a	C	n/a	n/a	n/a		n/a	n/a	n/a	n/a	n/a	n/a	n/a
I	n/a	C	n/a	n/a	n/a		C	I	I	C	C	C
C	C	n/a	n/a	C	n/a	C		C	C	n/a	C	C
n/a	C	C	n/a	n/a	n/a	C	C		C	I	I	C
C*	n/a	C	n/a	n/a	n/a	n/a	C	C		I	C	C
n/a	C	I	n/a	n/a	n/a	I	I	I	I		I	C
n/a	I	C	I	n/a	n/a	C	C	I	C	I		C
n/a	C	C	n/a	n/a	n/a	C	C	C	C	C	C	

* Compatible only with morphine doses of 1, 2, and 5 mg.

Use of Drug Formulas and Calculations

When giving drugs, you must be familiar with drug formulas and calculation methods to make sure your patient receives the prescribed drug in the correct dosage, strength, or flow rate. This appendix offers a quick review of ways to calculate the strength of a solution, drug dosages, and I.V. flow rates.

Calculating the Strength of a Solution

Most solutions are prepared in the required strength by the pharmacy or medical supply source.

But sometimes only a concentrated form is available, and you'll need to dilute the solution or solid to administer the prescribed strength.

When a solid form of a drug is used to prepare a solution, the drug must be completely dissolved. Solid drug forms, such as tablets, crystals, and powders, are considered 100% strength. (An exception to this is boric acid, which is only 5% at full strength.) The final diluted solution is stated in terms of liquid measurement. To prepare a solution, you'll need to add the prescribed solid or liquid form of the drug (the solute) to the prescribed amount of diluent (the solvent). Two of the most common clinical diluents are 0.9% Sodium Chloride Injection and Sterile Water for Injection.

You can use two formulas to calculate the strength of a solution, as shown in the examples below.

Method 1: Calculating percentage and volume

Use the following formula:

$$\frac{\textit{Weaker solution}}{\textit{Stronger solution}} = \frac{\textit{Solute}}{\textit{Solvent}}$$

Example: You need to dilute a stock solution of 100% strength to a 5% solution. How much solute will you need to add to obtain 500 ml of the 5% solution?

Calculate as follows:

$$\frac{5\ (\%)\ (\textit{Weaker solution})}{100\ (\%)\ (\textit{Stronger solution})} = \frac{X\ (\textit{g})\ (\textit{solute})}{500\ \textit{ml}\ (\textit{solvent})}$$

$$100\ \text{X} = (500)(5) \text{ or } 2{,}500$$

$$\text{X} = 25 \text{ g}$$

Answer: You'll need to add 25 g of solute to each 500 ml of solvent to prepare a 5% solution.

Method 2: Calculating percentage and volume

Use the following formula:

$$\frac{\text{(Desired strength)}}{\text{(Available strength)}} \times 100 \text{ ml (Total amount of desired solution)} = \text{X}\frac{0.25}{0.80} = 0.25$$

$$0.25 \times 100 \text{ (ml)} = \text{X}$$

$$\text{X} = 25 \text{ ml of } 80\% \text{ solution}$$

Example: You need to make 100 ml of a 20% solution, using an 80% solution. How much of the 80% solution must you add to the sterile water to yield a final volume of 100 ml of a 20% solution?

Calculate as follows:

$$\frac{20\ (\%)\ \text{(Desired strength)}}{80\ (\%)\ \text{(Available strength)}} \times 100 \text{ ml } (\textit{Total amount of desired solution}) = \text{X}\frac{0.25}{0.80} = 0.25$$

$$0.25 \times 100 \text{ (ml)} = \text{X}$$

$$\text{X} = 25 \text{ ml of } 80\% \text{ solution}$$

Answer: You'll need to add 25 ml of the 80% solution to the water to make a final volume of 100 ml of a 20% solution.

Calculating Drug Dosages

You may be required to calculate drug dosages when you need to administer a drug that's available only in one measure but prescribed in another. You should also be prepared to convert various units of measure, such as milligrams (mg) to grains (gr), and dry measurements to liquid. You can use three common methods of ratio and proportion to calculate drug dosages, as shown in the examples below.

CALCULATING ORAL DRUG DOSAGES

Example: You need to give a patient 0.25 mg of digoxin, which comes only in 0.125-mg tablets. How many tablets will you need to give him to attain the proper dosage?

Method 1: Using labeled amount of drug

In this method, true proportions between the drug label and the prescribed dose are used to determine ratio and proportion. The drug label, which states the amount of drug in one unit of measurement—in this case, 0.125 mg in each tablet of digoxin—is the first ratio, expressed as follows:

milligrams : tablets = milligrams : tablets

0.125 mg (amount of drug) : 1 tablet (unit of measure)

The prescribed dose—in this case, 0.25 mg—is the second ratio; it must be stated in the same order and units of measure as the first, as follows:

0.125 mg : 1 tablet = 0.25 mg : X (tablets)

Calculate as follows:

$$0.125\,X = 0.25\text{ mg}$$

$$X = \frac{0.25}{0.125}$$

$$X = 2$$

Answer: You'll need to give the patient 2 tablets of digoxin 0.125 mg.

Be sure to use critical thinking to assess whether your answer is correct. Because the amount of drug prescribed is greater than the amount of drug in 1 tablet, it's reasonable to expect the required number of tablets to be greater than one.

Method 2: Using an established formula

To determine the correct number of digoxin tablets to give using this method, use the following formula:

$$\frac{\textit{Prescribed dose}}{\textit{Dose available}} \times \text{Quantity (unit of measure)} = \text{X (unknown quantity to be given)}$$

Calculate as follows:

$$\frac{0.25}{0.125} = X$$

$$2 = X$$

Answer: You'll need to give the patient 2 tablets of digoxin 0.125 mg.

Method 3: Calculating according to proportion size

This method uses the same components as method #1, but the ratio is based on proportions according to size. To determine the correct number of digoxin tablets to give using this method, use the following formula:

$$\frac{\textit{Smaller}}{\textit{Larger}} = \frac{\textit{Larger}}{\textit{Smaller}}$$

Substitute 0.125 into the smaller part and 0.25 into the greater part of the first ratio. Critical thinking leads us to believe that you'll need more than 1 tablet of the weaker 0.125-mg strength to equal the stronger 0.25 mg. Set up the proportion as follows:

Calculate as follows:

$$\frac{0.125\ mg}{0.25\ mg} = \frac{1\ (tablet)}{X\ (tablets)}$$

$$0.125\ X = 0.25$$

$$X = \frac{0.25}{0.125}$$

$$X = 2\ \text{tablets}$$

Answer: You'll need to give the patient 2 tablets of digoxin 0.125 mg.

CALCULATING PARENTERAL DRUG DOSAGES

The same methods used for calculating oral drugs and solutions can be used for preparing parenteral injections.

Example: You need to administer a prescribed dose of 1 mg morphine sulfate from a unit-dose cartridge containing 4 mg/2 ml. How many milliliters will you need to give to equal the prescribed dose of 1 mg?

Method 1: Using labeled amount of drug

Using the same ratio as for oral drugs, the drug label—in this case, 4 mg—is the first ratio, and the prescribed dose—in this case, 1 mg—is the second ratio, expressed as follows:

4 mg (the amount of drug) : 2 ml (the unit of measure)

Calculate as follows:

$$4\ \text{mg} : 2\ \text{ml} = 1\ \text{mg}: X\ \text{ml}$$

$$4X = 2$$

$$X = \frac{2}{4}$$

$$X = 0.5\ \text{ml}$$

Answer: You'll need to give 0.5 ml of morphine sulfate to equal the prescribed dose of 1 mg.

Method 2: Using an established formula

Use this formula:

$$\frac{\textit{Prescribed dose}}{\textit{Dose available}} \times \text{Quantity (unit of measure)} = X\ \text{(unknown quantity to be given)}$$

Calculate as follows:

$$\frac{1\ mg}{4\ mg} \times 2\ \text{ml} = X\ \text{(number of ml)}$$

$$\frac{2}{4} = X$$

$$X = 0.5\ \text{ml}$$

Answer: You'll need to give 0.5 ml of morphine sulfate to equal the prescribed dose of 1 mg.

Method 3: Calculating according to proportion size

To determine the correct amount of morphine sulfate to give using this method, use the following formula:

smaller : greater = smaller : greater
milligrams : milligrams = milliliters : milliliters

Critical thinking leads us to believe that 1 mg is less than 4 mg and that you'll need less than 2 ml to give 1 mg of the drug; therefore, 1 mg goes into the smaller part of the first ratio, and X goes into the smaller part of the second ratio. Set up the proportion as follows:

$$1 \text{ mg} : 4 \text{ mg} = X \text{ (ml)} : 2 \text{ ml}$$

$$4X = 2$$

$$X = \frac{2}{4}$$

$$X = 0.5 \text{ ml}$$

Answer: You'll need to give 0.5 ml of morphine sulfate to equal the prescribed dose of 1 mg.

Calculating I.V. Flow Rates

When an I.V. solution is delivered by gravity, you must calculate the number of drops needed per minute for proper infusion. To calculate I.V. flow rates, you need to know three things:

- The drip factor—or the number of drops contained in 1 ml for the type of I.V. set you'll be using. This information is provided on the individual package label.
- The amount and type of fluid that you'll infuse as prescribed on the physician's order sheet
- The infusion duration time in minutes.

Once you've gathered this information, you can calculate the I.V. flow rate using the following equation:

$$\frac{\textit{Total number of ml}}{\textit{Total number of minutes}} \times \text{drip factor (gtt/ml)} = \text{flow rate (gtt/min)}$$

Example 1: If the physician prescribes 1,000 ml of D_{5W} to infuse over 10 hours, and the drip rate for your administration set is 15 drops (gtt)/ml, calculate as follows:

$$\frac{1{,}000 \text{ ml}}{10 \textit{ hours} \times 60 \textit{ minutes}} \times 15 \text{ gtt/m} = X \text{ gtt/minute}$$

$$\frac{1{,}000 \text{ ml}}{600 \text{ minutes}} \times 15 \text{ gtt/m} = X \text{ gtt/minute}$$

$$1.67 \text{ ml/minute} \times 15 \text{ gtt/m} = X \text{ gtt/minute}$$

$$25.05 \text{ gtt/minute} = X$$

Answer: To infuse, round off 25.05 to 25 gtt/min or according to your institution's policy.

Example 2: If the physician prescribes 500 ml of half-normal (0.45%) saline solution to infuse over 2 hours, and the drip rate for your administration set delivers 10 gtt/ml, calculate as follows:

$$\frac{500 \textit{ ml}}{2 \textit{ hours} \times 60 \textit{ minutes}} \times 15 \text{ gtt/m} = X \text{ gtt/minute}$$

$$\frac{1{,}000 \textit{ ml}}{120 \textit{ minutes}} \times 15 \text{ gtt/m} = X \text{ gtt/minute}$$

$$4.67 \text{ ml/minute} \times 15 \text{ gtt/m} = X \text{ gtt/minute}$$

$$41.7 \text{ gtt/minute} = X$$

Answer: To infuse, round off 41.7 to 42 gtt/min or according to your institution's policy.

Note: When preparing for I.V. administration using a controlled infusion device, the electronic flow-regulator will either count drops using an electronic eye or use a controlled pumping action to deliver the fluid in milliliters. Your final calculation will be based on the unit of measure used by the device: drops per minute or ml per hour.

Weights and Equivalents

The following three tables show approximate equivalents among systems of measurement.

Table 1 Liquid Equivalents Among Household, Apothecaries', and Metric Systems

HOUSEHOLD SYSTEM	APOTHECARIES' SYSTEM	METRIC SYSTEM
1 tsp	1 fluid dram	5 ml
1 tbs	0.5 fluid oz	15 ml
2 tbs (1 oz)	1 fluid oz	30 ml
1 cupful	8 fluid oz	240 ml
1 pint	16 fluid oz	473 ml
1 quart (qt)	32 fluid oz	946 ml (1 L)

Abbreviations: L=liter; ml=milliliter; oz=ounce; qt=quart; tbs=tablespoon; tsp=teaspoon

Table 2 Solid Equivalents Among Apothecaries' and Metric Systems

APOTHECARIES' SYSTEM	METRIC SYSTEM
15 gr	1 g (1,000 mg)
10 gr	0.6 g (600 mg)
7.5 gr	0.5 g (500 mg)
5 gr	0.3 g (300 mg)
3 gr	0.2 g (200 mg)
1.5 gr	0.1 g (100 mg)
1 gr	0.06 g (60 mg) or 0.065 g (65 mg)
0.75 gr	0.05 g (50 mg)
0.5 gr	0.03 g (30 mg)
0.25 gr	0.015 g (15 mg)
1/60 gr	0.001 g (1 mg)
1/100 gr	0.6 mg
1/120 gr	0.5 mg
1/150 gr	0.4 mg

Abbreviations: g=gram; gr=grain; mg=milligram

Table 3 Solid Equivalents Among Avoirdupois, Apothecaries', and Metric Systems

AVOIRDUPOIS	APOTHECARIES'	METRIC
1 gr	1 gr	0.065 g
15.4 gr	15 gr	1 g
1 oz	480 gr	28.35 g
437.5 gr	1 oz	31 g
1 lb	1.33 lb	454 g
0.75 lb	1 lb	373 g
2.2 lb	2.7 lb	1 kg

Abbreviations: g=gram; gr=grain; kg=kilograms; lb=pound; oz=ounce

Index

- Generic and alternate names: lowercase initial letter
- Trade names: uppercase initial letter
- Tables: *t* after page number

B

C

D

E

F

G

H

I

J

K

L

M

N

O

R

S

T

U